ExpertDDX
Pediatrics

SECOND EDITION

Merrow

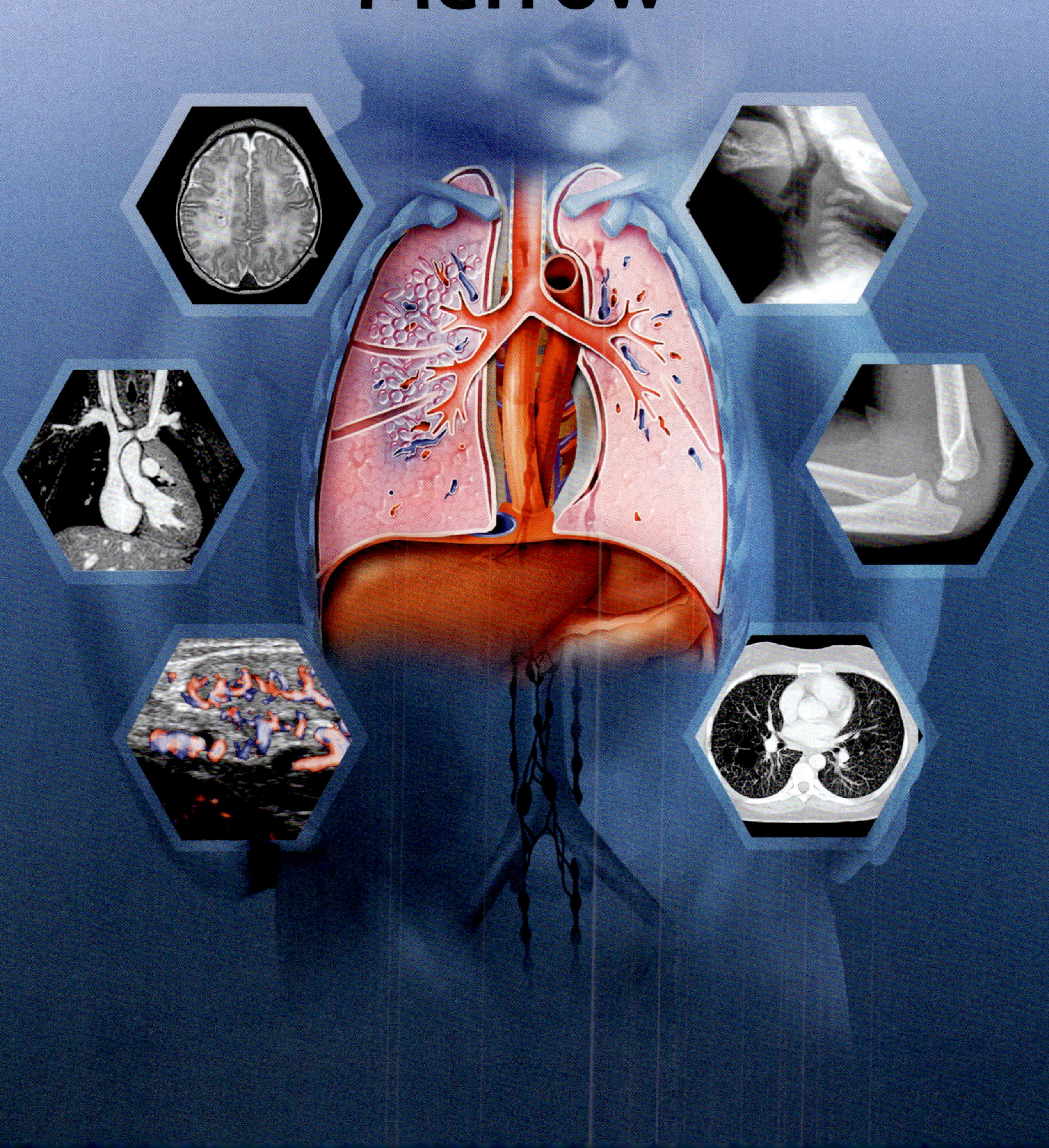

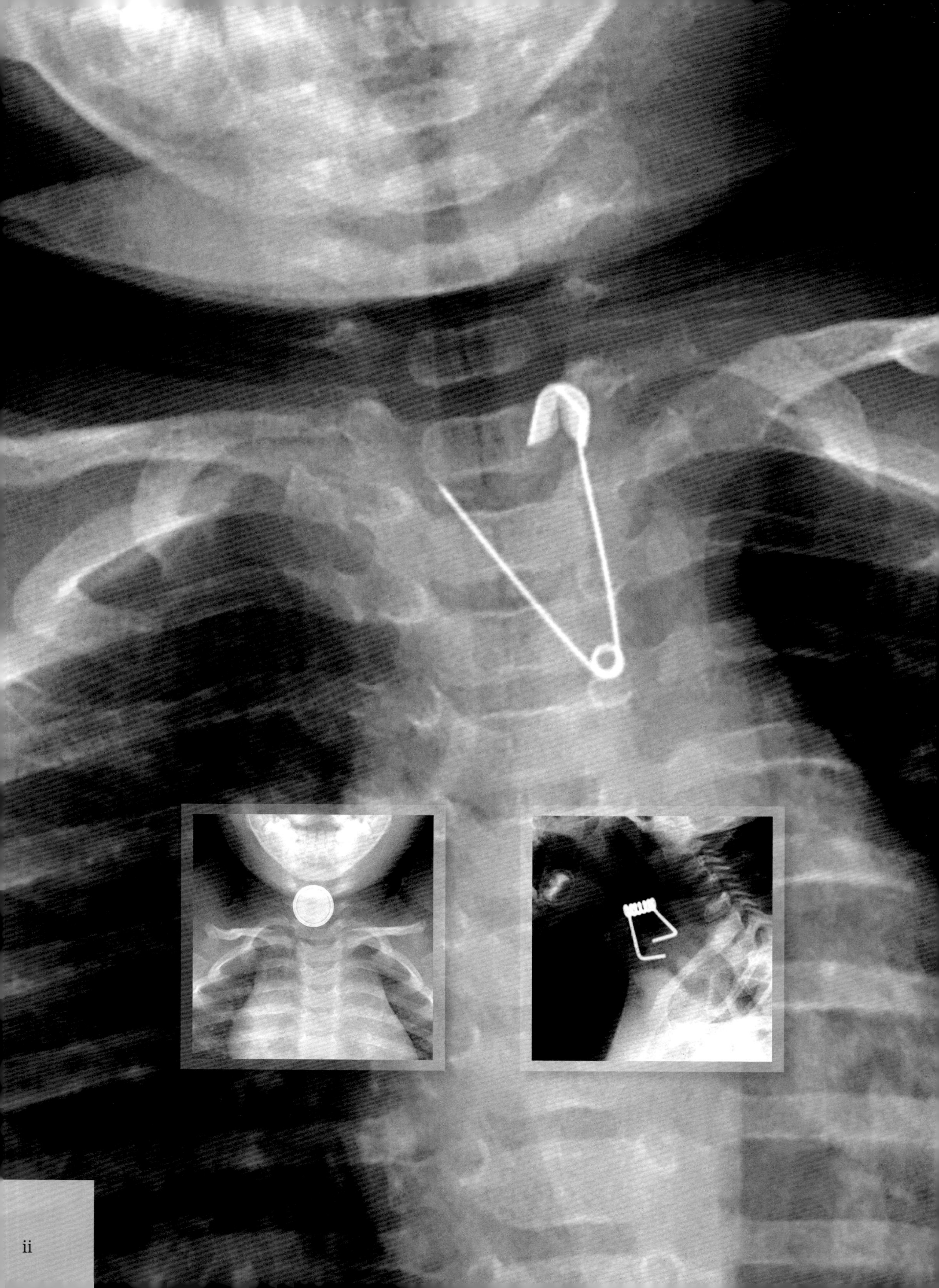

ExpertDDX Pediatrics

SECOND EDITION

A. Carlson Merrow, Jr., MD, FAAP
Corning Benton Chair for Radiology Education
Cincinnati Children's Hospital Medical Center
Associate Professor of Clinical Radiology
University of Cincinnati College of Medicine
Cincinnati, Ohio

Elsevier
1600 John F. Kennedy Blvd.
Ste 1800
Philadelphia, PA 19103-2899

EXPERTDDX: PEDIATRICS, SECOND EDITION

ISBN: 978-0-323-68177-3

Notices

Practitioners and researchers must always rely on their own experience and knowledge in evaluating and using any information, methods, compounds or experiments described herein. Because of rapid advances in the medical sciences, in particular, independent verification of diagnoses and drug dosages should be made. To the fullest extent of the law, no responsibility is assumed by Elsevier, authors, editors or contributors for any injury and/or damage to persons or property as a matter of products liability, negligence or otherwise, or from any use or operation of any methods, products, instructions, or ideas contained in the material herein.

Previous edition copyrighted 2010.

Library of Congress Control Number: 2019941281

Printed in Canada by TC Transcontinental, Beauceville, Quebec, Canada

Last digit is the print number: 9 8 7 6 5 4 3 2 1

Dedication

To Nan,

There is an intimacy of you and I where no interruption dare tread, where no calamity can take hold, where life is abundant and purposeful, and joy begets sustenance and wholeness, fight and adventure. I carry that with me every day…there are traces of it scattered throughout all of my work, and surely those are the best parts.

Thank you for sharing this life with me.

ACM

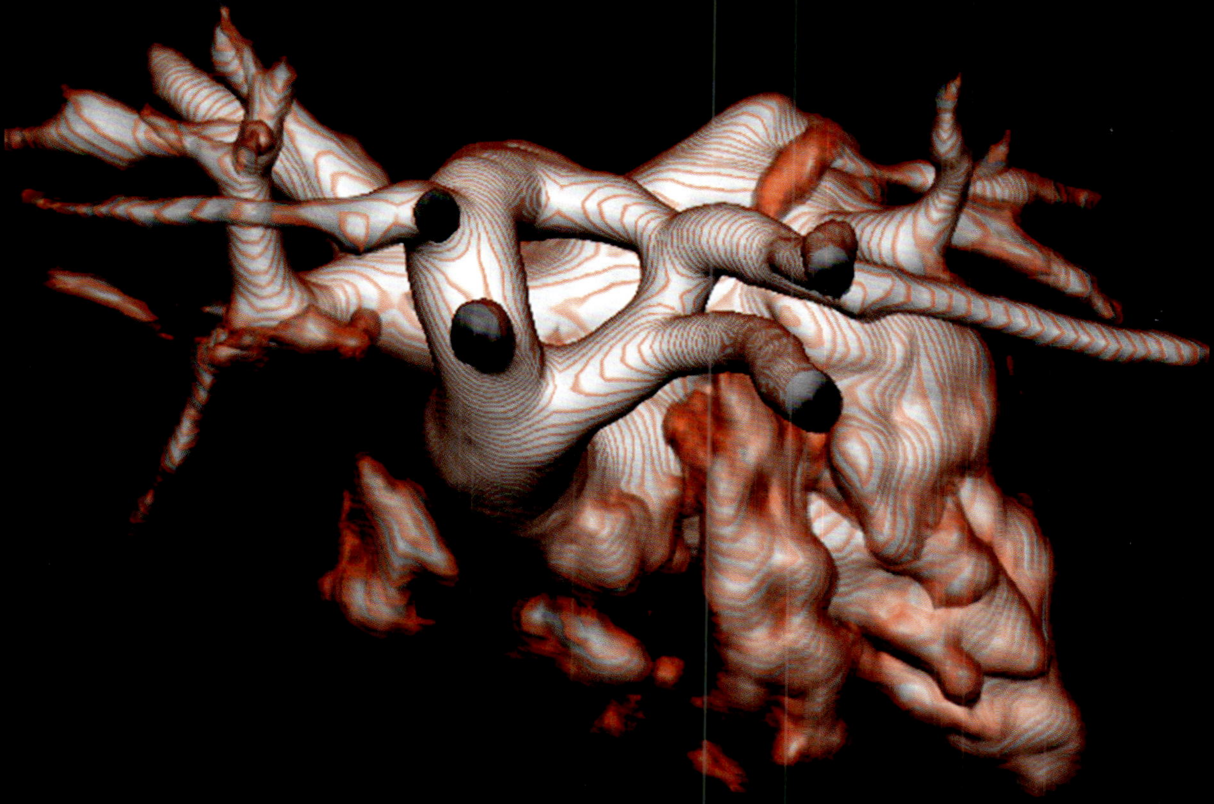

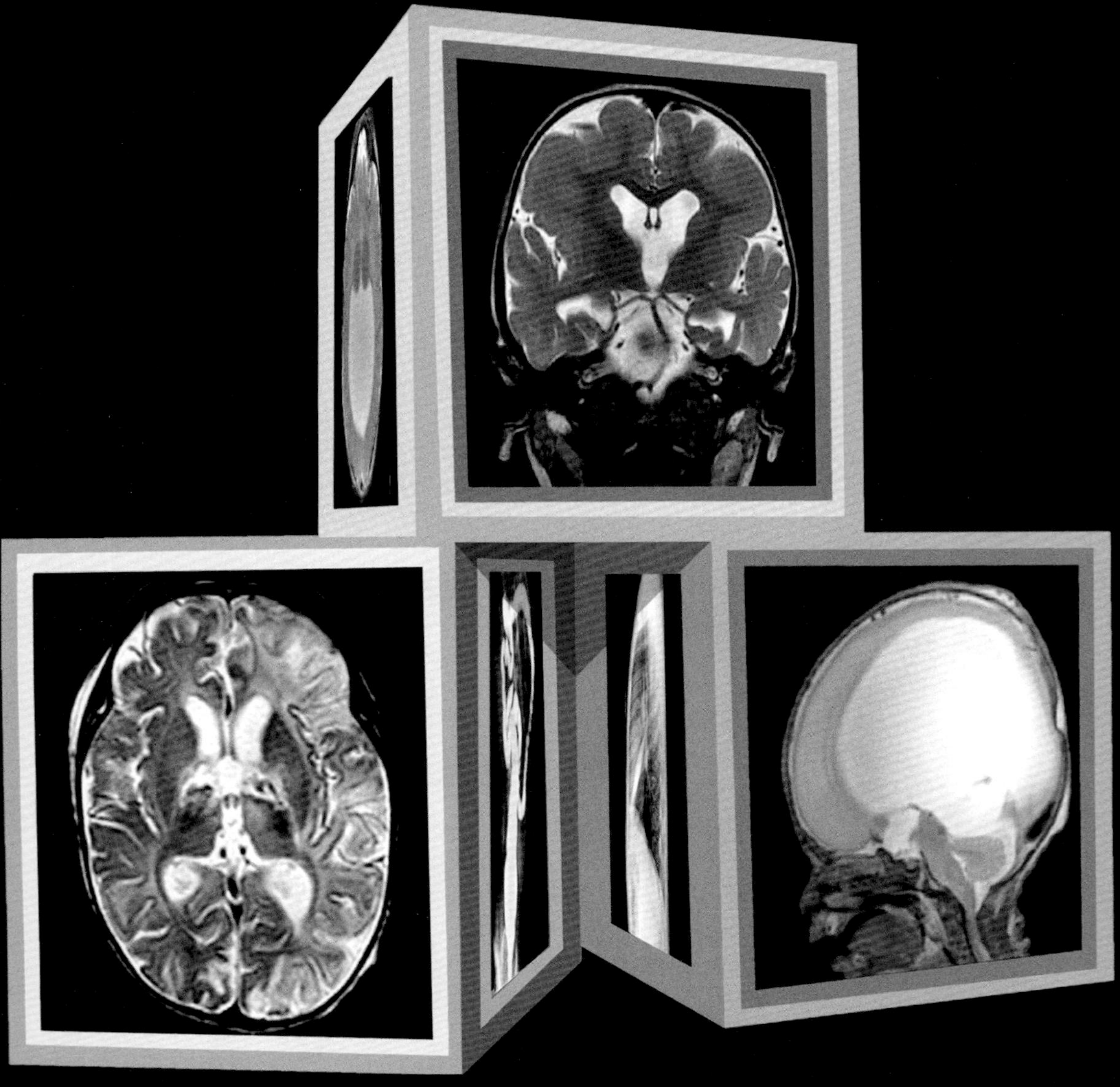

Contributing Authors

Michael R. Aquino, MD, MHSc
Pediatric Radiologist
Imaging Institute
Sections of Pediatric and Regional Radiology
Cleveland Clinic
Cleveland, Ohio

Bernadette L. Koch, MD
Associate Director of Radiology
Cincinnati Children's Hospital Medical Center
Professor of Clinical Radiology and Pediatrics
University of Cincinnati College of Medicine
Cincinnati, Ohio

Christopher Z. Lam, MD
Staff Body and Cardiac Radiologist
Department of Diagnostic Imaging
Hospital for Sick Children
Lecturer
Department of Medical Imaging
University of Toronto
Toronto, Ontario, Canada

Luke L. Linscott, MD
Pediatric Neuroradiologist
Primary Children's Hospital
Intermountain Pediatric Imaging
Adjunct Assistant Professor of Radiology
University of Utah School of Medicine
Salt Lake City, Utah

Arthur B. Meyers, MD
Cincinnati Children's Hospital Medical Center
Associate Professor of Radiology
University of Cincinnati College of Medicine
Cincinnati, Ohio

Emily S. Orscheln, MD
Staff Radiologist
Cincinnati Children's Hospital Medical Center
Assistant Professor of Radiology
University of Cincinnati College of Medicine
Cincinnati, Ohio

Additional Contributors

H. Christian Davidson, MD

H. Ric Harnsberger, MD

Steven J. Kraus, MD

Luke N. Ledbetter, MD

Kristine M. Mosier, DMD, PhD

Michael Nasser, MD

Sara M. O'Hara, MD, FAAP

Daniel Podberesky, MD

Karen L. Salzman, MD

Blair A. Winegar, MD

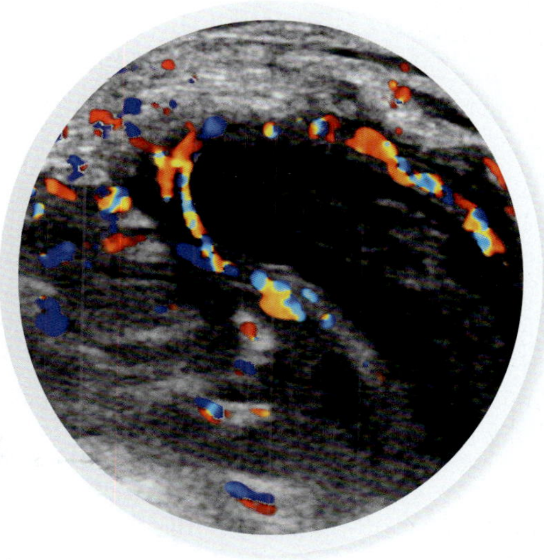

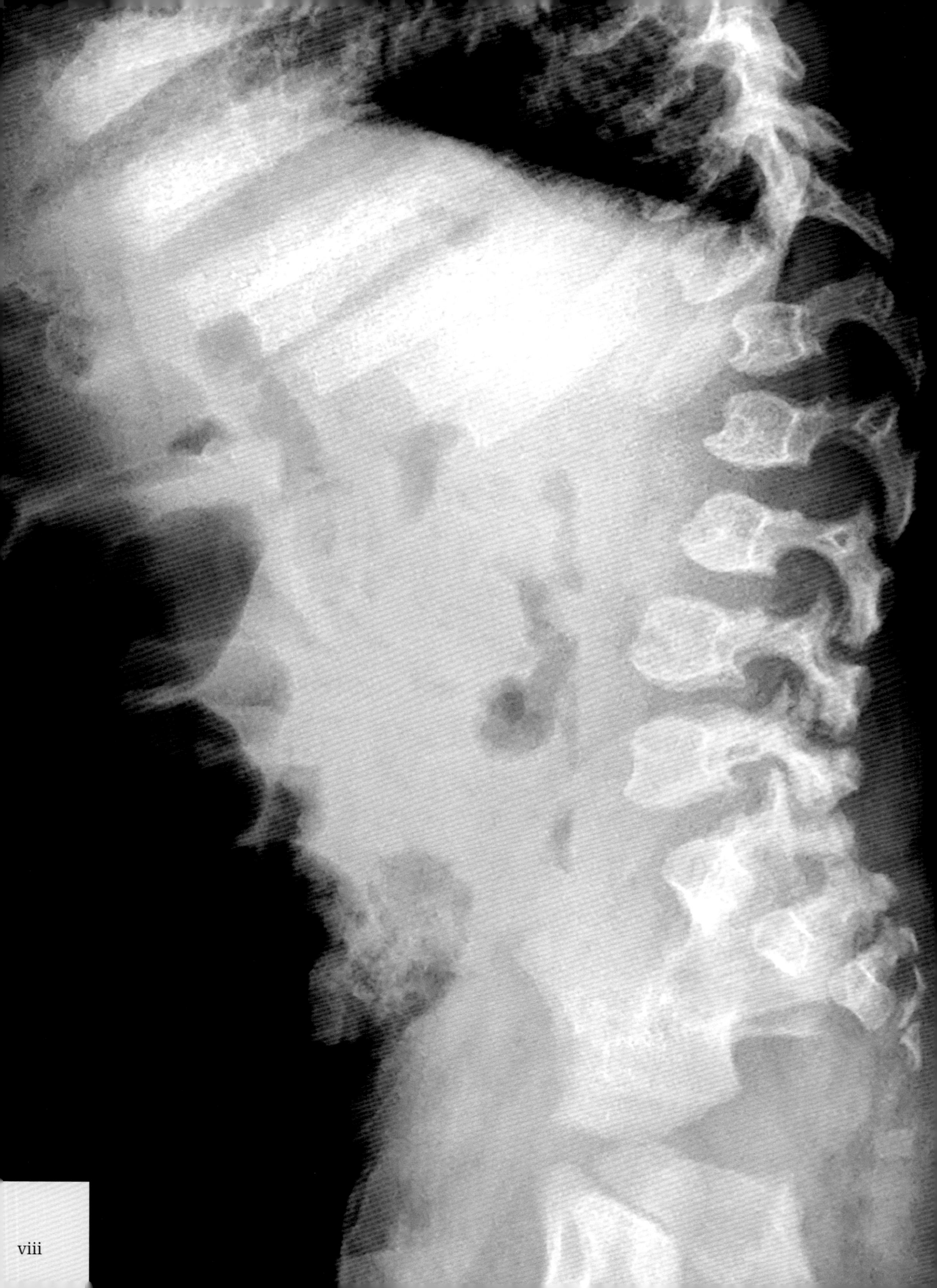

Preface

Welcome to the 2nd edition of *ExpertDDx: Pediatrics*. It is my honor and privilege to have led such an excellent team of pediatric radiologists in constructing a book that I believe will prove invaluable in your daily practice.

The capacity to craft a meaningful differential diagnosis remains, at least at this time, the skill of a human artisan, developed over many years, if not decades. To exquisitely articulate a narrow list of candidate pathologies provides critical direction for the clinician and patient, carrying great importance in the chain of care. But the valuable interpreter of images also knows to consider a broader spectrum of diseases intellectually before committing to a selective list of contenders in the radiologic report. This book generally embraces more extensive lists of entities that can produce characteristic radiologic findings, working through images and text to help you select the considerations most relevant to your patient's clinical and imaging scenario.

I hope that you find this thoroughly updated volume a useful guide in the realm of pediatric radiology, where the background of normal anatomy is rapidly changing, and the pathology can be uniquely sinister. Use it to expedite care and improve outcomes.

A thank you to all who contributed to this book, including authors and Elsevier staff (especially Nina!), but also spouses, families, teachers, and patients. The best care comes with deep passion, intense labor, and time that requires sacrifice. May there be great benefit for the children and families we serve.

A. Carlson Merrow, Jr., MD, FAAP
Corning Benton Chair for Radiology Education
Cincinnati Children's Hospital Medical Center
Associate Professor of Clinical Radiology
University of Cincinnati College of Medicine
Cincinnati, Ohio

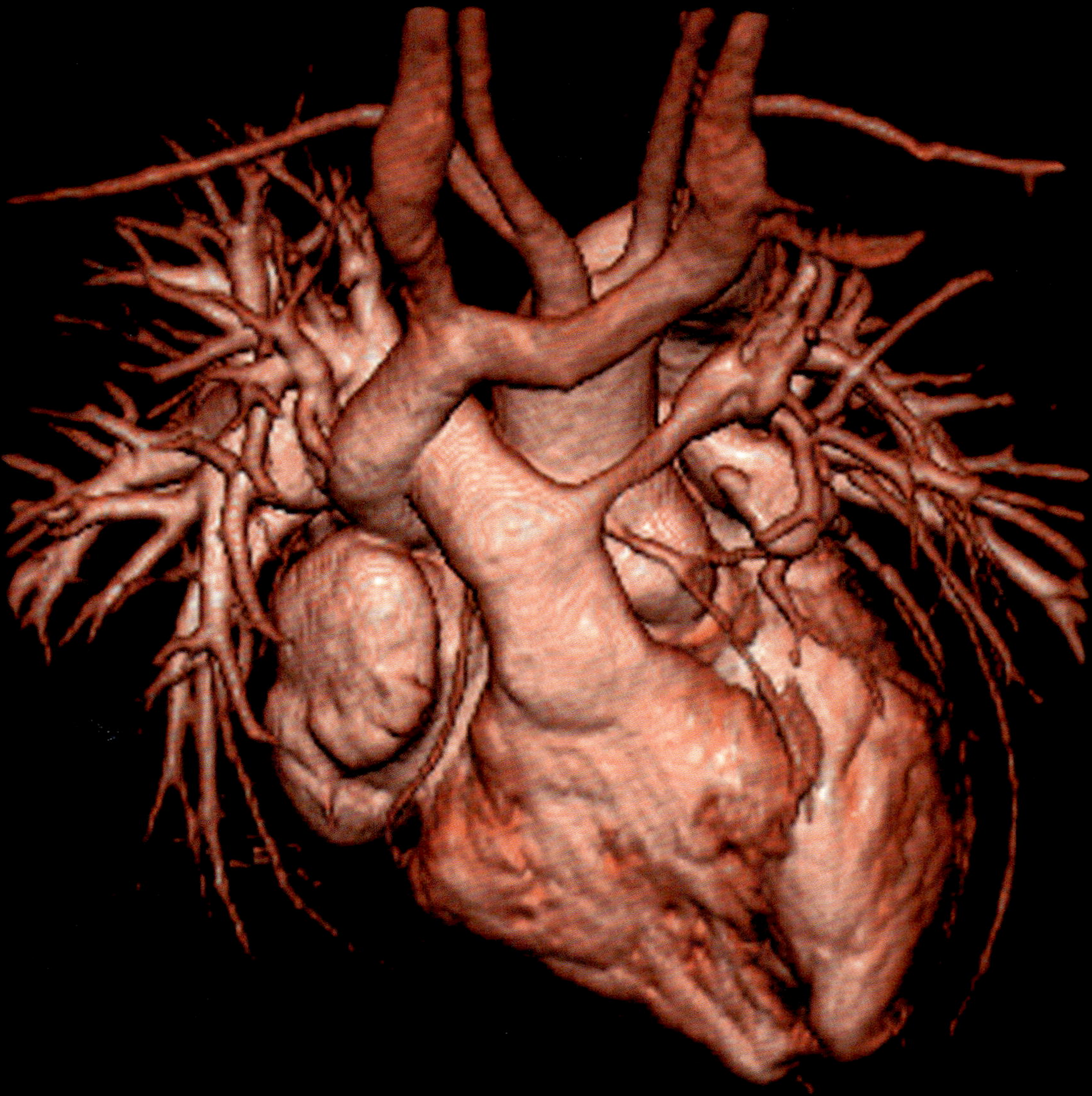

Acknowledgments

LEAD EDITOR

Nina I. Bennett, BA

TEXT EDITORS

Arthur G. Gelsinger, MA
Rebecca L. Bluth, BA
Terry W. Ferrell, MS
Megg Morin, BA

IMAGE EDITORS

Jeffrey J. Marmorstone, BS
Lisa A. M. Steadman, BS

ILLUSTRATIONS

Richard Coombs, MS
Lane R. Bennion, MS
Laura C. Wissler, MA

ART DIRECTION AND DESIGN

Tom M. Olson, BA

PRODUCTION COORDINATORS

Emily C. Fassett, BA
John Pecorelli, BS

ELSEVIER

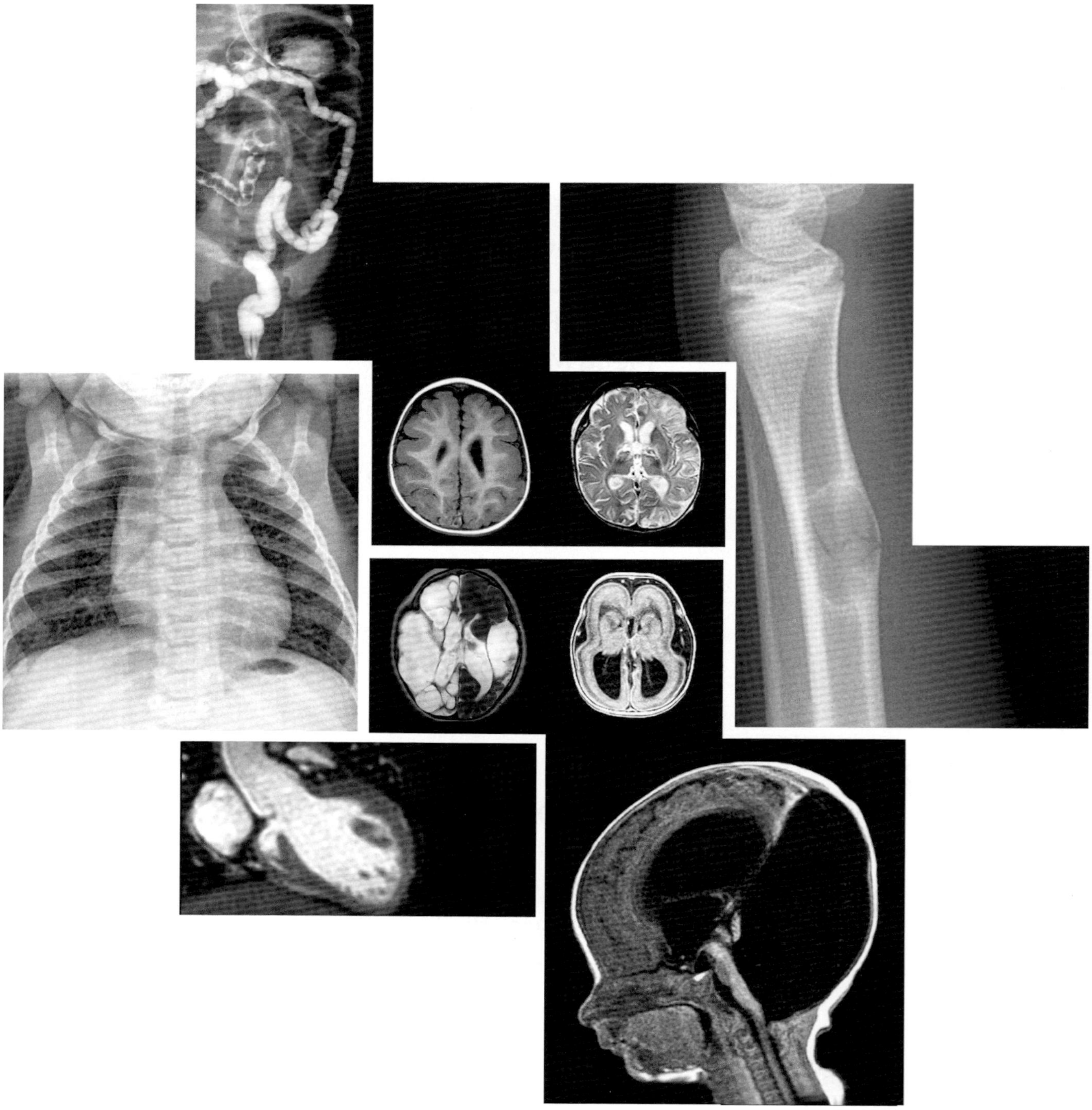

Sections

TABLE OF CONTENTS

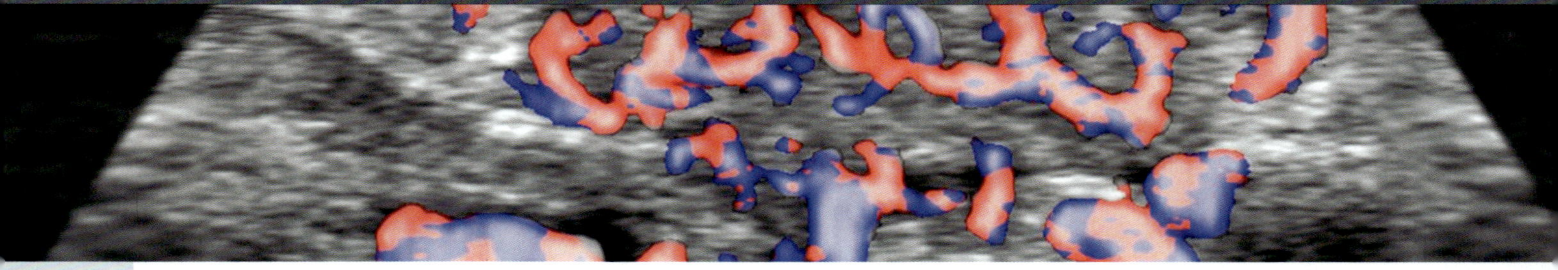

SECTION 1: CARDIAC

SECTION 2: CHEST

SECTION 3: GASTROINTESTINAL

TABLE OF CONTENTS

TABLE OF CONTENTS

TABLE OF CONTENTS

ExpertDDX

Pediatrics

SECOND EDITION

Merrow

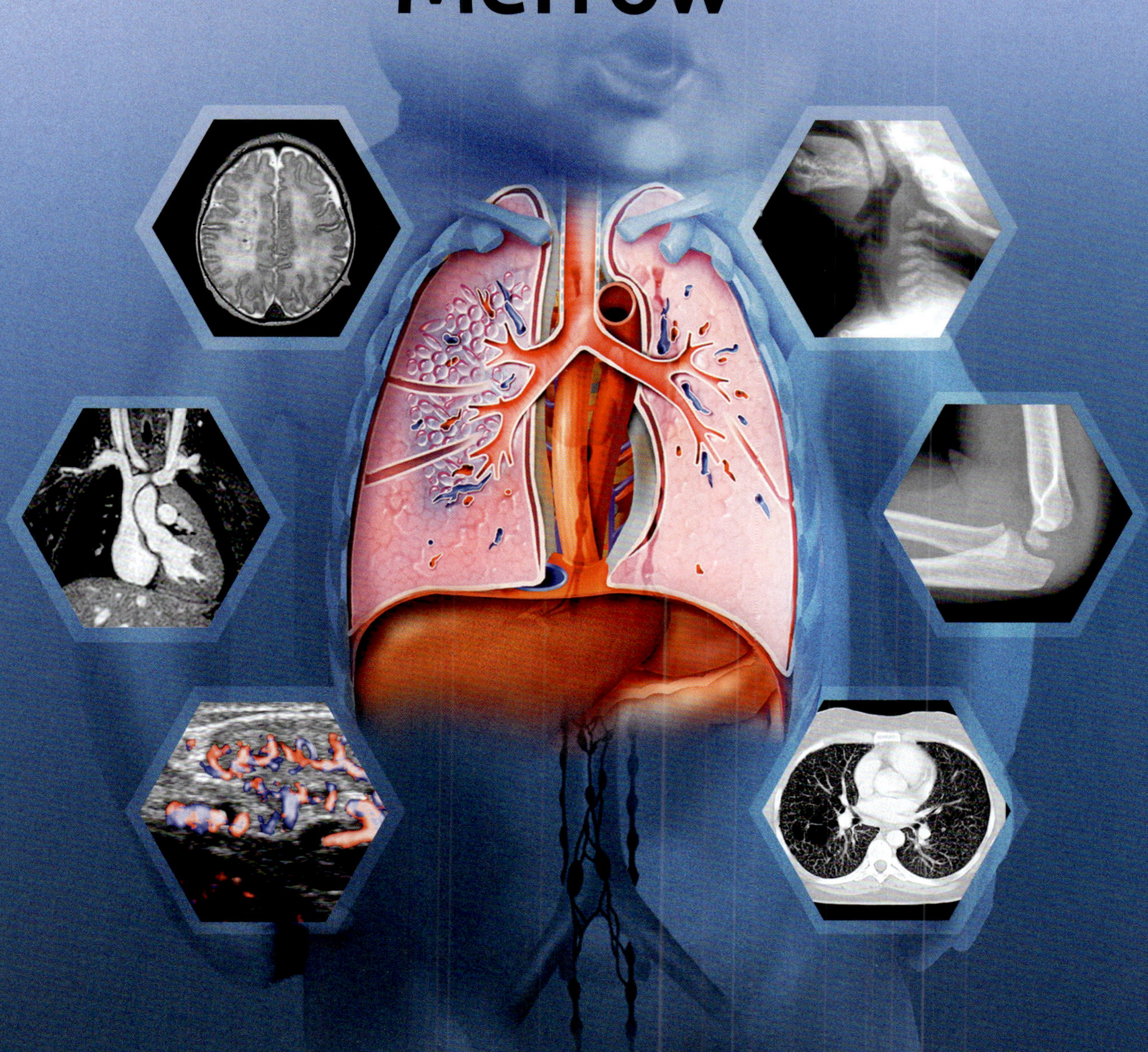

SECTION 1
Cardiac

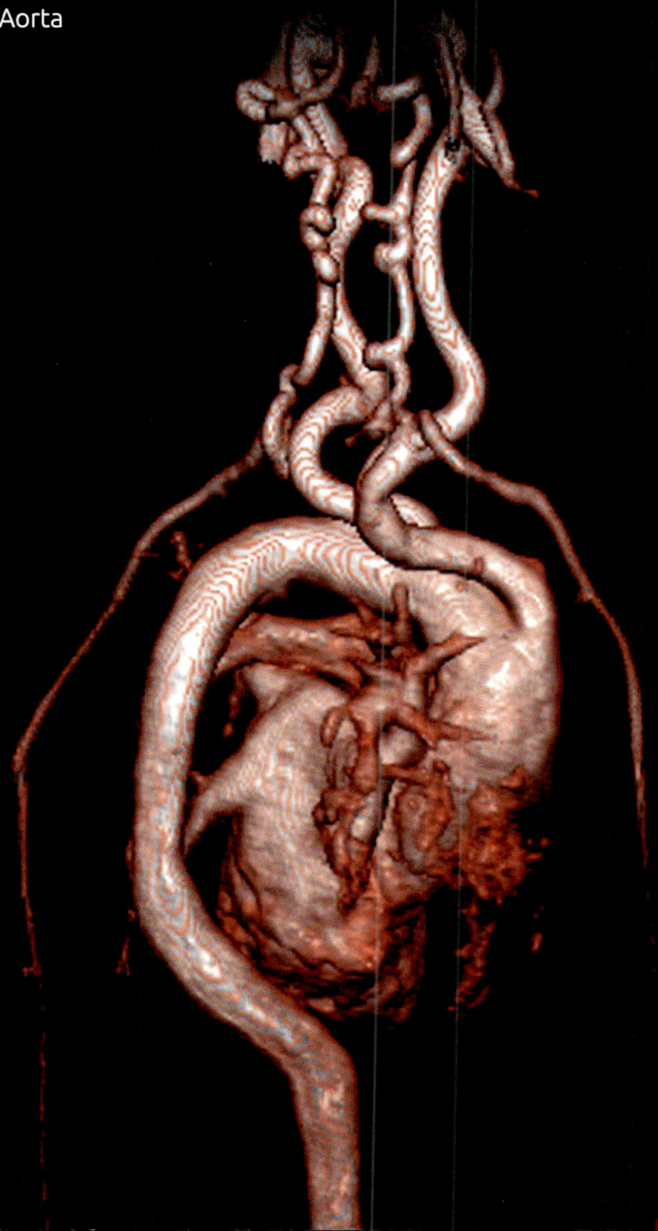

DIFFERENTIAL DIAGNOSIS

Common

- Intracardiac Shunt
- Vein of Galen Malformation
- Severe Anemia

Less Common

- Congenital or Infantile Hepatic Hemangiomas
- Arteriovenous Malformations
- Teratoma

Rare but Important

- Parkes-Weber Syndrome
- Chorioangioma

ESSENTIAL INFORMATION

Key Differential Diagnosis Issues

- Main causes
  - Intracardiac left-to-right shunt
  - Extracardiac left-to-right shunt
  - Severe anemia

Helpful Clues for Common Diagnoses

- **Intracardiac Shunt**
  - Heart failure is most common with ventricular level shunts
  - Radiographs: Cardiomegaly with increased pulmonary vascularity, superimposed interstitial edema, & air-trapping
  - **Ventricular septal defect (VSD)**
    - Most common congenital heart disease (CHD) in children (~ 50% of children with CHD); isolated defect in 20%
    - Classified based on location from perspective of right ventricle (RV) (with various systems proposed)
    - Perimembranous VSD: 70-80%
      - Defect in membranous septum & adjacent muscular septum, defined by tricuspid-mitral-aortic fibrous valvular continuity through defect
    - Muscular VSD: 2nd most common
      - Completely surrounded by ventricular myocardium
      - Often close spontaneously when small
    - Heart failure with large or multiple VSDs
    - Chamber enlargement: Left atrium (LA), left ventricle (LV), RV, pulmonary artery (PA)
  - **Atrioventricular septal defect (AVSD)**
    - a.k.a. endocardial cushion defect
    - Defined by common atrioventricular (AV) junction/annulus, typically with common AV orifice
    - May present at birth, depending on degree of shunting & AV regurgitation
    - Can have congestive heart failure, recurrent pulmonary infections, &/or early pulmonary hypertension
    - Strong association with trisomy 21; common in heterotaxy
    - Global chamber enlargement, greatest of right atrium (RA) & PA
- **Vein of Galen Malformation**
  - Fistula between deep choroidal arteries & median prosencephalic vein
  - Most common extracardiac cause of high-output heart failure in newborns
  - After birth, blood flow increases through malformation: Up to 80% of LV output may supply brain → increased cardiac output & heart failure
  - Intracranial findings
    - Large midline vascular anomaly at quadrigeminal plate cistern
    - Enlarged feeding arteries & draining veins
    - Ventriculomegaly
    - Areas of brain ischemia/infarction/volume loss
- **Severe Anemia**
  - **Sickle cell disease (SCD)**
    - Longstanding anemia leads to global cardiomegaly & heart failure
    - Physiologic contributions: High output of anemia, poor oxygen delivery to coronary arteries, possible underlying restrictive cardiomyopathy
    - More common in older children & adolescents
    - Many typical clues of SCD usually present (e.g., H-shaped vertebrae, infarcted spleen, etc.)
  - **β-thalassemia**
    - Severe anemia leads to global cardiomegaly & heart failure
    - Physiologic contributions: High output of anemia, elevated iron levels/deposition from transfusions
    - May manifest earlier in childhood

Helpful Clues for Less Common Diagnoses

- **Congenital or Infantile Hepatic Hemangiomas**
  - Benign endothelial neoplasm of neonates/infants
  - **Congenital hemangioma (CH)**
    - Present at birth, typically with no further growth postnatally
    - Subtypes: Rapidly involuting (RICH), noninvoluting (NICH), & partially involuting (PICH)
    - Most common is RICH: Almost entirely involuted by 14 months of age
    - Imaging
      - Internal heterogeneity due to fibrosis, Ca^{2+}, hemorrhage
      - Increased peripheral vascularity
      - Enlarged hepatic arteries & draining hepatic veins
    - Consumptive coagulopathy & high-output heart failure (from AV shunting) may occur
  - **Infantile hemangiomas (IH)**
    - Multiple hepatic lesions classified as multifocal or diffuse in distribution
      - May have cutaneous IH: Presence of 5 or more requires screening for hepatic IH
    - Not typically present at birth
    - Appear & rapidly grow in 1st few weeks/months of life (proliferative phase) & gradually involute over years (involutional phase)
      - Most stop growing by 8-12 months (can be up to 18 months)
      - 50% involute by 5 years of age, 90% involute by 9 years of age

- May have variable remnant fibrofatty tissue for remainder of life
  - Hypervascular progressive peripheral to central enhancement on dynamic CECT or T1 C+ MR
  - Diffuse form: Liver nearly completely replaced by numerous small to moderate-sized lesions
    - Aorta may be diminutive distal to celiac axis
    - May lead to hypothyroidism, heart failure, respiratory distress, liver failure, or abdominal compartment syndrome
- **Arteriovenous Malformations**
  - High-flow congenital lesions resulting from errors in vessel morphogenesis
  - Typical locations: Head, neck, extremities, liver
  - Lesions grow commensurate with child but may enlarge rapidly during times of hormonal stimulation
  - Tangle of flow voids with enlarged feeding arteries & draining veins
    - Early enhancement of veins due to shunting
- **Teratoma**
  - Germ cell tumor arising from pluripotent cells
  - Heterogeneous mixed solid-cystic mass
  - Typical locations: Sacrococcygeal region, neck, oropharynx, abdomen, retroperitoneum
  - Findings associated with increased risk for congestive heart failure
    - Larger lesions
    - Significant solid tissue component
    - Large feeding vessels/robust internal vascularity
    - Intralesional hemorrhage
    - Placentomegaly
    - Hydropic changes in fetus
  - Sacrococcygeal teratoma (SCT)
    - Type I: Entirely extrapelvic
    - Type II: Dumbbell shape, equal intrapelvic/extrapelvic
    - Type III: Primarily intrapelvic
    - Type IV: Entirely intrapelvic/abdominal
    - Early signs of high-output failure in fetus: Enlarged inferior vena cava (IVC) size, elevated descending aortic velocity, elevated combined cardiac output
  - Cervical teratoma
    - Differential consideration is lymphatic malformation if multicystic
    - Other considerations: Airway management, intracranial involvement

Helpful Clues for Rare Diagnoses

- **Parkes-Weber Syndrome**
  - Rare limb overgrowth syndrome associated with diffuse combined vascular malformation (capillary-arterial-venous anomaly with **high-flow** arteriovenous fistula/shunts)
  - Pitfall: Can be confused with Klippel-Trenaunay syndrome, which is characterized by limb overgrowth with diffuse combined **low-flow** vascular malformations
- **Chorioangioma**
  - Benign, rare hypervascular placental tumor
  - Consists of small caliber vascular structures & stroma
  - Often seen at base of umbilical cord with vascular supply arising near or from umbilical vessels
  - Potential fetal sequelae
    - Hydropic changes
    - Growth restriction

SELECTED REFERENCES

1. Masarone D et al: Pediatric heart failure: a practical guide to diagnosis and management. Pediatr Neonatol. 58(4):303-12, 2017
2. Merrow AC et al: 2014 Revised classification of vascular lesions from the International Society for the Study of Vascular Anomalies: radiologic-pathologic update. Radiographics. 36(5):1494-516, 2016
3. Niss O et al: Cardiomyopathy with restrictive physiology in sickle cell disease. JACC Cardiovasc Imaging. 9(3):243-52, 2016
4. Reddy YNV et al: High-output heart failure: a 15-year experience. J Am Coll Cardiol. 68(5):473-82, 2016

Intracardiac Shunt

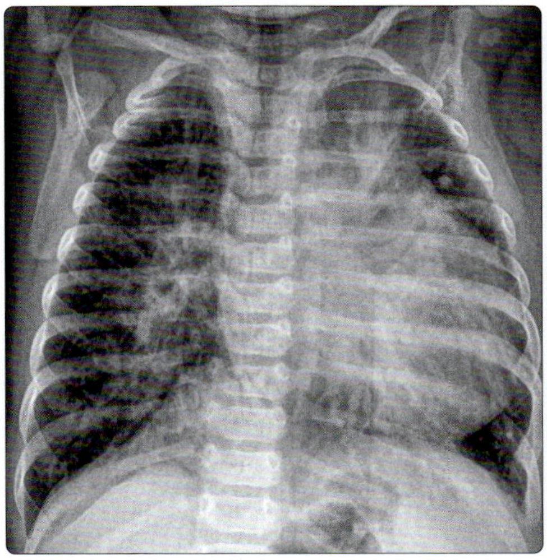

Intracardiac Shunt

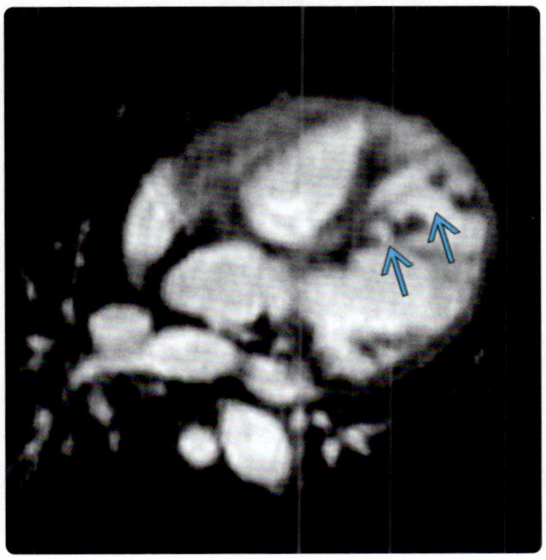

(Left) *PA radiograph in a 4 month old with heart failure with both a large ASD & VSD shows cardiomegaly with increased pulmonary vascularity, air-trapping, & central subsegmental atelectasis, typical of a L-to-R shunt. The vessels are indistinct, suggestive of superimposed interstitial edema due to heart failure.* **(Right)** *Axial oblique MRA MPR image in a 2 year old shows multiple moderate to large muscular VSDs ➡ (a "Swiss cheese" septum). Large or multiple VSDs can lead to high-output heart failure.*

(Left) *PA radiograph in a 6 year old shows globular cardiomegaly with a dilated main pulmonary artery, increased pulmonary vascularity, & superimposed edema, consistent with a large L-to-R shunt & heart failure.* **(Right)** *Four-chamber SSFP MR cine in the same patient shows a common atrioventricular junction with an associated primum ASD & inlet VSD, consistent with an AVSD. There is four-chamber dilation, greatest of the right-sided heart [right atrium (RA) & right ventricle (RV)].*

Intracardiac Shunt

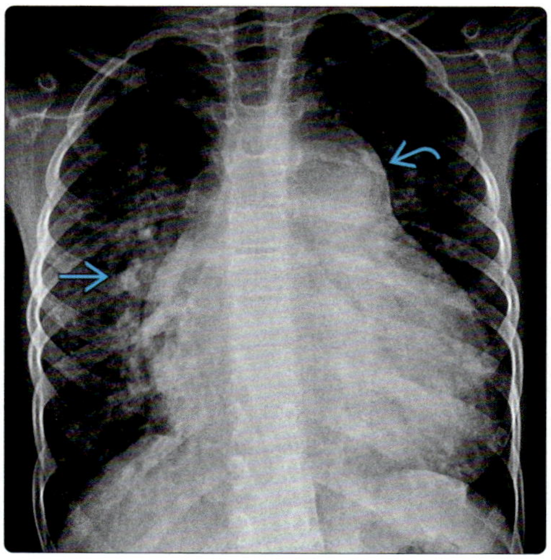

Intracardiac Shunt

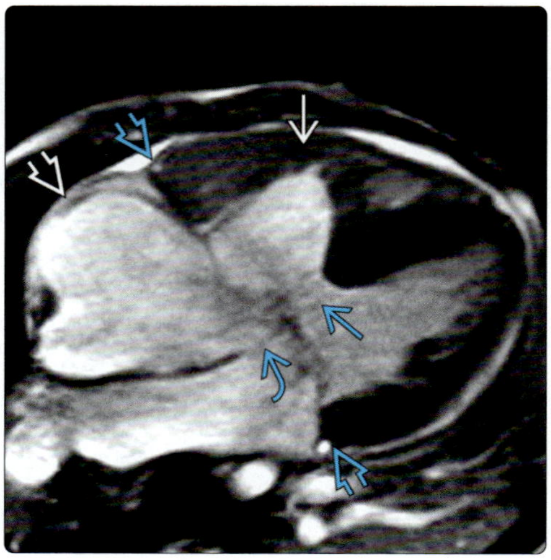

(Left) *AP radiograph in a 6 day old with heart failure shows cardiomegaly with increased pulmonary vascularity & mild superimposed interstitial edema.* **(Right)** *Axial T2 MR of the brain in the same patient shows a large intracranial flow void corresponding to high flow through a dilated persistent median prosencephalic vein, consistent with a vein of Galen malformation. Note the dilated & tortuous deep choroidal arteries, which have fistulous communications with the vein.*

Vein of Galen Malformation

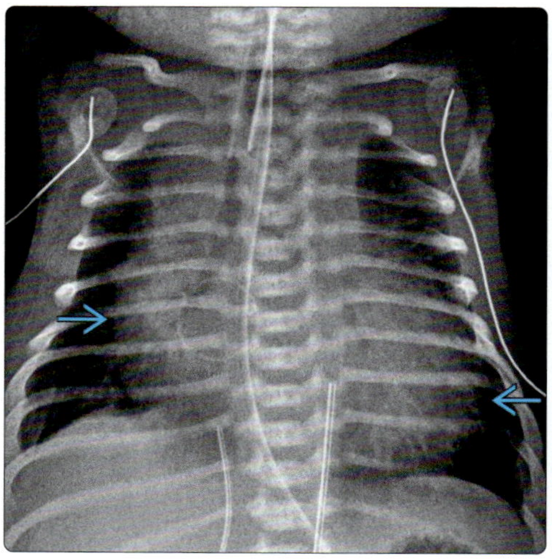

Vein of Galen Malformation

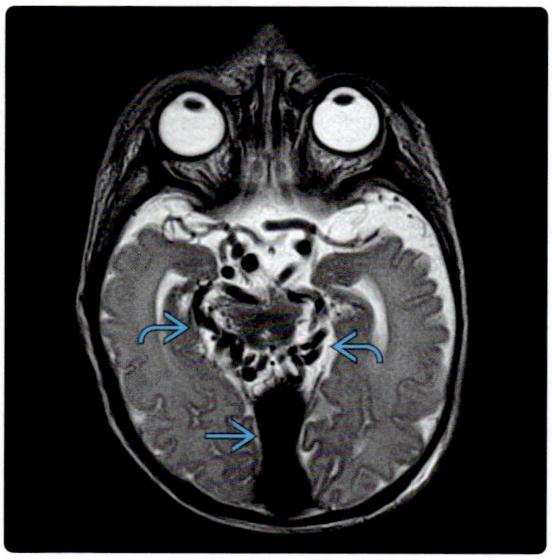

(Left) *Sagittal T1 MR in the same patient shows the large intracranial flow void of a dilated persistent median prosencephalic vein (typical of a vein of Galen malformation).* **(Right)** *Lateral angiogram with injection through the left vertebral artery in the same patient shows dilated & tortuous posterior choroidal arteries shunting via fistulae into a median prosencephalic vein. This is consistent with a vein of Galen malformation, which is the most common cause of extracardiac high-output heart failure in newborns.*

Vein of Galen Malformation

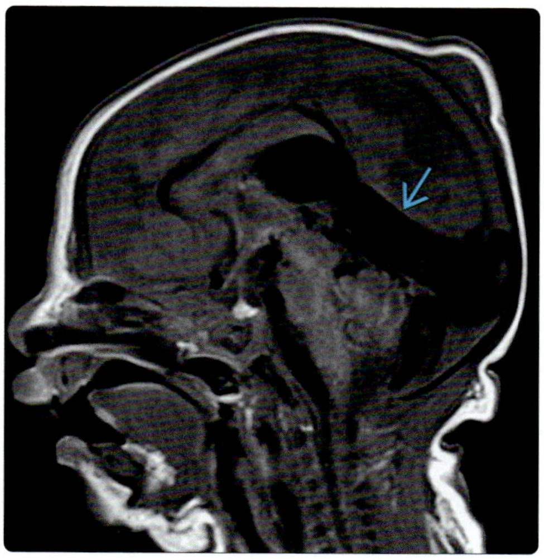

Vein of Galen Malformation

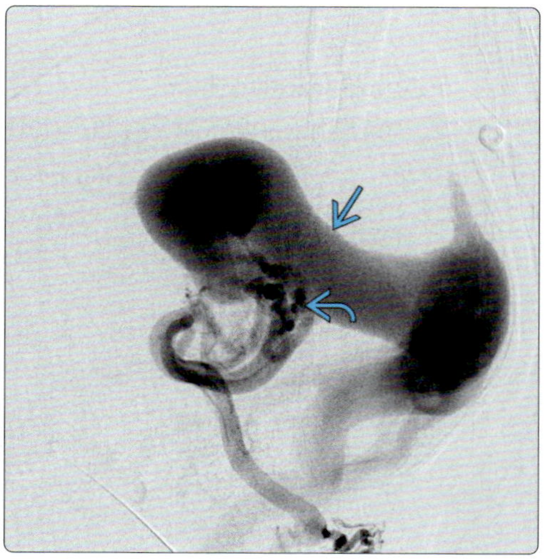

Severe Anemia

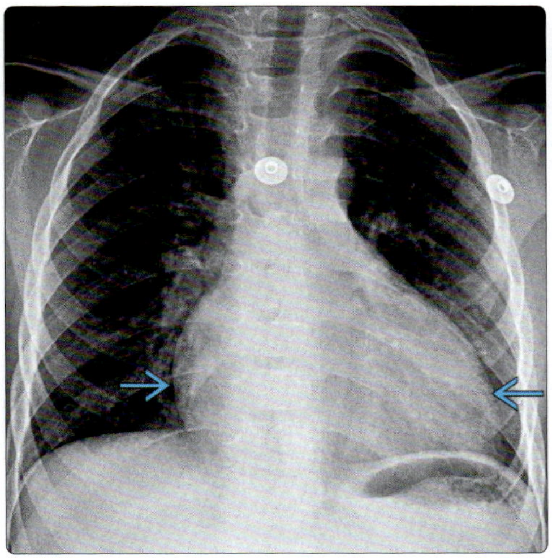

Severe Anemia

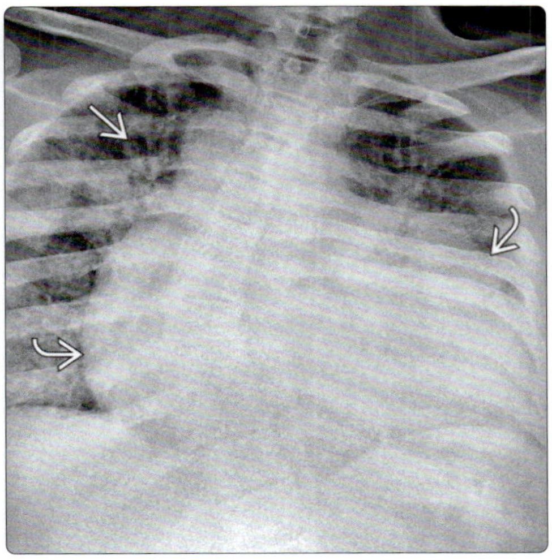

(Left) *PA radiograph in a 6 year old with sickle cell disease shows cardiomegaly due to the anemic state. However, there is no venous congestion or pulmonary edema at this time. Note the absence of a splenic shadow secondary to chronic infarction.* **(Right)** *AP radiograph shows marked cardiomegaly & pulmonary edema in this teenage female patient with advanced sickle cell disease & heart failure. She died from complications of the disease 1 month after this radiograph.*

Congenital or Infantile Hepatic Hemangiomas

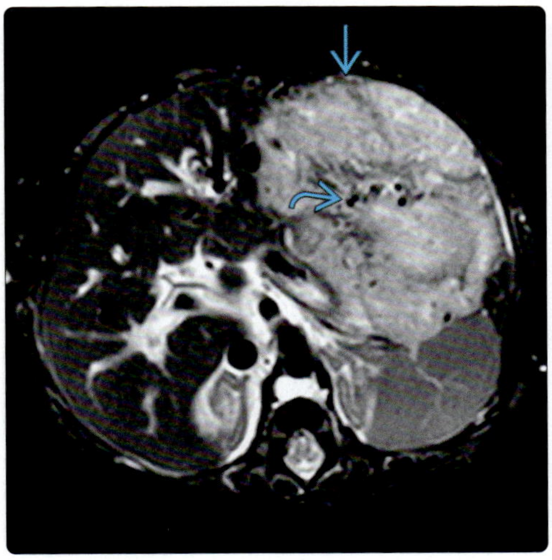

Congenital or Infantile Hepatic Hemangiomas

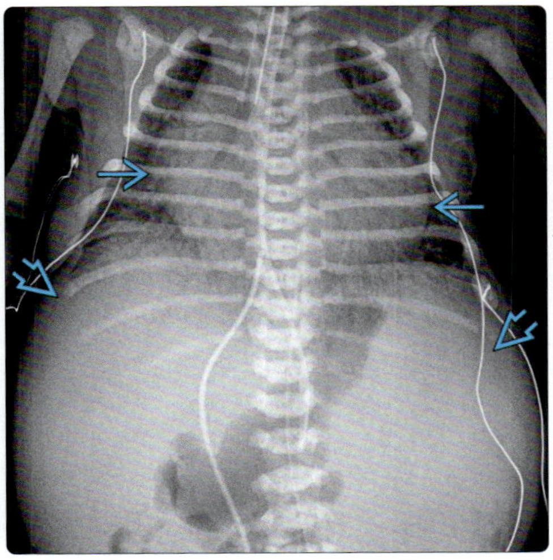

(Left) *Axial T2 FS MR in the same patient shows a large lobulated hyperintense left liver mass with multiple prominent flow voids, typical of a congenital hepatic hemangioma. Note the heterogeneity of the lesion.* **(Right)** *AP radiograph in a 7 day old shows severe cardiomegaly with increased pulmonary vascularity & superimposed interstitial edema. There is also an enlarged abdomen concerning for an abdominal mass.*

Congenital or Infantile Hepatic Hemangiomas

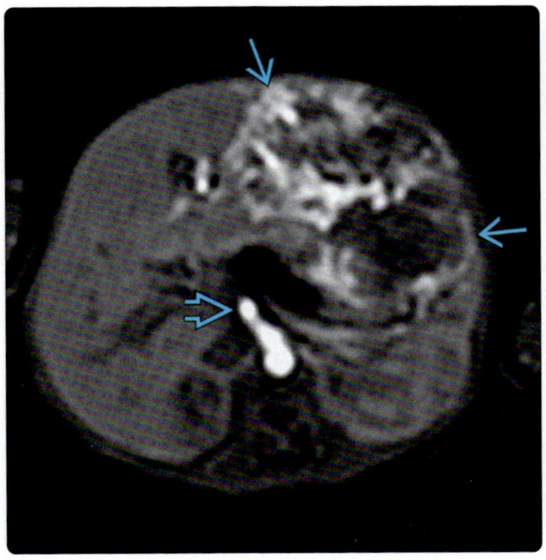

Congenital or Infantile Hepatic Hemangiomas

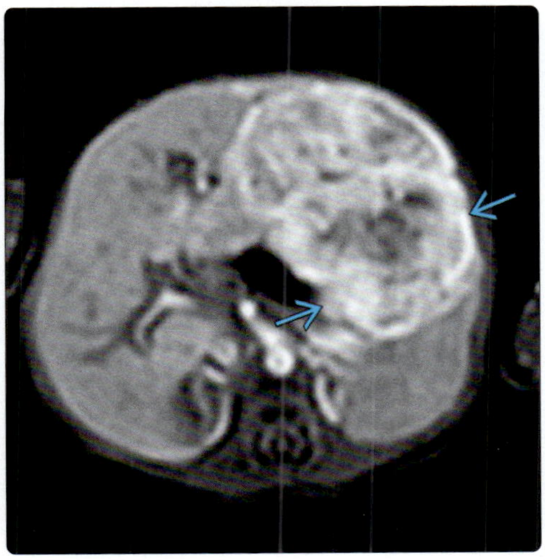

(Left) *Dynamic axial T1 C+ FS MR of the same patient in the early arterial phase shows early peripheral hyperenhancement of the mass. Also note the enlarged celiac axis (which supplies the lesion through the hepatic artery).* **(Right)** *Dynamic axial T1 C+ FS MR of the same patient in the parenchymal phase shows progressive enhancement of the central portions of the mass, typical of congenital hepatic hemangioma. All types of hepatic hemangiomas can lead to heart failure & cardiomegaly in the neonate.*

(Left) *Transverse ultrasound in a 9 week old shows an enlarged liver with multiple discrete lobulated hypoechoic masses →, typical of diffuse infantile hepatic hemangiomas.* **(Right)** *Axial arterial-phase CECT in the same patient shows diffuse infantile hepatic hemangiomas that have typical early peripheral hyperenhancement →. These lesions will progressively enhance centrally & may result in heart failure.*

Congenital or Infantile Hepatic Hemangiomas

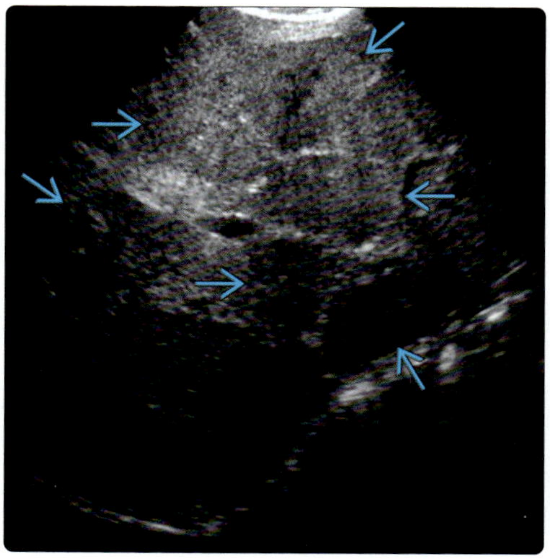

Congenital or Infantile Hepatic Hemangiomas

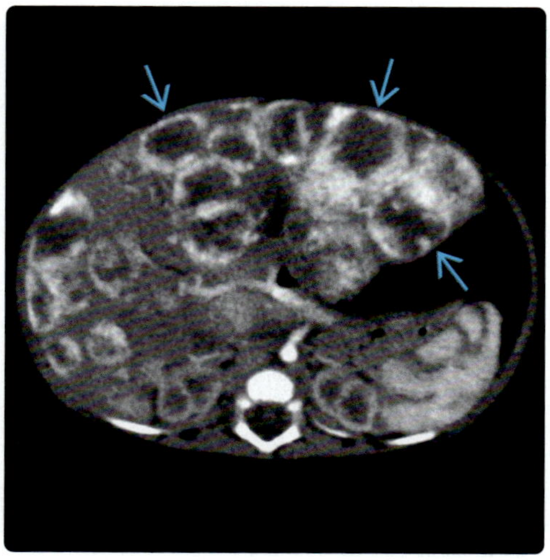

(Left) *AP radiograph shows mild cardiomegaly → & minimal edema in this 3 year old with a parotid gland arteriovenous malformation (AVM) who had clinical signs of congestive heart failure.* **(Right)** *Anterior catheter angiography in the same child shows the large right parotid gland AVM →, which is served primarily by the right external carotid artery & drained by the internal & external jugular veins. As in this case, vascular malformations with significant AV shunting can cause heart failure. This AVM was embolized.*

Arteriovenous Malformations

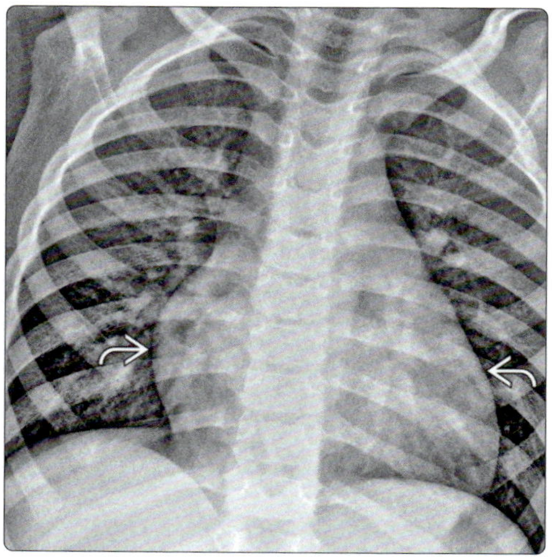

Arteriovenous Malformations

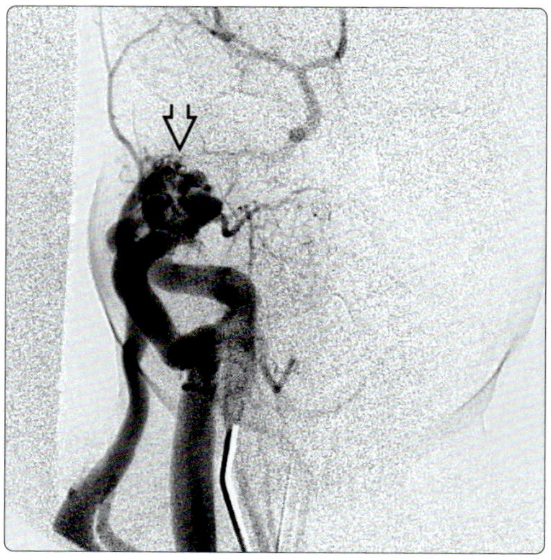

(Left) *Lateral decubitus radiograph of a newborn in heart failure shows a large sacrococcygeal mass → containing scattered internal Ca^{2+} →, consistent with a sacrococcygeal teratoma.* **(Right)** *Sagittal T2 MR in the same patient shows a heterogeneous dumbbell-shaped, mixed solid & cystic mass with internal → & external → components, consistent with a type II sacrococcygeal teratoma. Typically benign, the intraspinal extension → & extensive solid components increase risk of malignancy.*

Teratoma

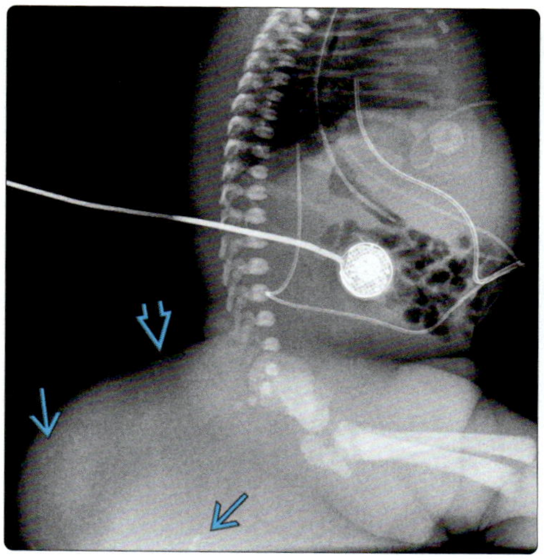

Teratoma

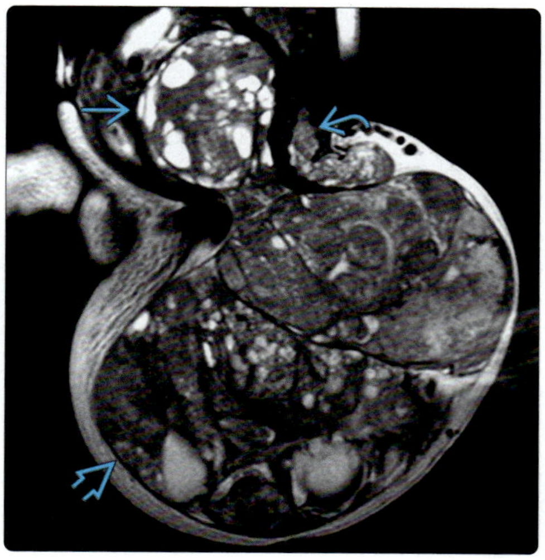

Parkes-Weber Syndrome

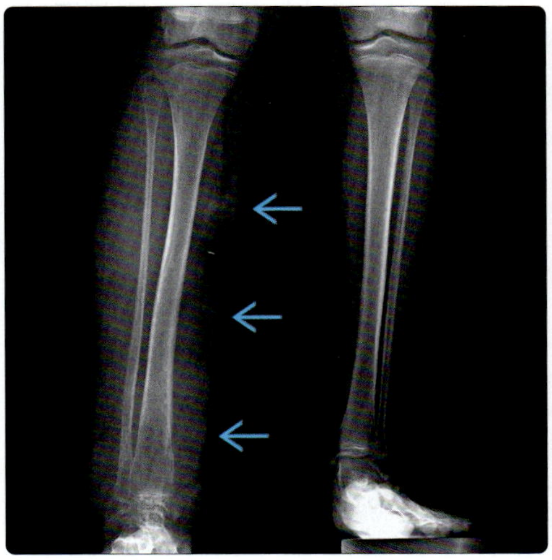

Parkes-Weber Syndrome

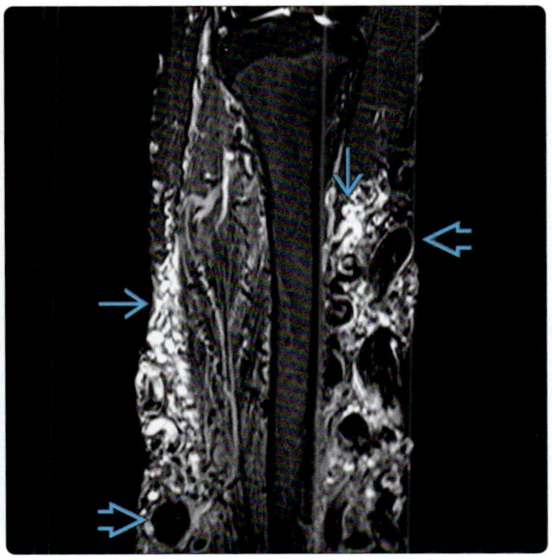

(Left) *Frontal standing radiograph in a 17 year old with Parkes-Weber syndrome shows bone hypertrophy & lobular soft tissue overgrowth of the right lower limb →, related to an extensive vascular malformation.* **(Right)** *Coronal STIR MR in the same patient shows an extensive, infiltrative vascular malformation with serpiginous T2-hyperintense vessels →. Additional tortuous flow voids ⇨ are consistent with high-flow components.*

Parkes-Weber Syndrome

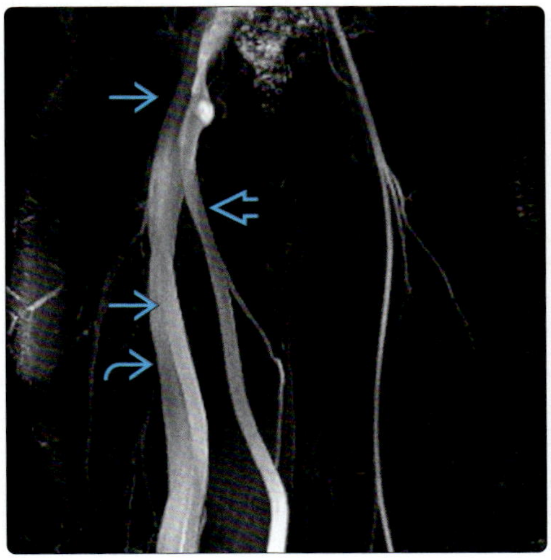

Parkes-Weber Syndrome

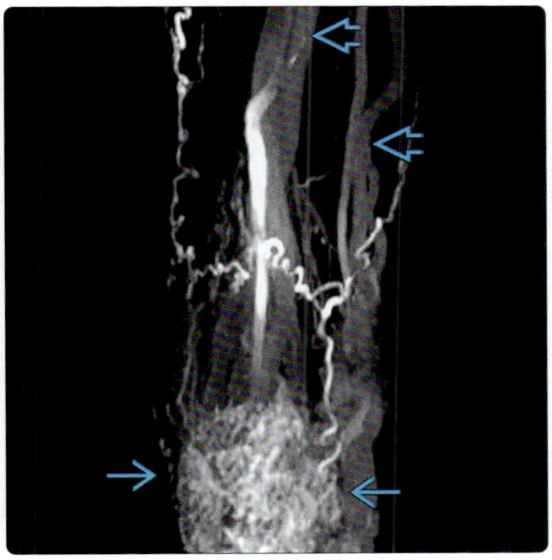

(Left) *Coronal late-arterial-phase MRA MIP in the same patient shows the markedly enlarged right external iliac & femoral arteries → relative to the left. There is early visualization of dilated right femoral ↪ & saphenous ⇨ veins, consistent with AV shunting.* **(Right)** *Coronal MRA MIP in the same patient shows the diffuse combined capillary-arterial-venous malformation with an extensive tangle of tortuous vessels →. Early filling of dilated veins is seen ⇨, consistent with extensive AV shunting, which was causing heart failure.*

Chorioangioma

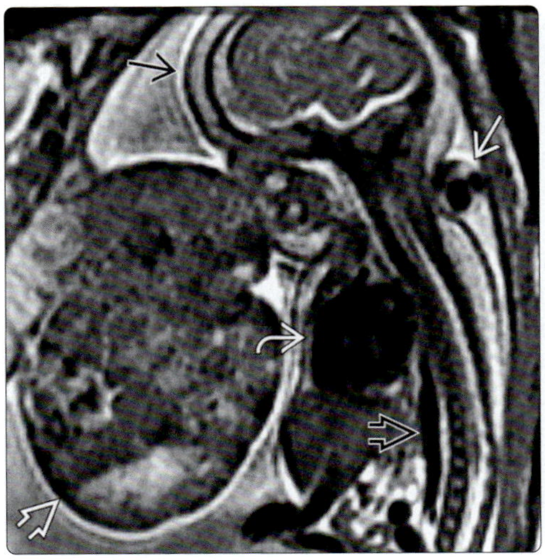

Chorioangioma

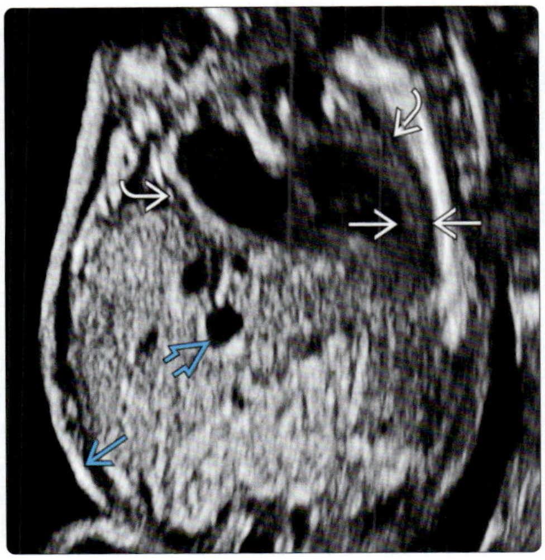

(Left) *Sagittal SSFSE T2 MR shows a large, heterogeneous placental mass ➡ affecting this 26-week-old fetus. Note the skin edema →, cord edema ➡, cardiomegaly ➡, & engorged aorta ⇨.* **(Right)** *Coronal prenatal ultrasound shows the same fetus with global cardiomegaly ➡ & thickened ventricular walls ➡. The umbilical vein is dilated ⇨, & there is skin edema →. Fetal echocardiography showed global ventricular dysfunction.*

DIFFERENTIAL DIAGNOSIS

Common

- Ebstein Anomaly
- Myocarditis
- Dilated Cardiomyopathy
- Pericardial Effusion

Less Common

- Pulmonary Atresia With Intact Ventricular Septum
- Tricuspid Valve Dysplasia
- High-Output Cardiac Failure
- Anomalous Left Coronary Artery From Pulmonary Artery
- Large Ventricular Level Shunt
  - Ventricular Septal Defect
  - Atrioventricular Septal Defect

Rare but Important

- Cardiac Tumors

ESSENTIAL INFORMATION

Key Differential Diagnosis Issues

- Neonate vs. older
  - Differential for massive cardiomegaly is typically considered in neonatal context
  - In children & adolescents, it can be due to acquired condition in previously healthy child or manifestation of underlying disease
- In neonate with cyanosis: Think congenital heart disease with severe tricuspid regurgitation
  - Enlarged heart is due to massively dilated right atrium (RA) from tricuspid regurgitation
  - Cardiac silhouette can fill nearly entire thorax
    - Wall-to-wall heart: Cardiac silhouette touches sides of thorax
    - Box-shaped heart: RA & right ventricle (RV) dilation leads to squaring of right & left superior heart borders, respectively
  - Differential: Ebstein anomaly, pulmonary atresia with intact ventricular septum (PA-IVS), & isolated tricuspid valve dysplasia (TVD) → definitive diagnosis by echocardiography
- In noncyanotic neonate: Consider heart failure, L → R shunt lesions, or pericardial effusion
  - Any form of left heart failure can result in noncyanotic severe cardiomegaly
    - Enlarged heart primarily due to dilated left ventricle (LV) & left atrium (LA), although chamber enlargement can be global
    - Differential includes: Dilated cardiomyopathy (DCM), myocarditis, high-output cardiac failure, or ischemic cardiomyopathy, such as with anomalous left coronary artery from pulmonary artery (ALCAPA)/anomalous right coronary artery from pulmonary artery (ARCAPA)
- Put together with pulmonary vascularity
  - Cyanotic with ↓ pulmonary vascularity: Ebstein anomaly, PA-IVS, TVD
  - Noncyanotic with pulmonary venous hypertension/edema: DCM, myocarditis, ALCAPA
  - Noncyanotic with normal or ↓ pulmonary vascularity: Pericardial effusion
  - Noncyanotic with ↑ pulmonary vascularity: Ventricular septal defect (VSD)/atrioventricular SD (AVSD) (young children), high-output cardiac failure from extracardiac arteriovenous shunting (neonate)

Helpful Clues for Common Diagnoses

- **Ebstein Anomaly**
  - Cyanotic lesion with (massive) cardiomegaly & ↓ pulmonary vascularity
  - Classic entity for wall-to-wall or box-shaped heart
  - Defined by apical displacement of septal & posterior tricuspid leaflets (> 8-mm/m² body surface area)
    - Anterior leaflet in normal position but large, redundant, & sail-like
    - Inlet portion of RV becomes incorporated into RA → "atrialization of RV"
    - Results in tripartite right heart → RA, atrialized RV, & functional RV (trabecular apex & outlet)
  - Broad spectrum of leaflet abnormality, ranging from mild (adult presentation) to severe (neonatal presentation)
    - Neonatal presentation is typically with severe tricuspid regurgitation, leading to massive dilation of RA & thus massive cardiomegaly
    - ↑ RA pressures lead to R → L shunt across patent foramen ovale or atrial septal defect, causing cyanosis
  - Commonly have conduction anomalies & arrhythmias
  - Poorer prognosis: Earlier gestational age, larger tricuspid annulus, pulmonary regurgitation
- **Myocarditis**
  - Noncyanotic
  - Typically of viral etiology in otherwise healthy children
  - Usually with normal heart size
  - Severe cardiomegaly with severe dysfunction → enlarged left heart chambers ± pericardial effusion
  - Clinically, can mimic acute myocardial infarction, although children more often present like heart failure
  - Diagnosis in children thus often presumptive & made on clinical basis (as distinct from adult population where coronary artery disease must be excluded)
  - MR can increase diagnostic confidence & may have role in prognostication (as some patients fully recover while others progress to DCM or develop arrhythmias)
- **Dilated Cardiomyopathy**
  - Noncyanotic with heart failure (pulmonary venous hypertension/edema)
  - Severe cardiomegaly from left-sided chamber dilation/dysfunction
    - Global chamber enlargement = worse prognosis
  - Most common etiologies: Prior viral myocarditis & genetic mutations, although specific etiology often cannot be confirmed (so labeled idiopathic)
    - Main question is often inflammatory DCM (from prior infectious myocarditis) vs. noninflammatory DCM
  - MR to assess chamber size & function; T2 mapping & late gadolinium enhancement may suggest etiology
- **Pericardial Effusion**
  - Noncyanotic with normal or ↓ pulmonary vascularity
  - Most common etiologies in children: Infectious or iatrogenic (trauma, surgery)
  - Radiographs insensitive unless large

- When large, consider bacterial pericarditis, malignancy, immune disorder
- o Frontal radiograph: Water bottle-shaped heart: Globular heart with disproportionate enlargement of silhouette near diaphragm (on upright films)
- o Lateral radiograph: Fat pad or Oreo cookie sign → separation of epicardial from pericardial fat by intervening pericardial fluid
- o Rapid development of effusion may cause cardiac tamponade with compression of cardiac chambers instead of cardiomegaly

Helpful Clues for Less Common Diagnoses

- **Pulmonary Atresia With Intact Ventricular Septum**
  - 1 of differentials for cyanotic neonate with wall-to-wall heart & ↓ pulmonary vascularity
  - Complete obstruction to RV outflow, although typically with well-developed confluent pulmonary arteries
  - Pulmonary flow depends on R → L interatrial shunt & L → R flow though ductus arteriosus
  - Rapid cyanosis develops with duct closure
  - RV typically is small & hypertrophied (prototypical hypoplastic right heart lesion)
  - Tricuspid valve is almost always abnormal (hypoplastic, dysplastic, ± Ebsteinoid)
  - Cardiomegaly depends on degree of tricuspid regurgitation & RA dilation
  - Aorta prominent due to ↑ left cardiac output
- **Tricuspid Valve Dysplasia**
  - Isolated TVD has valve hinge points in normal position (thus without Ebstein anomaly)
  - If severe tricuspid regurgitation → wall-to-wall heart
- **High-Output Cardiac Failure**
  - Noncyanotic with ↑ shunt vascularity & superimposed pulmonary venous hypertension/edema
  - Often seen with vascular malformations or neoplasms that allow arteriovenous shunting
    - Vein of Galen malformation: Most common extracardiac cause of high-output failure in newborns
    - Congenital or infantile hepatic hemangiomas
  - Can also see in older children with severe anemia
- **Anomalous Left Coronary Artery From Pulmonary Artery**
  - Noncyanotic with heart failure
  - Left coronary artery arises from pulmonary artery, leading to steal phenomenon
    - Retrograde flow in left coronary artery (supplied by right coronary collaterals) to pulmonary artery creates L → R shunt bypassing myocardium → ischemia
  - Cardiomegaly from left-sided chamber dilation
  - Severity of disease & age of presentation depend on degree of collateralization from right coronary artery
  - Cardiomegaly with pulmonary venous hypertension/edema in infant: Need to consider ALCAPA
  - ARCAPA can have similar findings (rare)
- **Large Ventricular Level Shunt**
  - VSD or AVSD
    - Noncyanotic with shunt vascularity (↑ pulmonary vascularity & hyperinflation/air-trapping)
    - Cardiac enlargement depends on defect & shunt size
      - VSD: LA, LV, & RV dilation; AVSD: Global dilation
    - With large shunt & severe cardiomegaly, often have superimposed heart failure with pulmonary edema
      - Compared to other causes of heart failure; however, features of shunt vascularity predominate

Helpful Clues for Rare Diagnoses

- **Cardiac Tumors**
  - Cardiac or pericardial tumors can cause enlarged cardiothymic silhouette
  - Most common cardiac tumors in children: Rhabdomyoma, fibroma, hemangioma, & malignancy
  - Requires advanced imaging ± biopsy for diagnosis

SELECTED REFERENCES

1. Canter CE et al: Diagnosis and treatment of myocarditis in children in the current era. Circulation. 129(1):115-28, 2014
2. Yoo SJ, MacDonald C, Babyn P (eds). Chest Radiographic Interpretation in Pediatric Cardiac Patients. New York, NY: Thieme Medical Publishers, 2010
3. Attenhofer Jost CH et al: Ebstein's anomaly. Circulation. 115(2):277-85, 2007

Ebstein Anomaly

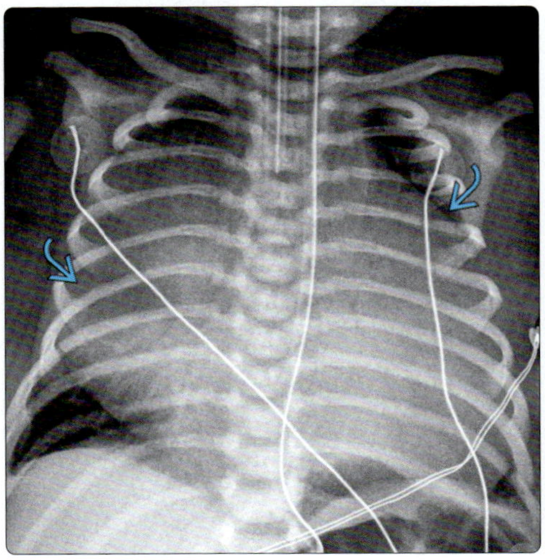

Ebstein Anomaly

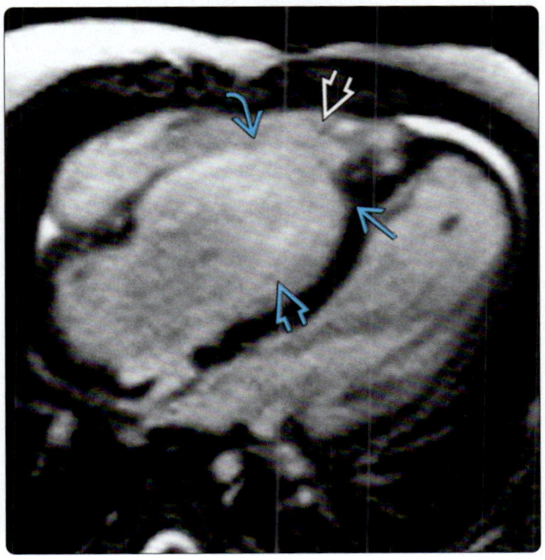

(Left) *AP radiograph in a cyanotic 3 day old with Ebstein anomaly shows massive cardiomegaly ➔ occupying nearly the entire thorax, with diminished pulmonary vascularity. The differential is PA-IVS & tricuspid valve dysplasia, which can also cause cyanosis & wall-to-wall heart due to RA dilation from severe tricuspid regurgitation.* **(Right)** *Four-chamber MR cine in a 4 month old shows apical displacement of the septal leaflet ➔, a redundant sail-like anterior leaflet ➔, & an atrialized RV ➔. Functional RV is small ➔.*

(Left) *Two-chamber MR cine in the same patient shows apical displacement of the posterior leaflet ➔ as well as an atrialized RV ⇨ & small functional RV ➡. (Right) Two-chamber MR cine in systole shows dephasing ↪ directed inferiorly from tricuspid regurgitation. The pathophysiology varies based on the degree of leaflet abnormality & associated defects. Severe valve dysplasia & regurgitation lead to massive cardiomegaly & early presentation, while milder forms present later with heart failure or arrhythmia.*

Ebstein Anomaly

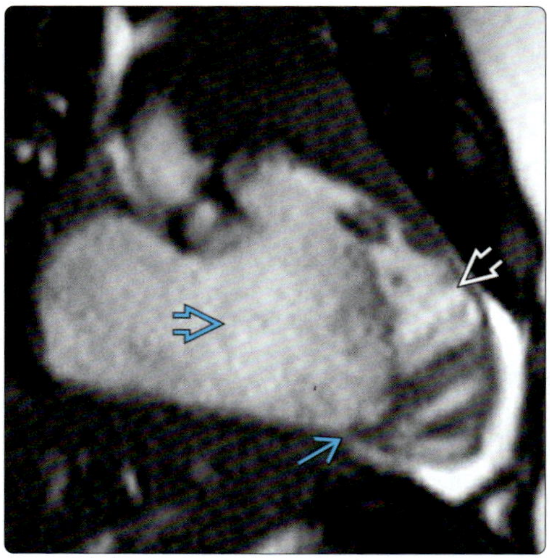

Ebstein Anomaly

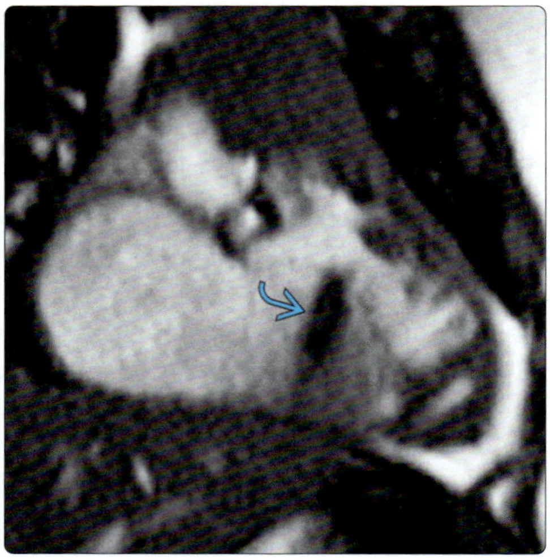

(Left) *Frontal radiograph in a 2 year old with respiratory distress shows cardiomegaly ➡, mild pulmonary congestion/edema ↪, & a small pleural effusion ➡. Blood samples grew Parvovirus.* **(Right)** *Short-axis delayed post-gadolinium phase-sensitive inversion recovery MR in a 16-year-boy with chest pain, elevated troponin, & ECG changes shows patchy epicardial late gadolinium enhancement of the lateral LV ➔ with associated myocardial edema, consistent with acute myocarditis.*

Myocarditis

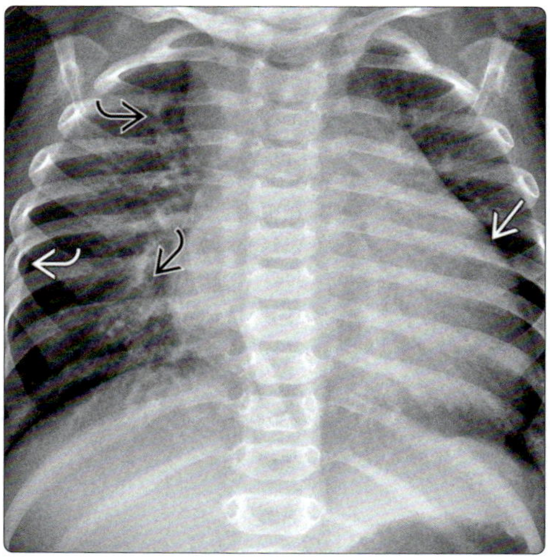

Myocarditis

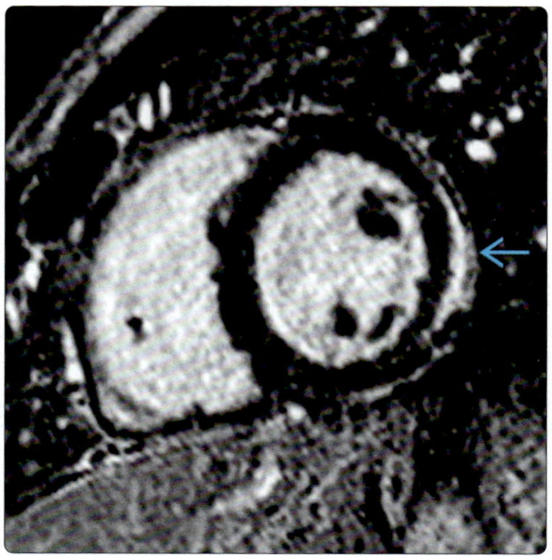

(Left) *Short-axis triple inversion recovery MR in the same patient shows patchy epicardial & myocardial edema of the LV free wall ➔, corresponding to areas of late gadolinium enhancement & consistent with acute myocarditis.* **(Right)** *PA radiograph in a 5-year-old girl shows cardiomegaly with splaying of the carina ➔, suggesting LA dilation. There is normal pulmonary vascularity with central interstitial edema ⇨, raising the possibility of left heart failure.*

Myocarditis

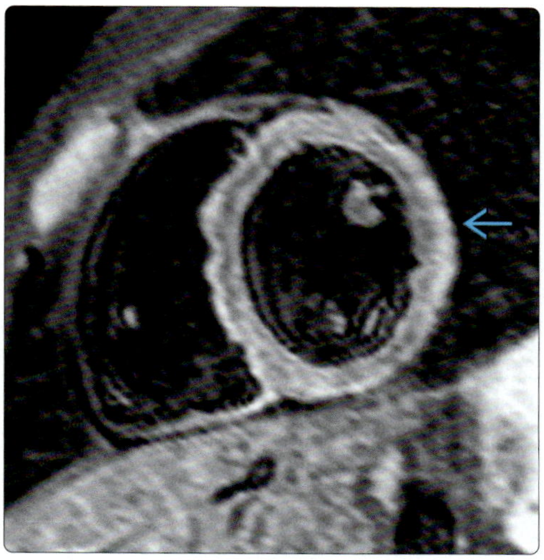

Dilated Cardiomyopathy

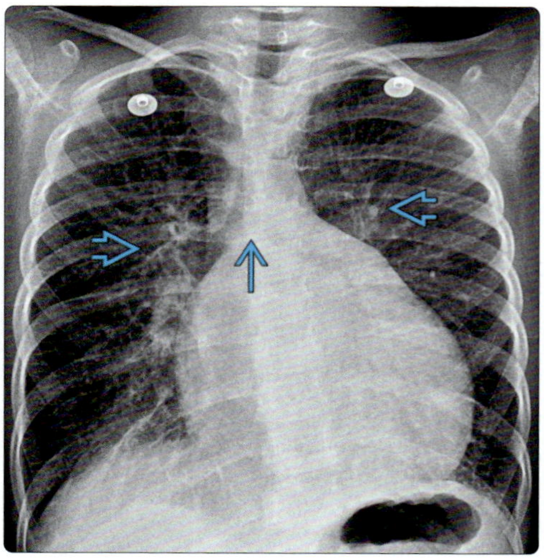

Dilated Cardiomyopathy

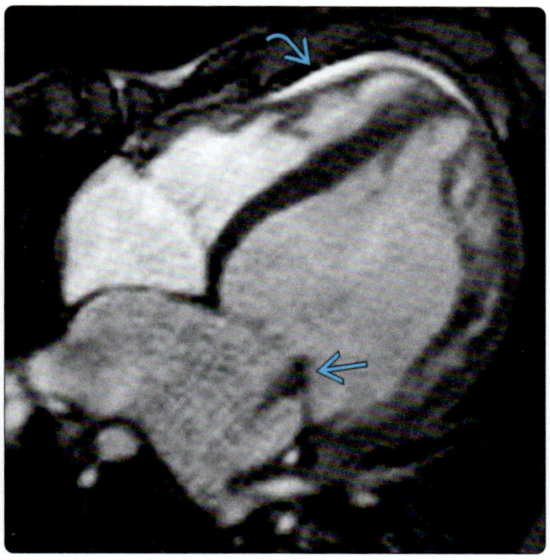

Dilated Cardiomyopathy

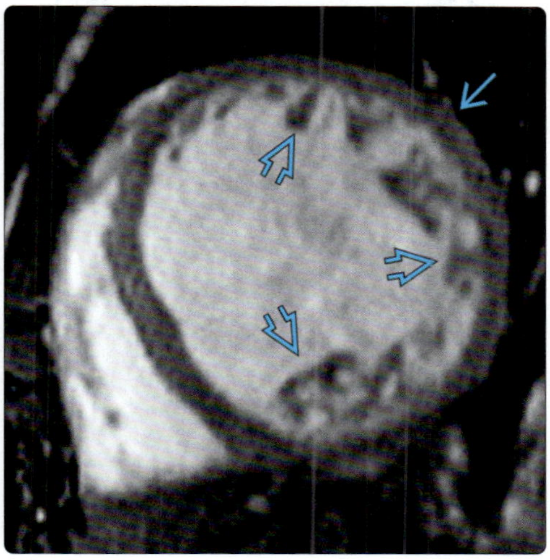

(Left) *Four-chamber MR cine in the same patient shows LA & LV dilation along with dephasing from mitral regurgitation. T2 mapping indicated diffuse myocardial edema (not shown), suggestive of dilated cardiomyopathy secondary to myocarditis. A small pericardial effusion is present.* **(Right)** *Short-axis MR cine in the same patient shows marked LV dilation with prominent trabeculations. Cardiac MR quantified LV size as 231 ml/m² with a severely diminished LV ejection fraction of 22%. The RV was normal.*

Dilated Cardiomyopathy

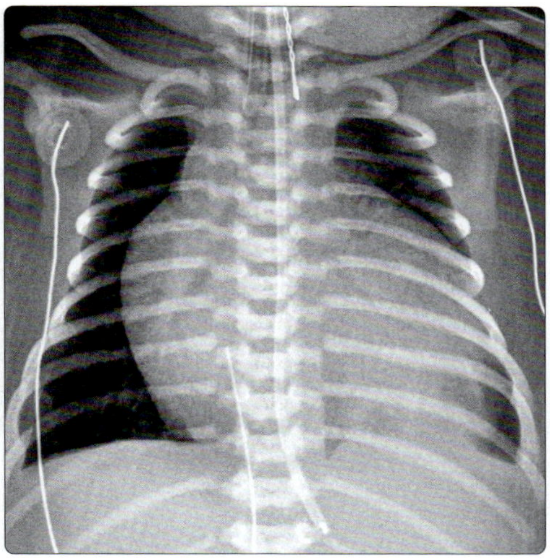

Dilated Cardiomyopathy

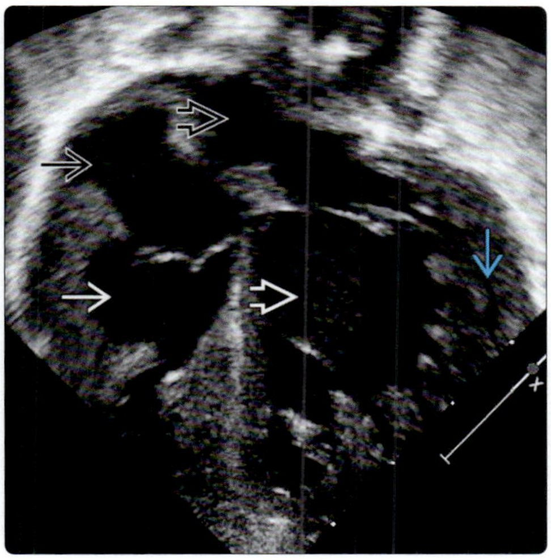

(Left) *AP radiograph in a 2 day old with dysmorphic features & heart failure shows massive cardiomegaly & normal pulmonary vascularity.* **(Right)** *Four-chamber echocardiography in the same patient shows biventricular dilation & hypertrophy, most consistent with severe cardiomyopathy secondary to a genetic inborn error of metabolism. This would not be considered a pure dilated cardiomyopathy. The RA, RV, LA, & LV are labeled. Note the severe hypertrophy of the ventricular myocardium.*

Pulmonary Atresia With Intact Ventricular Septum

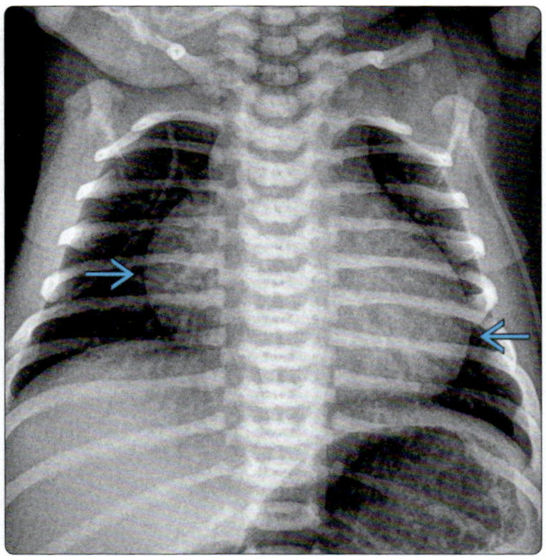

Pulmonary Atresia With Intact Ventricular Septum

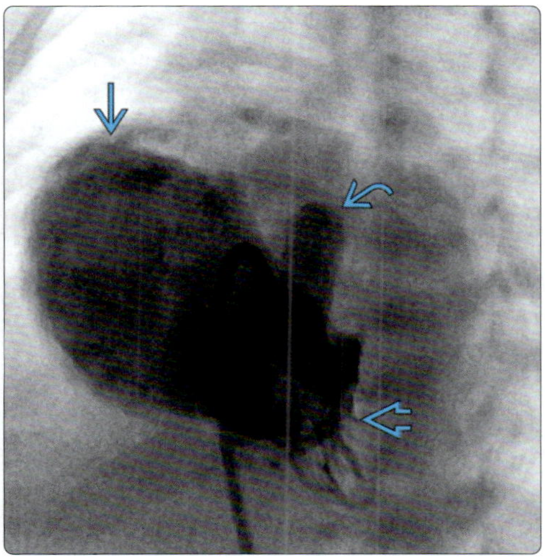

(Left) *AP radiograph in a cyanotic newborn with PA-IVS shows cardiomegaly with diminished pulmonary vascularity.* **(Right)** *Catheter angiogram in the same patient shows a hypoplastic hypertrophied RV, pulmonary atresia, & a dilated RA from tricuspid regurgitation. PA-IVS may have associated RV-coronary fistulae, which may preclude RV outflow decompression by pulmonary valvotomy if myocardial perfusion is dependent on RV pressure ("RV-dependent coronary physiology").*

(Left) *AP radiograph in a 6 day old shows massive cardiomegaly with increased pulmonary vascularity & mild superimposed interstitial edema.* **(Right)** *Axial T2 MR of the brain in the same patient shows a large intracranial flow void, corresponding to high flow through a dilated persistent median prosencephalic vein, consistent with a vein of Galen malformation. Also note the dilated & tortuous deep choroidal arteries, which have fistulous communications with the vein.*

High-Output Cardiac Failure

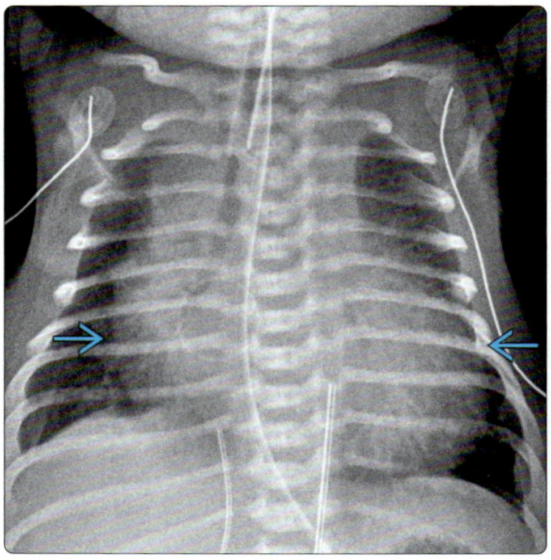

High-Output Cardiac Failure

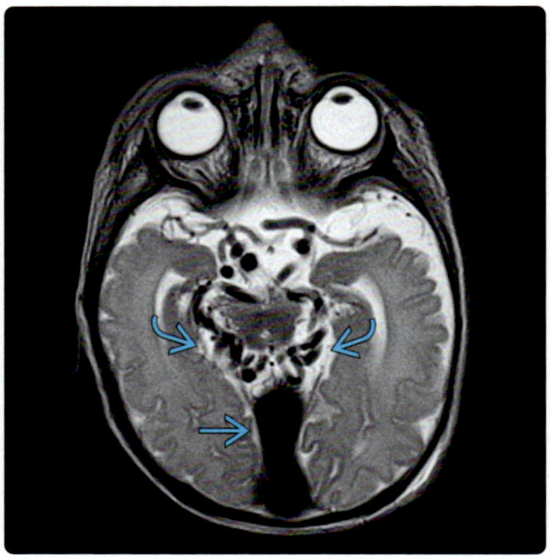

(Left) *AP radiograph in a 7 day old shows massive cardiomegaly with increased pulmonary vascularity & superimposed interstitial edema. There is also an enlarged abdomen, which is concerning for an abdominal mass.* **(Right)** *Axial T2 FS MR in the same patient shows a large lobulated hyperintense liver mass with multiple prominent flow voids, typical of a congenital hepatic hemangioma. Note the central heterogeneity of the lesion.*

High-Output Cardiac Failure

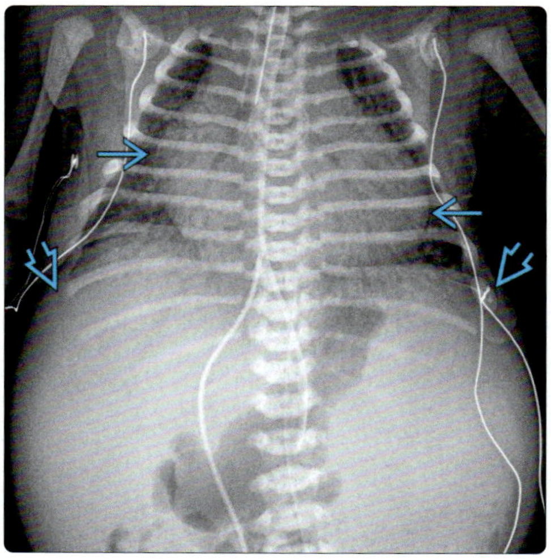

High-Output Cardiac Failure

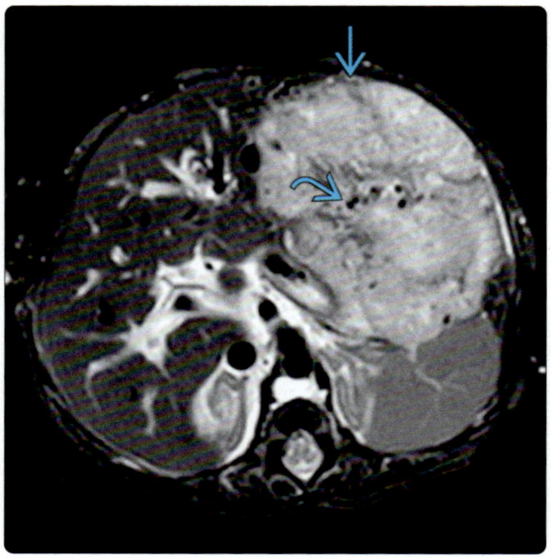

(Left) *Dynamic axial T1 C+ FS MR in the early arterial phase shows early peripheral hyperenhancement of the mass. Note that the enhancement is much earlier in the lesion than the hepatic parenchyma.* **(Right)** *Dynamic axial T1 C+ FS MR in the parenchymal phase shows progressive hyperenhancement of the central portions of the mass, typical of congenital hepatic hemangioma. All types of hepatic hemangiomas can lead to heart failure & massive cardiomegaly in a neonate.*

High-Output Cardiac Failure

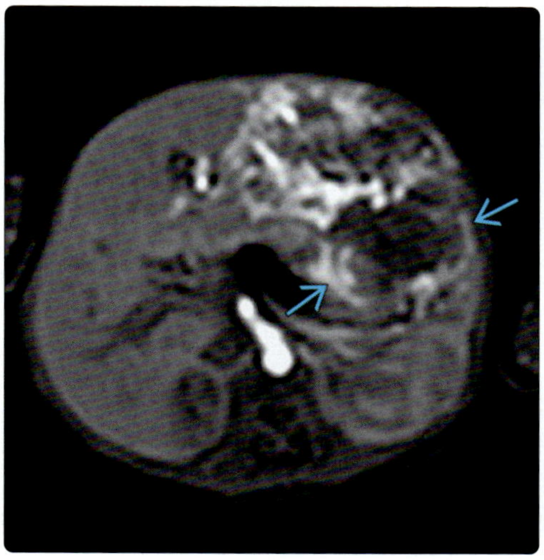

High-Output Cardiac Failure

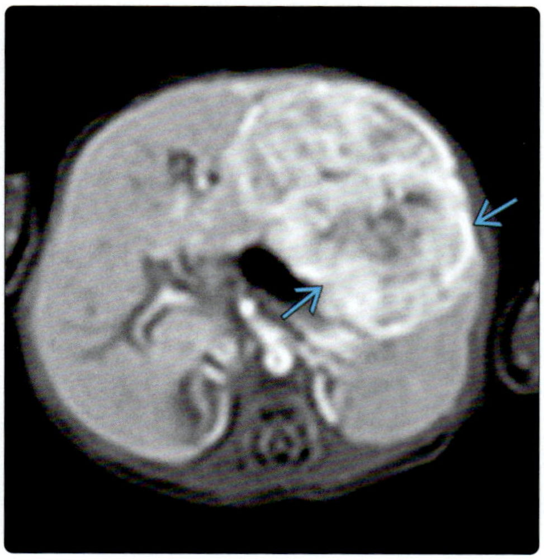

Anomalous Left Coronary Artery From Pulmonary Artery

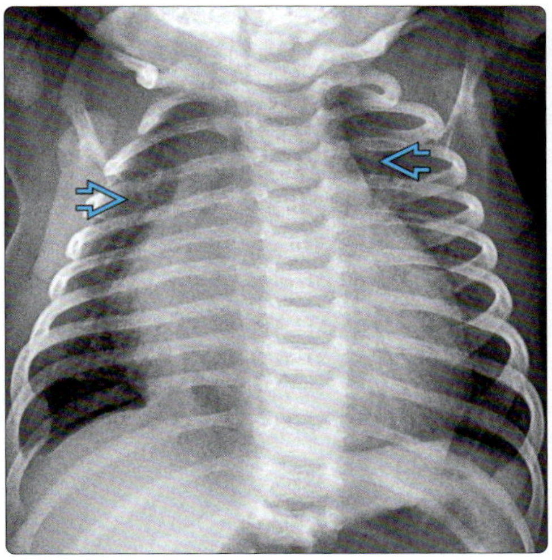

Anomalous Left Coronary Artery From Pulmonary Artery

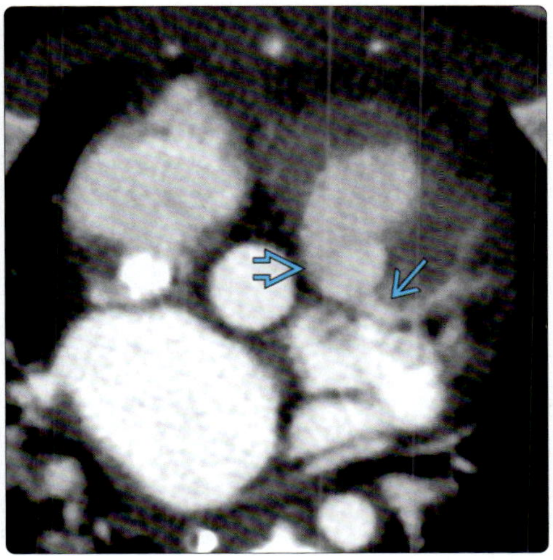

(Left) *PA radiograph in a 4-week-old girl shows cardiomegaly & mild venous congestion* ➩. *Echocardiography revealed ALCAPA with dilation of the LA & LV with severely reduced function (not shown).* **(Right)** *Axial oblique CECT MPR shows the left coronary artery* ➩ *arising from the main pulmonary artery* ➩. *Flow in the anomalous left coronary artery is retrograde into the pulmonary circulation, stealing from the right coronary via collaterals. This leads to myocardial ischemia & dilation.*

Atrioventricular Septal Defect

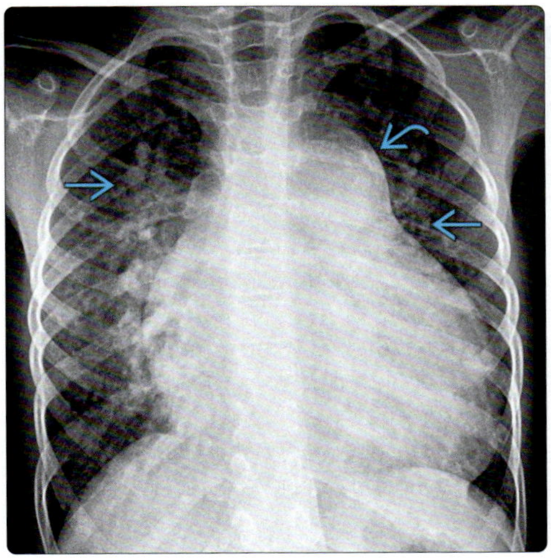

Atrioventricular Septal Defect

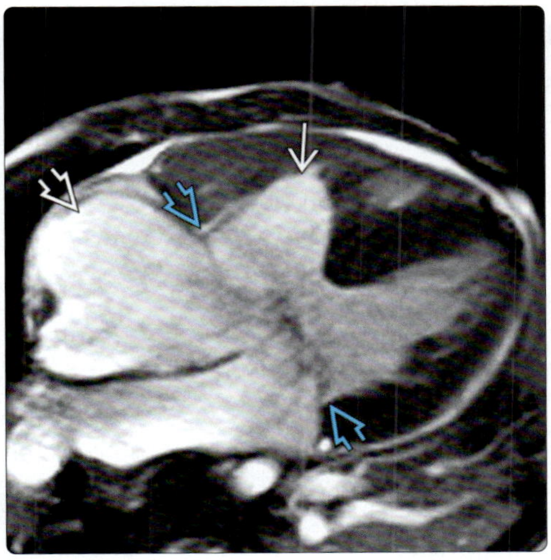

(Left) *PA radiograph in an acyanotic 6-year-old girl shows globular cardiomegaly with a dilated main pulmonary artery* ➩ *& increased pulmonary vascularity* ➩, *consistent with a large L → R shunt.* **(Right)** *Four-chamber MR cine in the same patient shows a complete balanced atrioventricular septal defect* ➩ *with 4-chamber dilation, greatest of the RA* ➔ *& RV* ➔.

Cardiac Tumors

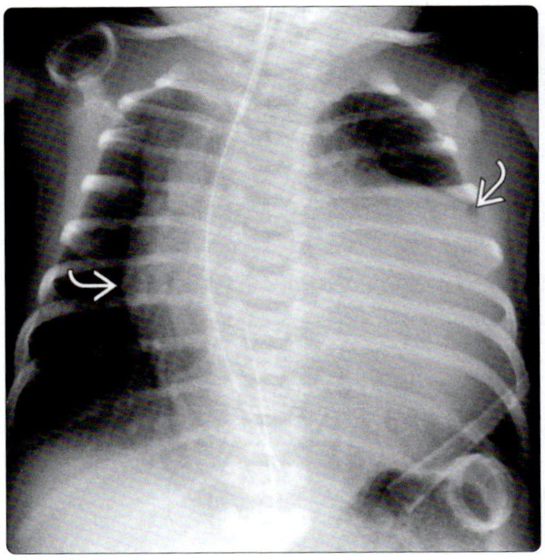

Cardiac Tumors

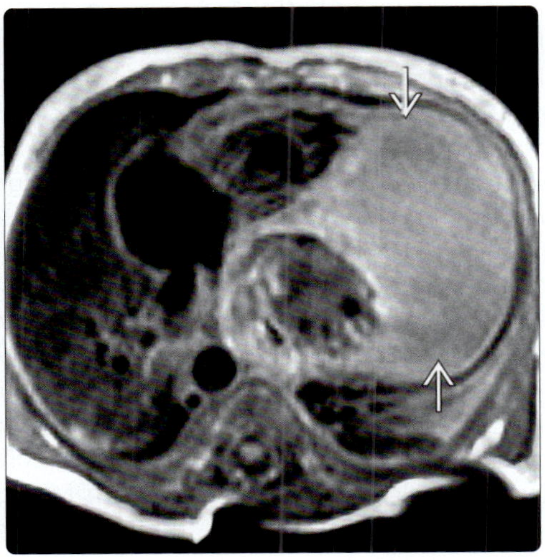

(Left) *Frontal radiograph shows severe cardiomegaly* ➔ *due to a massive LV rhabdomyoma in this infant with tuberous sclerosis. Note that the pulmonary vessels are normal in caliber.* **(Right)** *Axial T1 MR in the same child shows the homogeneous intermediate signal intensity myocardial rhabdomyoma* ➨. *This child's symptoms were treated with inotropic agents, & the lesion regressed spontaneously over time.*

DIFFERENTIAL DIAGNOSIS

Common

- Thrombus
- Rhabdomyoma
- Fibroma

Less Common

- Myxoma
- Hemangioma
- Teratoma
- Lipoma
- Pericardial Cyst
- Extracardiac Tumor or Malignancy

Rare but Important

- Purkinje Cell Tumor
- Papillary Fibroelastoma
- Primary Cardiac Malignant Tumor
  - Sarcoma
  - Lymphoma

ESSENTIAL INFORMATION

Key Differential Diagnosis Issues

- Primary cardiac tumors in children are rare
  - 90% are benign
- Fetal presentation: Arrhythmia, congestive heart failure (CHF), hydrops
- Childhood presentation: Arrhythmia, CHF, murmur, ventricular obstruction, sudden death
- MR features can often suggest specific histologic diagnosis
  - Malignancy usually cannot be completely excluded for highly vascular tumors
- Essential MR sequences: SSFP cine, T1 FSE/TSE ± FS, T2 FSE/TSE with FS, 1st-pass perfusion (FPP), & late gadolinium enhancement (LGE)

Helpful Clues for Common Diagnoses

- **Thrombus**
  - Most common cardiac mass
  - Location: Any chamber, mural or intraluminal, often in regions of stasis
    - Left atrial appendage in atrial fibrillation
    - Right atrium (RA) with central lines
    - Ventricles in areas of infarction
  - Acute thrombus: Homogeneously hypointense with no enhancement on all sequences
  - Organized thrombus: Can be heterogeneously iso-/hypointense with areas of peripheral enhancement
  - LGE sequence with long inversion time (600 ms): Thrombus is hypointense to myocardium
- **Rhabdomyoma**
  - Most common cardiac tumor in children
  - Benign hamartoma of myocardium
    - 50% have tuberous sclerosis complex
  - Almost all are diagnosed in utero or by 1 year of age
    - Most are diagnosed by echocardiography
  - Most regress spontaneously
  - Mural or intraluminal, attached to myocardium
  - Homogenously similar to myocardium; usually slightly T2 hyperintense
  - FPP: Hypointense
  - LGE: Absent or minimal heterogeneous enhancement
- **Fibroma**
  - 2nd most common cardiac tumor in children
    - Most common in surgical series & MR referral
    - Association with Gorlin syndrome & familial adenomatous polyposis
  - Benign, derived from fibroblasts with collagen
  - Rarely regress, may need resection
  - Solitary noncontractile intramyocardial ventricular mass (interventricular septum or free wall)
  - Central Ca^{2+} (20% by CT)
  - Typically iso-/hypointense on T1, T2, & FPP: Relative T2 hypointensity is rare for other tumors
  - Slow progressive enhancement
    - FPP: No enhancement
    - LGE: Characteristic avid heterogeneous enhancement ± central hypointense core due to diminished central blood supply

Helpful Clues for Less Common Diagnoses

- **Myxoma**
  - Most common benign cardiac tumor in adults, rare in children
    - Association with Carney syndrome (7%)
  - Myxoma cells are embedded in myxomatous matrix (high water content)
  - 80% with internal thrombus, hemorrhage, hemosiderin, or Ca^{2+}
  - Typically in left atrium (60-75%) & attached to interatrial septum near fossa ovalis but can be in any chamber
  - Pedunculated mobile mass with irregular borders
  - Heterogeneous, T1 hypointense, T2 hyperintense with progressive heterogeneous low-grade enhancement
  - Risk of tumor emboli
- **Hemangioma**
  - Benign vascular tumor
  - May be endocardial or intramyocardial in any chamber
  - T1: Iso- to hypointense
  - T2: Hyperintense, may be heterogeneous
  - FPP: Avid enhancement (differentiating from teratoma)
  - LGE: Iso- or mildly hyperintense, may be heterogeneous
  - Currently no validated imaging finding to differentiate benign from malignant hypervascular tumors (e.g., angiosarcoma), aside from frank invasion or metastases
- **Teratoma**
  - 2nd most common primary tumor in fetuses & neonates; otherwise, very rare
  - Typically pericardial rather than myocardial
    - Often with pericardial effusion
  - Commonly attached to base of pulmonary arteries (PAs) or aorta
  - May compress superior vena cava (SVC) or RA
  - Multilocular mixed solid & cystic mass
  - Heterogeneous, T1 iso-/hypointense, & T2 hyperintense
  - FPP: Hypointense (differentiating from hemangioma)
- **Lipoma**
  - Usually solitary; can be from any chamber

- Macroscopic fat signal on all sequences
- T1: Hyperintense with signal loss upon FS
- No enhancement on FPP or LGE imaging

- **Pericardial Cyst**
  - Benign congenital cystic lesion
  - Arises from pericardium without communication to pericardial space
  - Can be anywhere in mediastinum; most commonly at right cardiophrenic angle
  - Usually unilocular with signal characteristics of simple cyst: T1 hypointense, T2 hyperintense, no enhancement
    - Proteinaceous material can be T1 hyperintense
- **Extracardiac Tumor or Malignancy**
  - Extracardiac malignancy is much more common than primary cardiac malignancy
  - Presence of known malignancy at other site is most helpful
    - Leukemia, lymphoma, Wilms tumor, hepatoblastoma, neuroblastoma, Ewing sarcoma, osteoblastoma, testicular tumor
  - Spread to heart by lymphatics, direct invasion, or by SVC & inferior vena cava (IVC)
  - Heterogeneous, enhancing lesions without specific appearances
  - Look for pericardial involvement with effusion

Helpful Clues for Rare Diagnoses

- **Purkinje Cell Tumor**
  - Rare benign cardiac hamartoma in neonates & infants
  - Altered myocytes resembling histiocytes
  - Propensity to involve conduction system of ventricular myocardium → refractory ventricular arrhythmias
  - Limited literature on imaging appearance
  - Strong T1 hyperintensity that is iso- or hypointense on fat suppression
  - T2: Iso- to hypointense
  - FPP & LGE: No significant enhancement
- **Papillary Fibroelastoma**
  - Benign endocardial papilloma
  - Common in adults (mean age: 60 years); rare in children
  - Small pedunculated mobile mass from valve (90%)
  - Tends to arise from body of cardiac valves (therefore does not cause valvar dysfunction)
    - Compared to vegetations that tend to involve coaptation margins
  - T2 hypointense (due to fibrous content)
- **Primary Cardiac Malignant Tumor**
  - Very rare (data mainly from case reports)
  - 95% are sarcomas
    - Angiosarcoma, rhabdomyosarcoma, undifferentiated sarcoma, fibrosarcoma
    - Locally aggressive & infiltrative
      - Usually solitary heterogeneous, enhancing mass crossing tissue planes
      - May involve both cardiac & extracardiac structures
      - Look for pericardial involvement with effusion
  - Lymphoma
    - Rare in children
    - Defined as lymphoma restricted to only heart & pericardium
      - Secondary cardiac involvement by lymphoma via direct extension or hematogenous spread is much more common
    - Typically 1 or more masses involving right heart & > 1 chamber
    - T1 iso-/hypointense, T2 isointense to myocardium
    - Heterogeneous enhancement

SELECTED REFERENCES

1. Tzani A et al: Cardiac tumors in pediatric patients: a systematic review. World J Pediatr Congenit Heart Surg. 8(5):624-32, 2017
2. Ghadimi Mahani M et al: MRI of pediatric cardiac masses. AJR Am J Roentgenol. 202(5):971-81, 2014
3. Tao TY et al: Pediatric cardiac tumors: clinical and imaging features. Radiographics. 34(4):1031-46, 2014
4. Beroukhim RS et al: Characterization of cardiac tumors in children by cardiovascular magnetic resonance imaging: a multicenter experience. J Am Coll Cardiol. 58(10):1044-54, 2011

Thrombus

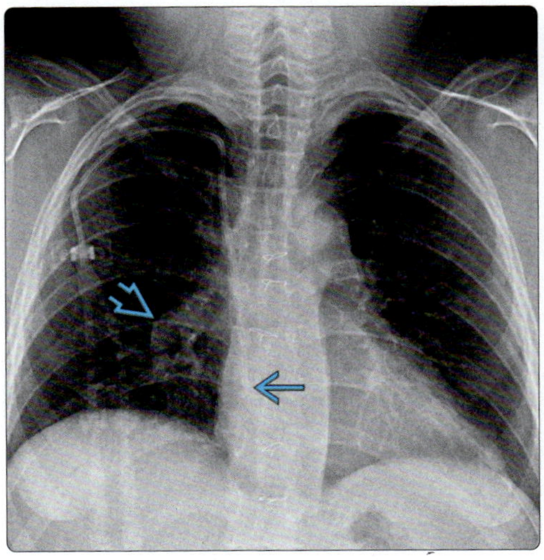

Thrombus

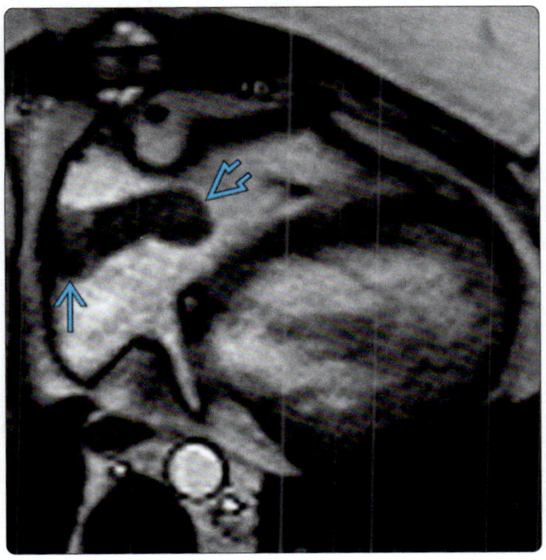

(Left) *PA radiograph, obtained for tachycardia in a 14-year-old female patient with a complex history, shows a right central venous catheter with its tip in the right atrium* ⇨*. In addition, there is dilation of the right lower lobe branch pulmonary artery near the segmental level* ⇨*, suspicious for pulmonary embolism.* **(Right)** *Axial SSFP MR in the same patient shows the right atrial catheter tip* ⇨ *with a pedunculated pericatheter mobile thrombus* ⇨*. This patient also had secondary segmental pulmonary emboli (not shown).*

(Left) *Axial SSFP MR in a 15 month old with tuberous sclerosis complex shows a small mass → arising from the right ventricular septum with similar signal intensity as myocardium, consistent with a rhabdomyoma.* **(Right)** *Short-axis late gadolinium enhancement PSIR MR in the same patient shows no delayed enhancement of the mass →. Rhabdomyomas appear similar to myocardium but are often slightly T2 hyperintense. Most are diagnosed by echo. There can be multiple lesions, & most regress.*

Rhabdomyoma

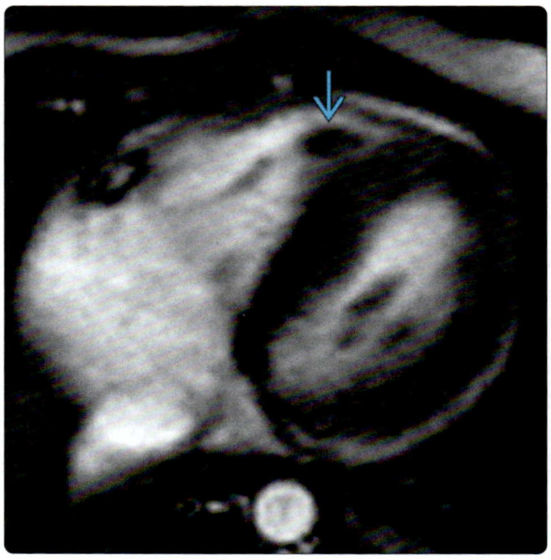

Rhabdomyoma

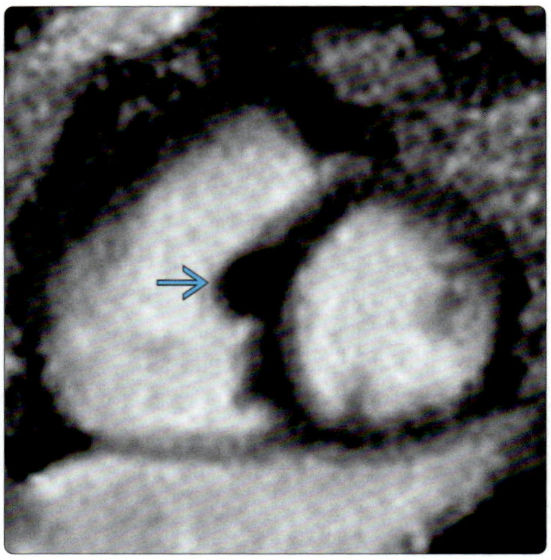

(Left) *Axial SSFP MR in a 2 year old shows a large hypointense right ventricular mass →, which obliterates the right ventricular cavity & bows the interventricular septum ⇨ to the left.* **(Right)** *Short-axis late gadolinium enhancement PSIR MR in the same patient shows avid delayed enhancement of the mass → with a central core of nonenhancement ⇨, classic for a fibroma. Fibromas are also characteristically T2 hypointense, which is rare for other tumors. Usually a thin rim of myocardium can be seen surrounding the mass.*

Fibroma

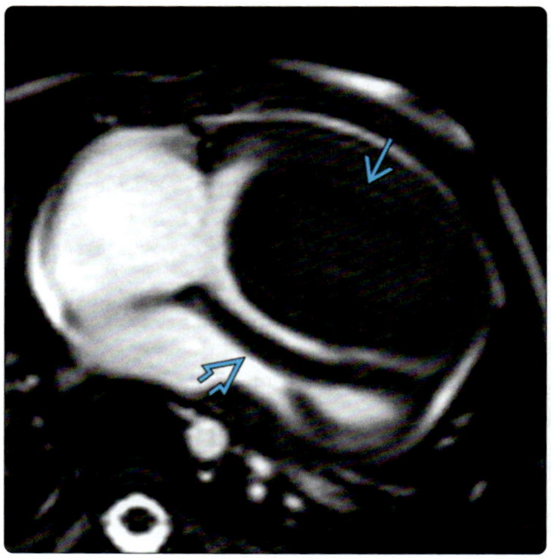

Fibroma

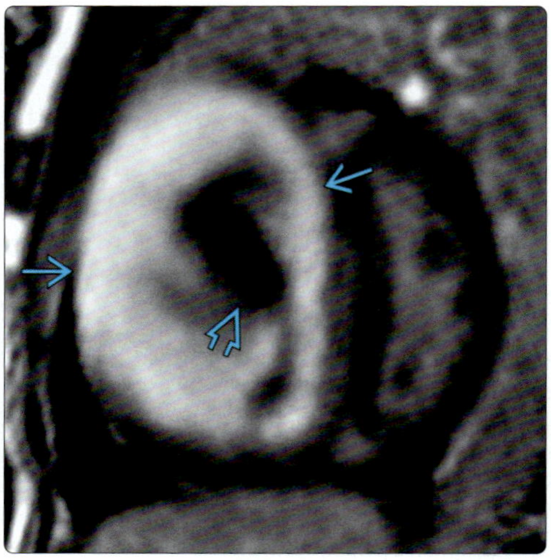

(Left) *Axial SSFP MR in a 6 week old shows a large, heterogeneous, solid & cystic pericardial mass ⇨ that compresses & displaces the heart posteriorly →. There is a moderate pericardial effusion ↪.* **(Right)** *Coronal T1 FS MR in the same patient again shows the large, solid-cystic mass ⇨ with areas of T1 hyperintensity →, representing proteinaceous or hemorrhagic components. A large, heterogeneous, solid-cystic pericardial mass in a neonate is consistent with a pericardial teratoma.*

Teratoma

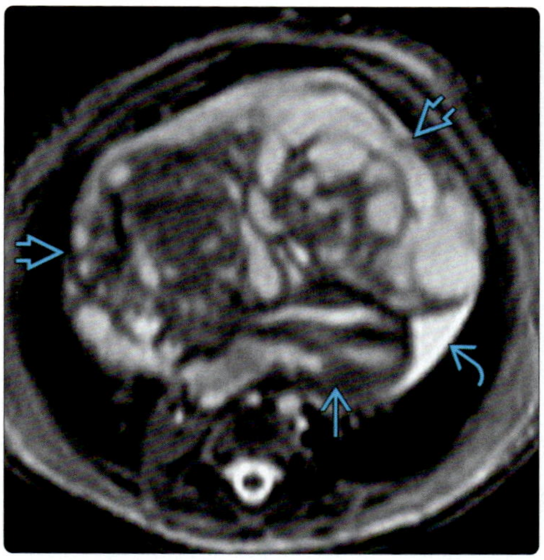

Teratoma

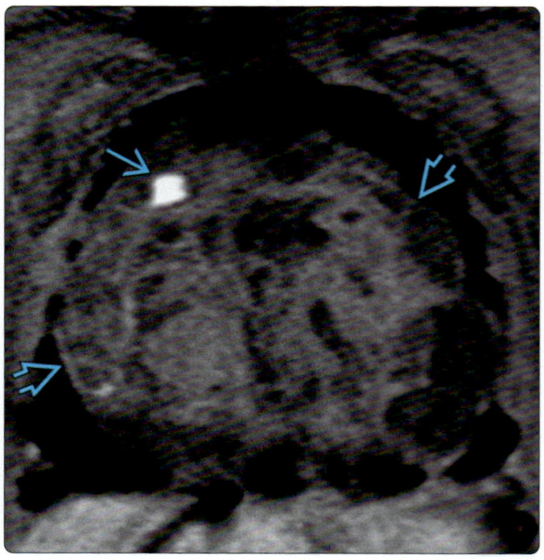

Lipoma

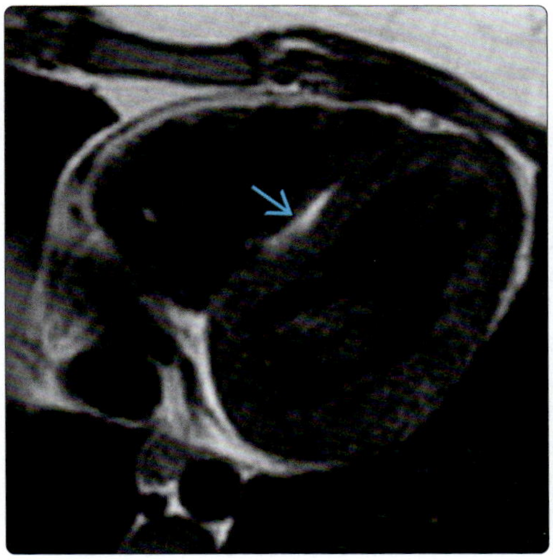

Pericardial Cyst

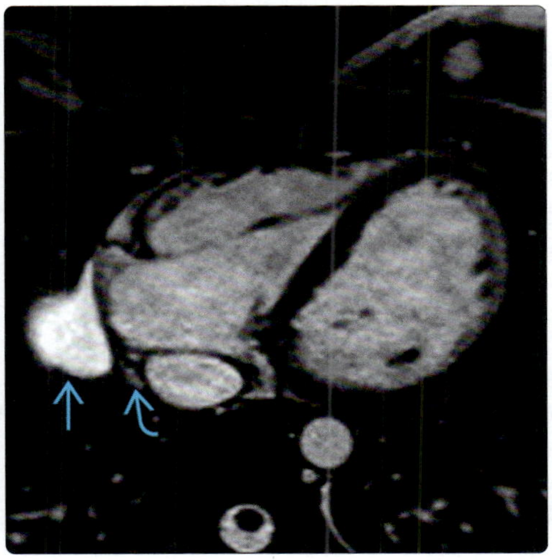

(Left) *Axial oblique T1 MR in a 17-year-old girl shows a thin region of hyperintensity within the interventricular septum. This focus follows the signal intensity of macroscopic fat, consistent with an intracardiac myocardial lipoma.* **(Right)** *Axial SSFP MR in a 16 year old shows an incidental, lobulated, cystic mass adjacent to the right atrium without internal septations, diagnostic for a pericardial cyst. Note the relationship with the pericardial fat. These cysts are invariably connected with the parietal pericardium.*

Extracardiac Tumor or Malignancy

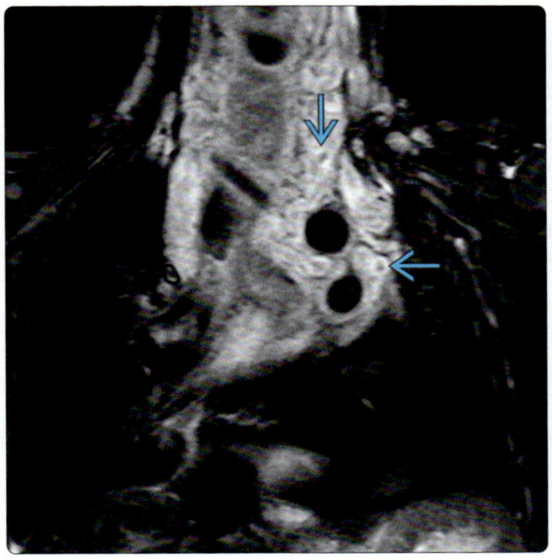

Extracardiac Tumor or Malignancy

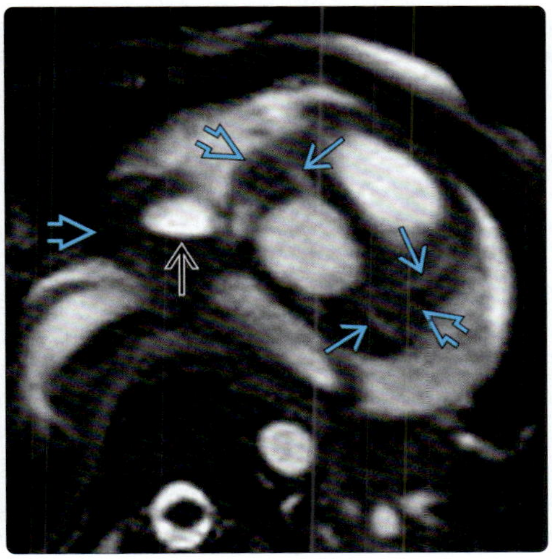

(Left) *Coronal STIR MR in a 2 year old with neurofibromatosis type 1 (NF1) shows confluent plexiform neurofibromas with extensive mediastinal & pericardial infiltration. There are characteristic lobulated & serpiginous contours of these lesions with multiple target signs.* **(Right)** *Axial SSFP MR in the same patient shows an intrapericardial tumor encasing the coronary arteries & SVC. Involvement of the heart from an extracardiac tumor/malignancy is much more common than a primary cardiac malignancy.*

Primary Cardiac Malignant Tumor

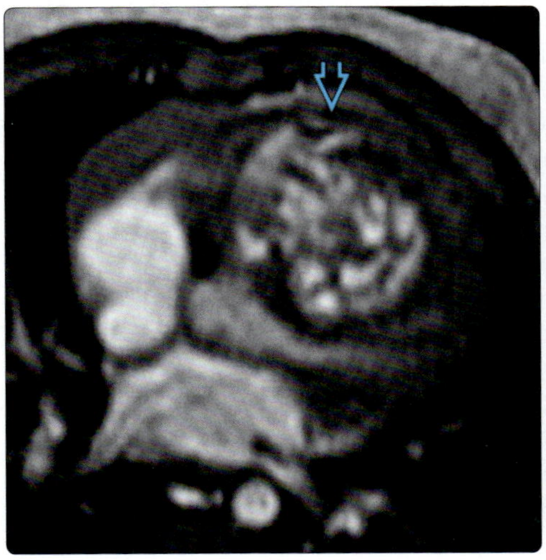

Primary Cardiac Malignant Tumor

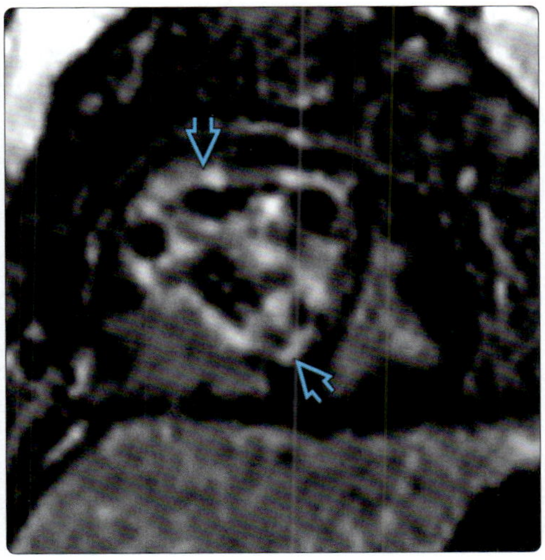

(Left) *Axial SSFP MR in a 3 year old with an elevated AFP level shows a heterogeneous, solid-cystic mass within the superior interventricular septum.* **(Right)** *Short-axis late gadolinium enhancement PSIR in the same patient shows that the tumor compromises the right ventricular lumen & has heterogeneous delayed enhancement of the solid components. This was a malignant intracardiac germ cell tumor. Primary pediatric cardiac malignancies are extremely rare, & data are mostly only from case reports.*

DIFFERENTIAL DIAGNOSIS

Common

- Atrial Septal Defect
- Ventricular Septal Defect
- Patent Ductus Arteriosus

Less Common

- Atrioventricular Septal Defect
- Partial Anomalous Pulmonary Venous Return

Rare but Important

- Vein of Galen Malformation
- Diffuse Infantile Hepatic Hemangiomas
- Congenital Hepatic Hemangioma
- Severe Anemia

ESSENTIAL INFORMATION

Key Differential Diagnosis Issues

- Radiographic appearance of ↑ pulmonary vascularity
  - Uniformly enlarged vessels at hila & within lungs
  - Sharp vessel margins (unless there is superimposed edema, atelectasis, or consolidation)
  - Convex bulge of main pulmonary artery (MPA) at left heart border
  - Descending interlobar right pulmonary artery (RPA) branch larger than trachea
  - Associated hyperinflation/air-trapping due to airway compression
  - Often not appreciable when pulmonary to systemic blood flow ratio (Qp:Qs) < 2:1
- ↑ vascularity typically related to left-to-right (L → R) shunt
  - Shunt causes right heart volume overload, ↑ blood flow to pulmonary arteries, & recirculation of oxygenated blood in lungs (acyanotic)
  - Definitive diagnosis usually by echocardiography
  - Classically, left-sided structures suggest level of shunt
    - Normal left atrium: Atrial septal defect (ASD) or partial anomalous pulmonary venous return (PAPVR)
      - Can see enlarged right atrium
    - Enlarged left atrium: Intact atrial septum with ventricular septal defect (VSD) or extracardiac shunt
    - Enlarged aorta: Supracardiac shunt [such as patent ductus arteriosus (PDA)]
  - Small L → R shunts often asymptomatic
  - Eisenmenger syndrome from long-term L → R shunt
    - Elevated pulmonary artery pressure → reversal of shunt, oxygen desaturation, & cyanosis
  - Helpful clinical features
    - Neonatal presentation of PDA in prematurity
    - Infantile presentation of ventricular shunt is usually with atrioventricular septal defect (AVSD) or left-sided obstructive lesion
    - ASD, VSD, PDA, PAPVR otherwise present older; VSD most common
    - Trisomy 21 & heterotaxy associated with AVSD
  - Other causes of acyanotic ↑ pulmonary vascularity include high-output cardiac states, such as from extracardiac shunting or severe anemia
    - Heart failure → cardiomegaly with indistinct vascular margins due to edema

Helpful Clues for Common Diagnoses

- **Atrial Septal Defect**
  - Isolated ASD: 6-10% of congenital heart disease (CHD)
    - Well tolerated through childhood, even if large
    - Indications for interventional/surgical closure
      - Degree of shunt (Qp:Qs > 2:1)
      - Right ventricular (RV) enlargement
  - Types: Secundum, primum, sinus venosus, coronary sinus
  - Secundum ASD (a.k.a. fossa ovalis defect): 80-90%
    - ≥ 1 hole in floor of fossa ovalis
    - Size of defect & sufficiency of rims determine candidacy for catheter-based closure
  - Primum ASD: Form of AVSD where bridging leaflets of common atrioventricular valve are attached to ventricular septal crest, allowing only interatrial shunting
  - Sinus venosus ASD
    - Located at sinus venosus (most posterior aspect of wall between right & left atria at caval insertions)
    - Superior type: At superior vena cava (SVC)-atrial junction; defect often also results in PAPVR of right upper pulmonary vein (85%)
    - Inferior type (rare): At inferior vena cava (IVC)-atrial junction; can be associated with PAPVR of right lower pulmonary vein
  - Coronary sinus defect
    - Defect of wall between coronary sinus & left atrium ("unroofed coronary sinus"); associated with left SVC
- **Ventricular Septal Defect**
  - Most common CHD in children, occurring in 50% of CHD; isolated defect in 20%
  - Classified based on location from perspective of RV (various systems proposed): 2 most common types are perimembranous & muscular
    - Atrioventricular conduction axis courses posteroinferior to perimembranous vs. anterosuperior to inlet muscular VSDs → important for surgical repair
  - Perimembranous VSD: 70-80% of VSDs
    - Defect in membranous septum & adjacent muscular septum, defined by tricuspid-mitral-aortic fibrous valvular continuity through defect
    - May extend to inlet or outlet
  - Muscular VSD
    - Completely surrounded by ventricular myocardium
    - Can be inlet, outlet, trabecular/apical, & multiple
    - If small, often close spontaneously
  - Secondary complications of VSDs
    - Adherent tricuspid valve tissue to VSD: Left ventricular (LV) → right atrial (RA) shunt
    - Subaortic ridge: Outflow stenosis
    - Aortic sinus prolapse through VSD: Aortic regurgitation
    - Dilation of right sinus of Valsalva with aortic-RV fistula
- **Patent Ductus Arteriosus**
  - Ductus arteriosus connects proximal descending aorta to pulmonary artery (typically proximal LPA)
  - Normally closes soon after birth (oxygen mediated)
    - Prostaglandins can help keep ductus arteriosus open
    - Indomethacin/ibuprofen help close duct
  - Main risk for PDA is prematurity, especially with concurrent respiratory distress & hypoxia

- Premature ductal tissue is less sensitive to oxygen-mediated constriction
- 65% of infants born < 28 weeks gestation have PDA
- Prevalence of > 80% in premature infants with significant lung disease
- Most cases are sporadic
- Untreated PDAs may lead to pulmonary hypertension
- Secondary complications of ductal aneurysm possible
- For some **cyanotic** CHDs, survival is dependent on PDA
  - Ductal-dependent systemic flow (R → L shunt): Hypoplastic left heart, critical aortic stenosis, interrupted aortic arch
  - Ductal-dependent pulmonary flow (L → R shunt): Pulmonary atresia, critical pulmonary stenosis

Helpful Clues for Less Common Diagnoses

- **Atrioventricular Septal Defect**
  - a.k.a. endocardial cushion defect
  - Defined by common atrioventricular junction/annulus, typically with common atrioventricular orifice
    - 5 leaflets: Superior bridging, left mural, inferior bridging, right mural, & right anterosuperior leaflets
    - Superior & inferior bridging leaflets may fuse → separate right & left atrioventricular orifices
    - Relationship of valve to ventricular septal crest determines degree of atrial & ventricular communication (variable)
    - "Complete" form: Bridging leaflets "free floating" ± chordal attachments to ventricular septal crest → all heart chambers communicate
  - Most severe radiographic findings with globular cardiomegaly, enlargement of all chambers, & markedly ↑ pulmonary vascularity with hyperinflation
  - May present at birth, depending on degree of shunting & atrioventricular regurgitation
  - Can have congestive heart failure, recurrent pulmonary infections, &/or early pulmonary hypertension
  - Strong association with trisomy 21; common in heterotaxy
- **Partial Anomalous Pulmonary Venous Return**
  - PAPVR on right > left
  - Right PAPVR: Usually right upper pulmonary vein to SVC; associated with sinus venosus ASD
  - Left PAPVR: Usually left upper pulmonary vein to left innominate vein; associated with secundum ASD
  - Total anomalous drainage of right lung to IVC-atrial junction is associated with scimitar syndrome
  - Isolated PAPVR of single vein is usually well tolerated

Helpful Clues for Rare Diagnoses

- **Vein of Galen Malformation**
  - Intracranial fistula between deep choroidal arteries & median prosencephalic vein
  - After birth, ↑ blood flow through malformation: Up to 80% of LV output may supply brain → ↑ cardiac output & heart failure
  - Most common extracardiac cause of high-output heart failure in newborns
- **Diffuse Infantile Hepatic Hemangiomas**
  - Enlarged liver nearly completely replaced by numerous small to moderate-sized lesions
    - Lesions show dynamic peripheral to central enhancement
  - May lead to high-output heart failure & respiratory distress
- **Congenital Hepatic Hemangioma**
  - Large solitary liver lesion with
    - Internal heterogeneity due to fibrosis, Ca^{2+}, hemorrhage
    - ↑ peripheral vascularity
    - Enlarged hepatic arteries & draining hepatic veins
  - Consumptive coagulopathy & high-output heart failure may occur

SELECTED REFERENCES

1. Robinson JD et al: Septal defects. In Coley BD et al: Caffey's Pediatric Diagnostic Imaging. 12th ed. Philadelphia: Elsevier Saunders. 737-43, 2013
2. Rojas CA et al: Ventricular septal defects: embryology and imaging findings. J Thorac Imaging. 28(2):W28–34, 2012
3. Rajiah P et al: Cardiac MRI: Part 1, cardiovascular shunts. AJR Am J Roentgenol. 197(4):W603-20, 2011
4. Rojas CA et al: Embryology and developmental defects of the interatrial septum. AJR Am J Roentgenol. 195(5):1100-4, 2010

Atrial Septal Defect

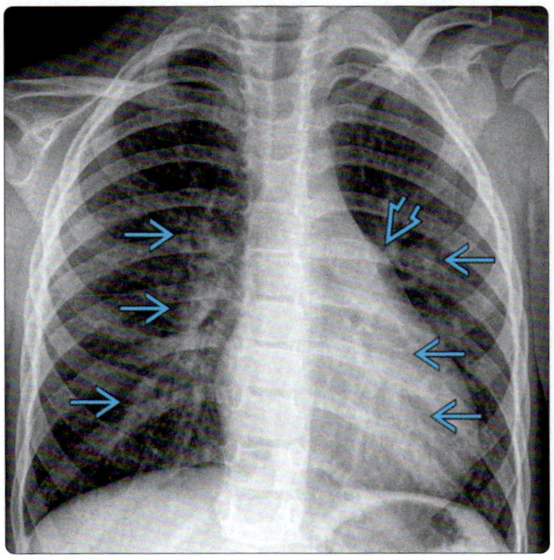

Atrial Septal Defect

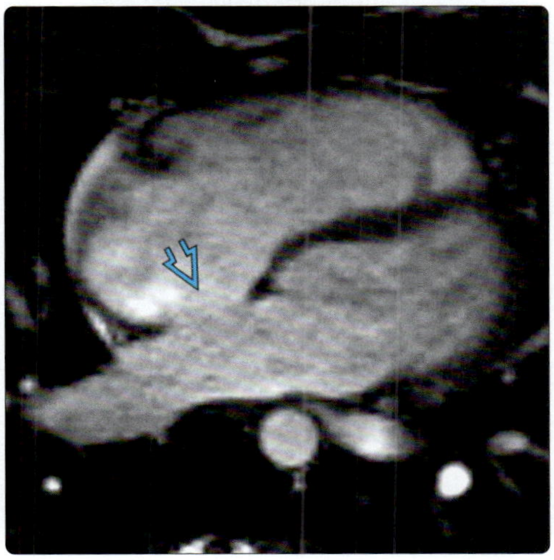

(Left) *PA radiograph in a 2-year-old girl with an ASD shows a normal heart size but a prominent MPA contour ⇨ & increased pulmonary vascularity ⇨. The LA is not dilated. Radiographic findings are often not appreciable with Qp:Qs < 2:1.* **(Right)** *Four-chamber MR SSFP in an asymptomatic 17 year old shows a large secundum ASD ⇨, which was well tolerated & found incidentally. Qp:Qs was correspondingly only 1.6:1; however, closure was indicated by the RA & RV enlargement. LA was not enlarged, as expected.*

(Left) *Four-chamber MRA MPR shows a superior sinus venosus ASD ➡ at the posterior aspect of the atrial septum at the SVC-atrial junction. This patient also had associated PAPVR of the RUPV (not shown). There is RA & RV dilation.* **(Right)** *PA radiograph in a 4-month-old girl with multiple VSDs shows ventricular enlargement with markedly increased pulmonary vascularity. The left lower lobe bronchus appears attenuated ➡ due to compression by an enlarged heart. There is associated basilar air-trapping ➡.*

Atrial Septal Defect

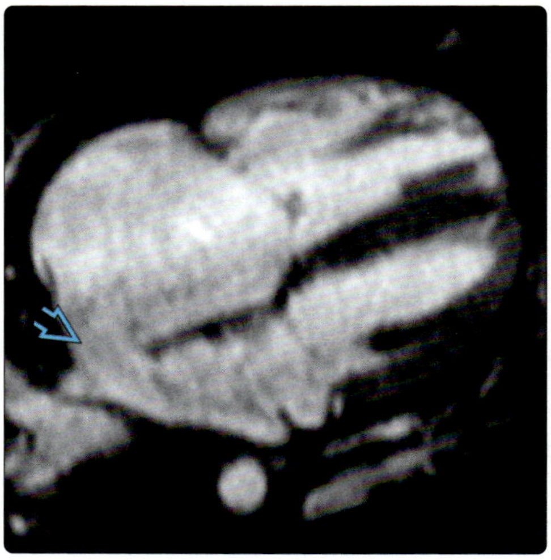

Ventricular Septal Defect

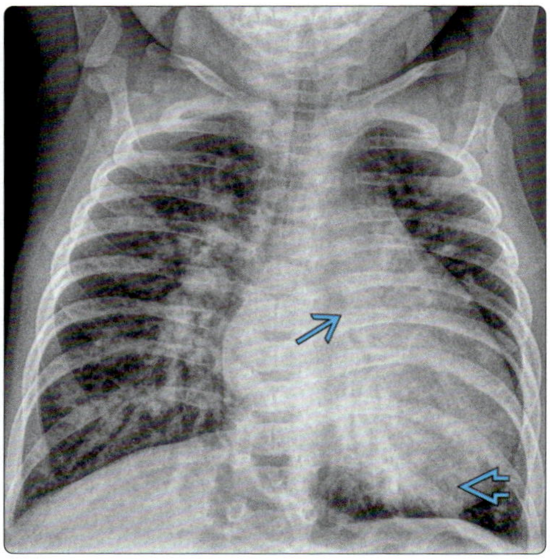

(Left) *Axial MR SSFP in a different patient shows multiple small muscular VSDs ➡ along the mid to apical trabecular septum. Small muscular VSDs are often restrictive & may spontaneously close due to normal myocardial growth & trabeculation.* **(Right)** *Axial oblique MRA MPR in a 2-year-old (ex-29-week premature) girl shows multiple moderate-to-large muscular VSDs ➡ (so-called Swiss cheese septum). She also had a large ASD (not shown), chronic lung disease of prematurity, & pulmonary hypertension.*

Ventricular Septal Defect

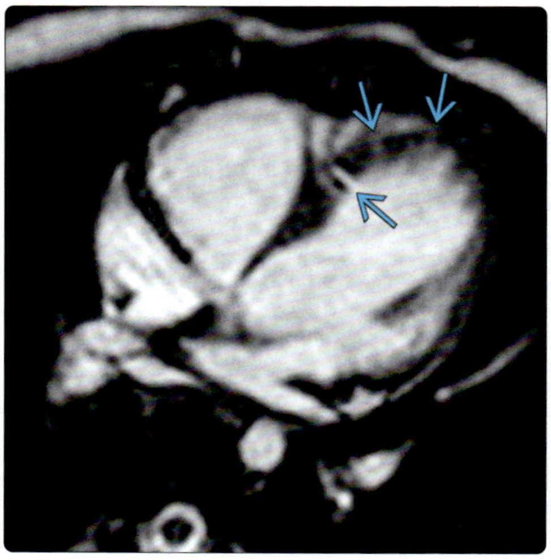

Ventricular Septal Defect

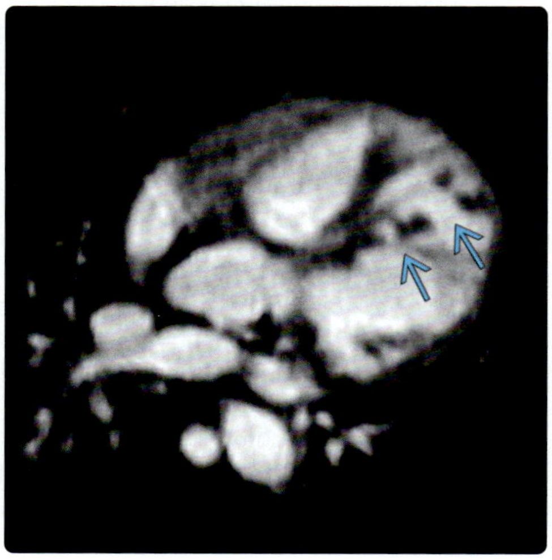

(Left) *Axial MR SSFP in a 6-month-old boy shows a perimembranous VSD ➡. The aortic sinuses are partially imaged ➡, depicting how the right coronary cusp may prolapse through the VSD, potentially causing aortic regurgitation.* **(Right)** *Short-axis MR SSFP shows the perimembranous VSD ➡ with tricuspid-aortic continuity ➡. The inlet septum is intact ➡. Note that the aortic, tricuspid, & mitral leaflets are visualized. This patient also had pulmonary vein stenosis, which has an association with VSDs & prematurity.*

Ventricular Septal Defect

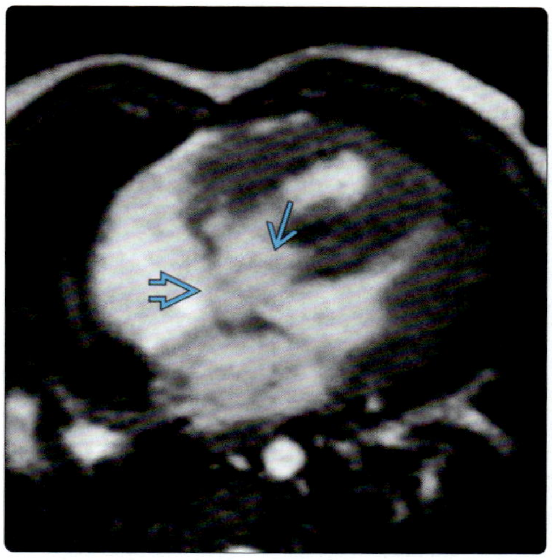

Ventricular Septal Defect

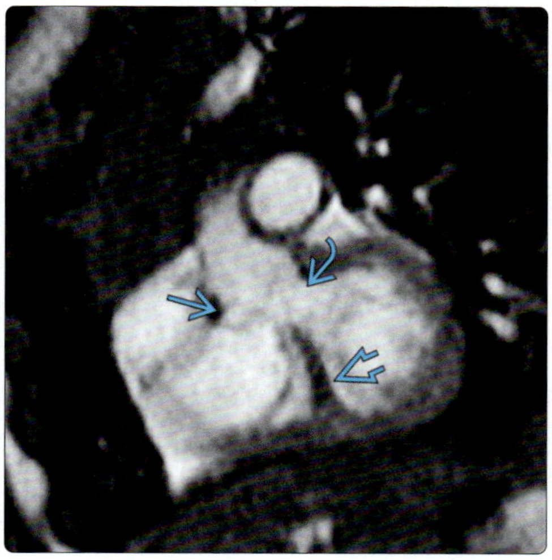

Patent Ductus Arteriosus

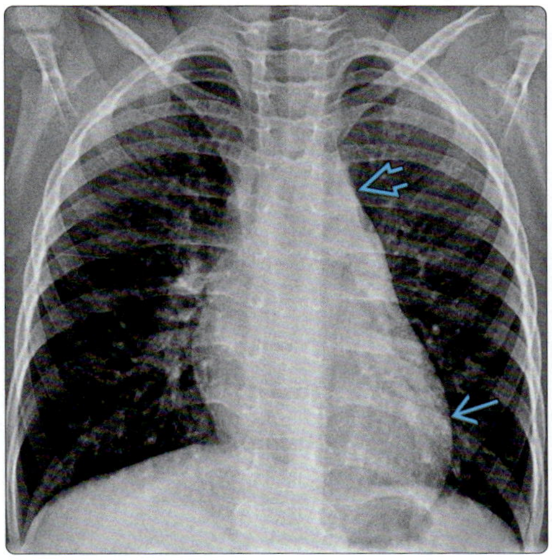

Patent Ductus Arteriosus

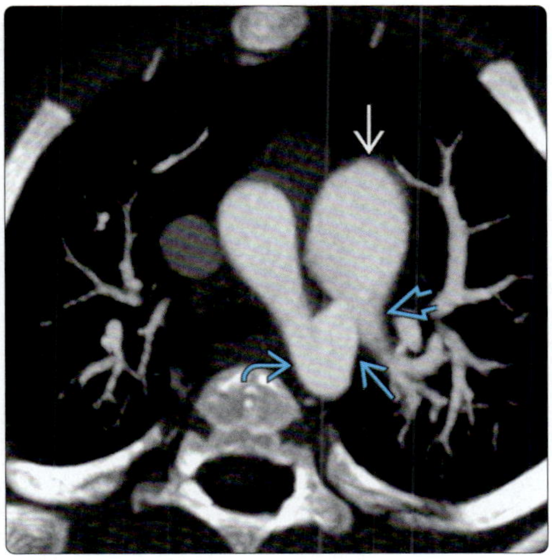

(Left) *PA radiograph in a 3-year-old girl with a PDA shows a prominent MPA with increased pulmonary vascularity. The splaying of the carina indicates LA dilation. There is also enlargement of both the LV & aorta. Aortic dilation suggests a supracardiac shunt, such as a PDA or aortopulmonary window.* **(Right)** *Axial-oblique CECT MIP in a 2-year-old boy shows a typical PDA coursing from the undersurface of the aortic arch to the distal MPA/proximal LPA. The MPA is enlarged.*

Patent Ductus Arteriosus

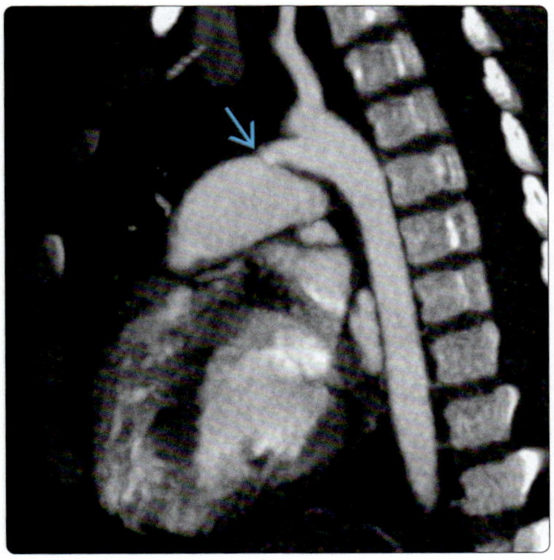

Patent Ductus Arteriosus

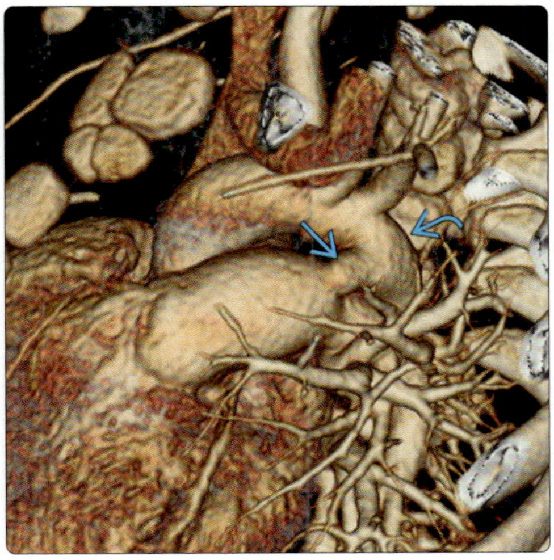

(Left) *Sagittal oblique CECT MIP shows the PDA with mild focal narrowing at the pulmonary end. The ductus arteriosus normally closes hours after birth (oxygen mediated). Prematurity & lung disease are risk factors for a PDA.* **(Right)** *Anterior oblique CECT 3D projection shows the PDA & its relation to the aortic arch & pulmonary arteries. An untreated PDA can lead to early pulmonary hypertension. PDAs can be closed by transcatheter intervention or surgery.*

Atrioventricular Septal Defect

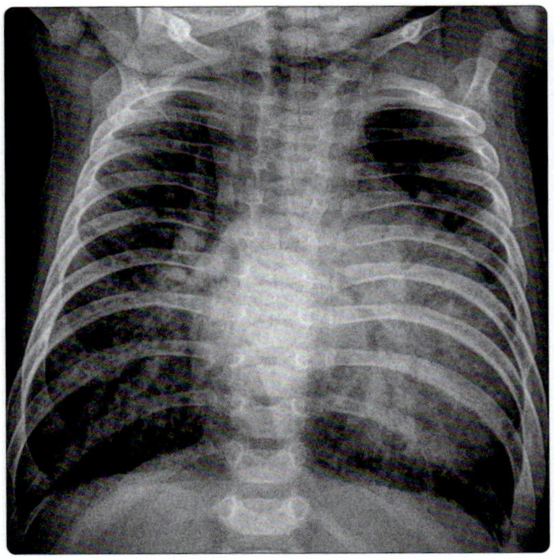

Atrioventricular Septal Defect

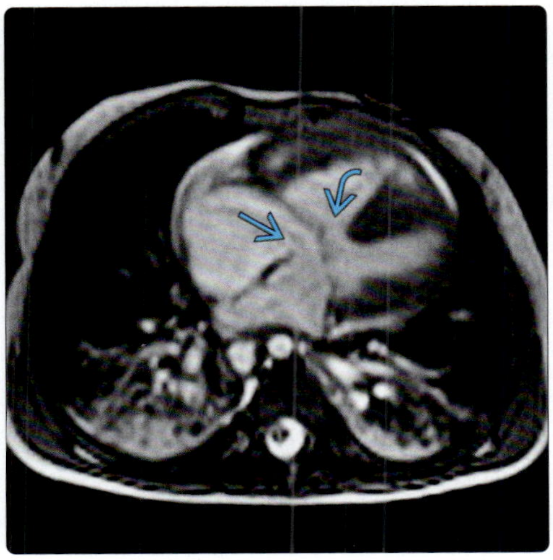

(Left) *PA radiograph in a 3-month-old girl with trisomy 21 & a complete AVSD shows globular cardiomegaly, a marked increase in pulmonary vascularity, & scattered air-trapping with subsegmental atelectasis, consistent with a large L-to-R shunt. The vessels are indistinct, suggestive of mild superimposed interstitial edema.* **(Right)** *Four-chamber MR SSFP in a 9-month-old boy with pulmonary hypertension shows a common AV junction, with an associated primum ASD & inlet VSD, consistent with a complete AVSD.*

(Left) *Short-axis MR SSFP in a patient with an AVSD shows a defect in the ventricular inlet septum . The outlet septum is intact .* **(Right)** *Coronal oblique MRA MIP in a 5-year-old girl shows anomalous drainage of multiple right pulmonary veins to the SVC . While some join high in the SVC (representing anomalous connections), others can be in near-normal locations but drain anomalously through an associated superior sinus venosus defect. Note the enlarged MPA .*

Atrioventricular Septal Defect

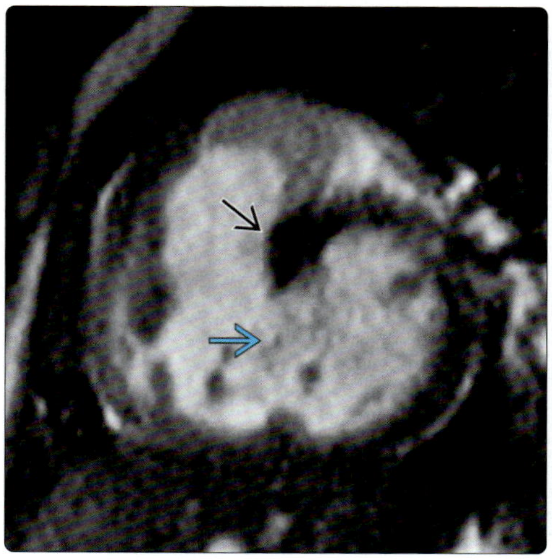

Partial Anomalous Pulmonary Venous Return

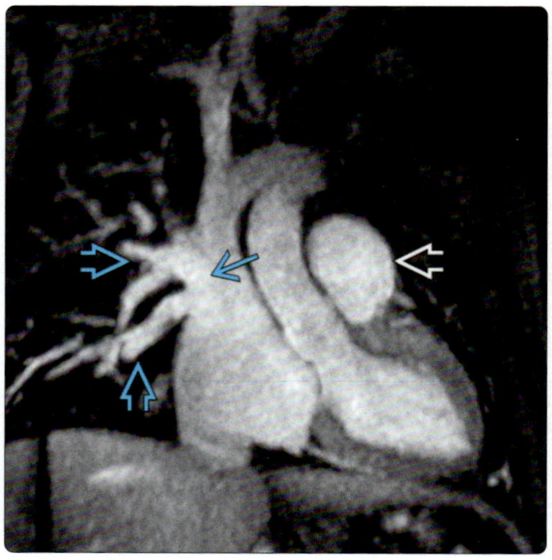

(Left) *Axial oblique MRA MPR shows an anomalous RUPV & a defect in the sinus venosus that allows communication between the SVC/RA junction to both the RUPV & LA . This pathophysiology can occur even when the RUPV is in the normal position.* **(Right)** *Sagittal oblique MRA MIP in the echographic view shows a defect in the superior sinus venosus , creating a sinus venosus ASD between the normal-sized LA & enlarged RA . The SVC has an overriding appearance. Note the enlarged RPA .*

Partial Anomalous Pulmonary Venous Return

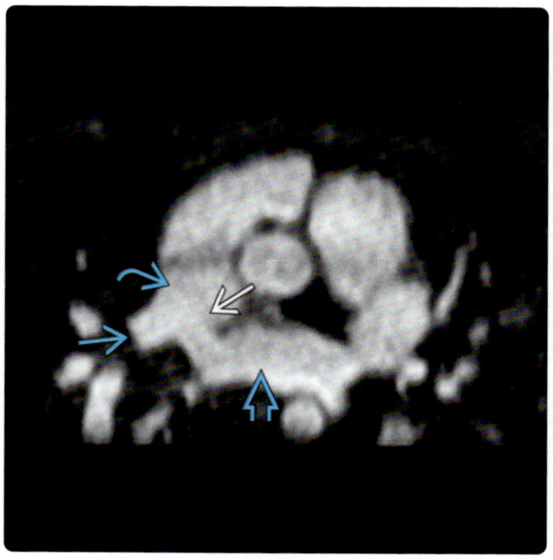

Partial Anomalous Pulmonary Venous Return

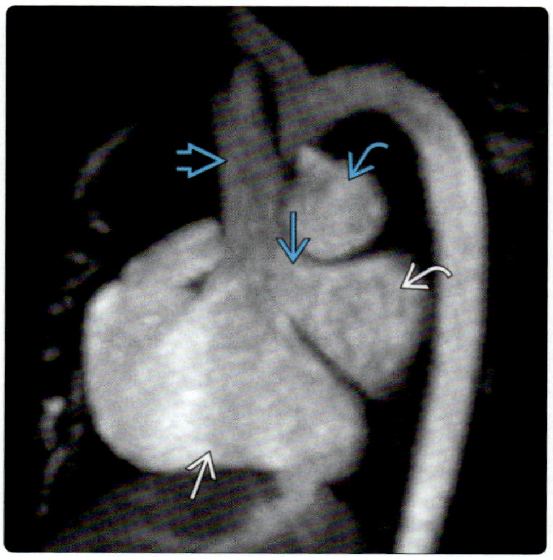

(Left) *Coronal oblique MRA MIP in a different patient shows anomalous connection of the right lower pulmonary vein to the IVC/RA junction.* **(Right)** *Sagittal oblique MRA MIP shows an associated inferior sinus venosus ASD . Note the enlarged RA & RPA , while the LA is normal in size. Isolated anomalous drainage of a pulmonary vein to the IVC-atrial junction is rare. More typically, anomalous drainage to this region is seen in association with scimitar syndrome.*

Partial Anomalous Pulmonary Venous Return

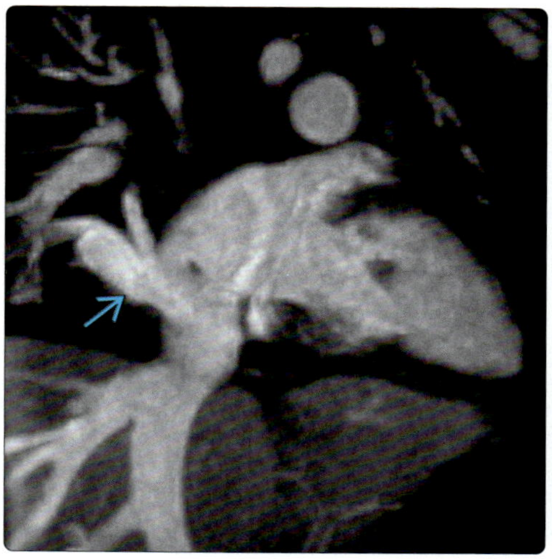

Partial Anomalous Pulmonary Venous Return

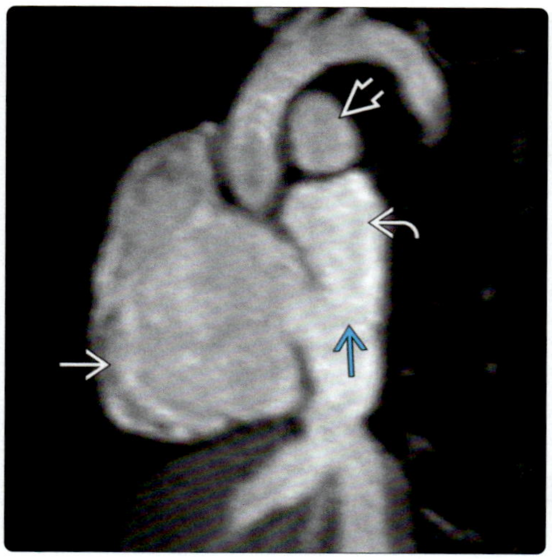

Partial Anomalous Pulmonary Venous Return

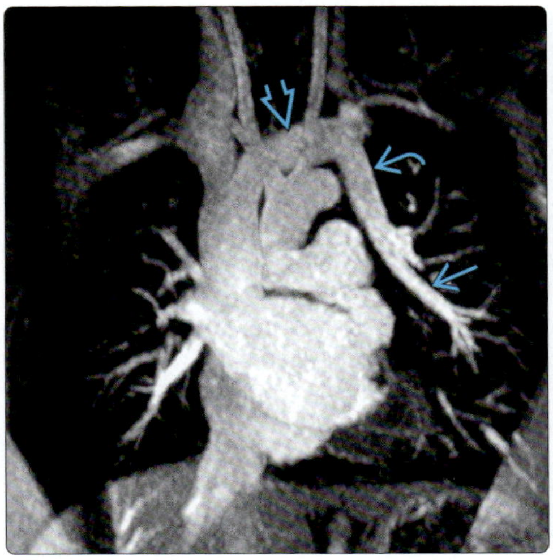

Partial Anomalous Pulmonary Venous Return

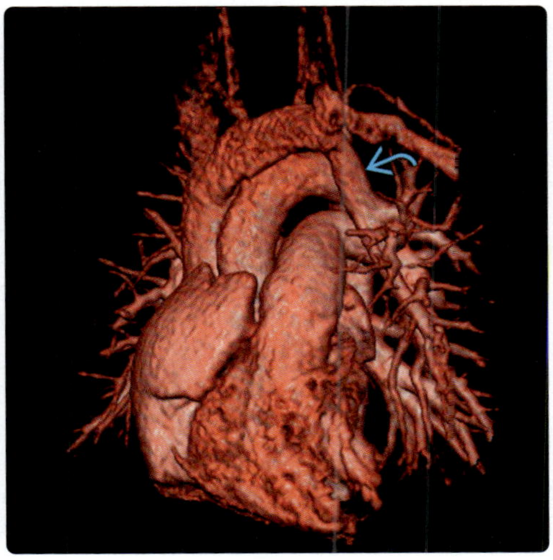

(Left) *Coronal oblique MRA MIP in an asymptomatic 10-year-old girl shows anomalous connection of the left upper pulmonary vein ➙ to the innominate vein ⇨ via a vertical vein ➚.* **(Right)** *Anterior oblique MRA 3D projection shows the same findings with anomalous connection of the LUPV to the innominate vein via a vertical vein ➚. The diagnosis was originally made after a heart murmur was heard at 18 months of age. MR showed only mild RV dilation & a Qp:Qs of 1.6:1, not meeting criteria for closure.*

Vein of Galen Malformation

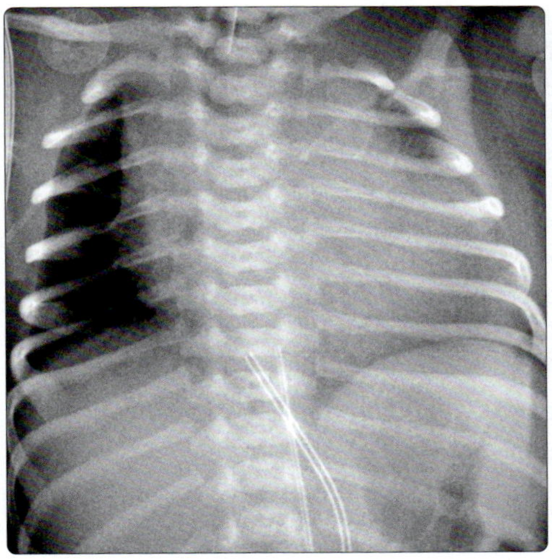

Vein of Galen Malformation

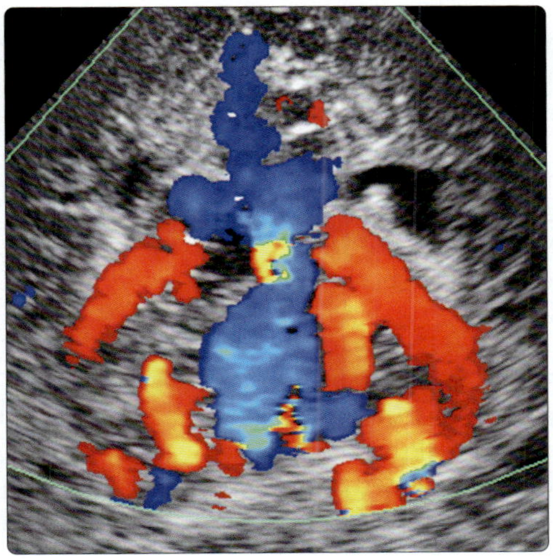

(Left) *AP radiograph of the chest in a newborn shows cardiomegaly due to a vein of Galen malformation (which occurs due to a direct communication between the deep choroidal arteries & the median prosencephalic vein).* **(Right)** *Coronal color Doppler US of the head shows abnormally enlarged arteries & veins due to a vein of Galen malformation. Vein of Galen malformations are the most common extracardiac cause of high-output cardiac failure in newborns.*

Diffuse Infantile Hepatic Hemangiomas

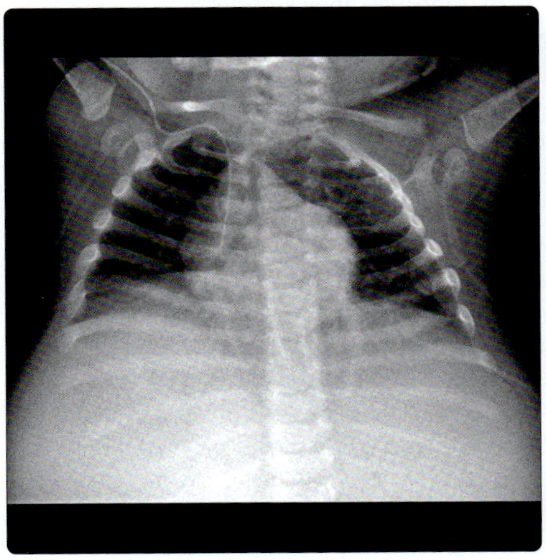

Diffuse Infantile Hepatic Hemangiomas

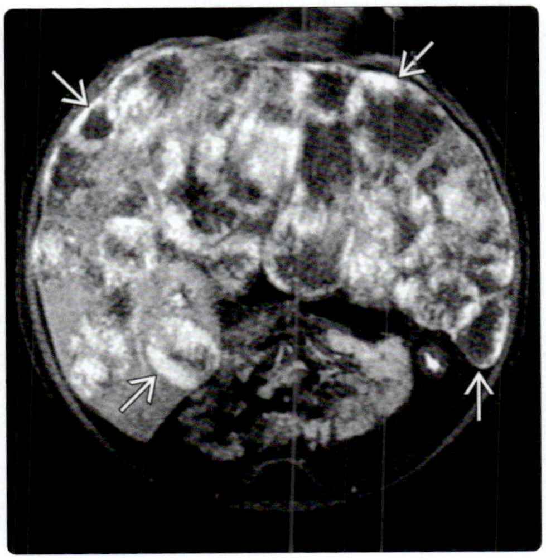

(Left) *AP radiograph of the chest shows mildly increased pulmonary vascularity & bulging of the upper abdomen. Infantile hepatic hemangiomas are the most common benign liver tumor in children.* **(Right)** *Coronal T1 C+ FS MR shows early peripheral enhancement of innumerable liver lesions ➡, which nearly replace the liver. Patients with diffuse infantile hemangiomas can present with hypothyroidism, high-output cardiac failure, liver failure, &/or abdominal distension.*

DIFFERENTIAL DIAGNOSIS

Common

- Tetralogy of Fallot

Less Common

- Ebstein Anomaly
- Pulmonary Atresia With Intact Ventricular Septum
- Tricuspid Atresia
- Transposition of Great Arteries

Rare but Important

- Other Complex Congenital Heart Disease With Severe Pulmonary Stenosis/Atresia

ESSENTIAL INFORMATION

Key Differential Diagnosis Issues

- Cyanotic heart disease: Deoxygenated blood enters systemic circulation (R → L shunt)
  - Most common causes (so-called 5 Ts): Tetralogy of Fallot (TOF), tricuspid valve anomalies (tricuspid atresia, Ebstein anomaly, tricuspid valve dysplasia/stenosis), transposition of great arteries (TGA), truncus arteriosus, total anomalous pulmonary venous return (TAPVR)
  - 2 main subtypes: Decreased vs. normal/increased pulmonary vascularity
- Cyanotic heart disease with **decreased** pulmonary vascularity: Underlying defect impedes pulmonary flow, usually from pulmonary stenosis or atresia (PS/PA)
  - Pulmonary flow dependent on L → R shunt through patent ductus arteriosus (PDA)
  - Rapid cyanosis develops with duct closure
  - Of DDxs, only classic TOF & PA with intact ventricular septum (PA/IVS) **by definition** have PS/PA
  - Severe Ebstein anomaly presenting in neonatal period commonly & classically also has decreased pulmonary vascularity from functional or anatomic critical PS/right ventricular (RV) outflow tract obstruction (RVOTO)
  - Tricuspid atresia, TGA, & other complex congenital heart disease (CHD) only have decreased pulmonary vascularity when there is additional PS/PA (or equivalent restriction to antegrade pulmonary flow); otherwise, flow is normal/increased
- Classic radiographic teaching: After determining that pulmonary vascularity is decreased, next consider heart size
  - Normal heart size: TOF
  - Cardiomegaly: Ebstein anomaly, PA/IVS
- In practice, echocardiography is used for diagnosis

Helpful Clues for Common Diagnoses

- **Tetralogy of Fallot (TOF)**
  - Most common cyanotic CHD in childhood
  - Fundamental defect is anterior, superior, & leftward malalignment of outlet septum causing RVOTO
  - Results in classic tetrad: 1) RVOTO, 2) RV hypertrophy, 3) ventricular septal defect (VSD), 4) aorta overriding VSD
  - Pathophysiology: Cyanosis from R → L shunt through VSD, proportional to degree of RVOTO
  - Variants
    - TOF with PA & major aortopulmonary collateral arteries (TOF/PA/MAPCAs)
      - a.k.a. PA with VSD & MAPCAs
      - Severe TOF without flow through pulmonary valve
      - Intrapericardial pulmonary arteries are severely diminutive & may not be confluent
      - Pulmonary circulation supplied via PDA &/or large congenital collaterals from aorta (MAPCAs)
    - TOF with absent pulmonary valve (TOF/APV)
      - TOF without functioning pulmonary valve tissue, allowing for severe pulmonary regurgitation
      - Increased volume of regurgitant flow back & forth through central pulmonary arteries
      - Aneurysmal main & branch pulmonary arteries may cause bronchial compression
      - Form of TOF with increased pulmonary vascularity & possible cardiomegaly
      - Respiratory symptoms predominate over cyanosis
    - "Pink" TOF
      - Mild PS with large VSD
      - Acts like isolated VSD: Acyanotic, increased vascularity, cardiomegaly
  - Radiographic appearance
    - Usually normal heart size
      - Cardiomegaly suggests TOF variant
    - Boot-shaped heart appearance
      - Leftward rotation of cardiac axis
      - Upturned apex from RV hypertrophy
      - Concave superior left heart border from absent/small main pulmonary artery (MPA)
      - Absent left aortic arch (as 25% have right arch)
      - Prominent ascending aorta (correlates with PS)
    - Caution: Vast majority of TOF does not have classic boot shape; also, other entities can mimic

Helpful Clues for Less Common Diagnoses

- **Ebstein Anomaly**
  - Apical displacement of septal & posterior tricuspid leaflets (> 8 mm/m² body surface area)
    - Inlet portion of RV becomes incorporated into right atrium (RA) → "atrialization of RV"
      - Tripartite right heart: RA, atrialized RV, & functional RV (with trabecular apex & outlet)
  - Broad spectrum in degree of leaflet abnormality ranging from mild (adults) to severe (neonates)
    - Neonatal presentation typically with severe tricuspid regurgitation (TR) → massive dilation of RA
      - Cardiomegaly in utero can lead to lung hypoplasia
    - Small functional RV can also have anatomically critical PS/RVOTO
      - "Functional PA" is possible wherein setting of severe TR & increased perinatal pulmonary vascular resistance, functional RV cannot generate adequate pressure to open pulmonary valve
      - Either scenario leads to classic presentation of decreased pulmonary vascularity & ductal-dependent pulmonary circulation in neonate
      - Elevated RA pressures lead to R → L shunt across patent foramen ovale (PFO) or atrial septal defect (ASD), causing cyanosis
    - Commonly have conduction anomalies & arrhythmias
  - Radiographic appearance

- Classic entity for "wall-to-wall" or box-shaped heart with decreased pulmonary vascularity
  - Massive cardiomegaly from enlarged RA due to severe TR
  - RA & RV dilation → squaring of right & left superior heart borders, respectively
  - DDx is PA/IVS or severe tricuspid valve dysplasia (as both have TR & massive RA dilation)

- **Pulmonary Atresia With Intact Ventricular Septum**
  - PA without VSD (completely distinct entity from TOF variant PA/VSD/MAPCAs)
  - Complete RVOTO, typically with well-developed confluent pulmonary arteries
  - Pulmonary flow depends on R → L interatrial shunt & L → R flow though PDA
  - RV typically small & hypertrophied (prototypical hypoplastic right heart lesion)
  - Tricuspid valve is almost always abnormal (hypoplastic, dysplastic, ± ebsteinoid)
  - Associated with coronary stenoses & RV fistulae
  - Radiographic appearance
    - Cardiomegaly depends on degree of TR & RA dilation
    - In DDx for cyanotic neonate with "wall-to-wall" heart & decreased pulmonary vascularity
- **Tricuspid Atresia**
  - Absent right atrioventricular (AV) communication
  - ASD or PFO always present, VSD common
  - Often with RVOTO or restrictive VSD, & thus decreased pulmonary vascularity
  - Concomitant TGA (30%)
  - Radiographic appearance
    - With pulmonary outflow obstruction: Normal heart size & decreased pulmonary vascularity
    - Without pulmonary outflow obstruction: Mild cardiomegaly & increased pulmonary vascularity
    - If ASD restrictive: RA dilation & marked cardiomegaly
    - Straight/concave right heart border if there is juxtaposition of right atrial appendage
      - Common association where right atrial appendage crosses to left
      - CT/MR: Fat extending into deep AV groove at site of atretic AV connection
- **Transposition of Great Arteries**
  - Ventriculoarterial discordance: Aorta arises from RV & MPA arises from left ventricle (LV)
  - Occurs with various forms of AV connections
    - AV concordance: RA-RV-aorta/left atrium (LA)-LV-MPA → complete TGA or D-TGA (aorta usually anterior & right of MPA)
    - AV discordance: RA-LV-aorta/LA-RV-MPA → congenitally corrected TGA or L-TGA (aorta usually anterior & left of MPA)
    - Univentricular AV connections (e.g., with tricuspid atresia)
  - 50% with VSD, LVOTO, or aortic obstructive lesion
  - Most common CHD with cyanosis on 1st day of life
  - Radiographic appearance
    - Neonates: Normal heart size & normal/decreased pulmonary vascularity
      - Increased pulmonary blood flow with decreased pulmonary vascular resistance over time is "classic"
    - Classic egg-on-string appearance
      - Superimposed, parallel great vessels & thymic stress/involution → narrow mediastinum of "string"
      - RA dilation over time → egg-on-side appearance

Helpful Clues for Rare Diagnoses

- **Other Complex Congenital Heart Disease With Severe Pulmonary Stenosis/Atresia**
  - Any other complex cyanotic CHD with PS/PA can have decreased pulmonary vascularity
  - Examples: Double-outlet RV, double-inlet LV, complex CHD with heterotaxy

SELECTED REFERENCES

1. Zucker EJ et al: Cyanotic congenital heart disease: essential primer for the practicing radiologist. Radiol Clin North Am. 55(4):693-716, 2017
2. Lee JY: Clinical presentations of critical cardiac defects in the newborn: decision making and initial management. Korean J Pediatr. 53(6):669-79, 2010
3. Yoo SJ et al: Chest Radiographic Interpretation in Pediatric Cardiac Patients. New York: Thieme Medical Publishers, 2010

Tetralogy of Fallot

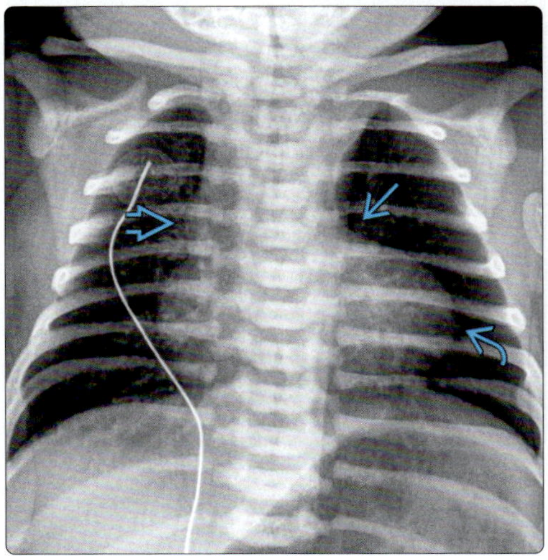

Tetralogy of Fallot

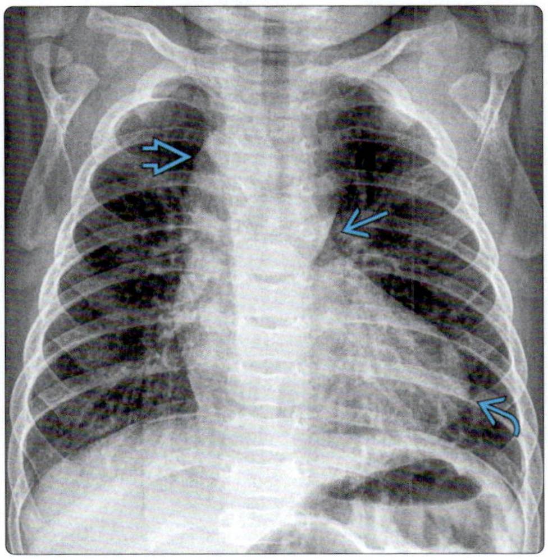

(Left) *AP radiograph in a 3 day old with tetralogy of Fallot (TOF) shows a boot-shaped heart due to an upturned apex ➢, small main pulmonary artery (MPA) ➡, & prominent ascending aorta ➡. The central pulmonary arteries (PAs) are diminutive, & there is ↓ pulmonary vascularity.* **(Right)** *PA radiograph in a 5 month old shows a boot-shaped heart with dextrorotation, an upturned apex ➢, concavity of the left superior heart border from a small MPA ➡, & a right arch ➡. There is ↓ pulmonary vascularity.*

(Left) *Coronal oblique CECT MIP (same patient) shows malalignment of the outlet septum causing multilevel RVOTO, pulmonary valvar stenosis & subvalvar muscular stenosis. There is right ventricular hypertrophy (RVH) from ↑ afterload, & the aorta overrides the ventricular septal defect (VSD) created by septal malalignment. The aortic arch is right sided.* **(Right)** *Sagittal oblique CECT MIP (same patient) better shows the aorta overriding a perimembranous VSD + RVH.*

Tetralogy of Fallot

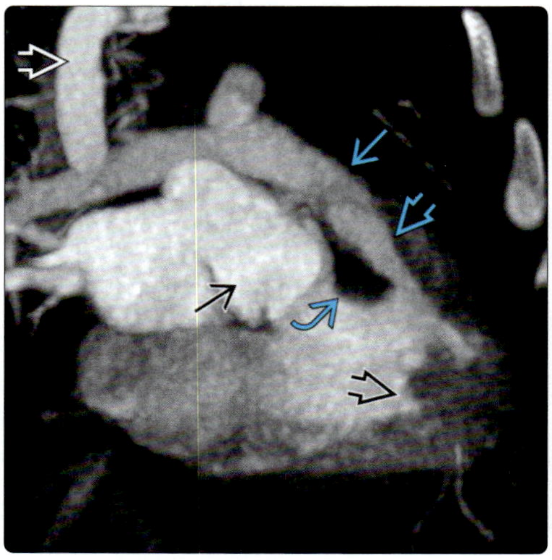

Tetralogy of Fallot

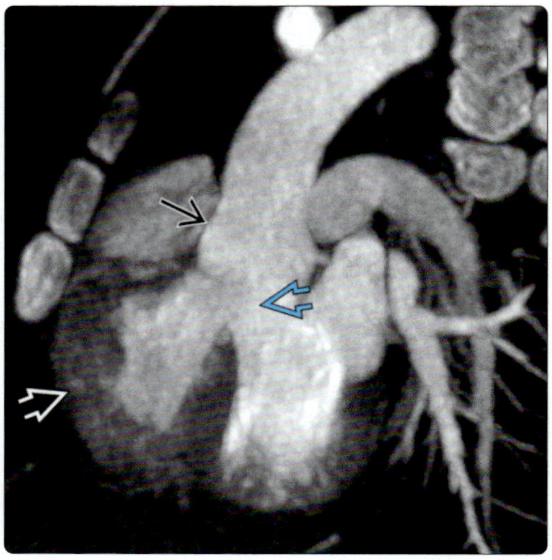

(Left) *Posteroanterior radiograph in a 3 month old with TOF shows an upturned apex, diminished MPA contour, & right aortic arch, creating a boot shape. There is also moderate cardiomegaly & ↑ pulmonary vascularity at the hilum with abnormal-appearing arborization, raising the possibility of TOF with pulmonary atresia & major aortopulmonary collateral arteries (MAPCAs).* **(Right)** *Axial oblique CECT MPR in the same patient shows pulmonary atresia with small confluent main & branch PAs.*

Tetralogy of Fallot

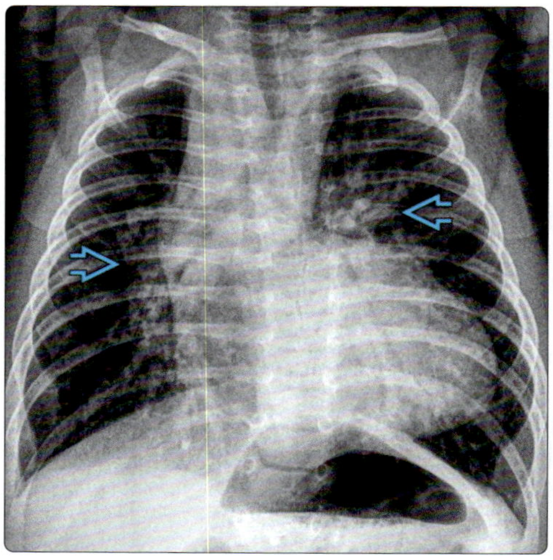

Tetralogy of Fallot

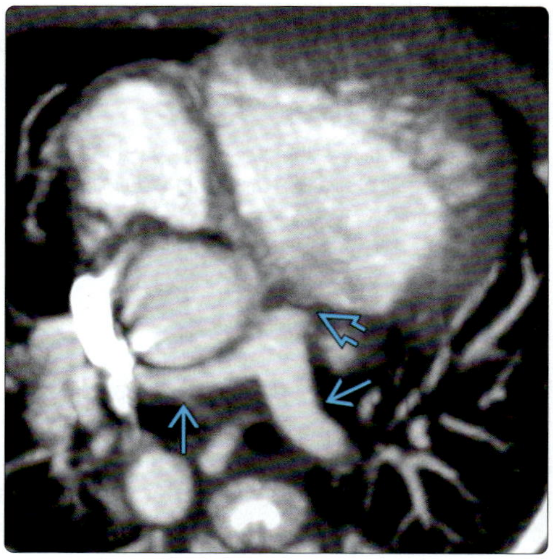

(Left) *Coronal oblique CECT MIP in the same patient shows multiple tortuous MAPCAs arising from the descending aorta.* **(Right)** *Posterior oblique 3D projection CECT in the same patient again shows multiple MAPCAs. Some connect to the branch PAs at the hilum, & others directly supply lung segments, an appearance termed arborization anomalies. Depending on size & whether the lung is dependent on MAPCA flow, these will be coiled or surgically reimplanted to the hilum in a unifocalization operation.*

Tetralogy of Fallot

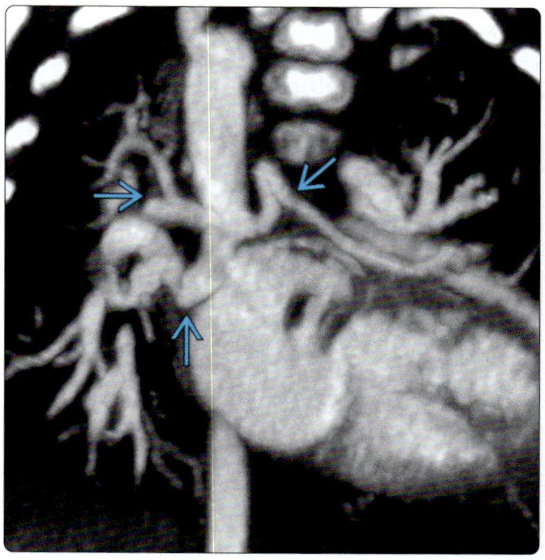

Tetralogy of Fallot

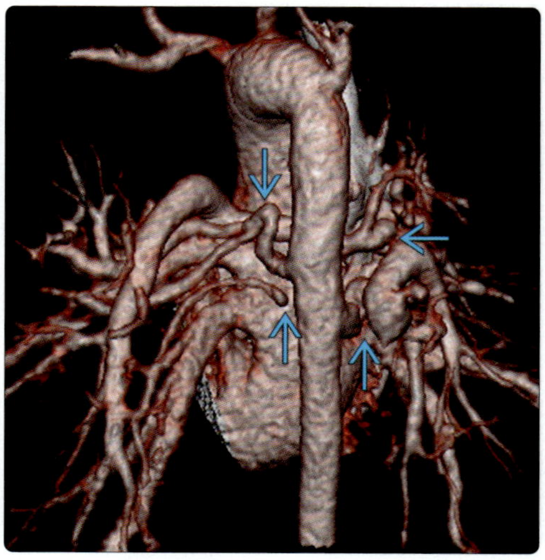

Tetralogy of Fallot

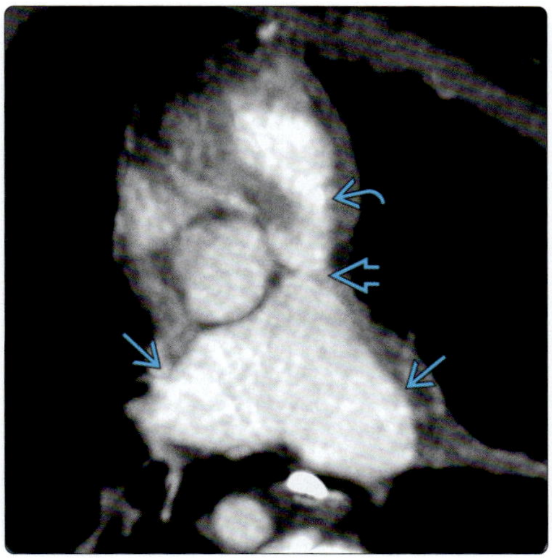

Tetralogy of Fallot

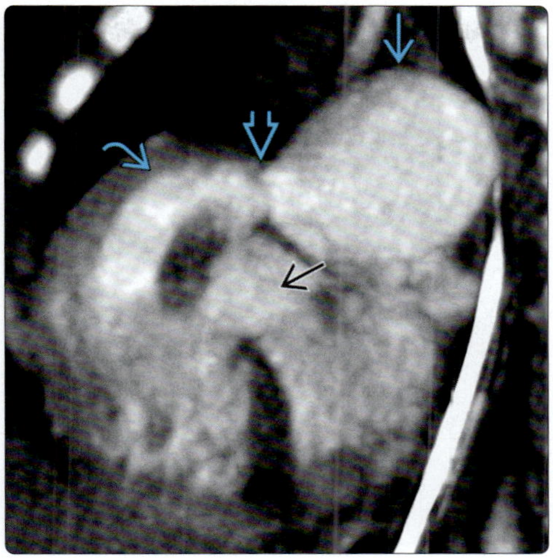

(Left) *Axial oblique CECT MPR in an 18 day old with TOF & an absent pulmonary valve (APV) shows incompetent rudimentary pulmonary valvar leaflets → that allow free regurgitation, resulting in aneurysmal dilation of main & branch PAs →. Note subvalvar muscular RVOT →.* **(Right)** *Sagittal CECT MPR in the same patient again shows rudimentary valvar tissue →, a dilated MPA →, & subvalvar RVOTO →. A perimembranous VSD is also evident →. TOF/APV is a form of TOF with enlarged central pulmonary vasculature.*

Ebstein Anomaly

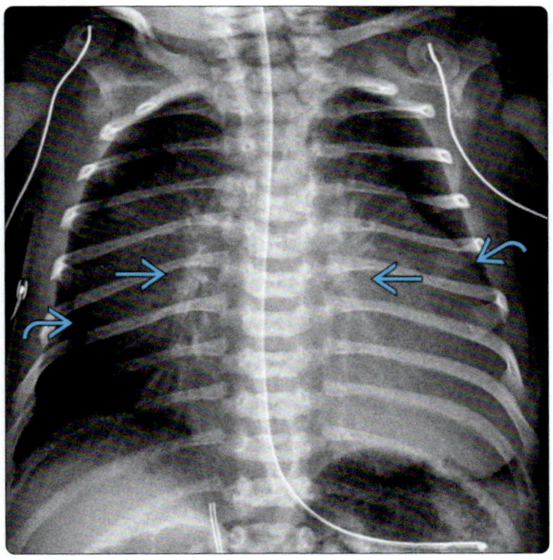

Ebstein Anomaly

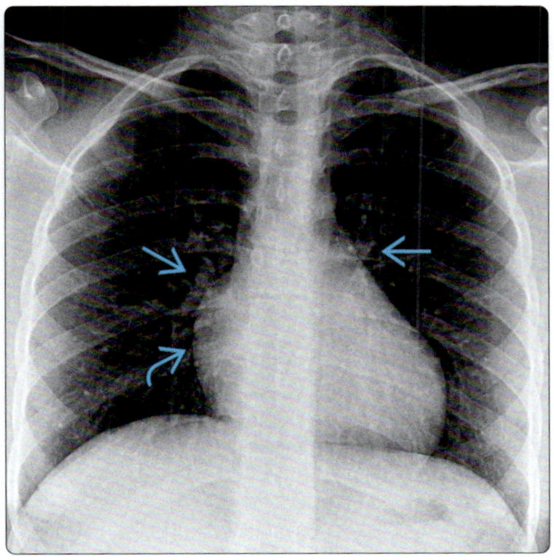

(Left) *AP radiograph in a 1 day old shows massive "wall-to-wall" cardiomegaly → with ↓ pulmonary vascularity →, consistent with Ebstein anomaly. Massive cardiomegaly is from severe tricuspid regurgitation leading to severe right atrium (RA) dilation. The ↓ vascularity is due to anatomic or functional PS/pulmonary atresia.* **(Right)** *PA radiograph in a 15 year old shows slight prominence of RA → & mildly small branch PAs →. The degree of valvar dysplasia is variable in Ebstein anomaly; if mild, radiographs can be near normal.*

Ebstein Anomaly

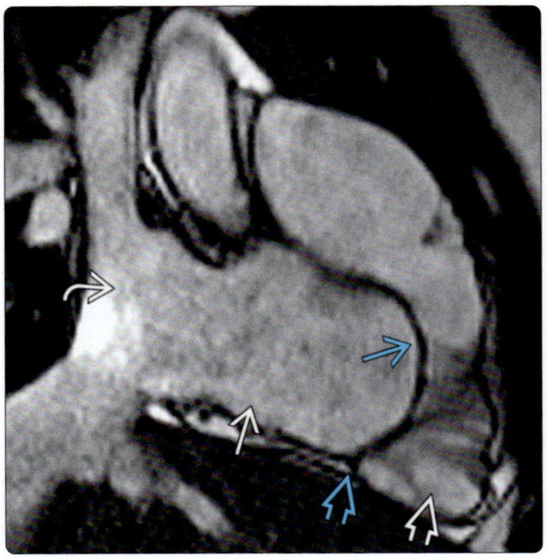

Ebstein Anomaly

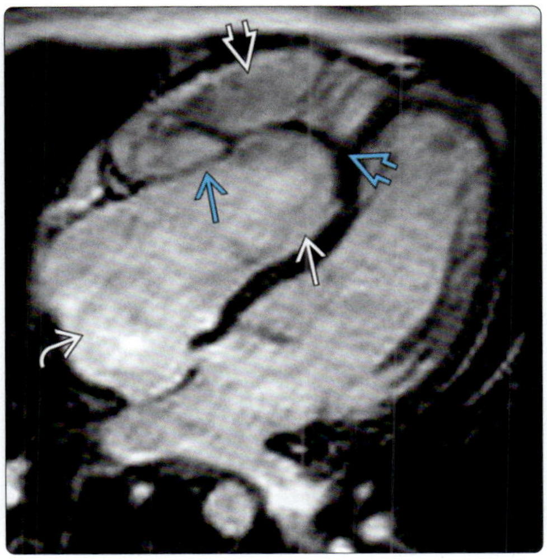

(Left) *Two-chamber SSFP MR in the same patient shows apical displacement of the septal & posterior leaflet hinge point → with a sail-like anterior leaflet →. The right heart is split into the functional right ventricle (RV) →, atrialized RV →, & RA →.* **(Right)** *Four-chamber SSFP MR shows apical displacement of the septal leaflet → with a sail-like anterior leaflet →, functional RV →, atrialized RV →, & RA →. There was only mild tricuspid regurgitation, resulting in milder symptoms & later presentation.*

(Left) *AP radiograph in a cyanotic newborn with pulmonary atresia with intact ventricular septum shows cardiomegaly with small central pulmonary vasculature . DDx includes any lesion with pulmonary obstruction & tricuspid regurgitation, such as Ebstein or tricuspid dysplasia.* **(Right)** *Angiogram (same patient) shows a hypoplastic hypertrophied RV , pulmonary atresia , & a dilated RA from tricuspid regurgitation . A catheter-based pulmonary valvotomy will be performed if coronary circulation not RV dependent.*

Pulmonary Atresia With Intact Ventricular Septum

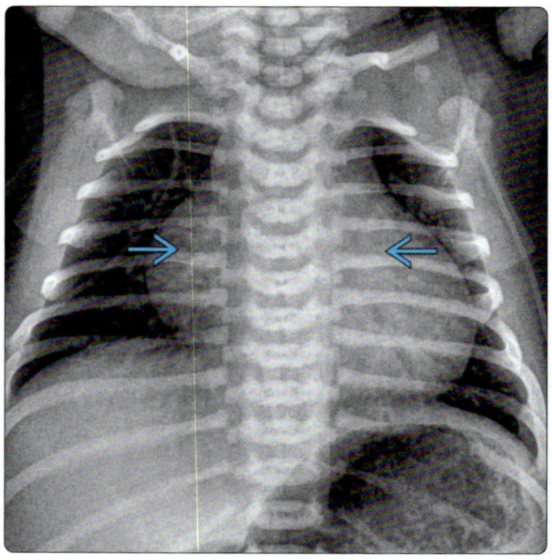

Pulmonary Atresia With Intact Ventricular Septum

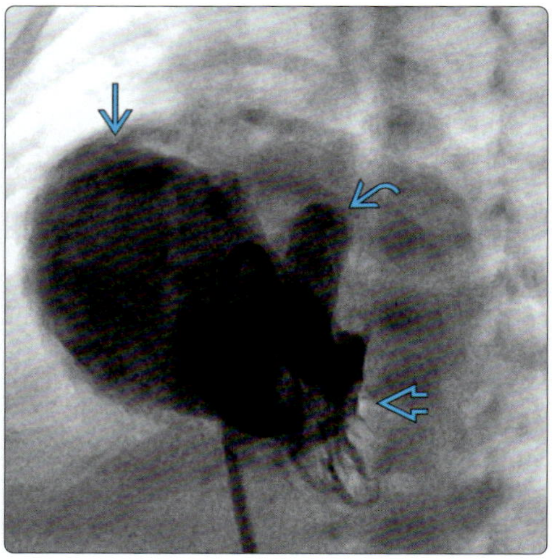

(Left) *PA radiograph in a 3 month old shows mild cardiomegaly & ↓ pulmonary vascularity . This appearance is nonspecific, but echo showed tricuspid atresia with a restrictive VSD & a small pulmonary valve.* **(Right)** *Four-chamber SSFP MR (same patient) at 3 years old (prior to Fontan) shows an absent right atrioventricular (AV) connection with pericardial fat extending deep into the AV groove , typical of tricuspid atresia. There is a restrictive VSD , small RV , & large postsurgical ASD , creating a common atrium.*

Tricuspid Atresia

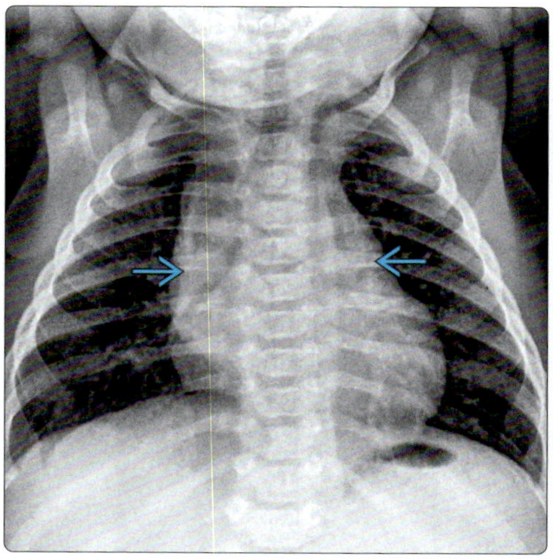

Tricuspid Atresia

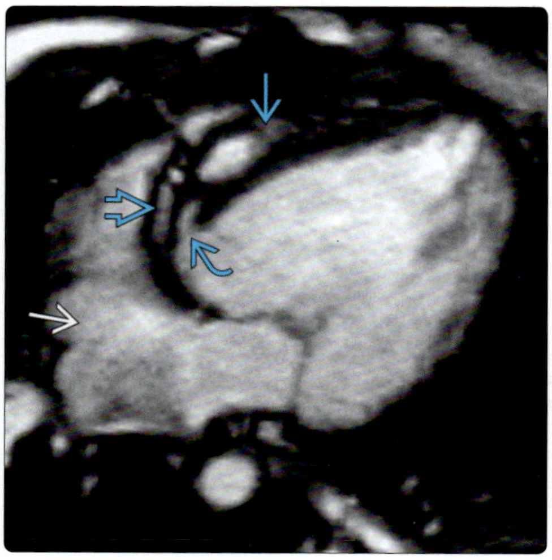

(Left) *Coronal oblique MRA MPR in the same patient shows the absent right AV connection , restrictive VSD , & small RV .* **(Right)** *Axial black blood MR in a 16 year old shows an absent right AV connection with pericardial fat extending into a deep right AV groove that reaches the crux of the heart, characteristic of tricuspid atresia. The right coronary vessels can extend into the right AV groove. Tricuspid atresia is also associated with malposed great vessels in 30%.*

Tricuspid Atresia

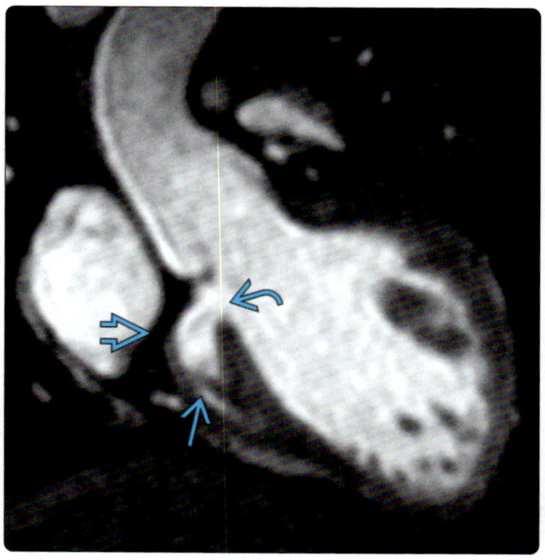

Tricuspid Atresia

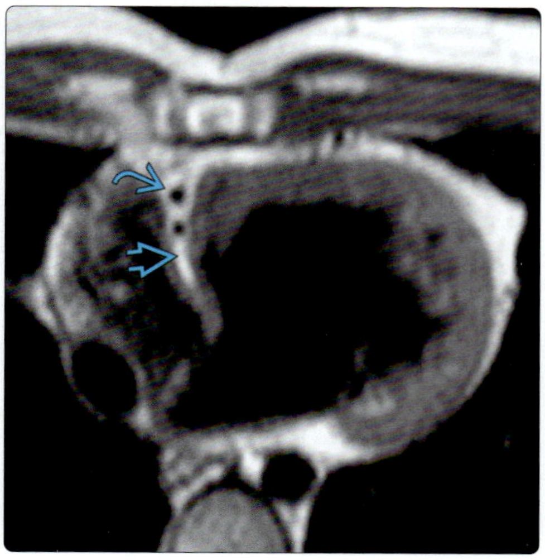

Transposition of Great Arteries

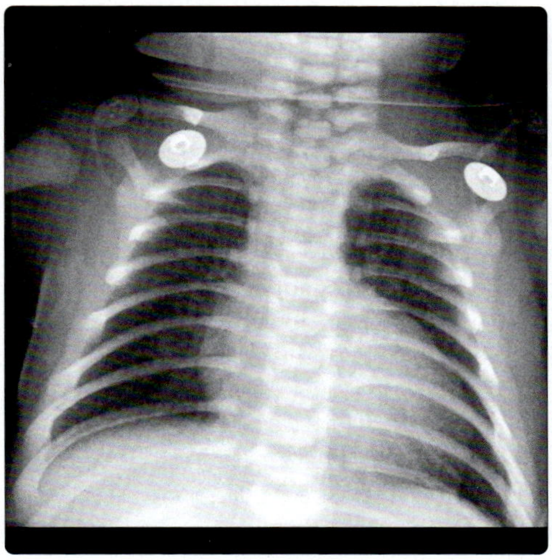

Transposition of Great Arteries

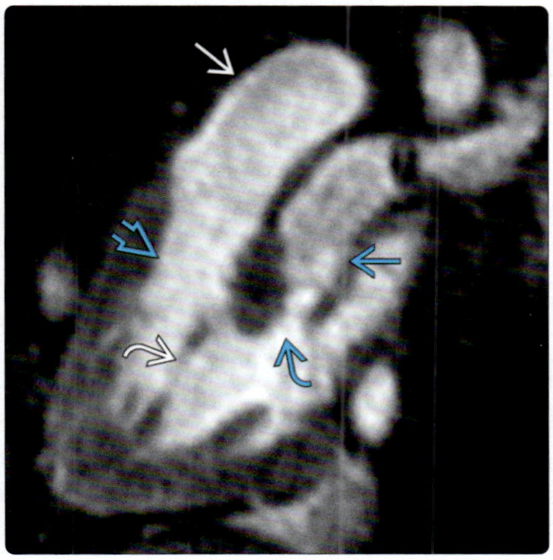

(Left) *AP radiograph shows a large heart with a narrow mediastinum & ↓ vascularity due to PS. Decreased pulmonary vascularity in TGA depends on the pulmonary vascular resistance & degree of pulmonary obstruction.* **(Right)** *Sagittal oblique MRA MPR in a 5 month old with complex TGA shows an anterior aorta → arising from the RV →, a smaller posterior MPA → with PS arising from the LV, muscular subvalvar stenosis →, & a large VSD →. A Blalock-Taussig shunt augmented pulmonary flow & grew the PAs.*

Transposition of Great Arteries

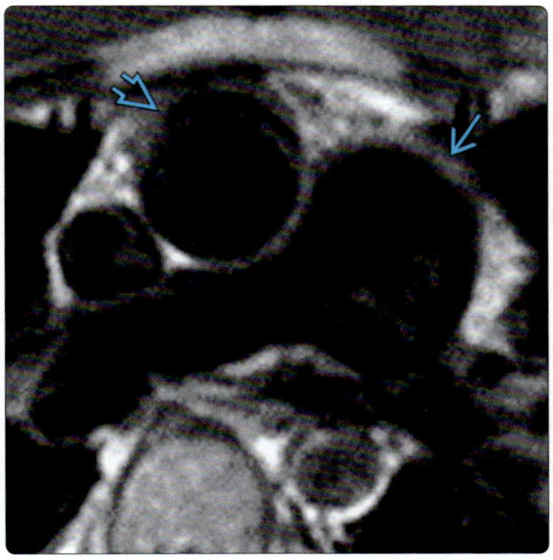

Other Complex Congenital Heart Disease With Severe Pulmonary Stenosis/Atresia

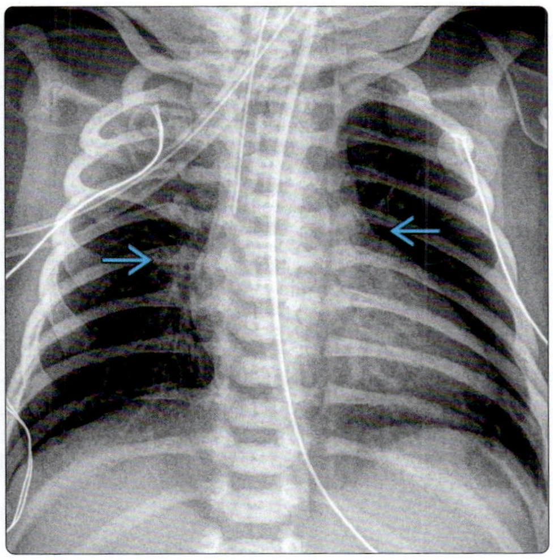

(Left) *Axial black blood MR in an 18 year old shows the aorta → anterior & right of MPA → (d-TGA), typical of complete transposition. Aorta anterior & left (l-TGA) is typical of congenitally corrected TGA. However, in practice, the orientation of malposed great vessels is variable in all conditions.* **(Right)** *AP radiograph in a cyanotic newborn with complex CHD shows nonspecific mild cardiomegaly with ↓ vascularity →. A low endotracheal tube is causing RUL atelectasis.*

Other Complex Congenital Heart Disease With Severe Pulmonary Stenosis/Atresia

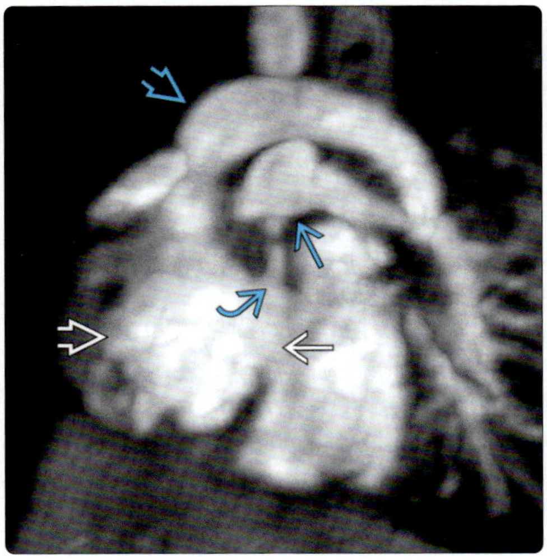

Other Complex Congenital Heart Disease With Severe Pulmonary Stenosis/Atresia

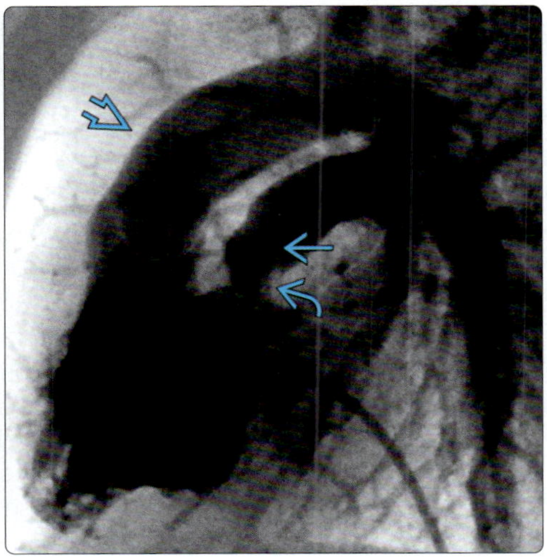

(Left) *Sagittal oblique MRA MIP (same patient) at 4 months old shows both great vessels arising from the RV →, consistent with double-outlet right ventricle (DORV). The great vessels are malposed with anterior aorta → & small posterior MPA → with an muscular subpulmonic obstruction →. Note unrestrictive VSD →.* **(Right)** *Lateral oblique angiogram shows DORV with an anterior aorta → & posterior MPA with PS → & subvalvar obstruction →.*

DIFFERENTIAL DIAGNOSIS

Common

- Transposition of Great Arteries

Less Common

- Total Anomalous Pulmonary Venous Return
- Truncus Arteriosus

Rare but Important

- Other Complex Congenital Heart Disease Without Pulmonary Stenosis/Atresia

ESSENTIAL INFORMATION

Key Differential Diagnosis Issues

- Cyanotic heart disease: Deoxygenated blood enters systemic circulation (R → L shunt)
- Most common causes (so-called 5 Ts): Tetralogy of Fallot, tricuspid valve anomalies (tricuspid atresia, Ebstein anomaly, tricuspid valve dysplasia/stenosis), transposition of great arteries (TGAs), truncus arteriosus, total anomalous pulmonary venous return (TAPVR)
- 2 main subtypes: ↓ vs. normal or ↑ pulmonary vascularity
- Cyanosis with **normal**/↑ pulmonary vascularity: Mixing of deoxy- & oxygenated blood independent of ductus arteriosus
    - Mixed blood preferentially enters lower resistance pulmonary circulation, causing ↑ pulmonary vascularity
    - Mixed blood that enters systemic circulation has lower oxygen saturation, causing cyanosis
- Congenital heart disease (CHD) with left-sided obstructions (hypoplastic left heart, coarctation, interrupted aortic arch) that depend on R → L patent ductus arteriosus (PDA) flow for systemic blood flow are also mildly cyanotic at birth with normal pulmonary vascularity
    - Best considered separately as presentations are dominated by systemic hypoperfusion & shock
- Imaging considerations
    - Normal chest radiograph does not exclude CHD
    - Classic radiographic appearances are not sensitive or specific
    - In practice, most lesions are known prenatally or diagnosed by echo soon after birth

Helpful Clues for Common Diagnoses

- **Transposition of Great Arteries**
    - Most common CHD with cyanosis on 1st day of life
    - Defined by ventriculoarterial discordance: Aorta arises from right ventricle (RV) & main pulmonary artery (MPA) arises from left ventricle (LV)
    - Complete TGA or D-TGA refers to TGA in setting of atrioventricular concordance: Right atrium (RA)-RV-aorta /left atrium (LA)-LV-MPA
        - Aorta usually lies anterior & to right of MPA (hence dextro-TGA)
    - Circulations are isolated in parallel
        - Deoxygenated systemic blood returns to RA, enters RV, exits aorta, back to RA
        - Oxygenated pulmonary blood returns to LA, enters LV, exits MPA, back to LA
    - Survival requires mixing of blood at atrial septal defect (ASD)/patent foramen ovale (PFO) & PDA (± VSD, present in ~ 40%)
        - Most blood is recirculated in parallel & "ineffective"
        - ASD/PFO: LA to RA shunt, source of effective systemic blood flow
        - PDA: Net aorta to pulmonary shunt, source of effective pulmonary blood flow
    - 2 main clinical types
        - TGA without VSD: Cyanosis within 1st week (severity depends on degree of mixing)
        - TGA with VSD: Minimal cyanosis; instead gets congestive heart failure by 4-8 weeks
    - Possible associated obstruction: RV or LV outflow obstruction, aortic obstructive lesions
    - Imaging appearance
        - Neonates: Normal heart size & pulmonary vascularity
        - ↑ pulmonary blood flow as ↓ pulmonary vascular resistance postnatally is classic pattern
        - However, can have ↓ pulmonary blood flow if there is pulmonary stenosis
        - Classic egg-on-string appearance
            - □ Superimposed, parallel great vessels & thymic stress/involution → narrow mediastinum of "string"
            - □ RA dilation over time → egg-on-side appearance
- Treatment
    - Early/temporary: Balloon atrial septostomy to improve mixing of blood
    - Complete repair: Jatene arterial switch operation (ASO), consisting of great artery translocation, including moving branch PAs anterior to aorta if necessary (Lecompte maneuver) & coronary reimplantation
    - Historic complete repair: Mustard or Senning atrial switch procedures (atrial baffles)

Helpful Clues for Less Common Diagnoses

- **Total Anomalous Pulmonary Venous Return**
    - Anomalous connection of all pulmonary veins to systemic veins or RA, bypassing LA
        - Usually all pulmonary veins drain to single site via confluence into vertical vein
    - Classified based on site of drainage
        - Supracardiac (50%): Left innominate, superior vena cava (SVC), or azygos vein; 50% obstructed
        - Cardiac (30%): RA or coronary sinus; 20% obstructed
        - Infracardiac (15%): Inferior vena cava (IVC), portal vein, left gastric vein; 90% obstructed (long length, diaphragmatic restriction, stenosis at anomalous connection, closure of ductus venosus)
        - Mixed (5%)
    - Interatrial R → L shunt is required for survival
    - Complete mixing of blood with identical oxygenation in all chambers
    - Associated with heterotaxy (usually right isomerism/asplenia)
    - Presentation
        - Obstructed: Marked cyanosis & low systemic output in 1st hours-days of life
        - Unobstructed: Like large L → R shunt with CHF symptoms at 4-6 weeks of life
    - Appearance

- Obstructed: Normal heart size with severe pulmonary edema ± lymphangiectasia, normal MPA/pulmonary vascularity, small aorta, thymic atrophy, hyperinflated lungs, pleural effusions
- Unobstructed: Moderate cardiomegaly (right-side enlargement) with ↑ pulmonary vascularity (mimics large L → R shunt)
- Snowman sign of supracardiac TAPVR: Dilated left vertical vein & SVC forms snowman head on frontal view; pretracheal density on lateral distinguishes from more anterior thymus
- MR or CT to define anatomy
- Postoperative risk of progressive or recurrent stenosis of repaired veins requires surveillance

- **Truncus Arteriosus**
  - Failure of outflow septation
  - Single common arterial trunk (with single semilunar valve) arises from heart & supplies systemic, pulmonary, & coronary circulations
  - Usually large subtruncal VSD of outlet septum
    - Occasionally extends to perimembranous region
    - Rarely remote VSD, multiple VSDs, or atrioventricular septal defect (AVSD)
  - Various classification systems, mainly based on pulmonary artery (PA) anatomy
  - Regardless of classification system used, key morphologic features to describe include
    - Pulmonary artery origins
      - Most commonly seen: Short distinct intrapericardial MPA segment giving rise to both PAs (but MPA segment is too short to surgically isolate)
      - Relationship to truncal sinuses & coronary origins
      - 1 PA may arise from PDA
    - Presence of interrupted aortic arch (10-15%), arch hypoplasia, or coarctation
    - Truncal valve dysplasia & function (trileaflet 60%, quadrileaflet 30%, range of 1-5 leaflets)
    - Coronary artery origins & course (anomalies in 5-20%)
  - Associations
    - Right aortic arch with mirror image branching (30%)
      - Highest association with right arch of any CHD (but most frequently seen CHD with right arch is TOF)
    - 22q11 deletion: Look for absent thymus, risk factor for late mortality from infection
  - Pathophysiology
    - Intracardiac mixing at VSD from similar ventricular pressures → cyanosis
    - Extracardiac preferential pulmonary flow at common trunk as ↓ pulmonary vascular resistance postnatally leads to ↑ pulmonary vascularity
    - Classified as cyanotic lesion, though pulmonary overcirculation & severe CHF predominates
  - Imaging appearance
    - Moderate to severe cardiomegaly with LA, RV, LV dilation (often at birth)
    - Oval heart shape: RA & RV dilation + absent right ventricular outflow tract (RVOT)
    - Can be boot-shaped & mediastinum may be narrow due to absent distinct MPA & absent thymus (22q11 or stress-induced), therefore commonly mimics other classic appearances
    - Suspect with moderate to severe cardiomegaly, oval shaped heart, small thymic shadow, & ↑ pulmonary vascularity
  - Hemitruncus & pseudotruncus are different entities that are not true truncus & are outdated terms that should no longer be used

Helpful Clues for Rare Diagnoses

- **Other Complex Congenital Heart Disease Without Pulmonary Stenosis/Atresia**
  - Any other complex cyanotic CHD without PS/PA can have normal or ↑ pulmonary vascularity
  - Examples: Double outlet right ventricle (DORV), double inlet left ventricle (DILV), complex CHD with heterotaxy

SELECTED REFERENCES

1. Zucker EJ et al: Cyanotic congenital heart disease: essential primer for the practicing radiologist. Radiol Clin North Am. 55(4):693-716, 2017
2. Files MD et al: Preoperative physiology, imaging, and management of transposition of the great arteries. Semin Cardiothorac Vasc Anesth. 19(3):210-22, 2015

Transposition of Great Arteries

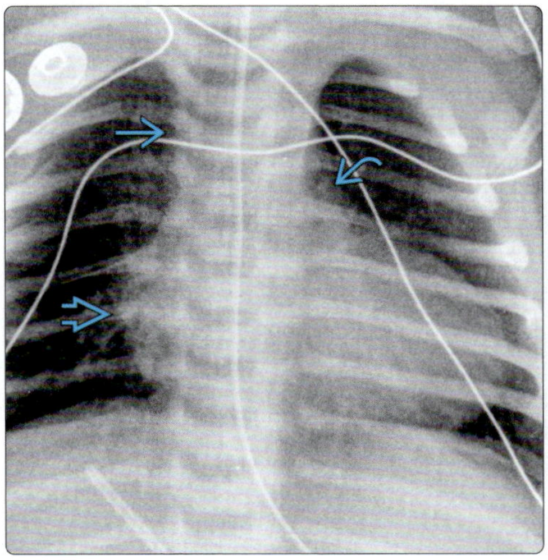

Transposition of Great Arteries

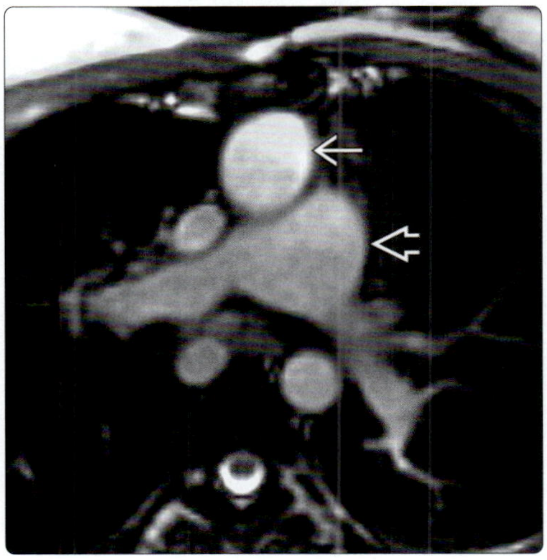

(Left) *AP radiograph in a cyanotic 7 day old shows increased pulmonary vascularity with an egg-on-a-string appearance of the cardiomediastinum, which is caused by a narrow mediastinum ⇨, loss of the normal main pulmonary artery (MPA) shadow ⇨, & mild dilation of the right atrium (RA) ⇨.* **(Right)** *Axial SSFP MR with TGA shows the aortic root ➡ anterior & to the right of the MPA ➡, coursing in parallel with loss of spiraling, which is the typical great vessel relationship in complete transposition.*

Transposition of Great Arteries

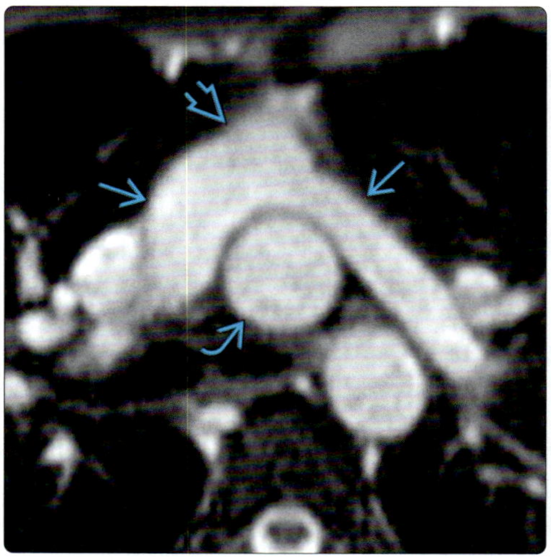

Transposition of Great Arteries

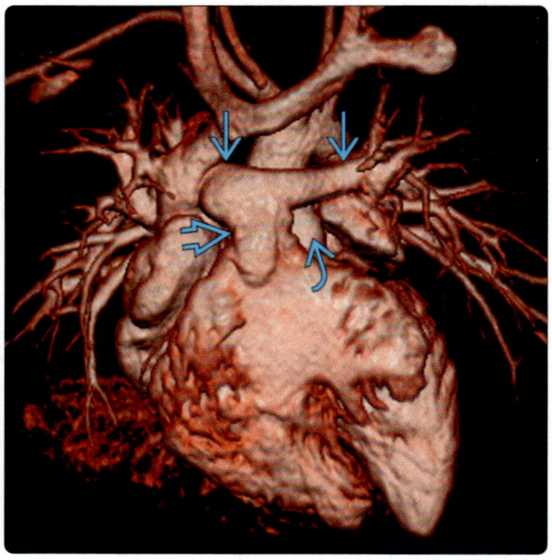

(Left) *Axial oblique MRA MPR in a 16 year old shows a post repair appearance of TGA after an arterial switch operation with the Lecompte maneuver, whereby the great vessel origins are switched, now with the MPA anterior & to the right of the aorta. The Lecompte maneuver also places the PAs anterior to the aorta. The coronaries are typically reimplanted during the procedure.* **(Right)** *Anterior MRA 3D projection in the same patient shows the MPA anterior to & the PAs draped across the aorta.*

Total Anomalous Pulmonary Venous Return

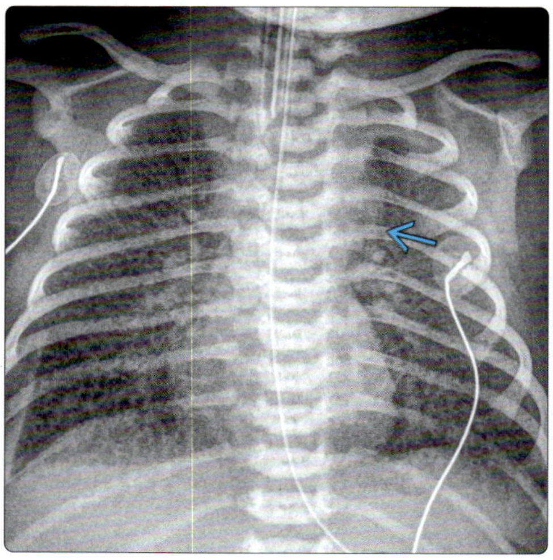

Total Anomalous Pulmonary Venous Return

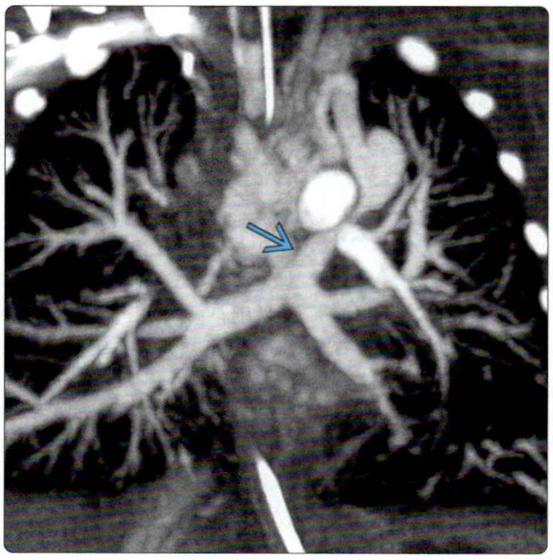

(Left) *AP radiograph in a 1 day old shows a snowman sign of supracardiac TAPVR due to a prominent vertical vein. The vertical vein needs to be dilated for this rare sign to be evident. The heart size is normal, & there is increased pulmonary vasculature with edema, consistent with an obstructed TAPVR. The fine interstitial reticulation is suspicious for lymphangiectasia.* **(Right)** *Coronal oblique CECT MIP in the same patient shows all pulmonary veins connecting to an obstructed vertical vein.*

Total Anomalous Pulmonary Venous Return

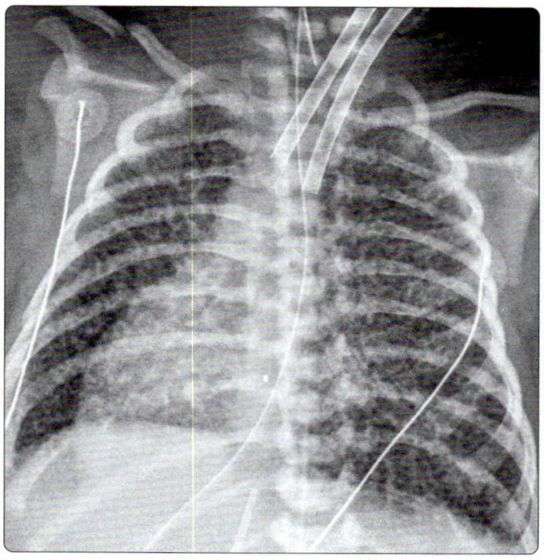

Total Anomalous Pulmonary Venous Return

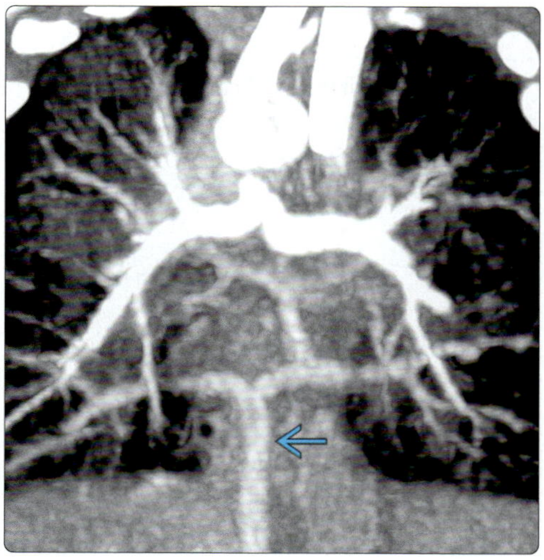

(Left) *AP radiograph in a 1 day old with dextrocardia & obstructed TAPVR on ECMO shows a normal heart size with pulmonary edema. The fine interstitial reticulation is suspicious for pulmonary lymphangiectasia, which can be seen in chronic pulmonary venous obstruction & carries a poor prognosis.* **(Right)** *Coronal CECT MIP in the same patient shows all pulmonary veins draining to a vertical vein that courses infradiaphragmatically, where it is obstructed (not shown). Infradiaphragmatic TAPVR is obstructed in 90%.*

Truncus Arteriosus

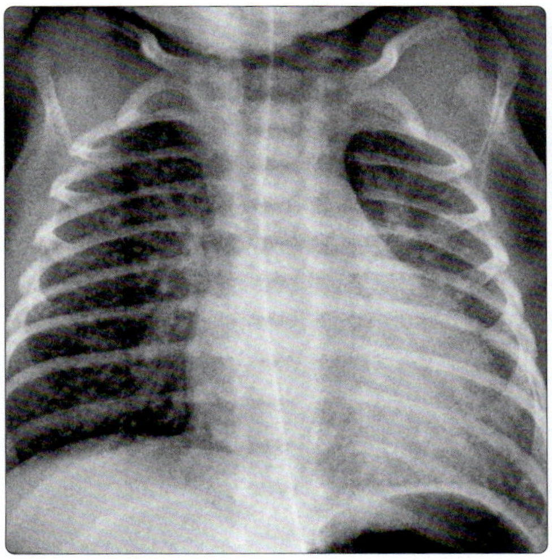

Truncus Arteriosus

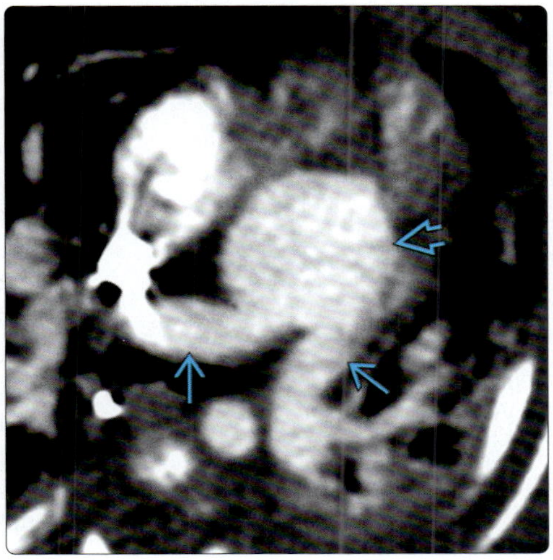

(Left) *AP radiograph in a cyanotic 5 day old shows nonspecific cardiomegaly & increased pulmonary vascularity. In practice, most radiographs of congenital heart disease (CHD) are nonspecific & definitive diagnosis requires echocardiography.* **(Right)** *Axial CECT in the same patient shows a single common arterial trunk arising equally from both ventricles & giving rise to closely adjacent right & left pulmonary arteries before continuing as the ascending aorta.*

Truncus Arteriosus

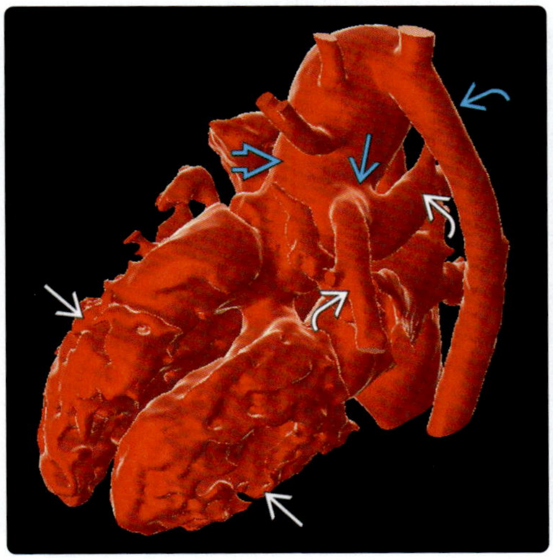

Truncus Arteriosus

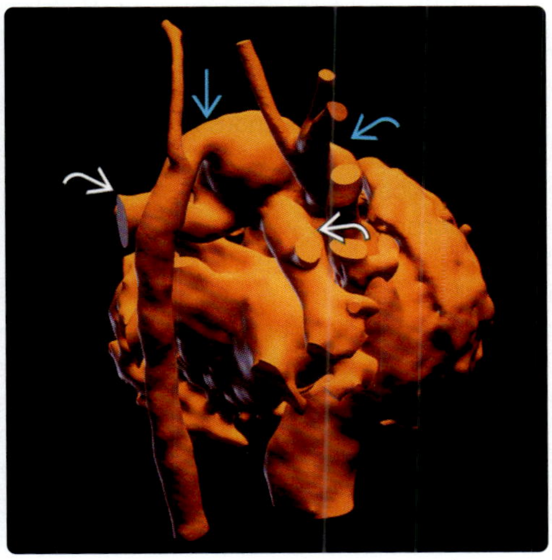

(Left) *Posterior CECT 3D projection in a patient with the most common form of truncus shows a common arterial trunk arising from both ventricles. There is a short MPA segment giving rise to both PAs, & there is a right aortic arch.* **(Right)** *Oblique CECT 3D projection in a patient with truncus shows that the common arterial trunk divides early into an interrupted aortic segment & a pulmonary segment that gives rise to the PAs. The descending aorta, which gives rise to the left subclavian, is supplied by a PDA.*

Other Complex Congenital Heart Disease Without Pulmonary Stenosis/Atresia

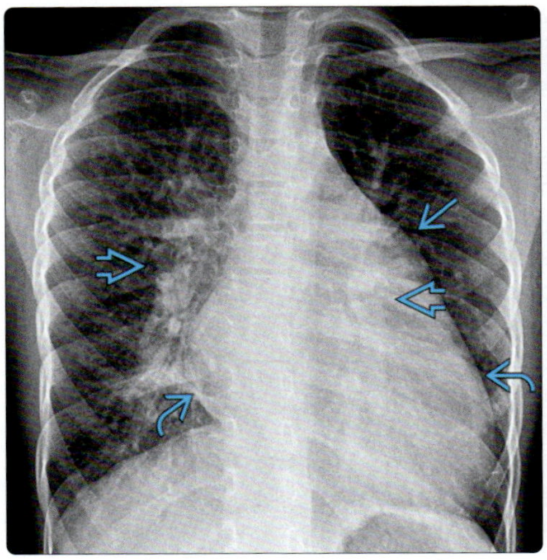

Other Complex Congenital Heart Disease Without Pulmonary Stenosis/Atresia

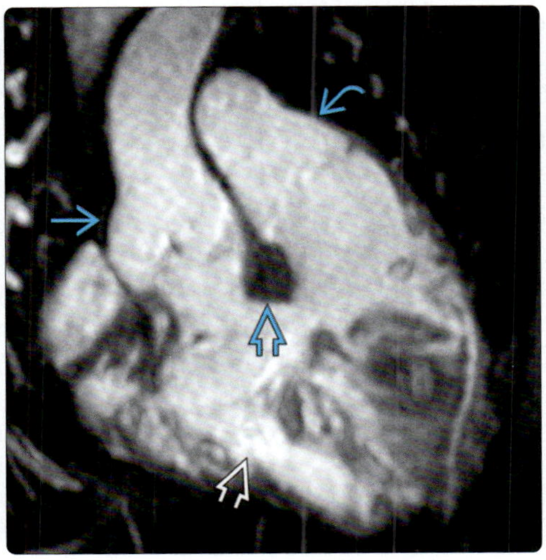

(Left) *PA radiograph in a 6 year old shows moderate cardiomegaly with an enlarged MPA & increased pulmonary vascularity.* **(Right)** *Coronal oblique MRA MIP in the same patient shows the aorta directly to the right of the MPA, both arising exclusively from the RV, typical of DORV. This patient had a dynamic subaortic stenosis caused by the subaortic infundibulum & prominent muscle bundles (not shown), which allowed minimal to no cyanosis, acting more like a L → R shunt.*

DIFFERENTIAL DIAGNOSIS

Common

- Atrial Septal Defect
- Pulmonary Arterial Hypertension

Less Common

- Atrioventricular Septal Defect
- Partial Anomalous Pulmonary Venous Return
- Restrictive Cardiomyopathy
- Dilated Cardiomyopathy

Rare but Important

- Ebstein Anomaly
- Pulmonary Atresia With Intact Ventricular Septum
- Tricuspid Valve Dysplasia
- Tricuspid Atresia

ESSENTIAL INFORMATION

Key Differential Diagnosis Issues

- Atria dilate in response to volume or pressure
- Main causes
  - L → R shunt into right atrium (RA)
    - Atrial septal defect (ASD), atrioventricular septal defect (AVSD), partial anomalous pulmonary venous return (PAPVR)
  - Secondary to right ventricular (RV) hypertension
    - Pulmonary hypertension, pulmonary atresia with intact ventricular septum (PA/IVS)
  - Secondary to right ventricular failure
    - Restrictive cardiomyopathy, dilated cardiomyopathy (DCM)
  - Tricuspid regurgitation/stenosis
    - Ebstein anomaly, PA/IVS, tricuspid valve dysplasia
- Chest radiograph
  - Frontal: Bulging of right heart border
    - Extending beyond medial 1/3 of right hemithorax, or
    - Occupying more than 1/2 of vertical distance between medial right clavicle & right hemidiaphragm
  - RA enlargement may not be detectable (e.g., most ASDs)
  - Pitfall: Normal RA may be displaced rightward by enlargement of another heart chamber
- Usually cannot determine etiology by radiograph alone

Helpful Clues for Common Diagnoses

- **Atrial Septal Defect**
  - Isolated ASD: 6-10% of congenital heart disease (CHD)
    - Most are well tolerated in childhood, even if large
    - Small ASDs can close spontaneously
    - Indications for interventional/surgical closure include degree of shunt (Qp:Qs > 2:1) & RV enlargement
  - L → R shunt → right heart volume overload → RA, RV, PA enlargement
  - Types of ASD
    - Secundum ASD (a.k.a. fossa ovalis defect): 80-90%
      - 1 or more holes in floor of fossa ovalis
      - Size of defect & sufficiency of rims determine candidacy for catheter-based closure
    - Primum ASD: Form of AVSD where bridging leaflets of common AV valve are attached to ventricular septal crest, allowing only interatrial shunting
    - Sinus venosus ASD
      - Located at sinus venosus (most posterior aspect of wall between right & left atria at caval insertions)
      - Superior type: At superior vena cava (SVC)-atrial junction; PAPVR of right upper pulmonary vein is often present (85%)
      - Inferior type (rare): At inferior vena cava (IVC)-atrial junction; ± PAPVR of right lower pulmonary vein
    - Coronary sinus ASD: Defect of wall between coronary sinus & left atrium (unroofed coronary sinus); associated with left SVC
- **Pulmonary Arterial Hypertension**
  - Defined by mean PA pressure > 25 mmHg at rest & > 30 mmHg during exercise with normal PA wedge pressure
  - In pediatrics, consider idiopathic, familial, pulmonary capillary hemangiomatosis, pulmonary venoocclusive disease, chronic L → R shunts, chronic pulmonary vein stenosis, chemotherapy, chronic lung disease of prematurity, or other lung disease
  - ↑ PA pressure & ↑ RV pressure → PA enlargement & RV hypertrophy
  - RA also sees ↑ pressure & dilates
    - Can be quantified on echo or MR & may be marker of adverse outcomes
    - Not detectable radiographically until late
  - Classic radiographic appearance: Dilated main & hilar pulmonary arteries with pruning & ↓ peripheral vascularity
  - CT: Consider when MPA:Ao diameter > 1.3 (if no CHD)

Helpful Clues for Less Common Diagnoses

- **Atrioventricular Septal Defect**
  - a.k.a. endocardial cushion defect
  - Defined by common AV junction/annulus, typically with common AV orifice
    - 5 leaflets: Superior bridging, left mural, inferior bridging, right mural, & right anterosuperior leaflets
    - Relationship of valve to atrial & ventricular septa determines degree of atrial & ventricular shunting
    - "Complete" form → all heart chambers communicate
  - Radiographs: Globular cardiomegaly, enlargement of all chambers, & markedly ↑ pulmonary vascularity with hyperinflation
  - May present at birth, depending on degree of shunting & AV regurgitation
  - Can have congestive heart failure, recurrent pulmonary infections, &/or early pulmonary hypertension
  - Strong association with trisomy 21; common in heterotaxy
- **Partial Anomalous Pulmonary Venous Return**
  - 1 or more (not all) pulmonary veins drain anomalously to systemic vein
  - L → R shunt → right heart volume overload → RA, RV, PA enlargement
  - Right PAPVR: Usually right upper pulmonary vein to SVC; associated with sinus venosus ASD
  - Left PAPVR: Usually left upper pulmonary vein to left innominate vein; associated with secundum ASD
  - Total anomalous drainage of right lung to inferior venocaval junction associated with scimitar syndrome
  - Isolated PAPVR of single vein is usually well tolerated

- Radiographs: Mild ↑ pulmonary vascularity with mild right heart dilation
  - Anomalous vessels may dilate & be seen on radiographs
- **Restrictive Cardiomyopathy**
  - Restricted ventricular diastolic filling with normal systolic function
  - Biventricular failure with normal or reduced ventricular sizes (by definition)
  - Biatrial dilation is characteristic
  - Usually idiopathic; can be caused by any condition with diffuse infiltration/deposition/fibrosis of myocardium
  - Imaging may be similar to constrictive pericarditis, except without pericardial thickening (> 4 mm)
- **Dilated Cardiomyopathy**
  - Ventricular dilation with poor function
    - Predominantly affects left heart, but if severe, can cause global dilation
  - Most common etiologies: Prior viral myocarditis & genetic mutations, although specific etiology often cannot be confirmed
    - Main question is often inflammatory DCM (prior viral myocarditis) vs. noninflammatory DCM
  - Radiographs: Cardiomegaly & pulmonary venous congestion
  - MR: Diffuse mid myocardial late gadolinium enhancement (LGE) is classic but rarely seen in children

Helpful Clues for Rare Diagnoses

- **Ebstein Anomaly**
  - Cyanotic lesion with RA dilation & ↓ pulmonary vascularity
  - Classic entity for wall-to-wall or box-shaped heart
  - Defined by apical displacement of septal & posterior tricuspid leaflets (> 8 mm/m² body surface area)
    - Anterior leaflet in normal position but large, redundant, & sail-like
    - Inlet portion of RV becomes incorporated into RA → "atrialization of RV"
    - Results in tripartite right heart: RA, atrialized RV, & functional RV (trabecular apex & outlet)
  - Broad spectrum of leaflet abnormalities, ranging from mild (adult presentation) to severe (neonates)
    - Neonates: Typically severe tricuspid regurgitation → massive dilation of RA & thus massive cardiomegaly
    - Elevated RA pressures lead to R → L shunt across patent foramen ovale (PFO) or ASD, causing cyanosis
  - Commonly have conduction anomalies & arrhythmias
  - Poorer prognosis: Earlier gestational age, larger tricuspid annulus, pulmonary regurgitation
- **Pulmonary Atresia With Intact Ventricular Septum**
  - Complete obstruction to RV outflow, although typically with well-developed confluent pulmonary arteries
  - RV is typically small & hypertrophied: Prototypical hypoplastic right heart lesion
  - Tricuspid valve is almost always abnormal: Hypoplastic, dysplastic, ± Ebsteinoid
  - RA dilation from tricuspid regurgitation & ↑ RV pressure
- **Tricuspid Valve Dysplasia**
  - Isolated tricuspid valve dysplasia with hinge points in normal position (thus without Ebstein anomaly)
  - However, radiograph looks exactly like Ebstein anomaly
  - Tricuspid regurgitation/stenosis → RA dilation
- **Tricuspid Atresia**
  - Absent right AV communication
  - Cyanotic heart lesion
  - ASD or PFO is always present; VSD is common
  - Often with RV outflow tract obstruction (OTO) or restrictive VSD, & thus decreased pulmonary vascularity
    - If no RVOTO: ↑ pulmonary vascularity
    - If ASD restrictive (small): RA dilation & cardiomegaly
  - Concomitant transposition of great arteries (30%)
  - CT/MR: Fat extending into deep AV groove at site of atretic AV connection

SELECTED REFERENCES

1. Deri A et al: Educational series in congenital heart disease: echocardiographic assessment of left to right shunts: atrial septal defect, ventricular septal defect, atrioventricular septal defect, patent arterial duct. Echo Res Pract. 5(1):R1-R16, 2018

Atrial Septal Defect

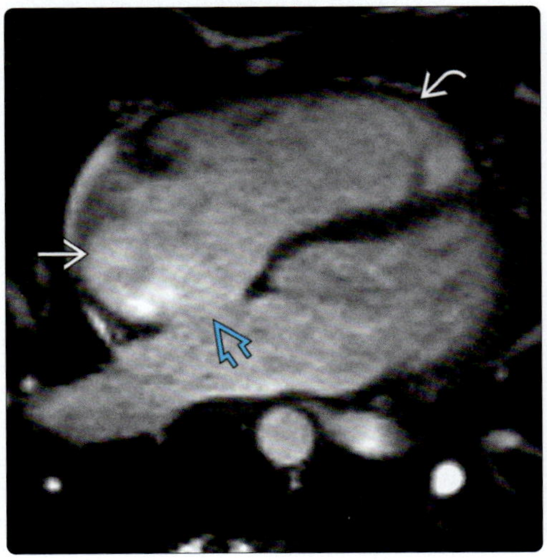

Atrial Septal Defect

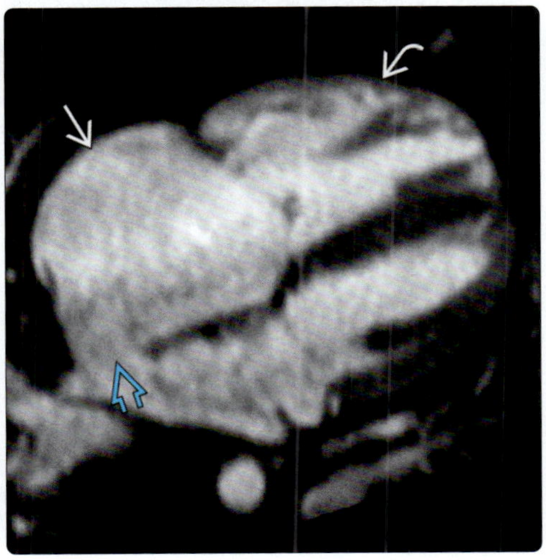

(Left) *Four-chamber SSFP MR in an asymptomatic 17 year old shows a large secundum ASD ➡, which was found incidentally. The Qp:Qs was only 1.6:1; however, closure was indicated by the RA ➡ & RV ➡ enlargement.* **(Right)** *Four-chamber MRA MPR shows a superior sinus venosus ASD ➡ at the posterior atrial septum at the SVC-atrial junction. Patient also had PAPVR of the right upper pulmonary vein (not shown). There is RA ➡ & RV ➡ dilation with a normal LA size, as expected for atrial level shunts.*

(Left) *PA radiograph in a 10-year-old girl with idiopathic pulmonary arterial hypertension shows dilated main & hilar pulmonary arteries with pruning & relatively decreased vascularity peripherally given the degree of central arterial dilation. There is only mild RA prominence.* **(Right)** *Coronal oblique CECT MIP in the same patient shows relatively small branch pulmonary arteries & veins relative to the dilated central pulmonary arteries.*

Pulmonary Arterial Hypertension

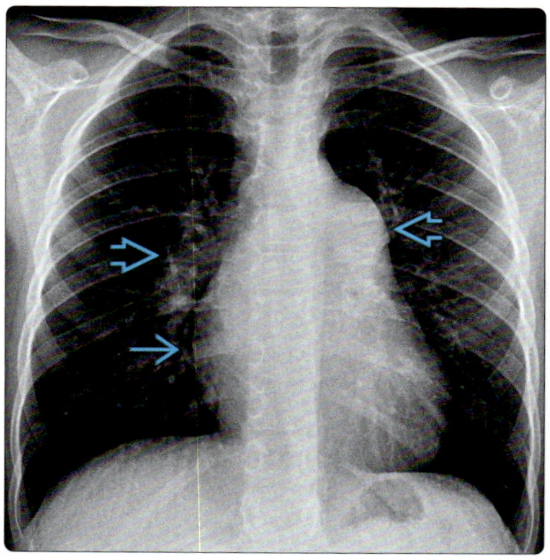

Pulmonary Arterial Hypertension

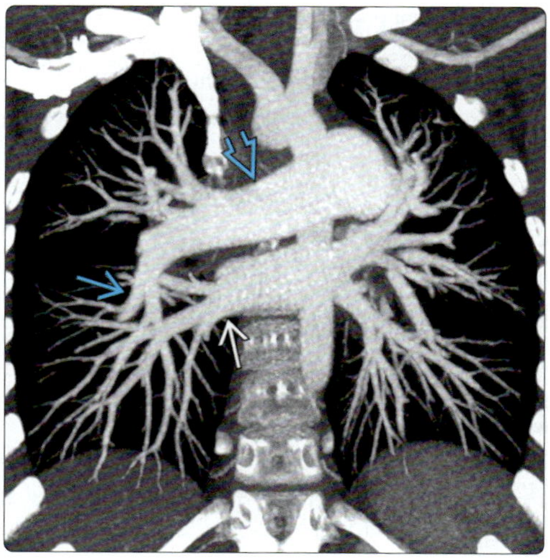

(Left) *Axial CECT in the same patient shows RV hypertrophy, which is in response to the elevated pulmonary vascular resistance. Diastolic RV dysfunction & right heart pressure overload can lead to RA dilation.* **(Right)** *PA radiograph in a 4 year old with pulmonary hypertension secondary to an ASD shows large central pulmonary arteries but less peripheral vascularity than expected. The RA is dilated. A decrease in peripheral vascularity over time in a L → R shunt may represent the development of pulmonary hypertension.*

Pulmonary Arterial Hypertension

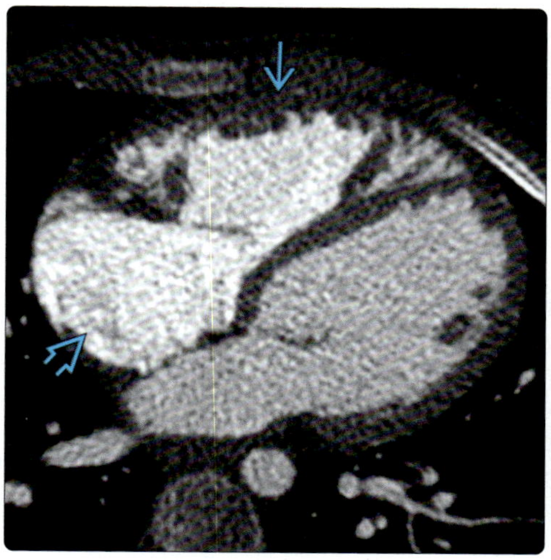

Pulmonary Arterial Hypertension

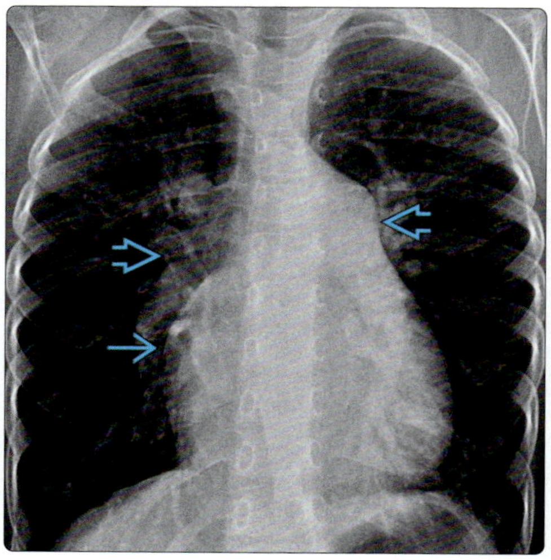

(Left) *Four-chamber SSFP MR in a 9 month old shows a common AV junction, a single large valve, & an associated primum ASD & inlet VSD, consistent with a complete AVSD. There is global chamber dilation, greatest of the RA.* **(Right)** *Coronal oblique MRA MIP in a 5 year old with PAPVR shows multiple right pulmonary veins draining to the SVC. While some join high to the SVC, others can be in essentially normal locations but drain anomalously through an associated superior sinus venosus defect.*

Atrioventricular Septal Defect

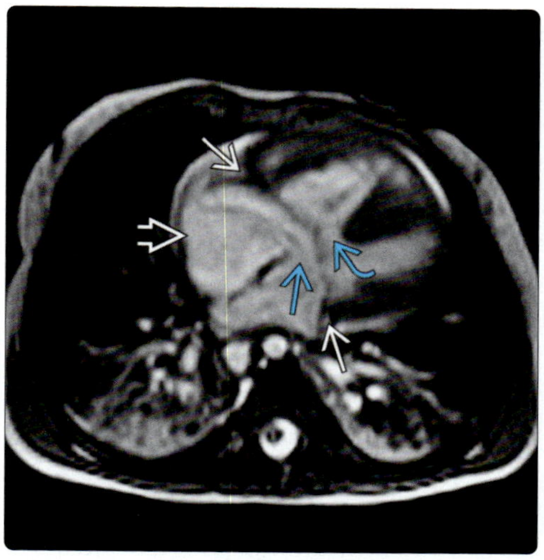

Partial Anomalous Pulmonary Venous Return

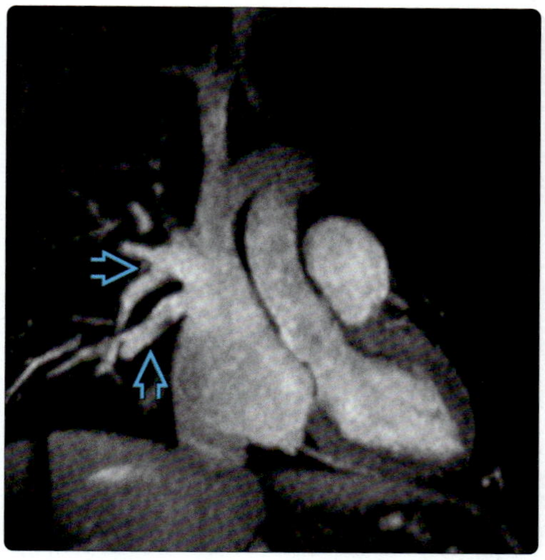

Restrictive Cardiomyopathy | **Restrictive Cardiomyopathy**

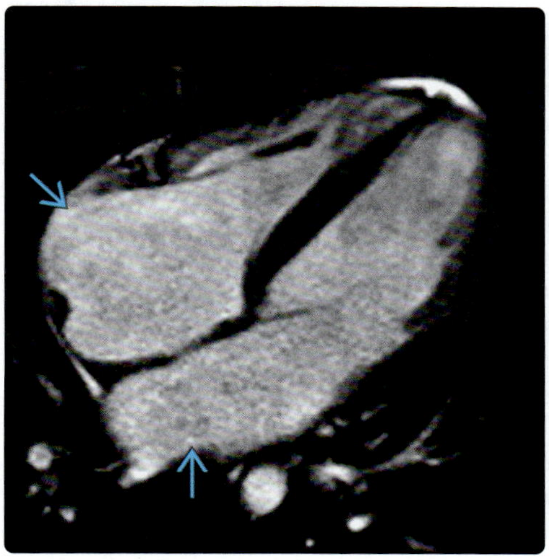

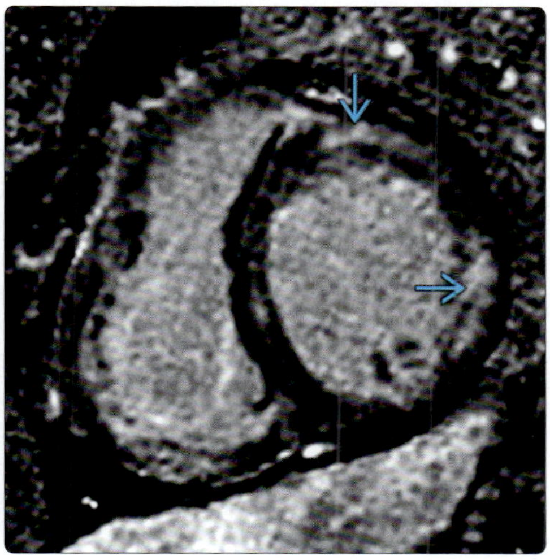

(Left) *Four-chamber SSFP MR in a 17 year old with a genetic restrictive cardiomyopathy (RCM) shows biatrial dilation → without ventricular dilation, characteristic of RCM.* **(Right)** *Short-axis LGE PSIR MR in the same patient shows moderate biventricular myocardial hypertrophy with extensive patchy delayed enhancement →, indicative of myocardial fibrosis. Associated diastolic dysfunction & impaired ventricular filling leads to biatrial dilation.*

Dilated Cardiomyopathy | **Dilated Cardiomyopathy**

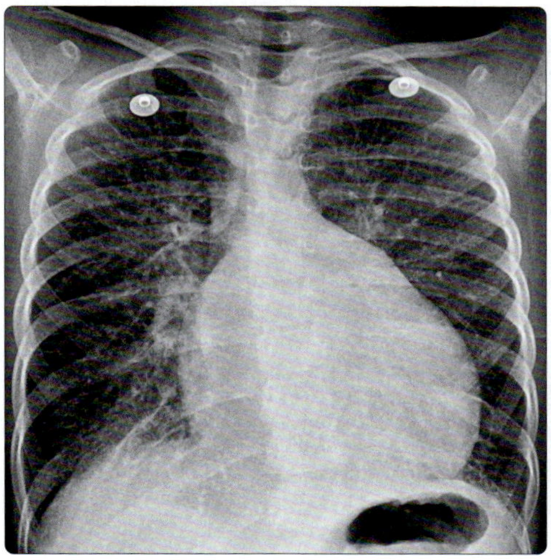

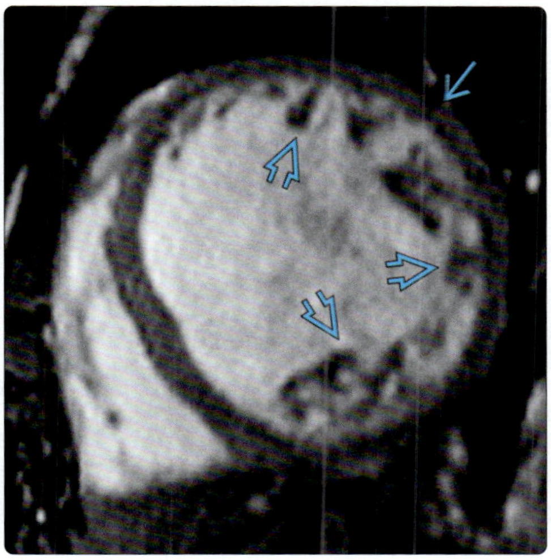

(Left) *PA radiograph in a noncyanotic 5 year old shows cardiomegaly with normal pulmonary vascularity & mild central interstitial edema, consistent with heart failure.* **(Right)** *Short-axis SSFP MR in the same patient shows marked LV dilation → with prominent trabeculations →. The overall picture was consistent with dilated cardiomyopathy (DCM) secondary to viral myocarditis. DCM typically affects the left heart structures but can result in global cardiomegaly (including RA dilation), which has a worse prognosis.*

Ebstein Anomaly | **Ebstein Anomaly**

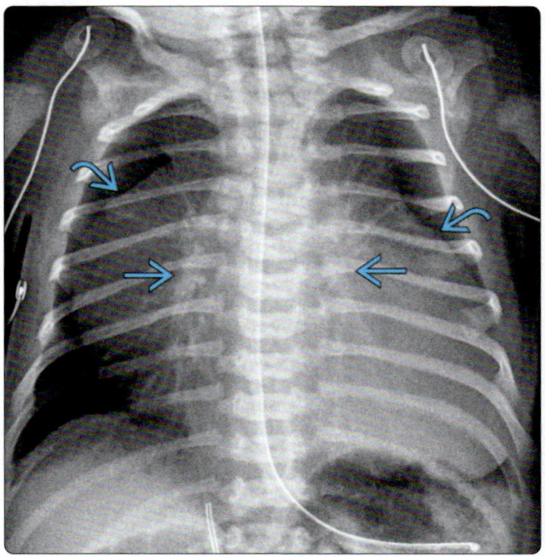

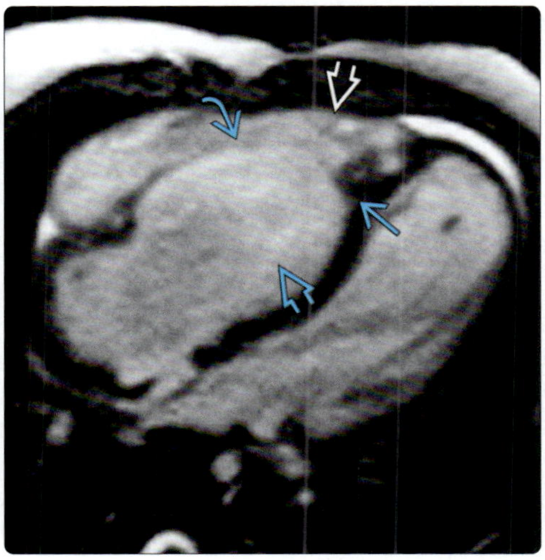

(Left) *AP radiograph in a 1 day old shows a wall-to-wall heart → with decreased pulmonary vascularity → due to Ebstein anomaly. The massive cardiomegaly is from severe tricuspid regurgitation, leading to severe RA dilation. The decreased vascularity is due to anatomic or functional PS/PA.* **(Right)** *Four-chamber SSFP MR in a 4 month old with Ebstein anomaly shows apical displacement of the septal leaflet →, a redundant sail-like anterior leaflet →, & the atrialized portion of the RV →. The functional RV is small →.*

DIFFERENTIAL DIAGNOSIS

Common

- Left-to-Right Shunts
- Pulmonary Regurgitation

Less Common

- Pulmonary Arterial Hypertension
- Right Ventricular Outflow Tract Obstruction
- Cardiomyopathy
  - Arrhythmogenic Right Ventricular Cardiomyopathy
  - Dilated Cardiomyopathy
  - Hypertrophic Cardiomyopathy
  - Ischemic Cardiomyopathy

Rare but Important

- Tricuspid Regurgitation

ESSENTIAL INFORMATION

Key Differential Diagnosis Issues

- Ventricles physiologically enlarge in 2 ways
  - Dilate in response to increased blood volume
    - Conventional meaning of enlargement
  - Hypertrophy in response to increased pressure
    - Contour change with only minimal change in size
- Main causes of dilation
  - Left-to-right shunts
  - Pulmonary regurgitation
  - Tricuspid regurgitation
  - Arrhythmogenic right ventricular cardiomyopathy (ARVC), dilated cardiomyopathy, ischemic cardiomyopathy
- Main causes of hypertrophy
  - Pulmonary arterial hypertension
  - Right ventricular outflow tract obstruction (RVOTO)
  - Hypertrophic cardiomyopathy
- Chest radiograph
  - Dilation: Loss of retrosternal clear space by dilated right ventricle (RV) & main pulmonary artery (MPA) (but cannot use if thymus is large)
    - Pitfall: RV dilation with leftward cardiac rotation can mimic appearance of left ventricle (LV) enlargement
  - Hypertrophy: Rounded, elevated cardiac apex (caused by leftward & superior deviation of cardiac axis)
    - Pitfall: Lordotic projection or hyperinflation can mimic appearance of elevated apex

Helpful Clues for Common Diagnoses

- **Left-to-Right Shunts**
  - All L → R shunts, except those beyond level of ventricles (i.e., PDA, aortopulmonary window) lead to volume overload of RV & eventual dilation
  - Most common: Atrial septal defect (ASD), ventricular septal defect (VSD), atrioventricular septal defect (AVSD)
  - Radiographs
    - Cardiomegaly
      - ASD: Mild right atrial (RA), RV, pulmonary artery (PA) enlargement
      - VSD: Left atrial (LA), LV, RV, PA enlargement (LA dilation suggests intact atrial septum)
      - AVSD: Global enlargement, greatest of RA & PA
    - Dilated PAs with increased pulmonary vascularity
      - Uniformly enlarged vessels at hila & within lungs
      - Convex bulge of MPA at left heart border
      - Descending RPA branch larger than trachea
    - Air-trapping due to vascular compression of small airways
    - Findings often not appreciable when pulmonary to systemic blood flow ratio (Qp:Qs) is < 2:1
  - Definitive diagnosis by echocardiography
  - One of main indications for repair of mild L → R shunts (such as ASD or partial anomalous pulmonary venous return) is presence of RV dilation
- **Pulmonary Regurgitation**
  - Pulmonary regurgitation volume overloads RV & leads to greatest degree of RV dilation
  - Can be congenital, but pulmonary regurgitation most commonly occurs after right ventricular outflow tract (RVOT) repair or intervention
    - Any type of nonvalve-sparing repair of Tetralogy of Fallot (TOF)
    - Any RV-PA conduit (such as for TOF or truncus)
    - Catheter balloon valvotomy ± stent for critical pulmonary stenosis (i.e., congenital pulmonary stenosis, TOF, pulmonary atresia with intact ventricular septum)
  - Follow-up of RV dilation in these scenarios is most common indication for pediatric cardiac MR
    - Degree of pulmonary regurgitation quantified by phase-contrast imaging
    - RV size quantified by cine imaging, as significant RV dilation is indication for mechanical pulmonary valve replacement

Helpful Clues for Less Common Diagnoses

- **Pulmonary Arterial Hypertension**
  - Defined by mean pulmonary arterial pressure > 25 mmHg at rest & > 30 mmHg during exercise, with normal pulmonary artery wedge pressure
  - In pediatrics consider: Idiopathic, familial, pulmonary venoocclusive disease/pulmonary capillary hemangiomatosis, chronic L → R shunts, chronic pulmonary vein stenosis, posttumoral therapy, chronic lung disease of prematurity, or other lung disease
  - Increased PA pressure & increased RV pressure → PA enlargement & RV hypertrophy
  - Classic radiographic appearance: Dilated main & hilar pulmonary arteries with decreased peripheral vascularity
  - CT: Consider when MPA:Ao diameter > 1.3 [if no congenital heart defect (CHD)]
- **Right Ventricular Outflow Tract Obstruction**
  - Leads to increased RV pressure & RV hypertrophy
  - **Congenital pulmonary stenosis**
    - Dysplastic pulmonary valve leaflets with normal-sized pulmonary annulus & PAs (unlike TOF)
    - May undergo balloon catheter valvotomy, which may create mixed stenosis/regurgitation
  - **Tetralogy of Fallot**
    - Anterior, superior, & leftward malalignment of outlet septum causing RVOTO
    - Results in classic tetrad: (1) RVOTO; (2) RV hypertrophy; (3) VSD; (4) aorta overriding VSD

- Cyanotic CHD with diminished pulmonary vascularity & relatively normal heart size
- Classic radiographic appearance: Boot-shaped heart
  - □ Leftward rotation of cardiac axis
  - □ Upturned apex from right ventricular hypertrophy
  - □ Concave superior left heart border from absent/small MPA
  - □ Absent left aortic arch contour if right aortic arch present (25%)
- Caution: Vast majority of TOF do not have boot shape; also, other entities can mimic
- After repair, physiology dominated by pulmonary regurgitation & RV dilation instead (though residual RVOTO may be present)

- **Post repair of CHD**
  - Any postoperative RVOT can have recurrent or residual stenosis, which can lead to RV hypertrophy
    - □ Subvalvar RVOT muscle bundles
    - □ Within RV-PA conduit
    - □ Residual hypoplastic or stenotic pulmonary arteries

- **Cardiomyopathy**
  - **Arrhythmogenic right ventricular cardiomyopathy**
    - Inherited cardiomyopathy with mutation in 1 of various desmosomal protein genes
    - Progressive epicardial to endocardial myocardial loss with fibrofatty replacement
      - □ Early regional involvement, progresses to global
      - □ Starts in subtricuspid & RVOT regions of RV free wall, along with LV posterolateral wall (displaced triangle of dysplasia)
    - Diagnosis important but challenging
      - □ Variable penetrance
      - □ 50-70% of carriers never express disease
      - □ Most children in concealed phase: Risk of sudden death despite normal morphology & function
    - Task Force Criteria (TFC) for diagnosis: Combination of major & minor criteria, including from MR
      - □ MR criteria: Regional RV wall motion abnormality + RV dilation or reduced RV ejection fraction
    - Considerations in pediatric population
      - □ Cardiac MR is most important contributor to diagnosis by TFC (unlike in adults)
      - □ RV wall motion abnormality is most important finding
      - □ Classic late-stage features in adults (such as late gadolinium enhancement & fatty replacement) are rare in children & are never seen without underlying wall motion abnormality
      - □ Cut-offs for RV dilation are based on adults & may not apply to adolescents, especially during puberty
  - **Dilated cardiomyopathy**
    - Ventricular dilation with poor function
      - □ Predominantly affects left heart, but if severe, can cause global dilation
    - Most common etiologies: Prior viral myocarditis or genetic mutations
    - Radiographs: Cardiomegaly & pulmonary venous congestion
    - MR: LGE is classic, rare in children
  - **Hypertrophic cardiomyopathy**
    - Most common hereditary cardiac disorder
    - Usually presents in adolescence or later
    - Asymmetric ventricular hypertrophy > 15 mm, typically of basal septum
    - ~ 30% get RV hypertrophy as well
    - MR: Can see patchy midwall LGE with predilection for RV insertion points
    - Risk of sudden cardiac death
  - **Ischemic cardiomyopathy**
    - RV ischemia rare, can be seen as result of CHD
    - RV failure results in RV dilation

Helpful Clues for Rare Diagnoses

- **Tricuspid Regurgitation**
  - Consider Ebstein anomaly or isolated tricuspid valve dysplasia
  - Severe tricuspid regurgitation volume overloads right heart → massive RA dilation & RV dilation

Left-to-Right Shunts

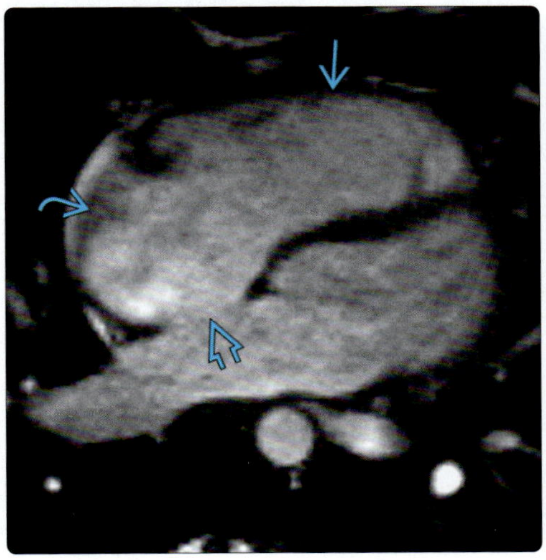

Left-to-Right Shunts

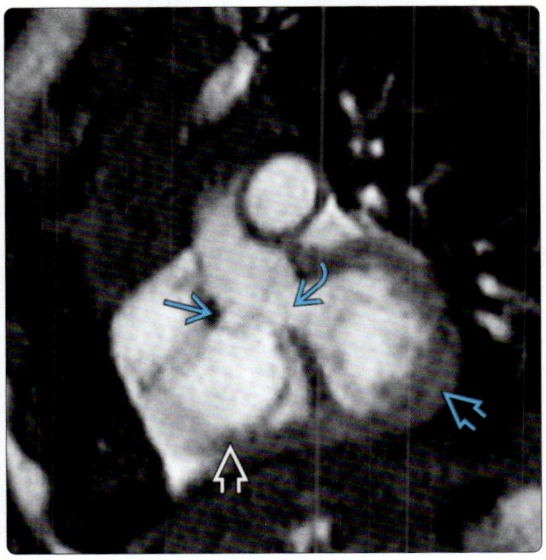

(Left) *Four-chamber SSFP MR in an asymptomatic 17 year old shows a large secundum atrial septal defect (ASD) ➡, which was well tolerated & found incidentally. ASD closure was indicated because of right atrial (RA) ➡ & right ventricular (RV) ➡ dilation. The left atrium (LA) was not enlarged, as expected.* **(Right)** *Short-axis SSFP MR in a 6 month old shows a perimembranous VSD ➡ with tricuspid-aortic continuity ➡. Volume overload from shunting between the LV ➡ & RV ➡ causes LA & biventricular dilation in VSDs.*

(Left) *PA radiograph in a 3 month old with trisomy 21 & a complete AVSD shows globular cardiomegaly, markedly increased pulmonary vascularity, & air-trapping, consistent with a large left-to-right shunt. The vessels are indistinct, suggestive of superimposed interstitial edema.* **(Right)** *Four-chamber SSFP MR in a 9 month old with pulmonary hypertension shows a common AV junction with an associated primum ASD & inlet VSD, consistent with a complete AVSD. There is dilation of the RA & RV.*

Left-to-Right Shunts

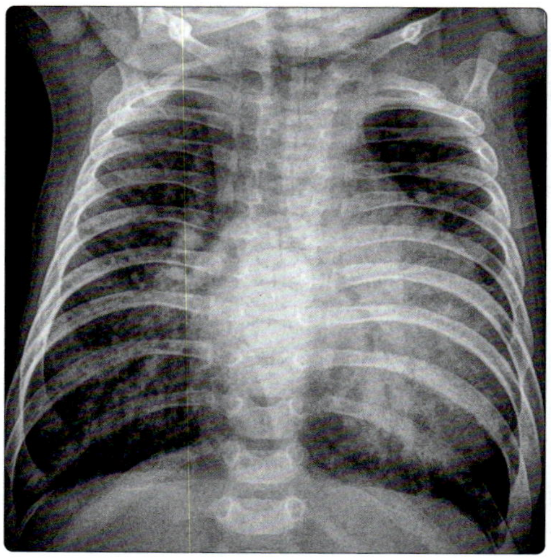

Left-to-Right Shunts

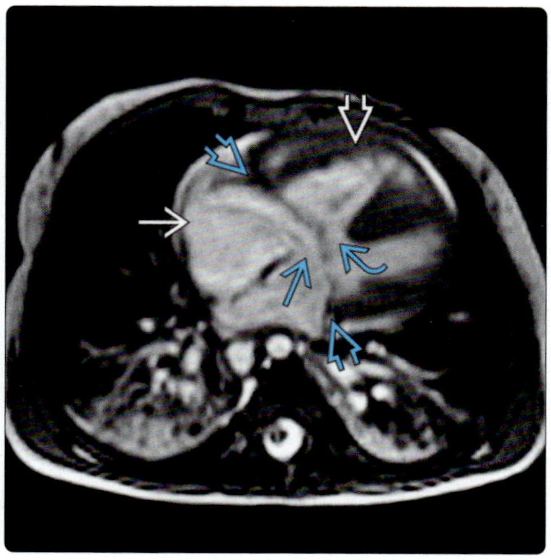

(Left) *RVOT SSFP MR in a 16 year old with TOF status post transannular patch repair shows a prominent MPA that allows free regurgitation into the RV.* **(Right)** *Four-chamber SSFP MR in the same patient shows the markedly enlarged RV. Septal flattening in diastole is a sign of RV volume overload. The increased volume leads to dilation of the RV & PAs. Diminished compliance of the RV can cause diastolic dysfunction & RA dilation. RV dilation is an indication for mechanical pulmonary valve replacement.*

Pulmonary Regurgitation

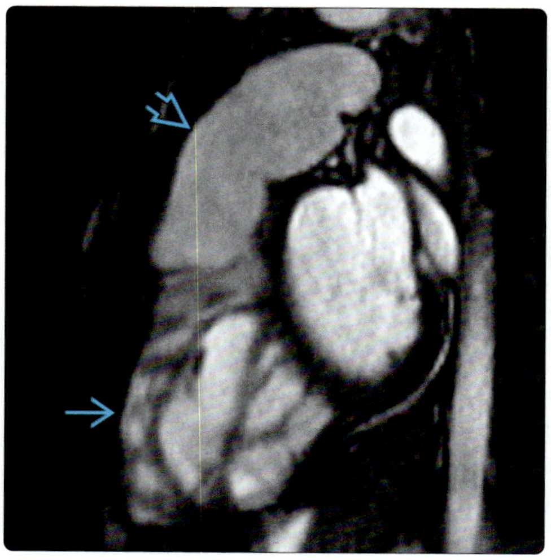

Pulmonary Regurgitation

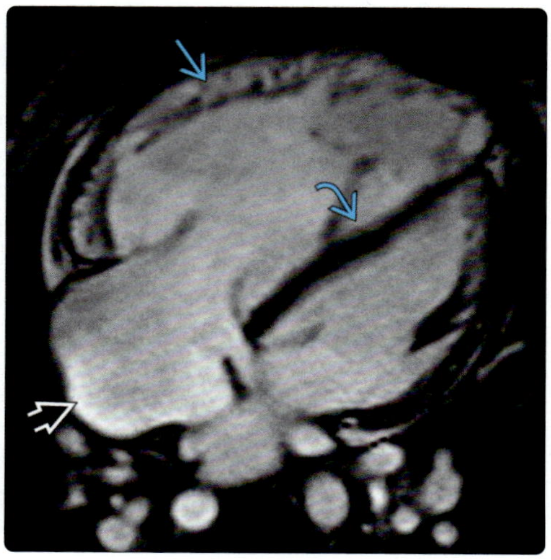

(Left) *PA radiograph in a 10-year-old girl with idiopathic pulmonary arterial hypertension shows dilated main & hilar pulmonary arteries with pruning & relatively decreased vascularity peripherally given the degree of central arterial dilation. There is mild upturning of the apex, suggestive of RV hypertrophy.* **(Right)** *Short-axis CECT in the same patient shows the RV hypertrophy in response to the elevated pulmonary vascular resistance. The RV myocardium is normally thin (but is as thick as the LV here).*

Pulmonary Arterial Hypertension

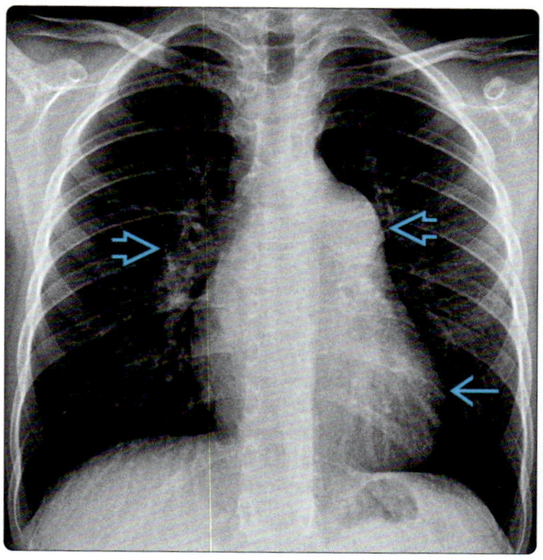

Pulmonary Arterial Hypertension

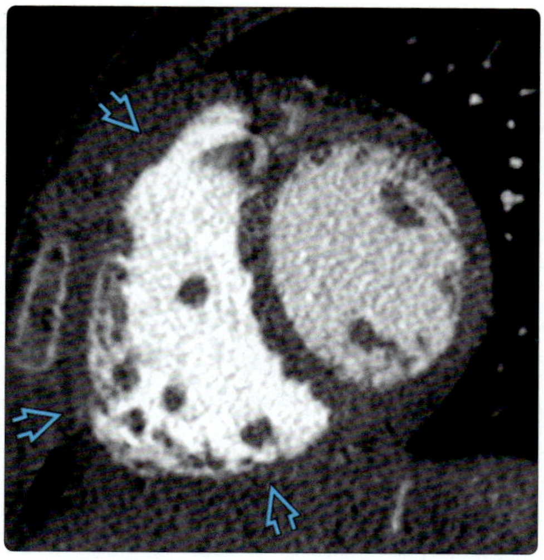

Right Ventricular Outflow Tract Obstruction

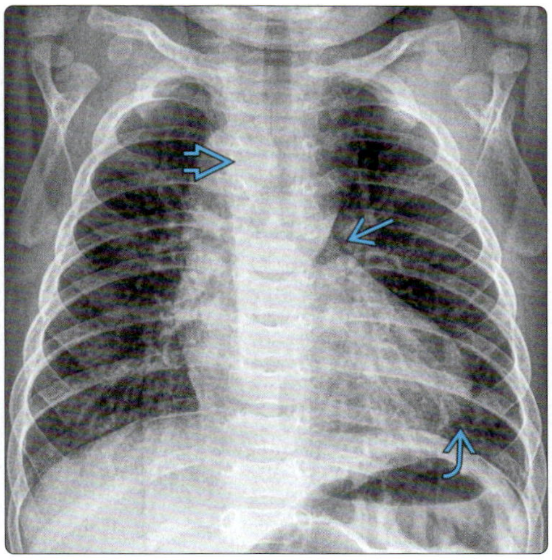

Right Ventricular Outflow Tract Obstruction

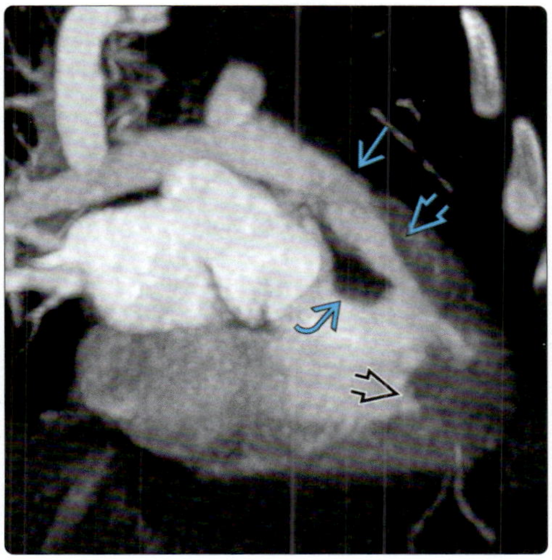

(Left) *PA radiograph in a 5 month old with TOF shows a boot-shaped heart with dextrorotation, an upturned apex, concavity of the left superior heart border from a small MPA, & right arch. There is decreased pulmonary vascularity.* **(Right)** *Coronal oblique CECT MIP in the same patient shows anterior & superior malalignment of the outlet septum, causing multilevel RVOTO with pulmonary valvar stenosis & subvalvar muscular stenosis. There is right ventricular hypertrophy (RVH) from increased afterload.*

Right Ventricular Outflow Tract Obstruction

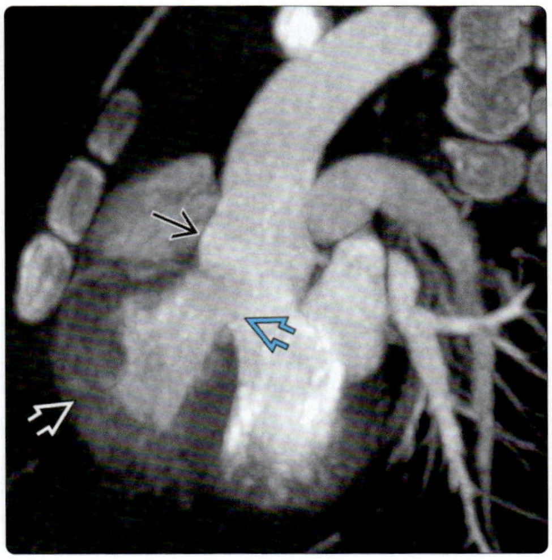

Right Ventricular Outflow Tract Obstruction

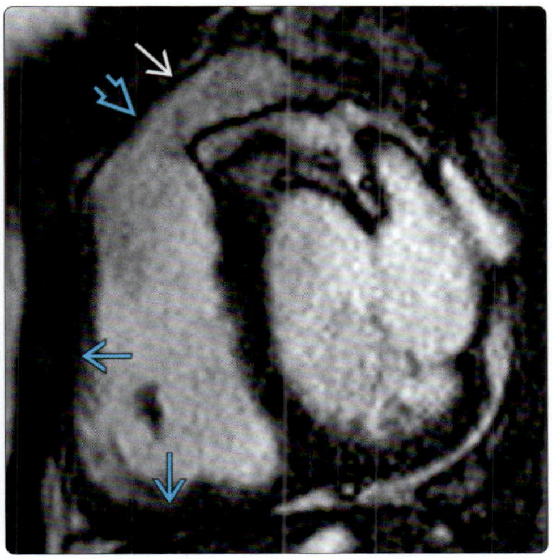

(Left) *Sagittal oblique CECT MIP in the same patient better shows the aorta overriding a perimembranous VSD + RVH.* **(Right)** *RVOT SSFP MR in a 15 year old with truncus arteriosus status post repair with an RV-PA conduit shows proximal conduit stenosis at the anastomosis. The stenosis leads leads to RV hypertrophy. Transcatheter intervention is usually the first option to relieve recurrent stenosis.*

Right Ventricular Outflow Tract Obstruction

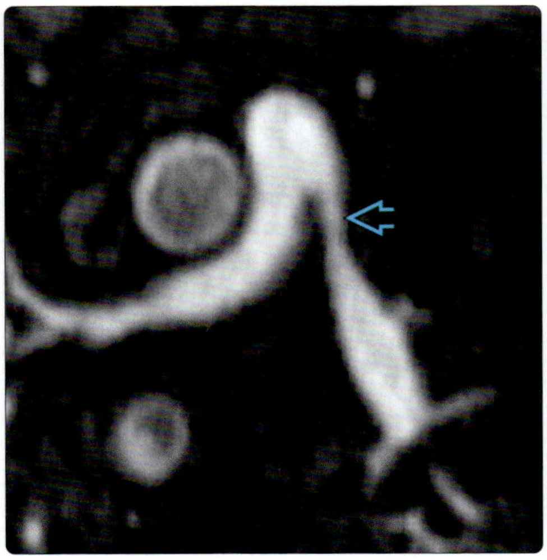

Right Ventricular Outflow Tract Obstruction

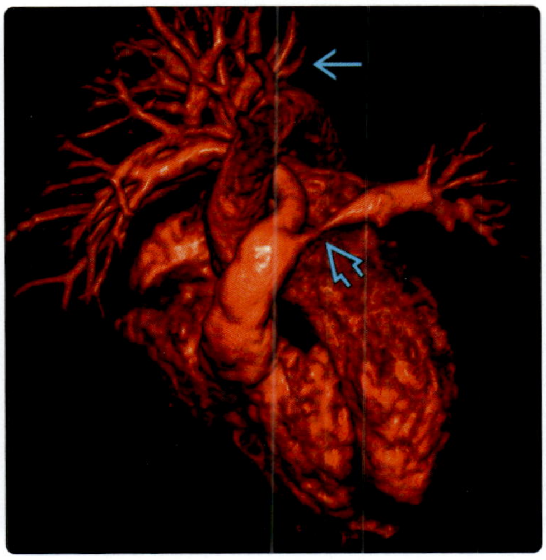

(Left) *Axial oblique MRA in the same patient shows additional severe segmental stenosis of the proximal LPA at the anastomosis with the distal conduit. This may further contribute to RV hypertrophy. There was also a right arch, which is seen in 30% of truncus arteriosus cases.* **(Right)** *MRA anterior oblique 3D projection in the same patient again shows the severe segmental LPA stenosis. Note the markedly increased blood flow to the right side, which was quantified on MR as 80% of total pulmonary blood flow.*

(Left) *Two-chamber SSFP MR in a 17 year old with right heart failure & arrhythmias shows RA → & RV → dilation. Pericardial effusion → & ascites → are present from right heart failure. MR findings contributed to a diagnosis of ARVC.* **(Right)** *Axial SSFP MR again shows the RA → & RV → dilation. The RV had global hypokinesia with an ejection fraction of 22% & severe dilation to 233 ml/m², meeting major criteria for ARVC. Notably, the heart & coronaries were anatomically normal.*

Arrhythmogenic Right Ventricular Cardiomyopathy

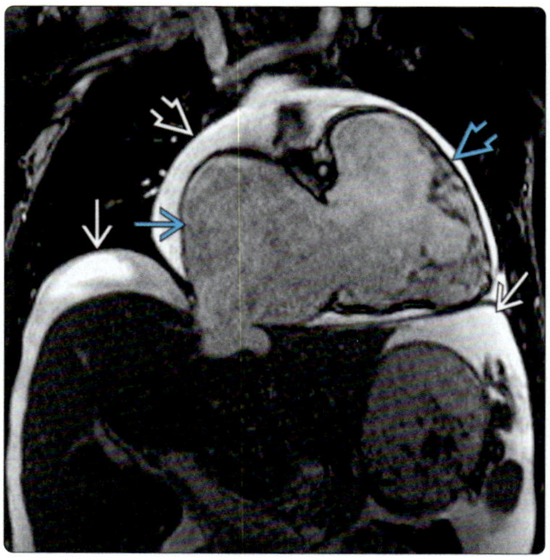

Arrhythmogenic Right Ventricular Cardiomyopathy

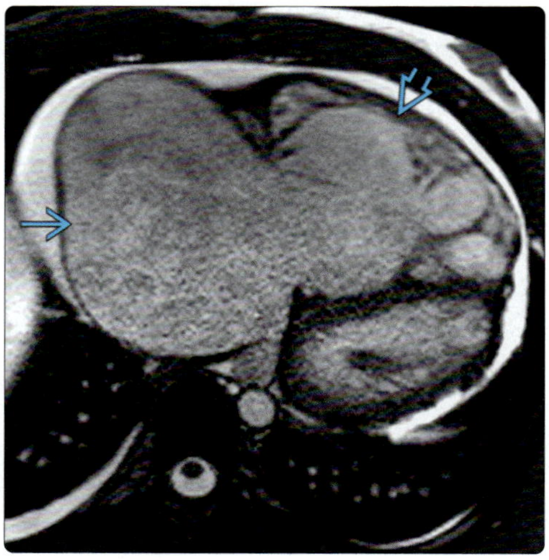

(Left) *Short-axis LGE PSIR MR in the same patient shows extensive LGE throughout the basal to mid RV free wall →. There is also LGE of the posterolateral LV →.* **(Right)** *Axial LGE PSIR MR again shows LGE of the RV free wall → & posterolateral LV →. This is the typical distribution of involvement in ARVC, known as the displaced triangle of dysplasia. LGE & LV involvement are not uncommon in adults with ARVC but are extremely rare in the pediatric population.*

Arrhythmogenic Right Ventricular Cardiomyopathy

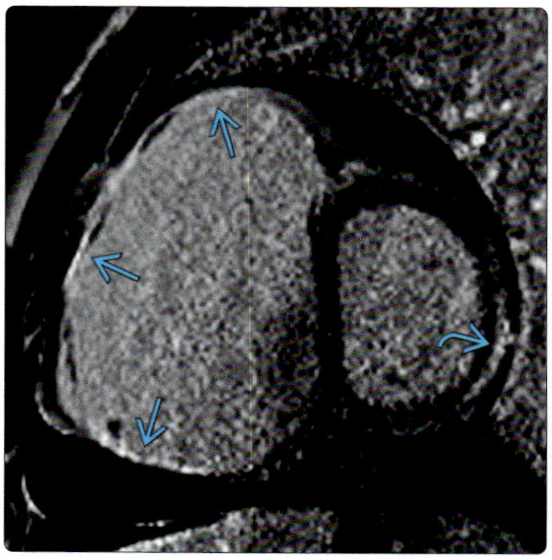

Arrhythmogenic Right Ventricular Cardiomyopathy

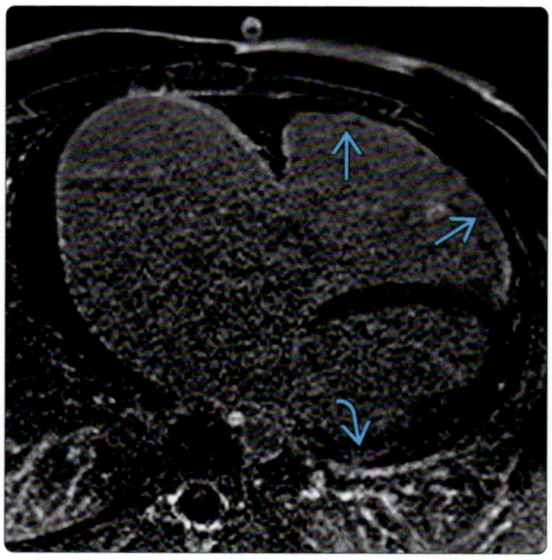

(Left) *AP radiograph in a 2 day old with dysmorphic features & heart failure shows massive cardiomegaly & normal pulmonary vascularity.* **(Right)** *Four-chamber echocardiogram in the same patient shows biventricular dilation & hypertrophy, most consistent with severe cardiomyopathy secondary to a genetic inborn error of metabolism. The RA →, RV →, LA →, & LV → are labeled. Note the severe hypertrophy of the ventricular myocardium →.*

Dilated Cardiomyopathy

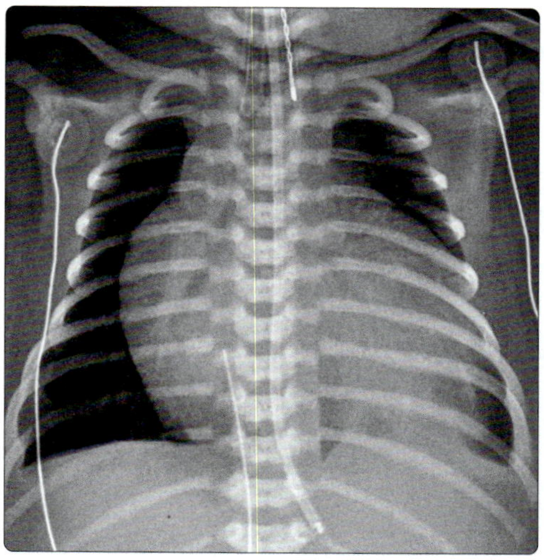

Dilated Cardiomyopathy

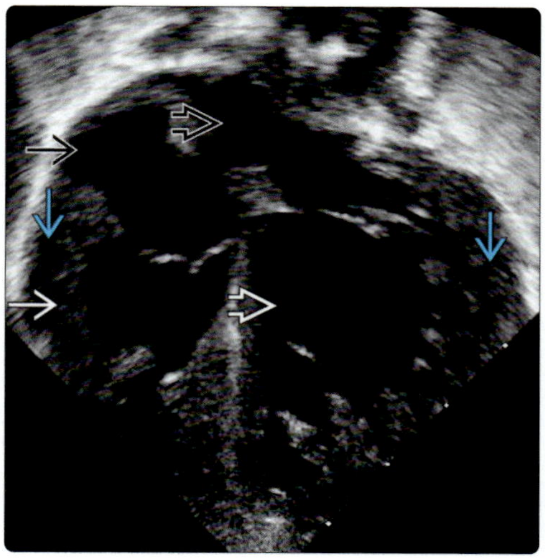

Hypertrophic Cardiomyopathy

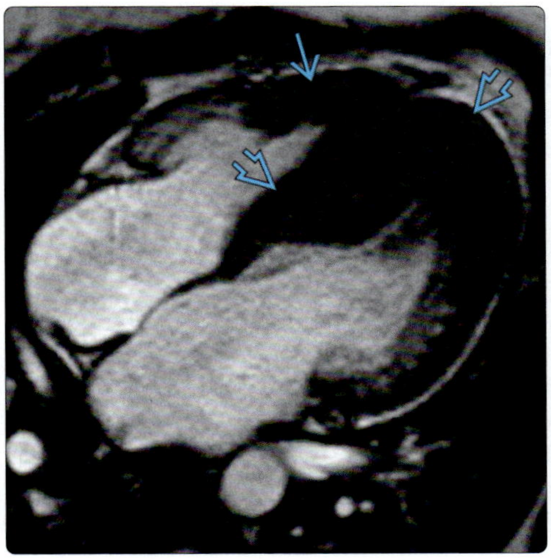

Hypertrophic Cardiomyopathy

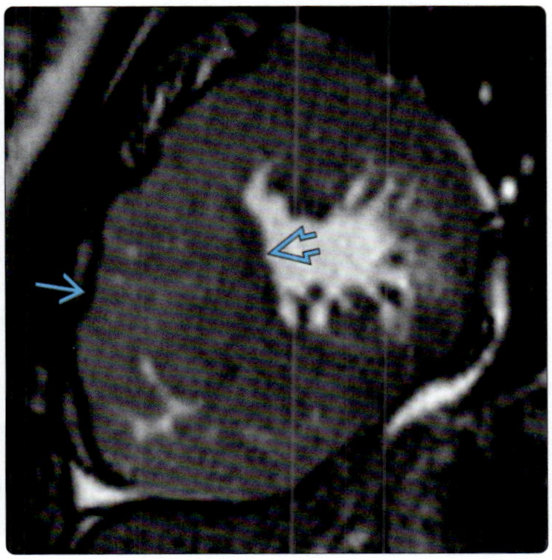

(Left) *Four-chamber SSFP MR in a 16 year old with hypertrophic cardiomyopathy (HCM) shows asymmetric LV hypertrophy of the midseptum & apex. There is also involvement of the RV, which is seen in ~ 30%. Hypertrophy is usually asymmetric in HCM.* **(Right)** *Short-axis SSFP C+ MR in the same patient shows asymmetric hypertrophy of the septal LV & RV. Hypertrophied segments in HCM are characterized by myocyte disarray, do not have normal contraction, & can cause sudden cardiac death.*

Ischemic Cardiomyopathy

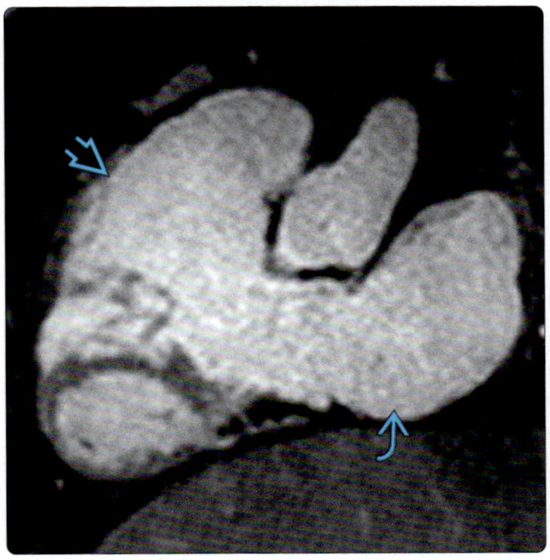

Ischemic Cardiomyopathy

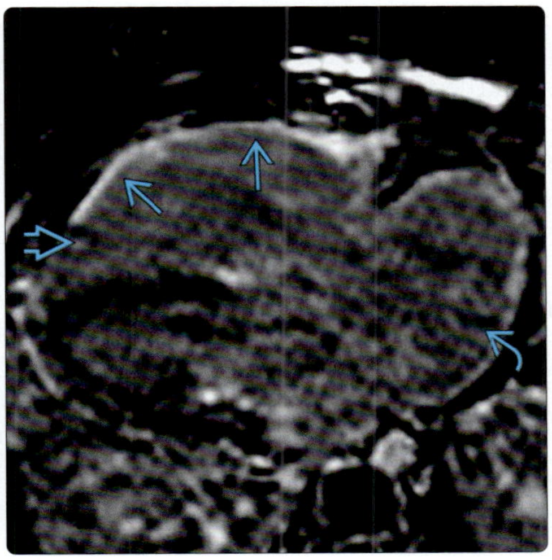

(Left) *Coronal MRA in a 10 year old with dextrocardia, double outlet right ventricle, & complex surgical history, now presenting with heart failure, shows dilation of the RV & RA.* **(Right)** *Axial LGE PSIR MR in the same patient shows the severe RA & RV dilation with extensive RV LGE. Heart failure in CHD is often multifactorial due to a range of myocardial insults accumulated over time, including cyanosis, cardiopulmonary bypass, pressure &/or volume overload, arrhythmia, & ischemia.*

Tricuspid Regurgitation

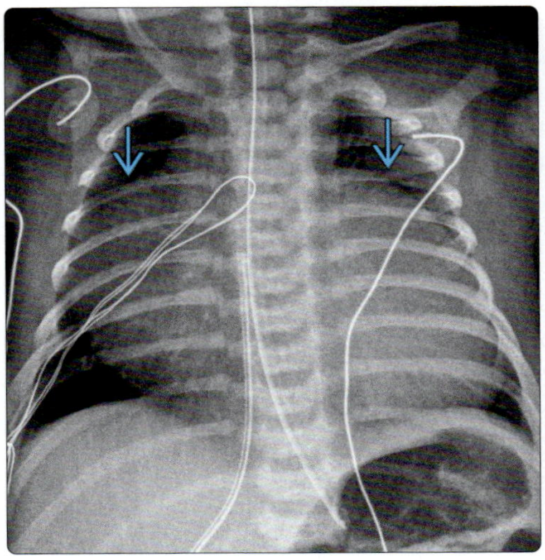

Tricuspid Regurgitation

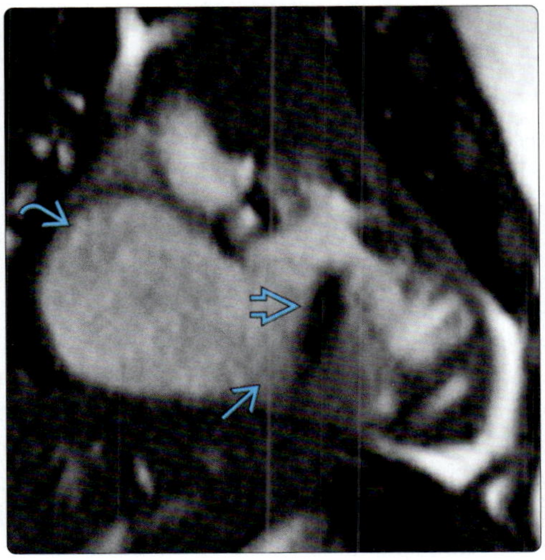

(Left) *AP radiograph in a 1 day old with isolated tricuspid valve dysplasia shows a wall-to-wall heart with squaring of the superior heart borders due to RA & RV outlet dilation. Volume overload of the right heart leads to both RA & RV dilation. Ebstein anomaly more commonly & classically produces this appearance.* **(Right)** *Two-chamber SSFP MR acquired in systole in a 4 month old with Ebstein anomaly shows a dephasing jet from tricuspid regurgitation, which causes dilation of the RA & atrialized RV.*

DIFFERENTIAL DIAGNOSIS

Common

- Tetralogy of Fallot
- Post Repair

Less Common

- Scimitar Syndrome
- Pulmonary Hypoplasia
- Peripheral Pulmonary Artery Stenosis
  - Williams Syndrome
  - Takayasu Arteritis
  - Alagille Syndrome
  - Connective Tissue Disorders
  - Congenital Rubella Syndrome

Rare but Important

- Ductal Origin of Pulmonary Artery

ESSENTIAL INFORMATION

Key Differential Diagnosis Issues

- Consider diffuse vs. focal abnormality
  - Diffusely small pulmonary artery (PA): Usually due to chronically ↓ pulmonary blood flow
    - Termed hypoplasia if congenital
  - Focal stenosis of branch or segmental PAs: Usually from inherited or congenital disease
  - Postoperative PAs can be diffusely small &/or have focal stenosis

Helpful Clues for Common Diagnoses

- **Tetralogy of Fallot**
  - Anterior, superior, & leftward malalignment of outlet septum, causing right ventricular outflow tract obstruction (RVOTO)
  - Results in classic tetrad: 1) RVOTO, 2) RV hypertrophy (RVH), 3) ventricular septal defect (VSD), 4) aorta overriding VSD
    - Main & branch PAs are often underdeveloped & small
  - Boot-shaped heart
    - Leftward rotation of cardiac axis
    - Upturned apex from RVH
    - Concave superior left heart border from small main PA (MPA)
    - Absent left aortic arch contour if right aortic arch is present (25%)
    - Prominent ascending aorta (correlates with pulmonic stenosis)
    - Caution: Vast majority of tetralogy of Fallot (TOF) do not have classic boot shape + other entities can mimic
  - After repair, branch PAs are at risk for persistent hypoplasia or focal stenosis at origins
  - TOF variant: TOF with pulmonary atresia & major aortopulmonary collateral arteries (TOF/PA/MAPCAs), a.k.a. pulmonary atresia with VSD & major aortopulmonary collateral arteries (PA/VSD/MAPCAs)
    - Severe TOF without flow through pulmonary valve
    - Intrapericardial PAs are severely diminutive & may not be confluent
    - Pulmonary circulation is supplied via patent ductus arteriosus (PDA) &/or large congenital collaterals from aorta (MAPCAs)
    - Repair requires "unifocalization" of MAPCAs to hilar branch PAs → at risk for stenosis
- **Post Repair**
  - Postoperative PAs can be diffusely small or have focal stenosis
  - Common examples
    - RV-PA conduits: Branch PAs can be hypoplastic or have focal stenosis at anastomosis
    - Arterial switch with Lecompte maneuver: Left PA often stretched over ascending aorta → can be small
    - Norwood operation: Reconstructed aortic arch can leave very little space for traversing left PA & left mainstem bronchus, either of which can be narrowed
    - Unifocalization or reimplanted PAs: Can have stenosis at sites of anastomosis

Helpful Clues for Less Common Diagnoses

- **Scimitar Syndrome**
  - a.k.a. hypogenetic right lung syndrome or congenital pulmonary venolobar syndrome
  - Variable combination of multiple abnormalities
    - Partial (1/3) or total (2/3) anomalous pulmonary venous connection of right lung
      - Typically connects to inferior vena cava (IVC) or IVC-right atrium (RA) junction
      - Can also connect to left atrium (LA) ("meandering pulmonary vein"), both IVC-RA & LA ("scimitar variant"), or rarely to superior vena cava ("upside-down scimitar syndrome")
      - Obstructed in 20%
      - If unobstructed, gets larger as it descends & collects more blood → looks like Turkish sword (scimitar)
    - Aberrant systemic arterial supply to right lower lung
      - > 70% from upper abdominal aorta
      - Involved lung may have dual arterial supply
    - Hypoplasia or aplasia of 1 or more right lung lobes
      - Lobation, segmentation, & fusion abnormalities
      - Abnormal bronchial branching
    - Right PA may be small or absent
    - Horseshoe or crossover lung
      - Right lower lung extends to left, demarcated by vertical fissure
    - Right hemidiaphragm abnormalities
  - Associated intracardiac defects (25%)
  - Infantile type: Pulmonary hypertension & heart failure
  - Adolescent type: Respiratory symptoms from right lung hypoplasia & airway abnormalities
  - Asymptomatic type: Incidentally seen on radiographs
- **Pulmonary Hypoplasia**
  - Hypoplastic lung, bronchus, & PA
  - Primary type: Congenital spectrum
    - Pulmonary aplasia: Absent lung & PA with rudimentary bronchus
    - Pulmonary agenesis: Absent lung, bronchus, & PA
  - Secondary type: Limitation of normal lung development by extrinsic compression
    - Diaphragmatic hernia, thoracic dystrophy, congenital lung malformations/masses, oligohydramnios

- **Peripheral Pulmonary Artery Stenosis**
  - Various congenital or inherited conditions can manifest with focal PA stenosis
  - Typically at origin of branch, lobar, or segmental PAs ± poststenotic dilation
  - **Williams syndrome**
    - Genetic elastin mutation
    - Numerous phenotypic features, classically: Hypercalcemia, mental retardation, elfin facies, ebullient personality
    - Cardiovascular abnormalities in 80%, mostly arterial stenoses; represent most common cause of death
      - Supravalvar aortic stenosis (most common)
      - Branch or peripheral PA stenosis (2nd most common)
      - Additional arterial stenoses: Aorta, head & neck vessels, coronary arteries, renal arteries
      - Associated arterial wall thickening
    - Systemic stenoses tend to be stable or progress; pulmonary stenosis tend to improve with growth
  - **Takayasu arteritis**
    - Chronic, idiopathic, granulomatous, large vessel vasculitis
      - Predominately of aorta & main branches
      - Less frequently of PAs or coronary arteries
    - Inflammation progresses from adventitia to intima
    - Wall thickening, stenosis (90%), mural thrombus, complete occlusion (30%), aneurysm (15%), & dissection (10%)
    - Childhood Takayasu has high morbidity & mortality
      - Hypertension in over 80% of pediatric patients
      - Diminished pulses with lower limb claudication in 10-35% of children
    - MR for angiography & vessel wall imaging
      - Active inflammation: Wall thickening, edema, & hyperenhancement
  - **Alagille syndrome**
    - Autosomal dominant genetic disorder
    - Variable expressivity of biliary, cardiac, ocular, & musculoskeletal anomalies with characteristic facies
    - Hallmark of disease: Paucity of intrahepatic bile ducts
      - 15-25% require liver transplant
    - Other characteristic major features
      - Peripheral pulmonary stenosis (76%)
      - Butterfly vertebral bodies
      - Ocular posterior embryotoxon
      - May be associated with complex congenital heart disease (CHD)
  - **Connective tissue disorders**
    - While more commonly presenting with vascular dilation, some connective tissue disorders, such as Cutis Laxa or Ehlers-Danlos Syndrome, can have peripheral PA stenosis
  - **Congenital rubella syndrome**
    - Now rare due to vaccination
    - Gestational age at infection determines outcome
      - > 80% risk of congenital defects if acquired in first 12 weeks of pregnancy
    - Cardiac defects: PDA, PA stenosis, PA hypoplasia
    - Classic abnormalities: Cataracts, heart defects, & sensorineural deafness

Helpful Clues for Rare Diagnoses

- **Ductal Origin of Pulmonary Artery**
  - PA arises from ipsilateral ductus arteriosus
  - Affected PA is usually hypoplastic
  - Upon ductal closure, PA becomes isolated
  - In past, has been called unilateral agenesis, absence, or interruption of PA
  - Can be solitary finding or seen with TOF or other CHD
  - Failure to treat may lead to lung hypoplasia, compensatory aortopulmonary collaterals, recurrent lung infections, & thoracic asymmetry with scoliosis

SELECTED REFERENCES

1. Agrawal H et al: Contralateral pulmonary hypertension following resuscitation of unilateral ductal origin of a pulmonary artery: a multi-institutional review. Pediatr Cardiol. 39(1):71-8, 2018
2. Russo RAG et al: Takayasu arteritis. Front Pediatr. 6:265, 2018

Tetralogy of Fallot

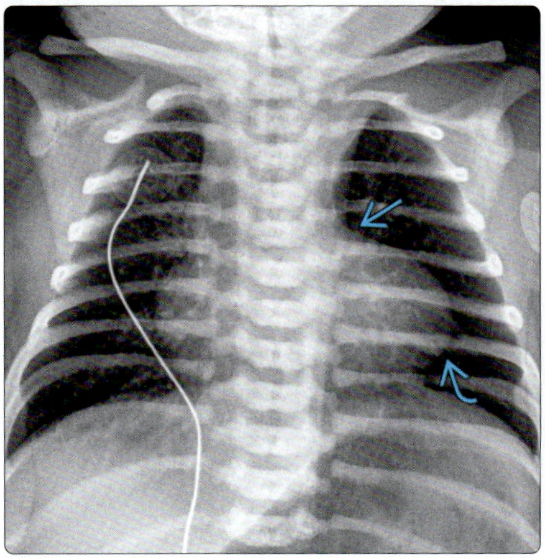

Tetralogy of Fallot

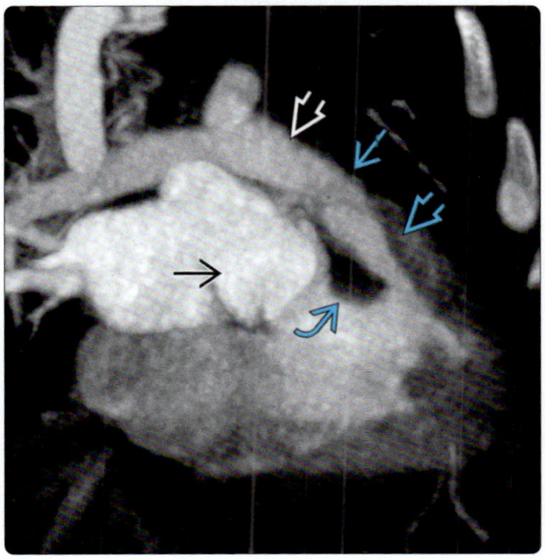

(Left) *AP radiograph in a 3 day old with Tetralogy of Fallot (TOF) shows a boot-shaped heart due to an upturned apex ➚ & small main pulmonary artery (MPA) ➙. There is ↓ pulmonary vascularity.* **(Right)** *Coronal oblique CECT MIP in a 5 month old with TOF shows anterior & superior malalignment of the outlet septum ➚, causing RVOTO with pulmonary valvar stenosis ➙ & subvalvar muscular stenosis ➙. The aorta ➙ is prominent relative to the small MPA ➡. Aortic flow & size are proportional to the stenosis.*

(Left) *Axial oblique CECT MPR in a 3 month old with TOF/PA/MAPCAs shows pulmonary atresia with small confluent main & branch PAs. The PAs in this TOF variant can be nonconfluent.* **(Right)** *Coronal oblique CECT MIP in the same patient shows multiple tortuous MAPCAs arising from the right-sided descending aorta. MAPCAs are highly variable in course & structure, often described as pulmonary "arborization anomalies". Defining the vascular distribution of each MAPCA is necessary prior to surgery.*

Tetralogy of Fallot

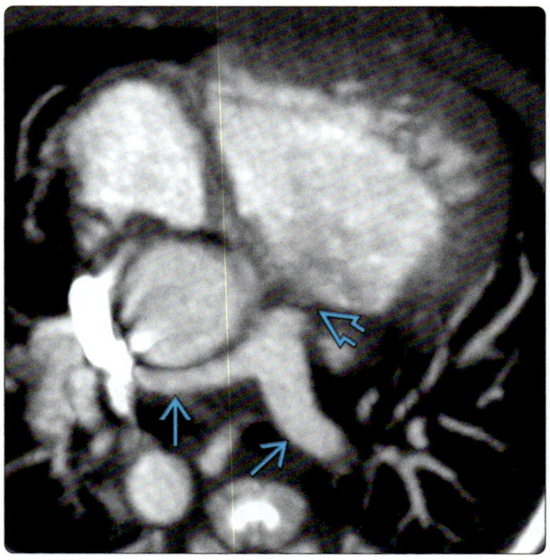

Tetralogy of Fallot

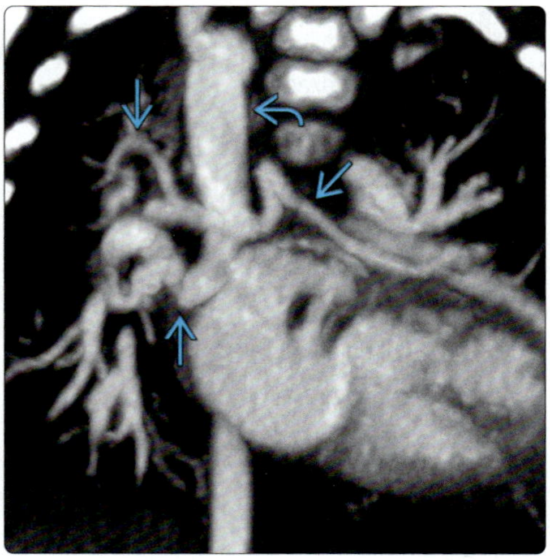

(Left) *Axial oblique MRA MPR in a 15 year old with truncus arteriosus status post repair with an RV-PA conduit shows severe segmental stenosis of the proximal LPA at the anastomosis with the distal conduit. There was also a right arch, which is seen in 30% of truncus arteriosus cases.* **(Right)** *MRA anterior oblique 3D projection in the same patient again shows the severe segmental LPA stenosis. Note the markedly increased blood flow to the right side, which was quantified on MR as 80% of total pulmonary blood flow.*

Post Repair

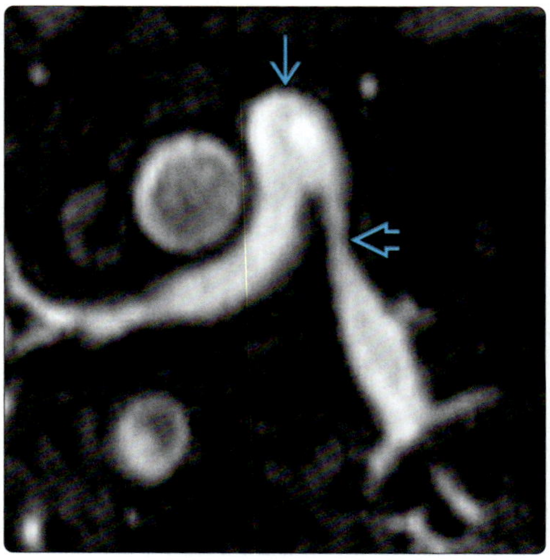

Post Repair

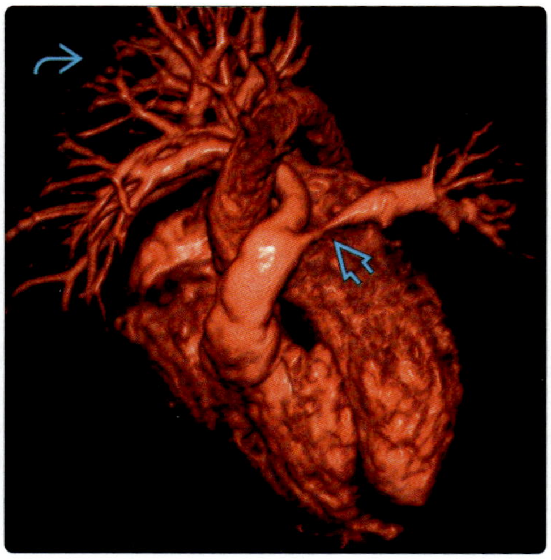

(Left) *Axial oblique MRA MPR in a 14 year old with transposition of the great arteries status post arterial switch operation with the Lecompte maneuver shows AP narrowing of the proximal LPA. The LPA is at risk of narrowing after an arterial switch as it is usually stretched across the aorta to reach its new position.* **(Right)** *Anterior inferior MRA 3D projection in the same patient again shows the LPA narrowing. There was asymmetric pulmonary blood flow with 79% to the right lung & 21% to the left lung.*

Post Repair

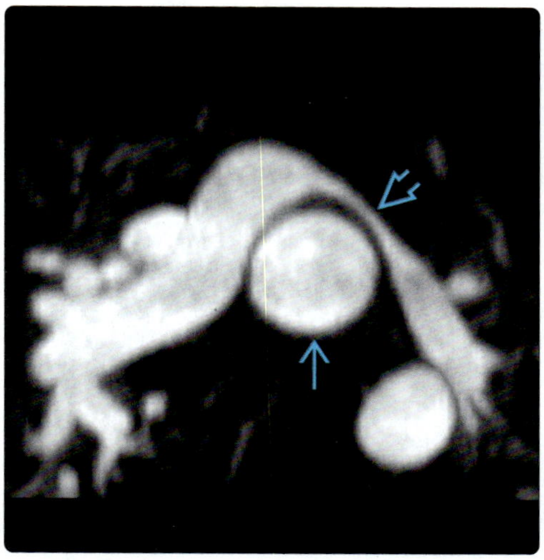

Post Repair

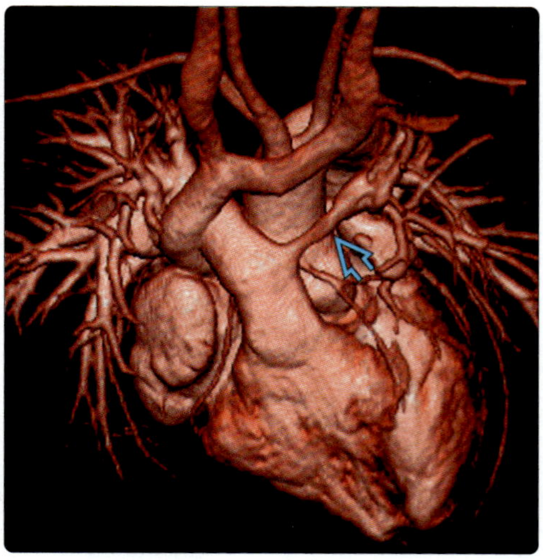

Scimitar Syndrome

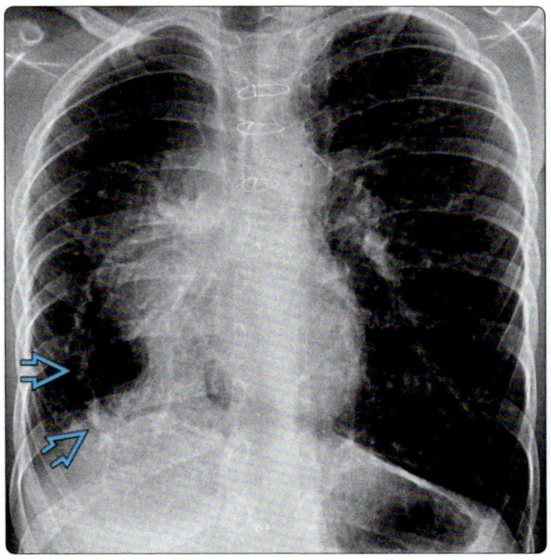

Scimitar Syndrome

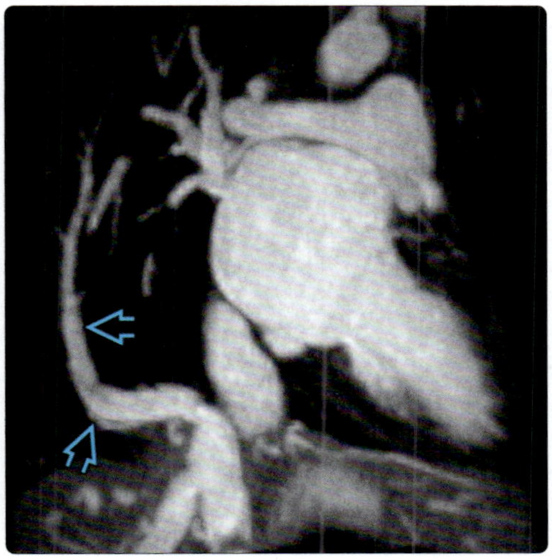

(Left) *PA radiograph in a 9 year old with scimitar syndrome shows a hypoplastic right lung with associated mediastinal shift to the right. There is a prominent vessel descending across the lower right hemithorax, consistent with a scimitar vein.* **(Right)** *Coronal oblique MRA MIP in the same patient again shows the anomalous pulmonary vein draining to the suprahepatic inferior vena cava. Unobstructed scimitar veins grow larger as they descend, giving the appearance of an upside down Turkish sword (scimitar).*

Scimitar Syndrome

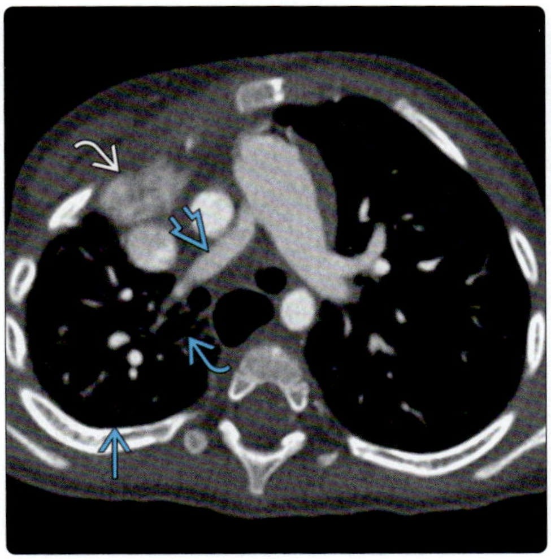

Scimitar Syndrome

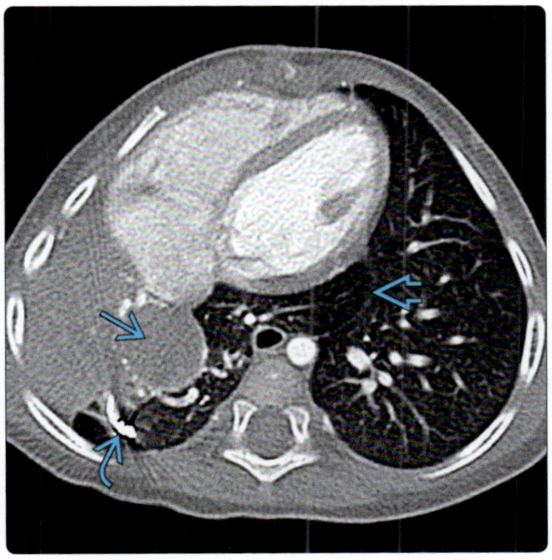

(Left) *Axial CECT in a 20 month old with scimitar syndrome shows a small RPA with a hypoplastic right lung & hemithorax with associated mediastinal shift & a tracheal branching anomaly.* **(Right)** *Axial CECT in the same patient shows a horseshoe or crossover lung along with a focal diaphragmatic anomaly. There are also coils from embolization of an aberrant systemic arterial supply to the lower right lung. Scimitar syndrome is comprised of a variable combination of multiple specific anomalies.*

Scimitar Syndrome

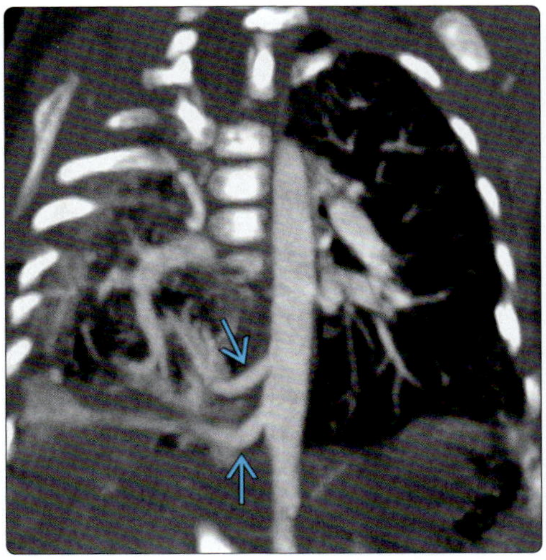

Pulmonary Hypoplasia

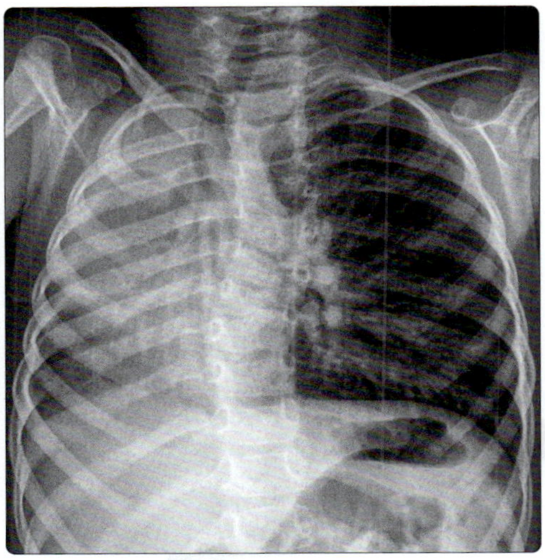

(Left) *Coronal oblique CECT MPR in the same patient at 20 days old shows 2 aberrant arteries providing systemic supply to the lower right lung via the descending aorta.* **(Right)** *PA radiograph in a 6 week old with primary pulmonary hypoplasia shows a small right hemithorax with mediastinal shift & dextroposition of the heart. There are also multiple contiguous mid thoracic vertebral segmentation anomalies with a focal scoliosis.*

(Left) *Axial oblique CECT MIP in the same patient shows a hypoplastic right lung & RPA.* **(Right)** *Coronal oblique CECT minIP in the same patient shows the hypoplastic lung & right main bronchus. Primary pulmonary hypoplasia is defined by a hypoplastic lung, PA, & bronchus. Pulmonary aplasia is an absent lung & PA with rudimentary bronchus. Pulmonary atresia is an absent lung, PA, & bronchus.*

Pulmonary Hypoplasia

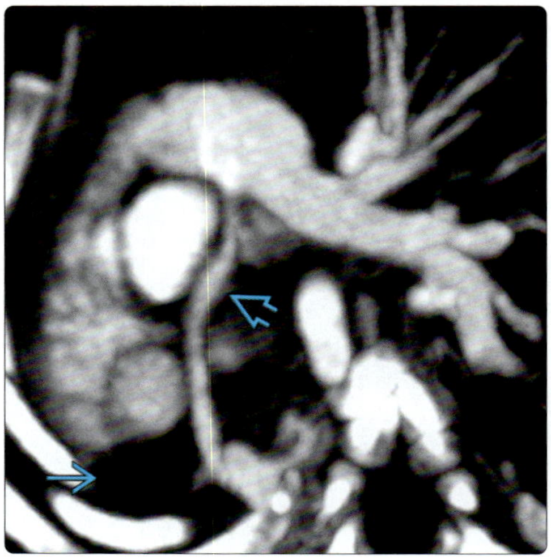

Pulmonary Hypoplasia

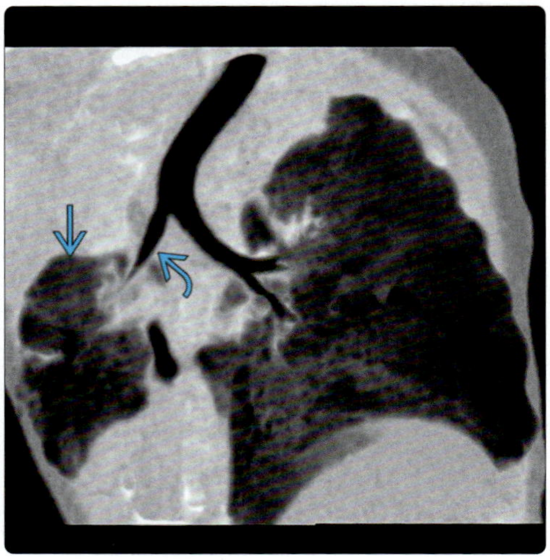

(Left) *Coronal oblique CECT MIP in a 5 month old shows multiple discrete peripheral pulmonary stenoses, common in Williams syndrome.* **(Right)** *Right anterior oblique catheter angiogram with direct injection into the right lower lobe PA in the same patient shows multiple peripheral pulmonary artery stenoses, typical in location at the segmental branch origins, with poststenotic dilation.*

Williams Syndrome

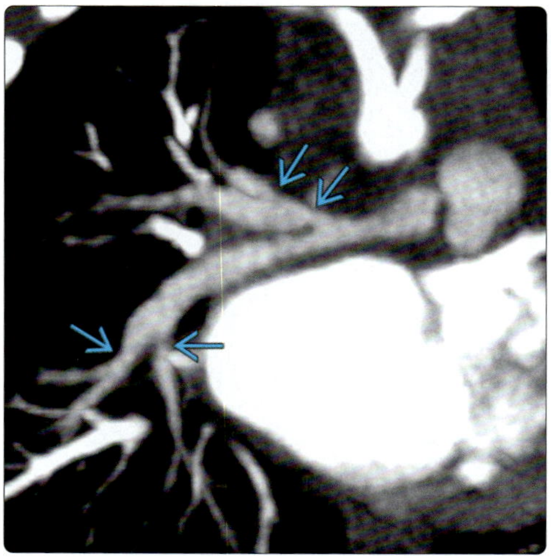

Williams Syndrome

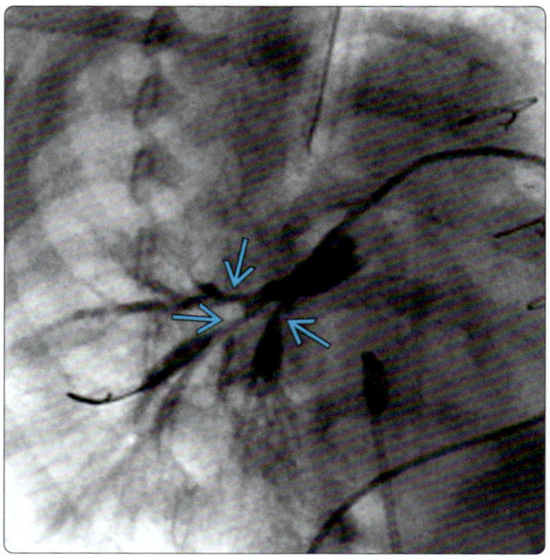

(Left) *Coronal oblique MRA MIP in a 13 year old with Takayasu arteritis shows long-segment narrowing of both common carotid arteries. In addition, there is peripheral pulmonary artery stenosis at branch origins.* **(Right)** *Axial T1 MR in a patient with Takayasu arteritis shows wall thickening of the ascending aorta, descending aorta, & RPA. Takayasu arteritis typically involves the aorta & great vessels but can also affect the PAs. MR can be used to assess for active inflammation of the vessel walls.*

Takayasu Arteritis

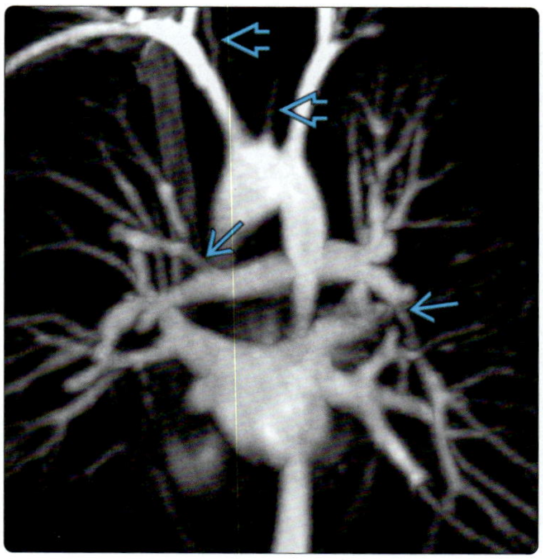

Takayasu Arteritis

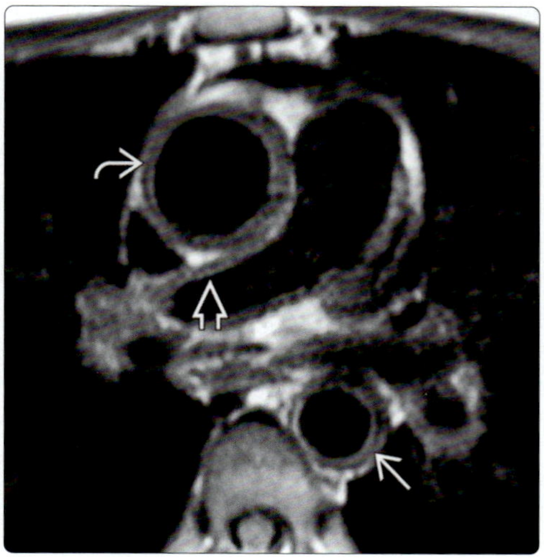

Alagille Syndrome

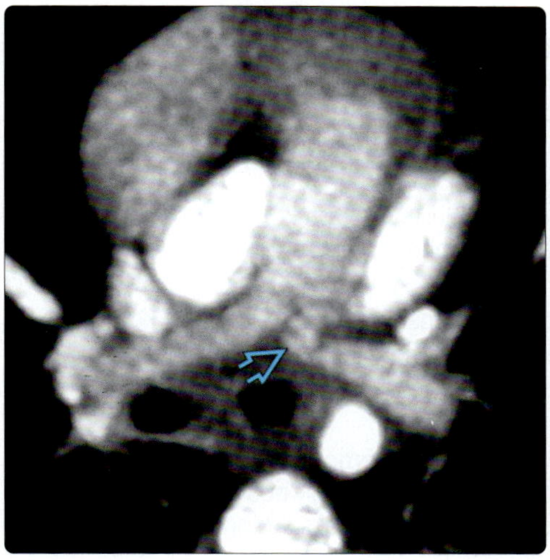

Alagille Syndrome

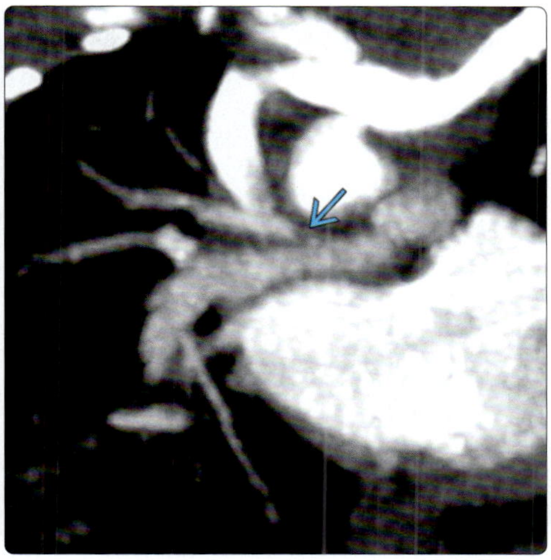

(Left) *Axial CECT in a 5 month old with Alagille syndrome shows a focal kink with narrowing of the proximal LPA ⇨, which is a common appearance of Alagille pulmonary disease on axial images.* **(Right)** *Coronal oblique CECT MPR in the same patient shows focal peripheral pulmonary stenosis at the right upper lobe branch PA ⇨. While the clinical course of Alagille syndrome is driven by the biliary disease, 76% of patients also have peripheral PA stenosis & may require intervention.*

Ductal Origin of Pulmonary Artery

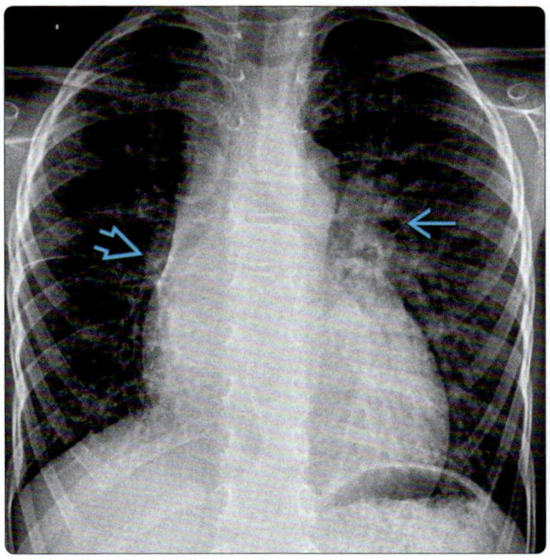

Ductal Origin of Pulmonary Artery

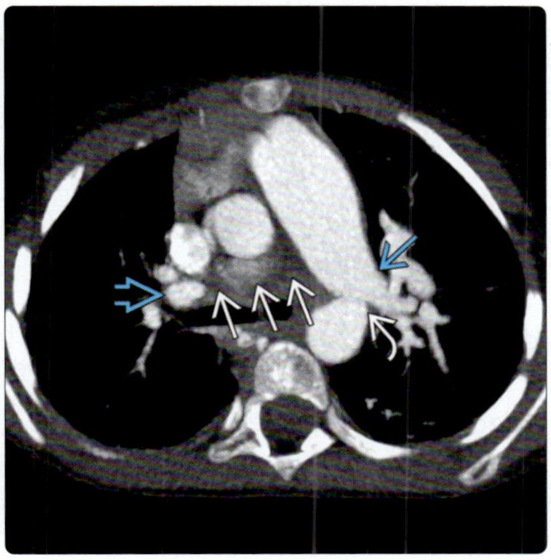

(Left) *PA radiograph in a 4 year old with a ductal origin of the RPA shows a small right lung that has relatively diminished pulmonary vascularity & a small RPA ⇨. The left lung pulmonary vascularity is increased ⇨.* **(Right)** *Axial oblique CECT MIP in the same patient shows a prominent LPA ⇨ with a small hilar RPA ⇨. There is absence of the intrapericardial RPA ➡. Note that the right lung is smaller than the left. There is also partial visualization of a left-sided patent ductus arteriosus (PDA) ➡.*

Ductal Origin of Pulmonary Artery

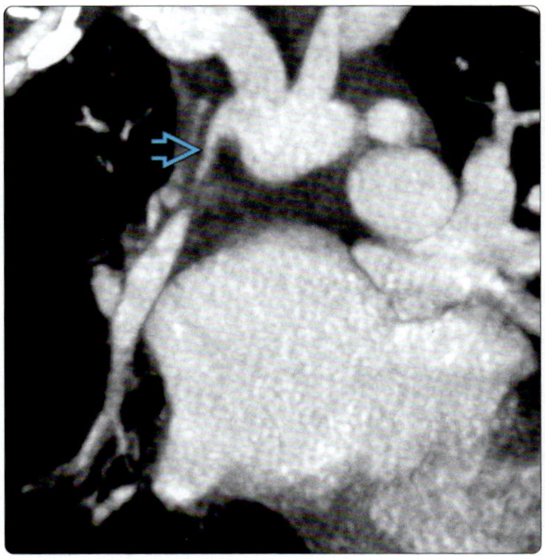

Ductal Origin of Pulmonary Artery

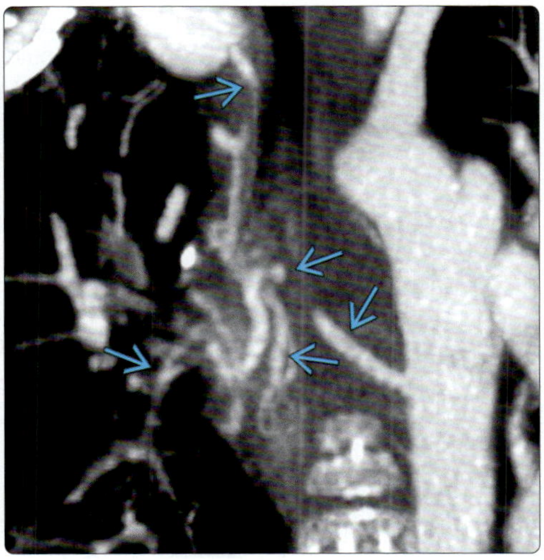

(Left) *Coronal oblique CECT MIP in the same patient shows that the hilar RPA is supplied by a right-sided PDA ⇨, which is severely stenotic.* **(Right)** *Coronal oblique CECT MIP in the same patient shows multiple tortuous aortopulmonary collaterals ⇨ that directly supply the right lung. The ductus supplying the hilar PA can close to a ligamentum & thus will not be visible. As such, this condition has been called unilateral agenesis, absence, or interruption of the PA in the past.*

DIFFERENTIAL DIAGNOSIS

Common

- Left-to-Right Shunts
- Pulmonary Arterial Hypertension

Less Common

- Pulmonary Valve Stenosis
- Pulmonary Thromboembolism

Rare but Important

- Absent Pulmonary Valve
- Mycotic Aneurysm
- Vasculitis
- Connective Tissue Disorder
- Complex Congenital Heart Disease

ESSENTIAL INFORMATION

Key Differential Diagnosis Issues

- Underlying causes
  - Increased &/or turbulent pulmonary blood flow
    - L → R shunts
    - Pulmonary valve stenosis
    - Absent pulmonary valve (APV)
    - Complex congenital heart disease (CHD)
  - Increased pulmonary pressure
    - Pulmonary arterial hypertension
    - Pulmonary thromboembolism
  - Vessel wall disease
    - Mycotic aneurysm
    - Connective tissue disorder
    - Vasculitis

Helpful Clues for Common Diagnoses

- **Left-to-Right Shunts**
  - All cardiac L → R shunts have increased blood flow to pulmonary arteries (PA), causing dilation
  - Radiographs: Characteristic shunt vascularity
    - Cardiomegaly, classically with specific pattern of chamber enlargement
      - Atrial septal defect (ASD): ↑ right atrium (RA), ↑ right ventricle (RV), ↑ ↑ PA
      - Ventricular septal defect (VSD): ↑ left atrium (LA), ↑ left ventricle (LV), ↑ RV, ↑ PA
      - Atrioventricular septal defect (AVSD): ↑ LA, ↑ LV, ↑ ↑ RA, ↑ RV, ↑ ↑ PA
      - Patent ductus arteriosus (PDA): ↑ LA, ↑ LV, ↑ aorta, ↑ PA
    - Enlarged central PA with diffusely increased pulmonary vascularity
      - Can have superimposed pulmonary edema, if severe
    - Air-trapping due to large vessels compressing pliable bronchioles
    - Findings often not appreciable when pulmonary:systemic blood flow ratio (Qp:Qs) is < 2:1
  - Definitive diagnosis by echocardiography
- **Pulmonary Arterial Hypertension**
  - Defined by mean pulmonary arterial pressure > 25 mm Hg at rest & > 30 mm Hg during exercise, with normal PA wedge pressure
  - In pediatrics, consider: Idiopathic, familial, pulmonary venoocclusive disease/pulmonary capillary hemangiomatosis, chronic L → R shunts, chronic pulmonary vein stenosis, prior tumoral therapy, chronic lung disease of prematurity, or other lung disease
  - Increased PA pressure & increased RV pressure → PA enlargement & RV hypertrophy
  - Radiographs
    - Dilated main & hilar PA with vascular pruning & decreased peripheral vascularity
  - CT
    - Consider when main pulmonary artery (MPA):Ao diameter > 1.3 (if no CHD or other explanation)
    - Should see RV hypertrophy
  - MR
    - Phase contrast: Can demonstrate hypertensive flow profile showing early systolic peak with multiple additional plateaus or peaks during deceleration phase of systole
      - If hypertension is unilateral, can show retrograde flow in ipsilateral PA (e.g., in chronic unilateral pulmonary vein stenosis)
    - Cine imaging: Septal flattening in systole is sign of pressure overload

Helpful Clues for Less Common Diagnoses

- **Pulmonary Valve Stenosis**
  - Dysplastic pulmonary valve leaflets with normal-sized pulmonary annulus
  - Can get poststenotic dilation of main PA
  - May eventually have mixed stenosis/regurgitation, either post balloon catheter valvotomy or from progressive valve dysplasia
    - Regurgitation contributes to PA dilation from volume overload
    - Will see RV hypertrophy from stenosis & RV dilation from regurgitation
  - Note: Tetralogy of Fallot (TOF), in contrast, has small pulmonary annulus & (usually) small PA
- **Pulmonary Thromboembolism**
  - PA obstruction from embolism or thrombus
  - Identifiable risk factor in 96-98% of children (unlike adults)
  - Risk factors: Central venous line, malignancy, lupus, renal disease, congenital thrombophilia, surgery, & trauma
    - Central venous lines are most common risk factor in children (80% of cases)
  - 30-60% have deep vein thrombosis
  - Chronic pulmonary embolism → right heart failure & pulmonary arterial hypertension

Helpful Clues for Rare Diagnoses

- **Absent Pulmonary Valve**
  - No functioning pulmonary valve tissue (i.e., either absent or rudimentary) → severe pulmonary regurgitation
  - Increased volume of regurgitant flow back & forth through central PA
  - Aneurysmal main & branch PA may cause bronchial compression
  - Usually occurs as TOF variant ("TOF/APV")
    - Form of TOF with ↑ pulmonary vascularity & possible cardiomegaly (unlike classic TOF with ↓ vascularity)

- Respiratory symptoms predominate over cyanosis
  - Rarely occurs as isolated condition
- **Mycotic Aneurysm**
  - Infection of arterial wall leading to weakening & dilation with possible aneurysm formation
  - PA mycotic aneurysms are strongly associated with CHD
    - Particularly with PDA or indwelling device
    - Consider in CHD with bacteremia & septic emboli
- **Vasculitis**
  - Behçet syndrome & Hughes-Stovin syndrome are rare vasculitides characterized by PA aneurysms
  - More common large & medium vessel vasculitides in children, such as Takayasu arteritis or Kawasaki disease, can rarely affect PA
    - These disorders more commonly lead to stenosis but can also cause dilation or aneurysms
    - Usually with coexistent systemic or coronary involvement
  - MR for angiography & vessel wall imaging
    - Active inflammation: Wall thickening, edema, & hyperenhancement
- **Connective Tissue Disorder**
  - Various connective tissue disorders (CTDs) have cardiovascular manifestations: Marfan, Ehlers-Danlos, Loeys-Dietz, & arterial tortuosity syndromes
  - Marfan & Loeys-Dietz patients eventually get MPA root dilation
    - Rarely rupture, but size correlates with disease severity
- **Complex Congenital Heart Disease**
  - Other complex CHDs can have prominent PA due to any combination of causes
    - Increased blood flow from L → R shunts
    - Regurgitation from incompetent valves or conduits
    - Asymmetric or turbulent flow from stenotic valves or shunts
    - Post PA surgery, especially unifocalization

SELECTED REFERENCES

1. Deri A et al: Educational series in congenital heart disease: echocardiographic assessment of left to right shunts: atrial septal defect, ventricular septal defect, atrioventricular septal defect, patent arterial duct. Echo Res Pract. 5(1):R1-16, 2018
2. Stark VC et al: The pulmonary artery in pediatric patients with Marfan syndrome: an underestimated aspect of the disease. Pediatr Cardiol. 39(6):1194-9, 2018
3. Caro-Domínguez P et al: Pulmonary arterial hypertension in children: diagnosis using ratio of main pulmonary artery to ascending aorta diameter as determined by multi-detector computed tomography. Pediatr Radiol. 46(10):1378-83, 2016
4. Kreibich M et al: Aneurysms of the pulmonary artery. Circulation. 131(3):310-6, 2015
5. Thacker PG et al: Pulmonary embolism in children. AJR Am J Roentgenol. 204(6):1278-88, 2015

Left-to-Right Shunts

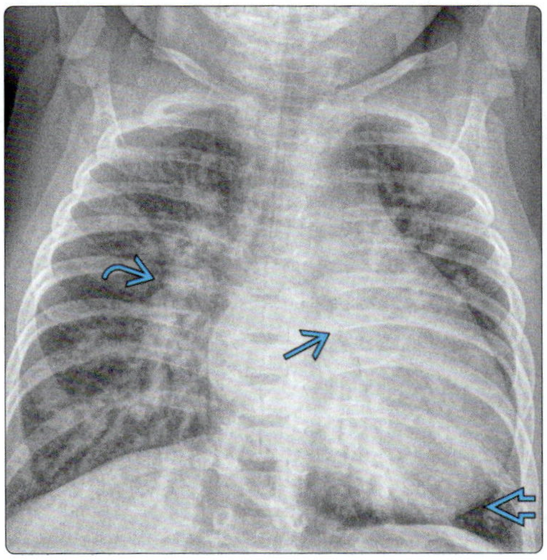

Left-to-Right Shunts

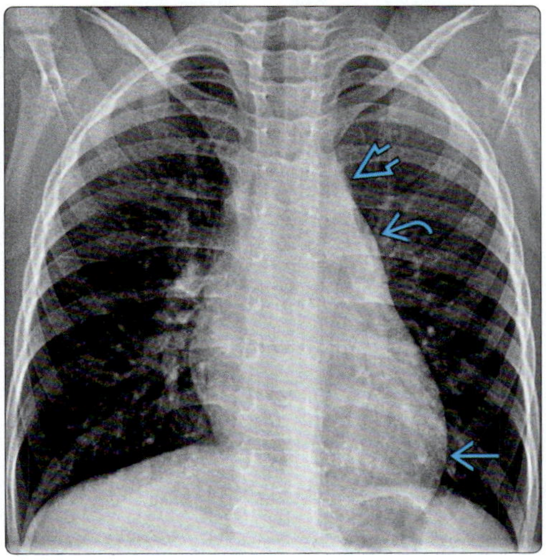

(Left) *PA radiograph in a 4 month old with multiple VSDs shows ventricular enlargement with markedly increased pulmonary vascularity ➡. The left lower lobe bronchus appears attenuated ➡ due to compression by an enlarged heart. There is associated basilar air-trapping ➡.* **(Right)** *PA radiograph in a 3 year old with a PDA shows a prominent MPA ➡ with increased pulmonary vascularity. There is also enlargement of both the LV ➡ & aorta ➡. The aortic dilation suggests a supracardiac shunt.*

(Left) *Axial oblique MRA MPR shows an anomalous right upper pulmonary vein (RUPV) ➡ & a sinus venosus atrial septal defect (ASD) ➡ that allows communication of the RUPV & LA ➡ to the superior vena cava (SVC)-RA junction ➡.* **(Right)** *Coronal oblique MRA MIP in a 5 year old shows anomalous drainage of multiple right PVs ➡ to the SVC ➡. Some join high (true anomalous connections), while others have a near-normal location but drain anomalously through a superior sinus venosus defect. Note the enlarged MPA ➡.*

Left-to-Right Shunts

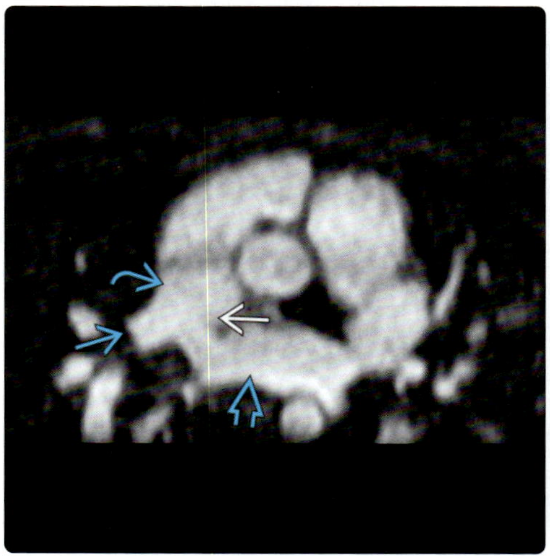

Left-to-Right Shunts

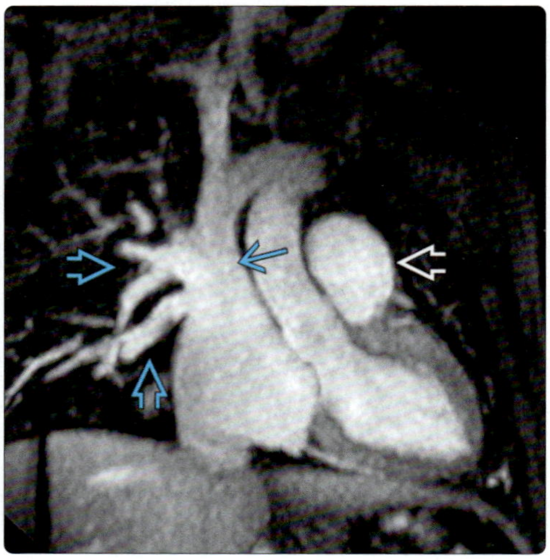

(Left) *PA radiograph in a 10-year-old girl with idiopathic pulmonary hypertension shows a dilated MPA & hilar PAs ➡ with pruning & relatively decreased vascularity peripherally, given the degree of central arterial dilation.* **(Right)** *Axial CECT in the same patient shows a dilated MPA ➡, much larger than the ascending aorta ➡. There is left main bronchus compression ➡. In the absence of congenital heart disease (CHD), an MPA to ascending aorta ratio of > 1.3 raises the possibility of pulmonary hypertension.*

Pulmonary Arterial Hypertension

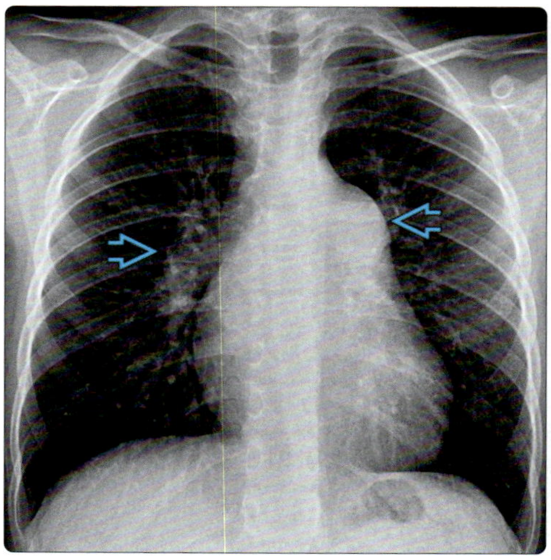

Pulmonary Arterial Hypertension

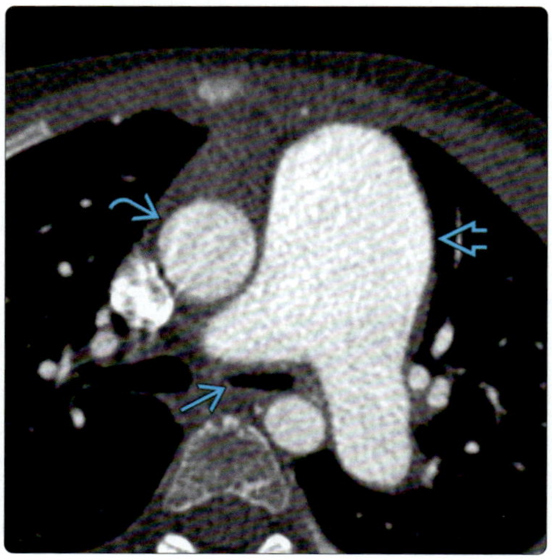

(Left) *Coronal oblique CECT MIP in the same patient shows small branch PAs ➡ & veins ➡ relative to the dilated central PA ➡.* **(Right)** *Axial CECT in the same patient shows right ventricle (RV) hypertrophy ➡ in response to the elevated pulmonary vascular resistance. RV dysfunction & right heart pressure overload can also lead to RA dilation ➡.*

Pulmonary Arterial Hypertension

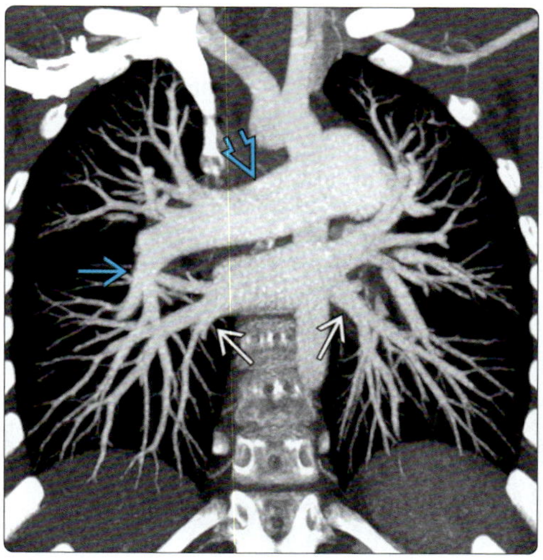

Pulmonary Arterial Hypertension

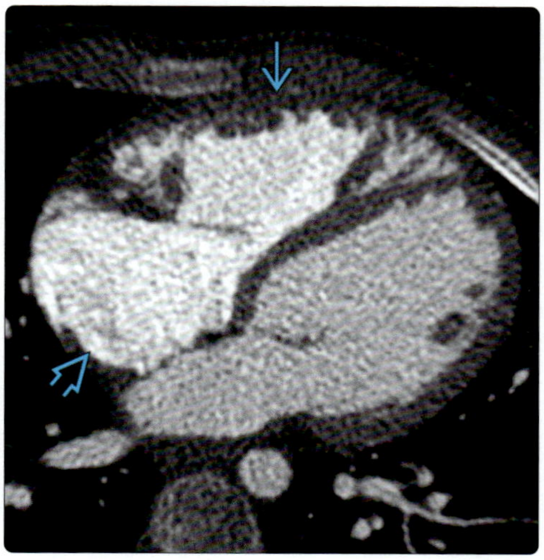

Prominent Pulmonary Artery

Pulmonary Arterial Hypertension

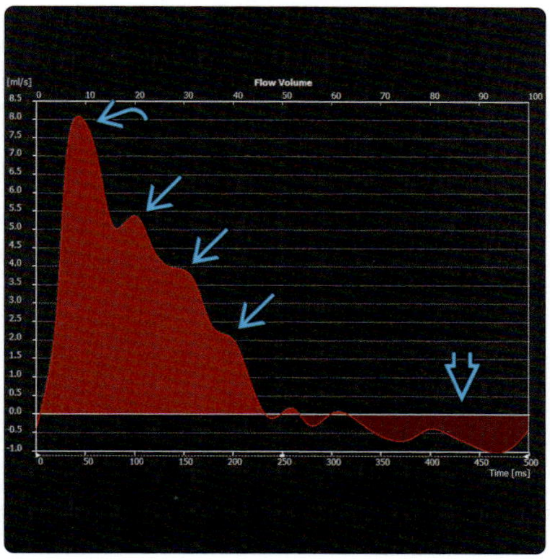

Pulmonary Valve Stenosis

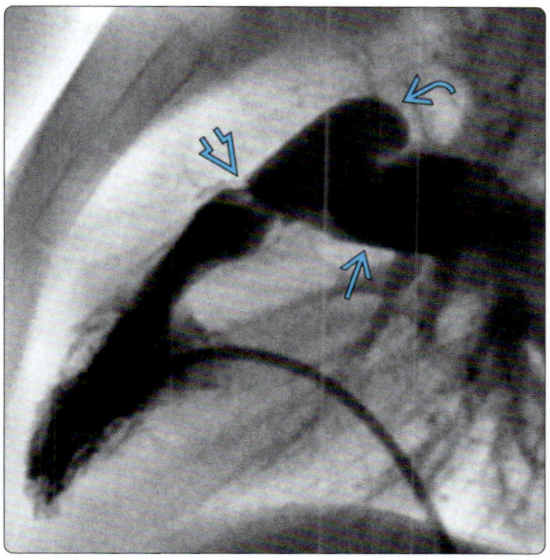

(Left) *MR phase-contrast RPA flow profile in a 4 month old shows a hypertensive waveform with an early sharp but diminished systolic peak & undulations throughout systole & diastole, which is retrograde. The undulations are reflected pressure waves from increased resistance.* **(Right)** *Lateral angiogram in a 20 month old with congenital pulmonary stenosis shows a dysplastic, stenotic pulmonary valve with poststenotic dilation of the PAs & a residual ductal stump.*

Pulmonary Valve Stenosis

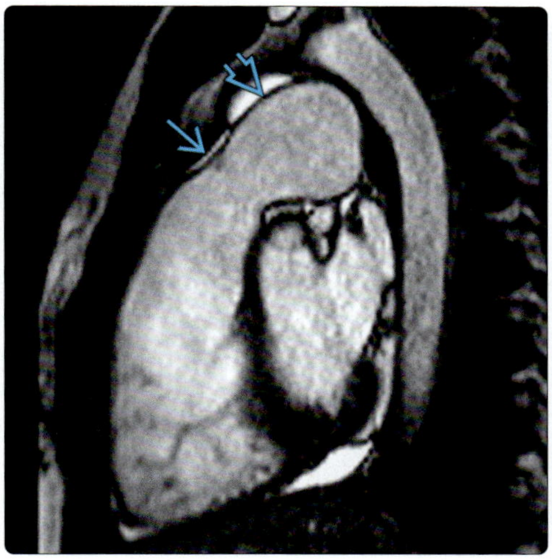

Pulmonary Valve Stenosis

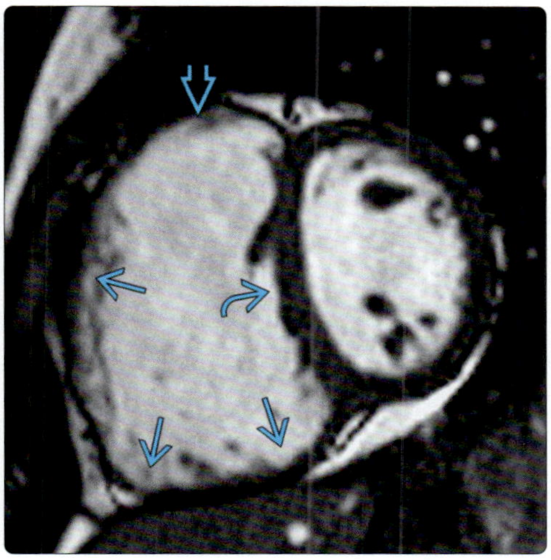

(Left) *RVOT SSFP MR in a 16 year old with pulmonary stenosis status post balloon pulmonary valvuloplasty as an infant (with residual mixed pulmonary stenosis/regurgitation) shows a prominent MPA with mild stenosis at the pulmonary valve.* **(Right)** *Short-axis SSFP MR in the same patient shows moderate RV dilation with mild hypertrophy. Septal flattening in diastole suggests volume overload. In most patients after balloon valvuloplasty, regurgitation dominates the clinical picture.*

Pulmonary Thromboembolism

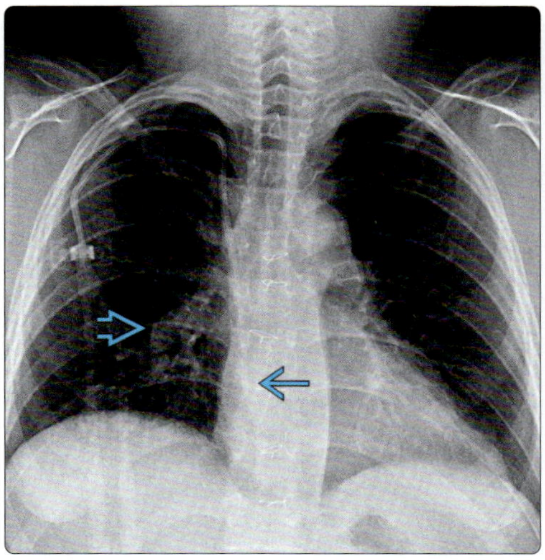

Pulmonary Thromboembolism

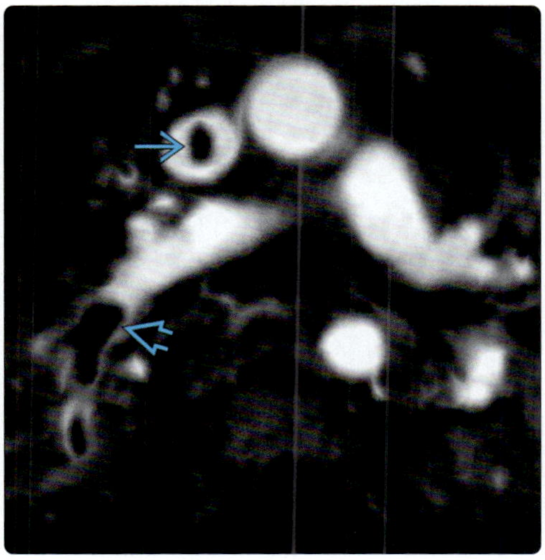

(Left) *PA radiograph, obtained for tachycardia in a 14-year-old female patient with a complex history, shows a right central venous catheter with its tip in the RA. There is also dilation of the right lower lobe branch PA, suspicious for pulmonary embolism (PE).* **(Right)** *Axial oblique MRA minIP in the same patient shows pericatheter thrombus & a branching pulmonary embolus with focal distension of the PA. Approximately 80% of PEs in children are from central venous lines.*

Absent Pulmonary Valve

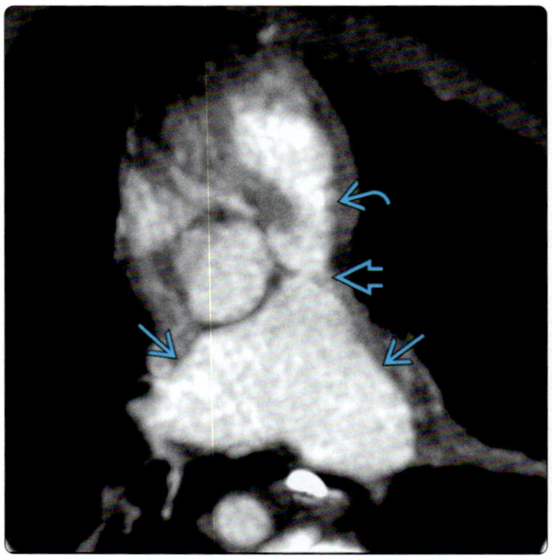

Absent Pulmonary Valve

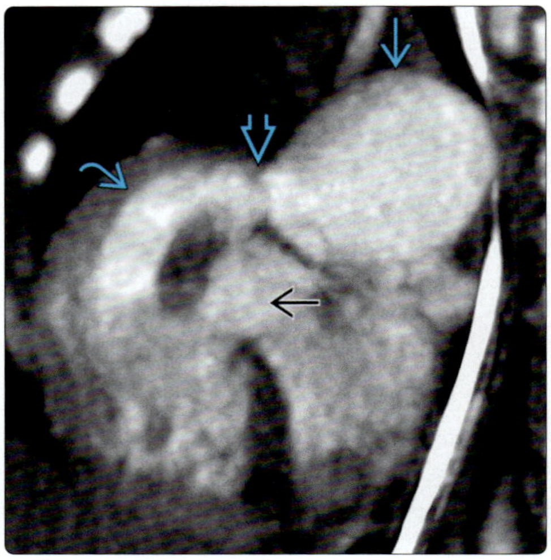

(Left) *Axial oblique CECT MPR in an 18 day old with TOF & an APV shows incompetent rudimentary pulmonary valvar leaflets → that allow free regurgitation, resulting in aneurysmal dilation of the MPA & branch PAs →. There is also subvalvar muscular RVOT obstruction →.* **(Right)** *Sagittal CECT MPR in the same patient again shows the rudimentary valvar tissue →, dilated MPA →, & RVOT obstruction →. The perimembranous VSD is also evident →. TOF/APV is a form of TOF with enlarged central pulmonary vasculature.*

Mycotic Aneurysm

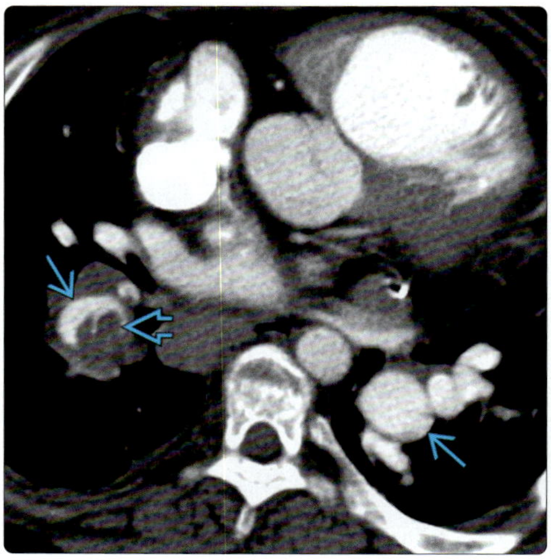

Mycotic Aneurysm

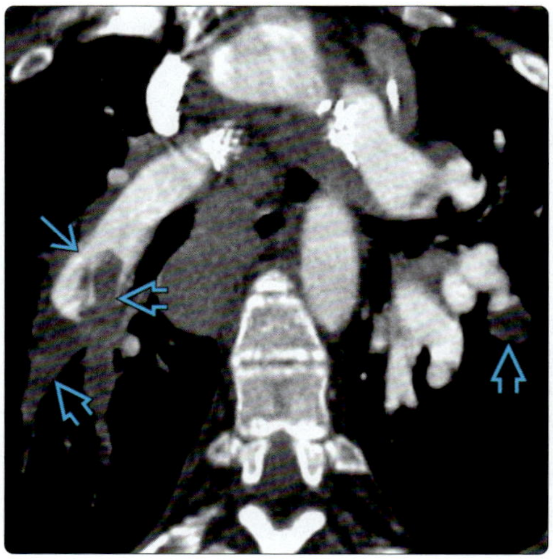

(Left) *Axial oblique CECT MPR in a 14 year old with TOF status post repair complicated by aspergillus pulmonary valve endocarditis shows septic thromboembolism → & mycotic aneurysm → formation of the bilateral PAs.* **(Right)** *Coronal oblique CECT MPR in the same patient shows septic thromboemboli → with a mycotic aneurysm →. Subsequent exams after treatment showed resolution of the emboli with persistent multifocal aneurysms of the PAs. CHD with indwelling devices, such as mechanical valves, are at risk of infection.*

Vasculitis

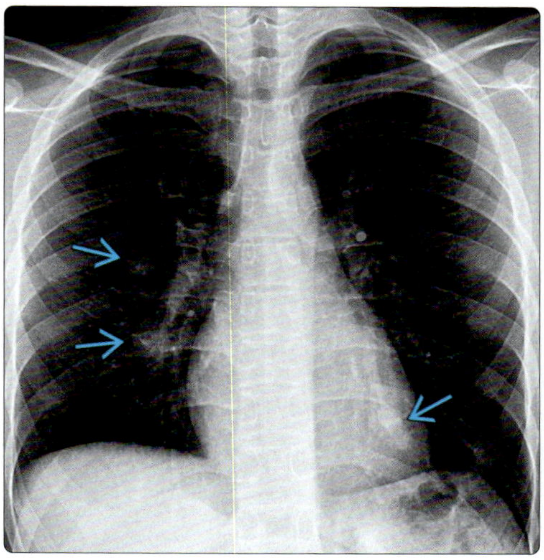

Vasculitis

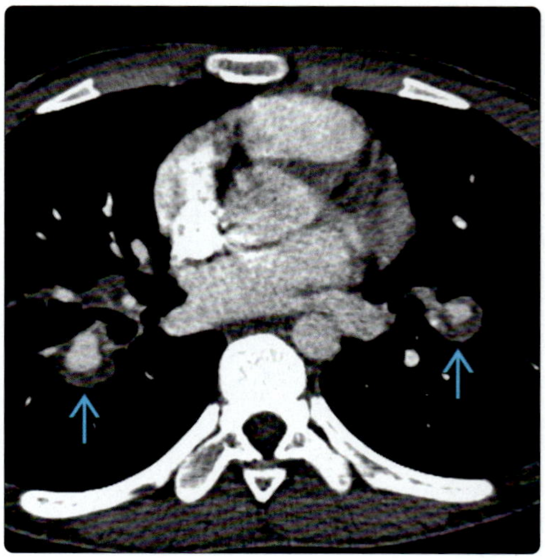

(Left) *PA radiograph in a 17 year old with Hughes-Stovin syndrome shows multiple PA aneurysms →.* **(Right)** *Axial oblique CECT MPR in the same patient shows 2 of the PA aneurysms → with associated vessel wall thickening &/or mural thrombus. Hughes-Stovin syndrome is a variant of Behçet syndrome, & both are rare vasculitides characterized by PA aneurysms.*

Vasculitis

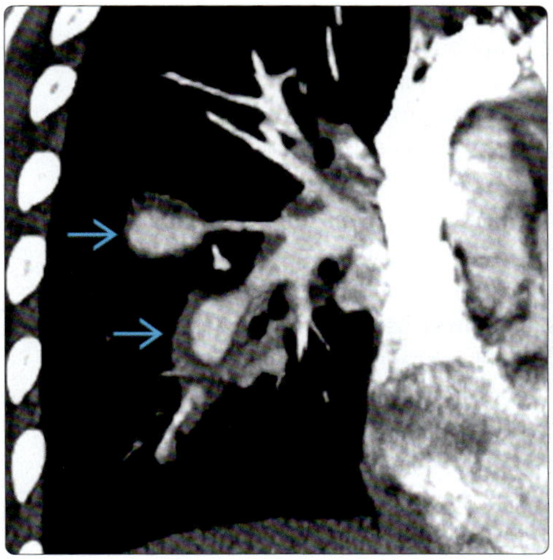

Vasculitis

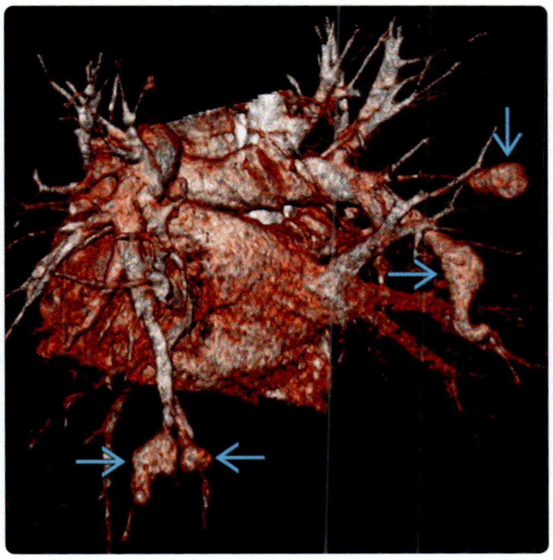

(Left) *Coronal oblique CECT MPR in the same patient again shows multifocal PA aneurysms ➡ with wall thickening &/or mural thrombus. MR can better assess wall thickening & active inflammation in vasculitis.* **(Right)** *Posterior oblique CECT 3D projection in the same patient again shows multifocal PA aneurysms ➡. Mycotic aneurysms would be in the differential if there was not an underlying diagnosis of Hughes-Stovin syndrome.*

Connective Tissue Disorder

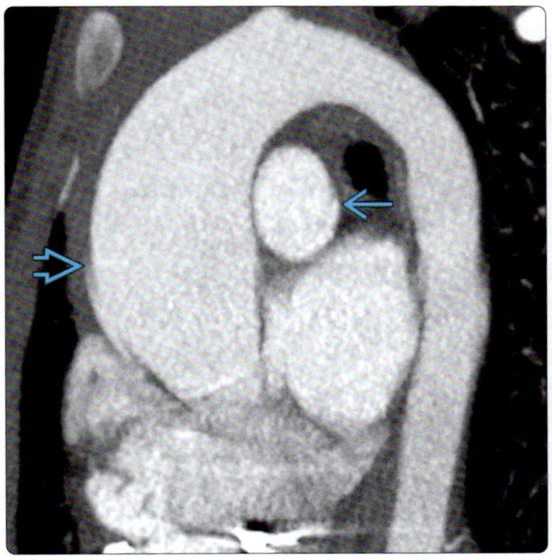

Connective Tissue Disorder

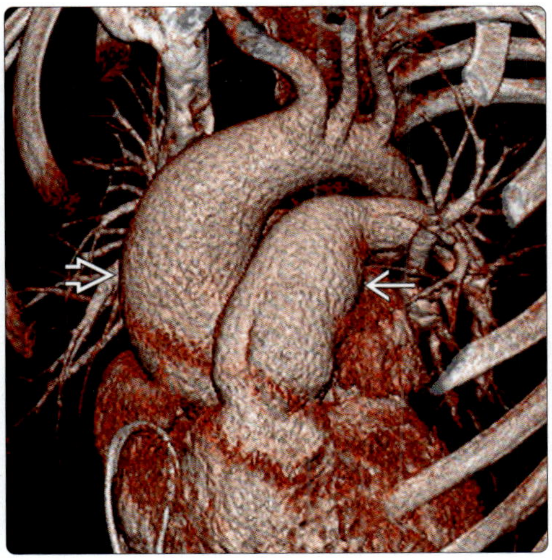

(Left) *Sagittal oblique CECT MIP in a 6 year old with Marfan syndrome shows marked dilation of the ascending aorta & aortic root ⇨ with effacement of the sinotubular junction. The right PA is also enlarged ➡.* **(Right)** *Anterior oblique CECT 3D projection in the same patient shows the dilated ascending aorta & aortic root ⇨ along with mild dilation of the MPA ➡. Despite dilation, the PA involvement rarely leads to dissection or rupture.*

Complex Congenital Heart Disease

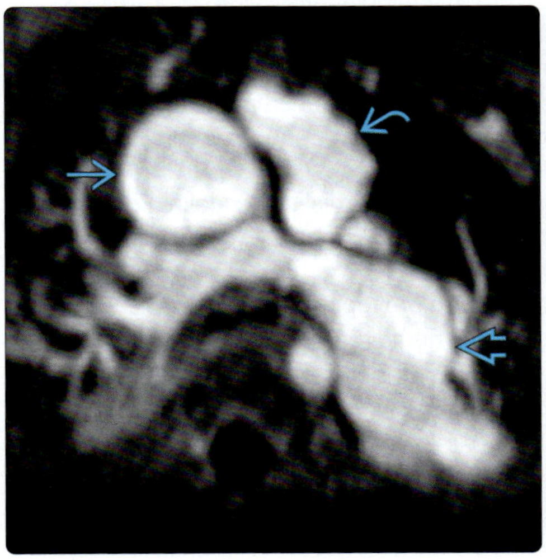

Complex Congenital Heart Disease

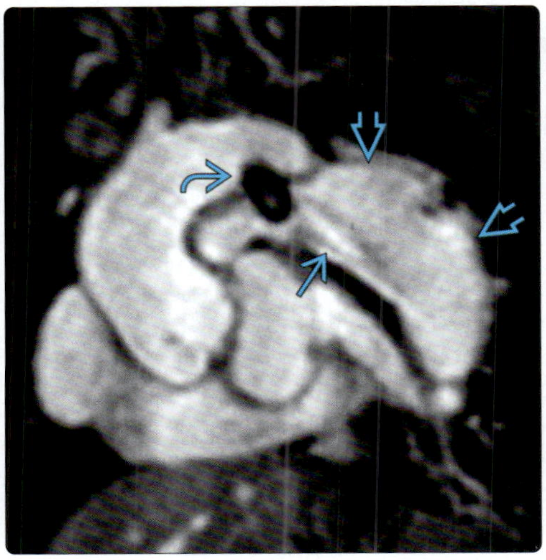

(Left) *Axial oblique MRA MIP in a 6 month old with pulmonary atresia & VSDs status post PDA stenting shows asymmetric aneurysmal dilation of the left PA ⇨. The aorta ➡ & a prominent left atrial appendage ↪ are also labeled.* **(Right)** *Coronal oblique MRA MIP in the same patient shows the dilated left PA ⇨. There is a turbulent flow jet ➡ directed from the PDA stent ↪ toward the left PA. The turbulent flow & increased L → R flow are likely responsible for the dilation.*

DIFFERENTIAL DIAGNOSIS

Common

- Left-to-Right Shunts With Intact Atrial Septum
  - Ventricular Septal Defect
  - Patent Ductus Arteriosus

Less Common

- Left Ventricular Failure
  - Dilated Cardiomyopathy
  - Hypertrophic Cardiomyopathy
  - Ischemic Cardiomyopathy
  - Restrictive Cardiomyopathy
- Left Ventricular Hypertension
  - Severe Aortic Stenosis
  - Severe Systemic Hypertension

Rare but Important

- Mitral Valve Stenosis
- Mitral Valve Regurgitation

ESSENTIAL INFORMATION

Key Differential Diagnosis Issues

- Atria dilate in response to volume or pressure
- 4 main causes
  - L → R shunts with intact atrial septum
  - Left ventricular (LV) failure
  - LV hypertension
  - Mitral valve disease
- Chest radiographic signs
  - Frontal: Splaying of carina (> 90°)
  - Frontal: Double density below carina
  - Frontal: Loss of flattened left atrial (LA) appendage segment between pulmonary arteries (PAs) & LV
  - Lateral: Posterior heart border extends beyond plane of trachea & reaches vertebral bodies
  - Lateral: Posterosuperior deviation of left main bronchus
  - Both: Posterolateral deviation of esophagus (R > L)
- LA morphology, size, & function are emerging as potential imaging biomarkers for various diseases

Helpful Clues for Common Diagnoses

- **Left-to-Right Shunts With Intact Atrial Septum**
  - LA dilation in L → R shunt implies intact atrial septum with level of shunt at ventricles or beyond [e.g., ventricular septal defect (VSD), patent ductus arteriosus (PDA), anteroposterior (AP) window, ruptured aortic sinus, coronary fistula]
    - ↑ pulmonary return leads to LA dilation
    - If there is interatrial communication [such as atrial septal defect (ASD)], LA is decompressed & not enlarged (but get RA dilation)
  - On radiographs, L → R shunts will also have ↑ pulmonary vascularity & air-trapping
  - **Ventricular septal defect**
    - Chamber enlargement: LA, right ventricle (RV), PA
    - Most common congenital heart disease (CHD) in children (~ 50% of children with CHD); isolated defect in 20%
    - Classified based on location from perspective of RV (various systems proposed): Perimembranous & muscular types are most common
    - Perimembranous VSD: 70-80% of VSDs
      - □ Defect in membranous septum & adjacent muscular septum, defined by tricuspid-mitral-aortic fibrous valvular continuity through defect
    - Muscular VSD
      - □ Completely surrounded by ventricular myocardium
      - □ Often close spontaneously when small
    - Holosystolic murmur on auscultation
  - **Patent ductus arteriosus**
    - Chamber enlargement: LA, LV, & ascending aorta
    - Ductus arteriosus connects proximal descending aorta to PA (typically proximal left PA)
    - Normally closes soon after birth (oxygen mediated)
    - Main risk is prematurity, especially with concurrent respiratory distress & hypoxia
      - □ Premature ductal tissue is less sensitive to oxygen-mediated constriction
      - □ 65% of infants born < 28-weeks gestation have PDA
      - □ Prevalence > 80% in premature infants with significant lung disease
    - Most cases are sporadic
    - Untreated may lead to pulmonary hypertension
    - Continuous machinery murmur at upper left sternal border

Helpful Clues for Less Common Diagnoses

- **Left Ventricular Failure**
  - Common causes of heart failure: CHD, viral myocarditis, cardiomyopathy
  - Any cause of chronic LV failure can lead to secondary left atrial enlargement
  - Radiograph: Also see LV dilation along with pulmonary venous hypertension or edema
    - Global cardiomegaly when severe
  - **Dilated cardiomyopathy**
    - Ventricular dilation with poor function
    - Most common etiologies: Prior viral myocarditis & genetic mutations, although specific etiology often cannot be confirmed (so labeled idiopathic)
      - □ Main question is often inflammatory dilated cardiomyopathy (DCM) (prior viral myocarditis) vs. noninflammatory DCM
    - MR: Diffuse mid myocardial late gadolinium enhancement (LGE) is classic but rarely seen in children
  - **Hypertrophic cardiomyopathy**
    - Most common hereditary cardiac disorder
    - Usually presents in adolescence or later
    - Asymmetric ventricular hypertrophy > 15 mm, typically of basal septum
    - LA dilation is multifactorial
      - □ LV dysfunction
      - □ Dynamic LV outflow tract (LVOT) obstruction from asymmetric septal hypertrophy &/or systolic anterior motion of mitral valve (SAM)
      - □ Mitral regurgitation if there is SAM

- MR: Can see patchy midwall LGE with predilection for RV insertion points
- Risk of sudden cardiac death
- **Ischemic cardiomyopathy**
  - Myocardial ischemia can lead to LV failure & left heart dilation
  - Common causes in children
    - Anomalous origin of left coronary artery from PA (ALCAPA)
    - Kawasaki disease → coronary artery aneurysms
- **Restrictive cardiomyopathy**
  - Restrictive ventricular diastolic filling with normal systolic function
  - Usually idiopathic, but any condition that can cause diffuse infiltration/deposition or fibrosis of myocardium can lead to restrictive cardiomyopathy
  - Biventricular failure with normal or reduced ventricular sizes (by definition)
  - Biatrial dilation is characteristic
  - Imaging may be similar to constrictive pericarditis, except without pericardial thickening (> 4 mm)

- **Left Ventricular Hypertension**
  - LV contraction against obstruction or equivalent physiology leads to increased LV pressure
  - Myocardium hypertrophies in response
  - When severe, impairs diastolic filling, leading to secondary LA dilation
  - Common causes: Severe aortic stenosis, severe systemic hypertension, aortic coarctation, hypertrophic cardiomyopathy with dynamic outflow obstruction
  - **Severe aortic stenosis**
    - Valvar (80%), subaortic (10-20%), or supravalvar (< 5%)
    - Valvar aortic stenosis in children is usually congenital with annular hypoplasia or abnormal cusp development
      - Most common is bicuspid aortic valve
    - Radiograph: Look for ascending aortic dilation, which may be due to combination of poststenotic dilation & intrinsic aortopathy
  - **Severe systemic hypertension**
    - Increasing prevalence of primary hypertension in pediatrics
      - Association with obesity & high salt intake
    - LV hypertrophy is finding of end-organ damage
      - Can be seen in up to 41% of children with hypertension
    - Secondary hypertension due to underlying disorder is more likely in younger children
      - Infants: Aortic coarctation, renal thrombosis or anomaly, chronic lung disease
      - Children: Renal parenchymal disease, renovascular disease/stenosis, endocrine disorders, tumors

Helpful Clues for Rare Diagnoses

- **Mitral Valve Stenosis**
  - Various congenital types of mitral valve stenosis
    - Typical type: 2 distinct papillary muscles, underdeveloped & closely spaced
    - Parachute mitral valve: All chordae tendineae connect to single papillary muscle
    - Mitral arcade: Elongated papillary muscles connect to anterior mitral leaflet (directly or via short chords)
  - Acquired stenosis from rheumatic heart disease (rare in developed countries)
  - Radiographs: LA enlargement with pulmonary venous hypertension or edema
- **Mitral Valve Regurgitation**
  - Systolic retrograde flow from LV to LA
  - Causes: Congenital, ischemia, traumatic rupture, endocarditis, rheumatic disease
  - Left heart volume overload leads to LA & LV enlargement

SELECTED REFERENCES

1. Norrish G et al: Risk factors for sudden cardiac death in childhood hypertrophic cardiomyopathy: a systematic review and meta-analysis. Eur J Prev Cardiol. 24(11):1220-30, 2017
2. Etesami M et al: Utility of late gadolinium enhancement in pediatric cardiac MRI. Pediatr Radiol. 46(8):1096-113, 2016
3. Maher KO et al: Aortic and mitral valve disease and left ventricular dysfunction in children. Pediatr Crit Care Med. 17(8 Suppl 1):S131-9, 2016

Ventricular Septal Defect

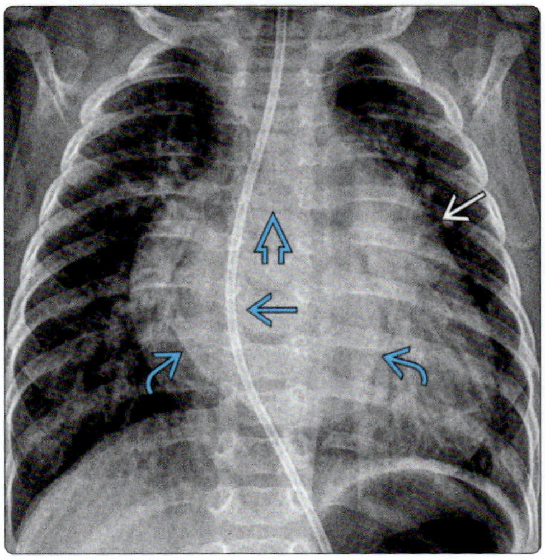

Ventricular Septal Defect

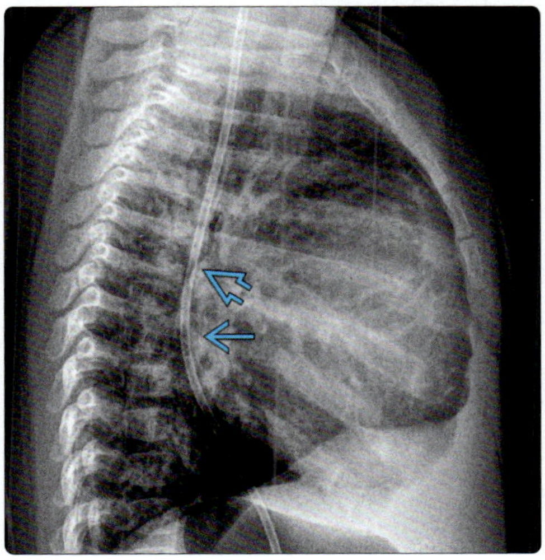

(Left) *PA radiograph in a 5 month old with a moderate VSD along with moderate mitral stenosis & regurgitation shows cardiomegaly with signs of LA enlargement, including splaying of the carina ➡, a double density ➡, deviation of the esophagus ➡, & loss of flattening between the PA & LV ➡. There is also increased pulmonary vascularity with superimposed pulmonary edema.* **(Right)** *Lateral radiograph in the same patient again shows LA enlargement with deviation of the left main bronchus ➡ & esophagus ➡.*

(Left) *PA radiograph in a 5 year old shows cardiomegaly with splaying of the carina →, consistent with LA dilation. Combined with normal pulmonary vascularity & mild central interstitial edema, these findings suggest left heart failure.* **(Right)** *Four-chamber SSFP MR in the same patient shows LA & LV dilation, along with a dephasing jet → from mitral regurgitation. The coronary arteries were normal, while T2 mapping indicated diffuse myocardial edema (not shown), consistent with DCM secondary to myocarditis.*

Dilated Cardiomyopathy

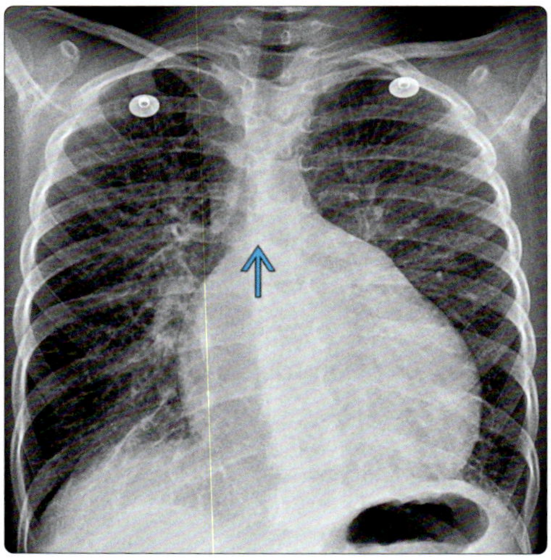

Dilated Cardiomyopathy

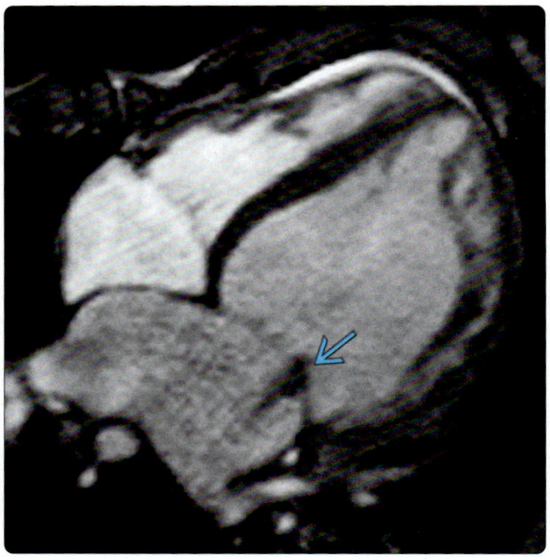

(Left) *Four-chamber SSFP MR in a 16 year old with HCM shows asymmetric septal → & apical hypertrophy of both the LV → & RV →. There is also LA dilation.* **(Right)** *Three-chamber SSFP C+ MR in systole shows dynamic LVOT obstruction from both septal hypertrophy → & systolic anterior motion of the mitral valve →. SAM allows for mitral regurgitation &, when combined with diastolic dysfunction from hypertrophy, leads to LA dilation. Note the patchy myocardial enhancement →, typical of HCM.*

Hypertrophic Cardiomyopathy

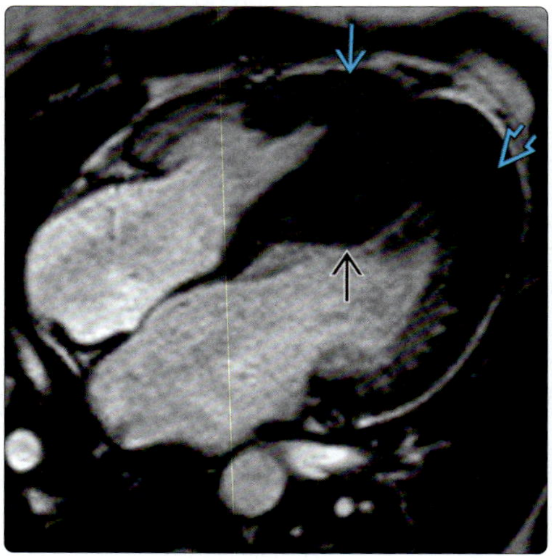

Hypertrophic Cardiomyopathy

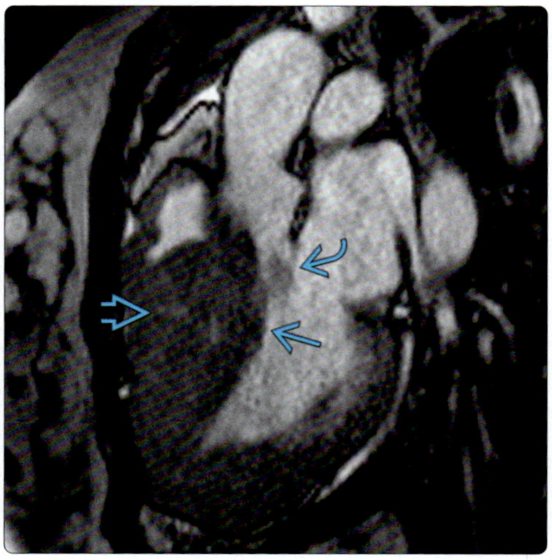

(Left) *PA radiograph in a 4 week old shows cardiomegaly & mild venous congestion. The differential for this appearance in an infant includes ALCAPA, DCM, myocarditis, or mitral regurgitation. Echocardiography revealed ALCAPA with LA & LV dilation & severely reduced function (not shown).* **(Right)** *Axial-oblique CECT MPR shows the left coronary artery → arising from the main pulmonary artery → (ALCAPA). There is also LA dilation → due to coronary steal with ischemic cardiomyopathy.*

Ischemic Cardiomyopathy

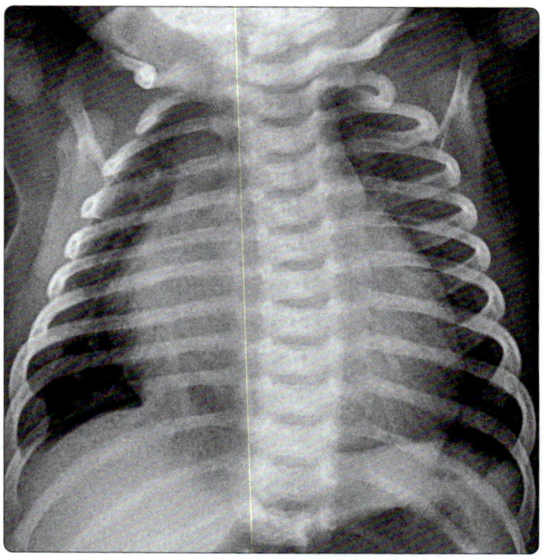

Ischemic Cardiomyopathy

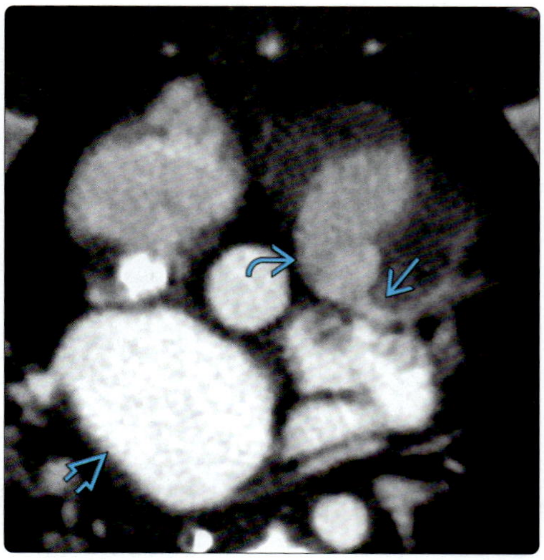

Restrictive Cardiomyopathy

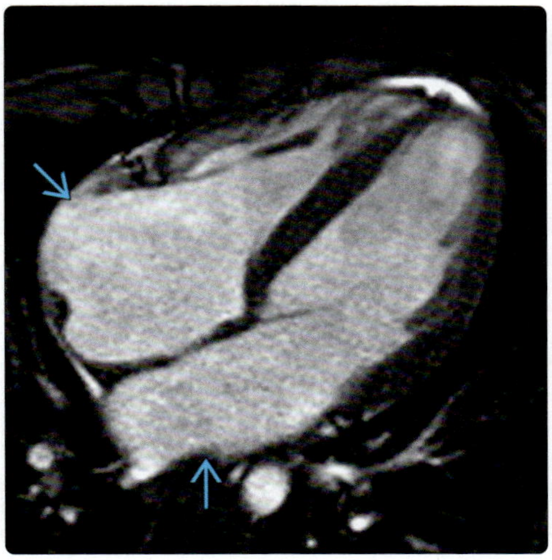

Restrictive Cardiomyopathy

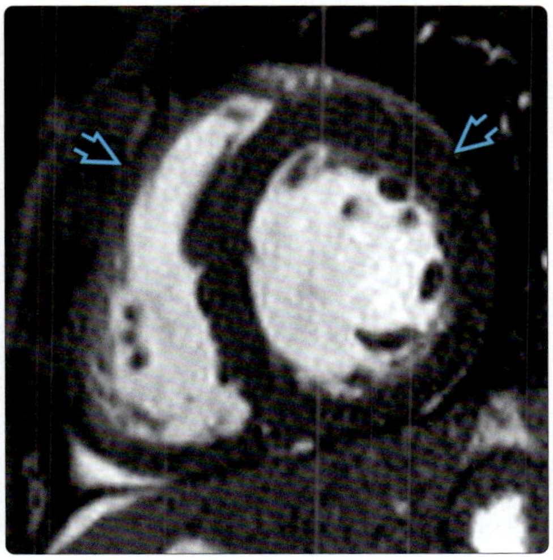

(Left) *Four-chamber SSFP MR in a 17 year old with a genetic restrictive cardiomyopathy (RCM) shows characteristic biatrial dilation without ventricular dilation.* **(Right)** *Short-axis SSFP MR in the same patient shows moderate diffuse myocardial hypertrophy of both ventricles. In RCM, diffuse myocardial infiltration or fibrosis leads to diastolic dysfunction with impaired filling & biatrial dilation. Systolic function is maintained. In contradistinction, constrictive pericarditis will also have pericardial thickening.*

Severe Aortic Stenosis

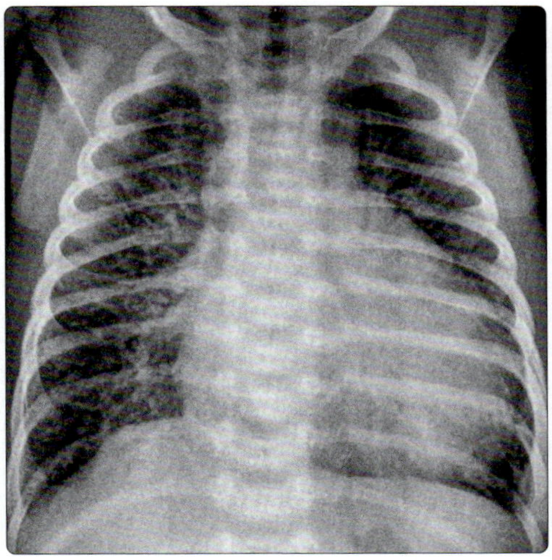

Severe Aortic Stenosis

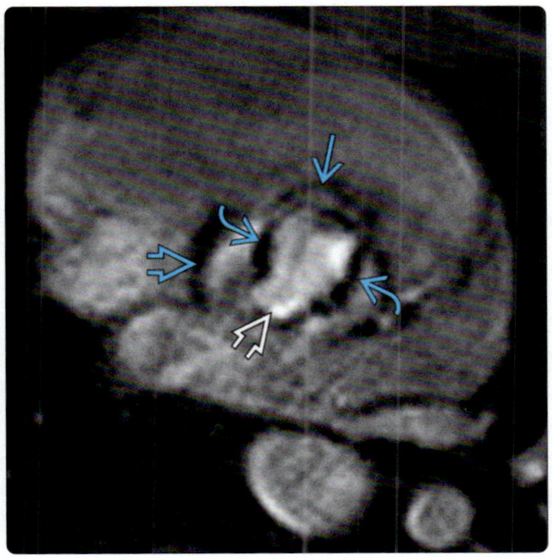

(Left) *PA radiograph in a 4-week-old boy shows moderate cardiomegaly with normal vascularity & moderate pulmonary edema, suggestive of left heart failure. Echocardiography showed a bicuspid aortic valve with severe stenosis & moderate LV dysfunction.* **(Right)** *Axial oblique GRE MR cine in the same patient at 10 years old shows the bicuspid aortic valve with fusion of the right & noncoronary cusps, thickened dysplastic valve leaflets, & a narrow restrictive opening.*

Mitral Valve Regurgitation

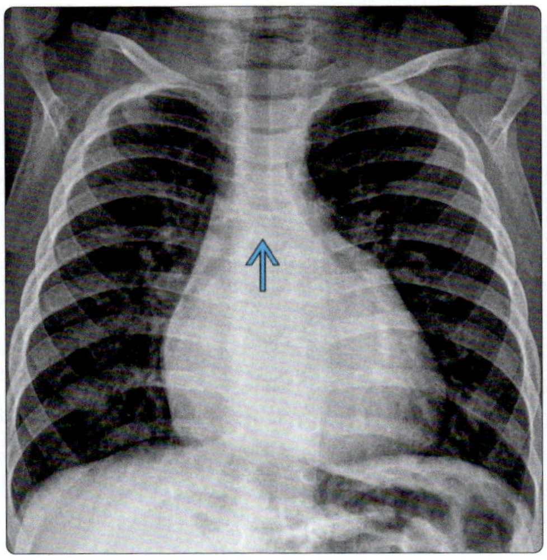

Mitral Valve Regurgitation

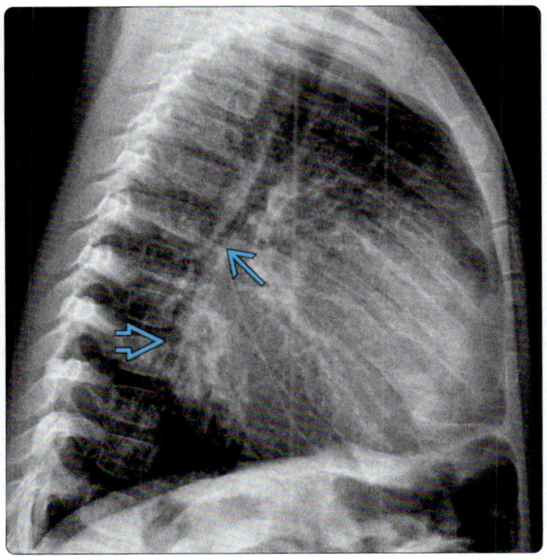

(Left) *PA radiograph in a 9-month-old girl with an arcade mitral valve causing severe stenosis & regurgitation shows cardiomegaly with splaying of the carina, consistent with LA dilation.* **(Right)** *Lateral radiograph in the same patient shows moderate cardiomegaly with signs of LA dilation, including posterior deviation of the left main bronchus & extension of the posterior heart border to the vertebral bodies. Both severe mitral stenosis & regurgitation led to LA dilation in this patient.*

DIFFERENTIAL DIAGNOSIS

Common

- Aortic Stenosis
- Hypoplastic Left Heart Syndrome
- Hypertropic Cardiomyopathy

Less Common

- Cor Triatriatum
- Supramitral Ring
- Mitral Valve Stenosis

Rare but Important

- Shone Complex
- Cardiac Mass

ESSENTIAL INFORMATION

Key Differential Diagnosis Issues

- Congenital left heart obstructive lesions encompass spectrum of disorders
- Caused by 1 or more lesions at level(s) of left atrium (LA), mitral valve, left ventricle (LV), or left ventricular outflow tract (LVOT) (subvalvar, at aortic valve, or supravalvar)
- Congenital lesions lead to underdevelopment of left-sided structures (as blood flow is required for growth)
  - Associated with aortic hypoplasia & obstructive aortic arch lesions (discussed separately)
  - Severe aortic valvar stenosis in utero leads to hypoplastic left heart syndrome
- Presentation depends on severity of lesion
  - Critical left heart obstruction presents when ductus arteriosus begins to close
    - Decreased systemic & coronary perfusion, acidosis, end-organ injury, & shock
      - Prostaglandins help keep ductus open: R → L shunt through PDA is required for systemic perfusion
  - Less severe left heart obstruction may present later
    - Failure to thrive, tachypnea, pulmonary congestion
- Myocardium hypertrophies in response to contraction against obstruction (increased afterload)

Helpful Clues for Common Diagnoses

- **Aortic Stenosis**
  - Valvar (80%), subaortic (10-20%), or supravalvar (< 5%)
  - Valvar aortic stenosis
    - In pediatrics, aortic stenosis is due to congenitally abnormal valve
      - Strong genetic component
    - Most common is bicuspid aortic valve (& most common type of congenital heart defect overall)
      - Conjoined right & left coronary cusps (70-80%)
      - Conjoined right & noncoronary cusps (15-25%)
      - Conjoined left & noncoronary cusps (< 5%)
    - ~ 50% have associated cardiac anomaly or coarctation
    - Degree of aortic stenosis is often progressive
    - Systemic circulation may depend on R → L PDA flow
    - Newborns can present with systemic hypoperfusion & cardiogenic shock as ductus arteriosus closes
    - Older children can present with early fatigue, chest pain, syncope, or systolic ejection murmur
    - Lifetime risk of aortopathy with ascending aortic dilation & dissection
    - Radiograph can be normal or show cardiomegaly, vascular congestion, & ascending aortic dilation
  - Subaortic stenosis
    - Discrete form: Fibromuscular ridge/membrane
      - Arises from ventricular septum & extends to anterior leaflet of mitral valve
    - Diffuse form: Long-segment muscular tunnel
    - Associated with perimembranous ventricular septal defect (VSD) with posterior malalignment of outlet septum
      - L → R shunt through VSD, combined with aortic stenosis, leads to decreased ascending aortic flow, often with arch hypoplasia, coarctation, or interrupted aortic arch
    - Usually not present at birth
    - May be due to abnormal underlying endothelial substrate stimulated to proliferate due to shear stress from chronic turbulence
    - Turbulent flow often damages aortic valve, leading to concurrent aortic regurgitation
    - Progressive course, often recurs after treatment
  - Supravalvar stenosis
    - Discrete narrowing at sinotubular junction
    - Strong association with genetic elastin mutation (classically Williams-Beuren syndrome)
    - Often with additional arterial hypoplasia or stenoses: Aorta, head & neck vessels, renal arteries, or pulmonary arteries (right, left, & segmental)
    - Significant arterial wall thickening: Can cause tethering of aortic valve leaflets & coronary ostial stenosis (typically LCA) → potential for myocardial ischemia & sudden death
    - In general, systemic stenoses tend to be stable or progress, but pulmonary stenoses tend to improve
- **Hypoplastic Left Heart Syndrome**
  - Spectrum of lesions defined by
    - Significant LV hypoplasia, including aortic or mitral valve atresia, stenosis, or hypoplasia, + ascending aorta & arch hypoplasia
    - Normally related great arteries
    - No atrioventricular septal defect
  - 3 major anatomic subtypes
    - Mitral atresia & aortic atresia (30%)
    - Mitral stenosis & aortic atresia (25%)
    - Mitral stenosis & aortic stenosis (45%)
  - Small LV is unable to support systemic circulation
  - Ductal dependent systemic circulation with 2 obligate shunts
    - L → R interatrial shunt (PFO/ASD) required to decompress pulmonary venous return
      - Complete mixing of blood in RA
    - R → L PDA flow required for systemic blood flow
      - Ascending aorta may only serve as conduit for retrograde flow to coronary arteries from PDA
  - Associated coarctation in 80%
  - Readily diagnosed in utero
  - Radiographs variable
    - Normal heart size to globular cardiomegaly

- Pulmonary vascularity is normal at birth with progressive increase over days
- If atrial septum is restrictive, signs of pulmonary venous obstruction occur, including pulmonary edema & fine reticulation of pulmonary lymphangiectasia
  - MR to quantify LV size & assess ascending aortic flow
    - Can see endocardial fibroelastosis on MR LGE imaging
  - Traditional staged palliation
    - Norwood operation with modified Blalock-Taussig shunt or RV-PA conduit at birth
    - Bidirectional cavopulmonary connection at 4-6 months
    - Fontan at 18-48 months
- **Hypertropic Cardiomyopathy**
  - Most common hereditary cardiac disorder
  - Asymmetric ventricular hypertrophy, typically of basal septum
  - May or may not have dynamic LVOT obstruction
    - Severe septal thickening → midcavitary obstruction
    - Systolic anterior motion of mitral valve
  - MR: Can see patchy midwall LGE with predilection for right ventricular insertion points
  - Risk of sudden cardiac death

Helpful Clues for Less Common Diagnoses

- **Cor Triatriatum**
  - Incomplete incorporation of common pulmonary vein confluence to LA
  - Pulmonary veins drain to accessory LA chamber, divided from LA by fibromuscular membrane, typically with small obstructive opening
    - Membrane is above orifice of LA appendage (unlike supramitral ring)
  - LA appears separated into smaller upper chamber, enclosed between pulmonary veins & cor triatriatum, & larger lower chamber of LA proper
  - Associated with ASD/PFO, usually through upper chamber
  - Variants include incomplete incorporation of only 1 side of common confluence or of single vein
    - Unilateral obstruction or long-segment pulmonary vein stenosis/hypoplasia
  - Main pathophysiology is pulmonary venous obstruction
- **Supramitral Ring**
  - Fibrous membrane above level of mitral valve annulus with narrow obstructed opening
    - Membrane is below orifice of LA appendage (unlike cor triatriatum)
  - Intimate relationship with mitral valve annulus; also close to circumflex coronary artery in atrioventricular groove
  - Often associated with other cardiac defects
- **Mitral Valve Stenosis**
  - Various congenital types of mitral valve stenosis
    - Typical type: 2 distinct papillary muscles, underdeveloped & closely spaced
    - Parachute mitral valve: All chordae tendineae connect to single papillary muscle
    - Mitral arcade: Elongated papillary muscles connect to anterior mitral leaflet (directly or via short chords)
  - Stenosis may be acquired from rheumatic heart disease
  - Radiograph shows LA enlargement with pulmonary venous hypertension or edema

Helpful Clues for Rare Diagnoses

- **Shone Complex**
  - Constellation of multiple left-sided obstructive lesions
  - Initial description had 4 anomalies
    - Supramitral ring, subaortic stenosis, parachute mitral valve, & aortic coarctation
    - Incomplete complex: Mitral valve anomaly with any other obstructive lesions of LVOT or thoracic aorta
- **Cardiac Mass**
  - Cardiac tumors can potentially obstruct LV lumen
  - Most common cardiac tumors in children: Rhabdomyoma, fibroma, hemangioma, & malignancy

SELECTED REFERENCES

1. Carr M et al: Educational series in congenital heart disease: congenital left-sided heart obstruction. Echo Res Pract. 5(2):R23-36, 2018
2. Ohye RG et al: Current therapy for hypoplastic left heart syndrome and related single ventricle lesions. Circulation. 134(17):1265-79, 2016

Aortic Stenosis

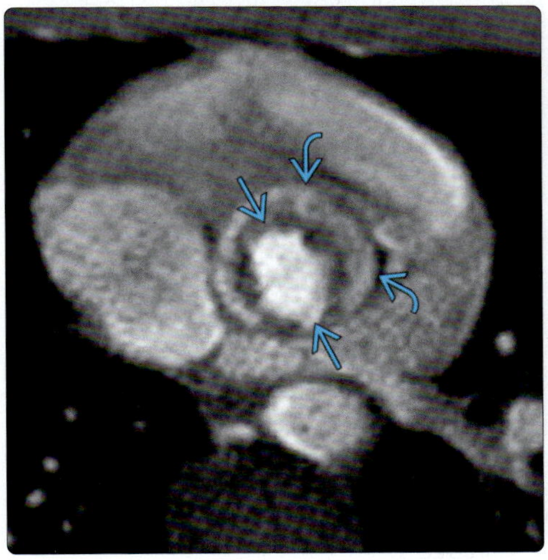

Aortic Stenosis

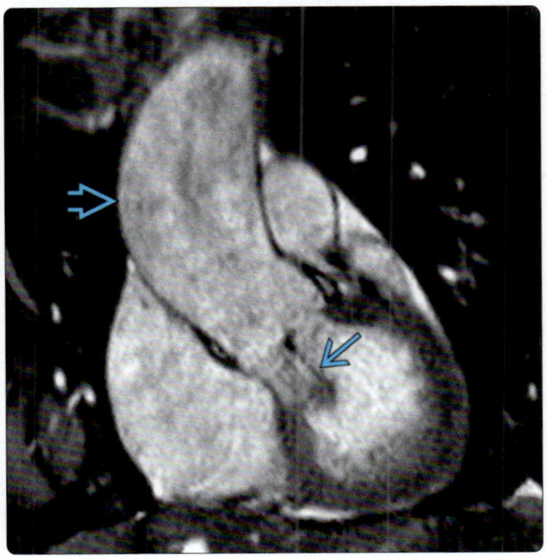

(Left) *Axial oblique GRE cine MR in a 15-year-old boy shows a thickened bicuspid aortic valve with fusion of the right & left coronary cusps ⇨, creating a stenotic elliptical opening ⇨.* **(Right)** *LVOT SSFP cine MR in the same patient shows jet-like dephasing from concurrent aortic regurgitation ⇨, which is also common in bicuspid aortic valve. Valvar dysfunction is slowly progressive in the pediatric population. The ascending aorta dilation ⇨ increases the risk of dissection & may be poststenotic &/or due to intrinsic aortopathy.*

(Left) *Three-chamber SSFP cine MR in a 9 year old shows a subaortic fibromuscular ridge* ➡ *causing a left ventricular outflow tract obstruction (LVOTO).* **(Right)** *LVOT SSFP cine MR in the same patient shows a turbulent dephasing jet* ➡ *that begins at the subaortic level in the region of the fibromuscular ridge & extends into the ascending aorta. The turbulent flow damages the aortic valve over time & can lead to concurrent aortic regurgitation.*

Aortic Stenosis

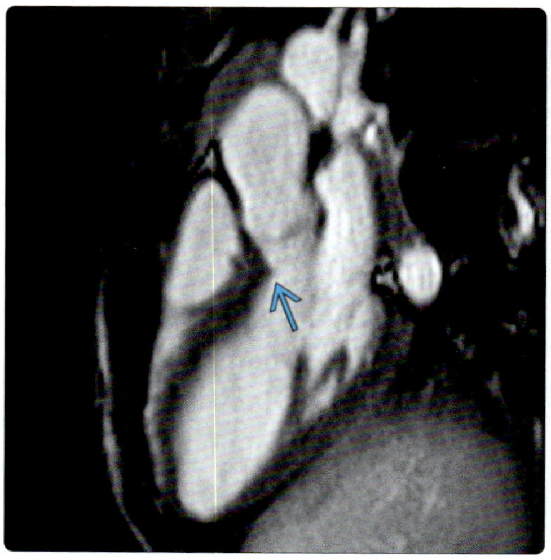

Aortic Stenosis

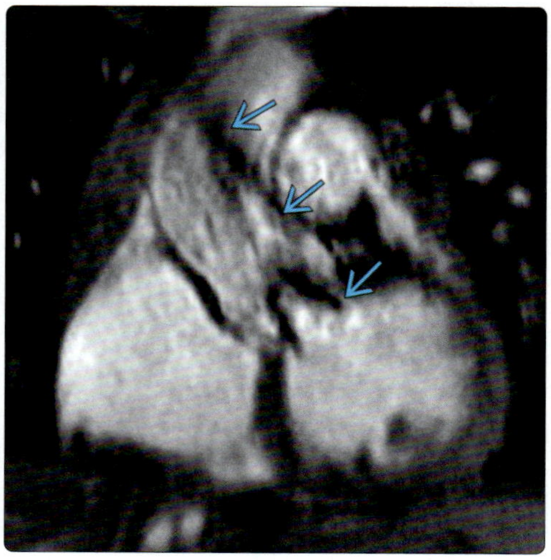

(Left) *Sagittal oblique CECT MIP in a 5 month old shows discrete supravalvar aortic stenosis at the sinotubular junction* ➡, *typical of Williams syndrome or related conditions with Elastin mutations. Wall thickening can cause coronary ostial stenosis.* **(Right)** *Coronal oblique CECT MIP in the same patient shows multiple discrete peripheral pulmonary stenoses* ➡, *also common in Williams syndrome. In general, systemic stenoses tend to be stable or progress, while pulmonary stenoses tend to improve with growth.*

Aortic Stenosis

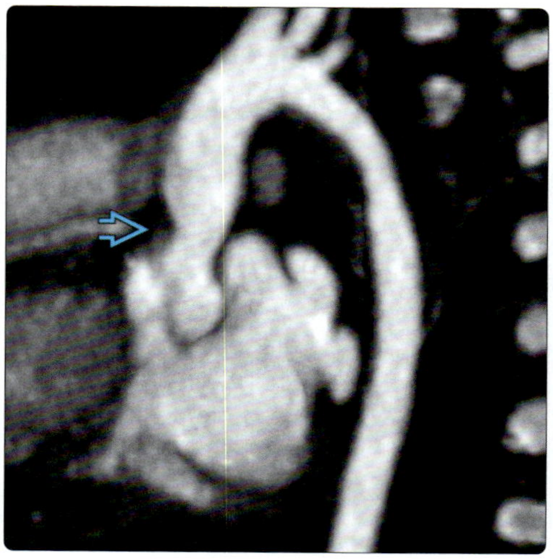

Aortic Stenosis

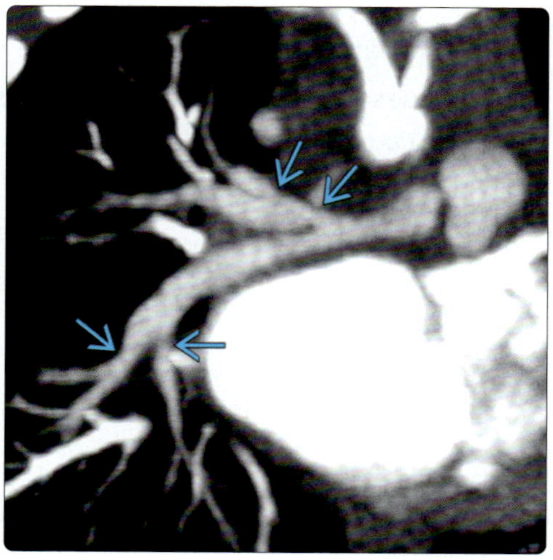

(Left) *AP radiograph in an 8 day old with HLHS (mitral stenosis/aortic stenosis) shows nonspecific mild cardiomegaly & increased pulmonary vascularity.* **(Right)** *Four-chamber SSFP cine MR in the same patient shows a small nonapex-forming LV* ➡ *& a dilated RV* ➡. *Note the tethered mitral valve leaflets* ➡ *with a turbulent flow jet* ➡ *from mitral stenosis compared to the normal opening of the tricuspid valve* ➡. *The LV size is borderline, which can be quantified by MR to evaluate for a biventricular vs. univentricular repair.*

Hypoplastic Left Heart Syndrome

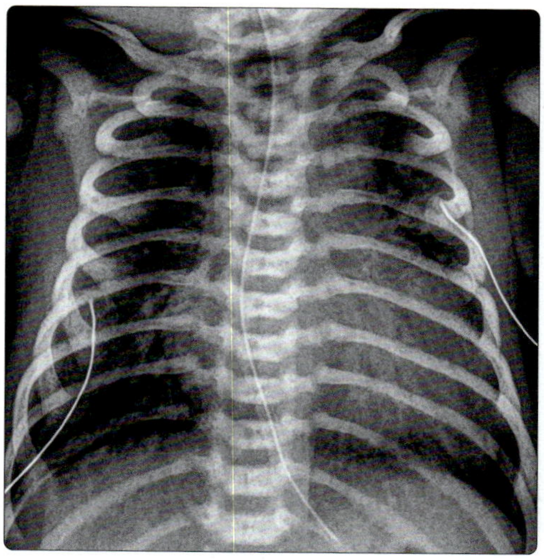

Hypoplastic Left Heart Syndrome

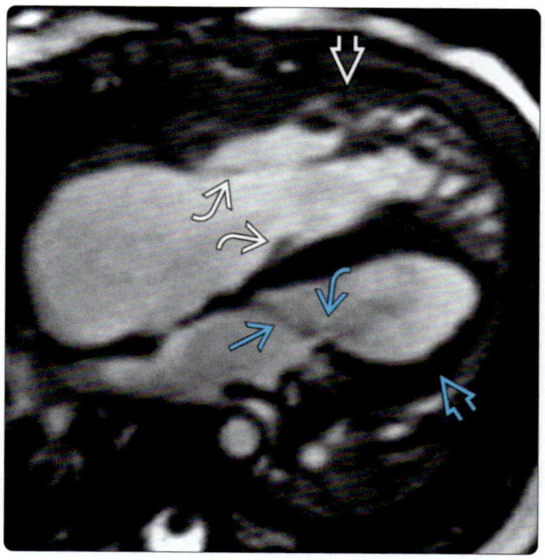

Hypoplastic Left Heart Syndrome

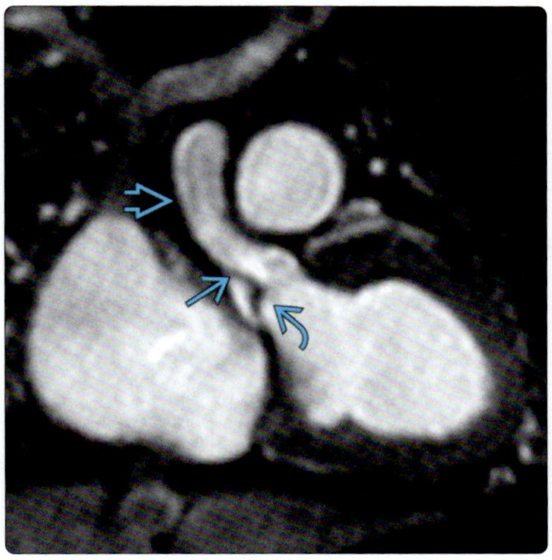

Hypoplastic Left Heart Syndrome

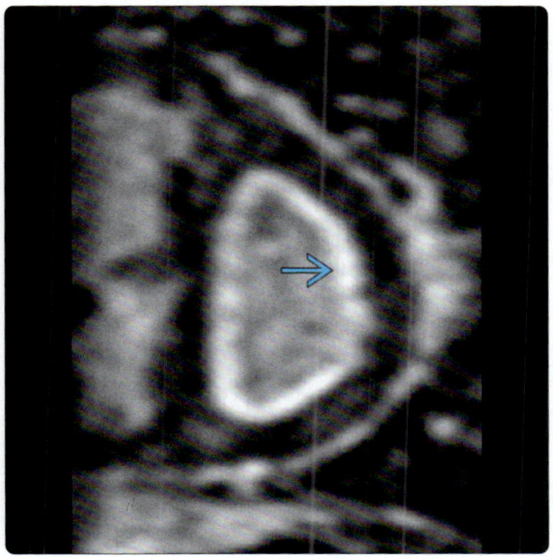

(Left) *Coronal oblique MRA MIP in the same patient at 4 months old shows a thickened stenotic aortic valve with a dephasing stenotic flow jet & small ascending aorta.* **(Right)** *Short-axis delayed MRA MIP shows circumferential endocardial late gadolinium enhancement in the LV, consistent with endocardial fibroelastosis. While the LV has grown, this patient was deemed not suitable for biventricular repair. The MR was performed for preoperative bidirectional cavopulmonary connection planning.*

Hypertropic Cardiomyopathy

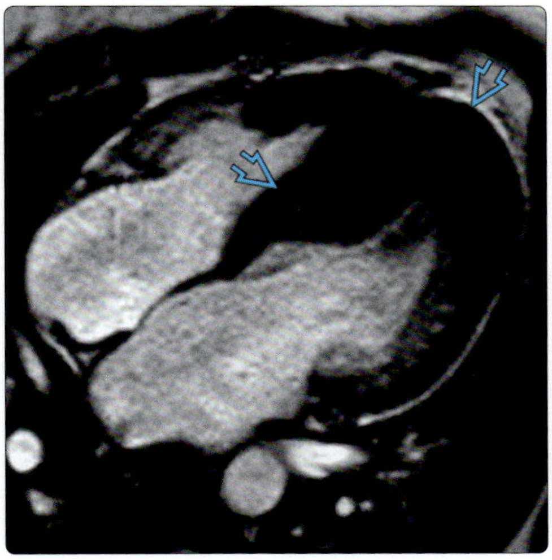

Hypertropic Cardiomyopathy

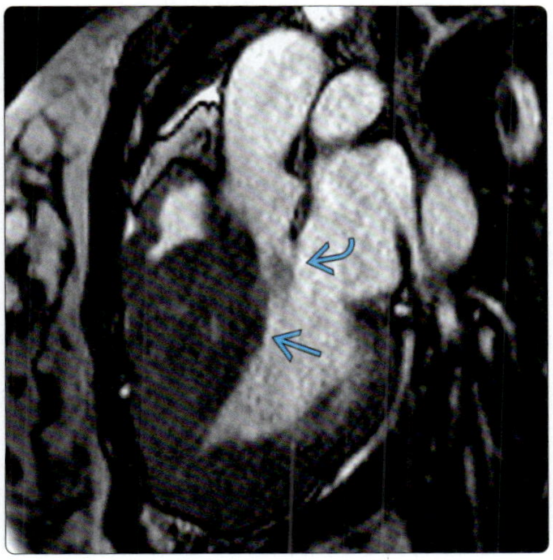

(Left) *Four-chamber SSFP cine MR in a 16 year old with HCM shows asymmetric LV hypertrophy of the midseptum & apex. Hypertrophy is usually asymmetric in HCM.* **(Right)** *Three-chamber SSFP C+ MR in systole shows dynamic LVOTO from both septal hypertrophy & systolic anterior motion of the mitral valve. In HCM, while the ejection fraction can be normal or high, the stroke volume & cardiac output are actually low due to a small cavity size. However, not all cases have a component of outlet obstruction.*

Hypertropic Cardiomyopathy

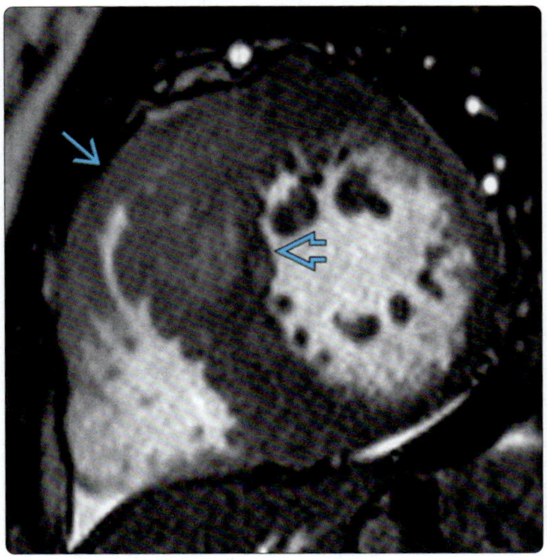

Hypertropic Cardiomyopathy

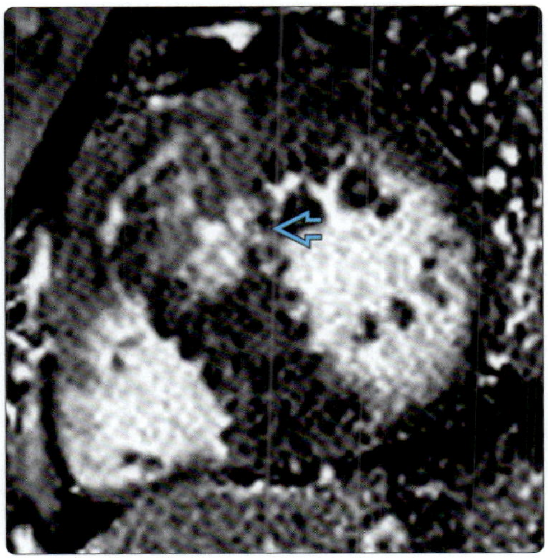

(Left) *Short-axis SSFP C+ MR in the same patient shows asymmetric hypertrophy of the septal LV & RV.* **(Right)** *Short-axis LGE PSIR MR in the same patient shows extensive patchy delayed enhancement of the interventricular septum, indicative of fibrosis. Hypertrophied segments in HCM are characterized by myocyte disarray & do not have normal contraction.*

(**Left**) *Short-axis SSFP C+ MR in a 15 year old with HCM shows hypertrophy of the interventricular septum.* (**Right**) *Short-axis LGE PSIR MR in the same patient shows mild LGE at the RV insertion points, which are the 1st areas to exhibit LGE in HCM. This case has a milder degree of fibrosis compared to the previous case. Areas of fibrosis can be substrates for fatal arrhythmias & sudden cardiac death. The extent of LGE has prognostic value & contributes to the decision to place an implantable cardioverter defibrillator.*

Hypertropic Cardiomyopathy

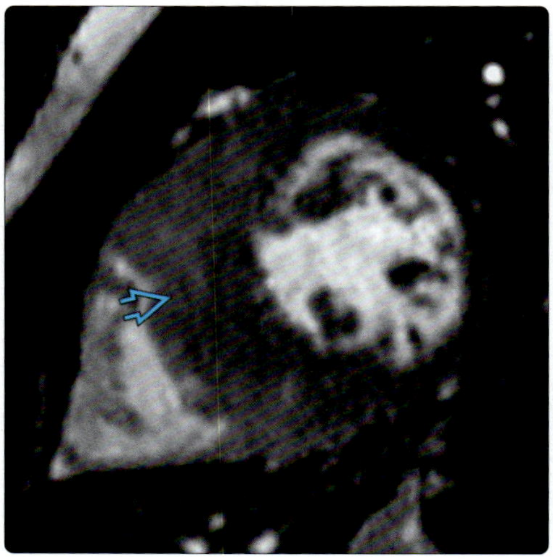

Hypertropic Cardiomyopathy

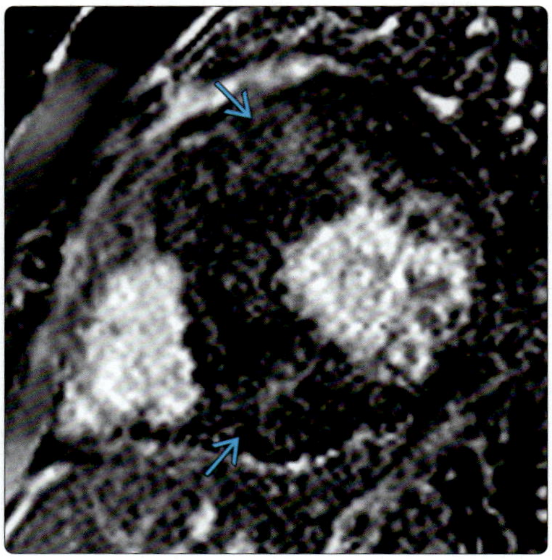

(**Left**) *Three-chamber GRE cine MR in systole in the same patient shows dynamic midcavitary/LVOTO from the septal hypertrophy & systolic anterior motion (SAM) of the mitral valve anterior leaflet. The SAM allows mitral valve regurgitation. The presence of a regurgitant jet can be a clue that SAM is present. A subvalvar dephasing jet is also seen in the outflow from the obstruction.* (**Right**) *LVOT GRE cine MR again shows midcavitary obstruction with a dephasing jet extending into the ascending aorta.*

Hypertropic Cardiomyopathy

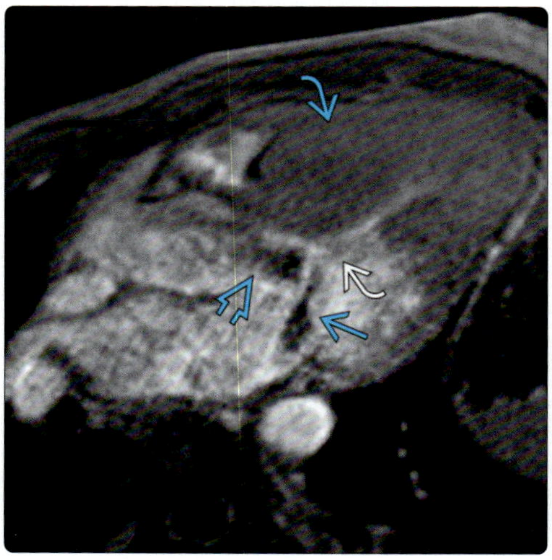

Hypertropic Cardiomyopathy

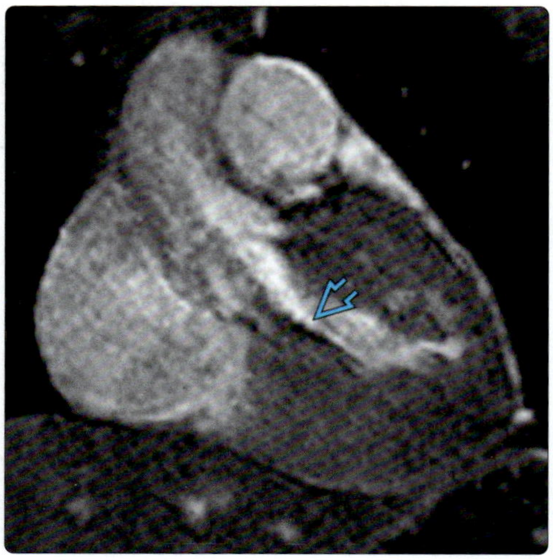

(**Left**) *Axial oblique SSFP MR in a 3 year old with cor triatriatum shows a thin transverse membrane in the LA, which separates the pulmonary veins from the LA proper, resulting in pulmonary venous obstruction. An ASD/PFO is often present that allows decompression of the upper chamber.* (**Right**) *Axial oblique CECT MPR in a 4 month old with cor triatriatum shows a transverse membrane above the orifice of the left atrial appendage (vs. below the orifice, which is typical of a supramitral ring).*

Cor Triatriatum

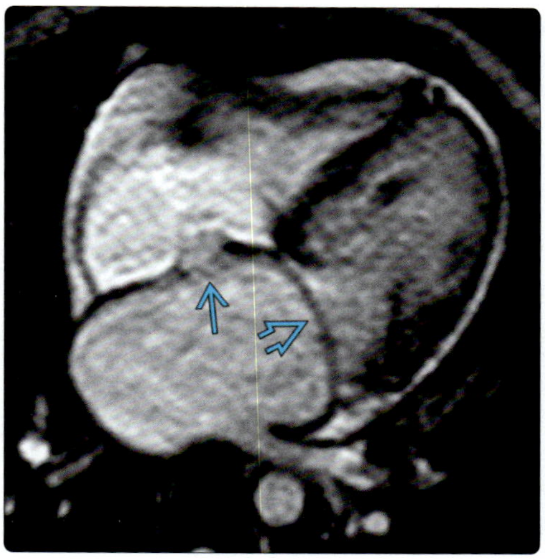

Cor Triatriatum

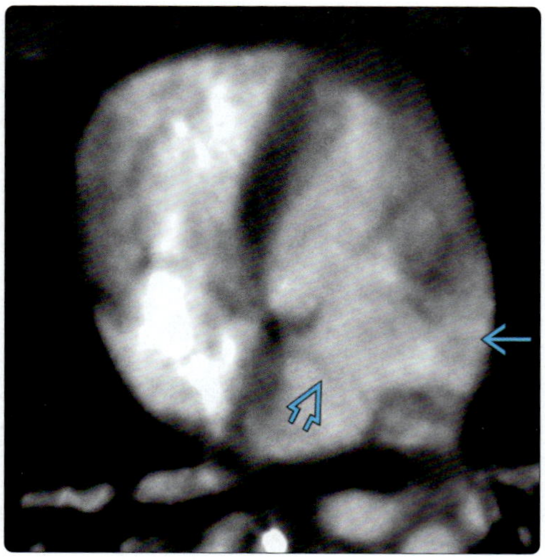

Mitral Valve Stenosis

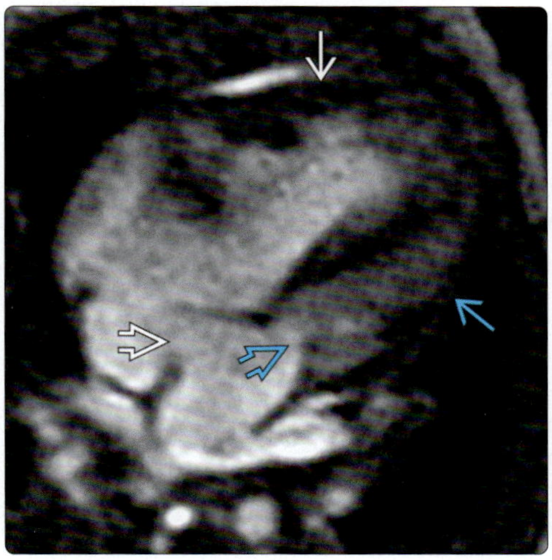

Mitral Valve Stenosis

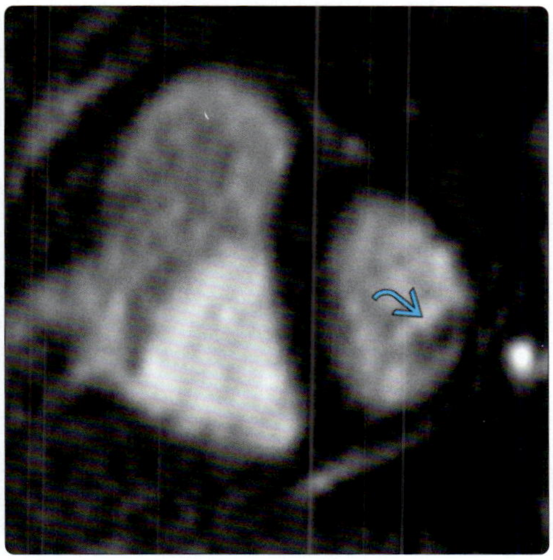

(Left) *Four-chamber SSFP cine MR in a 3 day old with complex congenital heart disease shows a small mitral valve with restricted motion of the leaflets ⇨ & a hypoplastic LV →. There is a large ASD ➡ with a dilated RV ➡.* **(Right)** *Short-axis SSFP MR in the same patient shows a single LV papillary muscle ↷, which, when combined with the previous image, is consistent with a parachute mitral valve. Normally, there are 2 papillary muscles of the mitral valve (anteromedial & posteromedial).*

Shone Complex

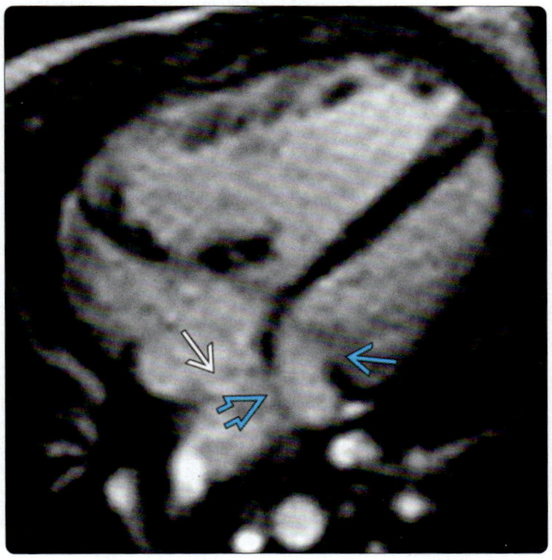

Shone Complex

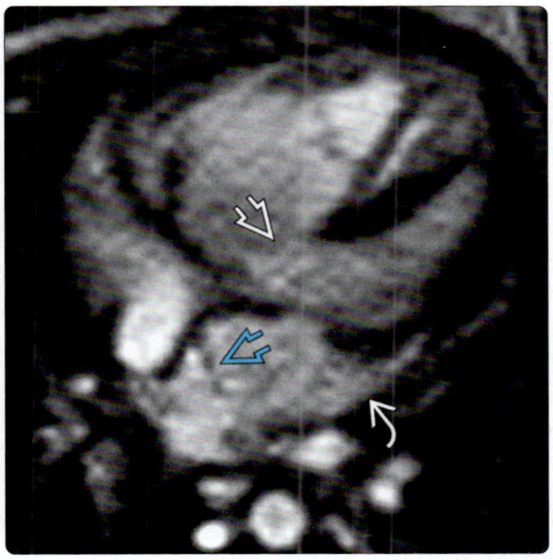

(Left) *Axial SSFP cine MR in a 3 day old with Shone complex shows a cor triatriatum ⇨, mitral stenosis →, & an ASD ➡ between the upper chamber & RA.* **(Right)** *Axial SSFP cine MR in the same patient again shows the cor triatriatum ⇨ (above the level of the left atrial appendage ➡) along with a large, perimembranous VSD ➡. Shone complex is defined by a mitral valve anomaly combined with other left-sided obstructions, classically supramitral ring, parachute mitral valve, subaortic stenosis, & coarctation.*

Shone Complex

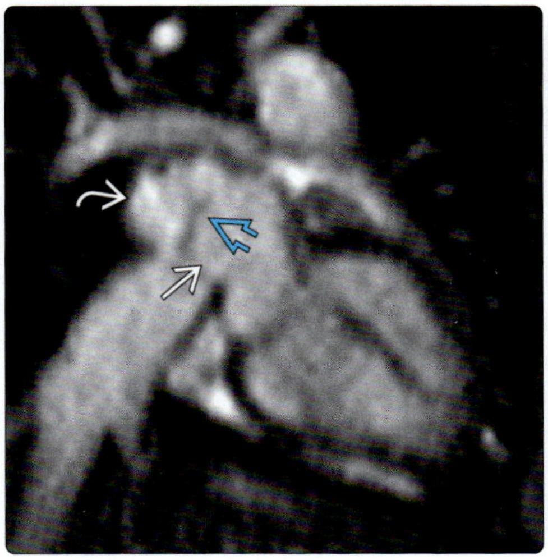

Shone Complex

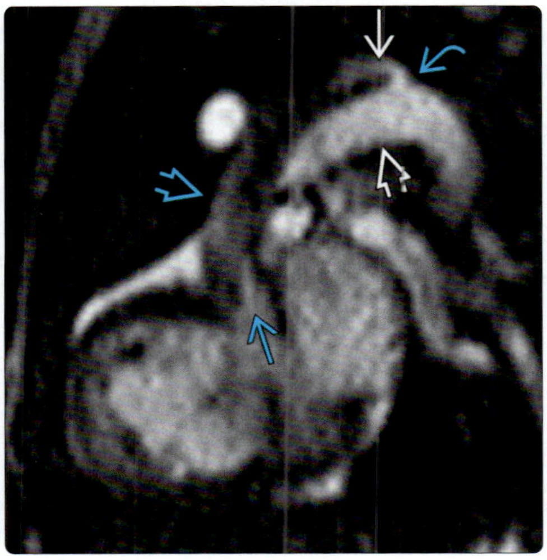

(Left) *Two-chamber SSFP cine MR again shows the cor triatriatum ⇨, which separates the LA into an upper chamber ➡ & lower chamber ➡.* **(Right)** *Sagittal oblique SSFP cine MR in the same patient shows a small ascending aorta ⇨ with a dephasing jet from aortic stenosis →. There is suggestion of a discrete coarctation ↷ with a tiny distal arch ➡. The descending thoracic aorta is supplied by a large PDA ➡. Multiple left-sided obstructions, as in this patient, are typical in Shone complex.*

DIFFERENTIAL DIAGNOSIS

Common

- Left Aortic Arch With Aberrant Right Subclavian Artery
- Double Aortic Arch

Less Common

- Right Aortic Arch With Aberrant Left Subclavian Artery
- Right Aortic Arch With Mirror-Image Branching

Rare but Important

- Cervical Aortic Arch
- Circumflex Aortic Arch
- Isolated Subclavian Artery
- Persistent 5th Arch

ESSENTIAL INFORMATION

Key Differential Diagnosis Issues

- Diverticulum of Kommerell
  - Diverticular outpouching of proximal descending aorta
  - Formed from flow through ductus arteriosus during fetal life
  - Indicates site of ligamentum ductus arteriosum
    - Almost always forms vascular ring
- Double aortic arch with dominant right arch & atretic left segment vs. right aortic arch with mirror-image branching
  - Common differential dilemma; helpful clues include
    - Arches are posteriorly directed, while brachiocephalic arteries are more anterior & laterally directed
    - Great vessels arise symmetrically in double aortic arch & asymmetrically in mirror-image branching
    - Presence of diverticulum of Kommerell almost always indicates double aortic arch
- Always evaluate for tracheobronchial compression/narrowing on radiographs, CT, or MR

Helpful Clues for Common Diagnoses

- **Left Aortic Arch With Aberrant Right Subclavian Artery**
  - Separate origin of right subclavian artery as last vessel from arch/proximal descending aorta, typically with retroesophageal course
  - Almost always without diverticulum of Kommerell at origin of aberrant right subclavian artery, therefore usually asymptomatic & incidental
    - Lack of diverticulum indicates ligamentum arteriosum is on same side as aortic arch → no vascular ring
  - Radiograph
    - Left aortic arch with possible indentation on posterior trachea on lateral view (but usually minimal if no diverticulum)
  - Esophagram
    - Frontal: Mild tubular impression on contrast column extending obliquely from left arch superiorly toward right shoulder
    - Lateral: Mild round posterior indentation caused by retroesophageal course of aberrant right subclavian artery
      - Only prominent if diverticulum present
  - CT & MR: Aberrant right subclavian artery arises as last vessel from aortic arch/proximal descending aorta & courses posterior to esophagus toward right
    - Look for AP compression of trachea
- **Double Aortic Arch**
  - Both limbs are usually complete, but one side may be hypoplastic, stenotic, or segmentally atretic
    - Stenosis or atresia is usually found distally after ipsilateral subclavian artery origin, in close proximity to ligamentum arteriosum
    - Atretic segment has persistent fibrous remnant (similar to ligamentum arteriosum), thus forming vascular ring
  - Most common morphology: Dominant (larger) right limb is more superior & posterior than left & courses behind esophagus before joining left limb posteriorly to form left-sided descending aorta
  - Symptoms usually present early
  - Radiograph
    - May show aortic knob (usually R > L) on both sides of superior mediastinum
      - Dominant right arch typically deviates trachea to left; more inferior left arch may shift trachea back to right
      - Trachea may show circumferential narrowing but typically more severe on right & posteriorly
    - Descending aorta can be seen on any side
      - Aortic knob & descending aorta on opposite sides should raise suspicion for double aortic arch or circumflex aortic arch
  - Esophagram
    - Frontal: Compression on both sides of esophagus at different levels
    - Lateral: Rounded posterior impression on esophagus
  - CT & MR
    - Demonstrate relative sizes of limbs & degree of associated tracheal narrowing
    - Site of arch stenosis or atresia suggests site of ligamentum arteriosum, which also must be excised
    - Diverticulum of Kommerell (in setting of atretic segment) or similar residual outpouching from undersurface of complete arch may be present, serving as another indicator of ligamentum arteriosum side
  - Rarely associated with intracardiac defects

Helpful Clues for Less Common Diagnoses

- **Right Aortic Arch With Aberrant Left Subclavian Artery**
  - Separate origin of right subclavian artery as last vessel from arch/proximal descending aorta, typically with retroesophageal course
    - Can more rarely lie anterior to esophagus or trachea
  - Look for diverticulum of Kommerell at origin of aberrant left subclavian artery → indicates left-sided ligamentum arteriosum to left pulmonary artery (LPA), completing vascular ring
  - Radiograph
    - Right aortic arch deviates trachea to left
    - Posterior wall of trachea indented by diverticulum of Kommerell
  - Esophagram
    - Frontal: Oblique impression on right side of esophagus directed superiorly toward left shoulder
    - Lateral: Posterior indentation caused by diverticulum of Kommerell

- CT & MR: Aberrant left subclavian artery arises as last vessel from arch/proximal descending aorta & courses posterior to esophagus toward left
  - Look for AP compression of trachea
- Low association (10%) with intracardiac defects

- **Right Aortic Arch With Mirror-Image Branching**
  - 3 vessels arise from right aortic arch in mirror image of normal left arch
    - Left brachiocephalic artery (most proximal)
    - Right common carotid artery
    - Right subclavian artery (most distal)
  - Vast majority of cases have right-sided ligamentum arteriosum → no vascular ring
    - Rarely can have left-sided ligamentum arteriosum but usually connects from LPA to left subclavian artery → no vascular ring
    - Extremely rarely, left-sided ligamentum arteriosum can connect from LPA to proximal descending aorta, forming ring
      - Diverticulum of Kommerell will be present
  - Radiograph
    - Right arch deviates trachea to left with descending aorta on right; usually lacks tracheal narrowing
  - High association (90%) with intracardiac defects
    - Most common: Tetralogy of Fallot, common arterial trunk (truncus arteriosus), or double-outlet right ventricle

Helpful Clues for Rare Diagnoses

- **Cervical Aortic Arch**
  - Arch extends above medial aspect of clavicles → may reach C2 level
  - Often has straightened or superiorly angulated course at midarch
  - Proposed embryogenesis: Persistence of 1st, 2nd, or 3rd pharyngeal arch
    - Normal aortic arch formed from 4th pharyngeal arch
  - May have associated symptomatic vascular ring
- **Circumflex Aortic Arch**
  - Descending aorta on opposite side of aortic arch
    - Arch crosses behind trachea & esophagus to descend on contralateral side
    - May cause posterior narrowing of trachea/esophagus, similar to vascular ring
- **Isolated Subclavian Artery**
  - "Isolation" refers to great vessel that is not connected to aortic arch proper (but may have atretic segment)
    - Most commonly involves subclavian artery
  - May be supplied by PDA or ipsilateral vertebral artery retrograde flow (subclavian steal)
- **Persistent 5th Arch**
  - Extrapericardial vessel arising from ascending aorta proximal or opposite to brachiocephalic artery origin
  - 2 main types
    - Systemic to systemic: Distal connection to dorsal aorta
      - 2 aortic arches on same side with superior-inferior relationship ("double barrel")
      - Superior arch is normal arch derived from 4th pharyngeal arch but may be obstructed (coarctation or interrupted)
    - Systemic to pulmonary: Distal connection to pulmonary arteries
      - Pathologic L → R shunt with pulmonary hypertension
      - Associated with critical right-sided obstruction

SELECTED REFERENCES

1. Hanneman K et al: Congenital variants and anomalies of the aortic arch. Radiographics. 37(1):32-51, 2017
2. Gould SW et al: Useful signs for the assessment of vascular rings on cross-sectional imaging. Pediatr Radiol. 45(13):2004-16, 2015
3. Schlesinger AE et al: Incomplete double aortic arch with atresia of the distal left arch: distinctive imaging appearance. AJR Am J Roentgenol. 184(5):1634-9, 2005
4. Yoo SJ et al: Fetal sonographic diagnosis of aortic arch anomalies. Ultrasound Obstet Gynecol. 22(5):535-46, 2003

Left Aortic Arch With Aberrant Right Subclavian Artery

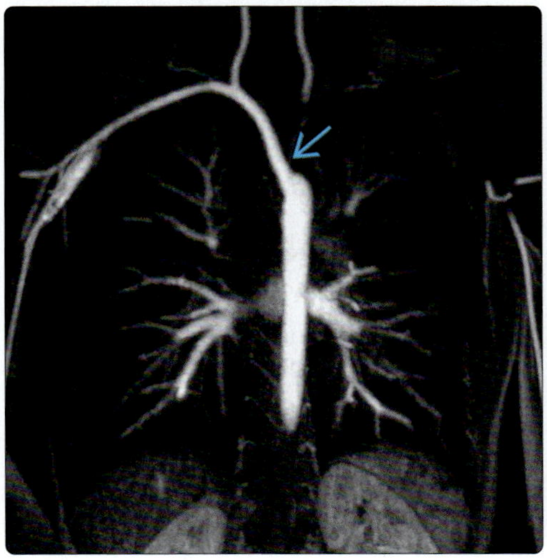

Left Aortic Arch With Aberrant Right Subclavian Artery

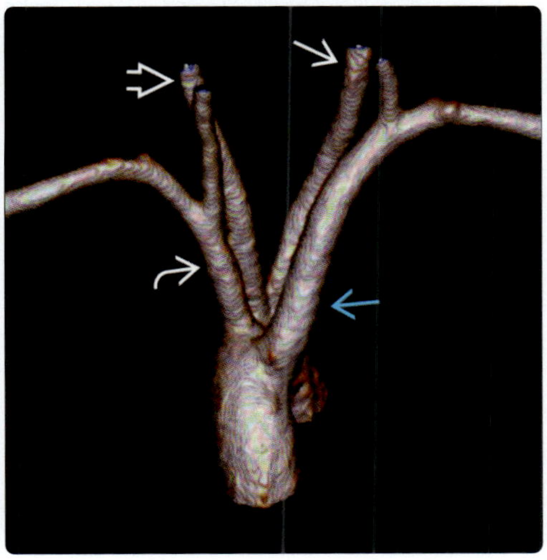

(Left) *Contrast-enhanced MRA in a 12-year-old asymptomatic boy shows an aberrant right subclavian artery ➙ arising from the proximal descending aorta. There is no diverticulum of Kommerell, which is typical of this entity & the absence of a vascular ring.* **(Right)** *Posterior MRA 3D projection in the same patient shows the aberrant right subclavian artery ➙ arising as the last branch of the aortic arch without a diverticulum of Kommerell. The right common carotid ➙, left common carotid ➙, & left subclavian ➙ arteries are noted.*

(Left) *PA radiograph in a 2 year old with respiratory distress upon playing or eating shows deviation of the trachea to the left by a dominant right aortic arch. There is also a lower rightward deviation of the trachea by a smaller left arch. As the aorta descends on the left, the findings suggest a double aortic or circumflex arch.* **(Right)** *Coronal T1 MR in the same patient shows the dominant right & smaller left arches, causing narrowing of the trachea.*

Double Aortic Arch

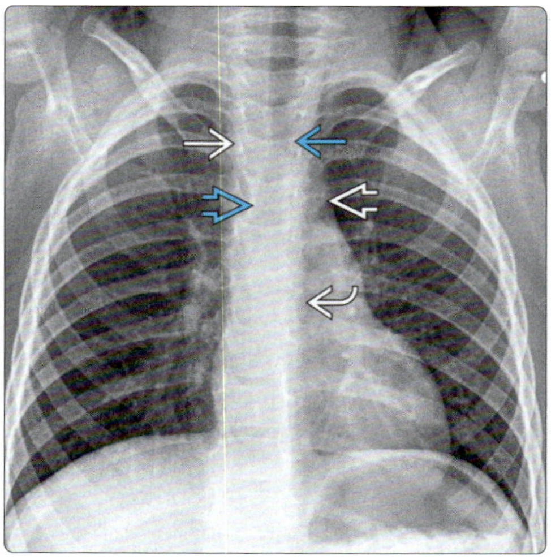

Double Aortic Arch

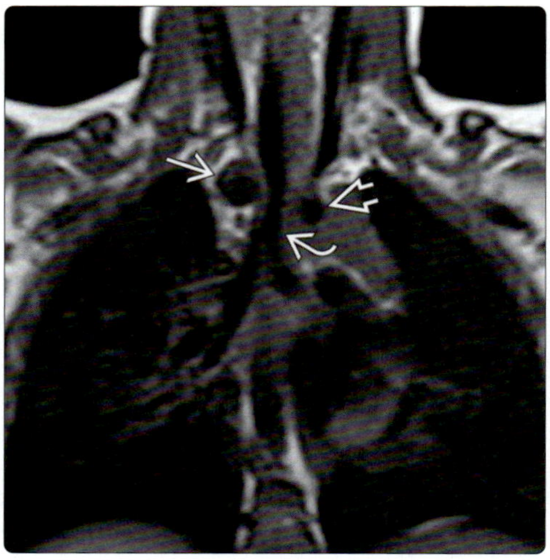

(Left) *Anterosuperior MRA 3D projection in the same patient shows the double aortic arch with a dominant right arch. The right common carotid, right subclavian, left common carotid, & left subclavian arteries arise symmetrically.* **(Right)** *Frontal (left) & lateral (right) esophagram images in a 10 week old show impressions on the esophagus by a dominant superior right arch & smaller lower left arch as well as a rounded posterior impression. The findings are consistent with a double aortic arch.*

Double Aortic Arch

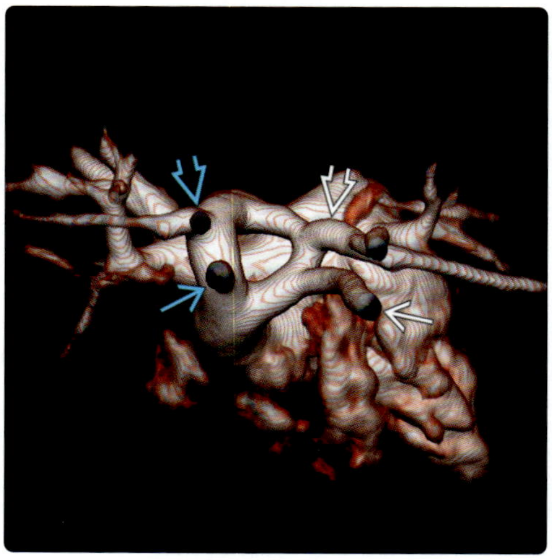

Double Aortic Arch

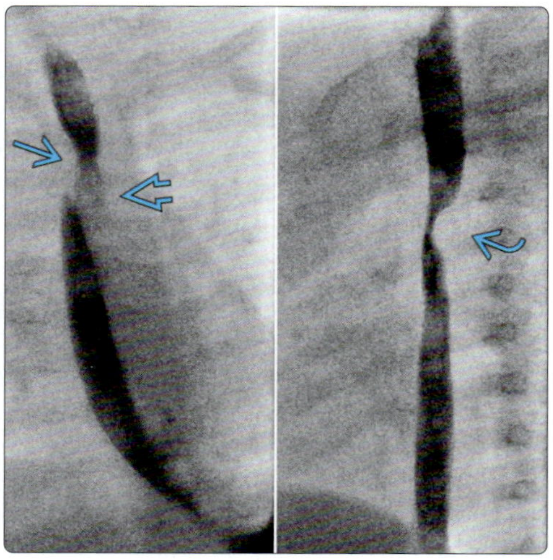

(Left) *Axial T1 MR in the same patient shows a dominant right arch & hypoplastic left arch. Both arches are posteriorly directed, encircling & narrowing the trachea.* **(Right)** *Coronal MR SSFP cine image in the same patient shows the right & left limbs of the double arch joining to continue as the descending aorta. There is focal stenosis of the distal left limb at the site of the ligamentum arteriosum.*

Double Aortic Arch

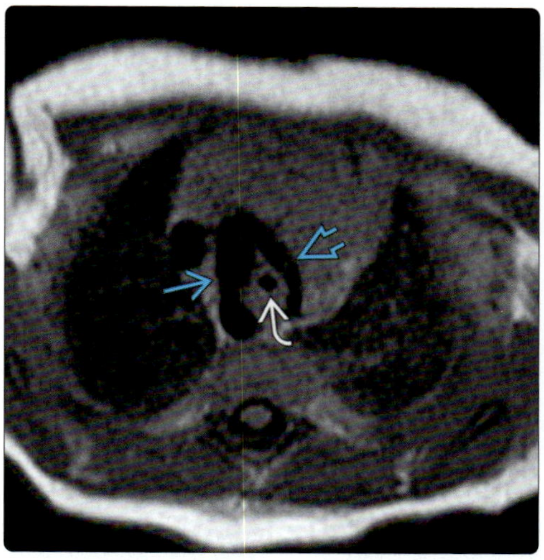

Double Aortic Arch

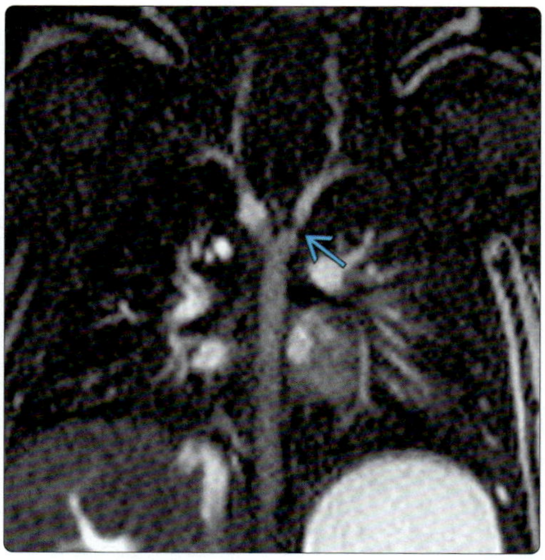

Right Aortic Arch With Aberrant Left Subclavian Artery

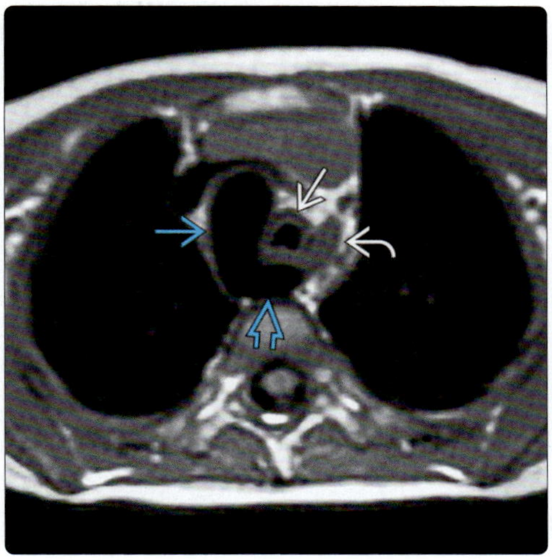

Right Aortic Arch With Aberrant Left Subclavian Artery

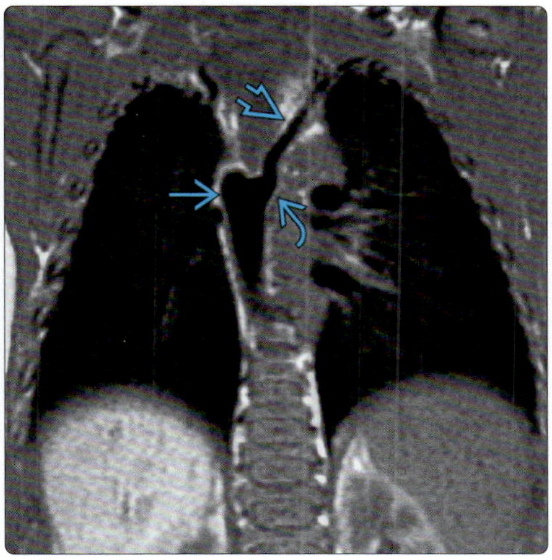

(Left) *Axial T1 MR shows a right-sided aortic arch & diverticulum of Kommerell, which gives rise to the aberrant left subclavian artery & passes posterior to the trachea & esophagus.* **(Right)** *Coronal T1 MR in the same patient shows a right-sided aortic arch with an aberrant left subclavian artery arising from a diverticulum of Kommerell.*

Right Aortic Arch With Aberrant Left Subclavian Artery

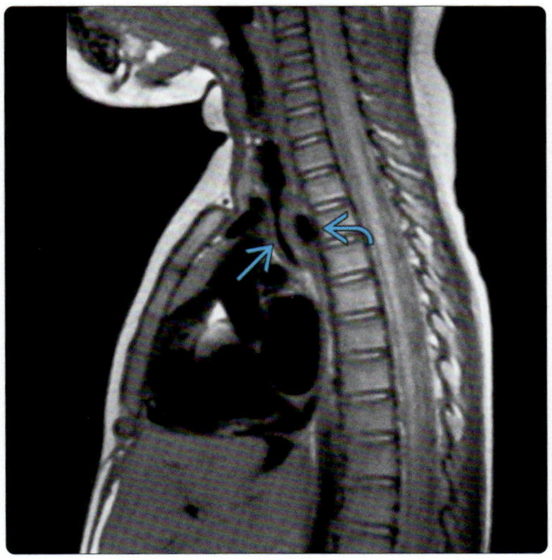

Right Aortic Arch With Aberrant Left Subclavian Artery

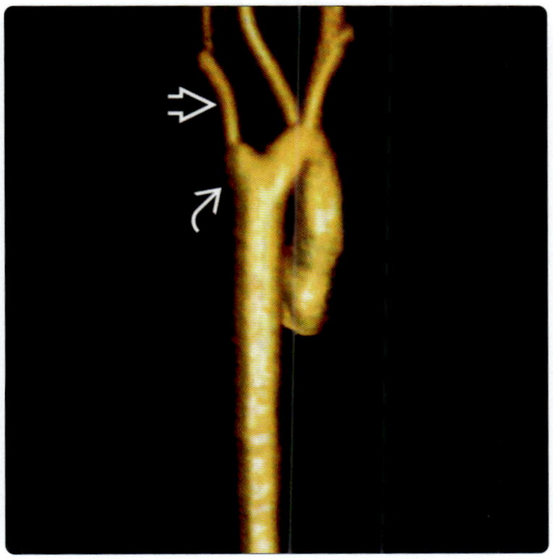

(Left) *Sagittal T1 MR shows a prominent diverticulum of Kommerell passing posterior to the trachea. There is a significant caliber change of the trachea as it courses anterior to the diverticulum.* **(Right)** *Posterior MRA 3D reconstruction in the same patient shows the prominent diverticulum of Kommerell giving rise to the aberrant left subclavian artery. A vascular ring is completed by a left-sided ligamentum arteriosum (not seen). The diverticulum itself also contributes to the symptoms.*

Right Aortic Arch With Mirror-Image Branching

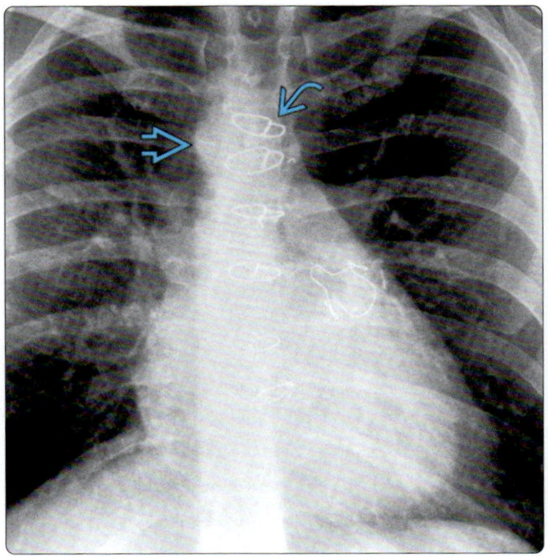

Right Aortic Arch With Mirror-Image Branching

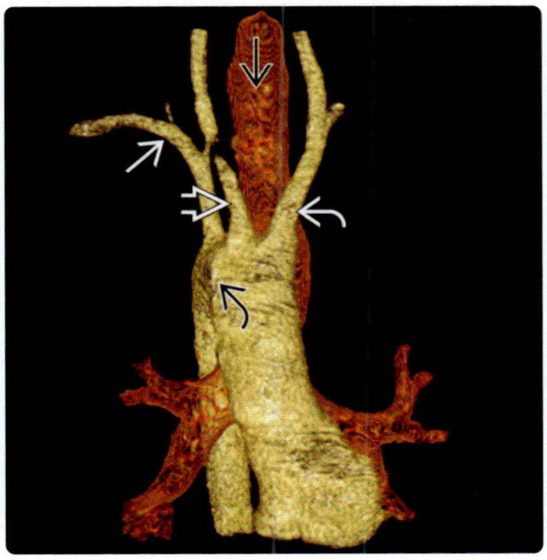

(Left) *PA radiograph shows a right arch displacing the trachea to the left. Note the evidence of prior cardiac surgery. There is a high correlation of right aortic arch mirror-image branching with congenital heart disease.* **(Right)** *Frontal 3D CTA reconstruction in the same patient shows the arch passing to the right of the trachea & descending on the right. The great vessels arise in the order of the left brachiocephalic artery, right common carotid artery, & finally the right subclavian artery.*

Right Aortic Arch With Mirror-Image Branching

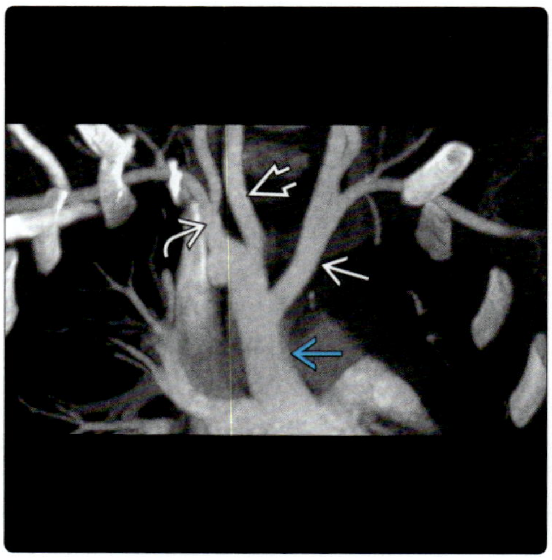

Cervical Aortic Arch

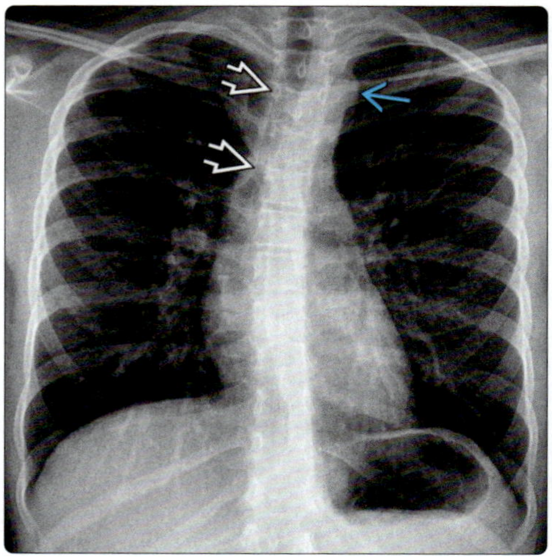

(Left) *Coronal CTA MIP shows a right aortic arch that descends on the right. The left brachiocephalic, right common carotid, & left subclavian arteries arise in a mirror-image pattern of a normal left arch. This patient also had tetralogy of Fallot.* **(Right)** *PA radiograph in a 13-year-old girl shows a left aortic arch extending above the medial aspect of the clavicles before descending on the left. There is long segment deviation of the trachea to the right.*

Cervical Aortic Arch

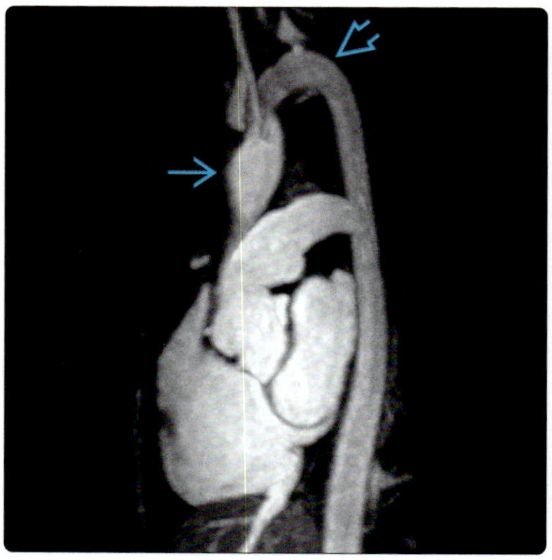

Cervical Aortic Arch

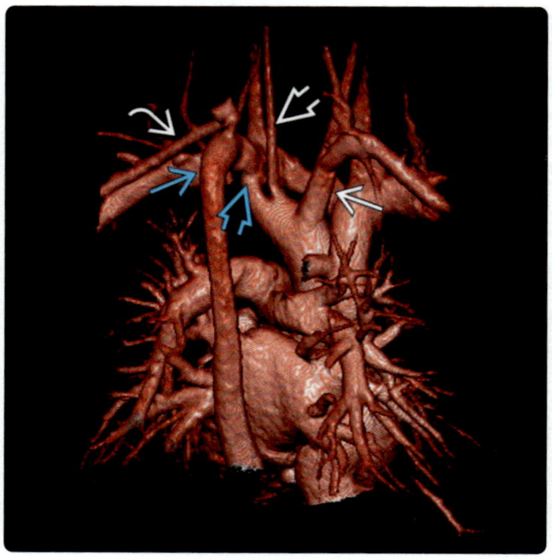

(Left) *Sagittal oblique MRA MIP in the same patient shows a tortuous ascending aorta with its apex at the midcervical level, consistent with a cervical left aortic arch.* **(Right)** *Posterior oblique MRA 3D projection in the same patient shows the cervical left aortic arch with abrupt superior angulation of the ascending aorta, which is common in this entity. There is a normal branching order of the right brachiocephalic, left common carotid, & left subclavian arteries.*

Cervical Aortic Arch

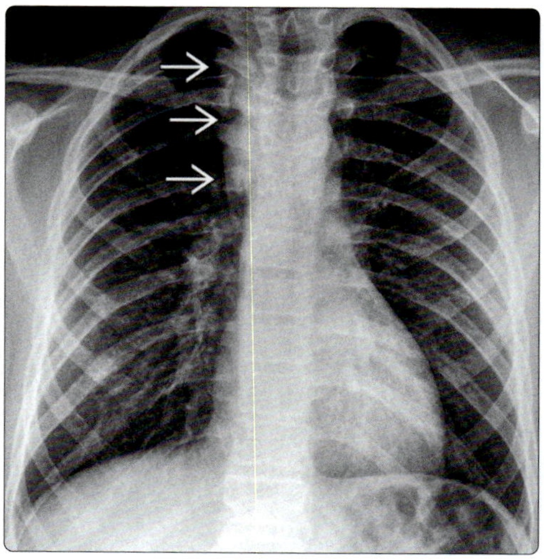

Cervical Aortic Arch

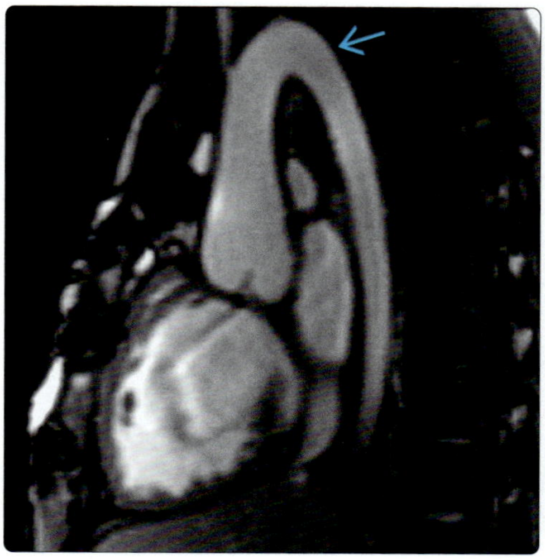

(Left) *PA radiograph shows a soft tissue density extending above the level of the clavicle into the superior mediastinum on the right. A cervical arch is more often right sided.* **(Right)** *Sagittal SSFP on MR shows a right-sided cervical arch that extends above the medial aspect of the clavicles.*

Circumflex Aortic Arch

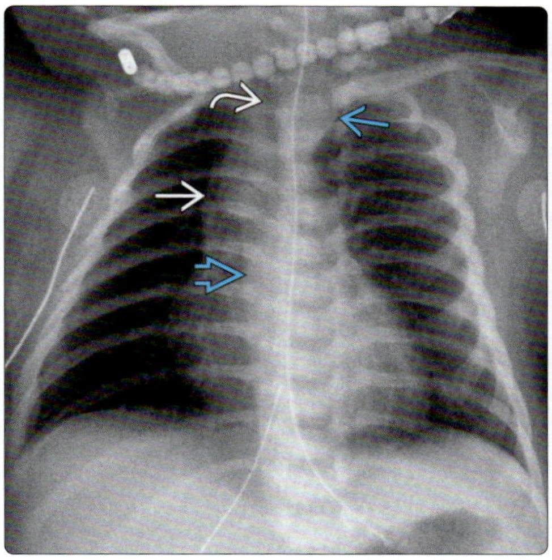

Circumflex Aortic Arch

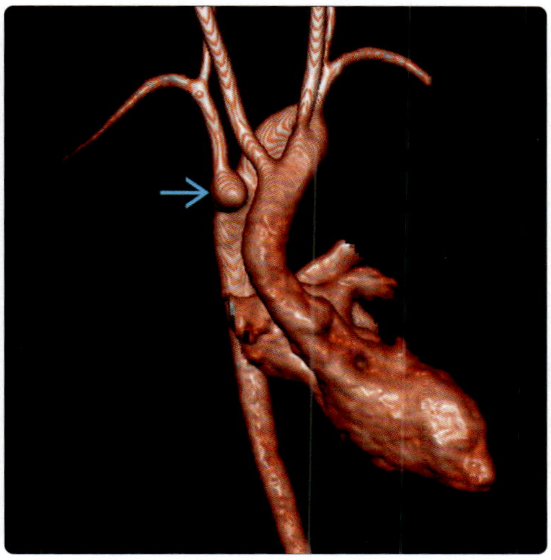

(Left) *AP radiograph in a 1-day-old girl with stridor shows a left arch → extending to the clavicular level, causing impression on the trachea →, with a tortuous ascending aorta → & right-sided descending aorta →. When the arch & descending aorta are on opposite sides, a vascular ring must be suspected.* **(Right)** *Anterior MRA 3D projection in the same patient at 6 years of age shows a left cervical & circumflex arch. Note also an aberrant right subclavian artery & diverticulum of Kommerell →.*

Isolated Subclavian Artery

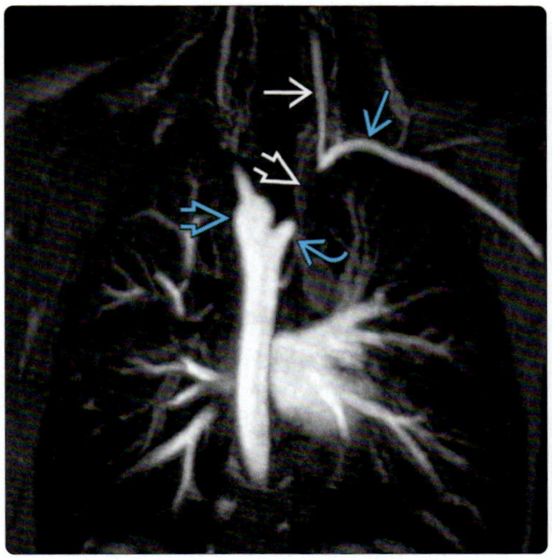

Isolated Subclavian Artery

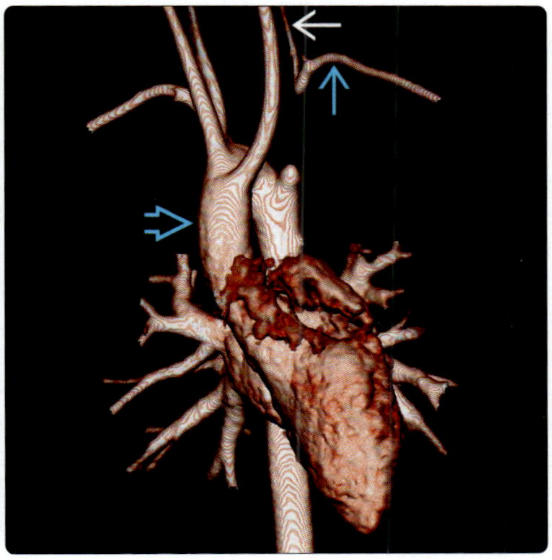

(Left) *Coronal MRA MIP in an 11-year-old girl shows a right aortic arch → with an isolated aberrant left subclavian artery → supplied retrograde via the left vertebral artery →. Note the apparent gap → between the aberrant left subclavian artery & diverticulum of Kommerell →.* **(Right)** *Anterior oblique MRA 3D projection in the same patient similarly shows a right aortic arch → with an isolated aberrant left subclavian artery → supplied retrograde via the left vertebral artery →.*

Persistent 5th Arch

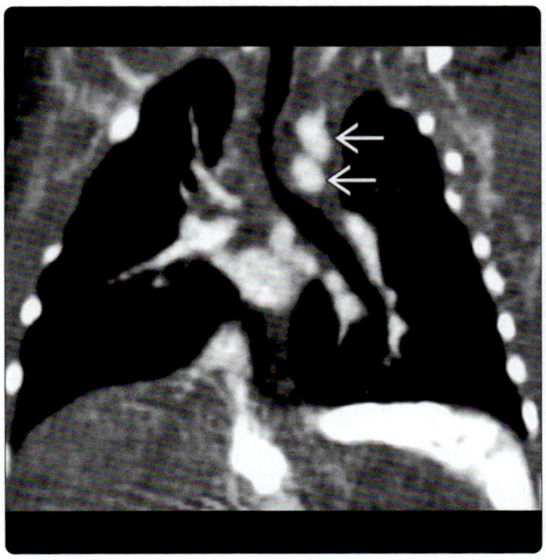

Persistent 5th Arch

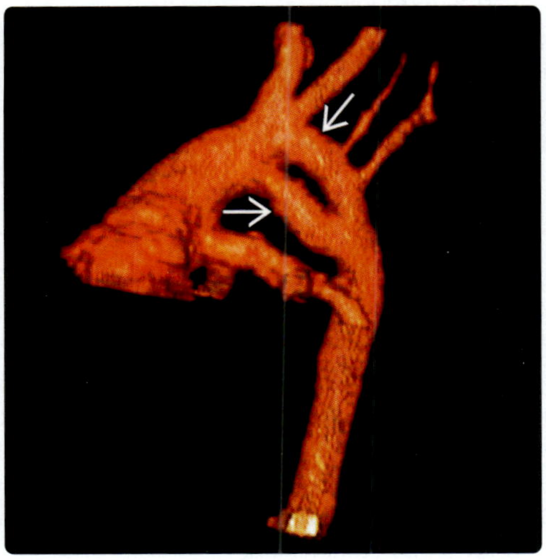

(Left) *Coronal CECT shows 2 aortic arches → to the left of the trachea, which have a superior-inferior relationship.* **(Right)** *Sagittal oblique CECT 3D reconstruction shows 2 aortic arches on the same side with a superior-inferior relationship →, consistent with the systemic-to-systemic type of persistent 5th arch. The superior arch can be obstructed by interruption or coarctation.*

Obstructive Aortic Arch Lesions

DIFFERENTIAL DIAGNOSIS

Common

- Aortic Coarctation
- Tubular Hypoplasia

Less Common

- Interrupted Aortic Arch

Rare but Important

- Aortic Atresia
- Persistent 5th Arch

ESSENTIAL INFORMATION

Key Differential Diagnosis Issues

- **Etiology of Obstructive Aortic Arch Lesions**
  - 3 proposed theories
    - Abnormal extension of contractile ductal tissue circumferentially around juxtaductal aorta creates coarctation when duct closes
    - Underlying left-sided obstructive intracardiac lesions cause decreased flow in aorta, especially at isthmus, causing decreased growth
    - Alterations in embryologic migration & growth of left 4th branchial arch (which forms distal aortic arch) & 7th intersegmental artery (which forms left subclavian artery), resulting in interrupted segments
  - Many cases likely represent interplay between all
  - Knowledge of proposed etiologies can explain morphology & help work out diagnosis in complex cases
- **Coarctation vs. Tubular Hypoplasia**
  - Coarctation: Focal narrowing near insertion of ductus arteriosus, often with proximal tapering of arch
  - Tubular hypoplasia: Diffuse uniform narrowing of arch, often with left ventricular (LV) outflow tract obstruction due to posterior malalignment of infundibular septum
  - May be seen together in complex congenital heart disease (CHD) or "'infantile" coarctation
- **Management Considerations**
  - Exact morphology influences choice between transcatheter vs. surgical treatment options
  - Conventional treatment for native obstruction is surgical repair, although there are evolving indications for transcatheter interventions
    - Choice ultimately depends on local institutional experience
  - Preferred surgical repair is end-to-end or extended end-to-end anastomosis
    - Patch augmentation may be required for tubular hypoplasia
  - Percutaneous balloon angioplasty is preferred option for restenosis
  - Percutaneous balloon angioplasty can also bridge to surgery in critically ill neonates who otherwise have increased surgical risk
  - Stent placement can be considered in larger children
  - Presence of tubular hypoplasia (vs. coarctation alone) may limit transcatheter possibilities

Helpful Clues for Common Diagnoses

- **Aortic Coarctation**
  - Focal shelf-like narrowing of thoracic aorta near insertion of ductus arteriosus distal to subclavian artery
  - Main etiology usually related to contractile ductal tissue extending circumferentially around juxtaductal aorta
  - Infants
    - Severe obstruction; presents early after ductus closes
      - Patent ductus allows blood to bypass coarctation
    - Moderate to marked cardiomegaly with congestive heart failure at ~ 1 week of life → strongly suggestive of coarctation
      - LV failure with enlargement of left atrium (LA), LV, & right ventricle (RV)
      - Pulmonary overcirculation with pulmonary hypertension & edema
      - Aorta is normal or small (no figure-of-3 sign)
      - No collaterals (therefore no rib notching)
    - Often associated with other CHDs that decrease antegrade flow through ascending aorta & increase right to left flow through patent ductus arteriosus (PDA)
      - Ventricular septal defects (VSDs)
      - Left-sided obstructive lesions (e.g., subaortic stenosis, mitral valve anomalies)
  - Children & adolescents
    - Milder degree of obstruction; presents later
      - Asymptomatic hypertension with arm-leg pressure differential
      - Absent or diminished lower extremity pulses
      - Leg discomfort on exertion
      - Incidental murmur
    - Development of collaterals from subclavian to intercostal arteries, bypassing coarctation
      - Rib notching: Rare in children < 7 years of age; arises from pressure erosion of intercostal collaterals along undersurface of 4th-8th ribs (1st-3rd ribs not involved as those intercostals arise above level of coarctation)
      - Rare: Aberrant right subclavian artery distal to coarctation leads to unilateral left-sided rib notching only
      - Dilated tortuous internal mammary arteries may cause scalloping of retrosternal soft tissues
    - Normal pulmonary vascularity & heart size, with possible prominent cardiac apex (LV hypertrophy)
    - Figure-of-3 sign: 3 components
      - Upper convexity of prominent aortic arch contour from prestenotic dilation
      - Central indentation from coarctation
      - Poststenotic dilation of descending thoracic aorta
    - Ascending aorta may be dilated when there is associated bicuspid aortic valve
  - Associations: Bicuspid aortic valve, Turner syndrome, circle of Willis berry aneurysms, PHACE syndrome
- **Tubular Hypoplasia**
  - Usually in infants
  - Diffuse uniform narrowing of arch & isthmus
  - Frequently occurs with coarctation but can be in isolation
  - Main etiology is usually related to decreased flow & thus growth

- Often associated with other lesions that decrease antegrade aortic flow, such as LV outflow tract obstruction
- Consider if arch diameter < 50% of ascending aorta or < 60% of descending aorta at diaphragm (assuming reference segments are normal)
  - Z-scores from age-matched controls also available
- Presence of tubular hypoplasia (vs. coarctation alone) affects surgical planning & may limit transcatheter possibilities

Helpful Clues for Less Common Diagnoses

- **Interrupted Aortic Arch**
  - Absent aortic arch segment of variable length
    - Complete discontinuity between ascending & descending aorta
    - Blood supply to descending aorta requires PDA
  - Main etiology is usually attributed to altered embryologic migration & growth of left 4th branchial arch (forms distal aortic arch) & 7th intersegmental artery (forms left subclavian artery)
  - 3 types
    - Type A (40%): Interruption distal to left subclavian artery, similar to coarctation
    - Type B (50-60%): Interruption between left carotid & left subclavian arteries
      - Often associated with intracardiac conotruncal anomaly causing subaortic obstruction & decreased ascending aortic flow
      - Commonly with 22q11.2 deletion syndrome & right aortic arch
    - Type C (5%): Interruption between brachiocephalic & left carotid arteries
  - VSD & PDA arealmost always present
  - Can have aberrant right subclavian artery distal to interruption
  - Other associations: Bicuspid aortic valve, mitral valve dysplasia, subaortic stenosis, truncus arteriosus, transposition of great arteries, aortopulmonary window, double-outlet RV

Helpful Clues for Rare Diagnoses

- **Aortic Atresia**
  - Imperforate fibrous strand of variable length
    - Aortic continuity maintained by fibrous cord
  - Typically occurs at ascending aorta or isthmus but any segment of aorta can be involved
- **Persistent 5th Arch**
  - a.k.a. ipsilateral double aortic arch, double lumen, or duplicated aortic arch
  - Extrapericardial vessel arising from ascending aorta proximal or opposite to brachiocephalic artery origin
  - Systemic-to-systemic type: Distal connection to dorsal aorta
    - 2 aortic arches on same side with superior-inferior relationship (double-barrel sign)
    - Often associated with coarctation or interruption of superior arch
    - May have different embryologic precursor (dorsal collateral) than systemic-to-pulmonary type
  - Systemic-to-pulmonary type: Distal connection to 6th aortic arch remnant (typically left pulmonary artery)

SELECTED REFERENCES

1. Hanneman K et al: Congenital variants and anomalies of the aortic arch. Radiographics. 37(1):32-51, 2017
2. Forbes TJ et al: Comparison of surgical, stent, and balloon angioplasty treatment of native coarctation of the aorta: an observational study by the CCISC (Congenital Cardiovascular Interventional Study Consortium). J Am Coll Cardiol. 58(25):2664-74, 2011
3. Matsui H et al: Anatomy of coarctation, hypoplastic and interrupted aortic arch: relevance to interventional/surgical treatment. Expert Rev Cardiovasc Ther. 5(5):871-80, 2007
4. Rigsby CK et al: Left Heart Lesions. In: Coley BD (ed). Caffey's Pediatric Diagnostic Imaging (12th edition), pp. 751-60, Philadelphia, PA: Elsevier Saunders, 2013
5. Epelman, M: Obstructive Lesions of the Aortic Arch. In: Yoo SJ, MacDonald C, Babyn P (eds). Chest Radiographic Interpretation in Pediatric Cardiac Patients, pp. 229-33, New York, NY: Thieme Medical Publishers. 2010

Aortic Coarctation

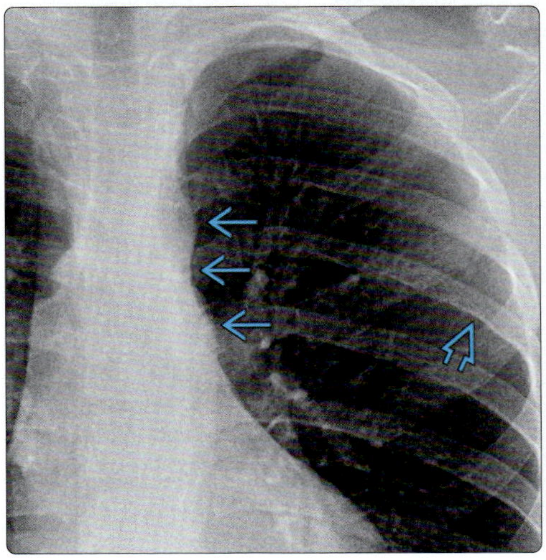

Aortic Coarctation

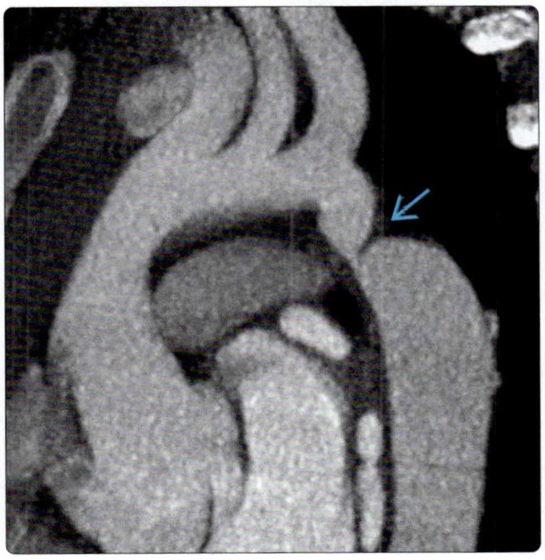

(Left) *PA radiograph in a 10-year-old boy with systemic hypertension shows a figure-of-3 sign ➡, consistent with aortic coarctation. There are foci of rib-notching along the undersurface of the ribs ➡ from intercostal collaterals feeding the descending aorta distal to the coarctation. Rib notching is typically not present in the first 3 ribs as these are proximal to the coarctation.* **(Right)** *Sagittal oblique CTA MIP in the same patient shows severe juxtaductal narrowing ➡ due to a posterior shelf, typical of coarctation.*

Aortic Coarctation

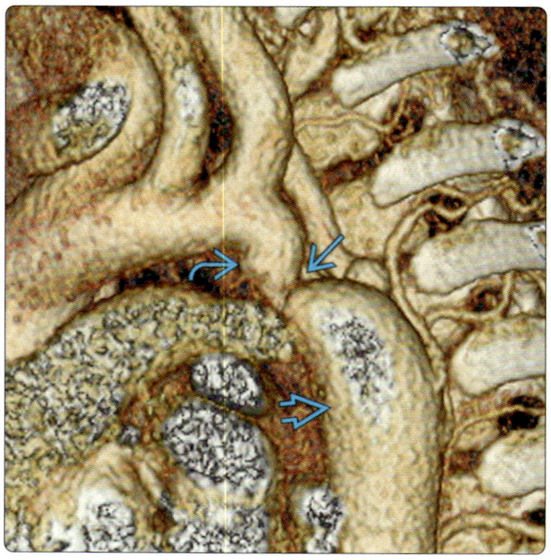

Aortic Coarctation

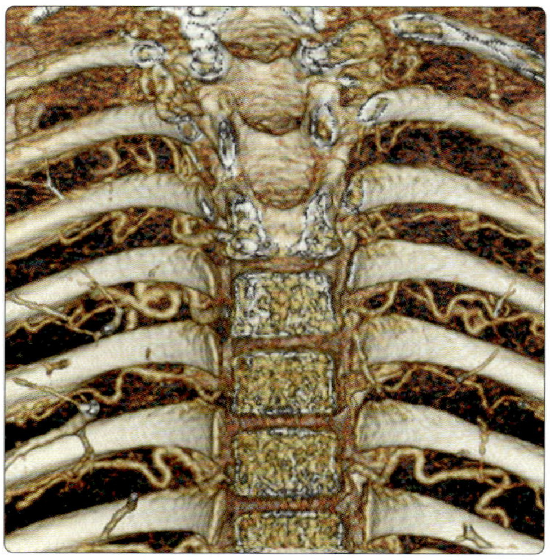

(Left) *Sagittal oblique CTA 3D projection in the same patient again shows the severe coarctation . Note mild associated tubular hypoplasia of the aortic arch along with poststenotic dilation of the descending aorta. Elongation & tortuosity of the isthmus can also be present.* **(Right)** *Coronal CTA 3D projection in the same patient shows the dilated & tortuous intercostal collaterals underlying the bilateral 4th & lower ribs.*

Tubular Hypoplasia

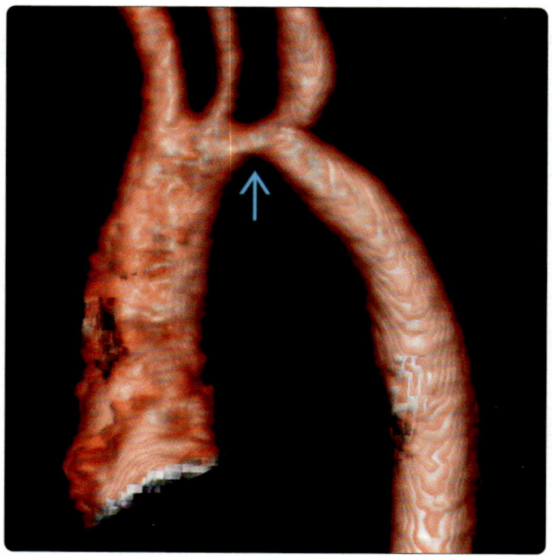

Tubular Hypoplasia

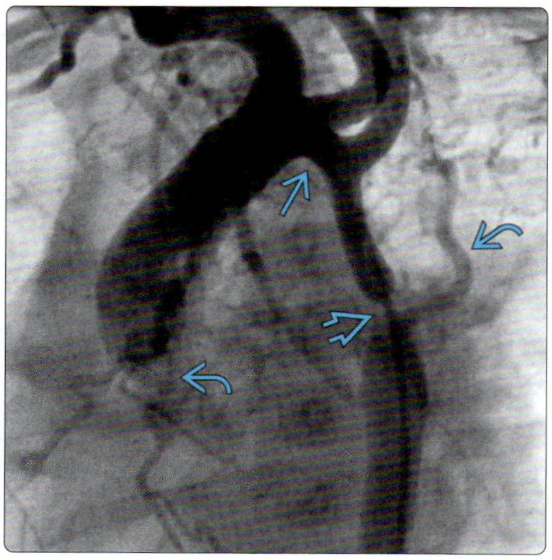

(Left) *Sagittal oblique MRA 3D projection in a 10- year-old boy with a murmur shows a short-segment uniform narrowing of the transverse arch without discrete stenosis, consistent with tubular hypoplasia of the aortic arch without coarctation.* **(Right)** *Sagittal oblique catheter angiogram in a 4-month-old boy with pallor, tachypnea, & respiratory impairment shows a severe coarctation along with tubular hypoplasia of an elongated & tortuous aortic arch/isthmus . Note the prominent collaterals .*

Interrupted Aortic Arch

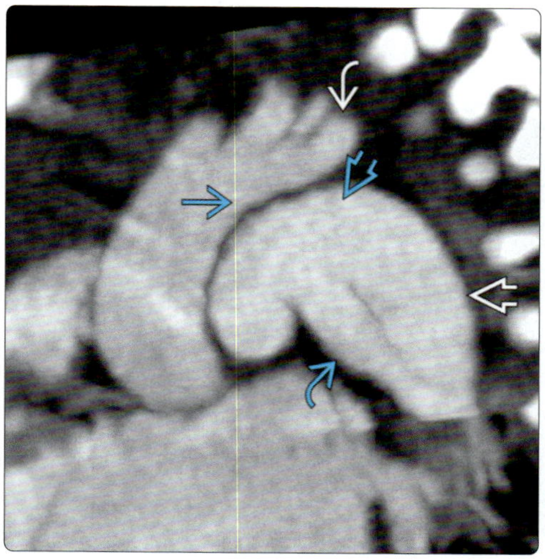

Interrupted Aortic Arch

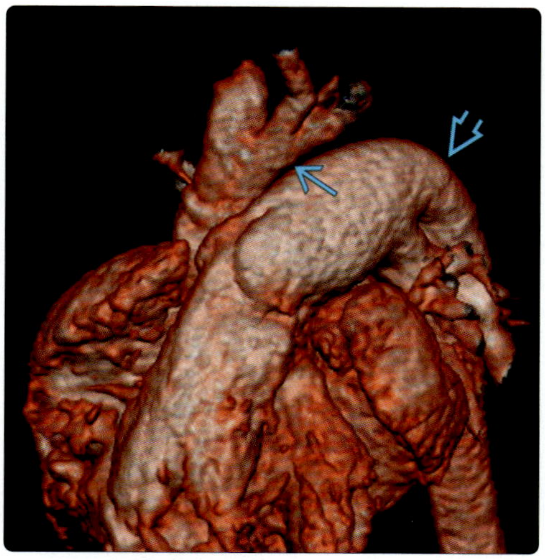

(Left) *Sagittal oblique CTA MIP in a 1-day-old girl shows discontinuity of the aorta distal to left subclavian artery , consistent with an interrupted aortic arch type A. The descending aorta is supplied by a large patent ductus arteriosus (PDA) . Note the left pulmonary artery .* **(Right)** *CTA 3D projection in the same patient shows the interrupted aortic arch with a large PDA supplying the descending aorta . This patient had other intracardiac left-sided obstructions, which are often seen in association with aortic obstructive lesions.*

Aortic Atresia

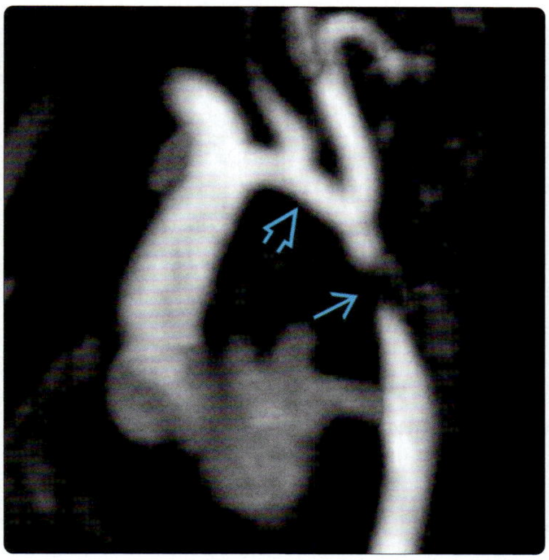

Aortic Atresia

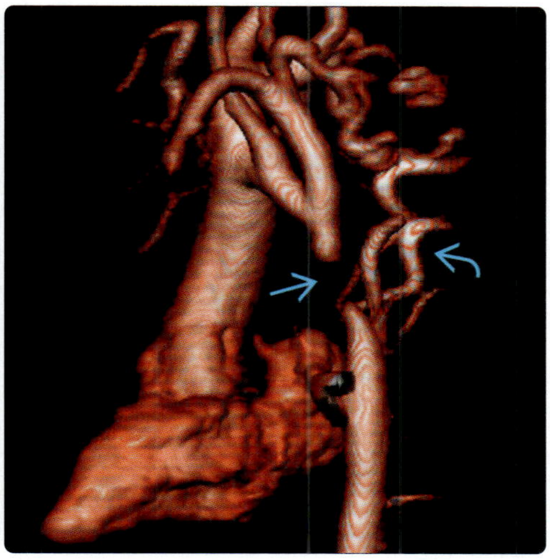

(Left) *Sagittal oblique MRA MIP in a 2-year-old girl with hypertension & an arm-leg blood pressure gradient shows lack of luminal opacification of a short segment of the proximal descending aorta, suspicious for aortic atresia, which was confirmed at surgery. There is also elongation & tubular hypoplasia of the aortic arch.* **(Right)** *Sagittal oblique MRA 3D projection in the same patient shows the proximal descending aorta obstruction with numerous bypassing collaterals.*

Persistent 5th Arch

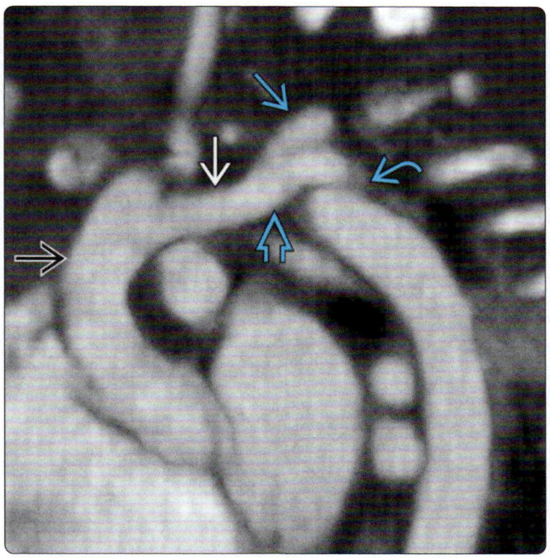

Persistent 5th Arch

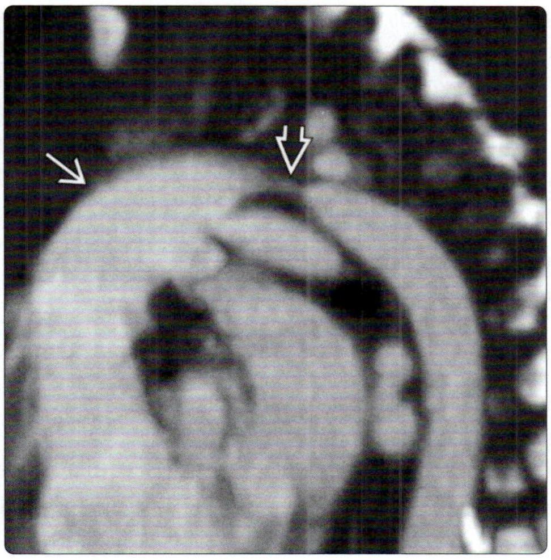

(Left) *Sagittal oblique CTA MIP in a 5-day-old syndromic boy shows a tortuous vessel arising from the ascending aorta, paralleling the main pulmonary artery (MPA) (not shown), & connecting to a distal arch, consistent with a persistent 5th arch. This gives rise to a left subclavian artery & shows focal juxtaductal narrowing like a coarctation.* **(Right)** *Sagittal oblique CTA MIP in the same patient shows the MPA & a tiny PDA. There was also an interrupted aortic arch (not shown).*

Persistent 5th Arch

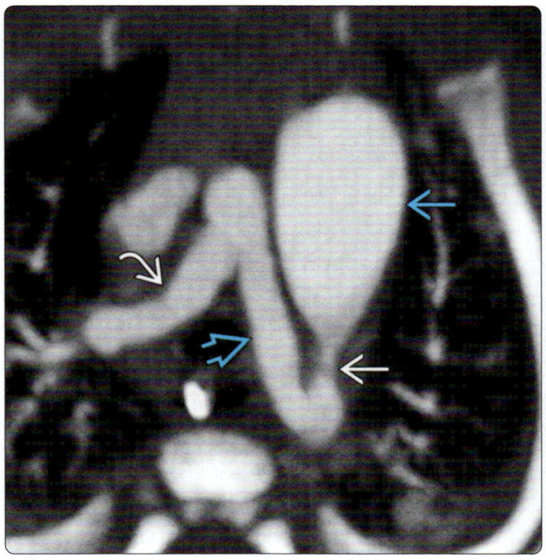

Persistent 5th Arch

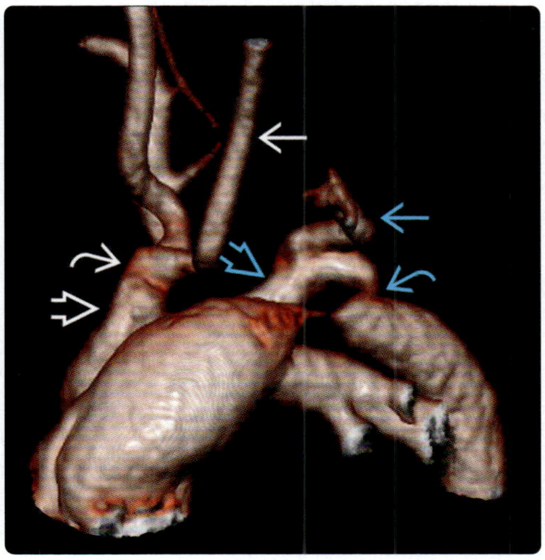

(Left) *Axial oblique CTA MIP in the same patient shows the persistent 5th arch & MPA at similar levels. The thread-like PDA & right brachiocephalic artery are also shown.* **(Right)** *CTA 3D projection in the same patient shows the interrupted aortic arch (type B) giving rise to the right brachiocephalic & left common carotid arteries. The persistent 5th arch arises from the ascending aorta & connects with the residual distal arch, which gives rise to the left subclavian artery & also has a discrete coarctation.*

DIFFERENTIAL DIAGNOSIS

Common

- Marfan Syndrome
- Bicuspid Aortic Valve
- Turner Syndrome

Less Common

- Ehlers-Danlos Syndrome
- Loeys-Dietz Syndrome

Rare but Important

- Trauma
- Mycotic Aneurysm
- Takayasu Arteritis
- Neurofibromatosis Type 1
- Tuberous Sclerosis Complex

ESSENTIAL INFORMATION

Key Differential Diagnosis Issues

- Genetic aortopathy underlies most pediatric aortic dilation
  - Genotyping is refining our understanding of syndromic & nonsyndromic aortopathies
- Connective tissue disorders are most common
  - Marfan syndrome (MFS)
  - Ehlers-Danlos syndrome (EDS)
  - Loeys-Dietz syndrome (LDS)
- Consider additional entities that also may exhibit connective tissue-like aortopathy
  - Bicuspid aortic valve (BAV)
  - Turner syndrome
  - Neurofibromatosis type 1 (NF1)
  - Tuberous sclerosis complex (TSC)
- Unlike adults, aortic dilation in children is less commonly acquired (such as from vasculitis, infection, or trauma)
- Congenital heart disease can also lead to aortic dilation (covered in other sections)

Helpful Clues for Common Diagnoses

- **Marfan Syndrome**
  - Autosomal dominant connective tissue disorder
  - Multisystem: Cardiovascular, ocular, & musculoskeletal; ± central nervous, pulmonary, dermatologic
  - Noncardiovascular features: Dural ectasia, ectopia lentis, pectus deformity, pes planus, scoliosis, protrusio acetabuli, arachnodactyly, bullae with pneumothorax
  - Cardiovascular manifestations: Dilation of aortic annulus, root, & ascending aorta
    - Effacement of sinotubular junction is classic description (tulip bulb appearance)
    - Risk for dissection
    - Dilation can also lead to aortic regurgitation
    - Can also get mitral valve prolapse, myocardial dysfunction; rarely pulmonary artery involvement
  - Death caused by aortic dissection, congestive heart failure, or valvular disease in > 90%
  - Indications for surgery in pediatric population are not well established; concerning features include
    - Severe aortic regurgitation
    - Dilation > 1 cm/year
    - Z-score > 3
- **Bicuspid Aortic Valve**
  - Most common cause of aortic stenosis & regurgitation
  - Typical morphology is nonseparation of 2 cusps of tricuspid aortic valve (rarely true bicuspid valve)
    - Conjoined right & left coronary cusps (70-80%)
    - Conjoined right & noncoronary cusps (15-25%)
    - Conjoined left & noncoronary cusps (< 5%)
  - Aortic root dilation is common
    - Morphology of cusp fusion & poststenotic flow pattern predict ascending aorta shape & dilation, supportive of mechanical mechanism
      - If regurgitation is present, increased blood flow volume also leads to dilation
    - However, dilation is common, even when valve is hemodynamically normal, suggestive of concomitant intrinsic aortopathy
    - Lifetime risk of dissection is higher than non-BAV patients with similar sized aortic aneurysms
  - High association with aortic coarctation
- **Turner Syndrome**
  - Monosomy of X chromosome (45 XO)
  - Characteristic features include short stature, webbed neck, lymphedema
  - Noncardiovascular imaging features: Osteoporosis, cervical vertebral hypoplasia, scoliosis, genu valgum, short metacarpals & metatarsals, renal anomalies, & gonadal dysgenesis
    - ± lymphatic malformation on prenatal ultrasound
  - Cardiovascular anomalies: BAV, aortic coarctation, aortic root dilation, aortic arch elongation, bilateral superior vena cava, & partial anomalous pulmonary venous return
    - Elevated risk of dissection (mean age ~ 30 years old)
    - Predisposing risk factors for dissection: BAV, aortic dilation, coarctation, hypertension, pregnancy

Helpful Clues for Less Common Diagnoses

- **Ehlers-Danlos Syndrome**
  - Spectrum of genetic disorders with defective collagen synthesis characterized by articular hypermobility, skin extensibility, & tissue fragility
    - 13 subtypes grouped into 5 groups (A-E) by causative molecular pathway
    - General features: Acrogeria, thin translucent skin, ecchymoses & hematomas; arterial, digestive, & obstetric ruptures
    - Vascular EDS (5%): Most severe form, characterized by cardiovascular complications (rare in other types)
  - Cardiovascular manifestations
    - Thoracoabdominal medium & large vessels
      - Discrete fusiform aneurysms of descending/abdominal aorta, iliac & cervical arteries, & branch arteries
      - Distribution much different than MFS (which involves ascending aorta)
    - Marked vessel friability: Risk of vessel rupture or dissection regardless of diameter
    - Minor trauma can lead to arteriovenous fistulas or pseudoaneurysms
  - Because of vessel wall friability, catheter or surgical intervention can be complicated by new aneurysms, rupture, or dissection

- **Loeys-Dietz Syndrome**
  - Autosomal dominant connective tissue disorder with dysregulation of TGF-β
  - Craniofacial features: Bifid uvula, cleft palate, hypertelorism, craniosynostosis, cervical spine instability
  - Also: Dural ectasia, joint laxity, scoliosis, pectus deformity
  - Vascular features: Arterial aneurysms & tortuosity with risk of dissection & rupture
  - Clinical overlap with MFS
    - LDS is more aggressive with abnormalities at younger age & faster progression
    - Aneurysms occur beyond aortic root (i.e., head & neck vessels, descending aorta, abdominal aorta)
    - LDS has higher risk of dissection & rupture (like vascular EDS but at smaller size & younger than MFS)
    - Look for arterial tortuosity, especially in head & neck
      - Vertebral tortuosity index is 1 imaging biomarker for cardiovascular prognosis in LDS
      - Differential: Arterial tortuosity syndrome
  - Lower threshold for surgery than MFS

Helpful Clues for Rare Diagnoses

- **Trauma**
  - Traumatic aortic injuries are uncommon in children
    - Iatrogenic dissection is most common
  - Imaging features of blunt thoracic aortic injury
    - Widened mediastinum on radiograph, ± rib fractures, left pleural effusion, apical cap, loss of aortic contour
    - 90% at aortic isthmus
      - Pseudoaneurysm
      - Intimal flap
      - Focal contour abnormality/sudden caliber change
      - Periaortic hematoma ± active extravasation
- **Mycotic Aneurysm**
  - Uncommon in children
  - Irregular, eccentric, &/or saccular aneurysm in unusual location with associated wall thickening/inflammation
  - Can occur in infants from umbilical arterial catheter
- **Takayasu Arteritis**
  - Chronic idiopathic granulomatous large vessel vasculitis
  - Predominately of aorta & main branches
  - Vessel wall inflammation, vascular stenosis (90%), mural thrombus, complete occlusion (30%), aneurysm (15%), & dissection (10%)
  - Childhood Takayasu has high morbidity & mortality
    - Greater involvement of abdominal aorta
    - Hypertension in > 80% of pediatric patients
    - Diminished pulses with lower limb claudication in 10-35% of children
  - MR for angiography & vessel wall imaging
    - Active inflammation: Wall thickening, edema, & hyperenhancement
- **Neurofibromatosis Type 1**
  - Autosomal dominant
  - Characteristic features: Café au lait macules, dermal neurofibromas, plexiform neurofibromas, & iris hamartomas
  - Vasculopathy is uncommon component of NF1
    - Medium & large vessels
    - Most common: Renal artery stenosis ± midaortic syndrome
    - Aneurysms & arteriovenous malformations can also occur
- **Tuberous Sclerosis Complex**
  - Autosomal dominant
  - Classic triad: Epilepsy, mental retardation, & adenoma sebaceum
  - Characterized by hamartomas of multiple organ systems
    - Cardiac rhabdomyomas & renal angiomyolipomas
  - Brain findings include subcortical tubers, subependymal nodules, & subependymal giant cell astrocytomas
  - Rare thoracic & abdominal aortic aneurysms

SELECTED REFERENCES

1. Zucker EJ: Syndromes with aortic involvement: pictorial review. Cardiovasc Diagn Ther. 8(Suppl 1):S71-81, 2018
2. Meester JAN et al: Differences in manifestations of Marfan syndrome, Ehlers-Danlos syndrome, and Loeys-Dietz syndrome. Ann Cardiothorac Surg. 6(6):582-94, 2017

Marfan Syndrome

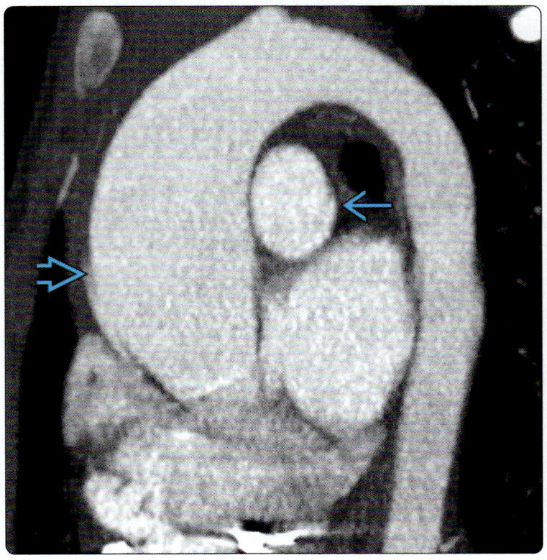

Marfan Syndrome

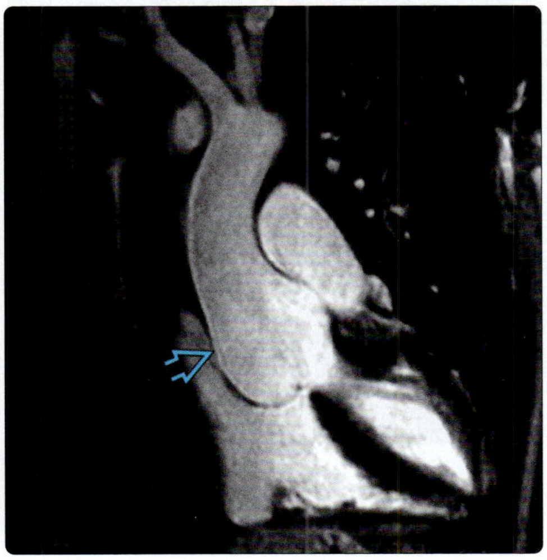

(Left) *Sagittal oblique CECT MIP in a 6 year old with Marfan syndrome shows marked dilation of the ascending aorta & aortic root* ➡ *with effacement of the sinotubular junction. The right pulmonary artery is also enlarged* ➡. **(Right)** *Coronal oblique MRA MIP in a 16-year-old boy with Marfan syndrome shows a dilated aortic root with effacement of the sinotubular junction* ➡, *creating the characteristic tulip bulb appearance. Aortic root dilation can lead to aortic valve regurgitation & increased risk for dissection.*

(Left) *Axial oblique GRE cine MR in a 15-year-old boy shows a thickened dysplastic bicuspid aortic valve with fusion of the right & left coronary cusps, creating a stenotic elliptical opening.* **(Right)** *Coronal oblique MRA MIP in the same patient shows ascending aortic dilation. Aortic dimensions must be monitored as patients with bicuspid aortic valve (BAV) have an increased risk of dissection compared to patients with a similar degree of aortic dilation but normal tricuspid aortic valves.*

Bicuspid Aortic Valve

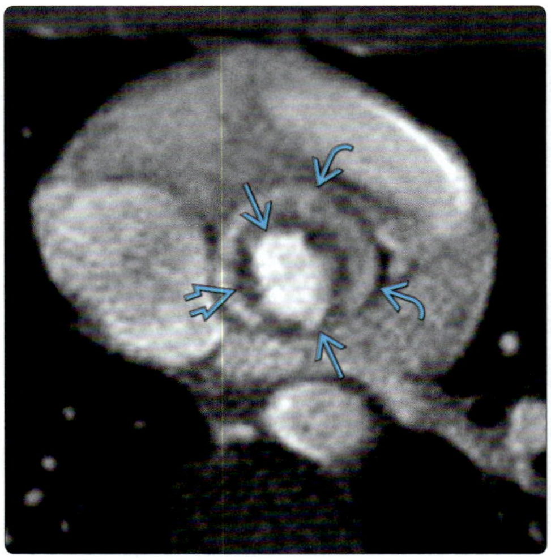

Bicuspid Aortic Valve

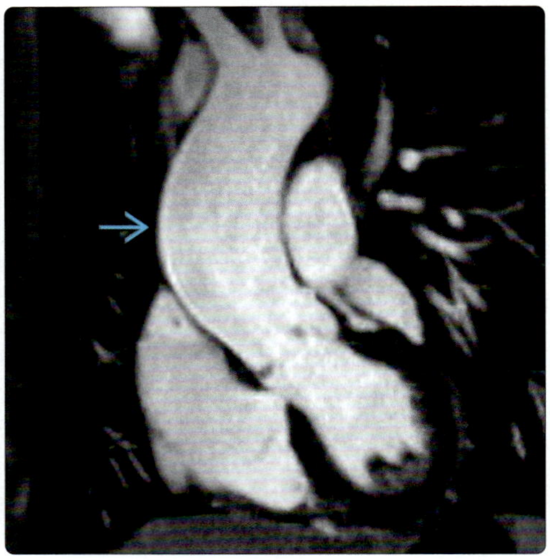

(Left) *Sagittal oblique black blood MR in a patient with Turner syndrome shows dilation of the ascending aorta & tubular hypoplasia of the aortic arch. BAV, aortic coarctation, & aortic dissection are the most common cardiovascular anomalies in Turner syndrome.* **(Right)** *Sagittal oblique SSFP MR in a patient with Turner syndrome shows dilation of the ascending aorta. Risk factors for dissection in Turner syndrome include hypertension, BAV, & coarctation.*

Turner Syndrome

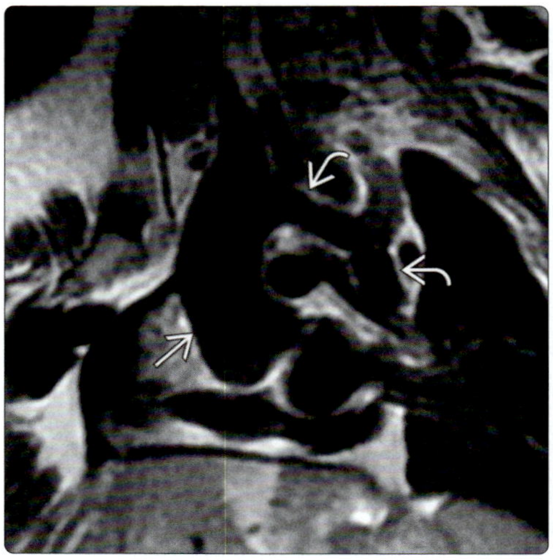

Turner Syndrome

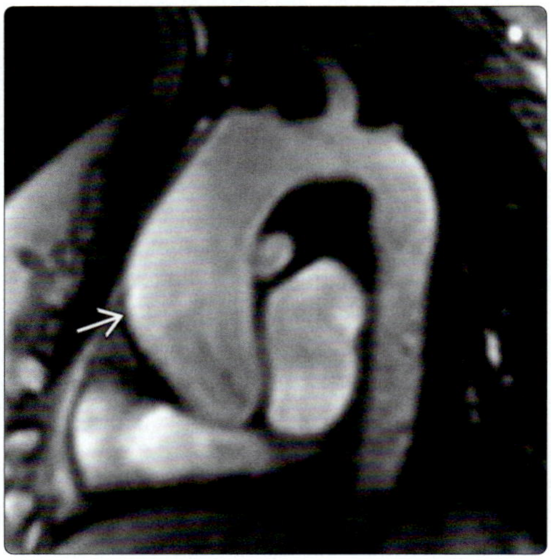

(Left) *Anterior oblique MRA 3D projection in a 15 year old with gene-confirmed vascular EDS shows a prominent ascending aorta. There is also increased tortuosity of the splenic artery. Tortuosity is more typical of LDS or arterial tortuosity syndrome.* **(Right)** *Axial NECT in a vascular EDS patient shows a hyperdense aortic wall, suspicious for intramural hematoma. Vascular EDS is associated with aneurysm, dissection, & arterial rupture, typically of the descending aorta or medium-sized vessels.*

Ehlers-Danlos Syndrome

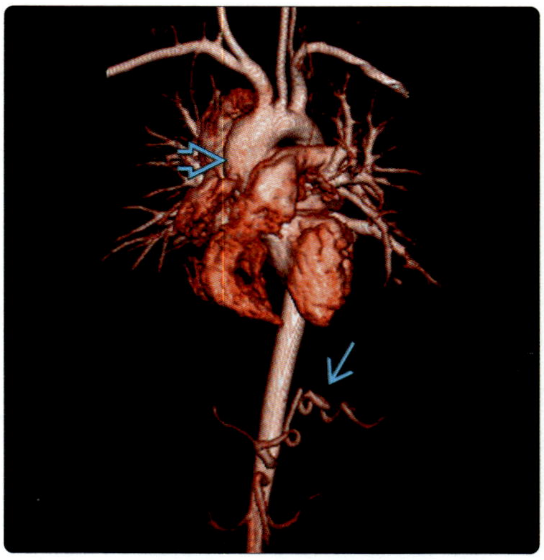

Ehlers-Danlos Syndrome

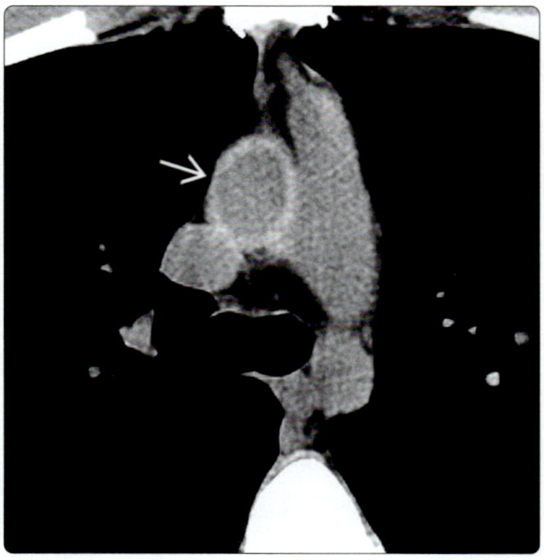

Loeys-Dietz Syndrome

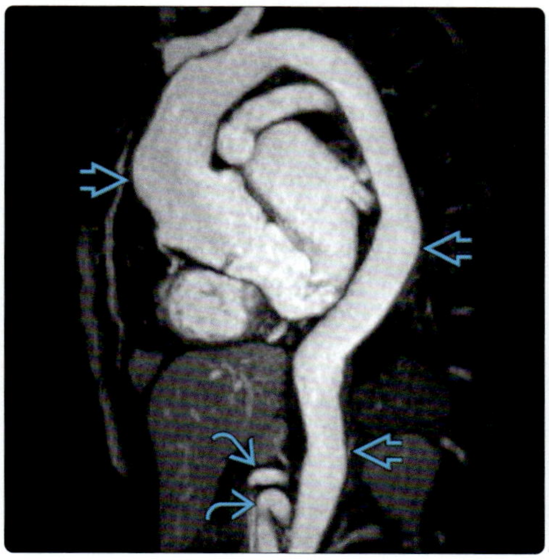

Loeys-Dietz Syndrome

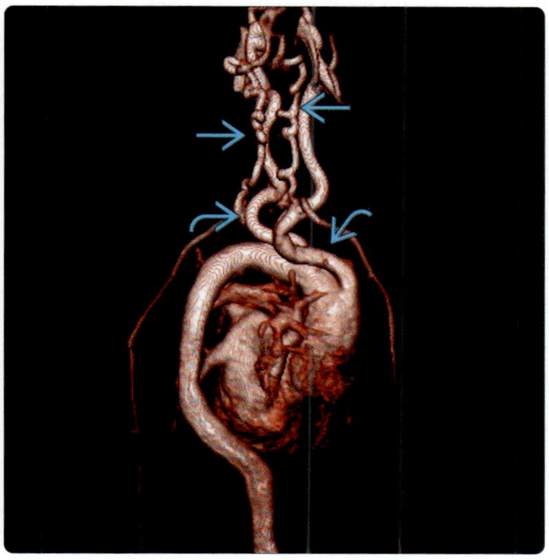

(Left) *Sagittal oblique MRA MIP in a 6 year old with LDS shows a markedly dilated & tortuous aorta. The splanchnic vessels are also dilated & tortuous.* **(Right)** *Posterior oblique MRA 3D projection in the same patient at 2 years earlier shows moderate tortuosity of the carotid arteries & the characteristic severe tortuosity of the vertebral arteries. The degree of vertebral tortuosity by imaging correlates with prognosis.*

Loeys-Dietz Syndrome

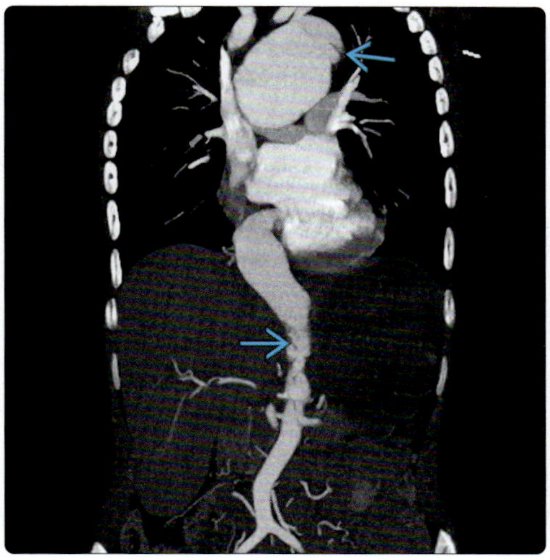

Loeys-Dietz Syndrome

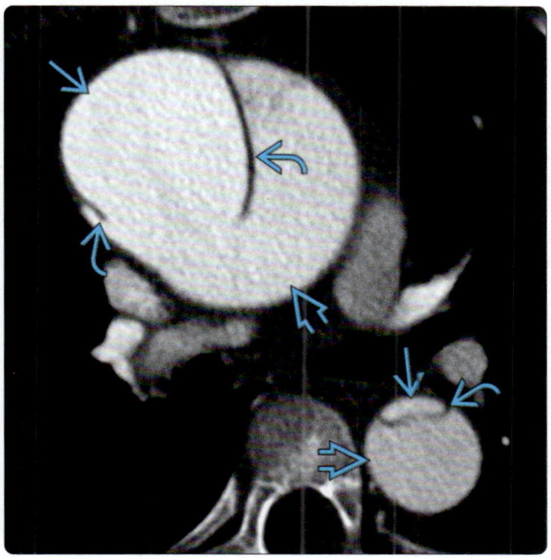

(Left) *Coronal CECT MIP in the same patient at 8 years old again shows a markedly dilated & tortuous aorta. There is now an acute dissection extending from the thoracic to abdominal aorta.* **(Right)** *Axial CECT in the same patient shows the site of aortic dissection in the ascending aorta with an intimal flap separating the smaller true lumen from the larger false lumen within the aortic wall. LDS patients have a high risk of aortic rupture or dissection.*

Loeys-Dietz Syndrome

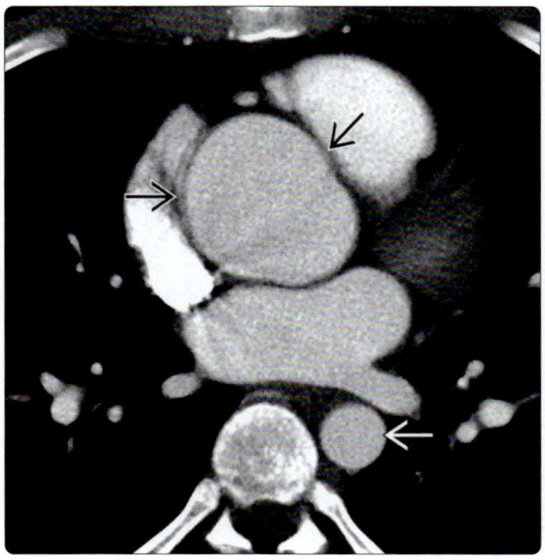

Loeys-Dietz Syndrome

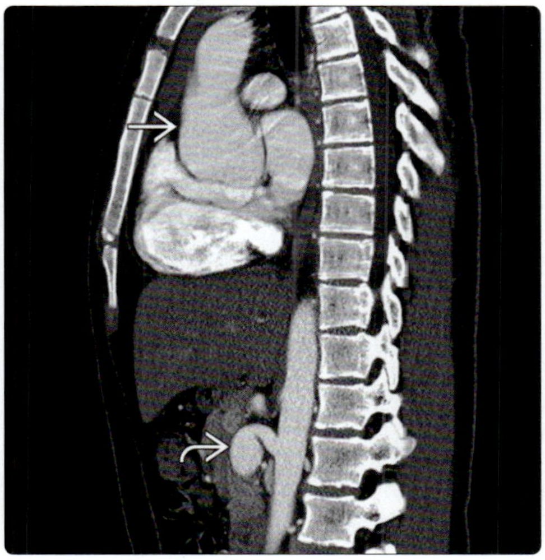

(Left) *Axial CECT in a patient with LDS shows marked dilation of the ascending aorta with a normal caliber descending aorta. LDS has craniofacial, musculoskeletal, & vascular anomalies. Other imaging features include dural ectasia, scoliosis, & pectus deformities.* **(Right)** *Sagittal CECT shows a markedly dilated ascending aorta along with aneurysm & tortuosity of the superior mesenteric artery. One of the main imaging differentials for tortuous arteries in infants & young children is arterial tortuosity syndrome.*

(Left) *AP radiograph in a 12 year old in a motor vehicle collision shows a widened mediastinum with rightward deviation of the trachea & esophagus, worrisome for aortic injury.* **(Right)** *Axial CECT in the same patient shows the typical appearance & location of a traumatic pseudoaneurysm at the aortic isthmus. The native lumen is posterior. There is periaortic hematoma & a small left hemothorax. Mortality is higher for thoracic aortic injury patients when the aortic contour is abnormal, as in this case.*

Trauma

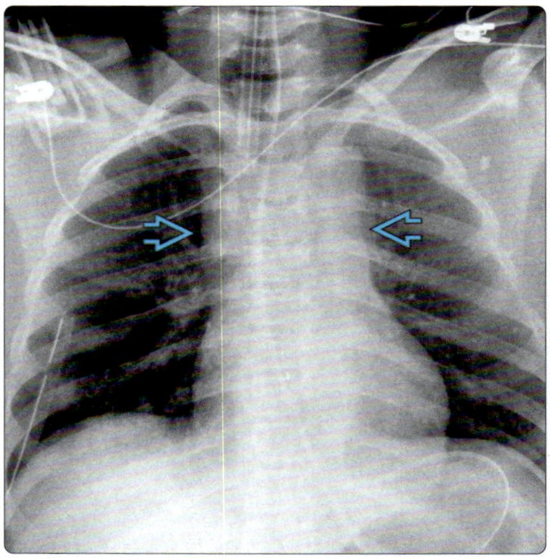

Trauma

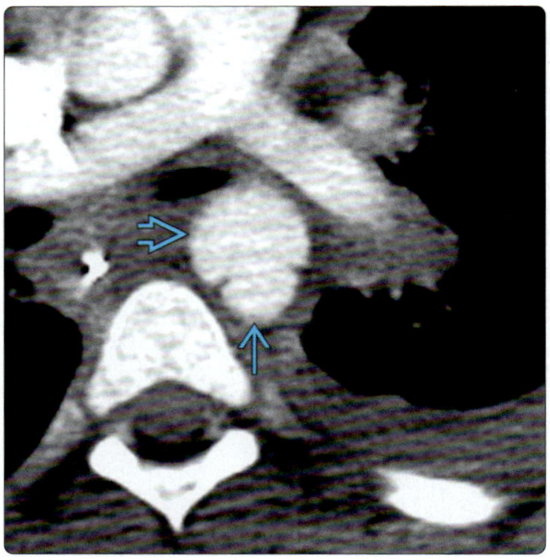

(Left) *Sagittal oblique CECT in the same patient shows the traumatic pseudoaneurysm at aortic isthmus. Traumatic pseudoaneurysms are usually larger, more irregular, & have acute rather than obtuse margins with the aorta as compared to the normal ductus diverticulum. A ductus diverticulum would also not show changes of a posterior aortic margin.* **(Right)** *AP radiograph after a motor vehicle crash shows widened mediastinum with loss of a normal aortic shadow.*

Trauma

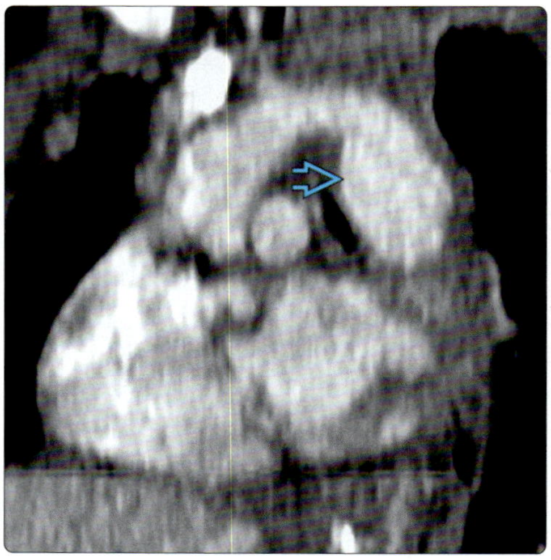

Trauma

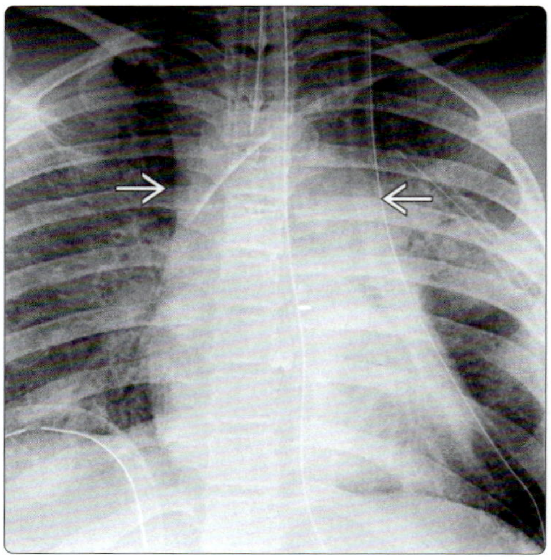

(Left) *Axial CECT in the same patient shows a focal aortic transection with active extravasation of contrast. Note the irregular contour of the aorta. Additional findings include a mediastinal hematoma & left hemothorax.* **(Right)** *Coronal CECT in the same patient shows irregularity of the wall with active extravasation from the descending thoracic aorta. Note the abrupt change to a normal caliber distally as well as a large periaortic hematoma.*

Trauma

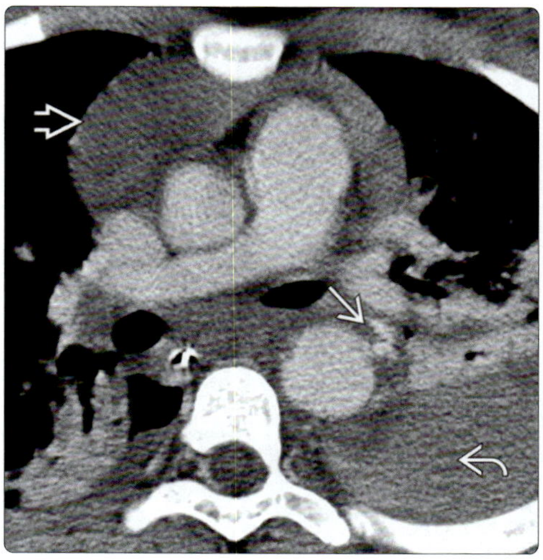

Trauma

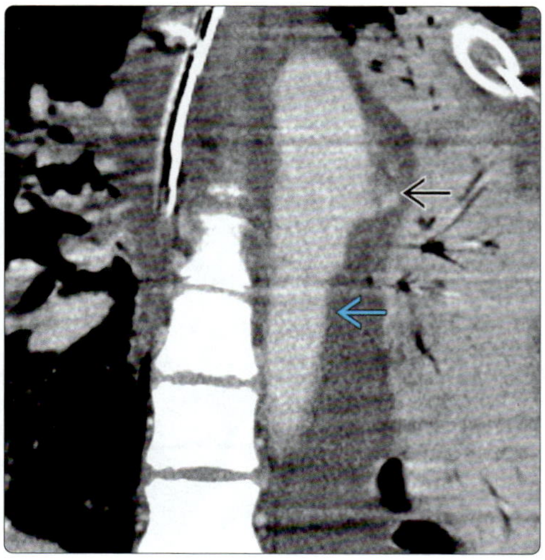

Mycotic Aneurysm

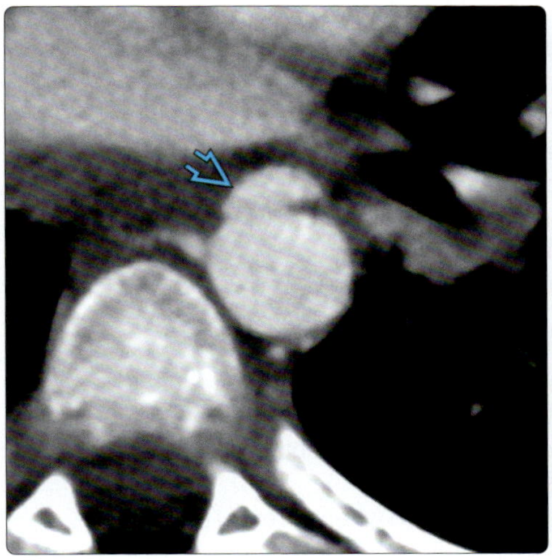

Takayasu Arteritis

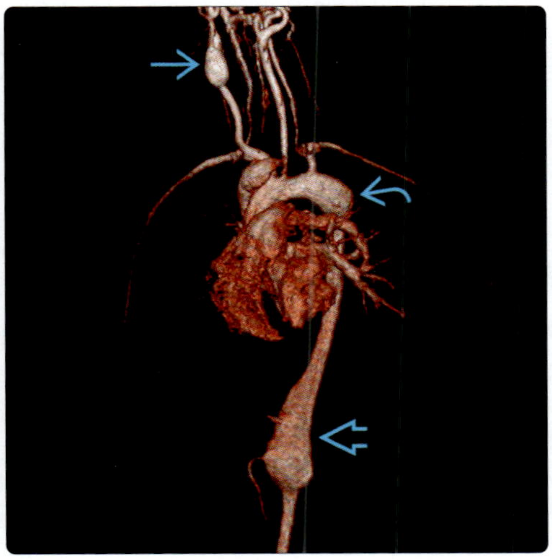

(Left) *Axial CECT in an 11 year old with sepsis shows irregular outpouching from the anterior aspect of the descending aorta due to a mycotic aneurysm.* **(Right)** *Sagittal oblique MRA 3D projection in a 12 year old with Takayasu arteritis shows aneurysms of the right common carotid artery, aortic isthmus, & abdominal aorta. While Takayasu arteritis more typically has stenoses, a recurrent cycle of intramural inflammation/hemorrhage & then healing can lead to aneurysm formation.*

Takayasu Arteritis

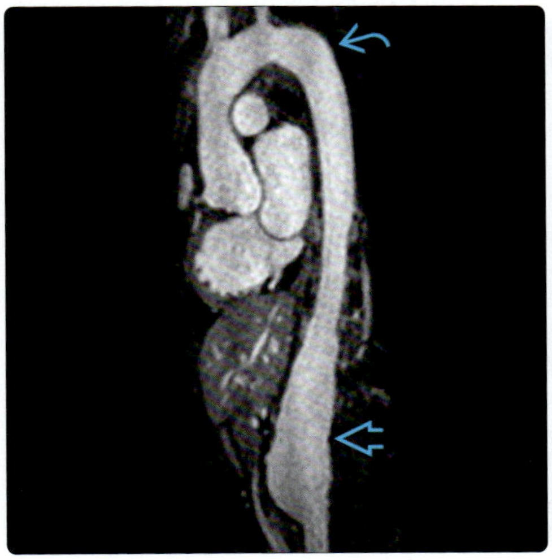

Takayasu Arteritis

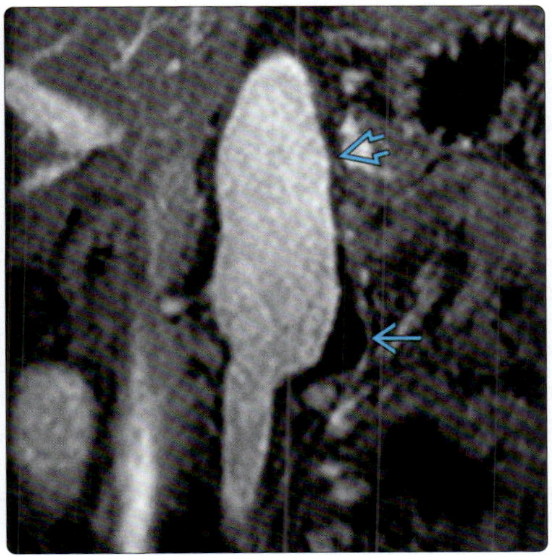

(Left) *Sagittal oblique MRA MIP in the same patient at 15 years of age again shows persistent aneurysmal dilation of the aortic isthmus & abdominal aorta.* **(Right)** *Coronal MRA in the same patient shows the large, irregular abdominal aortic aneurysm. Irregular eccentric hypointensity may represent intramural thrombus. Unlike adults, pediatric Takayasu arteritis commonly involves the abdominal aorta & branches, classically with middle aortic syndrome, resulting in renovascular hypertension.*

Takayasu Arteritis

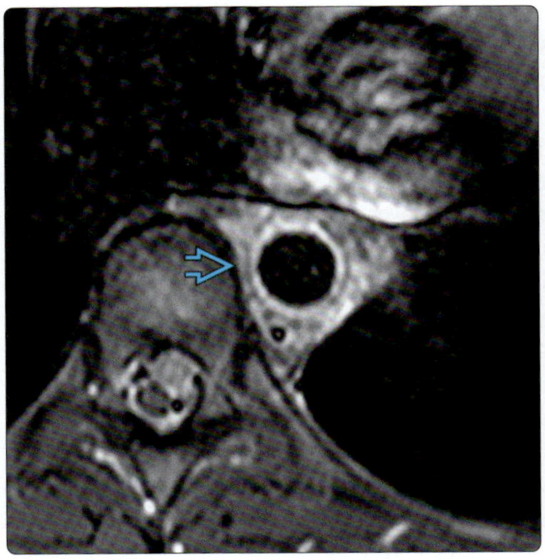

Takayasu Arteritis

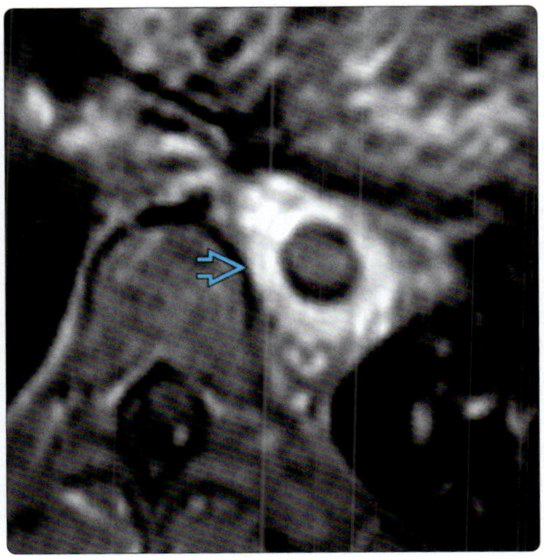

(Left) *Axial STIR MR in the same patient shows descending aortic wall thickening & edema as well as periaortic edema.* **(Right)** *Axial T1 C+ FS MR in the same patient at the same level shows descending aortic wall thickening & hyperenhancement. These findings are consistent with active inflammation. MR assessment of active wall inflammation directly affects how antiinflammatory medication is managed.*

DIFFERENTIAL DIAGNOSIS

Common

- Situs Inversus Totalis

Less Common

- Heterotaxy
  - Right-Sided Isomerism
  - Left-Sided Isomerism

ESSENTIAL INFORMATION

Key Differential Diagnosis Issues

- Situs anomalies reflect abnormalities of body lateralization
- Situs can be defined at 3 levels
  - Atrial appendages: Normal (solitus), inverted (inversus), right atrial isomerism (bilateral right atrial appendages), left atrial isomerism (bilateral left atrial appendages)
  - Bronchopulmonary relationship: Normal (solitus), inverted (inversus), right bronchopulmonary isomerism, left bronchopulmonary isomerism
  - Abdominal viscera: Normal (solitus), inverted (inversus), asplenia, polysplenia
- How to define structures
  - Right atrial appendage: Broad based & triangular with pectinate muscles extending to atrioventricular connection
  - Left atrial appendage: Tubular & finger-like with pectinate muscles distant from atrioventricular connection
    - Caution: Shape alone can be altered by hemodynamic factors; extent of pectinate muscles is purported overriding determinant feature
    - Note: Some argue true isomerism does not exist, & despite morphology, true right & left atria always exist in each person
      - In this school of thought, right atrium can always be defined as atrium that receives suprahepatic inferior vena cava (IVC)
  - Right bronchopulmonary morphology: Eparterial bronchus with trilobed lung
  - Left bronchopulmonary morphology: Hyparterial bronchus with bilobed lung
    - Clue for bronchopulmonary isomerism: Main bronchi are symmetric in length
      - Left main bronchus is normally 1.5-2.0x longer than right
  - Asplenia: No splenic tissue identified
  - Polysplenia: Multiple small spleens/splenules or single multilobulated spleen
    - Splenic tissue should be found along greater curvature of stomach (as gastrosplenic ligament maintains relationship) no matter where stomach lies
- Cardiac position is not reliable for determining situs (but discordance can suggest congenital heart disease)
- Gastric stomach bubble is often clue to abdominal visceral situs but can also be unreliable

Helpful Clues for Common Diagnoses

- **Situs Inversus Totalis**
  - All nonsymmetric organs (heart, lungs, liver, spleen, stomach) are exactly reversed from normal
  - Estimated occurrence = 0.01% of general population
  - 3-5% have congenital heart disease (compared to 0.6-0.8% for general population)
  - ~ 20% have primary ciliary dyskinesia (PCD)
    - Genetic disorder of mucociliary dysfunction & chronic otosinopulmonary disease
    - 50% have situs anomalies
    - Kartagener syndrome: Form of PCD with situs inversus, sinusitis &/or nasal polyposis, & bronchiectasis
      - 50% of PCD

Helpful Clues for Less Common Diagnoses

- **Heterotaxy**
  - Terminology
    - Heterotaxy: Any arrangement of situs other than situs solitus & situs inversus
    - Isomerism: Situation when normally asymmetric paired structures on opposite sides of left-right axis are morphologically symmetric mirror images of each other
    - Situs ambiguous: When components of situs solitus & inversus are in same patient (neither normal nor mirror-image arrangement)
      - Can be used when situs cannot be clearly defined at 1 level, though generally used synonymously with heterotaxy
      - Since situs can often be defined at each level, some argue against use of this term (i.e., just use heterotaxy)
  - No consensus on how to classify; traditionally have been grouped by either atrial appendage arrangement (right atrial isomerism/left atrial isomerism) or splenic status (asplenia/polysplenia)
    - ~ 20% of cases have discordant situs between atrial, bronchopulmonary, & abdominal visceral arrangements (as any combination is possible)
      - Cannot be classified into single category
    - Abdominal visceral arrangement is highly variable; sometimes cannot be defined simply as normal, inverted, asplenia, or polysplenia
    - Therefore, it is always best to systematically describe situs at each level
  - Nonetheless, atrial appendage arrangement remains best marker for constellation of congenital heart disease & associated findings
  - Groupings remain useful because of well-established anatomic & functional associations, though significant variation & overlap can exist within any individual patient
  - Associations common to all heterotaxy cases
    - High association with congenital heart disease, which is main factor in prognosis & management
    - Anomalous atrioventricular, ventriculoarterial, & venoatrial connections
      - Common entities: Intracardiac shunts, bilateral superior vena cava (SVC) (50%), anomalous pulmonary veins
      - Bilateral SVCs often connect to superior aspect of both atria (i.e., with either no coronary sinus or "unroofed" form)
      - Hepatic veins may connect directly to either atrium

- All cases of heterotaxy have abnormal splenic function, even in presence of normal-appearing solitary spleens
- May have intestinal malrotation & pancreatic abnormalities (e.g., annular pancreas, partial or complete pancreatic agenesis)

- CT/MR to define systemic & pulmonary venous connections along with other extracardiac anomalies
- **Right-sided isomerism**
  - More dire prognosis
  - Cardiac findings
    - 100% association with congenital heart disease
    - More severe cardiac disease with normal heart size & normal to decreased pulmonary vascularity (i.e., cyanotic congenital heart disease)
    - Single ventricle physiology in > 70%
    - Most common: Complete atrioventricular septal defect (AVSD), transposition or malposition of great arteries with bilateral infundibulum, pulmonary stenosis or atresia, & obstructed total anomalous pulmonary venous connections to systemic vein
    - May have supraventricular tachycardia as sinoatrial (SA) nodes may be bilateral (which are associated with right atria)
  - Pulmonary findings
    - Bilateral eparterial bronchi: Both upper lobe bronchi are posterosuperior to descending interlobar pulmonary arteries
    - Bilateral hypbrochial pulmonary arteries: Both interlobar pulmonary arteries course anteroinferior to right upper lobe bronchi
    - Bilateral trilobed lungs
    - Carina angle usually < 135°
  - Intraabdominal findings
    - Usually associated with asplenia (absent spleen)
    - Stomach is often paramidline
    - Symmetric midline liver
    - Malrotation is common
    - Abdominal aorta & IVC are often on same side in posterior-anterior orientation
- **Left-sided isomerism**
  - Significantly better prognosis
  - Cardiac findings
    - Less severe cardiac disease with cardiomegaly & normal to increased pulmonary vascularity (i.e., acyanotic with shunts)
    - Single-ventricle physiology in 25%, pulmonary obstruction in 30%
    - Most common: Complete or partial AVSD, normally related great vessels or double-outlet right ventricle (DORV) without subaortic infundibulum, intracardiac anomalous pulmonary veins
    - Interruption of IVC with azygos or hemiazygos continuation in 80% → look for dilated azygos vein
    - May have bradycardia with heart block (as SA node, which is associated with right atria, may be absent)
  - Pulmonary findings
    - Bilateral hyparterial bronchi: Both upper lobe bronchi branch inferior to pulmonary arteries
    - Bilateral epbronchial pulmonary arteries: Both pulmonary arteries course posteriorly, superior to main bronchi
    - Bilateral bilobed lungs
    - Carina angle usually > 135°
  - Intraabdominal findings
    - Usually associated with polysplenia (may be on right or left)
    - Indeterminate/variable stomach position
    - Midline or left-sided liver
    - Can have congenital portosystemic shunts
    - Can have biliary atresia
    - Malrotation may be present

SELECTED REFERENCES

1. Yim D et al: Disharmonious patterns of heterotaxy and isomerism: how often are the classic patterns breached? Circ Cardiovasc Imaging. 11(2):e006917, 2018

Situs Inversus Totalis

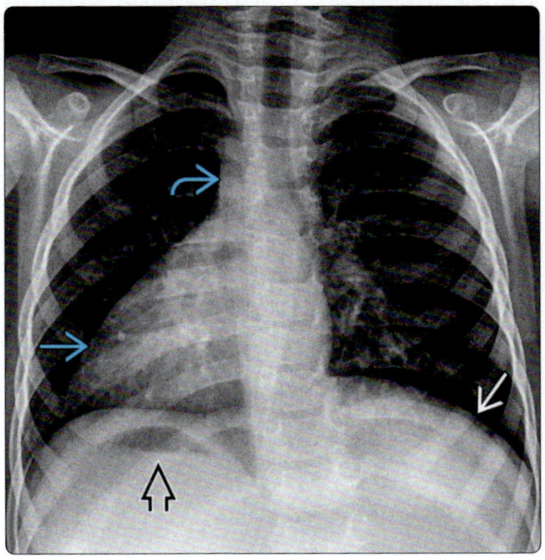

Situs Inversus Totalis

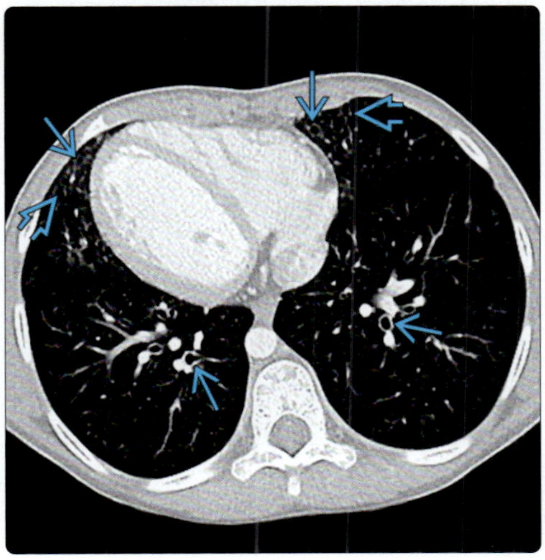

(Left) *PA radiograph in a 3 year old with primary ciliary dyskinesia shows situs inversus with dextroposition of the heart ➡, right aortic arch ➡, right-sided stomach bubble ➡, & left-sided liver shadow with higher left hemidiaphragm ➡.* **(Right)** *Axial CECT in the same patient at 7 years old shows mild lingular, left middle lobe, & bilateral lower lobe bronchiectasis ➡ with peribronchial thickening, tree-in-bud opacities ➡, & subsegmental atelectasis, reflecting chronic mucoid impaction ± infection.*

(Left) *AP radiograph in a 1 day old with right isomerism shows dextrocardia, a paramidline stomach, a large midline liver with midline UVC, & a UAC in a right descending aorta. There is diminished pulmonary vascularity.* **(Right)** *Four-chamber SSFP MR in a 2 year old with right isomerism shows bilateral, broad-based, triangular atrial appendages with pectinate muscles extending to the AV junction, consistent with right atrial appendage isomerism. Note a complete unbalanced RV-dominant AVSD.*

Right-Sided Isomerism

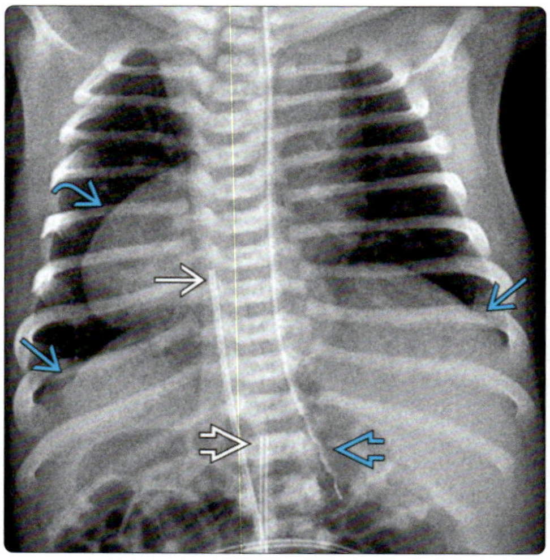

Right-Sided Isomerism

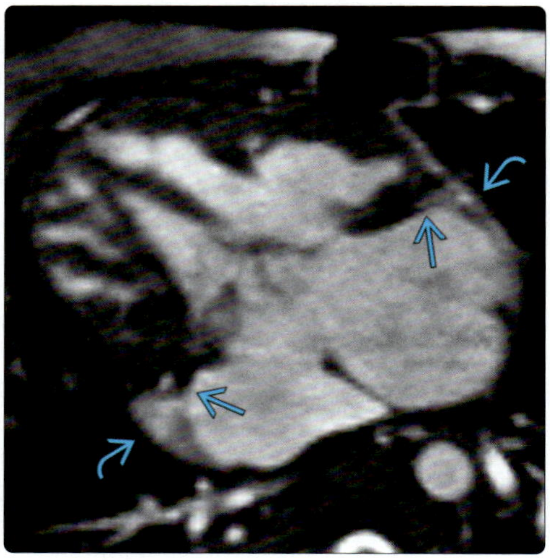

(Left) *Coronal oblique MRA MPR in the same patient shows right bronchopulmonary isomerism with bilateral eparterial bronchi, as bilateral upper lobe bronchi run superior to descending interlobar pulmonary arteries (PAs). The carina angle is < 135°.* **(Right)** *Axial SSFP MR shows a midline transverse liver, paramidline stomach, & asplenia. In this case, atrial, bronchopulmonary, & abdominal situs are all congruent with right isomerism.*

Right-Sided Isomerism

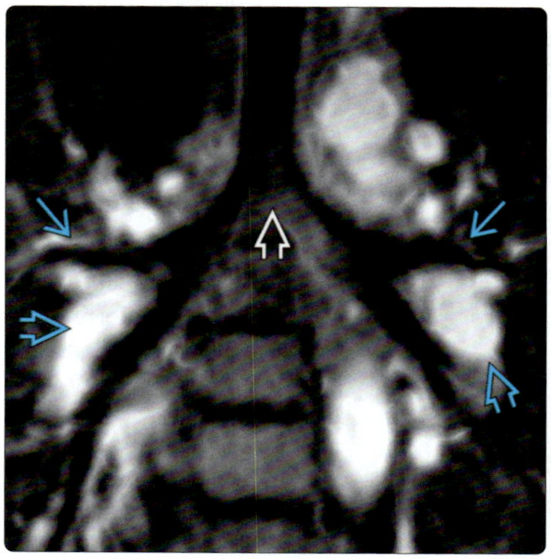

Right-Sided Isomerism

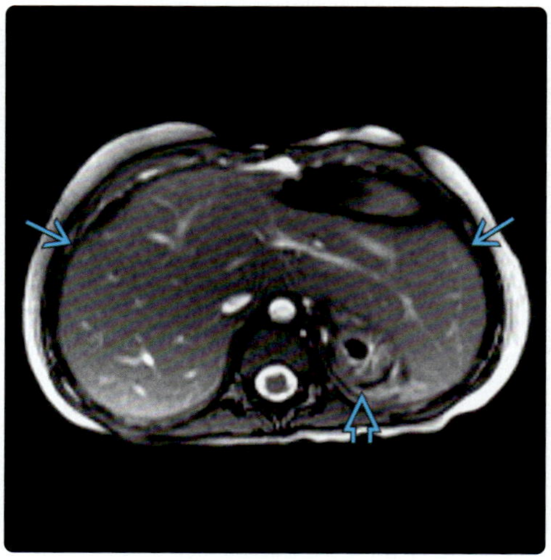

(Left) *Sagittal oblique MRA MIP in the same patient shows a malposed aorta anterior to the MPA with both arising from the RV (DORV). An MPA band & the LPA are shown.* **(Right)** *Posterior MRA 3D projection in a 1 day old with right isomerism shows all pulmonary veins connecting to a common posterior channel draining to the portal vein (infradiaphragmatic TAPVR). There was also TGA with pulmonary atresia & a tortuous PDA supplying the PAs. Note a large midline liver.*

Right-Sided Isomerism

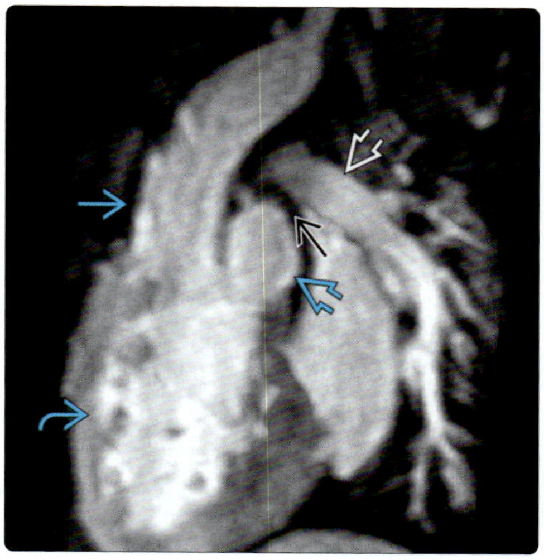

Right-Sided Isomerism

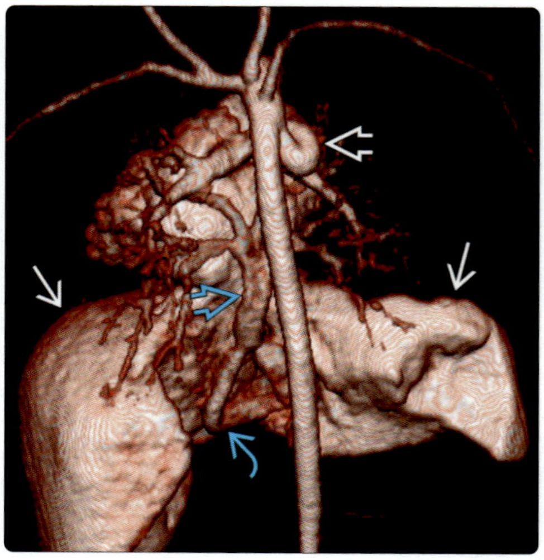

Left-Sided Isomerism

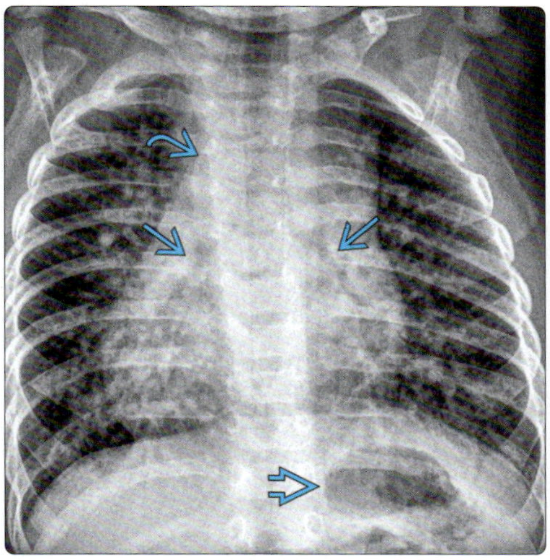

Left-Sided Isomerism

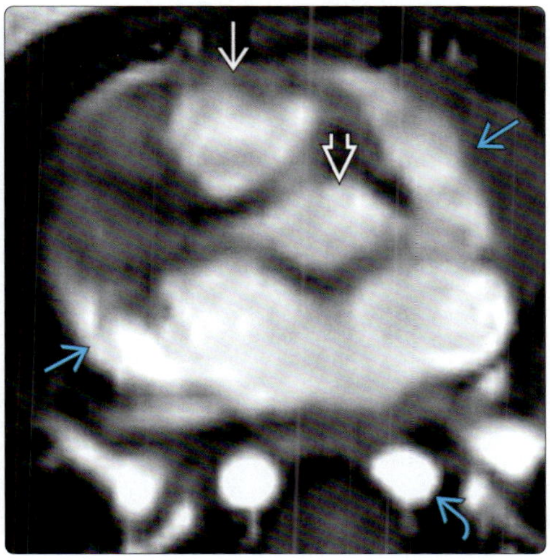

(Left) *PA radiograph in a 9 month old with left isomerism shows dextrocardia, increased (shunt) pulmonary vascularity, right aortic arch, symmetric-appearing bronchi, & left-sided stomach bubble.* **(Right)** *Axial SSFP MR in the same patient at 4 months of age shows dextrocardia with bilateral, tubular, finger-like atrial appendages, consistent with left atrial appendage isomerism. The aorta & MPA are normally related for an L-looped heart. Note the azygos continuation of an interrupted IVC.*

Left-Sided Isomerism

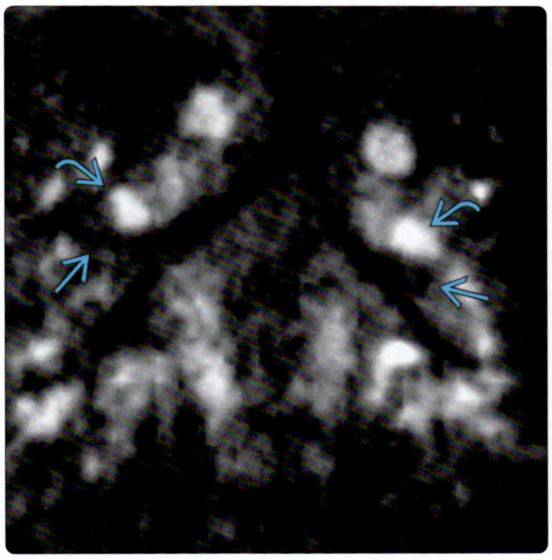

Left-Sided Isomerism

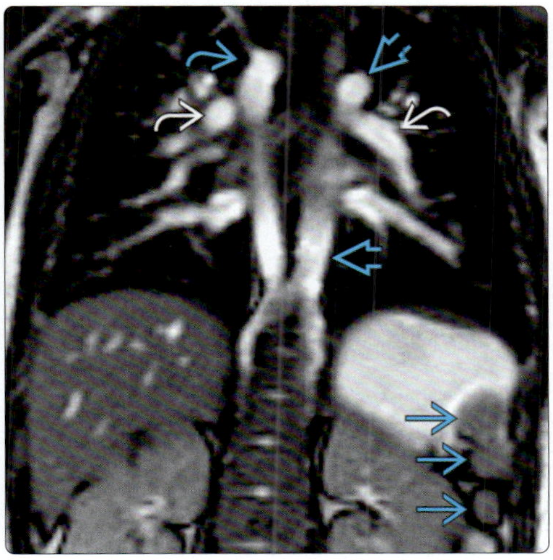

(Left) *Coronal oblique MRA MPR in the same patient shows bilateral hyparterial bronchi with the bilateral upper lobe bronchi coursing inferior to the bilateral branch PAs, which course posteriorly.* **(Right)** *Coronal SSFP MR in the same patient shows polysplenia, a right aortic arch descending on the right, an interrupted IVC with azygos continuation, & bilateral epbronchial PAs. Systemic evaluation of situs at each level is needed as situs can be discordant in a patient.*

Left-Sided Isomerism

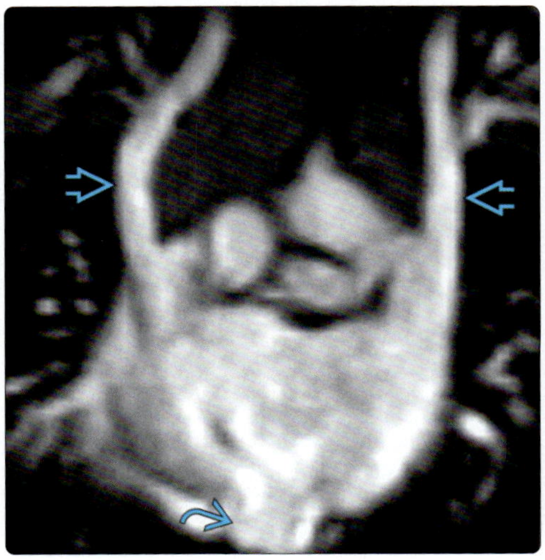

Left-Sided Isomerism

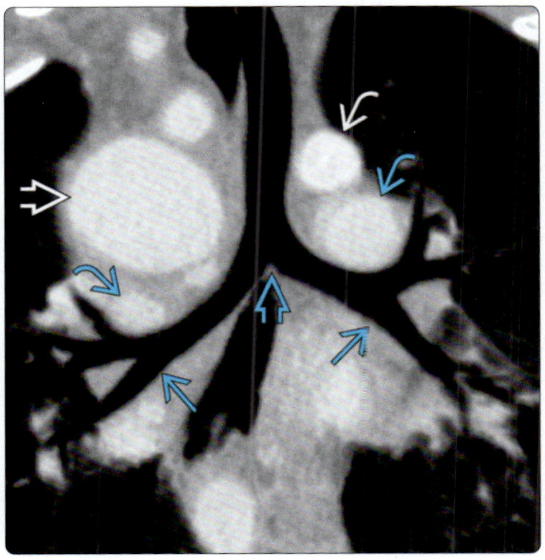

(Left) *Coronal oblique MRA MPR in the same patient shows bilateral SVCs connecting to the roof of the ipsilateral atrium with no (or "unroofed") coronary sinus & no connecting/bridging vein between the SVCs. Note a midline IVC.* **(Right)** *Coronal oblique CECT minIP in a 2 year old with left isomerism shows bilateral hyparterial bronchi with upper lobe bronchi coursing below the PAs. Note a wide carina angle, right aortic arch, & dilated azygos arch from an interrupted IVC with azygos continuation.*

SECTION 2

Chest

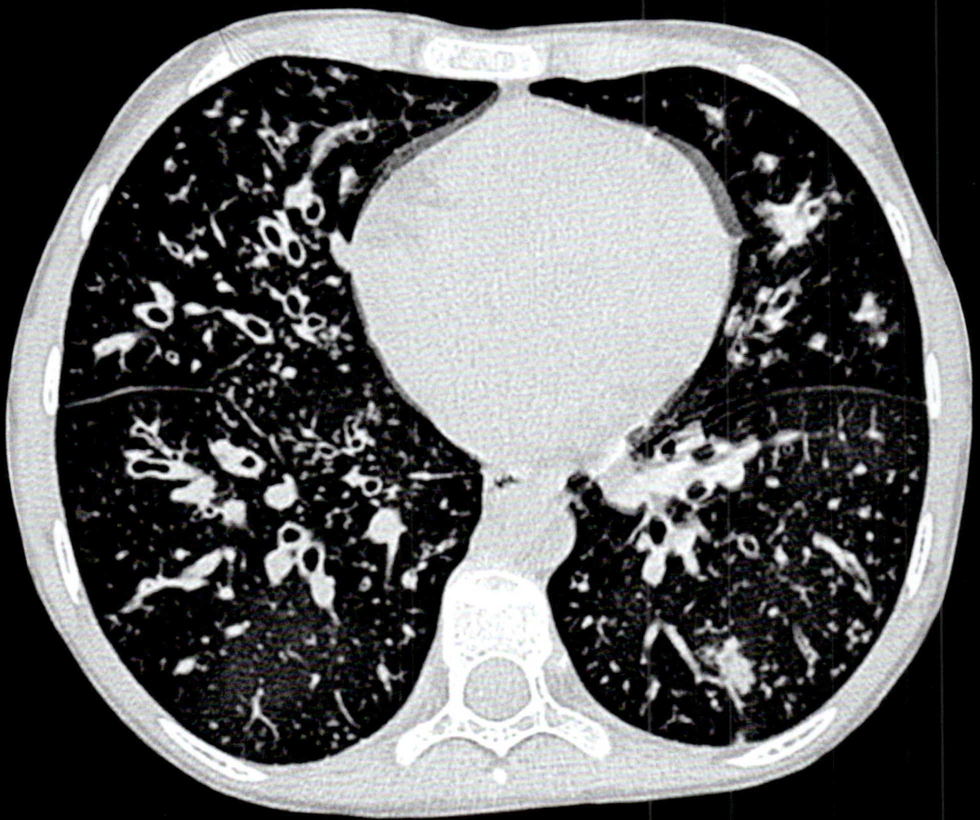

DIFFERENTIAL DIAGNOSIS

Common

- Surfactant Deficiency Disease
- Viral Pneumonia
- *Mycoplasma*

Less Common

- Aspergillosis
- Tuberculosis
- *Pneumocystis jiroveci*
- Lymphoproliferative Disease
- Pulmonary Langerhans Cell Histiocytosis

Rare but Important

- Sarcoidosis
- Systemic Lupus Erythematosus
- Pulmonary Venoocclusive Disease
- Lysosomal Storage Disorders
  - Gaucher Disease
  - Niemann-Pick Disease

ESSENTIAL INFORMATION

Key Differential Diagnosis Issues

- Interstitial thickening & multiple small nodules
  - Nonspecific pattern of disease

Helpful Clues for Common Diagnoses

- **Surfactant Deficiency Disease**
  - a.k.a. respiratory distress syndrome, hyaline membrane disease
  - Most common cause of morbidity in premature infants
    - Affects 15-30% of infants born at 32-36 weeks gestation
    - Rare in infants born > 36 weeks; possible in diabetic mothers
  - Decreased lung volumes & diffuse granular reticulonodular opacities
    - Findings are worst at 12-24 hours of life
    - Appearance changes after treatment with mechanical ventilation & administration of exogenous surfactant via endotracheal tube
      - Normalization of lung volumes
      - Alveoli can even become overdistended with bubbly lucencies
      - Uneven distribution of exogenous surfactant can lead to heterogeneous pattern of expansion & atelectasis
    - Complications of mechanical ventilation: Pulmonary interstitial emphysema, pneumomediastinum, pneumothorax
    - May progress to chronic lung disease of prematurity
- **Viral Pneumonia**
  - Most common cause of hospitalization in infants
    - Usually is self-limiting illness
  - Respiratory syncytial virus (RSV) is most common cause
    - Accounts for 28% of children hospitalized for community-acquired pneumonia in USA
  - Variable pattern of consolidation, ground-glass alveolar & interstitial opacities, nodules, bronchial wall thickening, & pleural effusions
    - CMV: Immunosuppressed, patchy & nodular ground-glass opacities
    - HPIV, RSV, HMPV, & influenza: Can have bronchial wall thickening with bronchovascular/multifocal opacities & centrilobular nodules
  - Risks for severe disease: Prematurity, age < 12 weeks, chronic lung disease, congenital heart disease, immunocompromised state
- **Mycoplasma**
  - Common cause of community-acquired pneumonia in children (10-30% of pediatric pneumonia)
    - Most common cause of pneumonia in children > 5 years old
  - More severe presentation in children < 5 years old
  - Bronchopneumonia, lobar consolidation; reticulonodular opacities in 52% (more common in lower lobes)
    - Classic CT appearance: Multifocal bronchovascular thickening with centrilobular nodules

Helpful Clues for Less Common Diagnoses

- **Aspergillosis**
  - Invasive & semiinvasive aspergillosis have small nodules that can appear reticulonodular on radiographs
  - Chronic pulmonary aspergillosis (semiinvasive)
    - Typically in patients with mild immunosuppression
    - Bronchopulmonary consolidation, nodules ± cavitation
  - Invasive aspergillosis
    - Usually occurs in severely immunocompromised
    - Patchy consolidation & nodules
      - Halo sign (early): Ground-glass opacity surrounding nodule or consolidation; highly suggestive in proper setting
      - Air crescent sign (late): Crescent of air in nodule or consolidation; indicates neutrophil recovery after initiation of treatment (good prognostic sign)
- **Tuberculosis**
  - Primary disease
    - More common in children than adults
    - Perihilar & paratracheal lymphadenopathy
      - Radiographic hallmark of disease, seen in 90% of children (but only 10-40% in adults)
      - Can compress airway (causing air-trapping or atelectasis)
      - Consolidation without lobar predilection
      - Ca^{2+} (6 months to 4 years after infection)
  - Progressive primary disease (primary tuberculosis that does not heal)
    - Cavitation: High bacterial load, highly contagious
    - Miliary infection (hematogenous spread)
      - Innumerable tiny nodules in random distribution; can appear reticulonodular on radiographs
      - More common in children & immunocompromised
    - Extrapulmonary spread
  - Postprimary disease (reinfection or reactivation)
    - Consolidation is typically of apical posterior segments of upper lobes & superior segments of lower lobes
    - Cavitation is common
    - Lymphadenopathy is uncommon
    - If immunocompromised, looks like progressive primary disease

- Pleural effusion/empyema
  - Can be seen in primary or postprimary disease
- **Pneumocystis jiroveci**
  - a.k.a., *Pneumocystis carinii*, *Pneumocystis* pneumonia (PCP)
  - Increased incidence with immunocompromised states
    - Traditionally, HIV was common cause but is now less frequently seen in developed countries
  - Bilateral perihilar interstitial infiltrates progressively coalescing to patchy ground-glass opacities
  - Pneumomediastinum & pneumothorax are possible late
  - Consolidation & nodules are less common
- **Lymphoproliferative Disease**
  - Spectrum of benign to malignant disorders
  - Variable appearance: Infiltrates, nodules, interstitial thickening, fibrosis, adenopathy
  - Includes lymphocytic interstitial pneumonia (LIP)
    - End stage of benign pulmonary lymphocytic hyperplasia
    - Response to viral infection (HIV, EBV, HHV-6), autoimmune disease (Sjögren), immunodeficiency, or idiopathic
    - Diffuse, symmetric, basal predominant, reticulonodular opacities
    - CT: Perilymphatic nodules, bronchovascular & septal thickening, ground-glass opacities, cysts
- **Pulmonary Langerhans Cell Histiocytosis**
  - Accumulation of Langerhans cells forming destructive bronchiolocentric granulomas
  - May be reactive response to unknown agent vs. neoplastic/monoclonal disease (evidence for both)
  - Often in setting of systemic Langerhans cell histiocytosis in children (unlike isolated pulmonary disease in adults from smoking)
  - Lung involvement is diffuse
    - Costophrenic angles are spared only in adults
  - See centrilobular pulmonary nodules (granulomas) that progress to irregular cysts
    - Airspace invasion leads to cavitation & formation of thick-walled cysts, progressing to thin-walled cysts
    - Multiple small nodules can appear reticulonodular on radiographs
    - Late findings: Confluent destructive parenchymal cystic change
  - Can present with spontaneous pneumothorax (10-20%)

Helpful Clues for Rare Diagnoses

- **Sarcoidosis**
  - Hilar & paratracheal adenopathy is most common thoracic finding in children
  - Parenchymal disease is uncommon in children
    - Bilateral perilymphatic nodules & mass-like opacities
    - Upper lobe & perihilar predominance
    - Lung fibrosis is extremely rare during pediatric age
- **Systemic Lupus Erythematosus**
  - Autoimmune multisystem disease
  - Most common thoracic manifestation is pleuritis
  - Can cause interstitial lung disease
- **Pulmonary Venoocclusive Disease**
  - Rare cause of pulmonary arterial hypertension
  - Occlusion of small pulmonary venules by intimal proliferation, collagen deposition, & fibrosis
  - Ill-defined centrilobular ground-glass micronodules, interstitial septal thickening, mediastinal & hilar lymphadenopathy
  - Important to raise possibility of pulmonary venoocclusive disease, as vasodilators can cause fatal pulmonary edema
- **Lysosomal Storage Disorders**
  - Gaucher disease & Niemann-Pick disease can have lung involvement that are similar in appearance
  - Diffuse reticulonodular pattern
  - CT: Inter- & intralobular septal thickening, ground-glass opacities, consolidation, bronchovascular thickening

SELECTED REFERENCES

1. Koo HJ et al: Radiographic and CT features of viral pneumonia. Radiographics. 38(3):719-39, 2018
2. Liszewski MC et al: Neonatal lung disorders: pattern recognition approach to diagnosis. AJR Am J Roentgenol. 210(5):964-75, 2018
3. Semple TR et al: Interstitial lung disease in children made easier...well, almost. Radiographics. 37(6):1679-703, 2017

Surfactant Deficiency Disease

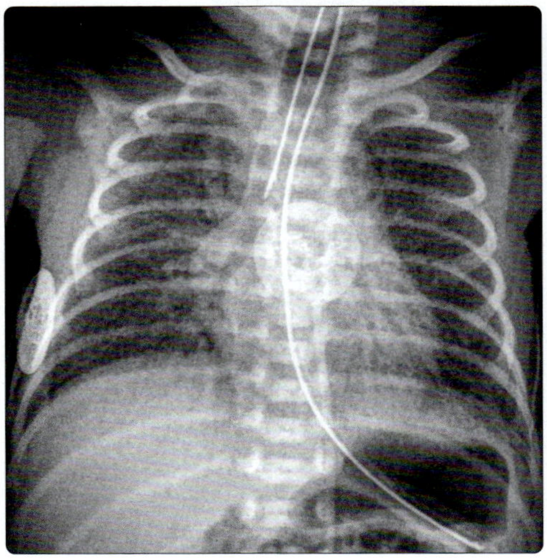

Surfactant Deficiency Disease

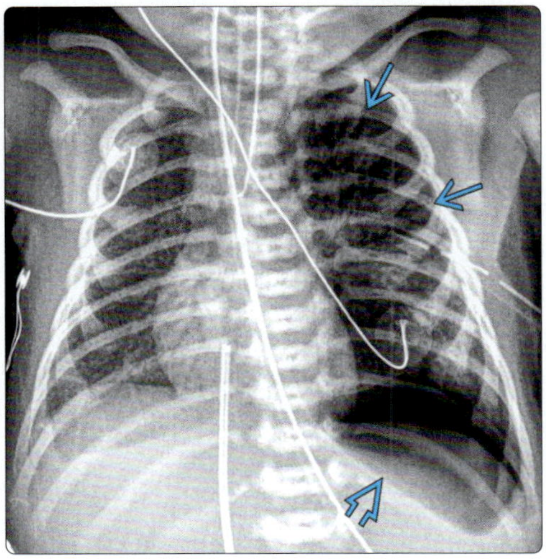

(Left) *AP radiograph in a premature newborn (26 weeks, 6 days gestational age) shows diffuse, hazy, granular opacities throughout the lungs, consistent with surfactant deficiency disease.* **(Right)** *AP radiograph in a premature 3 day old on mechanical ventilation shows left lung lucencies ➡ due to pulmonary interstitial emphysema. There is an associated left pneumothorax ➡ with depression of the hemidiaphragm & mediastinal shift. The right lung granular opacities are due to surfactant deficiency disease.*

(Left) *Axial CECT in a 14 year old with macrophage activation syndrome & disseminated CMV shows mild, patchy ground-glass opacities along with ill-defined ground-glass nodules →.* **(Right)** *Axial CECT in a 3 year old status post bone marrow transplant shows patchy & nodular ground-glass opacities →. Adenovirus was found in the blood. Viral pneumonias often show a variable pattern of consolidation, ground-glass opacities, interstitial thickening, & nodules.*

Viral Pneumonia

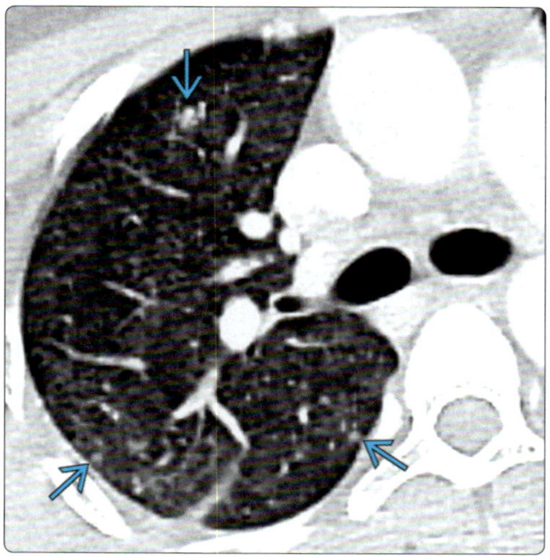

Viral Pneumonia

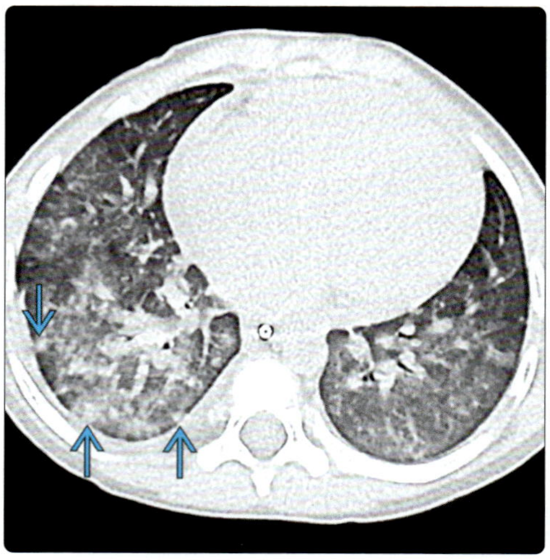

(Left) *AP radiograph of the chest shows a reticulonodular opacity in the right lower lobe →. Mycoplasma is the most common cause of pneumonia in children > 5 years of age.* **(Right)** *Axial CECT in the same patient shows further right lower lobe consolidation → along with lingular bronchovascular opacities & centrilobular nodules →. Mycoplasma was ultimately confirmed. Reticulonodular opacities are seen in ~ 50% of Mycoplasma infections & are more common in the lower lung.*

Mycoplasma

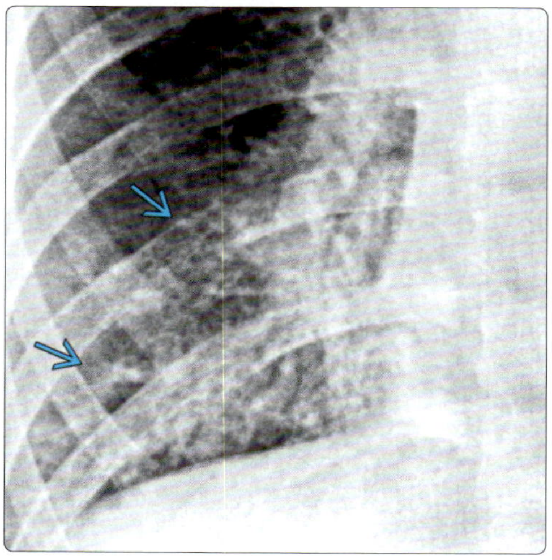

Mycoplasma

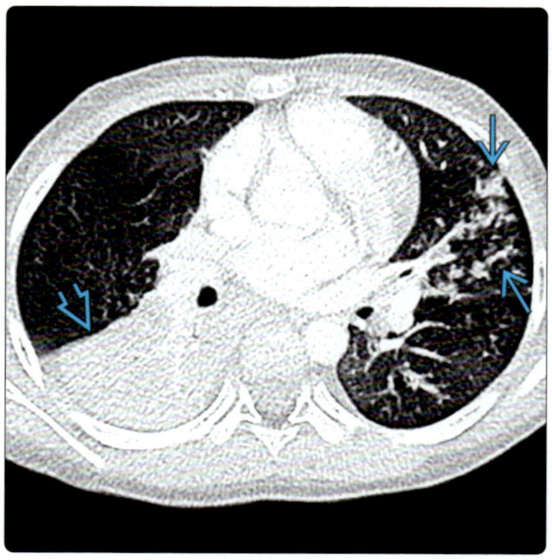

(Left) *PA radiograph in a 3 year old with chronic granulomatous disease shows bilateral lower lung reticulonodular opacities → along with mediastinal & hilar adenopathy →.* **(Right)** *Axial CECT in the same patient shows multiple small nodules → & infrahilar adenopathy → due to aspergillosis. There is also nonspecific, irregular interstitial thickening with distortion →. Chronic granulomatous disease is a classic congenital condition that is predisposed to aspergillus infections.*

Aspergillosis

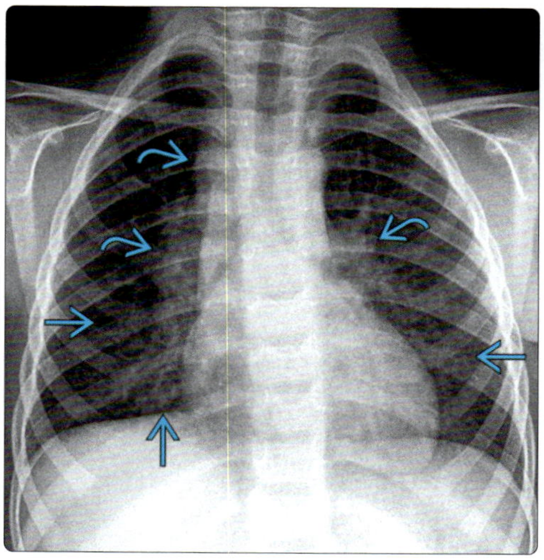

Aspergillosis

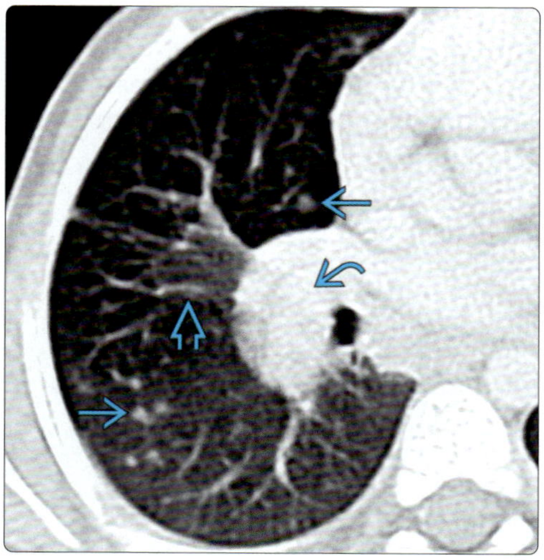

Tuberculosis

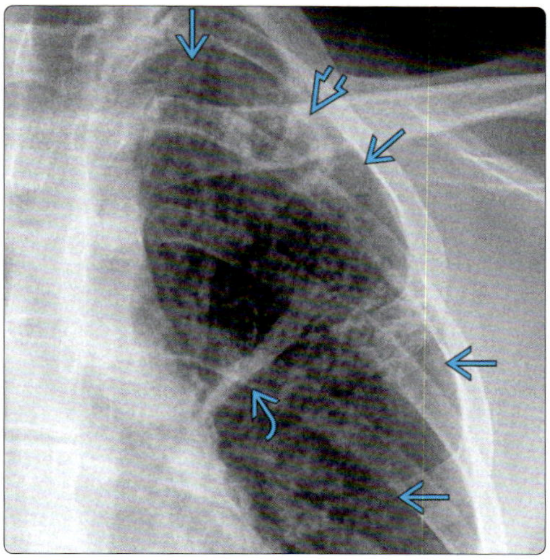

Tuberculosis

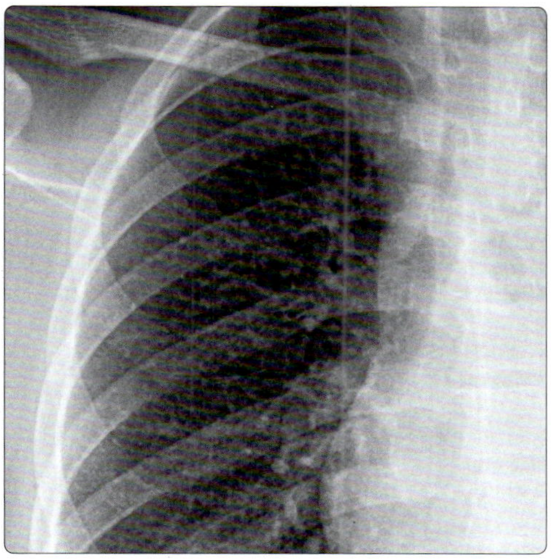

(Left) *PA radiograph in a 15 year old shows a reticulonodular opacity in the left upper lobe along with a cavitary lesion. There is also band-like atelectasis. This patient had disseminated tuberculosis (TB) with miliary disease in the lungs.* **(Right)** *PA radiograph in a 14 year old with TB meningitis shows a subtle reticulonodular pattern throughout the lungs, concerning for miliary TB. Miliary TB is due to hematogenous spread & can mimic a reticulonodular pattern on radiographs.*

Tuberculosis

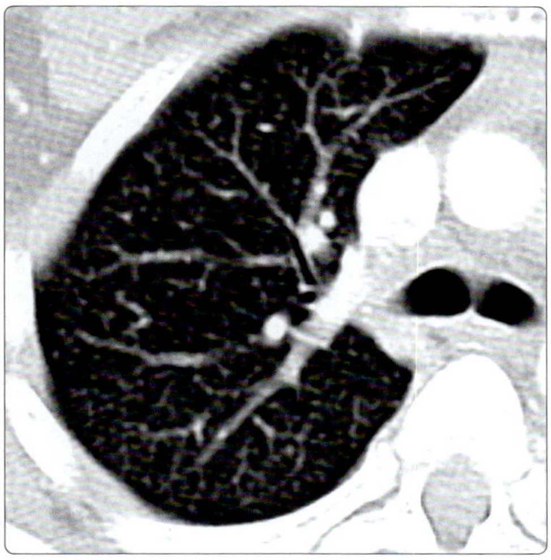

Tuberculosis

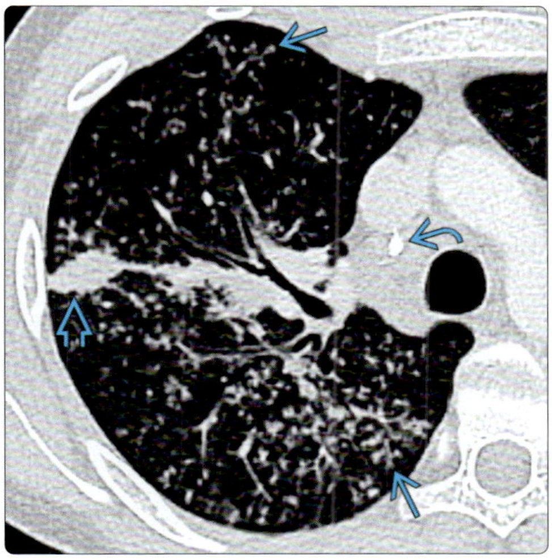

(Left) *Axial CECT in the same patient shows a fine miliary pattern of innumerable randomly distributed nodules, consistent with miliary TB.* **(Right)** *Axial CECT in a 14 year old from a country where TB is endemic shows irregular consolidation along with extensive tree-in-bud opacities, which can mimic a reticulonodular appearance on radiographs. Also note the dystrophic calcified hilar adenopathy. TB should be considered when tree-in-bud opacities are seen.*

Pneumocystis jiroveci

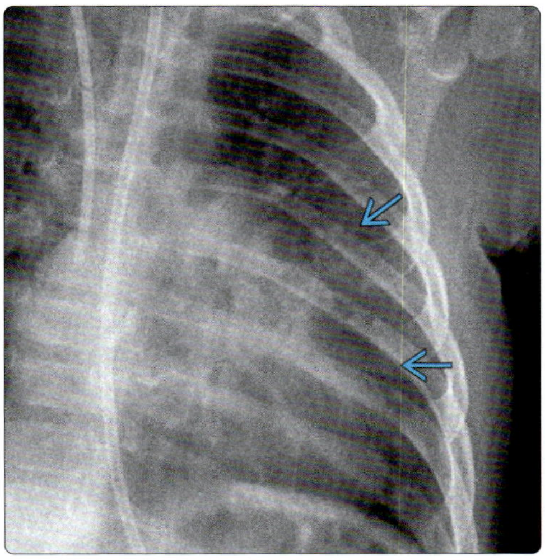

Pneumocystis jiroveci

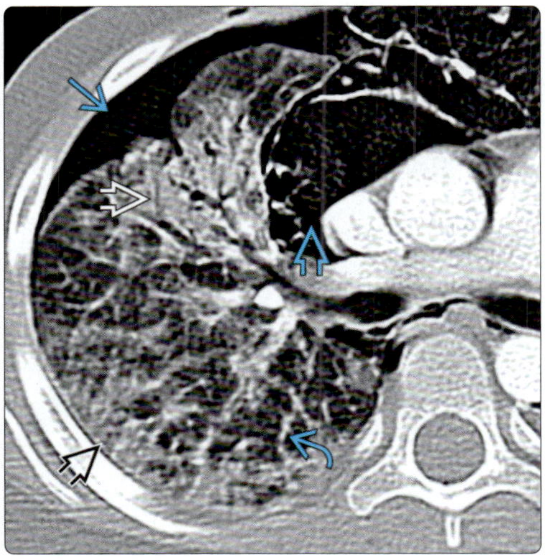

(Left) *PA radiograph in an 8 month old with severe combined immunodeficiency disease (SCID) shows a perihilar reticulonodular infiltrate among more confluent ill-defined opacities. SCID is a classic congenital condition predisposed to Pneumocystis infection.* **(Right)** *Axial CECT in a patient with Pneumocystis pneumonia shows a pneumothorax & pneumomediastinum. The lung shows consolidation with air bronchograms, ground-glass opacities, & septal thickening.*

(Left) *Axial CECT in a 10 year old with a lymphoproliferative disorder shows multiple lobulated pulmonary nodules & mediastinal & hilar adenopathy. Lymphoproliferative diseases encompass a spectrum of benign to malignant entities.* **(Right)** *Axial HRCT in a 15 year old shows tiny perilymphatic nodules, interstitial thickening, & innumerable tiny cystic spaces. Biopsy showed lymphocytic interstitial pneumonitis (LIP), which represents < 1% of childhood interstitial lung disease.*

Lymphoproliferative Disease

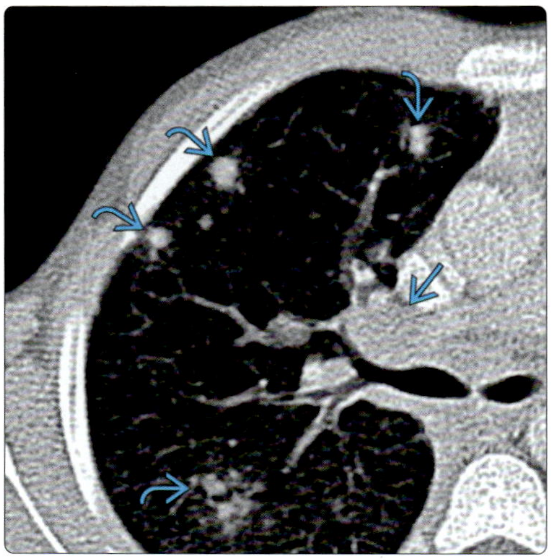

Lymphoproliferative Disease

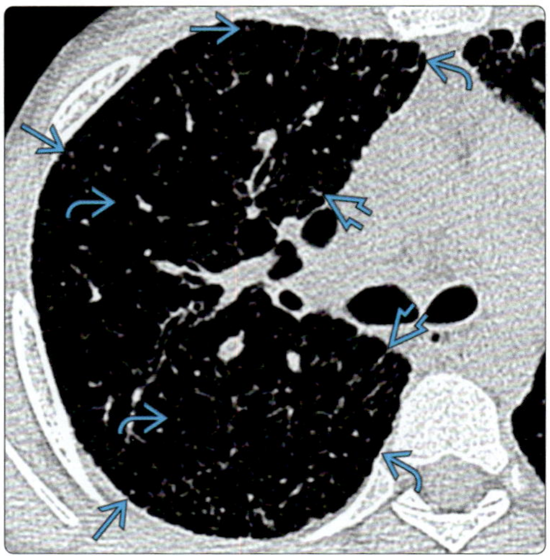

(Left) *AP radiograph of the chest shows thickened interstitial markings & multiple small nodules in a patient with a chest tube due to a spontaneous pneumothorax.* **(Right)** *Axial NECT in the same patient shows interstitial thickening & multiple nodules. A small pleural effusion is also present. Langerhans cell histiocytosis (LCH) in children is more commonly seen in the setting of multisystem disease rather than isolated pulmonary disease (like in adults from smoking).*

Pulmonary Langerhans Cell Histiocytosis

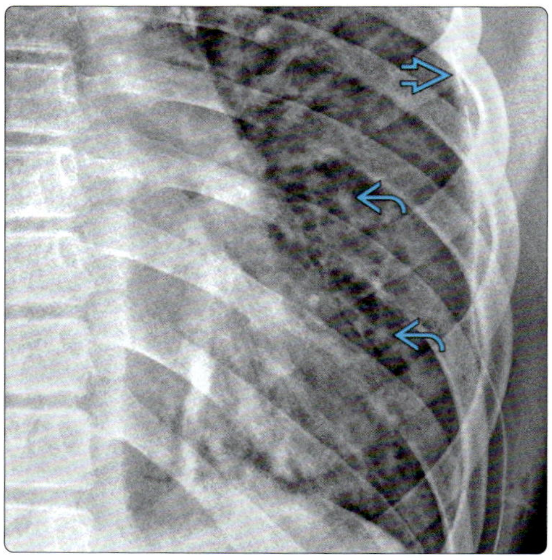

Pulmonary Langerhans Cell Histiocytosis

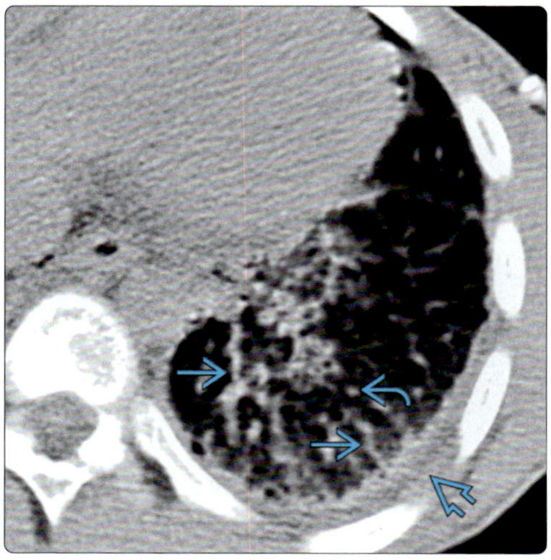

(Left) *PA radiograph in a 10 year old shows perihilar & upper lobe-predominant, hazy, ill-defined interstitial & airspace opacities along with a suggestion of reticulonodular infiltrates.* **(Right)** *Axial CECT in the same patient shows ground-glass opacities with associated irregular interstitial thickening & tiny perilymphatic nodules, representing pulmonary sarcoidosis. As in this case, pulmonary involvement in sarcoid has an upper lung & perihilar predominance.*

Sarcoidosis

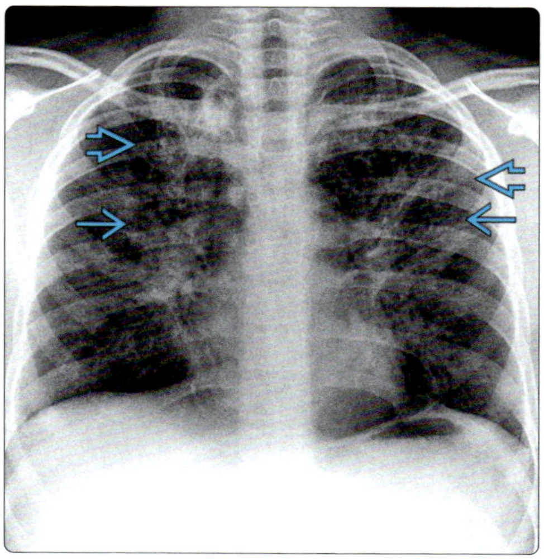

Sarcoidosis

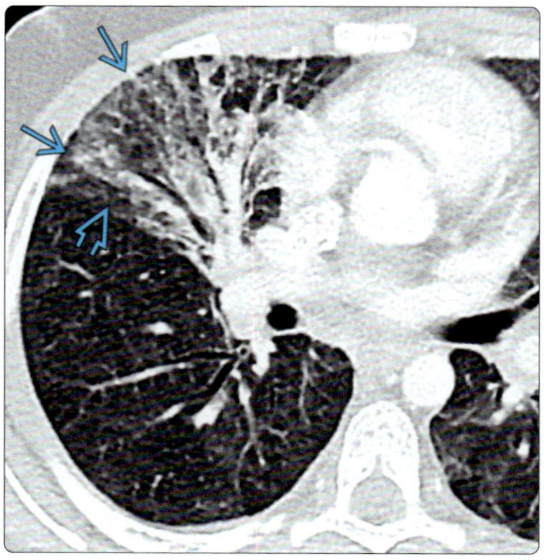

Systemic Lupus Erythematosus

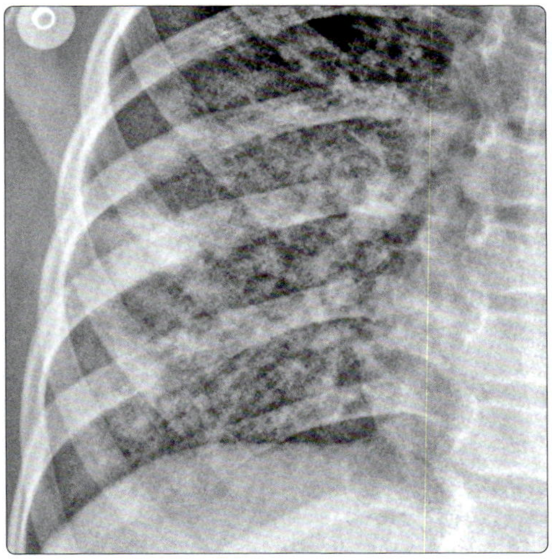

Systemic Lupus Erythematosus

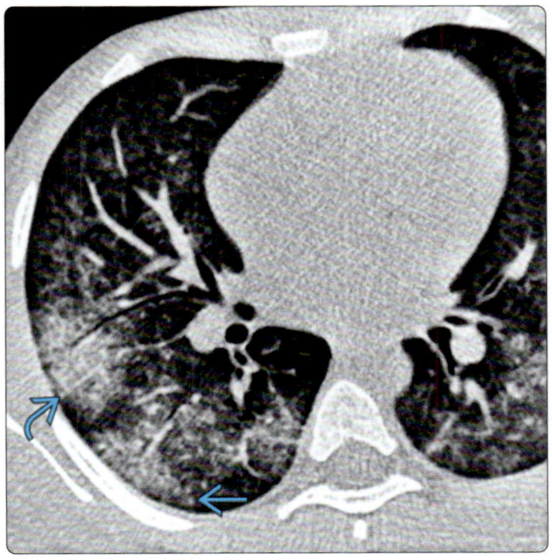

(Left) *AP radiograph of the chest shows a reticulonodular opacity in the right lung base. Systemic lupus erythematosus is an autoimmune disorder that can cause interstitial lung disease.* **(Right)** *Axial NECT in the same patient shows a reticulonodular opacity in the right lower lobe. There are areas of ground-glass opacity, septal thickening ➚, & small pulmonary nodules ➔. The most common thoracic manifestation of lupus is pleuritis.*

Pulmonary Venoocclusive Disease

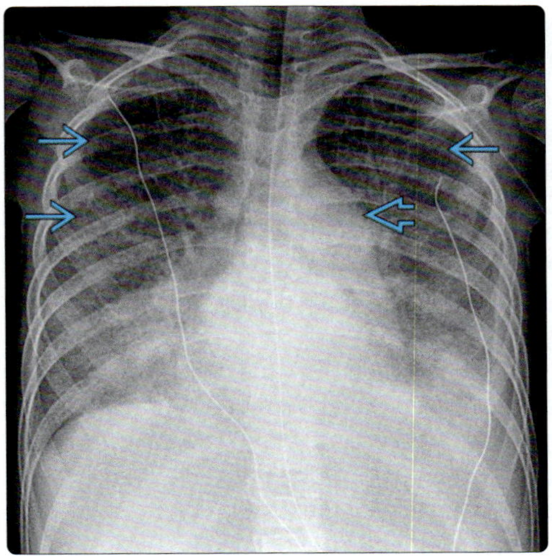

Pulmonary Venoocclusive Disease

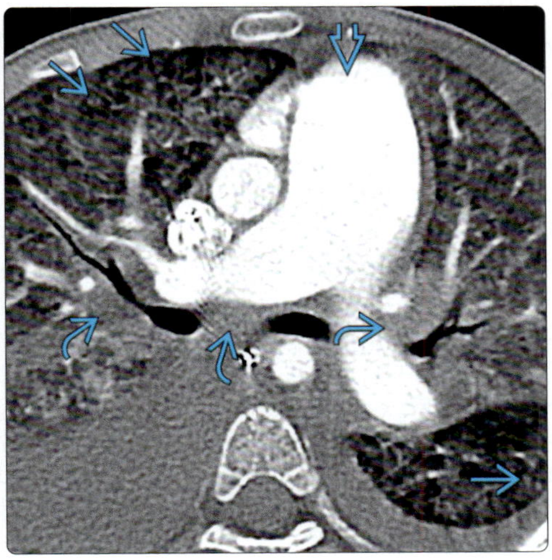

(Left) *PA radiograph in an 8 year old with pulmonary arterial hypertension shows an enlarged MPA ➯ & diffuse, hazy opacification with a subtle reticulonodular appearance of the lungs ➔.* **(Right)** *Axial CECT in the same patient shows an enlarged MPA ➯, diffuse ground-glass opacities, septal thickening, numerous centrilobular ground-glass micronodules ➔, bilateral pleural effusions, & mediastinal lymphatic congestion ➚. These findings are highly suspicious for PVOD. Vasodilators can be life threatening.*

Niemann-Pick Disease

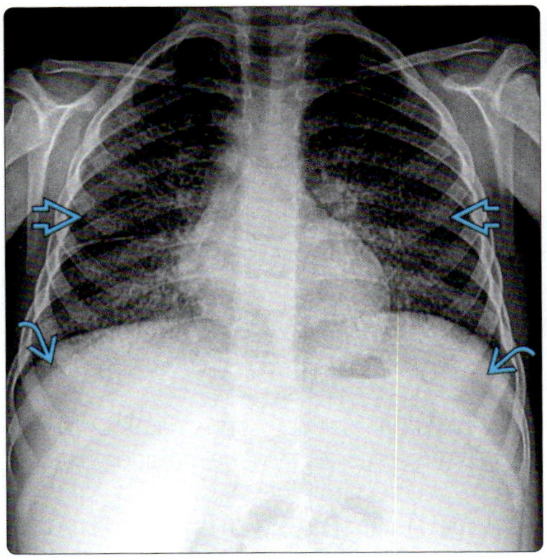

Niemann-Pick Disease

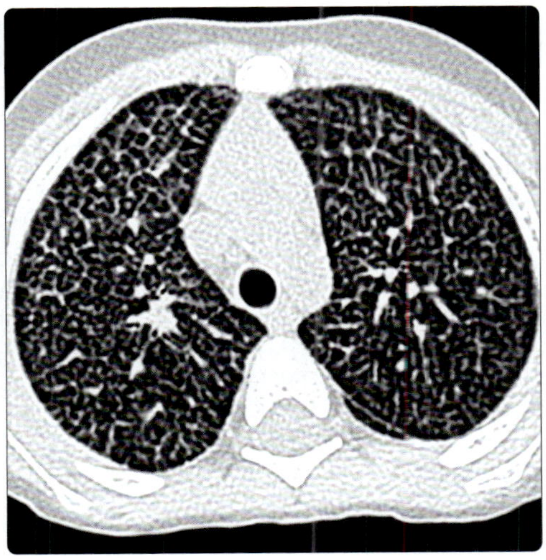

(Left) *PA radiograph in a 4 year old with Niemann-Pick disease shows diffuse reticulonodular opacities ➯ of the lungs. There is also hepatosplenomegaly ➚.* **(Right)** *Axial HRCT in the same patient shows diffuse, fine, nodular, inter- & intralobular septal thickening throughout the lungs. Niemann-Pick disease is an autosomal recessive lysosomal storage disorder with hepatosplenomegaly & variable CNS disease. Lung involvement is frequent in Niemann-Pick type B disease.*

DIFFERENTIAL DIAGNOSIS

Common

- Transient Tachypnea of Newborn
- Increased Pulmonary Vascularity
  - Left-to-Right Cardiac Shunts
- Surfactant Deficiency Disease

Less Common

- Pulmonary Interstitial Emphysema
- Meconium Aspiration Syndrome
- Neonatal Pneumonia

Rare but Important

- Childhood Interstitial Lung Disease
  - Surfactant Dysfunction Disorders
  - Neuroendocrine Cell Hyperplasia of Infancy
  - Pulmonary Interstitial Glycogenosis
- Total Anomalous Pulmonary Venous Return
- Congenital Pulmonary Lymphangiectasia

ESSENTIAL INFORMATION

Helpful Clues for Common Diagnoses

- **Transient Tachypnea of Newborn**
  - Delayed clearance of fetal lung fluid
  - More common with cesarean section, precipitous delivery, & maternal gestational diabetes
  - Resolves within 48-72 hours after birth
  - Diffuse interstitial opacities, especially perihilar, & trace pleural fluid (commonly seen in fissures)
- **Increased Pulmonary Vascularity**
  - Increased pulmonary arterial blood flow
  - Vessels can mimic irregular opacities
  - May be cyanotic or acyanotic condition
    - **Left-to-right cardiac shunts**
      - Acyanotic
      - May be intracardiac or extracardiac
      - Most common neonatal extracardiac shunt is vein of Galen malformation
- **Surfactant Deficiency Disease**
  - a.k.a. respiratory distress syndrome, hyaline membrane disease
  - Secondary to immaturity of lungs in premature infant
  - Most common cause of morbidity in premature infants
    - Up to 30% in infants born at 32- to 36-weeks gestation
    - Rare in infants born > 36 weeks, possible in diabetic mothers
  - Decreased lung volumes & diffuse hazy granular opacities
    - Findings worst at 12-24 hours of life
    - Appearance changes after treatment with mechanical ventilation & administration of exogenous surfactant via endotracheal tube
      - Normalization of lung volumes
      - Alveoli can even become overdistended with bubbly lucencies
      - Uneven distribution of exogenous surfactant can lead to heterogeneous pattern of expansion & atelectasis
  - Complications of mechanical ventilation: Pulmonary interstitial emphysema (PIE), pneumomediastinum, pneumothorax
  - May progress to chronic lung disease of prematurity

Helpful Clues for Less Common Diagnoses

- **Pulmonary Interstitial Emphysema**
  - Most common in patients with surfactant deficiency & resultant stiff lungs
  - Background lung disease + barotrauma from mechanical ventilation → alveolar rupture with air leak into interstitium
  - Circular & linear lucencies, may be branching; can rapidly develop between radiographs
    - Bilateral, unilateral, lobar, or segmental
    - Can progress to pneumomediastinum & pneumothorax
    - May resolve quickly with change in ventilator settings
- **Meconium Aspiration Syndrome**
  - Usually in term infant
  - Complication of fetal stress → defecation → aspiration of meconium
  - Relatively normal radiograph may worsen rapidly due to chemical pneumonitis
  - Lungs are generally hyperinflated with coarse irregular opacities, atelectasis, & regions of air-trapping
  - Complications: Pneumothorax (10-40%), PIE, superimposed pneumonia, persistent pulmonary hypertension
- **Neonatal Pneumonia**
  - Infection occurs shortly before, during, or shortly following birth
  - Classically caused by group B *Streptococcus;* however, *Staphylococcus epidermidis* is now more common
    - *Escherichia coli* is becoming most common in very low birth weight infants (< 1,500 gm)
  - Varied appearance on radiography
    - Normal lung volumes with ill-defined foci of consolidation are most classic, but opacification may also be diffuse
    - Pleural effusions more often seen than in surfactant deficiency disease (SDD) or meconium aspiration syndrome (MAS), which can point to diagnosis

Helpful Clues for Rare Diagnoses

- **Childhood Interstitial Lung Disease**
  - Current classification in infants
    - Diffuse developmental disorders
      - Group of diseases with abnormal development of lungs; near 100% mortality by 2 months
      - Types: Acinar dysplasia, congenital alveolar dysplasia, alveolar capillary dysplasia
    - Alveolar growth abnormalities
      - Secondary to other prenatal or postnatal conditions that affect lungs, but not by gene mutation directly involved in lung development
      - e.g., secondary pulmonary hypoplasia, chronic lung disease of prematurity, trisomy 21 lung disease
    - Surfactant dysfunction disorders & related abnormalities
      - Mutation in genes involved in production & metabolism of surfactant

- Specific conditions of unknown or poorly understood etiology
  - Neuroendocrine cell hyperplasia of infancy (NEHI)
  - Pulmonary interstitial glycogenosis (PIG)
  - NEHI & PIG may not be specific entities but represent common consequence of lung dysmaturation, which can be of various causes
- Besides NEHI, genetic testing or biopsy is often needed for ultimate diagnosis in infants
- Imaging: Variable combination of air-trapping, ground-glass opacities, consolidation, nodules, cysts, & irregular interstitial opacities
- **Surfactant dysfunction disorders**
  - Most caused by mutations in *SFTPB*, *SFTPC*, or *ABCA3*
  - Full term with diffuse hazy opacities similar to SDD
  - CT: Diffuse ground-glass opacities with interlobular septal thickening ("crazy paving")
  - *SFTPC* mutations are associated with cysts
- **Neuroendocrine cell hyperplasia of infancy**
  - Usually term infants with tachypnea, hypoxemia, wheezing ~ 3 months of age after initially well
  - Central ground-glass opacities, especially of right middle lobe & lingula (± air-trapping)
  - Imaging appearance is highly specific for NEHI & can be considered diagnostic (previously was considered 100% specific)
- **Pulmonary interstitial glycogenosis**
  - Preterm or term infants with tachypnea & hypoxemia between birth & 6 months of age
  - More commonly in conjunction with alveolar growth abnormality, congenital heart disease, or other process rather than isolated
  - Variable ground-glass opacities, reticular interstitial opacities, air-trapping, & cysts

- **Total Anomalous Pulmonary Venous Return**
  - Pulmonary venous return may be obstructed, especially in infracardiac type
    - Common draining vein courses through diaphragm & anastomoses with portal vein, returning to heart via hepatic circulation
  - Obstruction is less common in other (supracardiac & cardiac) types of anomalous venous return
  - Obstruction results in severe pulmonary edema ± pulmonary lymphangiectasia
  - Heart & aorta are small due to lack of venous return
  - Often with associated thymic atrophy, hyperinflated lungs, & pleural effusions
- **Congenital Pulmonary Lymphangiectasia**
  - Dilation of subpleural, interseptal, perivascular, & peribronchial pulmonary lymphatics
  - Can be primary or secondary
    - Primary type associated with trisomy 21 & Noonan syndrome
    - Secondary type due to chronic pulmonary venous obstruction in utero from congenital heart disease
      - Most commonly: Obstructed total anomalous pulmonary venous return (TAPVR) or hypoplastic left heart syndrome with restrictive atrial defect or intact atrial septum
  - Radiographs: Well-inflated lungs with fine reticular opacities
  - CT: Diffuse inter- & intralobular septal thickening with cobblestone lung surface
  - Fetal MR: T2-hyperintense lungs with fluid-filled, tubular branching structures extending from hila to lung periphery ("nutmeg" lung)
  - US: Lung surface irregularity with subpleural cystic-appearing foci
  - Chylous pleural effusions can be present

SELECTED REFERENCES

1. Bush A et al: Early onset children's interstitial lung diseases: discrete entities or manifestations of pulmonary dysmaturity? Paediatr Respir Rev. ePub, 2018
2. Liszewski MC et al: Neonatal lung disorders: pattern recognition approach to diagnosis. AJR Am J Roentgenol. 210(5):964-75, 2018
3. Lam CZ et al: Diagnosis of secondary pulmonary lymphangiectasia in congenital heart disease: a novel role for chest ultrasound and prognostic implications. Pediatr Radiol. 47(11):1441-51, 2017
4. Thacker PG et al: Current update on interstitial lung disease of infancy: new classification system, diagnostic evaluation, imaging algorithms, imaging findings, and prognosis. Radiol Clin North Am. 54(6):1065-76, 2016

Transient Tachypnea of Newborn | **Transient Tachypnea of Newborn**

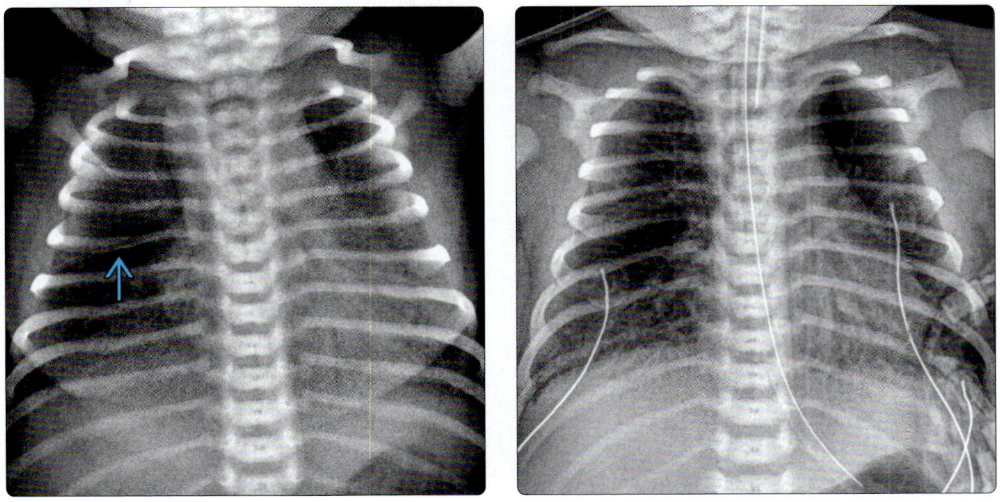

(Left) *AP radiograph in a term newborn with tachypnea & hypoglycemia due to maternal gestational diabetes, & delivered by elective cesarean section, shows diffuse interstitial opacities with trace right pleural fluid* ⇒. **(Right)** *AP radiograph in the same patient 1 day later shows improving interstitial opacities with persistent perihilar streakiness. The clinical history is typical of transient tachypnea of the newborn (TTN), & the improvement within 48-72 hours is diagnostic.*

(**Left**) *AP radiograph in a cyanotic 1 day old with transposition of the great arteries shows increased pulmonary vascularity, which will continue to increase as pulmonary vascular resistance drops after birth. Note the egg-on-a-string appearance.* (**Right**) *AP radiograph in an acyanotic 7 day old shows severe cardiomegaly with increased pulmonary vascularity. There is an enlarged abdomen due to a congenital hepatic hemangioma creating an extracardiac left-to-right shunt.*

Increased Pulmonary Vascularity

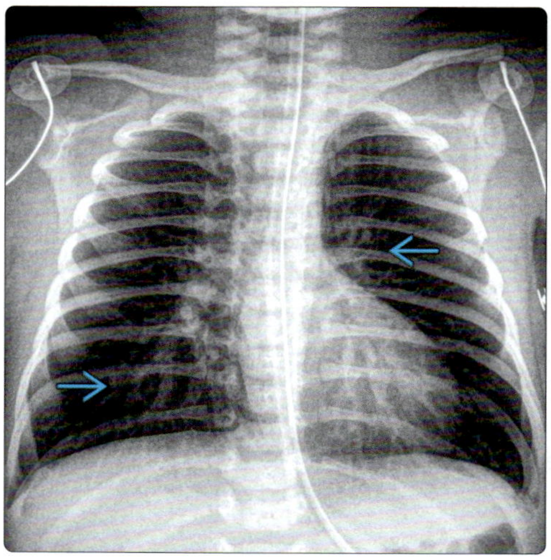

Increased Pulmonary Vascularity

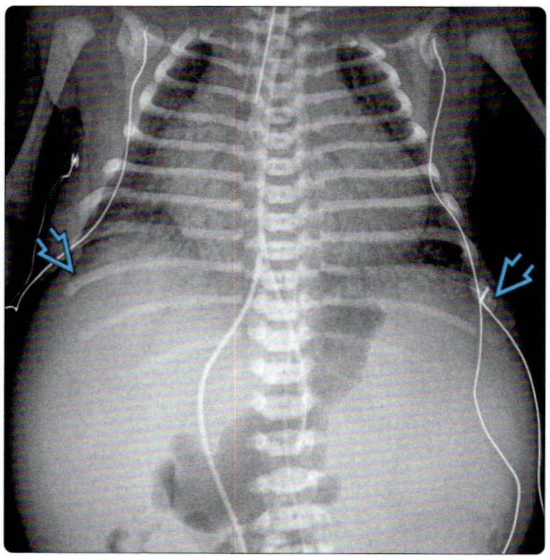

(**Left**) *AP radiograph in a premature newborn (26-weeks gestational age) shows diffuse hazy granular opacities throughout the lungs, consistent with surfactant deficiency disease (SDD).* (**Right**) *AP radiograph shows coarse irregular opacities throughout both lungs with a focal area of atelectasis in the left perihilar region. The patient is intubated, likely contributing to the relative lung hyperinflation in this patient with SDD. Chronic mechanical ventilation with supplemental oxygen can lead to chronic lung disease.*

Surfactant Deficiency Disease

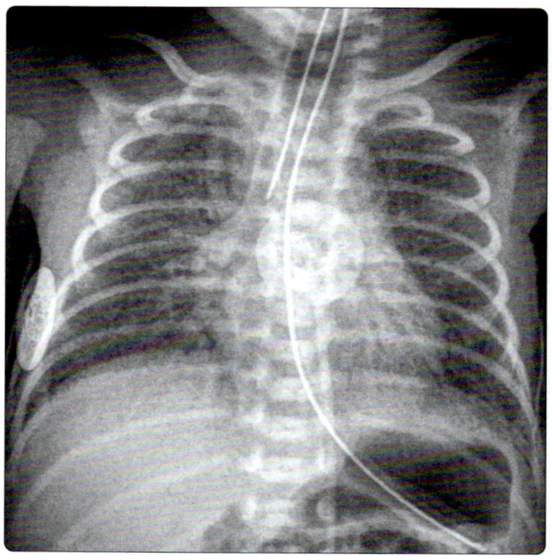

Surfactant Deficiency Disease

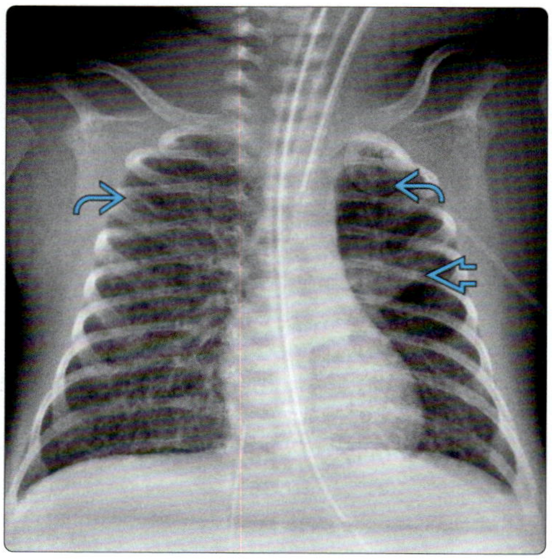

(**Left**) *AP radiograph in a premature 3 day old on mechanical ventilation shows left lung lucencies due to pulmonary interstitial emphysema. There is an associated left pneumothorax with depression of the hemidiaphragm & mediastinal shift. The right lung granular opacities are due to SDD.* (**Right**) *Axial NECT shows locules of air throughout the left lung interstitial spaces, consistent with pulmonary interstitial emphysema. This is a result of barotrauma from mechanical ventilation.*

Pulmonary Interstitial Emphysema

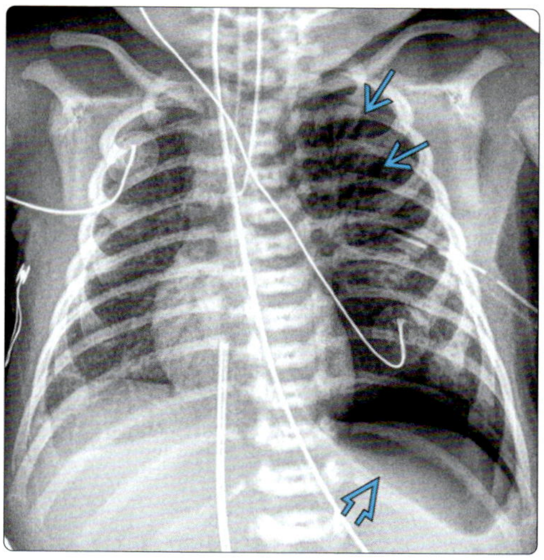

Pulmonary Interstitial Emphysema

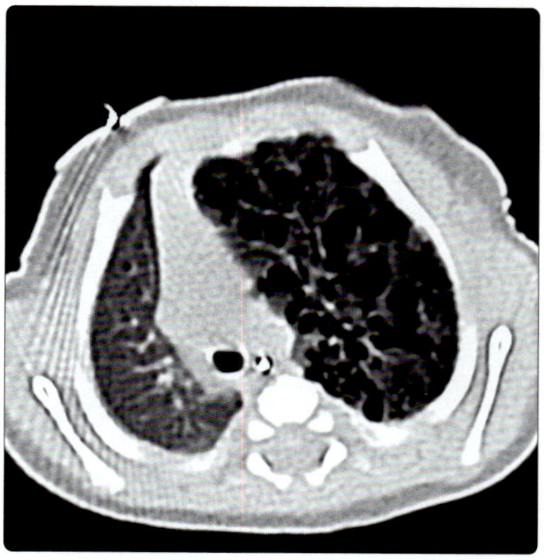

Meconium Aspiration Syndrome

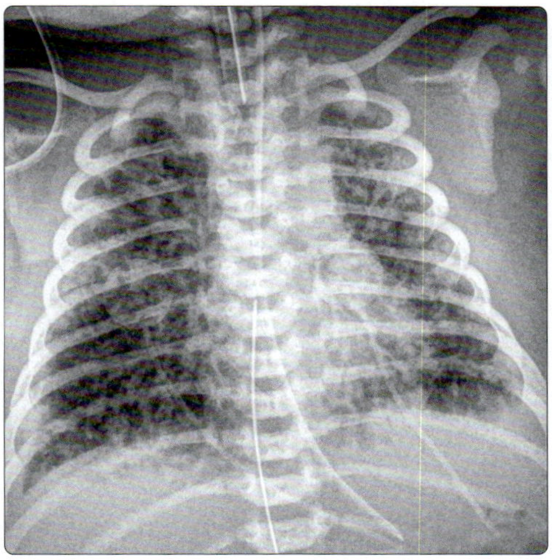

Meconium Aspiration Syndrome

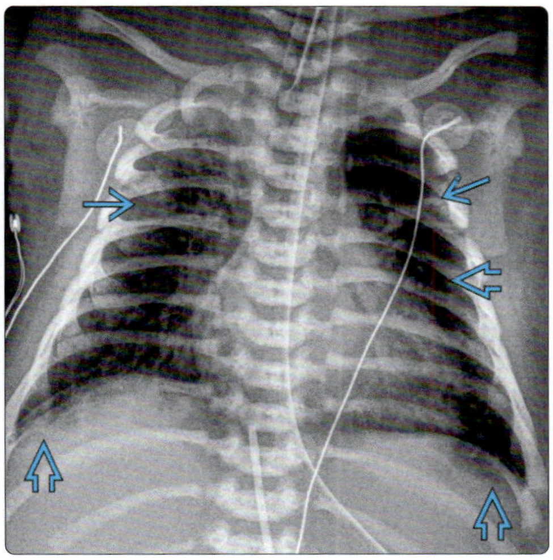

(Left) *AP radiograph in a term 1 day old with meconium aspiration & persistent pulmonary hypertension shows typical hyperinflated lungs with coarse irregular opacities & small bilateral pleural effusions.* **(Right)** *AP radiograph in a term 5 day old with hypoglycemia shows streaky irregular opacities ➡ with scattered air-trapping ➡, consistent with meconium aspiration. When provided, a clinical history of meconium-stained amniotic fluid is quite helpful in understanding the pathophysiology behind the image.*

Neonatal Pneumonia

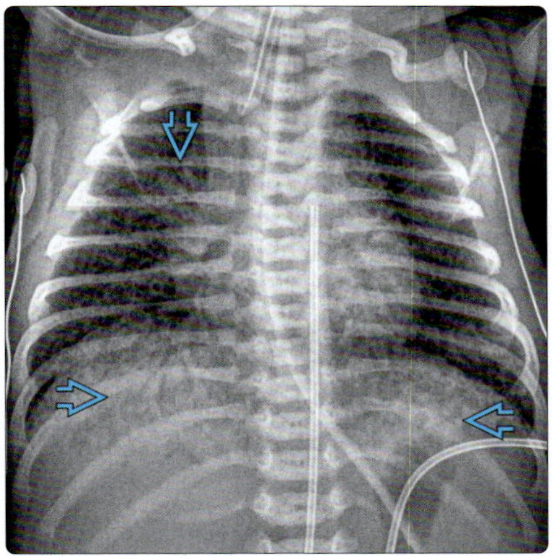

Neonatal Pneumonia

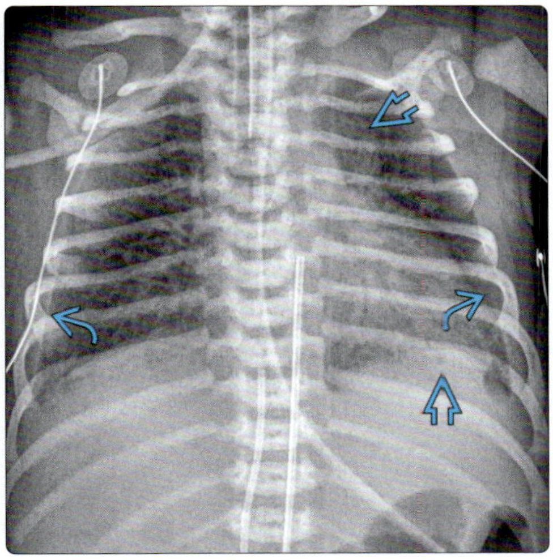

(Left) *AP radiograph in a 1 day old shows diffuse irregular lung opacities along with patchy confluent opacities ➡ due to neonatal pneumonia.* **(Right)** *AP radiograph in a 1 day old shows scattered irregular opacities, focal consolidations ➡, & bilateral pleural effusions ➡ secondary to neonatal pneumonia. Neonatal pneumonia can appear similar to many other neonatal conditions, & differentiation is usually clinical. Pleural effusions can be a clue.*

Surfactant Dysfunction Disorders

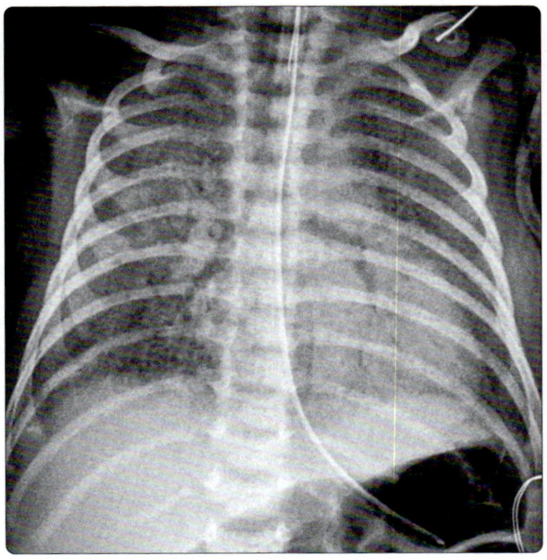

Surfactant Dysfunction Disorders

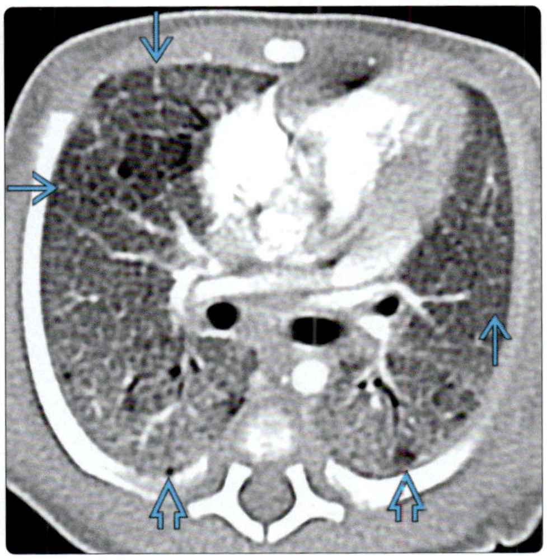

(Left) *AP radiograph in a 16 day old with respiratory failure shows patchy airspace opacities on a background of diffuse granular opacities.* **(Right)** *Axial CECT in the same patient shows diffuse ground-glass opacities with smooth septal thickening ➡ & scattered cysts or air-trapping ➡. This pattern is nonspecific but highly suggestive of surfactant dysfunction, which was confirmed on lung biopsy. Genetic testing revealed an SFTPB mutation.*

(Left) *AP radiograph in a 44 day old with tachypnea shows ill-defined airspace opacities of the bilateral upper lobes, right middle lobe, & lingula.* **(Right)** *Axial NECT in the same patient shows ground-glass opacities in the right middle lobe & lingula with right lower lobe air-trapping & otherwise relative lower lobe sparing. This pattern is highly specific for neuroendocrine cell hyperplasia of infancy (NEHI), & many would consider the diagnosis without biopsy.*

Neuroendocrine Cell Hyperplasia of Infancy

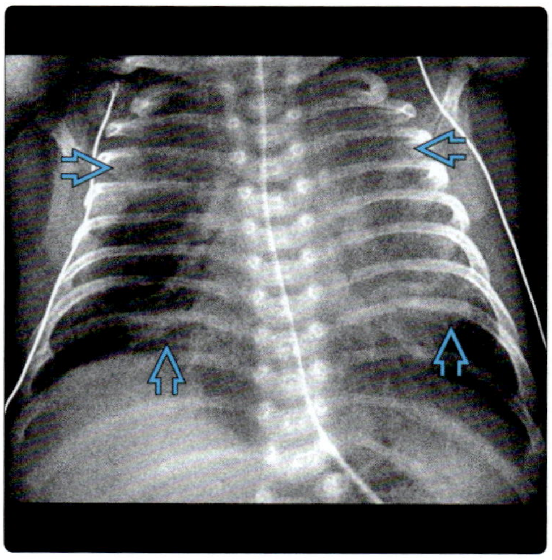

Neuroendocrine Cell Hyperplasia of Infancy

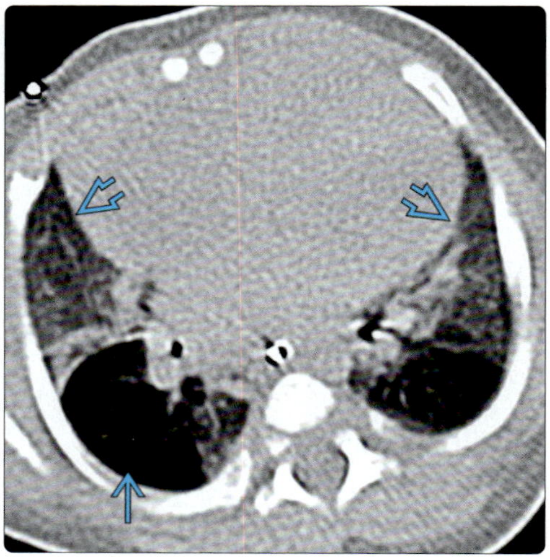

(Left) *AP radiograph in a 3 month old with persistent tachypnea & failure to thrive shows patchy ill-defined opacities with interspersed bubbly lucencies. This appearance is nonspecific & requires further work-up.* **(Right)** *Axial CECT in the same patient shows patchy geographic ground-glass opacities with scattered air-trapping &/or cystic-appearing lesions, some of which persisted as discrete cysts on follow-up. Lung biopsy revealed pulmonary interstitial glycogenosis.*

Pulmonary Interstitial Glycogenosis

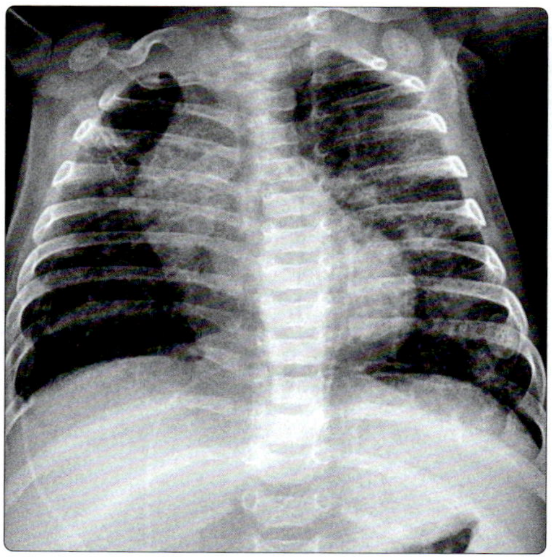

Pulmonary Interstitial Glycogenosis

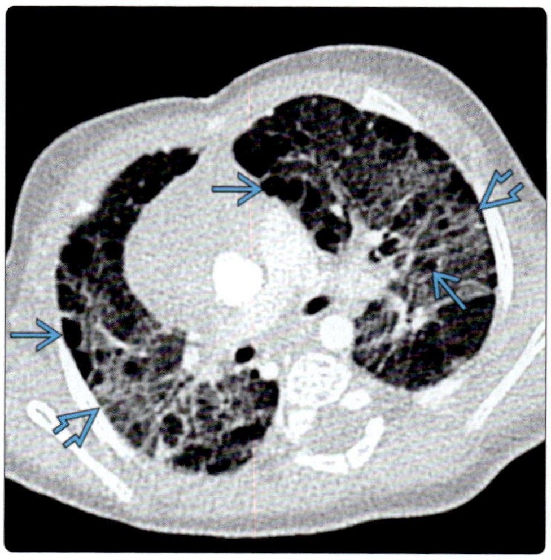

(Left) *AP radiograph in a 1 day old with right atrial isomerism & total anomalous pulmonary venous return shows increased pulmonary vascularity & mild interstitial edema. Note the left UVC in a midline liver, a right paramedian stomach, & bilateral right bronchial branching patterns.* **(Right)** *Coronal oblique CECT MIP in the same patient shows all pulmonary veins draining to a posterior vertical vein that courses infradiaphragmatic before connecting to the IVC (connection not shown).*

Total Anomalous Pulmonary Venous Return

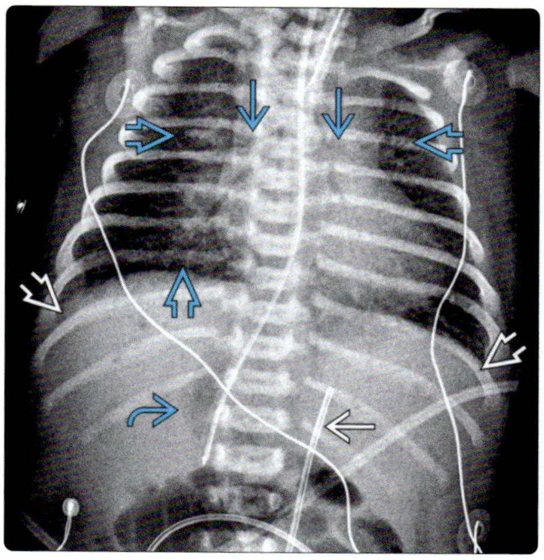

Total Anomalous Pulmonary Venous Return

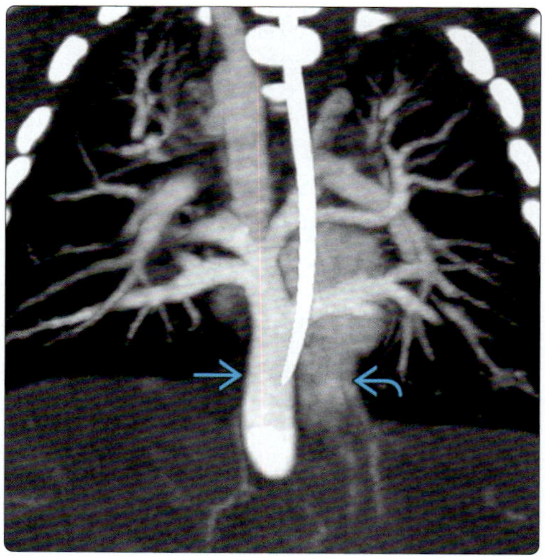

Congenital Pulmonary Lymphangiectasia

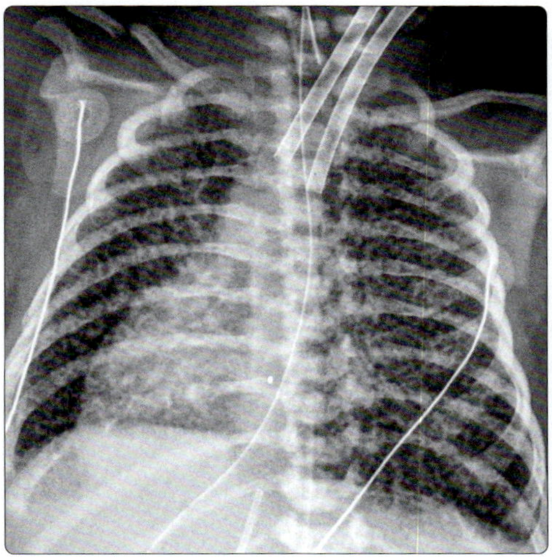

Congenital Pulmonary Lymphangiectasia

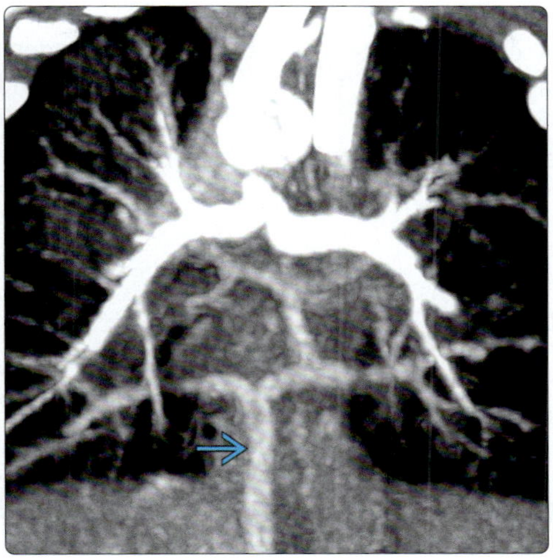

(Left) *AP radiograph in a 1 day old with dextrocardia & obstructed TAPVR on ECMO shows a normal heart size with pulmonary edema. The fine interstitial reticulation is suspicious for secondary pulmonary lymphangiectasia due to chronic pulmonary venous obstruction & carries a poor prognosis.* **(Right)** *Coronal CECT MIP in the same patient shows all pulmonary veins draining to a vertical vein → that courses infradiaphragmatically, where it is obstructed (not shown). Infradiaphragmatic TAPVR is obstructed in 90% of patients.*

Congenital Pulmonary Lymphangiectasia

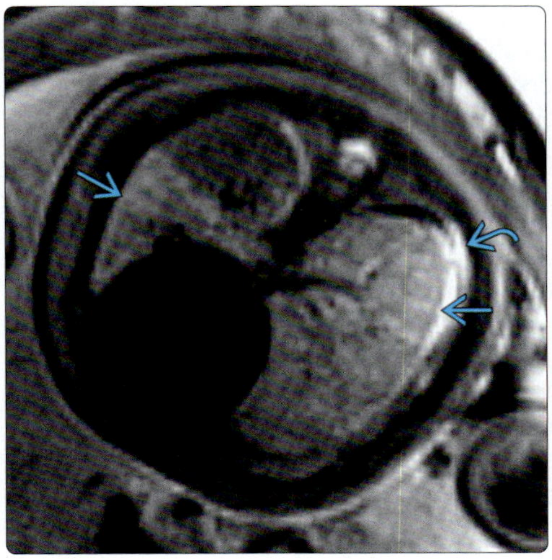

Congenital Pulmonary Lymphangiectasia

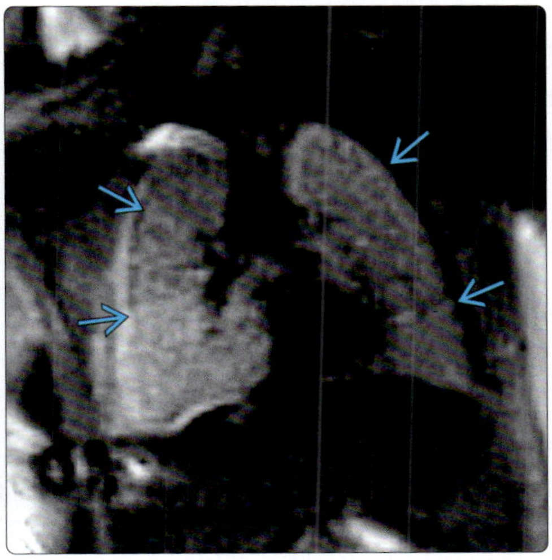

(Left) *Axial T2 SSFSE fetal MR in the same patient at 32-weeks gestation shows heterogeneous hyperintense lungs with fluid-filled, tubular branching structures extending from the hila to the periphery → along with a pleural effusion ↷.* **(Right)** *Coronal T2 SSFSE fetal MR in the same patient at 32-weeks gestation again shows hyperintense lungs with fluid-filled, tubular branching structures extending from the hila to the lung periphery →. This appearance is highly specific for pulmonary lymphangiectasia.*

Congenital Pulmonary Lymphangiectasia

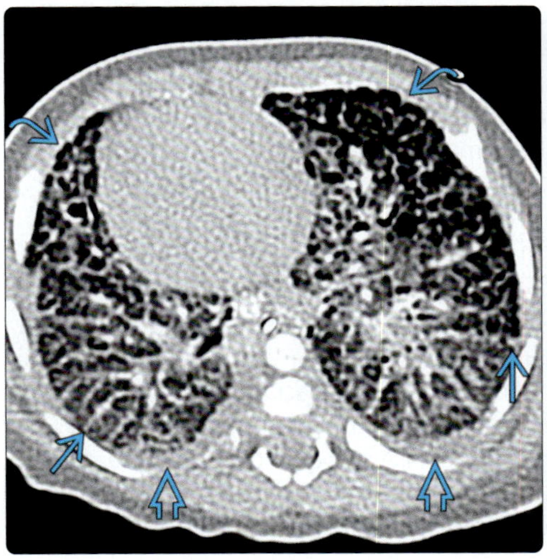

Congenital Pulmonary Lymphangiectasia

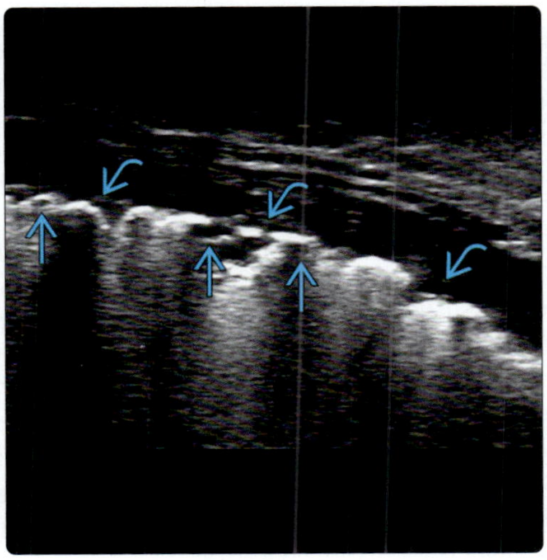

(Left) *Axial CECT in the same patient at 1 day old shows diffuse inter- & intralobular septal thickening → with a cobblestone lung surface ↷ & small pleural effusions ⇨, consistent with pulmonary lymphangiectasia.* **(Right)** *Transverse chest surface ultrasound in the same patient at 1 day old shows lung surface irregularity ↷ with subpleural cystic-appearing structures →, highly specific for pulmonary lymphangiectasia in the appropriate clinical setting. Primary & secondary types appear similar.*

DIFFERENTIAL DIAGNOSIS

Common

- Pulmonary Interstitial Emphysema
- Congenital Pulmonary Airway Malformation
- Congenital Diaphragmatic Hernia
- Chronic Lung Disease of Prematurity
- Cystic Fibrosis

Less Common

- Pneumatoceles
- Childhood Interstitial Lung Disease

Rare but Important

- Lymphangioleiomyomatosis
- Pulmonary Langerhans Cell Histiocytosis

ESSENTIAL INFORMATION

Key Differential Diagnosis Issues

- Various causes of bubbly lung appearance; age, clinical history, & extent of disease (unilateral vs. bilateral) are typically helpful
- CT may be necessary to narrow differential diagnosis

Helpful Clues for Common Diagnoses

- **Pulmonary Interstitial Emphysema**
  - Premature neonates
  - Background lung disease + barotrauma from mechanical ventilation → alveolar rupture with air leak into interstitium
  - Imaging: Reticular & cystic appearance (which can rapidly develop between radiographs)
    - Bilateral, unilateral, lobar, or segmental
    - Can progress to pneumomediastinum & pneumothorax
    - May resolve quickly with change in ventilator settings
- **Congenital Pulmonary Airway Malformation**
  - Previously known as cystic adenomatoid malformation (CCAM)
  - Hamartomatous proliferation of cystic & noncystic bronchiole-like tissue
    - At birth, communicates with abnormal cartilage- & gland-deficient bronchial tree
    - Stocker classification (0-4) based on level of airway maldevelopment (proximal to distal)
      - Type 0 (< 2%): Small lungs with severe acinar dysgenesis & large airway dysplasia; uniformly fatal
      - Type 1 (65%): Mainly ≥ 1 macrocysts (> 2 cm); may have air-fluid levels
      - Type 2 (10-15%): Multiple small cysts (0.5-2.0 cm)
      - Type 3 (5-8%): Innumerable microscopic cysts; appears solid
      - Type 4 (10-15%): Large peripheral cysts; unclear if distinct from type 1 pleuropulmonary blastoma
  - Imaging: Fluid-filled cysts at birth gradually fill with air
    - Types 1 & 2 can look like unilateral bubbly lung
    - Mass effect: Mediastinal shift, compressive atelectasis
    - Can coexist with other lung malformations, such as sequestration or bronchial atresia ("hybrid lesion")
      - Image by CTA through celiac axis to look for systemic arterial supply
  - Risk of recurrent infections
  - Small risk of malignancy development: Bronchoalveolar carcinoma, rhabdomyosarcoma
- **Congenital Diaphragmatic Hernia**
  - Bochdalek (90%): Posterolateral
    - Left 80-90%, right 10-15%, bilateral < 5%
  - Morgagni/ventral (10%): Retrosternal
  - Imaging: Bubbly bowel-like lucencies in hemithorax when stomach/bowel are involved
    - Lucencies in chest are contiguous from abdomen
    - Enteric tube may course into chest
    - Associated mass effect on mediastinum
    - Associated pulmonary hypoplasia & pulmonary hypertension: Major prognostic factors
  - Other associated cardiovascular, limb, central nervous, GI, GU, & genetic anomalies in 25-50%
- **Chronic Lung Disease of Prematurity**
  - a.k.a. bronchopulmonary dysplasia
  - Affects premature neonates with surfactant deficiency
  - Definition: Born < 32-weeks gestation with O_2 dependency > 28 days with failure at 36-weeks postmenstrual age to maintain O_2 saturation > 90% during trial of 21% inspired O_2
  - Risk factors: Fetal growth restriction, mechanical ventilation, high oxygen concentrations, postnatal sepsis
  - Imaging: Bubbly lung appearance begins ~ 2 weeks after birth
    - Hyperinflation & air-trapping
    - Cystic, bubbly lucencies
    - Coarse, band-like opacities (atelectasis & fibrosis)
  - Modern use of antenatal steroids, exogenous surfactant administration, & reduced ventilator/O_2 intensity → less inflammation & fibrosis
    - 1st see diffuse, hazy opacification progressing to coarse, interstitial opacities with air-trapping
- **Cystic Fibrosis**
  - Autosomal recessive multisystem disorder
  - Defects in gene for cystic fibrosis transmembrane conductance regulator (CFTR)
    - Encodes protein of cell membrane chloride channel
  - Leads to exocrine gland dysfunction in lungs, liver, pancreas, GI tract
    - Lungs: Thick secretions & impaired immunity
  - Lungs are normal at birth → chronic mucoid impaction → recurrent inflammation & infections → chronic structural lung damage (reinforcing cycle)
  - Imaging: Bronchiectasis (upper lobe predominance); cystic form can give bubbly lung appearance
    - Bronchial wall thickening, mucous plugging
      - Air-trapping with hypoperfusion (small airways disease)
      - Centrilobular nodular opacities (peripheral mucoid impaction &/or infectious/inflammatory debris)
    - Radiographs are insensitive for detection of early disease or for monitoring disease progression
    - CT (& emerging role of MR) for surveillance
      - Degree of bronchiectasis & small airways disease are important biomarkers of disease status
      - Lung changes can be independent of changes on pulmonary function tests

Helpful Clues for Less Common Diagnoses

- **Pneumatoceles**
  - Thin-walled cysts/cavities
  - May be secondary to trauma or infection/inflammation
  - Can resolve spontaneously, especially in young children
  - May become superinfected
  - When multiple, can appear as bubbly lungs
- **Childhood Interstitial Lung Disease**
  - a.k.a. diffuse parenchymal lung disease
  - Uncommon group of disorders
  - Can be diagnosed when there is diffuse lung disease & other more common entities have been excluded
    - Asthma, primary ciliary dyskinesia, cystic fibrosis, infection, recurrent aspiration
  - Can be idiopathic or secondary to known disorder (e.g., infection, drugs, exposure)
    - Possible association with systemic disease (e.g., connective tissue disease, vasculitis)
  - Current classification in infants
    - Diffuse developmental disorders
    - Alveolar growth abnormalities
    - Surfactant dysfunction disorders & related abnormalities
    - Specific conditions of unknown or poorly understood etiology
      - Neuroendocrine cell hyperplasia in infancy (NEHI)
      - Pulmonary interstitial glycogenosis (PIG)
  - Imaging
    - Variable combination of air-trapping, ground-glass opacities, consolidation, nodules, cysts, & linear/reticular opacities
    - PIG & surfactant dysfunction disorders more commonly have scattered air-trapping &/or cystic changes that can appear as bubbly lungs
    - Central ground-glass opacities, especially of right middle lobe & lingula (± air-trapping), are highly specific for NEHI
  - Besides NEHI, genetic testing or biopsy is often needed for ultimate diagnosis in infants

Helpful Clues for Rare Diagnoses

- **Lymphangioleiomyomatosis**
  - 2 subtypes: Tuberous sclerosis complex-associated & sporadic
  - Proliferation of low-grade neoplastic cells with smooth muscle-like & epithelioid-like populations
    - Metastatic from unknown primary tumor (possibly pelvic/uterine in origin & spread by lymphatics)
  - Results in small airway & lymphatic obstruction
  - Imaging: Randomly distributed thin-walled cysts with normal intervening parenchyma; CT minimum intensity projection (minIP) is quite helpful for cyst visualization
    - Can get upper & peripheral lung nodules: Multifocal micronodular pneumocyte hyperplasia
    - Can get chylous pleural effusions
    - Cyst rupture can lead to pneumothorax
- **Pulmonary Langerhans Cell Histiocytosis**
  - Accumulation of Langerhans cells forming destructive bronchiolocentric granulomas
    - May be reactive response to unknown agent vs. neoplastic/monoclonal disease (evidence for both)
  - Often occurs in setting of systemic Langerhans cell histiocytosis in children (unlike isolated pulmonary disease in adult smokers)
  - Imaging: Lung involvement is diffuse; costophrenic angles are spared in adults, not in children
    - Centrilobular pulmonary nodules (granulomas) progress to irregular cysts
      - Airspace invasion → cavitation & formation of thick-walled cysts → thin-walled cysts → confluent destructive parenchymal cystic change
    - Presents with spontaneous pneumothorax in 10-20%

SELECTED REFERENCES

1. Semple TR et al: Interstitial lung disease in children made easier…well, almost. Radiographics. 37(6):1679-703, 2017
2. Torre O et al: New insights in lymphangioleiomyomatosis and pulmonary Langerhans cell histiocytosis. Eur Respir Rev. 26(145), 2017
3. Tiddens HA et al: What did we learn from two decades of chest computed tomography in cystic fibrosis? Pediatr Radiol. 44(12):1490-5, 2014

Pulmonary Interstitial Emphysema

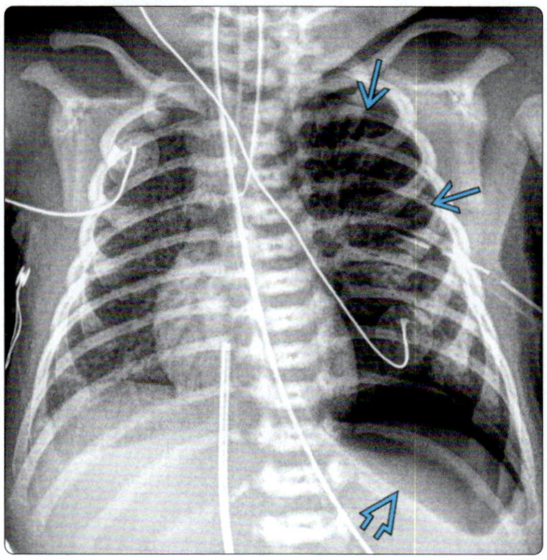

Pulmonary Interstitial Emphysema

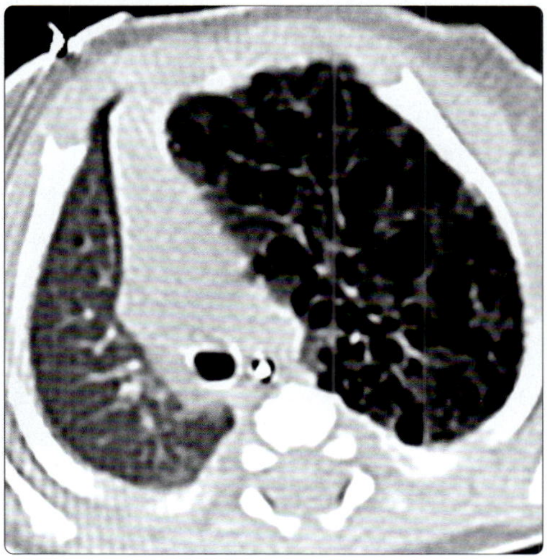

(Left) *AP radiograph in a premature 3 day old on mechanical ventilation shows left lung bubbly lucencies →, suspicious for pulmonary interstitial emphysema (PIE). There is an associated left pneumothorax ⇒ with depression of the hemidiaphragm & mediastinal shift. The right lung granular opacities are from surfactant deficiency disease.* **(Right)** *Axial NECT shows locules of air infiltrating through the left lung interstitial space, consistent with PIE. This is a result of barotrauma from mechanical ventilation.*

(Left) *PA radiograph in a 1 year old shows a bubbly right lower lung lesion that causes mass effect on the mediastinum & hemidiaphragm. Large congenital pulmonary airway malformations (CPAMs) can lead to secondary pulmonary hypoplasia.* **(Right)** *Axial CECT (same patient) shows a large right lower lobe lesion with cysts of variable size. A central solid-appearing focus with prominent vasculature was seen to arise from the abdominal aorta, representing a sequestration component ("hybrid lesion").*

Congenital Pulmonary Airway Malformation

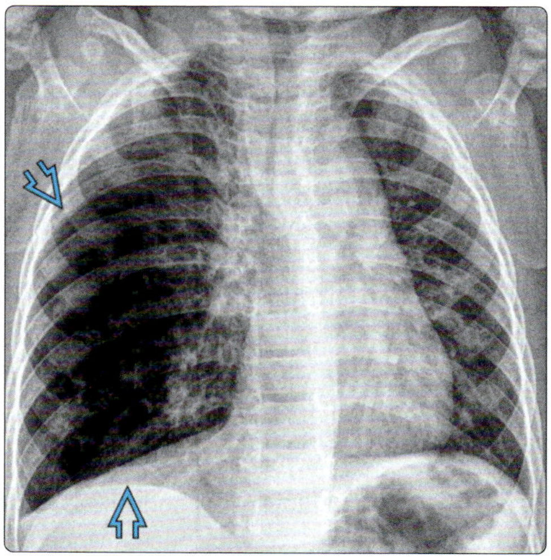

Congenital Pulmonary Airway Malformation

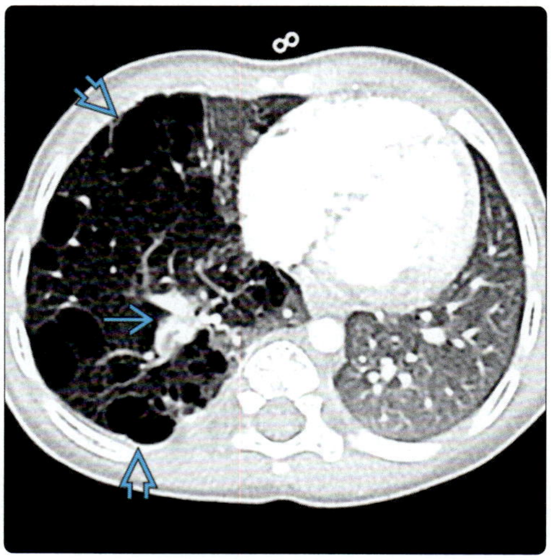

(Left) *AP radiograph in a newborn shows a bubbly mass in the left hemithorax, consistent with bowel in a left CDH. Note the abnormal courses of the enteric tube & umbilical venous catheter into the left hemithorax, suggestive of stomach & liver herniation, respectively.* **(Right)** *AP radiograph in a 6 week old, former 26-weeks-gestation infant, shows hyperinflated lungs with diffuse coarse reticular opacities & cystic bubbly lucencies, consistent with chronic lung disease of prematurity.*

Congenital Diaphragmatic Hernia

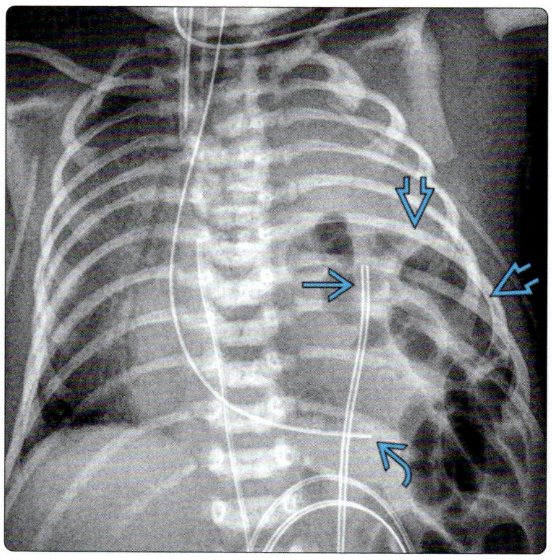

Chronic Lung Disease of Prematurity

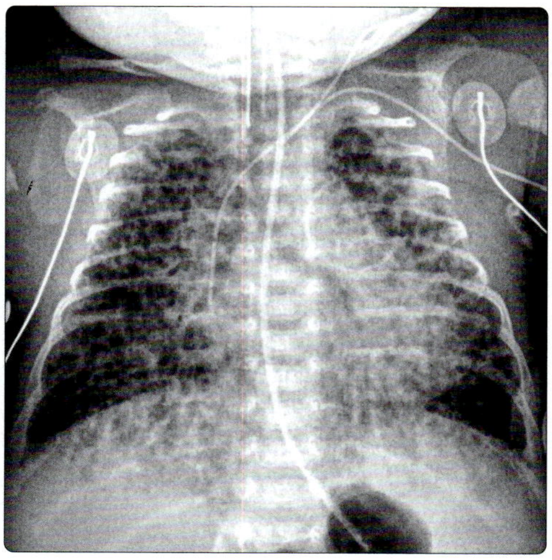

(Left) *PA radiograph in a 12 year old with severe CF recovering from a recent acute exacerbation of right lung pneumonia & empyema shows perihilar bubbly lucencies from bronchiectasis. There is also peribronchial thickening with tiny nodular opacities from mucous plugging & a right pleural effusion/thickening.* **(Right)** *Axial CECT (same patient) shows cystic bronchiectasis with bronchial wall thickening, nodular mucous plugging, & a pleural effusion with thickening from the recent empyema.*

Cystic Fibrosis

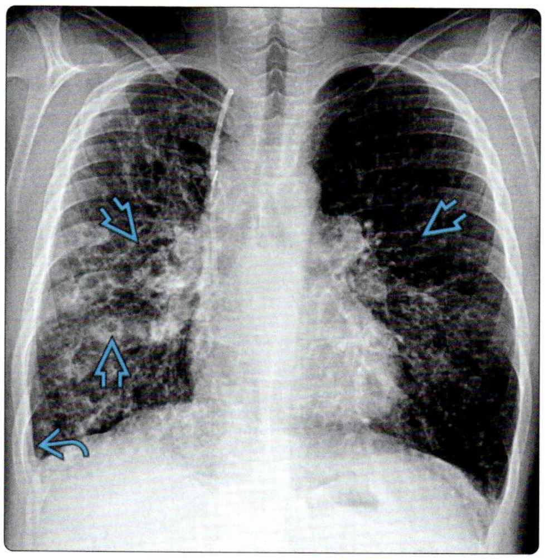

Cystic Fibrosis

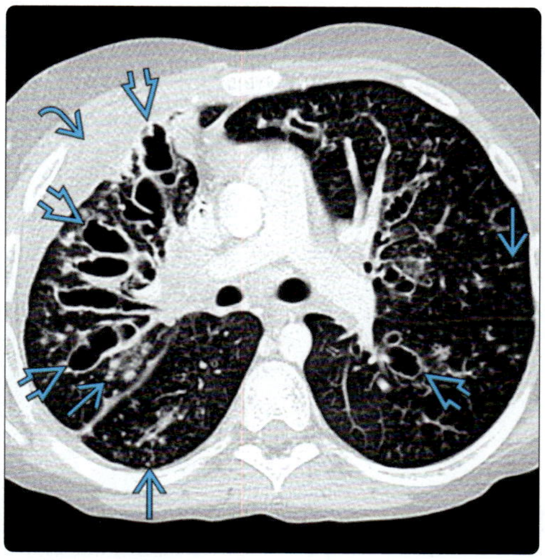

Pneumatoceles

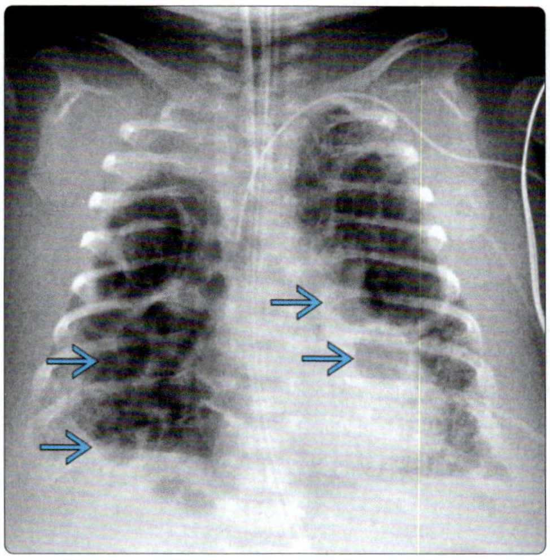

Childhood Interstitial Lung Disease

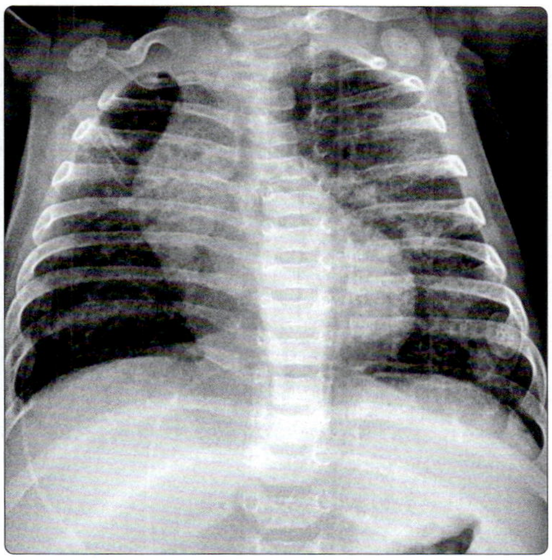

(Left) *Frontal radiograph shows bubbly lungs with multiple large cystic lucencies bilaterally ➡. The lucencies represent pneumatoceles in this 2 week old with pneumonia & sepsis. Pneumatoceles frequently resolve spontaneously in young children.* **(Right)** *AP radiograph in a 3 month old with persistent tachypnea & failure to thrive shows patchy ill-defined opacities with interspersed bubbly lucencies. This appearance is nonspecific & requires further work-up.*

Childhood Interstitial Lung Disease

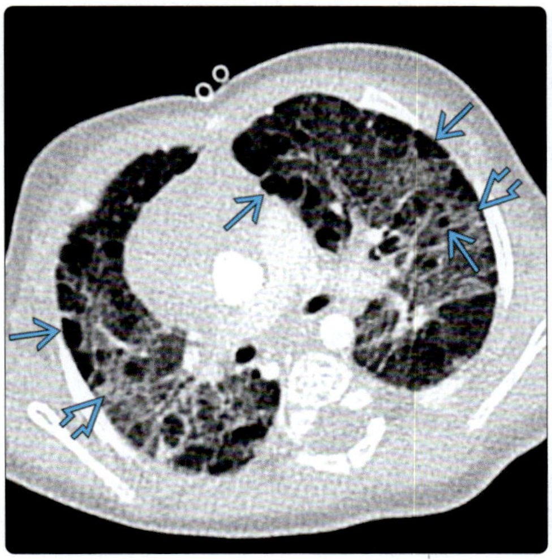

Lymphangioleiomyomatosis

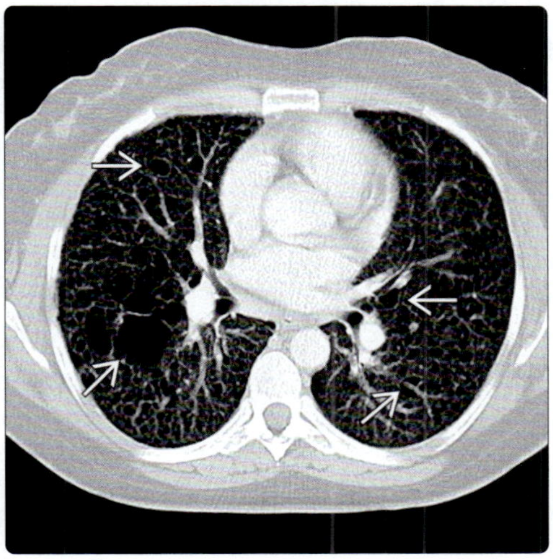

(Left) *Axial CECT in the same patient shows patchy geographic ground-glass opacities ➡ with scattered air-trapping &/or cystic-appearing lesions ➡, some of which persisted as discrete cysts on follow-up. Lung biopsy revealed pulmonary interstitial glycogenosis.* **(Right)** *Axial CECT shows innumerable parenchymal cysts of varying sizes ➡, creating a bubbly lung appearance. In this female adolescent with tuberous sclerosis complex, the appearance is consistent with lymphangioleiomyomatosis.*

Pulmonary Langerhans Cell Histiocytosis

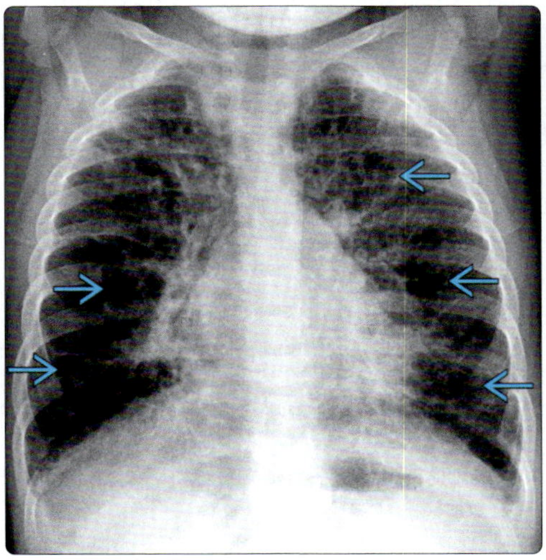

Pulmonary Langerhans Cell Histiocytosis

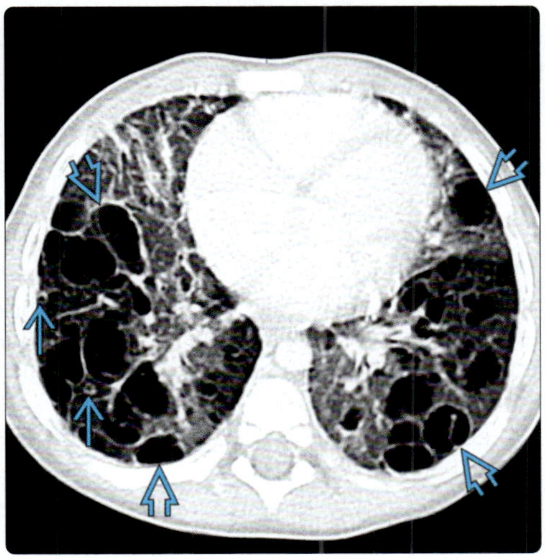

(Left) *PA radiograph in a 23 month old with respiratory distress shows a bubbly appearance of the lungs ➡ along with scattered coarse opacities.* **(Right)** *Axial CECT in the same patient shows numerous irregular lung cysts ➡. There are also cavitary nodules ➡. A biopsy of a cutaneous lesion confirmed the diagnosis of Langerhans cell histiocytosis (LCH). Pulmonary LCH (PLCH) is seen in ~ 25% of children at the presentation of multisystem LCH. Isolated PLCH represents < 10% of single-system LCH in children.*

Unilateral Hyperlucent Lung

DIFFERENTIAL DIAGNOSIS

Common

- Technical Factors
- Atelectasis
- Foreign Body Aspiration
- Pneumothorax

Less Common

- Swyer-James Syndrome
- Congenital Lung Malformation
- Pulmonary Sling
- Scimitar Syndrome
- Extrinsic Airway Compression by Mass

Rare but Important

- Pulmonary Agenesis/Aplasia/Hypoplasia
- Ductal Origin of Pulmonary Artery
- Poland Syndrome
- Endobronchial Tumor

ESSENTIAL INFORMATION

Key Differential Diagnosis Issues

- Must first determine if one lung is truly hyperlucent vs. contralateral lung being hyperdense
- Truly increased pulmonary lucency is most commonly due to air-trapping or hyperinflation
- Use systematic approach
    - Technical factors (rotation, lateral decentering)
    - Central airway obstruction
        - Foreign body aspiration
        - Extrinsic airway compression by mass
        - Endobronchial tumor
    - Lung abnormality
        - Atelectasis
        - Pneumothorax
        - Swyer-James syndrome
        - Congenital lung malformation
    - Vascular abnormality
        - Pulmonary sling
        - Scimitar syndrome
        - Pulmonary agenesis/aplasia/hypoplasia
        - Ductal origin of pulmonary artery
    - Chest wall abnormality
        - Poland syndrome
- Chest CT may be necessary in confusing cases

Helpful Clues for Common Diagnoses

- **Technical Factors**
    - Rotation: Most common cause of unilateral hyperlucent lung (1% all chest radiographs)
        - Side that patient rotates toward is hyperlucent (independent of AP or PA technique)
        - Look at clavicles & ribs to see if patient is rotated
    - Lateral decentering: Positioning of x-ray tube lateral to midline
        - Side closer to center of x-ray beam is hyperlucent
- **Atelectasis**
    - Collapse of lobe or entire lung leads to hyperinflation of remaining aerated lung, which will be hyperlucent
    - Direct signs: Shift of fissures, opacification of collapsed lung
    - Indirect signs: Elevation of ipsilateral hemidiaphragm, mediastinal/hilar shift toward collapse, crowding of ipsilateral pulmonary vessels & ribs, compensatory hyperinflation
- **Foreign Body Aspiration**
    - Food is most commonly aspirated foreign body
        - Most commonly peanuts
    - Most frequent from 6 months to 3 years of age
    - In children, air-trapping distal to obstruction occurs more commonly than atelectasis
    - Lateral decubitus radiographs: Failure of dependent lung to collapse in decubitus position suggests air-trapping
    - Fluoroscopy or expiratory images can also be utilized
    - 20-35% of children with foreign body aspiration may have normal radiographs
        - Need bronchoscopy if clinical concern persists
- **Pneumothorax**
    - Wide spectrum of etiologies in pediatric population
    - With spontaneous pneumothorax, consider
        - In neonates: Transthoracic pressure differential upon initial expansion of lungs with air
        - In teenagers: Rupture of apical blebs
    - Look for pleural line along margin of collapsing lung
        - Radiolucent space lacks pulmonary markings
    - In supine patients, anterior pneumothorax can cause appearance of unilateral hyperlucent lung
    - Look for findings of tension: Mediastinal shift, hemidiaphragm depression, etc.

Helpful Clues for Less Common Diagnoses

- **Swyer-James Syndrome**
    - Postinfectious obliterative bronchiolitis in childhood
        - Due to various lower respiratory tract infections: Adenovirus, respiratory syncytial virus, measles, pertussis, tuberculosis, *Mycoplasma*
    - Infection leads to bronchiolar inflammation & fibrosis
        - Reduced ventilation → compensatory hypoperfusion
        - Hyperexpansion/air-trapping of peripheral lung
    - Affected lung is small & hyperlucent with small hilum, attenuated pulmonary vascularity, bronchial wall thickening, bronchiectasis, & air-trapping
    - Chest CT can show involvement of both lungs, usually asymmetric (causing unilateral hyperlucent lung appearance)
- **Congenital Lung Malformation**
    - Spectrum of malformations of lung parenchyma & bronchovascular structures
        - Includes foregut duplication cyst, congenital pulmonary airway malformation (CPAM), bronchial atresia, congenital lobar overinflation (CLO), sequestration, scimitar syndrome, pulmonary sling, & pulmonary agenesis
    - Entities most strongly linked to obstruction of developing bronchus have intrinsic cystic or hyperinflated components & can present with unilateral hyperlucent lung (e.g., CPAM, bronchial atresia, CLO)
- **Pulmonary Sling**

- Left pulmonary artery arises from right pulmonary artery, then courses between trachea & esophagus to reach left hilum
  - Forms sling around trachea &/or right main bronchus
- Airway may be diffusely small or focally compressed, causing air-trapping & hyperlucency
  - Type 1: Normal carina position at T4-T5 level ± right tracheal bronchus
  - Type 2: Abnormal inferior carina at T6 level in inverted T shape ± right tracheal bronchus
    - Often with long segment inferior tracheal stenosis due to complete cartilaginous rings
- Variable degree of hyperinflation or hypoinflation depending on degree of obstruction & type of tracheobronchial branching pattern
  - Type 1: Often with right lung hyperinflation
  - Type 2: Often with bilateral hyperinflation

- **Scimitar Syndrome**
  - a.k.a. hypogenetic right lung syndrome or congenital pulmonary venolobar syndrome
  - Variable combination of multiple abnormalities
    - Partial or total anomalous pulmonary venous connection of right lung, typically to inferior vena cava
      - If unobstructed, gets larger as it descends & collects more blood → looks like Turkish sword (scimitar)
    - Aberrant systemic arterial supply to right lower lung
      - Right pulmonary artery may be small or absent
    - Hypoplasia or aplasia of 1 or more right lung lobes
      - Compensatory hyperinflation of contralateral lung, appearing hyperlucent
    - Horseshoe or cross-over lung
    - Right hemidiaphragm abnormalities
    - Associated intracardiac defects (25%)
- **Extrinsic Airway Compression by Mass**
  - Any mass in mediastinum or hila may compress tracheobronchial tree
    - Foregut duplication cysts
    - Lymphadenopathy
    - Neoplasm
  - Chest CT is usually necessary to see mass

Helpful Clues for Rare Diagnoses

- **Pulmonary Agenesis/Aplasia/Hypoplasia**
  - Congenital spectrum
    - Agenesis: Absent lung, pulmonary artery, & bronchus
    - Aplasia: Absent lung & pulmonary artery with rudimentary blind-ending bronchus
    - Hypoplasia: Hypoplastic lung, pulmonary artery, & bronchus
  - Other associated congenital anomalies are frequent
  - Compensatory hyperexpansion of contralateral lung occurs
  - Also consider secondary lung hypoplasia: Limitation of normal lung development by extrinsic compression or decreased expansion
    - Diaphragmatic hernia, thoracic dystrophy, congenital lung malformations/masses, oligohydramnios
- **Ductal Origin of Pulmonary Artery**
  - Pulmonary artery arises from ipsilateral ductus arteriosus
    - Affected pulmonary artery is usually hypoplastic
    - In past, has been called unilateral "agenesis," "absence," or "interruption" of pulmonary artery
  - Upon ductal closure, pulmonary artery becomes isolated
  - Can get small ipsilateral hypovascular (hyperlucent) lung with contralateral hyperexpansion
- **Poland Syndrome**
  - Absent/underdeveloped unilateral chest wall
    - Absent/atrophic pectoralis musculature
    - Less attenuating overlying tissue → unilateral hyperlucency
  - Associations: Ipsilateral syndactyly, Sprengel deformity, rhizomelia, absent nipple/breast, dextrocardia
- **Endobronchial Tumor**
  - Consider carcinoid tumor (80%), mucoepidermoid carcinoma, myofibroblastic tumor, papilloma, adenoid cystic carcinoma, & metastases
  - Obstruction can cause air-trapping & hyperlucent lung; more commonly see lobar collapse or consolidation

Technical Factors

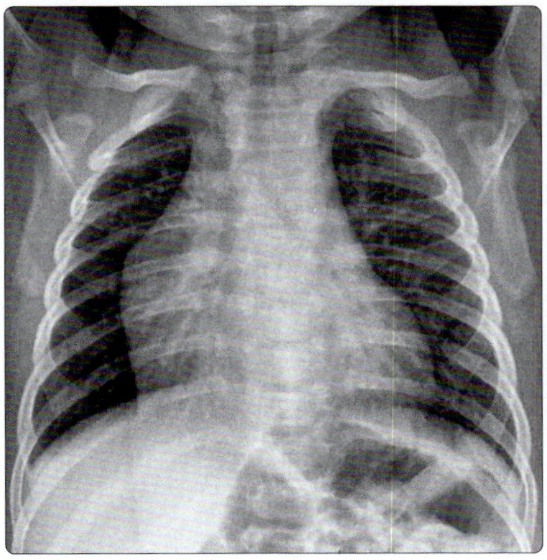

Atelectasis

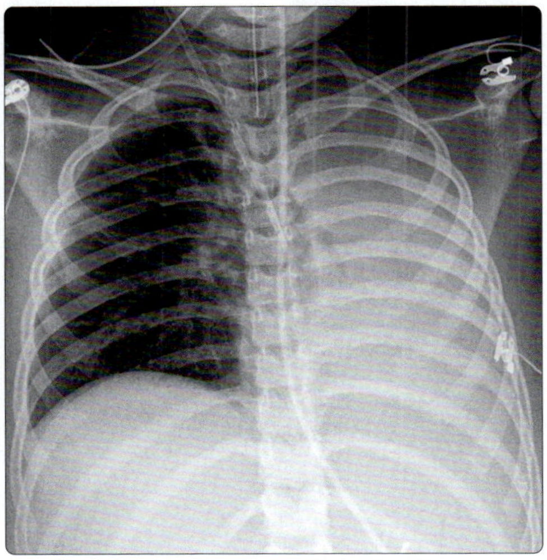

(Left) *PA radiograph in a 3 month old shows the right posterior ribs appearing longer than the left as well as the left medial clavicle appearing closer to midline than the right, indicating rightward rotation that is causing hyperlucency of the right lung. Note that the cardiothymic shadow is also shifted to the right.* **(Right)** *AP radiograph in a 9 year old with hemophagocytic lymphohistiocytosis shows complete collapse of the left lung with compensatory hyperinflation & resultant hyperlucency of the right lung.*

(Left) *PA radiograph in a 19 month old with wheezing shows hyperlucency of the left lower lung.* **(Right)** *Left lateral decubitus radiograph in the same patient shows a lack of left lower lung collapse despite the left side being down, suggesting left lower lobe air-trapping. Bronchoscopy revealed an aspirated walnut in the left main bronchus. Note that 20-35% of children with foreign body aspiration may have normal radiographs. Therefore, bronchoscopy is needed if there is persistent clinical concern.*

Foreign Body Aspiration

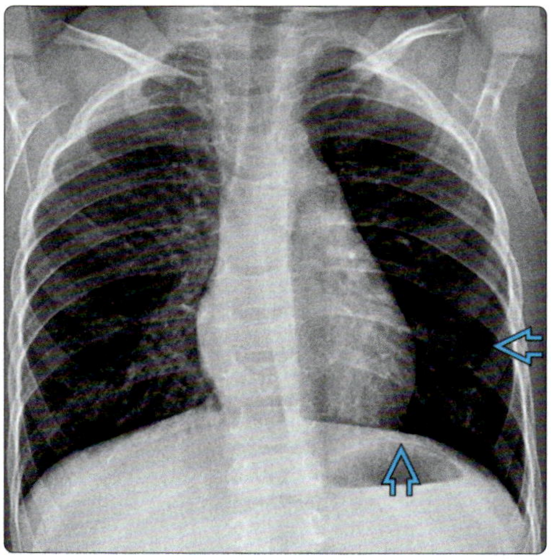

Foreign Body Aspiration

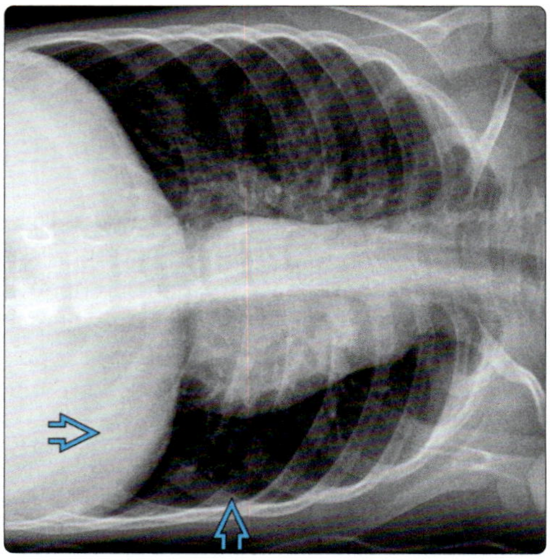

(Left) *PA radiograph in a 17 year old shows a hyperlucent left hemithorax with a distinct pleural line & a lack of lung markings peripherally, consistent with a moderate pneumothorax.* **(Right)** *PA radiograph in 6 year old shows a smaller, hyperlucent left lung with attenuated pulmonary vascularity, along with bilateral peribronchial thickening, consistent with Swyer-James syndrome.*

Pneumothorax

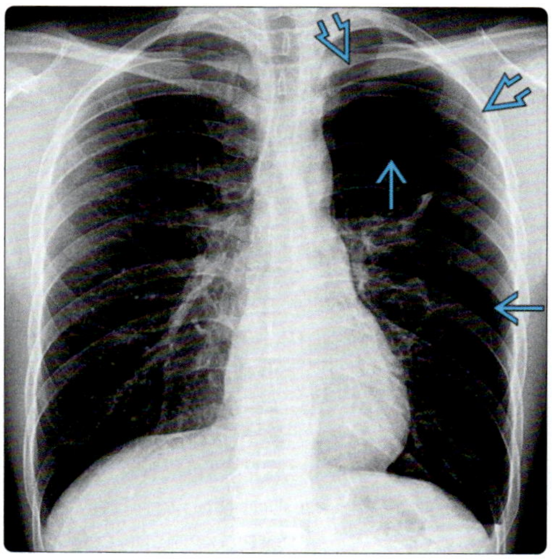

Swyer-James Syndrome

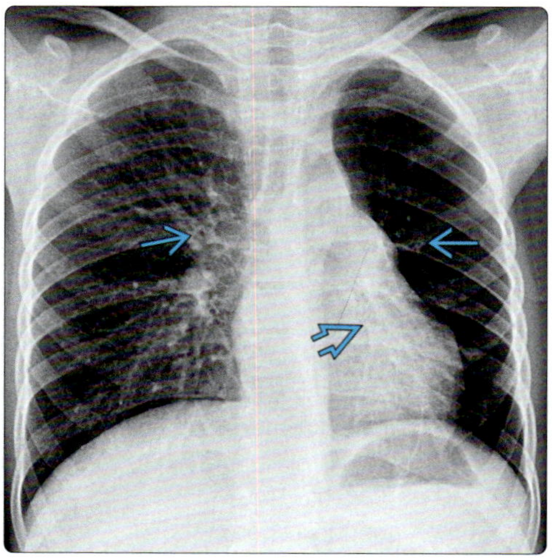

(Left) *Axial CECT in the same patient at 3 years old shows a smaller, hyperlucent left lung with peribronchial thickening & nodular/tree-in-bud lingular opacities from mucoid impaction/inflammation. Note the similar but less severe findings on the right. Both lungs are often involved, though asymmetrically.* **(Right)** *PA radiograph in a 3 month old with known bronchial atresia shows hyperlucency of most of the right hemithorax with air-trapping & mediastinal mass effect.*

Swyer-James Syndrome

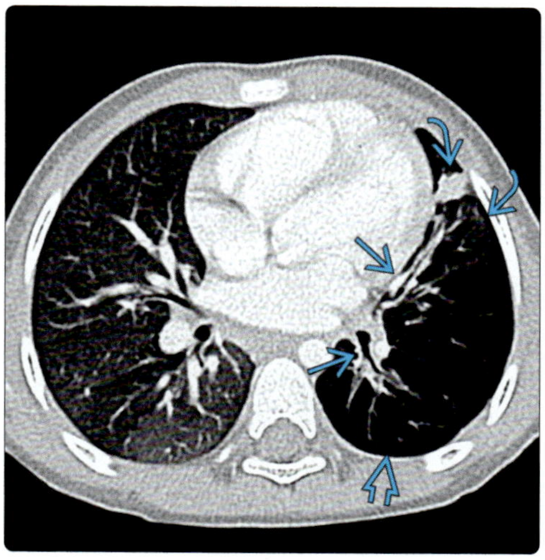

Congenital Lung Malformation

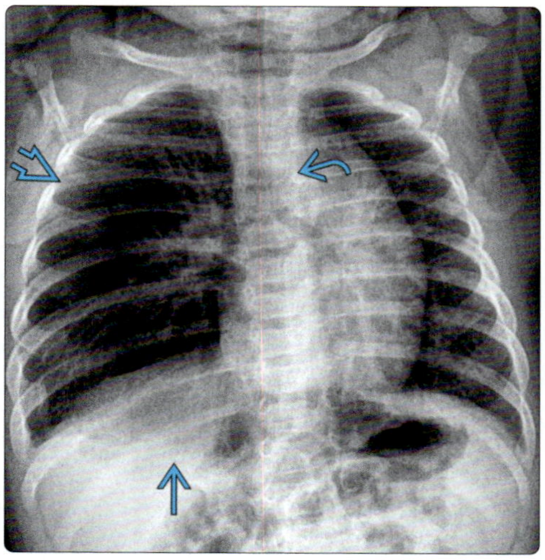

Congenital Lung Malformation

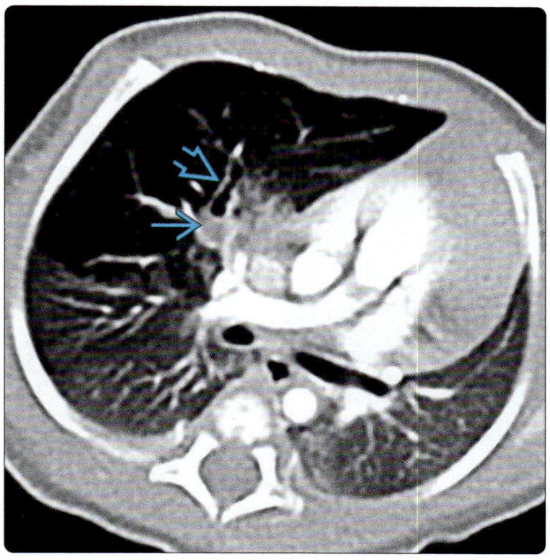

Pulmonary Sling

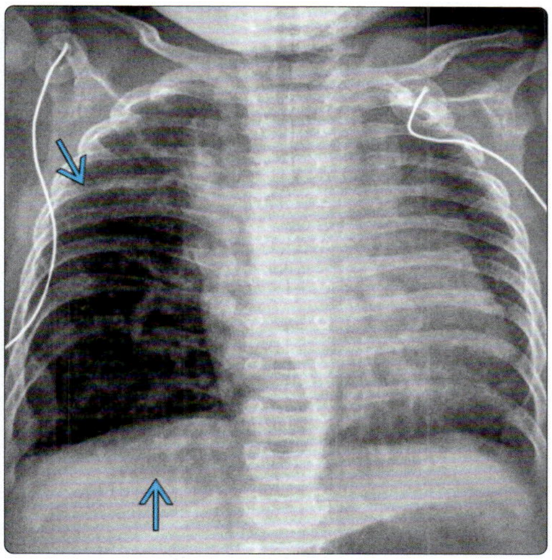

(Left) *Axial CECT in the same patient with bronchial atresia shows the atretic right middle lobe bronchus with mucoid impaction & dilation distal to the atresia. The right middle lobe is hyperinflated with reduced vascularity. Any congenital lung malformation with cysts or hyperinflation can appear as a hyperlucent hemithorax, though a focal lesion is more commonly seen.* **(Right)** *PA radiograph in a 3 month old with an ASD, VSD, & pulmonary sling shows increased pulmonary vascularity with a hyperlucent right lower lung.*

Pulmonary Sling

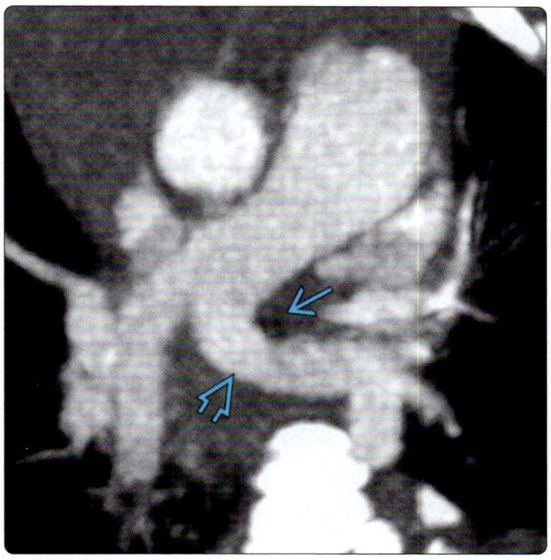

Pulmonary Sling

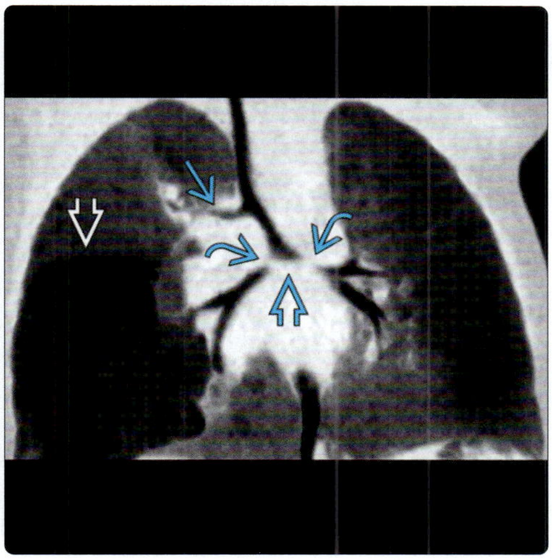

(Left) *Axial oblique CECT MIP in the same patient shows a pulmonary sling coursing behind an attenuated round trachea.* **(Right)** *Coronal oblique CECT minIP in the same patient shows a type 2 inferior carina with a tracheal bronchus. The sling causes compression of both main bronchial origins with air-trapping & hyperlucency of the right middle lobe.*

Scimitar Syndrome

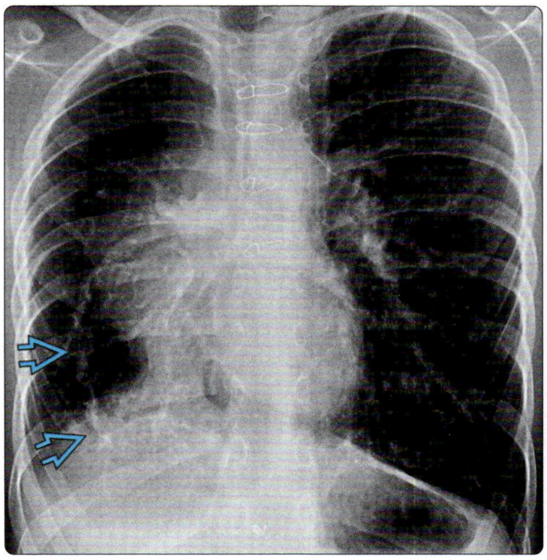

Scimitar Syndrome

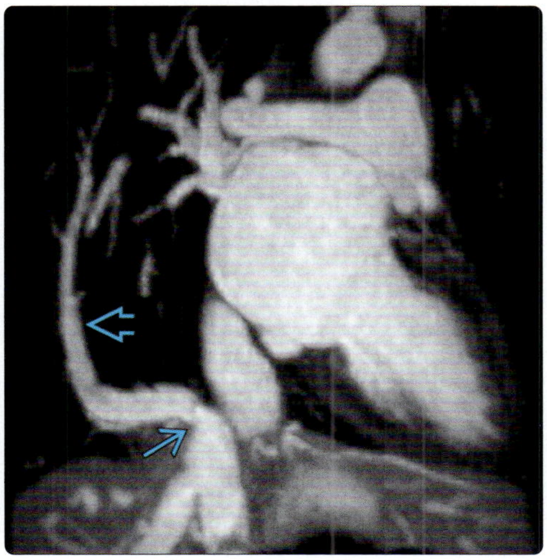

(Left) *PA radiograph in a 9 year old with scimitar syndrome shows a hypoplastic right lung with associated mediastinal shift to the right. A scimitar vein descends across the lower right hemithorax. There is compensatory hyperinflation & relative lucency of the left hemithorax.* **(Right)** *Coronal oblique MRA MIP in the same patient shows the anomalous pulmonary vein draining to the suprahepatic IVC. Unobstructed scimitar veins grow larger as they descend, appearing similar to an upside down Turkish sword (scimitar).*

(Left) *Frontal radiograph in a 3 year old with dyspnea & cough shows hyperlucency & hyperexpansion of the right lung. There is an abnormal soft tissue density bulge at the upper right mediastinal border with displacement of the trachea, suspicious for a mass.* **(Right)** *Coronal CECT in the same patient demonstrates the hyperlucent, hyperinflated right lung & the mediastinal mass, which compressed the right main bronchus (not shown). Surgical pathology demonstrated fibrosing mediastinitis.*

Extrinsic Airway Compression by Mass

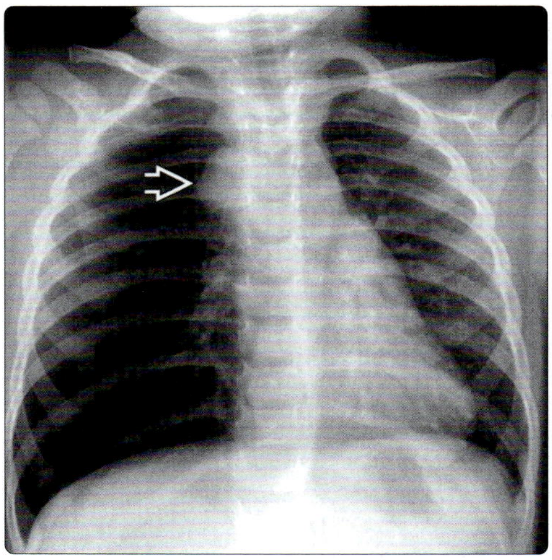

Extrinsic Airway Compression by Mass

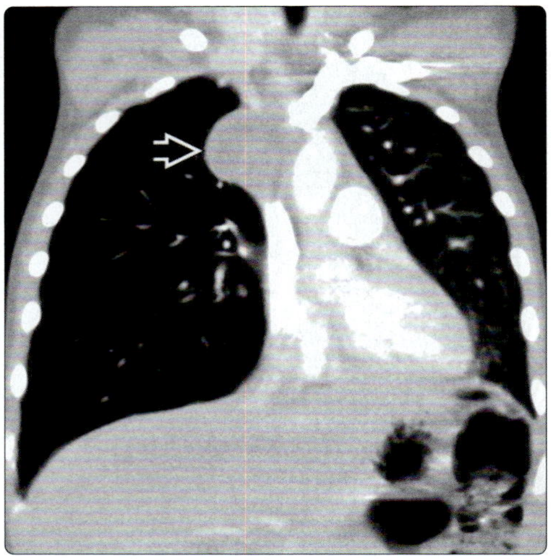

(Left) *PA radiograph in a 6 week old with primary pulmonary hypoplasia shows a small right hemithorax with mediastinal shift & dextroposition of the heart. The left hemithorax is relatively hyperlucent. There are also multiple contiguous midthoracic vertebral segmentation anomalies with a focal scoliosis.* **(Right)** *Axial oblique CECT MIP in the same patient shows a hypoplastic right lung & right pulmonary artery (RPA).*

Pulmonary Agenesis/Aplasia/Hypoplasia

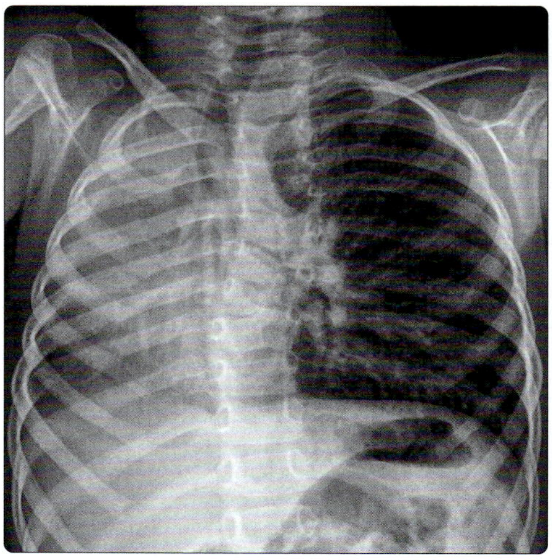

Pulmonary Agenesis/Aplasia/Hypoplasia

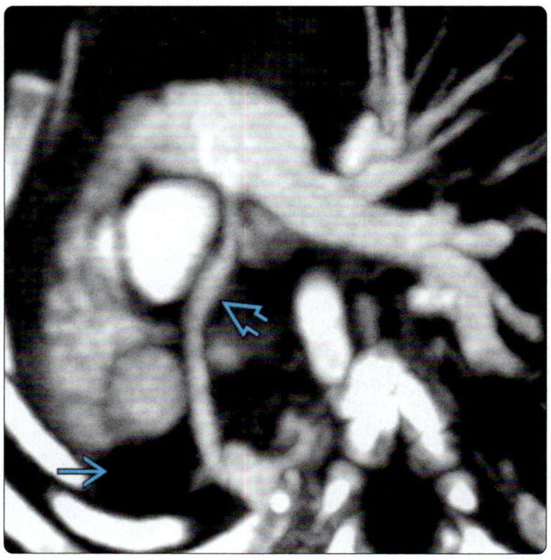

(Left) *Coronal oblique CECT minIP shows the hypoplastic lung & right main bronchus. Primary pulmonary hypoplasia is defined by a hypoplastic lung, artery, & bronchus. Pulmonary aplasia is an absent lung & artery with rudimentary bronchus. Pulmonary atresia is an absent lung, artery, & bronchus.* **(Right)** *PA radiograph in a 4 year old with a ductal origin of the RPA shows a smaller hyperlucent right lung with relatively diminished pulmonary vascularity. The left lung has increased pulmonary vascularity.*

Pulmonary Agenesis/Aplasia/Hypoplasia

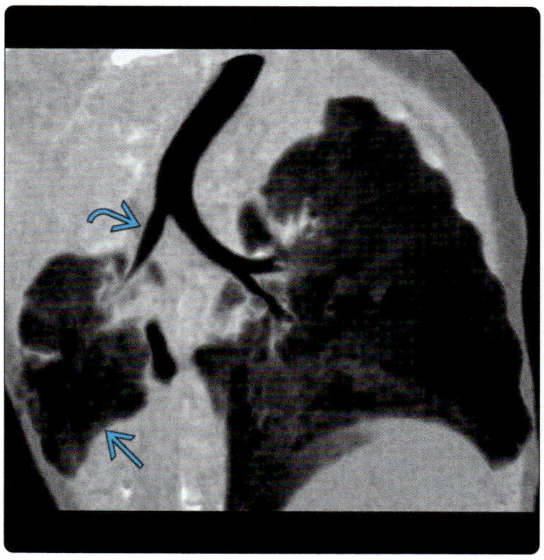

Ductal Origin of Pulmonary Artery

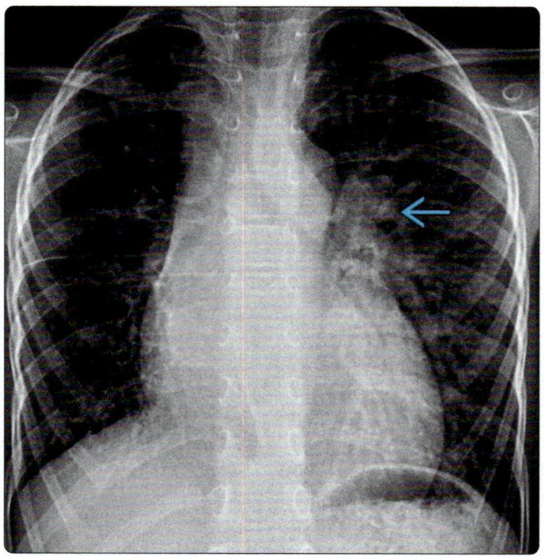

Ductal Origin of Pulmonary Artery

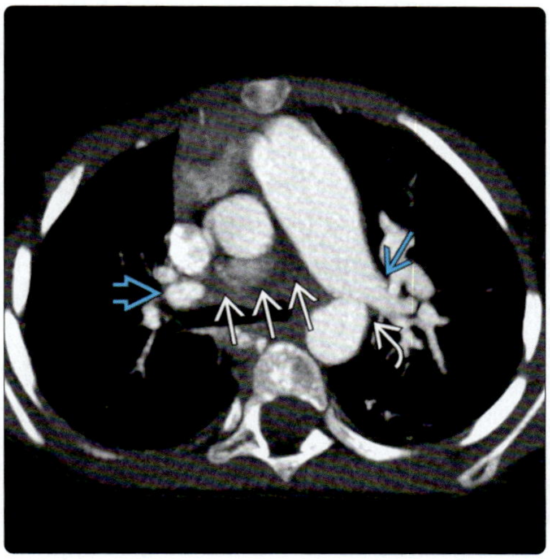

Ductal Origin of Pulmonary Artery

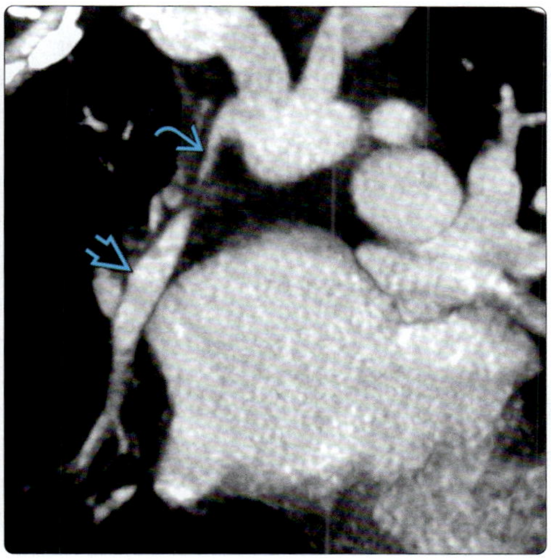

(Left) *Axial oblique CECT MIP in the same patient shows a prominent left pulmonary artery (LPA) with a small hilar RPA. There is absence of the intrapericardial RPA. Note that the right lung is smaller than the left. There is also partial visualization of a left-sided PDA.* **(Right)** *Coronal oblique CECT MIP in the same patient shows that the hilar RPA is supplied by a right-sided patent ductus arteriosus (PDA) that is severely stenotic.*

Poland Syndrome

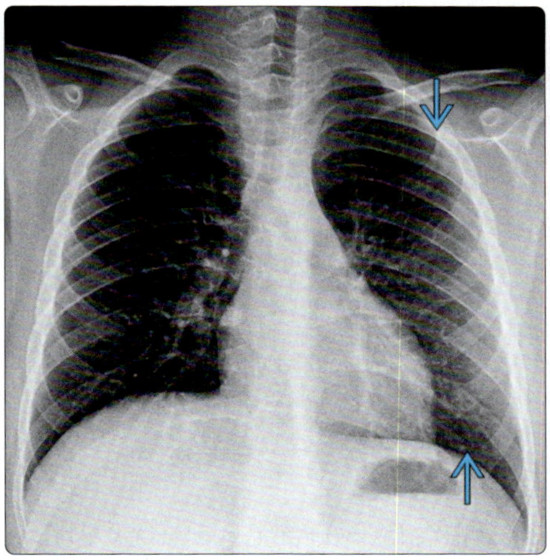

Poland Syndrome

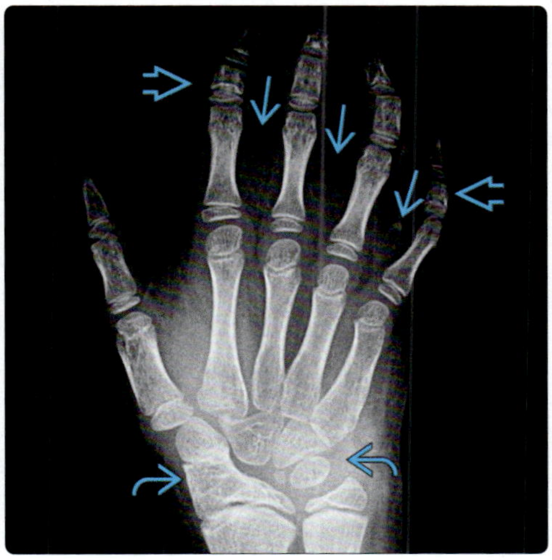

(Left) *PA radiograph shows right hemithorax hyperlucency with loss of the normal lateral density gradient of chest musculature & soft tissue (as seen on the left). Poland syndrome should be considered in the asymptomatic patient. Ipsilateral chest wall deformities & dextrocardia may also be seen.* **(Right)** *PA radiograph of the right hand shows short middle phalanges, partial syndactyly, & dysplastic carpal bones. Ipsilateral upper limb skeletal anomalies may be seen in Poland syndrome.*

Endobronchial Tumor

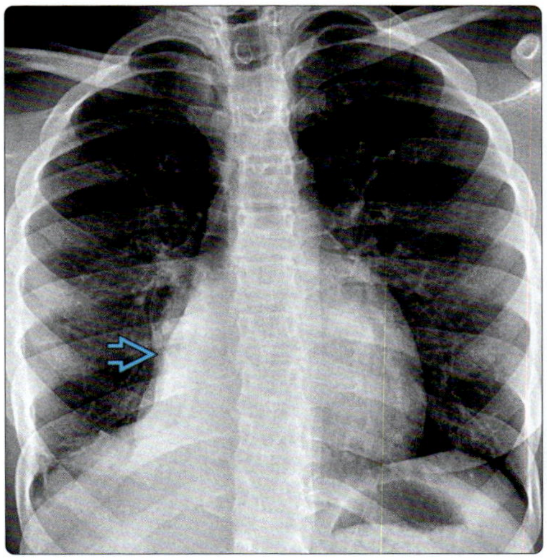

Endobronchial Tumor

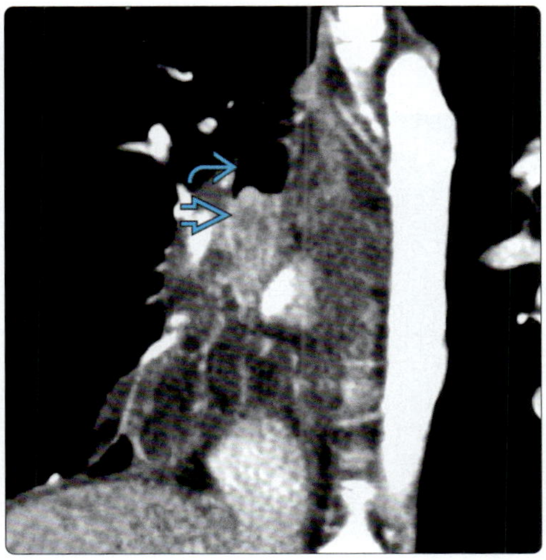

(Left) *PA radiograph in a 13 year old shows right lower lobe collapse.* **(Right)** *Coronal CECT in the same patient shows an enhancing mass filling the dilated right lower lobar bronchus, causing right lower lobe collapse & consolidation. Biopsy revealed a carcinoid tumor, which comprises 80% of endobronchial tumors in children. When not completely obstructive, regional air-trapping can occur, creating a hyperlucent appearance. However, collapse & consolidation are more common, as in this patient.*

DIFFERENTIAL DIAGNOSIS

Common

- Technical Factors
- Asthma
- Congenital Heart Disease

Less Common

- Foreign Body Aspiration

Rare but Important

- Obliterative Bronchiolitis
- Emphysema

ESSENTIAL INFORMATION

Key Differential Diagnosis Issues

- Look for clues of hyperaeration: Narrow cardiomediastinal silhouette, depressed hemidiaphragms, increased retrosternal airspace

Helpful Clues for Common Diagnoses

- **Technical Factors**
  - Overexposed chest radiograph attenuates pulmonary markings, resulting in hyperlucent appearance of lungs
  - Good inspiratory effort can result in bilateral, hyperinflated, hyperlucent lungs
- **Asthma**
  - Chronic reversible hyperresponsiveness of airways leads to airflow obstruction
  - Acute exacerbation: Airway inflammation from environmental triggers due to pathologic immune-mediated response
  - Imaging is indicated only when patient is not responding to therapy & concern exists for complications (barotrauma, pneumonia)
  - Chest radiograph may show bilateral hyperinflated, hyperlucent lungs; can be normal
- **Congenital Heart Disease**
  - Severe cyanosis can lead to bilateral hyperinflation due to reflex hyperventilation
    - Cyanotic disease with decreased pulmonary vascularity accentuates this appearance
      - Tetralogy of Fallot, pulmonary atresia, tricuspid atresia, Ebstein anomaly
  - Vascular rings can compress airway, leading to diffuse or regional hyperinflation
  - Left-to-right shunts & interstitial edema also cause air-trapping but will not be hyperlucent due to increased vascularity &/or edema

Helpful Clues for Less Common Diagnoses

- **Foreign Body Aspiration**
  - Food is most common
  - Most frequent from 6 months to 3 years of age
  - Tracheal foreign body may cause bilateral air-trapping & hyperlucent lungs
  - Esophageal foreign body can cause edema leading to tracheal compression & bilateral hyperlucent lungs
  - Fluoroscopy, inspiratory/expiratory images, or lateral decubitus radiographs can be utilized
  - 20-35% of children with foreign body aspiration may have normal radiographs
    - Bronchoscopy is required if clinical concern persists

Helpful Clues for Rare Diagnoses

- **Obliterative Bronchiolitis**
  - a.k.a. constrictive bronchiolitis or bronchiolitis obliterans
  - Bronchial inflammation results in airway obstruction
  - Causes: Post infectious, lung transplant (rejection or graft-vs.-host), bone marrow transplant (graft-vs.-host), connective tissue disorders, toxic fumes, drug related
  - Hyperlucent lungs with diminished pulmonary vascularity
  - CT: Mosaic attenuation (inspiratory) & air-trapping (expiratory) ± bronchial wall thickening, bronchiectasis, centrilobular nodules
- **Emphysema**
  - Rare in children
  - Can be seen with Marfan syndrome, cutis laxa, & α-1-antitrypsin deficiency
  - Typically panacinar/panlobular

Technical Factors

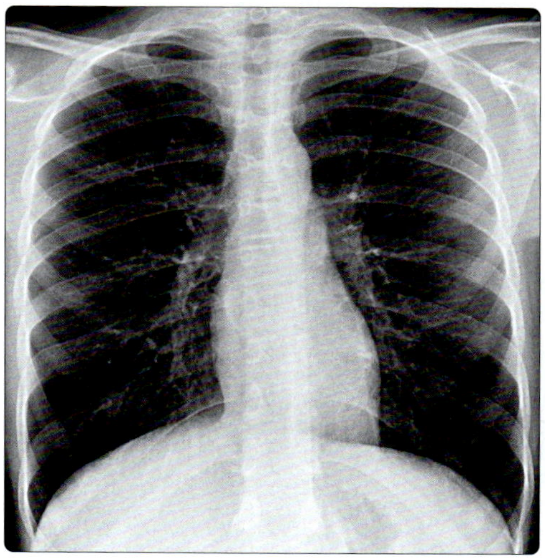

Asthma

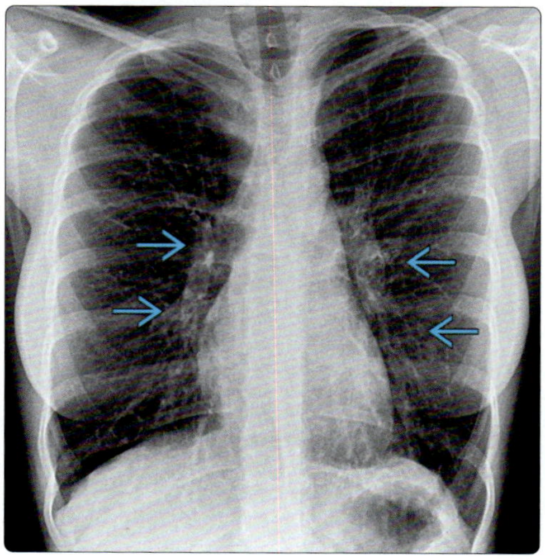

(Left) *PA radiograph in an 11 year old shows bilateral hyperlucent lungs due to robust inspiration. Note the narrowed cardiomediastinum. The exam is otherwise normal.* **(Right)** *PA radiograph in a 13 year old with asthma who presented with chest pain & wheezing shows bilateral hyperinflated lungs along with mild central peribronchial & interstitial thickening ➔, consistent with an acute exacerbation with small airways inflammation.*

Congenital Heart Disease

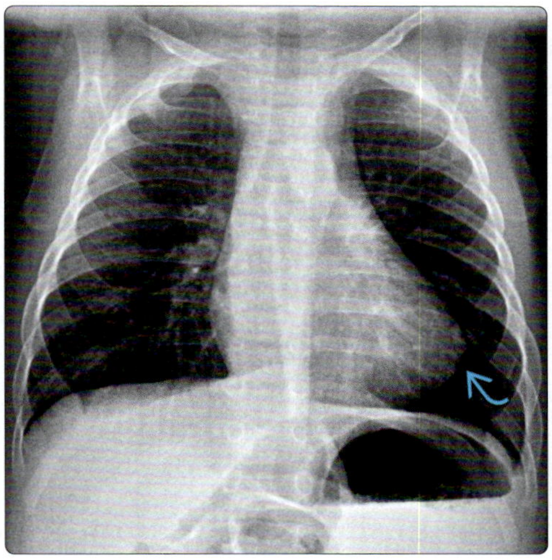

Foreign Body Aspiration

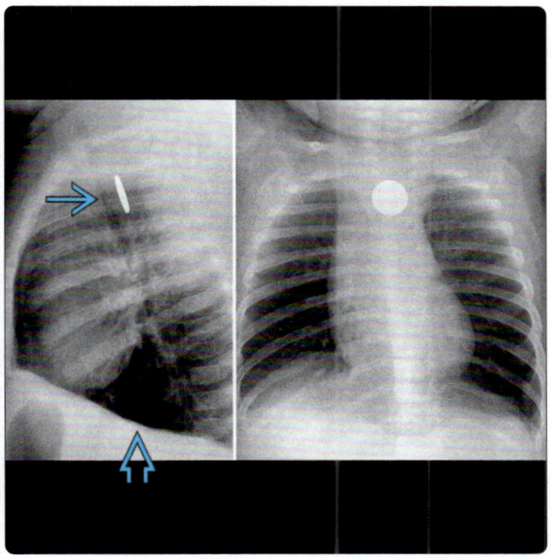

(Left) *PA radiograph in a 6 month old with tetralogy of Fallot shows diminished pulmonary vascularity & bilateral hyperlucent, hyperinflated lungs from cyanosis. There is an upturned apex ↷ from right ventricular hypertrophy.* **(Right)** *Lateral & frontal radiographs in a 1 year old show a swallowed coin stuck in the proximal esophagus. The associated edema causes tracheal narrowing → with resultant hyperlucency & hyperexpansion of the lungs. Note the flattened diaphragm ⇨.*

Obliterative Bronchiolitis

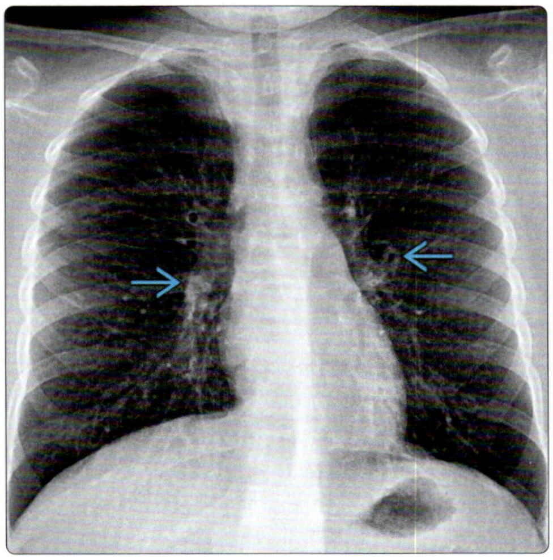

Obliterative Bronchiolitis

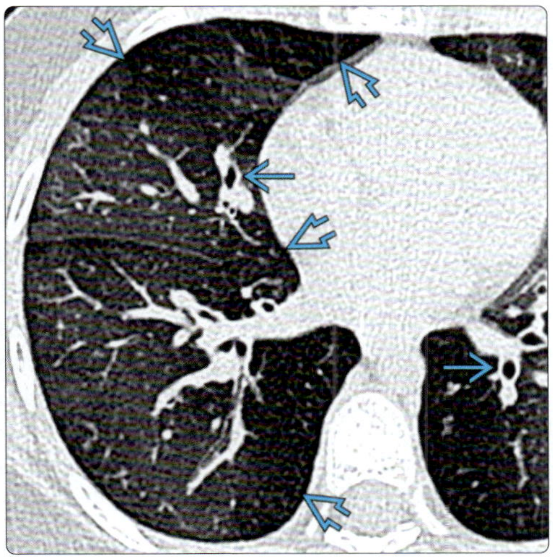

(Left) *PA radiograph in an 11 year old status post bone marrow transplant shows bilateral hyperinflated lungs with peribronchial thickening →.* **(Right)** *Axial expiratory NECT in the same patient shows bronchial wall thickening → with bilateral mosaic attenuation due to regional expiratory air-trapping ⇨, consistent with obliterative bronchiolitis. This reflects graft-vs.-host disease in a patient after bone marrow transplant & is often referred to as bronchiolitis obliterans syndrome.*

Emphysema

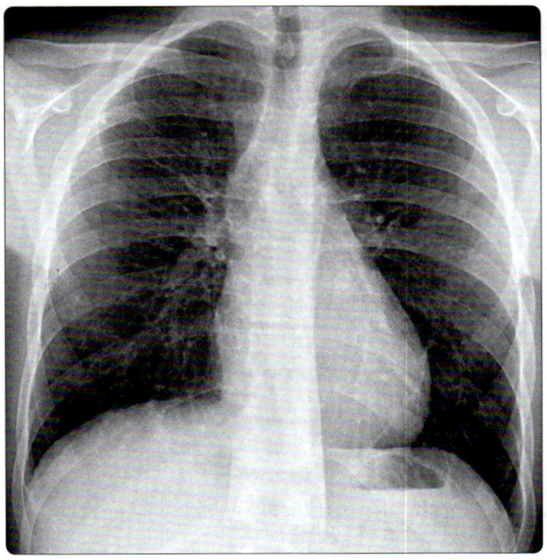

Emphysema

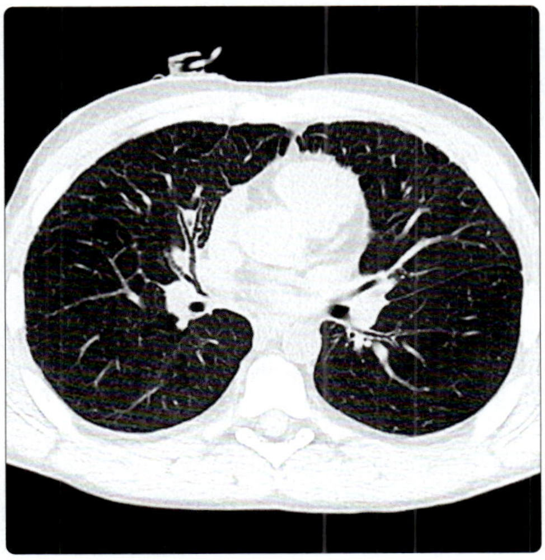

(Left) *PA radiograph in a 16 year old with a complex history shows bilateral hyperlucent lungs with diminished peripheral vascularity.* **(Right)** *Axial CECT in the same patient shows diffuse parenchymal hypoattenuation with a paucity of vessels, consistent with panlobular emphysema. This was likely related to a combination of secondary pulmonary hypoplasia, chronic lung disease, & recurrent infections. Panlobular emphysema can be difficult to detect on radiographs, which may appear normal.*

DIFFERENTIAL DIAGNOSIS

Common

- Pneumonia With Cavitary Necrosis
- Pulmonary Abscess
- Aspergillus Infection
- Pneumatocele
- Tuberculosis
- Congenital Pulmonary Airway Malformation

Less Common

- Septic Emboli

Rare but Important

- Metastatic Disease
- Granulomatosis With Polyangiitis
- Tracheobronchial Papillomatosis

ESSENTIAL INFORMATION

Key Differential Diagnosis Issues

- Cavitary lesions in children are most frequently infectious or congenital in nature
- History is very helpful, but CT is frequently necessary to narrow considerations

Helpful Clues for Common Diagnoses

- **Pneumonia With Cavitary Necrosis**
  - Complication of lobar pneumonia
    - Severely ill children
    - *Streptococcus* & *Staphylococcus* are most common
  - Radiographs may underestimate degree of necrosis
  - Variable number of thin-walled cavities
    - Contain fluid &/or air
    - Lack enhancing border
    - Show adjacent consolidation
    - Loss of surrounding lung architecture with decreased parenchymal enhancement
  - Look for other complications of pneumonia
    - Pleural effusion/empyema
    - Bronchopleural fistula
    - Pulmonary abscess
      - Thick, enhancing wall (unlike cavitary necrosis)
  - Typically resolves completely with nonsurgical treatment
    - Interventional therapy can be harmful
- **Pulmonary Abscess**
  - Frequently due to anaerobic infection from aspiration
    - Others: *Streptococcus*, *Staphylococcus*, fungi, mycobacteria, & parasites
  - More commonly seen in immunocompromised children
  - Irregularly shaped cavity with internal air-fluid level
    - Size of air-fluid level is similar on frontal & lateral views
  - Thick, shaggy, enhancing rind (unlike nonenhancing thin wall in cavitary necrosis)
  - Look for other signs of infection (consolidation, pleural effusion/empyema, cavitary necrosis)
  - Typically resolves with IV antibiotics without drainage
- **Aspergillus Infection**
  - Spectrum of 4 main pulmonary syndromes broadly dependent on immune status
    - Allergic bronchopulmonary aspergillosis: Hypersensitivity to *Aspergillus*
    - Aspergilloma: Immunocompetent
    - Chronic pulmonary aspergillosis (semiinvasive aspergillosis): Mildly immunosuppressed
    - Invasive aspergillosis: Severely immunocompromised
  - Aspergilloma
    - Colonization of existing lung cavity in patients of normal immunity → fungal ball (mycetoma)
      - Can form in any preexisting cavity (TB, cystic fibrosis, bullae, etc.)
      - No pulmonary invasion
    - Ball in cavity creates air crescent sign
    - Fungal ball within cavity may move to dependent location with change in patient position
    - Thickening of cavity wall ± adjacent pleura (may be 1st radiographic sign of disease)
  - Chronic pulmonary aspergillosis (semiinvasive aspergillosis)
    - Typically in patients with mild immunosuppression
    - May have cavitary necrosis
    - Shows bronchopulmonary consolidation ± cavitation
- **Pneumatocele**
  - Thin-walled cyst/cavity
  - Sequela of prior parenchymal insult (trauma, infection)
  - Often resolves spontaneously, especially in younger children
  - May become superinfected
- **Tuberculosis**
  - Infection with *Mycobacterium tuberculosis*
  - Appearance related to immune response
    - Immune status
    - Uninfected vs. previously infected
  - Primary disease
    - More common in children than adults
    - Perihilar & paratracheal lymphadenopathy
      - Radiographic hallmark of disease, seen in 90% of children (only 10-40% in adults)
      - Can compress airway (causing air-trapping or atelectasis)
    - Consolidation without lobar predilection
    - Ca^{2+} (6 months to 4 years after infection)
  - Progressive primary disease (primary TB that does not heal)
    - Cavitation: High bacterial load, highly contagious
    - Miliary infection (hematogenous spread)
      - Innumerable tiny nodules in random distribution
      - More common in children & immunocompromised
    - Extrapulmonary spread
  - Postprimary disease (reinfection or reactivation)
    - Consolidation typically of apical posterior segments of upper lobes & superior segments of lower lobes
    - Cavitation is common
    - Lymphadenopathy is uncommon
    - If immunocompromised, looks like progressive primary disease
  - Pleural effusion/empyema
    - Can be seen in primary or postprimary disease
- **Congenital Pulmonary Airway Malformation**

- Cystic types may develop infection & appear as cavity with air-fluid levels

Helpful Clues for Less Common Diagnoses

- **Septic Emboli**
  - Can reach lungs from variety of sources
    - Infected central lines
    - Peripheral septic thrombophlebitis
    - Infected heart valves
  - Immunocompromised patients at increased risk
  - Multiple nodules ± cavitation
    - Cavities with thick & thin walls representing various stages of evolution
    - Typically peripherally located
    - May see draining or feeding vessel
  - Look for associated consolidation or pleural effusions
  - Lemierre syndrome
    - Oropharyngeal infection → septic thrombophlebitis of jugular vein → septic pulmonary emboli

Helpful Clues for Rare Diagnoses

- **Metastatic Disease**
  - Most common cavitating lung metastases are from adult neoplasms
    - Squamous cell (lung, head & neck, esophagus, cervical)
    - Adenocarcinoma (colon, rectum)
  - Very rare in children
    - Can be seen with metastatic sarcomas (fibrosarcoma, osteosarcoma)
    - Has been reported with Wilms
  - Can be thin- or thick-walled depending on type of primary malignancy
  - History of primary neoplasm is helpful
  - May be difficult to differentiate from infectious cavitary lesions
- **Granulomatosis With Polyangiitis**
  - a.k.a. Wegener granulomatosis
  - Necrotizing small & medium-sized vessel vasculitis with granulomatous inflammation
  - Classical triad of involvement
    - Upper respiratory tract: Recurrent epistaxis, sinusitis, otitis media
      - Most common manifestation in children
    - Lower respiratory tract: Lung nodules with cavitation, pulmonary hemorrhage, & airway strictures
    - Renal glomerulonephritis: Hematuria
  - Lung nodules with cavitation occur in ~ 50%
    - Usually thick-walled with irregular inner margin
    - Perinodular ground-glass (alveolar hemorrhage)
    - 5 mm to 10 cm in size
    - Tend to be multiple
  - Associated chest findings
    - Pulmonary hemorrhage
    - Airway strictures
      - Subglottic stenosis in 10-20% of children
- **Tracheobronchial Papillomatosis**
  - Benign squamous papillomas of respiratory tract
  - Infection with human papilloma virus types 6 & 11
    - For juvenile-onset type, is usually acquired during vaginal delivery
  - 2/3 are diagnosed prior to age 5
  - Most commonly presents with hoarseness or voice change (as vocal cords are usually 1st affected)
  - Airway papillomas (nodular or sessile)
  - Lower airway & lung involvement in < 5%
    - Nodules with cavitation, often thin walled
      - Lower & posterior lung predominance
      - Superinfection: Air-fluid levels
    - Complications: Postobstructive collapse & pneumonia
  - Increased risk of squamous cell carcinoma

SELECTED REFERENCES

1. Jariwala MP et al: Primary vasculitis in childhood: GPA and MPA in childhood. Front Pediatr. 6:226, 2018
2. Lichtenberger JP 3rd et al: Primary lung tumors in children: radiologic-pathologic correlation from the radiologic pathology archives. Radiographics. 38(7):2151-72, 2018
3. Andronikou S et al: Computed tomography in children with community-acquired pneumonia. Pediatr Radiol. 47(11):1431-40, 2017

Pneumonia With Cavitary Necrosis

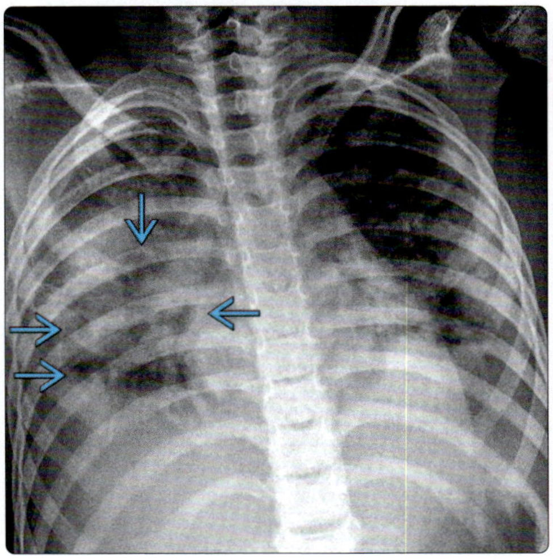

Pneumonia With Cavitary Necrosis

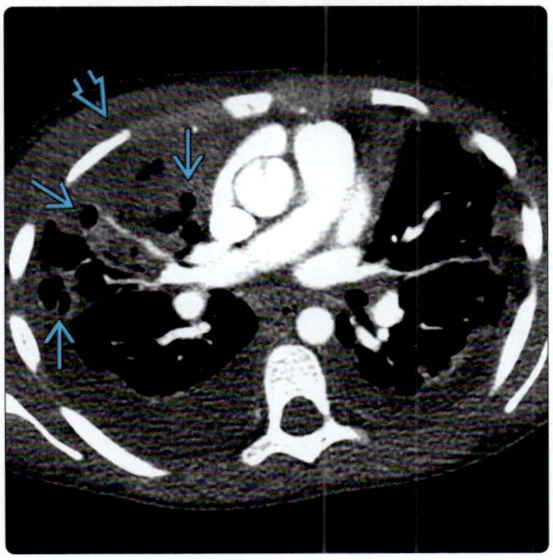

(Left) *AP radiograph in a 7 year old with MSSA bacteremia shows patchy multifocal airspace opacities with irregular lucencies ➔, suggestive of pneumonia with cavitary necrosis.* **(Right)** *Axial CECT in the same patient shows thin-walled cavitation ➔ amidst hypoattenuating consolidation, consistent with cavitary necrosis. Areas of cavitation do not become air-filled until communicating with aerated lung. Note the other signs of infection, including the bilateral pleural effusions with possible empyema necessitans ➲.*

(Left) *PA radiograph in a 6 year old with complicated pneumonia shows a cavitary mass in the left lower lung with an air-fluid level, suspicious for an abscess. Other signs of infection are present, including right upper lung consolidation & a right pleural effusion.* **(Right)** *Lateral radiograph in the same patient shows the cavitary mass in the posterior lower lobe with air-fluid level, similar in size to the frontal view & consistent with an abscess. Pulmonary abscesses usually resolve with IV antibiotics alone.*

Pulmonary Abscess

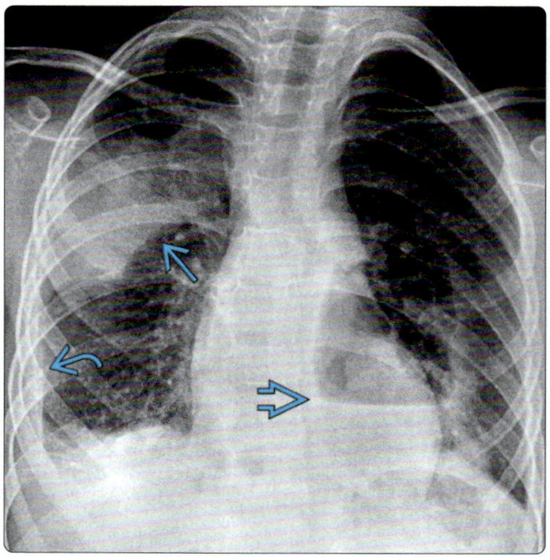

Pulmonary Abscess

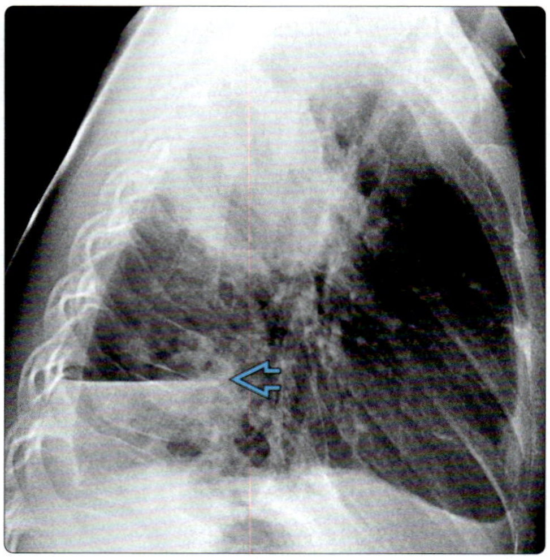

(Left) *Axial CECT in the same patient shows the left lower lobe cavitary lesion with a thick irregular wall & an internal air-fluid level, consistent with a pulmonary abscess.* **(Right)** *Axial CECT in the same patient shows an additional heterogeneous, predominantly hypodense right upper lobe mass with pockets of air & thick irregular peripheral thickening, suggestive of a developing wall along a focus of necrosis (i.e., a developing pulmonary abscess).*

Pulmonary Abscess

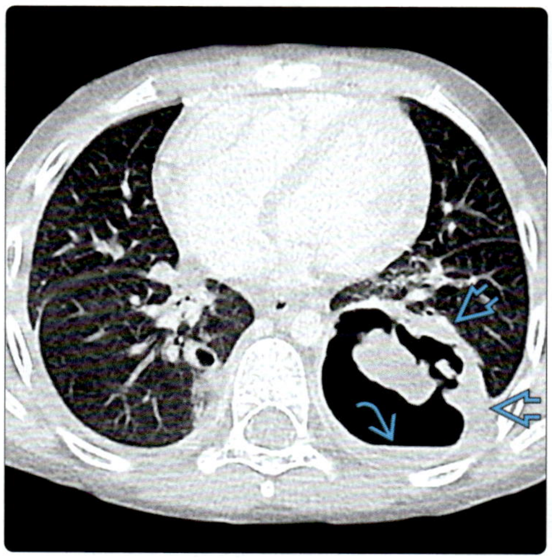

Pulmonary Abscess

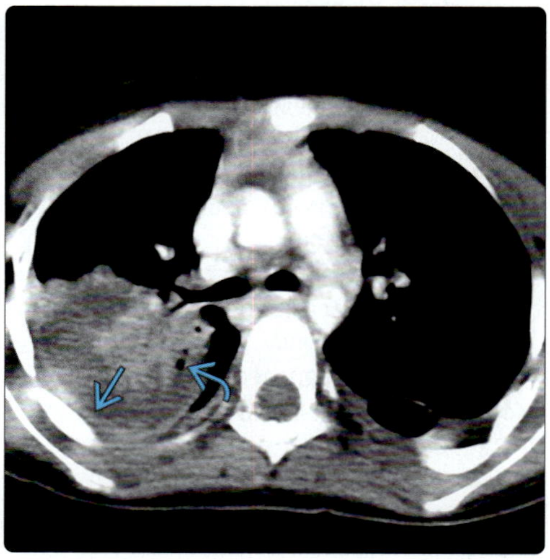

(Left) *PA radiograph in a 17 year old with cystic fibrosis shows an irregular mass in the left upper lobe with pockets of internal air, suggestive of cavitation. Note the peribronchial thickening & scattered nodular opacities (mucus plugging) due to cystic fibrosis.* **(Right)** *Axial CECT in the same patient shows the cavitary mass with irregular wall, associated linear scarring, & peripheral crescentic pockets of air (air-crescent sign), indicative of an aspergilloma. This lesion arose from a focal area of cystic bronchiectasis.*

Aspergillus Infection

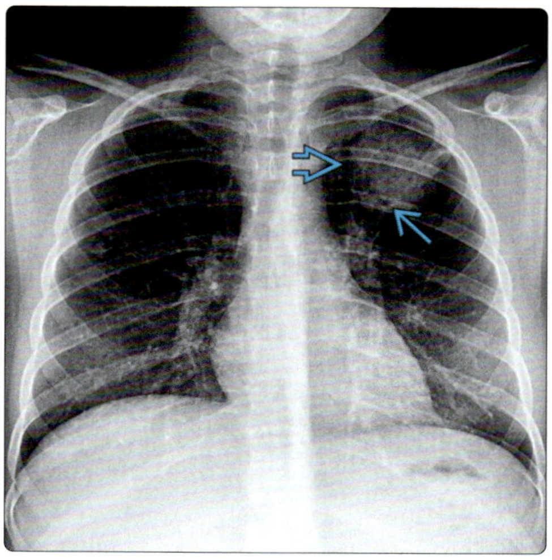

Aspergillus Infection

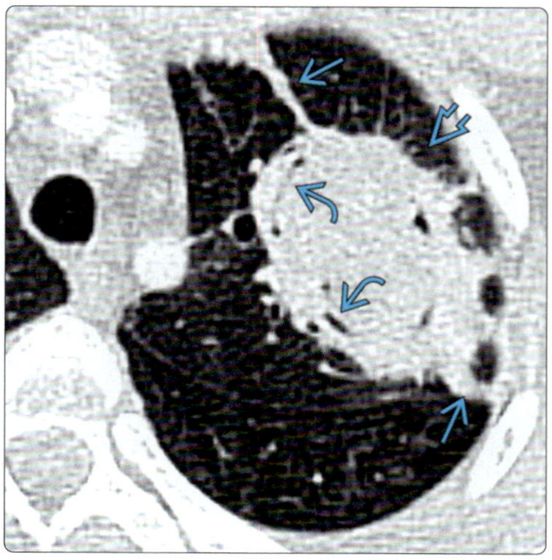

Aspergillus Infection

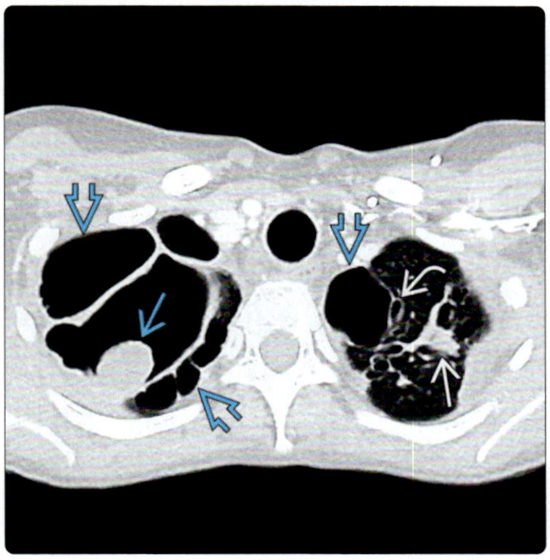

Aspergillus Infection

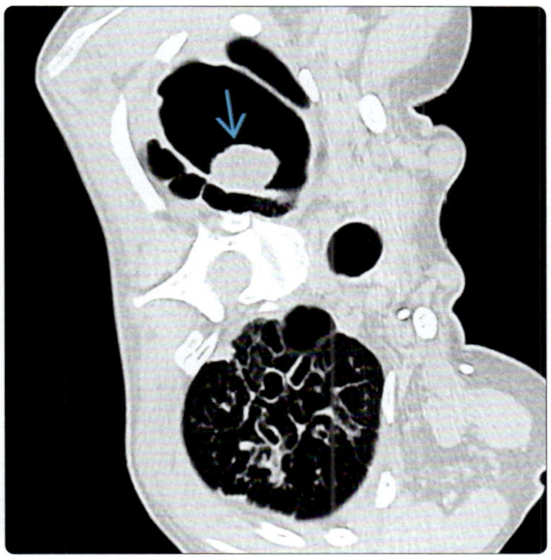

(Left) *Axial CECT in a 17 year old with severe cystic fibrosis shows biapical subpleural cystic changes, including one with a fungal ball, consistent with an aspergilloma. Note the regional bronchiectasis & scarring.* **(Right)** *Axial NECT in the same patient in the left lateral decubitus position shows movement of the fungal ball into a dependent location, confirming the diagnosis. Most mycetomas are aspergillomas (& the terms are often used interchangeably).*

Aspergillus Infection

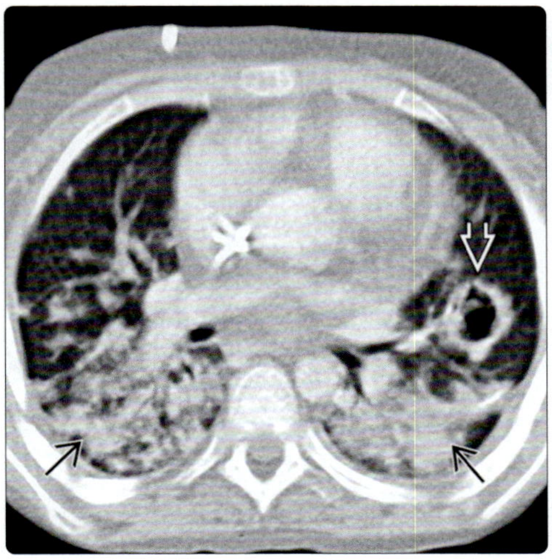

Pneumatocele

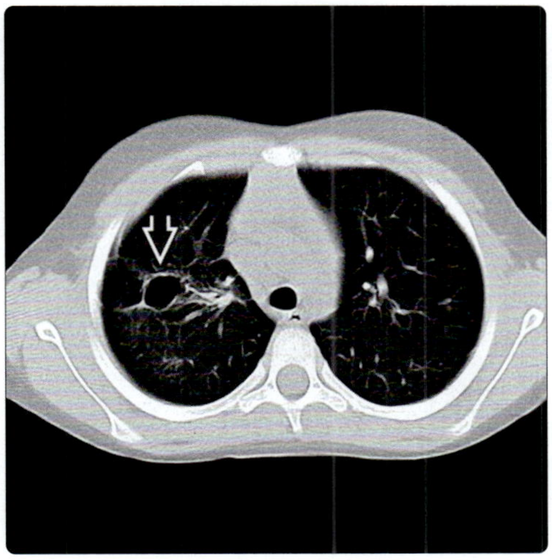

(Left) *Axial CECT in a 10 year old with Fanconi anemia & respiratory infection shows a thick-walled cavitary mass plus lower lobe predominant consolidation. Biopsy showed chronic necrotizing pulmonary aspergillosis.* **(Right)** *Axial NECT in a 7 year old with a remote history of right upper lobe pneumonia shows a well-defined, thin-walled parenchymal cavity, consistent with a pneumatocele related to the previous infection. There is surrounding parenchymal scarring.*

Tuberculosis

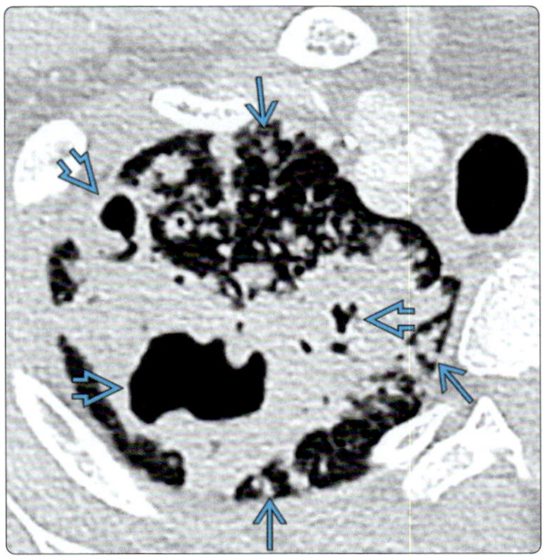

Tuberculosis

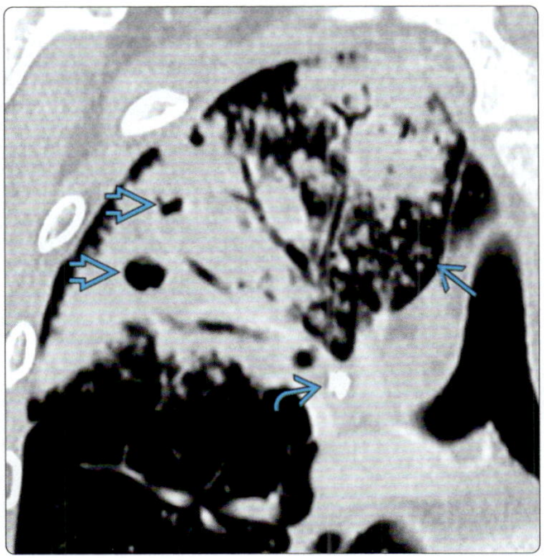

(Left) *Axial CECT in a 14 year old from a country where TB is endemic shows right upper lobe consolidation with areas of irregular cavitation along with tree-in-bud opacities, consistent with pulmonary TB.* **(Right)** *Coronal CECT in the same patient again shows the cavitary consolidation & tree-in-bud opacities. Also note the dystrophic calcified hilar adenopathy. Childhood TB is generally paucibacillary; therefore, the diagnosis of intrathoracic TB often depends on imaging.*

(Left) *PA radiograph in a 14 month old shows a multilobulated mass in the right lower lung with both gas & fluid densities.* **(Right)** *Axial CECT in the same patient shows a lung lesion with cysts of varying size, some of which are filled with fluid. There is adjacent air-trapping. When a congenital pulmonary airway malformation (CPAM) contains fluid-filled cysts or solid-appearing components, the appearance can mimic a cavitary mass. Note that increasing fluid content within CPAM cysts can be due to infection.*

Congenital Pulmonary Airway Malformation

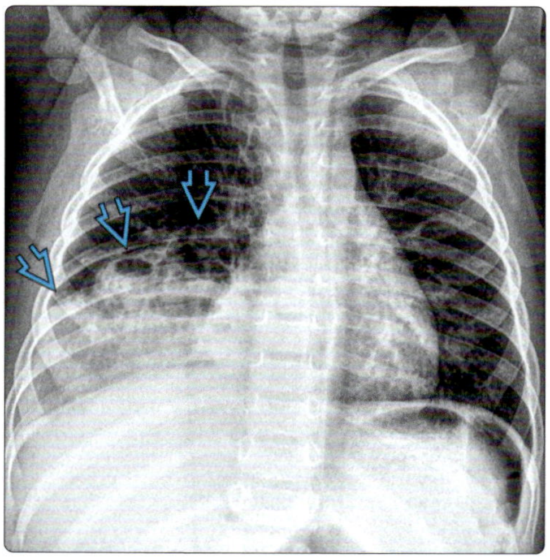

Congenital Pulmonary Airway Malformation

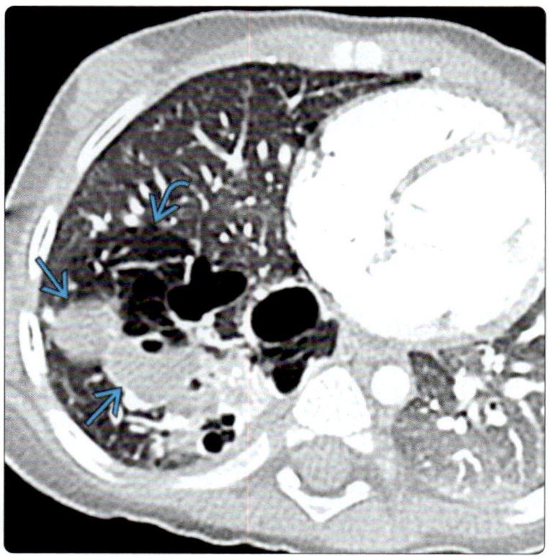

(Left) *Coronal CECT MIP in the same patient shows a systemic artery supplying this mass, making this a hybrid lesion with both sequestration & CPAM components. CPAMs are the most common congenital lung malformation & can coexist with other malformations, such as sequestration or bronchial atresia.* **(Right)** *Axial CECT in a 12 year old shows a large right upper lobe cavitary lesion with air-fluid levels. Pathology confirmed an infected CPAM. CPAMs are at risk for recurrent infection (& rarely malignancy).*

Congenital Pulmonary Airway Malformation

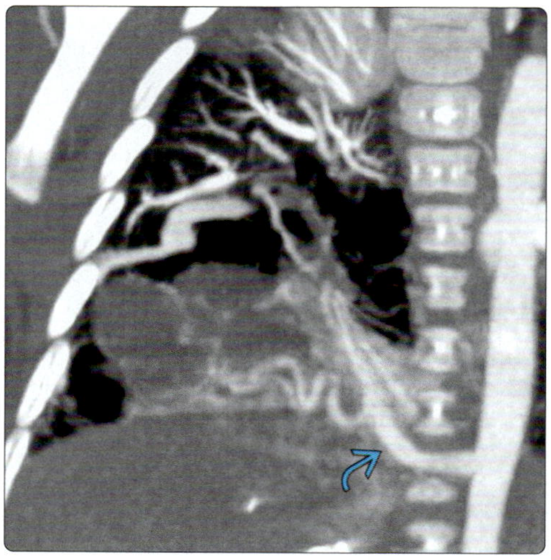

Congenital Pulmonary Airway Malformation

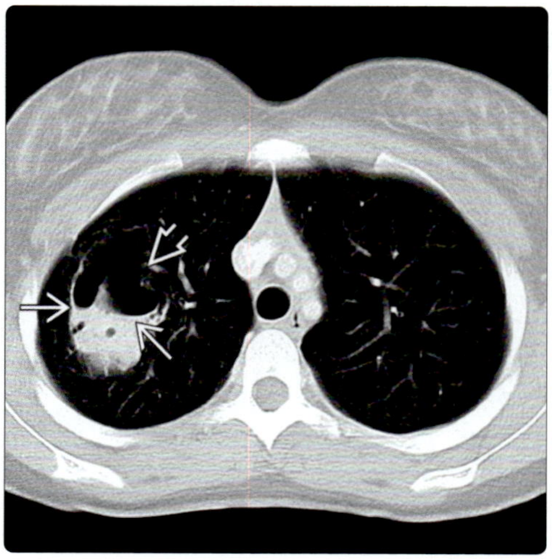

(Left) *Axial CECT in a 17 year old with Lemierre syndrome shows multiple pulmonary nodules, some with cavitation, consistent with septic emboli. Despite the feeding vessel sign, pulmonary arteries typically course closely around septic emboli, while vessels associated with the center of septic emboli are pulmonary veins.* **(Right)** *Axial CECT in a 16 year old with known osteosarcoma shows multiple randomly distributed pulmonary nodules, some of which have cavitation, consistent with metastatic disease.*

Septic Emboli

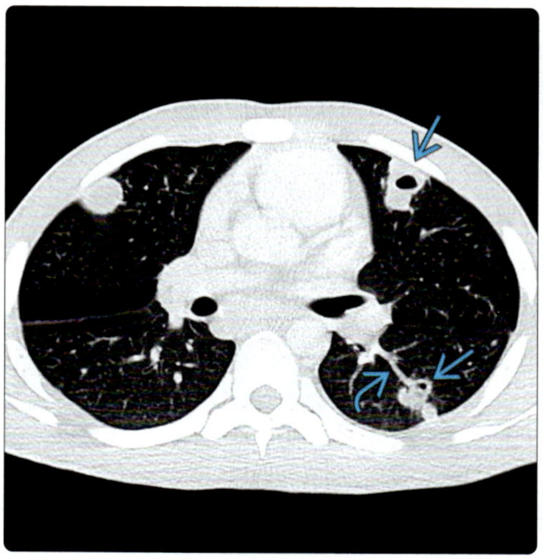

Metastatic Disease

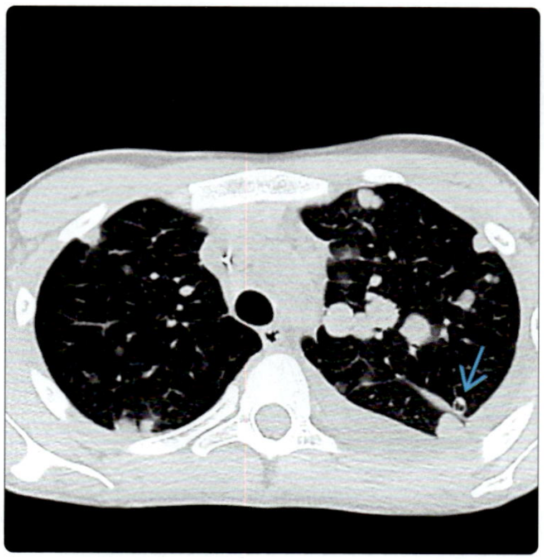

Granulomatosis With Polyangiitis

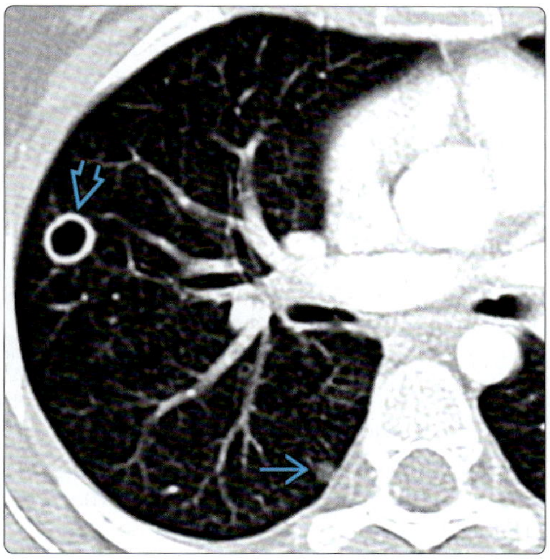

Granulomatosis With Polyangiitis

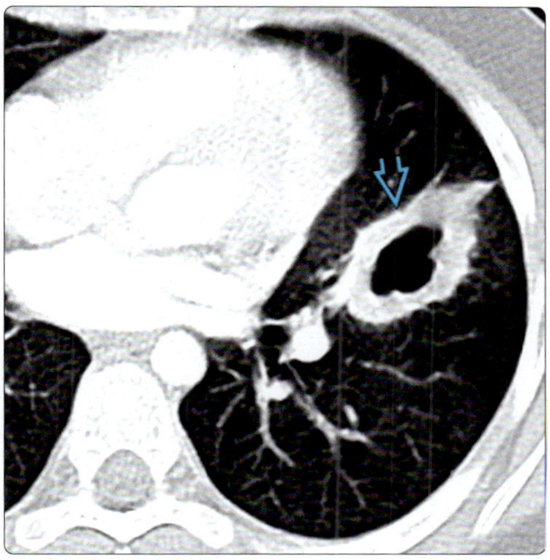

(Left) *Axial CECT in a 10 year old with known granulomatosis with polyangiitis (GPA) shows multiple lung nodules →, including one with cavitation →.* **(Right)** *Axial CECT in the same patient shows another cavitary lung nodule →. Note that this cavitary nodule has a thick wall with irregular inner margin. Other potential features of nodules in GPA include ground-glass halos from hemorrhage or air-fluid levels if secondarily infected. Pulmonary hemorrhage may be the initial manifestation of lower respiratory involvement.*

Granulomatosis With Polyangiitis

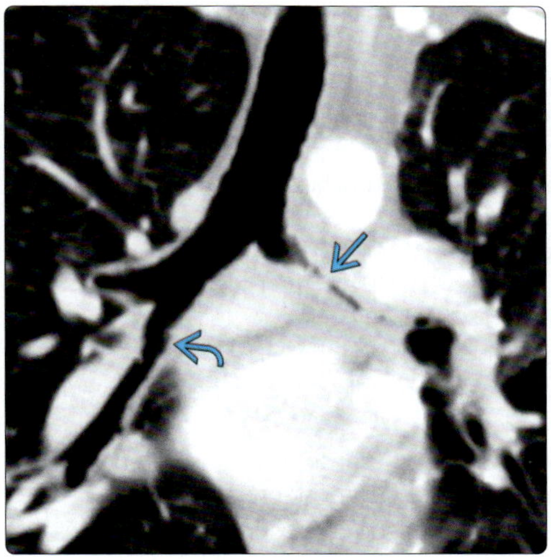

Tracheobronchial Papillomatosis

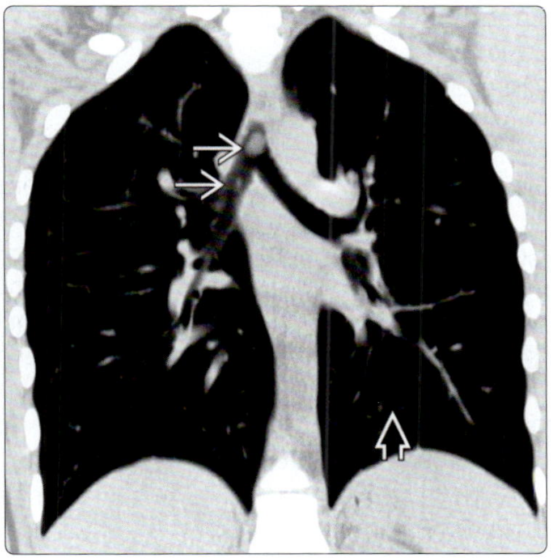

(Left) *Coronal CECT in the same patient at 14 years old shows irregular wall thickening & narrowing of the left main bronchus →. Similar milder changes are seen in the right lower lobar bronchus →. Airway involvement in GPA can be smooth or irregular & may be circumferential.* **(Right)** *Coronal NECT in a 13 year old with tracheobronchial papillomatosis shows a thin-walled cavity in the left base →. Note also the papillomas within the trachea & right main bronchus →.*

Tracheobronchial Papillomatosis

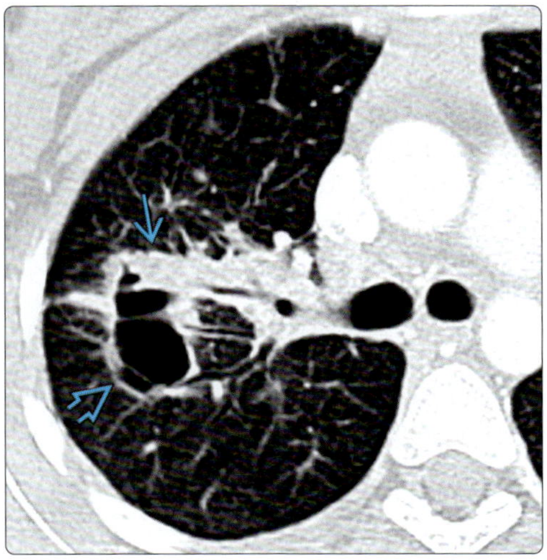

Tracheobronchial Papillomatosis

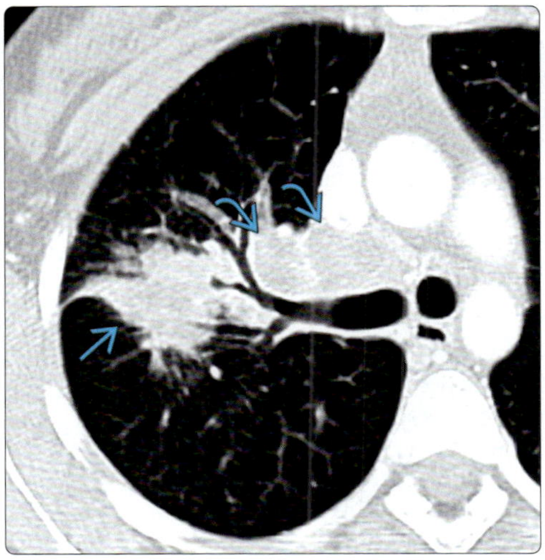

(Left) *Axial CECT in a 15 year old with tracheobronchial papillomatosis shows an irregular cavitary lesion → along with nonspecific regional bronchovascular thickening →.* **(Right)** *Short-term follow-up axial CECT in the same patient shows solid growth into the cavity → from a closely adjacent nodule (not shown). There is also new hilar & mediastinal lymphadenopathy →. Biopsy confirmed squamous cell carcinoma. Rapid growth of nodules in tracheobronchial papillomatosis should raise suspicion for malignancy.*

DIFFERENTIAL DIAGNOSIS

Common

- Congenital Pulmonary Airway Malformation
- Congenital Lobar Overinflation
- Congenital Diaphragmatic Hernia
- Pneumatocele
- Pulmonary Abscess

Less Common

- Lung Contusion With Laceration
- Loculated Pneumothorax
- Bulla
- Bronchial Atresia

Rare but Important

- Traumatic Diaphragmatic Hernia
- Pleuropulmonary Blastoma

ESSENTIAL INFORMATION

Key Differential Diagnosis Issues

- Lucent lung masses in children are most frequently due to congenital or infectious etiologies
- History is very helpful, but CT is frequently necessary to narrow differential
- Note on congenital lung malformations
  - Spectrum of malformations of lung parenchyma & bronchovascular structures
    - Includes foregut duplication cyst, congenital pulmonary airway malformation (CPAM), bronchial atresia, congenital lobar overinflation (CLO), sequestration, scimitar syndrome, pulmonary sling, & pulmonary agenesis
  - Etiology may be combination of proposed theories
    - (1) Defective budding of tracheobronchial tree from primitive foregut (e.g., foregut duplication cysts)
    - (2) Obstruction of developing bronchus with variation in severity, timing, & location
    - (3) Underlying vascular anomaly
    - (4) Genetic
  - Entities most strongly linked to obstruction of developing bronchus have intrinsic cystic or hyperinflated components & can present with lucent lung mass (e.g., CPAM, CLO, bronchial atresia)
  - Some entities will have mix of airway, parenchymal, & vascular anomalies (e.g., sequestration, scimitar syndrome, pulmonary sling)
  - Hybrid Lesion: Mixture of different lesions by imaging &/or histology
    - Traditional example is CPAM with anomalous systemic arterial supply (like bronchopulmonary sequestration)
    - Could also be used for lesions with component of bronchial atresia or CLO-like air-trapping

Helpful Clues for Common Diagnoses

- **Congenital Pulmonary Airway Malformation**
  - Previously known as congenital cystic adenomatoid malformation (CCAM)
  - Most common congenital lung malformation (30-40%)
  - Due to hamartomatous proliferation of cystic & noncystic bronchiole-like tissue
    - Communicates with abnormal cartilage- & gland-deficient bronchial tree at birth
  - Thought to be caused by intrauterine airway obstruction
  - Appears prenatally as fluid-filled cysts that progressively fill with air after delivery
  - Stocker classification (0-4) based on level of airway maldevelopment (proximal to distal)
    - Type 0 (< 2%): Small lungs with severe acinar dysgenesis & large airway dysplasia; uniformly fatal
    - Type 1 (65%): Mainly 1 or more macrocysts (> 2 cm)
      - May have air-fluid levels postnatally
    - Type 2 (10-15%): Multiple small cysts (0.5-2.0 cm)
    - Type 3 (5-8%): Innumerable microscopic cysts
      - Appears solid
    - Type 4 (10-15%): Large peripheral cysts
      - Controversy as to whether this represents distinct entity from type 1 pleuropulmonary blastoma (PPB): Indistinguishable by imaging; pathologic diagnosis is challenging
  - Evidence of associated mass effect
    - Mediastinal shift, compressive atelectasis
  - Can coexist with other pulmonary malformations, such as sequestration, bronchial atresia (hybrid lesion)
    - Image upper abdomen through celiac axis to look for systemic arterial supply CTA
  - Recurrent infection risk
  - Small malignancy risk: Bronchioalveolar carcinoma, rhabdomyosarcoma
  - Reports of type 4 CPAM were likely type 1 PPB → erroneous reports of PPB arising from CPAM
- **Congenital Lobar Overinflation**
  - Overinflation of 1 or more lobes
    - Left upper > right middle > right upper > > lower lobes
    - Multifocal in only ~ 5%
  - Air-trapping caused by intrinsic or extrinsic bronchial luminal narrowing during development
    - Various causes: Absent/dysplastic cartilage, mucosal fold/web, inspissated mucus, bronchial kinking, foregut duplication cysts, vascular compression
  - In 1st hours to days of life: Fluid-density lobar or segmental opacification from retained fetal fluid
  - Progressive hyperlucency & expansion thereafter
    - Mass effect can lead to respiratory compromise
  - ~ 15% have associated congenital heart disease
- **Congenital Diaphragmatic Hernia**
  - Bochdalek (90%): Posterolateral
    - Left 80-90%, right 10-15%, bilateral < 5%
  - Morgagni/ventral (10%): Retrosternal
  - Right-sided hernias may just involve liver
  - Bubbly bowel-like lucencies in chest when stomach/bowel involved
    - Enteric tube may course into chest
  - Associated mass effect on mediastinum
  - Associated pulmonary hypoplasia & pulmonary hypertension → major prognostic factors
  - Other associated cardiovascular, limb, central nervous, GI, GU, &/or genetic anomalies in 25-50%
- **Pneumatocele**
  - Thin-walled cyst

- Can be secondary to infection or trauma (including iatrogenic barotrauma)
- Frequently resolves spontaneously in young children
- **Pulmonary Abscess**
  - Can be due to anaerobic infection from aspiration
    - Others: *Staphylococcus, Streptococcus,* fungi, mycobacteria, & parasites
  - Irregularly-shaped lucent mass with internal air-fluid level
    - Size of air-fluid level similar on frontal & lateral
    - Thick, shaggy, enhancing rind
  - Look for other signs of infection
    - Pleural effusion/empyema
    - Lung consolidation
  - Typically resolves with IV antibiotics without drainage

Helpful Clues for Less Common Diagnoses

- **Lung Contusion With Laceration**
  - Penetrating or blunt trauma with large shearing forces can result in laceration
  - Commonly associated with pneumothorax
  - Appears as thin-walled lucent lung cavity filled with air &/or fluid
  - Complications: Bronchopleural fistula, pulmonary abscess, pneumatocele, air embolism
- **Loculated Pneumothorax**
  - May mimic lucent lung mass
  - Typically found within fissure or in subpulmonic location
  - CT will confirm pleural rather than parenchymal source
- **Bulla**
  - Thin-walled pulmonary parenchymal air-filled space
  - Commonly seen with emphysema
    - α-1-antitrypsin in children/adolescents
    - Idiopathic
  - Can be seen with connective tissue disorders such as Marfan syndrome
  - Superinfection: Look for air-fluid level
  - Can rupture & cause pneumothorax
- **Bronchial Atresia**
  - Noncommunication of segmental/subsegmental bronchus with central airway
    - May result from in utero vascular insult
  - Left upper > left lower > right middle lobe
  - Appears as central tubular/branching density due to mucoid impaction of bronchus distal to atresia
    - Finger in glove appearance
  - Distal lung is hyperinflated with decreased vascularity
    - Air-trapping of distal lung from collateral air drift
  - Can coexist with other pulmonary malformations, such as CPAM or sequestration

Helpful Clues for Rare Diagnoses

- **Traumatic Diaphragmatic Hernia**
  - Due to blunt or penetrating trauma
  - Left > right (liver protective)
  - High incidence of concomitant injuries
  - Plain radiographs may be insensitive
    - Distorted or elevated diaphragm
    - Abdominal contents in thorax
  - CT signs: Discontinuity of hemidiaphragm, dependent viscera sign, collar sign
- **Pleuropulmonary Blastoma**
  - Rare malignant childhood tumor
  - Typically appears as large mass in peripheral lung involving visceral pleura with effusion & mediastinal shift
  - 3 types; lesion evolves from type 1 to type 3 (with progressively worse prognosis)
    - Type 1: Large, air-filled, multilocular cystic mass
    - Type 2: Large, air-filled, cystic & solid mass
    - Type 3: Solid pulmonary mass
  - *DICER1* mutation in 2/3 (tumor predisposition syndrome)
    - PPB, cystic nephroma, pineoblastoma, embryonal rhabdomyosarcoma, ovarian sex cord-stromal tumors
  - May be indistinguishable from CPAM
    - Prenatal 2nd trimester detection, lung hyperinflation, systemic arterial supply (sequestration component), or asymptomatic patient favors CPAM

Congenital Pulmonary Airway Malformation

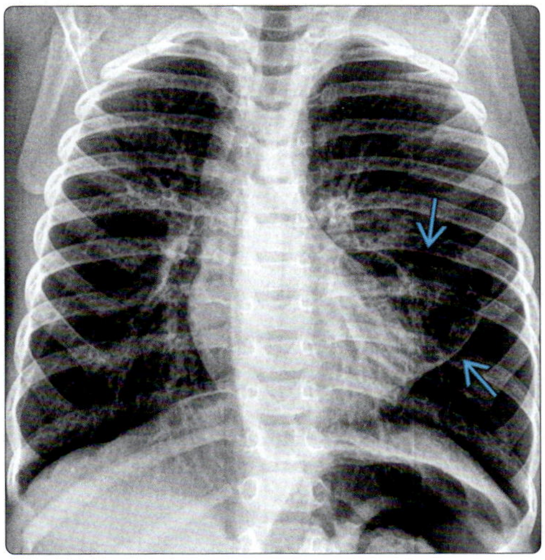

Congenital Pulmonary Airway Malformation

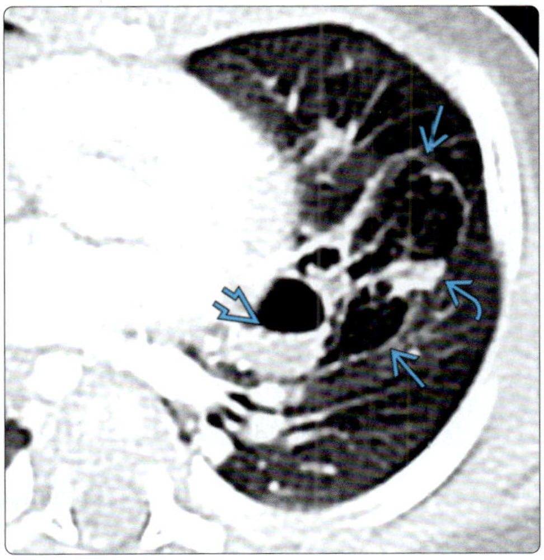

(Left) *PA radiograph in an 18 month old with a prenatally diagnosed lung lesion shows a lucent focus in the lingula causing mild mass effect on the heart & regional vasculature.* **(Right)** *Axial CECT in the same patient at 3 months of age shows a lingular congenital pulmonary airway malformation (CPAM) predominantly composed of small cysts. Note that there are some foci suggestive of fluid-filled cysts, solid tissue, or microcystic components. There is also an air-fluid level in a larger central cyst, which is not uncommon.*

(Left) *Coronal CECT in the same patient again demonstrates a multicystic lesion, consistent with a CPAM. CPAMs are at risk for recurrent infection (& rarely malignancy).* **(Right)** *PA radiograph in a 1 year old shows a lucent right lower lung mass with suggestion of multiple internal cystic components. It causes mass effect on the mediastinum & diaphragm. Large CPAMs can lead to secondary pulmonary hypoplasia.*

Congenital Pulmonary Airway Malformation

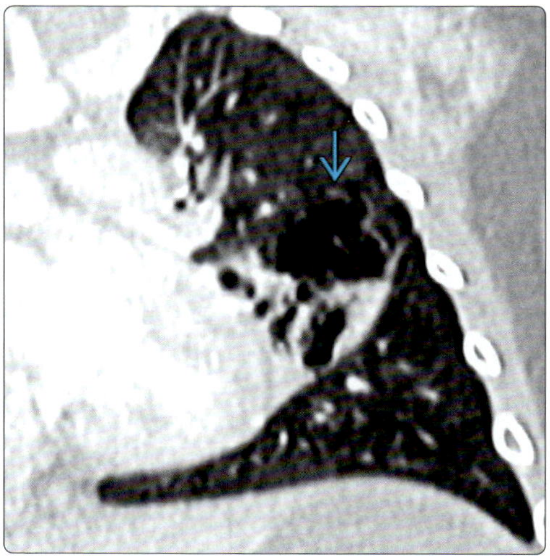

Congenital Pulmonary Airway Malformation

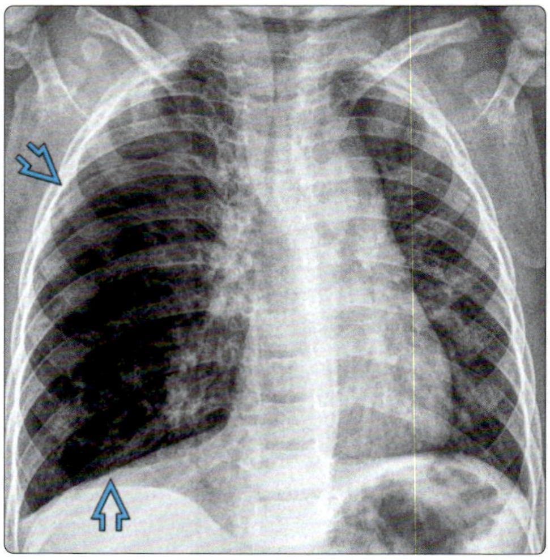

(Left) *Axial CECT in the same patient shows a large right lower lobe lesion with cysts of variable size. There is a central component with solid-appearing tissue & prominent vascularity.* **(Right)** *Coronal CECT MIP in the same patient shows that the central solid-appearing component has systemic arterial supply from a prominent tortuous vessel that arises from the descending aorta, consistent with a hybrid lesion containing both CPAM & bronchopulmonary sequestration components.*

Congenital Pulmonary Airway Malformation

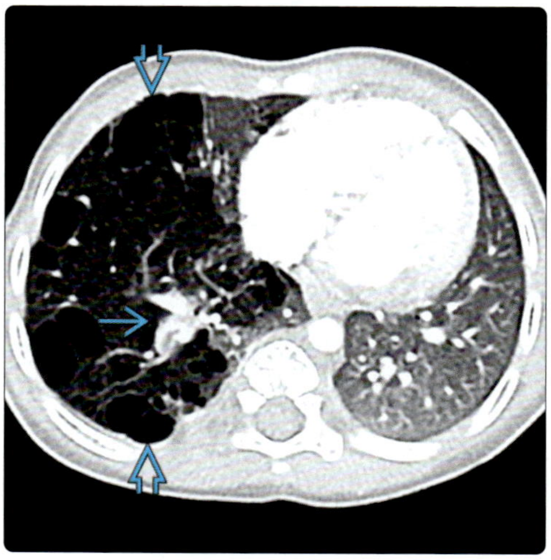

Congenital Pulmonary Airway Malformation

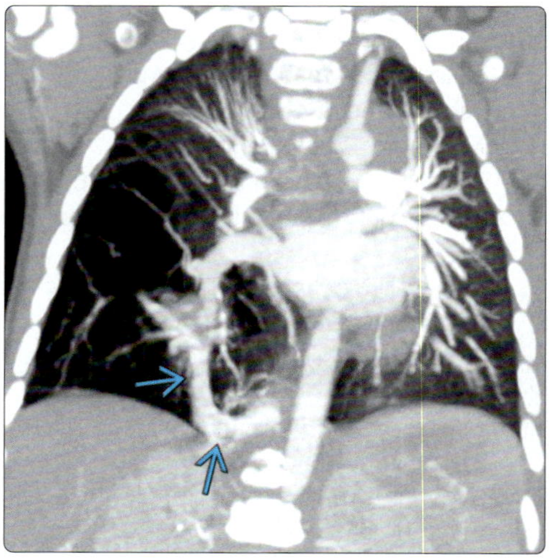

(Left) *PA radiograph in a 4 month old shows an incidental finding of hyperinflation vs. a lucent lung mass in the right lower lung.* **(Right)** *Axial CECT in the same patient shows relative overinflation & hyperlucency of the entire right middle lobe with mediastinal shift to the left. There is apparent kinking & narrowing of the right middle lobe bronchus as it courses underneath the right pulmonary artery (not shown). The findings are consistent with congenital lobar overinflation.*

Congenital Lobar Overinflation

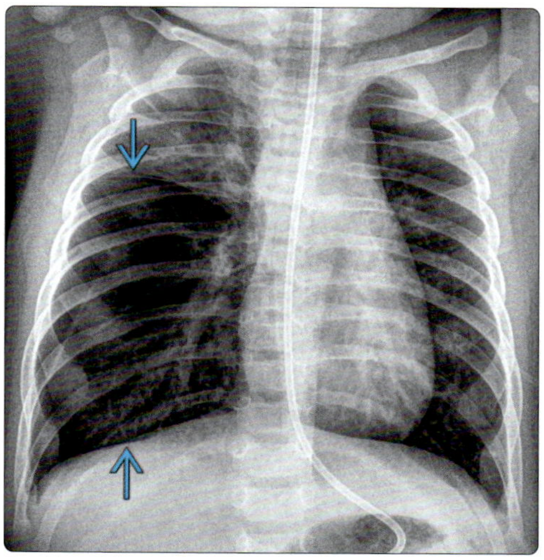

Congenital Lobar Overinflation

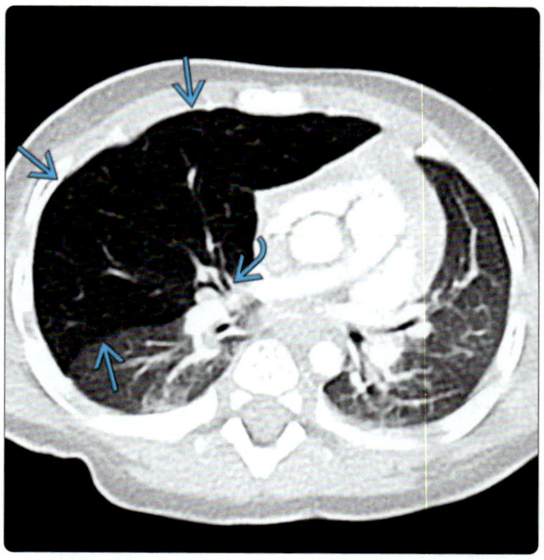

Congenital Diaphragmatic Hernia

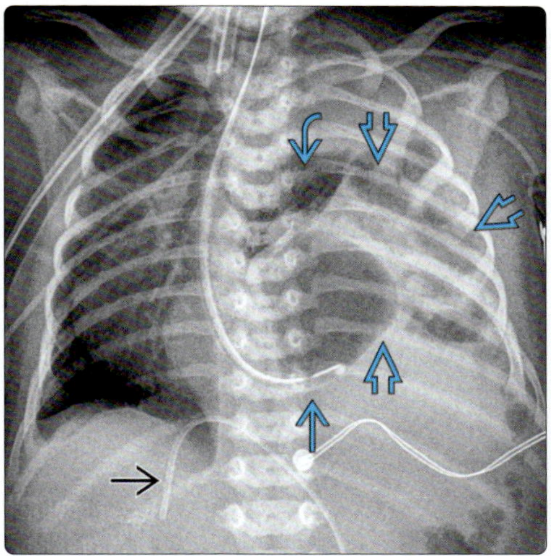

Congenital Diaphragmatic Hernia

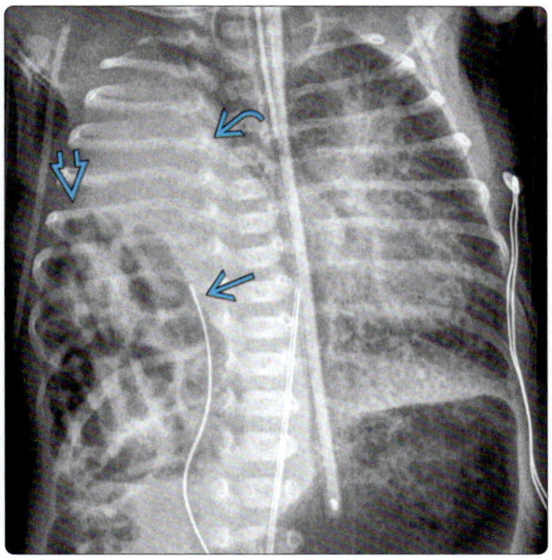

(Left) *AP radiograph in a newborn shows bubbly lucencies in the left hemithorax ➔, typical of bowel in a left CDH. The enteric tube courses into the herniated stomach ➔. There is mass effect with a small aerated left lung ➔ & mediastinal shift. The UVC is malpositioned ➔.* **(Right)** *AP radiograph in a 5 day old shows bubbly lucencies in the right hemithorax ➔, consistent with a right CDH containing bowel. The UVC also courses into the right hemithorax ➔ due to liver herniation ➔.*

Congenital Diaphragmatic Hernia

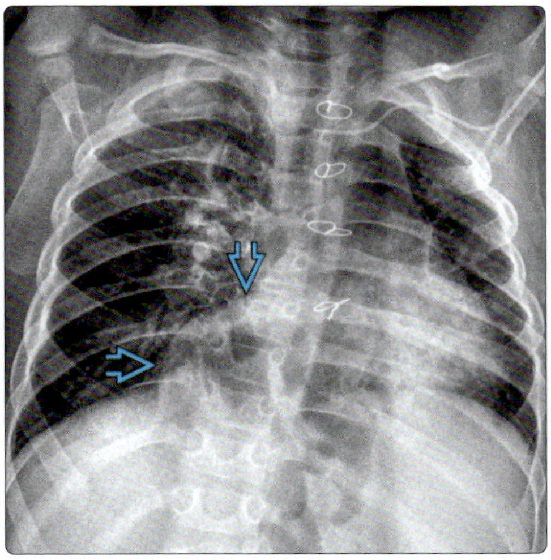

Congenital Diaphragmatic Hernia

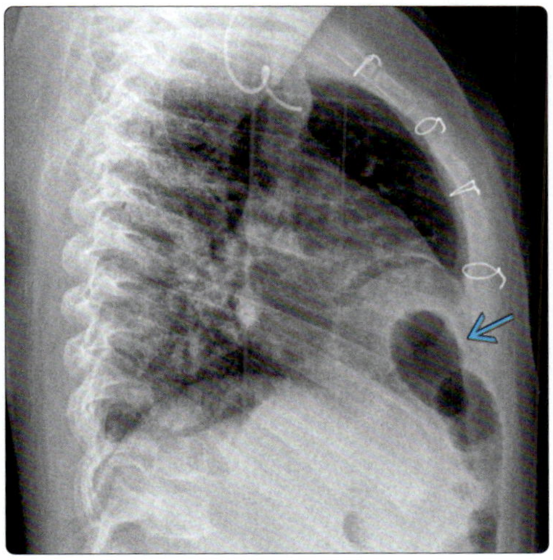

(Left) *PA radiograph in a 19 month old with trisomy 21 status post repair of an AVSD shows a mixed lucent & soft tissue density mass at the right cardiophrenic angle ➔.* **(Right)** *Lateral radiograph in the same patient shows the retrosternal mass containing bowel-like lucencies ➔, consistent with a Morgagni hernia. While most Morgagni hernias are isolated defects, there is a rare association with trisomy 21. The differential for an anterior diaphragmatic hernia is the rare central tendon hernia that occurs in midline.*

Pneumatocele

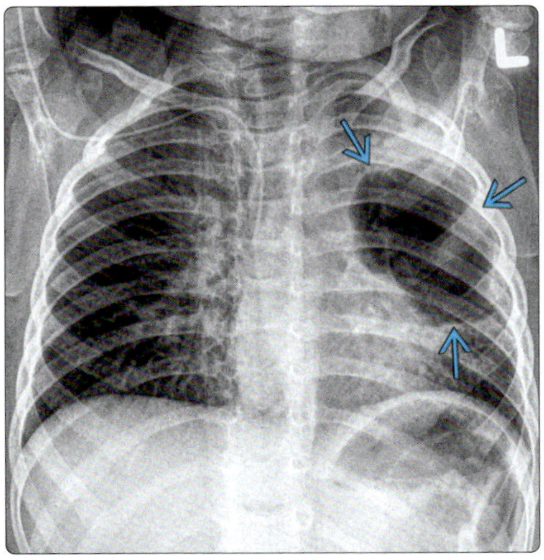

Pneumatocele

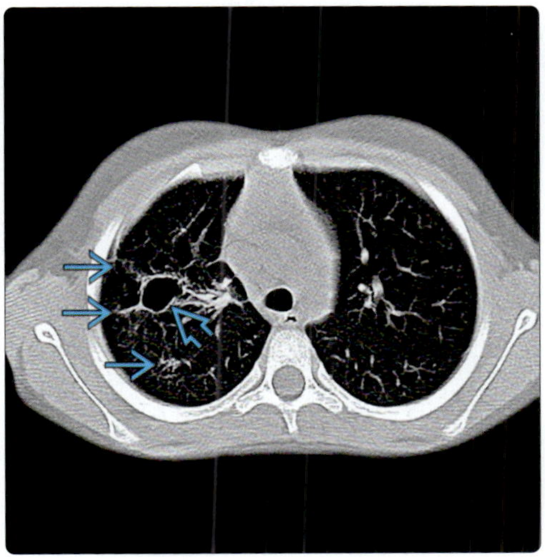

(Left) *PA radiograph in an 18 month old with a history of ALL & Pseudomonas pneumonia shows a lucent lesion in an area of prior left upper lobe consolidation ➔, consistent with a postinfectious pneumatocele.* **(Right)** *Axial NECT in a 7 year old with prior right upper lobe pneumonia shows a well-defined, thin-walled parenchymal cyst in the right upper lobe ➔, consistent with a postinfectious pneumatocele. Note the wispy areas of surrounding parenchymal scars ➔.*

(Left) *PA radiograph in a 6 year old with complicated pneumonia shows a lucent mass in the left lower lobe with an air-fluid level, suspicious for an abscess. Other signs of infection are present, including right upper lung consolidation & a right pleural effusion.* **(Right)** *Lateral radiograph in the same patient shows the lucent mass in the posterior lower lobe with an air-fluid level, similar in size to the frontal radiograph & consistent with an abscess. Pulmonary abscesses usually resolve with IV antibiotics alone.*

Pulmonary Abscess

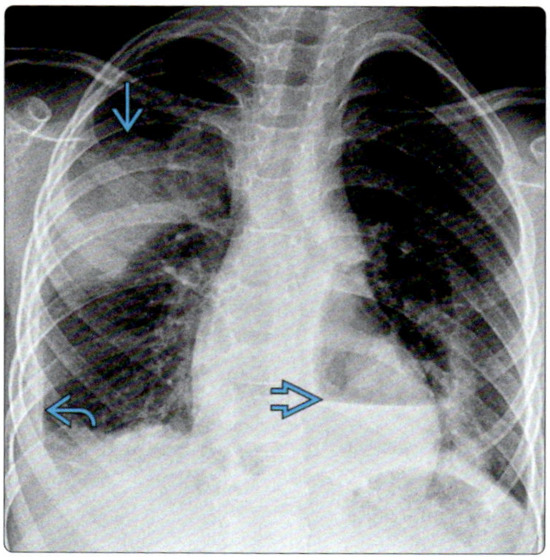

Pulmonary Abscess

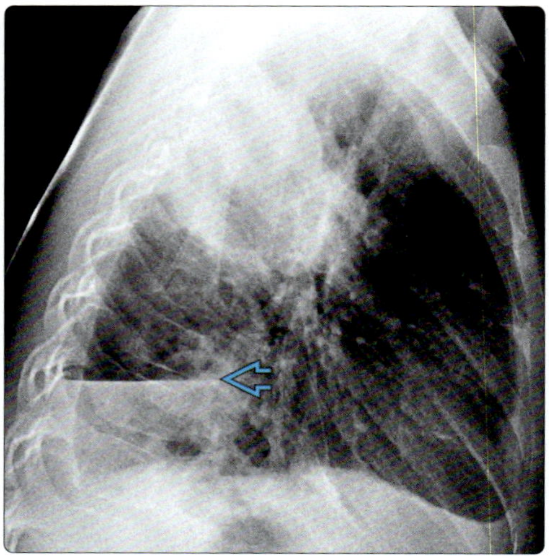

(Left) *Axial CECT in the same patient shows the left lower lobe cavitary lesion with a thick irregular wall & internal air-fluid level, consistent with an abscess.* **(Right)** *Axial CECT in a 4 year old hit by a car shows a diffuse left upper lobe contusion with a central lucent lesion, consistent with a pulmonary laceration. This child also had multiple rib fractures & a pneumothorax. Pulmonary lacerations imply a more severe multi-system trauma & are associated with a mortality rate of up to 40%.*

Pulmonary Abscess

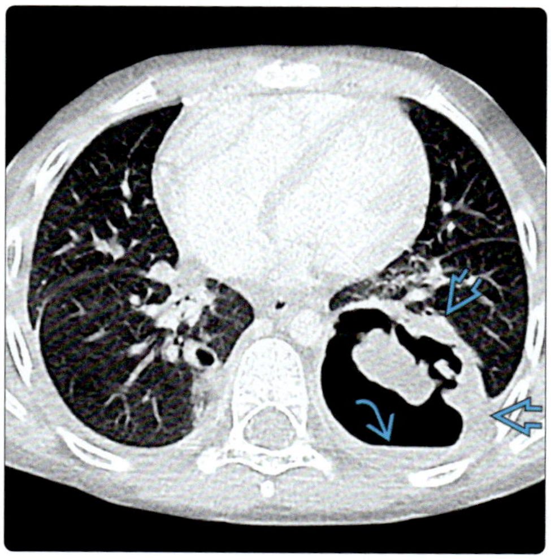

Lung Contusion With Laceration

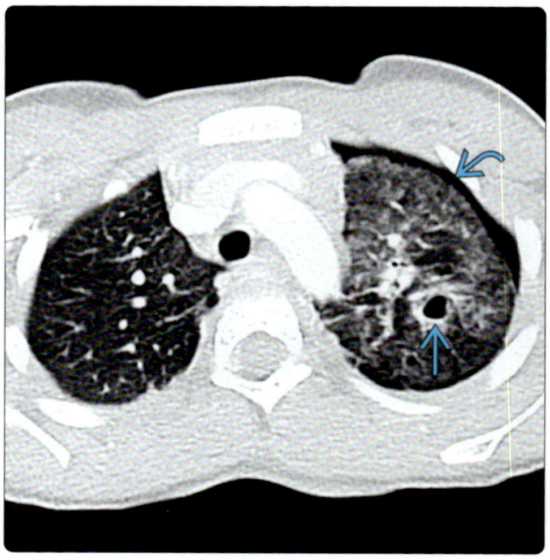

(Left) *AP radiograph shows lucent lesions in the right apex & lateral base, consistent with a loculated pneumothorax in this 5 day old with a partially evacuated neonatal pneumothorax. Pneumothoraces can be difficult to see when loculated (or in supine infants).* **(Right)** *Coronal CECT in a 3 year old shows a large idiopathic bulla within the right lung causing mass effect on the right upper lobe & leftward mediastinal shift. A type 1 pleuropulmonary blastoma (PPB) would be in the DDx for this appearance.*

Loculated Pneumothorax

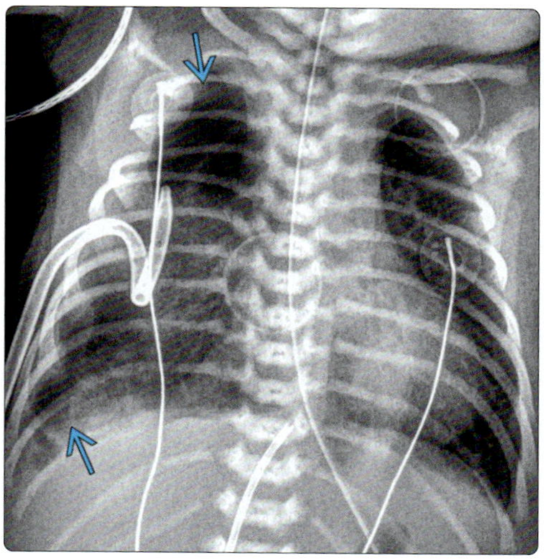

Bulla

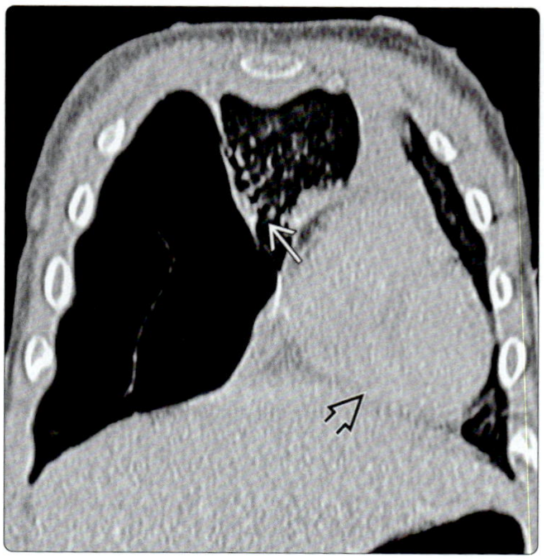

Bronchial Atresia

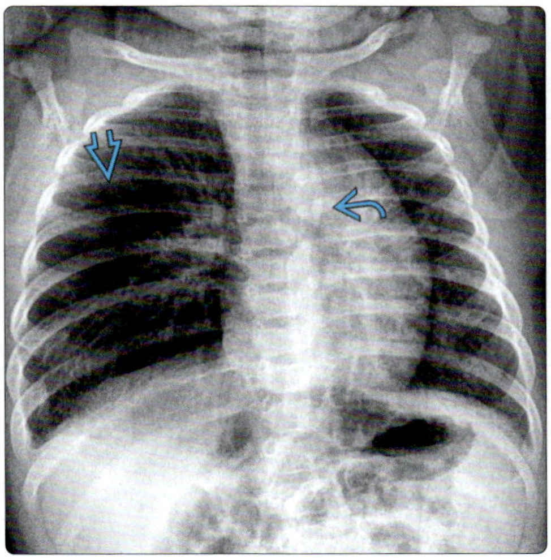

Bronchial Atresia

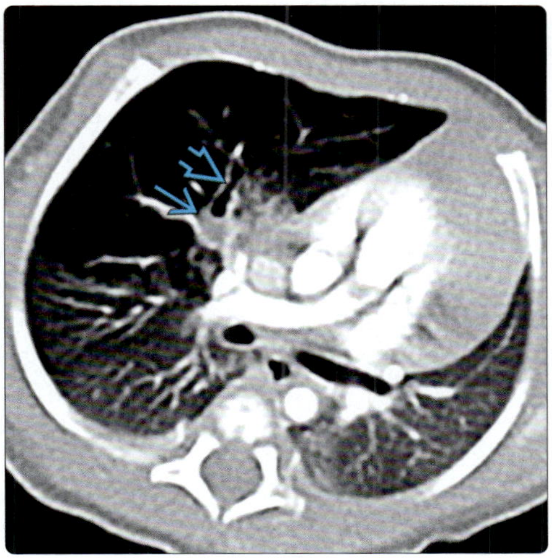

(Left) *PA radiograph in a 3 month old shows a mass-like lucency within the right hemithorax ⇨ (due to hyperinflation & air-trapping of the right middle lobe) causing mediastinal mass effect ↷.* **(Right)** *Axial CECT in the same patient shows an atretic right middle lobe bronchus with mucoid impaction ⇨ & dilation ⇨ distal to the atresia. The right middle lobe is hyperinflated with reduced vascularity. These findings are consistent with bronchial atresia.*

Traumatic Diaphragmatic Hernia

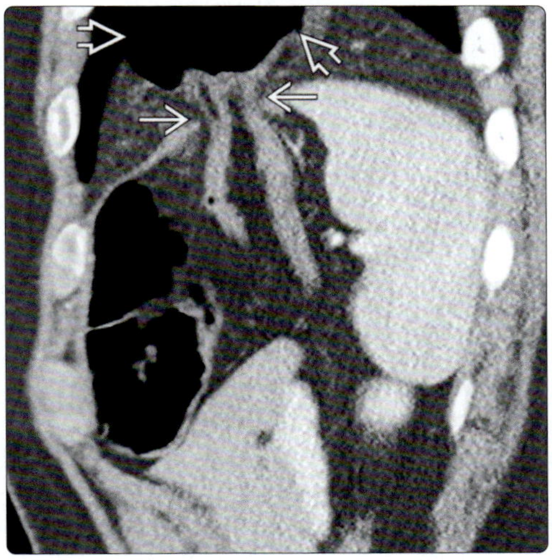

Pleuropulmonary Blastoma

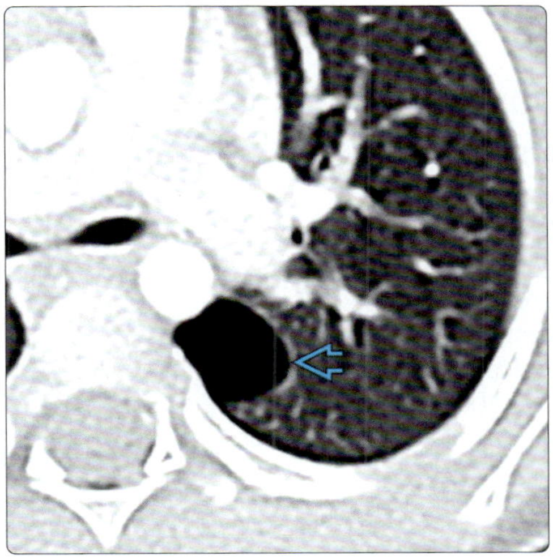

(Left) *Sagittal CECT shows a lucent mass ➡ in the left hemithorax that is surrounded by fat. This abnormality communicates with the abdomen via a defect in the diaphragm ➡ that was due to a stab wound.* **(Right)** *Axial CECT in a 3 year old with a DICER1 tumor predisposition syndrome shows a lucent subpleural lung mass ⇨ that was a type 1 PPB. Type 1 PPB cannot be distinguished at imaging from benign cystic lesions such as CPAM. In a patient with DICER1, any lung cyst should be considered a PPB until proven otherwise.*

Pleuropulmonary Blastoma

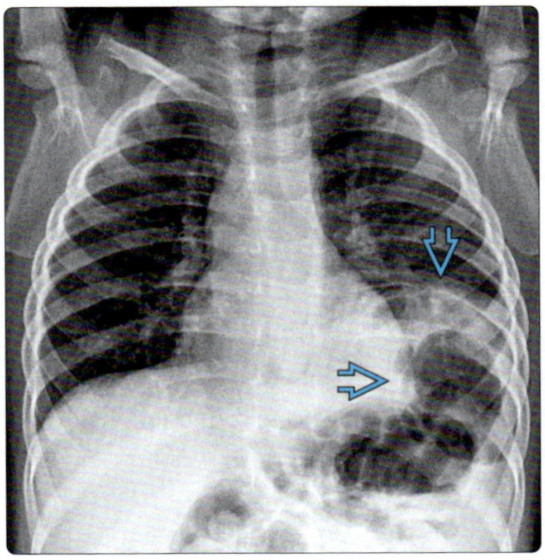

Pleuropulmonary Blastoma

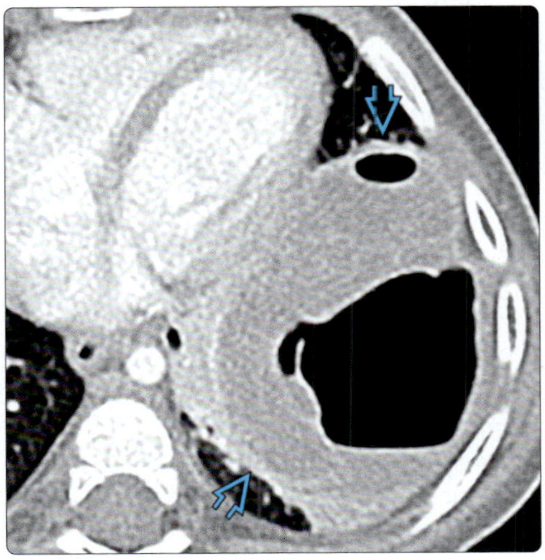

(Left) *PA radiograph in a 23 month old with DICER1 shows a heterogeneous solid & cystic mass in the left lower lung ⇨.* **(Right)** *Axial CECT in the same patient shows a mixed solid-cystic mass ⇨ involving the pleura, consistent with a type 2 PPB in this patient with DICER1. Despite the large size, PPBs rarely invade the chest wall. This lesion was identified on screening whole body MR, which some have endorsed for use in cancer predisposition syndromes.*

Round Lung Mass

DIFFERENTIAL DIAGNOSIS

Common

- Round Pneumonia

Less Common

- Overlying Artifact
- Lung Abscess/Cavitary Necrosis
- Fungal Infection
- Congenital Lung Malformation
  - Bronchogenic Cyst
  - Congenital Pulmonary Airway Malformation
  - Bronchopulmonary Sequestration
- Extrapulmonary Neoplasm
  - Chest Wall Lesion
  - Neuroblastoma
- Retrocaval Thymus

Rare but Important

- Metastases
- Loculated Pleural Fluid (Pseudocyst)
- Primary Lung Neoplasm
  - Pleuropulmonary Blastoma

ESSENTIAL INFORMATION

Key Differential Diagnosis Issues

- Consider round pneumonia
  - < 8 years of age, solitary lesion, soft tissue density (without air-fluid levels)
  - Fever & cough are often present
  - Treat with antibiotics & follow-up with radiographs
    - CT is not indicated to evaluate for other potential causes of mass in this clinical scenario
- Consider posterior mediastinal (e.g., neuroblastoma) or chest wall lesion
  - Look for underlying rib erosion or destruction
- Consider overlying artifact
  - Look for sharp margins & unnatural geographic shapes (too round)

Helpful Clues for Common Diagnoses

- **Round Pneumonia**
  - Most common solitary round "lung mass" in child
  - Mean age is 5 years; less common after 8 years
    - Thought to be related to poorly developed collateral circulation in early life
    - Round lesions seen after 8 years of age should have increased suspicion for other underlying causes
  - Most commonly appears as solitary lesion (98%) with well-defined borders (70%)
  - More common posteriorly (83%) & in lower lobes (65%)
  - Mean diameter = 3.8 cm
  - Air bronchograms help confirm airspace consolidation
  - Tend to resolve on follow-up imaging (95.0%) rather than progression to lobar pneumonia (4.6%)
  - May have abdominal pain rather than chest symptoms

Helpful Clues for Less Common Diagnoses

- **Overlying Artifact**
  - Should always be considered as potential cause of any round lung radiodensity
  - Often will be unusually round (or other geometric shape), suggesting unnatural cause
    - Common causes include hair braids, buttons, shirt pocket contents, monitor leads, & other devices
- **Lung Abscess/Cavitary Necrosis**
  - Abscesses are uncommon in otherwise healthy children
    - Most commonly occur with underlying immunodeficiency or complex medical disorders
    - Thick, irregular enhancing wall
    - Can appear as round lung mass if no air-fluid level is present
  - Cavitary necrosis is complication of pneumonia with variable thin-walled cavities
    - Contains fluid &/or air
    - Lacks enhancing border
    - Loss of surrounding lung architecture with decreased parenchymal enhancement
    - Shows adjacent consolidation
  - Both typically resolve with intravenous (IV) antibiotics without drainage
- **Fungal Infection**
  - Uncommon in otherwise healthy children
  - Most commonly occurs with underlying immunodeficiency or complex medical disorders
    - Impaired immune function from chemotherapy or conditioning for stem cell transplant
    - Severe combined immunodeficiency disease is predisposed to *Pneumocystis jirovecii* pneumonia
    - Chronic granulomatous disease is predisposed to invasive aspergillosis
  - Typically multifocal, clustered, poorly defined nodules with variable, ill-defined consolidation
- **Congenital Lung Malformation**
  - Spectrum of malformations of lung parenchyma & bronchovascular structures
  - Includes foregut duplication cyst, congenital pulmonary airway malformation (CPAM), bronchial atresia, lobar overinflation, sequestration, scimitar syndrome, pulmonary sling, & pulmonary agenesis
  - Now recognized that many have mixture of different lesions by imaging &/or histology → "hybrid lesion"
    - Traditional example is CPAM with anomalous systemic arterial supply (sequestration-like components)
    - Could also be used for lesions with component of bronchial atresia or overinflation-like air-trapping
  - **Bronchogenic cyst**
    - Much less common than round pneumonia
    - Most are hilar or mediastinal (around central airways) rather than in parenchyma
    - Are typically unilocular & fluid-filled (no air-fluid levels) unless infection leads to wall breakdown
    - Can see mass effect
  - **Congenital pulmonary airway malformation**
    - Filled with fluid prenatally & in early in life → progressively fills with air after delivery (& may show air-fluid levels)
    - Usually multicystic
  - **Bronchopulmonary sequestration**
    - Nonfunctioning lung tissue disconnected from bronchial tree
    - Vascular supply from systemic artery is key feature

- Intralobar & extralobar types
  - Intralobar: Shares pleura of affected lobe; drainage is usually via pulmonary vein
  - Extralobar: Separate pleural covering; drainage is usually via systemic vein
- Both usually occur in lower lungs; extralobar type can be infradiaphragmatic or mediastinal
- Solid on initial imaging in postnatal period
  - Intralobar type may show gradual aeration from collateral flow or CPAM components
  - Extralobar type does not aerate unless in communication with foregut

- **Extrapulmonary Neoplasm**
  - **Chest wall lesion**
    - Rib lesion can appear as round lung lesion on chest radiograph
    - Entities include enchondroma, osteochondroma, aneurysmal bone cyst, fibrous dysplasia, Langerhans cell histiocytosis, Ewing sarcoma, osteosarcoma
    - Look for rib destruction or erosion
  - **Neuroblastoma**
    - In young child (< 5 years of age), posterior mediastinal mass is neuroblastoma until proven otherwise
    - Will often be obvious posterior mediastinal mass, particularly when in inferior chest
    - Can appear as round lesion when large & at apex; can be difficult at times to determine anatomic location
      - Look for associated rib erosion/destruction to identify lesion as posterior mediastinal mass
    - Often have Ca^{2+}
- **Retrocaval Thymus**
  - Extension of thymus between superior vena cava & trachea into right paratracheal location
  - Most common aberrant location of thymus
  - Can have appearance as mass on chest radiograph or CT
  - Lesion should be contiguous with & appear similar to normal thymus on all modalities

Helpful Clues for Rare Diagnoses

- **Metastases**
  - Usually multifocal, though dominant lesion may appear solitary
- **Loculated Pleural Fluid (Pseudocyst)**
  - Fluid can become loculated in pleural fissures & present as round-appearing mass on frontal view
  - Fairly uncommon in children
- **Primary Lung Neoplasm**
  - Pleuropulmonary blastoma (PPB), infantile fibrosarcoma (primary bronchopulmonary fibrosarcoma), fetal lung interstitial tumor, inflammatory myofibroblastic tumor, neuroendocrine tumor, various carcinomas
  - **Pleuropulmonary blastoma**
    - Rare primary malignancy of childhood
    - Can appear as round mass but is more typically diagnosed late, appearing as large mass filling hemithorax, often with associated pleural disease
    - 3 types: PPB evolves from type 1 to type 3 (with progressively worse prognosis)
      - Type 1: Large, air-filled, multilocular cystic mass
      - Type 2: Large, air-filled, cystic & solid mass
      - Type 3: Solid pulmonary mass
    - *DICER1* mutation in 2/3 (tumor predisposition syndrome)
      - PPB, cystic nephroma, pineoblastoma, embryonal rhabdomyosarcoma, ovarian sex cord-stromal tumors
    - May be indistinguishable from CPAM
      - Prenatal 2nd trimester detection, lung hyperinflation, systemic arterial supply (sequestration component), or asymptomatic patient favors CPAM

SELECTED REFERENCES

1. Lichtenberger JP 3rd et al: Primary lung tumors in children: radiologic-pathologic correlation from the radiologic pathology archives. Radiographics. 38(7):2151-72, 2018
2. Restrepo R et al: Imaging of round pneumonia and mimics in children. Pediatr Radiol. 40(12):1931-40, 2010

Round Pneumonia

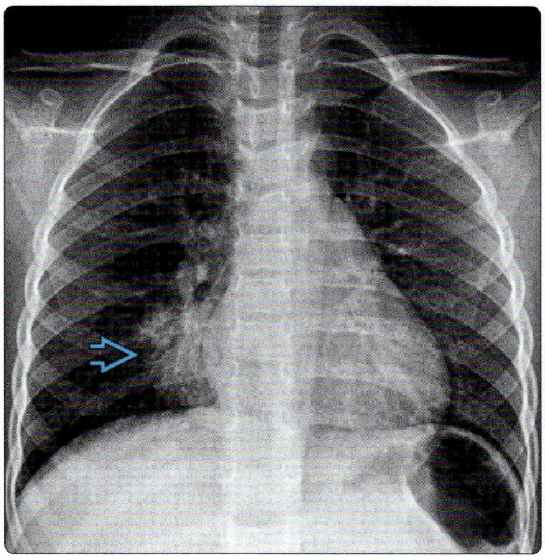

Round Pneumonia

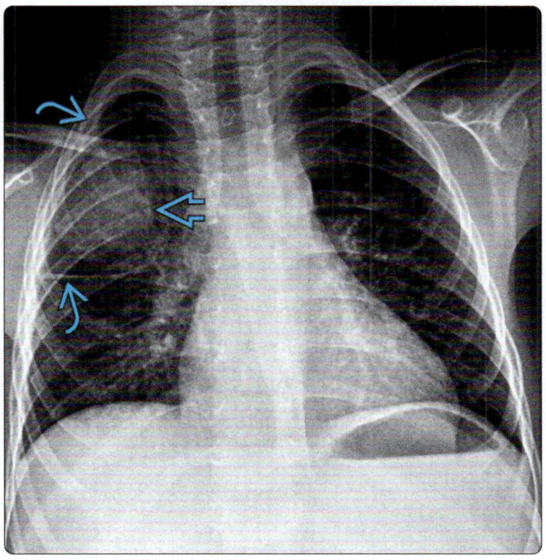

(Left) *PA radiograph in a 4 year old with cough & fever shows a rounded right lower lobe consolidation ➔ with air bronchograms, consistent with a round pneumonia.* **(Right)** *PA radiograph in a 4 year old with cough & fever shows a right upper lobe rounded consolidation ➔, consistent with a round pneumonia. There is a small associated right pleural effusion ➔. Follow-up radiographs showed complete resolution of the opacity. Round pneumonia is less common after 8 years of age due to the development of collateral channels.*

(Left) *AP radiograph in a 2 year old with a posterior fossa tumor shows a rounded artifact overlying the left hemithorax due to an ECG lead. Artifacts often appear as geometric shapes with well-defined borders.* **(Right)** *Frontal radiograph of the chest in a patient with cavitary necrosis complicating a pneumonia shows new central lucency in the right midlung in an area of previous consolidation. Areas of cavitation do not become air filled until communicating with aerated lung.*

Overlying Artifact

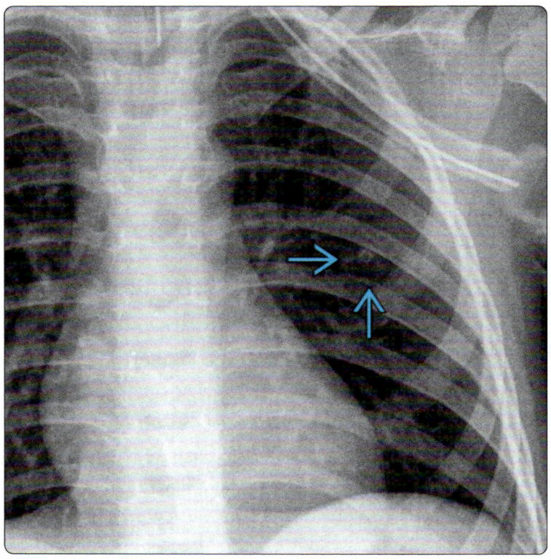

Lung Abscess/Cavitary Necrosis

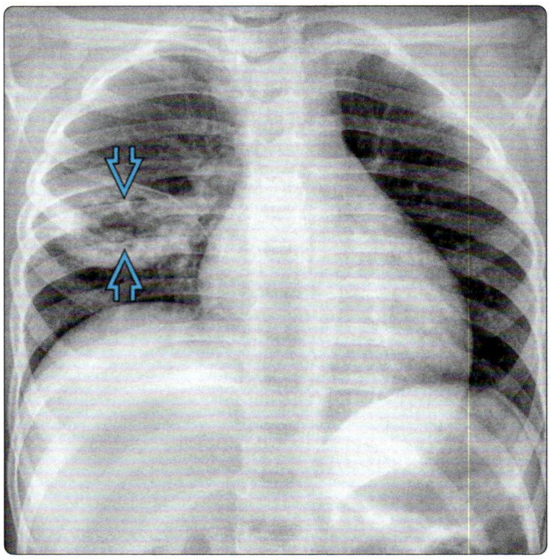

(Left) *Axial CECT in the same patient shows a multiseptated cavitary lesion with a nonenhancing wall. These lesions usually resolve with antibiotics alone & do not require drainage.* **(Right)** *PA radiograph in a 17 year old with relapsed leukemia & fever shows a rounded mass in the right lower lung. Fungal infection is most commonly seen in patients immunocompromised by chemotherapy or conditioning for stem cell transplant. The most common organism in these scenarios is aspergillus causing invasive Aspergillosis.*

Lung Abscess/Cavitary Necrosis

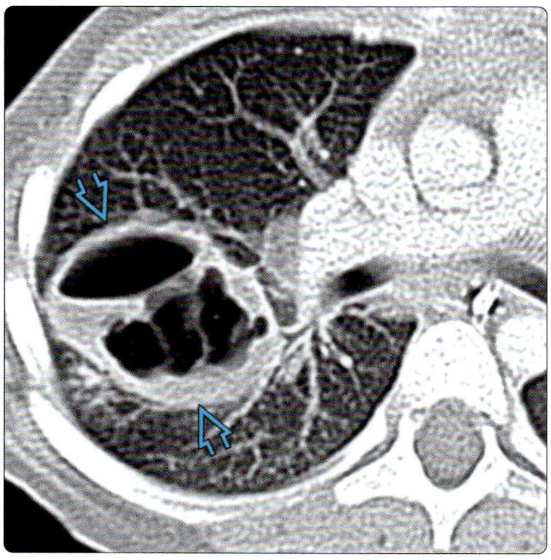

Fungal Infection

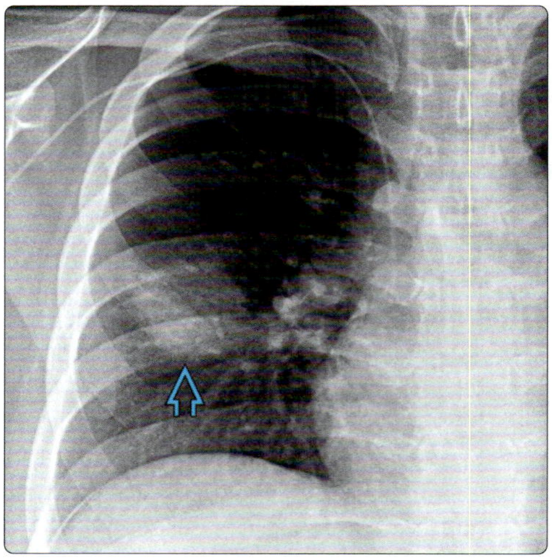

(Left) *Axial CECT in the same patient shows a round area of consolidation with a surrounding ground-glass halo, consistent with invasive aspergillosis. Multiple variable-sized nodules or patchy areas of consolidation can be present in invasive aspergillosis. The ground-glass halos represent hemorrhage & are highly suggestive of the diagnosis.* **(Right)** *Axial CECT in the same patient after starting antifungal treatment shows an air crescent sign, indicating improvement. The ground-glass hemorrhagic components have resolved.*

Fungal Infection

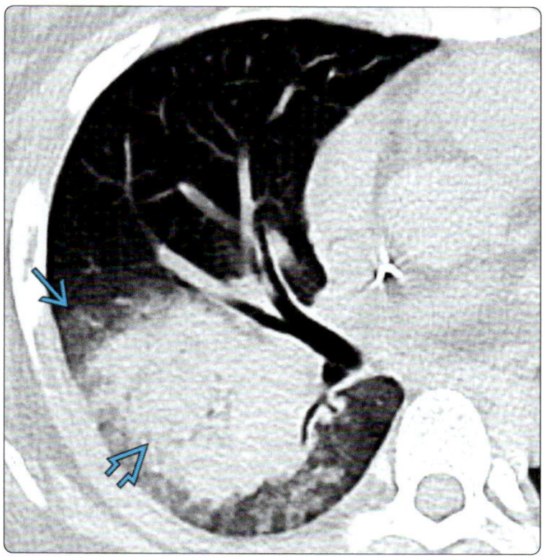

Fungal Infection

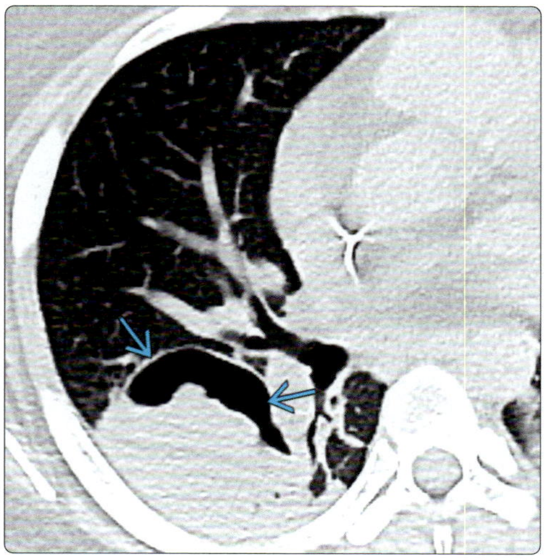

Bronchogenic Cyst

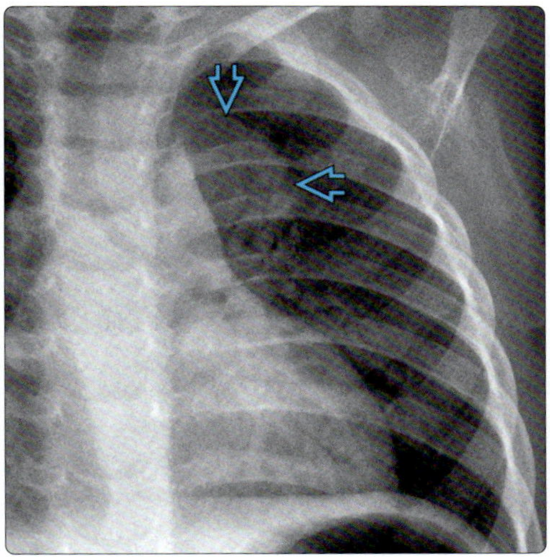

Bronchogenic Cyst

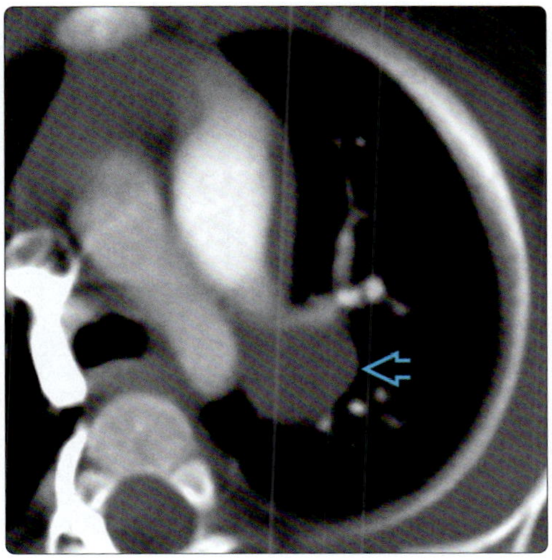

(Left) *PA radiograph in a 2 year old shows a rounded opacity in the medial left upper lung.* **(Right)** *Axial CECT in the same patient shows a corresponding thin-walled, cystic-appearing lesion in the left hilum, most consistent with a bronchogenic cyst. Bronchogenic cysts are usually closely related to the central airways, & mass effect on the airway can cause atelectasis or air-trapping. Surgical resection is usually recommended due to the risk of infection (& rarely malignancy).*

Congenital Pulmonary Airway Malformation

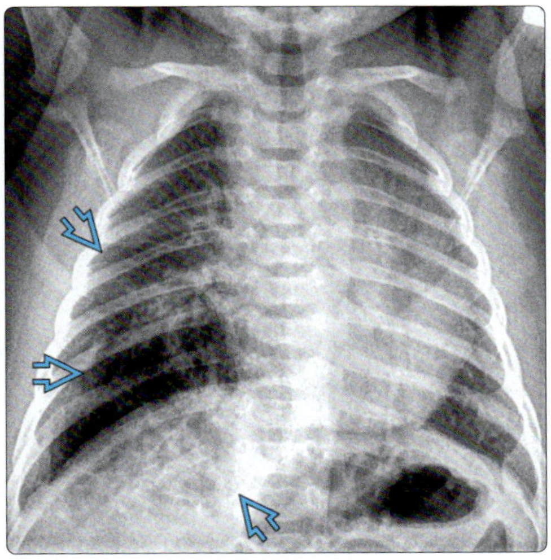

Congenital Pulmonary Airway Malformation

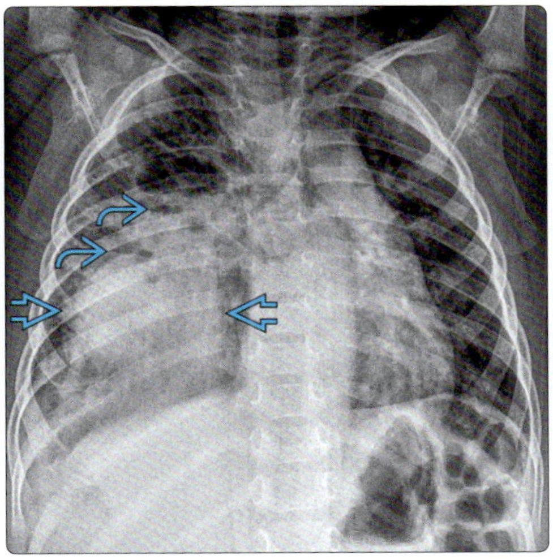

(Left) *PA radiograph in a 56 day old shows a multicystic lucent mass in the right lower lung , which was a congenital pulmonary airway malformation (CPAM).* **(Right)** *PA radiograph in the same patient at 15 months old now shows fluid filling portions of the right lower lung lesion due to superinfection, creating a rounded right lower lung mass containing air-fluid levels . Resection is recommended if feasible for CPAMs due to the risk of infection (& rarely malignancy).*

Bronchopulmonary Sequestration

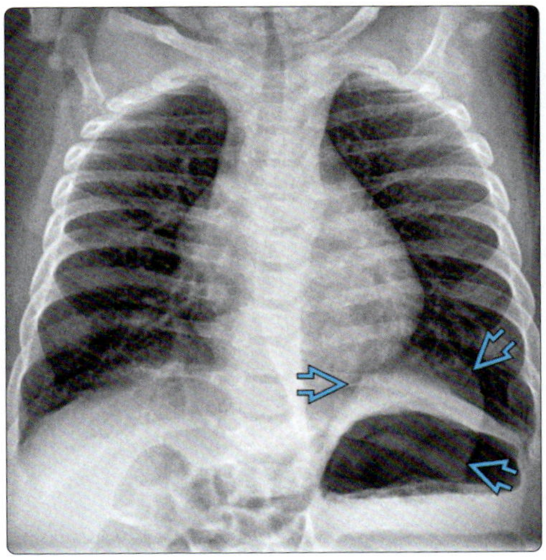

Bronchopulmonary Sequestration

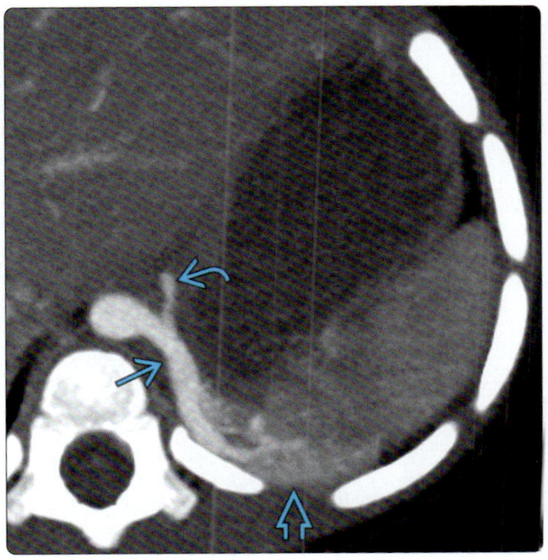

(Left) *AP radiograph in an asymptomatic 3 month old shows a rounded opacity in the left lower lobe with the appearance & location being suspicious for a bronchopulmonary sequestration.* **(Right)** *Axial CECT in the same patient shows an enhancing left lower lung mass abutting the diaphragm. There is prominent systemic arterial supply from the abdominal aorta along with systemic venous drainage to the portal vein (not shown). The findings are consistent with an extralobar sequestration.*

Chest Wall Lesion

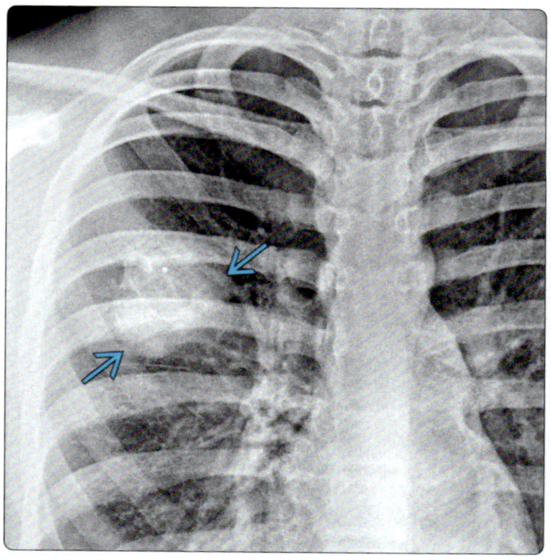

Chest Wall Lesion

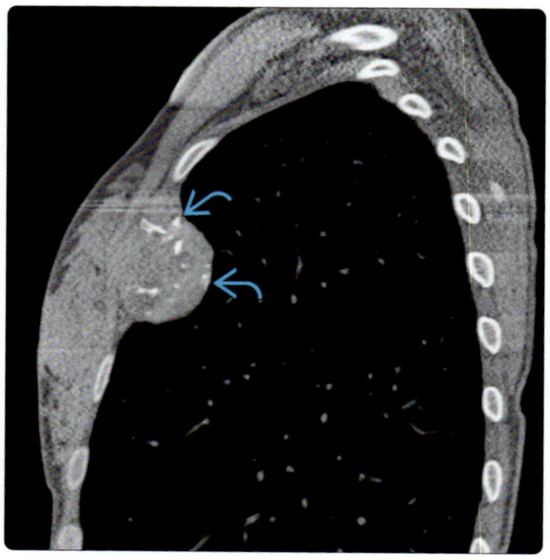

(Left) *Frontal radiograph shows an enchondroma of the rib as a rounded, somewhat lobulated density. Note the appearance of the adjacent anterior 3rd rib, which is a clue to the chest wall origin of this lesion. Also note the metallic "BB" placed on the region of the palpable lesion during a physical examination.* **(Right)** *Sagittal NECT in the same patient shows the enchondroma of the anterior right 3rd rib. Note the chondroid matrix & loss of a normal rib at this level (compared to the adjacent ribs).*

Neuroblastoma

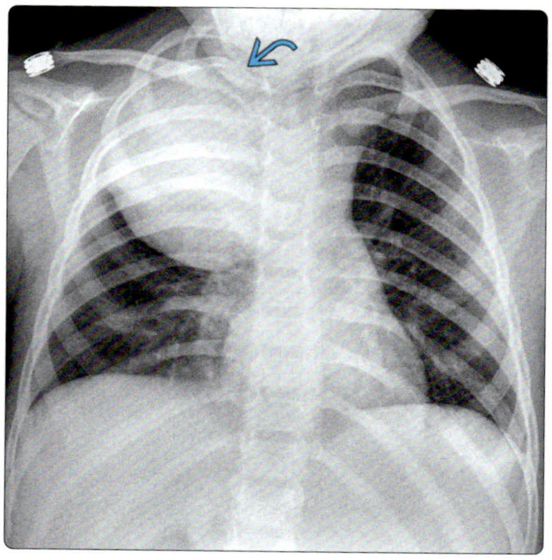

Neuroblastoma

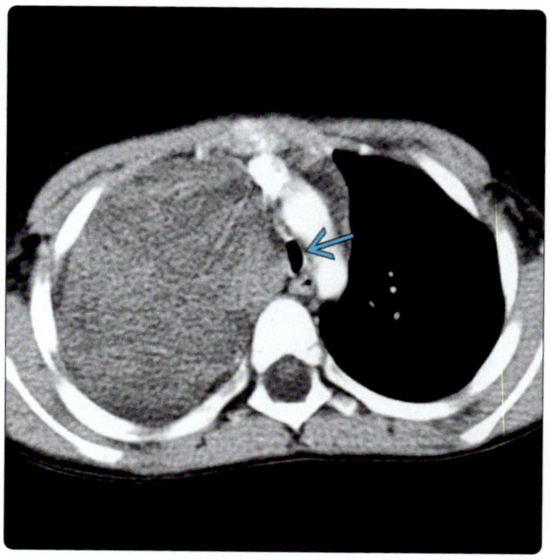

(Left) *Frontal radiograph shows a large, round, soft tissue density mass overlying the apex of the right hemithorax. Note the widening of the interspace between the right 3rd & 4th ribs, as compared to the same interspace on the left. There is also erosion of the posterior right 3rd rib.* **(Right)** *Axial NECT in the same patient shows a large mass filling the superior right hemithorax. Note the mediastinal shift to the left & compression of the trachea.*

Neuroblastoma

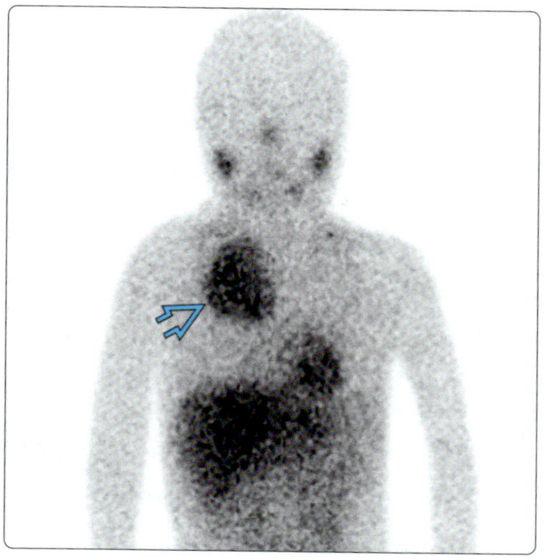

Neuroblastoma

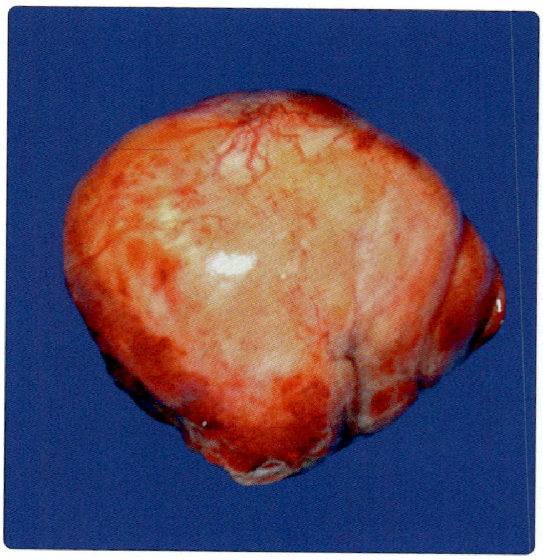

(Left) *Frontal MIBG scintigraphy in the same patient shows increased uptake in the lesion, consistent with neuroblastoma. Note the normal activity in the salivary glands, heart, & liver. No osseous metastases are seen.* **(Right)** *Gross pathology in the same patient shows the round, encapsulated mass representing a resected neuroblastoma. Neuroblastoma can occur anywhere along the sympathetic chain & is the most common extracranial solid tumor in children.*

Retrocaval Thymus

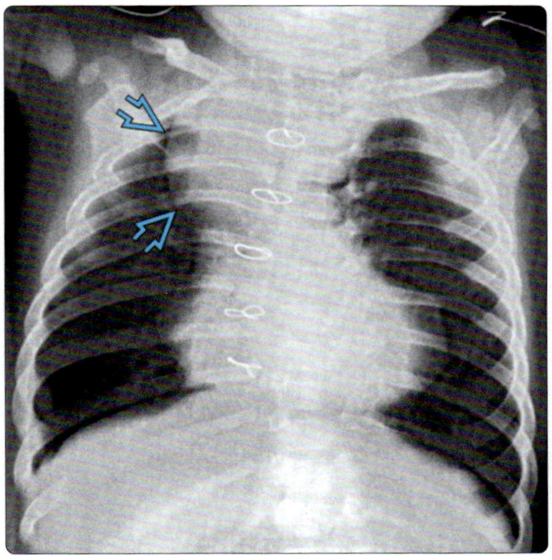

Retrocaval Thymus

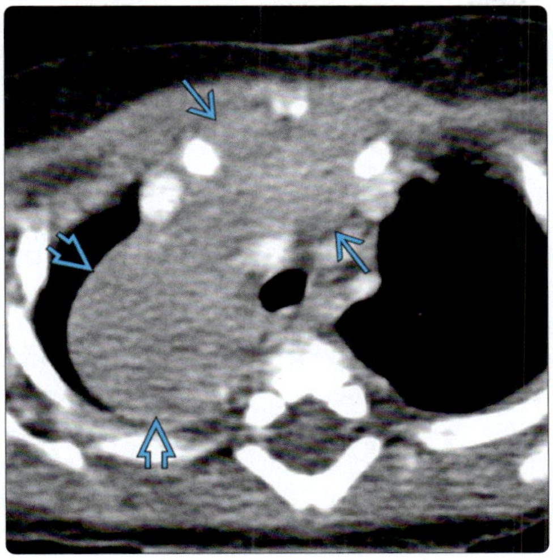

(Left) *Frontal radiograph in a child with a history of cardiac surgery shows a right superior mediastinal mass. Note the sternotomy wires.* **(Right)** *Axial CECT in the same child shows a homogeneous right paratracheal mass. The mass is contiguous & isodense with the thymus. Also note the characteristic lack of vessel or airway compression. The thymus had been small on the immediate preoperative radiograph, making this appearance consistent with thymic rebound hyperplasia in a retrocaval thymus.*

Loculated Pleural Fluid (Pseudocyst)

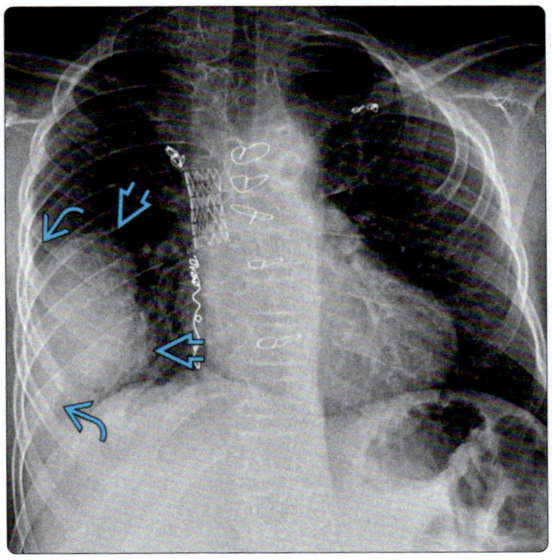

Loculated Pleural Fluid (Pseudocyst)

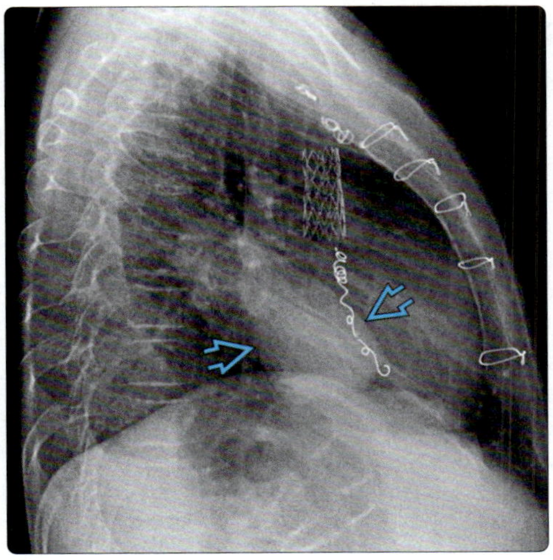

(Left) *PA radiograph in a 9 year old with complex congenital heart disease status post failed Fontan with takedown shows a chronic loculated right pleural effusion simulating a lung mass on the PA projection. The broad-based interface with the chest wall & associated lateral effusion are clues to the diagnosis.* **(Right)** *Lateral radiograph in the same patient shows that the mass is actually loculated fluid within the major fissure.*

Pleuropulmonary Blastoma

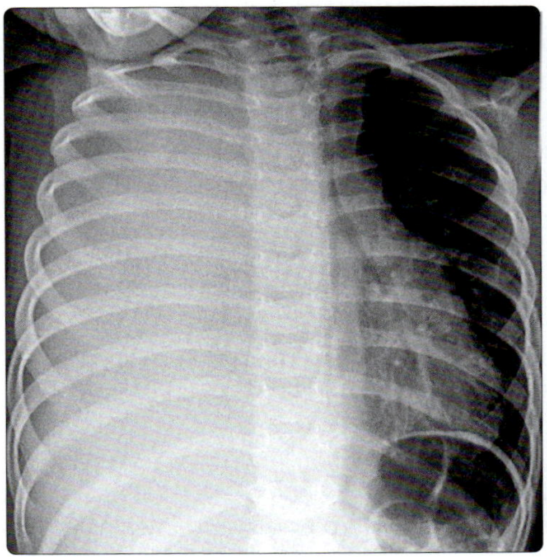

Pleuropulmonary Blastoma

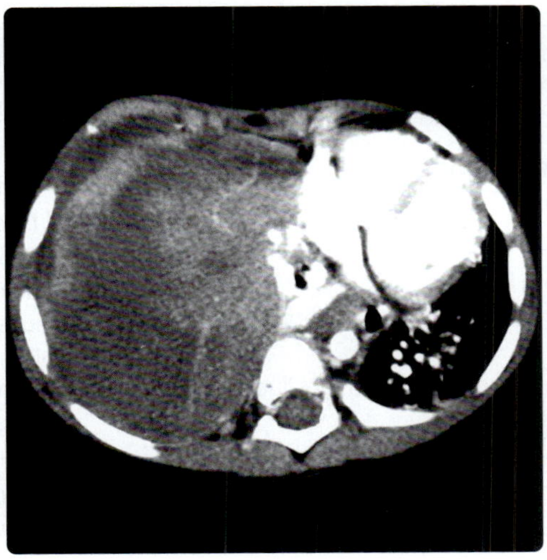

(Left) *PA radiograph in a 3 year old with a 2-day history of fever shows complete opacification of the right hemithorax with mediastinal shift.* **(Right)** *Axial CECT in the same patient shows a large, solid, heterogeneously enhancing mass filling the right hemithorax. This appearance is typical for a type 3 pleuropulmonary blastoma. Subsequent genetic testing revealed the DICER1 tumor predisposition syndrome.*

DIFFERENTIAL DIAGNOSIS

Common

- Fungal Infection
- Mycoplasma Infection

Less Common

- Tuberculosis
- Viral Infection
- Septic Emboli
- Aspiration
- Metastatic Disease
- Lymphoproliferative Disease
  - Posttransplant Lymphoproliferative Disorder
  - Primary Pulmonary Lymphoma
- Pulmonary Langerhans Cell Histiocytosis
- Granulomatosis With Polyangiitis

Rare but Important

- Sarcoidosis
- Hypersensitivity Pneumonitis

ESSENTIAL INFORMATION

Key Differential Diagnosis Issues

- Distribution
  - Centrilobular (bronchovascular spread with subpleural sparing): Infection, aspiration, vasculitis, hypersensitivity pneumonitis (HP)
    - Tree in bud: Infection (mycobacteria, bronchopneumonia, fungal), aspiration, mucus plugging (e.g., cystic fibrosis)
  - Random (hematogenous spread, extending to pleura): Metastases, miliary infection [tuberculosis (TB), fungal], Langerhans cell histiocytosis (LCH)
  - Perilymphatic: Sarcoidosis, lymphangitic spread of tumor
- Cavitary nodules: Septic emboli, *Aspergillus*, granulomatosis with polyangiitis (GPA), papillomatosis
- Patient demographic/clinical considerations
  - High-risk TB population
  - Regional endemic fungal infections
  - Immunocompromised patient
- Many primary neoplasms metastasize to lung; primary tumor is typically known when lung metastases are detected in children

Helpful Clues for Common Diagnoses

- **Fungal Infection**
  - Histoplasmosis
    - Common in midwestern USA
    - Variable appearance: Multiple nodules or ill-defined airspace opacities
    - Mediastinal/hilar lymphadenopathy with gradual Ca^{2+}
    - Pulmonary nodules often calcify
  - *Candida*
    - Typically in multiple underlying medical conditions
    - Variable pattern: Nodules, segmental consolidation, ± cavitation
    - Look for other systemic disease: Spleen, liver, bloodstream, sinuses
  - *Aspergillosis*
    - Chronic pulmonary aspergillosis (semiinvasive)
      - □ Typically in patients with mild immunosuppression
      - □ Bronchopulmonary consolidation, nodules ± cavitation
    - Invasive aspergillosis
      - □ Typically in severely immunocompromised
      - □ Patchy consolidation & nodules
      - □ Halo sign (early): Ground-glass attenuation (of hemorrhage) surrounding nodule or consolidation; highly suggestive in proper setting
      - □ Air crescent sign (late): Crescent of air in nodule or consolidation; indicates neutrophil recovery after initiation of treatment (good prognostic sign)
  - Coccidioidomycosis
    - Highly variable appearance: Nodules, infiltrates, or thin-walled cavities
    - Pleural effusions & adenopathy are possible
- **Mycoplasma Infection**
  - Wide spectrum of radiologic & clinical presentations
    - Typically in older school-aged children
    - Bronchopneumonia, lobar consolidation, reticulonodular opacities
    - Multifocal bronchovascular thickening with centrilobular nodules

Helpful Clues for Less Common Diagnoses

- **Tuberculosis**
  - Primary disease (more common in children)
    - Perihilar & paratracheal lymphadenopathy
      - □ Radiographic hallmark of disease; seen in 90% of children (but only 10-40% of adults)
      - □ Can compress airway → air-trapping or atelectasis
    - Consolidation without lobar predilection
    - Ca^{2+} (6 months to 4 years after infection)
  - Progressive primary disease (primary without healing)
    - Cavitation, miliary disease, extrapulmonary spread
  - Postprimary disease (reinfection or reactivation)
    - Consolidation typically of apical posterior segments of upper lobes & superior segments of lower lobes
    - Cavitation is common
    - Lymphadenopathy is uncommon
  - Cavitary TB: High bacterial load, highly contagious
  - Miliary infection (hematogenous spread)
    - Innumerable tiny nodules in random distribution
    - More common in children & immunocompromised
  - Pleural effusion/empyema
    - Can be seen in primary or postprimary disease
- **Viral Infection**
  - Variable pattern of consolidation, ground-glass opacities, nodules, bronchial wall thickening, hyperinflation, & pleural effusions
  - Childhood viruses that more commonly have nodules
    - CMV: Immunosuppressed; patchy & nodular ground-glass opacities
    - Human parainfluenza virus (HPIV), respiratory syncytial virus (RSV), human metapneumovirus (HMPV), & influenza: All can have bronchial wall thickening with bronchovascular/multifocal opacities & centrilobular nodules
    - Human papillomavirus (HPV): Endobronchial spread of laryngeal papillomatosis with bilateral, lower lobe-predominant, varying-sized nodules that may cavitate

- **Septic Emboli**
  - Common organisms: *Staphylococcus*, *Streptococcus*
  - Search for underlying source: Soft tissue infection, osteomyelitis, central line infection, endocarditis
  - Multiple nodules ± cavitation
    - Cavities with thick & thin walls representing various stages of evolution
    - Typically peripheral & basilar predominant
    - Despite well-known feeding vessel sign, arteries typically course closely around septic emboli, while veins lie directly in center of nodules
- **Aspiration**
  - Often in children with complex chronic conditions
  - Central lower & dependent lung-predominant consolidation & atelectasis
  - Centrilobular nodules & tree-in-bud opacities
- **Metastatic Disease**
  - Wilms tumor: In addition to lung nodules, may see extension into renal vein, inferior vena cava (IVC), right atrium
  - Ewing sarcoma
  - Rhabdomyosarcoma
  - Osteosarcoma: Nodules may be ossified & can lead to pneumothorax or hemothorax
- **Lymphoproliferative Disease**
  - **Posttransplant lymphoproliferative disorder**
    - Spectrum ranging from lymphoid hyperplasia to poorly differentiated lymphoma
    - Thoracic posttransplant lymphoproliferative disorder (PTLD) is most common after lung transplant
    - Lung mass, nodules, effusions, or adenopathy
  - **Primary pulmonary lymphoma**
    - Rare
    - Lung nodules in Hodgkin > non-Hodgkin types
    - Variable pattern of round nodules or ill-defined opacities, typically with mediastinal/hilar adenopathy
- **Pulmonary Langerhans Cell Histiocytosis**
  - Often occurs in setting of systemic LCH in children (unlike isolated pulmonary disease in adult smokers)
  - Imaging: Lung involvement is diffuse; costophrenic angles are spared in adults, not in children
    - Centrilobular pulmonary nodules (granulomas) progress to irregular cysts
      - Airspace invasion → cavitation & formation of thick-walled cysts → thin-walled cysts → confluent destructive parenchymal cystic change
    - Presents with spontaneous pneumothorax in 10-20%
- **Granulomatosis With Polyangiitis**
  - a.k.a. Wegener granulomatosis
  - Necrotizing small & medium-sized vessel vasculitis with granulomatous inflammation
  - Classic triad of involvement
    - Upper respiratory tract (most common in children): Recurrent epistaxis, sinusitis, otitis media
    - Lower respiratory tract: Lung nodules with cavitation, pulmonary hemorrhage, airway strictures (subglottic stenosis in 10-20% of children)
    - Renal glomerulonephritis (hematuria)
  - Lung nodules with cavitation in ~ 50%
    - Multiple basilar-predominant, 0.5- to 10.0-cm thick-walled nodules with irregular inner margin & perinodular ground-glass opacity (alveolar hemorrhage)

Helpful Clues for Rare Diagnoses

- **Sarcoidosis**
  - Bilateral perilymphatic nodules & mass-like opacities
    - Upper lobe & perihilar predominance
  - Hilar & paratracheal adenopathy
- **Hypersensitivity Pneumonitis**
  - History of specific dust exposures is key
  - Centrilobular ground-glass opacities
  - Diffuse ground-glass opacification in acute phase

SELECTED REFERENCES

1. Koo HJ et al: Radiographic and CT features of viral pneumonia. Radiographics. 38(3):719-39, 2018

Fungal Infection

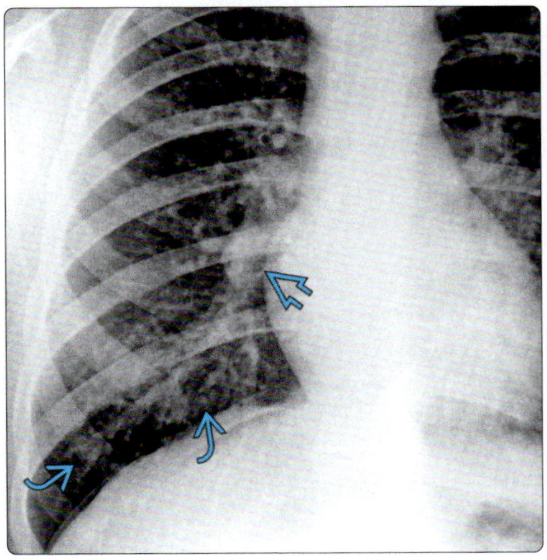

Fungal Infection

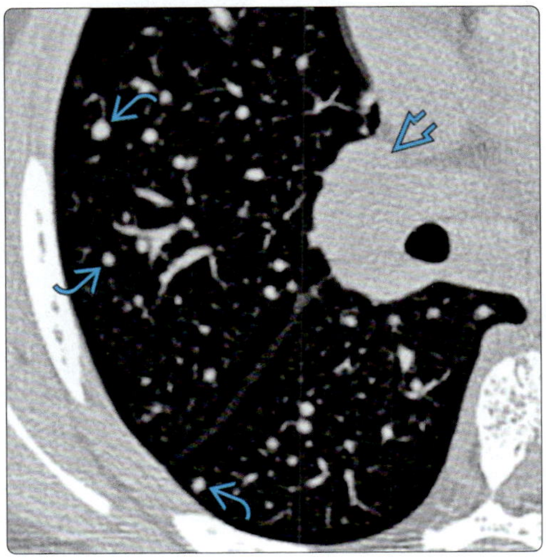

(Left) *AP radiograph in a 15 year old with biopsy-proven histoplasmosis shows numerous small, indistinct, nodular opacities* ➔ *& right hilar adenopathy* ➔. **(Right)** *Axial CECT in the same patient shows a typical appearance of a fungal infection with multiple small pulmonary nodules* ➔ *at the lung base. Right hilar adenopathy* ➔ *is redemonstrated. Histoplasmosis is the most common mycosis in North America, endemic in the Mississippi, Ohio, & St. Lawrence river valleys.*

Fungal Infection

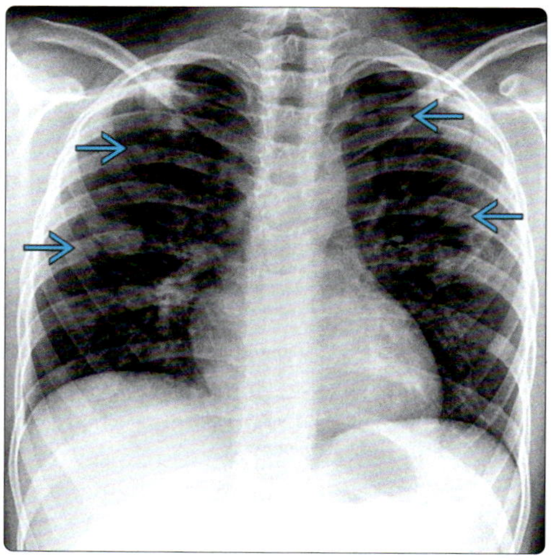

Fungal Infection

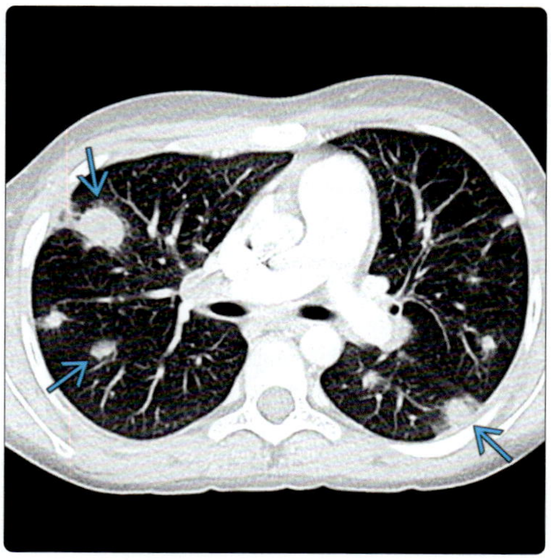

(Left) *PA radiograph in a 13 year old with chronic granulomatous disease shows numerous pulmonary nodules* →. **(Right)** *Axial CECT in the same patient shows multiple nodules with ground-glass halos* →*, consistent with invasive aspergillosis. Chronic granulomatous disease is a congenital immunodeficiency classically associated with aspergillosis, although aspergillosis is more frequently seen in children with acquired impairments of immune function (as from chemotherapy or conditioning for stem cell transplant).*

Mycoplasma Infection

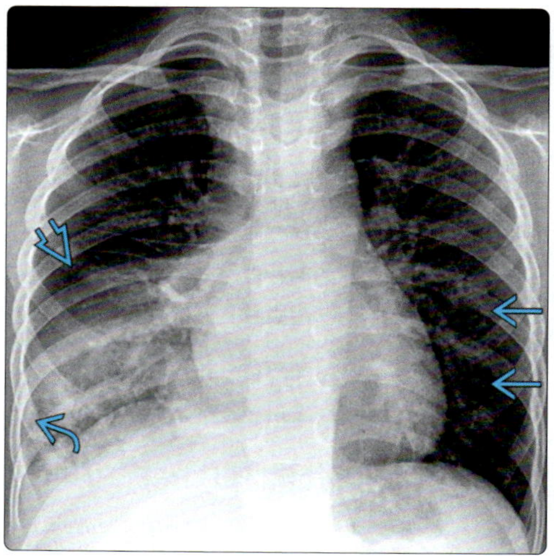

Mycoplasma Infection

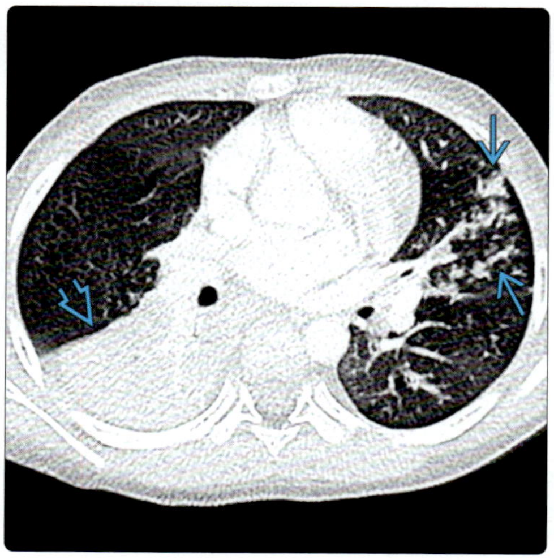

(Left) *PA radiograph in a 4 year old with pneumonia that was not improving despite antibiotics shows right lower lung hazy consolidation* ⇒ *& a pleural effusion* ↷*. There are also left lower lung reticulonodular opacities* →*, which raise the possibility of Mycoplasma.* **(Right)** *Axial CECT in the same patient shows the right lower lobe consolidation* ⇒ *along with lingular bronchovascular opacities & centrilobular nodules* →*. Mycoplasma was ultimately confirmed.*

Tuberculosis

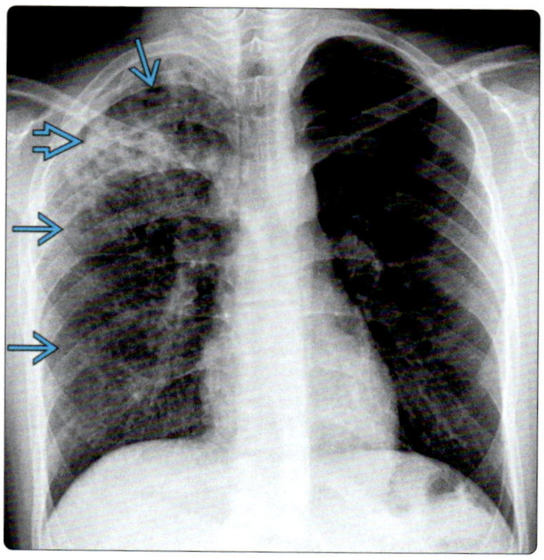

Tuberculosis

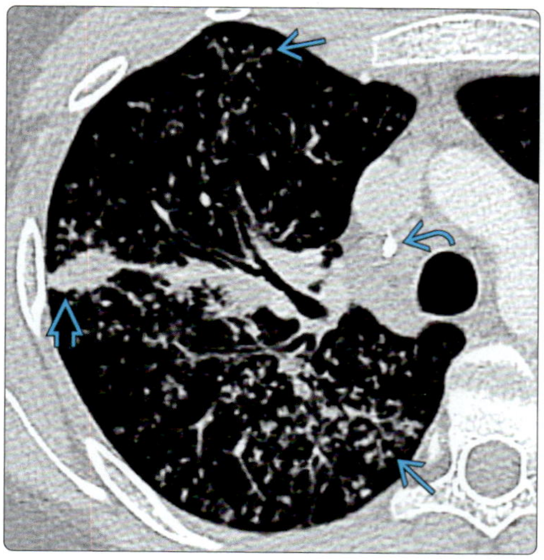

(Left) *PA radiograph in a 14 year old from a country where tuberculosis (TB) is endemic shows cavitary right upper lobe consolidation* ⇒ *along with reticulonodular opacities throughout the right lung* →*, consistent with pulmonary TB.* **(Right)** *Axial CECT in the same patient shows irregular consolidation* ⇒ *along with extensive tree-in-bud opacities* →*, which were creating the reticulonodular appearance on radiographs. Also note the dystrophic calcified hilar adenopathy* ↷*. TB should be considered when tree-in-bud opacities are seen.*

Viral Infection

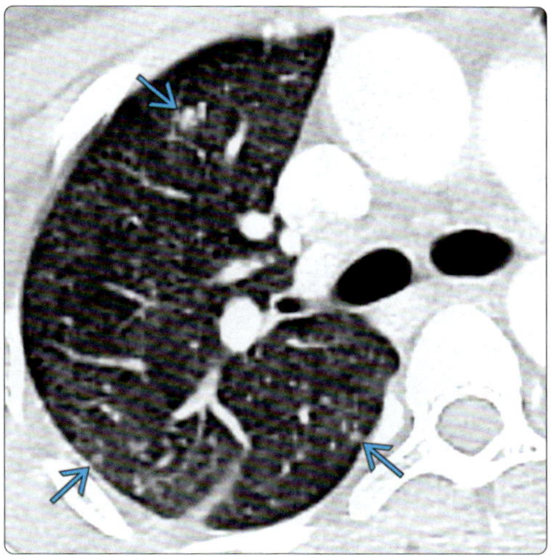

Viral Infection

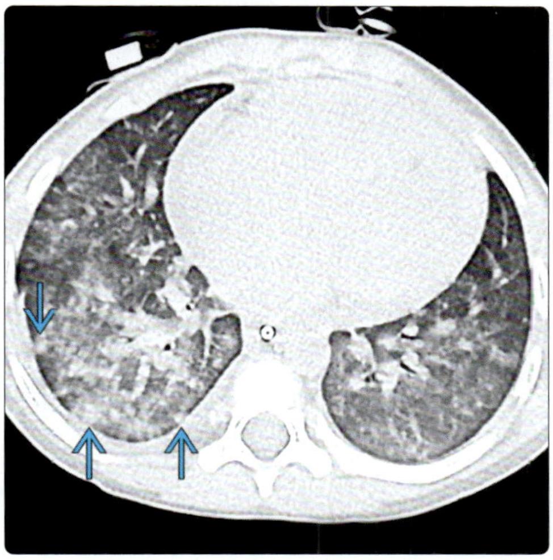

(Left) *Axial CECT in a 14 year old with macrophage activation syndrome & disseminated CMV shows mild, patchy ground-glass opacities throughout the lungs along with ill-defined ground-glass nodules.* **(Right)** *Axial CECT in a 3 year old status post bone marrow transplant shows patchy & nodular ground-glass opacities. Adenovirus was found in the blood. Viral pneumonias often show a variable pattern of consolidation, ground-glass opacities, interstitial thickening, & nodules.*

Septic Emboli

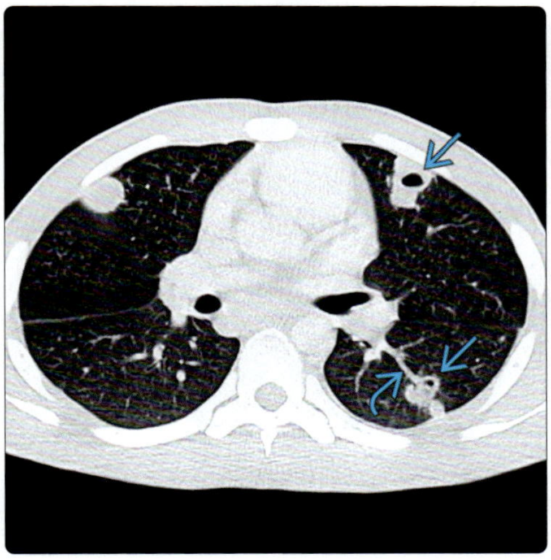

Aspiration

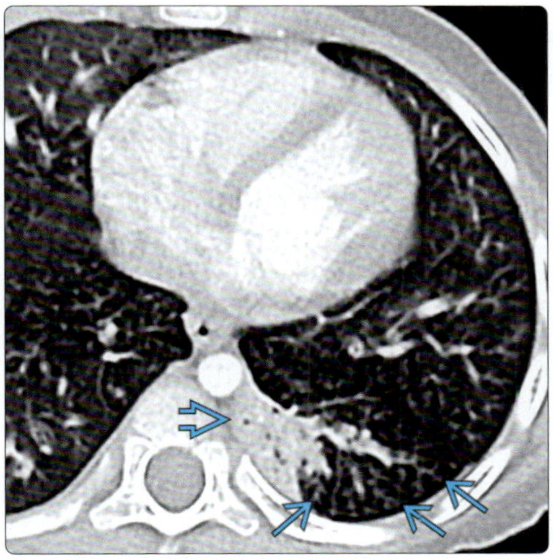

(Left) *Axial CECT in a 17 year old with Lemierre syndrome shows multiple pulmonary nodules, some with cavitation, consistent with septic emboli. Despite the feeding vessel sign, pulmonary arteries typically course closely around septic emboli, while vessels associated with the center of septic emboli are pulmonary veins.* **(Right)** *Axial CECT in a 2 year old with central hypotonia & gastroesophageal reflux shows left lower lobe tree-in-bud opacities & segmental atelectasis from chronic microaspiration.*

Metastatic Disease

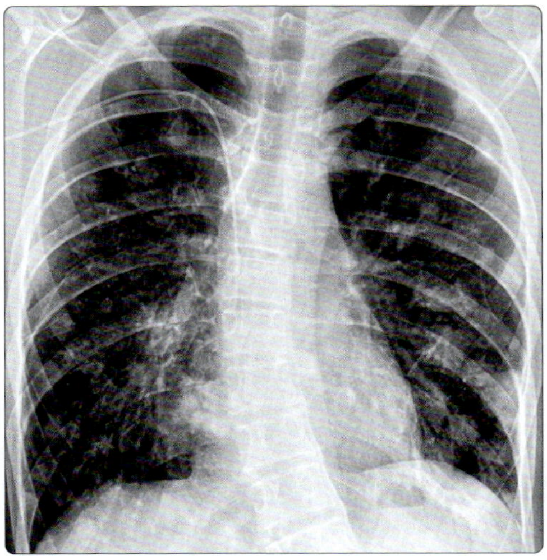

Metastatic Disease

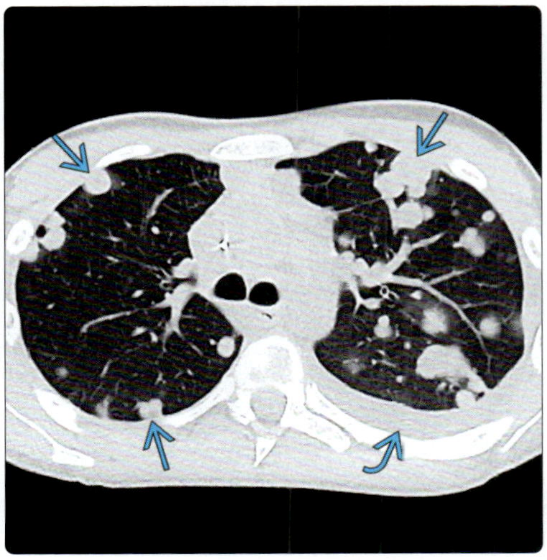

(Left) *PA radiograph in a 16 year old with osteosarcoma shows multiple nodular pulmonary metastases.* **(Right)** *Axial CECT in the same patient shows randomly distributed pulmonary nodules & a small left pleural effusion, consistent with metastatic disease. Approximately 20% of osteosarcoma patients have metastases at diagnosis, with pulmonary metastases comprising 80-90% of these. Metastasectomy is the treatment of choice if complete surgical resection of all metastatic lesions is feasible (not this case).*

(Left) *PA radiograph in a 13 year old with papillary thyroid carcinoma shows innumerable small pulmonary nodules, consistent with miliary metastases.* **(Right)** *Axial CECT in the same patient shows innumerable randomly distributed pulmonary nodules, consistent with hematogenous miliary metastases. The most common primary tumors to metastasize to the lungs in children are rhabdomyosarcoma, osteosarcoma, Wilms tumor, Ewing sarcoma, neuroblastoma, & hepatoblastoma.*

Metastatic Disease

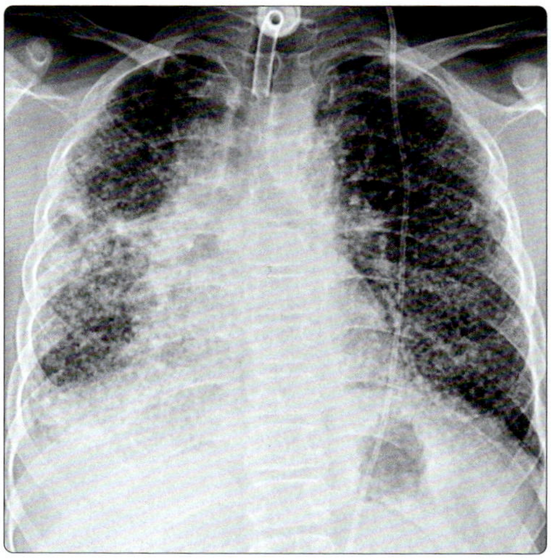

Metastatic Disease

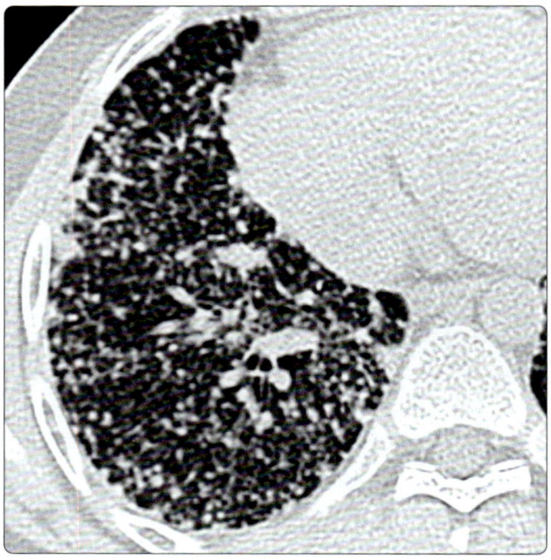

(Left) *PA radiograph in an 8 year old status post lung transplant shows bilateral, ill-defined nodular opacities →.* **(Right)** *Axial CECT in the same patient shows right lower lobe nodules → with regional ill-defined ground-glass opacities & a small pleural effusion ↪, consistent with posttransplant lymphoproliferative disorder (PTLD). The majority of PTLD is related to Ebstein-Barr virus infection, & the abdomen is the most common site of occurrence. Thoracic PTLD is most common after lung transplant.*

Posttransplant Lymphoproliferative Disorder

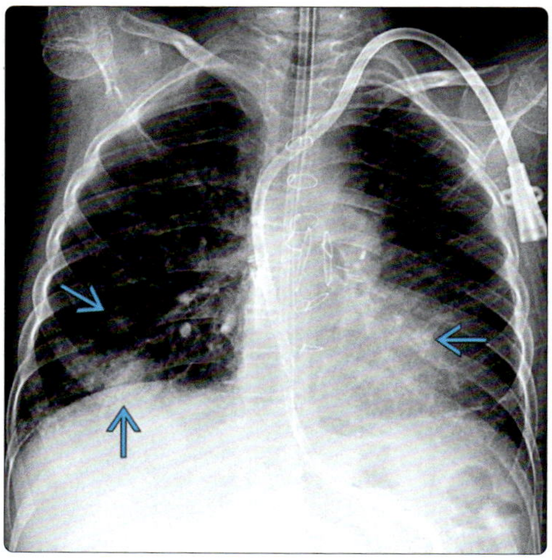

Posttransplant Lymphoproliferative Disorder

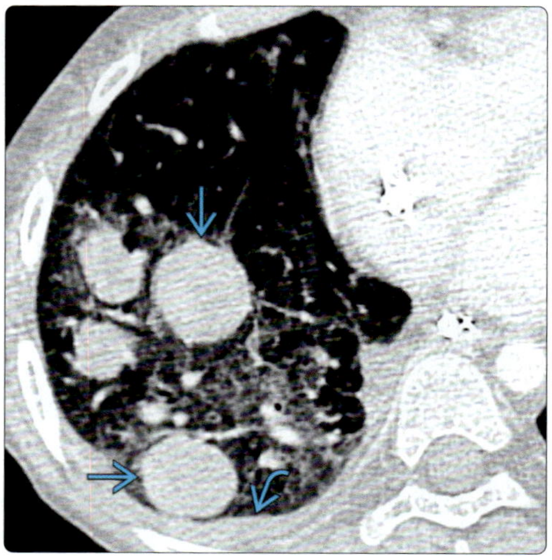

(Left) *Axial CECT shows numerous confluent bronchovascular nodules →, some with air bronchograms. Biopsy revealed lymphoma.* **(Right)** *Axial CECT in a 23 month old with respiratory distress shows numerous irregular lung cysts ⇨. There are also cavitary nodules →. A biopsy of a cutaneous lesion confirmed the diagnosis of Langerhans cell histiocytosis (LCH). Pulmonary LCH is seen in ~ 25% of children at the presentation of multisystem LCH. Isolated PLCH represents < 10% of single-system LCH in children.*

Primary Pulmonary Lymphoma

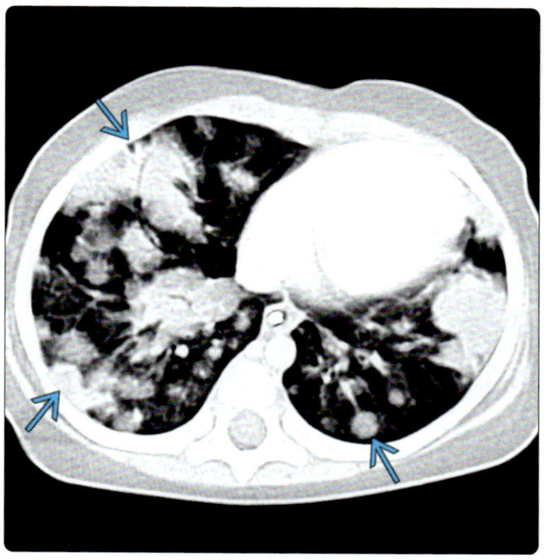

Pulmonary Langerhans Cell Histiocytosis

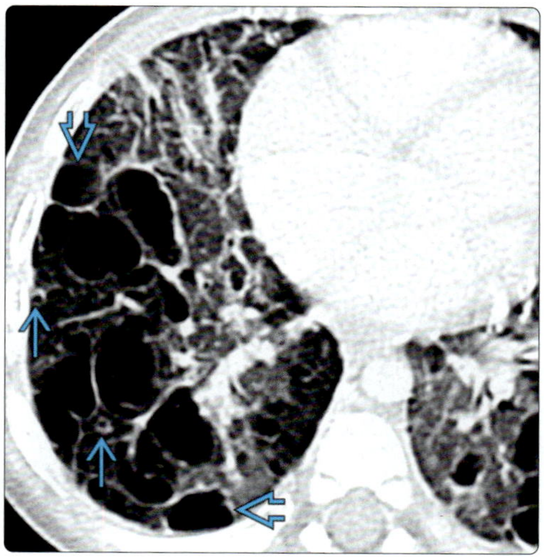

Granulomatosis With Polyangiitis

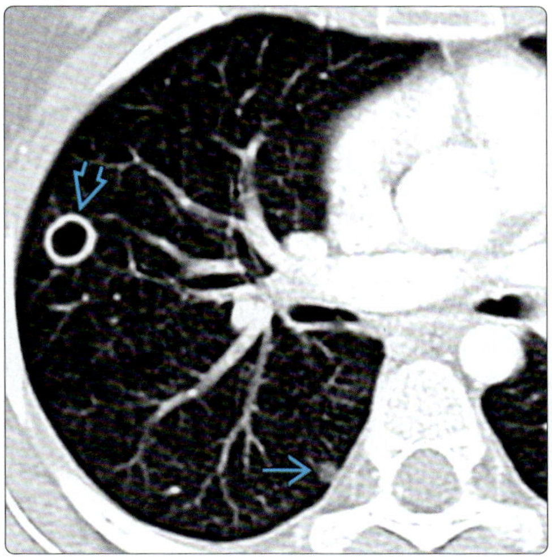

Granulomatosis With Polyangiitis

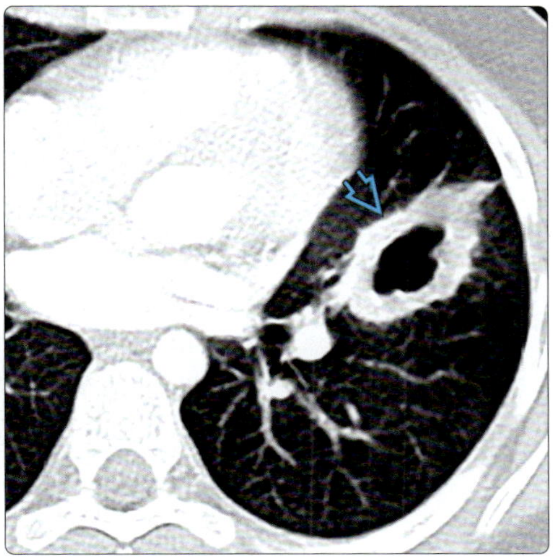

(Left) *Axial CECT in a 10 year old with known granulomatosis with polyangiitis (GPA) shows multiple lung nodules →, including one with cavitation ⇨.* **(Right)** *Axial CECT in the same patient shows another cavitary lung nodule ⇨. Note that this cavitary nodule has a thick wall with an irregular inner margin. Other potential features of nodules in GPA include ground-glass halos (from hemorrhage) or air-fluid levels (if secondarily infected). Pulmonary hemorrhage may be the initial manifestation of lower respiratory involvement.*

Sarcoidosis

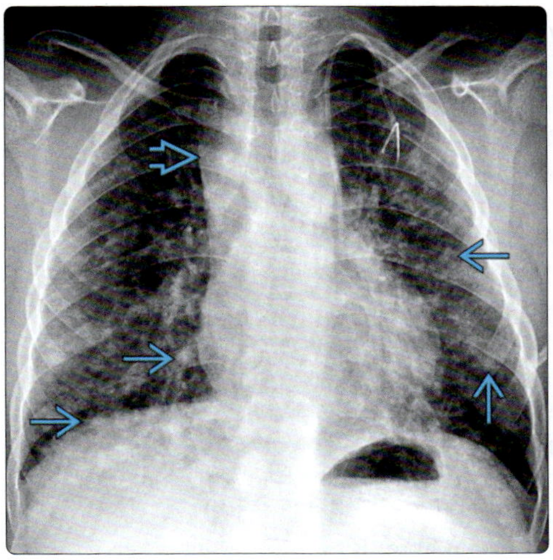

Sarcoidosis

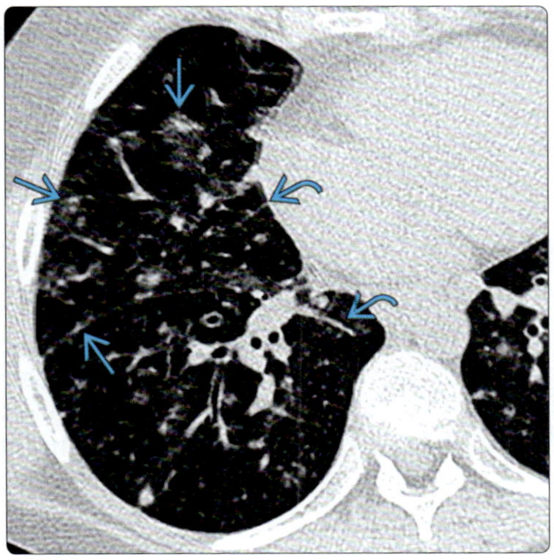

(Left) *PA radiograph in a 14 year old with chronic cough shows multiple small, ill-defined nodules → on a background of alveolar ground-glass & interstitial reticular opacities. The right paratracheal thickening ⇨ is suspicious for lymphadenopathy.* **(Right)** *Axial NECT in the same patient shows multiple perilymphatic nodules → with associated ground-glass opacities & interstitial thickening ↪ (more so on other slices).*

Sarcoidosis

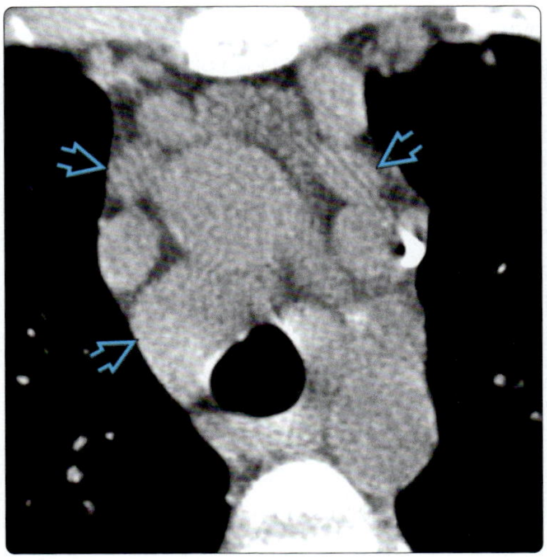

Hypersensitivity Pneumonitis

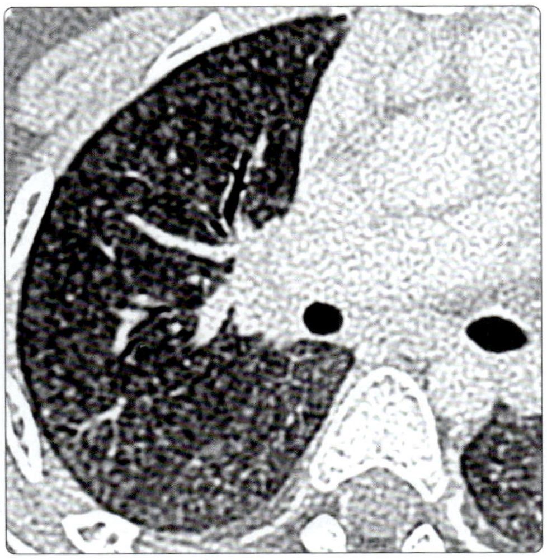

(Left) *Axial NECT in the same patient shows paratracheal & prevascular lymphadenopathy ⇨. Biopsy revealed sarcoidosis. Hilar & paratracheal adenopathy is the most common thoracic finding in pediatric sarcoidosis, whereas lung involvement is uncommon.* **(Right)** *Axial CECT in a 7 year old with shortness of breath & a pet bird in the house reveals multiple small, centrilobular ground-glass nodules, consistent with hypersensitivity pneumonitis. Symptoms improved after prednisone & removal of the pet bird.*

DIFFERENTIAL DIAGNOSIS

Common

- Infectious Pneumonia
- Aspiration Pneumonia
- Pulmonary Edema
- Atelectasis
- Pleural Effusion

Less Common

- Pulmonary Contusion
- Pulmonary Hemorrhage
- Pulmonary Infarct
- Lymphoma
- Near Drowning
- Congenital Lung Malformation

Rare but Important

- Hydrocarbon Aspiration
- Hypersensitivity Pneumonitis
- Pulmonary Alveolar Proteinosis
- Cryptogenic Organizing Pneumonia
- Lymphoid Hyperplasia
- Radiation Pneumonitis
- Pleuropulmonary Blastoma
- Inflammatory Myofibroblastic Tumor
- Posttransplant Lymphoproliferative Disorder

ESSENTIAL INFORMATION

Key Differential Diagnosis Issues

- Opacity on radiographs is created by blood, pus, protein, water, &/or cells
- Age, presentation, & past history direct differential: Infectious, trauma, congenital, malignancy, etc.

Helpful Clues for Common Diagnoses

- **Infectious Pneumonia**
  - Lung consolidation ± air bronchograms
  - Typically poorly defined or "fluffy"; may be round in patients < 8 years of age
  - Not associated with volume loss
  - Mass effect should suggest parapneumonic effusion (or, less likely, underlying mass)
- **Aspiration Pneumonia**
  - Consider in patients with seizure, history of emesis or gastroesophageal reflux, abnormal modified barium swallow studies, history of facial or neck surgery
  - Most common sites: Right lower lobe if patient is upright; posterior segments of upper lobes & superior segments of lower lobes if patient is supine
- **Pulmonary Edema**
  - Cardiogenic or noncardiogenic (neurogenic, renal or hepatic disorders, toxins, etc.) disorders result in
    - Increased hydrostatic gradient
    - Low oncotic pressure
    - Increased capillary permeability
  - Interstitial edema → alveolar edema → consolidation
  - Batwing perihilar opacities, Kerley lines, pleural effusions
- **Atelectasis**
  - Airspace collapse resulting in volume loss with elevation of diaphragm, ipsilateral mediastinal shift, retraction of fissure toward collapse
  - Can be lobar, segmental, subsegmental, or plate-like
  - Commonly seen with viral respiratory infection, mucus plugging, aspirated foreign body, postoperative status

Helpful Clues for Less Common Diagnoses

- **Pulmonary Contusion**
  - Hemorrhage & edema in alveoli & interstitium due to traumatic alveolar capillary damage
    - Nonsegmental peripheral consolidative or ground-glass opacity with subpleural sparing
  - May not be evident in first 4-6 hours
  - Resolves in 7-10 days
  - Look for other signs of trauma: Pneumothorax, fractures, etc.
- **Pulmonary Hemorrhage**
  - Common causes in children: Infection, cystic fibrosis, Goodpasture syndrome, Wegener granulomatosis, trauma, iatrogenic
  - May present with hemoptysis, anemia
- **Pulmonary Infarct**
  - Peripheral, wedge-shaped consolidation with decreased or absent enhancement
  - Pulmonary embolus is most common cause
    - Radiographic clues of pulmonary embolus
      - Hampton hump: Pleural-based, peripheral, wedge-shaped consolidation
      - Westermark sign: Oligemia
      - Fleischner sign: Prominent central pulmonary artery
  - Other etiologies could include vasculitis, iatrogenic embolization of nontarget tissue during treatment of pulmonary arteriovenous malformation (AVM)
- **Lymphoma**
  - Consider with chronic consolidation or multifocal opacities unresponsive to antibiotics
  - Non-Hodgkin lymphoma is most frequent
  - Look for associated lymphadenopathy, splenomegaly, constitutional symptoms (fever, night sweats, weight loss)
- **Near Drowning**
  - Drowning is 2nd most common cause of accidental death in children
  - Hypoxemia occurs secondary to aspiration or laryngospasm
  - Pulmonary edema pattern may have delayed appearance
    - Edema typically resolves fairly rapidly
- **Congenital Lung Malformation**
  - Spectrum of cystic, solid, or mixed lesions
  - Develop as sequelae of in utero airway obstruction → tracheobronchial & pulmonary maldevelopment
  - Commonly identified on prenatal ultrasound
  - On postnatal radiographs
    - Congenital lobar overinflation may present as confluent opacity early due to retained fetal fluid
    - Pulmonary sequestration presents as persistent basilar opacity with systemic arterial supply
    - Congenital pulmonary airway malformation can present as cystic &/or solid lesion

Helpful Clues for Rare Diagnoses

- **Hydrocarbon Aspiration**
  - Gasoline, kerosene, lighter fluid
  - Severe chemical pneumonitis
  - Patchy consolidation develops over several hours
  - Pneumatocele(s) may develop
- **Hypersensitivity Pneumonitis**
  - a.k.a. extrinsic allergic alveolitis
  - Type 3 immune response to environmental antigen
    - Moldy hay, dust, pigeon droppings
  - Reticulonodular opacities on radiographs
  - Consolidation may occur during acute/subacute phase
  - CT may demonstrate ground-glass opacities, centrilobular nodules, & consolidation
- **Pulmonary Alveolar Proteinosis**
  - Various disorders resulting in abnormal accumulation of surfactant within alveoli
  - Perihilar consolidation
  - "Crazy paving" on CT
    - Ground-glass opacities & septal thickening
  - Diagnosis via bronchoalveolar lavage
- **Cryptogenic Organizing Pneumonia**
  - Granulation tissue in bronchioles & alveolar inflammation
  - Patchy alveolar consolidation, ground-glass opacification, centrilobular nodules
  - Diagnosis via tissue biopsy
- **Lymphoid Hyperplasia**
  - Nonneoplastic proliferation of polymorphic lymphoid cells & germinal centers
  - Nonspecific nodular or mass-like area of consolidation, focal > diffuse
  - Adenopathy
- **Radiation Pneumonitis**
  - Typically requires at least 4,500 rads
  - Acute: 1-8 weeks after radiation
    - Patchy consolidation confined to radiation port
  - Chronic: 9-12 months after radiation & beyond
    - Consolidation & fibrosis/scarring
    - Bronchiectasis
- **Pleuropulmonary Blastoma**
  - Most common primary lung malignancy in children; typically found < 6 years of age
  - Cystic, solid, or mixed lesion
    - Cystic lesions are more likely in infants
    - Solid lesions typically present later
  - Risk factors & findings predictive of pleuropulmonary blastoma (PFB) > congenital lung malformation (CLM): *DICER1* mutation, pneumothorax, more complex solid & cystic areas, not visualized on prenatal ultrasound performed at 30 weeks or less
- **Inflammatory Myofibroblastic Tumor**
  - May occur in lung or chest wall
  - May present with cough, fever, chest pain, hemoptysis
  - Lower lobe predominant peripheral, lobulated mass
  - Ca^{2+} in 15%
- **Posttransplant Lymphoproliferative Disorder**
  - Consider in transplant recipients with new lung masses &/or consolidation ± lymphadenopathy
  - Most common within 1 year of transplant
  - Related to EBV infection
  - Look for other sites of involvement: Lymphadenopathy, splenomegaly, low-density liver lesions

SELECTED REFERENCES

1. Lichtenberger JP 3rd et al: Primary lung tumors in children: radiologic-pathologic correlation from the radiologic pathology archives. Radiographics. 38(7):2151-72, 2018
2. Sirajuddin A et al: Primary pulmonary lymphoid lesions: radiologic and pathologic findings. Radiographics. 36(1):53-70, 2016

Infectious Pneumonia

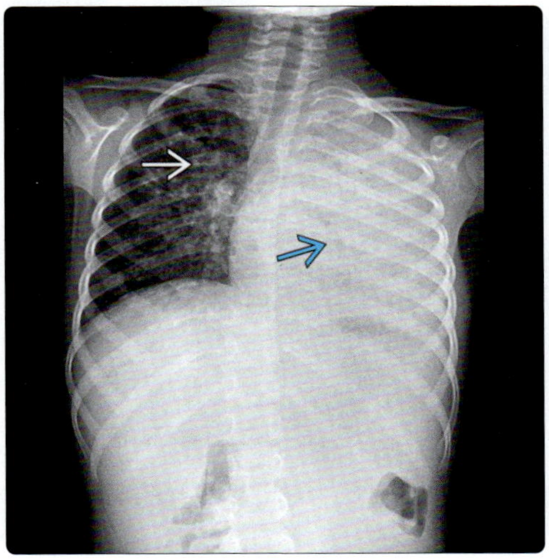

Infectious Pneumonia

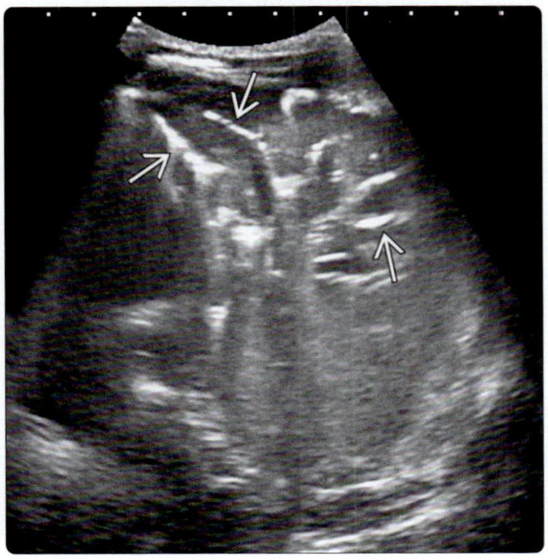

(Left) *PA radiograph shows near-complete opacification of the left hemithorax with air bronchograms ➡ in an 8 year old with infectious pneumonia. Patchy airspace & interstitial opacities are also seen in the right lung ➡.* **(Right)** *Transverse US of the left hemithorax in the same patient shows branching linear echogenicities ➡, consistent with sonographic air bronchograms in the consolidated left lung. A small to moderate simple pleural effusion was also identified (not shown).*

(**Left**) *Frontal radiograph shows right lower lobe opacities* ➡ *in an 8 year old with seizures & multiple episodes of aspiration pneumonia.* (**Right**) *Frontal radiograph from a 1 year old with pulmonary hypertension & edema shows an enlarged cardiac silhouette & diffuse pulmonary opacities with air bronchograms. Scattered Kerley B lines are noted peripherally* ➡*.*

Aspiration Pneumonia

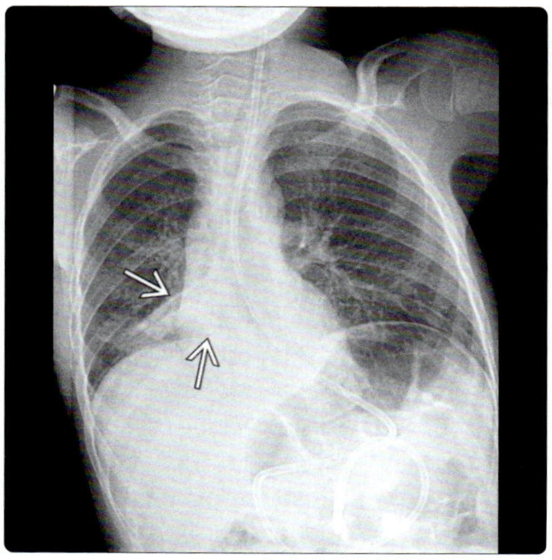

Pulmonary Edema

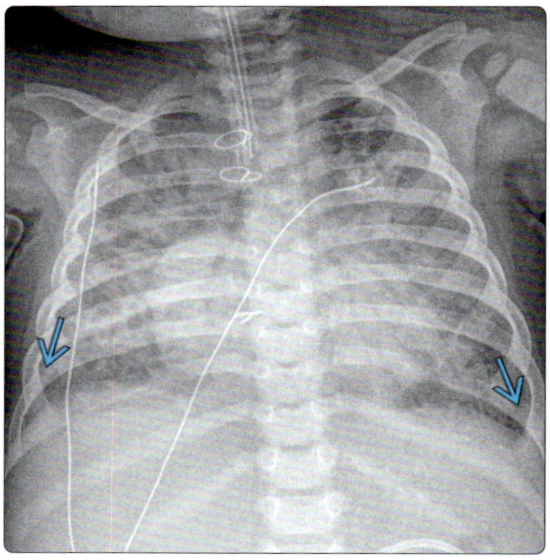

(**Left**) *Frontal radiograph shows extensive left lower lobe atelectasis* ➡ *with volume loss & leftward mediastinal shift* ➡ *in this 2 year old who aspirated a peanut.* (**Right**) *AP radiograph shows pleural & parenchymal opacities, consistent with a moderate to large right pleural effusion* ➡ *& adjacent air-space disease, in this 12 year old with shortness of breath.*

Atelectasis

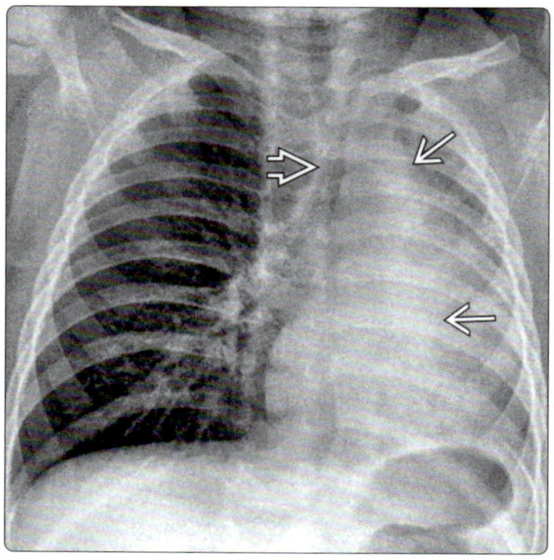

Pleural Effusion

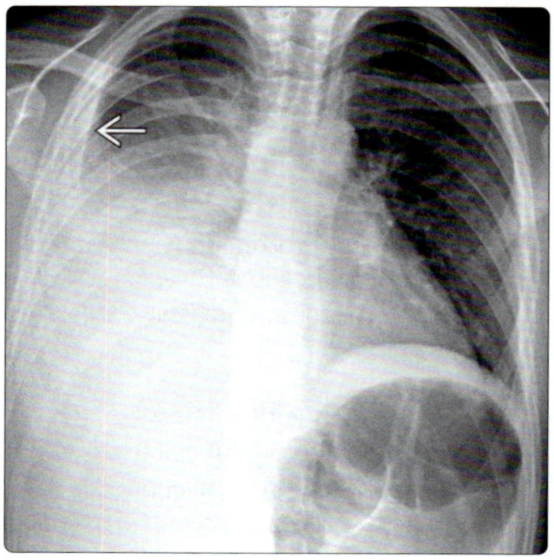

(**Left**) *Sagittal US from the same patient demonstrates a moderate to large pleural effusion* ➡ *without septations or other complexity.* (**Right**) *Axial CECT in a trauma patient shows confluent density in the left lower lobe* ➡*. Note the thin crescentic lucency adjacent to the chest wall* ➡*. This finding of subpleural sparing is frequently seen in pulmonary contusions.*

Pleural Effusion

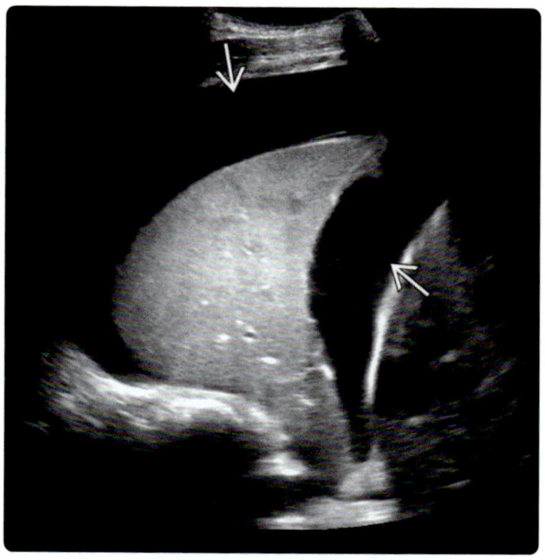

Pulmonary Contusion

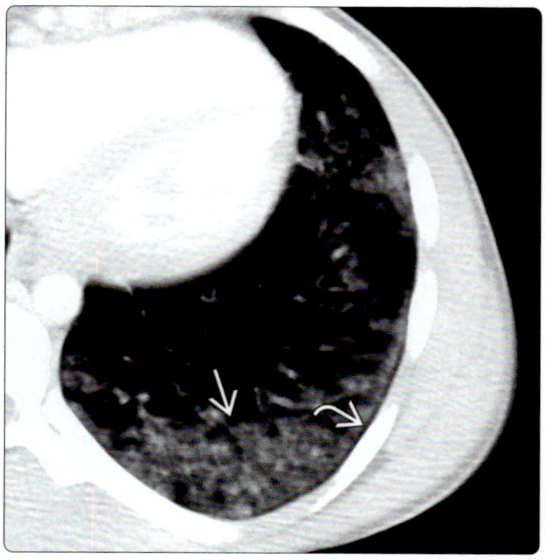

Pulmonary Hemorrhage

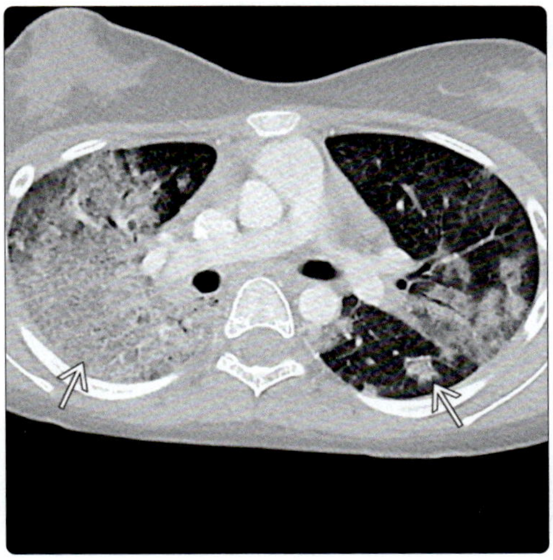

Pulmonary Infarct

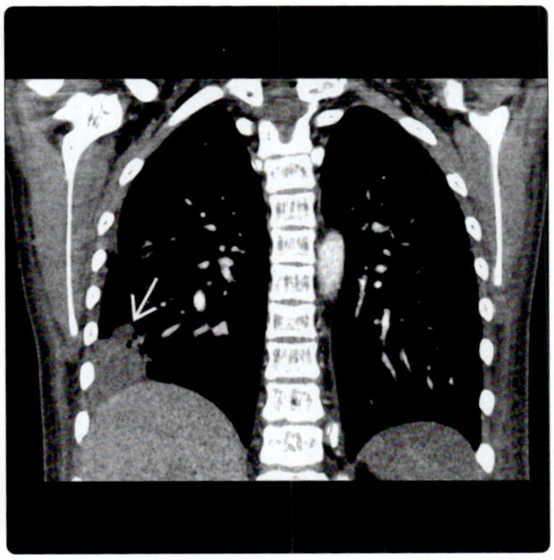

(Left) *Axial CECT from a 9 year old with pulmonary capillaritis demonstrates diffuse ground-glass opacity in the right lung & similar patchy foci in the left lung, consistent with hemorrhage* ➡*. Interlobular septal thickening is also noted in these regions, particularly on the right.* **(Right)** *Coronal CECT shows a wedge-shaped nonenhancing density, consistent with a pulmonary infarct* ➡*, in a 12 year old with a right lower lobe pulmonary embolus (not shown).*

Lymphoma

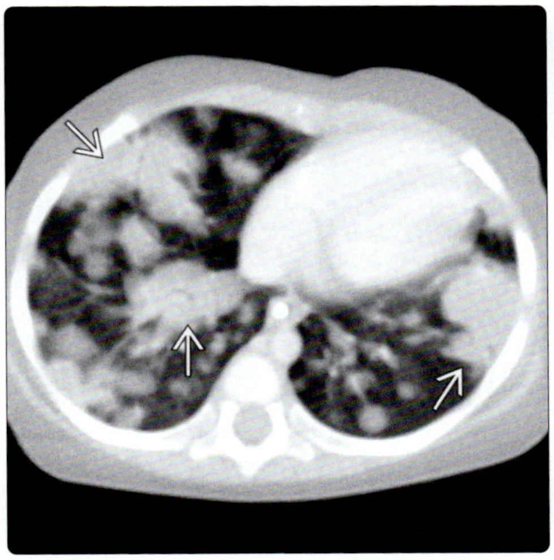

Near Drowning

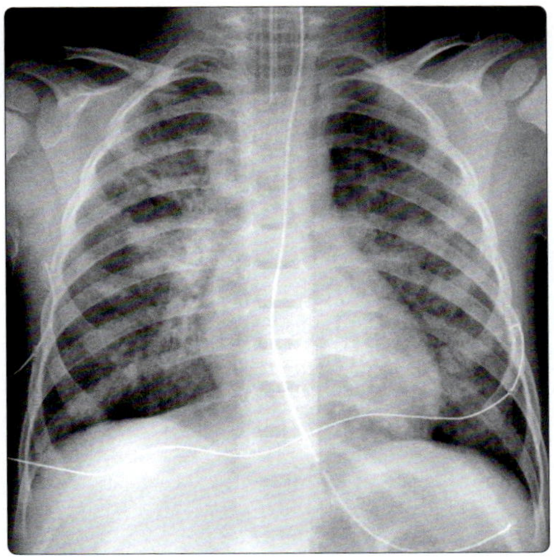

(Left) *Axial CECT from a 1 year old demonstrates irregular foci of consolidation* ➡ *amidst multiple round nodules, due to pulmonary lymphoma. Multiple chronic masses or regions of consolidation that are nonresponsive to antibiotics should raise suspicion for lymphoma.* **(Right)** *Frontal radiograph shows nonspecific bilateral fluffy airspace opacification in this intubated 2-year-old patient 1 day after a near-drowning event. There is no cardiomegaly, & there are no pleural effusions.*

Congenital Lung Malformation

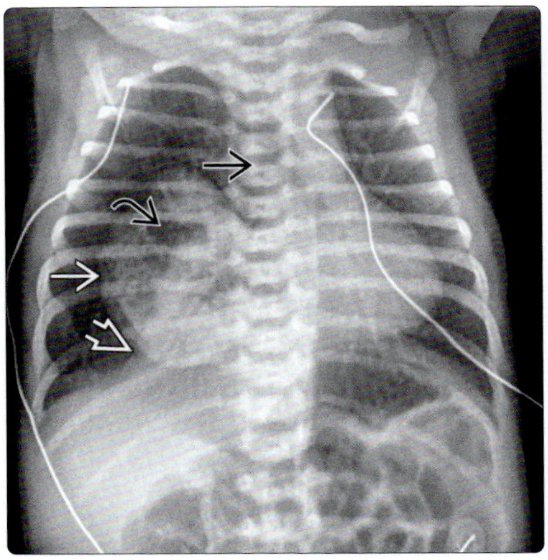

Congenital Lung Malformation

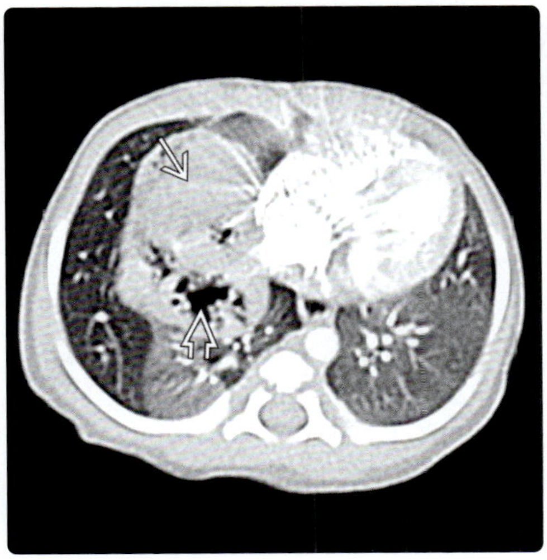

(Left) *AP radiograph shows a large, round opacity* ➡ *with associated right lower lobe collapse* ➡ *& mediastinal shift* ⇨ *in this 6 day old with a prenatally diagnosed lesion. Cystic foci* ↷ *are identified within the lesion, suggesting a CPAM.* **(Right)** *Axial CECT from the same patient confirms the presence of a solid* ➡ *& gas-filled cystic* ➡ *mass, consistent with a CPAM.*

(Left) *Frontal radiograph obtained on a 1 year old with a history of lamp oil aspiration shows patchy & confluent areas of consolidation in the bilateral lung bases.* **(Right)** *Axial NECT shows bilateral lower lobe septal thickening, ground-glass opacities, centrilobular nodules, & a small focus of consolidation ➔. Bronchoalveolar lavage confirmed hypersensitivity pneumonitis in this 8-year-old patient.*

Hydrocarbon Aspiration

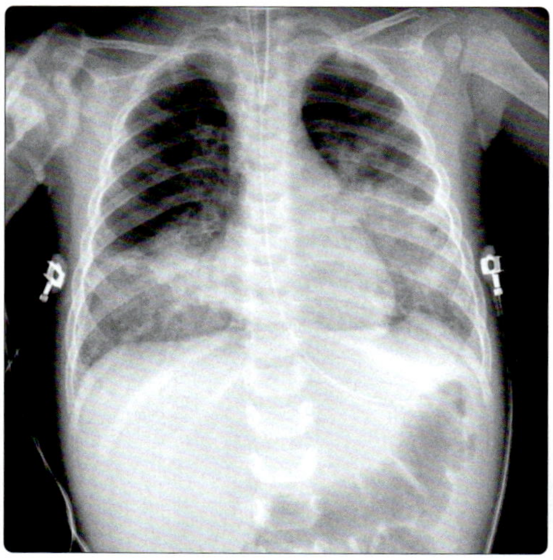

Hypersensitivity Pneumonitis

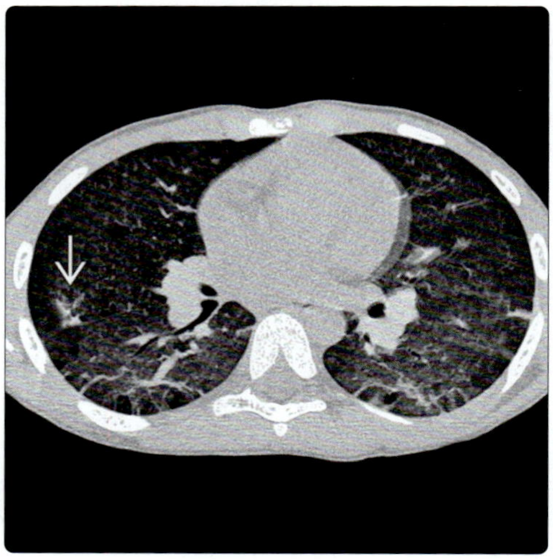

(Left) *Axial CECT shows a dependent gradient of increasingly dense ground-glass opacities throughout both lungs in a 15 month old with worsening respiratory status & confirmed pulmonary alveolar proteinosis.* **(Right)** *Axial NECT shows relatively symmetric confluent peribronchovascular nodular consolidation with scattered air bronchograms ⇨. Biopsy showed findings of cryptogenic organizing pneumonia in this 7 year old.*

Pulmonary Alveolar Proteinosis

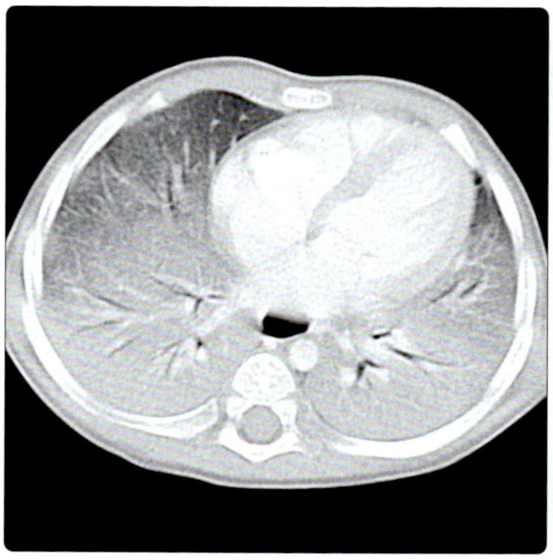

Cryptogenic Organizing Pneumonia

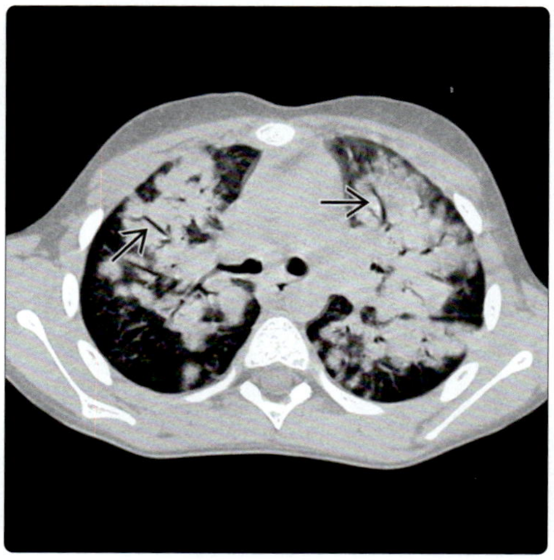

(Left) *Frontal radiograph shows relatively symmetric bibasilar areas of nodular consolidation in this patient with lymphoid hyperplasia. There is also mediastinal widening ➔, consistent with adenopathy.* **(Right)** *Coronal CECT shows well-demarcated consolidation in the right upper lung with volume loss, bronchiectasis ⇨, & chest wall deformity in this 19 year old status post radiation therapy for an upper right chest wall Ewing sarcoma.*

Lymphoid Hyperplasia

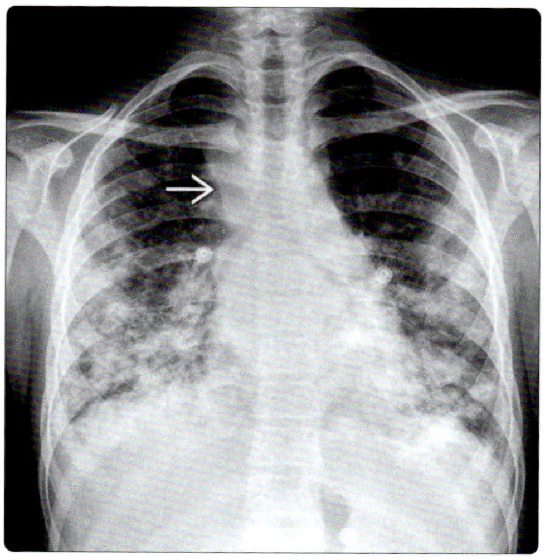

Radiation Pneumonitis

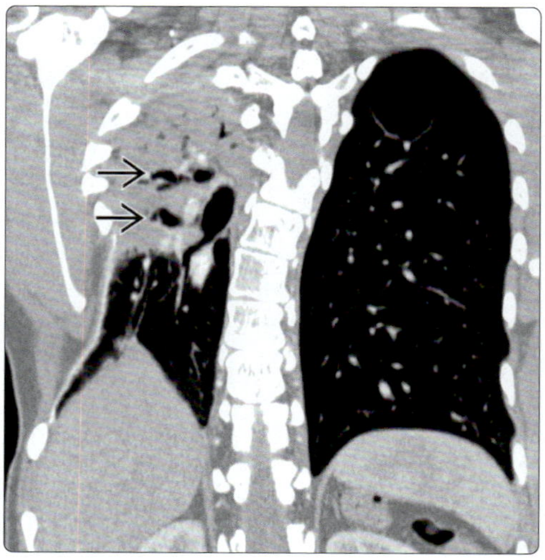

Pleuropulmonary Blastoma

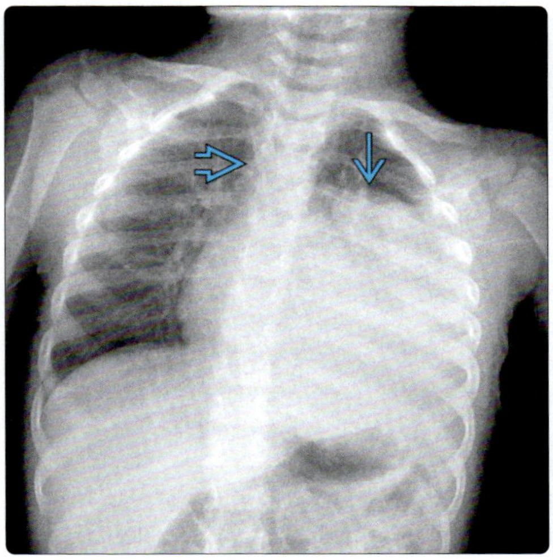

Pleuropulmonary Blastoma

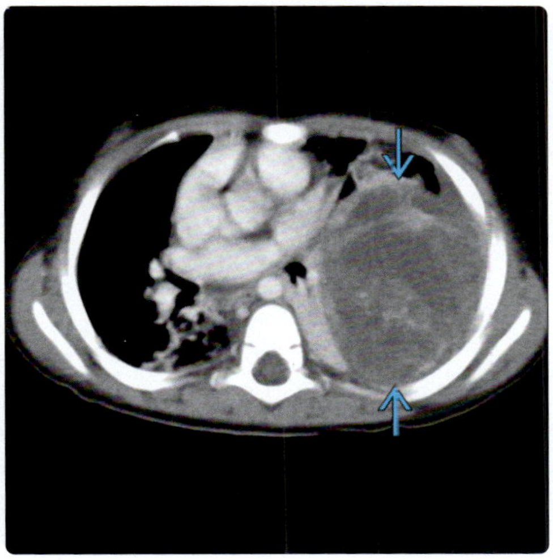

(Left) *Frontal radiograph in a 3 year old with fever shows opacification of most of the left hemithorax. There is a rounded margin to the opacity superiorly* ⇨*, & a mild rightward mediastinal shift* ⇨ *is noted.* **(Right)** *Axial CECT from the same patient demonstrates a heterogeneous soft tissue mass* ⇨ *of the left hemithorax, proven to be a pleuropulmonary blastoma in this 3 year old with a DICER1 mutation. The solid appearance suggests a type III pleuropulmonary blastoma.*

Inflammatory Myofibroblastic Tumor

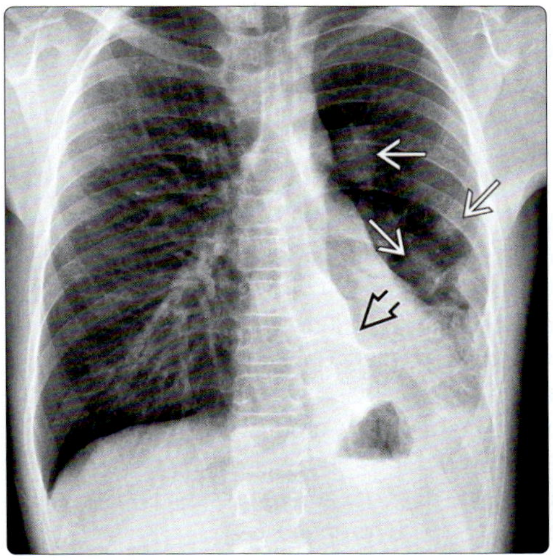

Posttransplant Lymphoproliferative Disorder

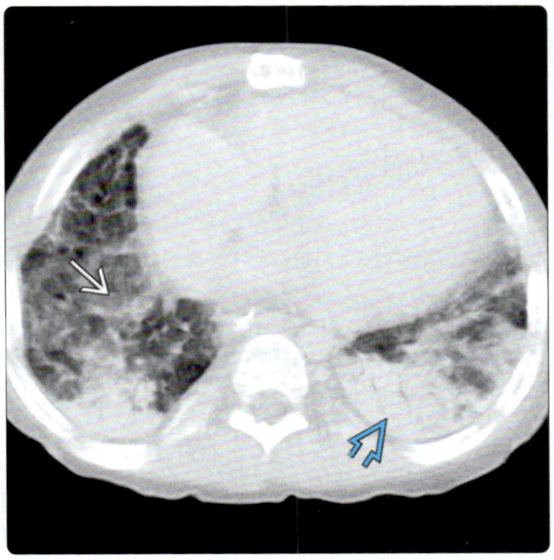

(Left) *Frontal radiograph shows a medial pleural-based mass* ⇨*, as well as multiple nodular foci of pulmonary consolidation* ➡*, in this adolescent with a biopsy-proven inflammatory myofibroblastic tumor.* **(Right)** *Axial CECT depicts diffuse ground-glass opacities* ➡ *& basilar consolidation* ⇨ *that were persistent over several studies in this 14 year old with a history of a heart transplant. Biopsy confirmed the diagnosis of PTLD, which can present as areas of consolidation in < 10% of cases.*

Posttransplant Lymphoproliferative Disorder

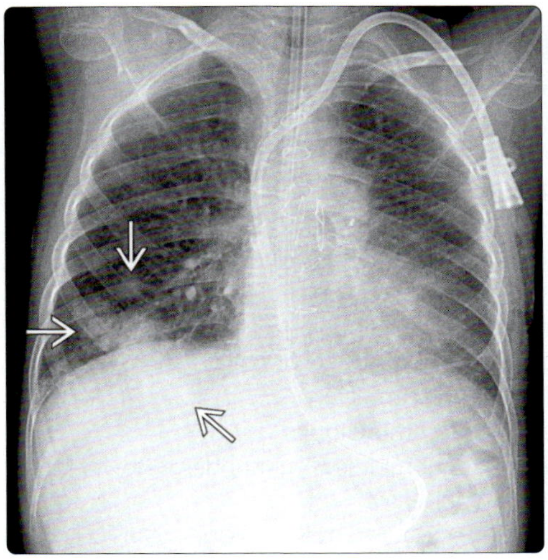

Posttransplant Lymphoproliferative Disorder

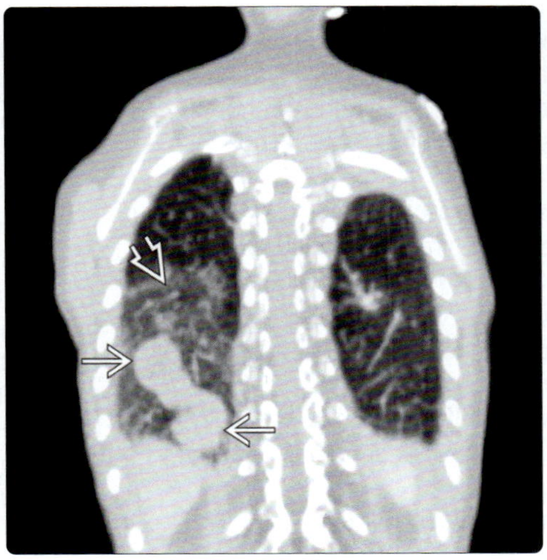

(Left) *Frontal radiograph from an 8 year old with a history of a lung transplant demonstrates right lower lobe consolidation with areas of nodular opacity* ➡*, concerning for infection or PTLD.* **(Right)** *Coronal CECT in the same patient shows a typical appearance of PTLD with multiple round masses* ➡ *& additional surrounding ground-glass opacities* ➡*.*

DIFFERENTIAL DIAGNOSIS

Common

- Normal Thymus
- Congenital Pulmonary Airway Malformation
- Bronchopulmonary Sequestration
- Congenital Diaphragmatic Hernia

Less Common

- Congenital Lobar Overinflation
- Foregut Duplication Cyst
- Lymphatic Malformation
- Bronchial Atresia
- Neuroblastoma

Rare but Important

- Pleuropulmonary Blastoma
- Pericardial Teratoma
- Mesenchymal Hamartoma
- Infantile Fibrosarcoma

ESSENTIAL INFORMATION

Key Differential Diagnosis Issues

- Neonatal lung masses are most commonly due to in utero developmental anomalies: Spectrum of malformations of lung parenchyma & bronchovascular structures
- Mediastinal & chest wall masses can mimic lung masses
- Prenatal US & MR provide excellent characterization of congenital chest masses & their relationships to heart, spine, airway, & chest wall
  - MR allows calculation of lung volumes with assessment of pulmonary hypoplasia, which informs survival
- Postnatal CTA provides preoperative evaluation

Helpful Clues for Common Diagnoses

- **Normal Thymus**
  - Most common anterior mediastinal mass in infants
  - Changes in appearance with age
    - Most prominent in infancy with convex margins
      - Stress of illness in neonatal ICU patients may cause reduced thymic volume
    - Gradually decreases in size with concave margins in later childhood & teenage years
  - May be asymmetric across midline; can extend inferiorly to drape over heart, superiorly into neck, or posteriorly between great vessels & trachea
    - No mass effect on airway or vessels
  - Radiographs: Homogeneous with mildly undulating margins; often slightly lucent to cardiac silhouette
  - US: Hypoechoic with diffuse "dot-dash" echoes
  - CT/MR: Homogeneous appearance on CT & MR with mild uniform homogeneous enhancement
- **Congenital Pulmonary Airway Malformation (CPAM)**
  - Previously known as congenital cystic adenomatoid malformation (CCAM)
  - Most common congenital lung malformation (30-40%)
  - Due to hamartomatous proliferation of cystic & noncystic bronchiole-like tissue
  - Appears prenatally as fluid-filled cysts that progressively fill with air after delivery
  - Stocker classification (0-4) based on level of airway maldevelopment (proximal to distal)
    - Type 0 (< 2%): Small lungs with severe acinar dysgenesis & large airway dysplasia; uniformly fatal
    - Type 1 (65%): Mainly 1 or more macrocysts (> 2 cm)
      - May have air-fluid levels postnatally
    - Type 2 (10-15%): Multiple small cysts (0.5-2.0 cm)
    - Type 3 (5-8%): Innumerable microscopic cysts
      - Appears solid
    - Type 4 (10-15%): Large peripheral cysts
  - Evidence of associated mass effect
    - Mediastinal shift, compressive atelectasis
  - Can coexist with other pulmonary malformations, such as sequestration, bronchial atresia (hybrid lesion)
    - CTA: Cover through celiac axis to look for systemic arterial supply
  - Carries recurrent infection risk
  - Small malignancy risk: Bronchioalveolar carcinoma, rhabdomyosarcoma
    - Reports of type 4 CPAM were likely type 1 pleuropulmonary blastoma (PPB) → erroneous reports of PPB arising from CPAM
- **Bronchopulmonary Sequestration**
  - Nonfunctioning lung disconnected from bronchial tree
  - Vascular supply from systemic artery is key feature
  - Intralobar & extralobar types
    - Intralobar: Shares pleura of affected lobe; drainage is usually via pulmonary vein
    - Extralobar: Separate pleural covering; drainage is usually via systemic vein
  - Both usually occur in lower lungs; extralobar type can be infradiaphragmatic or mediastinal
  - Radiographs: Solid on initial imaging in postnatal period
    - Intralobar type may show gradual aeration from collateral flow or CPAM components
    - Extralobar type does not aerate unless it is in communication with foregut
- **Congenital Diaphragmatic Hernia**
  - Bochdalek (90%): Posterolateral
    - Left 80-90%, right 10-15%, bilateral < 5%
  - Morgagni/ventral (10%): Retrosternal
  - Right-sided hernias may just involve liver
  - Radiographs: Bubbly bowel-like lucencies in chest when stomach/bowel are involved
    - Degree of bowel gas distention varies between radiographs
    - Enteric tube may course into chest
    - Umbilical venous catheter is often deviated due to liver herniation
  - Associated pulmonary hypoplasia & pulmonary hypertension → major prognostic factors
- **Congenital Lobar Overinflation**
  - Overinflation of 1 or more lobes
    - Left upper > right middle > right upper >> lower lobes; multifocal in only ~ 5%
  - Due to air-trapping caused by intrinsic or extrinsic bronchial luminal narrowing during development
  - Radiographs: In 1st hours to days of life, fluid-density lobar or segmental opacification from retained fetal fluid
    - Progressive hyperlucency & expansion thereafter

Helpful Clues for Less Common Diagnoses

- **Foregut Duplication Cyst**
  - Includes bronchogenic, esophageal, & neurenteric cysts
    - Bronchogenic cysts are most commonly subcarinal, precarinal, or paratracheal (middle mediastinum)
    - Esophageal cysts are intimately associated with esophagus
    - Neurenteric cysts lie at junction between posterior & middle mediastinum
      - Extend into or communicate with spinal canal
      - Associated with congenital vertebral defects
  - US/CT/MR: All are usually round with smooth wall & thin peripheral enhancement
    - 50% appear as simple fluid-filled cysts
    - Otherwise variable appearance due to proteinaceous or hemorrhagic contents or superinfection
- **Lymphatic Malformation**
  - Congenital error of vessel morphogenesis
  - Grows commensurate with patient; may show rapid enlargement from infection, trauma, or hormones
  - May be focal or transspatial (extending across tissue planes); often involves neck, chest wall, &/or axilla
  - US/MR: Thin-walled, fluid-filled multiloculated mass with only peripheral & septal enhancement
    - May contain fluid-fluid levels or foci of T1 shortening due to blood products
- **Bronchial Atresia**
  - Noncommunication of segmental/subsegmental bronchus with central airway
  - Left upper > left lower > right middle lobe
  - Radiographs/CT: Appears as central tubular/branching density due to mucoid impaction of bronchus distal to atresia ("finger in glove")
    - Distal lung is hyperinflated with decreased vascularity
- **Neuroblastoma**
  - Most common posterior mediastinal mass in young
    - Can occur anywhere along sympathetic chain
  - Radiograph: Elongated oval mass with tapered borders in paraspinal location
    - Can appear as round lesion when large & at apex
    - Homogeneously solid ± fine or chunky Ca^{2+} (30%)
    - ± separation or erosion of ribs or enlargement of neural foramina
  - CT: Better demonstrates Ca^{2+} (80-90% of neuroblastoma)
  - MR: Better demonstrates intraspinal extension
  - Nuclear medicine imaging: I-123 MIBG is mainstay for diagnosis & assessing response to therapy

Helpful Clues for Rare Diagnoses

- **Pleuropulmonary Blastoma**
  - Rare malignant childhood tumor
  - Typically appears as large mass in peripheral lung involving visceral pleura with effusion & mediastinal shift
  - 3 types; lesion evolves from type 1 to type 3 over time (with progressively worse prognosis)
    - Type 1: Large, air-filled, multilocular cystic mass
      - Only type reported in newborns
    - Type 2: Large, air-filled, cystic & solid mass
    - Type 3: Solid pulmonary mass
  - May be indistinguishable from CPAM
    - Prenatal 2nd trimester detection, lung hyperinflation, systemic arterial supply (sequestration component), or asymptomatic patient favors CPAM
- **Pericardial Teratoma**
  - US/CT/MR: Heterogeneous mixed solid & cystic mass, ± Ca^{2+} &/or fat; often has pericardial effusion
- **Mesenchymal Hamartoma**
  - Most commonly presents in infancy
  - Radiographs/CT: Large mass with bizarre distortion & erosion of multiple adjacent ribs; rarely multifocal
    - Majority have internal mineralization with septal Ca^{2+}
  - CT/MR: Often have secondary aneurysmal bone cyst with fluid-fluid levels
- **Infantile Fibrosarcoma**
  - May arise from chest wall or lung
  - MR: Hemorrhagic components may be T1 hyperintense
    - Heterogeneous enhancement
  - More favorable prognosis than adult fibrosarcoma

Normal Thymus

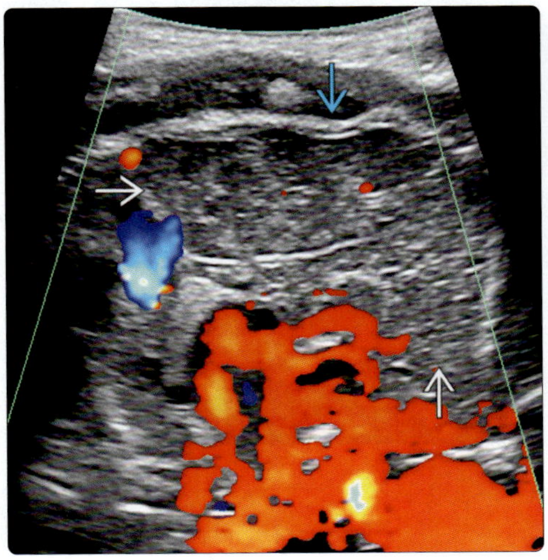

Normal Thymus

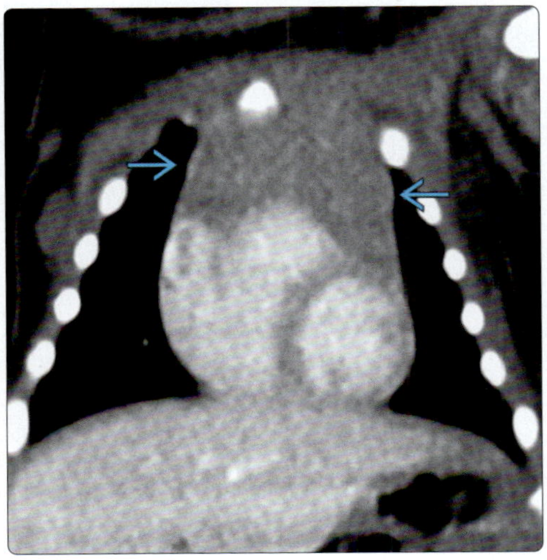

(Left) *Transverse color Doppler US of the upper chest in a newborn shows hypoechoic tissue ➡ anterior to the great vessels that has undulating margins ⇒ & diffuse "dot-dash" echoes, typical of the thymus. Note the lack of vascular compression by the thymus.* **(Right)** *Coronal CECT in the same patient shows the homogeneous thymic tissue draped over the heart with mildly convex margins ⇒. Note that the thymus can normally be even larger than this in infants, filling much of the central chest*

(Left) *Frontal radiograph in a neonate shows a bubbly mass in the left hemithorax with mixed areas of lucency & soft tissue density. The cysts are of varying size & were stable on serial radiographs. Note the rightward mediastinal shift, including the enteric tube. The diaphragm is intact.* **(Right)** *Axial CECT in the same patient shows a multiloculated cystic lung mass with internal air-fluid levels. Surgical pathology confirmed a type 1 congenital pulmonary airway malformation (CPAM).*

Congenital Pulmonary Airway Malformation

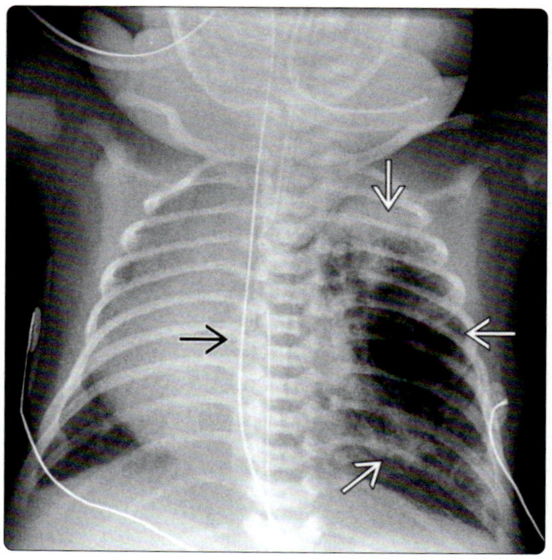

Congenital Pulmonary Airway Malformation

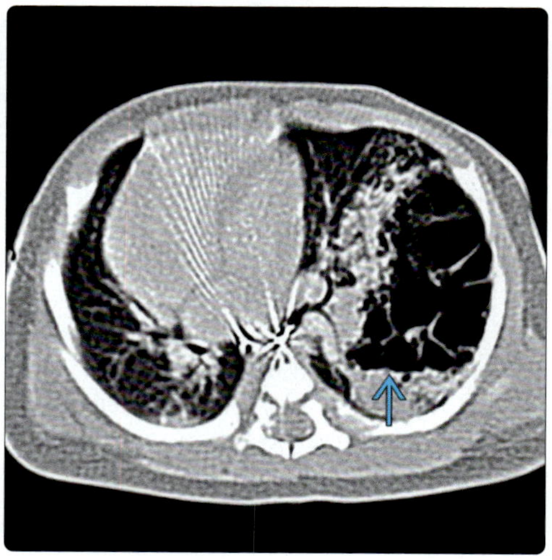

(Left) *Coronal SSFSE T2 MR in a 34-week gestation fetus shows a large multicystic mass filling most of the right hemithorax, shifting the heart & thymus to the left with compression of the left lung. Resection at delivery confirmed a type 1 CPAM.* **(Right)** *Axial CECT in an infant shows a large right lower lobe lesion with cysts of variable size. A central solid-appearing focus with prominent vasculature was seen to arise from the abdominal aorta, representing a sequestration component (hybrid lesion).*

Congenital Pulmonary Airway Malformation

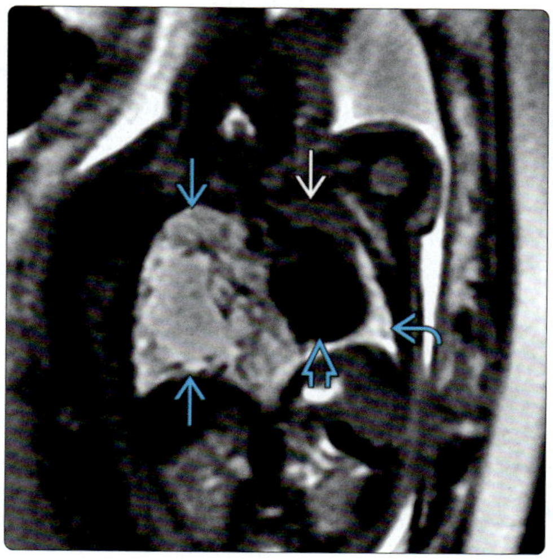

Congenital Pulmonary Airway Malformation

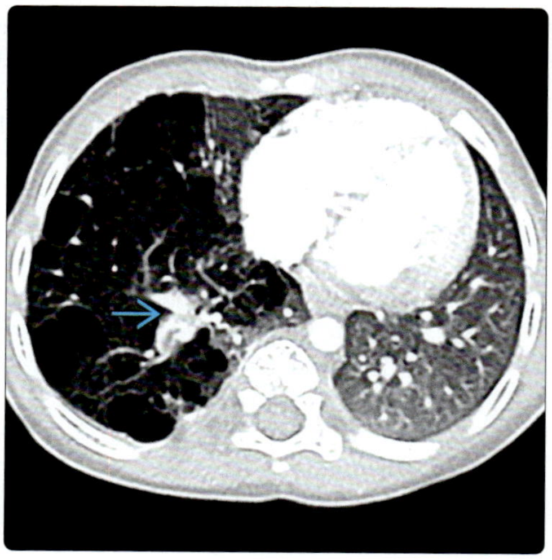

(Left) *AP radiograph in an asymptomatic 3 month old shows a rounded opacity in the left lower lobe with the appearance & location being suspicious for a bronchopulmonary sequestration.* **(Right)** *Axial CECT in the same patient shows an enhancing left lower lung mass abutting the diaphragm. There is prominent systemic arterial supply from the abdominal aorta, along with systemic venous drainage to the portal vein (not shown). The findings are consistent with an extralobar sequestration.*

Bronchopulmonary Sequestration

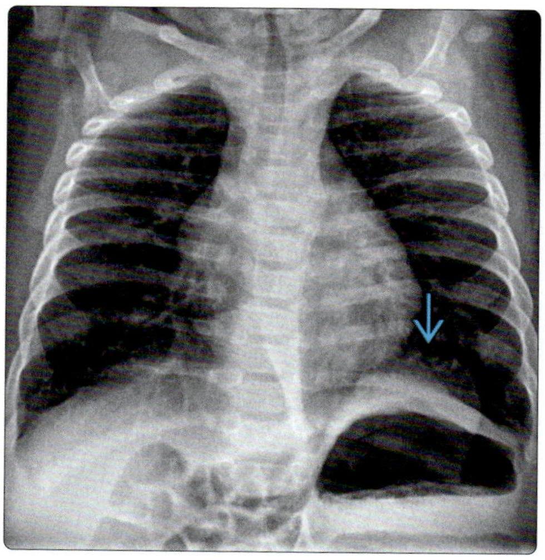

Bronchopulmonary Sequestration

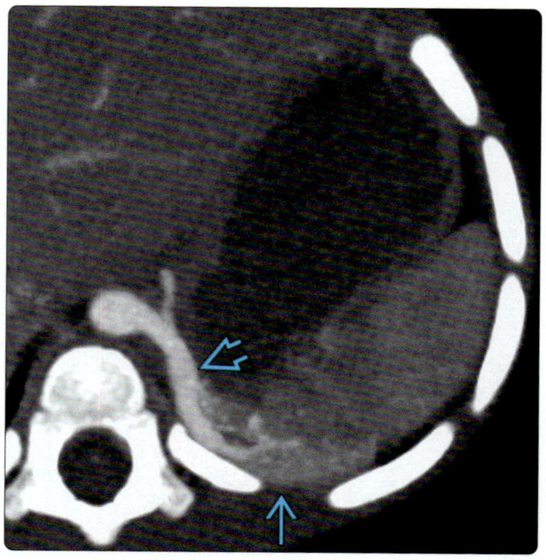

Congenital Diaphragmatic Hernia

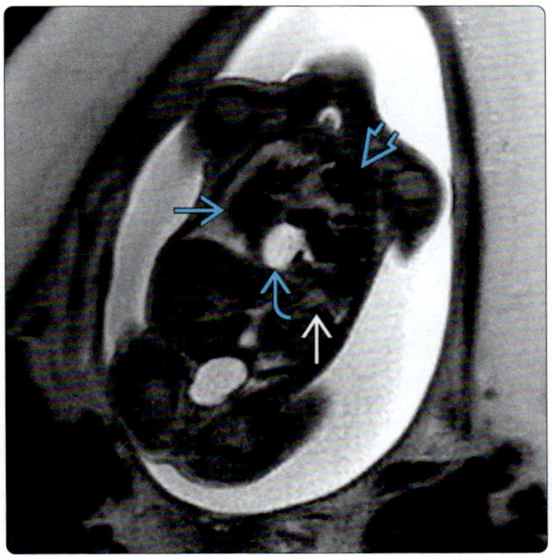

Congenital Diaphragmatic Hernia

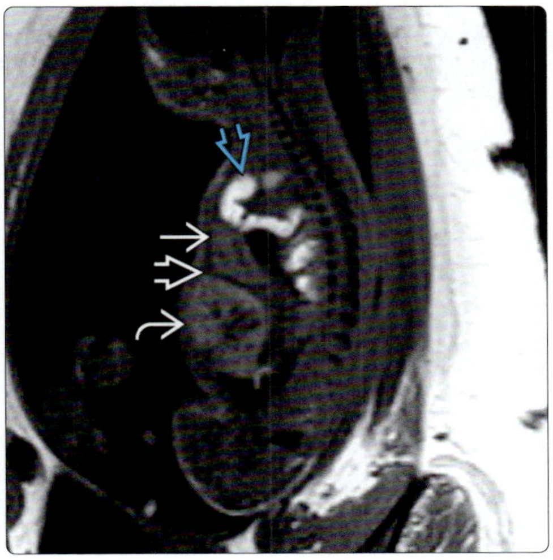

(Left) *Coronal SSFSE T2 MR in a 32-week fetus shows a large left congenital diaphragmatic hernia (CDH) with stomach, bowel, & liver extending into the chest. The heart is shifted to the right.* **(Right)** *Sagittal T1 MR in the same fetus shows the left hemithorax filled with bowel & a portion of the liver that herniated through the posterior defect. Most of the liver remains in the abdomen below the intact anterior left hemidiaphragm.*

Congenital Diaphragmatic Hernia

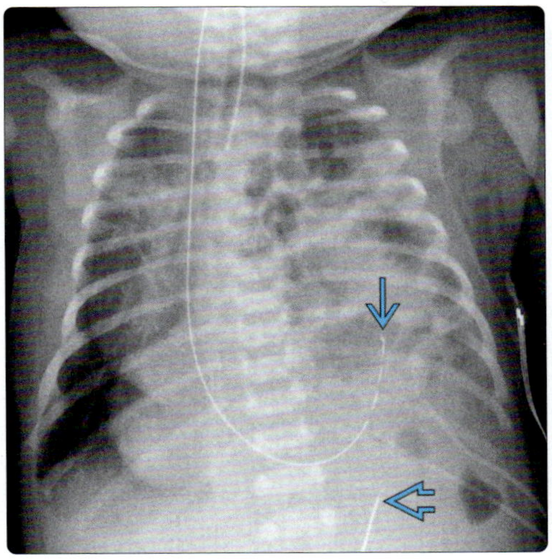

Congenital Diaphragmatic Hernia

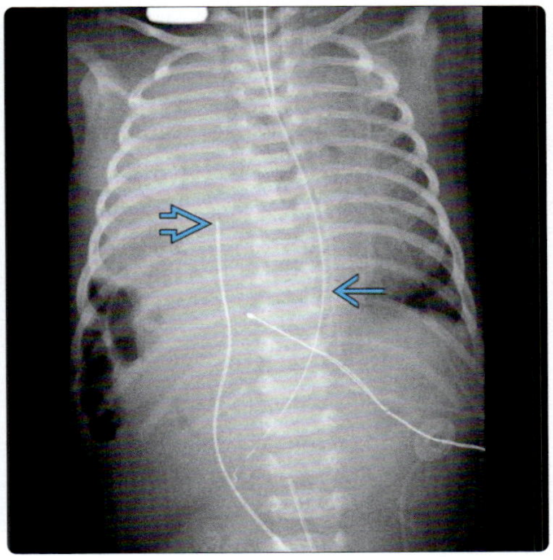

(Left) *AP radiograph in the same patient at delivery shows the left hemithorax filled with gas-distended bowel. Note the "reverse J" nasogastric (NG) tube appearance in the herniated stomach. The umbilical venous catheter (UVC) is deviated by left hepatic lobe herniation.* **(Right)** *AP radiograph shows a right CDH with right hemithorax opacification by herniated liver & bowel. Note the leftward deviation of the NG tube & high rightward position of the UVC due to right liver herniation.*

Congenital Lobar Overinflation

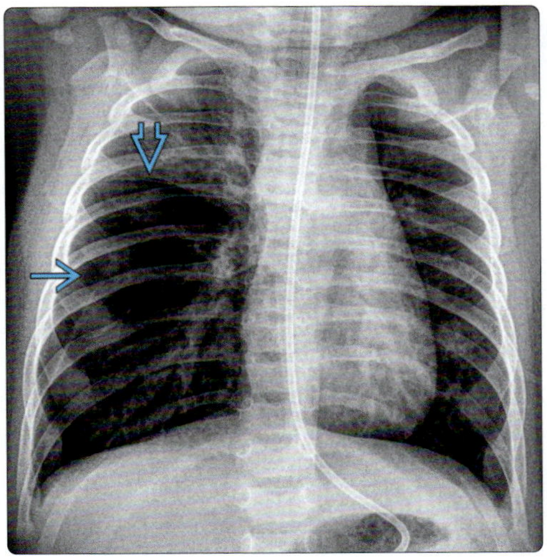

Congenital Lobar Overinflation

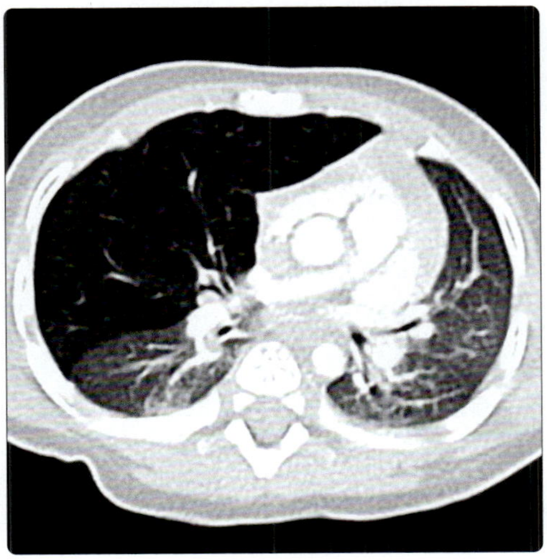

(Left) *PA radiograph in a 4 month old shows an incidental finding of hyperinflation vs. a lucent lung mass in the right lower lung. Note the elevated minor fissure.* **(Right)** *Axial CECT in the same patient shows overinflation & hyperlucency of the entire right middle lobe with mediastinal shift to the left. There was apparent kinking & narrowing of the right middle lobe bronchus as it coursed underneath the right pulmonary artery (not shown). The findings are consistent with congenital lobar overinflation.*

(Left) *PA radiograph shows a rounded opacity along the medial left upper lung.* **(Right)** *Axial CECT in the same patient shows a corresponding thin-walled, cystic-appearing lesion in the left hilum, most consistent with a bronchogenic cyst. Bronchogenic cysts are usually closely related to the central airways, & mass effect on the airway can cause atelectasis or air-trapping. Surgical resection is usually recommended due to the risk of infection (& rarely malignancy).*

Foregut Duplication Cyst

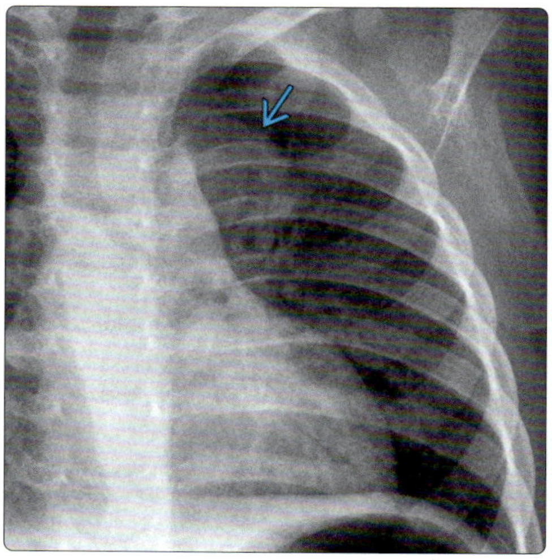

Foregut Duplication Cyst

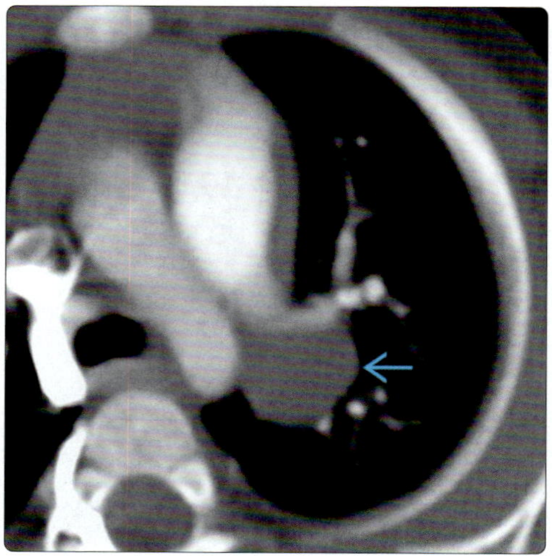

(Left) *AP radiograph in a newborn shows marked expansion of the right chest/abdominal wall soft tissues with right apical pleural thickening & mediastinal widening.* **(Right)** *Axial T2 FS (top) & T1 C+ FS (bottom) MR images in the same patient show a large, predominantly macrocystic lymphatic malformation infiltrating the chest wall, pleural, & mediastinal soft tissues. Note the typical multicystic appearance with thin rim enhancement, fluid-fluid levels, & lack of vascular compression.*

Lymphatic Malformation

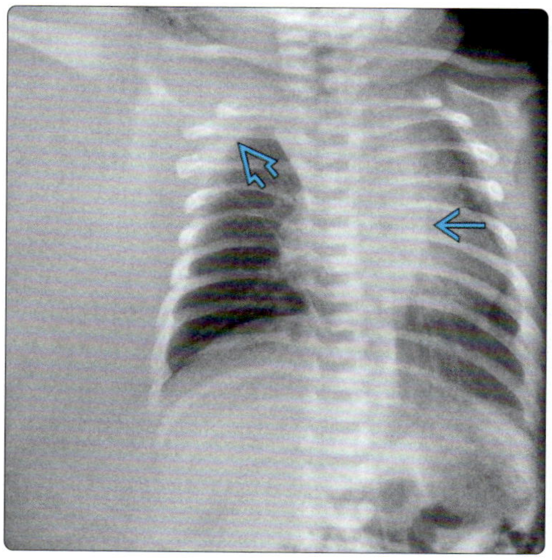

Lymphatic Malformation

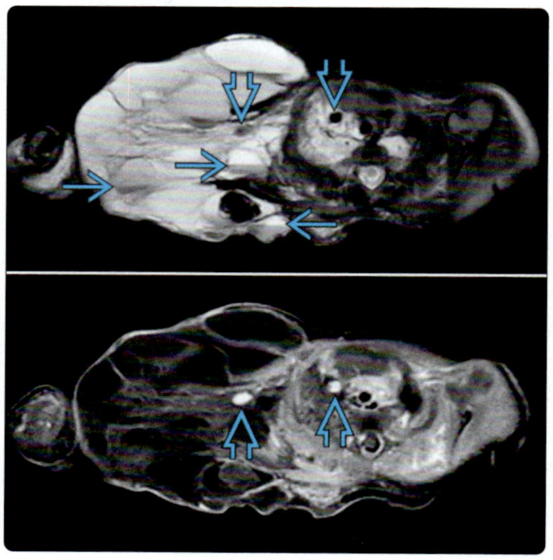

(Left) *PA radiograph in a 3 month old shows a mass-like lucency within the right hemithorax due to hyperinflation & air-trapping of the right middle lobe with mediastinal mass effect.* **(Right)** *Axial CECT in the same patient shows an atretic right middle lobe bronchus with mucoid impaction & dilation distal to the atresia. The right middle lobe is hyperinflated with reduced vascularity. These findings are consistent with bronchial atresia.*

Bronchial Atresia

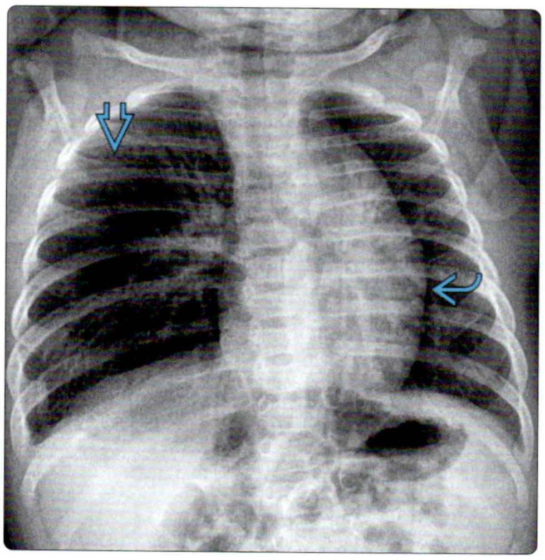

Bronchial Atresia

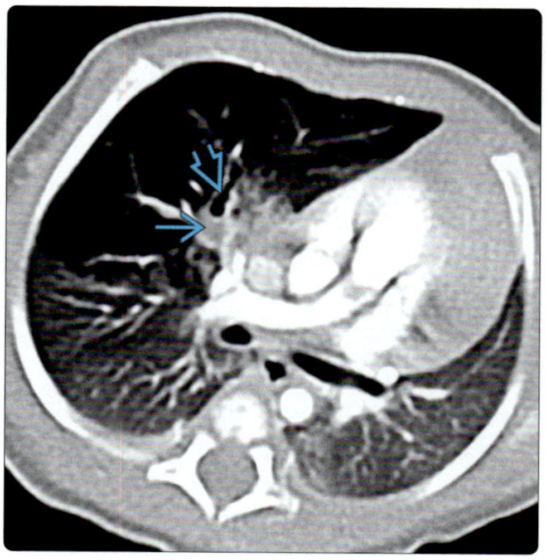

Neuroblastoma

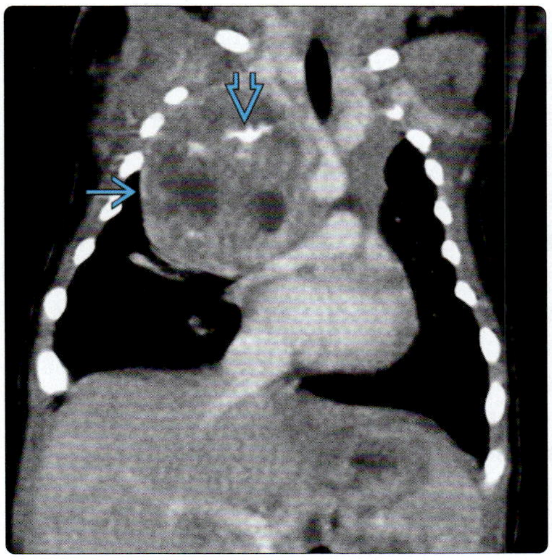

Pleuropulmonary Blastoma

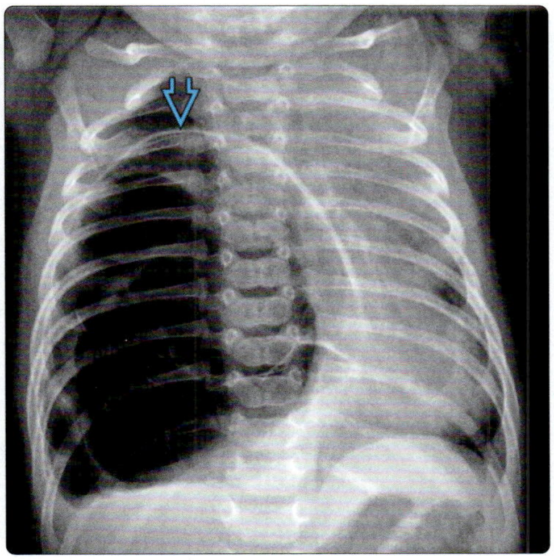

(Left) *Coronal CECT shows a well-circumscribed 6-cm mass in the right apex of a neonate. Note the Ca^{2+} & mediastinal shift. The findings are typical of neuroblastoma.* **(Right)** *Frontal radiograph shows a large lucent mass occupying the right hemithorax & causing marked leftward mediastinal shift. Surgical pathology demonstrated a type 1 pleuropulmonary blastoma (PPB) in this 1 month old. Note that this imaging appearance is not able to be differentiated from a type 1 CPAM.*

Pericardial Teratoma

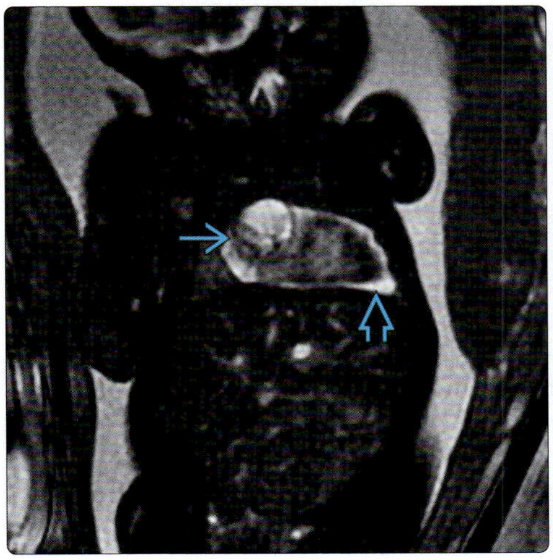

Pericardial Teratoma

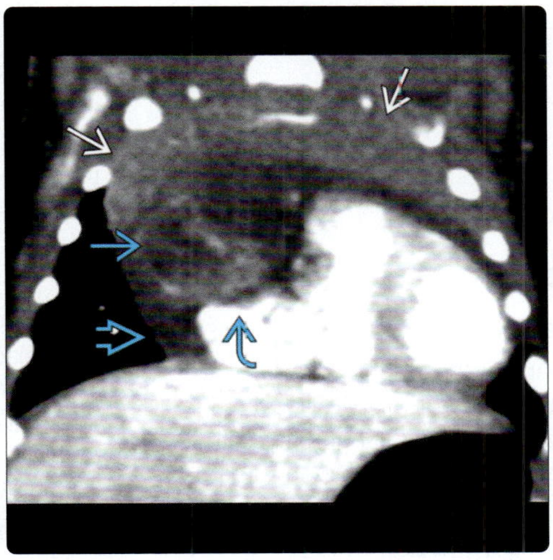

(Left) *Coronal SSFP MR in a 31-week fetus shows a heterogeneous mixed solid & cystic mass along the right atrium. A pericardial effusion is noted.* **(Right)** *Coronal CECT in the same patient after delivery shows a heterogeneous 3-cm mass that contained fluid & fat components. There is mass effect on the right atrium as well as a pericardial effusion. Note the normal thymus splayed over the heart.*

Mesenchymal Hamartoma

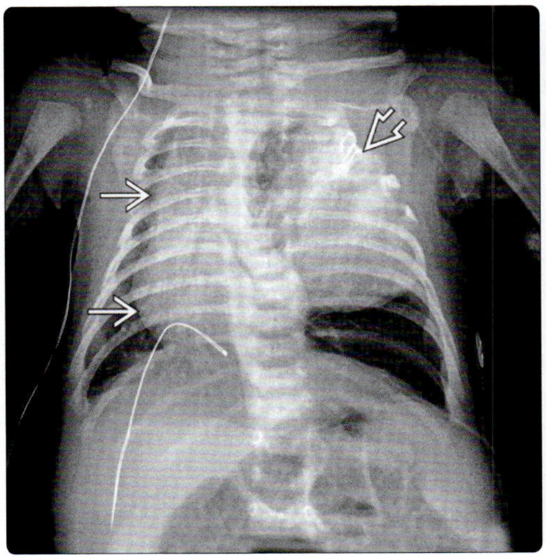

Mesenchymal Hamartoma

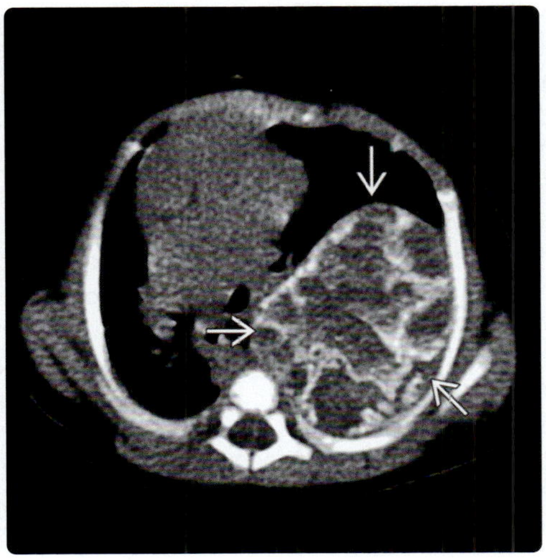

(Left) *Frontal radiograph shows a large left upper hemithorax mass with bizarre distortion of multiple adjacent ribs. Note the rightward mediastinal shift in this 3-week-old neonate.* **(Right)** *Axial NECT in the same patient shows septal Ca^{2+} of the large mass. Additional images showed fluid-fluid levels in many of the cystic foci, typical of a mesenchymal hamartoma.*

Chest Wall Mass

DIFFERENTIAL DIAGNOSIS

Common

- Normal Variants
- Infantile Hemangioma
- Healing Rib Fractures

Less Common

- Accessory Breast Tissue
- Venous Malformation
- Lymphatic Malformation
- Ewing Sarcoma
- Neuroblastoma
- Langerhans Cell Histiocytosis
- Rhabdomyosarcoma
- Plexiform Neurofibromas
- Fibrous Dysplasia
- Osteochondroma
- Enchondroma
- Infection
- Desmoid
- Infantile Myofibroma

Rare but Important

- Osteosarcoma
- Aneurysmal Bone Cyst
- Dermoid
- Mesenchymal Hamartoma of Chest Wall

ESSENTIAL INFORMATION

Key Differential Diagnosis Issues

- Helpful clinical & imaging features: Age, bone vs. soft tissue origin, solid vs. cystic mass, unifocal vs. multifocal
- Certain lesions favor ribs: Ewing sarcoma, Langerhans cell histiocytosis, fibrous dysplasia, enchondroma, aneurysmal bone cyst (ABC), mesenchymal hamartoma

Helpful Clues for Common Diagnoses

- **Normal Variants**
  - Most likely diagnosis in children with asymptomatic palpable anterior chest wall mass
    - Typically painless unless protuberance leads to repetitive injury to that site
    - Occur in up to 1/3 of children
  - Possibilities include: Asymmetric costal cartilage (± bifid rib), tilted sternum, accessory cartilage rests, etc.
    - Protuberance of cartilage may be due to underlying scoliosis or pectus deformities
- **Infantile Hemangioma**
  - Benign vascular neoplasm of capillaries
  - Appear in 1st weeks to months of life, grow rapidly in 1st year, involute slowly over subsequent years
  - Mass remains clinically soft throughout life cycle
  - Subcutaneous lesions without characteristic cutaneous stigmata are more likely to be imaged
  - Discrete lobulated compressible mass, typically isolated to subcutaneous tissues
    - Patchy regions of ↑ & ↓ echogenicity
    - Doppler shows high vessel density (> 5/cm²) with abundant low-resistance arterial waveforms
    - Rapid uniform enhancement with contrast
- **Healing Rib Fractures**
  - Most child abuse victims are < 1 year of age
  - Abuse can fracture any portion of rib but posterior medial rib fractures are most specific for abuse
  - Subacute rib fractures form palpable prominent callus
  - Identification of unsuspected rib fractures should initiate process of investigation, including skeletal survey

Helpful Clues for Less Common Diagnoses

- **Accessory Breast Tissue**
  - Most commonly found in axilla
  - Hypoechoic lobules intermixed with echogenic fat; similar to normal breast tissue deep to nipple
    - ± continuity with normal breast tissue
  - Often presents with hormonal stimulation (e.g., puberty)
- **Venous Malformation**
  - Present at birth, grows proportionate to child
    - May rapidly enlarge with trauma, infection, or during periods of hormonal stimulation
  - Collection of low flow serpentine structures that demonstrate gradual enhancement; often transspatial
    - Discrete mass vs. scattered vessels (or both)
    - True phleboliths are essentially diagnostic
      - ▫ Round Ca^{2+} on US/CT; low signal on MR
      - ▫ Thrombus (without Ca^{2+}) may show T1 shortening
    - Fluid-fluid levels are common due to stagnant blood
- **Lymphatic Malformation**
  - Present at birth & grows proportionate to child
    - May rapidly enlarge with trauma, infection, or during periods of hormonal stimulation
  - Circumscribed vs. infiltrative transspatial multicystic mass
    - Macrocysts: > 1 cm; thin enhancing septa with varying complexity of internal fluid; no central enhancement
    - Microcysts: < 1 cm; may appear solid & enhancing
  - Commonly involves axilla, neck, pleura, & mediastinum
  - Multifocal bone lesions may occur in systemic forms
- **Ewing Sarcoma**
  - Most common in teenage years; very rare < 5 years old
  - Arises from rib, scapula, clavicle, spine, or soft tissues
    - Classic Askin tumor arises from chest soft tissues
  - Involved bone: Lucent, expanded, & permeated with cortical loss & aggressive periosteal reaction
  - Associated soft tissue mass is often large
- **Neuroblastoma**
  - Tumor of sympathetic chain primitive neural crest cells
  - Thoracic presentation: Mean age of 25 months
    - Abdominal: 15-17 months
  - Round, elongated, or lobulated paraspinal mass ± Ca^{2+}
  - Look for rib erosion &/or splaying or pedicle changes with extension into spinal canal
- **Langerhans Cell Histiocytosis**
  - Benign neoplastic clonal proliferation
  - Common flat bone lesion with variety of appearances
  - Most common imaging features
    - "Punched-out" lytic lesion, frequently with well-defined (possibly sclerotic or T2-hypointense) margins
    - ± periosteal reaction, but not spiculated; often absent
    - Enhancing soft tissue fills bone defect but does not extend significantly beyond bone
    - Variable surrounding marrow & soft tissue edema

- **Rhabdomyosarcoma**
  - Most common pediatric soft tissue malignancy
  - Affects any pediatric age range, but is rarely congenital
  - Often well-circumscribed, firm, & round mass
    - Rarely invades bone & deeper soft tissues
  - Vascularity & enhancement range from minimal to moderate; rarely intense
  - Typically restricts diffusion due to cellularity
- **Plexiform Neurofibromas**
  - Seen exclusively in neurofibromatosis type 1 (NF1)
  - Lobulated soft tissue masses tracking along nerves
  - Cross section of individual lesion shows target appearance: T2-hyperintense rim, T2-hypointense center
  - Variable enhancement, often central
- **Fibrous Dysplasia**
  - Isolated or multifocal benign bone lesions
  - Often bubbly with lucent & expansile components
  - Classic appearance is ground glass matrix (think smudged or frosted glass) on CT or radiographs
  - MR: Hyperintense T2 signal & enhancement if active
- **Osteochondroma**
  - Benign protuberant bone growth (exostosis)
  - Isolated vs. multiple hereditary forms
  - Sessile (with broad base) or pedunculated (with narrow stalk); U-shaped rim of sclerosis en face
  - Flowing corticomedullary continuity with bone of origin
  - Complications: Fracture, irritation of overlying tissues, neurovascular impingement, or malignancy (rare)
    - Internal rib lesion may cause hemo/pneumothorax
- **Enchondroma**
  - Benign cartilaginous lesion; classically lucent & expansile with endosteal scalloping in short tubular bones
  - Rib (& digit) lesions may be exophytic/surface lesions
  - ± chondroid matrix (ring & arc Ca^{2+})
- **Infection**
  - May involve bone, joint, &/or soft tissues
    - Isolated rib osteomyelitis is uncommon
  - Rim-enhancing collection with irregular walls & central diffusion restriction suggest abscess
- **Desmoid**
  - a.k.a. aggressive fibromatosis
  - Benign but infiltrative/locally aggressive lesion
  - Variable MR signal intensity, but frequently has low T1/T2 signal components due to collagen
    - High T2 signal & enhancement suggest more active cellular components
- **Infantile Myofibroma**
  - Nondescript benign soft tissue mass of infants
  - Variable size & heterogeneity; often causes bizarre remodeling of adjacent bone
    - ± Ca^{2+}, low T2 signal components, enhancement
      - May show outer rim of enhancement only
  - If multifocal, bone lesions are typically expansile & lytic, often symmetric in metadiaphyses
    - Visceral lesions portend worse prognosis

Helpful Clues for Rare Diagnoses

- **Osteosarcoma**
  - Aggressive bone malignancy, most common in teenagers
  - Less common in axial skeleton than Ewing sarcoma
  - Variable lytic & sclerotic components with cortical permeation/destruction & aggressive periosteal reaction
    - Cloud-like osteoid matrix is classic in both bone lesion & overlying soft tissue mass
- **Aneurysmal Bone Cyst**
  - Classic expansile bubbly lucent lesion with numerous thin internal septa & fluid-fluid levels
- **Dermoid**
  - Unilocular thick-walled cystic lesion, often presternal
- **Mesenchymal Hamartoma of Chest Wall**
  - Most commonly presents in infancy
  - Large soft tissue mass with bizarre distortion & erosion of multiple adjacent ribs; rarely multifocal
  - Majority have internal mineralization with septal Ca^{2+}
  - Often have secondary ABC with fluid-fluid levels

Normal Variants

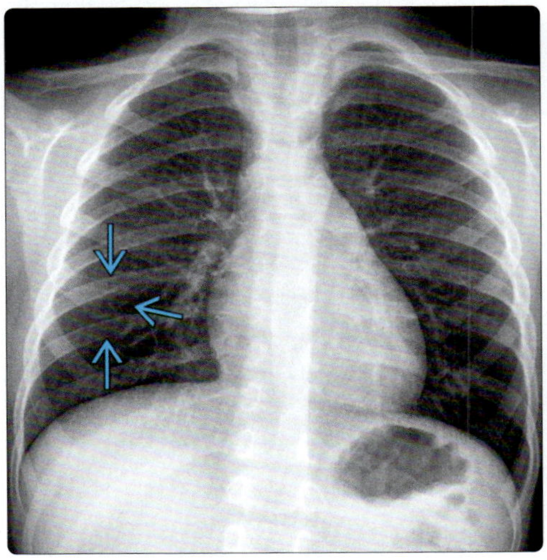

Normal Variants

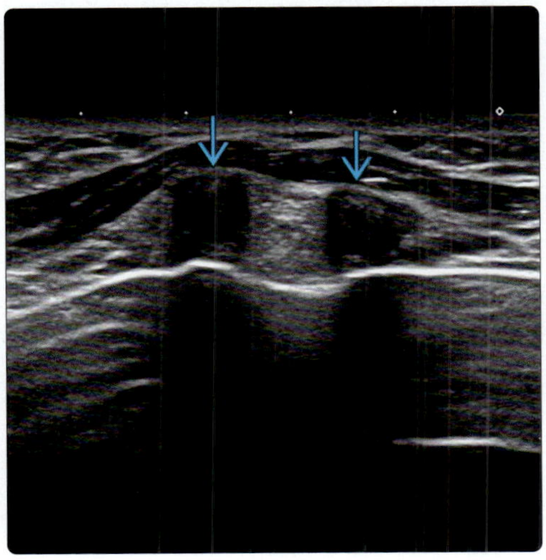

(Left) *PA radiograph in a 5 year old with a chest wall bump shows a bifid right 5th rib anteriorly ➡. These chest wall variants are commonly asymptomatic & often overlooked on imaging.* **(Right)** *Longitudinal US of a 15 year old at a site of chest wall protuberance shows splayed bifid costal cartilages ➡ that separated & reunited lateral & medial to this image, respectively.*

Normal Variants

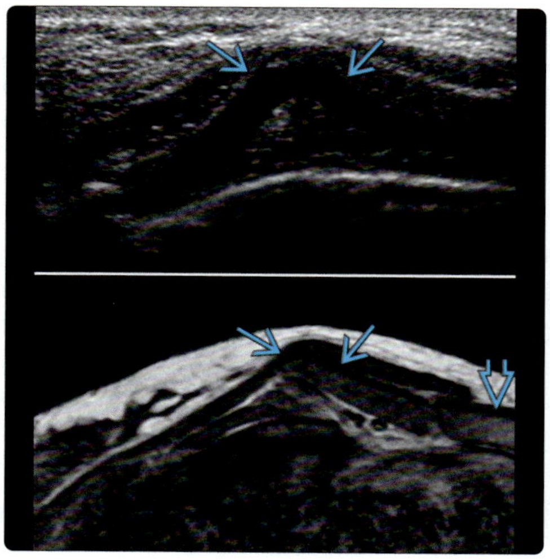

Infantile Hemangioma

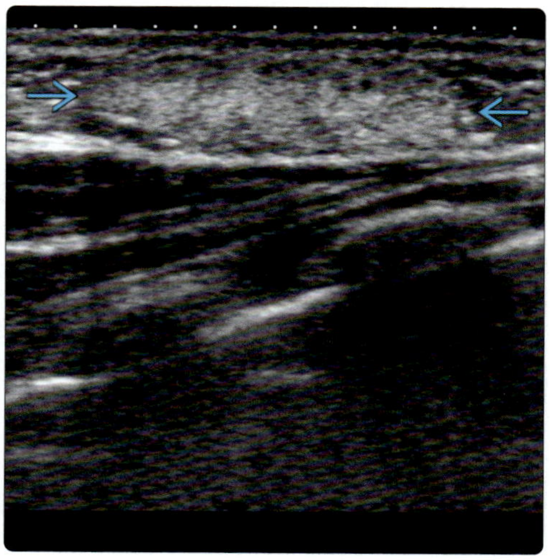

(Left) *Transverse US (top) & axial T1 MR (bottom) images in a 16 year old with a chest wall bump show anterior protuberance of an angulated costal cartilage → secondary to an unusual bifid rib configuration. Note the ossified sternum medially ⇨.* **(Right)** *Longitudinal US in a 6 month old with a new compressible soft tissue mass shows an elongated lesion in the subcutaneous fat with mixed increased & decreased echogenicity →. No large vessels are seen by grayscale imaging.*

Infantile Hemangioma

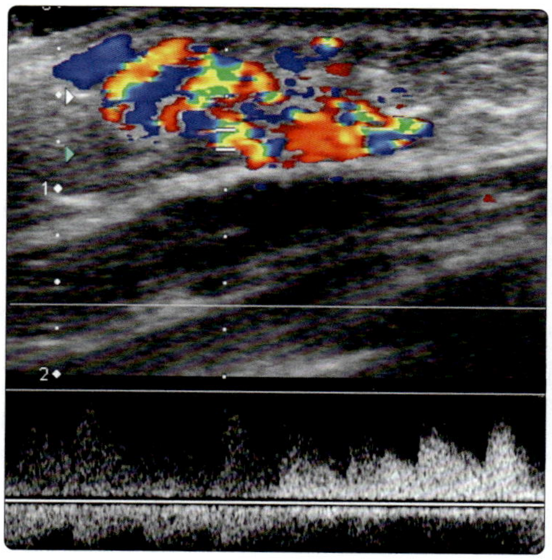

Infantile Hemangioma

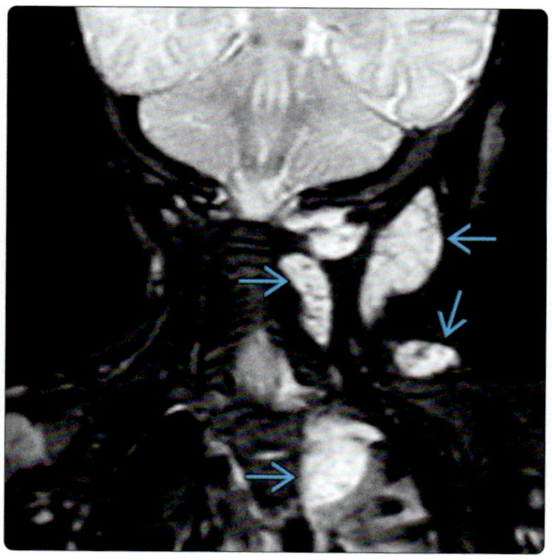

(Left) *Longitudinal color Doppler US in the same patient shows a high vessel density in the mass (> 5 vessels/cm²) with abundant low resistance arterial flow, typical of an infantile hemangioma.* **(Right)** *Coronal STIR MR in a 2 month old with PHACE syndrome shows numerous lobulated high signal intensity masses → of the soft tissues due to infantile hemangiomas. These lesions demonstrated typical early uniform enhancement on postcontrast sequences (not shown).*

Healing Rib Fractures

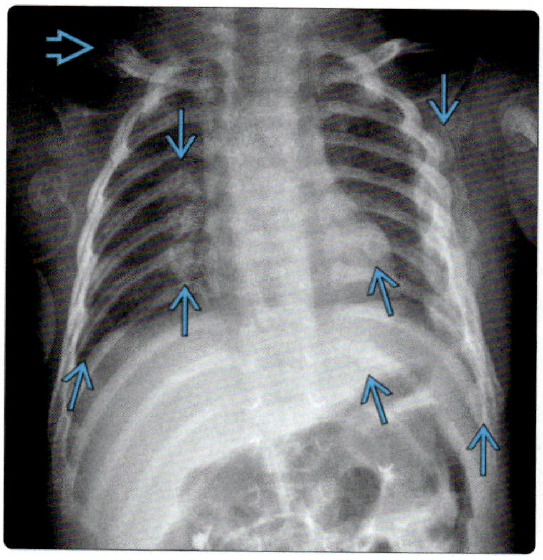

Healing Rib Fractures

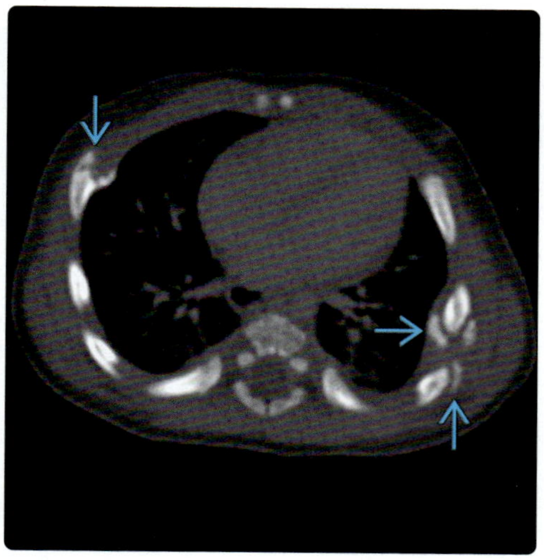

(Left) *AP radiograph in a 2 month old being evaluated for child abuse shows numerous healing rib fractures with abundant callus formation →. A healing clavicle fracture is also present ⇨.* **(Right)** *Axial CECT in the same patient shows bulbous callus formation at many healing rib fractures →. Such callus is often palpable & may be the only physical exam finding of abuse. This patient also had severe intracranial injuries.*

Venous Malformation

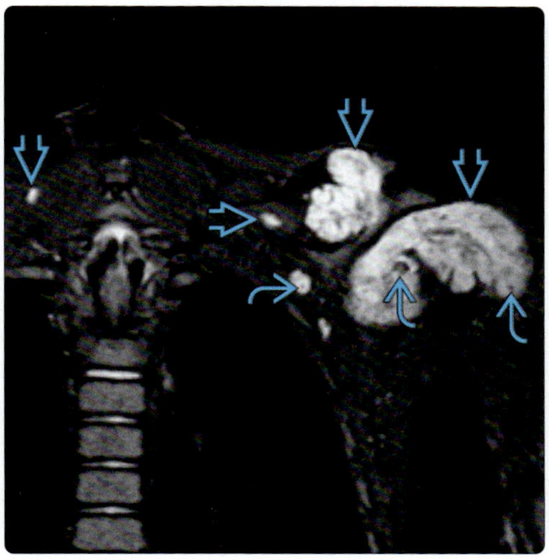

Lymphatic Malformation

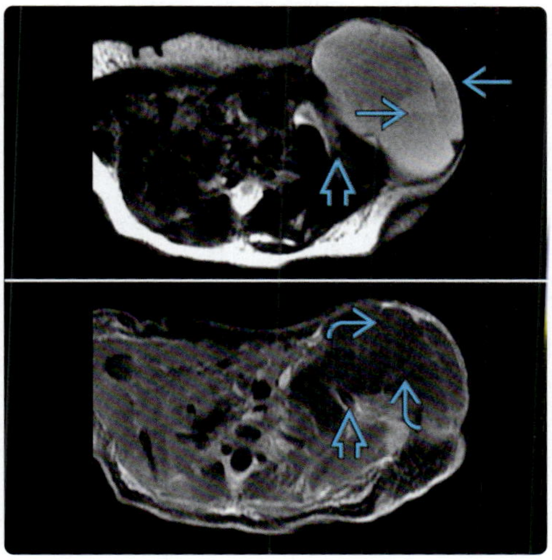

(Left) *Coronal STIR MR in an 18 month old with blue rubber bleb nevus syndrome shows multiple lobulated fluid signal intensity intramuscular masses of the upper chest. Small round low-signal foci were due to phleboliths.* **(Right)** *Axial T2 (top) & T1 C+ FS (bottom) MR images in a newborn show a large multiloculated cystic mass of the lower neck & upper chest wall surrounding the clavicle. There is only enhancement of multiple thin septations, & several internal fluid levels are due to layering blood products.*

Ewing Sarcoma

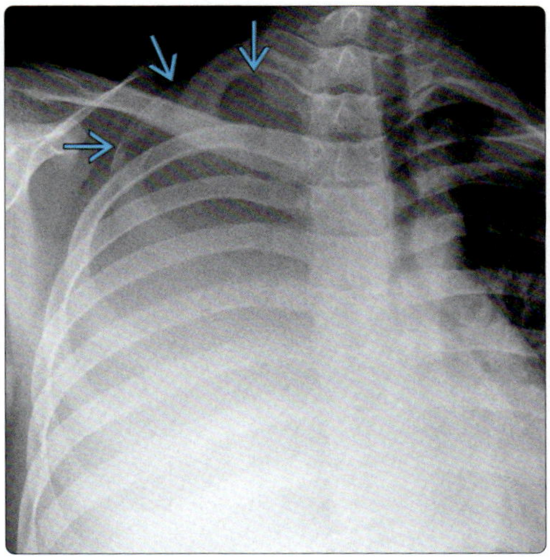

Ewing Sarcoma

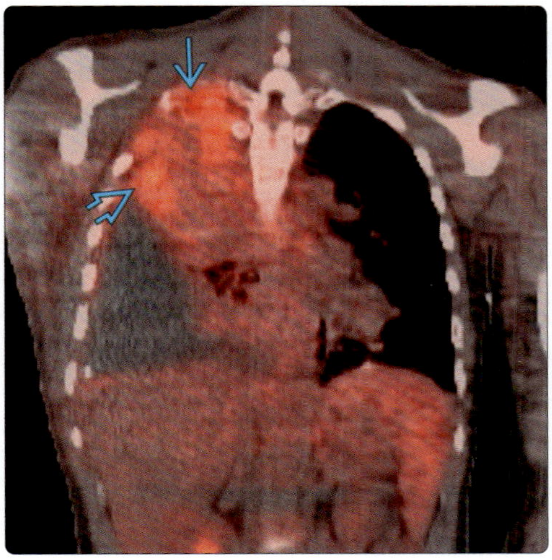

(Left) *PA radiograph in a 15 year old with pain & shortness of breath shows opacification of the right hemithorax with leftward mediastinal shift. There is permeation, expansion, & lysis of the right 2nd rib.* **(Right)** *Coronal FDG PET/CT in the same patient shows increased metabolic activity in the right 2nd rib as well as the emanating soft tissue mass. A large pleural effusion is also present. Ewing sarcoma was confirmed at biopsy.*

Neuroblastoma

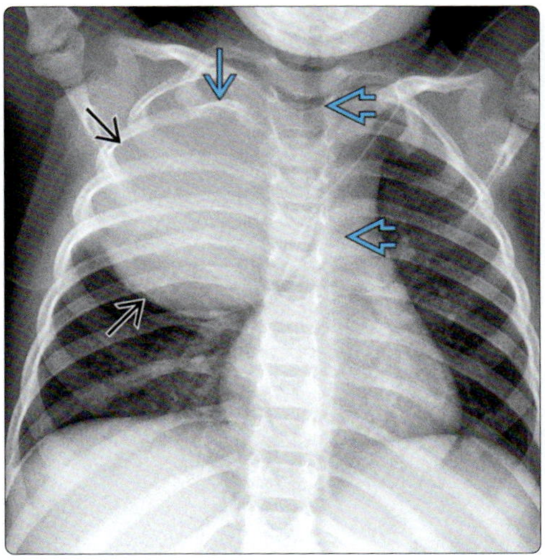

Neuroblastoma

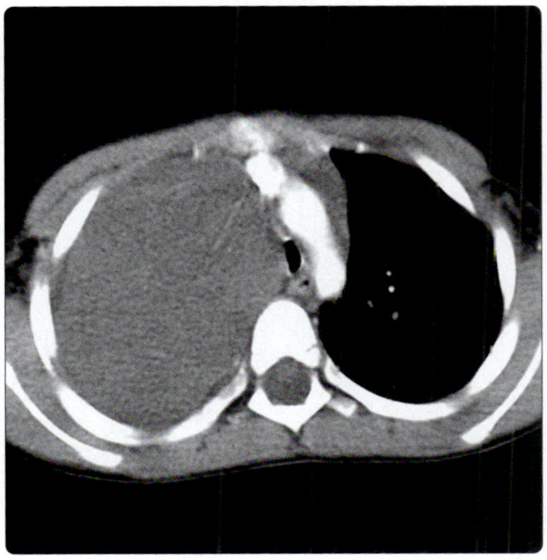

(Left) *AP radiograph in a toddler shows a soft tissue mass at the right apex with associated rib splaying & erosions. These findings are typical of a paraspinal neuroblastoma. Also note the leftward mediastinal shift.* **(Right)** *Axial CECT in the same child shows a large homogeneous mass in the superior right hemithorax with mediastinal shift to the left & compression of the trachea. While not seen in this case, neuroblastomas often show calcification on CT.*

(Left) *AP radiograph in a 2 year old with pain shows lucency & expansion of the posterior right 7th rib ⇨.* **(Right)** *Sagittal T1 C+ FS MR in the same patient shows an enhancing lesion expanding & disrupting the posterior rib ⇨ with surrounding soft tissue edema ⇨. Langerhans cell histiocytosis is more commonly frankly lytic without expansion of the affected bone.*

Langerhans Cell Histiocytosis

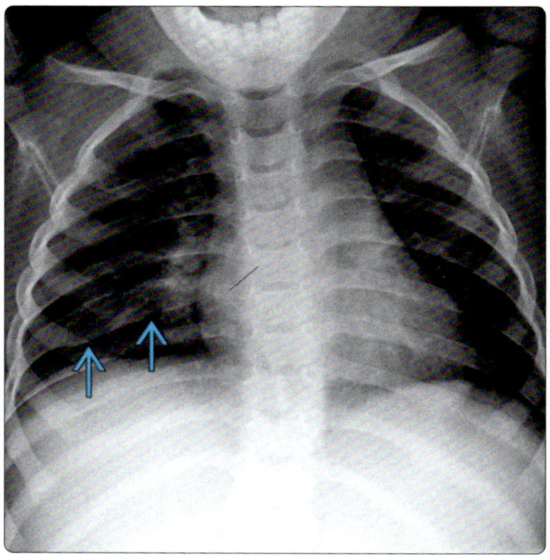

Langerhans Cell Histiocytosis

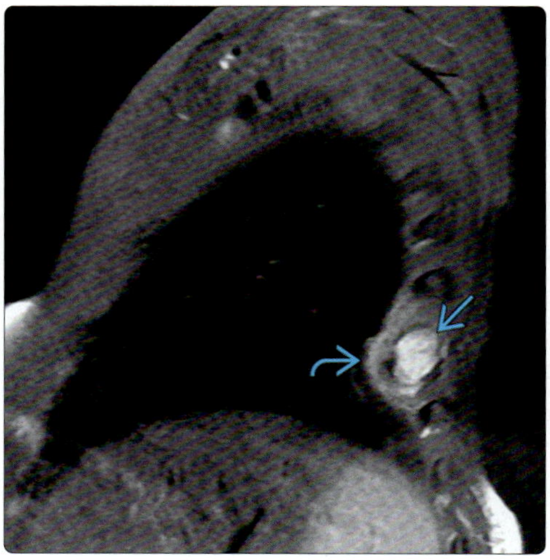

(Left) *Axial CECT in a 21 month old shows a relatively nonenhancing solid soft tissue mass ⇨ of the chest wall with deeper invasion ⇨. Biopsy confirmed a rhabdomyosarcoma.* **(Right)** *Coronal STIR MR in a 17 year old with neurofibromatosis type 1 shows numerous lobulated high signal intensity lesions of the chest wall, arms, & retroperitoneum along the courses of nerves. Many lesions show the typical target sign of plexiform neurofibromas with hypointense centers ⇨.*

Rhabdomyosarcoma

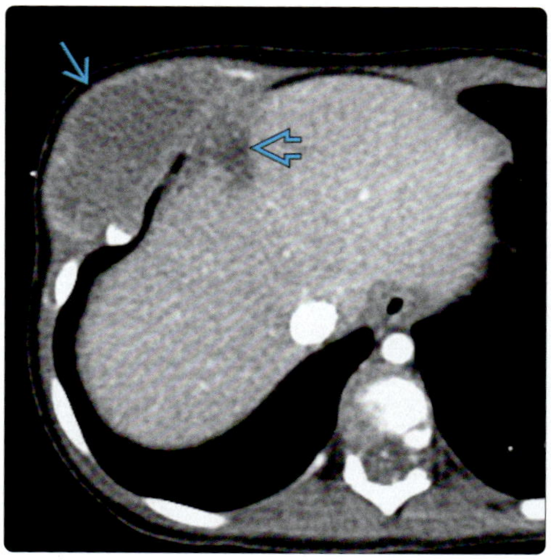

Plexiform Neurofibromas

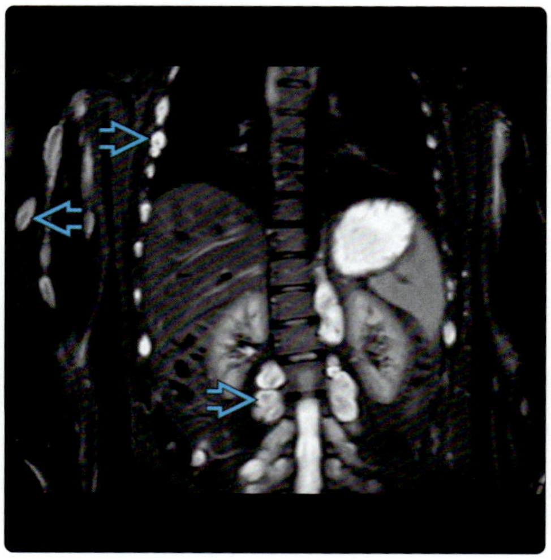

(Left) *Axial NECT in a 15 year old with multifocal fibrous dysplasia shows a classic mildly expansile lesion of the right 8th rib with a ground-glass matrix ⇨. An additional bubbly lucent focus ⇨ is seen in the 6th rib.* **(Right)** *Transverse color Doppler US in a 16 year old with a painful protuberance shows apparent lobulation of the anterior rib ⇨ with an overlying avascular hypoechoic mass ⇨.*

Fibrous Dysplasia

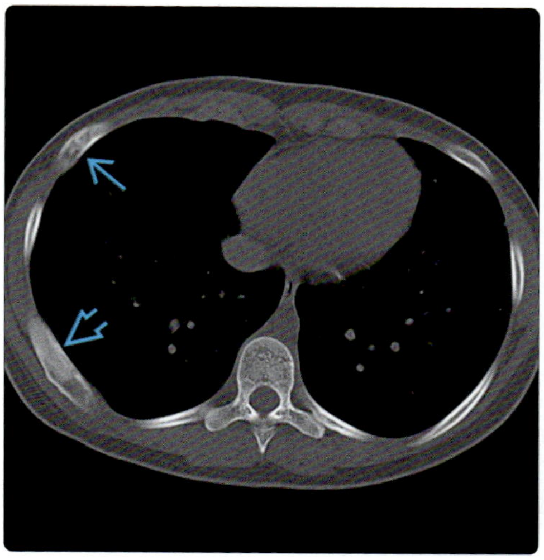

Osteochondroma

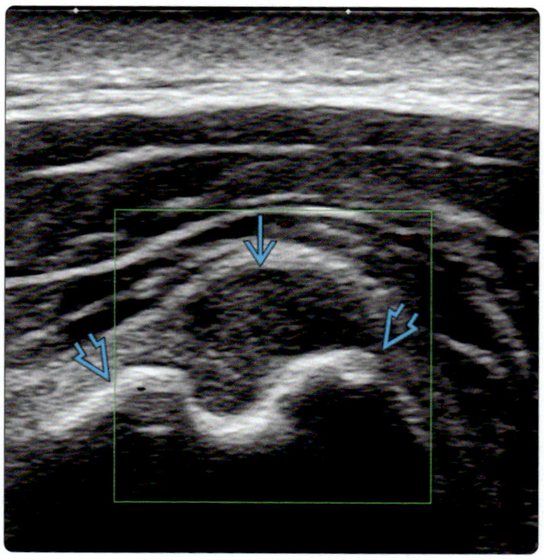

Osteochondroma

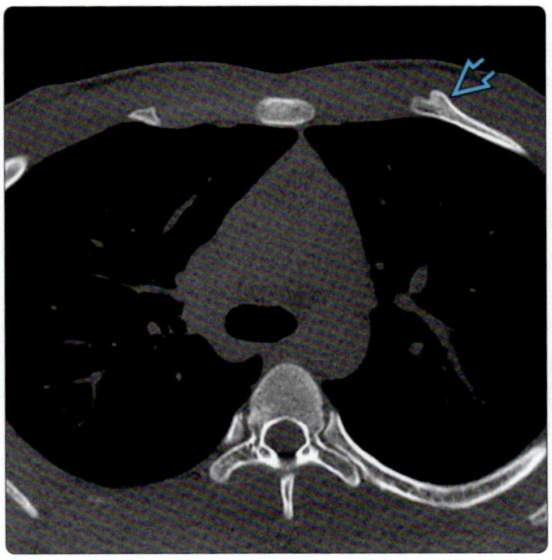

Infection

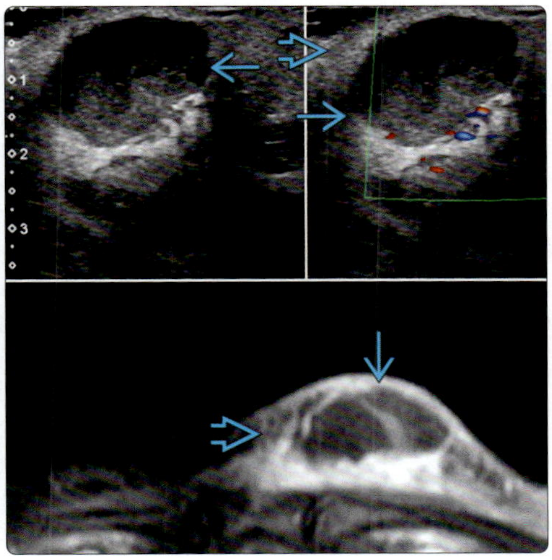

(Left) *Axial NECT in the same patient shows an exostosis ⇨ with corticomedullary continuity from the underlying rib. The hypoechoic focus on US was due a to cartilage cap. Unlike this case, rib osteochondromas pointing inward can lead to hemo/pneumothorax.* **(Right)** *US & axial T1 C+ FS MR in a 2 year old show an avascular mass with enhancing wall ⇨ & surrounding soft tissue inflammation ⇨. Swirling internal echoes were seen upon compression, consistent with fluid. The abscess was due to Actinomyces.*

Desmoid

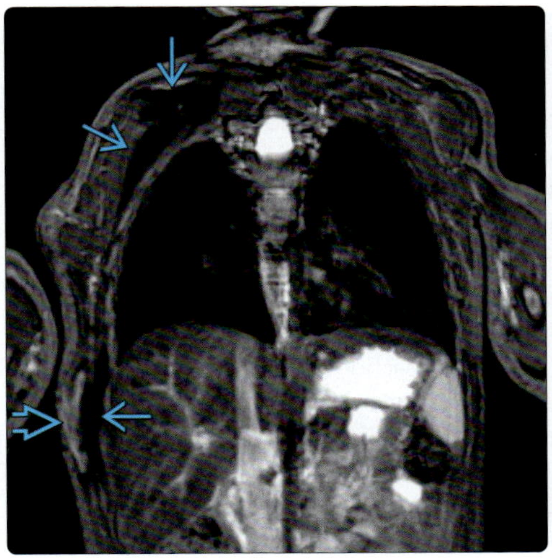

Osteosarcoma

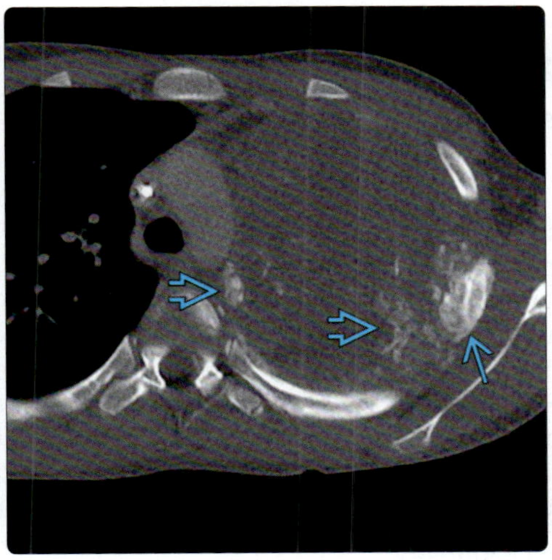

(Left) *Coronal STIR MR in a 30 month old shows 2 elongated soft tissue lesions of the chest wall, both of which contain very low signal intensity components ⇨ due to collagen in fibromatosis. The more inferior lesion also has a higher signal superficial component ⇨, which is more typical of an active cellular lesion.* **(Right)** *Axial CECT in a 14 year old with chest pain shows a destructive lesion of a lateral left rib ⇨. Abnormal soft tissue fills the left hemithorax & demonstrates abundant osteoid formation ⇨ from an osteosarcoma.*

Dermoid

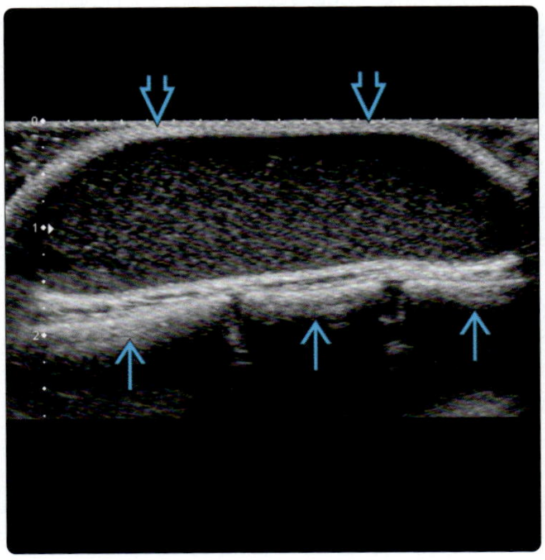

Mesenchymal Hamartoma of Chest Wall

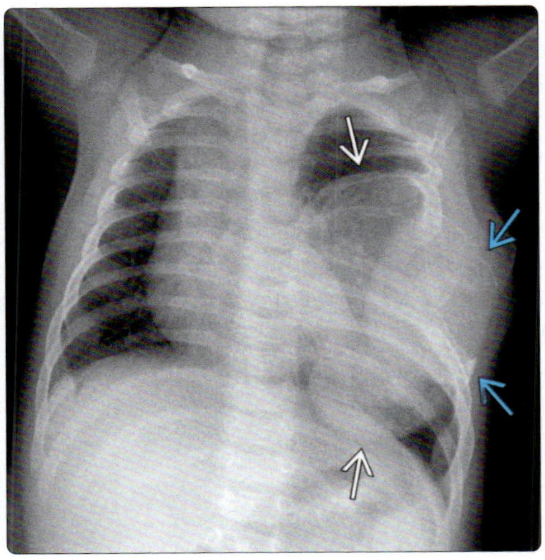

(Left) *Longitudinal US of the chest in a 4 year old shows a well-defined elongated, unilocular thick-walled collection ⇨ anterior to the sternal ossification centers ⇨. Swirling internal debris was noted upon compression. Resection confirmed a dermoid.* **(Right)** *AP radiograph in an infant shows a large soft tissue mass ➡ distorting multiple ribs in bizarre ways ⇨ (including erosion, splaying, & expansion). The findings are typical of a mesenchymal hamartoma.*

DIFFERENTIAL DIAGNOSIS

Common

- Chest Wall Asymmetry/Rib Fusion Anomaly
- Healing Fracture

Less Common

- Osteochondroma
- Fibrous Dysplasia
- Chronic Recurrent Multifocal Osteomyelitis
- Osteomyelitis (Pyogenic)
- Langerhans Cell Histiocytosis
- Ewing Sarcoma
- Enchondroma
- Aneurysmal Bone Cyst
- Metastasis

Rare but Important

- Lymphoma/Leukemia
- Osteosarcoma
- Osteoblastoma
- Lymphatic Anomalies

ESSENTIAL INFORMATION

Key Differential Diagnosis Issues

- Flat bones
  - Skull/face (e.g., occipital, parietal, frontal, nasal)
  - Chest wall/shoulder girdle (e.g., ribs, sternum, scapula)
    - Clavicle is technically long bone, but clavicular tumors are more typical of flat vs. long bone lesions
  - Pelvis (e.g., ilium, ischium, pubis)
- Flat bones typically function to protect internal organs (e.g., skull → brain, ribs/sternum → heart/lungs)
- Red marrow persists in many flat bones through childhood
- Aggressive lesion in pediatric flat bone: Strongly consider Langerhans cell histiocytosis (LCH) or Ewing sarcoma

Helpful Clues for Common Diagnoses

- **Chest Wall Asymmetry/Rib Fusion Anomaly**
  - Painless palpable chest wall "mass" common in children
    - Often erroneously thought to be new/rapidly growing
    - Most are due to asymmetries of rib cartilages
    - Others may be rib fusion anomalies (e.g., bifid rib)
    - Can be confirmed with radiographs &/or ultrasound
    - CT/MR is typically **not** needed, particularly if painless
- **Healing Fracture**
  - Healing flat bone fracture with callus can mimic mass
  - Should be differentiated from pathologic fracture
  - Rib, sternal, & scapular fractures in young children are very concerning for nonaccidental injury (i.e., child abuse)

Helpful Clues for Less Common Diagnoses

- **Osteochondroma**
  - Common benign bone lesion arising from displaced growth cartilage
  - Most common in long bone metaphyses (70%); less common in ribs, scapula, pelvis
  - Pedunculated or sessile with cortical & medullary continuity to parent bone
    - May appear as U-shaped rim of sclerosis when viewed en face
  - Cartilage cap thickness is variable during childhood
  - Malignant degeneration is very rare in childhood
    - Growth after skeletal maturity or pain raises concern for malignant degeneration
      - Pain is more commonly due to exostosis fracture or irritation of overlying soft tissues
- **Fibrous Dysplasia**
  - Monostotic or polyostotic expansile lesion with endosteal scalloping & lucent to ground-glass matrix
  - McCune-Albright: Precocious puberty, café au lait spots, & polyostotic fibrous dysplasia
- **Chronic Recurrent Multifocal Osteomyelitis**
  - Multifocal nonpyogenic inflammatory bone lesions with relapsing/remitting course
  - Most common sites: Tibia, femur, spine, pelvis, clavicle
    - Medial clavicular lesion strongly suggest of chronic recurrent multifocal osteomyelitis (CRMO)
  - Radiographic features may be mixed at presentation
    - Acute: Lytic lesion (usually in metaphysis near physis)
    - Late: Progressive adjacent sclerosis
    - Recurrence: New lytic areas or periosteal reaction
  - MR shows increased T2 signal & enhancement of lesion & surrounding marrow
    - ± soft tissue & periosteal inflammation
    - ± reactive adjacent joint effusion/synovitis
    - No abscess
- **Osteomyelitis (Pyogenic)**
  - Microbial infection of bone
  - Most common organism: *Staphylococcus aureus*
  - Radiographic changes may take up to 10-14 days
    - Earlier: Soft tissue swelling
    - Later: Periosteal reaction & lytic lesions
- **Langerhans Cell Histiocytosis**
  - Idiopathic proliferation of atypical Langerhans cells
  - Axial skeleton lesions
    - Well-defined lytic skull lesion(s) without sclerotic rim
    - One of most common causes of vertebra plana
  - Appendicular skeleton lesions
    - Variable nonaggressive to aggressive appearance
    - Frank osteolysis ("punched-out" lytic lesion) is typical
  - MR shows enhancing tissue filling bone defect without substantial extraosseous extension
    - May show low T2 signal rim at bone-lesion margin with surrounding marrow edema but relatively little soft tissue inflammation
  - LCH should be considered in differential diagnosis for most aggressive pediatric bone lesions due to variable appearance
- **Ewing Sarcoma**
  - Age: Classically 10-25 years old, but 2-10 year age range is not uncommon
    - 90% before age 20 years
  - Ewing sarcoma family of tumors (ESFT)
    - Includes: Skeletal & extraskeletal Ewing sarcoma
    - Askin tumor: Extraskeletal Ewing sarcoma that occurs in chest wall/thoracopulmonary region
      - Classically arises in chest wall soft tissues; less commonly from bone or periphery of lung
      - May invade pleural space, ribs, lung

   - If teenager presents with opacified hemithorax & permeative destruction of 1 rib, favor Askin tumor
- Greater propensity for flat bones & diaphyses vs. other primary bone malignancies
- Ill-defined, lytic, permeative bone lesion with aggressive periosteal reaction (lamellated, "onion skin," interrupted)
  - May create "ghost" of flat bone with entire bone expanded, permeated, & demineralized
  - Often has large soft tissue component, particularly in pelvis

- **Enchondroma**
  - Most common: Small tubular hand/foot bones & ribs
    - Typically central diaphysis in long bones
  - Well-defined lucent lesion with chondroid matrix, endosteal scalloping, marginal sclerosis
    - Chondroid matrix may be visible as punctate foci, arcs, or rings of Ca^{2+}
    - ± mild expansile remodeling of bone
- **Aneurysmal Bone Cyst**
  - Cystic bone lesion with blood-filled spaces
    - Can occur de novo as primary lesion
    - Also secondary to other bone tumors
  - Expansile, septated lesion ± periosteal reaction
    - Fluid-fluid levels seen on CT & MR with thin septations
  - Most commonly occur in metaphyses of long bones
  - Less commonly occur in flat bones
- **Metastasis**
  - Osseous metastases in children
    - Neuroblastoma, lymphoma/leukemia, & sarcomas are most common
    - Medulloblastoma & clear cell sarcoma of kidney are uncommon but classic
  - Metastatic bone disease typically looks similar regardless of type of malignancy
    - Lytic/permeative lesions; less likely sclerotic or mixed
    - MR shows well-defined lesions of variable size against normal T1 fatty yellow marrow
      - Neuroblastoma & leukemia/lymphoma may have more diffuse & confluent marrow replacement

Helpful Clues for Rare Diagnoses

- **Lymphoma/Leukemia**
  - Usually disseminated disease
  - Lymphoma may rarely be primary of bone
    - Typically radiolucent & permeative with interrupted periosteal reaction
    - ± regions of sclerosis
- **Osteosarcoma**
  - Most common malignant primary bone tumor in children & young adults
  - Rarely occurs in flat bones
  - Ill-defined tumor with cloud-like osteoid matrix, cortical destruction, & aggressive periosteal reaction
    - Osteoid matrix extending from bone lesion into overlying soft tissues is virtually pathognomonic
- **Osteoblastoma**
  - Benign osseous lesion with osteoid production
  - Related to osteoid osteoma (but > 1.5 cm)
  - Often found in vertebral column
  - Expansile & lucent with cortex usually preserved ± internal Ca^{2+}
- **Lymphatic Anomalies**
  - May be focal or part of more extensive process
    - Generalized lymphatic anomaly (GLA) shows multifocal cystic bone lesions ± soft tissue & splenic lesions, ± chylous effusions
    - Gorham-Stout disease shows aggressive osteolysis, often at multiple adjacent bones, due to microcystic lymphatic malformation

SELECTED REFERENCES

1. Bloem JL et al: Bone and soft tissue tumors of hip and pelvis. Eur J Radiol. 81(12):3793-801, 2012
2. Girish G et al: Imaging review of skeletal tumors of the pelvis malignant tumors and tumor mimics. ScientificWorldJournal. 2012:240281, 2012
3. Girish G et al: Imaging review of skeletal tumors of the pelvis--part I: benign tumors of the pelvis. ScientificWorldJournal. 2012:290930, 2012
4. Nam SJ et al: Imaging of primary chest wall tumors with radiologic-pathologic correlation. Radiographics. 31(3):749-70, 2011

Chest Wall Asymmetry/Rib Fusion Anomaly

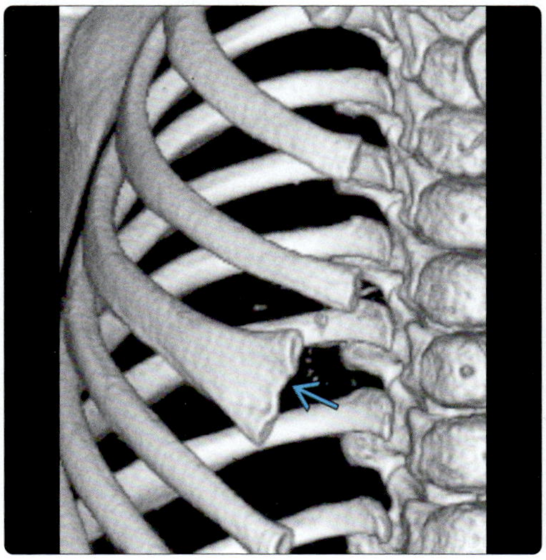

Healing Fracture

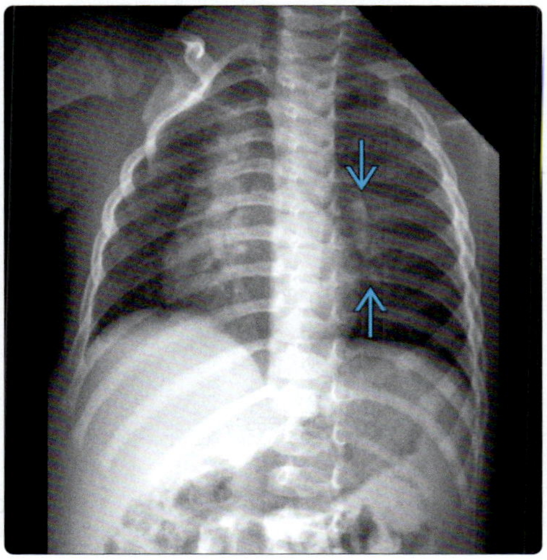

(Left) *Anterior 3D projection of a bone CT from a 4-year-old boy with a palpable chest wall abnormality shows a bifid 4th right rib ⇒. Rib anomalies are common, occurring in up to 3% of the population.* **(Right)** *Anterior oblique radiograph in a 4-month-old girl shows healing posterior left 6th, 7th, & 8th rib fractures ⇒ with callus formation at the fracture sites. Posterior rib fractures have a high specificity for nonaccidental injury. A child advocacy work-up confirmed that this child was abused.*

(Left) *Lateral radiograph in a 6-year-old boy with a palpable left chest wall mass shows a subtle ossific density* ⇨ *projecting over 1 of the ribs.* **(Right)** *Axial bone CT in the same patient shows an exophytic bony lesion extending from the anterior aspect of a left rib. The lesion has cortical* ⇨ *& medullary* ➡ *continuity with the underlying bone that is characteristic of osteochondromas (a.k.a. exostoses). If rib osteochondromas project inward, they can cause pleural irritation & hemopneumothorax.*

Osteochondroma

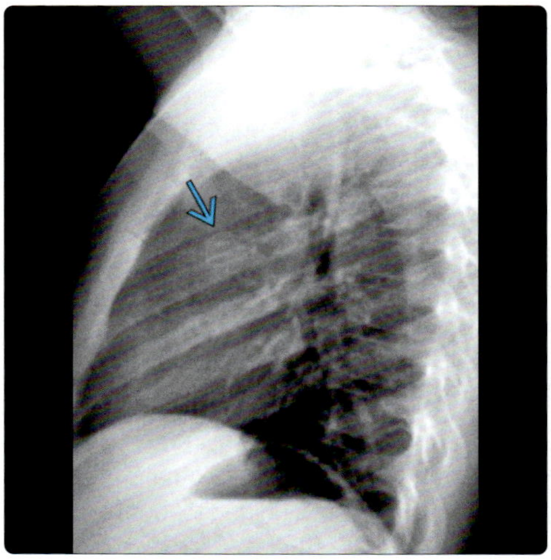

Osteochondroma

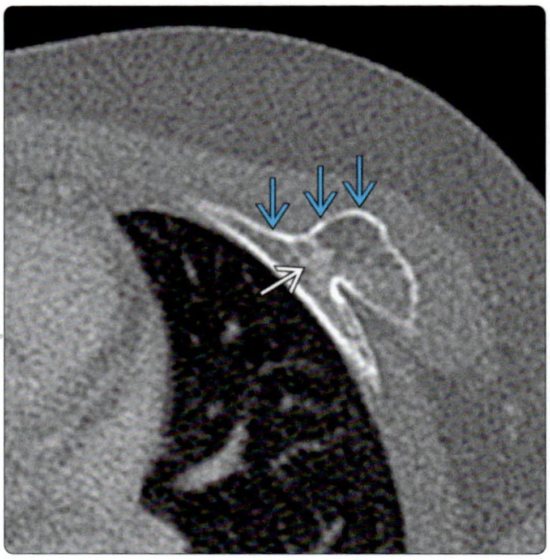

(Left) *Axial T2 FS (left) & T1 C+ FS (right) MR images in a patient with fibrous dysplasia show heterogeneity of an anterior 6th-rib lesion* ⇨ *with intermediate to low T2 signal in an 8th-rib lesion* ⇨*. Enhancement is present within both lesions* ⇨*, typical of active disease.* **(Right)** *Axial bone CT in the same patient shows internal heterogeneity of the right anterior 6th-rib lesion* ⇨ *while the 8th-rib lesion* ⇨ *shows the classic ground-glass internal matrix of fibrous dysplasia.*

Fibrous Dysplasia

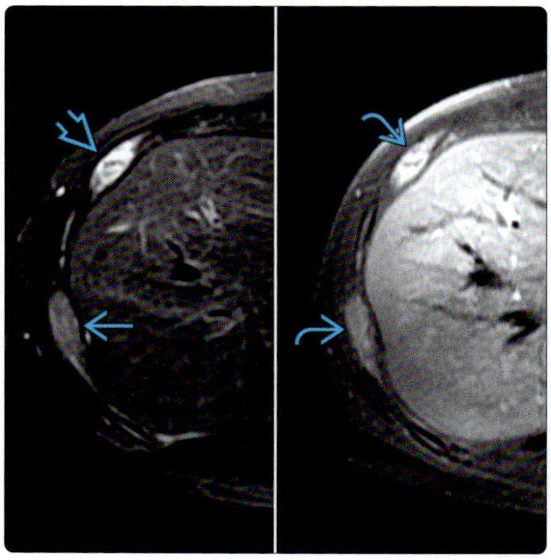

Fibrous Dysplasia

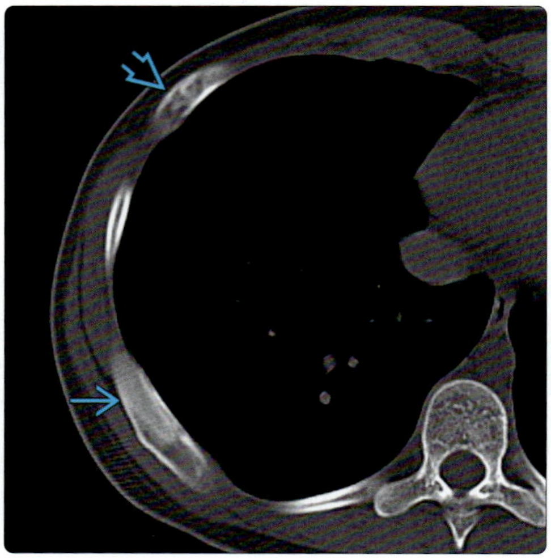

(Left) *AP radiograph (top) in a 4-year-old girl with right clavicle pain shows expansion & permeation of the right medial clavicle* ⇨*. Coronal STIR MR (bottom) shows increased marrow signal with periosteal reaction* ⇨ *& adjacent soft tissue inflammation* ⇨*. She also had other bone lesions (not shown) typical of CRMO.* **(Right)** *Sagittal oblique T2 FS MR in a 1 year old with chest wall swelling & redness shows a large abscess* ⇨ *originating from an infected 5th rib* ⇨*. MRSA was confirmed upon drainage.*

Chronic Recurrent Multifocal Osteomyelitis

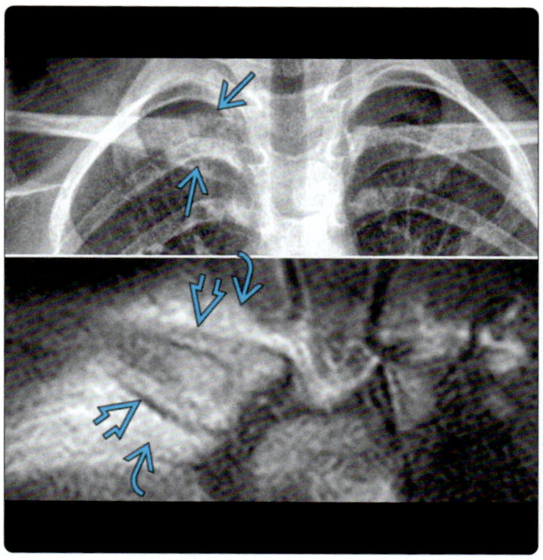

Osteomyelitis (Pyogenic)

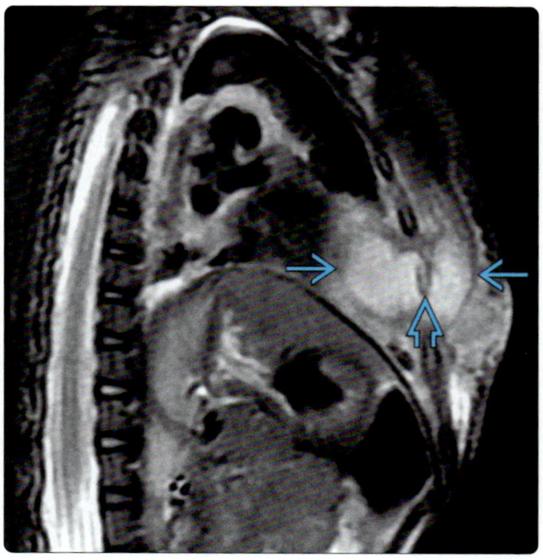

Langerhans Cell Histiocytosis

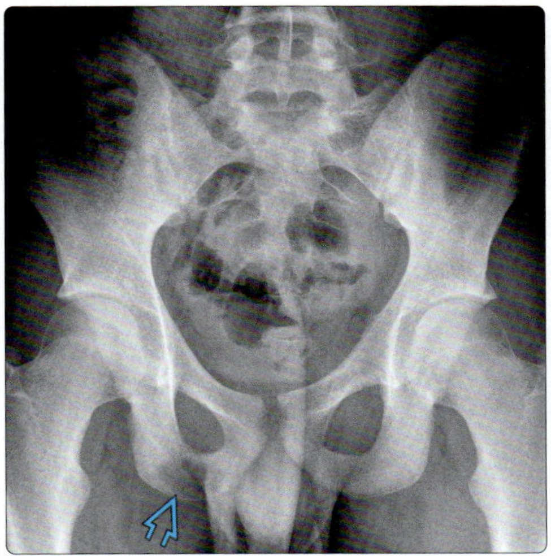

Langerhans Cell Histiocytosis

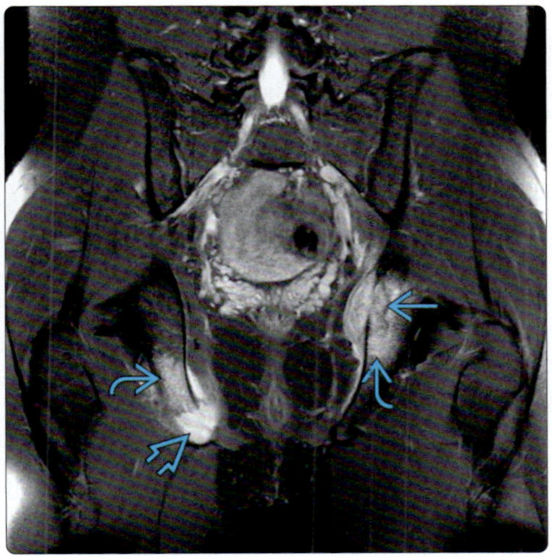

(Left) *AP radiograph in a 15 year old with hip pain shows a lucent lesion with a wide zone of transition in the right ischium .* **(Right)** *Coronal T2 FS MR in the same patient shows destructive lesions in the right & left ischial bones extending into the overlying soft tissues & producing moderate surrounding marrow edema . Langerhans cell histiocytosis was confirmed on biopsy.*

Ewing Sarcoma

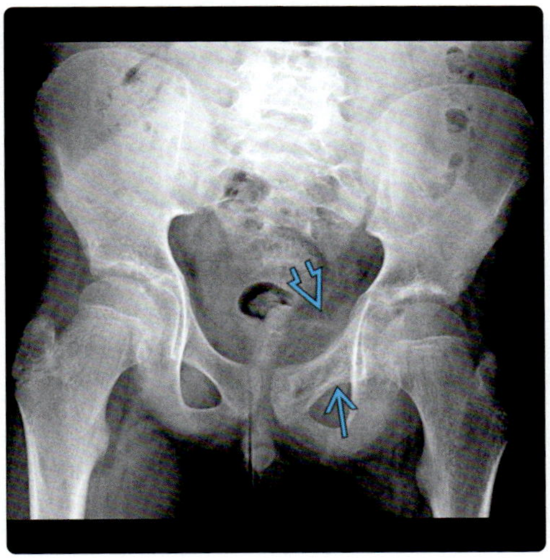

Ewing Sarcoma

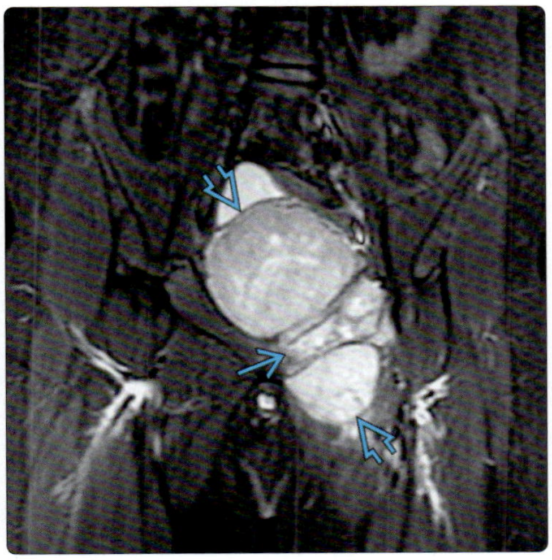

(Left) *AP radiograph in a 10-year-old boy with left hip pain shows expansion & mottling of the left superior pubic ramus with associated periosteal reaction . A soft tissue mass displaces the obturator fat pad .* **(Right)** *Coronal T2 FS MR in the same child shows a permeative, mildly expansile tumor in the right superior pubic ramus with large soft tissue components extending superiorly & inferiorly. Pathology confirmed the diagnosis of a Ewing sarcoma.*

Ewing Sarcoma

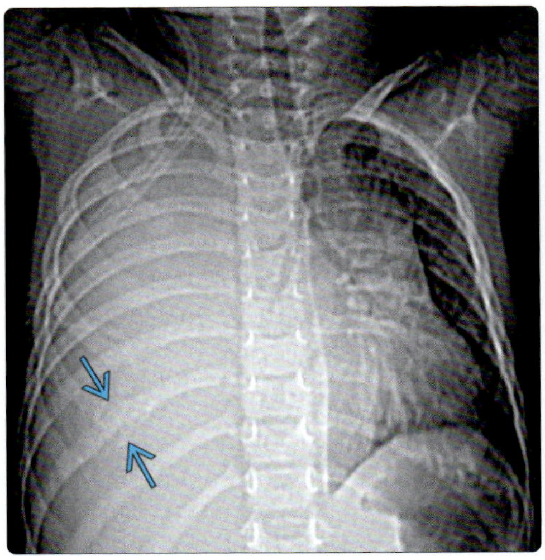

Ewing Sarcoma

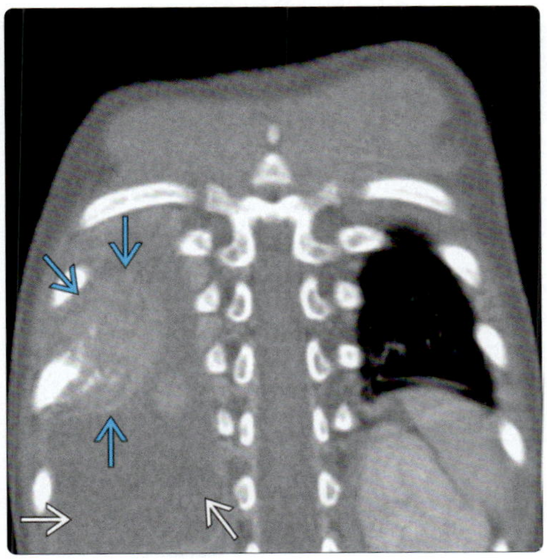

(Left) *Scout CT in a 2 year old with respiratory distress shows opacification of the right hemithorax with leftward shift of the mediastinum. Note the aggressive, expansile lesion in the right 9th rib .* **(Right)** *Coronal reformatted CT in the same patient shows an expansile, destructive right 9th-rib mass . The tumor invaded the right pleural space with an associated large pleural effusion . Chest wall Ewing sarcomas (a.k.a. Askin tumors) classically arise from the soft tissues rather than the rib.*

(Left) *Frontal radiograph shows a rounded mass ⇨ inseparable from an anterior rib with suggestion of internal* Ca^{2+}*. The palpable mass was noticed a few days prior.* **(Right)** *Axial NECT in the same patient shows an irregular, expanded, cupped anterior rib ➡ at the costochondral junction. Note the small* Ca^{2+} *↪ within the soft tissue mass ⇨. This mass was pathologically proven to be an enchondroma.*

Enchondroma

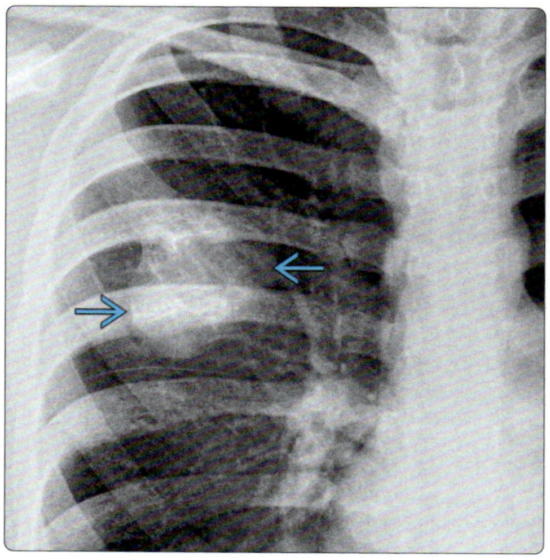

Enchondroma

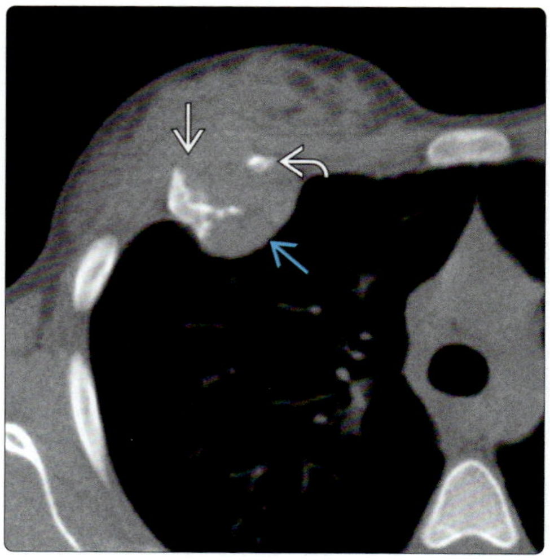

(Left) *Scout CT in a 10 year old with a left upper chest wall mass shows an expansile lesion arising from the anterior right 2nd rib ⇨.* **(Right)** *Sagittal T2 FS MR in the same child shows an expansile lesion of the right 2nd rib that is predominately cystic. Note the layering fluid-fluid levels within the lesion ⇨ typical of an aneurysmal bone cyst.*

Aneurysmal Bone Cyst

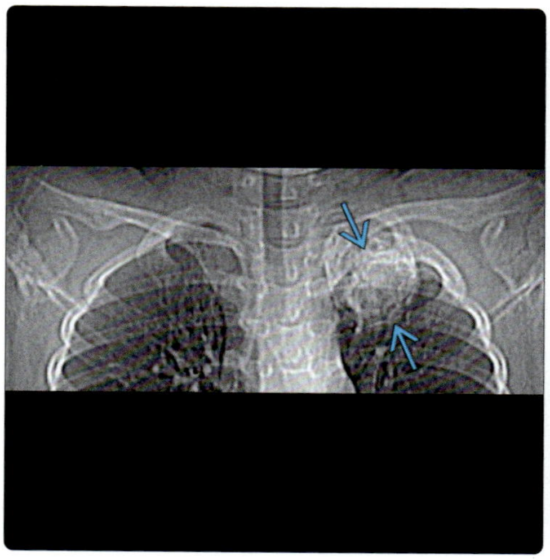

Aneurysmal Bone Cyst

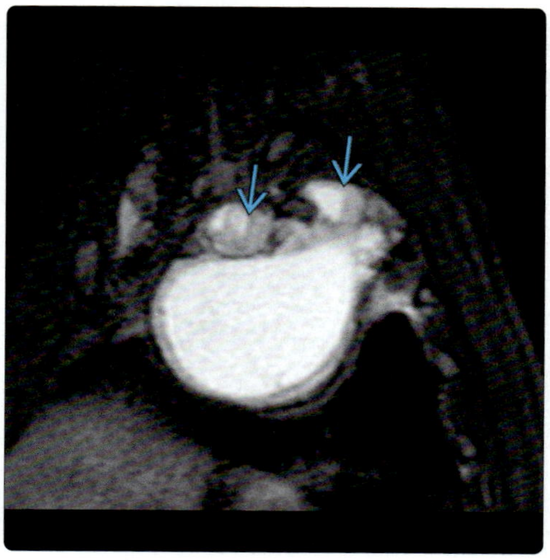

(Left) *Coronal T2 FS (left) & T1 (right) MR images in a 4 year old who presented with left hip pain & a limp show diffuse marrow replacement ⇨ that is most commonly due to leukemia or neuroblastoma in children.* **(Right)** *Axial CECT of the abdomen in the same child shows a midline mass ⇨ that is encasing the aorta & renal arteries & invading the renal hilum ⇨. These findings are characteristic of neuroblastoma, which typically presents with an abdominal mass but can present with pain from osseous metastases.*

Metastasis

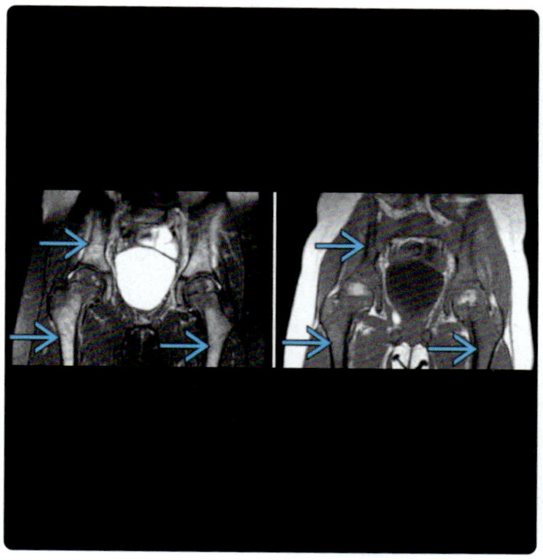

Metastasis

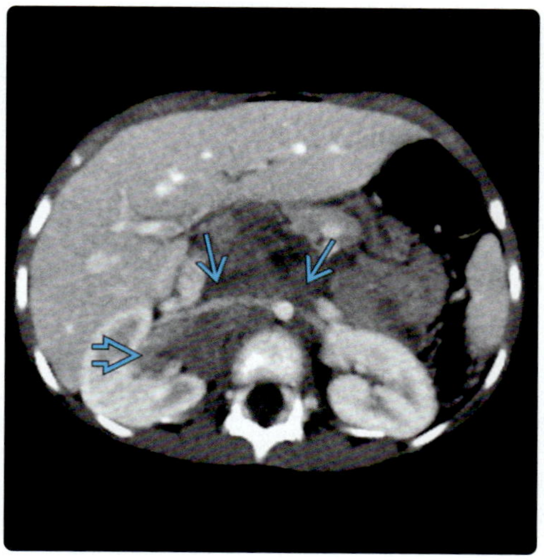

Metastasis

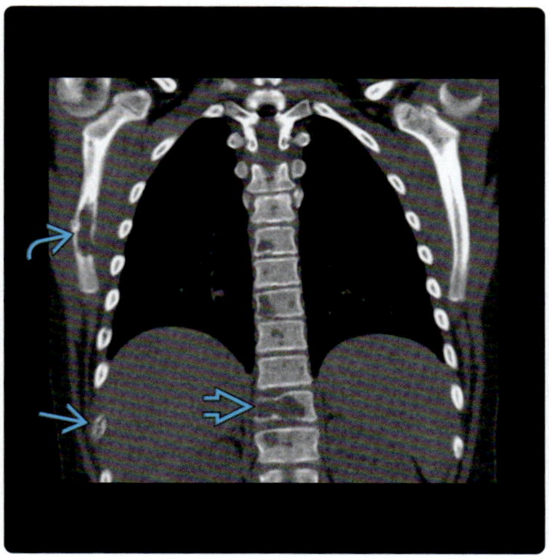

Osteosarcoma

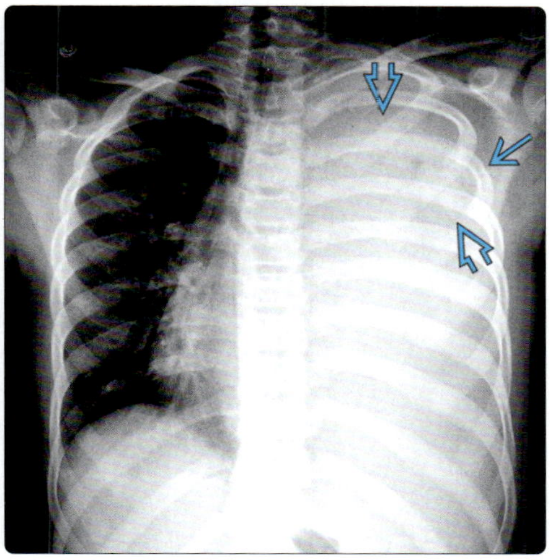

(Left) *Coronal NECT of the chest in a 12 year old with metastatic rhabdomyosarcoma shows multiple lytic lesions throughout the vertebral bodies, right 9th rib, & right scapula. Note the pathologic fracture of the 10th vertebral body.* **(Right)** *Frontal radiograph in a 14 year old shows complete left hemithorax opacification with rightward mediastinal shift. There are subtle destructive changes of the left 4th rib with intrathoracic foci of osteoid matrix due to an osteosarcoma.*

Osteoblastoma

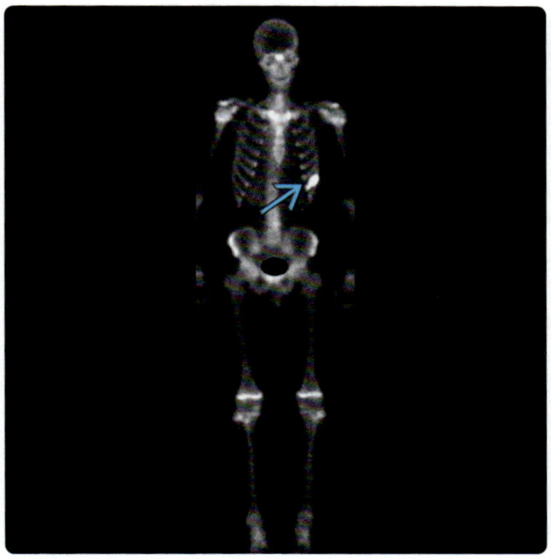

Osteoblastoma

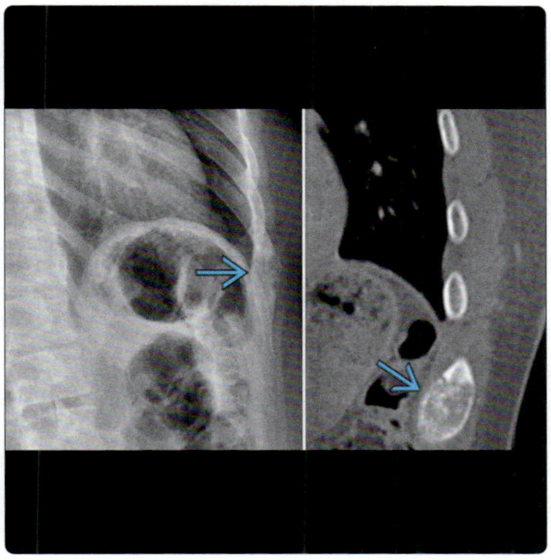

(Left) *Anterior Tc-99m nuclear bone scan in a 15 year old with left rib pain shows an area of increased radiotracer uptake in the right 6th anterior rib due to an osteoblastoma.* **(Right)** *Oblique radiograph (left) & coronal reformatted CT (right) of the left ribs in a patient with pain show an expansile lesion of the right 7th rib. Internal Ca^{2+} can be seen on both the radiograph & the CT. Biopsy proved osteoblastoma.*

Lymphoma/Leukemia

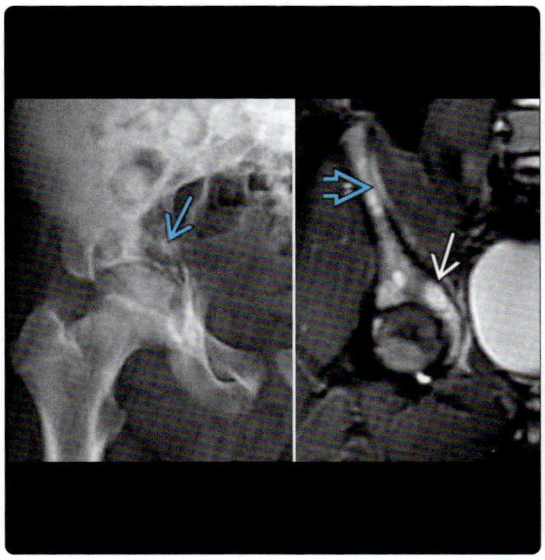

Lymphatic Anomalies

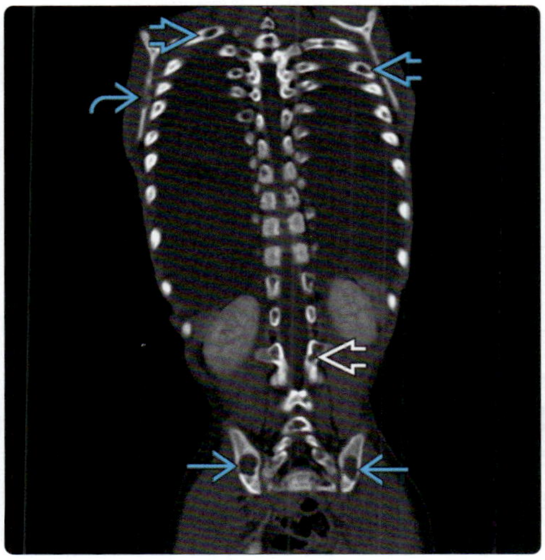

(Left) *Radiograph (left) of the right hip in a 14 year old shows an aggressive right acetabular lesion. Coronal STIR MR (right) shows lesions in the acetabulum & right ilium. Biopsy revealed lymphoma.* **(Right)** *Coronal CECT of a 4 year old with shortness of breath shows large, bilateral pleural effusions & numerous osseous lytic lesions, including the scapula, ribs, vertebrae, & iliac bones. Splenic lesions were also noted (not shown). Generalized lymphatic anomaly was ultimately confirmed.*

DIFFERENTIAL DIAGNOSIS

Common

- Surfactant Deficiency Disease
- Meconium Aspiration Syndrome
- Pulmonary Interstitial Emphysema
- Asthma
- Pulmonary Hypoplasia
- Pneumomediastinum (Mimic)
- Iatrogenic Pneumothorax
- Spontaneous Pneumothorax
- Trauma
- Artifact (Mimic)

Less Common

- Cystic Fibrosis
- Langerhans Cell Histiocytosis
- Tuberous Sclerosis Complex

Rare but Important

- Cystic Lung Lesion (Mimic)
- Ex Vacuo Pneumothorax
- Metastatic Neoplasm
- Infection
- Marfan Syndrome
- Ehlers-Danlos Syndrome

ESSENTIAL INFORMATION

Key Differential Diagnosis Issues

- History is extremely helpful in determining possible source of pneumothorax
  - Trauma, asthma, recent instrumentation
- Appearance of pneumothorax depends on position of patient & amount of pleural gas
  - In supine patient, air collects anteromedially
    - Sharp, well-delineated cardiac & mediastinal borders
  - In upright patient, air collects laterally & apically
    - Radiolucent space lacking pulmonary vascular markings
    - Curvilinear white pleural line is visible
- Size of pneumothorax is difficult to accurately estimate on chest radiograph
- Signs of tension pneumothorax
  - Depressed/inverted hemidiaphragm
  - Contralateral shift of mediastinum
  - Expansion of spaces between ribs
- Expiratory, decubitus, & cross-table lateral views may all aid in diagnosis in equivocal cases
  - Ultrasound may also be useful, demonstrating lack of "lung sliding"
- Mimics of pneumothorax: Skin folds, external materials, pneumomediastinum, & air-filled lung lesion

Helpful Clues for Common Diagnoses

- **Surfactant Deficiency Disease**
  - Premature neonates
  - Extensive granular opacities with hypoinflation
  - Air leak from alveolar rupture can lead to pneumothorax
- **Meconium Aspiration Syndrome**
  - History of meconium-stained amniotic fluid is helpful
  - Coarse interstitial & patchy opacities with hyperinflation
  - Pneumothorax may result from air-trapping & alveolar rupture
- **Pulmonary Interstitial Emphysema**
  - Due to barotrauma from mechanical ventilation in premature neonates, often with surfactant deficiency
  - Alveolar rupture results in pneumothorax & interstitial gas
    - Reticular & cystic parenchymal lucencies
- **Asthma**
  - Airway narrowing & mucous plugging lead to air-trapping & alveolar rupture
  - History of asthma exacerbation is helpful
  - ± hyperinflation, peribronchial thickening
- **Pulmonary Hypoplasia**
  - Potter syndrome in newborn
    - Fetal urinary anomalies → oligohydramnios → pulmonary hypoplasia & typical abnormal facies
  - Pneumothorax may result from progressive air leaks &/or mechanical ventilation
- **Pneumomediastinum (Mimic)**
  - Air localized to mediastinum from ruptured alveolus or aerodigestive tract
  - Central lucencies with pleural line lateral to main pulmonary artery & aortic arch
  - Vertical lucencies tracking on either side of superior mediastinum into neck
  - May result in spinnaker sail sign, continuous diaphragm sign, ring around artery sign
- **Iatrogenic Pneumothorax**
  - Mechanical ventilation
  - Instrumentation, such as central line placement or thoracentesis
  - Resection of space-occupying mass leaves gas-filled cavity that eventually fills with fluid
- **Spontaneous Pneumothorax**
  - May affect healthy newborns
  - Other major population is teenage males
    - Often due to rupture of apical blebs
      - Coronal reformatted CT of lung apices is typically diagnostic
      - Blebs can be resected to prevent recurrence
- **Trauma**
  - Pneumothorax may result from blunt or penetrating trauma
  - May also result from rupture of pneumatocele from old trauma
  - Motor vehicle crashes, falls, & sports injuries are common etiologies
  - Other signs of trauma: Fractures, pulmonary contusions, mediastinal injuries, pleural effusions
- **Artifact (Mimic)**
  - Skin fold
    - Line extends beyond thoracic cavity into soft tissues
    - Lung markings are still visible laterally
  - Shadows under upper ribs
    - Companion shadows: Due to tangential imaging of parietal pleura & extrapleural soft tissues

- Costal groove: Line from groove in rib in which intercostal arteries & veins run
- Mach effect
  - Edge-enhancement at border between objects of different density
- Consider decubitus or cross-table lateral view in equivocal cases

Helpful Clues for Less Common Diagnoses

- **Cystic Fibrosis**
  - Chronic mucous thickening leads to bronchiectasis, bronchial wall thickening, mucus plugging, hyperinflation, prominent hila
  - Can lead to airway obstruction & alveolar rupture
  - Superimposed infection increases pneumothorax risk
  - Pneumothorax indicates poor prognosis
- **Langerhans Cell Histiocytosis**
  - Small pulmonary nodules & parenchymal lung cysts
  - Apical reticulonodular pattern
  - Lung cysts may rupture & result in pneumothorax
  - Pulmonary involvement is seen in up to 50% of patients with pulmonary Langerhans cell histiocytosis
    - Look for osseous, thymic, hepatic, & splenic involvement
- **Tuberous Sclerosis Complex**
  - Lymphangioleiomyomatosis with small parenchymal cysts & chylous pleural effusion
  - Pneumothorax in ~ 70%
  - Cerebral subependymal nodules & giant cell astrocytomas, renal angiomyolipomas, cardiac rhabdomyomas

Helpful Clues for Rare Diagnoses

- **Cystic Lung Lesion (Mimic)**
  - Features suggesting underlying lung lesion
    - Curvilinear septations in otherwise lucent hemithorax
      - Congenital pulmonary airway malformation (CPAM), pleuropulmonary blastoma (PPB)
    - Lucency conforms to lobar configuration
      - Congenital lobar overinflation
  - May have mass effect with mediastinal shift & hemidiaphragm depression
  - Placement of chest tube creates undesirable bronchopleural fistula
- **Ex Vacuo Pneumothorax**
  - Occurs adjacent to rapidly developing atelectasis, especially of right upper lobe
    - Abrupt decrease of pleural pressure releases nitrogen from pleural capillaries
    - Gas collects only around collapsed lobe
  - Treated by bronchoscopy with reexpansion of lobe, not chest tube
- **Metastatic Neoplasm**
  - Pneumothorax may occur in presence of metastases, especially when present on pleural surface
  - Seen in children with osteosarcoma & Wilms tumor
- **Infection**
  - Any infection that causes alveolar destruction can lead to pneumothorax
  - Most common with tuberculosis & *Pneumocystis*
- **Marfan Syndrome**
  - Autosomal dominant connective tissue disorder
  - Associations: Aortic aneurysms, kyphoscoliosis, arachnodactyly
- **Ehlers-Danlos Syndrome**
  - Connective tissue disorder
  - Findings similar to Marfan syndrome; more likely to have subcutaneous Ca^{2+} & heterotopic ossification

SELECTED REFERENCES

1. Piccolo CL et al: Diagnostic imaging in pediatric thoracic trauma. Radiol Med. 122(11):850-65, 2017
2. Feinberg A et al: Can congenital pulmonary airway malformation be distinguished from type I pleuropulmonary blastoma based on clinical and radiological features? J Pediatr Surg. 51(1):33-7, 2016
3. Varkki S et al: Isolated pulmonary Langerhans cell histiocytosis. Indian J Pediatr. 80(8):700-3, 2013

Surfactant Deficiency Disease

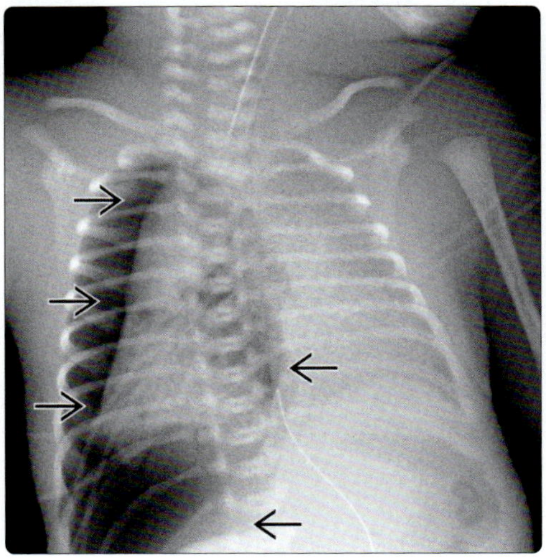

Meconium Aspiration Syndrome

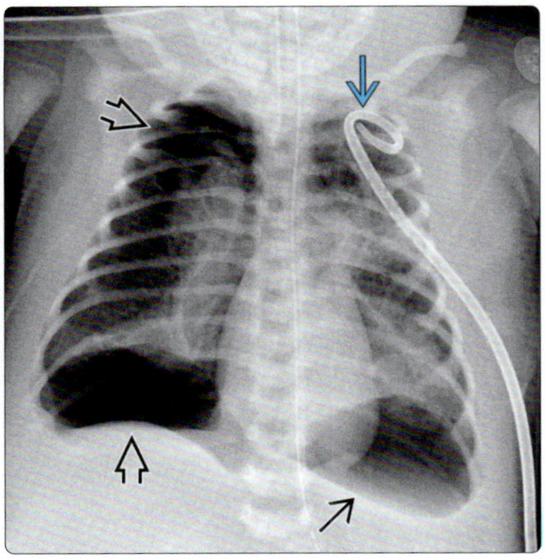

(Left) *AP radiograph shows a large right tension pneumothorax → in this premature neonate with surfactant deficiency disease. Note the granular opacities throughout the lungs.* **(Right)** *AP radiograph shows large bilateral pneumothoraces in this neonate with meconium aspiration. Note the bilateral coarse interstitial lung opacities. The left pneumothorax is localized inferiorly → after placement of a catheter superiorly →. The right pneumothorax → is under tension with depression of the diaphragm.*

(Left) *Frontal radiograph shows a left pneumothorax ⇨ in this premature neonate with pulmonary interstitial emphysema. Note the typical bubbly lucencies throughout the left lung.* **(Right)** *Upright frontal radiograph shows a left apical pneumothorax in a 14 year old suffering an asthma attack. Note the white pleural line ➡ & lack of pulmonary markings superolateral to this line.*

Pulmonary Interstitial Emphysema

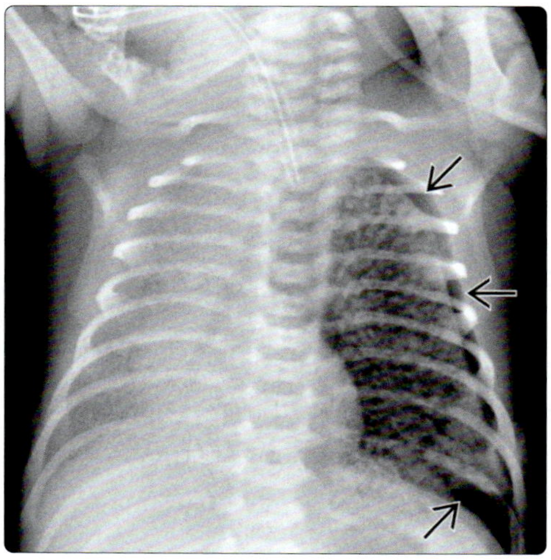

Asthma

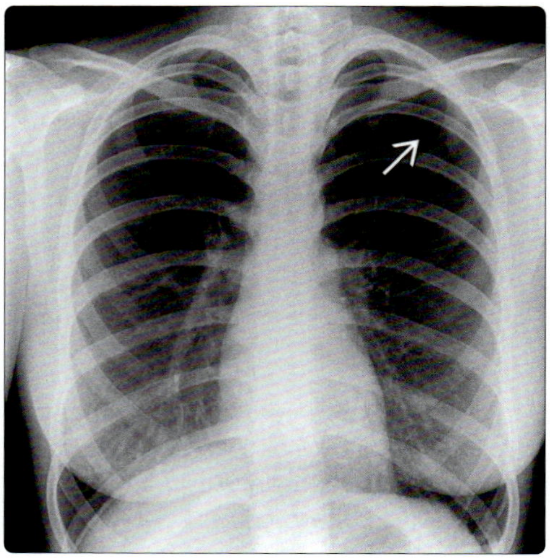

(Left) *AP radiograph in a neonate with Potter syndrome shows a moderate right pneumothorax ➡ with partial collapse of the lung as well as shift of the mediastinum to the left ➡, evidence of tension.* **(Right)** *AP radiograph in a newborn shows a sharply circumscribed lucency ⇨ tracking along the superior cardiac margins, crossing the midline, & elevating the thymic lobes ⇨. This is a typical appearance for pneumomediastinum in a neonate. Note the malpositioned endotracheal tube.*

Pulmonary Hypoplasia

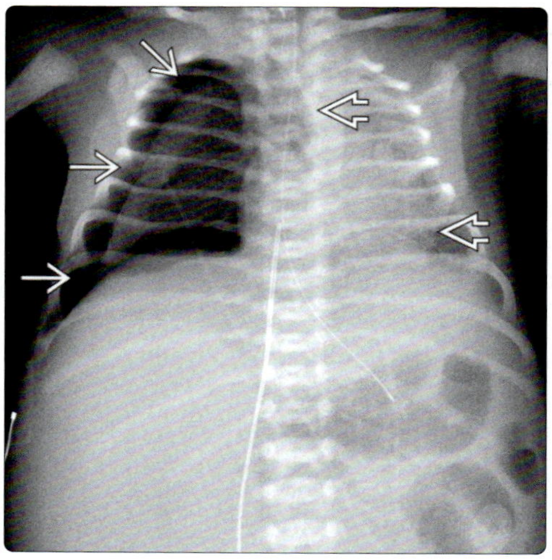

Pneumomediastinum (Mimic)

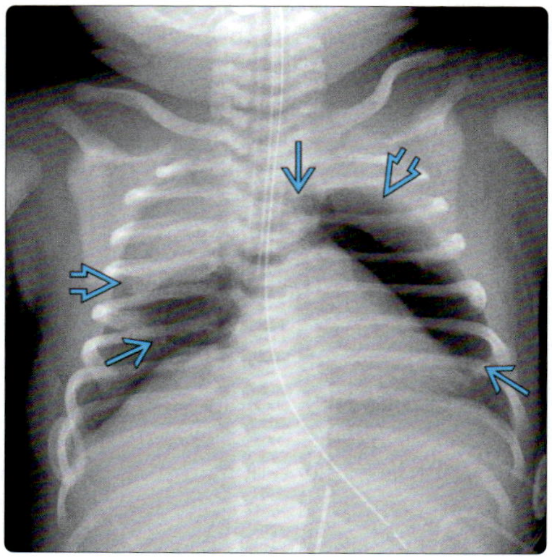

(Left) *AP radiograph shows a small anteromedial right pneumothorax ⇨ in this infant after bilateral chest tube placements for pleural fluid drainage. Note the sharp, well-demarcated right cardiac border ⇨.* **(Right)** *Frontal radiograph shows a small right apical pneumothorax ⇨ in this 10-year-old patient following central line placement by a right subclavian vein approach.*

Iatrogenic Pneumothorax

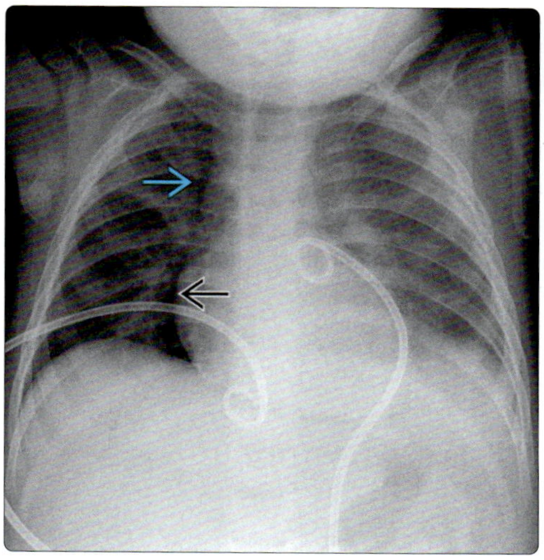

Iatrogenic Pneumothorax

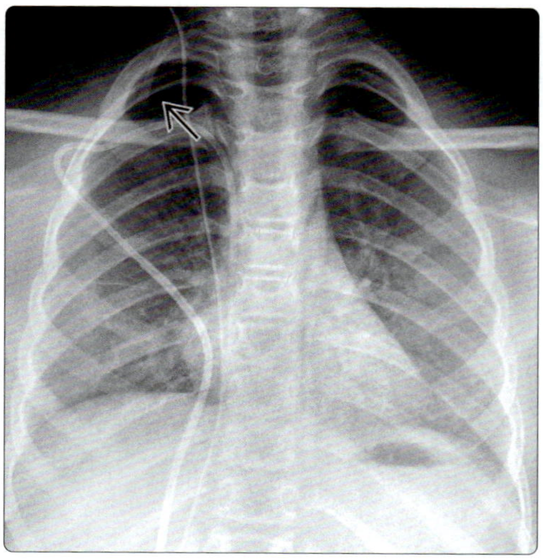

Spontaneous Pneumothorax

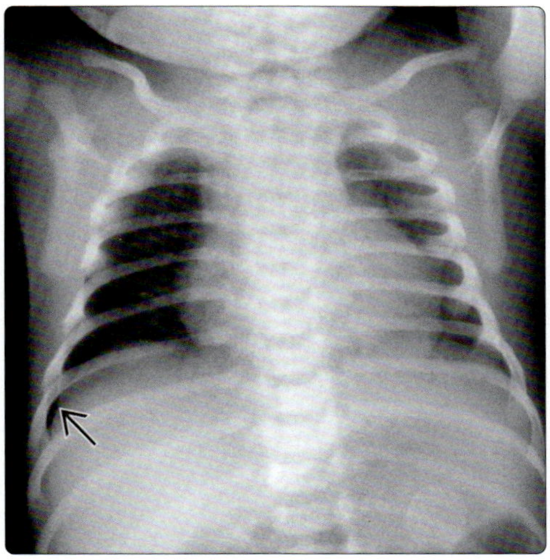

Spontaneous Pneumothorax

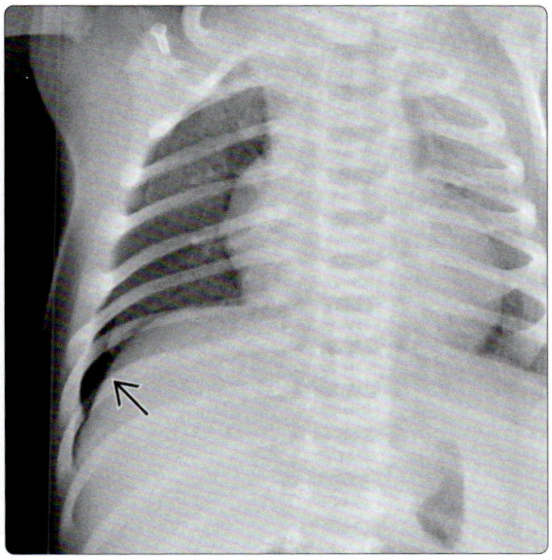

(Left) *Frontal radiograph shows a deep right costophrenic angle ⇨. In a supine patient, pleural gas may collect at the anterior base. When this air collects laterally, it abnormally deepens the costophrenic angle.* **(Right)** *Left lateral decubitus radiograph in the same patient better demonstrates the deep right costophrenic angle ⇨ secondary to an anterolateral pneumothorax. No cause was determined in this newborn.*

Spontaneous Pneumothorax

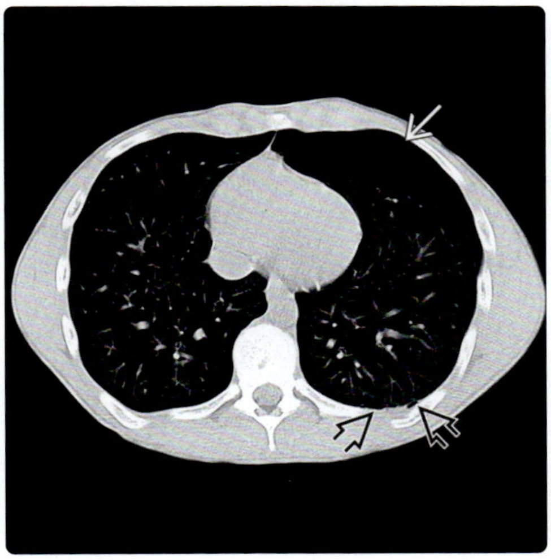

Spontaneous Pneumothorax

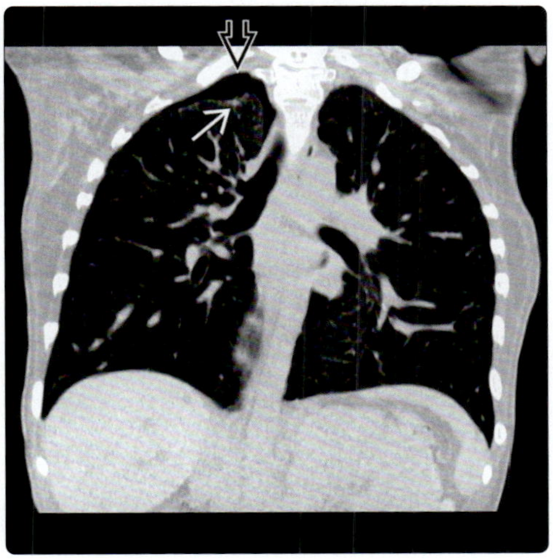

(Left) *Axial NECT shows a small to moderate left pneumothorax ➡, the result of spontaneous rupture of tiny pleural blebs ⇨ in this 17-year-old patient.* **(Right)** *Coronal NECT shows a small right apical pneumothorax ⇨ in this 16-year-old patient. Note the collapsed tiny apical pleural blebs that likely underwent spontaneous rupture ➡. As most blebs leading to spontaneous pneumothorax occur at the apices, the NECT can be targeted to this level.*

Trauma

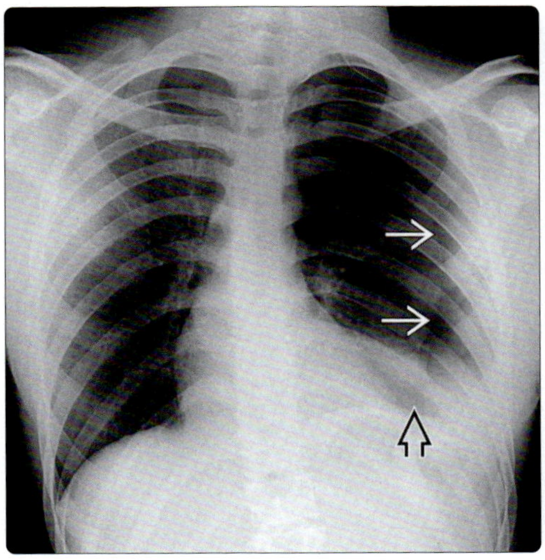

Trauma

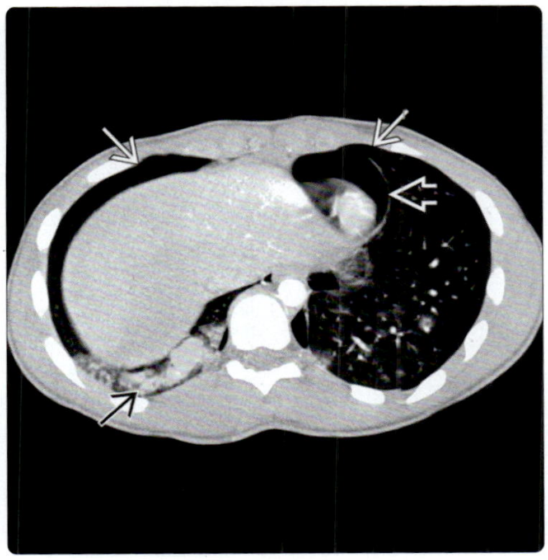

(Left) *Frontal radiograph shows a moderate to large left pneumothorax in this 16 year old following a stab wound. Note the white pleural line ➡ & lack of pulmonary markings beyond this line. The left basilar opacity ⇨ was a combination of atelectasis & pleural fluid.* **(Right)** *Axial CECT shows bilateral small pneumothoraces ➡, pneumomediastinum ➡, & pulmonary contusions ⇨ in this 17-year-old patient after a motor vehicle crash.*

(Left) *AP radiograph shows curvilinear increased lucency along the right ➔ & left ➔ heart borders. This 10 year old was status post biopsy of a right upper lobe nodule ➔. Follow-up imaging confirmed that the lucency was due to Mach effect, not pneumothorax.* **(Right)** *Frontal radiograph shows a linear interface over the right hemithorax ➔. Note the presence of lung markings lateral to this interface as well as the absence of a distinct white pleural line. A decubitus view confirmed that this was a skin fold.*

Artifact (Mimic)

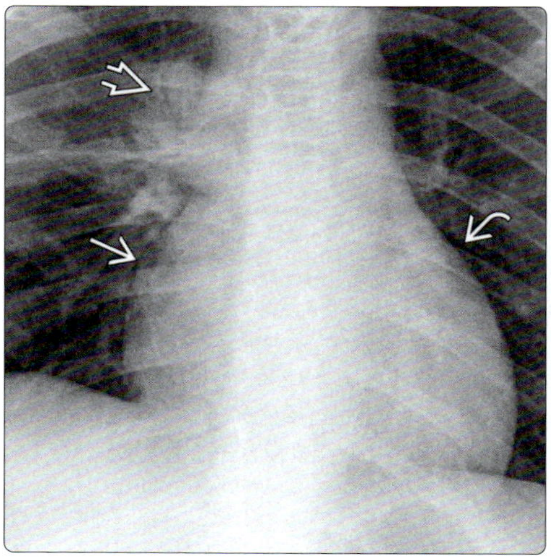

Artifact (Mimic)

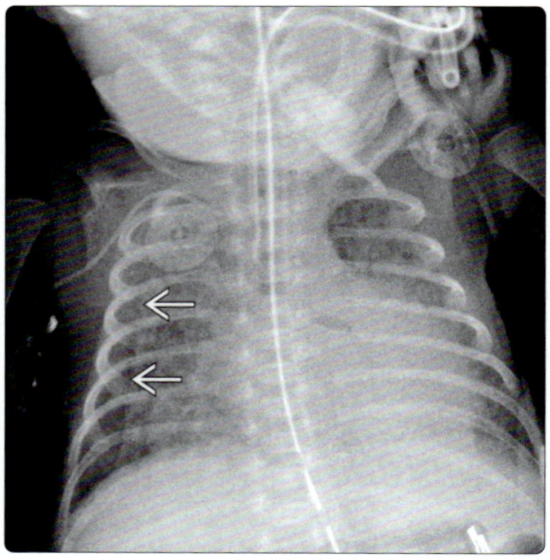

(Left) *Coronal NECT shows diffuse reticulonodular parenchymal lung disease ➔, multiple calcified lymph nodes ➔, & small bilateral pneumothoraces ➔ in this 16-year-old patient with Langerhans cell histiocytosis.* **(Right)** *Axial NECT shows a small anterior left pneumothorax ➔ in this adolescent patient with tuberous sclerosis complex. Note the innumerable small parenchymal lung cysts ➔ bilaterally, consistent with lymphangioleiomyomatosis.*

Langerhans Cell Histiocytosis

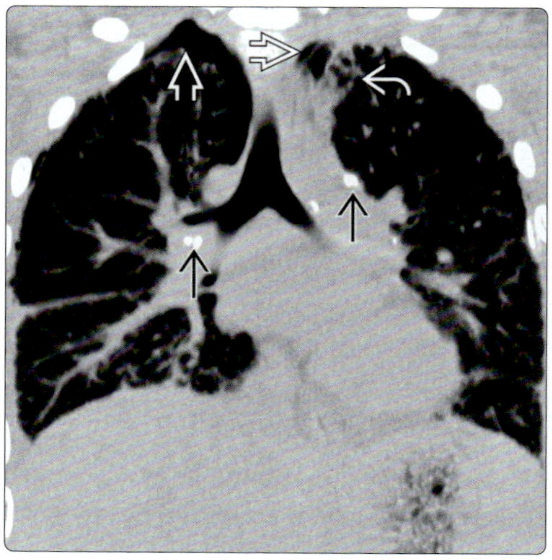

Tuberous Sclerosis Complex

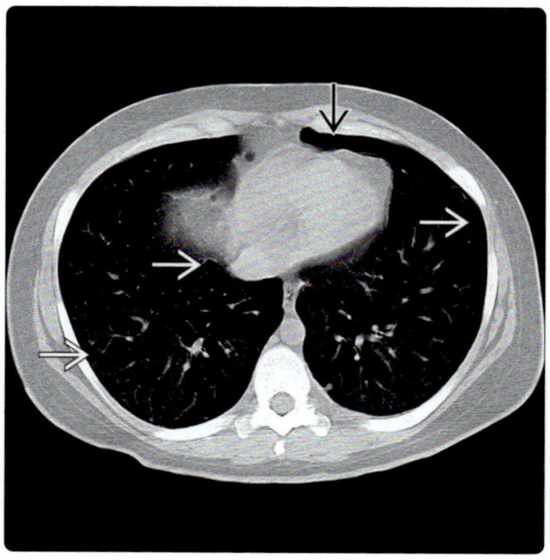

(Left) *PA radiograph for scoliosis in an otherwise asymptomatic 15 year old shows a lucent left upper lobe lesion ➔ that mimics a pneumothorax. Note the subtle septations ➔ in the lesion. There is no significant mass effect.* **(Right)** *Coronal NECT in the same patient shows multiple thin septations ➔ within the cystic lung lesion. There is distortion/hypoplasia of the left upper lobe but no mediastinal mass effect. A type I congenital pulmonary airway malformation (CPAM) was confirmed at resection.*

Cystic Lung Lesion (Mimic)

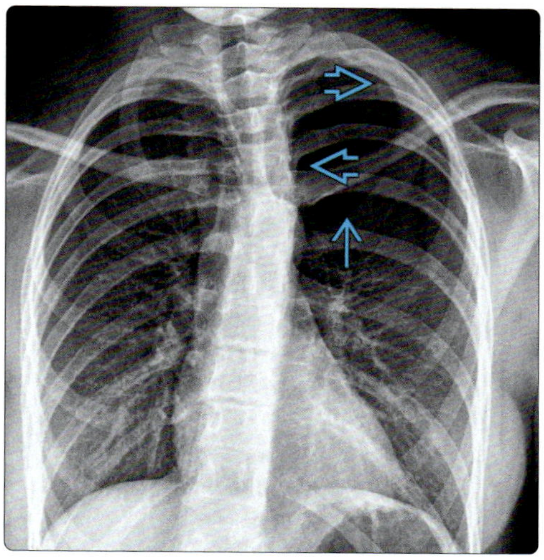

Cystic Lung Lesion (Mimic)

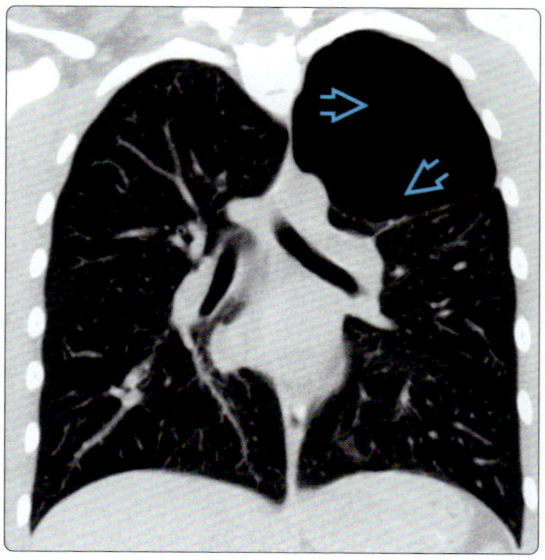

Ex Vacuo Pneumothorax

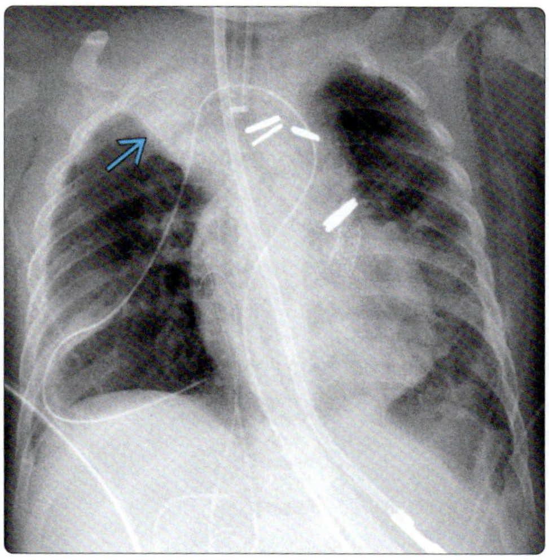

Ex Vacuo Pneumothorax

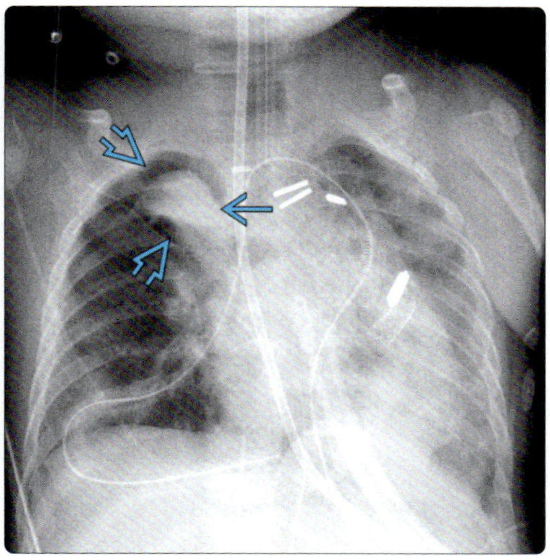

(Left) *Postoperative AP radiograph in a 4 month old with complex congenital heart disease shows complete atelectasis of the right upper lobe* ➔. **(Right)** *AP radiograph in the same patient 24 hours later shows a focal pneumothorax* ➔ *surrounding the collapsed right upper lobe* ➔. *Note that the pneumothorax does not extend inferiorly along the other lobes. The correct treatment for an ex vacuo pneumothorax is reexpansion of the lung, not placement of a chest tube.*

Metastatic Neoplasm

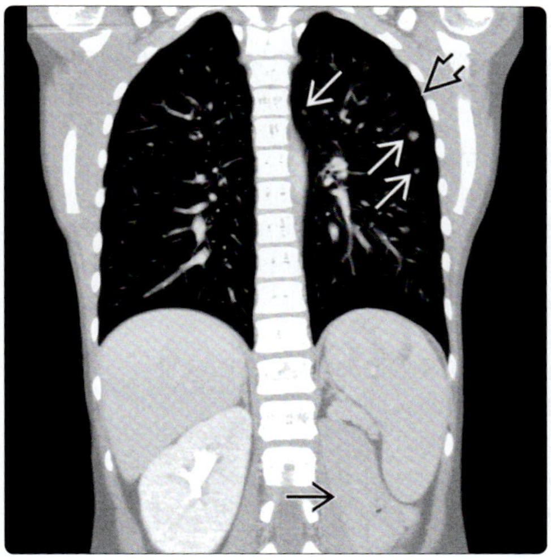

Infection

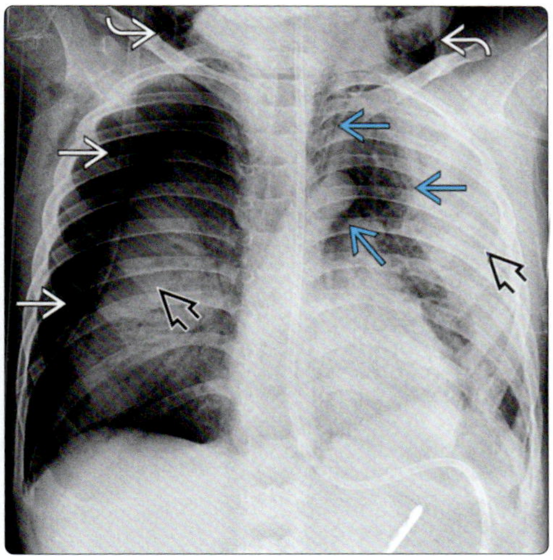

(Left) *Coronal CECT shows a small left pneumothorax* ➔ *& 3 small pulmonary nodules* ➔ *in the left lung. Note the absence of the left kidney* ➔ *in this patient with metastatic Wilms tumor status post nephrectomy.* **(Right)** *Frontal radiograph shows pneumomediastinum* ➔*, subcutaneous emphysema* ➔*, & a right pneumothorax* ➔*. Note the dense consolidative lung disease* ➔ *with air bronchograms in this 6 year old with Pneumocystis pneumonia.*

Infection

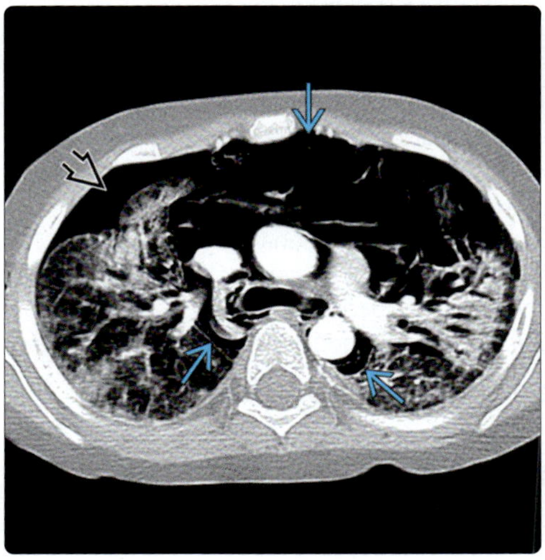

Marfan Syndrome

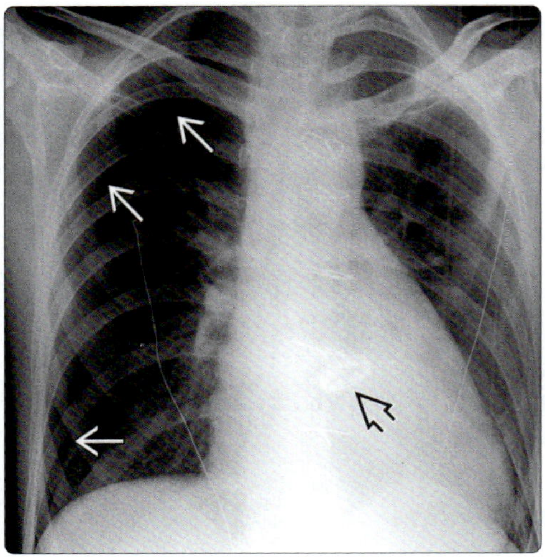

(Left) *Axial CECT of the same patient shows extensive pneumomediastinum* ➔ *& a right pneumothorax* ➔ *associated with scattered areas of parenchymal consolidation & ground-glass opacities.* **(Right)** *Frontal radiograph shows a right-sided pneumothorax* ➔ *in this 18-year-old patient with Marfan syndrome. Note the median sternotomy wires & prosthetic aortic valve* ➔*, clues to the presence of cardiac disease.*

DIFFERENTIAL DIAGNOSIS

Common

- Asthma
- Straining Against Closed Glottis
- Aspiration
- Blunt Chest Trauma
- Iatrogenic
- Surfactant Deficiency Disease
- Pulmonary Interstitial Emphysema

Less Common

- Infection
- Extension of Pneumoperitoneum or Pneumoretroperitoneum

Rare but Important

- Esophageal Perforation
- Illicit Drug Use

ESSENTIAL INFORMATION

Key Differential Diagnosis Issues

- Potential sources for pneumomediastinum
  - Trachea & bronchi
  - Lungs
  - Esophagus
  - Pleural space
  - Head/neck
  - Peritoneal space
  - Retroperitoneal space
- Helpful radiographic signs in pneumomediastinum
  - Thymic spinnaker sail sign: Elevation of thymus in young child by large amount of pneumomediastinum
  - Continuous diaphragm sign: Air trapped posterior to pericardium outlines superior midline diaphragm
  - Ring around artery sign: Air surrounding pulmonary artery branch
  - Air in inferior pulmonary ligament: Retrocardiac extension of pneumomediastinum
  - Double wall sign: Intramural gas along proximal airways
  - Naclerio V sign: Air outlines lateral margin of descending aorta & extends laterally along left hemidiaphragm
  - Associated pneumothorax, pneumopericardium, or subcutaneous emphysema
- Pneumomediastinum is frequently asymptomatic & self-limited
- History is extremely helpful in determining possible source of pneumomediastinum
  - Is there trauma history?
  - Is there history of recent instrumentation?
  - Is patient asthmatic?
- Contrast esophagram is rarely helpful: Majority are negative in setting of blunt trauma or spontaneous pneumomediastinum

Helpful Clues for Common Diagnoses

- **Asthma**
  - Airway narrowing & mucous plugging lead to air-trapping & alveolar rupture
  - Lungs may be normal or hyperinflated
- **Straining Against Closed Glottis**
  - History is helpful
    - Vomiting
    - Giving birth
    - Weight lifting
  - No specific imaging features
- **Aspiration**
  - May lead to air-trapping & alveolar rupture
  - Meconium aspiration
    - History of meconium-stained amniotic fluid
    - Coarse interstitial & patchy opacities with hyperinflation
  - Foreign body aspiration
    - Peanuts are most common in children
    - Frequency of right vs. left bronchial tree involvement is equal in young children
      - Right > left bronchial tree involvement is seen in older children & adults
    - Unilateral hyperinflation > atelectasis
    - Decubitus views can be helpful if radiolucent foreign body is suspected
      - Dependent side should decrease in volume
      - Nondependent side should increase in volume
      - Suspect obstructing foreign body in ipsilateral bronchial tree if dependent side does not decrease in volume
- **Blunt Chest Trauma**
  - Motor vehicle crash, fall, sports injury
  - Due to alveolar rupture &/or tracheobronchial injury
  - Other signs of trauma may be present
    - Fractures
    - Pulmonary contusions
    - Mediastinal injuries
    - Pleural effusions
- **Iatrogenic**
  - Mechanical ventilation
  - Instrumentation can result in
    - Tracheobronchial injury
    - Esophageal injury
  - May be seen in postoperative patients
- **Surfactant Deficiency Disease**
  - Premature neonates with diffuse granular opacities
  - Air leak from alveolar rupture can lead to pneumomediastinum
- **Pulmonary Interstitial Emphysema**
  - Premature infants
  - Barotrauma from mechanical ventilation → alveolar rupture with air leak into pulmonary interstitium
  - Reticular & cystic pulmonary lucencies intermixed with background granular opacities
  - Can progress to pneumomediastinum & pneumothorax

Helpful Clues for Less Common Diagnoses

- **Infection**
  - Mycoplasma pneumonia
    - Common cause of community-acquired pneumonia in children
    - Bronchopneumonia, lobar consolidation; reticulonodular opacities in 52% (more common in lower lobes)

- ☐ Classic CT appearance: Multifocal bronchovascular thickening with centrilobular nodules
  - Can be complicated by alveolar destruction & rupture leading to pneumomediastinum
- o *Pneumocystis* pneumonia
  - Classically seen with HIV/AIDS
  - Bilateral perihilar interstitial infiltrates progressively coalesce to patchy ground-glass opacities
    - ☐ Consolidation & nodules are less common
  - Can result in parenchymal lung cysts, which can rupture & lead to pneumomediastinum
- o Viral bronchiolitis
  - Most common: Respiratory syncytial virus, adenovirus, human metapneumovirus, influenza virus, & parainfluenza virus
  - Bronchiolar inflammation → edema & increased mucus production → airway obstruction → alveolar rupture → pneumomediastinum
  - Background of peribronchial cuffing & hyperinflation are typically present

- **Extension of Pneumoperitoneum or Pneumoretroperitoneum**
  - o No direct constant communication between peritoneal space & mediastinum
  - o Direct communication does exist between retroperitoneal space & mediastinum
    - Esophageal hiatus
    - Aortic hiatus
  - o Pneumomediastinum can result from extension of peritoneal or retroperitoneal gas
    - Perforation of hollow viscous
    - Laparoscopy

Helpful Clues for Rare Diagnoses

- **Esophageal Perforation**
  - o Iatrogenic is most common cause
  - o Other causes
    - Vomiting/retching
    - Penetrating trauma
    - Foreign bodies
    - Toxic ingestion
  - o Lack of serosa increases vulnerability to tear
  - o Reflux esophagitis increases risk
  - o Look for associated pleural effusion
- **Illicit Drug Use**
  - o Various mechanisms purported with different agents

SELECTED REFERENCES

1. Gasser CR et al: Pediatric spontaneous pneumomediastinum: narrative literature review. Pediatr Emerg Care. 33(5):370-74, 2017
2. Richer EJ et al: Are esophagrams indicated in pediatric patients with spontaneous pneumomediastinum? J Pediatr Surg. 51(11):1778-81, 2016
3. Tortajada-Girbés M et al: Spontaneous pneumomediastinum and subcutaneous emphysema as a complication of asthma in children: case report and literature review. Ther Adv Respir Dis. 10(5):402-9, 2016
4. Bejvan SM et al: Pneumomediastinum: old signs and new signs. AJR. 166:1041-8, 1996

Asthma

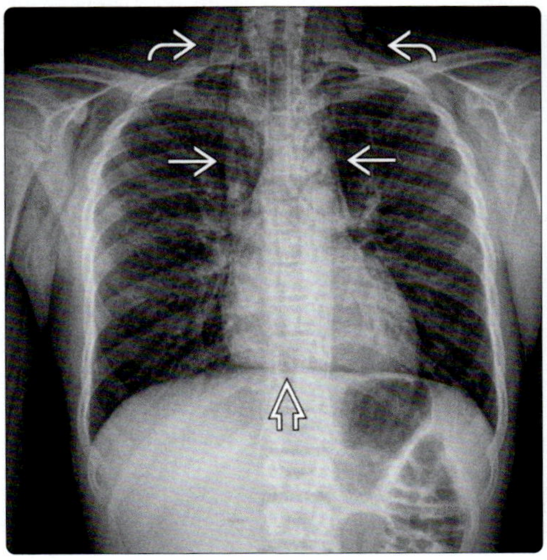

Straining Against Closed Glottis

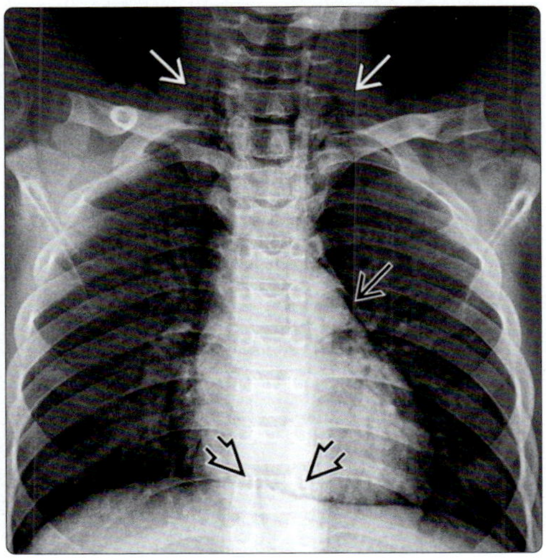

(Left) *AP radiograph obtained on a 14 year old with an asthma exacerbation demonstrates lucency infiltrating & expanding the mediastinum ➡. There is a continuous diaphragm sign ⇨. Subcutaneous emphysema is also noted ↪.* **(Right)** *Frontal radiograph shows curvilinear air along the left mediastinal border ⇨ with a continuous diaphragm sign inferiorly ⇨. There is also subcutaneous emphysema ➡ in the neck in this 9 year old with vomiting.*

(Left) *AP radiograph in a newborn with meconium aspiration shows pneumomediastinum* → *with air tracking across the midline just above the heart & elevating the thymic lobes* →. **(Right)** *Left-side down decubitus view of a 2-year-old patient demonstrates persistent hyperinflation of the left lung* →. *There is pneumomediastinum with elevation of the thymus* → *& subcutaneous emphysema* →. *An aspirated foreign body was removed from the left main bronchus.*

Aspiration

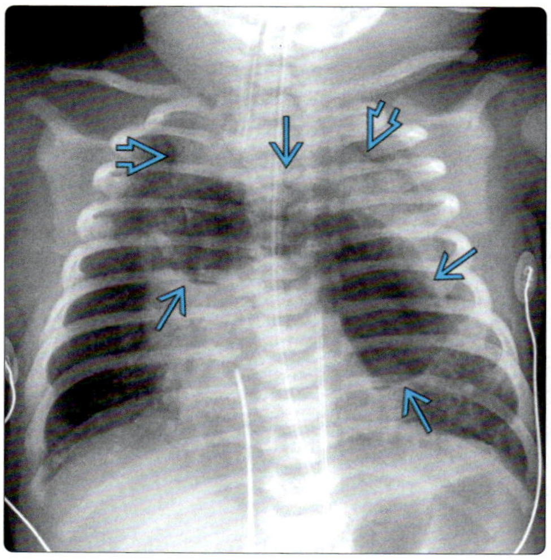

Aspiration

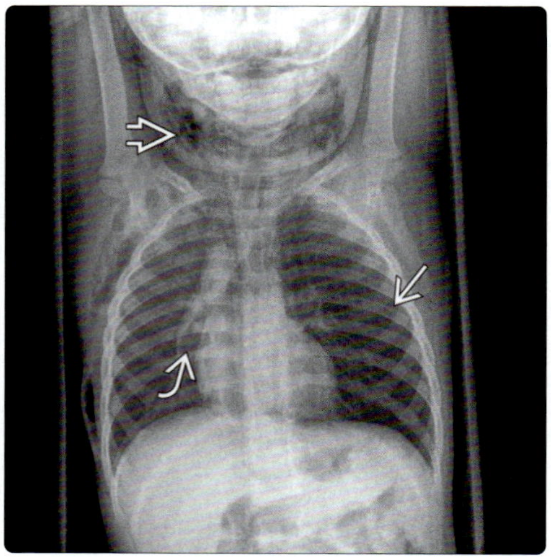

(Left) *AP radiograph shows pneumomediastinum* → *in this 13-year-old patient status post motor vehicle collision. Other findings of trauma include a right clavicle fracture* →, *lung contusion* →, *& subcutaneous emphysema* →. **(Right)** *Axial CECT image from a 5 year old after a bicycle accident shows pneumomediastinum* →, *pulmonary contusions* →, *& subcutaneous emphysema* →.

Blunt Chest Trauma

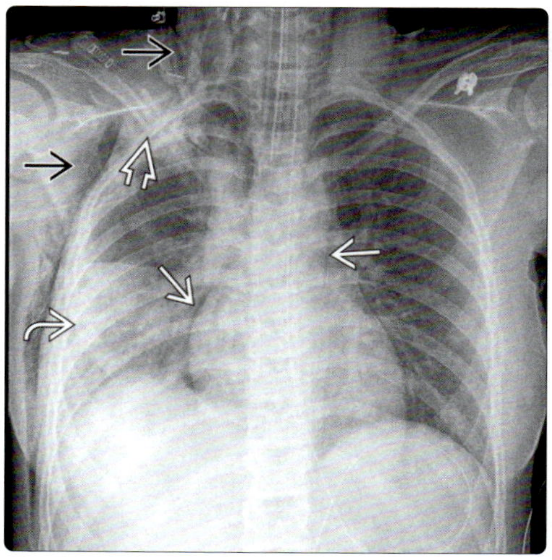

Blunt Chest Trauma

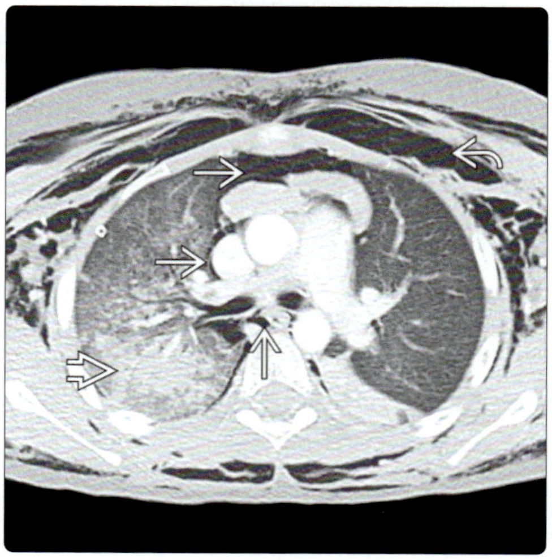

(Left) *Frontal radiograph shows pneumomediastinum with air extending along the inferior pulmonary ligament* → *in this 6-month-old postoperative patient with a tracheostomy. There is a small right pneumothorax* → *as well.* **(Right)** *AP radiograph shows lucency surrounding the mediastinum* → *in this premature 3 day old. Diffuse granular opacities consistent with known surfactant deficiency disease are also seen.*

Iatrogenic

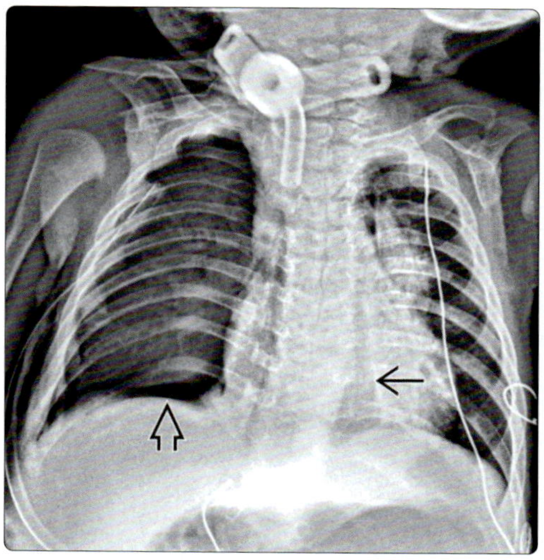

Surfactant Deficiency Disease

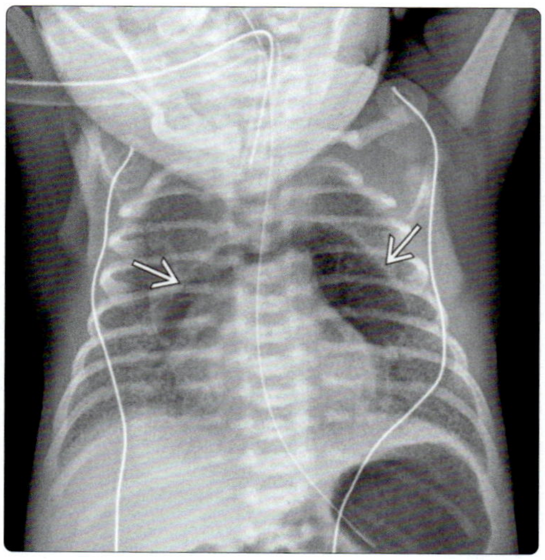

Pulmonary Interstitial Emphysema

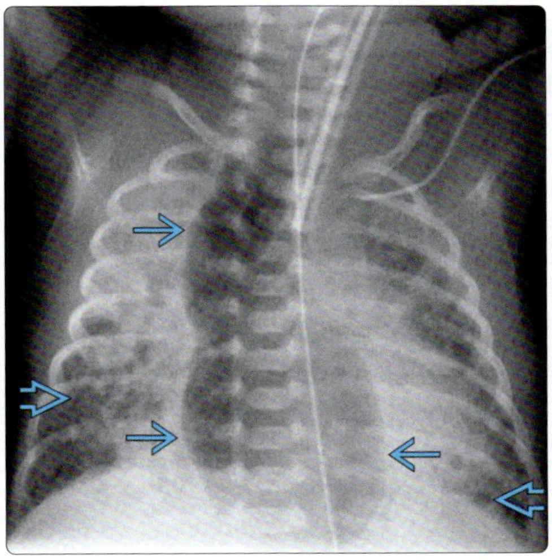

Infection

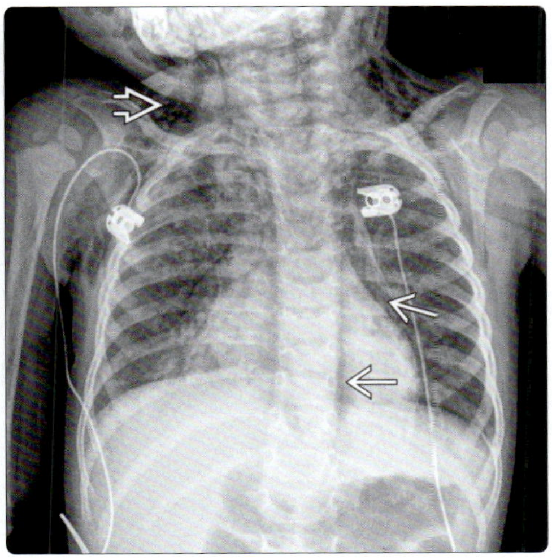

(Left) *AP radiograph in a 9-day-old premature infant with surfactant deficiency shows a large posterior mediastinal air collection →. Note the cystic bubbly lucencies → in the lungs, typical of pulmonary interstitial emphysema.* **(Right)** *Frontal radiograph of a 1 year old with respiratory syncytial virus bronchiolitis demonstrates pneumomediastinum →, subcutaneous emphysema →, & peribronchial cuffing.*

Infection

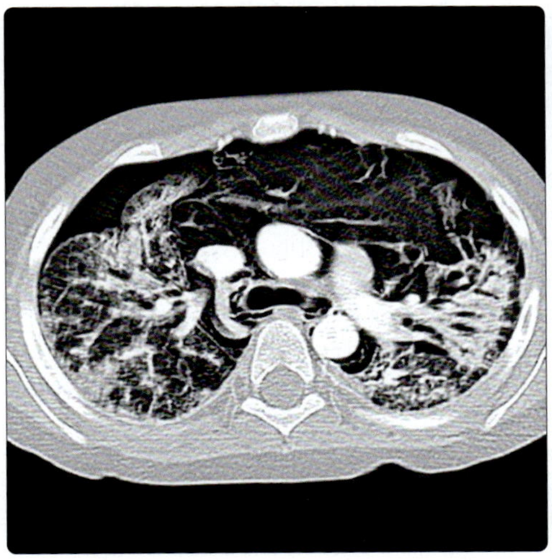

Extension of Pneumoperitoneum or Pneumoretroperitoneum

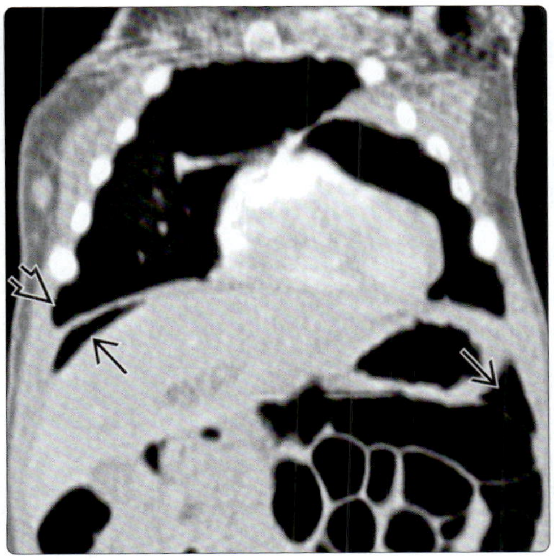

(Left) *Axial CECT shows pneumomediastinum & pneumothorax. There are diffusely scattered areas of airspace density, which indicate nonspecific underlying pulmonary parenchymal disease, in this 6 year old with Pneumocystis pneumonia.* **(Right)** *Coronal CECT shows pneumomediastinum that presumably extended from the pneumoperitoneum → in this 8-week-old abused child with a pancreatic laceration & duodenal injury (not shown). There is a tiny right pneumothorax →.*

Esophageal Perforation

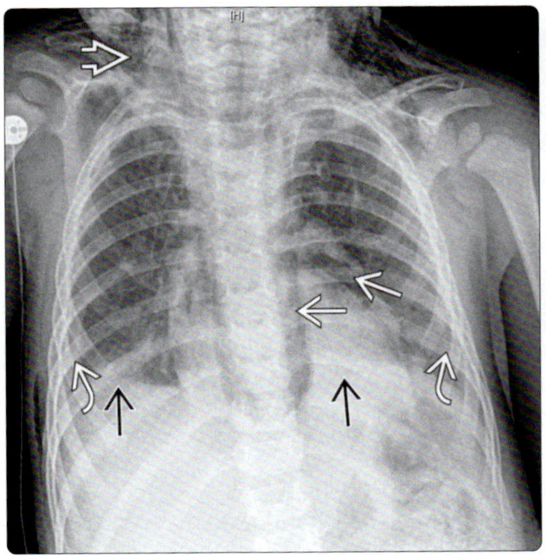

Esophageal Perforation

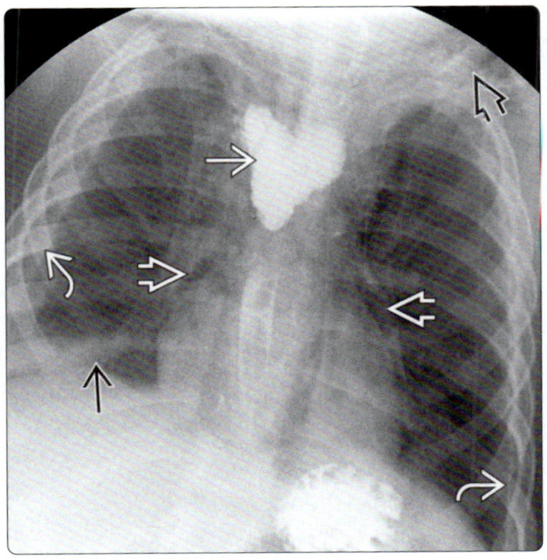

(Left) *AP radiograph demonstrates pneumomediastinum →, subcutaneous emphysema →, basilar opacities →, & small bilateral effusions → in this 3 year old with concern for esophageal perforation status post removal of a coin from the esophagus.* **(Right)** *Frontal esophagram in the same patient confirms esophageal perforation with a large volume of extraluminal contrast →. Again note the pneumomediastinum →, bilateral effusions →, basilar opacities →, & subcutaneous emphysema →.*

DIFFERENTIAL DIAGNOSIS

Common

- Normal Thymus
- Lymphoma
- Infectious Lymphadenopathy

Less Common

- Foregut Duplication Cyst
- Lymphatic Malformation
- Neuroblastoma
- Thymic Cyst
- Germ Cell Tumor
- Trauma
- Congenital or Acquired Cardiovascular Pathology
- Neurofibromatosis Type 1

Rare but Important

- Thyroid Carcinoma
- Thymoma

ESSENTIAL INFORMATION

Key Differential Diagnosis Issues

- Normal pediatric mediastinum is wider than in adults due to thymus, particularly in first 5 years of life
- Location of pediatric mediastinal lesions
  - Anterior: Thymus, thymus-related pathology, lymphoma, germ cell tumor
  - Middle: Lymphadenopathy, vascular pathologies, foregut duplication cysts
  - Posterior: Neurogenic tumors

Helpful Clues for Common Diagnoses

- **Normal Thymus**
  - Most common mediastinal "mass" in neonates & infants
    - Quadrilateral shape or sail-shaped
  - Thymus increases in weight until adolescence when it begins to involute
    - Gradually becomes triangular-shaped in adolescence
  - May decrease in size during illness/stress & increase in size with recovery (hyperplasia/"rebound")
  - Visible by radiograph until ~ 5 years of age
    - Usually more prominent on right side; may mimic upper lobe consolidation
    - More lucent than heart
    - Borders are typically undulating along ribs
    - Appearance may change with respiration
    - Causes no mass effect on airway
  - "Dot-dash" echoes throughout thymus on US
  - Homogeneous appearance on CT & MR
- **Lymphoma**
  - Incidence increases with age
    - 25% of cancers in children 15-19 years old
    - Most common mediastinal mass in teenagers
  - Hodgkin lymphoma (HL): More common in teens; non-HL (NHL): More common < 10 years of age
  - HL involves contiguous nodal groups; NHL is more commonly extranodal
  - Mediastinal disease is common in HL & NHL
    - Often causes tracheal & superior vena cava (SVC) compression
    - Consider leukemia in younger patients
  - Pleural effusion is frequent
- **Infectious Lymphadenopathy**
  - Organism depends on geographic location
  - Common causes: Tuberculosis (TB), histoplasmosis, coccidioidomycosis, & blastomycosis
    - TB & histoplasmosis may have lymph nodes with low-attenuation centers on CECT in acute phase
    - Lymph node Ca^{2+} in old disease
  - Enlarged lymph nodes can compress SVC

Helpful Clues for Less Common Diagnoses

- **Foregut Duplication Cyst**
  - May have bronchial or esophageal origin
  - Most common location: Paratracheal or subcarinal
  - Round or oval mass with smooth contour
  - Homogeneous appearance
    - Typically of simple fluid but complex with high protein content, hemorrhage, or infection
    - Wall of cyst is thin & does not enhance unless complicated by infection
  - May lead to bronchial compression → atelectasis or hyperinflation
- **Lymphatic Malformation**
  - Transspatial lymph-containing multilocular endothelial-lined lesions with thin internal septations
  - Most common in neck, mediastinum, & axilla
  - Size of individual cysts (> 1 cm vs. < 1 cm) determines treatment options: Macrocystic vs. microcystic
    - Lesions often have both components
  - Grows commensurate with patient; may rapidly enlarge with trauma, infection, or hormonal stimulation
    - Simple-appearing fluid becomes more complex
  - Rim & septations will enhance; thickness (& surrounding tissue edema) increases with inflammation
  - Lesions usually encase & separate vessels without significant compression
  - Most are asymptomatic; can develop dyspnea or dysphagia if sufficiently large
- **Neuroblastoma**
  - Up to 20% found in posterior mediastinum
  - Mean age of 25 months (older than abdominal neuroblastoma)
  - Ovoid, bulging paraspinal mass ± Ca^{2+} & rib or pedicle splaying & erosion
  - Mediastinal nodal involvement is uncommon
- **Thymic Cyst**
  - Cystic remnant of thymopharyngeal duct; occurs anywhere between pyriform sinus & anterior mediastinum
  - May arise directly from mediastinal thymus or be connected by fibrous cord
  - Usually unilocular with dominant cyst
  - Mural nodularity or adjacent soft tissue may represent aberrant thymic tissue
  - Most present at 2-15 years of age
    - Most are asymptomatic; can develop neck swelling, dyspnea, or dysphagia if sufficiently large
- **Germ Cell Tumor**

- Primary tumor originates from germ cells that fail to complete migration from urogenital ridge
- Metastatic occurs from primary gonadal tumor source
- Increased levels of α-fetoprotein & β-HCG
- Types: Teratoma, seminoma, nonseminomatous germ cell tumor (NSGCT)
  - Teratoma: Solid & cystic with fat & Ca^{2+}
    - Accounts for 60% of mediastinal germ cell tumors
  - Seminoma: Homogeneous soft tissue mass
  - NSGCT: Heterogeneous soft tissue mass; hemorrhage & necrosis are common

- **Trauma**
  - Traumatic aortic injuries are uncommon but occur in teens > younger children
    - Consider iatrogenic trauma as well
  - Mediastinal hematoma is cause of mediastinal widening
  - Prominent or indistinct aortic knob on chest radiography ± left pleural effusion
  - Periaortic hematoma, aortic contour abnormality, &/or active extravasation on chest CTA
  - Associated injuries are common
- **Congenital or Acquired Cardiovascular Pathology**
  - Aortic valve stenosis
    - Results in poststenotic dilation
    - Can be valvular (most common), subaortic, or supravalvular
    - Associated with Turner syndrome, bicuspid aortic valve, & coarctation of aorta
  - Aneurysm
    - Connective tissue disorders: Marfan, Ehlers-Danlos, Loeys-Dietz syndromes
      - Dilation of sinus of Valsalva & ascending aorta
      - Other systemic manifestations
    - Vasculitis: Takayasu arteritis
      - Large vessel vasculitis of aorta & main branches; more commonly shows wall thickening
    - Mycotic aneurysm: Infection of vessel wall; can occur in infants secondary to umbilical arterial catheter
  - Total anomalous pulmonary venous return (TAPVR)
    - Supracardiac (type 1) snowman appearance on chest radiograph with shunt vascularity
  - Postoperative complication of cardiovascular surgery
    - Hematoma, seroma, pseudoaneurysm, mediastinitis/infection
- **Neurofibromatosis Type 1**
  - Common autosomal dominant disorder
  - Classic clinical findings of café au lait spots, axillary freckling, & dermal or plexiform neurofibromas
  - Plexiform neurofibromas can occur along any nerves; distributions & severity can be quite variable
    - May infiltrate or compress hollow organs
  - Target appearance in cross section on MR & US
    - Loss of targetoid appearance, discordant growth, cysts, &/or peripheral enhancement should raise concern for malignant peripheral nerve sheath tumor

Helpful Clues for Rare Diagnoses

- **Thyroid Carcinoma**
  - Thyroid nodules in 1.5% of children; majority are benign
    - Must be evaluated in light of TI-RADS scoring
    - Concerning features: Solid, hypoechoic, taller than wide, irregular margins or extension beyond thyroid, microCa^{2+}
  - Extremely rare to cause pediatric mediastinal widening
    - Irregular anterior/superior mediastinal mass with Ca^{2+}; heterogeneous lymph nodes with Ca^{2+} & cystic foci
  - Increased risk with multiple endocrine neoplasia, radiation exposure; mutations of *PTEN*, *DICER1*, or *APC*
- **Thymoma**
  - Asymptomatic or symptoms from mass effect or paraneoplastic syndrome (40%)
  - Soft tissue mass; may have thin peripheral capsular Ca^{2+}, cystic components, & necrosis
  - Invasive form may have irregular margins, chest wall involvement, & pleural extension
  - Associated with myasthenia gravis

Normal Thymus

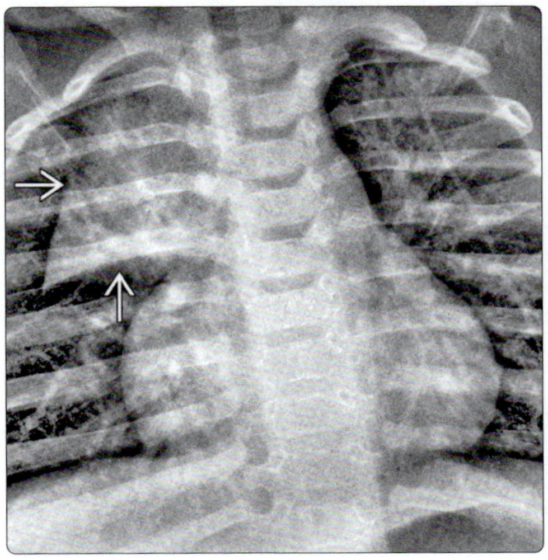

Normal Thymus

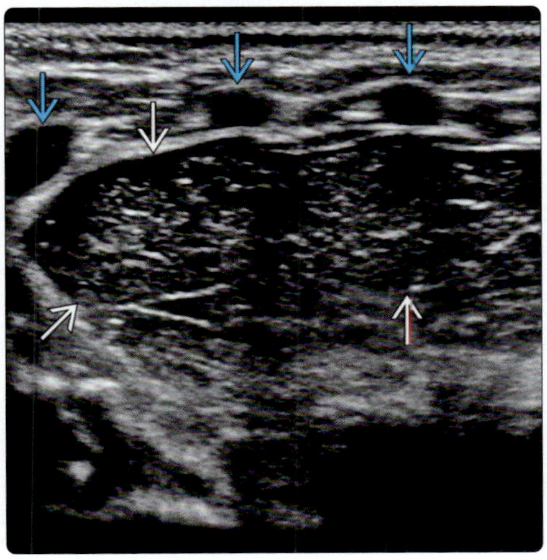

(Left) *PA radiograph of the chest shows a sail-like appearance of the normal thymus ➡. The lateral border of the thymus typically has an undulating contour along the anterior lateral chest wall.* **(Right)** *Longitudinal ultrasound shows the normal thymus ➡ just deep to the anterior ribs ➡. Sonographically, the thymus is hypoechoic with multiple linear & punctate "dot-dash" echogenic foci. Ultrasound can help distinguish a normal thymus from a mediastinal mass.*

(Left) *Frontal chest radiograph demonstrates lobular widening of the mediastinum in this 13-year-old patient who presented with positional dyspnea.* **(Right)** *Axial CECT from the same patient confirms a lobulated anterior mediastinal soft tissue mass, typical of lymphoma. There is mass effect on the underlying mediastinal structures. This can result in superior vena cava (SVC) syndrome, which limits blood return to the heart via the SVC.*

Lymphoma

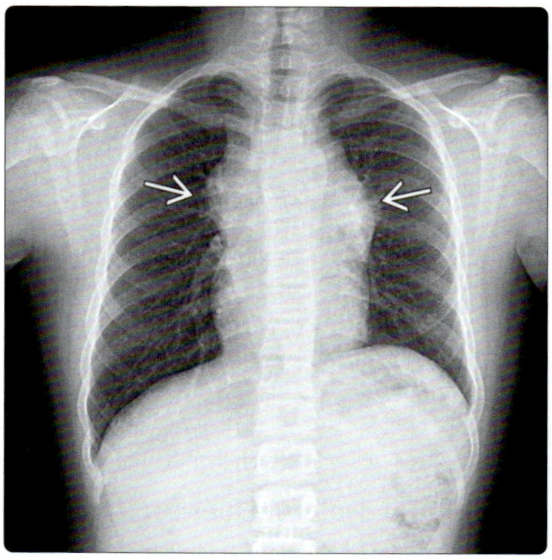

Lymphoma

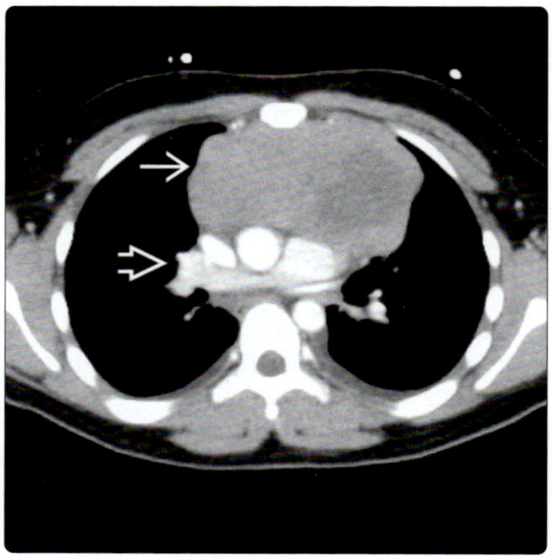

(Left) *FDG PET/CT in the same patient confirms an FDG-avid anterior mediastinal mass, consistent with the diagnosis of lymphoma.* **(Right)** *Frontal radiograph in a 16 year old with shortness of breath for 3 months shows prominence of the mediastinum with left hilar & right midlung opacities.*

Lymphoma

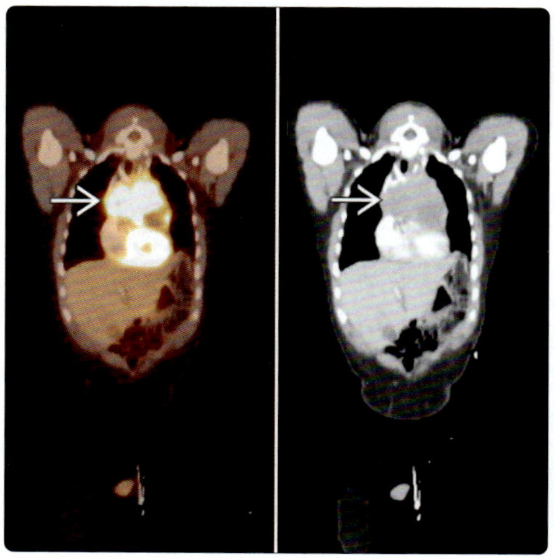

Infectious Lymphadenopathy

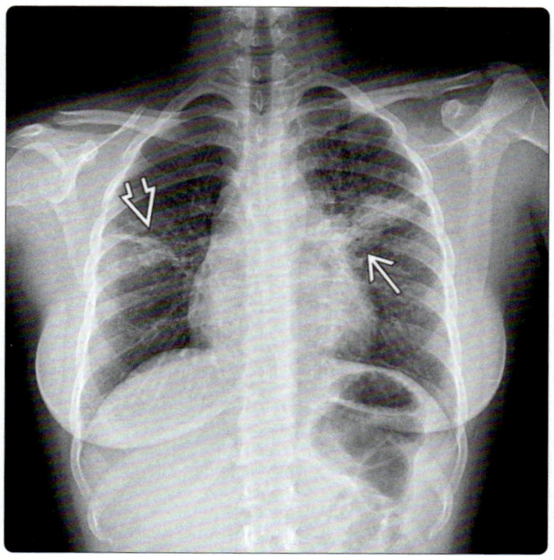

(Left) *Axial CECT in the same patient shows a heterogeneous mass in the anterior mediastinum due to a conglomeration of lymph nodes. There is an adjacent small fluid collection with a focus of gas concerning for an abscess. Also note the left lung consolidation. Pathology was positive for tuberculosis.* **(Right)** *Axial CECT shows a circular, low-density mass in the pretracheal region. The mass has a thin, enhancing wall but otherwise shows fluid density, characteristic of a bronchogenic cyst.*

Infectious Lymphadenopathy

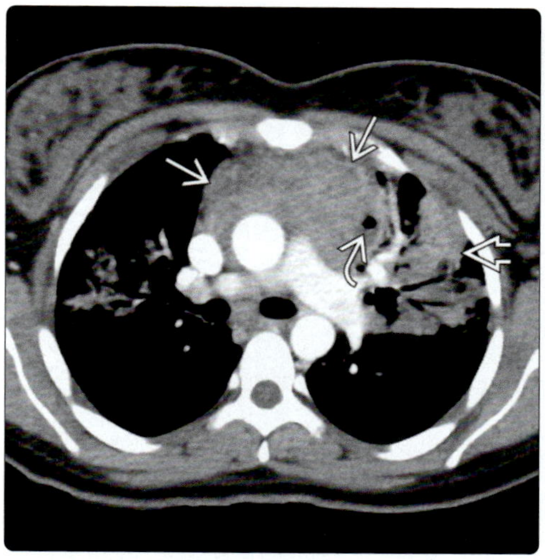

Foregut Duplication Cyst

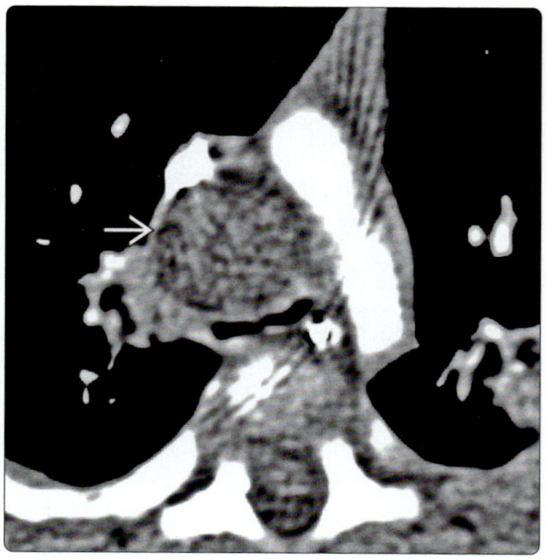

Lymphatic Malformation

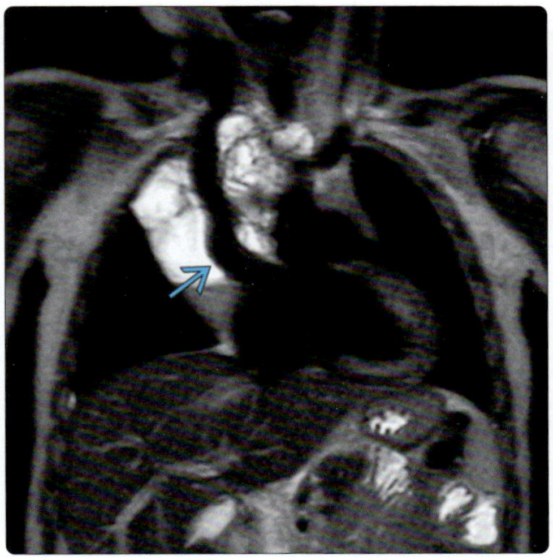

Thymic Cyst

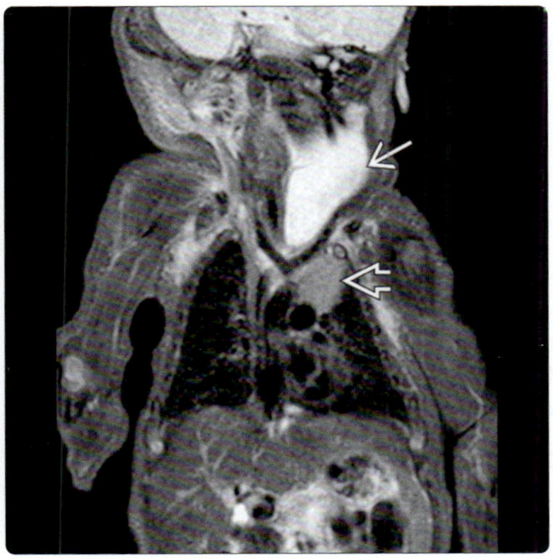

(Left) *Coronal T2 SSFSE MR of a 2 year old with recent respiratory distress shows a multilobulated cystic mass of the mediastinum surrounding & displacing (but not effacing) the SVC. There are macrocysts & microcysts in this lesion. No significant enhancement was seen after contrast (not shown), typical of a lymphatic malformation.* **(Right)** *Coronal STIR MR in a 6 day old with a thymic cyst shows a unilocular cystic mass in the left neck extending into the superior mediastinum to abut the thymus.*

Germ Cell Tumor

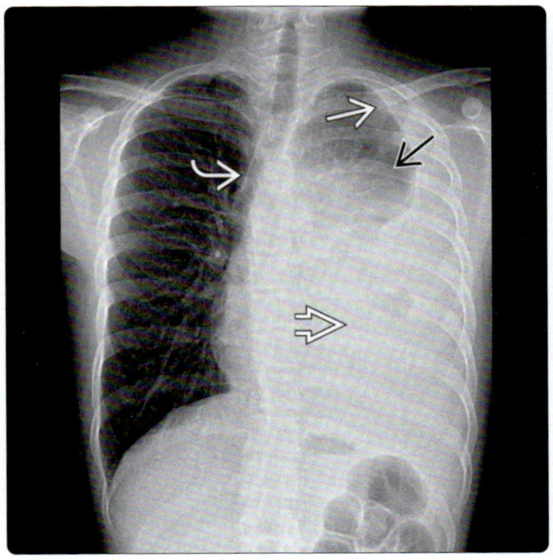

Germ Cell Tumor

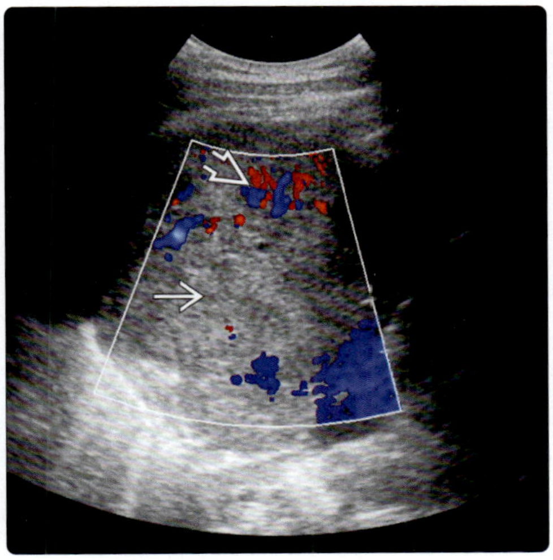

(Left) *Frontal chest radiograph in a 16 year old demonstrates a moderate left pleural effusion, a suggestion of mediastinal widening, & a confluent mid to lower left lung opacity. There is mild mediastinal shift to the right.* **(Right)** *Color Doppler ultrasound performed in the same patient to evaluate the pleural effusion also identifies a heterogeneous soft tissue mass with internal vascularity.*

Germ Cell Tumor

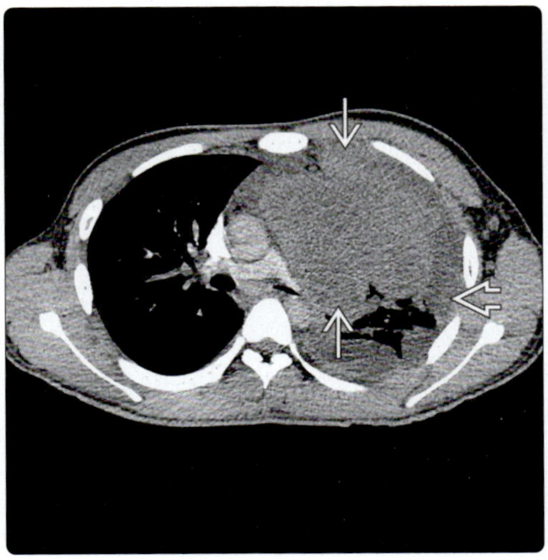

Germ Cell Tumor

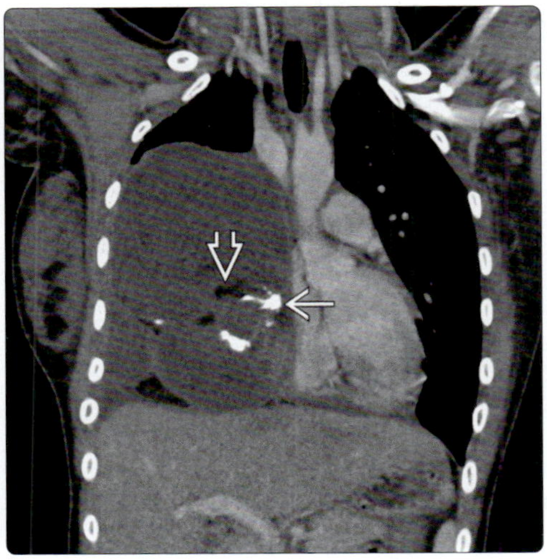

(Left) *Axial CECT performed in the same patient demonstrates an anterior mediastinal mass & left pleural effusion. The mass was subsequently identified as a yolk sac tumor.* **(Right)** *Coronal CECT shows a mediastinal mass consistent with a teratoma in a 16-year-old female patient. The mass has areas of varying density, consistent with Ca^{2+} & fat.*

(Left) *AP radiograph of the chest shows a widened mediastinum, left apical cap of pleural fluid, & large right pneumothorax. Traumatic aortic injuries are uncommon in children but become more frequent as they enter the late teen years.* **(Right)** *Axial CECT shows a mediastinal hematoma & left hemothorax. In older children & adults, the thymus normally has concave borders, whereas mediastinal hematomas often cause convex mediastinal borders.*

Trauma

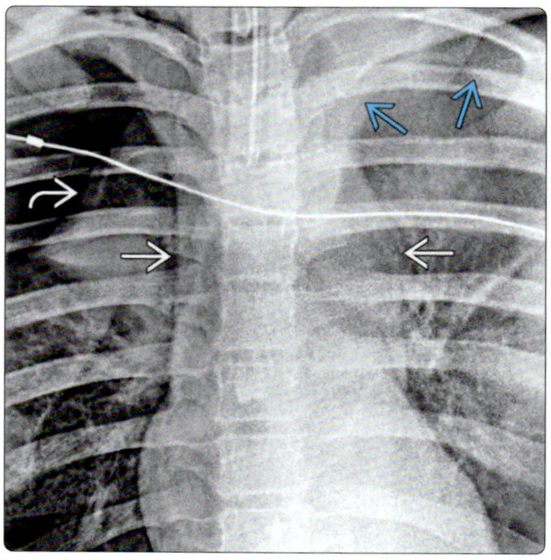

Trauma

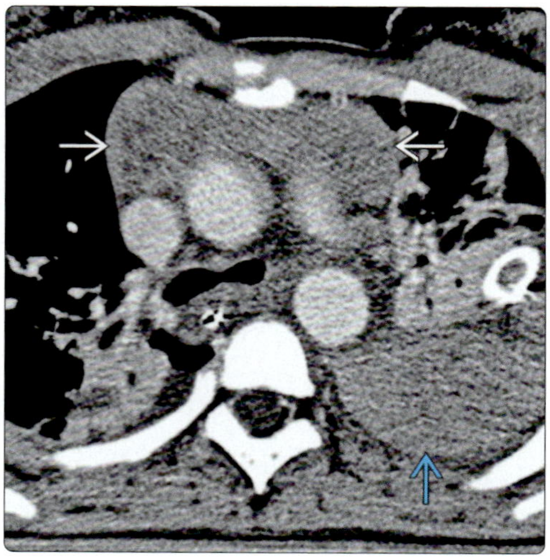

(Left) *Frontal chest radiograph in a 5 month old with Loeys-Dietz syndrome (LDS) depicts widening of the mediastinum, subtle concavity at the right margin of the trachea, & tortuosity of the descending aorta.* **(Right)** *Coronal SSFP MR in the same patient depicts dilation of the aortic sinus & ascending aorta. LDS tends to be more aggressive than Marfan syndrome with an earlier age of onset & more rapid progression, including dissection & rupture. Tortuous cervical arteries are typical.*

Congenital or Acquired Cardiovascular Pathology

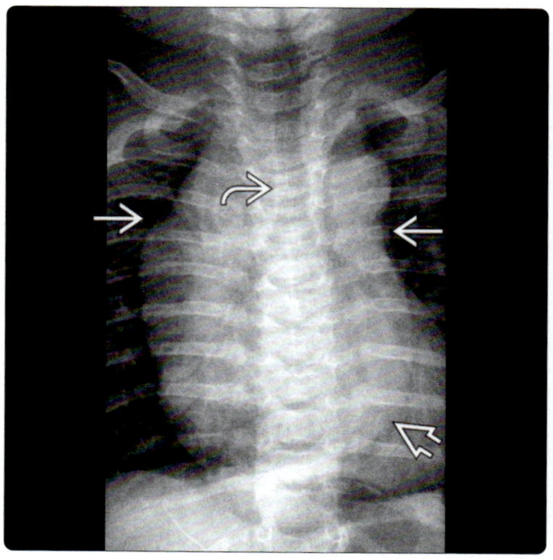

Congenital or Acquired Cardiovascular Pathology

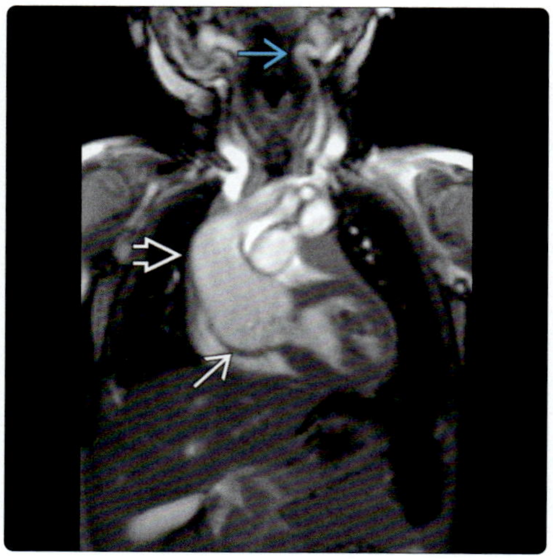

(Left) *Portable frontal radiograph in an 8 month old status post truncus arteriosus repair, postoperative day 2, shows new mediastinal widening.* **(Right)** *Axial CECT from the same patient depicts a mildly heterogeneous, nonenhancing anterior mediastinal collection. This collection had a Hounsfield unit measurement that was consistent with a hematoma.*

Congenital or Acquired Cardiovascular Pathology

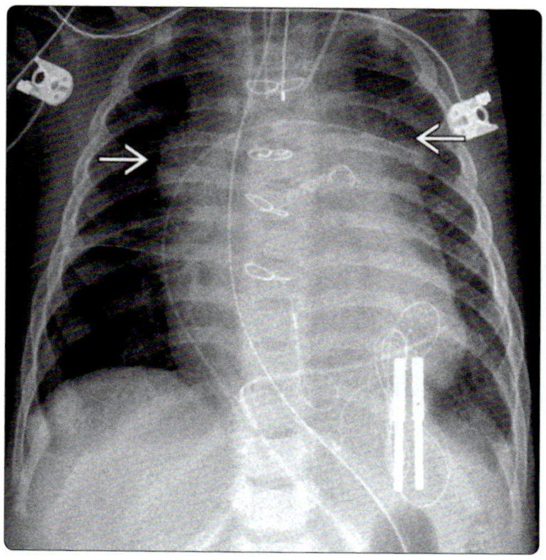

Congenital or Acquired Cardiovascular Pathology

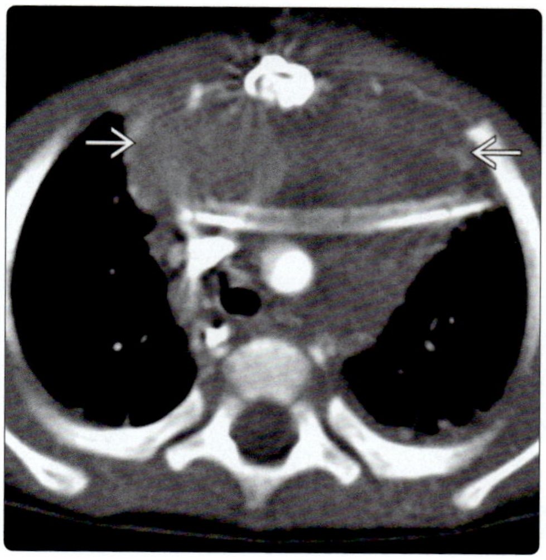

Neurofibromatosis Type 1

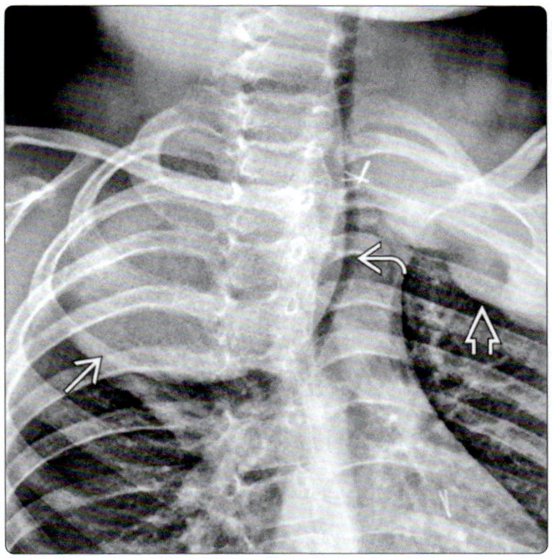

Neurofibromatosis Type 1

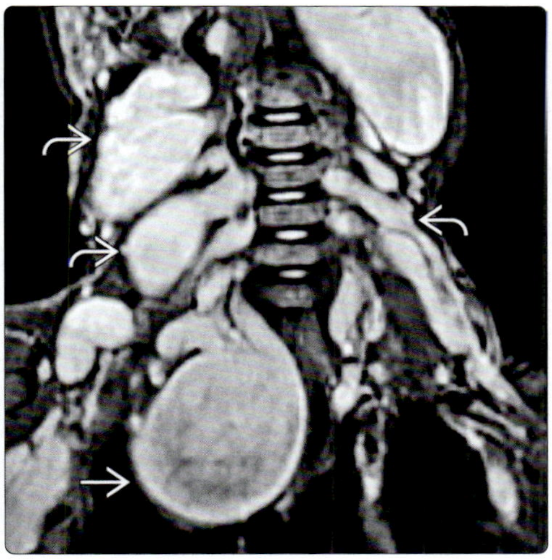

(Left) *PA radiograph of the chest shows a large mass in the upper right hemithorax/mediastinum, displacing the trachea to the left. A lobulated mass is also present in the left apex. These findings were due to plexiform neurofibromas in neurofibromatosis type 1 (NF1).* **(Right)** *Coronal STIR MR shows a large plexiform neurofibroma at the right apex/upper mediastinum. There are extensive lobulated neurofibromas along every cervical nerve.*

Thyroid Carcinoma

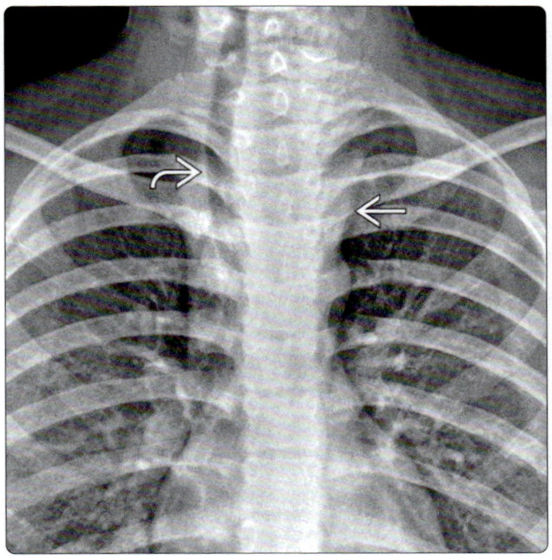

Thyroid Carcinoma

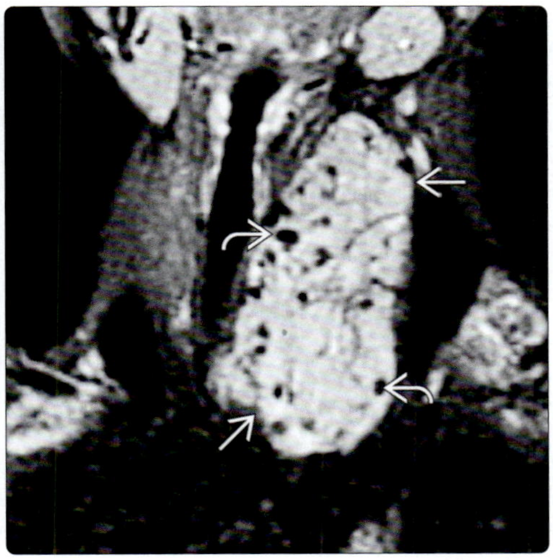

(Left) *PA radiograph of the chest shows a mass in the upper mediastinum displacing the trachea to the right. Thyroid carcinoma is uncommon in children, although it is the most common pediatric endocrine tumor.* **(Right)** *Coronal STIR MR shows an unusually large & solid, but hyperintense thyroid carcinoma in the left neck with extension to the upper mediastinum. The mass has multiple internal flow voids due to increased vascularity.*

Thymoma

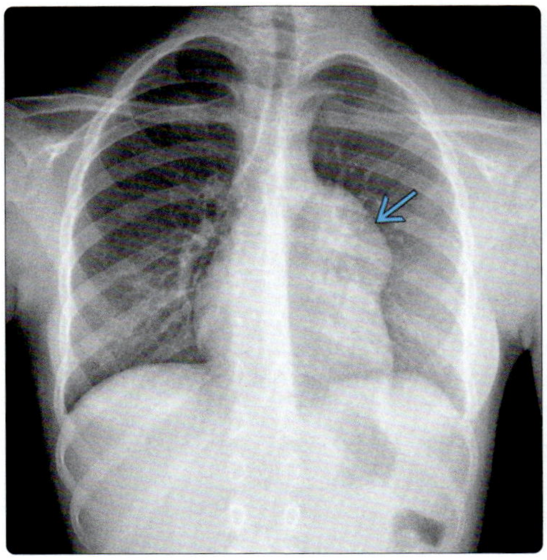

Thymoma

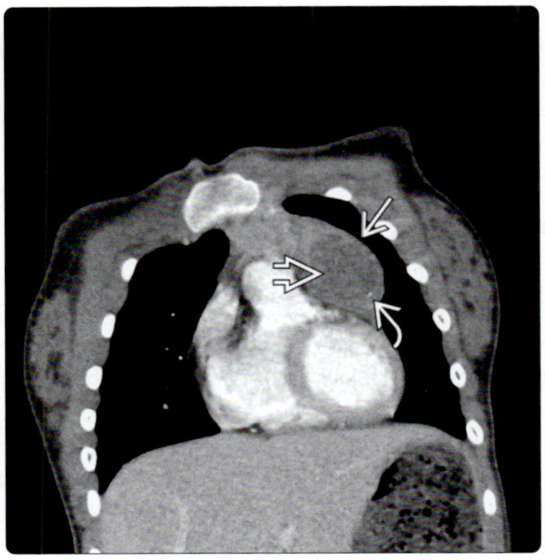

(Left) *Frontal radiograph in a 12 year old demonstrates an abnormal prominent convexity of the left mediastinal border, suggesting a mass.* **(Right)** *Coronal CECT from the same patient shows a corresponding left mediastinal mass with a complex cystic component & subtle linear Ca^{2+}. The mass was diagnosed as a thymoma at pathology. This tumor is quite uncommon in children.*

DIFFERENTIAL DIAGNOSIS

Common

- Normal Thymus (Mimic)
- Rebound Thymic Hyperplasia (Mimic)
- Lymphoma

Less Common

- Germ Cell Tumor
- Lymphatic Malformation

Rare but Important

- Congenital Thymic Cyst
- Langerhans Cell Histiocytosis
- Thymoma
- Lipomatous Tumor
    - Lipoma
    - Thymolipoma
- Morgagni Hernia

ESSENTIAL INFORMATION

Key Differential Diagnosis Issues

- International Thymic Malignancy Interest Group 3: Compartment mediastinal classification system based on CT
- Anterior mediastinum (prevascular compartment)
    - Boundaries: Sternum (anterior), anterior pericardium to pulmonary veins (posterior), & parietal mediastinal pleura (lateral)
    - Contents: Thymus, fat, lymph nodes, left brachiocephalic vein
- Middle mediastinum (visceral compartment)
    - Boundaries: Posterior margin of prevascular compartment (anterior), 1 cm posterior to anterior cortex of vertebral bodies (posterior), & parietal mediastinal pleura (lateral)
    - Contents: Heart, superior vena cava (SVC), thoracic aorta, intrapericardial pulmonary arteries, thoracic duct, trachea, carina, esophagus, & lymph nodes
- Posterior mediastinum (paravertebral compartment)
    - Boundaries: Posterior margin of visceral compartment (anterior) & lateral margins of vertebral transverse processes (posterolateral)
    - Contents: Thoracic spine & paravertebral soft tissues
- Superior & inferior boundaries are thoracic inlet & diaphragm for all compartments

Helpful Clues for Common Diagnoses

- **Normal Thymus (Mimic)**
    - Most common anterior mediastinal mass in infants
    - Changes in appearance with age
        - Most prominent in infancy with quadrilateral shape & convex margins
        - Gradually becomes triangular-shaped in later childhood & teenage years
        - Thymus increases in weight until adolescence, when it begins to involute
        - Visible on frontal radiograph until ~ 5 years of age
    - May be asymmetric across midline
    - Can extend inferiorly to drape over heart, superiorly into neck, or posteriorly between great vessels & trachea
    - Key imaging features
        - Sail sign: Looks like nautical sail
        - Notch sign: Indentation between thymus & cardiac silhouette
        - Wave sign: Undulations caused by anterior ribs
        - Mildly lucent relative to heart
        - No mass effect on adjacent vasculature or airway
        - Change in shape with phase of respiration (pliable)
        - Homogeneous appearance on CT & MR with mild, uniform, homogeneous enhancement
        - Ultrasound often characteristic: Hypoechoic with diffuse linear & punctate "dot-dash" echoes
- **Rebound Thymic Hyperplasia (Mimic)**
    - Thymic size can vary in states of wellness vs. stress
        - May decrease in size during illness/stress & then increase in size with recovery
        - Scenarios include recovery from burns, surgery, cessation of corticosteroids, & after chemotherapy
        - Thymic hyperplasia can occur anytime between 1-12 months after chemotherapy
    - Maintains normal parenchymal appearance & triangular or trapezoidal shape on all modalities
    - Also maintains normal gross architecture & histologic appearance
- **Lymphoma**
    - Most common anterior mediastinal pathology in children
    - Distorts shape of thymus, which assumes lobulated or biconvex contour
    - Mass effect on trachea & vessels may be primary clue to differentiate from normal thymus
    - Mass usually crosses midline
    - May be homogeneous or heterogeneous, lobulated soft tissue mass on CECT & MR
        - Typically more heterogeneous than normal thymus, even if only mild
    - May become necrotic & heterogeneous upon treatment or growth beyond blood supply
    - Rarely calcifies before treatment; 5% calcify after
    - May be associated with involvement of lymph nodes in hila or other mediastinal compartments
        - PET best identifies involved nodes & distant disease
    - Pleural & pericardial involvement is not uncommon (15%), especially effusions; lung involvement is unusual
    - SVC effacement is common; invasion & occlusion may cause SVC syndrome

Helpful Clues for Less Common Diagnoses

- **Germ Cell Tumor**
    - 2nd most common extragonadal site after sacrococcygeal region
    - Occurs within or near thymus
    - Majority are mature teratomas (60%); seminoma is next most common
    - Lobulated or smooth contours on radiography; constituent elements may be identified, especially Ca^{2+}
    - Intrinsic elements are better identified on CT
        - Homogeneous or heterogeneous soft tissue
        - Fluid/cysts
        - Macroscopic fat
        - Coarse calcified components (25%)
    - May be well demarcated or inseparable from vessels

- Most commonly unilateral but may cross midline
- Invasion of adjacent structures, necrosis, or hemorrhage suggest malignancy
- **Lymphatic Malformation**
  - Congenital error of vessel morphogenesis
  - Usually detected prenatally or as neonate
  - Grows commensurate with patient; may show rapid enlargement due to infection, trauma, or hormonal stimulation
  - Thin-walled, fluid-filled, multiloculated mass with only peripheral & septal enhancement
    - May contain fluid-fluid levels or foci of T1 shortening due to blood products
  - May be focal or transspatial (extending across tissue planes); often involves neck, chest wall, &/or axilla
  - May be associated with more generalized lymphatic disorder (including splenic & bone lesions)

Helpful Clues for Rare Diagnoses

- **Congenital Thymic Cyst**
  - Cystic remnant of thymopharyngeal duct
  - Usually in lateral infrahyoid neck between carotid artery & jugular vein but can extend to anterior mediastinum
  - Usually smooth & thin walled; can have mural nodularity
    - May rarely have partial wall Ca^{2+}
  - May contain proteinaceous or hemorrhagic contents
- **Langerhans Cell Histiocytosis (LCH)**
  - Thymic LCH is common in multisystem disease
    - Typically occurs in very young patients
  - Most commonly presents as diffuse enlargement
  - Contour may be smooth or lobulated
  - Involved thymus is heterogeneous on CECT & MR
    - Irregular Ca^{2+} & cystic lesions may be present
      - Ca^{2+} are usually subtle in comparison to germ cell tumors & are usually only visible on CT
  - Enlarged, involved gland can displace trachea & great vessels, unlike normal thymus
  - Appearance of thymus reverts to normal with therapy
- **Thymoma**
  - < 1% of pediatric mediastinal masses
  - Invasive & noninvasive types
  - Associated with myasthenia gravis & other paraneoplastic syndromes in children & adults
  - May have Ca^{2+} (30%)
  - Invasive type: Irregular, heterogeneous mass with necrosis & hemorrhage with ipsilateral pleural dissemination
  - Noninvasive type: Small & homogeneous mass
- **Lipomatous Tumor**
  - **Lipoma**
    - Similar composition as subcutaneous fat
    - Relatively radiolucent to other soft tissues
    - Asymptomatic
  - **Thymolipoma**
    - Rare benign mass comprised of normal thymic tissue interspersed with fat
    - Nonenhancing soft tissue is interwoven within fat in whorled configuration
- **Morgagni Hernia**
  - Anteromedial parasternal defect of diaphragm, adjacent to xiphoid process
  - 90% occur on right side → right cardiophrenic angle mass on radiography
  - More commonly asymptomatic than Bochdalek type of congenital diaphragmatic hernia
  - Contents of hernia are variable but most commonly contain omentum with liver & bowel being less common
    - Contents determine radiographic appearance
    - Nature of contents is more easily assessed on CT & MR
  - Occasionally diagnosed on barium study

SELECTED REFERENCES

1. Carter BW et al: ITMIG classification of mediastinal compartments and multidisciplinary approach to mediastinal masses. Radiographics. 37(2):413-36, 2017
2. Thacker PG et al: Imaging evaluation of mediastinal masses in children and adults: practical diagnostic approach based on a new classification system. J Thorac Imaging. 30(4):247-67, 2015
3. Ranganath SH et al: Mediastinal masses in children. AJR Am J Roentgenol. 198(3):W197-216, 2012

Normal Thymus (Mimic)

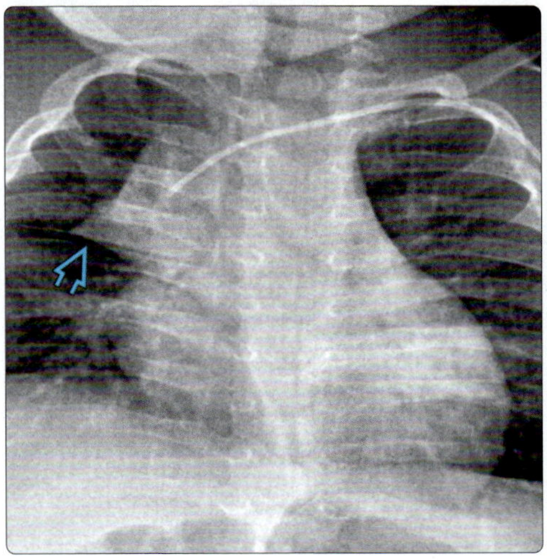

Normal Thymus (Mimic)

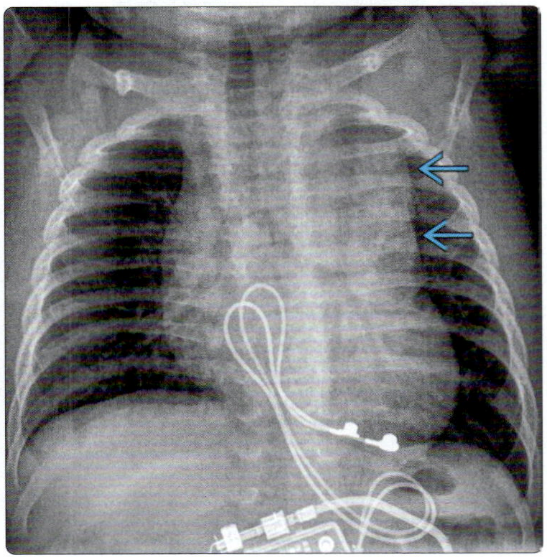

(Left) *AP radiograph in a 7-month-old former premature infant shows a triangular-shaped inferolateral margin ➡ of the right superior mediastinal border, consistent with the sail sign of a normal thymus.* **(Right)** *Frontal radiograph in a 3 month old with a pacemaker secondary to complete heart block shows left mediastinal prominence with an undulating border ➡, consistent with a wave sign caused by a pliable normal thymus abutting the anterior ribs. A normal thymus is the most common anterior mediastinal mass in infants.*

(Left) *Axial CECT in a 13 year old before treatment of an abdominal anaplastic lymphoma shows a small, triangular-shaped normal thymus* ➾. **(Right)** *Axial CECT in the same patient after completion of chemotherapy shows posttreatment rebound hyperplasia of the now larger, quadrilateral-shaped thymus* ➾. *The thymus can atrophy to 40% of its normal size during stress but can rebound to up to 50% larger after treatment, usually within 9 months.*

Rebound Thymic Hyperplasia (Mimic)

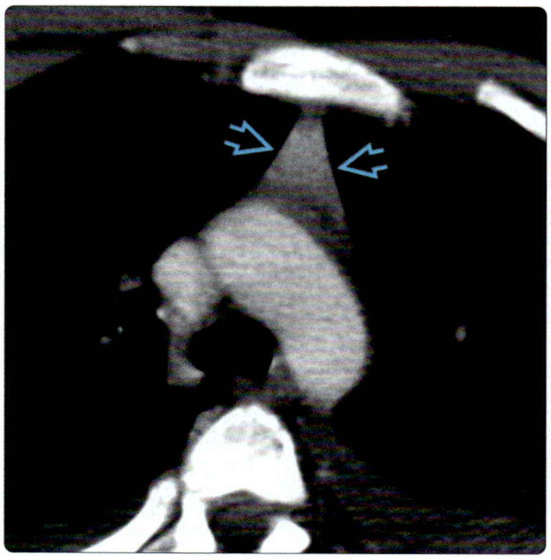

Rebound Thymic Hyperplasia (Mimic)

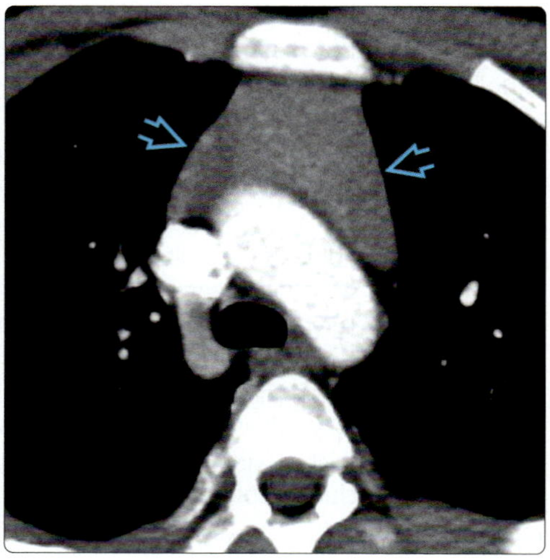

(Left) *PA radiograph in a 12 year old with head & neck swelling shows a multilobulated mediastinal mass* ➾ *that is similar in density to the heart.* **(Right)** *Axial CECT in the same patient shows a heterogeneous, lobulated anterior mediastinal mass* ➾ *engulfing the aorta & great vessels. There is severe narrowing of the superior vena cava (SVC)* ➙*, resulting in SVC syndrome. Concentrated contrast from an upper arm injection opacifies collateral vessels* ➚ *that are bypassing the SVC.*

Lymphoma

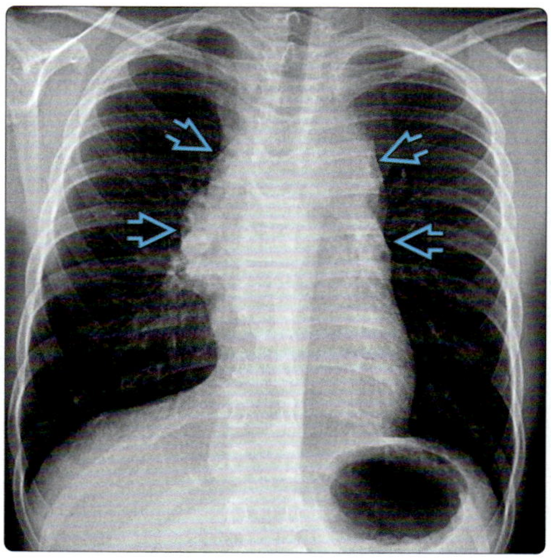

Lymphoma

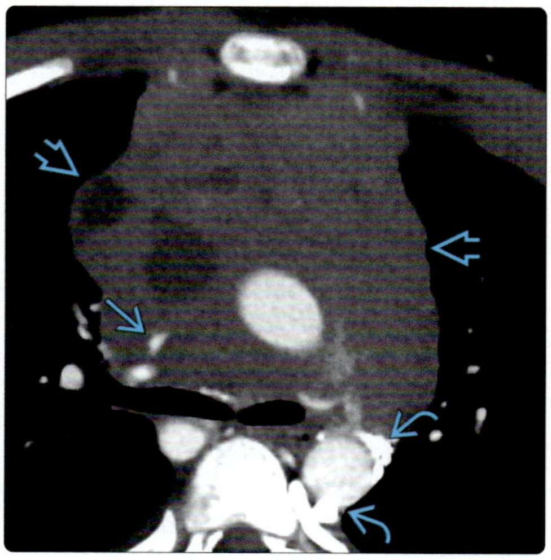

(Left) *PA radiograph in a 15 year old with constitutional symptoms shows a lobulated mediastinal mass* ➾ *along with a left pleural effusion* ➚ *& left lower lobe collapse* ➙. *Pleural effusions are common in lymphoma.* **(Right)** *Coronal FDG PET/CT in the same patient shows intense FDG uptake in multifocal conglomerate nodal masses* ➾. *When lymphoma is suspected, PET/CT should be used for staging.*

Lymphoma

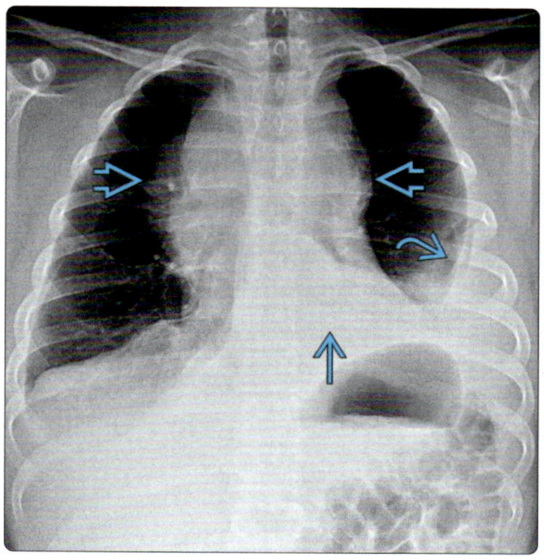

Lymphoma

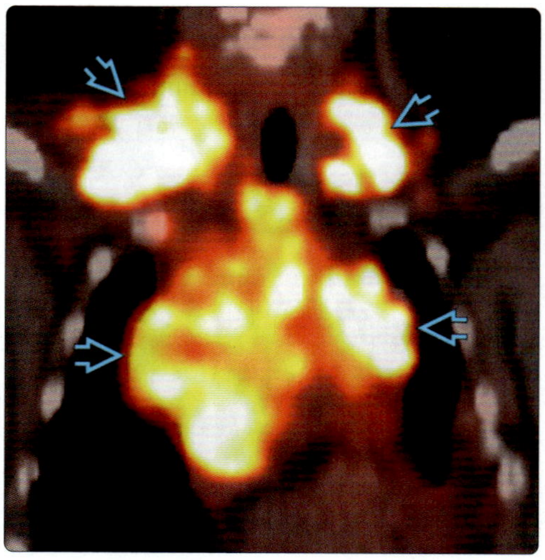

Germ Cell Tumor

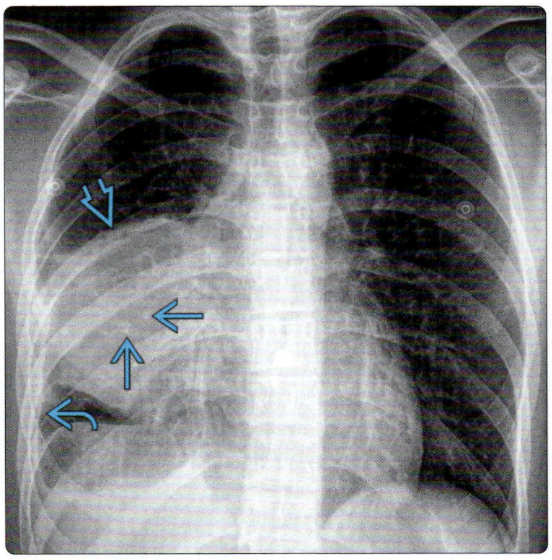

Germ Cell Tumor

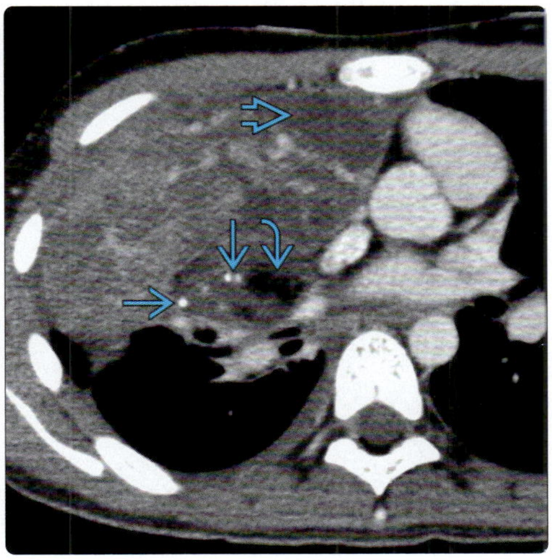

(Left) *PA radiograph in a 16 year old with fatigue, arm numbness, & elevated a-fetoprotein shows a right cardiomediastinal mass with suggestion of faint Ca^{2+} & an associated small right pleural effusion.* **(Right)** *Axial CECT in the same patient shows a heterogeneous anterior mediastinal mass with enhancing solid, fluid, macroscopic fatty, & calcified components, consistent with a germ cell tumor. Note the mass effect on the mediastinal vessels.*

Lymphatic Malformation

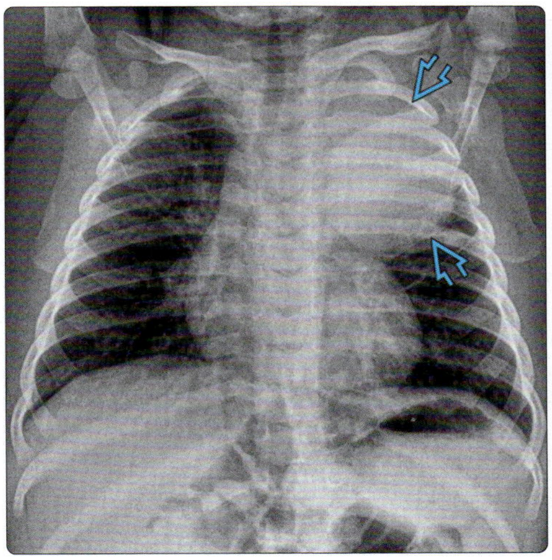

Lymphatic Malformation

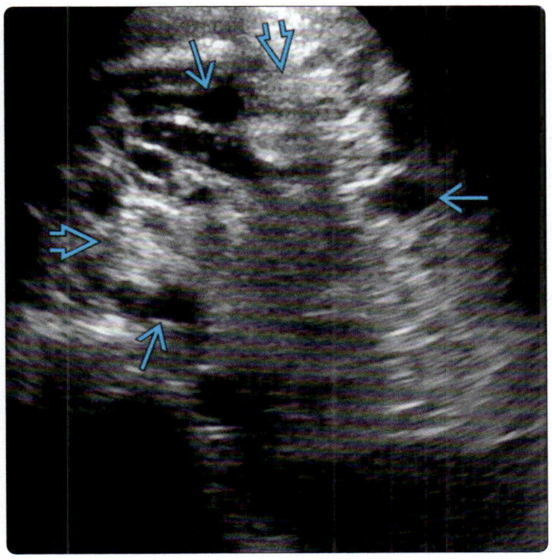

(Left) *PA radiograph in a 15 month old with recurrent cough & difficulty feeding shows a left upper hemithorax mass. Note the rightward tracheal shift but lack of bone abnormalities.* **(Right)** *Ultrasound in the same patient shows an extensive lesion with both macrocystic & microcystic components. No significant internal vascular flow was seen by color Doppler (not shown). Findings are suspicious for a lymphatic malformation.*

Lymphatic Malformation

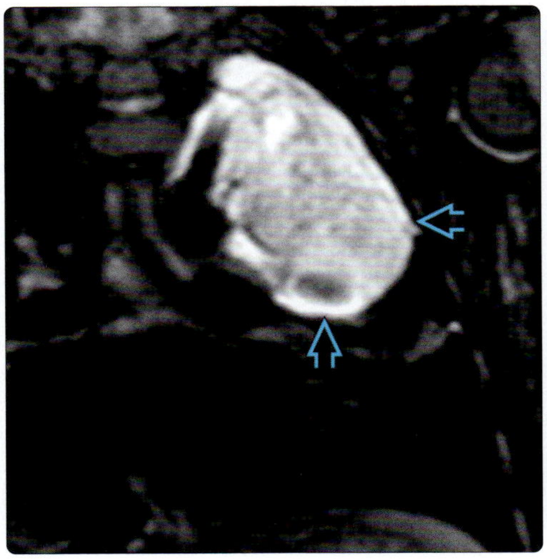

Lymphatic Malformation

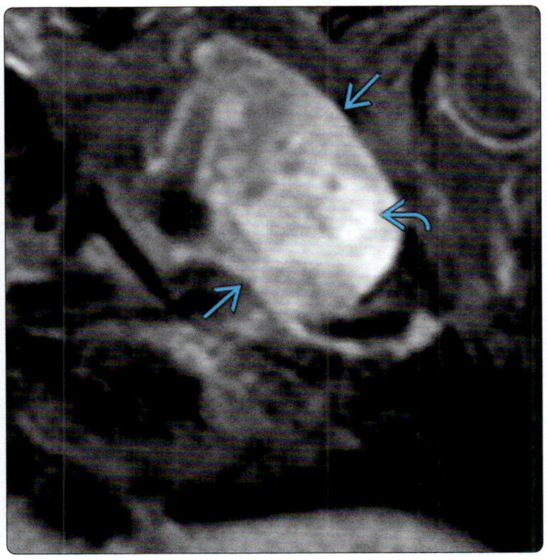

(Left) *Coronal STIR MR in the same patient shows a multiseptated cystic lesion.* **(Right)** *Delayed coronal T1 C+ FS MR in the same patient shows macrocystic septal enhancement with more solid-appearing enhancement in microcystic components. Note that some areas had intrinsic T1 hyperintensity (not shown) due to blood products &/or proteinaceous content.*

(Left) *AP radiograph shows a narrowed trachea that is deviated to the right in this neonate who presented with respiratory distress.* **(Right)** *Axial CECT in the same patient shows a cystic mass extending into the anterior mediastinum in the expected location of the thymus. This cyst has an enhancing rim, & the trachea is deviated to the right. Thymic cysts, which grow into the neck, typically extend between the jugular vein & the carotid artery.*

Congenital Thymic Cyst

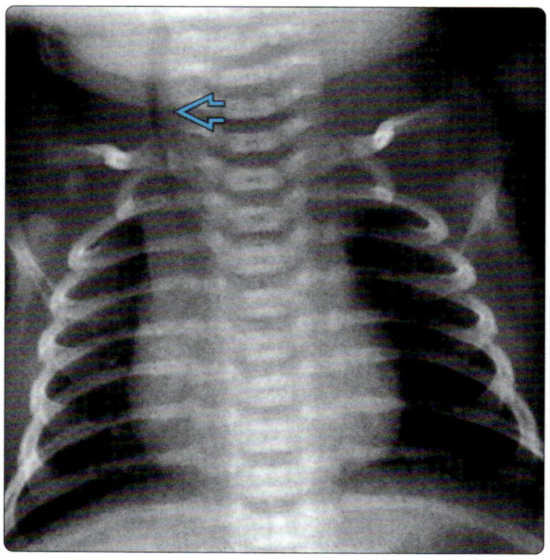

Congenital Thymic Cyst

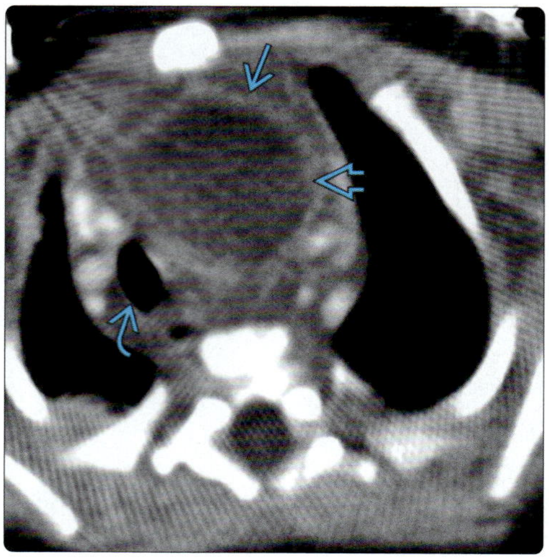

(Left) *AP radiograph shows a convex appearance to both sides of the mediastinum in a young child. The mediastinum should have straighter margins. The patient also had osseous lesions, consistent with Langerhans cell histiocytosis (LCH).* **(Right)** *Axial CECT in the same patient shows a mass in the anterior mediastinum extending into the middle mediastinum. The mass demonstrates some lacy* Ca^{2+} *anteriorly.*

Langerhans Cell Histiocytosis

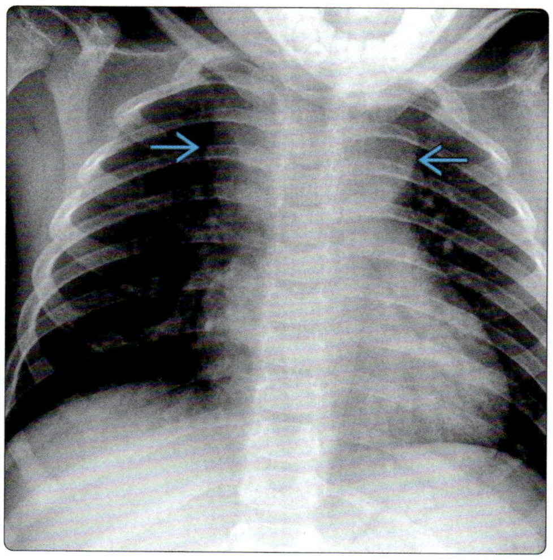

Langerhans Cell Histiocytosis

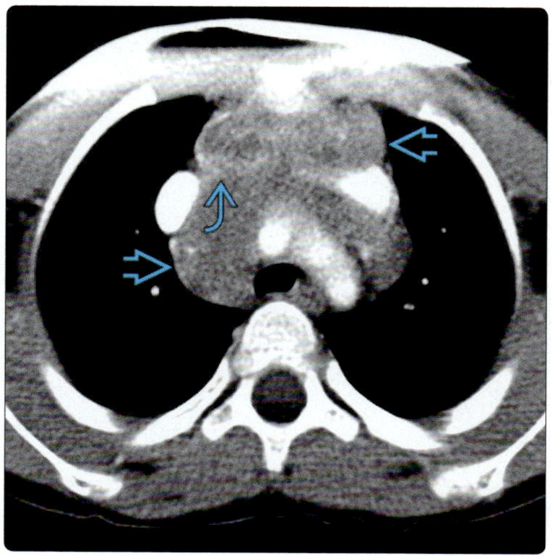

(Left) *Axial NECT in a young child shows a bulky mass in the anterior mediastinum. The mass causes lobulated enlargement of the thymus, which is heterogeneous, with foci of lace-like* Ca^{2+} *& low-attenuation cystic foci. The thymus is frequently involved in LCH when there are multiple organs involved.* **(Right)** *Axial NECT in the same patient shows involvement of the lung parenchyma with small cysts. Rupture of a peripheral cyst can lead to a pneumothorax.*

Langerhans Cell Histiocytosis

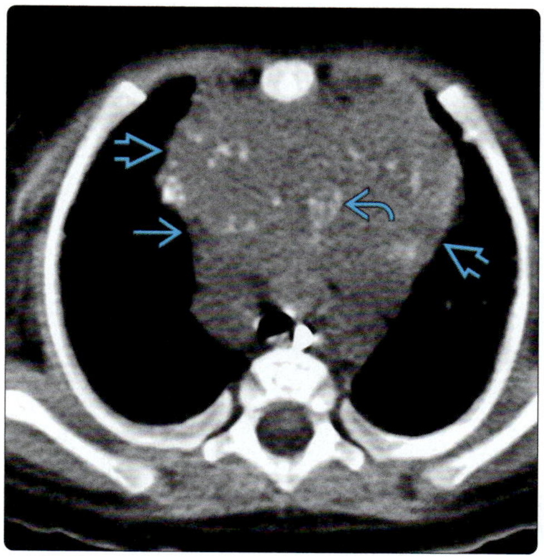

Langerhans Cell Histiocytosis

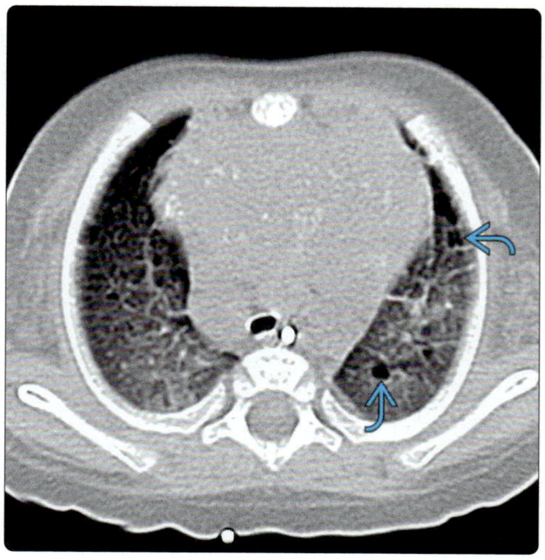

Thymoma

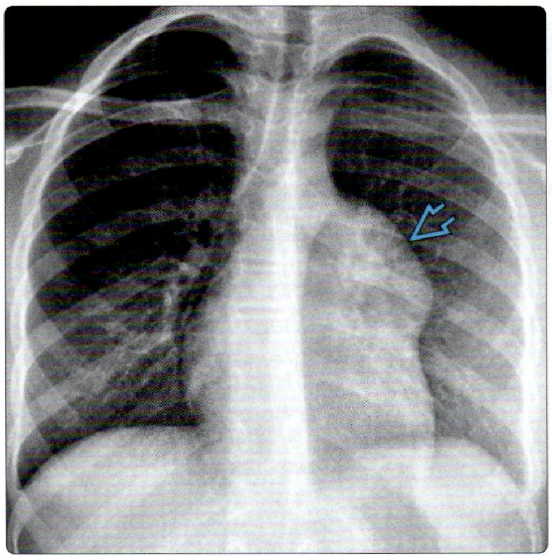

Thymoma

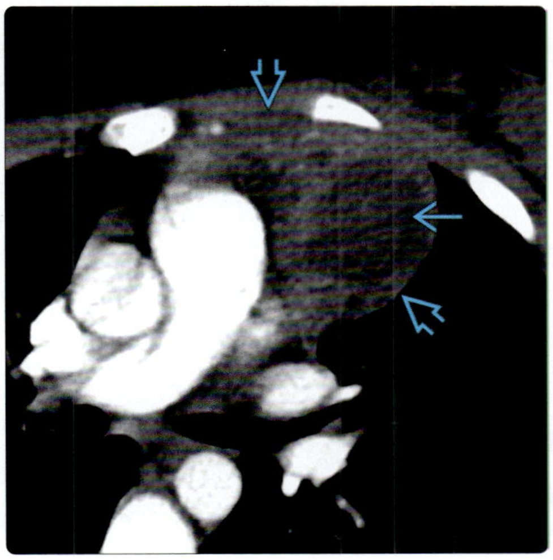

(Left) *PA radiograph in an 11 year old with left back pain for 1 week shows a left mediastinal mass ➔.* **(Right)** *Axial CECT in the same patient shows a heterogeneous anterior mediastinal mass ➔ with low-attenuation areas ➔ representing necrosis or cystic change. Biopsy revealed a thymoma. Thymoma often metastasizes to the ipsilateral pleura. Pleural involvement by thymoma rarely produces an effusion. Similar to adults, thymomas in children are associated with paraneoplastic syndromes such as myasthenia gravis.*

Lipomatous Tumor

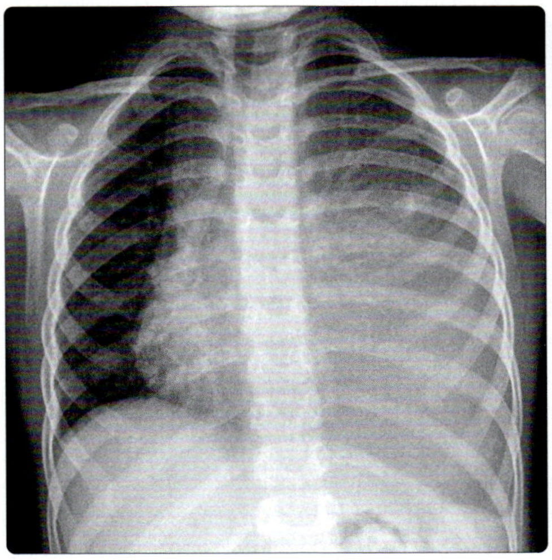

Lipomatous Tumor

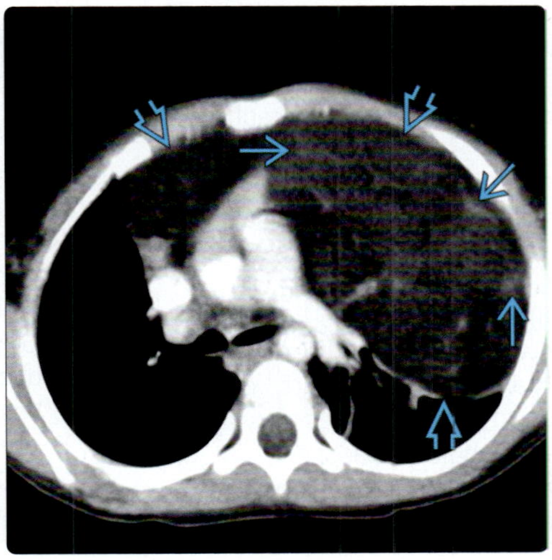

(Left) *PA radiograph in a 5 year old with an upper respiratory tract infection shows incidental opacification of the left hemithorax that is relatively low in density compared to soft tissue. There is associated mediastinal shift.* **(Right)** *Axial CECT in the same patient shows a large anterior mediastinal mass ➔ predominantly composed of macroscopic fat with scattered amorphous soft tissue components ➔. Surgical pathology revealed a lipoma-like lipoblastoma. Lipomatous tumors of the anterior mediastinum are rare.*

Morgagni Hernia

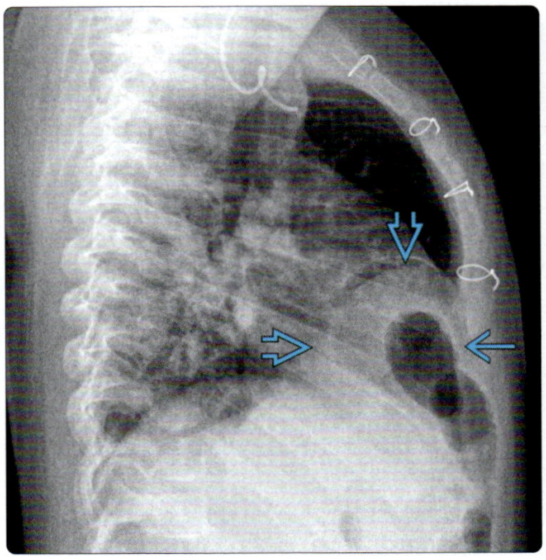

Morgagni Hernia

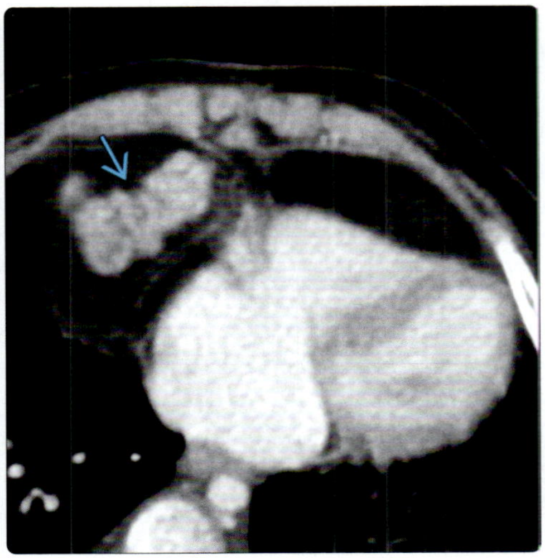

(Left) *Lateral radiograph in a 19 month old with trisomy 21 status post repair of an atrioventricular septal defect shows an anterior mediastinal mass ➔ containing bowel-like lucencies ➔, consistent with a Morgagni hernia.* **(Right)** *Axial CECT in the same patient at 22 months old shows intraabdominal fat & bowel ➔ herniating into the anteromedial thorax at the costophrenic margin, consistent with a Morgagni hernia. While most Morgagni hernias are isolated defects, there is a rare association with trisomy 21.*

DIFFERENTIAL DIAGNOSIS

Common

- Lymphoma
- Foregut Duplication Cyst

Less Common

- Lymphadenopathy
- Vascular Lesion

Rare but Important

- Postoperative Complications
- Pericardial Lesions
- Malignant Tumors

ESSENTIAL INFORMATION

Key Differential Diagnosis Issues

- International Thymic Malignancy Interest Group 3: Compartment mediastinal classification system based on CT
- Anterior mediastinum (prevascular compartment)
  - Boundaries: Sternum (anterior), anterior pericardium to pulmonary veins (posterior), & parietal mediastinal pleura (lateral)
  - Contents: Thymus, fat, lymph nodes, left brachiocephalic vein
- Middle mediastinum (visceral compartment)
  - Boundaries: Posterior margin of prevascular compartment (anterior), 1 cm posterior to anterior cortex of vertebral bodies (posterior), & parietal mediastinal pleura (lateral)
  - Contents: Heart, superior vena cava (SVC), thoracic aorta, intrapericardial pulmonary arteries, thoracic duct, trachea, carina, esophagus, & lymph nodes
- Posterior mediastinum (paravertebral compartment)
  - Boundaries: Posterior margin of visceral compartment (anterior) & lateral margins of vertebral transverse processes (posterolateral)
  - Contents: Thoracic spine & paravertebral soft tissues
- Superior & inferior boundaries are thoracic inlet & diaphragm for all compartments

Helpful Clues for Common Diagnoses

- **Lymphoma**
  - Usually occurs with confluent multicompartment disease that involves anterior mediastinum
  - Most commonly involves paratracheal > hilar > subcarinal nodal groups
  - Homogeneous or heterogeneous soft tissue attenuation & signal intensity on CT & MR
  - May compress or invade SVC, esophagus, tracheobronchial tree, or pericardium
    - SVC more often compressed without associated obstruction, but invasion may lead to SVC syndrome
    - Bronchial involvement may lead to lobar collapse
    - Pericardial involvement can result in pericardial effusion
- **Foregut Duplication Cysts**
  - Include bronchogenic, esophageal, & neurenteric cysts
  - Bronchogenic cysts are most commonly subcarinal, precarinal, or paratracheal
    - Lung collapse or hyperlucency may result from bronchial compression
  - Esophageal cysts are typically intimately associated with esophagus
  - Neurenteric cysts extend to posterior mediastinum
    - Failure of separation of gastrointestinal tract from primitive neural crest
    - Extend into or communicate with spinal canal
    - Associated with congenital vertebral defects
  - All are usually round with smooth wall & thin peripheral enhancement
    - 50% appear as simple fluid-filled cysts
    - Otherwise variable appearance due to proteinaceous/hemorrhagic contents or superimposed infection

Helpful Clues for Less Common Diagnoses

- **Lymphadenopathy**
  - Usually related to infection in pediatric population
    - However, many metastatic lesions commonly lead to middle mediastinal lymphadenopathy
  - Most common inciting organism depends on geographic location
  - Consider primary tuberculosis (TB), histoplasmosis, coccidioidomycosis, & blastomycosis
    - TB & histoplasmosis may have lymph nodes with low-attenuation centers on CECT during acute phase
    - Ca^{2+} of lymph nodes indicates more remote disease
- **Vascular Lesion**
  - Most commonly due to congenital anomalies of aorta & its branches
    - Convexity to right of trachea on radiograph may be due to right aortic arch or double aortic arch
    - Posterior impression/anterior bowing of trachea on lateral radiograph may be due to
      - □ Diverticulum of Kommerell related to aberrant subclavian artery
      - □ Passage of aorta across midline posterior to trachea & esophagus in double or circumflex aortic arch
  - Dilation of ascending aorta
    - Convexity along right mediastinal border on chest radiograph; may be due to
      - □ Congenital aortic valvar stenosis (with bicuspid aortic valve)
      - □ Connective tissue disorders (Marfan, Loeys-Dietz, or vascular Ehlers-Danlos syndromes)
  - Dilation of pulmonary arteries is less common
    - Convexity in aortopulmonary window on radiographs due to
      - □ L → R shunts
      - □ Pulmonary arterial hypertension
      - □ Pulmonary valve stenosis
      - □ Massive pulmonary thromboembolism
  - May also involve azygous vein & anomalous pulmonary venous drainage
    - Azygous vein enlargement leads to convexity above right main bronchus
      - □ Most commonly from azygous continuation of inferior vena cava (IVC)
      - □ May also be secondary to obstruction of SVC

- Supracardiac total anomalous pulmonary venous return leads to snowman appearance of mediastinum on radiograph
- All pathologies are best seen on CTA or MR

Helpful Clues for Rare Diagnoses

- **Postoperative Complications**
  - Some fluid is always present in operative bed following cardiac surgery
    - Usually resolves within days with gradual decrease in size of mediastinum
  - Concern should be raised if radiographs demonstrate increased widening of mediastinum
  - May be due to hematoma, seroma, or infection
    - Hematoma may be associated with pseudoaneurysm at surgical site
      - Contrast protrusion from vessel lumen on CTA
      - Blood products, thrombus, &/or flow void with pulsation artifact on MR
- **Pericardial Lesions**
  - Pericardial effusion
    - Enlargement of cardiac silhouette with water bottle configuration on radiography
    - Lungs are usually clear
    - Fat pad sign on lateral chest radiograph is rarely seen due to relative lack of fat in mediastinum in pediatric population
    - May be secondary to infection (most commonly viruses), recent surgery or trauma, or related to neoplasia (lymphoma)
  - Pericardial cyst
    - Benign congenital cystic lesion
    - Arises from pericardium, usually without communication to pericardial space
    - Rounded convexity, most commonly in right cardiophrenic angle on radiography
    - Usually unilocular with characteristics of simple cyst
  - Pericardial tumors are uncommon
    - Teratoma is most common, seen in neonates & infants
      - Often heterogeneously cystic & solid
      - Associated pericardial effusion is common
- **Malignant Tumors**
  - Both primary & secondary malignant tumors are very rare, excluding lymphoma
  - Consider carcinoid, melanoma, rhabdomyosarcoma, malignant germ cell tumors, or squamous cell carcinoma in patients with respiratory papillomatosis

SELECTED REFERENCES

1. Carter BW et al: ITMIG Classification of mediastinal compartments and multidisciplinary approach to mediastinal masses. Radiographics. 37(2):413-36, 2017
2. Thacker PG et al: Imaging evaluation of mediastinal masses in children and adults: practical diagnostic approach based on a new classification system. J Thorac Imaging. 30(4):247-67, 2015
3. Ranganath SH et al: Mediastinal masses in children. AJR Am J Roentgenol. 198(3):W197-216, 2012

Lymphoma

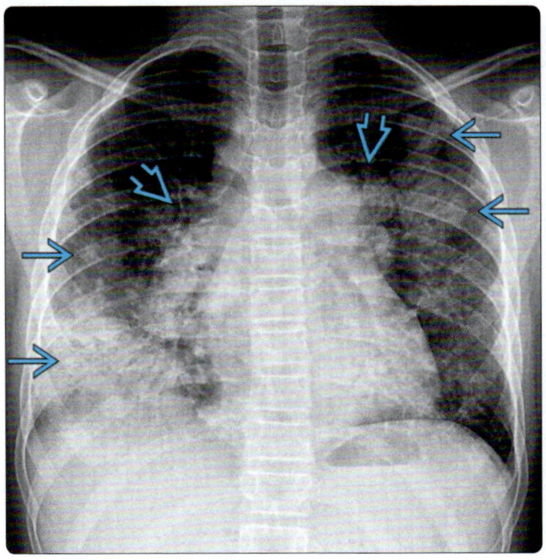

Lymphoma

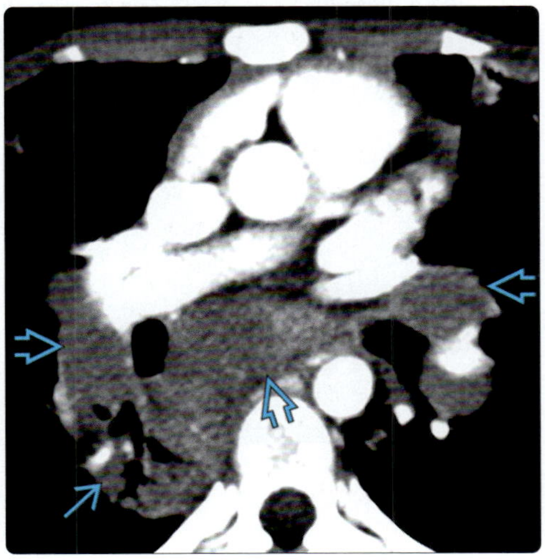

(Left) *PA radiograph in an 11 year old with a cough & weight loss shows multilobulated hilar masses ➡ along with multifocal round & confluent lung opacities ➡. The findings are worrisome for mediastinal & pulmonary lymphoma.* **(Right)** *Axial CECT in the same patient shows bulky subcarinal & hilar adenopathy ➡ along with airspace consolidation ➡. Lymphoma can be centered in the middle mediastinum but more commonly occurs as confluent disease extending from the anterior mediastinum.*

(Left) *Axial CECT in the same patient shows multiple bronchovascular round lung masses → along with adenopathy ⇨, consistent with mediastinal & pulmonary lymphoma. Primary pulmonary lymphoma is rare & can manifest as bronchovascular nodules or ill-defined opacities, commonly with mediastinal adenopathy.* **(Right)** *Coronal FDG PET/CT in the same patient shows FDG uptake in the mediastinal & pulmonary lesions →. PET/CT is the imaging modality of choice for initial staging & follow-up of lymphoma.*

Lymphoma

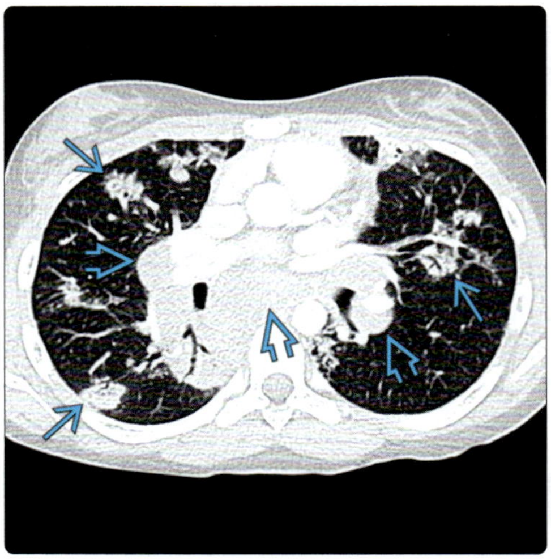

Lymphoma

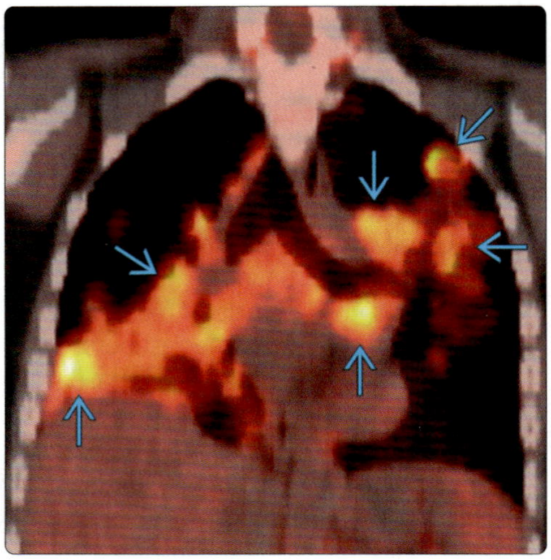

(Left) *Axial CECT in a 4 year old with dysphagia shows a simple-appearing subcarinal/hilar cystic lesion ⇨ with a thin wall & no solid components, typical of a bronchogenic cyst. The mass abuts the esophagus →.* **(Right)** *Coronal CECT in the same patient again shows the duplication cyst ⇨ as a simple-appearing cystic lesion with a thin wall & no solid components, intimately associated with the esophagus →. Esophageal duplication cysts typically occur in the distal 1/3 of the esophagus.*

Foregut Duplication Cyst

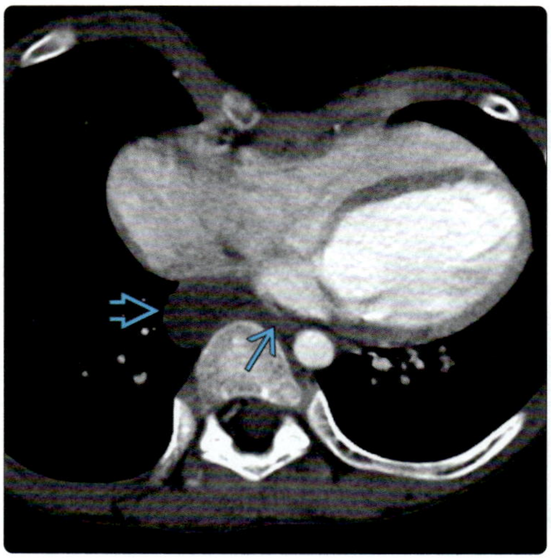

Foregut Duplication Cyst

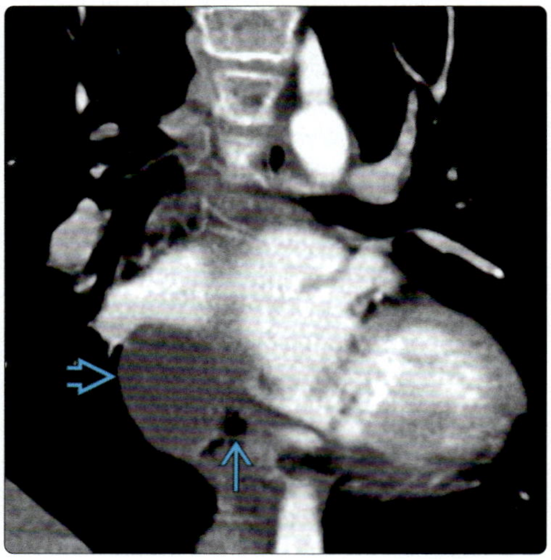

(Left) *Axial CECT shows a heterogeneous mass ↪ in the pretracheal region that compresses the trachea → & displaces the superior vena cava (SVC) anteriorly ⇨.* **(Right)** *Axial CECT shows the same mass more inferiorly ↪, causing compression of the right & left main bronchi →. The narrowing of the right main bronchus is causing air-trapping in the right lung, which is low in attenuation & hyperinflated ⇨. These lymph nodes were enlarged due to a Histoplasma infection.*

Lymphadenopathy

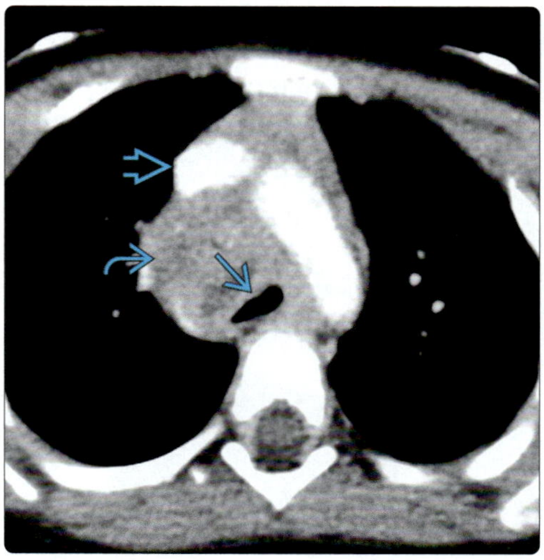

Lymphadenopathy

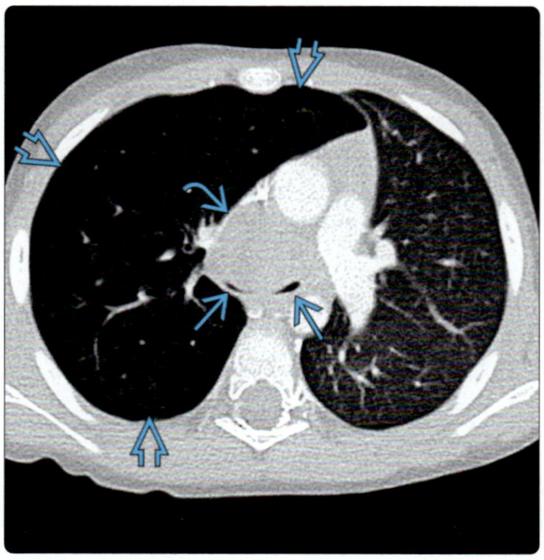

Lymphadenopathy

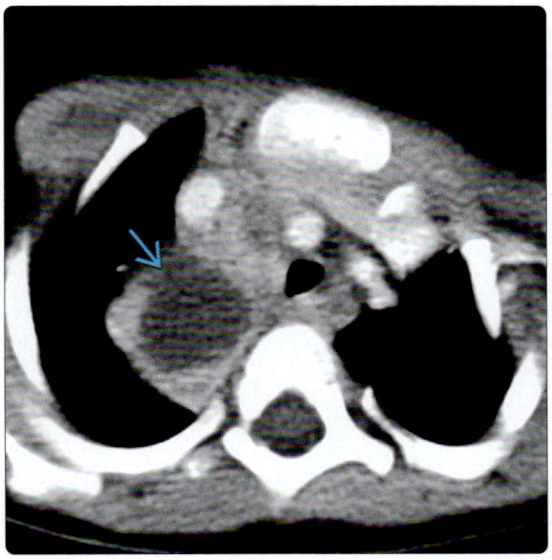

Lymphadenopathy

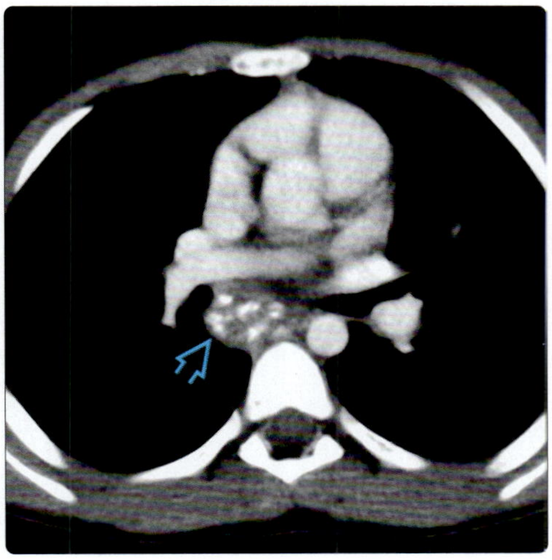

(Left) *Axial CECT shows low-attenuation nodes → in the right paratracheal region. Note the enhancing rim. Worldwide, tuberculosis (TB) is the most common infectious cause for this appearance.* **(Right)** *Axial CECT shows coarse Ca^{2+} of subcarinal lymph nodes →. These are commonly seen in cases of remote infection with the fungus Histoplasma capsulatum, the organism that causes histoplasmosis. Ca^{2+} of lung parenchymal nodules is often seen in such cases as well.*

Vascular Lesion

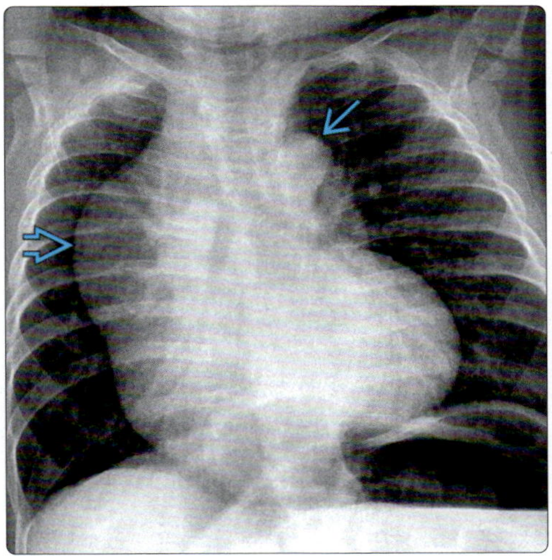

Vascular Lesion

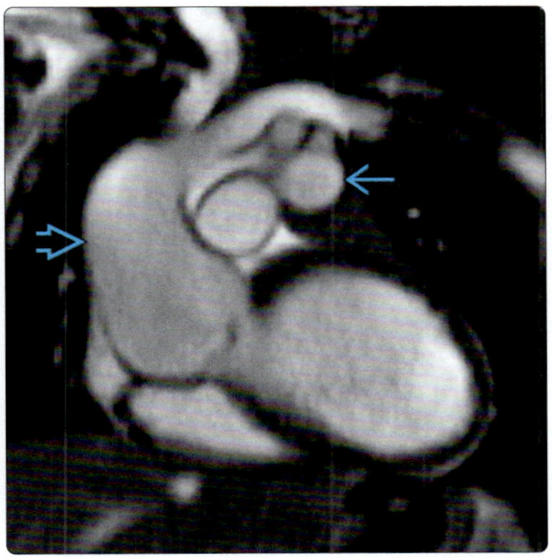

(Left) *Frontal radiograph in a 1 year old with Loeys-Dietz syndrome shows an abnormal mass-like contour to the right superior mediastinum → & a prominent aortic knob →. In a patient with Loeys-Dietz, this is consistent with a dilated & tortuous aorta.* **(Right)** *Left ventricular outflow tract SSFP cine MR in the same patient shows the dilated & tortuous ascending aorta → & arch →. There is effacement of the aortic sinotubular junction, typical of connective tissue aortopathies. Patients with Loeys-Dietz syndrome are at high risk for dissection.*

Vascular Lesion

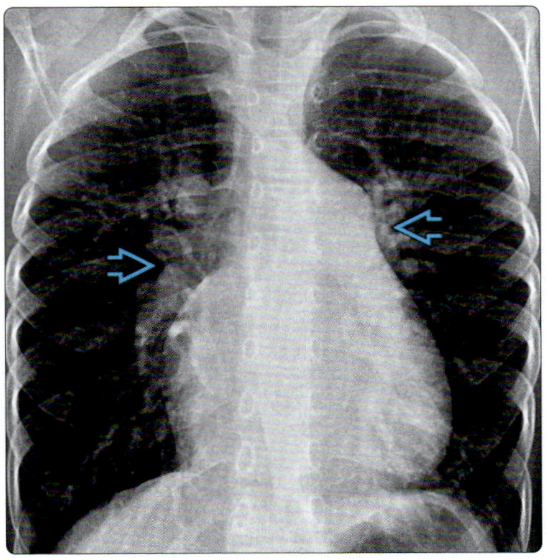

Vascular Lesion

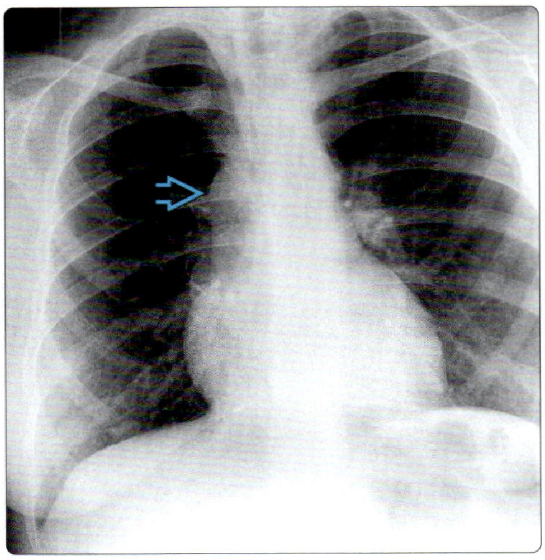

(Left) *PA radiograph in a 4 year old with pulmonary hypertension secondary to an ASD shows large central pulmonary arteries → but less peripheral vascularity than expected. Decreasing peripheral vascularity in a L → R shunt over time may represent the development of pulmonary hypertension.* **(Right)** *AP radiograph shows an abnormal convexity → above the right main bronchus with thickening of the right paratracheal stripe. This patient had obstruction of the inferior vena cava, resulting in an enlarged azygous vein.*

Vascular Lesion

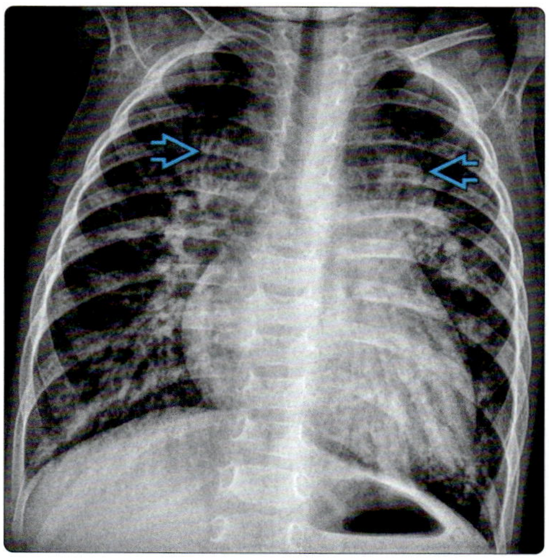

Vascular Lesion

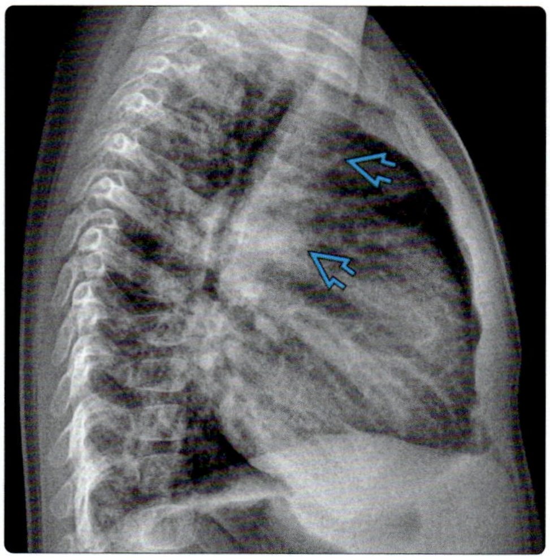

(Left) *PA radiograph in a 1 year old shows a rounded contour to the mediastinum ⇨ along with ↑ pulmonary vascularity & mild interstitial edema.* **(Right)** *Lateral radiograph in same patient shows pretracheal density ⇨, confirming that this mass lies in the middle mediastinum & is not thymus. This appearance is known as the snowman sign, which is seen in unobstructed supracardiac total anomalous pulmonary venous return from dilation of an anomalous left-sided vertical vein & right-sided SVC due to ↑ blood flow.*

Postoperative Complications

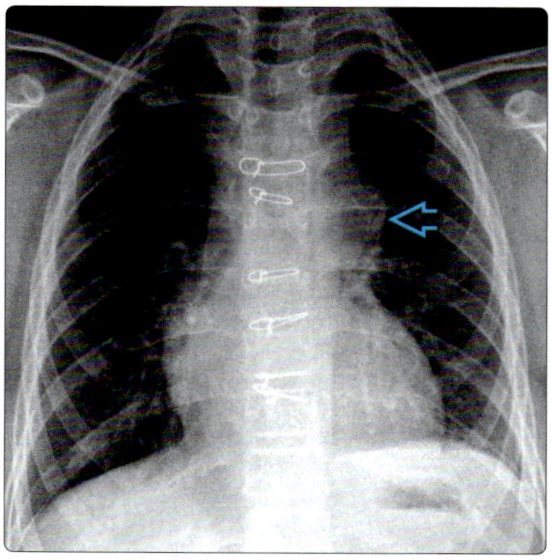

Postoperative Complications

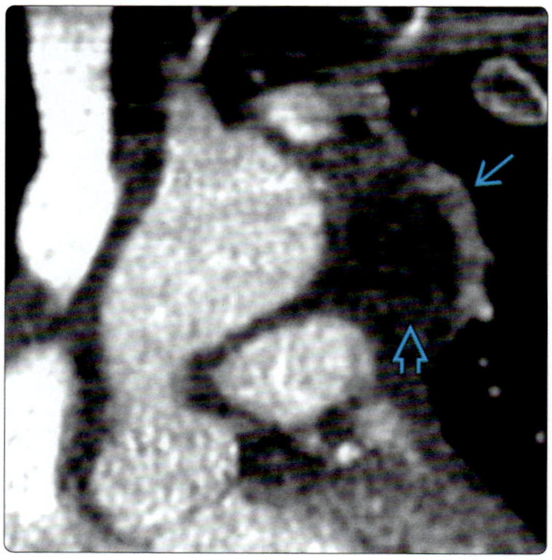

(Left) *PA radiograph in a 9 year old after discharge for a coarctation repair shows a new round, mass-like opacity of the left superior mediastinum ⇨. A hematoma or pseudoaneurysm needs to be considered.* **(Right)** *Coronal CECT (same patient) shows that the contour anomaly is related to postsurgical loculated mediastinal fluid/seroma ⇨, along with adjacent compressive atelectasis →. Increasing mediastinal widening after cardiac surgery should raise concern for hematoma, seroma, or infection.*

Postoperative Complications

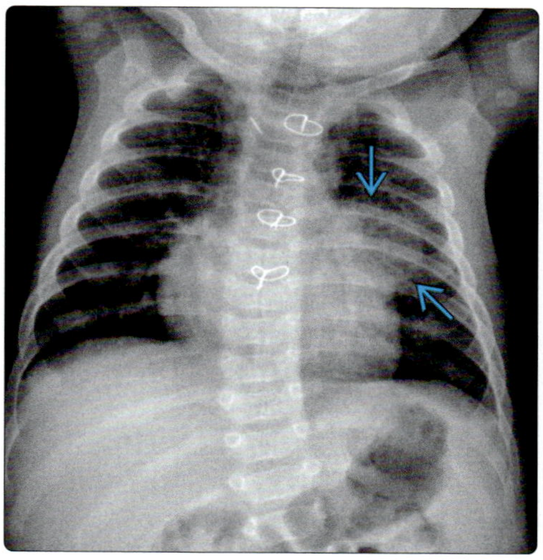

Postoperative Complications

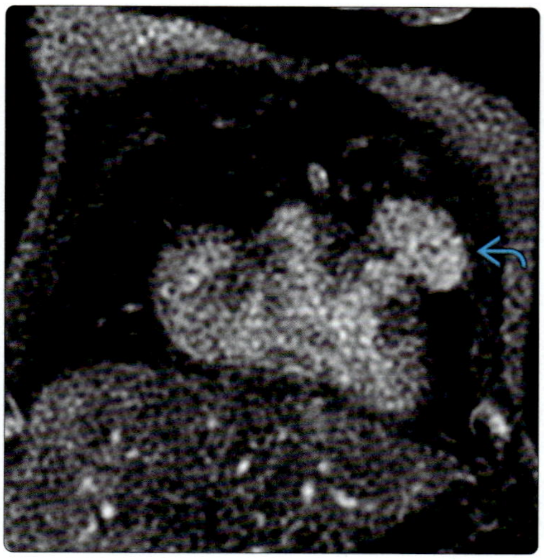

(Left) *Postoperative AP radiograph shows a new round opacity → adjacent to the left heart border. Preoperative radiographs had not demonstrated a mass.* **(Right)** *Coronal MRA shows filling of this lesion with blood ↪. This mass was due to a leak that developed after a corrective procedure for hypoplastic left heart syndrome. Pseudoaneurysms should always be considered as a cause of a new mass in patients with prior vascular surgery.*

Pericardial Lesions

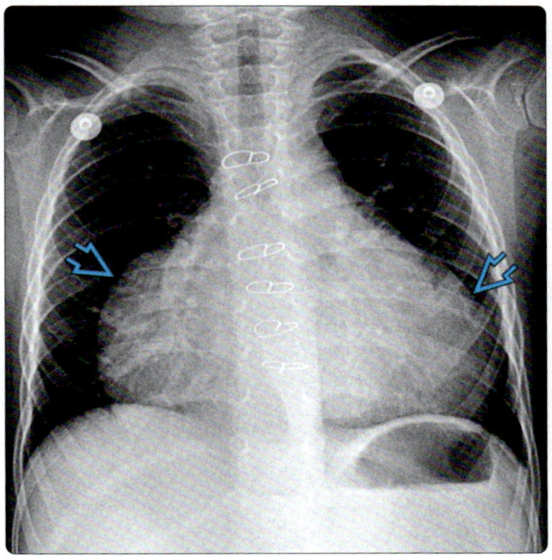

Pericardial Lesions

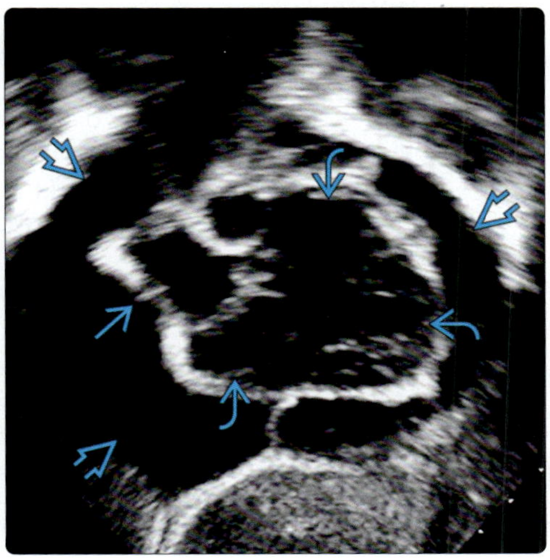

(Left) *PA radiograph in a 3 year old with hypoplastic left heart syndrome status post Fontan completion shows severe enlargement of the cardiac silhouette in a water bottle appearance, consistent with a large pericardial effusion.* **(Right)** *Subxiphoid coronal echocardiogram in the same patient shows the large pericardial effusion causing contour deformity of the right atrium, which can potentially impair filling & lead to cardiac tamponade. Note the dilated single right ventricle.*

Pericardial Lesions

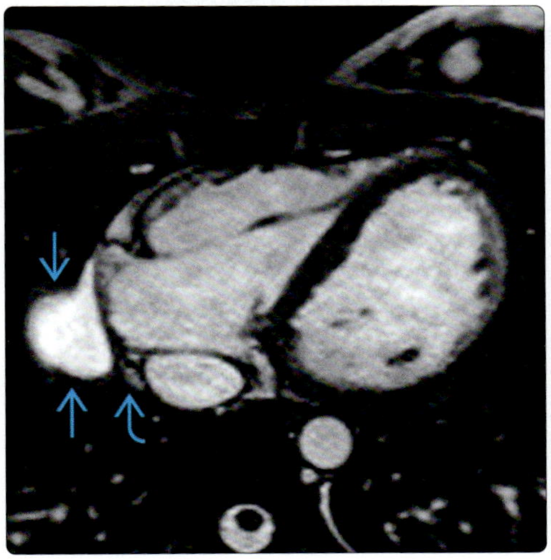

Pericardial Lesions

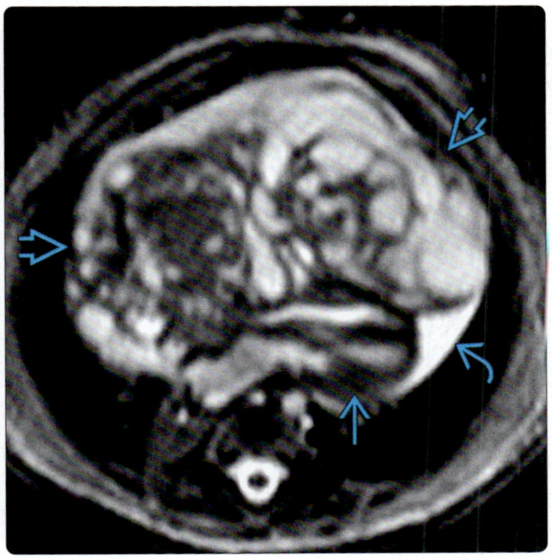

(Left) *Axial SSFP MR in a 16 year old shows an incidental lobulated cystic mass adjacent to the right atrium without internal septations, diagnostic for a pericardial cyst. Note the relationship with the pericardial fat. These cysts are connected with the parietal pericardium.* **(Right)** *Axial SSFP MR in a 6 week old shows a large, heterogeneous, solid & cystic pericardial teratoma that compresses & displaces the heart posteriorly. There is a moderate pericardial effusion.*

Malignant Tumors

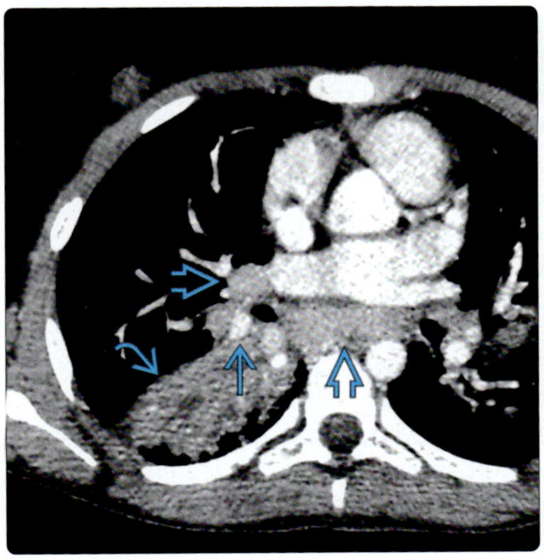

Malignant Tumors

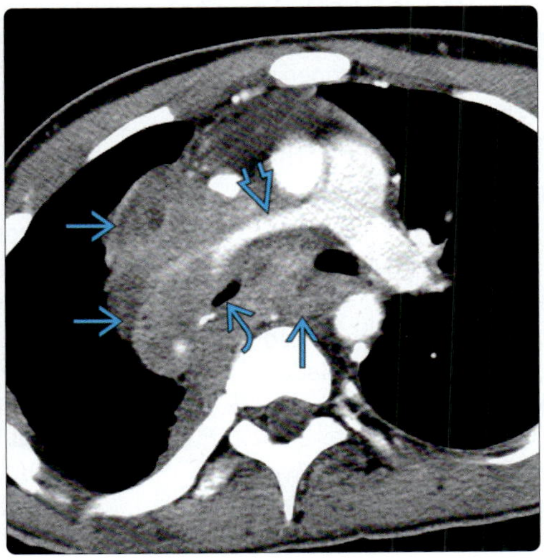

(Left) *Axial CECT shows an enhancing mass in the right lower lobe bronchus with associated hilar & mediastinal lymphadenopathy, consistent with a carcinoid tumor. Collapse of the right lower lobe is also present.* **(Right)** *Axial CECT shows extensive middle mediastinal adenopathy in a patient with malignant melanoma. The right main pulmonary artery is narrowed, as is the right main bronchus. At another level, the tumor extended into a neural foramen.*

Posterior Mediastinal Mass

DIFFERENTIAL DIAGNOSIS

Common

- Neural Crest Tumors
- Lymphoma

Less Common

- Nerve Sheath Tumors
- Foregut Duplication Cysts

Rare but Important

- Meningocele
- Paraspinal Abscess
- Extramedullary Hematopoiesis
- Musculoskeletal Tumor

ESSENTIAL INFORMATION

Key Differential Diagnosis Issues

- International Thymic Malignancy Interest Group 3: Compartment mediastinal classification system based on CT
- Anterior mediastinum (prevascular compartment)
  - Boundaries: Sternum (anterior), anterior pericardium to pulmonary veins (posterior), & parietal mediastinal pleura (lateral)
  - Contents: Thymus, fat, lymph nodes, left brachiocephalic vein
- Middle mediastinum (visceral compartment)
  - Boundaries: Posterior margin of prevascular compartment (anterior), 1 cm posterior to anterior cortex of vertebral bodies (posterior), & parietal mediastinal pleura (lateral)
  - Contents: Heart, superior vena cava (SVC), thoracic aorta, intrapericardial pulmonary arteries, thoracic duct, trachea, carina, esophagus, & lymph nodes
- Posterior mediastinum (paravertebral compartment)
  - Boundaries: Posterior margin of visceral compartment (anterior) & lateral margins of vertebral transverse processes (posterolateral)
  - Contents: Thoracic spine & paravertebral soft tissues
- Superior & inferior boundaries are thoracic inlet & diaphragm for all compartments
- 90% of posterior mediastinal tumors are neurogenic
  - Posterior mediastinal mass in young child should be considered neuroblastoma (NB) until proven otherwise

Helpful Clues for Common Diagnoses

- **Neural Crest Tumors**
  - Includes NB, ganglioneuroblastoma (GNB), & ganglioneuroma (GN) (spectrum)
    - NB: Malignant with immature, undifferentiated sympathetic cells; occurs in younger population (median age < 2 years)
    - GNB: Intermediate between NB & GN
    - GN: Most mature & least aggressive; occurs in older population (median age ~ 7 years)
  - 20% of NB occurs in posterior mediastinum
    - Can occur anywhere along sympathetic chain
  - Radiograph: Elongated oval mass with tapered borders in paraspinal location
    - Homogeneously solid ± fine or chunky Ca^{2+} (30%)
    - ± separation or erosion of ribs or enlargement of neural foramina
    - Can appear more round at apex
  - CT: Better demonstrates Ca^{2+} (80-90% of NB, ~ 50% of GN)
  - MR: Better demonstrates intraspinal extension
  - Nuclear medicine imaging
    - I-123 MIBG: Mainstay for diagnosis & assessing response to therapy
    - PET/CT: Most useful if tumor is non-MIBG avid
- **Lymphoma**
  - Typically occurs in children > 5 years of age
  - Nearly always associated with sites in other mediastinal compartments
    - Isolated posterior mediastinal lymphoma is uncommon
  - Often encases & compresses brachiocephalic veins & SVC, deviates & compresses trachea
  - Look for disease in hila, lungs, axillae, pleural space, neck, & upper abdomen

Helpful Clues for Less Common Diagnoses

- **Nerve Sheath Tumors**
  - Includes schwannoma (neurilemoma), localized neurofibroma, plexiform neurofibroma, & malignant peripheral nerve sheath tumor (MPNST)
  - Radiographs: Sharply defined, round, smooth, or lobulated paraspinal masses
    - May see rib remodeling/splaying, neural foraminal enlargement, or posterior vertebral body scalloping
  - CT: Mild heterogeneous enhancement (iso- to hypoenhancing to muscle)
  - MR: Low to intermediate on T1; intermediate to high on T2; variable enhancement
  - Neurofibromas may have T2 target appearance: High signal peripherally & intermediate signal centrally
    - Most commonly seen in neurofibromatosis type 1 (NF1); look for associated scoliosis, dural ectasia, & meningoceles
      - □ May be visible along intercostal nerves & in skin & subcutaneous tissues
      - □ Can distort ribs, giving them ribbon-like appearance
    - Plexiform neurofibromas are extensive, lobulated, infiltrative tumors that may extend into middle mediastinum & other compartments
      - □ Pathognomonic of NF1
  - MPNSTs in children usually arise from preexisting neurofibroma in setting of NF1
    - Clues to transformation: Rapid enlargement, heterogeneous enhancement, central necrosis, perilesional edema, or intratumoral cysts
      - □ PET may be best tool to detect malignant transformation
- **Foregut Duplication Cysts**
  - Include bronchogenic, esophageal, & neurenteric cysts
  - Bronchogenic cysts are most commonly subcarinal, precarinal, or paratracheal (middle mediastinum)
  - Esophageal cysts are typically intimately associated with esophagus
    - Can extend to posterior mediastinum

- Neurenteric cysts lie at junction between posterior & middle mediastinum
  - Failure of separation of gastrointestinal tract from primitive neural crest
  - Extend into or communicate with spinal canal
  - Associated with congenital vertebral defects
- All are usually round with smooth wall & thin peripheral enhancement
  - 50% appear as simple fluid-filled cysts
  - Show otherwise variable appearance due to proteinaceous/hemorrhagic contents or superinfection

Helpful Clues for Rare Diagnoses

- **Meningocele**
  - Herniation of leptomeninges through intervertebral foramen
  - May be anterior, lateral, or dorsal
  - Majority associated with NF; vertebral & rib anomalies are common
  - Associated with other spinal anomalies; may lead to kyphosis or scoliosis
  - CT: Fluid attenuation
  - MR: Low on T1, high on T2; no enhancement
- **Paraspinal Abscess**
  - Discitis is more common in preschool children vs. vertebral osteomyelitis in older children
  - *Staphylococcus aureus* is most common pyogenic organism; tuberculosis is most common worldwide
  - Discitis & osteomyelitis
    - Disc space narrowing with indistinct end plates
    - Paravertebral soft tissue mass with rim enhancement
  - Tuberculosis
    - Disc space narrowing often occurs later than in pyogenic osteomyelitis
    - Gibbus deformity
- **Extramedullary Hematopoiesis**
  - 1 or more lobulated soft tissue masses in lower thoracic paraspinal region, typically in setting of chronic severe anemia
  - CT: Homogeneous soft tissue attenuation
  - MR: Homogeneous signal with mild to moderate enhancement; look for red marrow reconversion in spine
  - May have expanded ribs & vertebral bodies
- **Musculoskeletal Tumor**
  - Some primary (e.g., rhabdomyosarcoma) & secondary (i.e., metastatic) tumors can occur at nearly any site in body

SELECTED REFERENCES

1. Carter BW et al: ITMIG classification of mediastinal compartments and multidisciplinary approach to mediastinal masses. Radiographics. 37(2):413-36, 2017
2. Thacker PG et al: Imaging evaluation of mediastinal masses in children and adults: practical diagnostic approach based on a new classification system. J Thorac Imaging. 30(4):247-67, 2015
3. Ranganath SH et al: Mediastinal masses in children. AJR Am J Roentgenol. 198(3):W197-216, 2012

Neural Crest Tumors

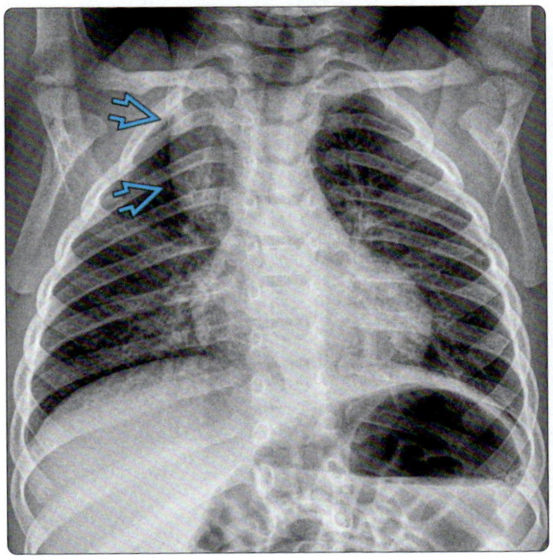

Neural Crest Tumors

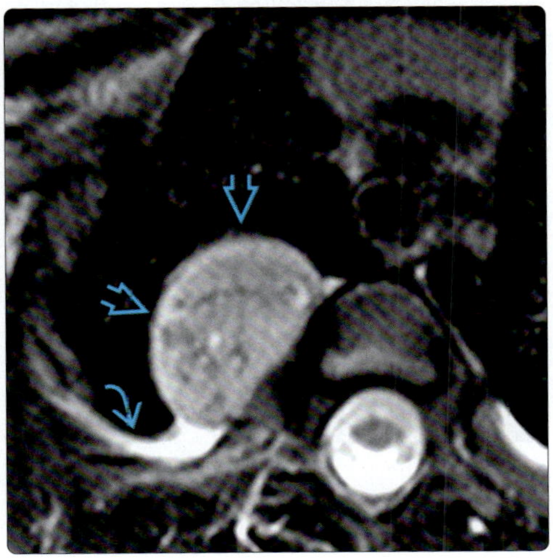

(Left) *PA radiograph in a 16-month-old male patient with weight loss, developmental regression, & new-onset opsoclonus shows a right mediastinal mass ➡.* **(Right)** *Axial T2 FS MR in the same patient shows an ovoid, heterogeneous intermediate signal intensity right paraspinal mass ➡, consistent with a neuroblastoma. There is a small right pleural effusion ↪. MR best detects any intraspinal extension through the neural foramina (not seen here), which is an image-defined risk factor for staging.*

(Left) *PA radiograph in a 6 month old with respiratory distress shows a posterior mediastinal mass containing amorphous Ca^{2+}. Note the rib erosion & remodeling, a clue to the posterior mediastinal location. There is also a moderate right pleural effusion.* (Right) *Axial CECT in the same patient shows a large posterior mediastinal mass with amorphous Ca^{2+} & associated rib erosion, consistent with a neuroblastoma. Ca^{2+} are common in neural crest tumors.*

Neural Crest Tumors

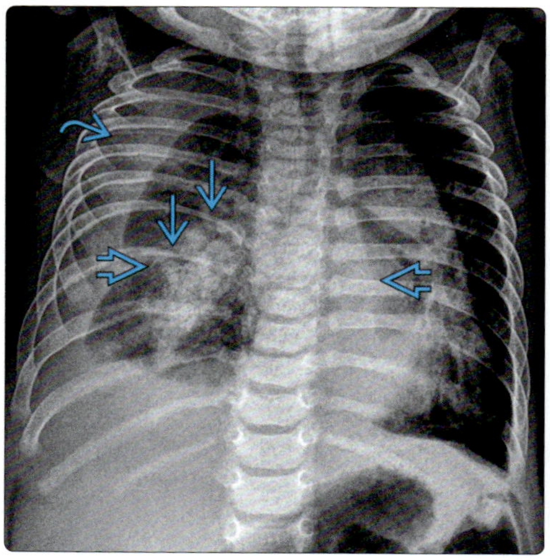

Neural Crest Tumors

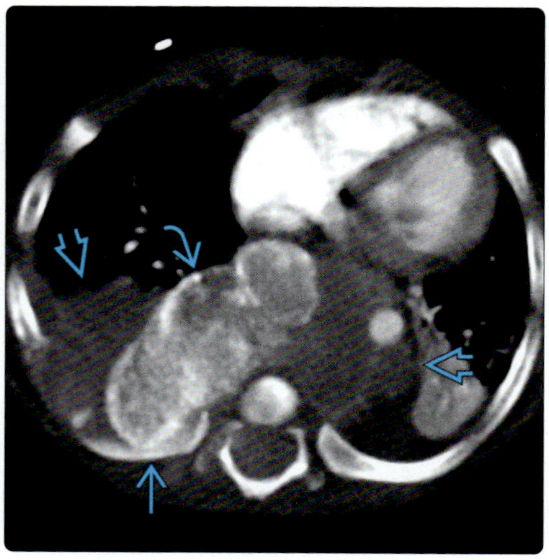

(Left) *PA radiograph in a 2 year old with chest pain shows an oblong convexity along the right mediastinum.* (Right) *Axial CECT in the same patient shows a right paraspinal posterior mediastinal mass with scattered stippled Ca^{2+}. Any posterior mediastinal mass in a young child should be considered neuroblastoma until proven otherwise. In this case, surgical pathology revealed a ganglioneuroblastoma, which is an intermediate-grade neuroblastic tumor.*

Neural Crest Tumors

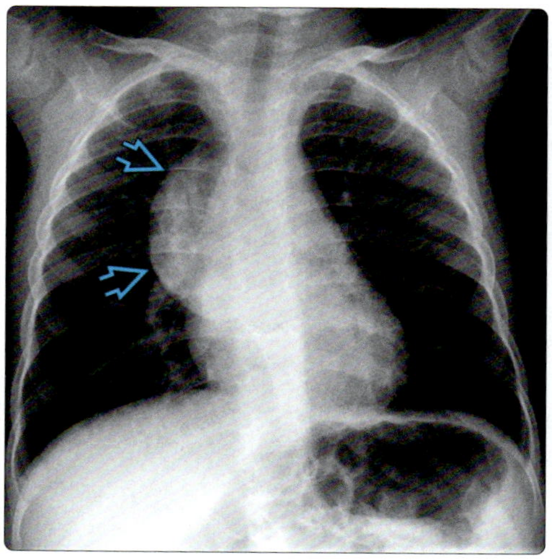

Neural Crest Tumors

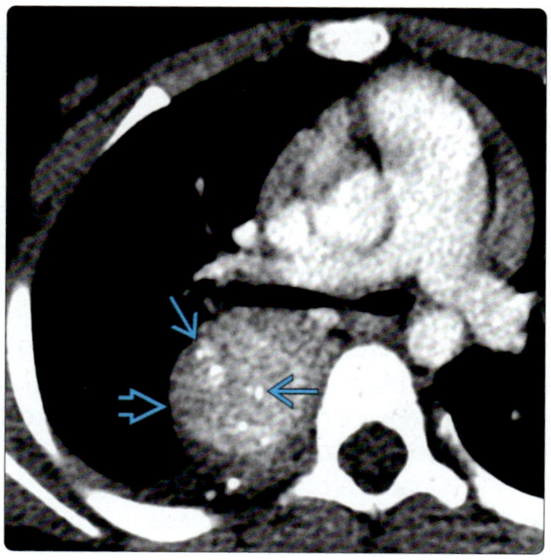

(Left) *Coronal CECT in the same patient shows the right paraspinal mass with scattered stippled Ca^{2+} & areas of necrosis/cystic change. Neuroblastic tumors typically have an oblong shape spanning multiple vertebral levels in craniocaudal dimension.* (Right) *Frontal projection MIBG in the same patient shows intense MIBG uptake in the mass. MIBG scans are a mainstay for staging & posttreatment surveillance of neuroblastic tumors.*

Neural Crest Tumors

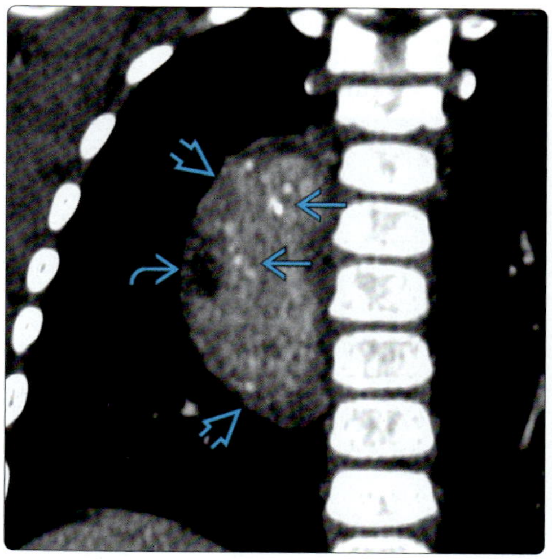

Neural Crest Tumors

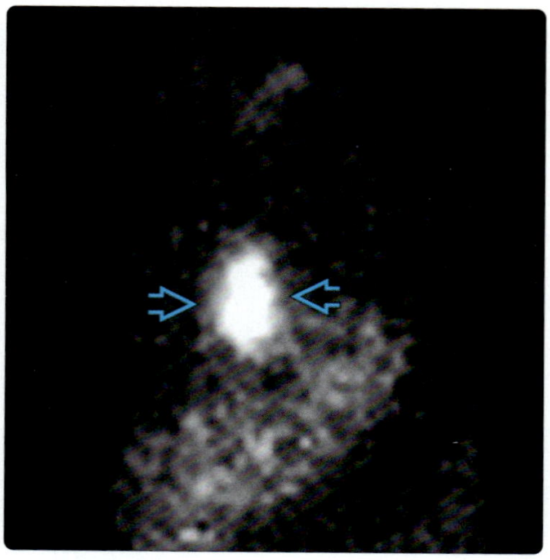

Lymphoma

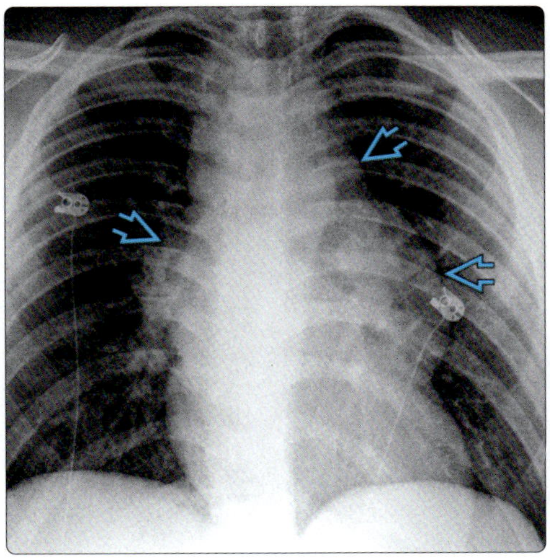

Lymphoma

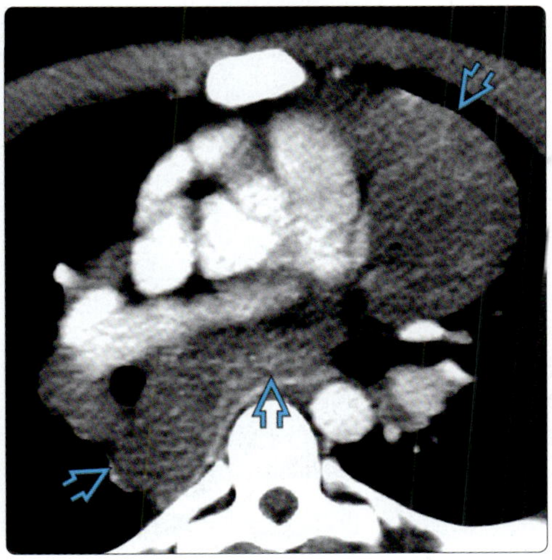

(Left) *PA radiograph in a 16 year old with fever, weight loss, & night sweats shows a lobulated mediastinal & hilar mass, suspicious for lymphoma.* **(Right)** *Axial CECT in the same patient shows multiple lobulated masses of the anterior, middle, & posterior mediastinum. Isolated involvement of the posterior mediastinum by lymphoma is uncommon, though the non-Hodgkin types are most likely to involve the posterior mediastinum.*

Nerve Sheath Tumors

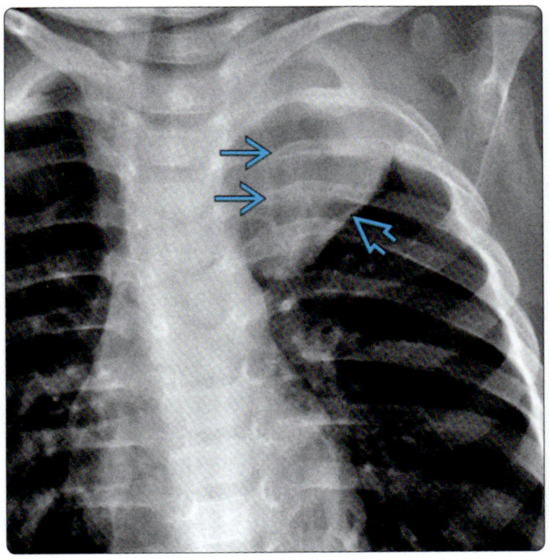

Nerve Sheath Tumors

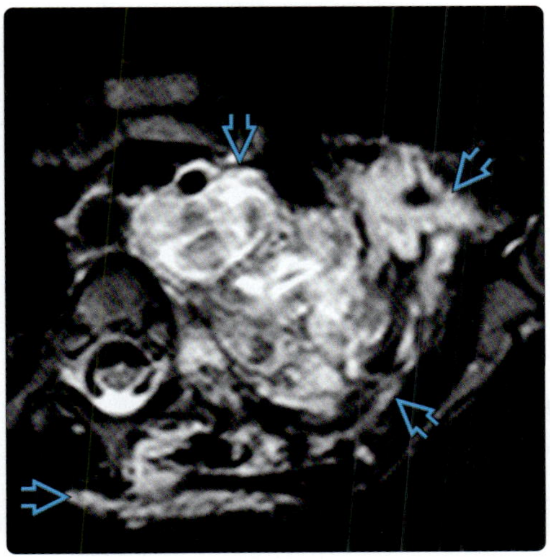

(Left) *PA radiograph in a 21 month old with neurofibromatosis type 1 (NF1) shows an incidental mass in the left upper hemithorax. Posterior rib remodeling confirms a posterior location.* **(Right)** *Axial T2 FS MR in the same patient shows an extensive left paraspinal plexiform neurofibroma infiltrating the mediastinum, axilla, & paraspinal soft tissues. Plexiform neurofibromas represent tortuous lobulated expansions of long nerve segments, occurring almost exclusively in NF1 patients.*

Nerve Sheath Tumors

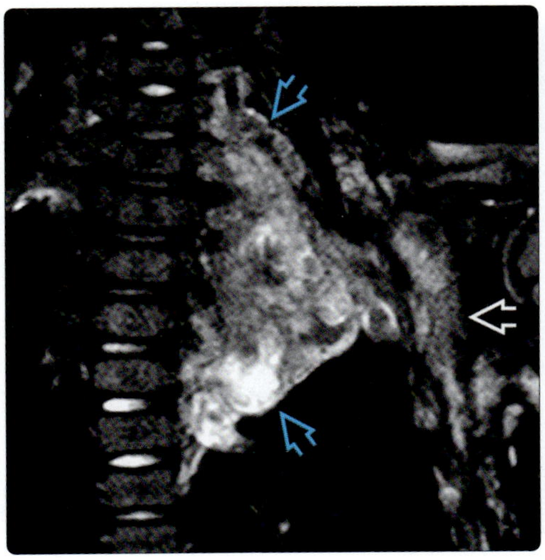

Nerve Sheath Tumors

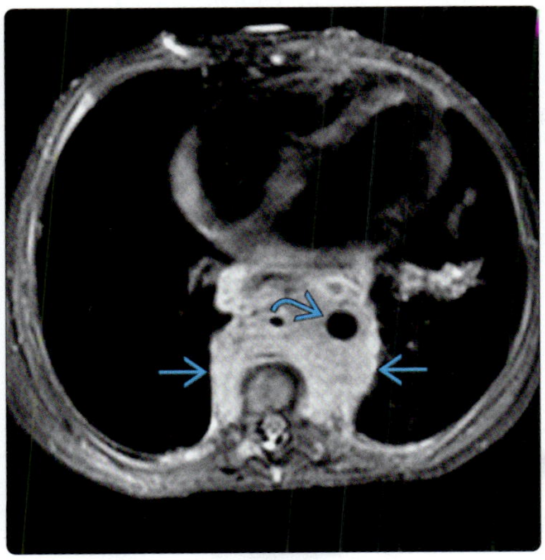

(Left) *Coronal STIR MR in the same patient shows the broad-based left paraspinal plexiform neurofibroma with chest wall extension. Neurofibromas often have a target appearance in cross section with peripheral hyperintensity & central low to intermediate intensity.* **(Right)** *Axial STIR MR shows a lobulated, hyperintense paraspinal mass. This plexiform neurofibroma infiltrates the mediastinum & elevates the aorta away from the spine.*

(Left) *Axial T1 MR in an infant shows a dumbbell-shaped cyst with intraspinal & mediastinal components. The waist of the cystic lesion traverses an associated vertebral segmentation anomaly.* **(Right)** *Sagittal T2 SSFSE MR in the same patient shows the cyst with intraspinal & mediastinal components traversing a vertebral segmentation anomaly. This is consistent with a neurenteric cyst. Progressive neurological decline can occur from cord compression.*

Foregut Duplication Cysts

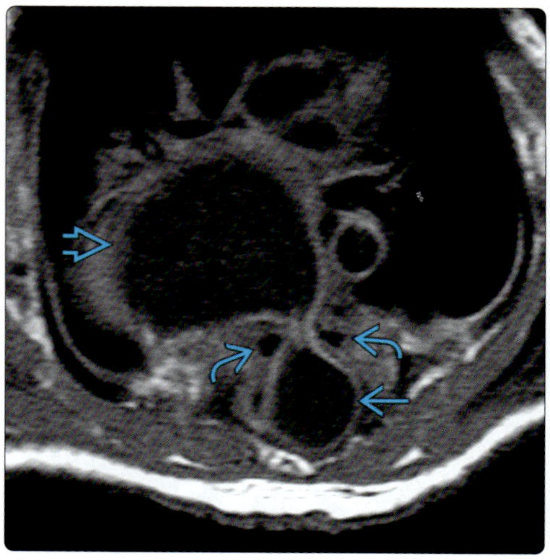

Foregut Duplication Cysts

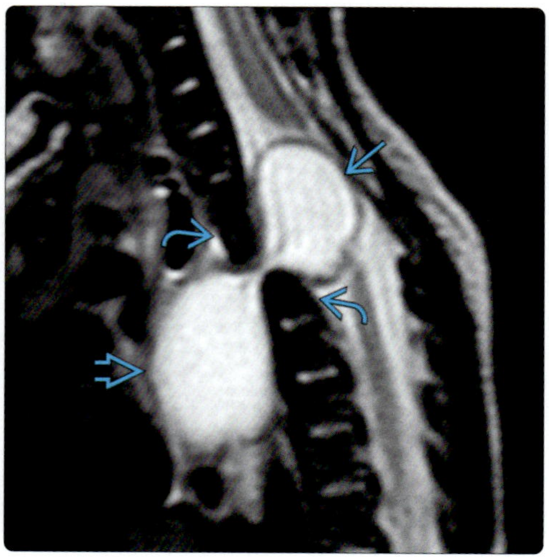

(Left) *Axial T2 MR shows a meningocele extending through an expanded neural foramen. There is also a meningocele component that extends dorsally within the spinal canal, compressing & anteriorly displacing the thecal sac & spinal cord.* **(Right)** *Axial CECT shows a large fluid-density mass extending from the spinal canal via expanded neural foramina in a patient with NF1, consistent with a large thoracic meningocele.*

Meningocele

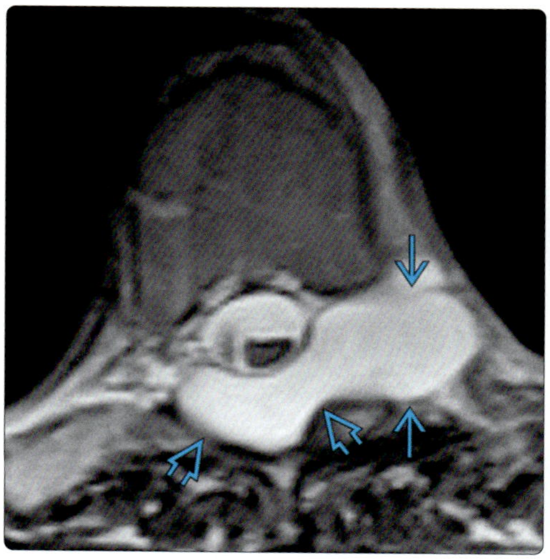

Meningocele

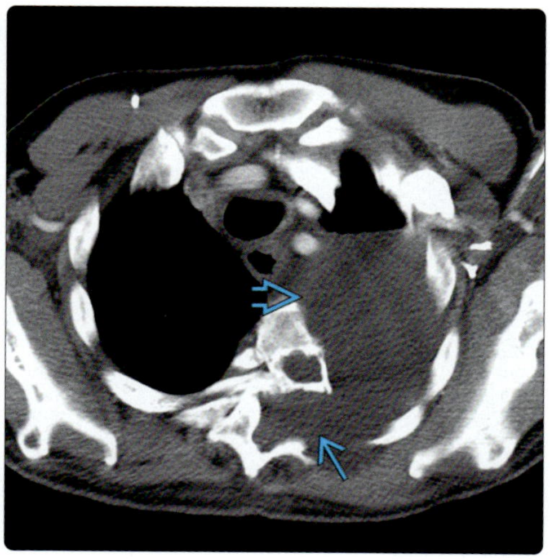

(Left) *Axial CECT in a 1 year old with Staphylococcus aureus bacteremia & meningitis shows a complex multiseptated paraspinal fluid collection with thick, enhancing rim & displaced vertebral bone destruction, consistent with a paraspinal abscess.* **(Right)** *Coronal T1 C+ FS MR in the same patient shows the complex paraspinal abscess with a thick, enhancing rim. Bacterial paraspinal abscesses usually originate from vertebral osteomyelitis &/or discitis.*

Paraspinal Abscess

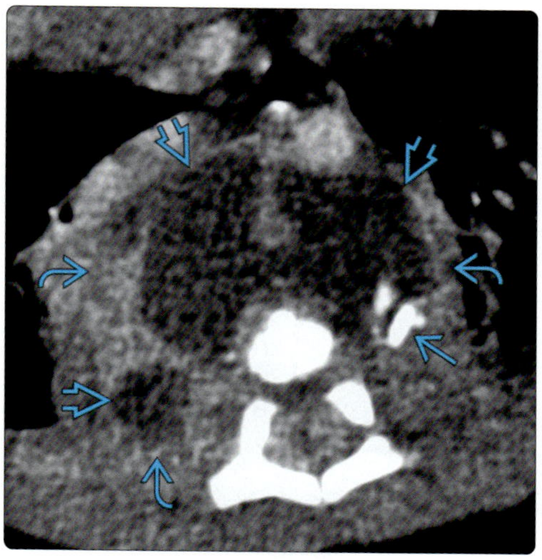

Paraspinal Abscess

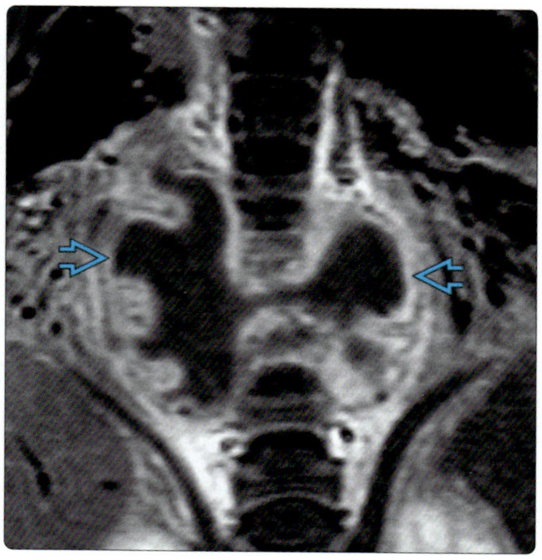

Paraspinal Abscess

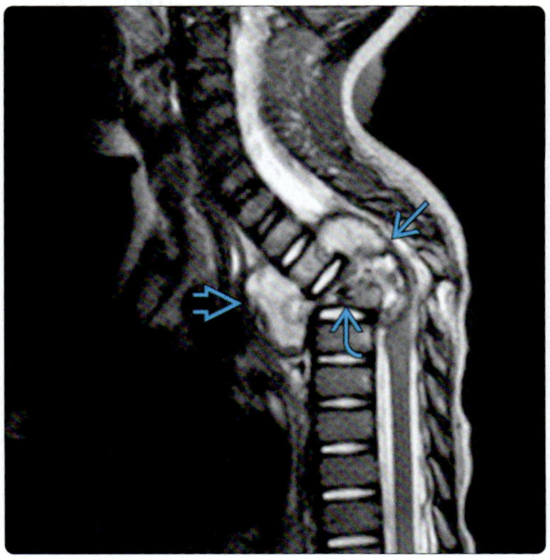

Paraspinal Abscess

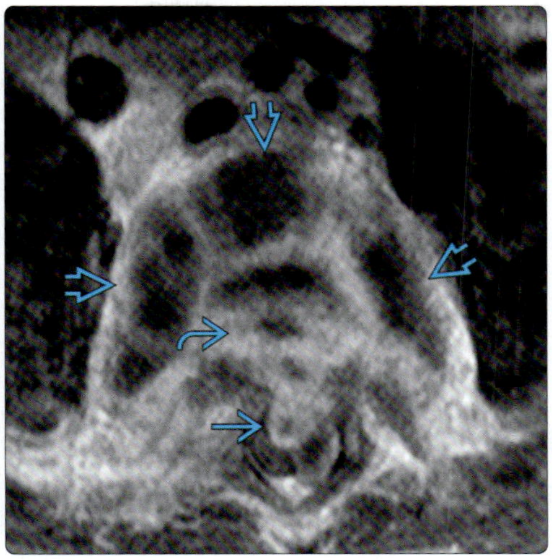

(Left) *Sagittal T2 MR shows thoracic spinal tuberculosis with kyphotic deformity & large epidural & paraspinal abscesses. A focal gibbus deformity is present with near-complete destruction of an intervertebral disc & 2 adjacent vertebral bodies.* **(Right)** *Axial T1 C+ FS MR shows large paravertebral abscesses with an intraspinal component. There is also abnormal enhancement of the vertebral body. Tuberculosis is the most common cause of infectious spondylitis worldwide.*

Extramedullary Hematopoiesis

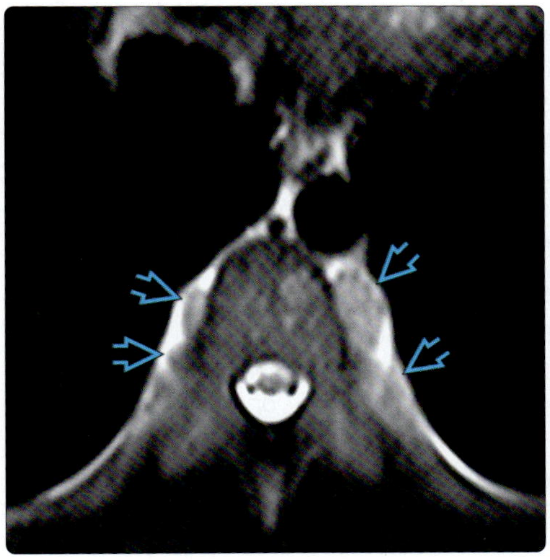

Extramedullary Hematopoiesis

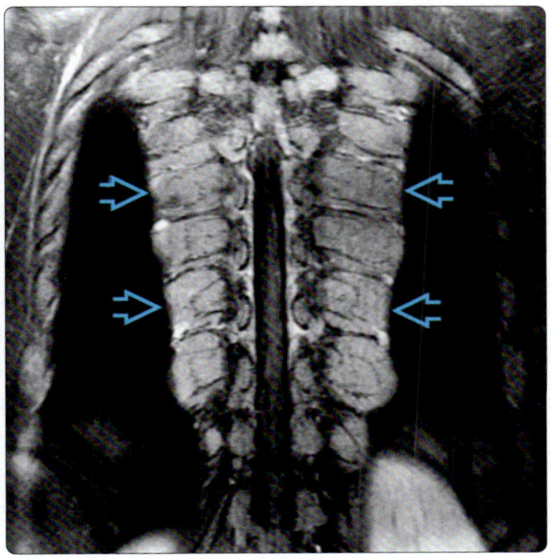

(Left) *Axial T2 FS MR in a 17 year old with β-thalassemia on chronic transfusion therapy shows multiple lobulated paraspinal masses, most consistent with extramedullary hematopoiesis given the clinical history.* **(Right)** *Coronal T1 C+ FS MR shows diffuse, mild to moderate enhancement of bilateral paraspinal masses, typical of extramedullary hematopoiesis. The masses are recruited tissue that produces red blood cells.*

Musculoskeletal Tumor

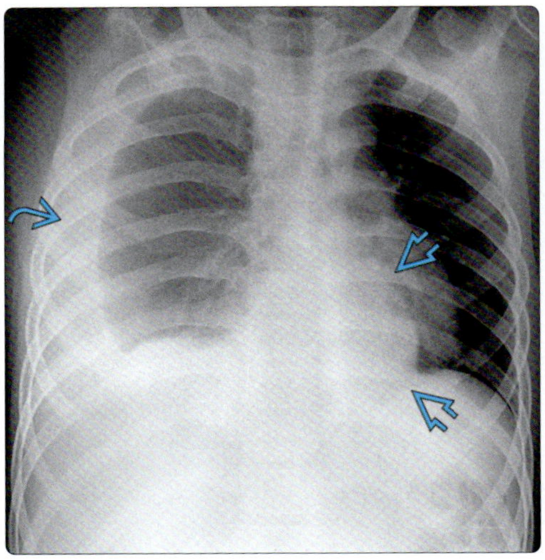

Musculoskeletal Tumor

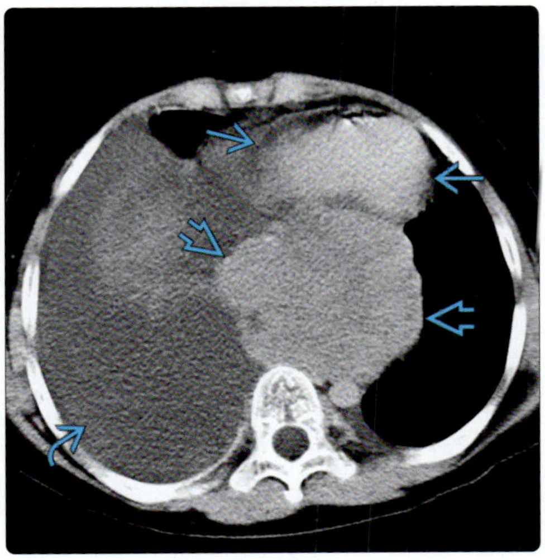

(Left) *Frontal radiograph shows a soft tissue mass predominantly to the left of midline. A large right-sided pleural effusion is present. The heart is displaced slightly into the left hemithorax.* **(Right)** *Axial CECT in the same patient shows a large mildly heterogeneous soft tissue mass in the middle mediastinum with mild extension to the posterior mediastinum. The heart is displaced anteriorly. There is an associated large right pleural effusion. Pathology demonstrated a rhabdomyosarcoma.*

DIFFERENTIAL DIAGNOSIS

Common

- Anastomotic Stricture
- Vascular Ring

Less Common

- Caustic Ingestion
- Eosinophilic Esophagitis
- Gastroesophageal Reflux

Rare but Important

- Congenital Esophageal Stenosis
- Epidermolysis Bullosa

ESSENTIAL INFORMATION

Key Differential Diagnosis Issues

- Medical & surgical history
- Location of stricture
- Clinical examination

Helpful Clues for Common Diagnoses

- **Anastomotic Stricture**
  - History of repaired esophageal atresia
  - Narrowing is located at level of anastomosis
  - Proximal esophagus often remains dilated
  - Generalized esophageal dysmotility is typical
  - Mild postthoracotomy lateral rib changes persist at 1-2 levels; usually right sided unless patient has right aortic arch (which dictates left approach)
- **Vascular Ring**
  - Right aortic arch with aberrant left subclavian artery
    - Trachea shifted slightly to left
    - Oblique impression on right side of proximal esophagus (directed from right inferior to left superior) on frontal view
    - Posterior indentation on lateral esophagram
  - Double aortic arch
    - Indentations on both sides of esophagus on frontal view (may be at slightly different levels) with posterior indentation on lateral view
  - Pulmonary sling
    - Left pulmonary artery arises from proximal right pulmonary artery
    - Passes between trachea & esophagus, causing anterior impression on lateral esophagram

Helpful Clues for Less Common Diagnoses

- **Caustic Ingestion**
  - History is key
  - Acute: Ulceration → perforation → pneumomediastinum
  - Chronic: Cicatrization & scarring → long segment stricture (smooth or irregular)
- **Eosinophilic Esophagitis**
  - Chronic dysphagia & chest pain; often presents as teenager with recurrent sensation of food becoming stuck at certain level
  - Specific degree of eosinophilia on biopsy
  - Esophagram
    - 50% normal
    - Reflux & abnormal motility in many
    - Ringed esophagus with mucosal irregularity seen less frequently in pediatrics
- **Gastroesophageal Reflux**
  - Dysmotility is most common
  - Mucosal irregularity typically occurs in distal esophagus
  - Concentric, smooth, tapered distal stricture

Helpful Clues for Rare Diagnoses

- **Congenital Esophageal Stenosis**
  - Caused by tracheobronchial remnants in esophageal wall, fibromuscular hypertrophy, or membranous webs
  - Results in short, smooth distal esophageal stricture
- **Epidermolysis Bullosa**
  - Excessive skin fragility → extensive skin blisters
  - Involvement of GI tract leads to scarring/strictures

(Left) *Oblique fluoroscopic esophagram prior to dilation in a 6 year old with repaired esophageal atresia & tracheoesophageal fistula demonstrates focal stenosis at the site of anastomosis in the proximal esophagus ➔. The esophagus typically shows chronic dysmotility in these cases.* **(Right)** *Oblique lateral esophagram shows focal stenosis at the upper esophagus with proximal dilation in this 18 month old with a history of esophageal atresia repair ➔. The proximal esophagus often remains dilated in these cases.*

Anastomotic Stricture

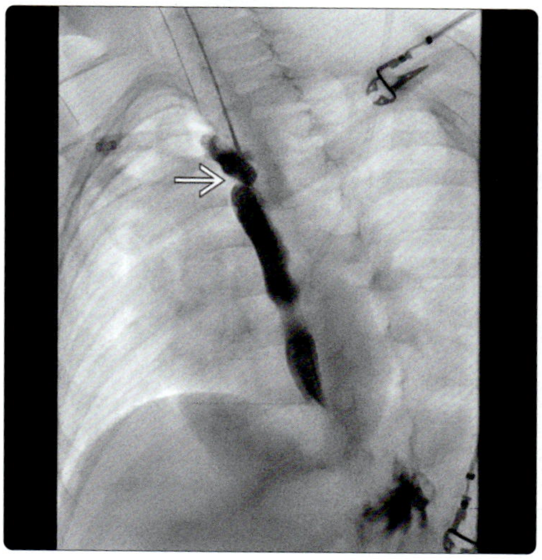

Anastomotic Stricture

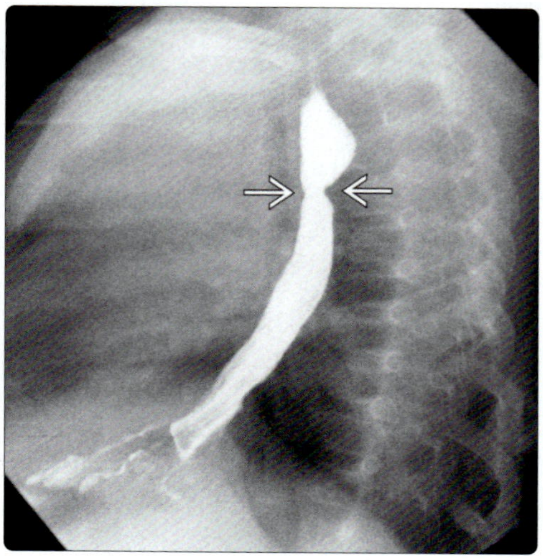

Vascular Ring

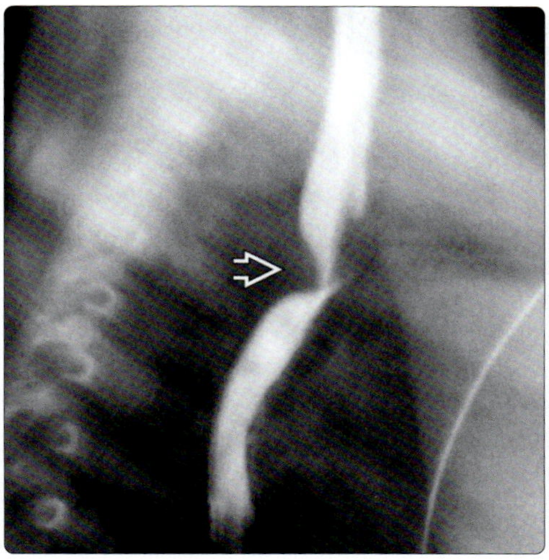

Caustic Ingestion

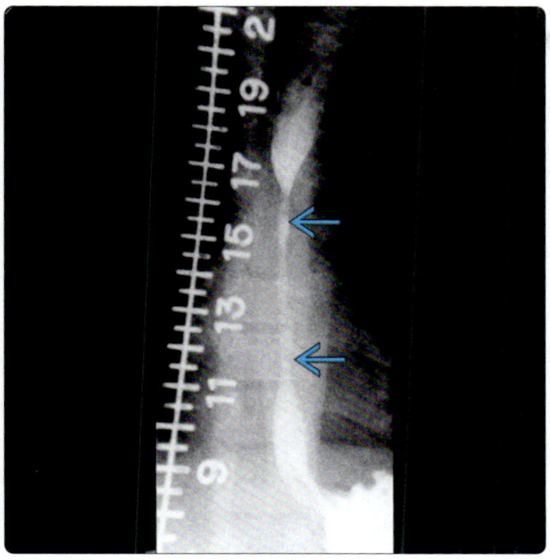

(Left) *Lateral fluoroscopic image from an upper GI study in a patient with a double aortic arch shows posterior indentation on the esophagus . A right aortic arch with aberrant left subclavian artery can also have a similar appearance on this view, though the frontal view may provide more specific clues.* **(Right)** *Frontal esophagram shows a long segment of smooth stricture involving the mid to distal esophagus in this 7 year old with a history of caustic ingestion.*

Eosinophilic Esophagitis

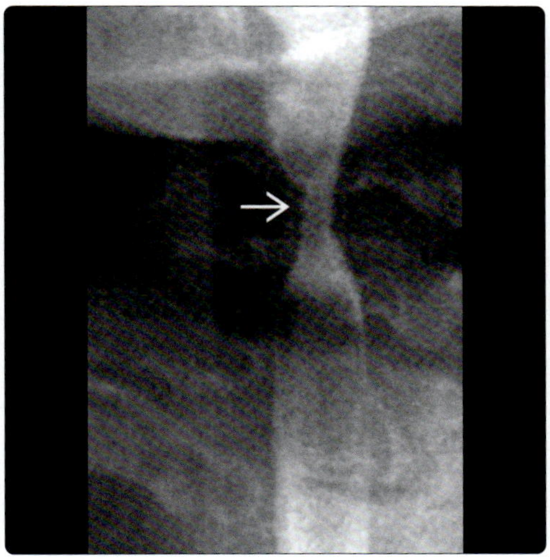

Gastroesophageal Reflux

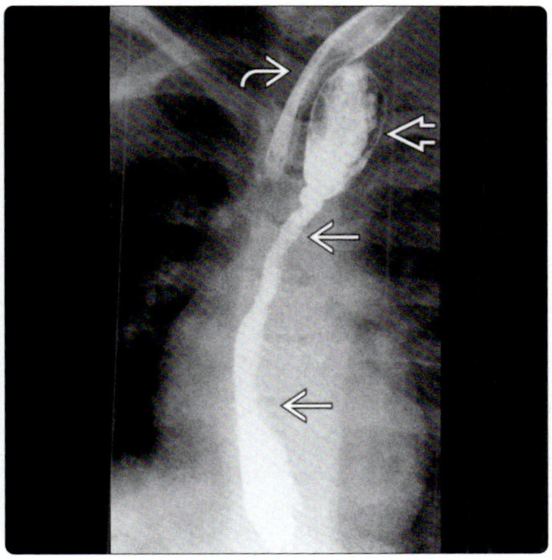

(Left) *Frontal esophagram obtained in a 12 year old with known eosinophilic esophagitis demonstrates a focally narrowed & ringed-appearance of the esophagus . Note that the esophagram can be normal in ~ 50% of cases of eosinophilic esophagitis.* **(Right)** *Frontal upper GI study in an 11 year old with severe gastroesophageal reflux shows a narrow-caliber esophagus with irregularity & proximal dilation . Also note the aspirated barium within the trachea .*

Congenital Esophageal Stenosis

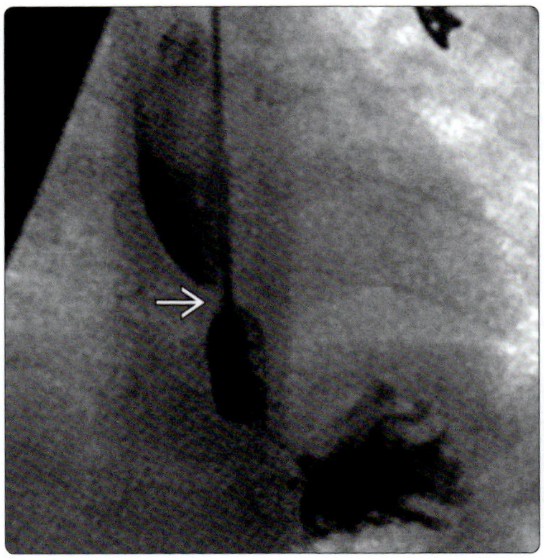

Epidermolysis Bullosa

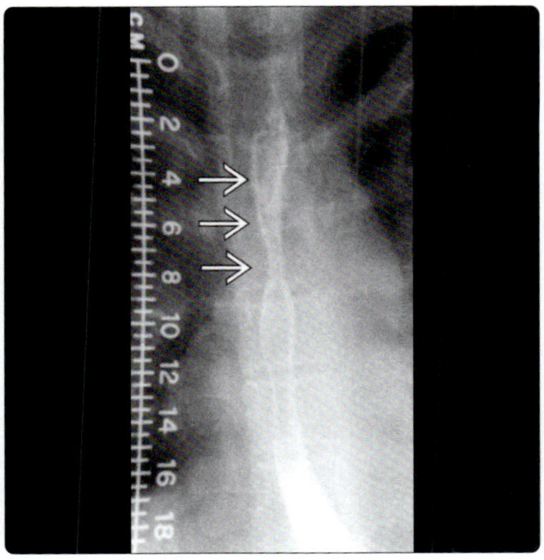

(Left) *Frontal image from a pullback esophagram in a 6 month old with congenital esophageal stenosis demonstrates short, smooth, severe narrowing of the distal esophagus . Congenital stenosis of the distal esophagus is typically due to fibromuscular thickening or a tracheobronchial cartilage remnant.* **(Right)** *Frontal esophagram shows a short segment esophageal stricture in this 15 year old with epidermolysis bullosa. Strictures most commonly involve the proximal esophagus in this population.*

Esophageal Extrinsic Impressions

DIFFERENTIAL DIAGNOSIS

Common

- Aortic Arch
- Left Main Bronchus
- Left Atrium

Less Common

- Right Aortic Arch With Aberrant Left Subclavian Artery
- Left Aortic Arch With Aberrant Right Subclavian Artery
- Double Aortic Arch

Rare but Important

- Pulmonary Sling
- Bronchogenic Cyst
- Gastrointestinal Duplication Cyst
- Neurogenic Tumors

ESSENTIAL INFORMATION

Key Differential Diagnosis Issues

- 2 main groups: Vascular structures or masses
- May be incidental or present with dysphagia
  - Complete vascular ring or sling: May present with stridor due to tracheal impingement
  - Vascular etiology: Less likely to cause isolated dysphagia
- Chest radiograph
  - 1st step in work-up of stridor/respiratory symptoms
  - Must evaluate position & contour of trachea
    - Is aortic arch right or left sided?
    - Is descending aorta right or left sided?
    - Is there symmetry in lung aeration?
- Esophagram
  - Historically used to diagnose vascular rings & slings
  - Cross-sectional imaging is current study of choice
    - Esophagrams still ordered when radiographic findings are subtle & dysphagia symptoms predominate
- CT/MR
  - Directly delineates vascular anatomy & relationship with trachea & esophagus
  - Characterizes mass, if present

Helpful Clues for Common Diagnoses

- **Aortic Arch**
  - Esophagram
    - Frontal projection: Smooth crescentic impression on lateral aspect of proximal esophagus
      - □ Correlates to position of right vs. left aortic arch on radiograph (typically at T3-T4 level)
- **Left Main Bronchus**
  - Esophagram
    - Smooth tubular impression across midesophagus just below aortic arch
    - Frontal projection: Oblique impression mirroring course of left mainstem bronchus
    - Lateral projection: Smooth crescentic impression on anterior esophagus just below level of aortic arch
- **Left Atrium**
  - Esophagram
    - Lateral projection: Broad, smooth, crescentic impression on anterior aspect of lower esophagus

Helpful Clues for Less Common Diagnoses

- **Right Aortic Arch With Aberrant Left Subclavian Artery**
  - Usually has diverticulum of Kommerell: Focal outpouching at base of aberrant subclavian artery
    - Diverticulum of Kommerell is main structure causing significant impression on esophagus
    - Indicates presence of left ligamentum arteriosum, which completes vascular ring
      - □ May compress trachea; symptomatic stridor in 5%
  - Radiographs
    - Frontal: Right aortic arch deviates trachea to left
    - Lateral: Posterior indentation on trachea by diverticulum of Kommerell
  - Esophagram
    - Frontal: Oblique impression on right side of proximal esophagus directed from right inferior to left superior
    - Lateral: Smooth, rounded impression on posterior aspect of proximal esophagus caused by diverticulum of Kommerell
  - CT/MR
    - Aberrant left subclavian artery arises as last vessel from arch/proximal descending aorta & courses posterior to esophagus toward left
    - Look for AP compression of trachea
  - Low association with intracardiac defects (10%)
- **Left Aortic Arch With Aberrant Right Subclavian Artery**
  - Aberrant right subclavian artery arises as last vessel from aortic arch/proximal descending aorta & courses posterior to esophagus toward right
  - Almost always without diverticulum of Kommerell at origin of aberrant right subclavian artery, therefore usually asymptomatic & incidental
    - Lack of diverticulum indicates ligamentum arteriosum is on same side as aortic arch → no vascular ring
  - Esophagram
    - Impressions are opposite of those seen in right aortic arch with aberrant left subclavian artery
    - Since no diverticulum/ring, impressions are mild
- **Double Aortic Arch**
  - Most common morphology: Larger right limb more superior & posterior than left, coursing behind esophagus before joining left limb posteriorly to continue as left-sided descending aorta
  - Radiographs
    - May show aortic knobs (usually R > L) on both sides of superior mediastinum
    - Dominant right arch typically deviates trachea to left; more inferior left arch may shift trachea back to right
      - □ Trachea may have straight midline position
    - Trachea may show circumferential narrowing, but narrowing typically more severe on right & posteriorly
    - Descending aorta can be seen on any side
      - □ Aortic knob & descending aorta on opposite sides should raise suspicion for double aortic arch or circumflex aortic arch
  - Esophagram
    - Frontal: Compression on both sides of esophagus at different levels
      - □ Right arch is typically larger & more cranial
    - Lateral: Smooth, rounded impression on posterior aspect of proximal esophagus

- CT/MR
  - Complete vascular ring encircles trachea & esophagus
  - Origins of head & neck vessels are symmetric with separate anterior carotid artery & posterior subclavian artery arising from each limb

Helpful Clues for Rare Diagnoses

- **Pulmonary Sling**
  - Left pulmonary artery (LPA) arises from right pulmonary artery, coursing between trachea & esophagus to reach left hilum
  - Anomalous LPA forms sling around trachea &/or proximal right bronchus
  - 2 main types
    - Type 1: Normal carina position at T4-T5 level ± right tracheal bronchus
    - Type 2: Abnormal inferior carina at T6 level in inverted T shape, ± right tracheal bronchus
      - More common
      - Sometimes called pseudocarina, with right main stem bronchus called bridging bronchus
      - Often with long segment inferior tracheal stenosis due to complete cartilaginous rings
  - Radiographs
    - Look for abnormal tracheobronchial pattern with low carina around T6
    - Variable degree of hyperinflation or hypoinflation depending on degree of obstruction & type of tracheobronchial branching pattern
      - Type 1: Often shows right lung hyperinflation
      - Type 2: Often shows bilateral hyperinflation
    - Lateral: Round soft tissue density of LPA sling between midtrachea & esophagus
  - Esophagram
    - Essentially only vascular ring with smooth rounded impression on anterior aspect of midesophagus & posterior aspect of air-filled trachea
  - CT/MR
    - Round, small trachea in cross section (instead of oval) suggests complete cartilaginous rings, though difficult to assess with confidence in neonates
    - Inspiratory & expiratory imaging can assess for associated tracheobronchomalacia
- **Bronchogenic Cyst**
  - Radiographs
    - Round, well-defined, soft tissue or fluid density mass in middle mediastinum
    - Typically paratracheal, carinal, or hilar
    - Rarely causes mass effect on trachea with air-trapping or atelectasis
  - Esophagram
    - Incidental smooth, rounded, external impression
  - CT/MR
    - Thin-walled cystic lesion of variable internal signal/attenuation, depending on internal contents
- **Gastrointestinal Duplication Cysts**
  - ~ 18% of GI duplication cysts are esophageal
  - Radiographs
    - Well-defined soft tissue mediastinal mass
  - Esophagram
    - Rounded or tubular impression on esophagus
    - Rarely see communication with esophageal lumen
  - CT/MR
    - Cystic lesion contiguous with esophagus
- **Neurogenic Tumors**
  - e.g., neuroblastoma, plexiform neurofibromas
  - Radiographs
    - Round/ovoid paraspinal mass or elevation of paraspinal stripe
    - ± bone changes: Rib erosion/splaying, pedicle changes, scoliosis
  - CT/MR
    - ± Ca^{2+}, spinal canal invasion, aortic encasement/lifting

SELECTED REFERENCES

1. Backer CL et al: Vascular rings. Semin Pediatr Surg. 25(3):165-75, 2016
2. Gould SW et al: Useful signs for the assessment of vascular rings on cross-sectional imaging. Pediatr Radiol. 45(13):2004-16, 2015
3. Fordham LA: Imaging of the esophagus in children. Radiol Clin North Am. 43(2):283-302, 2005

Aortic Arch

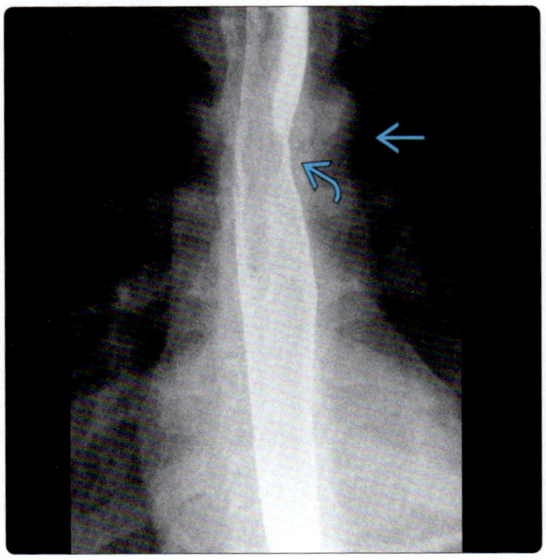

Left Main Bronchus

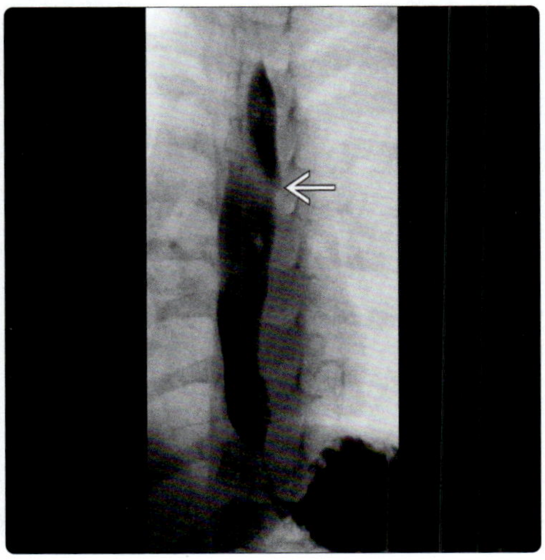

(Left) *Frontal esophagram in a 15 year old shows a smooth, crescentic impression on the left lateral aspect of the proximal thoracic esophagus ➩. This normal impression is caused by a left aortic arch ➩.* **(Right)** *Frontal esophagram demonstrates an oblique tubular impression on the esophagus ➡ by the left main bronchus. This impression is located below the aortic arch & follows the course of the lucent left main bronchus.*

(Left) *Lateral double-contrast esophagram in a 17 year old shows a normal crescentic impression on the anterior esophagus by the lucent left main bronchus. The gaseous distention of the esophagus shows how it cascades around the bronchus. The trachea is noted more proximally.* **(Right)** *Lateral esophagram shows a normal broad, smooth, crescentic impression on the anterior lower esophagus caused by the left atrium. A higher anterior extrinsic impression is caused by the left main bronchus.*

Left Main Bronchus

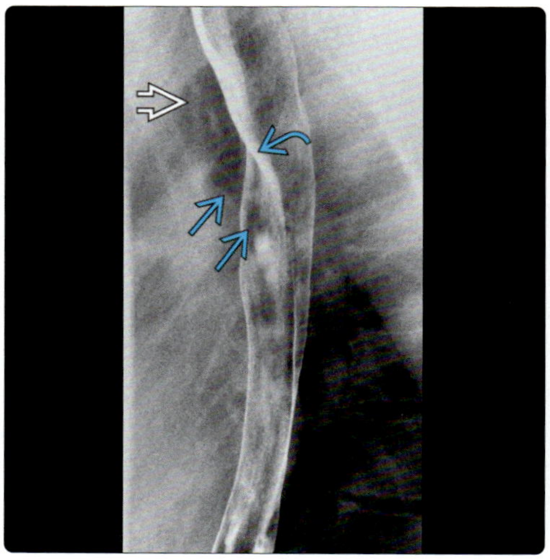

Left Atrium

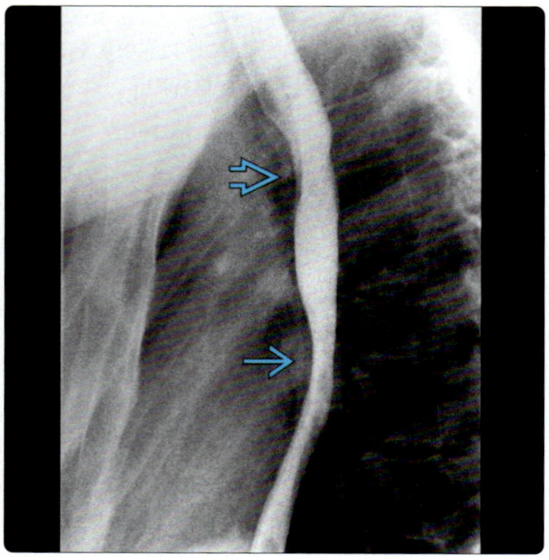

(Left) *Frontal esophagram in an 11 year old with dysphagia shows an oblique impression on the right lateral aspect of the proximal esophagus that is directed obliquely from right inferior to left superior, along with a right arch.* **(Right)** *Lateral esophagram in the same patient shows a round impression on the posterior aspect of the esophagus due to a diverticulum of Kommerell at the origin of the aberrant left subclavian artery from the right aortic arch.*

Right Aortic Arch With Aberrant Left Subclavian Artery

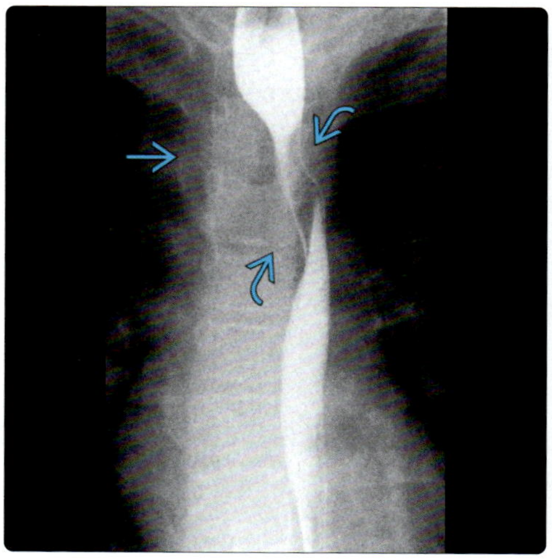

Right Aortic Arch With Aberrant Left Subclavian Artery

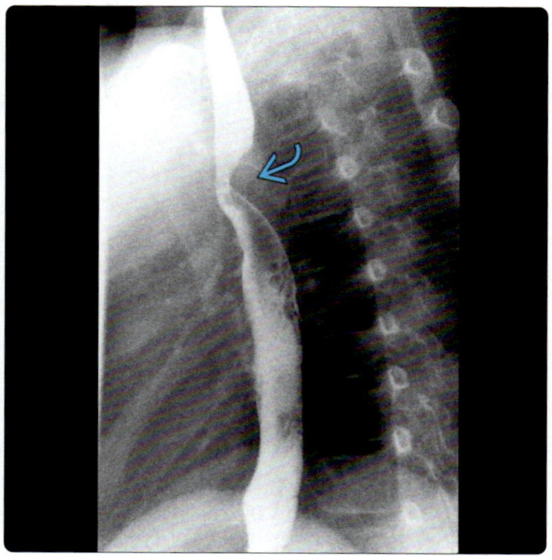

(Left) *Axial CECT MIP in the same patient shows a right arch with a large diverticulum of Kommerell at the base of the aberrant left subclavian artery, which courses behind the esophagus. The left common carotid artery is also seen.* **(Right)** *Coronal CECT MIP shows the right arch, diverticulum of Kommerell, aberrant left subclavian artery, & descending aorta. A diverticulum denotes the presence of a left ligamentum arteriosum, completing a vascular ring.*

Right Aortic Arch With Aberrant Left Subclavian Artery

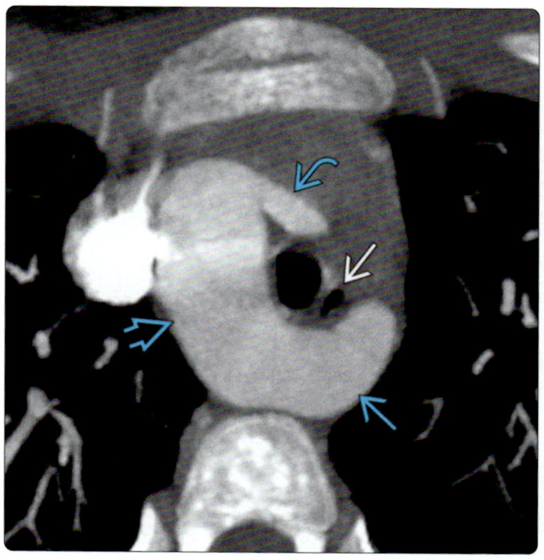

Right Aortic Arch With Aberrant Left Subclavian Artery

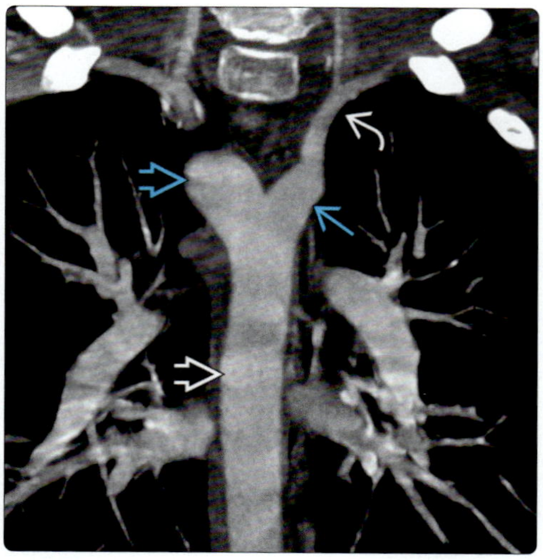

Right Aortic Arch With Aberrant Left Subclavian Artery

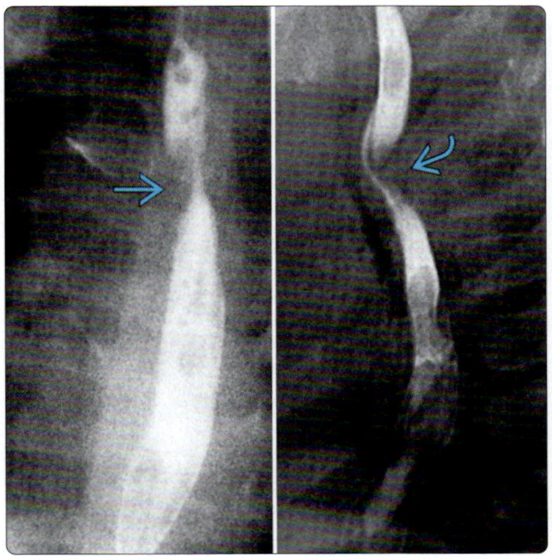

Right Aortic Arch With Aberrant Left Subclavian Artery

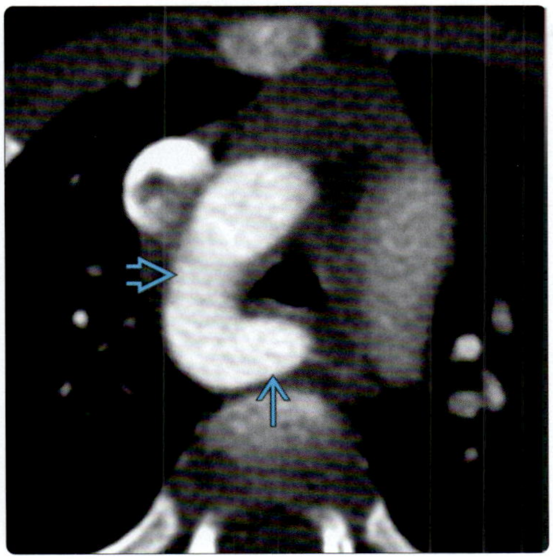

(Left) *Frontal (left) & lateral (right) esophagram images in a 53 week old with intermittent vomiting show an impression* ➔ *on the proximal esophagus directed obliquely from right inferior to left superior on the frontal image, which corresponds to a posterior impression* ➔ *on the lateral view, consistent with a right aortic arch with an aberrant left subclavian artery.* **(Right)** *Axial CECT in the same patient shows the typical appearance of a right arch* ➔ *with an aberrant left subclavian artery & diverticulum of Kommerell* ➔.

Left Aortic Arch With Aberrant Right Subclavian Artery

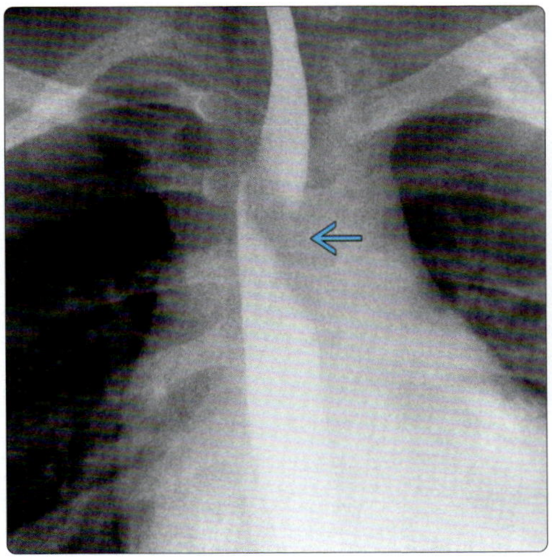

Left Aortic Arch With Aberrant Right Subclavian Artery

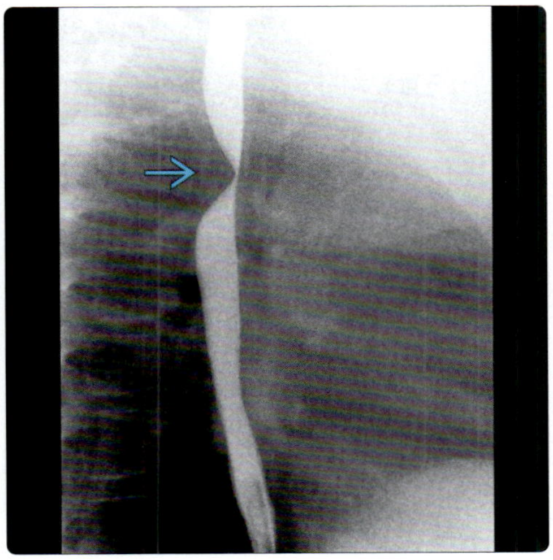

(Left) *Frontal esophagram in a 10 year old with dysphagia shows an oblique impression on the proximal esophagus* ➔ *from left inferior to right superior.* **(Right)** *Lateral esophagram in the same patient shows a posterior impression* ➔ *on the esophagus at the same level. The findings are consistent with a left arch with an aberrant right subclavian artery. In this entity, there is usually a left ligamentum arteriosum, meaning no vascular ring or diverticulum of Kommerell. Therefore, it is usually incidental.*

Left Aortic Arch With Aberrant Right Subclavian Artery

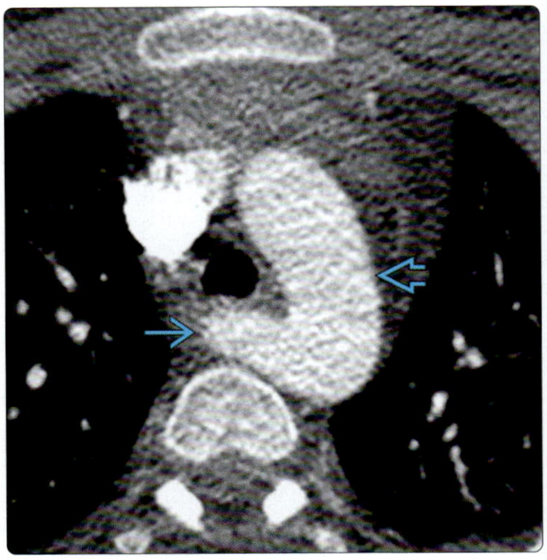

Left Aortic Arch With Aberrant Right Subclavian Artery

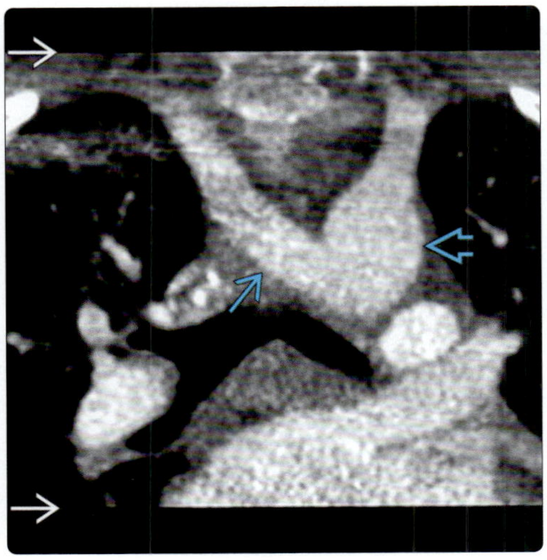

(Left) *Axial CECT in the same patient shows the left arch* ➔ *with aberrant right subclavian artery* ➔. **(Right)** *Coronal CECT in the same patient shows the left arch* ➔ *with an aberrant right subclavian artery* ➔. *The course of the aberrant subclavian artery mirrors the defect on the frontal esophagram. Note that dose can be reduced in CT for preoperative vascular ring assessment by using lower mA & limited scan coverage* ➔.

(Left) *Frontal esophagram in a 22 month old with dysphagia shows extrinsic impressions on both sides of the proximal esophagus, consistent with a double aortic arch. Typically, the right arch is larger & higher, while the left arch is smaller & lower.* **(Right)** *Lateral esophagram in the same patient shows a rounded posterior impression at the same level, which reflects the dominant right arch looping behind the esophagus when the aorta descends on the left vs. a diverticulum of Kommerell when the aorta descends on the right.*

Double Aortic Arch

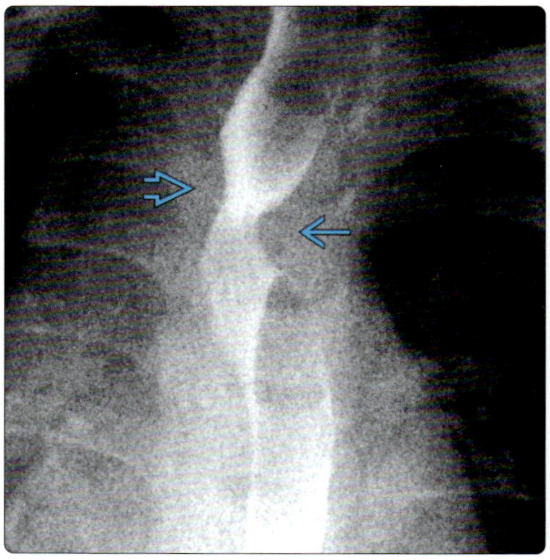

Double Aortic Arch

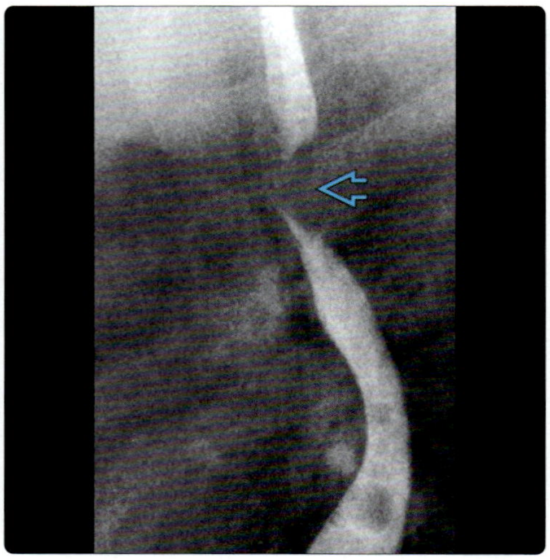

(Left) *Coronal CECT minIP in the same patient shows the dominant right arch & part of the smaller left arch with mild narrowing of the trachea.* **(Right)** *Posterior oblique CECT 3D projection in the same patient shows the double arch & reveals distal atresia of the left arch. A vascular ring is maintained by fibrous continuity at the atretic site, along with a left ligamentum (as evidenced by a diverticulum of Kommerell).*

Double Aortic Arch

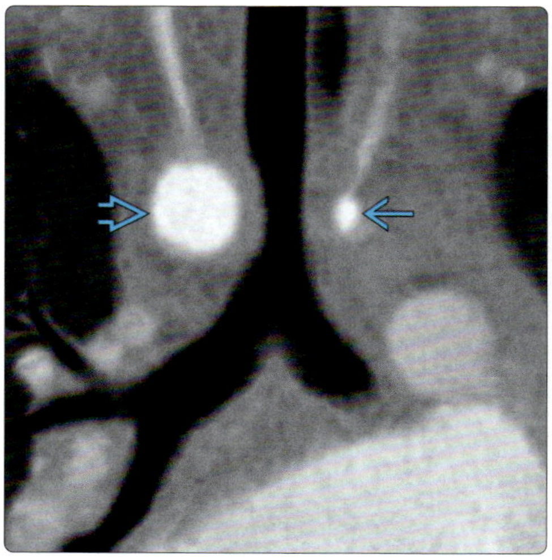

Double Aortic Arch

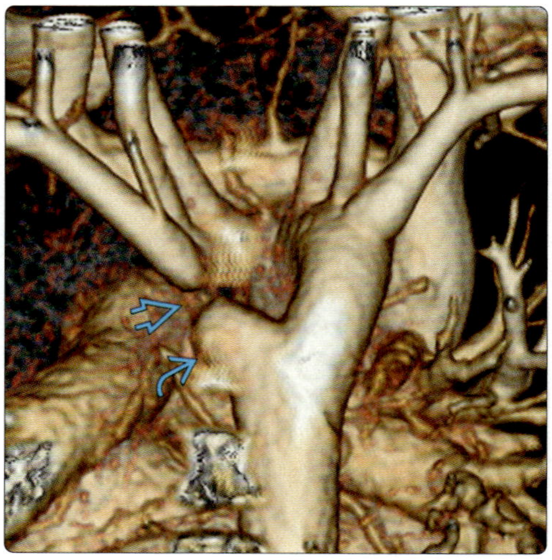

(Left) *Axial oblique CECT MIP in an 11 week old shows a left pulmonary artery (LPA) sling that arises from the proximal right pulmonary artery & courses between the trachea & esophagus.* **(Right)** *Sagittal oblique CECT minIP in the same patient shows the LPA sling coursing between the trachea & esophagus. Note how the sling causes a contour deformity on the anterior esophagus & posterior trachea.*

Pulmonary Sling

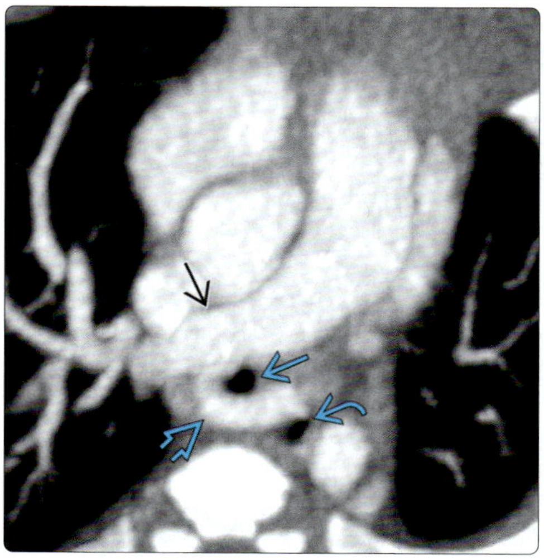

Pulmonary Sling

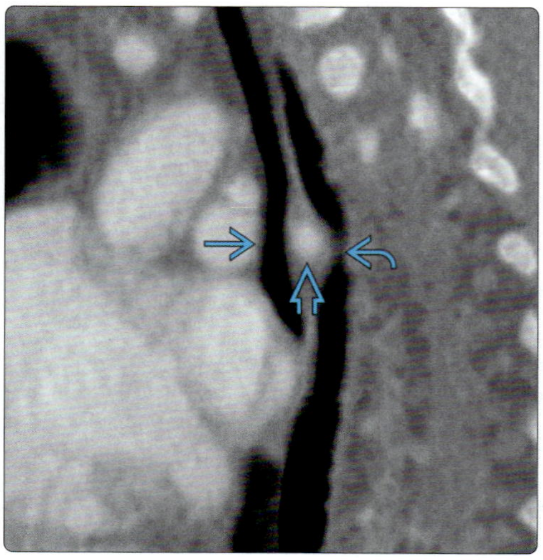

Pulmonary Sling

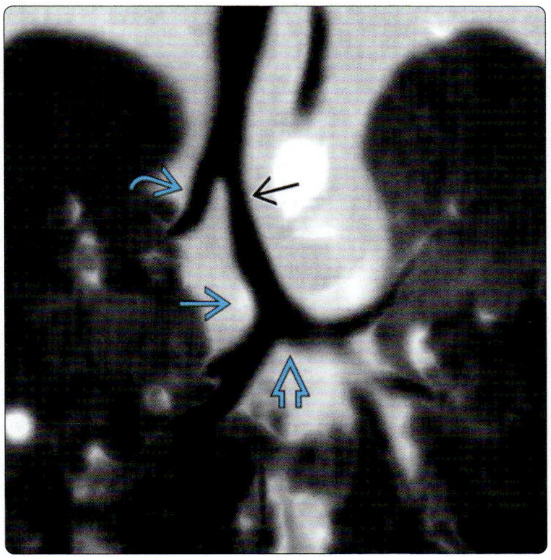

Bronchogenic Cyst

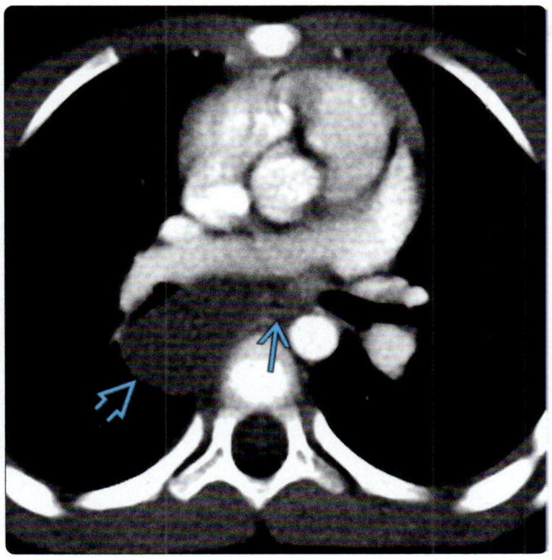

(Left) *Coronal oblique CECT minIP in a 7 day old shows a typical airway configuration in LPA slings with a low & wide carina & tracheal bronchus. The small LPA sling is at the carina. A low-lying carina in an LPA sling is associated with complete tracheal rings & stenosis of the intermediate segment.* **(Right)** *Axial CECT in a 4 year old shows a simple-appearing subcarinal/hilar cystic lesion with a thin wall & no solid components, typical of a bronchogenic cyst. The mass abuts the esophagus.*

Gastrointestinal Duplication Cyst

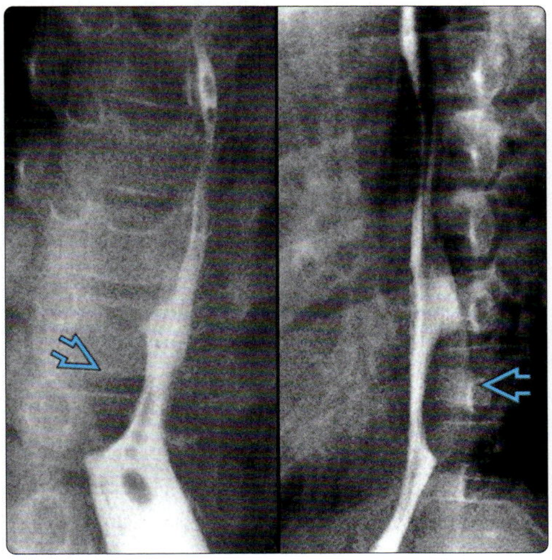

Gastrointestinal Duplication Cyst

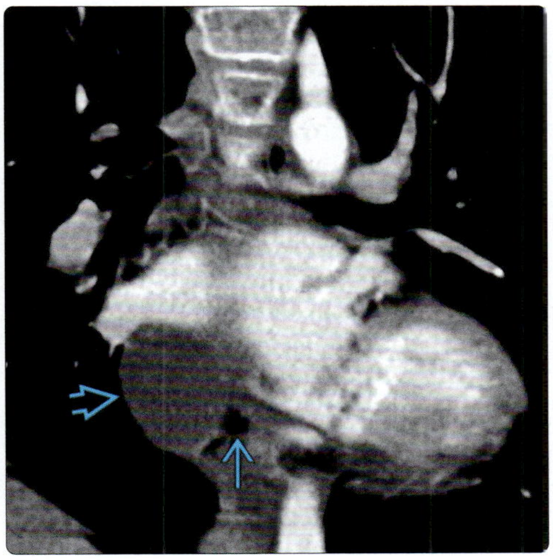

(Left) *Frontal (left) & lateral (right) esophagram images in a 7 year old show a rounded impression on the lower esophagus with a claw sign, likely due to an esophageal duplication cyst (which rarely communicate with the esophageal lumen).* **(Right)** *Coronal CECT in the same patient confirms the esophageal duplication cyst as a simple-appearing cystic lesion with thin wall & no solid components, intimately associated with the esophagus.*

Neurogenic Tumors

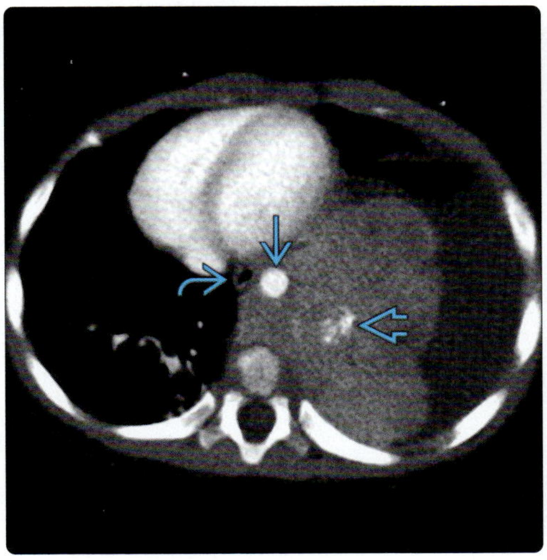

Neurogenic Tumors

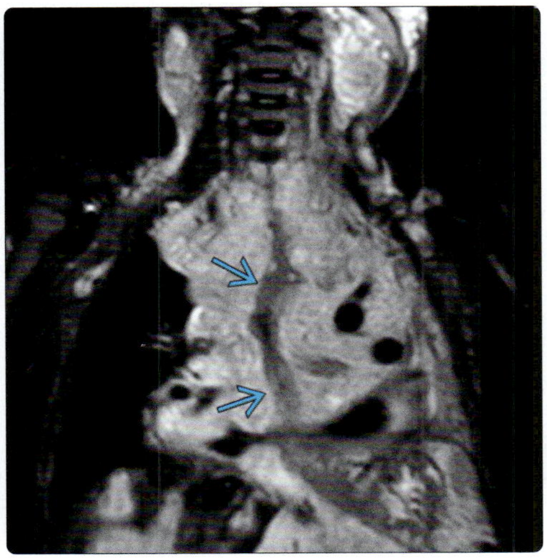

(Left) *Axial CECT in a 7 month old shows a large, lobulated paraspinal soft tissue mass lifting the aorta & esophagus away from the spine, typical of neuroblastoma. Calcifications are seen in up to 90% of these tumors by CT.* **(Right)** *Coronal STIR MR in a 7 year old with neurofibromatosis type 1 shows extensive plexiform neurofibromas in the mediastinum, neck, & upper abdomen. The esophagus is encased, distorted, & infiltrated in this severe case.*

SECTION 3

Gastrointestinal

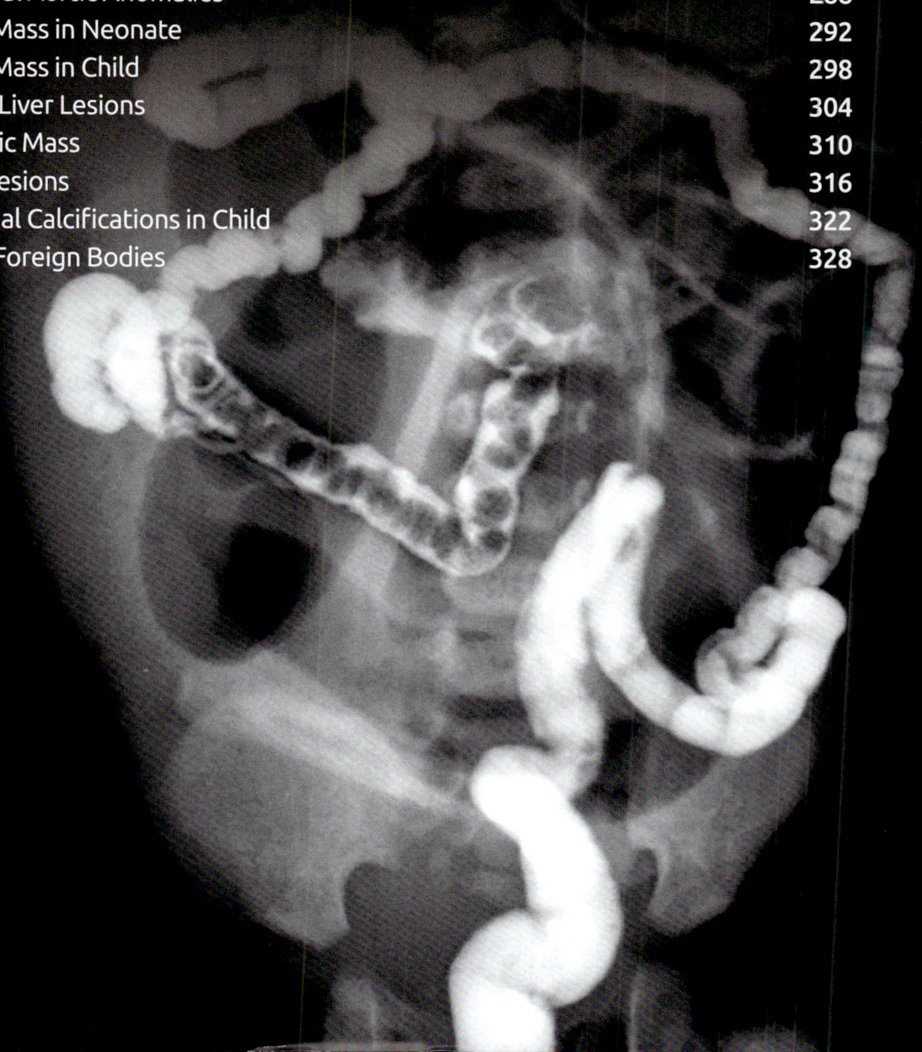

DIFFERENTIAL DIAGNOSIS

Common

- Esophageal Atresia
- Duodenal Atresia, Web, or Stenosis
- Midgut Volvulus
- Hypertrophic Pyloric Stenosis

Less Common

- Jejunal Atresia
- Ladd Bands
- Annular Pancreas
- Internal Hernia

Rare but Important

- Preduodenal Portal Vein
- Gastric Volvulus
- Pyloric Atresia

ESSENTIAL INFORMATION

Key Differential Diagnosis Issues

- Many neonatal bowel obstructions are diagnosed prenatally by US &/or MR
- Clinical clues to underlying diagnosis
  - Age of presentation (hours vs. days vs. weeks of life)
  - Acute onset after tolerating feeds vs. never tolerating
  - Bilious vs. nonbilious emesis
- Extent of bowel gas provides clue to level of obstruction
  - Isolated esophageal atresia (EA) → gasless abdomen
  - Pyloric atresia → "single bubble"
  - Duodenal atresia (DA) → "double bubble" without distal gas
  - Midgut volvulus (MGV) vs. duodenal stenosis/web (DS/DW) → duodenal dilation with distal gas + bilious emesis
  - Jejunal atresia → "triple bubble" without distal gas
- Degree of dilation can suggest chronic vs. acute
  - Very dilated bulbous segment suggests chronic longstanding in utero obstruction
  - Mild dilation favors more recent onset
- Note that atresias are congenital complete obstructions without distal gas; forms of atresia include
  - Intact membrane across lumen
  - Fibrous cord separating blind ends
  - Completely disconnected blind ends
- Note that classic radiographic clues require obstructed segments to be gas filled; recent vomiting or nasogastric suction may decompress dilated bowel
- Normal bowel gas pattern does not exclude MGV (surgical emergency)
  - Bilious emesis in neonate should be evaluated with upper GI series (UGI) with rare exception

Helpful Clues for Common Diagnoses

- **Esophageal Atresia**
  - Difficulty swallowing secretions, choking with feeds
    - Inability to pass nasogastric tube to stomach
  - Fluid distention of proximal esophagus on fetal imaging
    - High T2 signal in distended pouch on fetal MR; may decompress intermittently
    - Anechoic fluid distention of pouch on fetal US
    - Small stomach; polyhydramnios after 20 weeks
  - Air-filled esophageal pouch on newborn radiograph
    - Nasogastric tube tip does not reach distal esophagus
  - Most have associated tracheoesophageal fistula (TEF)
    - Fistula usually lies just above carina, extending anterior & superior from esophagus toward trachea
    - Distal bowel gas is present due to distal esophageal communication with trachea
    - Gasless abdomen if EA is isolated (without fistula)
  - 50-75% have associated anomalies
    - VACTERL association in 10-20% (vertebral, anorectal, cardiac, renal, limb anomalies)
    - Trisomy 18, trisomy 21 (isolated EA)
- **Duodenal Atresia, Web, or Stenosis**
  - Most common upper bowel obstruction in neonate
  - DA is often diagnosed prenatally
  - Dilated, round stomach & proximal duodenum → "double bubble" on fetal imaging
    - Anechoic & fluid filled on US
    - High T2 signal on MR
      - □ Proximal obstructions will generally have fluid signal in dilated segments, not high T1 signal
  - Air-filled "double bubble" with no distal gas on neonatal radiograph
    - With classic "double bubble" radiograph, no further imaging is required to confirm DA
    - If duodenum is only mildly distended (not rounded), cannot exclude MGV (especially if there is any distal gas) → perform UGI
  - > 50% have associated anomalies
    - Biliary anomalies are common; up to 33% have annular pancreas
    - Up to 33% have Down syndrome
    - Up to 28% have malrotation
  - DW & DS have shared pathophysiology with DA
    - Variable presentation depending on size of web fenestration or degree of stenosis
    - May present later or with nonbilious emesis
      - □ Typically have bowel gas distal to obstruction
- **Midgut Volvulus**
  - 50% present in 1st week of life, 90% in first 12 months
  - Bilious emesis, often after initially tolerating feeds
    - Bilious emesis is not specific for MGV, as it is also seen in other proximal & distal obstructions
    - Only confirms that obstruction is distal to ampulla of Vater
  - Narrow fixation of small bowel mesentery in malrotation allows twisting of midgut around superior mesenteric artery (SMA) → bowel obstruction & ischemia
  - 3 classic bowel gas patterns seen in MGV
    - Normal
    - Proximal obstruction: Mild dilation of stomach & proximal duodenum with presence of distal gas
    - Ischemic ileus: Late finding with diffuse dilation of bowel loops
  - UGI: Tapered (beak) appearance of distal D2 or D3 + narrowing of twisted distal duodenum/proximal jejunum in corkscrew configuration
    - Abnormal position of duodenojejunal junction

- Normally lies at or to left of left vertebral pedicle at level of duodenal bulb on frontal projection with posterior D2-D4 course on lateral projection
  - If contrast does not pass beyond "beak" in D2/D3, cannot exclude MGV (i.e., must go to surgery)
  - US: Twisting ("whirlpool") of mesenteric vessels & bowel about SMA
- **Hypertrophic Pyloric Stenosis**
  - Nonbilious projectile emesis occurs at 2-12 weeks of age (i.e., not congenital)
  - US: Thickened pyloric muscle (> 3 mm of single wall) & elongated pyloric channel (> 15 mm)
  - UGI: String sign of minimal barium in narrowed & elongated pyloric channel + hyperperistaltic "caterpillar stomach"

Helpful Clues for Less Common Diagnoses

- **Jejunal Atresia**
  - Complete occlusion of jejunal lumen
    - Likely due to in utero ischemic event
    - More likely to have additional atresias
  - Dilated, fluid-filled proximal bowel on fetal imaging
  - "Triple bubble" on neonatal radiographs with proximal jejunal atresia
    - Dilated, air-filled stomach, duodenum, & proximal jejunum without distal gas
  - Associations with gastroschisis, cystic fibrosis, malrotation
- **Ladd Bands**
  - Fibrous bands found in patients with malrotation due to attempted fixation of bowel in setting of shortened mesenteric fixation
    - May result in obstruction, often at D2
- **Annular Pancreas**
  - Band of pancreatic tissue surrounds D2
  - Neonatal presentation is often preampullary obstruction with nonbilious emesis
  - Almost always associated with duodenal narrowing with severity dictating timing of presentation
  - Similar radiographic & UGI findings as DA, DW, DS
  - CECT & MR can visualize abnormal pancreatic tissue
- **Internal Hernia**
  - Transmesenteric hernia is most common in neonates
    - Congenital mesenteric defect near ileocecal valve or ligament of Treitz
  - UGI findings are often subtle & nonspecific, but associated abnormalities may be identified
  - Reported associations with malrotation, jejunal/ileal atresias, intestinal duplications, Hirschsprung disease

Helpful Clues for Rare Diagnoses

- **Preduodenal Portal Vein**
  - Portal vein lies anterior to duodenum & pancreas
  - Observed in 3-5% of patients with another cause of congenital duodenal obstruction
    - Rarely reported as primary cause of obstruction
  - Similar radiographic & UGI findings to DA, DW, DS
- **Gastric Volvulus**
  - Organoaxial, mesenteroaxial, or combined
    - Organoaxial morphology may be seen as incidental transient finding without obstruction in neonates
  - Radiographs show distended rounded stomach in abdomen or thorax
  - UGI for further evaluation
    - Organoaxial: Greater curvature superior to lesser curvature, pylorus at level of gastric cardia
    - Mesenteroaxial: Pylorus superior to fundus, pylorus near or overlying gastroesophageal junction
  - Often associated with diaphragmatic hernias
    - Bochdalek, Morgagni, hiatal, or paraesophageal
    - Absent/deficient ligamentous fixation of stomach
- **Pyloric Atresia**
  - "Single bubble" on radiographs with no distal gas
  - Associations (30-50%) with epidermolysis bullosa, hereditary multiple intestinal atresias (HMIA)/multiple intestinal atresia with immunodeficiency (MIAI)

SELECTED REFERENCES

1. Maxfield CM et al: A pattern-based approach to bowel obstruction in the newborn. Pediatr Radiol. 43(3):318-29, 2013

Esophageal Atresia

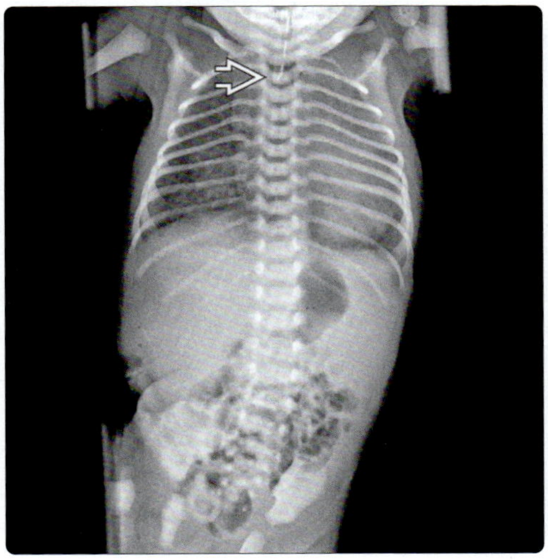

Esophageal Atresia

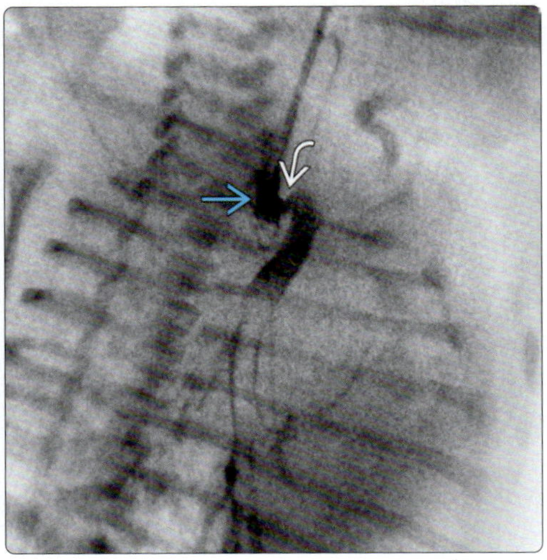

(Left) *AP radiograph shows a nasogastric tube tip overlying the thoracic inlet ➔ due to esophageal atresia (EA). The presence of abdominal gas confirms the existence of a tracheoesophageal fistula (TEF).* **(Right)** *Oblique esophagram in a 9 day old with Down syndrome & a prenatally diagnosed EA shows a proximal TEF ➔, the least common type of EA-TEF. Prior to this study, the patient had greater-than-expected output from the tube in the proximal esophageal pouch ➔.*

Duodenal Atresia, Web, or Stenosis

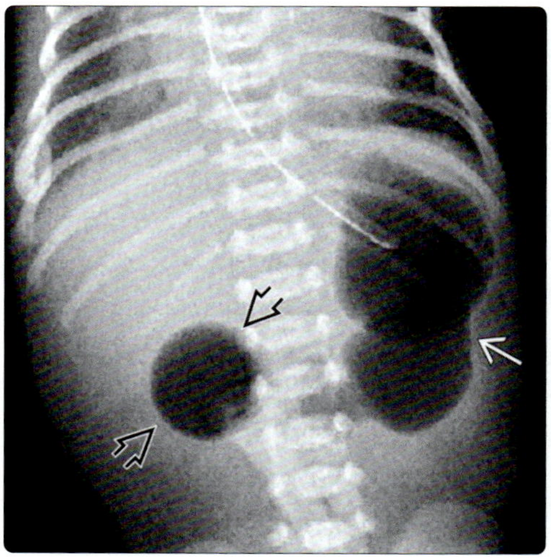

Duodenal Atresia, Web, or Stenosis

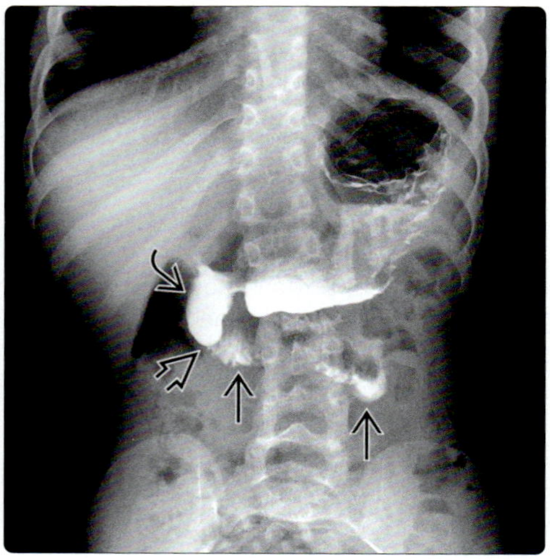

(Left) *AP abdominal radiograph of a newborn shows a dilated stomach ➡ & a bulbous, dilated proximal duodenum ⇨ with no distal bowel gas, consistent with duodenal atresia (DA).* **(Right)** *Upright upper GI (UGI) in this older child with a long history of vomiting shows dilation of the 2nd duodenal segment ↪, a windsock appearance of the obstructed segment ⇨ (due to a web), & decompression of the distal duodenum & proximal jejunum →.*

Duodenal Atresia, Web, or Stenosis

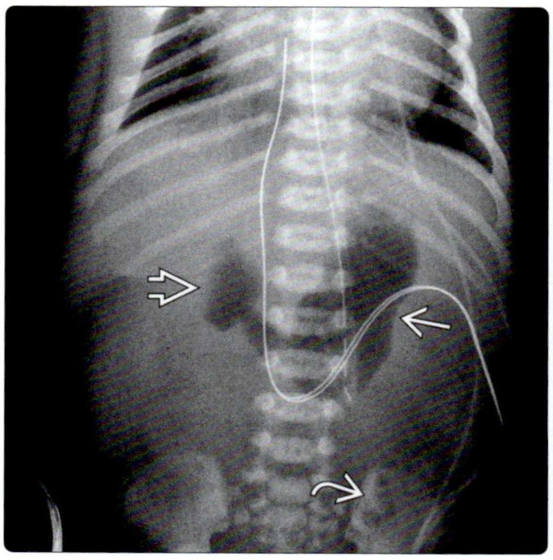

Duodenal Atresia, Web, or Stenosis

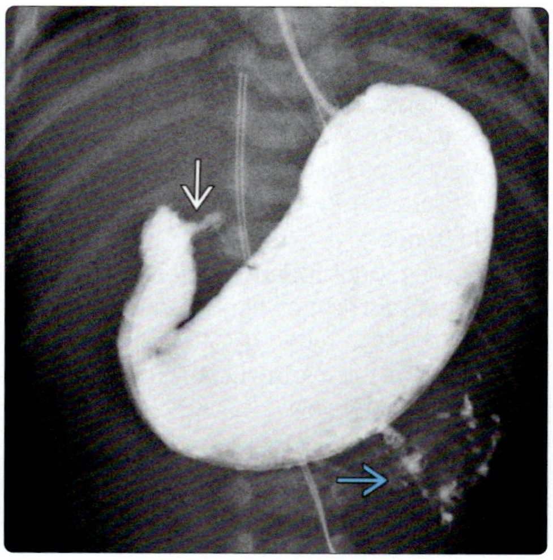

(Left) *AP radiograph in a 5 day old with bilious emesis shows a dilated stomach ➡ & nonspherical dilated proximal duodenum ➡. There is a small amount of distal bowel gas ➡. The differential diagnosis includes duodenal stenosis or web, midgut volvulus, or (rarely) DA with anomalous biliary anatomy allowing air to pass beyond the atretic segment.* **(Right)** *Supine UGI series shows an abrupt narrowing in the proximal duodenum ➡ with contrast passing distally ➡. Stenosis was confirmed at surgery.*

Midgut Volvulus

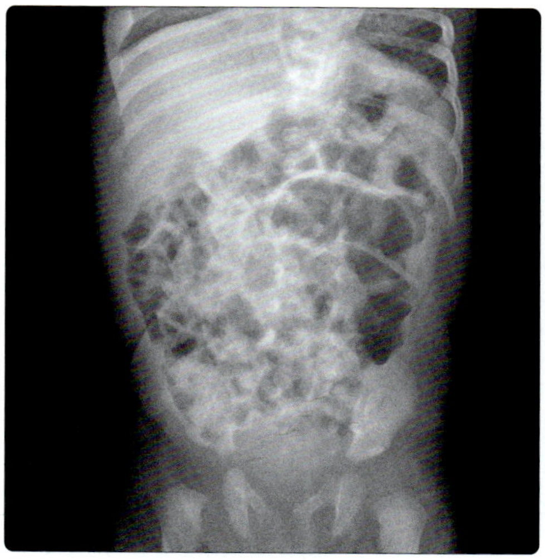

Midgut Volvulus

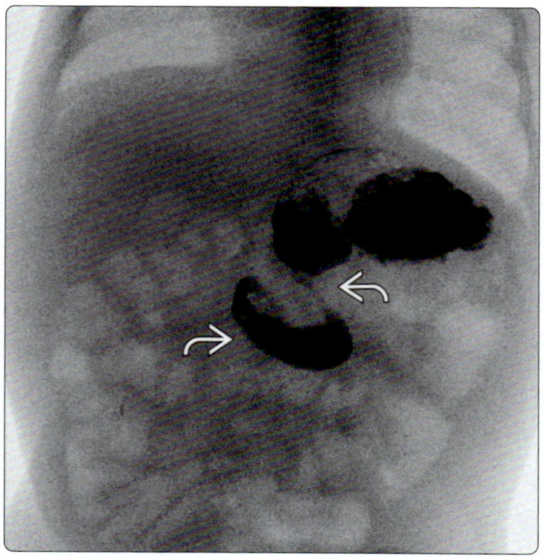

(Left) *AP radiograph in a 17 day old with a 1-week history of bilious emesis demonstrates a nonobstructive bowel gas pattern. There were no air-fluid levels on the decubitus view (not shown). Note that a normal abdominal radiograph does not exclude malrotation with midgut volvulus.* **(Right)** *Subsequent UGI series in the same patient shows the characteristic corkscrew configuration of the duodenum ➡ in malrotation with midgut volvulus.*

Midgut Volvulus

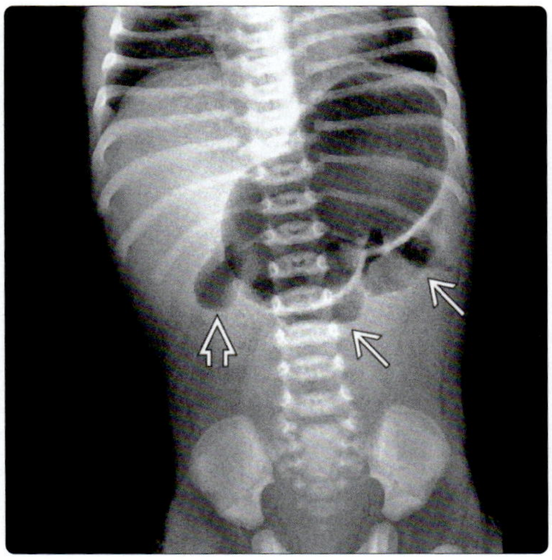

Midgut Volvulus

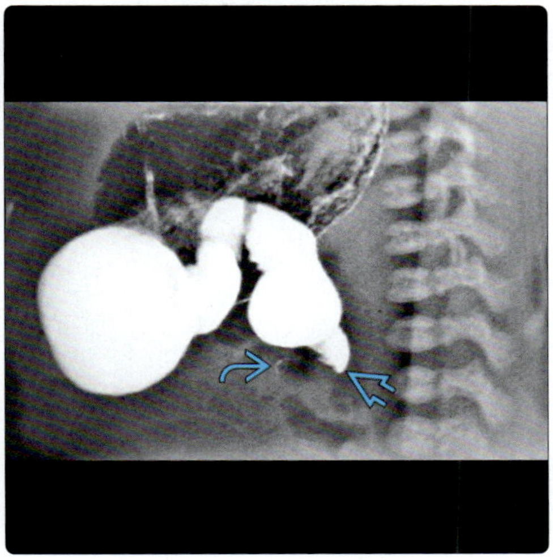

(Left) *AP radiograph shows a dilated air-filled stomach & less distended duodenum with small amounts of distal gas. This is an abnormal pattern in a 2-day-old infant who presented with bilious vomiting (as gas should be scattered throughout the bowel by this time).* **(Right)** *Lateral UGI shows duodenal dilation to the distal D2 segment with an abrupt taper/beak at the leading edge of the contrast bolus. A narrowed twisted segment is suggested distal to this level.*

Midgut Volvulus

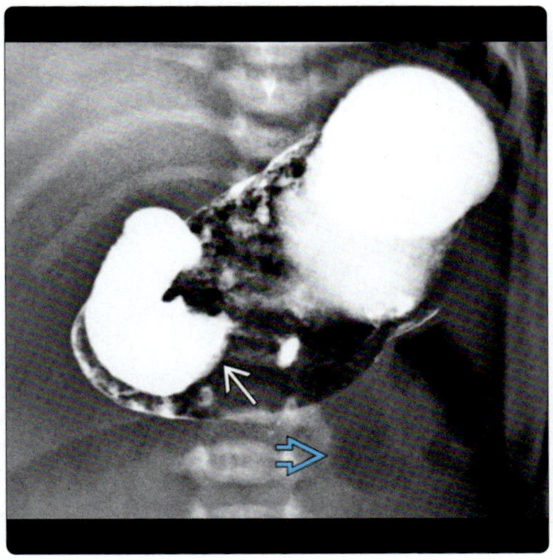

Midgut Volvulus

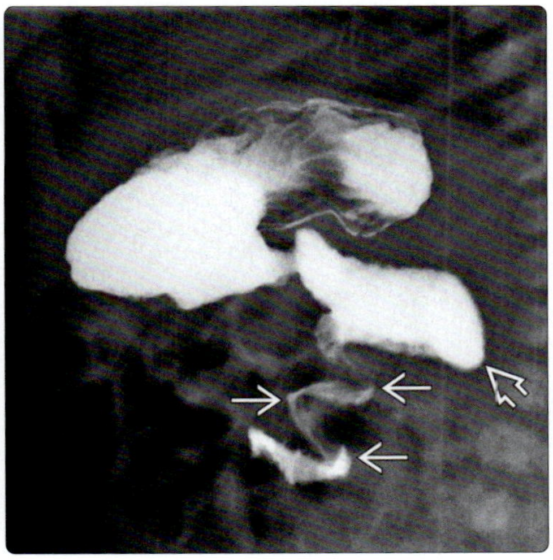

(Left) *Frontal UGI shows proximal duodenal dilation with a tapered D3 segment. Note the distal bowel gas. This appearance represents midgut volvulus until proven otherwise. Surgery confirmed malrotation with volvulus in this case.* **(Right)** *Lateral UGI shows the classic corkscrew appearance of a midgut volvulus. The proximal duodenum is mildly distended but tapers rapidly at the level of the twist.*

Hypertrophic Pyloric Stenosis

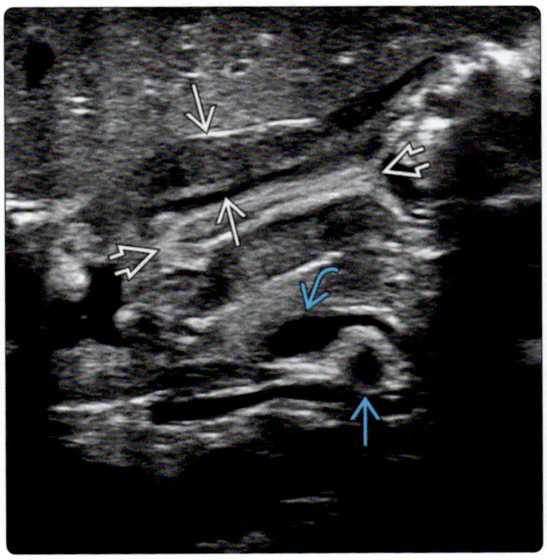

Hypertrophic Pyloric Stenosis

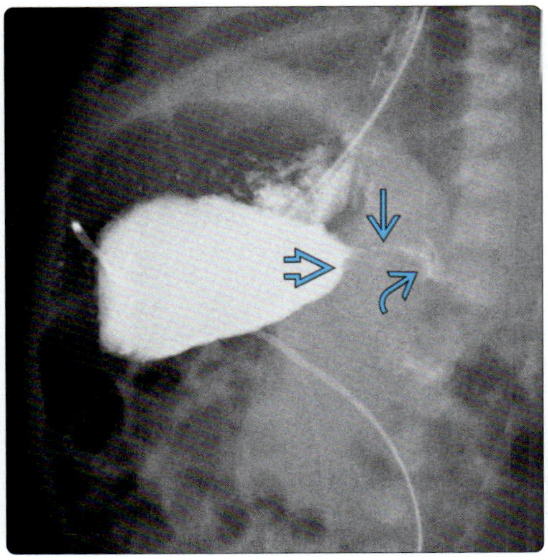

(Left) *Oblique US shows a thickened hypoechoic pyloric muscle (4 mm) with an elongated channel (24 mm) in this 23 day old with projectile emesis. Note the normal relationship of the SMA & SMV, which is often abnormal in the setting of malrotation.* **(Right)** *Right lateral decubitus UGI in a 1 month old with nonbilious vomiting shows a thin "string" of contrast traversing a narrowed & elongated pyloric channel. The pyloric muscle makes a bulbous impression on the contrast in the antrum & duodenum.*

(Left) *AP radiograph in a newborn with jejunal atresia shows a few dilated loops of gas-filled bowel, more than expected with a duodenal obstruction. Mass effect on the bowel loops & Ca^{2+} in the left abdomen suggest a large meconium pseudocyst due to in utero perforation, which was confirmed by US (not shown).* **(Right)** *Coronal SSFSE T2 MR shows a dilated fetal stomach & proximal small bowel loops. Jejunal atresia was confirmed at repair shortly after delivery.*

Jejunal Atresia

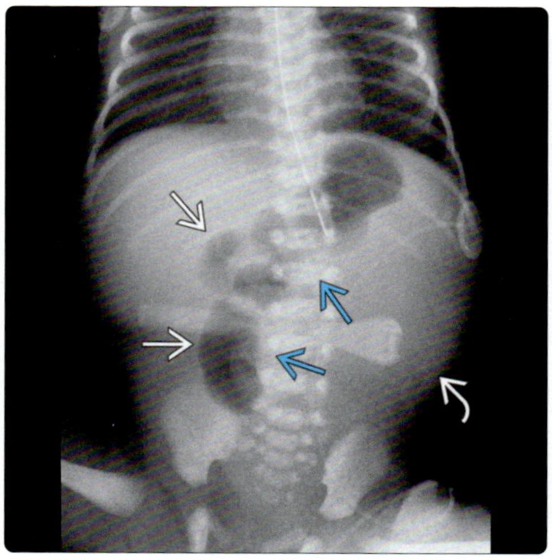

Jejunal Atresia

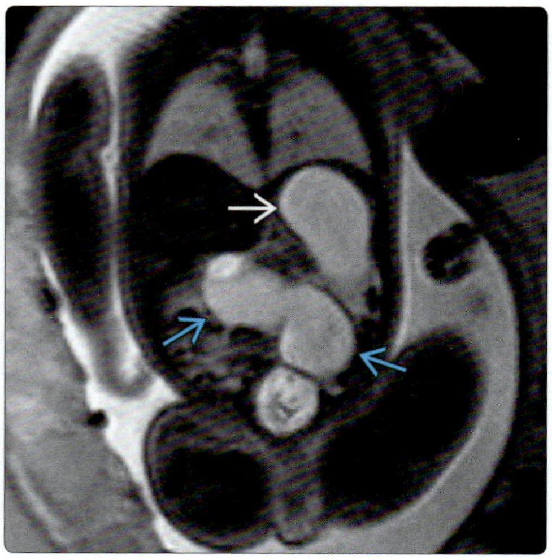

(Left) *Supine UGI in a 1 month old with bilious emesis shows a dilated proximal duodenum with abrupt tapering & no distal contrast passage. Malrotation & obstructing Ladd bands were found at surgery. Note that this appearance could be seen with midgut volvulus or a web.* **(Right)** *AP radiograph of a newborn who presented with bilious vomiting shows a rounded air collection in the midabdomen in the expected location of the duodenum. The distal gas suggests either a partial or acute-onset (i.e., since birth) obstruction.*

Ladd Bands

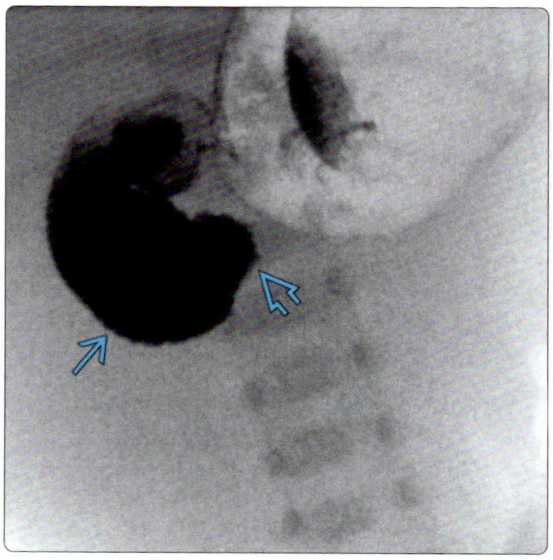

Annular Pancreas

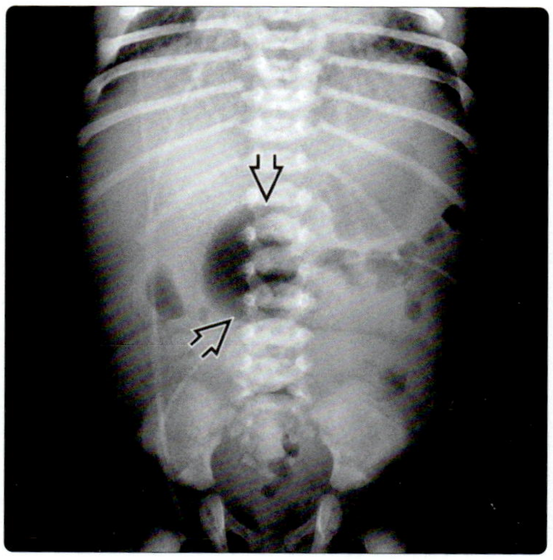

(Left) *Frontal UGI in the same patient shows a dilated proximal duodenum with no distal contrast. Surgery confirmed an annular pancreas, which often occurs in conjunction with duodenal stenosis.* **(Right)** *Coronal MRA in a 6 month old shows pancreatic tissue surrounding a narrowed D2 segment, consistent with an annular pancreas.*

Annular Pancreas

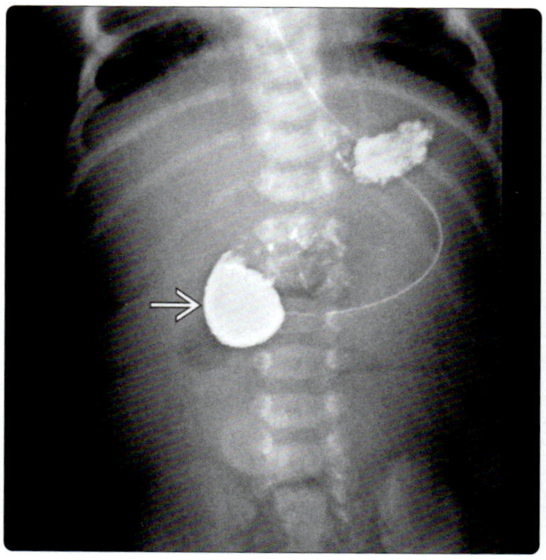

Annular Pancreas

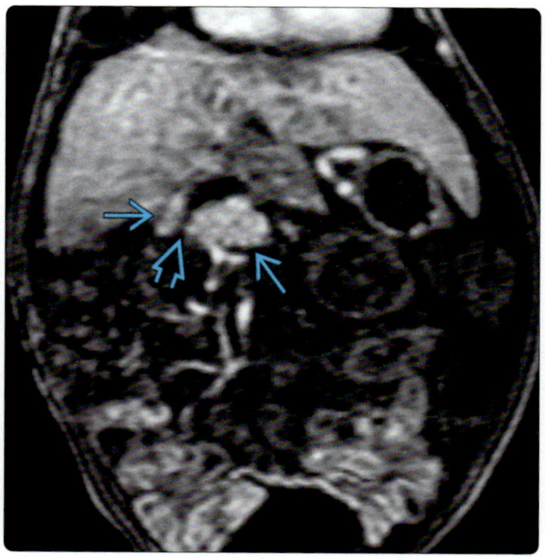

Preduodenal Portal Vein

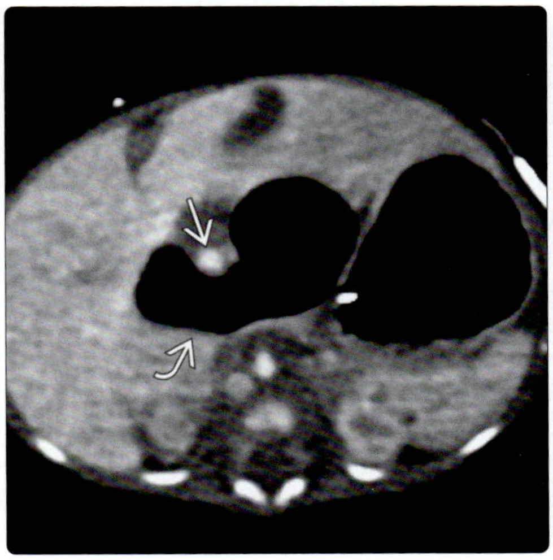

Gastric Volvulus

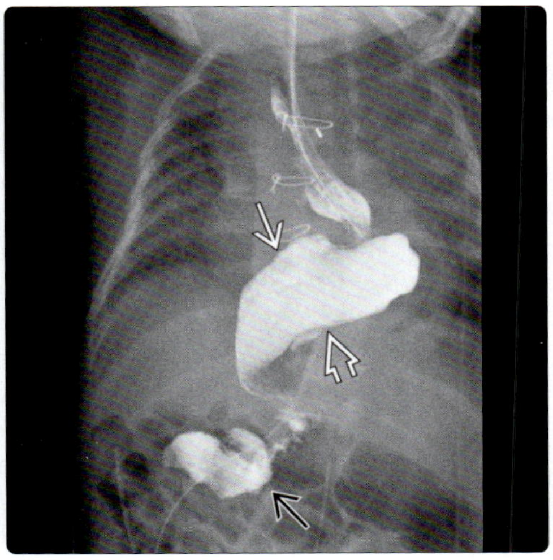

(Left) *Axial CTA performed for congenital heart disease in a 4 week old shows a preduodenal portal vein* →. *The duodenum is patulous* →, *sequela of a previously repaired coexistent duodenal web.* **(Right)** *Supine UGI series in an infant with an abnormal feeding tube course shows that the greater curvature of the stomach* → *was superior to the lesser curvature* →, *indicating an organoaxial gastric volvulus in the setting of a hiatal hernia. Malrotation* → *was also confirmed. Neither finding was obstructive.*

Gastric Volvulus

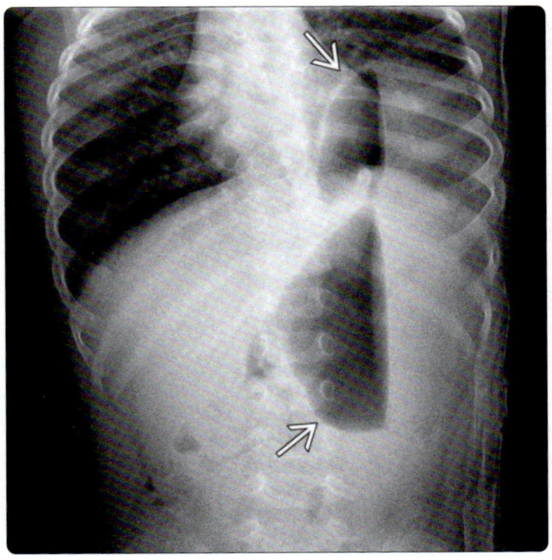

Gastric Volvulus

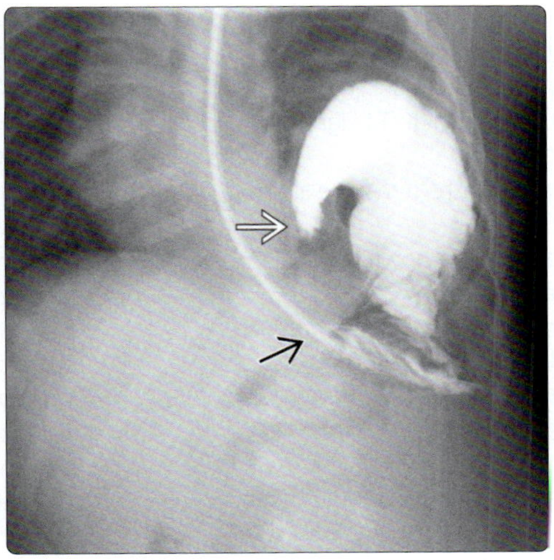

(Left) *Left decubitus radiograph in a 6 month old shows air-fluid levels in the dilated stomach* →, *a portion of which is herniated into the inferior left hemithorax. The infant presented acutely with vomiting & fever, but there was reportedly poor feeding since birth.* **(Right)** *Subsequent supine UGI series shows a mesenteroaxial gastric volvulus with the pylorus* → *lying superior to the gastroesophageal junction* →. *A predisposing Bochdalek hernia was confirmed intraoperatively.*

Pyloric Atresia

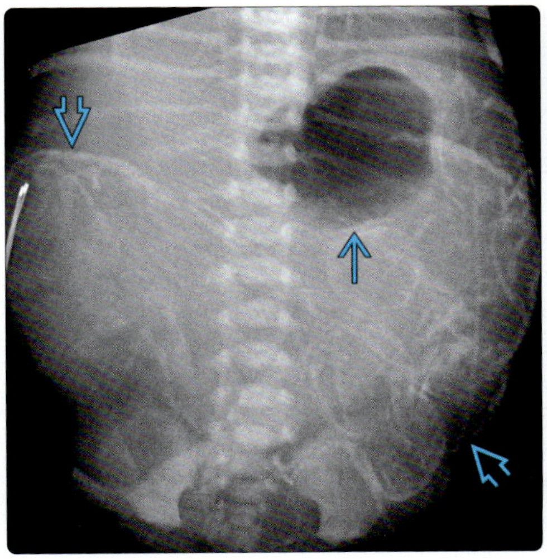

Pyloric Atresia

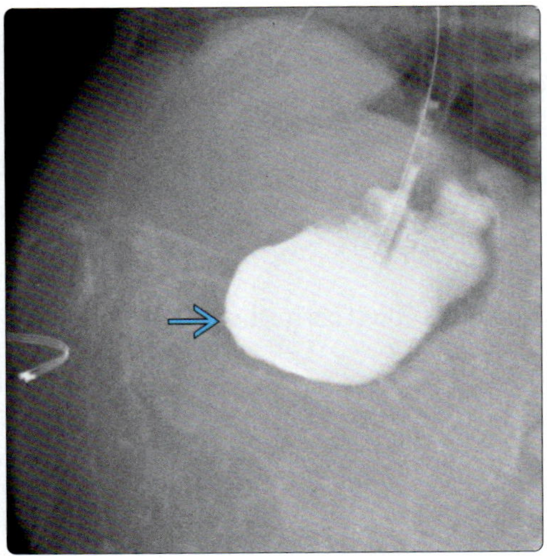

(Left) *AP radiograph in a newborn with a prenatally diagnosed bowel obstruction (with numerous dilated loops seen on fetal imaging) shows a "single bubble" in the left upper quadrant* → *with no distal bowel gas. Numerous bowel* Ca^{2+} *are noted* →. **(Right)** *Right lateral decubitus UGI in the same patient shows no contrast emptying from the stomach* →. *Numerous atresias were found throughout the GI tract in this patient with hereditary multiple intestinal atresias (HMIA) who eventually showed immunodeficiency.*

DIFFERENTIAL DIAGNOSIS

Common

- Hirschsprung Disease
- Meconium Plug Syndrome
- Necrotizing Enterocolitis (Mimic)

Less Common

- Meconium Ileus
- Jejunoileal Atresia
- Midgut Volvulus (Mimic)
- Inguinal Hernia

Rare but Important

- Anorectal Malformation
- Colonic Atresia
- Omphalomesenteric Duct Remnant

ESSENTIAL INFORMATION

Key Differential Diagnosis Issues

- Typically presents with bilious emesis, failure to pass meconium, &/or abdominal distention in first 48 hours
  - May be suspected prenatally: Dilated bowel, ascites or localized fluid collections, abnormal Ca^{2+}
    - Distal obstructions often show high T1 signal meconium in dilated loops
    - Expected rectal meconium pattern may be absent after 20 weeks; ± microcolon
- Abdominal radiographs: Many dilated bowel loops
  - If no air-fluid levels, suspect meconium ileus
  - Ca^{2+}: Intraluminal suggests anorectal malformation, multiple atresias, or total colonic Hirschsprung disease (HD); peritoneal may be due to any bowel perforation
  - If mass effect is seen, suspect complications of meconium ileus
  - Disproportionately dilated loop favors colonic or ileal atresia
- Findings of water soluble contrast enema (WSCE) limit DDx: Colonic vs. small bowel (SB) process
  - Rectosigmoid (RS) ratio < 1: HD
  - Sigmoid transition: Meconium plug syndrome or HD
  - Interrupted small distal colon: Colonic atresia
  - Microcolon: Meconium ileus, ileal atresia
  - If WSCE is normal, consider upper GI (UGI) to exclude midgut volvulus
    - UGI may be requested 1st with bilious emesis

Helpful Clues for Common Diagnoses

- **Hirschsprung Disease**
  - Often presents with newborn distal bowel obstruction & failure to pass meconium
    - May present later with chronic constipation
  - Absence of enteric ganglion cells results in spasmodic aperistaltic small caliber segment
    - Aganglionic segment extends retrograde from anus for variable length
      - Histologic transition zone lies where normal nerves are encountered
    - Results in functional obstruction
  - WSCE: RS ratio < 1
    - Transition from small distal to dilated proximal colon is most commonly seen at sigmoid (short-segment HD)
      - Transition is often missed if very distal (at anorectal verge): Enema is often interpreted as normal
      - Radiologic transition zone is not necessarily equivalent to histologic transition zone, especially in long-segment HD
  - Other supporting (but variable) WSCE findings
    - Distal colonic spasm with irregular contractions
    - Colitis with mucosal irregularity
    - Delayed evacuation
  - Total colonic HD
    - Small colon without transition ± intraluminal ileal Ca^{2+}
    - Colon may be short & "question mark" in shape
  - Ultimately, WSCE can not exclude diagnosis of HD; rectal biopsy is appropriate with high clinical suspicion
- **Meconium Plug Syndrome**
  - Poorly named: Not due to abnormal meconium
  - a.k.a. neonatal small left colon syndrome or functional immaturity of colon
  - No recognized pathologic findings
  - WSCE: RS ratio > 1
    - Small left colon with transition to dilated bowel near splenic flexure; ± colonic meconium pellets
    - Meconium often evacuates during & after enema
  - Associations: Maternal diabetes or Mg^{2+} therapy
  - Resolves in several days ± therapeutic enemas
    - Consider early biopsy to exclude long-segment HD
- **Necrotizing Enterocolitis (Mimic)**
  - Primarily disorder of premature neonatal bowel (especially of very low birth weight, < 1,500 g infants) due to infection &/or ischemia
  - Onset typically occurs after 1-3 weeks of life
  - Patient develops feeding intolerance, abdominal distention & discoloration, bradycardia, bloody stools
  - Classic radiographic appearance: Focal or generally dilated "unfolded" fixed loops with wall thickening, pneumatosis, portal venous gas, free air
  - US: May demonstrate absent peristalsis, wall thickening or thinning, ↑ or ↓ vascularity, pneumatosis, portal venous gas, free air, complex fluid
  - WSCE: Not performed acutely; obtained if delayed strictures are suspected

Helpful Clues for Less Common Diagnoses

- **Meconium Ileus**
  - Poorly named: Not ileus but true obstruction
    - Abnormally thick meconium causes obstruction at distal ileum
  - Strong association with cystic fibrosis
  - Complicated meconium ileus (~ 50%): Superimposed segmental volvulus, atresia, necrosis, &/or perforation
  - Radiographs show multiple dilated air-filled loops
    - Typical of simple meconium ileus
    - ± "soap bubble" densities in right lower quadrant (due to gas in impacted meconium)
      - Air-fluid levels are less likely than other distal obstructions due to thick meconium
    - Gasless abdomen or mass effect with bowel displacement suggests complicated meconium ileus

- Peritoneal Ca^{2+} indicates meconium peritonitis (due to in utero bowel perforation)
  - Free air is rarely seen at birth
- WSCE: Microcolon with RS ratio > 1
  - Contrast refluxes into terminal ileum (TI), which is filled with abnormal meconium; may reflux proximally into dilated loops
    - If simple/uncomplicated, serial therapeutic enemas with higher osmolality contrast may be used to loosen meconium & relieve obstruction
- Possible US findings
  - Solid echogenic meconium in obstructed loops
  - ± peritoneal Ca^{2+}, complex ascites, or meconium pseudocyst if complicated by perforation

- **Jejunoileal Atresia**
  - Complete occlusion of lumen due to membrane, blind ends with intervening fibrous cord, or disconnected ends
    - Likely due to in utero ischemic event
    - Jejunal atresia may cause distal obstruction pattern if it involves distal jejunum, has multiple atresias, or has long segment of discontinuity
  - Radiographs show multiple dilated air-filled loops
    - May have focal disproportionately dilated loop
    - ± air-fluid levels within bowel loops
    - Gasless abdomen suggests bowel perforation
  - WSCE: Microcolon with RS ratio > 1
    - Variable contrast reflux into ileum depending on level of atresia, not reaching dilated loops
      - No filling defects in ileum
  - Association with gastroschisis, meconium ileus/cystic fibrosis, malrotation
- **Midgut Volvulus (Mimic)**
  - May cause ischemic ileus with diffuse bowel dilation
  - WSCE: Normal caliber colon with RS ratio > 1
    - Position of colon, particularly cecum, is abnormal
    - WSCE should not be exam of choice in ill-appearing neonate with bilious emesis
  - UGI: "Corkscrew" beyond tapered dilated proximal duodenum is classic
  - CECT/US: "Whirlpool" of twisted bowel & mesenteric vessels around superior mesenteric artery (SMA); may result in effacement of superior mesenteric vein/SMA with ↓ bowel wall enhancement
- **Inguinal Hernia**
  - Radiographs may show gas in inguinal canal/scrotum
    - Not necessarily obstructive

Helpful Clues for Rare Diagnoses

- **Anorectal Malformation**
  - Imperforate anus or anteriorly located stenotic rectal orifice on physical exam in male patients
  - Anterior stenotic rectal orifice or single perineal orifice on physical exam in female patients
  - Radiographs: Numerous dilated loops
    - Intraluminal Ca^{2+} if urine & meconium mix due to fistula from distal colon to bladder or urethra
      - ± air in bladder or vagina due to fistula
    - Prone cross-table lateral view (or US) to evaluate pouch to anus distance
      - Best if patient is > 24 hours old
      - Useful if fistula level is not clinically apparent (~ 5%)
  - Associations: Down syndrome, Currarino triad, VACTERL, OEIS, caudal regression
- **Colonic Atresia**
  - Least common intestinal atresia
  - May affect any segment of colon
  - Radiographs often show disproportionately dilated loop of proximal colon
  - WSCE: Small distal colon with abrupt halt to contrast passage at level of atresia
- **Omphalomesenteric Duct Remnant**
  - Embryologic structure from yolk sac to primitive midgut
  - Remnants along course from umbilicus to ileum: Diverticulum (i.e., Meckel), sinus tract, cyst, fibrous band
    - Remnant at ileum may serve as point for volvulus
  - WSCE: Usually normal caliber colon; may see medial deviation of cecum & reflux of contrast into beak-shaped obstructed TI
  - CECT: Distal SB obstruction without clear etiology

Hirschsprung Disease

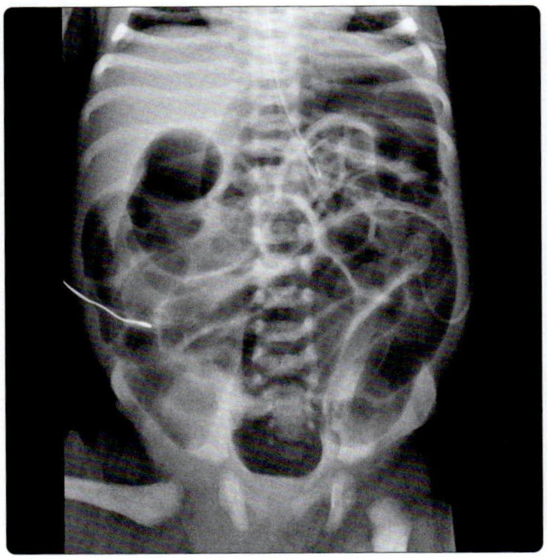

Hirschsprung Disease

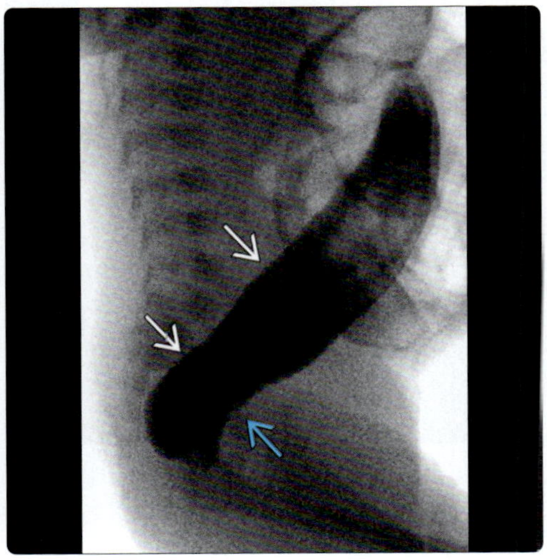

(Left) *AP radiograph in a 1 day old with vomiting shows diffuse dilation of gas-distended bowel loops, suggesting a distal obstruction.* **(Right)** *Lateral view from the subsequent water soluble contrast enema (WSCE) shows a rectosigmoid (RS) ratio < 1 ➡, typical of Hirschsprung disease (HD). Subtle irregularity of the anterior rectal wall ➡ is likely due to spasm, also commonly seen in HD. Intraoperatively, there was a short affected segment with the histologic transition zone in the rectum.*

Hirschsprung Disease

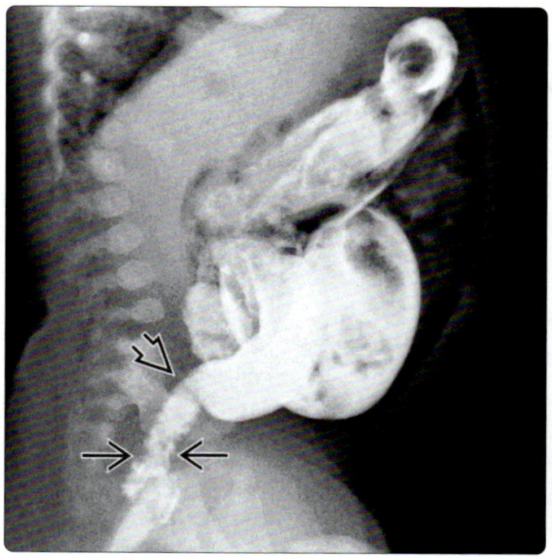

Hirschsprung Disease

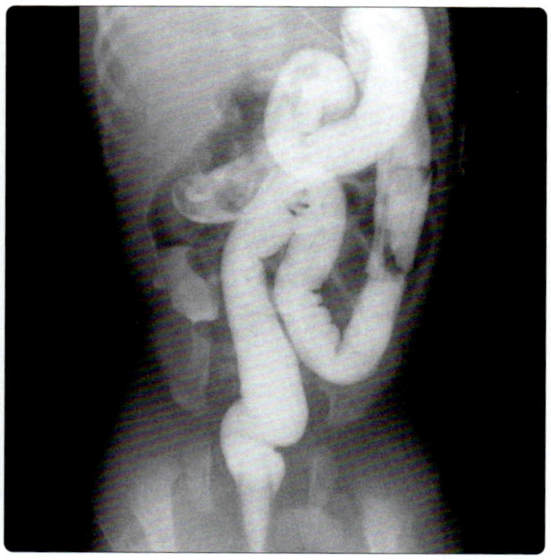

(Left) *Lateral WSCE in a neonate with infrequent stooling shows a narrow rectum with transition ➩ to the dilated colon at the RS junction, consistent with HD. Note the spasm ➔ in the distal segment.* **(Right)** *Frontal WSCE in a 1 day old with a family history of HD who was found to have a distal obstructive gas pattern on the preceding abdominal radiograph shows a mildly small caliber colon diffusely, but not a microcolon, without a clear transition. Total colonic HD was confirmed intraoperatively.*

Hirschsprung Disease

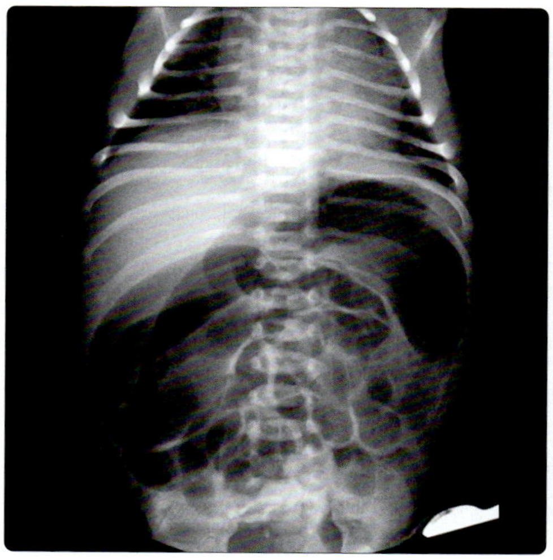

Hirschsprung Disease

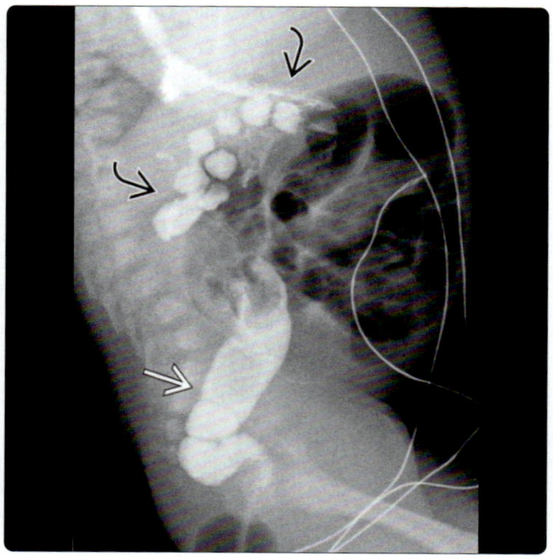

(Left) *AP radiograph in a 1 day old with bilious emesis & abdominal distention shows numerous dilated bowel loops throughout the abdomen in a distal obstructive pattern.* **(Right)** *Initial lateral image from a subsequent WSCE demonstrates an equivocal RS ratio ➡. Contrast from a preceding upper GI is also seen ➩, which was performed first to exclude malrotation & midgut volvulus.*

Hirschsprung Disease

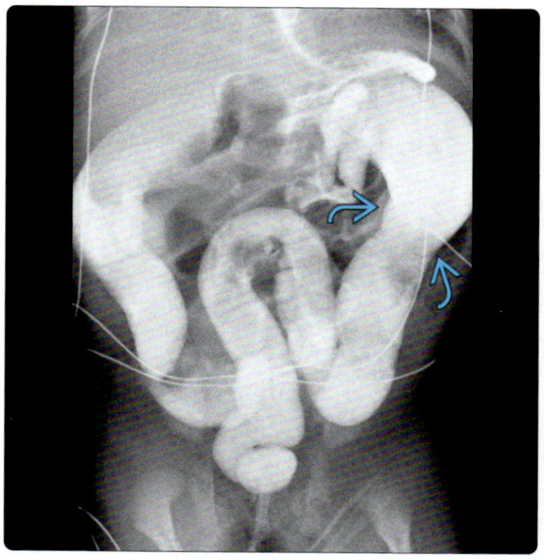

Meconium Plug Syndrome

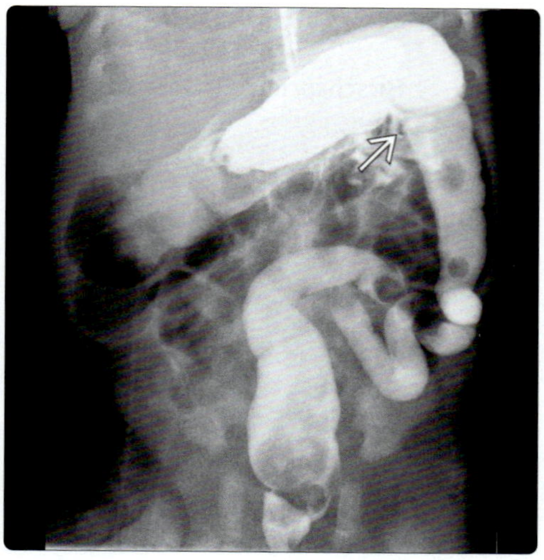

(Left) *Frontal view in the same patient shows a transition to dilated colon at the splenic flexure ➩. Rectal biopsy showed HD, & the histologic transition zone was ultimately confirmed at the splenic flexure.* **(Right)** *Frontal WSCE in a 1 day old with emesis shows a gradual transition at the splenic flexure ➡ from small sigmoid & descending segments to transverse colon; however, the RS ratio was > 1. There was passage of meconium during the exam & the patient improved within a few days, as expected with meconium plug syndrome.*

Meconium Plug Syndrome

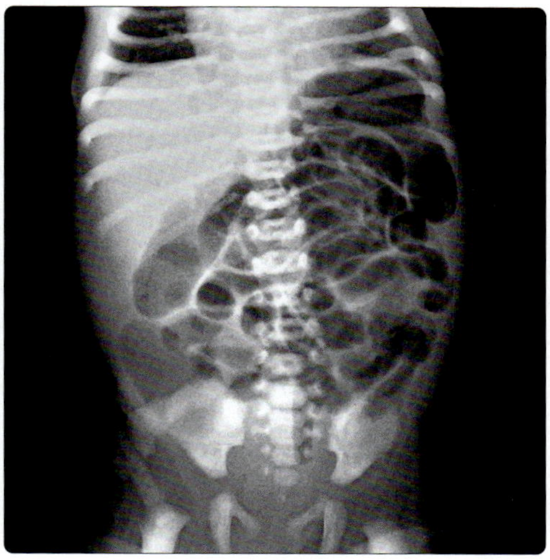

Meconium Plug Syndrome

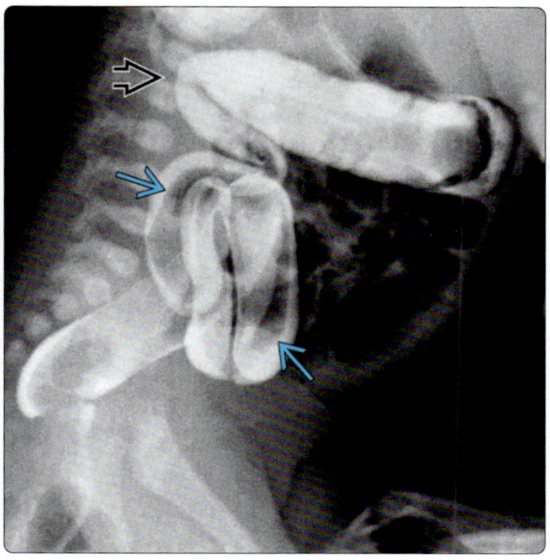

(Left) *AP radiograph in a 2-day-old infant shows multiple air-filled dilated loops of bowel, consistent with a neonatal distal intestinal obstruction.* **(Right)** *Lateral WSCE in the same patient shows a RS ratio > 1, a small left colon, a transition to dilated colon at the splenic flexure ➩, & multiple large tubular meconium plugs → in the entire colon, typical of meconium plug (a.k.a. small left colon) syndrome.*

Meconium Plug Syndrome

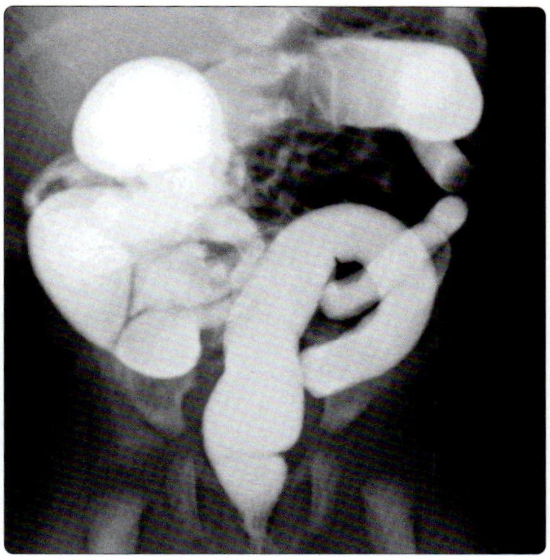

Meconium Ileus

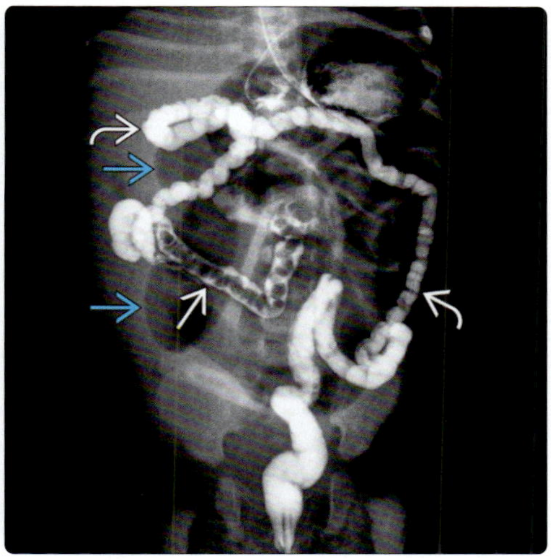

(Left) *Frontal WSCE subsequently performed in the same infant shows that the meconium plugs seen on the earlier study have passed. In many cases of meconium plug syndrome, the enema is curative.* **(Right)** *Frontal WSCE in a newborn shows a microcolon ➡ with meconium pellets lined up in the terminal ileum in a pearls-on-a-string ➡ appearance. Note the dilated loops of a small bowel obstruction → in this patient with meconium ileus.*

Meconium Ileus

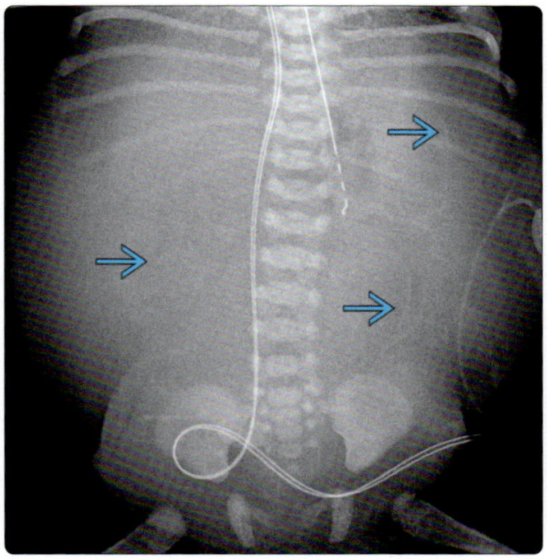

Meconium Ileus

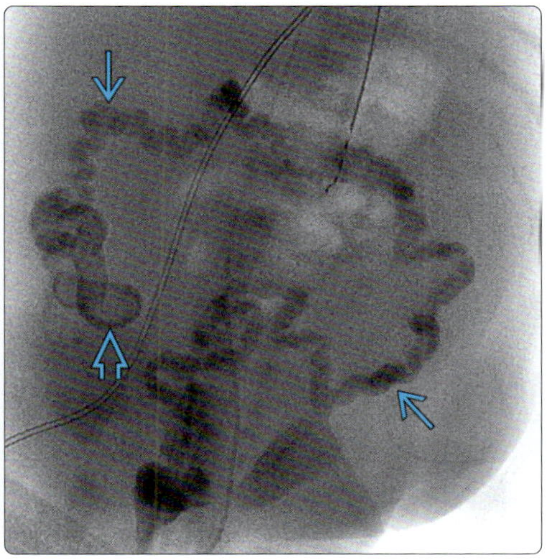

(Left) *AP radiograph in a newborn shows a distended & nearly gasless abdomen with numerous curvilinear Ca^{2+} along the peritoneum →. This patient had a meconium ileus complicated by volvulus, leading to in utero perforation. Large complex ascites was noted on ultrasound (not shown).* **(Right)** *Frontal WSCE in the same newborn shows a microcolon → with abnormal meconium filling the terminal ileum →. The RS ratio is > 1 (normal). Cystic fibrosis was subsequently confirmed.*

Jejunoileal Atresia

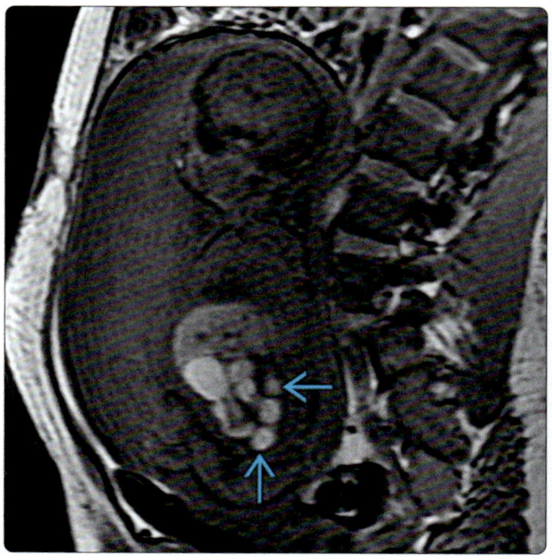

Jejunoileal Atresia

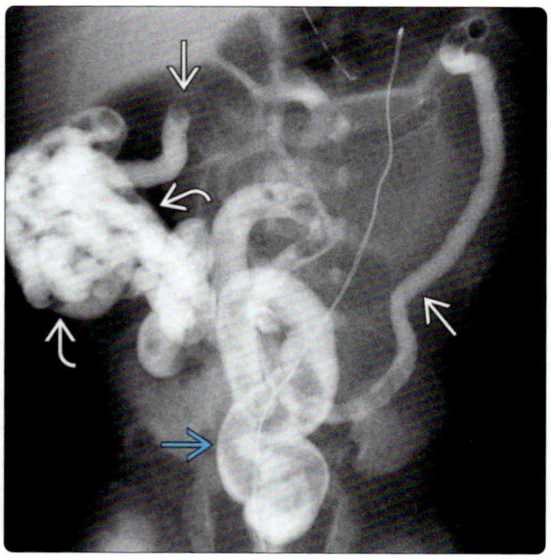

(Left) *Sagittal T1 fetal MR performed at 30-weeks gestation shows numerous dilated bowel loops containing T1-hyperintense meconium, typical of a congenital distal bowel obstruction.* **(Right)** *Frontal WSCE performed shortly after birth in the same patient demonstrates a microcolon with a normal RS ratio. There is filling of numerous small caliber distal ileal loops that do not contain meconium pellets. Intraoperatively, an atretic segment was encountered in the distal jejunum.*

Midgut Volvulus (Mimic)

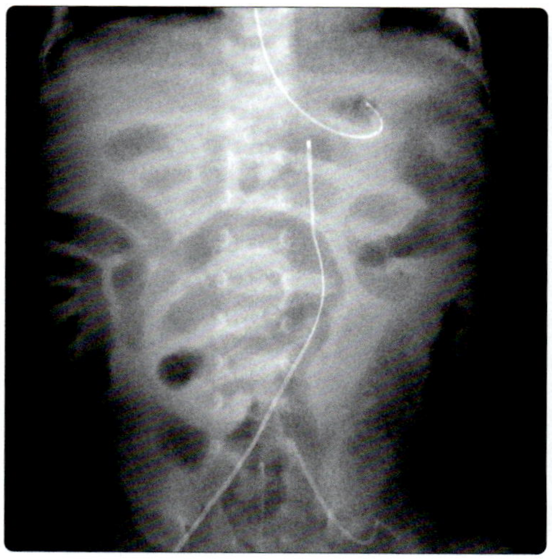

Midgut Volvulus (Mimic)

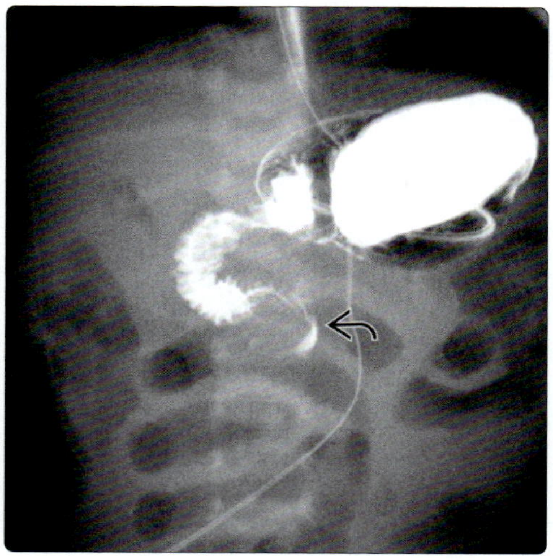

(Left) *Frontal scout image from an upper GI in a 3 week old with bilious emesis demonstrates multiple mildly dilated bowel loops throughout the abdomen. Bowel wall thickening is also seen, likely reflecting an ischemic ileus, which is typically a later finding in midgut volvulus.* **(Right)** *Frontal view from the subsequent upper GI series demonstrates the abnormal course of the duodenum with narrowing & twisting, consistent with malrotation & midgut volvulus.*

Anorectal Malformation

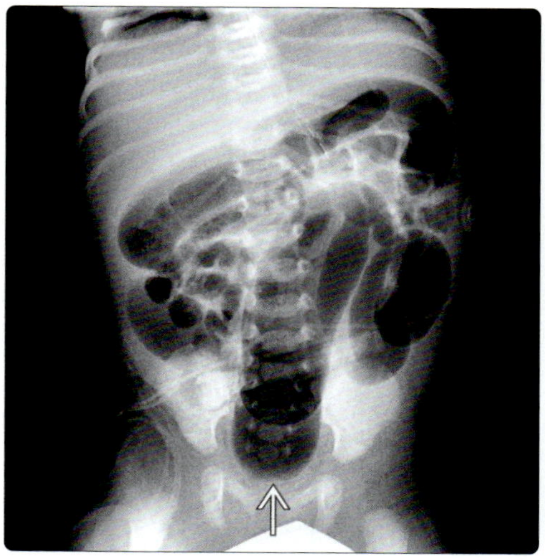

Anorectal Malformation

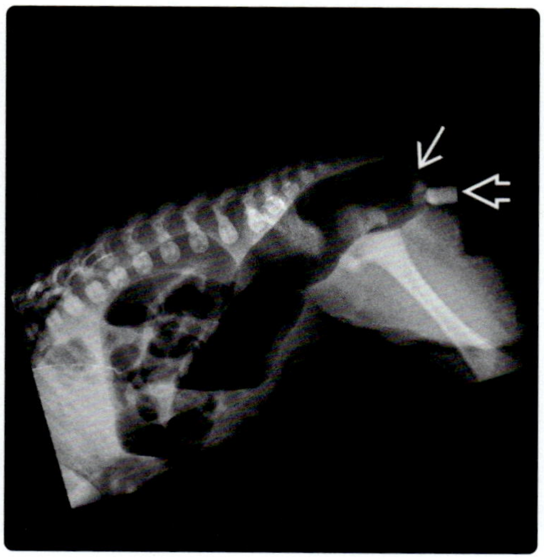

(Left) *AP radiograph in a 1-day-old boy who had no anal opening on the perineum shows multiple dilated bowel loops, consistent with distal obstruction all the way to the rectum in this patient with an anorectal malformation (ARM).* **(Right)** *Prone cross-table lateral radiograph shows a dilated air-filled rectum very close to the expected location of the anal sphincter (marker), consistent with a low ARM. This positioning is used to fully distend the rectum with air when the level of ARM is clinically occult.*

Anorectal Malformation

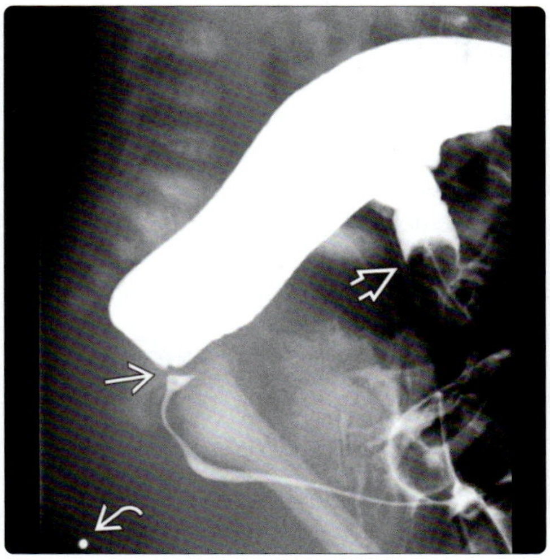

Colonic Atresia

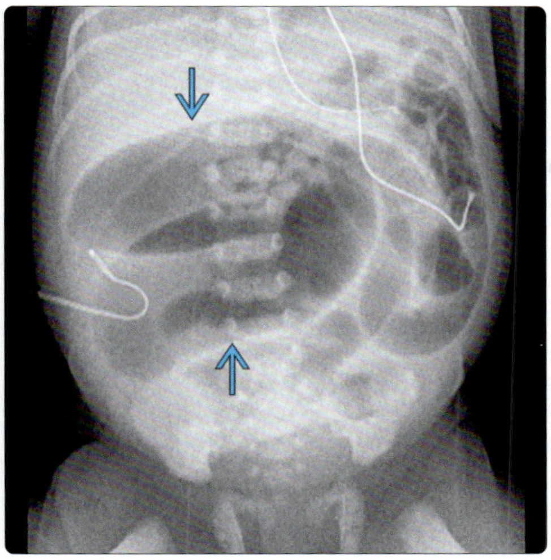

(Left) *Distal colostogram in a 7 day old with an ARM status post diverting colostomy shows a rectourethral fistula . To achieve adequate pressure to visualize the fistula, a balloon was carefully inflated to occlude the mucous fistula . Note the marker for the expected anal opening .* **(Right)** *AP radiograph in a newborn with vomiting shows numerous dilated bowel loops. There is a disproportionately dilated loop , suggesting colonic atresia. A WSCE (not shown) demonstrated a microcolon abruptly ending in the right abdomen.*

Colonic Atresia

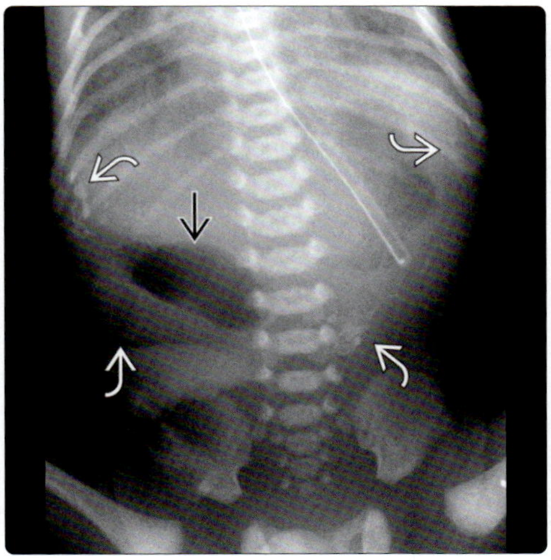

Colonic Atresia

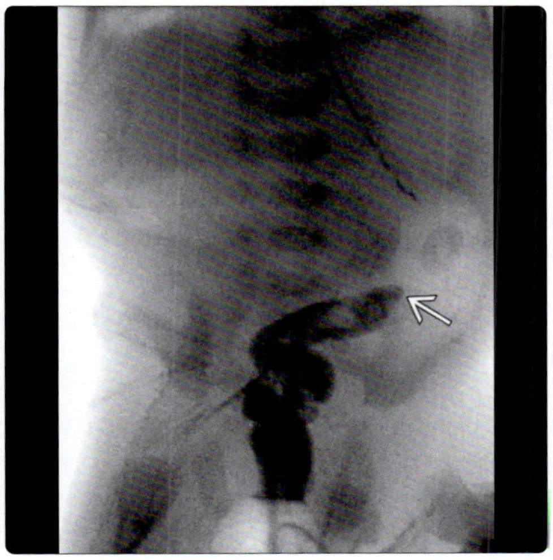

(Left) *AP radiograph in a newborn with a suspected in utero bowel perforation shows scattered peritoneal Ca^{2+} confirming meconium peritonitis. There is an overall paucity of bowel gas with a dilated loop visible over the right midabdomen.* **(Right)** *Frontal WSCE showed that contrast was unable to pass proximal to the sigmoid colon . Colonic atresia, multiple jejunoileal atresias, & multiple meconium pseudocysts were identified intraoperatively.*

Omphalomesenteric Duct Remnant

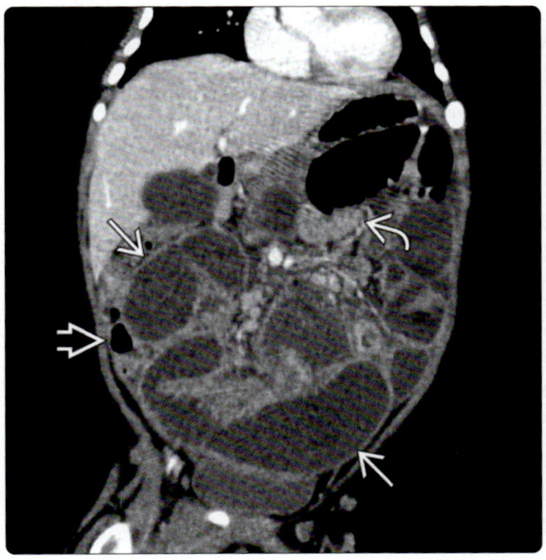

Omphalomesenteric Duct Remnant

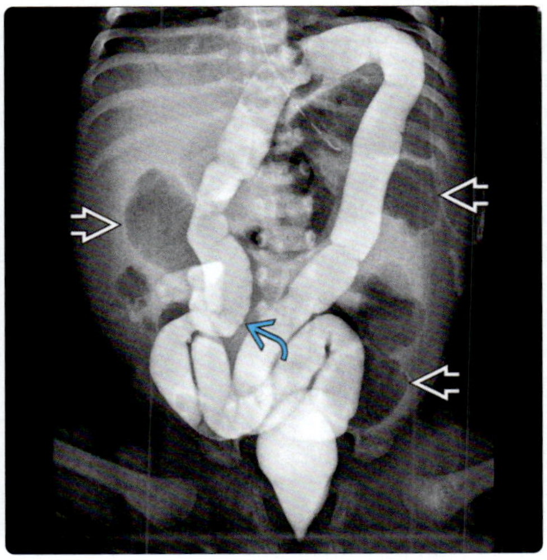

(Left) *Coronal CECT in a 6 month old with a small bowel obstruction shows multiple dilated small bowel loops , several nondilated small bowel loops , & a nondilated colon . At surgery, a segmental volvulus related to an omphalomesenteric duct remnant was found.* **(Right)** *Frontal WSCE shows an obstruction secondary to an omphalomesenteric duct remnant. There is a normal RS ratio with a mildly small colon. The cecum is positioned medially .*

DIFFERENTIAL DIAGNOSIS

Common

- Ileal Atresia
- Meconium Ileus
- Meconium Plug Syndrome
- Hirschsprung Disease
- Defunctionalized Colon

Less Common

- Jejunal Atresia
- Colonic Atresia
- Ileal Duplication Cyst
- Omphalomesenteric Duct Remnant

Rare but Important

- Megacystis-Microcolon-Intestinal Hypoperistalsis Syndrome

ESSENTIAL INFORMATION

Key Differential Diagnosis Issues

- Definition: Microcolon refers to small caliber of colon on contrast enema, typically in newborns
  - Distal (not proximal) congenital bowel obstructions typically lead to microcolon
- Clinical features: Consider patient age (including gestational age), timing of symptom onset, & history of prior ileostomy/colostomy
  - Most entities present in newborn period with bilious emesis, abdominal distention, &/or failure to pass meconium
- Imaging
  - Radiographs of newborn
    - Classically show distal obstruction pattern with numerous dilated, gas-filled bowel loops
    - In utero perforation may lead to Ca^{2+} along peritoneal lining (meconium peritonitis) or in localized collection (meconium pseudocyst)
      - Perforation typically seals as atresia or stenosis in utero, making free air uncommon on initial radiographs
  - Water-soluble contrast enema (WSCE)
    - Length of colon overall: Normal vs. short
    - Length of small caliber colon: Diffuse vs. distal only with transition to proximal dilation
    - Caliber of rectum vs. sigmoid: > 1 (normal) or < 1 (abnormally small rectum)
    - Visualization of distal ileum: Freely opacified by contrast enema vs. demonstrating filling defects vs. not able to be opacified
  - Ultrasound may be useful if newborn radiographs suggest mass effect on bowel
    - Complex localized collection or free fluid suggests perforation
    - Impacted meconium or obstructing duplication cyst may appear mass-like
  - Fetal imaging may provide clues
    - T1-bright meconium often accumulates in dilated loops if distal obstruction is present

Helpful Clues for Common Diagnoses

- **Ileal Atresia**
  - In utero ischemic event leads to variations of bowel wall interruption (from membrane to intervening fibrous cord to complete discontinuity)
  - Radiographs: Distal obstruction pattern
    - ± air-fluid levels within bowel loops
  - WSCE: Diffuse microcolon with little or no meconium in small-caliber distal small bowel
    - Reflux of contrast abruptly halts at atresia
    - Normal rectosigmoid ratio (> 1)
- **Meconium Ileus**
  - Not actually ileus (as abnormally thick meconium obstructs distal small bowel)
  - Most cases are secondary to cystic fibrosis (CF)
    - 15% of CF patients have meconium ileus (MI) at birth
  - 50% of cases are complicated by segmental volvulus, ischemia, perforation, or atresia
  - Radiographs: Distal obstruction pattern
    - ± "soap bubble" densities in lower abdomen due to gas intermixed with impacted abnormal meconium in ileum
    - Few or no air-fluid levels due to thick meconium
    - Paucity of bowel gas, soft tissue mass, or Ca^{2+} suggests complicated MI
  - Ultrasound
    - Useful if complication is suspected
      - Complex free or localized fluid confirms meconium peritonitis
      - Ca^{2+} may be seen over liver surface or along cyst lining
    - Impacted meconium may form heterogeneous mass within bowel
      - Contents may contain echogenic foci of gas & do not swirl with compression
  - WSCE: Diffuse microcolon
    - Normal rectosigmoid ratio (> 1)
    - Contrast classically refluxes into terminal ileum (TI), outlining impacted pellets of abnormal meconium ("pearls on string")
    - Contrast may then enter dilated loops
    - However, contrast may not pass proximal to distal obstructing meconium
      - Cannot differentiate this appearance from ileal atresia
- **Meconium Plug Syndrome**
  - a.k.a. neonatal small left colon, functional immaturity of colon
  - No proven underlying pathology (i.e., meconium is normal & does not cause obstruction in this poorly understood entity)
  - Often occurs in premature infant or with history of maternal magnesium administration
  - Radiographs: Distal obstruction pattern
  - WSCE: Small distal colon
    - Normal rectosigmoid ratio (> 1)
    - Transition to dilated proximal colon in left upper quadrant near splenic flexure
    - Meconium plugs may be scattered in colon, proximal or distal to transition
- **Hirschsprung Disease**
  - Lack of ganglion cells in distal colon; extends retrograde for variable lengths (i.e., may involve entire colon)

- Rarely aganglionosis involves entire intestine (total intestinal Hirschsprung)
  - Radiographs: Distal obstruction pattern
    - ± distal ileal intraluminal Ca^{2+}
  - WSCE: Affected distal colon is typically small (i.e., rectosigmoid ratio < 1)
    - Total colonic Hirschsprung disease may show normal colon, short colon with question mark configuration, or diffuse microcolon
- **Defunctionalized Colon**
  - Clinical history of prior disease requiring ostomy
    - Necrotizing enterocolitis (NEC), spontaneous intestinal perforation, bowel ischemia, complicated inflammatory bowel disease, etc.
  - WSCE: Small diameter of residual colon distal to ostomy (due to chronic disuse)
    - Rectosigmoid ratio usually > 1
    - Normal diameter is usually regained after ostomy takedown

Helpful Clues for Less Common Diagnoses

- **Jejunal Atresia**
  - May cause microcolon if
    - Atresia lies in distal jejunum
    - Atresia is of unusual length
    - Multiple atresias are present
- **Colonic Atresia**
  - Ischemic event similar to other nonduodenal atresias
  - Radiographs: Distal bowel obstruction
    - Disproportionate dilation of 1 or 2 bowel loops, typically in right abdomen
  - WSCE: Distal microcolon terminating at level of colonic atresia
- **Ileal Duplication Cyst**
  - Radiographs: Rounded mass (or paucity of bowel gas) noted amidst dilated bowel loops
  - Ultrasound: Duplication cyst classically shows "gut signature" trilaminar wall (though this is not specific)
    - Peristalsis is highly suggestive
    - Cyst may extrinsically compress bowel or serve as lead point for intussusception
- **Omphalomesenteric Duct Remnant**
  - Rare cause of distal bowel obstruction at any age
  - WSCE: May show medial deviation & beaked appearance of cecum or TI

Helpful Clues for Rare Diagnoses

- **Megacystis-Microcolon-Intestinal Hypoperistalsis Syndrome**
  - Rare, often fatal condition, usually in females
  - Similar features to prune-belly syndrome with abdominal wall laxity
  - Radiographs: Distal obstruction pattern
    - Megacystis may displace bowel loops
  - Upper GI: Malrotation, lack of peristalsis
  - WSCE: Microcolon; may lie in left abdomen due to malrotation

SELECTED REFERENCES

1. Gunderman PFR et al: Fetal MRI in management of complicated meconium ileus: prenatal and surgical imaging. Prenat Diagn. 38(9):685-91, 2018
2. Rattan KN et al: Gastrointestinal duplication presenting as neonatal intestinal obstruction: an experience of 15 years at Tertiary Care Centre. J Neonatal Surg. 6(1):5, 2017
3. Maxfield CM et al: A pattern-based approach to bowel obstruction in the newborn. Pediatr Radiol. 43(3):318-29, 2013
4. Puri P et al: Variants of Hirschsprung disease. Semin Pediatr Surg. 21(4):310-8, 2012
5. Sinha CK et al: Neonatal Meckel's diverticulum: spectrum of presentation. Pediatr Emerg Care. 25(5):348-9, 2009

Ileal Atresia

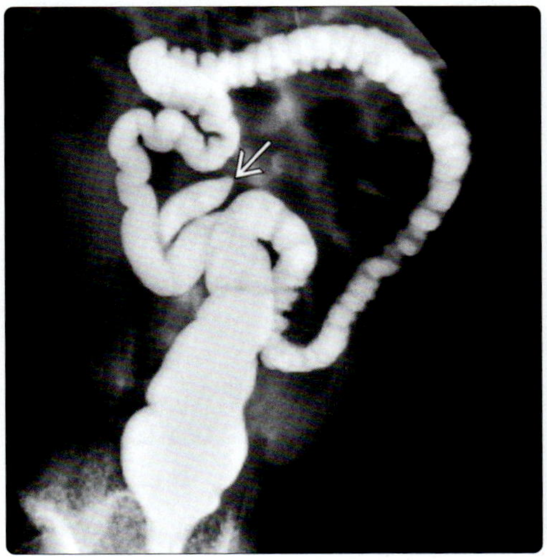

Ileal Atresia

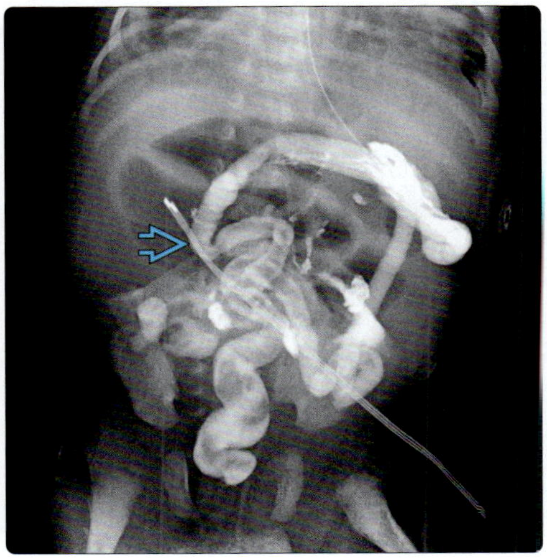

(Left) *Supine frontal WSCE shows a normal rectosigmoid ratio in a microcolon containing no significant meconium. The reflux of contrast abruptly terminated in the terminal ileum ➡. Ileal atresia was confirmed at surgery.* **(Right)** *Supine frontal WSCE in a newborn with bilious emesis shows a microcolon with a normal rectosigmoid ratio (> 1). The proximal colon is shifted medially ➡ by dilated small bowel loops. A preceding upper GI showed normal midgut rotation. Surgery confirmed a distal ileal atresia.*

(Left) *Supine frontal WSCE in a newborn shows a microcolon with a normal rectosigmoid ratio (> 1). The normal-caliber terminal ileum is filled with impacted meconium ➔. Unopacified dilated small bowel loops are noted in the background.* **(Right)** *Supine frontal WSCE in a newborn shows a microcolon with reflux of contrast into the terminal ileum, which is of normal caliber & filled with impacted meconium ➔. This constellation of findings is characteristic of meconium ileus.*

Meconium Ileus

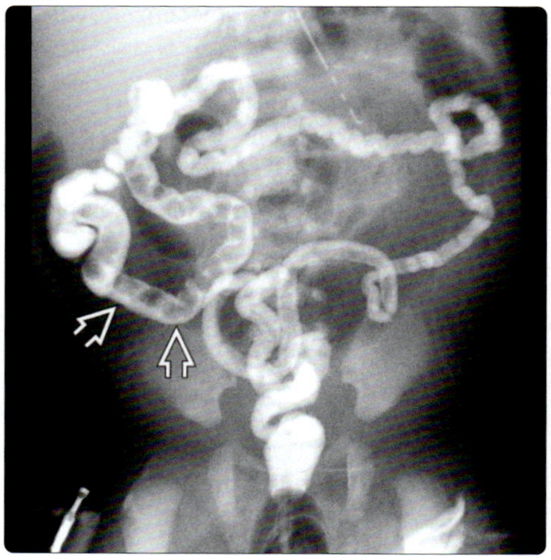

Meconium Ileus

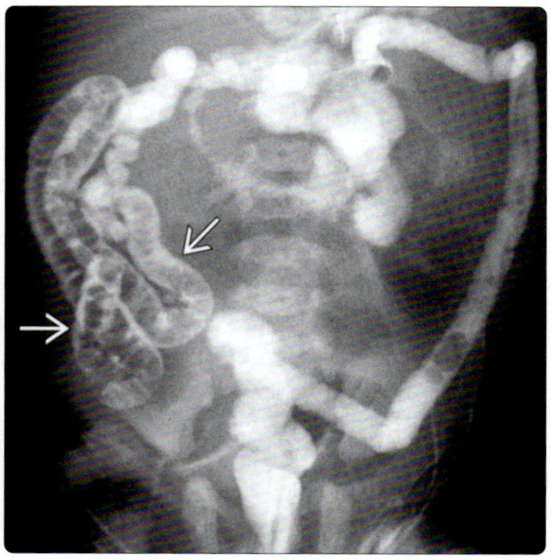

(Left) *AP radiograph in a newborn with emesis shows scattered dilated bowel loops. "Soap bubble" density ➔ is seen in the left abdomen due to impacted abnormal meconium causing a meconium ileus in this patient.* **(Right)** *AP radiograph in a newborn with abdominal distention shows multiple dilated, gas-filled bowel loops with an obstructing round mass ➔ in the right abdomen.*

Meconium Ileus

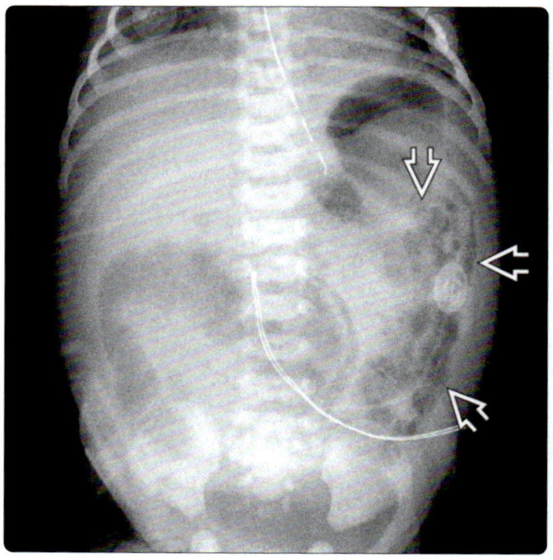

Meconium Ileus

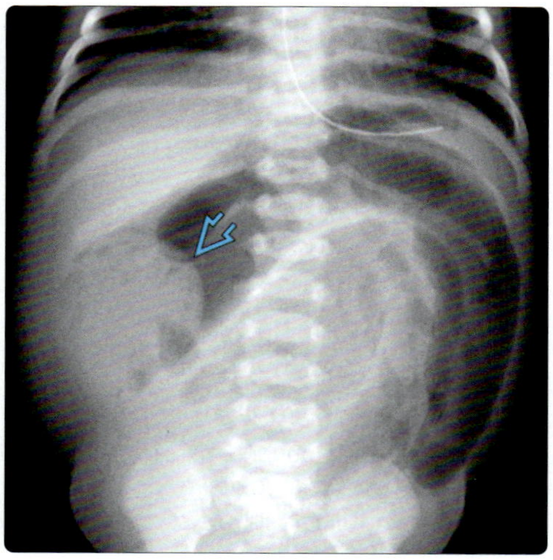

(Left) *Longitudinal ultrasound in the same patient shows a dilated, thick-walled bowel loop ➔ filled with a ball of abnormal meconium. The echogenic foci ➔ are due to gas intermixed with the meconium. Scattered free fluid was also noted, concerning for an associated complication.* **(Right)** *Supine frontal WSCE in the same patient shows a microcolon with a normal rectosigmoid ratio. The dilated bowel loops could not be opacified. A meconium ileus complicated by ischemia was found at surgery.*

Meconium Ileus

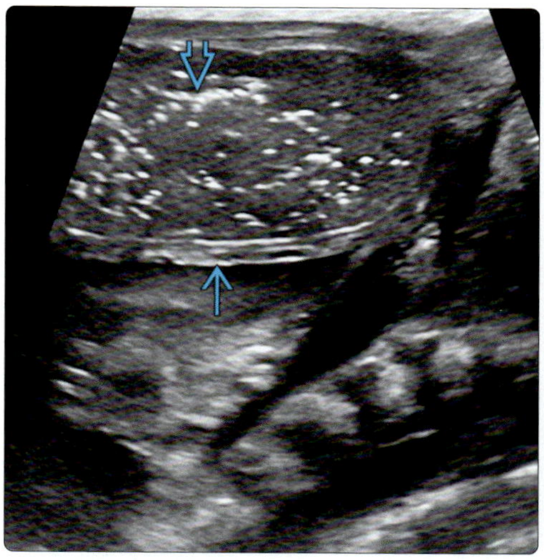

Meconium Ileus

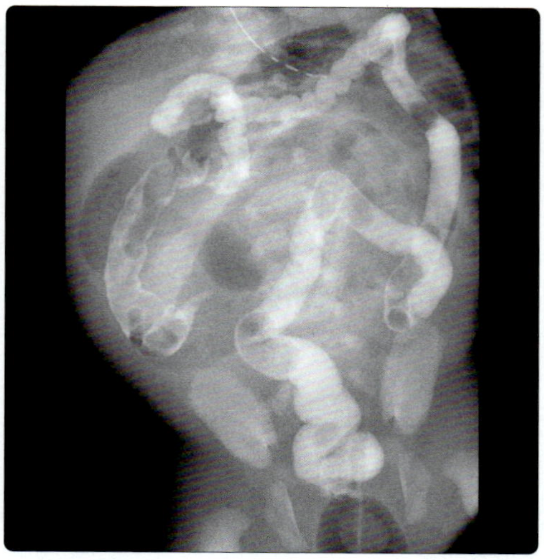

Meconium Plug Syndrome

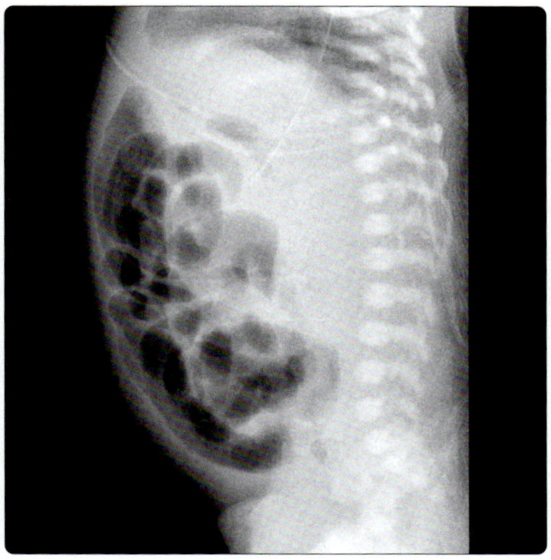

Meconium Plug Syndrome

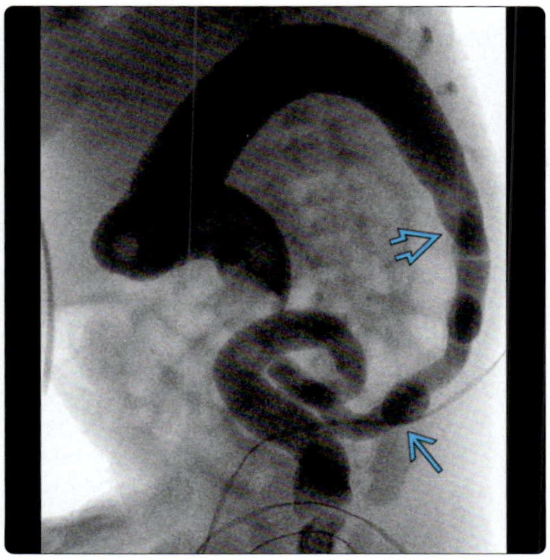

(Left) *Cross-table lateral radiograph in a newborn with distention & emesis shows numerous dilated bowel loops with air-fluid levels, consistent with a distal obstruction.* **(Right)** *Supine frontal WSCE in the same patient shows a small-caliber distal colon* ⇨ *with a normal rectosigmoid ratio (> 1). There is gradual transition to a mildly dilated proximal colon near the splenic flexure* ⇨*. While Hirschsprung disease could have this appearance, bowel function recovered after the enema, typical of meconium plug syndrome.*

Hirschsprung Disease

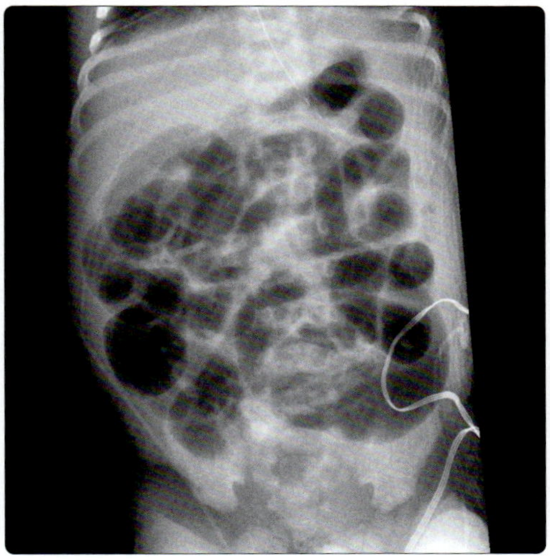

Hirschsprung Disease

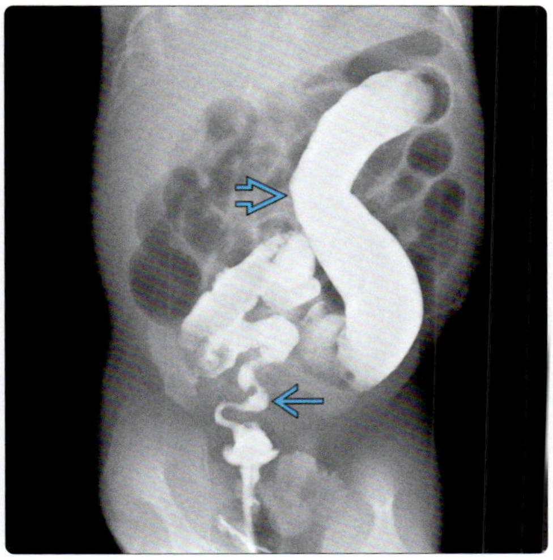

(Left) *Left-side-down decubitus radiograph in a newborn with emesis shows numerous dilated bowel loops throughout the abdomen, typical of a distal obstruction. There is no free intraperitoneal air.* **(Right)** *Supine frontal WSCE in the same patient shows a small distal colon* ⇨ *with an abnormal rectosigmoid ratio (< 1). There is transition to a mildly dilated descending colon* ⇨ *at the proximal sigmoid level. HD was confirmed on biopsy.*

Defunctionalized Colon

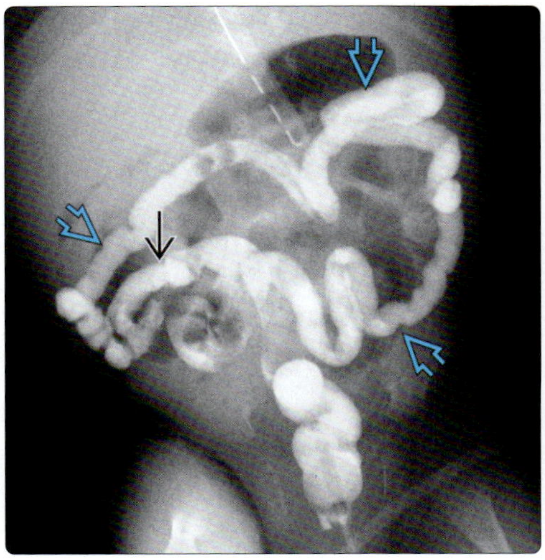

Defunctionalized Colon

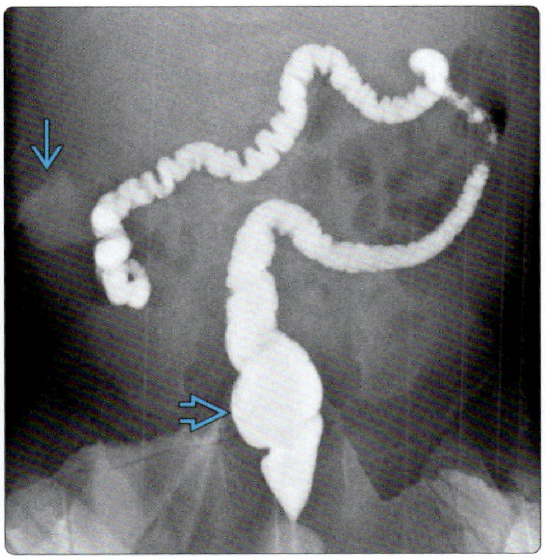

(Left) *Supine frontal WSCE shows a normal rectosigmoid ratio with a small colon* ⇨ *& a normal terminal ileum* → *in a patient with an ileostomy for perforated NEC. An enema was performed prior to ileostomy takedown to exclude a colonic stricture.* **(Right)** *Supine frontal WSCE shows a diffusely small-caliber colon in a former 25-week gestation premature infant with a history of spontaneous intestinal perforation. The patient has had an ostomy* ⇨ *for 4 months, resulting in an unused small colon. Note the normal rectum* ⇨*.*

(Left) *Supine frontal radiograph in a newborn with emesis & abdominal distention shows numerous dilated bowel loops of similar caliber, save a disproportionately dilated loop ⇨ in the right abdomen.* **(Right)** *Supine frontal WSCE in the same patient shows a small-caliber distal colon with a normal rectosigmoid ratio (> 1). Contrast could not be refluxed into the more proximal colon. Colonic atresia was confirmed at surgery.*

Colonic Atresia

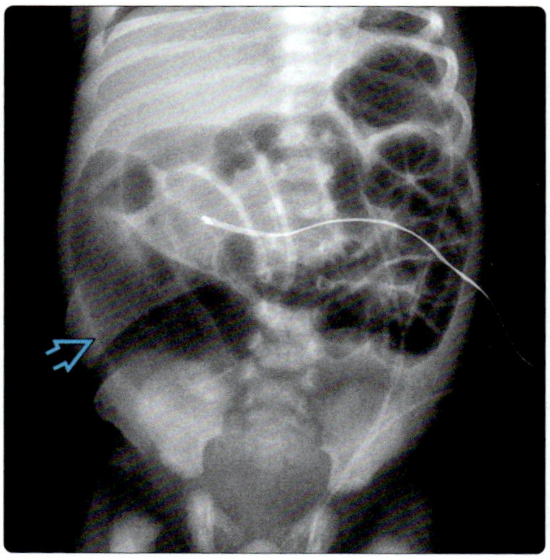

Colonic Atresia

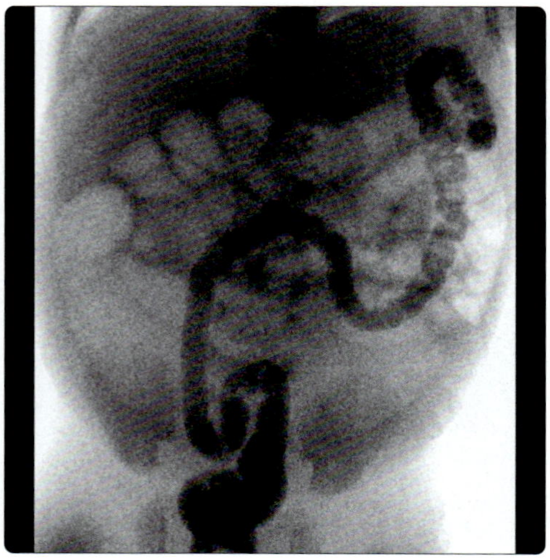

(Left) *AP radiograph in a newborn with abdominal distention shows numerous gas-filled, dilated bowel loops with a disproportionately dilated loop → in the right abdomen.* **(Right)** *Lateral WSCE in the same patient shows a small distal colon with a normal rectosigmoid ratio (> 1). No contrast could be refluxed further into the colon. Note the dilated, gas-filled loops filling the remainder of the abdomen. Colonic atresia was found at surgery.*

Colonic Atresia

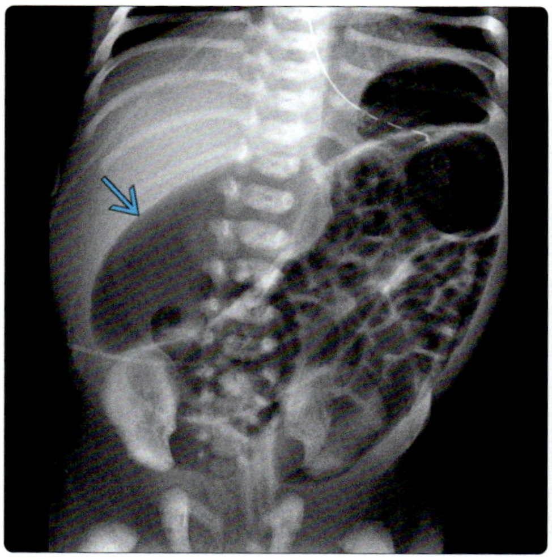

Colonic Atresia

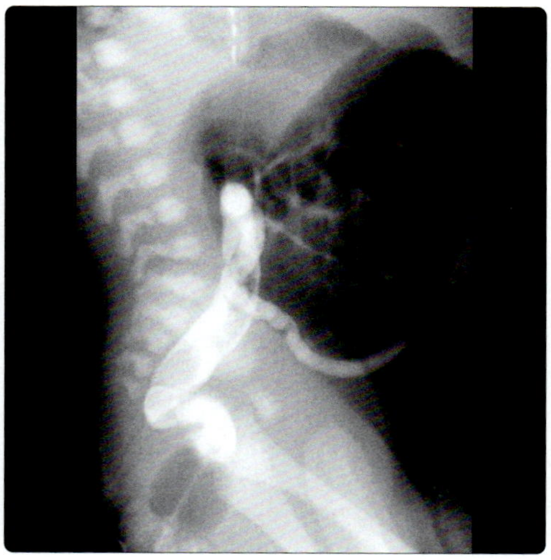

(Left) *AP radiograph in a 5 month old with a new onset of emesis shows dilated small bowel loops centrally with a paucity of bowel gas in the left abdomen.* **(Right)** *Transverse ultrasound in the same patient shows a well-circumscribed, round cyst in the left lower quadrant. The cyst has a trilaminar or "gut signature" wall → that is not specific but does favor a GI duplication cyst. This duplication cyst originated from the ileum.*

Ileal Duplication Cyst

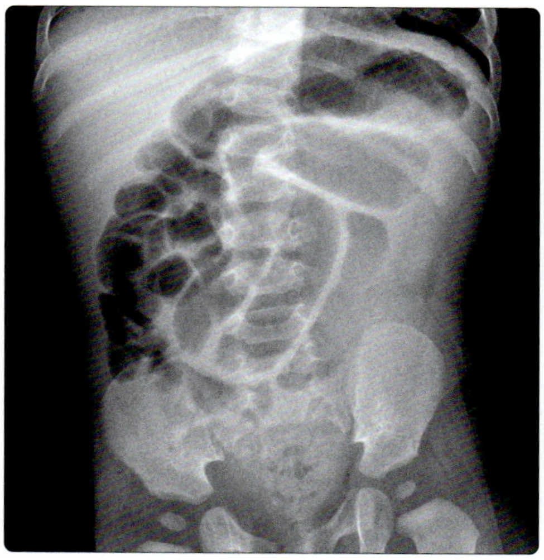

Ileal Duplication Cyst

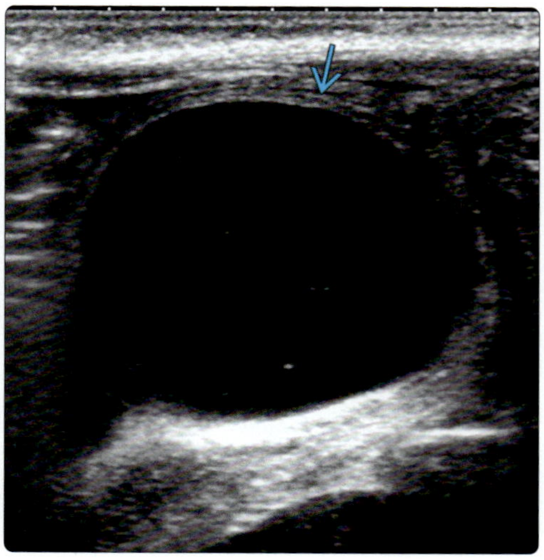

Omphalomesenteric Duct Remnant

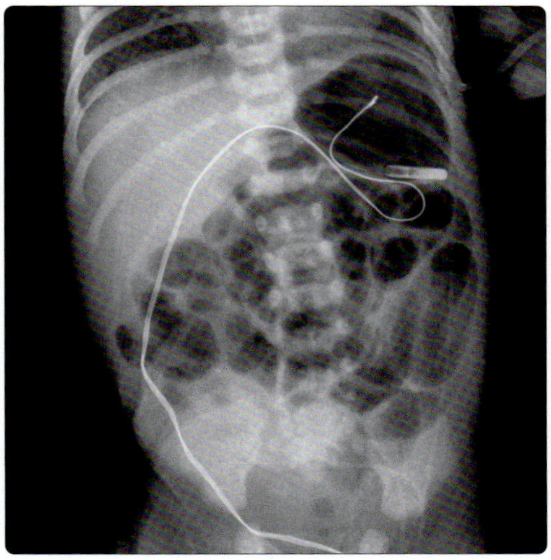

Omphalomesenteric Duct Remnant

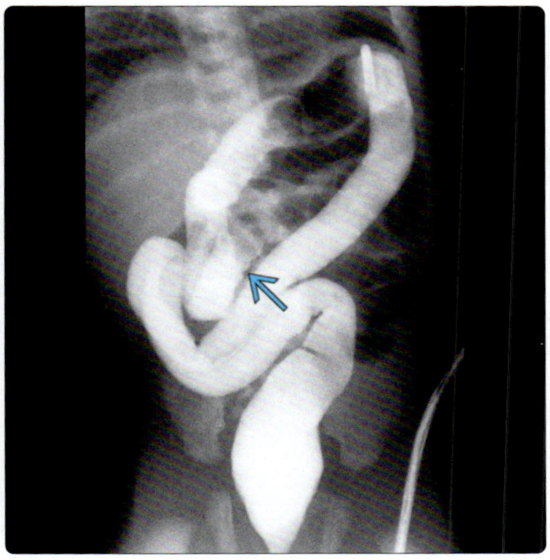

(Left) *AP radiograph in a 4 day old with distention & failure to pass meconium demonstrates numerous dilated bowel loops, typical of a distal obstruction.* **(Right)** *Supine WSCE in the same patient shows a mildly small colon diffusely with a normal rectosigmoid ratio (> 1). There is medialization of the cecum →, which is nonspecific but has been reported with obstructions due to omphalomesenteric duct remnants.*

Megacystis-Microcolon-Intestinal Hypoperistalsis Syndrome

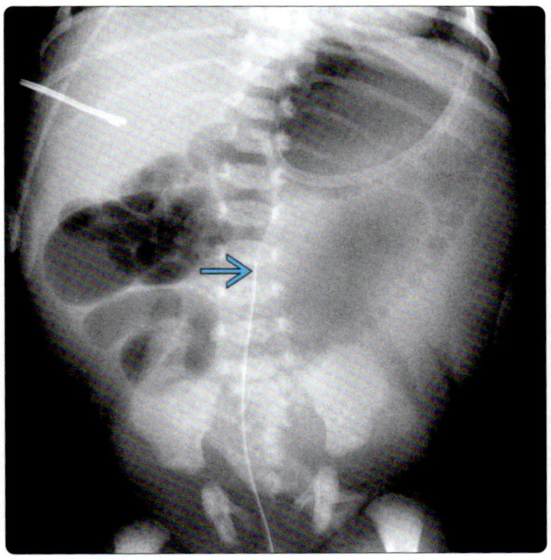

Megacystis-Microcolon-Intestinal Hypoperistalsis Syndrome

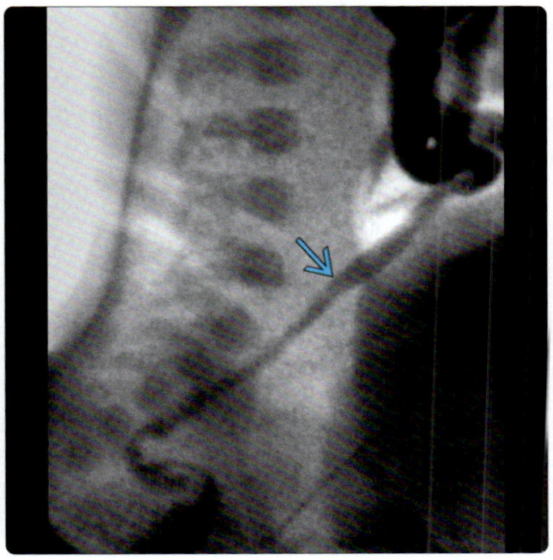

(Left) *AP radiograph of a 2 day old with failure to pass meconium & vomiting shows multiple dilated bowel loops. Note the high position of the bladder catheter →, suggesting megacystis.* **(Right)** *Lateral contrast enema in the same patient shows a very small colon →. A subsequent upper GI series confirmed malrotation in this female patient who was ultimately diagnosed with megacystis-microcolon-intestinal hypoperistalsis syndrome (MMIHS).*

Megacystis-Microcolon-Intestinal Hypoperistalsis Syndrome

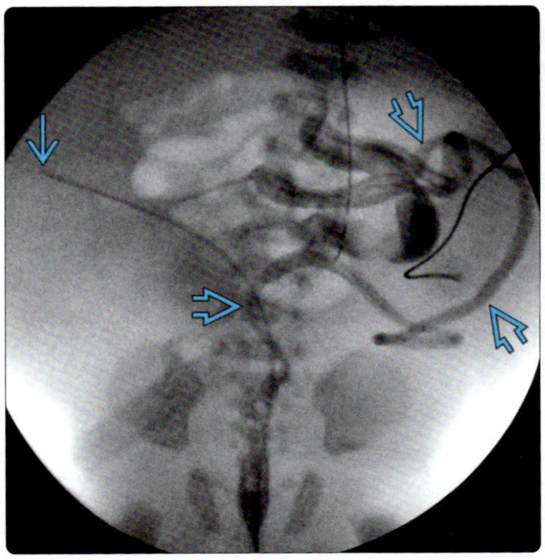

Megacystis-Microcolon-Intestinal Hypoperistalsis Syndrome

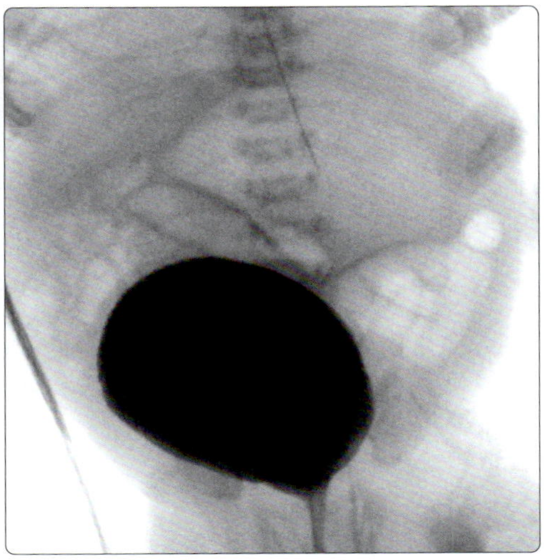

(Left) *Supine frontal WSCE in a female newborn shows a catheter in the bladder → extending high & lateral due to megacystis. A microcolon ⇨ lies almost entirely in the left abdomen due to malrotation in this patient with MMIHS.* **(Right)** *Supine frontal VCUG in the same patient shows filling of a large, round urinary bladder, consistent with megacystis.*

DIFFERENTIAL DIAGNOSIS

Common

- Aerophagia
- Ileus
- Hypertrophic Pyloric Stenosis
- Midgut Volvulus
- Duodenal Atresia, Stenosis, or Web

Less Common

- Duodenal Hematoma
- Bezoar
- Gastroparesis

Rare but Important

- Gastric Volvulus
- Gastric Duplication Cyst
- Pyloric Atresia

ESSENTIAL INFORMATION

Key Differential Diagnosis Issues

- Important clinical considerations
  - Age of patient
  - Duration & nature of symptoms (such as pain, vomiting, distention, respiratory distress)
  - History of recent procedure or trauma
  - Color of emesis
    - Bilious (suggesting obstruction beyond ampulla of Vater) vs. nonbilious (preampullary obstruction)
    - Bloody vs. nonbloody
- Important imaging considerations
  - Radiographs: Often primary modality for investigating pediatric emesis [except for suspected hypertrophic pyloric stenosis (HPS)]
    - Moderate to marked dilation of stomach
      - Shape & position of stomach are also important
    - Assessment of gas beyond pylorus is critical
      - Volume & distribution of gas
      - Caliber of bowel loops

Helpful Clues for Common Diagnoses

- **Aerophagia**
  - Common cause of distended stomach in young children
    - Swallowed air is often associated with crying or respiratory symptoms
    - Positive pressure ventilation via mask or laryngeal mask airway may also distend stomach/bowel
  - Stomach & bowel will typically show similar degrees of distention in aerophagia with overall nonobstructive pattern
    - Stomach dilation can be temporarily disproportionate
- **Ileus**
  - Lack of peristalsis → functional obstruction
  - Numerous causes: Postoperative, opioids, metabolic, ischemic, etc.
  - Generalized gaseous dilation of stomach & bowel with air-fluid levels
    - No transition point
    - Vomiting or nasogastric tube may decompress
- **Hypertrophic Pyloric Stenosis**
  - Presents with nonbilious projectile vomiting
  - Age range: 2-12 weeks (i.e., not congenital)
  - Radiographs classically (but not always) demonstrate paucity of bowel gas beyond stomach
    - Caterpillar sign: Hyperperistaltic stomach with undulations of wall
    - Duodenum not dilated
  - US is preferred diagnostic modality
    - Thickened pyloric muscle (single wall > 3 mm), elongated pyloric channel (> 15 mm); static morphology during exam (unlike spasm)
    - Minimal to no passage of fluids from stomach into duodenal bulb
  - Upper GI series (UGI)
    - "String of contrast" passing through narrowed & elongated channel
    - Hypertrophied muscle creates impression on contrast-filled gastric antrum & duodenal bulb
    - Caterpillar sign: Distended hyperperistaltic stomach undulating in real time
- **Midgut Volvulus**
  - Classically presents with bilious emesis in infant (90% < 12 months of age)
  - Radiographs are nonspecific & range from normal to proximal obstruction to ischemic ileus (rare)
  - UGI demonstrates mild to moderate dilation of stomach & proximal duodenum
    - Abrupt taper (or beak) of contrast is often seen near D2/D3 junction ± "corkscrew" of twisted & narrowed bowel just beyond taper
      - Degree of bowel narrowing in "corkscrew" is variable
    - Distal bowel is decompressed
    - Duodenojejunal junction does not show normal location to left of spine at level of duodenal bulb (on frontal image)
    - Midgut volvulus cannot be excluded if contrast does not pass beyond proximal duodenal taper/beak
  - US may show dilated D2 with D3 coursing anterior to superior mesenteric artery as it tapers & enters "whirlpool" twist of bowel & vessels
  - Surgical emergency: Can lead to ischemia/infarction
- **Duodenal Atresia, Stenosis, or Web**
  - Failure of luminal recanalization during embryogenesis
    - Duodenal atresia, stenosis, & web are continuum
  - Duodenal atresia is often diagnosed prenatally
    - Presentation of web & stenosis varies depending on degree of stenosis or size of web fenestration
  - Radiographs show "double bubble" of dilated stomach & rounded, dilated duodenal bulb with complete absence of distal gas; UGI is not necessary with classic appearance
    - Duodenal stenosis or web will have some distal gas
      - UGI performed to exclude midgut volvulus
  - Fluoroscopic findings
    - Duodenal atresia: UGI is not usually performed
    - Duodenal stenosis: Focal change in caliber in proximal duodenum
    - Duodenal web: With later presentation, may have windsock appearance of stretched web extending to distal duodenum

Helpful Clues for Less Common Diagnoses

- **Duodenal Hematoma**
  - Most common cause is blunt abdominal trauma
    - "Handle bar" injury, child abuse
    - Other causes: Biopsy, bleeding disorder, Henoch-Schönlein purpura
  - Most commonly located in D2 or D3
    - May be in lumen, wall, or paraduodenal tissues
  - Radiograph may show gastric distention with variable distal bowel gas
  - UGI may show extrinsic compression of lumen or coiled-spring appearance of clot expanding lumen
  - CECT/US shows ovoid or circumferential heterogeneous or homogeneous mass with luminal narrowing
    - Acute hematoma is high in attenuation/echogenicity & decreases with time
    - ± distention of stomach & proximal duodenum
    - Signs of perforation include extraluminal air, extraluminal contrast, & retroperitoneal fluid
- **Bezoar**
  - Obstructive mass of indigestible material
    - Hair, medications, inspissated milk (infant formula), vegetable material
  - Mottled-appearing filling defect in distended stomach
    - Food debris may have similar appearance
  - Bezoar is compliant & conforms to contour of stomach
  - UGI may help to further delineate bezoar size & extent; contrast may enter interstices of bezoar
- **Gastroparesis**
  - Delayed gastric emptying in absence of mechanical obstruction
  - Causes include: Idiopathic, type 1 diabetes, opioids, postviral, postsurgical, neuromuscular disorders, metabolic, etc.
  - Nuclear medicine gastric emptying study confirms
  - UGI: Dilated, hypoperistaltic stomach with retained food/fluid after fasting
  - CTA/Doppler: Reported association with median arcuate ligament syndrome (MALS)

Helpful Clues for Rare Diagnoses

- **Gastric Volvulus**
  - Often associated with diaphragm abnormalities
  - Radiographs show distended stomach in abdomen or thorax with abnormal configuration
  - Organoaxial volvulus
    - Rotation of stomach along longitudinal axis
    - Greater curvature of stomach lies superior to lesser curvature
    - May be transient incidental finding in neonates
  - Mesenteroaxial volvulus
    - Rotation of stomach along craniocaudal axis
    - Pylorus lies superior to fundus in left upper quadrant
      - 2 air-fluid levels on radiographs: Higher one is antrum, lower one is fundus
    - Antrum may show beaking on UGI due to twisting
- **Gastric Duplication Cyst**
  - Duplication cysts can occur anywhere along GI tract
    - Gastric is uncommon (7%)
  - Most present < 1 year of age, F > M
    - Obstruction, pain, bleeding, or ulceration
  - Usually associated with greater curvature & posterior gastric wall
  - Classic duplication cysts demonstrate "bowel signature" on US with trilaminar wall
    - ± peristalsis of cyst wall
  - UGI may show extrinsic mass effect on stomach
- **Pyloric Atresia**
  - Presents with nonbilious emesis (vs. prenatal diagnosis)
  - "Single bubble" on radiographs with no distal gas
  - No normal pyloric opening seen on US or UGI
  - Associations (30-50%): Epidermolysis bullosa, hereditary multiple intestinal atresias (HMIA)

SELECTED REFERENCES

1. Maxfield CM et al: A pattern-based approach to bowel obstruction in the newborn. Pediatr Radiol. 43(3):318-29, 2013
2. Otjen JP et al: Usual and unusual causes of pediatric gastric outlet obstruction. Pediatr Radiol. 42(6):728-37, 2012

Aerophagia

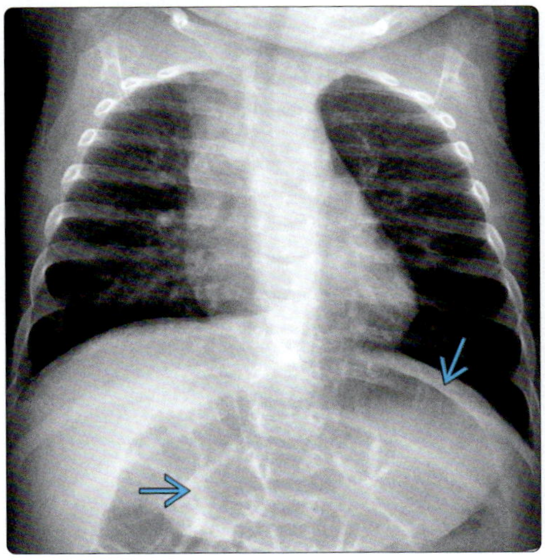

Hypertrophic Pyloric Stenosis

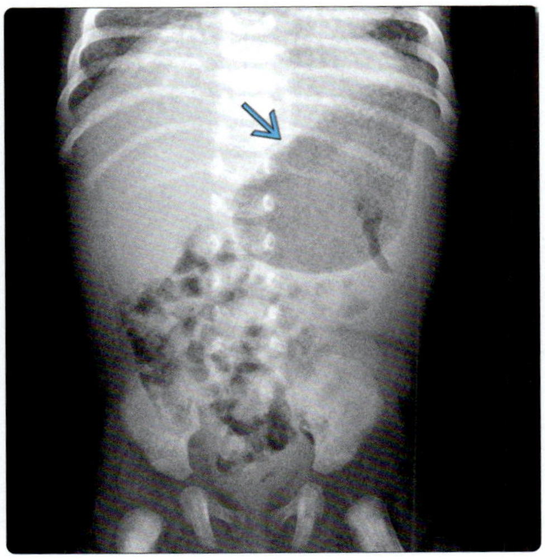

(Left) *Supine AP radiograph of the chest in a 7 month old with bronchiolitis shows moderate dilation of the stomach → & other gas-filled loops of bowel, a common appearance of air swallowing in patients with coughing or respiratory distress.* **(Right)** *AP radiograph in a 4 week old with hypertrophic pyloric stenosis (HPS) shows a mildly dilated gas-filled stomach → with a normal bowel gas pattern distally. Radiographs are not sensitive or specific for HPS.*

(Left) *Oblique US of a 4 week old with vomiting shows a thickened hypoechoic pyloric muscle with elongation of the pyloric channel & distention of the stomach. The persistence of this appearance throughout the exam is consistent with HPS.* **(Right)** *Right lateral decubitus upper GI image in a 5 week old with HPS shows a "string" of contrast passing through the narrowed pyloric channel. The hypertrophied muscle bulges into the stomach & duodenal bulb.*

Hypertrophic Pyloric Stenosis

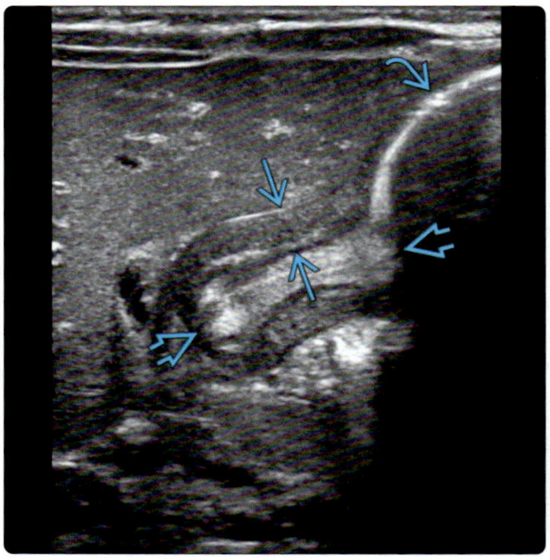

Hypertrophic Pyloric Stenosis

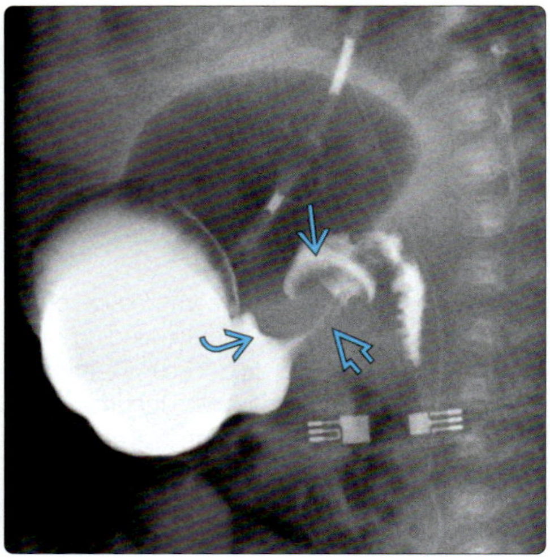

(Left) *AP radiograph in a 6 day old with bilious vomiting shows a dilated stomach & little distal bowel gas.* **(Right)** *Right lateral decubitus upper GI image in the same patient shows an abnormal anterior course of D3 with a twisted corkscrew appearance of midgut volvulus. Radiographs may be normal or have a proximal or distal obstructive pattern in the setting of midgut volvulus (with the latter being due to ischemic ileus).*

Midgut Volvulus

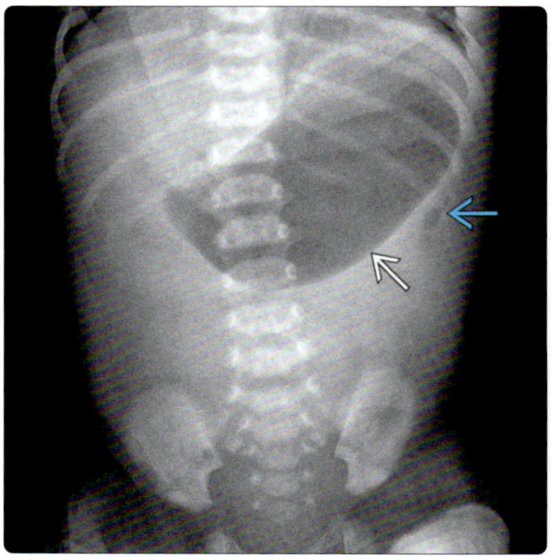

Midgut Volvulus

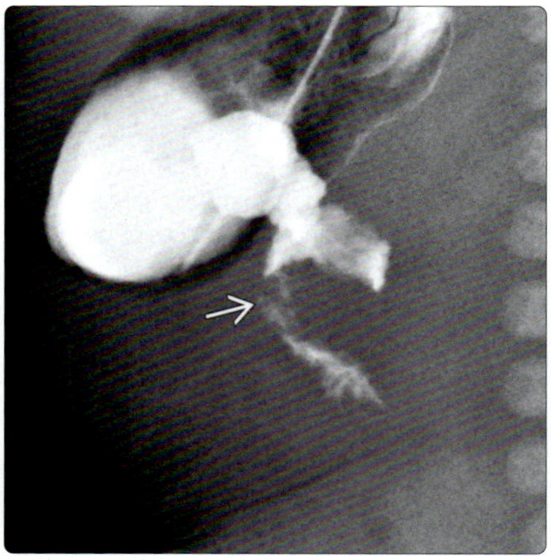

(Left) *AP radiograph in a newborn demonstrates the classic double-bubble sign of duodenal atresia with a dilated stomach, round dilated proximal duodenum, & no distal bowel gas. If a nasogastric tube is placed to suction, the stomach & duodenum may be decompressed.* **(Right)** *Axial CECT demonstrates circumferential thickening of D2 after a bicycle handle bar injury to the abdomen. There is also a focal laceration. Duodenal hematomas may cause obstruction.*

Duodenal Atresia, Stenosis, or Web

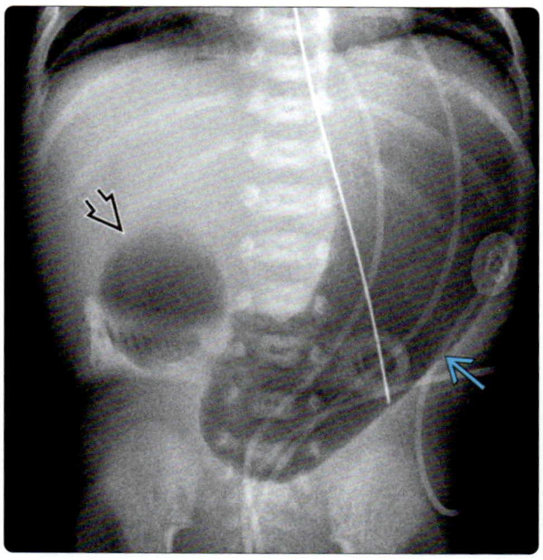

Duodenal Hematoma

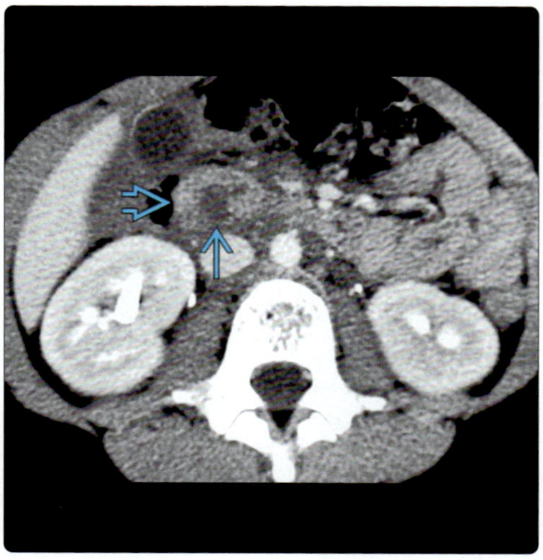

Bezoar

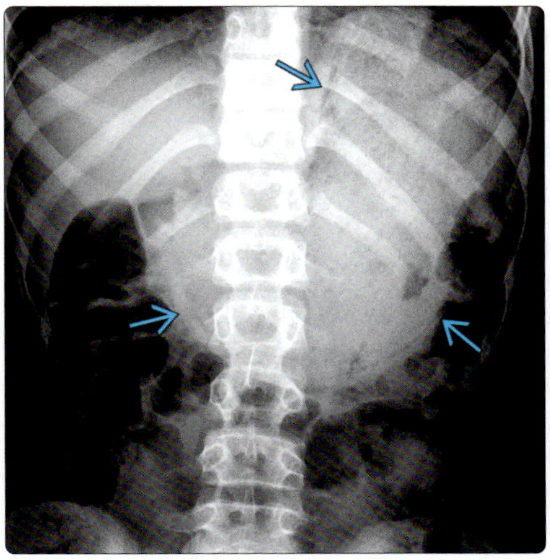

Bezoar

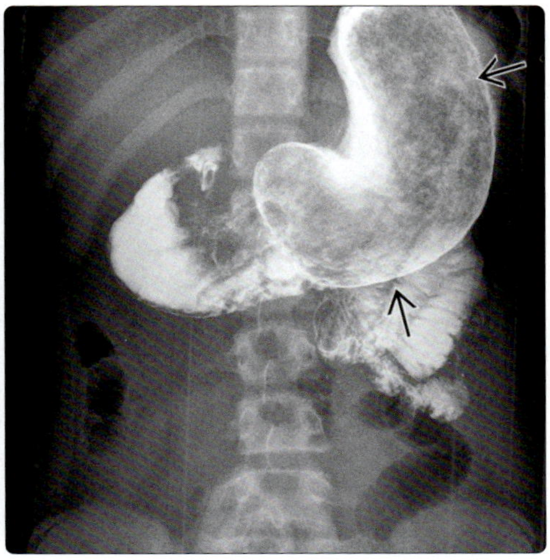

(Left) *AP radiograph shows a dilated stomach with a mottled appearance of the gastric contents in this 10-year-old girl with a known trichobezoar. The bezoar was removed by surgery.* **(Right)** *Frontal upper GI image in a 15-year-old patient with trichotillomania shows contrast outlining a large filling defect that distends the stomach & conforms to the gastric contours, consistent with a trichobezoar.*

Gastric Volvulus

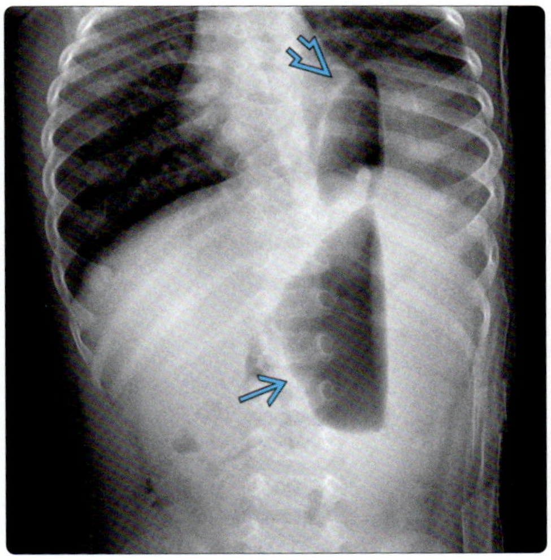

Gastric Volvulus

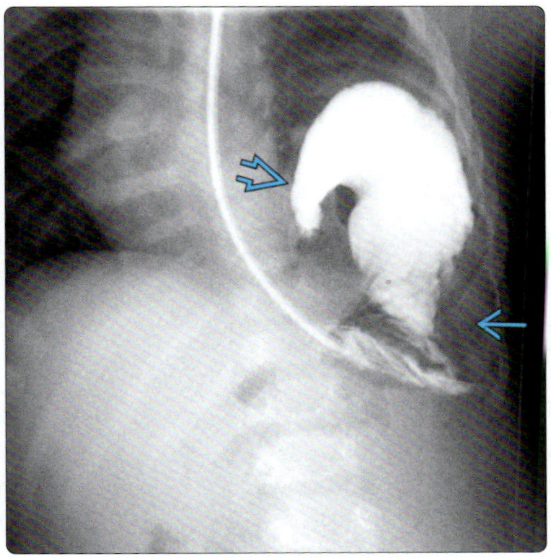

(Left) *Left decubitus radiograph in a 6 month old shows dilation of the stomach with an abnormal configuration. The portion herniated into the left hemithorax corresponds to the gastric antrum, while the lower portion is the gastric fundus. Diaphragmatic hernias predispose to gastric volvulus.* **(Right)** *Frontal upper GI image in the same patient shows an abnormal position of the pylorus superior to the gastric fundus, due to a mesenteroaxial volvulus. The stomach is now decompressed by a nasogastric tube.*

Gastric Duplication Cyst

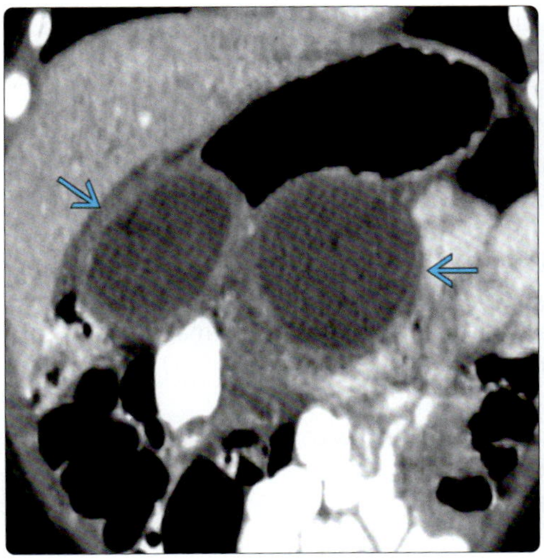

Pyloric Atresia

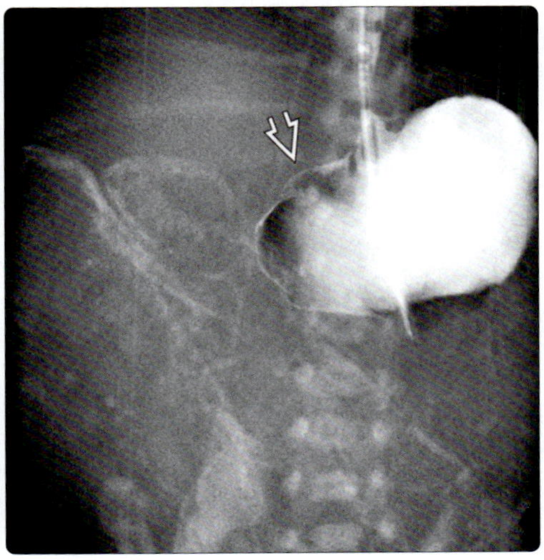

(Left) *Coronal CECT in a 9 month old with vomiting shows 2 cystic lesions at the gastric antrum. Intraoperatively, these were found to represent a dumbbell-shaped gastric duplication cyst.* **(Right)** *Frontal upper GI image in a newborn with hereditary multiple intestinal atresias (HMIA) shows contrast filling, but not passing beyond, the stomach. Intraluminal calcifications are seen in numerous dilated bowel loops. Immunodeficiency ultimately developed in this patient, which is common in HMIA.*

DIFFERENTIAL DIAGNOSIS

Common

- Malrotation & Midgut Volvulus
- Ladd Bands
- Duodenal Atresia/Stenosis/Web

Less Common

- Jejunal Atresia/Stenosis (Mimic)
- Superior Mesenteric Artery Syndrome
- Duodenal Hematoma
- Bezoar
- Gastrointestinal Duplication Cyst

Rare but Important

- Annular Pancreas
- Stricture
- Compression by Other Masses
- Compression by Other Vascular Structures

ESSENTIAL INFORMATION

Key Differential Diagnosis Issues

- Imaging work-up is based on age symptoms, medical/surgical history, ± radiographic pattern
  - Bilious vomiting occurs if obstruction lies beyond ampulla of Vater
    - Not specific, but typically triggers urgent work-up for midgut volvulus (MGV) in neonates/infants due to potentially catastrophic consequences of delayed diagnosis
  - Number of dilated, gas-filled bowel loops on radiographs typically ↑ with more distal obstruction

Helpful Clues for Common Diagnoses

- **Malrotation & Midgut Volvulus**
  - Malrotation: Abnormal midgut rotation & fixation in utero results in abnormal positions of bowel
    - Several variants; those with narrow mesenteric root (from distal duodenum to cecum) are prone to MGV
  - MGV: Twisting of malrotated bowel; surgical emergency
    - May result in obstruction, ischemia, & bowel necrosis; can lead to short gut syndrome or shock/death
    - Must be excluded in patients with bilious emesis
  - Radiograph: Normal does not exclude MGV
    - Proximal obstruction: Distention of stomach through 2nd duodenum with ↓ (but typically not absent) distal gas
    - Ischemic ileus: Diffusely distended & featureless loops → mimics distal obstruction
  - Upper GI (UGI): Duodenojejunal junction normally lies to left of left-sided pedicles at vertical level of duodenal bulb on supine image
    - Abnormal position suggests malrotation
    - Abrupt beaking/tapering of contrast with distal swirl ("corkscrew") is classic for MGV, typically at D2/D3
      - If twist is completely obstructive, contrast will not pass beyond level of beak (which can mimic web/stenosis; determination must be made in OR)
    - Given typical acute nature of MGV with emesis, proximal duodenal dilation is usually only mild
  - US/CECT: Malrotation shows reversal of superior mesenteric artery (SMA)-superior mesenteric vein (SMV) relationship + failure of D3 to pass dorsal to SMA
    - MGV: Whirlpool sign of twisted bowel & vessels along SMA axis on color⁾⁾ Doppler US; ± abrupt cutoff of SMV, possibly SMA
- **Ladd Bands**
  - Peritoneal bands due to abnormal bowel rotation; bands cross duodenum & obstruct
  - Imaging findings are nonspecific but show malrotation + narrowing/transition at site of bands
- **Duodenal Atresia/Stenosis/Web**
  - Failure of recanalization of lumen in utero rather than vascular insult (as with more distal atresias)
    - Most common at D2 distal to ampulla of Vater
  - Atresia presents on prenatal imaging or in 1st few days after delivery; stenosis or web may present later
  - Radiograph: Dilated, air-filled stomach & duodenum with no distal bowel gas = double-bubble sign of atresia
    - Often quite bulbous from chronic in utero obstruction
    - May be absent if patient just vomited or if stomach is decompressed by nasogastric tube
    - Presence of distal bowel gas with less pronounced proximal dilation favors web, stenosis, or MGV
  - UGI: Not indicated if radiograph is classic for duodenal atresia
    - Stenosis: Proximal dilation with focal narrowing, potentially due to annular pancreas
    - Web: Windsock appearance ± pinhole aperture
      - If contrast fails to pass D2/D3 in setting of distal bowel gas, patient must go to OR to exclude MGV
  - Associated with other anomalies
    - Down syndrome (25%), vertebral or rib anomalies (> 33%), congenital heart disease; assess for VACTERL sequence anomalies
    - Other GI anomalies: Malrotation, pancreatic & biliary anomalies, Meckel diverticulum, other atresias, GI duplications (25%)

Helpful Clues for Less Common Diagnoses

- **Jejunal Atresia/Stenosis (Mimic)**
  - Presents in 1st few days of life
  - Radiograph: "Triple bubble" vs. dilation of more loops (depending on level of obstruction)
  - UGI: Contrast does not pass beyond point of obstruction
    - May not be indicated with classic history & radiograph
  - Contrast enema: Will show microcolon if atresia lies in distal jejunum, if > 1 atresia is present, or if long segment of bowel is absent
    - Even with classic proximal obstruction, risk of other atresias may lead to request for enema
- **Superior Mesenteric Artery Syndrome**
  - Mid D3 compressed by SMA
  - Presents in older children with recent history of weight loss, postprandial pain, & emesis
  - UGI: Proximal duodenum is often mildly distended
    - Delay in passage of contrast through D3 with back & forth motion proximally
    - Contrast column halts at vertical linear extrinsic compression caused by SMA

- Contrast progresses with patient rotation that moves SMA & duodenum off of spine
- US/CT: Most studies involve adult populations; range of normal measurements in children vary widely
  - Acute SMA-aorta angle (< 25°)
  - ↓ distance between anterior wall of aorta & posterior wall of SMA at mid duodenum (< 8 mm)

- **Duodenal Hematoma**
  - Presenting history of blunt > penetrating trauma
    - Handlebar injury, motor vehicle collision
    - Consider child abuse if < 2 years old with delayed presentation & history inconsistent with injury
  - Relevant medical history: Bleeding disorder, anticoagulation, Henoch-Schönlein purpura, recent endoscopic procedure + biopsy
  - Radiographs: Nonspecific proximal obstruction
  - UGI: Eccentric/circumferential luminal narrowing if hematoma is intramural or extrinsic
    - Expansion of duodenal lumen with coiled spring appearance if hematoma is intraluminal
  - US/CECT/MR: Avascular intraluminal, intramural, &/or paraduodenal collection
    - Nonenhancing; attenuation of 40-70 HU on CECT
    - Variable echogenicity on US, ↓ with time; nonenhancing; variable T1 & T2 signal on MR
- **Bezoar**
  - Indigestible materials accumulate in stomach > bowel, causing obstruction
  - Most common types
    - Trichobezoar (hair): Most common in young female patients; alopecia is frequent
    - Phytobezoar (indigestible food components): Most common in adults; fruit & vegetable fibers common
    - Lactobezoar (concretion of milk/formula & mucous proteins): Most common in infants
      - GI tract capacity overwhelmed: Vomiting & diarrhea → dehydration → excessive water resorption → lactobezoar; ± erroneous preparation of formula
  - Radiographs/UGI: Filling defect in stomach may show interstices of bezoar outlined by gas/contrast
  - US: Broad, hyperechoic arc with dirty posterior shadow
  - CT: Circumscribed intraluminal mass, often with concentric ring architecture
- **Gastrointestinal Duplication Cyst**
  - Occurs anywhere along GI tract: Ileum > jejunum > duodenum
  - Presents with obstruction, intussusception, GI bleeding
  - US: Cystic mass + bowel wall signature (echogenic inner mucosal & outer serosal layers with middle hypoechoic muscular layer)
    - Peristalsis is rarely seen but is highly suggestive
  - CECT: May have ↑ attenuation with proteinaceous or hemorrhagic contents
  - Nuclear medicine: Uptake of Tc-99m pertechnetate radiotracer if cyst contains gastric mucosa

Helpful Clues for Rare Diagnoses

- **Annular Pancreas**
  - Congenital anomaly
  - UGI: Circumferential narrowing of D2 on UGI
  - US, CECT, MR: D2 encircled by pancreatic tissue
- **Stricture**
  - Nonspecific luminal narrowing + proximal dilation; due to prior inflammation, surgery, or necrotizing enterocolitis
- **Compression by Other Masses**
  - Lymphoma, choledochal cyst, pancreatic pseudocyst, etc.
    - Lymphoma may be intramural or extrinsic
  - Mass effect with partial obstruction is typical
- **Compression by Other Vascular Structures**
  - Partial obstruction of duodenum by preduodenal portal vein or replaced right hepatic artery

SELECTED REFERENCES

1. Brinkley MF et al: Congenital duodenal obstruction: causes and imaging approach. Pediatr Radiol. 46(8):1084-95, 2016
2. Tackett JJ et al: Malrotation: Current strategies navigating radiologic diagnosis of a surgical emergency. World J Radiol. 6(9):730-6, 2014
3. Arthurs OJ et al: Nutcracker and SMA syndromes: what is normal SMA angle in children? Eur J Radiol. 81(8):e854-61, 2012

Malrotation & Midgut Volvulus

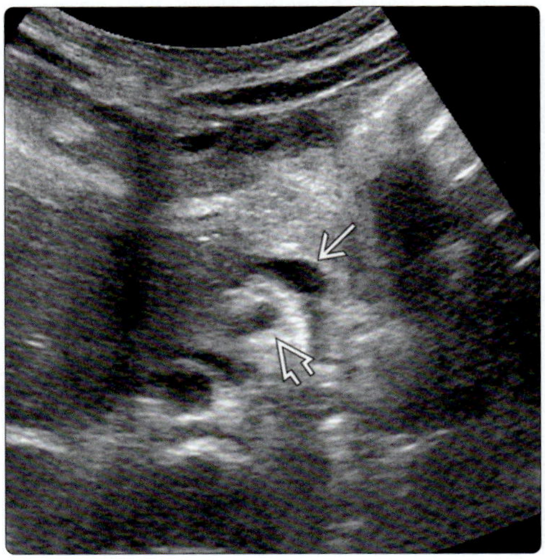

Malrotation & Midgut Volvulus

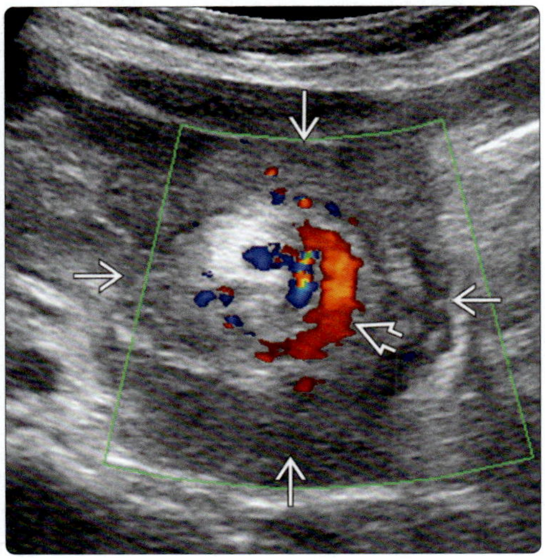

(Left) *Transverse US from a 9 month old with bilious vomiting shows an abnormal superior mesenteric artery (SMA)-superior mesenteric vein (SMV) relationship with the SMV ➡ anterior & to the left of the SMA ➡.* **(Right)** *Color Doppler US obtained more caudally in the same patient demonstrates a mass-like appearance of the twisted mesentery & bowel ➡ with a swirling whirlpool sign ➡ of vessels, typical of midgut volvulus. This swirling is most apparent on real time superior to inferior transducer sweeps.*

(Left) *Axial CECT in a 3 year old with a history of heterotaxy shows a dilated D2 segment with rapid tapering of D3 as it courses anterior to & twists around the SMA & SMV. Note the dilated stomach in the right upper quadrant.* **(Right)** *More caudal axial CECT in the same patient with heterotaxy shows continued twisting of the proximal bowel inferiorly along the mesenteric axis due to malrotation with a superimposed midgut volvulus.*

Malrotation & Midgut Volvulus

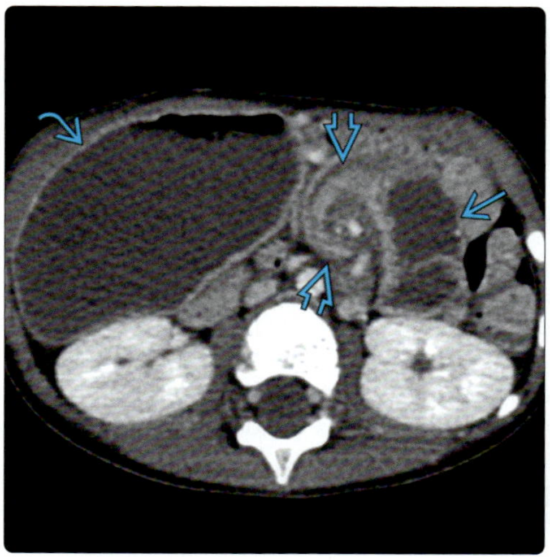

Malrotation & Midgut Volvulus

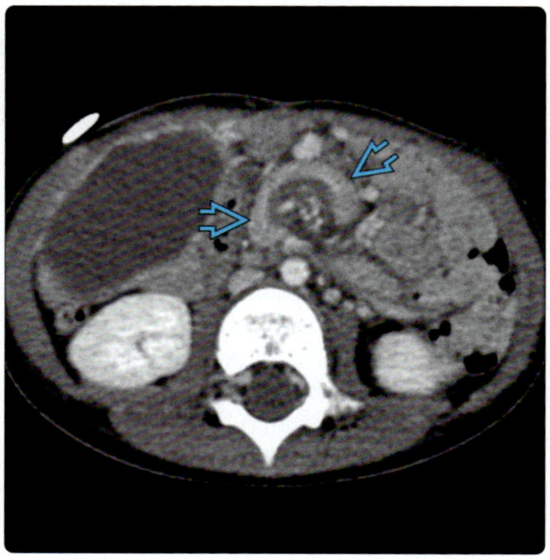

(Left) *Lateral upper GI image shows the corkscrew sign of midgut volvulus. The proximal duodenum is only mildly dilated, & the twist begins at the D3 level.* **(Right)** *Frontal radiograph in a newborn shows a dilated stomach & duodenal bulb (D1), together demonstrating the classic double-bubble sign of duodenal atresia. Note that there is no distal bowel gas. The appearance is consistent with a longstanding in utero obstruction of the duodenum.*

Malrotation & Midgut Volvulus

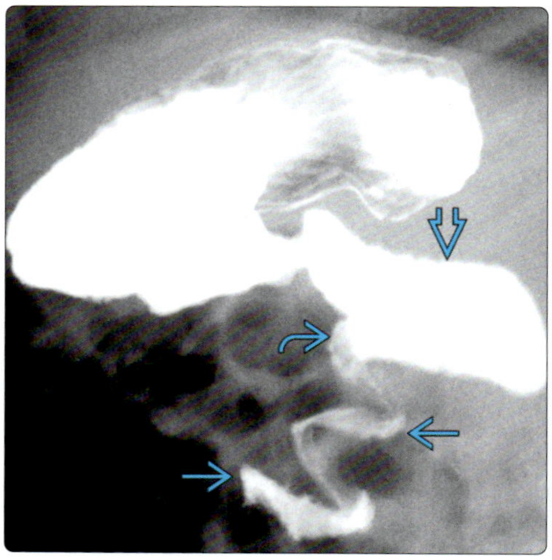

Duodenal Atresia/Stenosis/Web

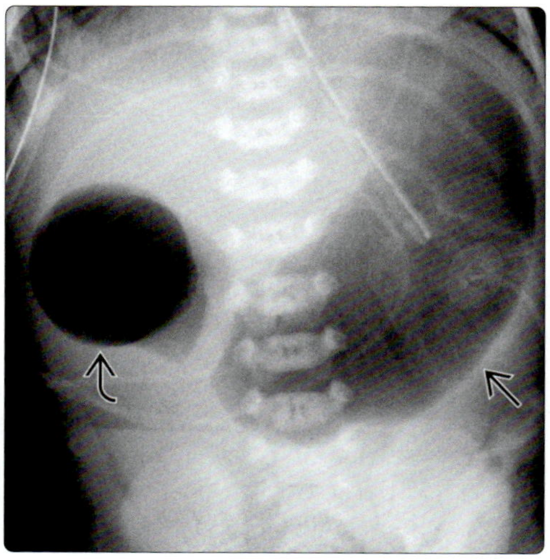

(Left) *Frontal radiograph of the abdomen from a 1 day old demonstrates a double-bubble appearance of the stomach & proximal duodenum (D1) with a lack of distal bowel gas. Surgery confirmed the diagnosis of duodenal atresia.* **(Right)** *Frontal view obtained during an upper GI image in a 38 day old with trisomy 21 depicts dilation of D2 with a tiny amount of contrast passing through a small aperture in a proven duodenal web. Bowel gas is seen distally.*

Duodenal Atresia/Stenosis/Web

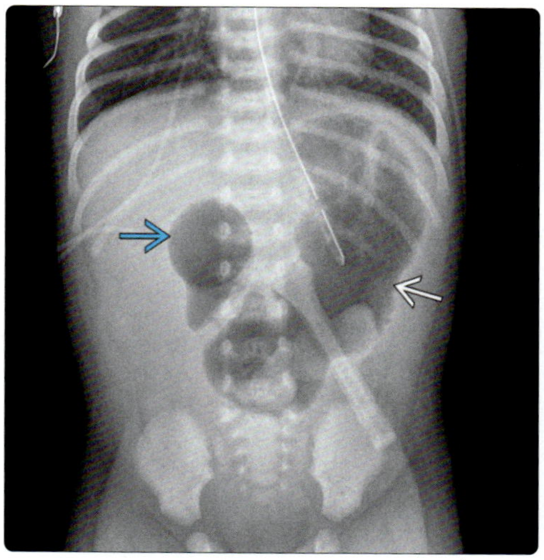

Duodenal Atresia/Stenosis/Web

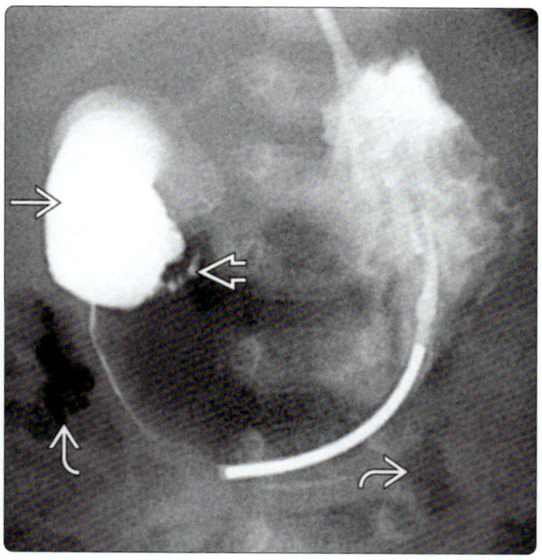

Duodenal Atresia/Stenosis/Web

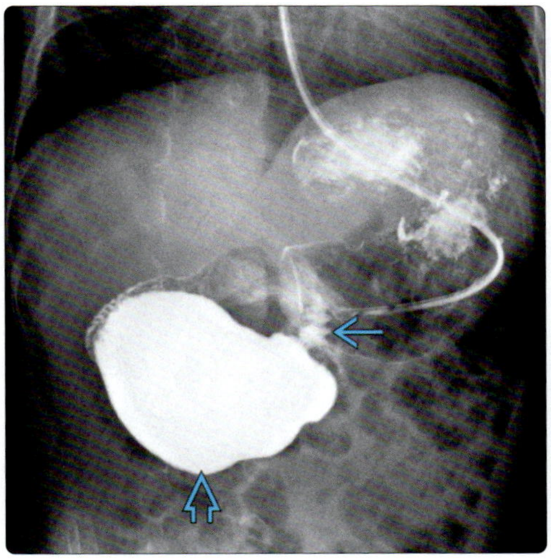

Duodenal Atresia/Stenosis/Web

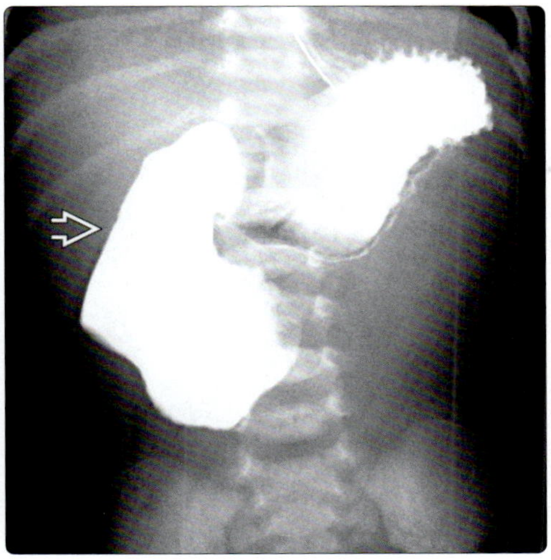

(Left) *LPO upper GI image in an 11 month old with vomiting shows dilation of the D2 & D3 segments ⇨ with abrupt transition to a small-caliber D4 segment →. Note the lack of twisting at this transition, confirming that there is no midgut volvulus. An underlying web was surgically resected.* **(Right)** *Frontal upper GI image shows a dilated duodenum ➔ secondary to a surgically proven web in D3. The size of the duodenum supports a chronic intermittent or partial obstruction as a single acute event would not enlarge the duodenum to this degree.*

Jejunal Atresia/Stenosis (Mimic)

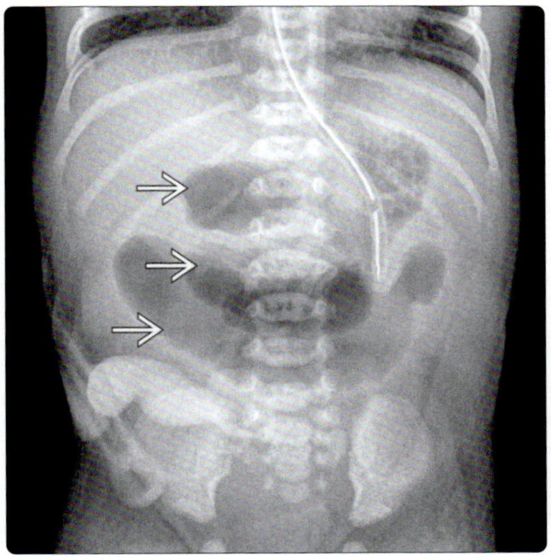

Jejunal Atresia/Stenosis (Mimic)

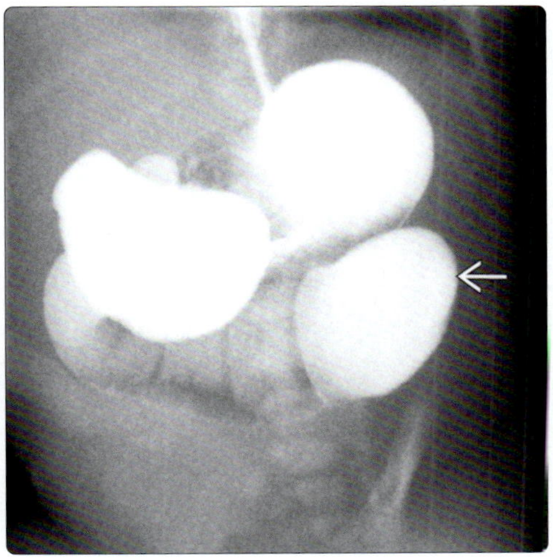

(Left) *AP radiograph in a newborn with bilious emesis shows dilation of a few proximal bowel loops ➔ (extending beyond the level of the duodenum) without distal bowel gas in this newborn with jejunal atresia.* **(Right)** *Supine frontal upper GI image in the same patient shows a bulbous blind-ending loop of proximal small bowel ➔ in the left upper quadrant due to an atretic jejunal loop. Note the lack of distal bowel gas, consistent with a congenital obstruction.*

Jejunal Atresia/Stenosis (Mimic)

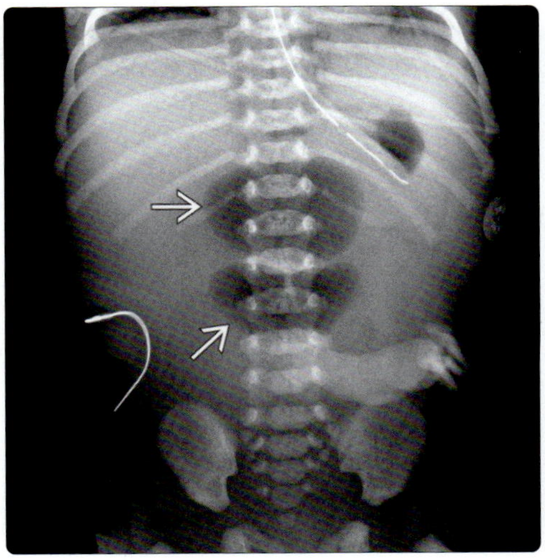

Superior Mesenteric Artery Syndrome

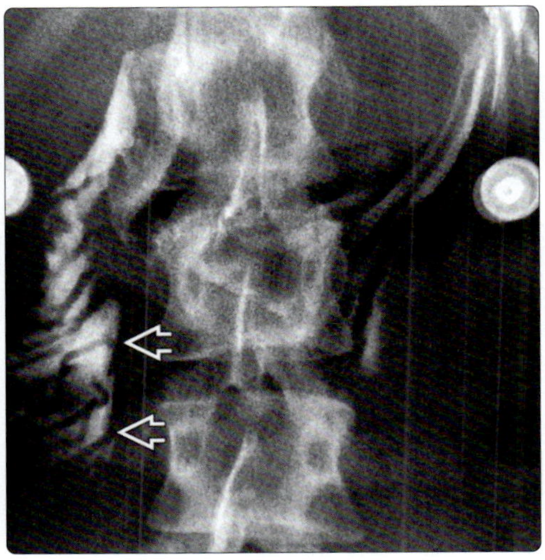

(Left) *AP radiograph shows several distended loops of bowel in the central abdomen ➔ due to jejunal atresia in a newborn with bilious emesis. Note the absence of distal bowel gas.* **(Right)** *Supine frontal upper GI image shows contrast material in the stomach & proximal duodenum, terminating abruptly as the contrast encounters a vertically oriented focus of extrinsic compression ➔ (due to the SMA). This 18-year-old woman presented with weight loss & vomiting after spine surgery.*

(Left) *Coronal CECT in a 20 year old with weight loss, vomiting, & delayed gastric emptying shows dilation of the contrast-filled stomach & duodenum up to the level of the SMA.* **(Right)** *Sagittal CECT MIP in the same patient shows narrowing of D3 between the SMA & aorta at the level of the spine. There is associated narrowing of the aortomesenteric angle & aortomesenteric distance, consistent with SMA syndrome.*

Superior Mesenteric Artery Syndrome

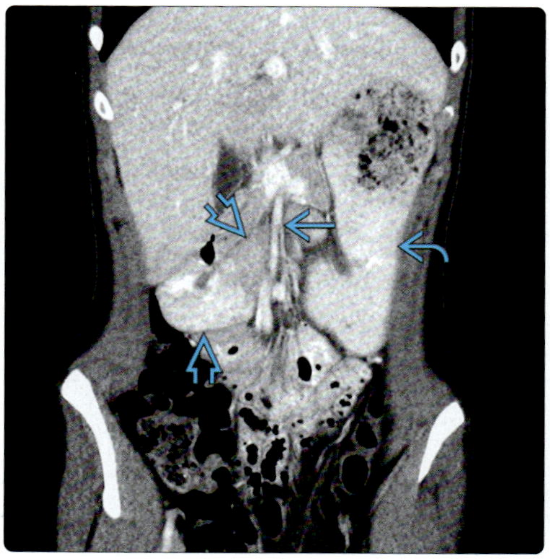

Superior Mesenteric Artery Syndrome

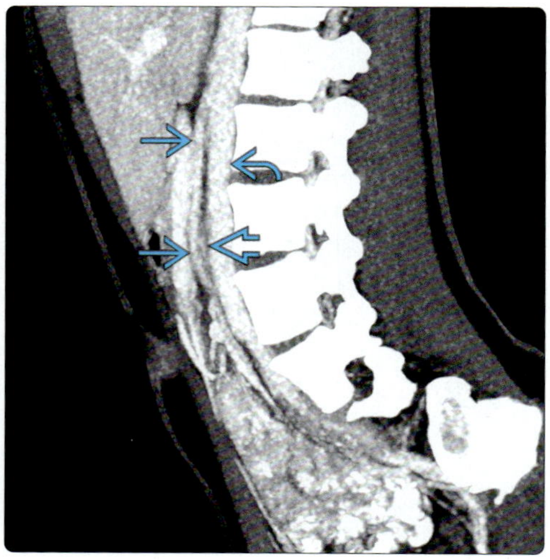

(Left) *Coronal CECT from a 12 year old with bilious vomiting status post endoscopy demonstrates heterogeneous high-attenuation material in the bowel wall extending from D2 to D4, consistent with hematoma. There is resultant narrowing of the lumen, causing obstruction.* **(Right)** *Lateral view obtained during an upper GI in the same patient shows a luminal filling defect from the duodenal hematoma, obstructing the further passage of contrast.*

Duodenal Hematoma

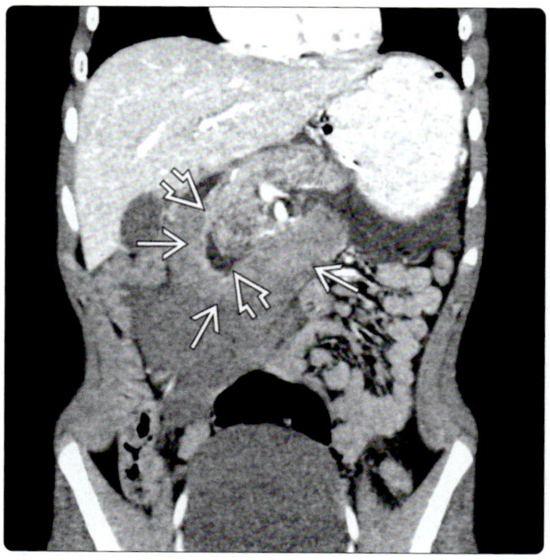

Duodenal Hematoma

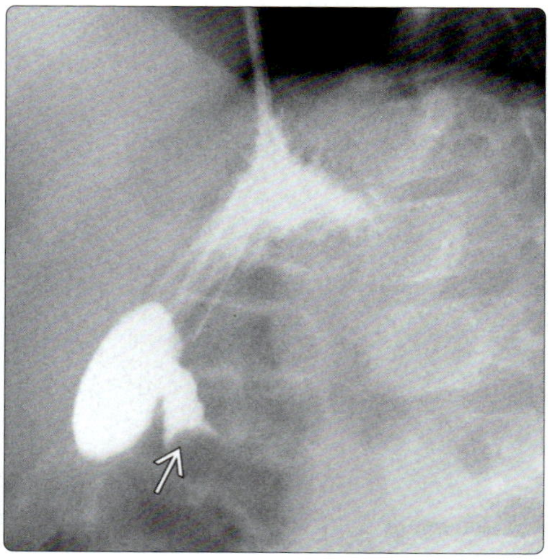

(Left) *Frontal view from an upper GI in a teenager shows a long filling defect extending through the duodenum & into the proximal jejunum. The bowel is dilated with mildly thickened folds. The filling defect was due to a trichobezoar.* **(Right)** *Axial CECT shows a thick-walled duplication cyst associated with the 2nd portion of the duodenum. Note the enhancing mucosa & lower attenuation muscular wall.*

Bezoar

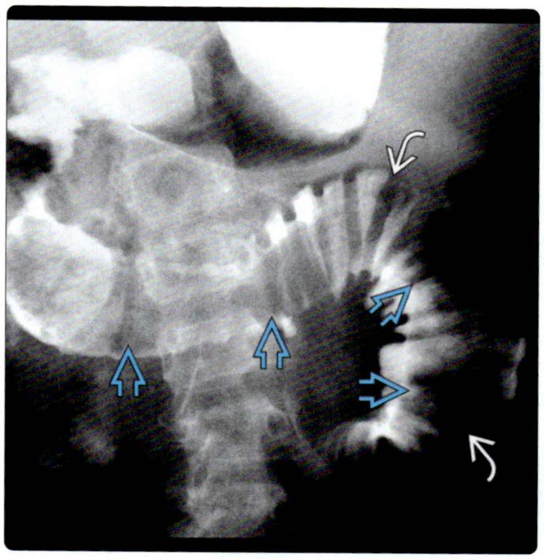

Gastrointestinal Duplication Cyst

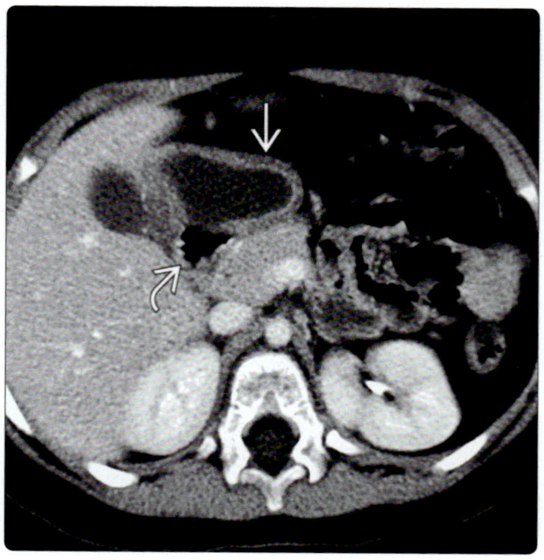

Gastrointestinal Duplication Cyst

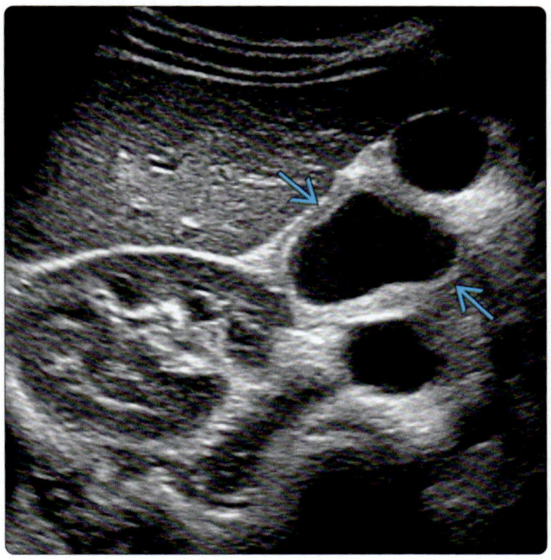

Gastrointestinal Duplication Cyst

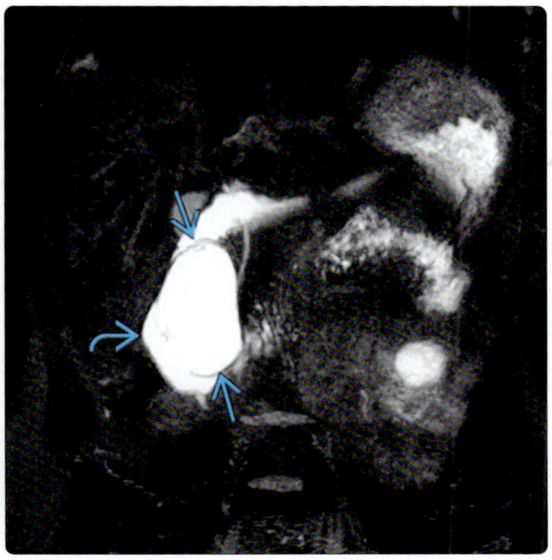

(Left) *Transverse US in an 11 year old with upper abdominal pain shows a well-circumscribed cystic lesion with a trilaminar or "gut signature" wall ➔, typical of a duplication cyst.* **(Right)** *Coronal MRCP MIP image in the same patient shows the elongated cyst ➔ protruding into the D2 lumen ➔. Surgical resection confirmed a duodenal duplication cyst.*

Annular Pancreas

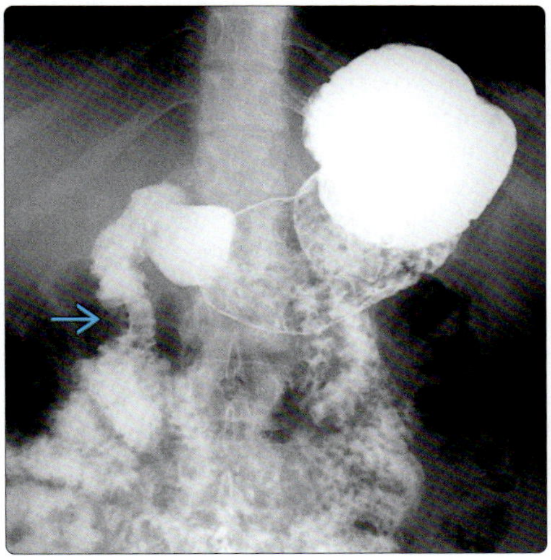

Annular Pancreas

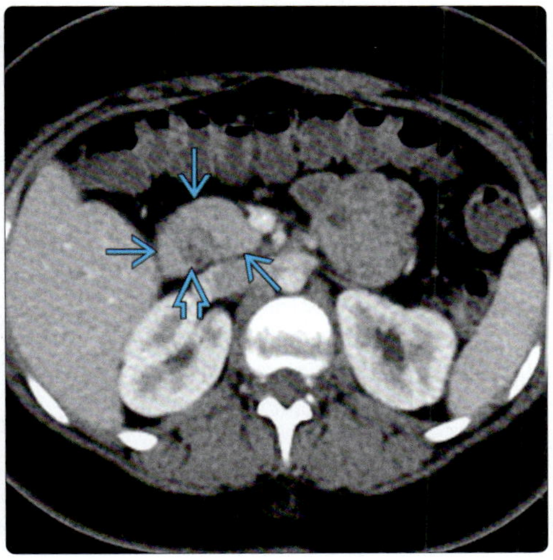

(Left) *Supine frontal upper GI in an 11 year old shows a filling defect ➔ at the lateral D2 lumen, though contrast passed beyond this level without difficulty.* **(Right)** *Axial CECT in the same patient shows narrowing of the D2 lumen ➔ due to encasement by pancreatic tissue ➔ (annular pancreas). Varying degrees of duodenal obstruction may be seen in such cases.*

Compression by Other Masses

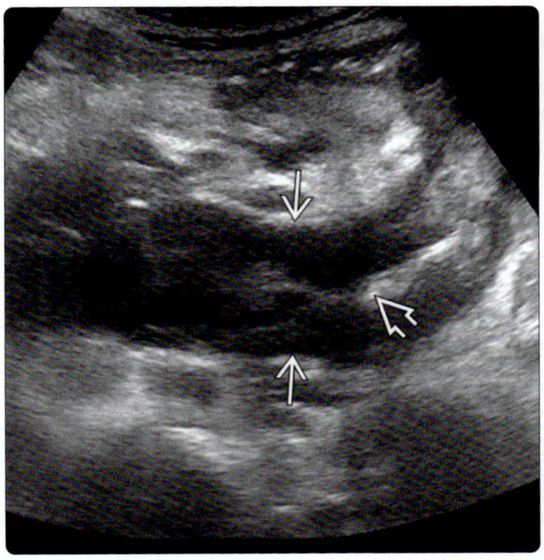

Compression by Other Masses

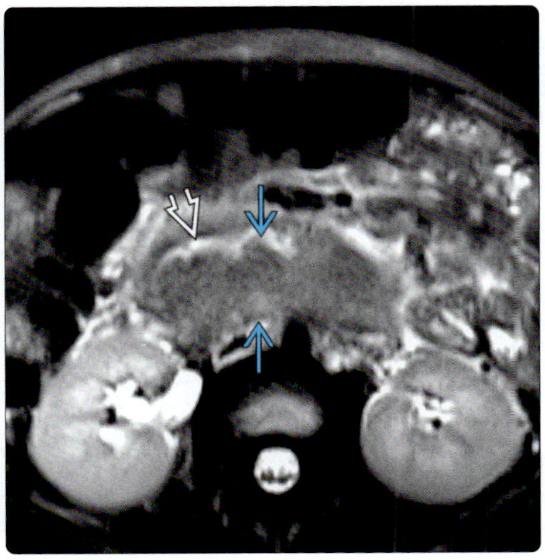

(Left) *Transverse US in a 9 year old with hematemesis demonstrates marked hypoechoic bowel wall thickening ➡ involving the distal D2 & D3 segments with narrowing of the lumen ➡.* **(Right)** *Axial T2 SSFSE MR in the same patient shows wall thickening at D3 with decreased T2 signal intensity ➔ & a narrowed lumen ➡. Biopsy confirmed lymphomatous infiltration of the bowel wall.*

DIFFERENTIAL DIAGNOSIS

Common

- Adhesions
- Enteritis (Mimic)
- Appendicitis
- Ileus (Mimic)
- Inguinal Hernia
- Ileocolic Intussusception
- Malrotation With Midgut Volvulus

Less Common

- Meckel Diverticulum
- Duodenal Web or Stenosis
- Stricture
- Distal Intestinal Obstruction Syndrome
- Stomal Obstruction
- Superior Mesenteric Artery Syndrome
- Internal Hernia
- Ladd Bands
- Chronic Intestinal Dysmotility (Mimic)
- Bezoar

Rare but Important

- Obstructing Mass
- Hypoperfusion Complex (Mimic)

ESSENTIAL INFORMATION

Key Differential Diagnosis Issues

- Some obstructions tend to present in specific age range
  - Atresias: 1st few days of life (or prenatally), not beyond
  - Midgut volvulus: Most present in 1st year of life
  - Ileocolic intussusception: 6 months to 3 years of life
  - Appendicitis: Less common under 2 years of age but more likely to have delayed diagnosis with complications

Helpful Clues for Common Diagnoses

- **Adhesions**
  - Prior history of abdominal surgery &/or inflammation
  - CECT: Abrupt transition from dilated to nondilated bowel, often with focal angulation, kink, or tethering
- **Enteritis (Mimic)**
  - Focal or diffusely gas- &/or fluid-distended loops of bowel without clear transition point
  - Dependent colonic fluid levels are highly suggestive
  - ± wall thickening, hyperenhancement, hyperperistalsis
- **Appendicitis**
  - May lead to focal or generalized ileus (depending on extent of abdominal inflammation) or partial obstruction
  - US/CECT/MR: Appendix appears as dilated fluid-filled blind-ending tubular structure in right lower quadrant with inflammation of surrounding fat; ± appendicolith
    - May be decompressed if perforated; look for adjacent gas &/or localized fluid collections
    - Inflammation of adjacent bowel is typically only present if appendix has ruptured
- **Ileus (Mimic)**
  - Diminished/absent peristalsis → functional failure of bowel without mechanical obstruction
  - Numerous causes: Inflammatory, postoperative, ischemic, metabolic, pharmacologic, septic
- **Inguinal Hernia**
  - Palpable lump in groin ± pain, dilated bowel; inability to reduce if incarcerated
  - Radiographs: Gas extends abnormally into inguinal canal (± scrotum); ± obstructive bowel gas pattern
    - ± herniated mesentery/bowel on US/CECT
- **Ileocolic Intussusception (ICI)**
  - Telescoping of proximal bowel segment into distal bowel segment
    - Most commonly due to regional adenitis/idiopathic
    - May be secondary to pathologic lead point
      - e.g., duplication cyst, bowel hematoma, etc.
  - Presents with currant jelly stools, crampy abdominal pain, intermittent fussiness, emesis, right-sided mass; usually between 6 months to 3 years of age
  - Radiographs: Not sensitive or specific; may show
    - Absence of colonic gas in right abdomen
    - Focal or generalized dilation of small bowel (SB) loops
    - Rounded mass of intussusceptum in right upper or mid abdomen
      - May have target appearance of trapped lucent fat
      - May be outlined by crescent of gas
  - US: Cross section shows classic target sign due to layers of intussuscepted bowel, lymph nodes, fat, & vessels trapped in intussuscipiens; mean diameter of ICI is 2.6 cm
  - Enteroenteric (SB-SB) intussusceptions are more common but are usually incidental & transient
    - US: Typically only see bowel layers without trapped fat or lymph nodes; mean diameter is 1.5 cm
    - Length > 3.5 cm or pathologic lead point with signs of obstruction may indicate need for surgery
- **Malrotation With Midgut Volvulus**
  - Abnormal rotation of midgut → narrow mesenteric fixation → predisposition to bowel twisting → obstruction &/or ischemia
  - Classically present with bilious emesis in infants
  - Typical malrotation findings
    - D3 passes anterior to superior mesenteric artery (SMA) instead of posterior
    - Duodenal-jejunal junction does not lie left of spine or at height of duodenal bulb
    - Cecum often lies high & medial; entire colon may be in left abdomen
  - Typical midgut volvulus findings
    - Classic radiographic appearances: Normal, proximal obstruction with distal gas, or ischemic ileus
    - Upper GI series (UGI): Mild dilation of stomach & proximal duodenum with abrupt taper ("beak") of D2/D3; bowel distal to beak is narrowed & twisted ("corkscrew")
    - US: Abnormal SMA/SMV relationship with swirling of bowel & vessels around SMA ("whirlpool")
    - CECT: Whirlpool twisting of bowel/vessels
      - ± abrupt cutoff of SMV (± SMA), midgut ischemia

Helpful Clues for Less Common Diagnoses

- **Meckel Diverticulum**
  - Omphalomesenteric duct remnant: Embryologic structure from yolk sac to primitive midgut

- Remnants include Meckel diverticulum, sinus tract, cyst, fibrous band
  - ▫ Remnant may serve as obstructing band, lead point for ICI, or site of volvulus
- WSCE: Usually normal caliber colon; may see medial deviation of cecum & reflux of contrast into beak-shaped obstructed terminal ileum
- CECT: Distal SB obstruction without clear etiology; Meckel is rarely visualized unless inflamed

- **Duodenal Web or Stenosis**
  - Incomplete failure of in utero lumen recanalization
  - Often presents beyond neonatal period, depending on size of opening at web/stenosis
  - Radiographs: Distended, air-filled stomach & duodenum, less pronounced than classic duodenal atresia; variable amounts of distal bowel gas
  - UGI: Windsock appearance of web ± pinhole aperture
  - May be associated with annular pancreas
- **Stricture**
  - Luminal narrowing with proximal dilation
  - Secondary to inflammatory bowel disease, postoperative change, prior necrotizing enterocolitis, etc.
- **Distal Intestinal Obstruction Syndrome**
  - Abdominal manifestation of cystic fibrosis (meconium ileus equivalent in older child)
    - Accumulation of viscous fecal material in distal ileum → proximal dilation
- **Stomal Obstruction**
  - Ostomy with decreased output
  - Dilated bowel extends to level of stoma without other transition point
- **Superior Mesenteric Artery Syndrome**
  - Occurs in older children with recent history of weight loss, postprandial pain, & emesis
  - D3 compressed by SMA, leading to stomach & proximal duodenal dilation
    - UGI: Contrast obstructs at vertically-oriented extrinsic compression (SMA) on D3 while supine
      - ▫ Rolling patient will move SMA/bowel off of spine & facilitate contrast passage
    - US/CECT: Acute SMA-aorta angle (< 25°) &/or ↓ distance between aorta & SMA (< 8 mm)
      - ▫ Normal measurements in children vary widely
- **Internal Hernia**
  - Protrusion of bowel loops through congenital or acquired peritoneal/mesenteric defect
  - Location: Paraduodenal, pericecal, foramen of Winslow, transmesenteric, transmesocolic, intersigmoid, retroanastomotic
- **Ladd Bands**
  - Peritoneal bands associated with malrotation may obstruct proximal SB
- **Chronic Intestinal Dysmotility (Mimic)**
  - Generalized dilation with diminished function
  - Many causes, e.g., gastroschisis, postinfectious, etc.
- **Bezoar**
  - Indigestible materials accumulate & cause obstruction
    - Trichobezoar (hair): Most common in female patients
    - Lactobezoar (concretion of milk/formula)
  - Radiographs: Distention of stomach by mottled material
    - This appearance is more commonly due to normal recent food ingestion
  - UGI: Intraluminal filling defect with contrast extending between interstices; material can embolize distally
  - US: Broad, hyperechoic superficial arc with posterior acoustic shadowing
  - CECT: Circumscribed intraluminal mass, often with concentric ring architecture

Helpful Clues for Rare Diagnoses

- **Obstructing Mass**
  - Differential depends on age, history, imaging features
    - e.g., lymphoma, duplication cyst, hematoma, etc.
- **Hypoperfusion Complex (Mimic)**
  - Shock (hypovolemic, neurogenic, cardiac, sepsis)
  - Diffuse wall thickening with hyperenhancing accentuated folds & fluid distention
  - Flat IVC, ascites, ± ↑ enhancement of adrenals, kidneys, pancreas, & vessels

Adhesions

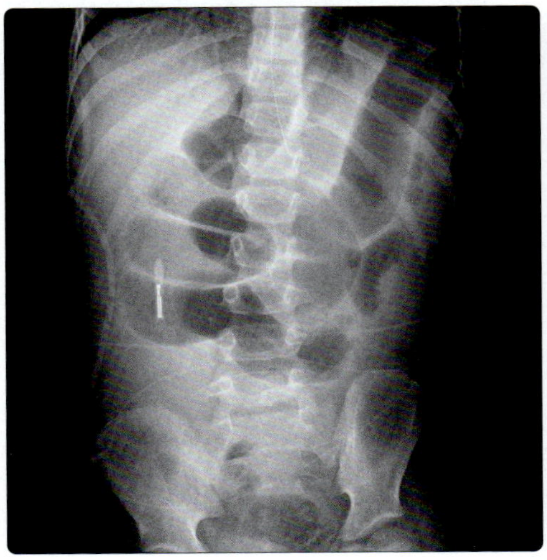

Adhesions

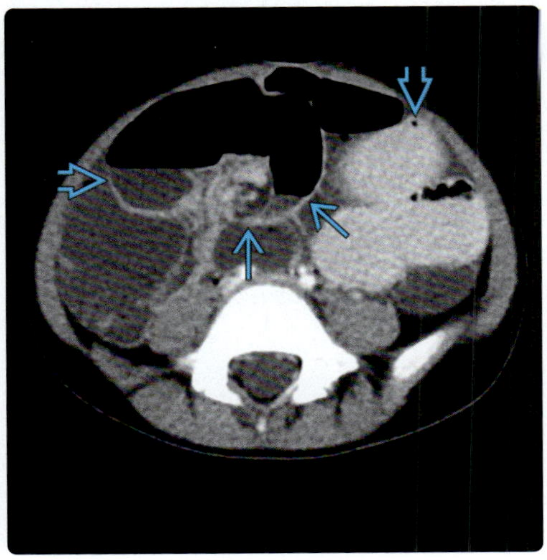

(Left) *AP radiograph in a 7 year old with vomiting shows multiple dilated small bowel (SB) loops with a paucity of colonic gas. A Meckel diverticulum had been resected years prior to this presentation.* **(Right)** *Axial CECT in the same patient shows multiple dilated SB loops ⇨ with focal tapering → at the transition point along the posterior aspect of the mesenteric vessels. While this appearance could suggest a volvulus, only adhesions were found at surgery.*

Enteritis (Mimic)

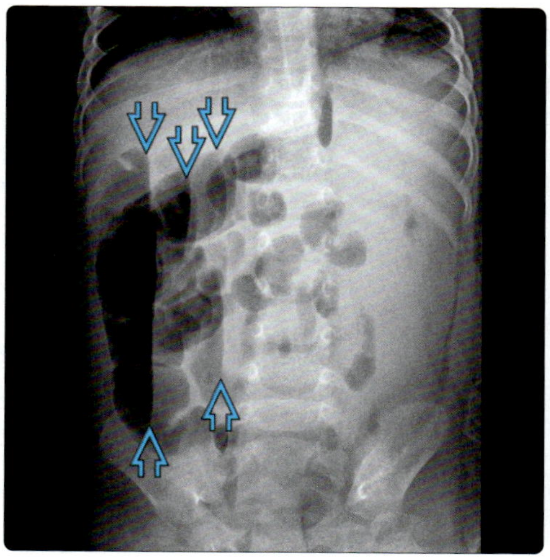

Appendicitis

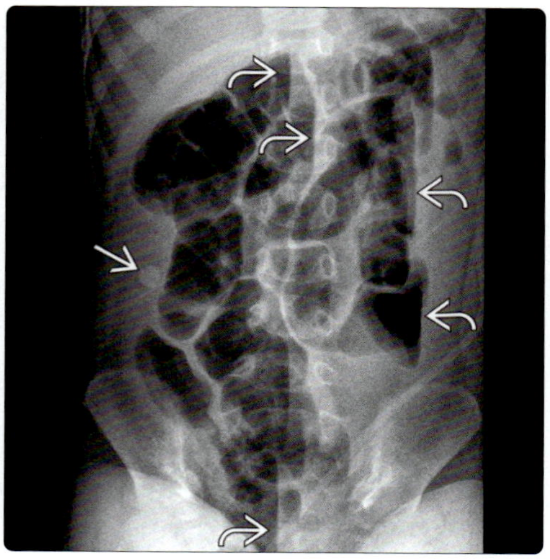

(Left) *Left decubitus radiograph in a 2 year old with vomiting shows gaseous distention of large > SB. There are numerous intraluminal fluid levels, predominantly colonic. This appearance is most commonly due to gastroenteritis.* **(Right)** *Left decubitus radiograph in a 2 year old with fever & pain shows mild dilation of gas-filled bowel diffusely. Many loops contain fluid levels, suggesting generalized inflammation &/or ileus. Note the appendicolith on the right. Appendicitis was confirmed at surgery.*

Ileus (Mimic)

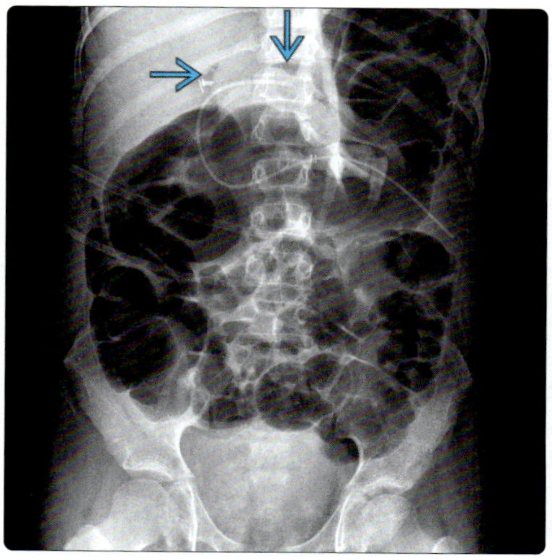

Inguinal Hernia

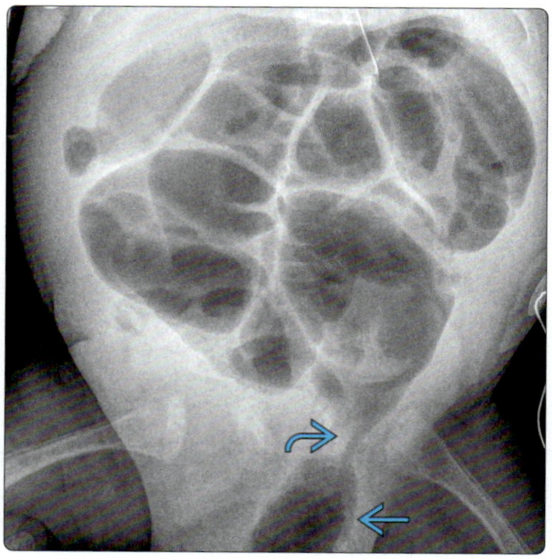

(Left) *AP radiograph in a 10 year old status post cholecystectomy in the last several days shows generalized dilation & gaseous distention of bowel, typical of a postoperative ileus. Residual small amounts of free air are noted, within normal limits for the recent surgery.* **(Right)** *AP radiograph of a 7-day-old infant with abdominal distention shows a gas-filled loop of bowel extending through the inguinal canal into the scrotum with dilation of the proximal bowel.*

Ileocolic Intussusception

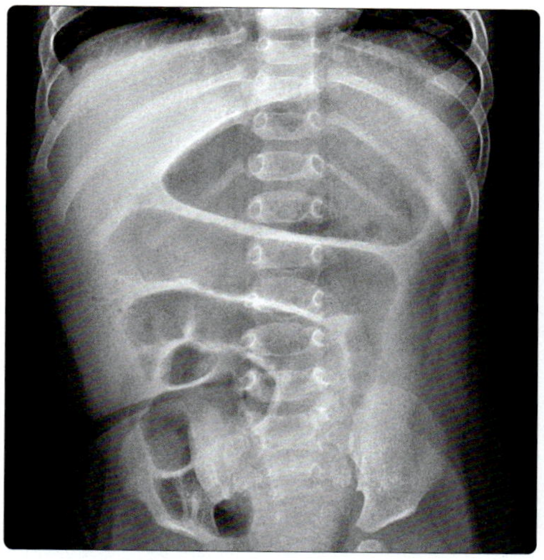

Ileocolic Intussusception

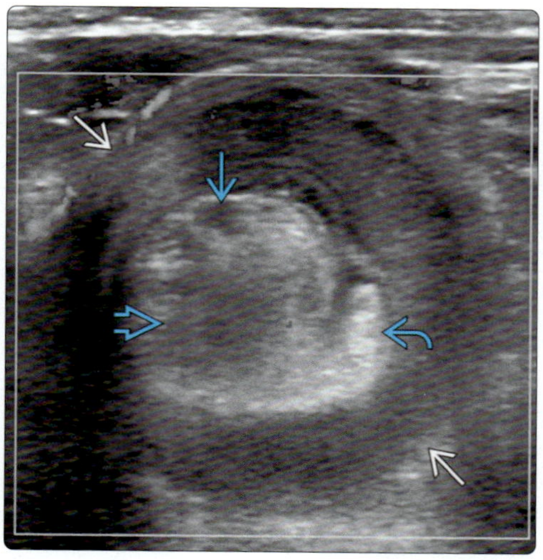

(Left) *AP radiograph shows multiple dilated loops of SB in a 6 month old who presented with abdominal distention. There is a paucity of colonic gas.* **(Right)** *Transverse US in the same patient shows an ileocolic intussusception with visualization of the target sign. Echogenic fat, hypoechoic lymph nodes, & bowel are noted in the intussusceptum. This intussusception was successfully reduced with an air enema.*

Malrotation With Midgut Volvulus

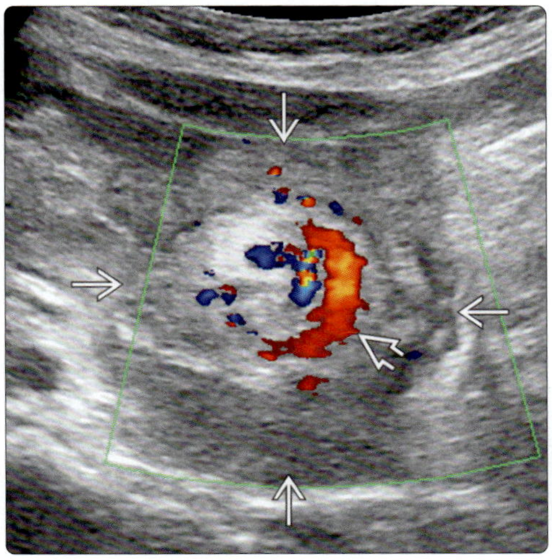

Malrotation With Midgut Volvulus

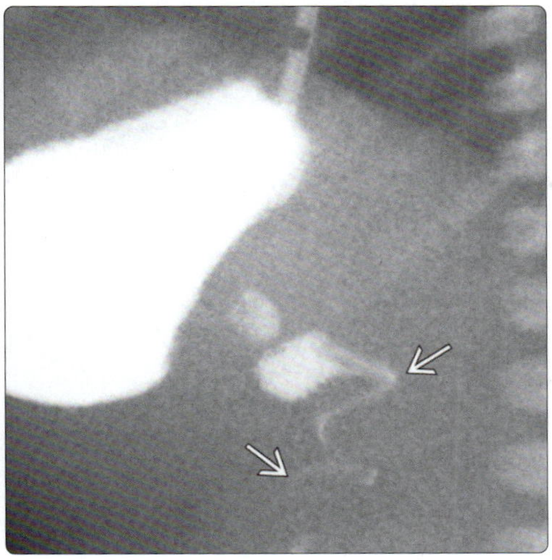

(Left) *Color Doppler US in a 9 month old with bilious emesis demonstrates a mass-like appearance of the mesentery ➡ with a whirlpool sign ➡, consistent with midgut volvulus. The swirling of bowel & vessels was best seen with real-time sweeps.* **(Right)** *Lateral UGI image in a 2 day old with bilious emesis depicts a corkscrew appearance of narrowed & twisted duodenum ➡, consistent with midgut volvulus.*

Meckel Diverticulum

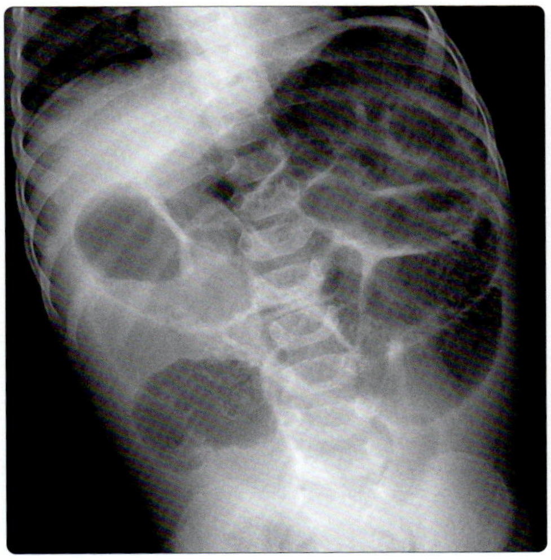

Duodenal Web or Stenosis

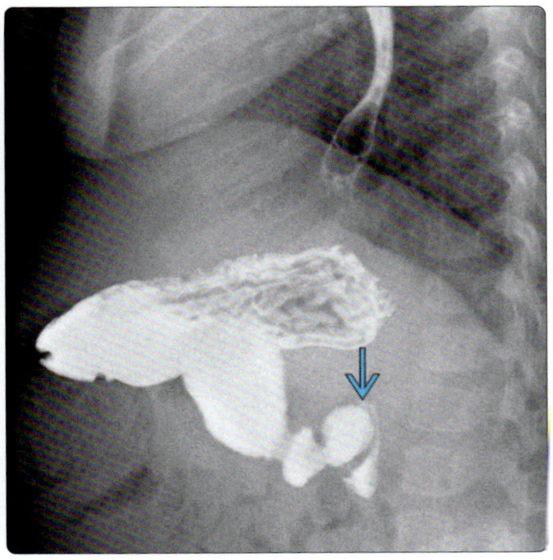

(Left) *AP radiograph in an 18 month old with vomiting & distention shows numerous dilated SB loops throughout the abdomen, most notable on the left. A volvulus secondary to a Meckel diverticulum was found at surgery.* **(Right)** *Right lateral decubitus UGI in a 14 month old with intermittent vomiting shows a thin curvilinear filling defect ➡ at the junction of the 1st & 2nd duodenum. The filling defect shows convexity towards the smaller caliber 2nd duodenum. A web was confirmed at surgery.*

Stricture

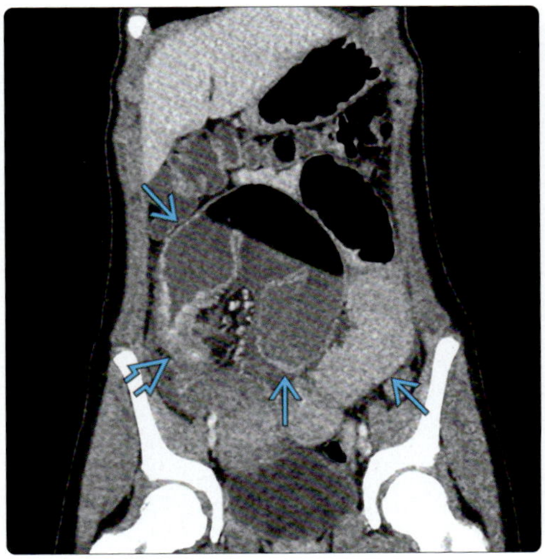

Stricture

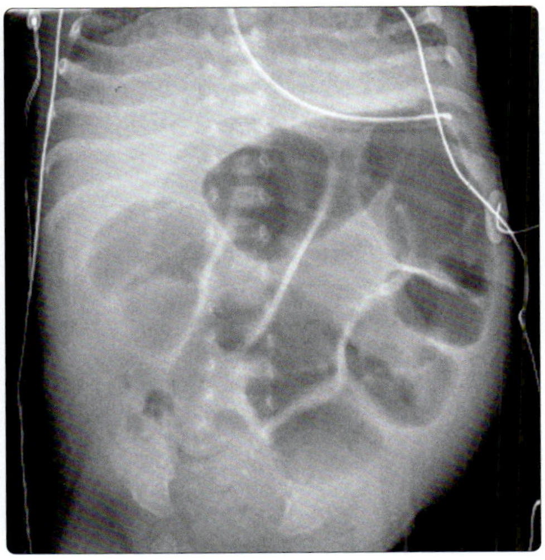

(Left) *Coronal oblique CECT in a 12 year old with Crohn disease shows dilation of SB ➡ secondary to a distal ileal stricture ➡.* **(Right)** *AP radiograph in an infant with a history of necrotizing enterocolitis several weeks prior shows new dilation of multiple SB loops. Further work-up identified a stricture of the distal ileum.*

(Left) *AP radiograph in a 13 year old with abdominal distention & decreased ileostomy output shows marked SB dilation. The stoma is seen in the left lower quadrant.* **(Right)** *Axial CECT in the same 13 year old shows marked bowel dilation extending to the level of the stoma. An attempt to pass a Foley catheter was unsuccessful, suggesting an obstruction at the level of the fascia.*

Stomal Obstruction

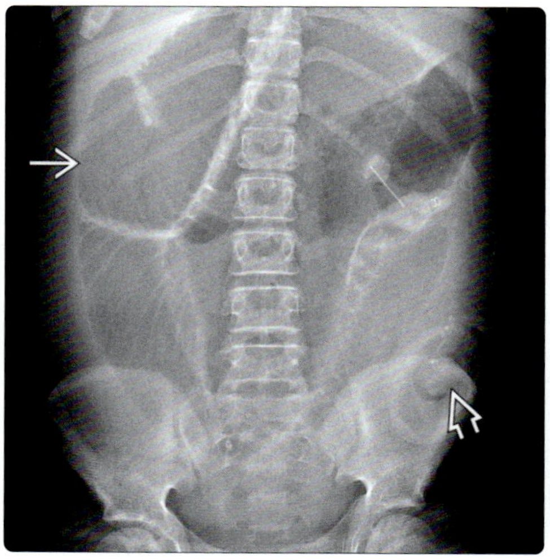

Stomal Obstruction

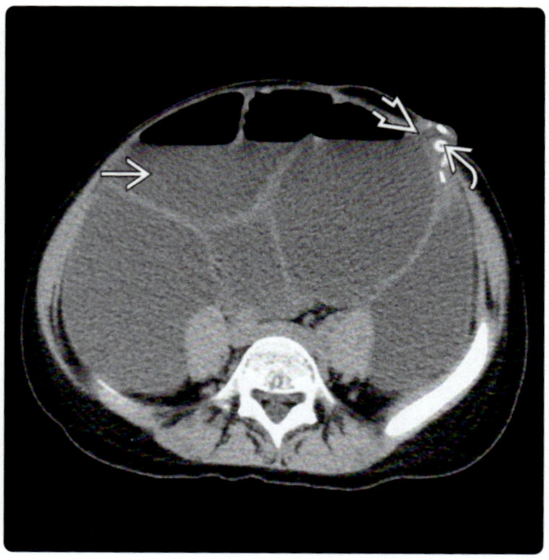

(Left) *Right decubitus stomagram in a 6 year old with an ileostomy due to Hirschsprung disease shows dilation of the contrast-filled bowel up to the level of the stoma. Contrast did not empty from the stoma despite vigorous peristalsis of these loops consistent with obstruction at the fascial plane.* **(Right)** *LPO UGI in a child with intermittent pain & distention shows a circumscribed collection of SB loops. A right paraduodenal internal hernia was found at surgery.*

Stomal Obstruction

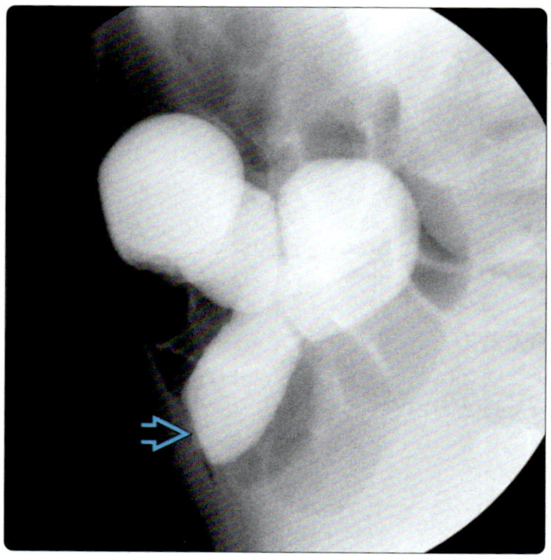

Internal Hernia

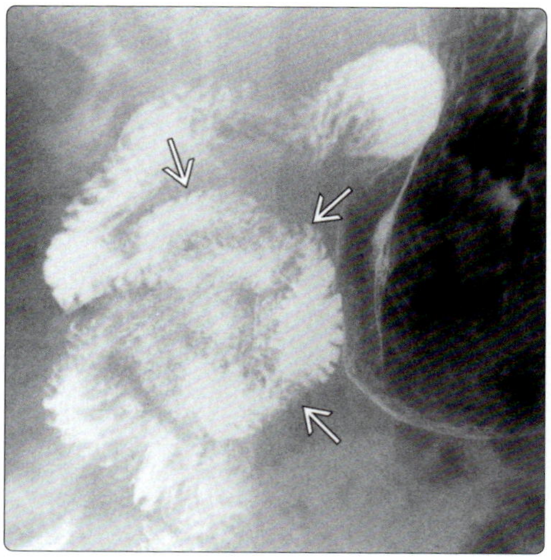

(Left) *Axial CECT in a 12 year old with pain shows a medial cecum at a focus of suggested mesenteric twisting. There is engorgement of adjacent vessels, dilation of left SB loops, & lateralization of right SB loops. A transmesenteric hernia was found at surgery.* **(Right)** *Supine UGI in a 1 month old with vomiting shows mild dilation of D1/D2 with an abrupt beak at the D2/D3 junction. No contrast passed distally, raising concern for MGV. Surgery revealed malrotation with obstructing Ladd bands but no MGV.*

Internal Hernia

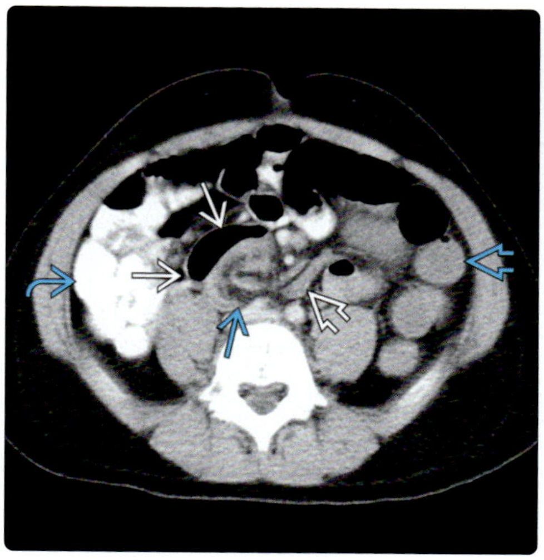

Ladd Bands

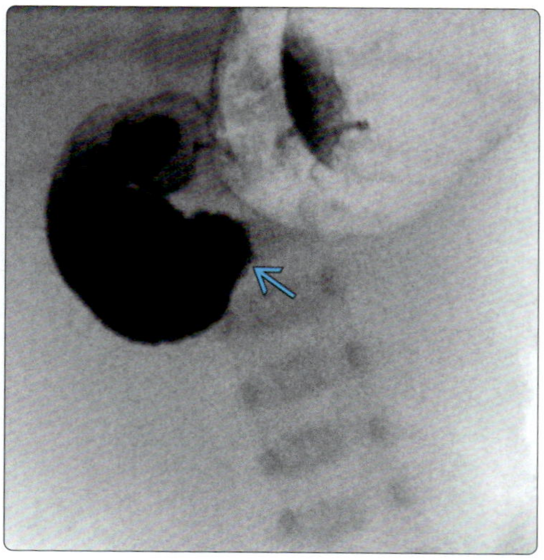

Bezoar

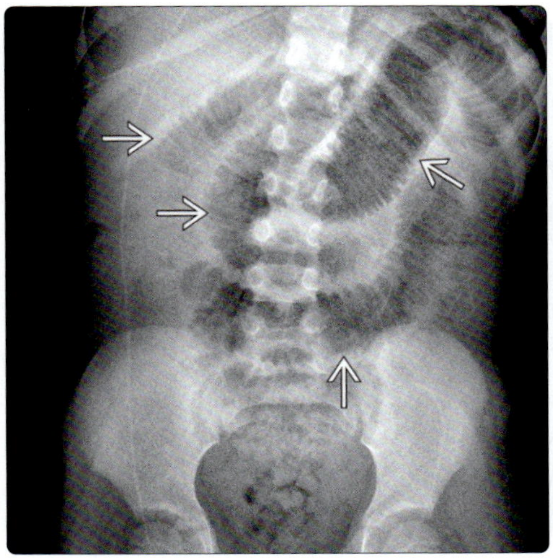

Bezoar

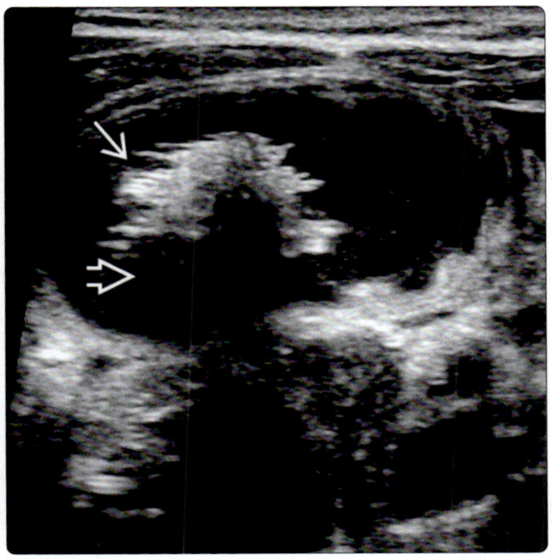

(Left) *AP radiograph of a 7 year old with pain, emesis, & alopecia shows multiple dilated SB loops →, concerning for obstruction.* **(Right)** *Transverse ultrasound from the same patient shows a mass impacted in the distal ileum. The mass has a broad, echogenic, arc-like surface → with dense posterior acoustic shadowing → & was found to be a trichobezoar at surgery.*

Obstructing Mass

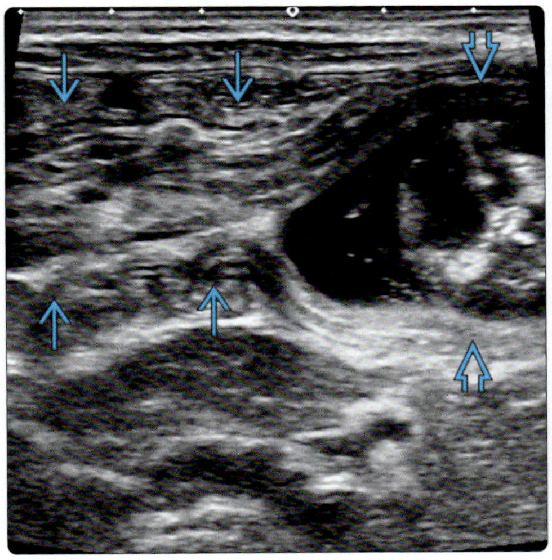

Obstructing Mass

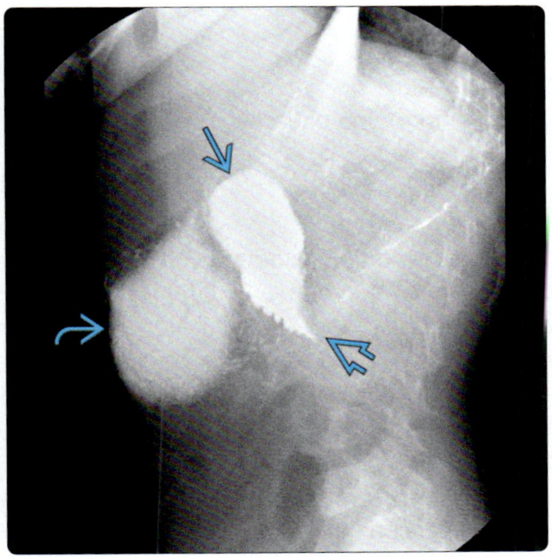

(Left) *Longitudinal ultrasound of the right abdomen in a 16 month old with fussiness shows an ileocolic intussusception → with a pathologic lead point of an enteric duplication cyst →.* **(Right)** *Right lateral decubitus UGI in a 5 year old with vomiting after a duodenal biopsy shows dilation of the stomach → & proximal duodenum →. There is tapering of D2 due to extrinsic compression →. US showed an avascular mass consistent with a hematoma.*

Obstructing Mass

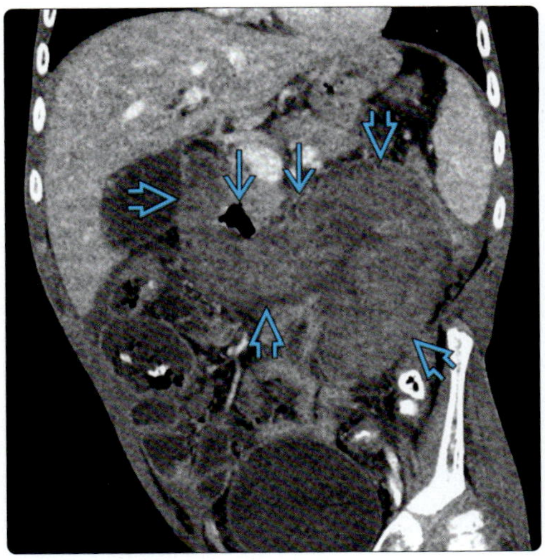

Hypoperfusion Complex (Mimic)

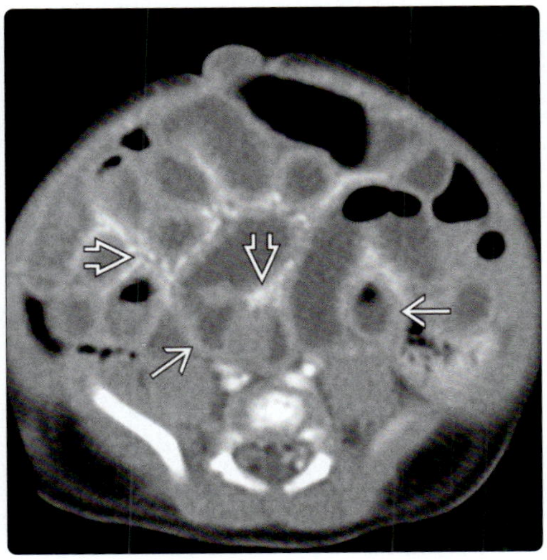

(Left) *Coronal CECT in a 12 year old with chronic immunodeficiency & new hematemesis shows a large intramural hematoma → extending from D2 into the proximal jejunum. There is variable effacement of the bowel lumen → by this mass.* **(Right)** *Axial CECT of a 2 month old with cardiogenic shock shows diffusely abnormal SB, which is dilated & fluid-filled with mildly thickened hyperenhancing walls →. Also note the intense enhancement of the mesenteric vessels →.*

DIFFERENTIAL DIAGNOSIS

Common

- Infectious Enteritis
- Necrotizing Enterocolitis
- Distal Bowel Obstruction

Less Common

- Henoch-Schönlein Purpura
- Celiac Disease
- Distal Intestinal Obstruction Syndrome
- Hypoperfusion Complex

Rare but Important

- Bowel Ischemia
- Graft-vs.-Host Disease

ESSENTIAL INFORMATION

Helpful Clues for Common Diagnoses

- **Infectious Enteritis**
  - Most not imaged unless symptoms are atypical, another disease is being excluded, or patient at risk for complications
    - Immunosuppression/compromise ↑ risk
  - Imaging: Bowel wall & fold thickening, hyperemia, hypo-/hyperperistalsis, fluid distention of loops
    - Location of involvement varies with organism
- **Necrotizing Enterocolitis**
  - Prematurity (< 1,500 g, < 32-weeks gestation), bloody stools, feeding intolerance, distended abdomen
  - Imaging: Pneumatosis, portal venous gas, fixed distended bowel loops, absent/reduced peristalsis, bowel wall thickening/thinning, fluid collections, free air
- **Distal Bowel Obstruction**
  - Mechanical blockage of bowel
    - Common newborn etiologies: Atresias, midgut volvulus, Hirschsprung disease, meconium ileus
    - Common childhood etiologies: Appendicitis, adhesions, inguinal hernia, intussusception, Meckel diverticulum, midgut volvulus (AAIIMM)
  - Imaging: Transition point from dilation to collapse

Helpful Clues for Less Common Diagnoses

- **Henoch-Schönlein Purpura**
  - Purpuric rash on extremities, hematuria, proteinuria, GI bleeding, arthralgias
  - Imaging: Bowel wall thickening due to hemorrhage (may be multifocal), small bowel-small bowel intussusceptions, ↑ renal parenchymal echogenicity, scrotal wall edema
- **Celiac Disease**
  - Pain, diarrhea, malabsorption, ↑ tissue transglutaminase & IgA endomysial antibodies
  - Imaging: Reversal of jejunal-ileal fold pattern (↓ in jejunum, ↑ in ileum), wall thickening, mesenteric lymph nodes, multiple intussusceptions, splenic atrophy
- **Distal Intestinal Obstruction Syndrome**
  - Patient with cystic fibrosis & bowel obstructions
  - Imaging: Accumulation of viscous fecal material at distal ileum (most common) with proximal dilation
- **Hypoperfusion Complex**
  - Shock (hypovolemic, neurogenic, cardiac, sepsis)
  - Imaging: Diffuse wall thickening, hyperenhancement with accentuated folds, fluid distention
    - Flat inferior vena cava, ascites, ± ↑ enhancement of adrenals, kidneys, pancreas, & vessels

Helpful Clues for Rare Diagnoses

- **Bowel Ischemia**
  - Arterial compromise, venous insufficiency, low-flow state
  - Imaging: Vascular distribution, bowel wall thickening or thinning, abnormal mucosal enhancement (absent, ↑, or ↓), mesenteric edema, pneumatosis, portal venous gas
    - Look for midgut volvulus or occlusive thrombus
- **Graft-vs.-Host Disease**
  - History of allogeneic bone marrow or stem cell transplant
  - Imaging: Diffuse bowel wall thickening, mild fluid distention, "mucosal" hyperenhancement (likely granulation tissue due to mucosal sloughing), featureless lumen ribbon sign

(Left) *Cross-table lateral radiograph of a 7-day-old premature infant with necrotizing enterocolitis depicts diffuse bubbly & curvilinear lucencies* → *outlining the gas-distended bowel, consistent with pneumatosis. No free air is seen at this time.* **(Right)** *Supine frontal radiograph of a 7-day-old premature infant shows a small bowel obstruction secondary to bowel herniating through the inguinal canal* → *into the scrotum* →.

Necrotizing Enterocolitis

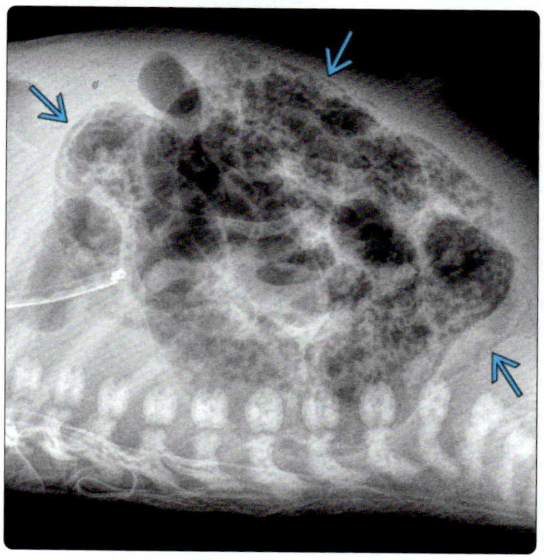

Distal Bowel Obstruction

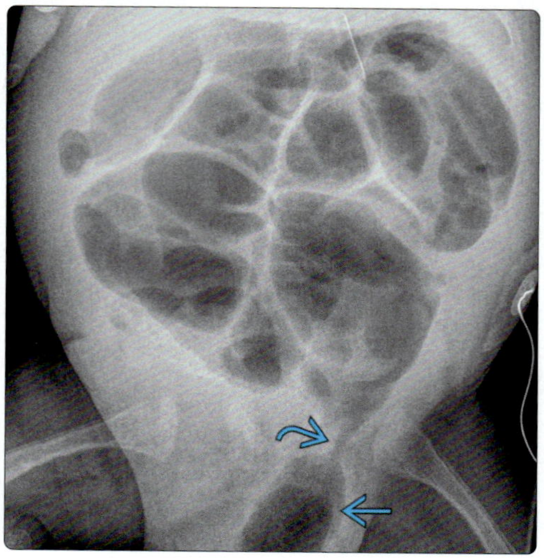

Henoch-Schönlein Purpura

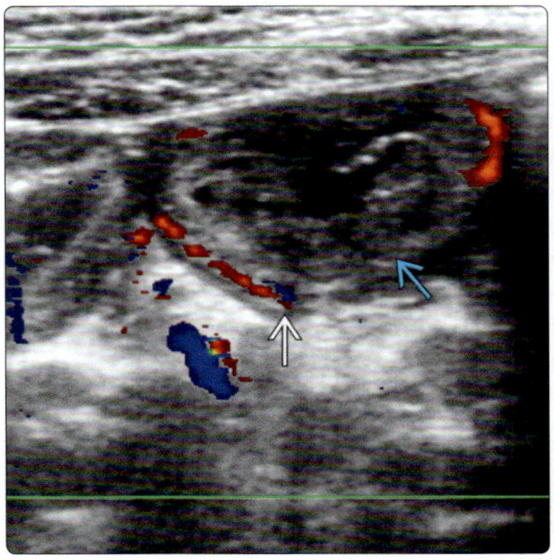

Celiac Disease

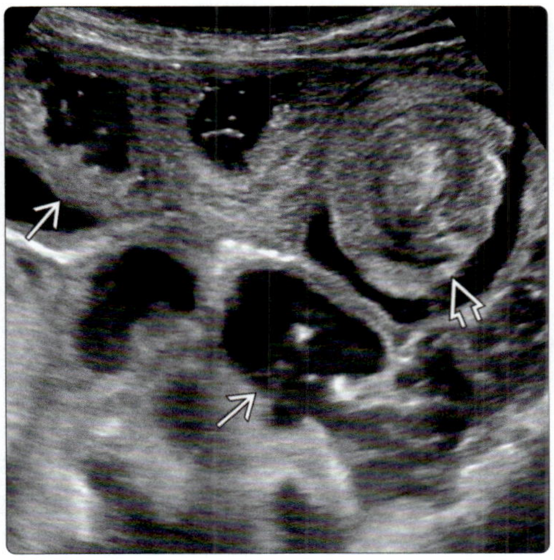

(Left) *Transverse color Doppler US demonstrates small bowel wall thickening & hyperemia in a 4 year old with Henoch-Schönlein purpura that presented with abdominal pain & intussusception.* **(Right)** *Transverse US from a 2 year old with abdominal pain & distention shows multiple fluid-distended, thick-walled loops of bowel. Multiple small bowel-small bowel intussusceptions were also identified. The patient was determined to have celiac disease during further work-up.*

Distal Intestinal Obstruction Syndrome

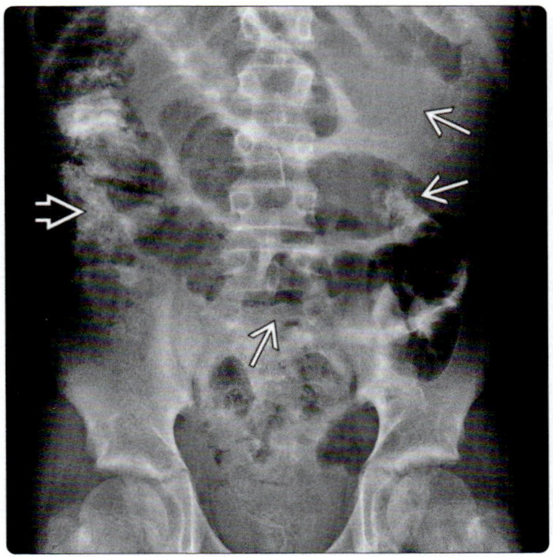

Hypoperfusion Complex

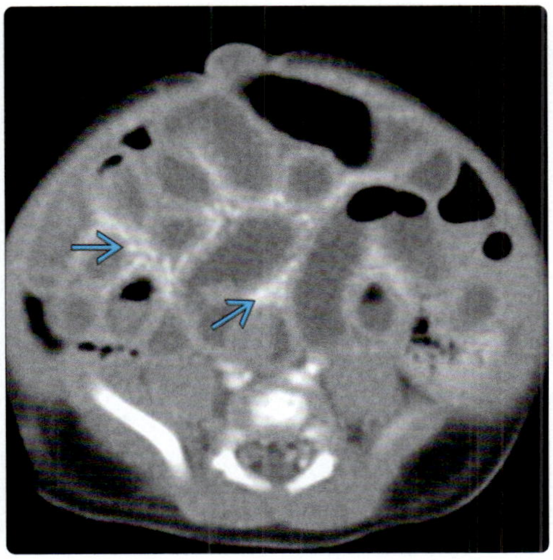

(Left) *Abdominal radiograph in a 14 year old with cystic fibrosis & distal intestinal obstruction syndrome shows multiple dilated small bowel loops. Contrast is seen in the cecum & ascending colon from the prior enema.* **(Right)** *Axial CECT of a 2-month-old boy with cardiogenic shock shows diffusely abnormal small bowel, which is dilated, fluid filled, & mildly hyperenhancing. Also note the intense enhancement of the mesenteric vessels.*

Bowel Ischemia

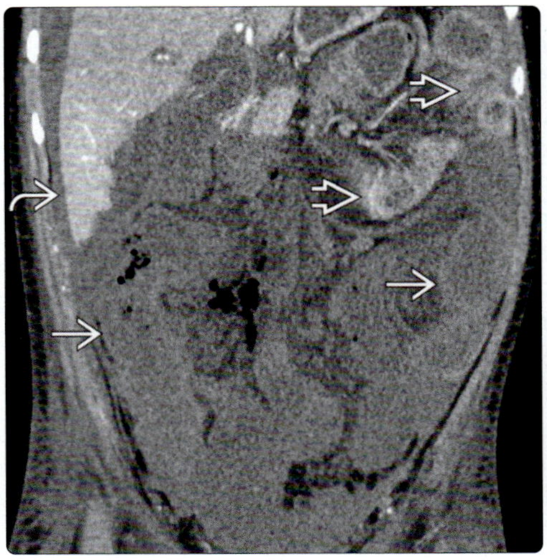

Graft-vs.-Host Disease

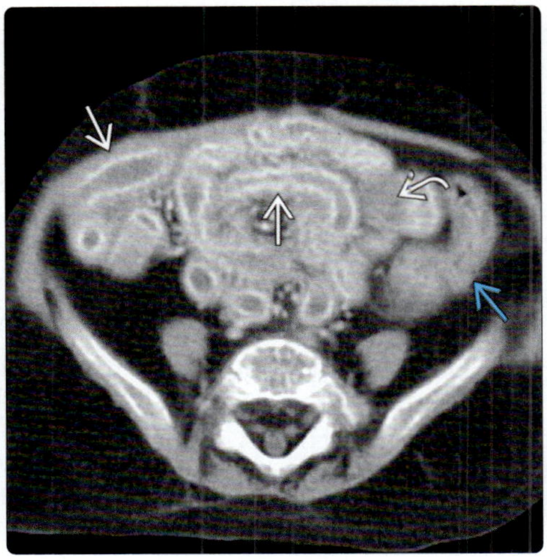

(Left) *Coronal CECT in an 11 year old with multisystem organ failure shows lack of wall enhancement of most of the bowel with adjacent stranding & ascites. Note few enhancing jejunal loops. SMA & IMA were largely occluded (not shown).* **(Right)** *Axial CECT from a 4 year old with a history of a bone marrow transplant shows wall thickening & luminal enhancement of small > large bowel. There is also infiltration of the mesentery. UGI series showed ribbon-like bowel, consistent with GVHD.*

DIFFERENTIAL DIAGNOSIS

Common

- Appendicitis
- Ovarian Cyst
- Infectious Enteritis/Colitis
- Urinary Tract Infection
- Ileocolic Intussusception
- Inguinal Hernia
- Ovarian Torsion
- Midgut Volvulus
- Inflammatory Bowel Disease
- Pancreatitis
- Urinary Tract Calculus

Less Common

- Obstruction by Adhesions
- Foreign Body Ingestion
- Meckel Diverticulum
- Henoch-Schönlein Purpura
- Distal Intestinal Obstruction Syndrome
- Child Abuse
- Pelvic Inflammatory Disease
- Cholecystitis

Rare but Important

- Gastric Volvulus
- Colonic Volvulus
- Wandering Spleen
- Splenic Sequestration

ESSENTIAL INFORMATION

Key Differential Diagnosis Issues

- Age, sex, & location of pain can be quite helpful
  - Neonatal processes are considered separately
- Bilious vs. nonbilious emesis
  - Bilious: Any bowel obstruction distal to sphincter of Oddi, but greatest concern is for midgut volvulus (MGV)
- Number of dilated loops
  - Implies proximal vs. distal obstructive etiologies
- Vital signs & laboratory studies
  - Fever, ↑ WBC, ↑ ESR, ↑ CRP, ↑ fecal calprotectin → infectious/inflammatory etiologies
  - Abnormal urinalysis → urinary tract etiologies
  - ↑ LFT/↑ bilirubin → biliary etiology
  - ↑ amylase & ↑ lipase → pancreatitis
  - ↑ lactate → concern for bowel ischemia

Helpful Clues for Common Diagnoses

- **Appendicitis**
  - RLQ pain, fever, ↓ appetite, + Rovsing & obturator signs, emesis, ↑ WBC
  - Enlarged, noncompressible, blind-ending, tubular structure arising from cecum + adjacent fat inflammation
    - ± appendicolith, adjacent fluid collection
- **Ovarian Cyst**
  - Simple cyst: Round, avascular, ↑ through transmission
  - Hemorrhagic cyst: Uniform echoes vs. lace-like retracted clot vs. layering debris
  - Cyst > 5 cm: ↑ risk for ovarian torsion
- **Infectious Enteritis/Colitis**
  - Very common but not necessarily imaged
  - Radiographs frequently show colonic air-fluid levels
  - US may show many fluid-filled hyperperistalsing bowel loops, ± prominent mesenteric lymph nodes
- **Urinary Tract Infection**
  - Dysuria, enuresis, fever, irritability, foul-smelling urine
  - High fever & flank pain ↑ likelihood of pyelonephritis
    - Focal renal edema with blurring of corticomedullary differentiation, variable change in echogenicity, & ↓ enhancement/perfusion
    - ± bladder wall & urothelial thickening, bladder debris, vesicoureteral reflux
- **Ileocolic Intussusception**
  - Currant jelly stools, crampy abdominal pain, emesis, right-sided abdominal mass
  - Radiographs are not sensitive or specific
    - May show paucity of colonic gas in right abdomen, round mass in right/upper abdomen ± entrapped lucent fat or surrounding crescent of air
  - US: Target sign of intussusception in cross section with mean diameter of 2.6 cm
    - Compared to 1.5-cm mean diameter in small bowel-small bowel (SB-SB) intussusception, which also usually lacks entrapped fat or lymph nodes
- **Inguinal Hernia**
  - Palpable inguinal lump; incarceration suspected if unable to be reduced + pain & obstruction
  - Radiographs show gas extending into inguinal region with obstructive bowel gas pattern
  - US/CECT may show abnormal fluid, bowel wall thickening, & ↓ enhancement/flow with ↓ peristalsis, suggesting ischemia
- **Ovarian Torsion**
  - Enlarged ovary, often > 5-12x contralateral side
  - Heterogeneous parenchyma with peripheral follicles
    - Can mimic mass with only 1 normal ovary visualized
  - May be displaced to midline or contralateral side
  - Flow may be preserved due to dual blood supply or torsion/detorsion
- **Midgut Volvulus**
  - Bilious emesis; rarely presents with ischemic ileus/shock
  - Upper GI (UGI) shows mild dilation of stomach & proximal duodenum with abrupt taper or "beak" at D2/D3
    - Contrast passing beyond beak shows narrowing & twisting ("corkscrew" on UGI & "whirlpool" on US)
- **Inflammatory Bowel Disease**
  - Crohn disease (CD) & ulcerative colitis (UC)
    - CD: Transmural skip lesions anywhere from mouth to anus; most common at terminal ileum/cecum
    - UC: Contiguous proximal extension from anus
  - Pain, diarrhea, weight loss, bloody stool
  - Bowel wall thickening & hyperenhancement, luminal narrowing, engorged vasa recta
- **Pancreatitis**
  - Vomiting, pain, ↑ amylase & lipase
  - Acute interstitial edematous: Enlargement with relatively normal enhancement + adjacent inflammation
  - Acute necrotizing: Regions of moderately to severely ↓ enhancement
  - Gradual organization of fluid collections

- **Urinary Tract Calculus**
  - Shadowing echogenic focus with twinkling artifact on Doppler at renal pelvis or ureter; if obstructed, look for
    - Dilation of renal pelvis & ureter above stone
    - Absence of ureteral jet in urinary bladder

Helpful Clues for Less Common Diagnoses

- **Obstruction by Adhesions**
  - History of prior surgery or inflammation
  - May see abrupt caliber change/kink of bowel
- **Foreign Body Ingestion**
  - Variable density; many are nonradiopaque
  - Echogenic shadowing focus with unusual shape/margin on US or filling defect on fluoroscopic contrast study
  - Button batteries & magnets are of particular concern
- **Meckel Diverticulum**
  - Variable presentations: GI bleeding, obstruction, &/or pain with inflammation
  - Blind-ending tubular structure arising from distal ileum; may be seen if inflamed; often not seen with obstruction
  - Positive Tc-99m pertechnetate scan with GI bleeding
- **Henoch-Schönlein Purpura**
  - Purpuric rash on extremities, hematuria, proteinuria, GI bleeding, arthralgias
  - Bowel wall thickening (may be multifocal), SB-SB intussusceptions, ↑ renal parenchymal echogenicity, scrotal wall edema/hyperemia
- **Distal Intestinal Obstruction Syndrome**
  - Abnormally thickened meconium of cystic fibrosis may lead to distal SB obstruction
- **Child Abuse**
  - History inconsistent with fracture or child's stage of development, patterned burns/bruises
  - Classic metaphyseal lesions, posterior rib fractures, fractures of varying age
  - ↑ LFTs may indicate need for abdominal CT
    - Most common injuries: Proximal SB, pancreas, liver
- **Pelvic Inflammatory Disease**
  - Sexually active female patients, cervical motion tenderness, vaginal discharge, fever
    - RUQ pain with Fitz-Hugh-Curtis syndrome
  - Pyosalpinx, tuboovarian abscess, complex free fluid
- **Cholecystitis**
  - High rate of chronic cholecystitis in children with gallstones but otherwise normal gallbladder by US
  - Acute cholecystitis is much less common than adults

Helpful Clues for Rare Diagnoses

- **Gastric Volvulus**
  - Retching, epigastric distention, inability to pass NG tube
  - Pylorus at or above level of gastroesophageal junction (mesenteroaxial)
  - Greater curvature above lesser curvature (organoaxial)
  - Abnormal orientation of stomach, may appear round when supine; diaphragm abnormalities are common
- **Colonic Volvulus**
  - More common with disabled patients with chronic constipation/dysmotility
  - Suspect if patient with chronic bowel dilation presents with acutely worsened pain & dilation
    - Focal marked dilation of bowel loop, ± coffee bean appearance with sigmoid volvulus
    - "Beak" on water-soluble contrast enema
    - CECT may show beak & twisted vessels/mesentery
- **Wandering Spleen**
  - Spleen absent from usual position in LUQ due to lax or absent splenic ligaments
  - Risk of torsion of long vascular pedicle
- **Splenic Sequestration**
  - Patients with hemoglobinopathies
  - Abdominal pain, acute splenic enlargement, drop in hemoglobin > 2 g/dL

SELECTED REFERENCES

1. Hijaz NM et al: Managing acute abdominal pain in pediatric patients: current perspectives. Pediatric Health Med Ther. 8:83-91, 2017
2. Naffaa L et al: Imaging of acute pelvic pain in girls: ovarian torsion and beyond. Curr Probl Diagn Radiol. 46(4):317-29, 2017
3. Chang PT et al: Diagnostic errors of right lower quadrant pain in children: beyond appendicitis. Abdom Imaging. 40(7):2071-90, 2015

Appendicitis

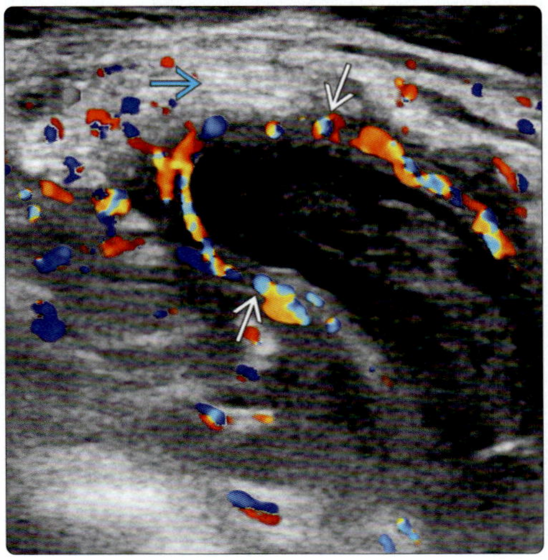

Appendicitis

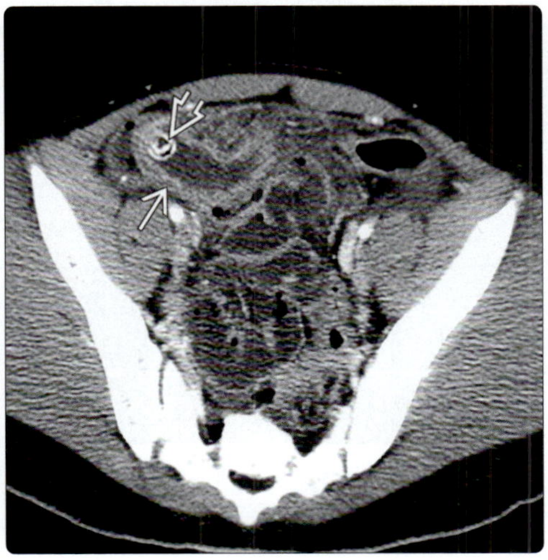

(Left) *Longitudinal color Doppler US shows an enlarged, hyperemic appendix ➡ with adjacent echogenic fat ➡ in a 5-year-old boy with RLQ pain, consistent with acute appendicitis.* **(Right)** *Axial CECT shows a dilated, thick-walled, blind-ending fluid-filled tubular structure ➡ containing a lamellated appendicolith ➡ in the RLQ, consistent with acute appendicitis.*

(Left) *Transverse US in a 16-year-old girl with right abdominal pain shows an ovoid, well-circumscribed, 6-cm cystic lesion of the right ovary with lace-like internal contents & no vascularity on Doppler (not shown). This hemorrhagic ovarian cyst had resolved by the follow-up exam.* **(Right)** *Longitudinal color Doppler US in a 7 year old with a urinary tract infection (UTI) shows ↑ echogenicity & ↓ perfusion of the upper pole of the right kidney, consistent with pyelonephritis.*

Ovarian Cyst

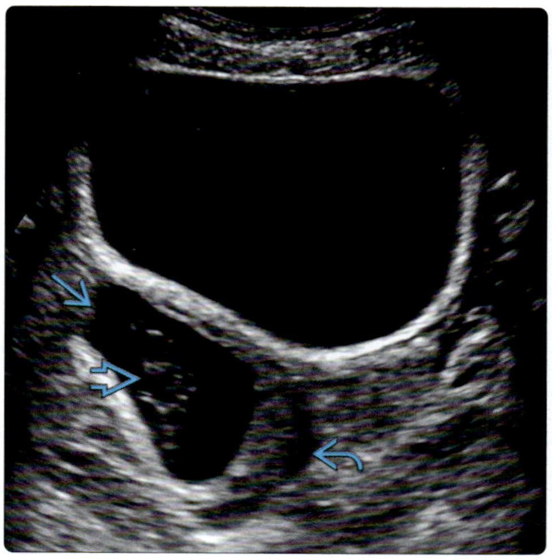

Urinary Tract Infection

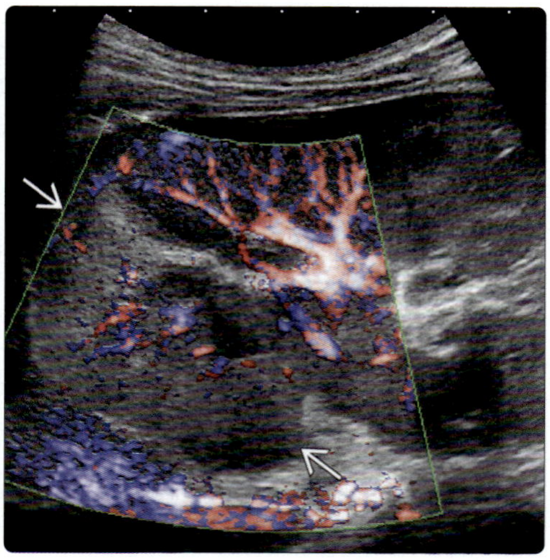

(Left) *Transverse US in a 6 month old with intermittent pain shows a rounded, 3-cm, RUQ mass with a target sign, consistent with an ileocolic intussusception. The hypoechoic foci are due to entrapped bowel & lymph nodes surrounded by echogenic fat.* **(Right)** *Supine frontal radiograph of a 7-day-old premature infant with abdominal distention shows a gas-filled loop of bowel extending through the inguinal canal into the scrotum with dilation of the proximal bowel.*

Ileocolic Intussusception

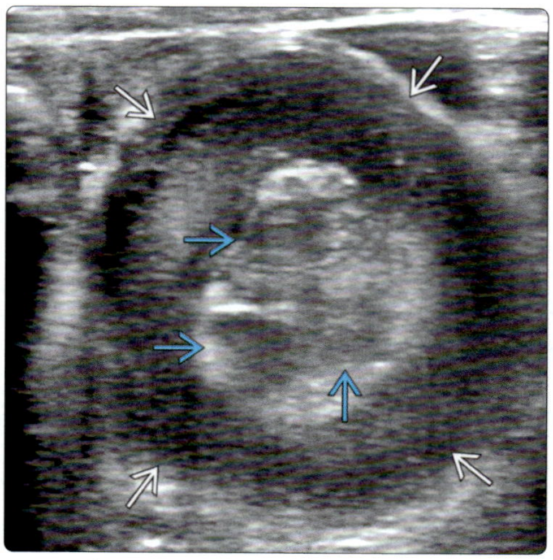

Inguinal Hernia

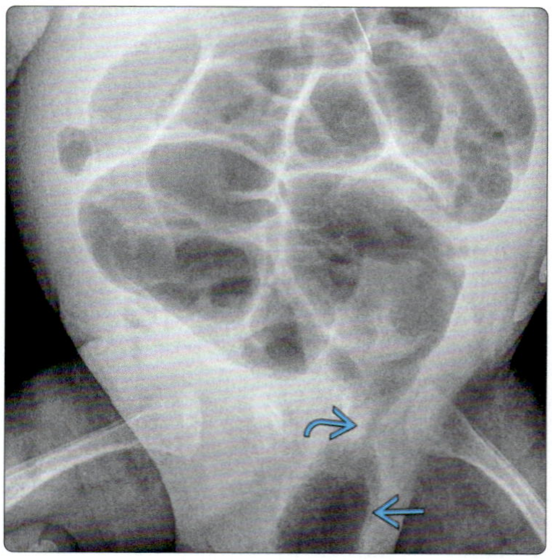

(Left) *Longitudinal color Doppler US in a 10 month old with an irreducible lump in the right inguinal region depicts an avascular loop of bowel traversing the inguinal canal into the scrotum, concerning for a strangulated inguinal hernia.* **(Right)** *Transverse color Doppler US in a 13-year-old girl with abdominal pain shows an enlarged, heterogeneous right ovary with a lack of internal flow, consistent with ovarian torsion. Several small peripheral follicles are noted.*

Inguinal Hernia

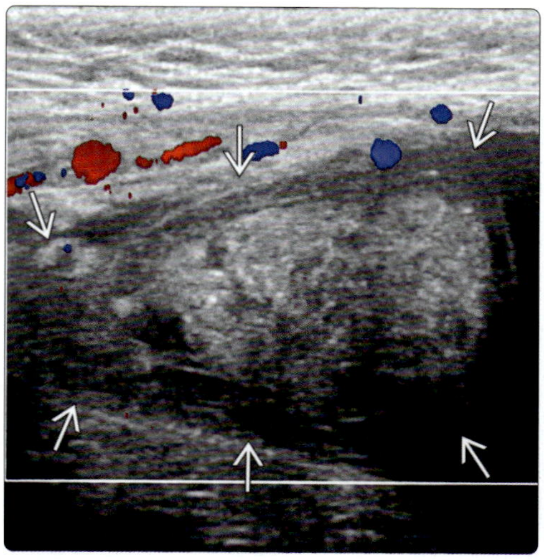

Ovarian Torsion

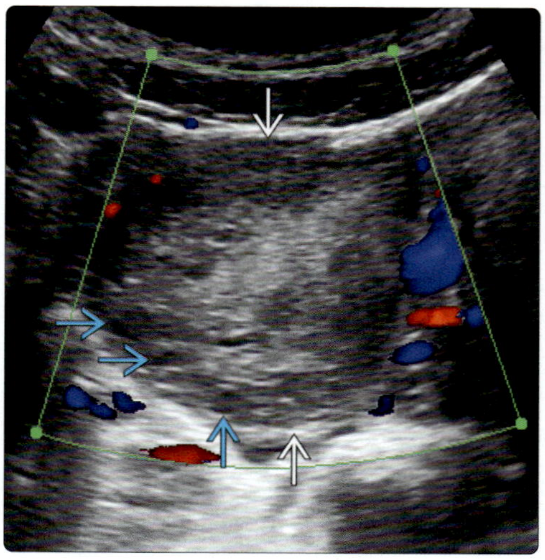

Midgut Volvulus

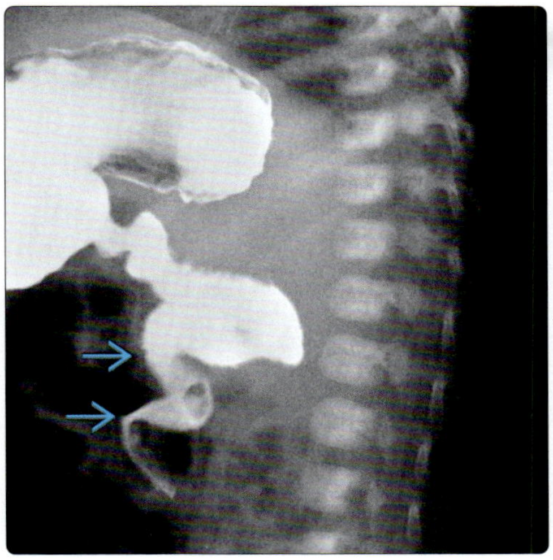

Inflammatory Bowel Disease

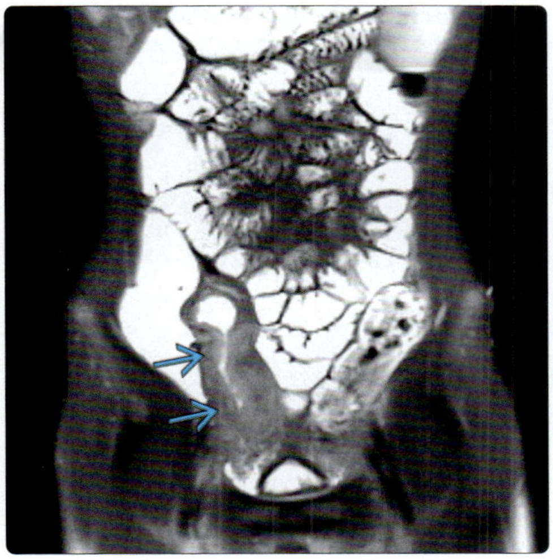

(Left) *Lateral right-side-down upper GI (UGI) in an infant with bilious emesis shows the typical corkscrew appearance of the duodenum → due to midgut volvulus superimposed on intestinal malrotation.* **(Right)** *Coronal T2 FS MR enterography in a 13 year old with Crohn disease shows ↑ T2 signal intensity of the thickened wall of the terminal ileum → with luminal narrowing & surrounding inflammation.*

Pancreatitis

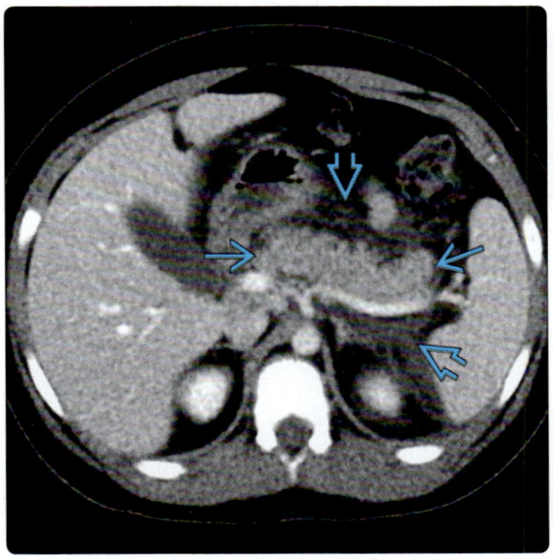

Urinary Tract Calculus

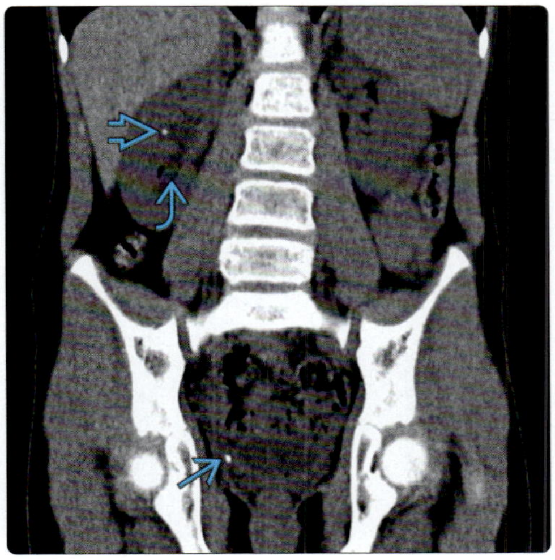

(Left) *Axial CECT in a 10 year old with acute pain, guarding, & elevated lipase shows a mildly enlarged but homogeneously enhancing pancreas → with surrounding inflammation ⇨, consistent with acute interstitial edematous pancreatitis.* **(Right)** *Coronal NECT in an 11 year old with right flank pain shows a 3-mm calculus at the right ureterovesical junction →. Mild right hydroureteronephrosis → was present, & additional calyceal calculi ⇨ were noted.*

Foreign Body Ingestion

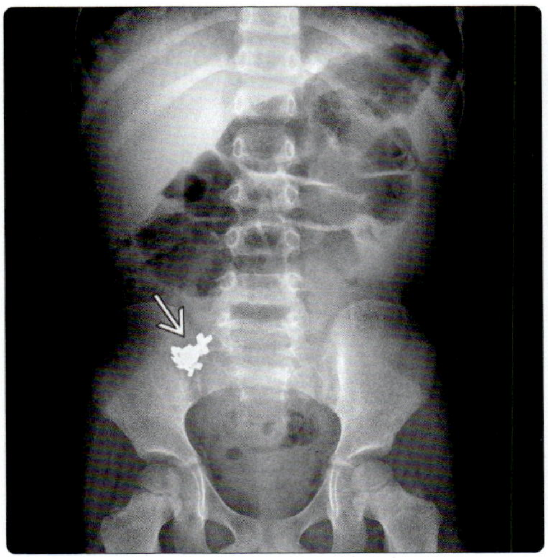

Meckel Diverticulum

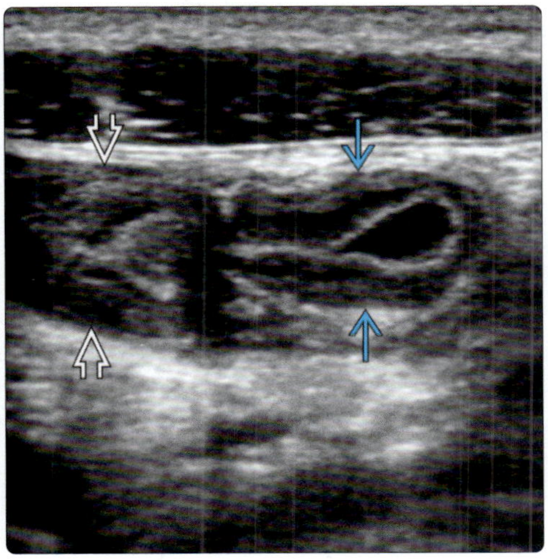

(Left) *Frontal radiograph shows a cluster of magnets ➡ in the abdominal RLQ. Attraction of the magnets (which were initially separated in adjacent loops of bowel) caused pressure erosions & perforation.* **(Right)** *Longitudinal US shows a Meckel diverticulum → as a blind-ending tubular structure with "gut signature" arising from the terminal ileum ➡ in a 14 year old. These diverticula may become inflamed, lead to bleeding, or cause obstruction.*

(Left) *Transverse color Doppler US in a 4 year old with Henoch-Schönlein purpura shows multiple loops of small bowel (SB) with wall thickening. Transient SB-SB intussusceptions were also noted (not shown). The patient presented with abdominal pain & a purpuric rash on his lower extremities.* **(Right)** *Axial CECT shows dilated, thick-walled, hyperenhancing loops of SB ➡ with free intraperitoneal fluid ➡. These findings preceded the classic skin lesions of Henoch-Schönlein purpura.*

Henoch-Schönlein Purpura

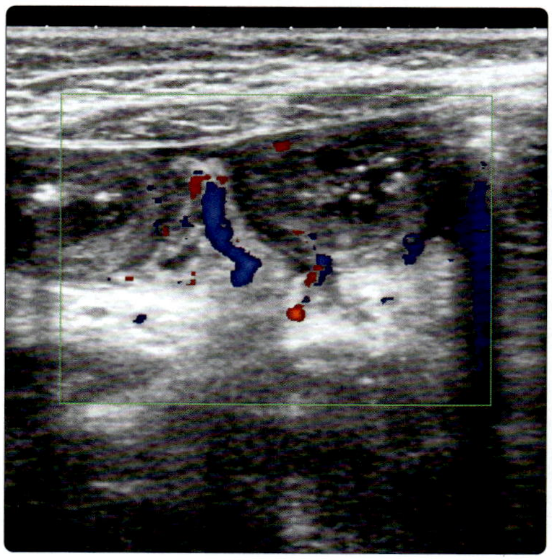

Henoch-Schönlein Purpura

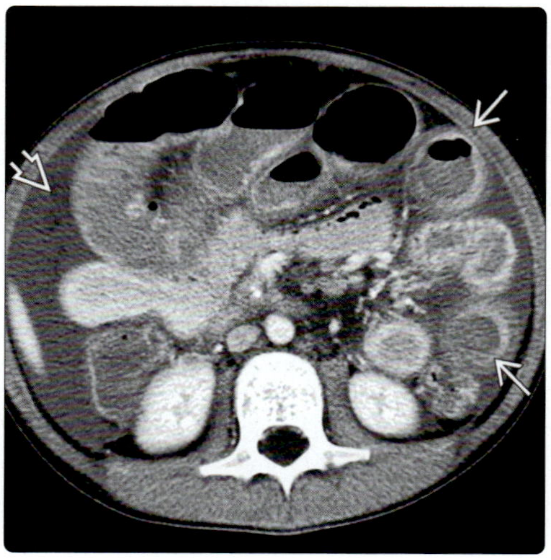

(Left) *Frontal radiograph in a 2-year-old child with cystic fibrosis (CF), pain, & vomiting shows multiple dilated loops of SB ➡ with fecal loading in the right abdomen ➡, suggesting DIOS given the medical history.* **(Right)** *Supine frontal water-soluble contrast enema in the same patient shows fecal loading extending into the distal ileum ➡, consistent with DIOS. Serial, relatively high osmolar contrast enemas, with adequate monitoring & IV hydration, can be used to relieve such obstructions in CF patients.*

Distal Intestinal Obstruction Syndrome

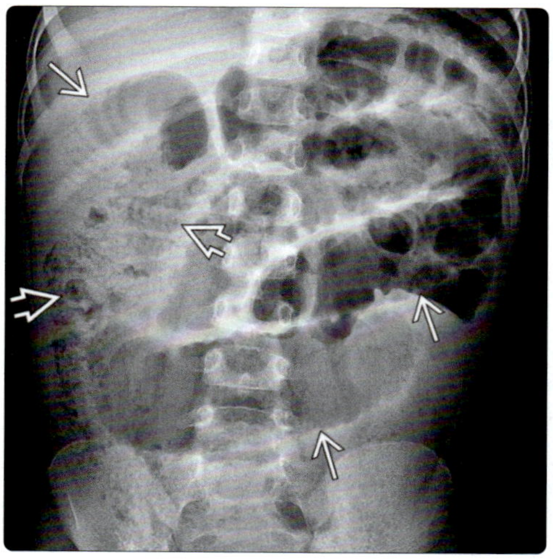

Distal Intestinal Obstruction Syndrome

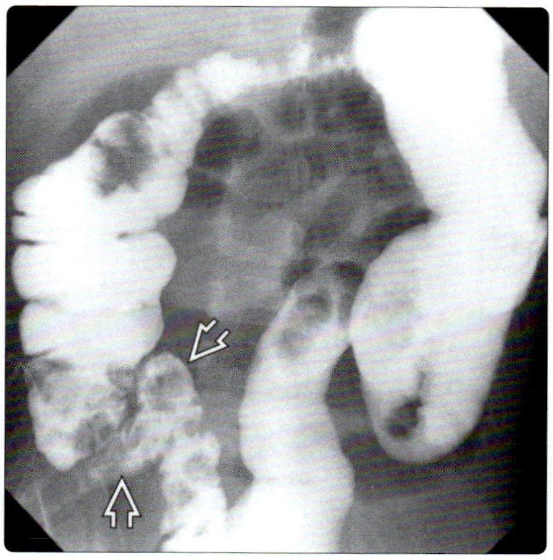

(Left) *Axial CECT shows a healing rib fracture ➡, hemoperitoneum ➡, pneumoperitoneum ➡, & a heterogeneously enhancing liver with laceration ➡ in a young child with suspected physical abuse. Note the hyperenhancing adrenal glands ➡ & collapsed IVC ➡ due to hypoperfusion complex. Duodenal & jejunal perforations were found at surgery.* **(Right)** *Longitudinal color Doppler US in a 15-year-old girl with months of pain & dysuria shows a thick-walled, 6-cm cystic mass of the right adnexa.*

Child Abuse

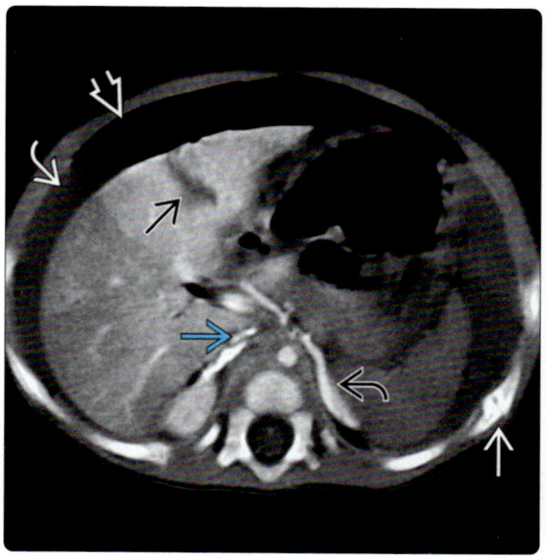

Pelvic Inflammatory Disease

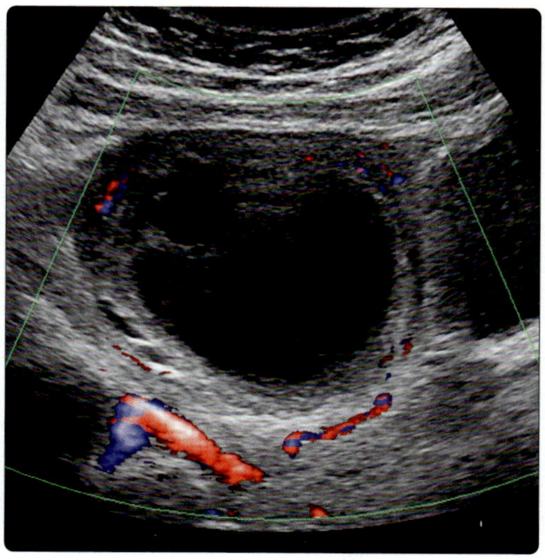

Pelvic Inflammatory Disease

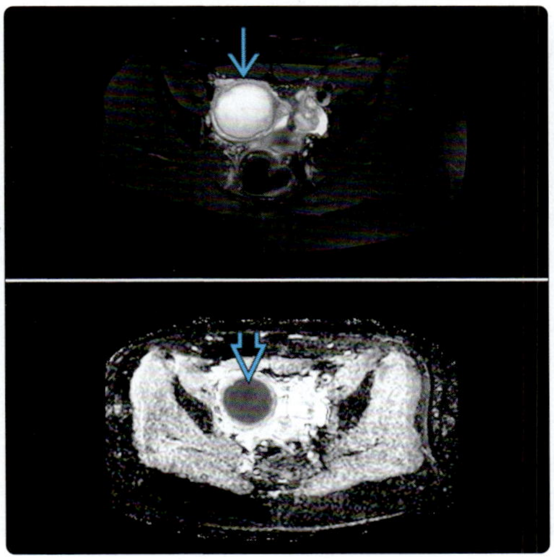

Pelvic Inflammatory Disease

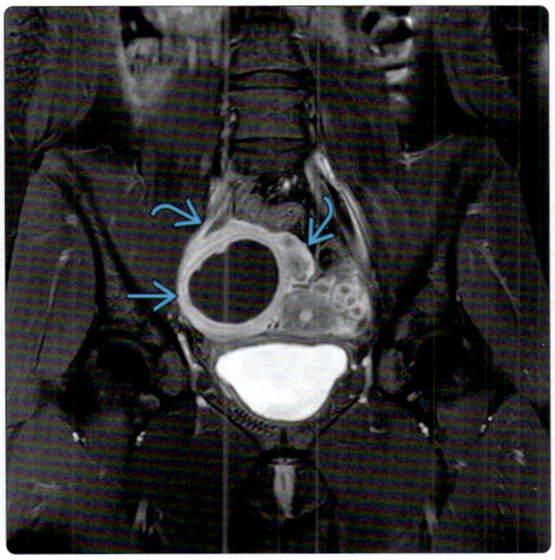

(Left) *Axial T2 FS (top) & ADC map (bottom) MR images in the same patient show a thick, T2-hypointense rim to the collection with diffusion restriction of the central contents suggesting abscess.* **(Right)** *Coronal T1 C+ FS MR in the same patient shows diffuse, thick rim enhancement of the collection with mild inflammation of the surrounding tissues. Tuboovarian abscess was confirmed at surgery with adhesions to multiple adjacent structures.*

Cholecystitis

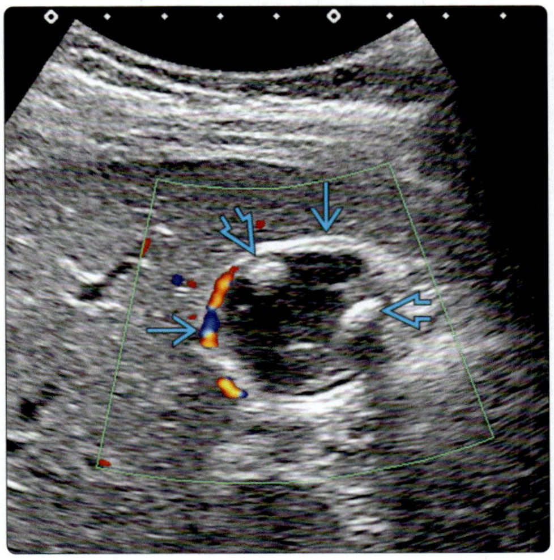

Gastric Volvulus

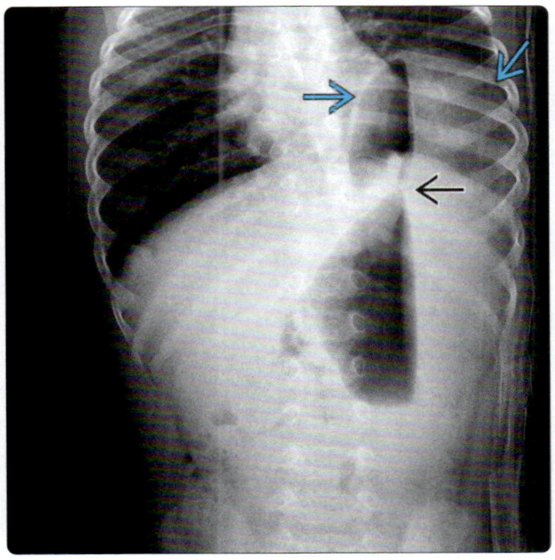

(Left) *Transverse color Doppler US in a 14 year old with RUQ pain shows a distended gallbladder with a mildly thickened & hyperemic wall. The echogenic filling defects with posterior acoustic shadowing are consistent with stones. Acute on chronic cholecystitis was found at resection.* **(Right)** *Left decubitus radiograph shows a midgastric body twist in a 6 month old with mesenteroaxial gastric volvulus who presented with nonbilious emesis. This entity is frequently associated with diaphragmatic hernias.*

Colonic Volvulus

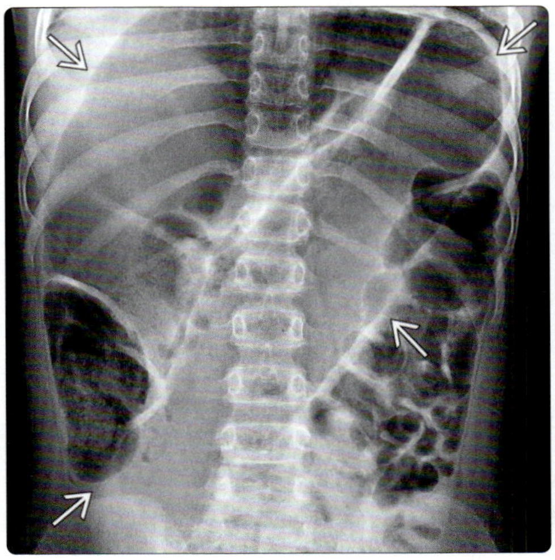

Wandering Spleen

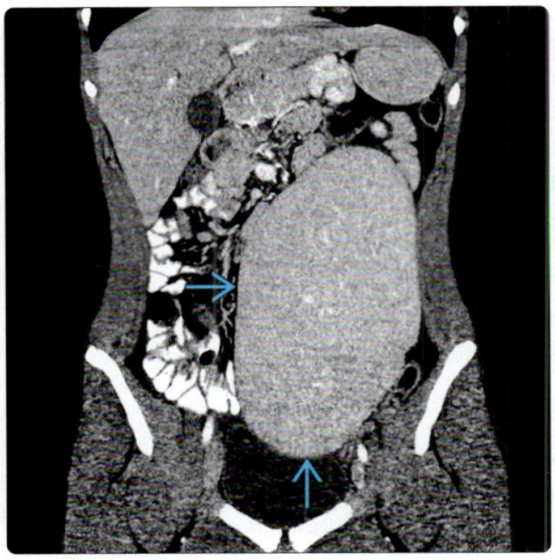

(Left) *Supine abdominal radiograph of a 9 year old with abdominal distention, pain, & emesis shows marked colonic distention with a coffee bean sign. A volvulus of redundant sigmoid colon was seen at surgery.* **(Right)** *Coronal CECT shows a massively enlarged spleen in the lower anterior abdomen in this teenager with pain. The pathology report described extensive venous congestion, probably from intermittent torsion given the clinical presentation.*

DIFFERENTIAL DIAGNOSIS

Common

- Appendicitis
- Infectious Enteritis & Enterocolitis
- Ileocolic Intussusception
- Mesenteric Adenitis
- Crohn Disease

Less Common

- Obstructing Renal/Ureteral Calculus
- Hemorrhagic Ovarian Cyst
- Ovarian Torsion
- Pyelonephritis
- Pneumonia
- Omental Infarct
- Epiploic Appendagitis
- Meckel Diverticulum

Rare but Important

- Neutropenic Colitis
- Pelvic Inflammatory Disease
- Ectopic Pregnancy

ESSENTIAL INFORMATION

Key Differential Diagnosis Issues

- Sex, age, medical history, & CBC limit differential

Helpful Clues for Common Diagnoses

- **Appendicitis**
  - Uncommon < 2 years of age
  - Fever, decreased appetite, positive Rovsing & obturator signs, emesis, leukocytosis
  - Imaging: Blind-ending tubular structure arising from cecum inferior to terminal ileum (TI)
    - Differentiates from TI & Meckel diverticulum
    - > 6-mm diameter with fluid-distended noncompressible lumen plus surrounding inflammatory fat stranding/increased echogenicity
    - ± appendicolith, wall irregularity &/or hyperemia, adjacent fluid collection
    - Inflammatory changes centered & most severe at appendix; TI & cecum not typically thickened without perforated appendicitis
- **Infectious Enteritis & Enterocolitis**
  - Viral > bacterial > parasitic (in developed countries)
  - Organisms with predilection for affecting particular segments of bowel
    - Proximal small bowel: *Giardia, Strongyloides, Mycobacterium avium-intracellulare, Cryptosporidium*
    - Distal small bowel: *Yersinia, Salmonella, Campylobacter, Shigella, Anisakis*
    - TI & cecum: Typhlitis, tuberculosis, amebiasis
    - Right colon: *Yersinia, Salmonella, Entamoeba histolytica*
  - Imaging: Bowel wall & fold thickening, hyperemia, hypo-/hyperperistalsis, fluid levels (particularly in colon)
  - Positive stool cultures &/or ova/parasite tests
  - Neutropenia & immunosuppression increase risk
- **Ileocolic Intussusception**
  - Clinical triad: Currant jelly stool, intermittent abdominal pain, emesis
  - Age of ~ 3 months to 3 years; if outside this range, consider lead point/mass
  - Imaging: Ultrasound highly sensitive & specific
    - Target sign in short axis, pseudokidney sign in longitudinal axis
      - Layers of intussuscepted bowel, mesenteric fat, lymph nodes, blood vessels
    - Target sign mean diameter of 2.6 cm vs. 1.5 cm in small bowel-small bowel intussusception
    - Right-sided abdominal soft tissue mass & air crescent sign on radiographs
- **Mesenteric Adenitis**
  - Likely due to viral etiologies
  - Imaging: Classic definition is cluster of ≥ 3 enlarged lymph nodes, each ≥ 5 mm in size (in short axis)
    - Nodes retain normal architecture with fatty hilum
      - Note that prominent mesenteric & right lower quadrant (RLQ) lymph nodes are common in children
    - ± ↑ echogenicity of RLQ fat
    - Must see normal appendix; diagnosis of exclusion
    - Associated bowel wall thickening is uncommon & necessitates further work-up
- **Crohn Disease**
  - Abdominal pain, diarrhea, weight loss
  - Anemia, leukocytosis, ↑ CRP, ↑ ESR, ↑ fecal calprotectin, p-ANCA(-), ASCA(+), HLA-B27
  - Imaging: Bowel wall thickening, mural stratification, mucosal hyperenhancement, engorged vasa recta
    - Concurrent appendix involvement is common; isolated appendix involvement is rare
    - Skip lesions, occurring anywhere along GI tract (mouth to anus); TI most common
    - Complications include strictures, fistulae, abscesses
  - Extraintestinal manifestations: Peripheral arthritis, ankylosing spondylitis, sacroiliitis, ocular inflammation, erythema nodosum, pyoderma gangrenosum

Helpful Clues for Less Common Diagnoses

- **Obstructing Renal/Ureteral Calculus**
  - Intermittent colicky pain (may radiate to groin/scrotum), hematuria
  - Imaging: Echogenic shadowing focus in urinary tract with associated collecting system dilation
    - Twinkling artifact on Doppler
    - Absent ipsilateral ureteral jet
    - Delayed nephrogram on CT; surrounding fat stranding
- **Hemorrhagic Ovarian Cyst**
  - More common than ovarian torsion
  - Imaging: Avascular ovarian cystic mass
    - Variable appearance depending on age of blood products
      - May be uniform, have layering debris level, or have reticular lace-like echogenicity due to retracted echogenic clot
    - Majority show increased through transmission
    - Normal ovarian tissue (with normal flow) is often splayed by cyst
      - However, cysts > 5 cm are at increased risk of superimposed torsion
    - Resolves on short-term follow-up

- **Ovarian Torsion**
  - Imaging: Enlarged ovary, > 5x contralateral side
    - Torsed ovary will not be < 20 mL in volume in postpubertal patient
    - Heterogeneous parenchyma with peripheral follicles; may not be recognizable as ovary
      - Underlying cyst or dermoid is common
    - May be displaced to midline or contralateral side
      - Pelvic mass in female patient with acute pain & inability to identify 2 normal ovaries is torsion until proven otherwise
    - Flow may be preserved due to dual blood supply or torsion/detorsion
      - May be asymmetric to normal side
- **Pyelonephritis**
  - Infected urine, fever, flank pain
  - Imaging: Increased or decreased parenchymal echogenicity, typically at pole kidney
    - Loss of corticomedullary differentiation
    - Striated nephrogram or wedge-shaped hypoenhancing area
    - Regional decreased perfusion on Doppler
    - ± abscess (may mimic small cystic or heterogeneous infiltrative mass)
- **Pneumonia**
  - Lower lobe pneumonia may present as abdominal pain
  - Imaging: Scrutinize lung bases for round or fluffy opacity on all studies
- **Omental Infarct**
  - Imaging: Triangular or ill-defined soft tissue mass with increased echogenicity/density
    - Typical location at RLQ
- **Epiploic Appendagitis**
  - Imaging: Hyperechoic oval mass adjacent to colonic wall; may appear similar to omental infarct
    - Fat density with hyperattenuating rim on CT
- **Meckel Diverticulum**
  - Occult or frank lower GI bleeding, abdominal pain, vomiting
  - Imaging: Blind-ending tubular structure arising from distal ileum, ± inflammation &/or obstruction
    - Actual diverticulum may not be visualized
    - Focal radiotracer uptake with Tc-99m pertechnetate scan if causing bleeding

Helpful Clues for Rare Diagnoses

- **Neutropenic Colitis (Typhlitis)**
  - Neutropenic patient, typically with absolute neutrophil count < 500 cells/μL
  - Most common at right colon but can involve other areas of colon or small bowel
  - Imaging: Bowel wall thickening & pericolonic inflammatory changes
    - ± pneumatosis
- **Pelvic Inflammatory Disease**
  - Sexually active female patient, cervical motion tenderness, vaginal discharge, fever
    - Consider abuse as underlying cause in younger children with pelvic inflammatory disease (PID)
  - Imaging: May be normal early in disease
    - Prominent ovaries adherent to uterus in salpingo-oophoritis
    - Pyosalpinx, tuboovarian abscess, complex free fluid
    - Pelvic floor inflammatory change & stranding
- **Ectopic Pregnancy**
  - β-HCG positive sexually active female patient with pain & vaginal bleeding
  - Serial β-HCG to differentiate ectopic from early/failing intrauterine pregnancy (IUP) or demise if no IUP is visualized
  - Imaging: Pseudogestational sac, heterogeneous mass, tubal ring sign, hemoperitoneum

SELECTED REFERENCES

1. Hijaz NM et al: Managing acute abdominal pain in pediatric patients: current perspectives. Pediatric Health Med Ther. 8:83-91, 2017
2. Ullah I et al: Epiploic appendagitis: a rare cause of chronic right lower quadrant pain in a child. J Pediatr. 182:400-400.e1, 2017
3. Chang PT et a : Diagnostic errors of right lower quadrant pain in children: beyond appendicitis. Abdom Imaging. 40(7):2071-90, 2015

Appendicitis

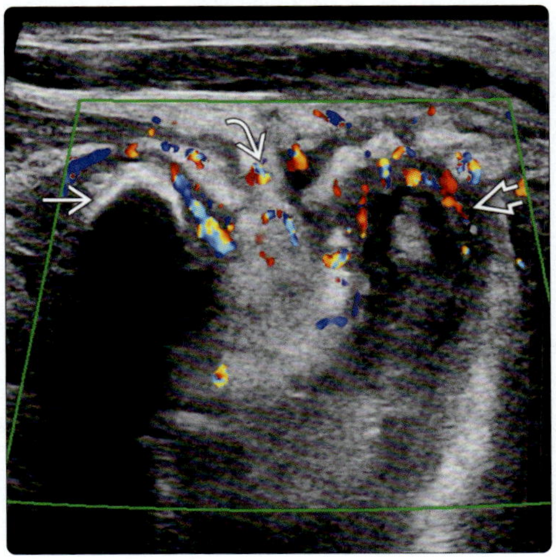

Appendicitis

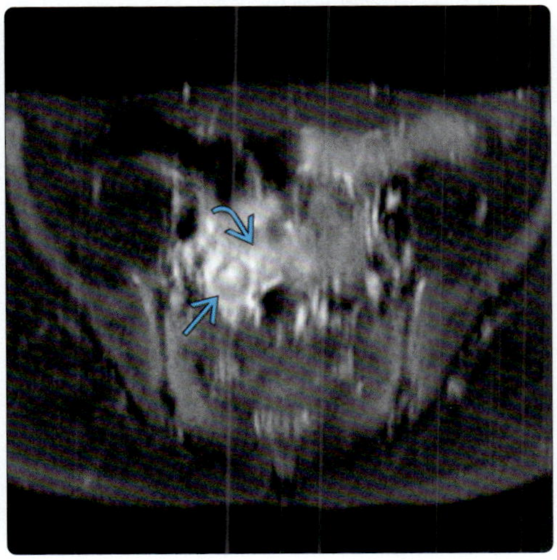

(Left) *Transverse color Doppler ultrasound from a 5 year old with right lower quadrant (RLQ) pain shows a shadowing appendicolith ➡ & an enlarged, hyperemic appendiceal tip ➡ distally. The periappendiceal fat is thickened, echogenic, & hyperemic ➡.* **(Right)** *Axial T2 FS MR from a 13 year old with leukocytosis, RLQ pain, & vomiting shows increased signal intensity of the enlarged appendix ➡ & periappendiceal tissues ➡, consistent with appendicitis.*

(Left) *Axial CECT shows a dilated & hyperemic appendix* ➔*, measuring 11 mm in diameter. There is mild inflammation of the surrounding fat* ➔ *+ a small amount of free intraperitoneal fluid* ➔*.* **(Right)** *Axial CECT shows RLQ colonic wall thickening* ➔ *as compared to a normal colonic wall in the left abdomen* ➔*. This teenager's stool culture was positive for Salmonella. Infectious enteritis/enterocolitis is more frequently imaged by ultrasound in children, usually to exclude other etiologies.*

Appendicitis

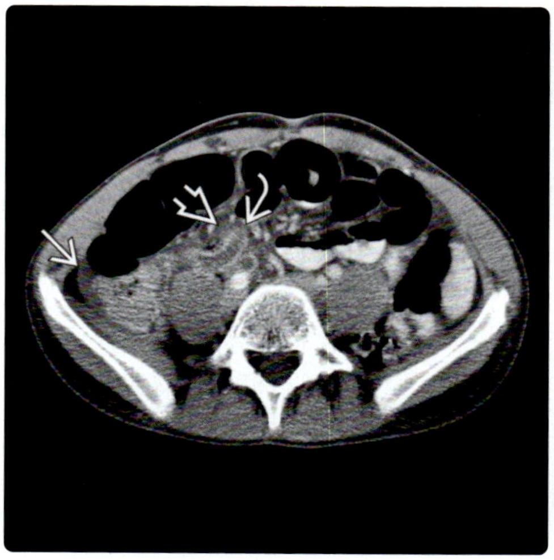

Infectious Enteritis & Enterocolitis

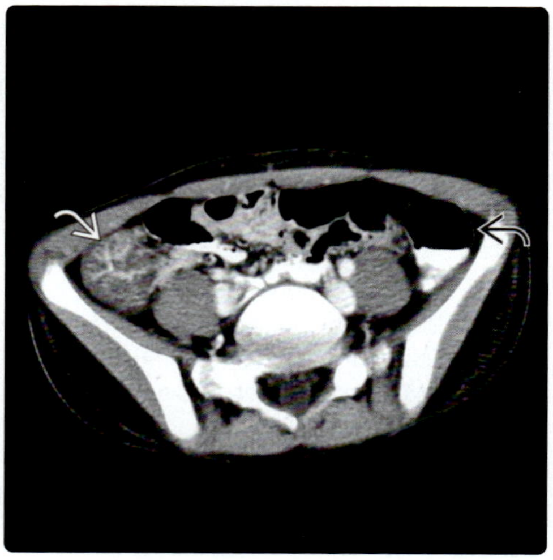

(Left) *Transverse ultrasound from a 3 year old with intermittent abdominal pain demonstrates a RLQ mass with a target sign* ➔ *(due to layers of intussuscepted bowel, fat, vessels, & lymph nodes within the outer intussuscipiens). The mean diameter of the intussusception is 2.6 cm when ileocolic.* **(Right)** *Supine air enema image obtained during reduction of the ileocolic intussusception in the same patient shows the filling defect of the intussusceptum* ➔*, now pushed retrograde to the right colon.*

Ileocolic Intussusception

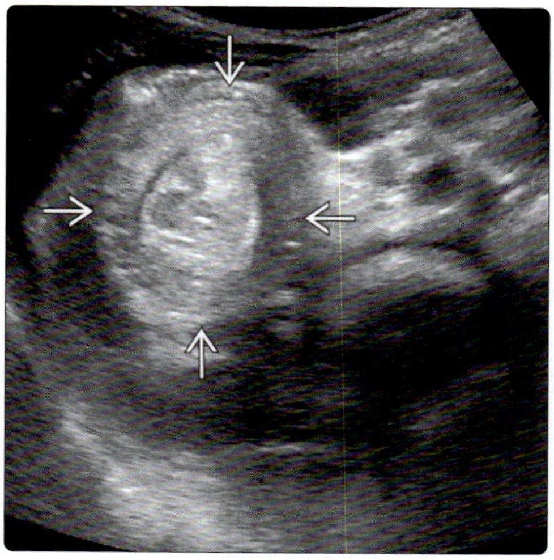

Ileocolic Intussusception

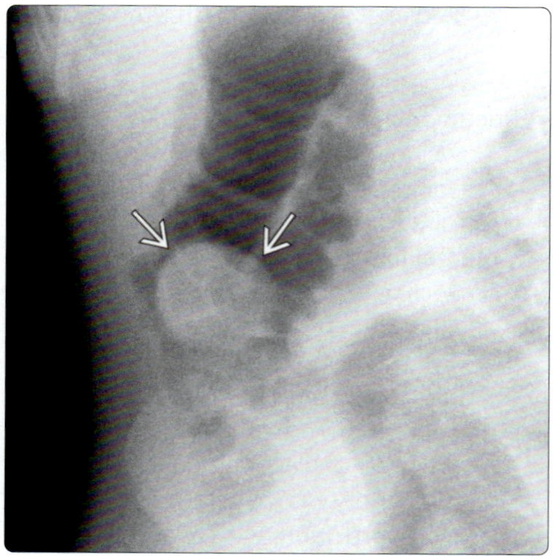

(Left) *Axial ultrasound shows a cluster of prominent lymph nodes* ➔ *in the RLQ. This qualifies as mesenteric adenitis with > 3 lymph nodes at ≥ 5 mm in short-axis diameter. In the absence of a visible adjacent source of inflammation, this is most likely reactive to viral inflammation.* **(Right)** *Coronal T2 FS MR enterography in a 13 year old with Crohn disease shows thickening of the terminal ileum with luminal narrowing & increased signal in the bowel wall* ➔ *& surrounding tissues.*

Mesenteric Adenitis

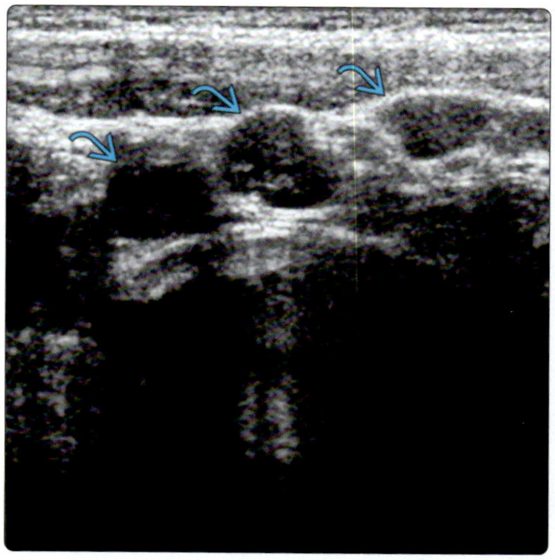

Crohn Disease

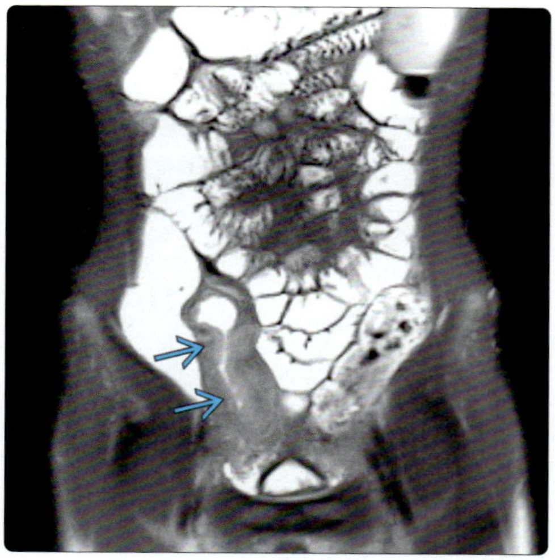

Obstructing Renal/Ureteral Calculus

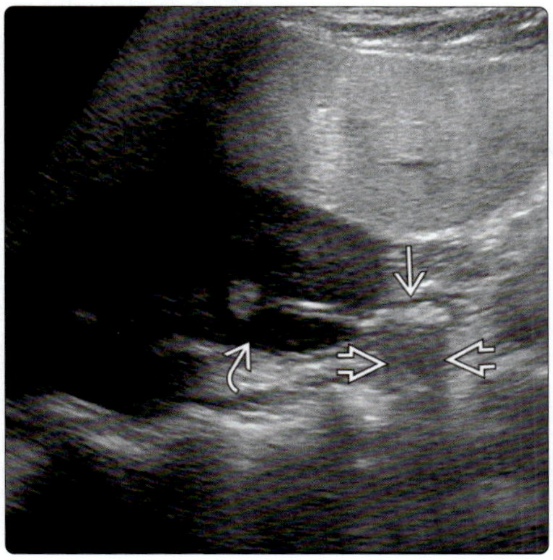

Obstructing Renal/Ureteral Calculus

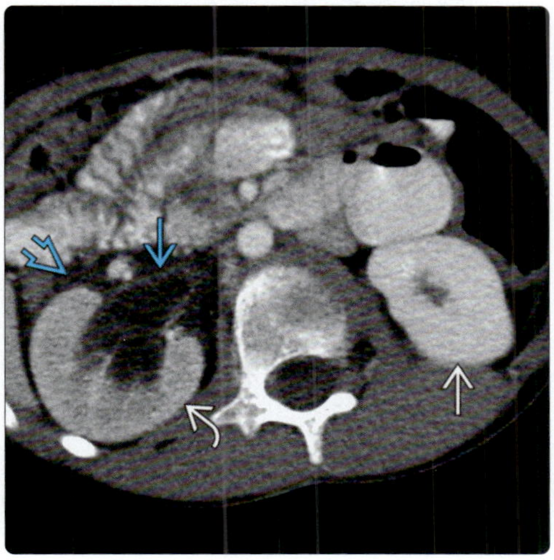

(Left) *Transverse ultrasound from a 17 year old with colicky abdominal pain shows an echogenic stone with posterior acoustic shadowing at the proximal ureter with associated collecting system dilation.* **(Right)** *Axial CECT shows an obstructed, enlarged right kidney with delayed parenchymal enhancement relative to the left kidney. Note the collecting system dilation & perinephric fluid. A 1-cm midureteral calculus (not shown) was identified on this study.*

Hemorrhagic Ovarian Cyst

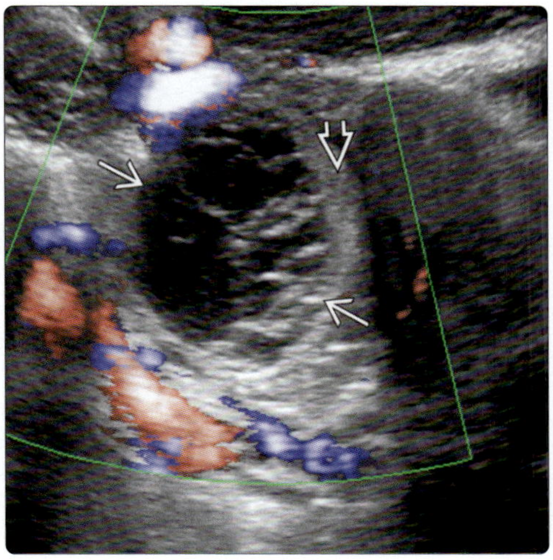

Ovarian Torsion

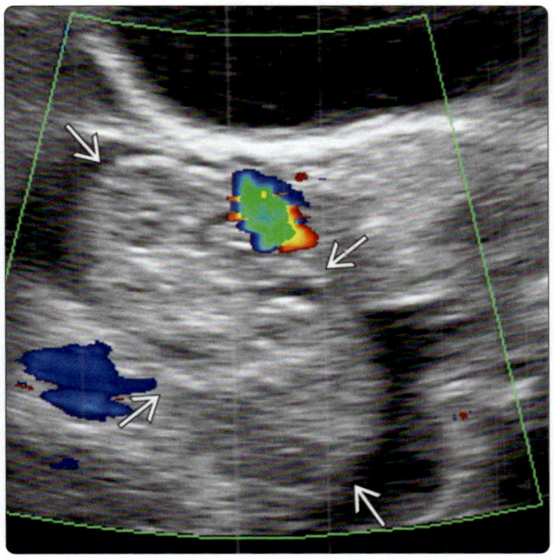

(Left) *Transverse color Doppler ultrasound from a 16-year-old female patient with RLQ pain shows an avascular cystic mass in the right ovary with a reticular lace-like pattern, consistent with a hemorrhagic cyst. A rim of ovarian parenchyma is noted. This cyst resolved on follow-up imaging.* **(Right)** *Transverse color Doppler ultrasound depicts an enlarged right ovary without flow in a 15-year-old female patient with ovarian torsion. The right ovary volume was 34 mL, compared to < 5 mL on the left.*

Ovarian Torsion

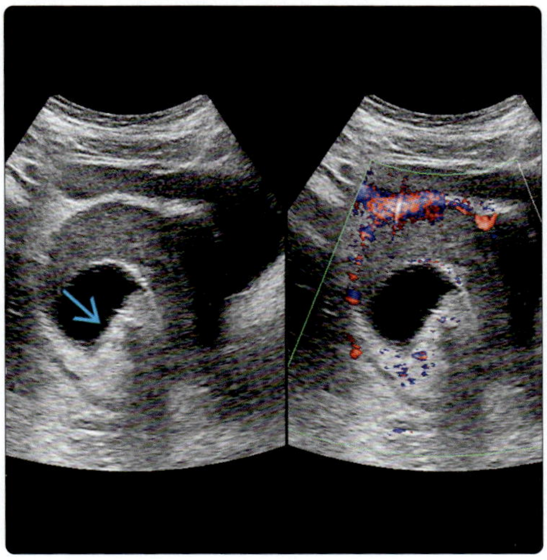

Ovarian Torsion

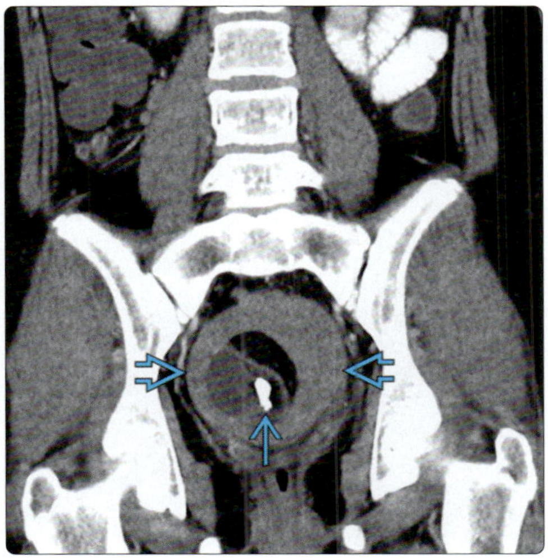

(Left) *Transverse grayscale (left) & color Doppler (right) ultrasound images in a 13 year old with RLQ pain show an avascular mass in the pelvic midline containing a debris-fluid level. While a normal right ovary was seen (not shown), no left ovary could be identified.* **(Right)** *Coronal CECT in the same patient shows that the round mass contains fluid, fat, & Ca^{2+}, consistent with a dermoid. The mass lies within a torsed left ovary.*

(**Left**) *Longitudinal color Doppler ultrasound in a 7 year old with pyelonephritis demonstrates increased parenchymal echogenicity of the upper pole* ➡ *with diminished corticomedullary differentiation & perfusion.* (**Right**) *Axial CECT shows patchy, wedged-shaped foci of hypoenhancement of the right kidney* ➡ *(a.k.a. striated nephrogram), commonly seen with acute pyelonephritis. No abscess or perinephric fluid was detected on this study.*

Pyelonephritis

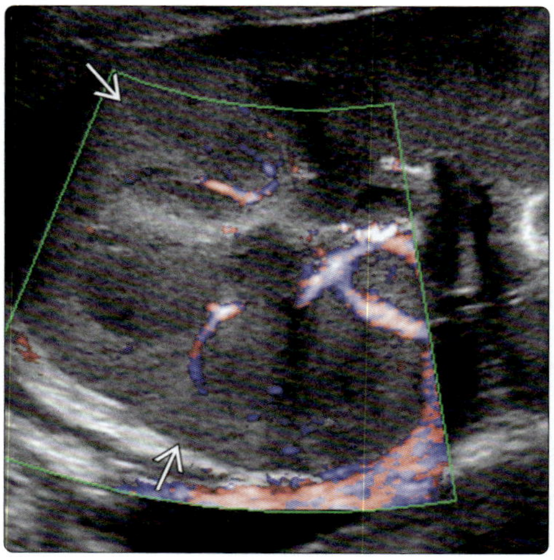

Pyelonephritis

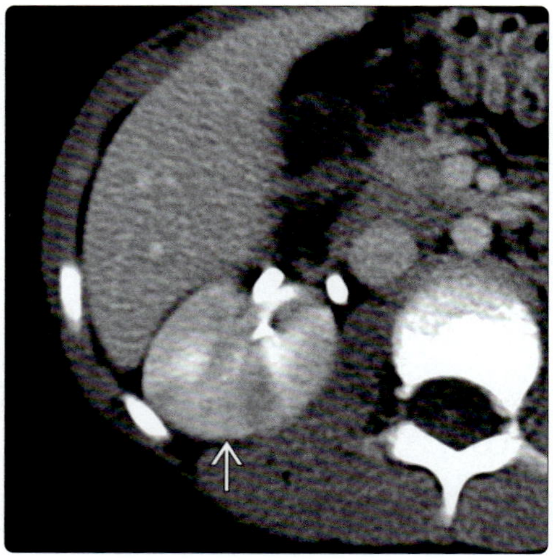

(**Left**) *Upright radiograph shows an ovoid opacity* ➡ *at the medial right lung base, hiding behind the hemidiaphragm. There is no rib splaying or erosion to suggest a neuroblastoma. This was, in fact, a right lower lobe pneumonia in a child who presented with abdominal pain.* (**Right**) *Axial CECT from an 8 year old depicts an ill-defined area of increased attenuation* ➡ *between the anterior abdominal wall & colon, consistent with an omental infarction.*

Pneumonia

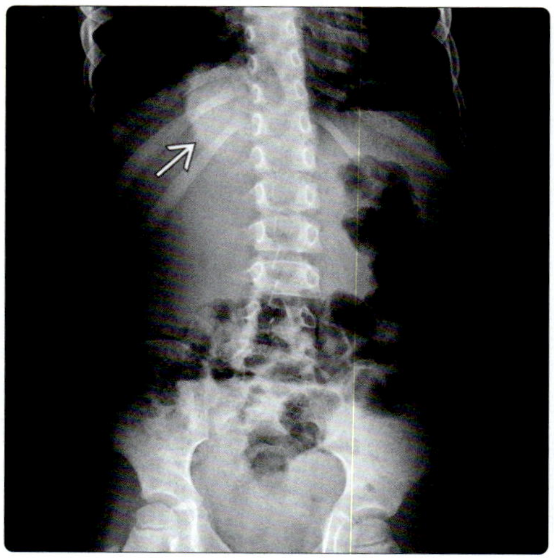

Omental Infarct

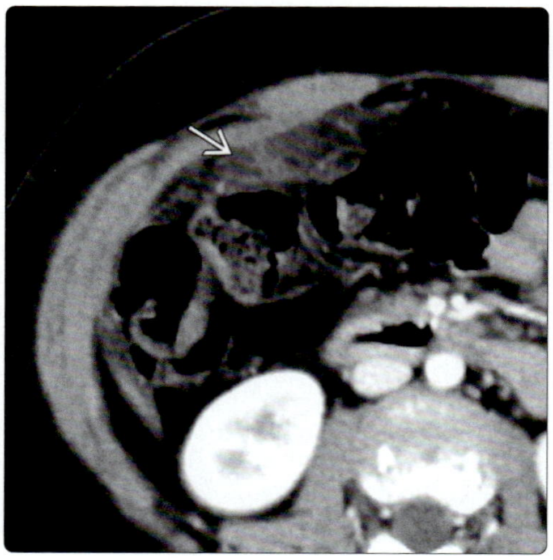

(**Left**) *Transverse ultrasound of the RLQ at a site of tenderness shows a focus of echogenic fat* ➡*, consistent with epiploic appendagitis in an 8 year old with RLQ pain.* (**Right**) *Axial CECT shows a small, oval mass* ➡ *adjacent to the sigmoid colon. It has a fat density core & an enhancing rim with inflammation of the adjacent mesenteric fat, consistent with epiploic appendagitis.*

Epiploic Appendagitis

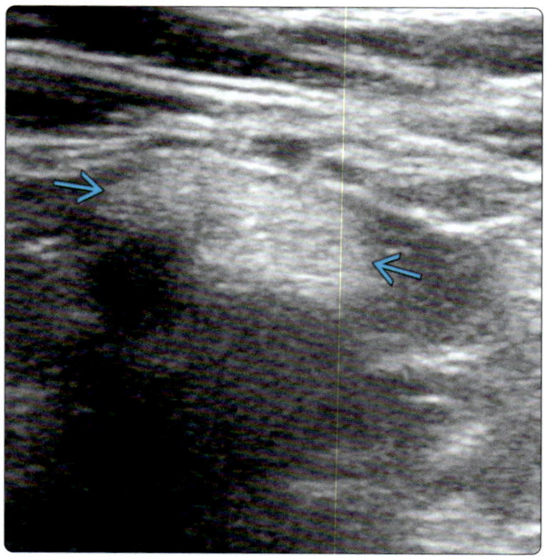

Epiploic Appendagitis

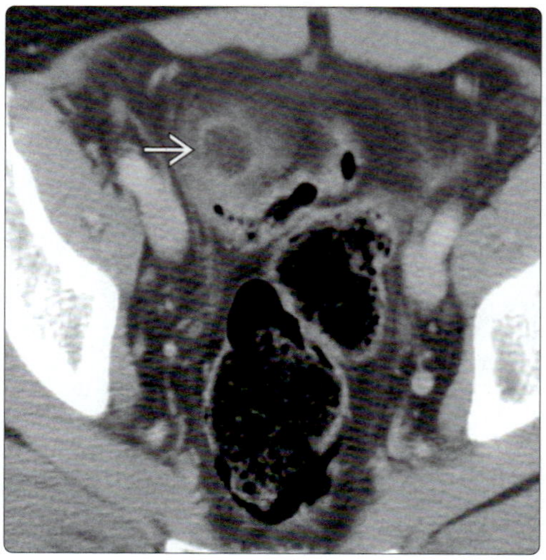

Meckel Diverticulum

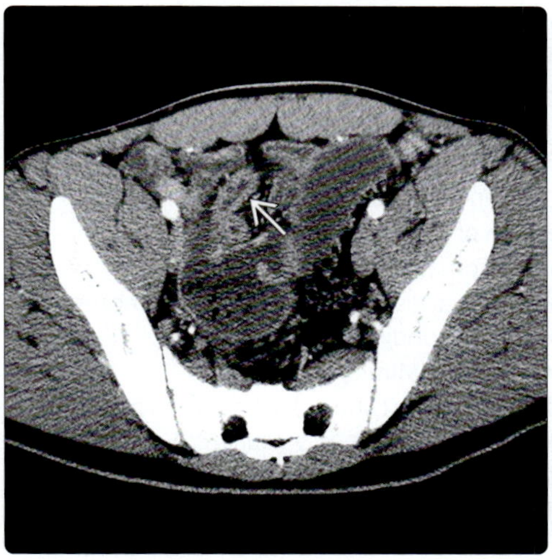

Meckel Diverticulum

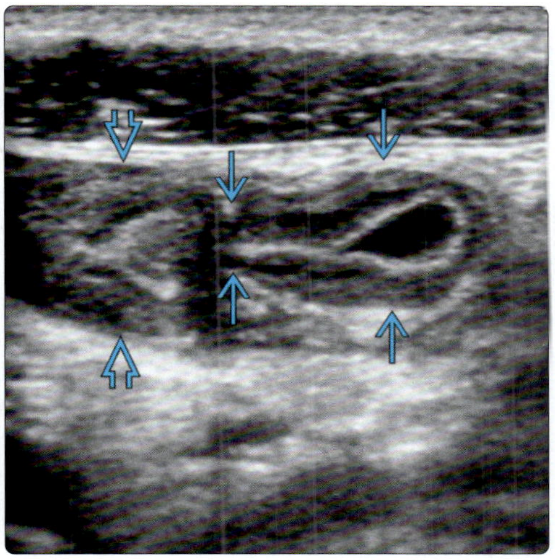

(Left) *Axial CECT shows a blind-ending tubular structure with thickened walls in the RLQ. A normal appendix, not shown here, was also present. A Meckel diverticulum was identified at surgery. These frequently present with GI bleeding, bowel obstruction, or inflammation.* **(Right)** *Longitudinal ultrasound shows a Meckel diverticulum as a blind-ending tubular structure with "gut signature" arising from the terminal ileum in a 14 year old with a history of intussusception.*

Neutropenic Colitis

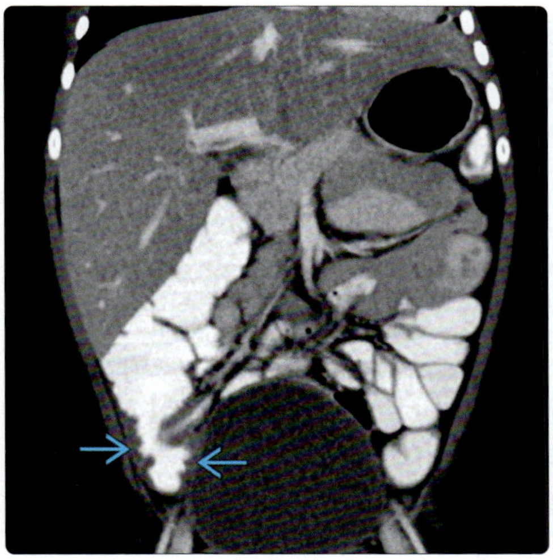

Neutropenic Colitis

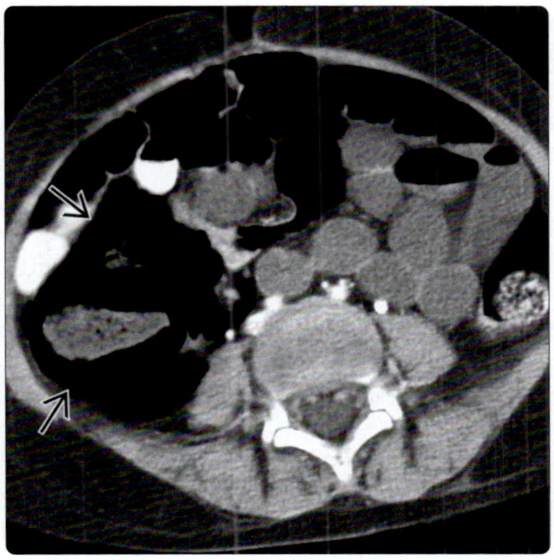

(Left) *Coronal CECT in a 2 year old with leukemia, febrile neutropenia, & pain shows wall thickening & irregularity of the cecum in the RLQ, consistent with neutropenic colitis.* **(Right)** *Axial CECT in a patient with leukemia shows gas circumferentially within the wall of the ascending colon, consistent with pneumatosis. No bowel wall thickening, abscess, or ascites was detected in this child to suggest ischemia. Note that benign pneumatosis from steroids could also have this appearance.*

Pelvic Inflammatory Disease

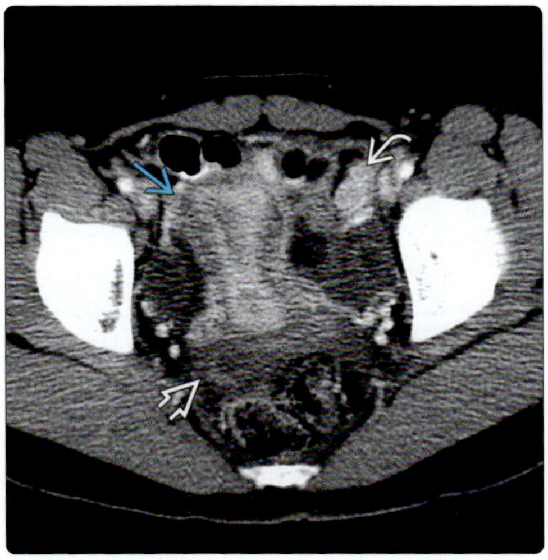

Ectopic Pregnancy

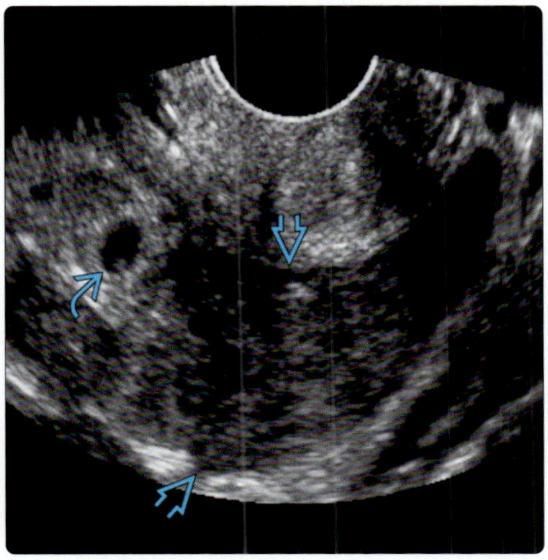

(Left) *Axial CECT shows an inflamed, edematous uterus as well as a thickened, hyperenhancing left fallopian tube. A portion of a posterior cul-de-sac abscess is also seen in this patient with pelvic inflammatory disease.* **(Right)** *Transverse transvaginal ultrasound shows a thick-walled extrauterine gestational sac as well as a large, heterogeneous, predominantly hypoechoic acute hematoma in the cul-de-sac.*

DIFFERENTIAL DIAGNOSIS

Common

- Acute Purulent Appendicitis
- Lymphoid Hyperplasia

Less Common

- Inflammatory Bowel Disease
- Fecal Distention of Appendix (Mimic)
- Meckel Diverticulitis (Mimic)
- Ileocolic Intussusception
- Cystic Fibrosis
- Burkitt Lymphoma

Rare but Important

- Necrotizing Enterocolitis
- Mucocele

ESSENTIAL INFORMATION

Helpful Clues for Common Diagnoses

- **Acute Purulent Appendicitis**
    - Fever, anorexia, nausea, vomiting, right lower quadrant (RLQ) tenderness are typical ± elevated WBC
    - Diameter of noncompressible appendix are typically > 6 mm, but specificity increases significantly with
        - Periappendiceal fat infiltration & fluid; ± appendiceal hyperemia, fecalith, fluid-filled lumen
    - Terminal ileum & cecum are not usually thickened in absence of appendiceal perforation
- **Lymphoid Hyperplasia**
    - Hypoechoic wall (lamina propria) of appendix is usually < 1 mm in thickness
    - Wall thickening often occurs with other illnesses (e.g., gastroenteritis, mesenteric adenitis)
    - May also occur with viral "pink" appendicitis & classic purulent appendicitis
    - Lack of surrounding inflammatory change makes superimposed operative purulent appendicitis unlikely

Helpful Clues for Less Common Diagnoses

- **Inflammatory Bowel Disease**
    - Intermittent diarrhea, pain, bloody stools, anal fissures
    - Crohn disease or ulcerative colitis may involve appendix
        - Isolated appendiceal disease is rare; disproportionate involvement of terminal ileum &/or cecum is typical
        - Look for fistula, abscess, mesenteric vessel engorgement, fat proliferation
- **Fecal Distention of Appendix (Mimic)**
    - Usually asymptomatic
    - Echogenic material distends lumen of noncompressible appendix; no surrounding inflammation
- **Meckel Diverticulitis (Mimic)**
    - Inflamed, blind-ending tubular structure can mimic appendix (but is less commonly visualized)
    - More often presents with GI bleeding or obstruction
- **Ileocolic Intussusception**
    - Appendix is often abnormal due to underlying viral inflammation & lymphoid hyperplasia ± edema
    - Abnormal appendix may serve as lead point or rarely intussuscept in isolation
    - Inflammation from perforated appendicitis can mimic ileocolic intussusception but is typically limited to RLQ
- **Cystic Fibrosis**
    - Rate of appendicitis lower in cystic fibrosis (CF) than healthy population
    - Noninflamed appendix is usually > 6 mm in diameter in CF; no surrounding inflammation should be seen
- **Burkitt Lymphoma**
    - Bulky nodal masses with regions of marked bowel wall thickening, often without luminal narrowing
        - Appendix often involved, may not be discernible
    - Other visceral lesions (e.g., kidney) are usually present

Helpful Clues for Rare Diagnoses

- **Necrotizing Enterocolitis**: Neonatal appendiceal perforation may represent localized necrotizing enterocolitis; rarely suspected preoperatively
- **Mucocele**: Chronic cystic dilation of appendix
    - Layers of mucoid material: Onion skin sign

(Left) *Transverse ultrasound of the abdominal right lower quadrant (RLQ) in an 11 year old with 2 days of pain & vomiting shows a noncompressible, 9-mm diameter appendix with induration of the surrounding fat & mild periappendiceal fluid.* **(Right)** *Longitudinal color Doppler ultrasound in the same patient shows dilation of the hyperemic fluid-filled appendix, irregularity of the echogenic mucosal lining, & edema of the adjacent fat. Acute purulent appendicitis was confirmed at surgery.*

Acute Purulent Appendicitis

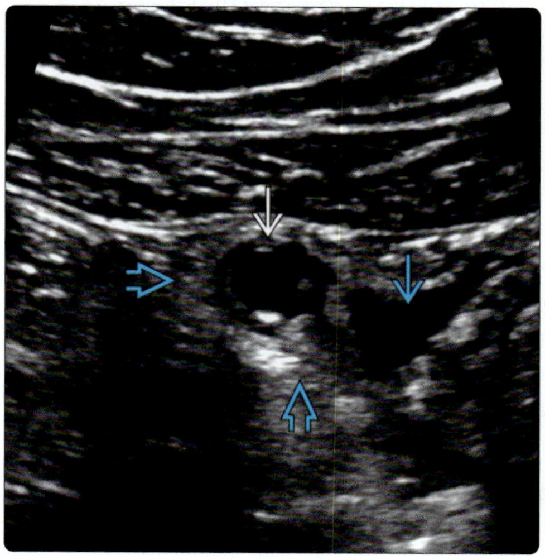

Acute Purulent Appendicitis

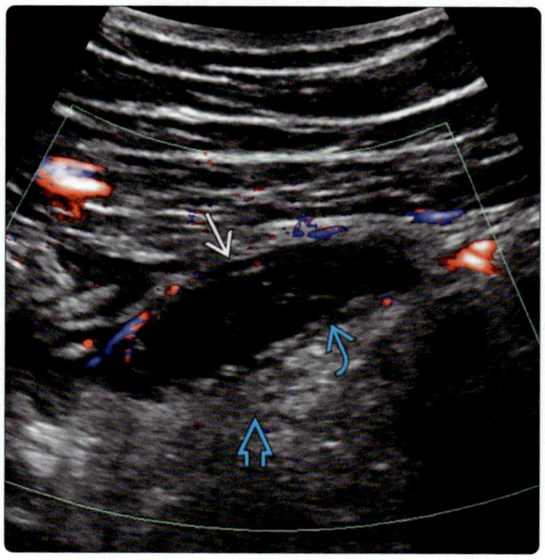

Lymphoid Hyperplasia

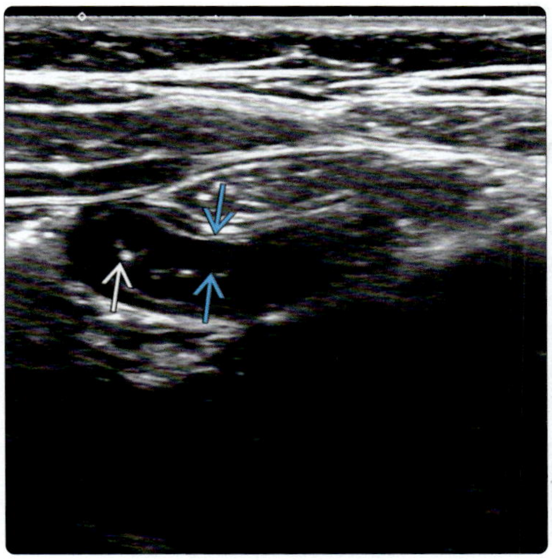

Inflammatory Bowel Disease

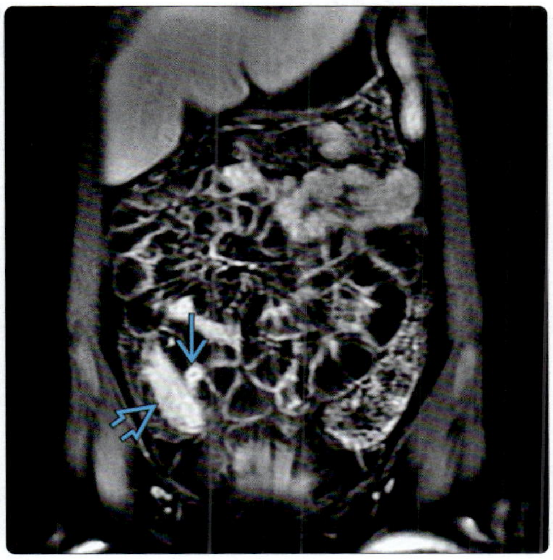

(Left) *Transverse ultrasound in a 5 year old with RLQ pain shows wall thickening of the appendix at > 2 mm ➔. The appendiceal lumen, with echogenic contents, is collapsed ➔, & there is no surrounding inflammation. The overall diameter was 6 mm. The patient was managed conservatively without complication.* **(Right)** *Coronal T1 C+ FS MR in a 16 year old with 2 months of abdominal pain & a perianal fissure shows abnormal thickening of the terminal ileum ➔ & adjacent appendix ➔. Biopsies confirmed Crohn disease.*

Fecal Distention of Appendix (Mimic)

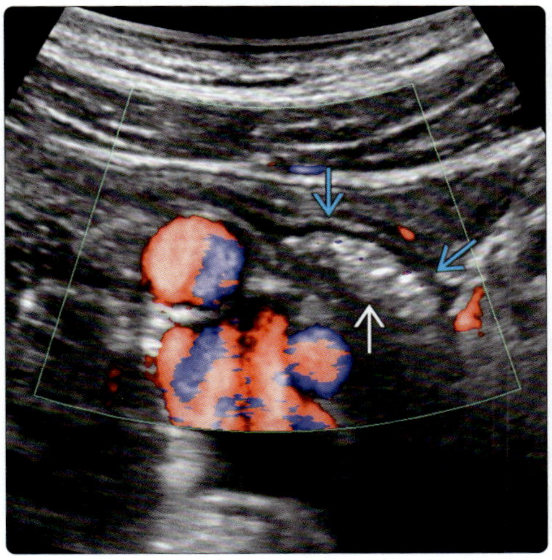

Meckel Diverticulitis (Mimic)

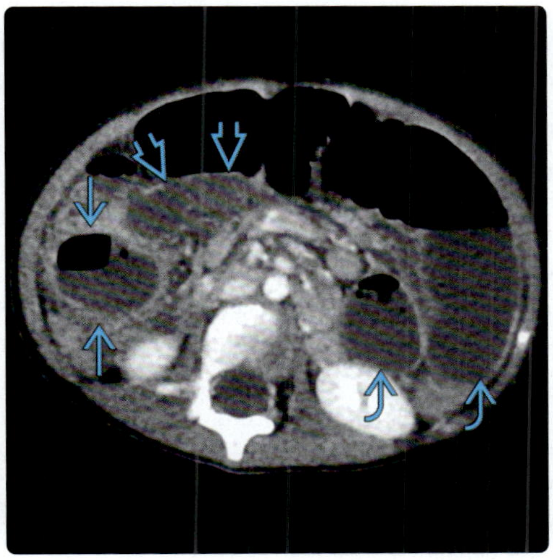

(Left) *Transverse color Doppler ultrasound in a patient with RLQ pain shows a noncompressible, 8-mm appendix ➔ diffusely distended by echogenic fecal material ➔. No surrounding inflammation was seen. The patient was managed conservatively without complication.* **(Right)** *Axial CECT in a 5 year old with pain & vomiting shows an abscess ➔ contiguous with a fluid-distended, blind-ending tubular structure ➔ that was found to be a perforated Meckel diverticulum. Note the small bowel obstruction ➔.*

Cystic Fibrosis

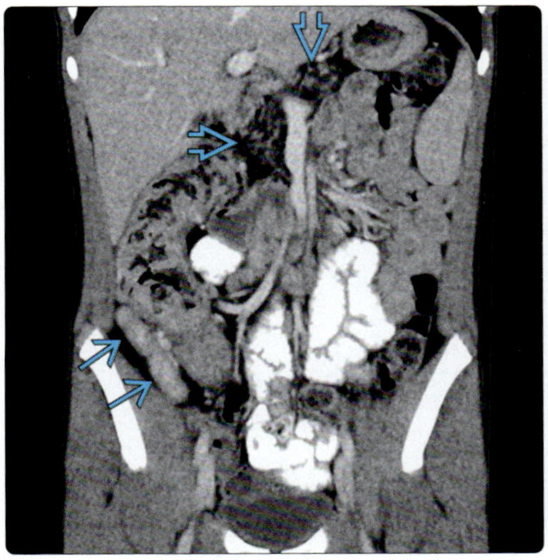

Burkitt Lymphoma

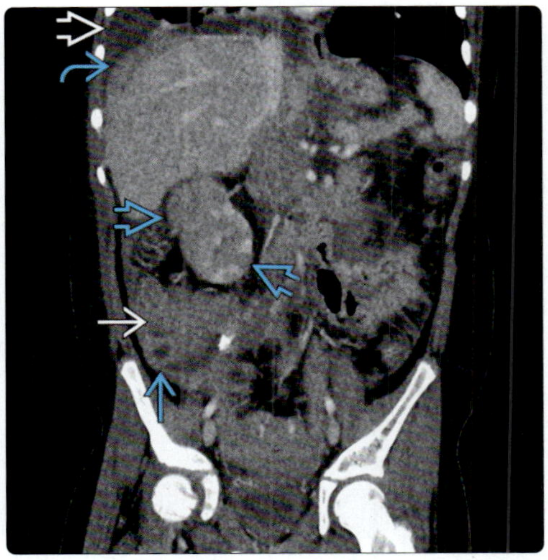

(Left) *Coronal CECT in a 10 year old with cystic fibrosis (CF) & a palpable mass (due to a stool ball) shows a common appendiceal appearance in CF: Dilation without surrounding inflammation ➔. The pancreatic fatty replacement ➔ is also typical of CF.* **(Right)** *Coronal CECT in an 8 year old with abdominal pain shows an abnormal appendix ➔ within an infiltrative lymphomatous mass ➔. Involvement of the kidneys ➔, diaphragm ➔, & pleura ➔ was also noted.*

DIFFERENTIAL DIAGNOSIS

Common

- Idiopathic Ileocolic Intussusception
- Ileocolic Intussusception With Lead Point
- Small Bowel-Small Bowel Intussusception
- Edematous Ileocecal Valve (Mimic)

Less Common

- Perforated Appendicitis (Mimic)
- Meckel Diverticulum (Mimic)
- Hypertrophic Pyloric Stenosis (Mimic)

Rare but Important

- Lymphoma (Mimic)

ESSENTIAL INFORMATION

Key Differential Diagnosis Issues

- Size, location, & presence of central mesenteric fat & lymph nodes differentiate small bowel-small bowel (SB-SB) from ileocolic intussusception
  - Sweeping through entirety of intussusception on ultrasound, including uninvolved proximal & distal bowel, will help discern types & mimics

Helpful Clues for Common Diagnoses

- **Idiopathic Ileocolic Intussusception**
  - Most common between 3 months & 3 years of age
  - Almost always located in right abdomen, though may extend into left abdomen & pelvis
    - Normal insertion of terminal ileum at cecum not seen
  - Target sign size (diameter of intussusception) > 2 cm
    - > 3 cm is more specific for ileocolic type
  - Lymph nodes & mesenteric fat seen in intussusceptum
    - Fat core diameter:outer wall thickness ratio > 1
- **Ileocolic Intussusception With Lead Point**
  - < 3 months old or > 3 years old raises suspicion
  - Focal mass or bowel wall abnormality may or may not be identified prospectively on imaging
    - Meckel diverticulum, intestinal polyp, enteric duplication cyst, intramural hematoma, lymphoma
  - Difficult or failed reduction at enema is common
- **Small Bowel-Small Bowel Intussusception**
  - Usually < 2 cm in diameter
  - Little fat & lymph nodes in intussusceptum
    - Fat core diameter:wall thickness ratio < 1
  - Most often idiopathic & transient
    - Length > 3.5 cm is more likely to require intervention
- **Edematous Ileocecal Valve (Mimic)**
  - Filling defect persists in medial cecum after successful air enema reduction of intussusception
  - Aperistaltic donut sign: Broad hypoechoic rim & echogenic center, lacks invaginated mesentery

Helpful Clues for Less Common Diagnoses

- **Perforated Appendicitis (Mimic)**
  - Blind-ending tubular structure arises from cecum
  - Look for surrounding indurated/echogenic fat
  - ± complex fluid collection with swirling debris
- **Meckel Diverticulum (Mimic)**
  - Blind-ending tubular structure arises from antimesenteric border of ileum; can appear cyst-like
- **Hypertrophic Pyloric Stenosis (Mimic)**
  - Age: 3 weeks to 3 months
  - Presents with projectile, nonbilious emesis
  - Thickening of pyloric muscle & elongation of channel persist throughout ultrasound
    - Found focally at junction of stomach & duodenum

Helpful Clues for Rare Diagnoses

- **Lymphoma (Mimic)**
  - Bowel wall thickening > 1 cm ± bulky mass
  - ± other lymph node conglomerates, visceral masses, & splenomegaly

SELECTED REFERENCES

1. Edwards EA et al: Intussusception: past, present and future. Pediatr Radiol. 47(9):1101-08, 2017
2. Kitazono MT et al: Intussusception: edematous ileocecal valve mimicking incomplete reduction. Pediatr Emerg Care. 28(3):300-1, 2012

(Left) *Transverse right abdominal ultrasound in an 8 year old with pain shows a target sign → with abundant mesenteric fat → & lymph nodes → centrally, consistent with an ileocolic intussusception.* **(Right)** *Longitudinal ultrasound of the right abdomen shows focal hypoechoic bowel wall thickening → serving as a lead point for an ileocolic intussusception →. Pathology demonstrated a non-Hodgkin lymphoma.*

Idiopathic Ileocolic Intussusception

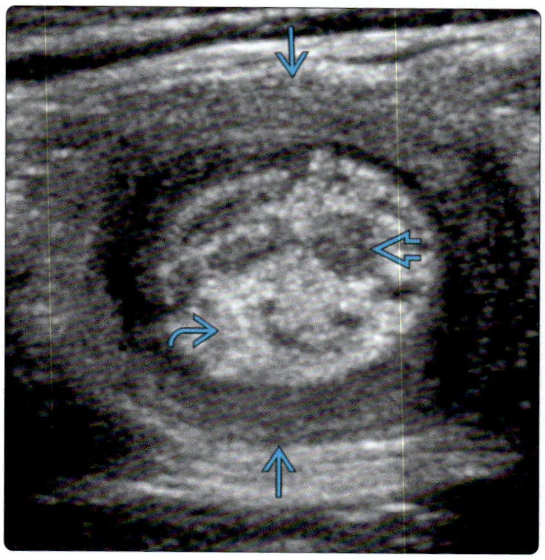

Ileocolic Intussusception With Lead Point

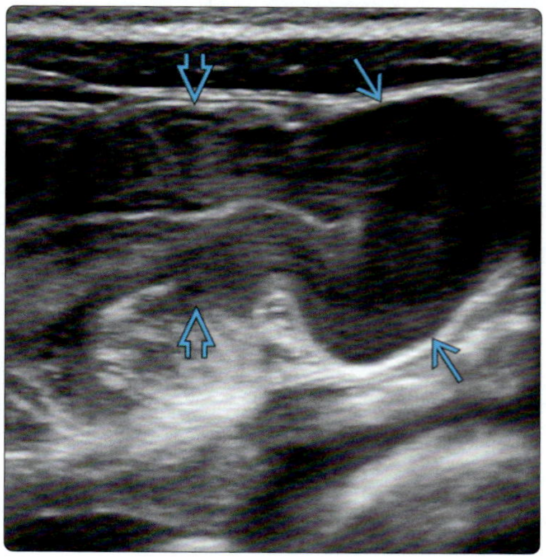

Ileocolic Intussusception With Lead Point

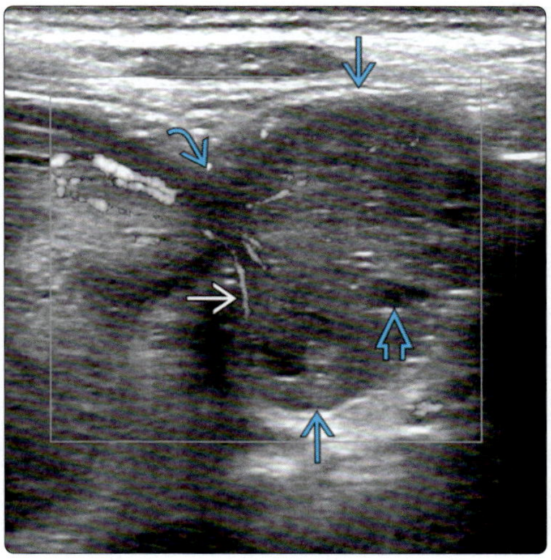

Ileocolic Intussusception With Lead Point

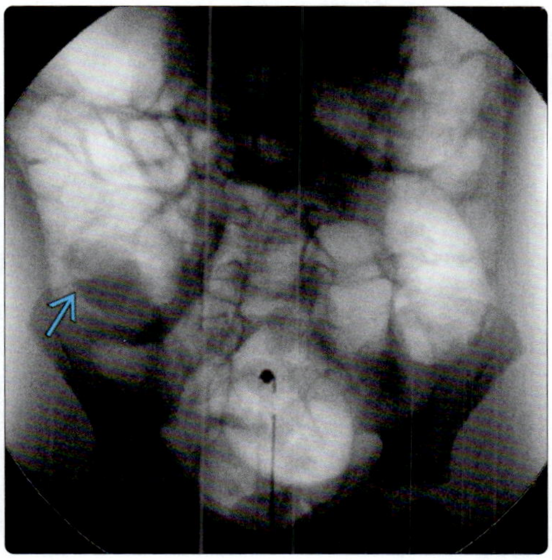

(Left) *Longitudinal ultrasound in a 3 year old shows a pedunculated lead point mass at the head of an intussusceptum. The mostly solid mass contains peripheral cysts & internal vascularity. Resection ultimately confirmed a juvenile polyp.* **(Right)** *Supine air enema image from the same patient demonstrates a persistent filling defect in the cecum status post reduction, consistent with the juvenile polyp. An edematous ileocecal valve is typically more round & medial.*

Small Bowel-Small Bowel Intussusception

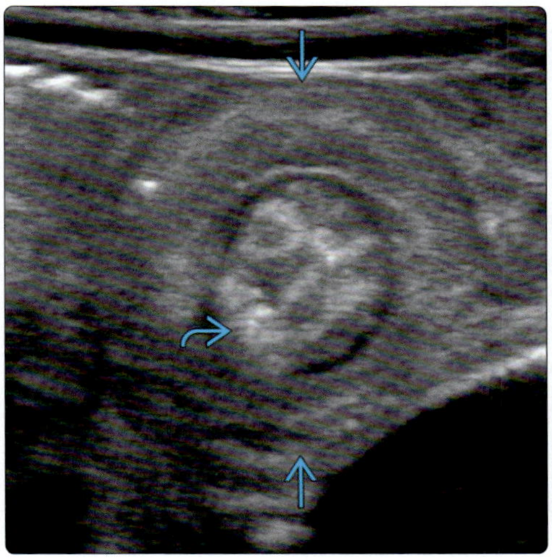

Perforated Appendicitis (Mimic)

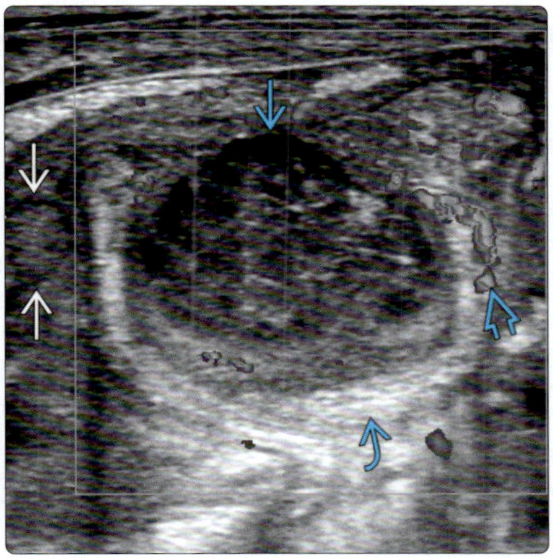

(Left) *Transverse ultrasound in a 7 year old with diarrhea shows a target sign with a diameter < 2 cm & minimal central echogenic fat, consistent with a small bowel-small bowel intussusception.* **(Right)** *Transverse ultrasound in a 2 year old (diagnosed with an intussusception on a preceding outside ultrasound, not shown) demonstrates a complex fluid collection with surrounding echogenic fat & hyperemia, mimicking a target sign. This image confirmed perforated appendicitis (partially visualized) with abscess.*

Hypertrophic Pyloric Stenosis (Mimic)

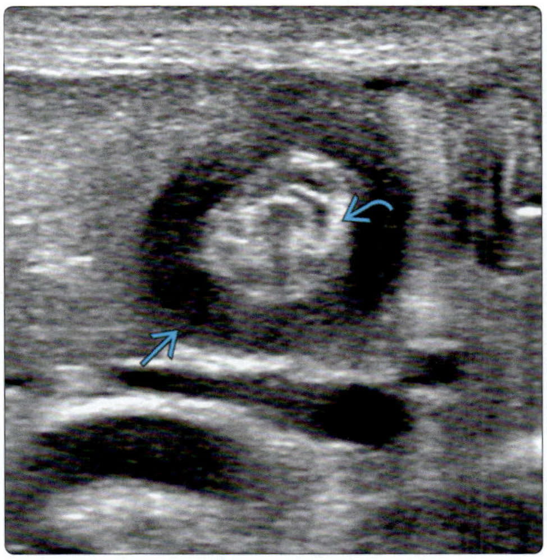

Lymphoma (Mimic)

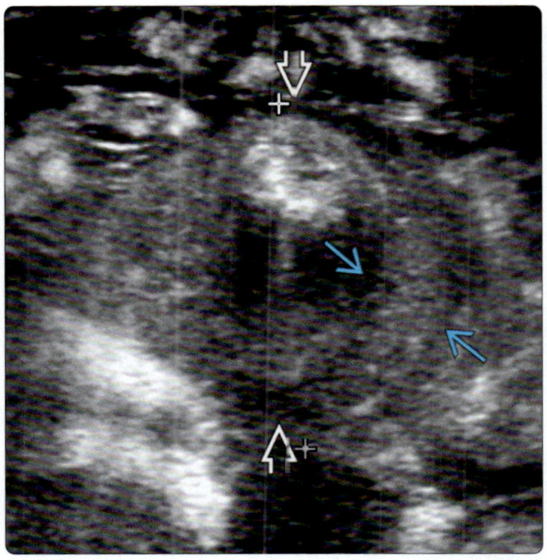

(Left) *Transverse ultrasound in a 4 week old with projectile emesis shows, in cross section, a thickened pyloric muscle & central echogenic mucosa, mimicking the appearance of an intussusception.* **(Right)** *Transverse ultrasound from an 8 year old with pain demonstrates a target-like appearance, mimicking an intussusception, though none was found during an air enema. The findings were due to marked appendiceal wall thickening > 1 cm. Non-Hodgkin lymphoma of the appendix was found at surgery.*

DIFFERENTIAL DIAGNOSIS

Common

- Crohn Disease
- Ulcerative Colitis
- Infectious Colitis
- Necrotizing Enterocolitis
- Cow's Milk Protein Allergy

Less Common

- Pseudomembranous Colitis
- Neutropenic Colitis
- Ischemic Colitis

Rare but Important

- Lymphoma (Mimic)
- Graft-vs.-Host Disease

ESSENTIAL INFORMATION

Key Differential Diagnosis Issues

- Age, medical history, & distribution limit considerations

Helpful Clues for Common Diagnoses

- **Crohn Disease**
  - Transmural involvement anywhere from mouth to anus, most common in terminal ileum
  - Skip lesions, penetrating disease (e.g., fistulae & abscesses), stricturing disease (e.g., proximal dilation), engorged vasa recta, fibrofatty proliferation
- **Ulcerative Colitis**
  - Contiguous involvement extends proximally from anus
  - Not transmural (i.e., no penetrating disease); loss of haustra, mural stratification, pseudopolyps
- **Infectious Colitis**
  - Nonspecific bowel wall thickening with varying distribution depending on infectious organism
- **Necrotizing Enterocolitis**
  - Prematurity (< 1,500 g, < 32 weeks gestation), bloody stools, feeding intolerance, distended abdomen
  - Pneumatosis, portal venous gas (PVG), fixed distended bowel loops, decreased peristalsis, bowel wall thickening or thinning, pneumoperitoneum, fluid collections
- **Cow's Milk Protein Allergy**
  - Primarily clinical diagnosis of newborns & infants
  - Bowel wall thickening & hyperemia most common at descending & sigmoid colon; irregularity & luminal narrowing at rectum may mimic Hirschsprung disease
  - Resolves after removal of cow's milk allergen from diet

Helpful Clues for Less Common Diagnoses

- **Pseudomembranous Colitis**
  - *Clostridium difficile* usually after antibiotic use
  - Typically pancolitis with bowel wall thickening > 10 mm
  - Accordion sign: Oral contrast between thickened haustra
- **Neutropenic Colitis**
  - Absolute neutrophil count < 500 cells/μL
  - Bowel wall thickening (low attenuation on CECT), pericolic inflammation, pneumatosis (more common than in other colitides after neonatal period); most commonly affects right colon
- **Ischemic Colitis**
  - Arterial compromise, venous insufficiency, shock
    - Midgut volvulus, thrombosis
  - Vascular distribution, bowel wall thinning or thickening, abnormal mucosal enhancement (absent, increased, or decreased), mesenteric edema, pneumatosis, PVG

Helpful Clues for Rare Diagnoses

- **Lymphoma (Mimic)**
  - Marked focal or diffuse hypoechoic bowel wall thickening; commonly involves terminal ileum
  - ± obstruction, intussusception, cavitation, perforation
  - ± adenopathy, other visceral lesions (e.g., kidneys, liver, lung)
- **Graft-vs.-Host Disease**
  - History of allogenic bone marrow or stem cell transplant
  - Diffuse intestinal wall thickening, mild fluid distention, featureless "mucosal" hyperenhancement (though mucosa often sloughed), lumen ribbon sign

Crohn Disease

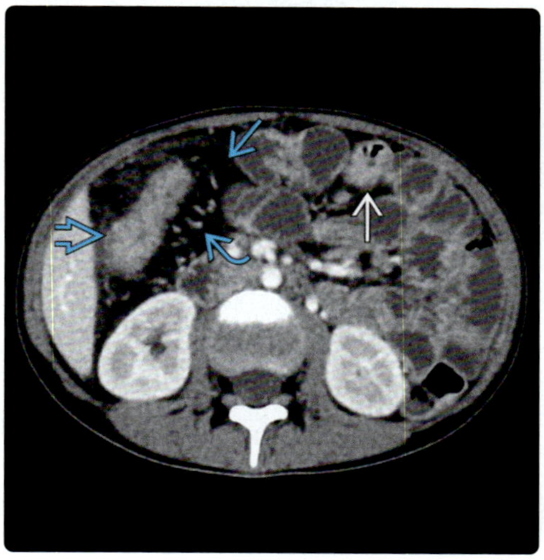

Ulcerative Colitis

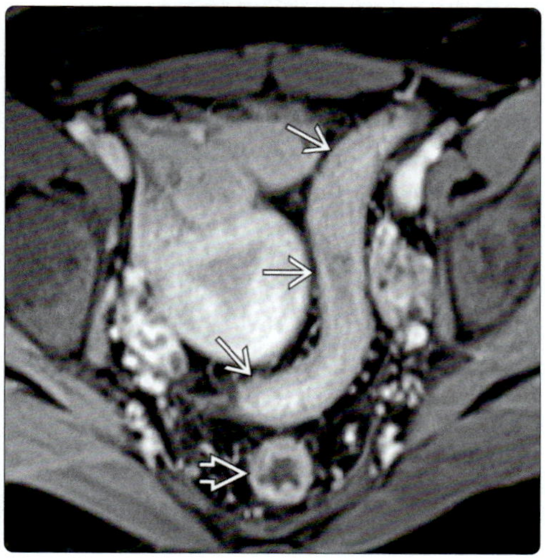

(Left) *Axial CECT in a 14 year old with pain & diarrhea shows hepatic flexure thickening with surrounding fatty proliferation, fat stranding, & vascular engorgement. There was contiguous involvement of the TI (not shown), along with skip lesions, typical of Crohn disease.* **(Right)** *Axial T1 C+ FS MR demonstrates wall thickening, increased enhancement, & loss of haustral folds of the sigmoid colon & rectum. These findings were contiguous, extending proximally from the anus, typical of ulcerative colitis.*

Necrotizing Enterocolitis

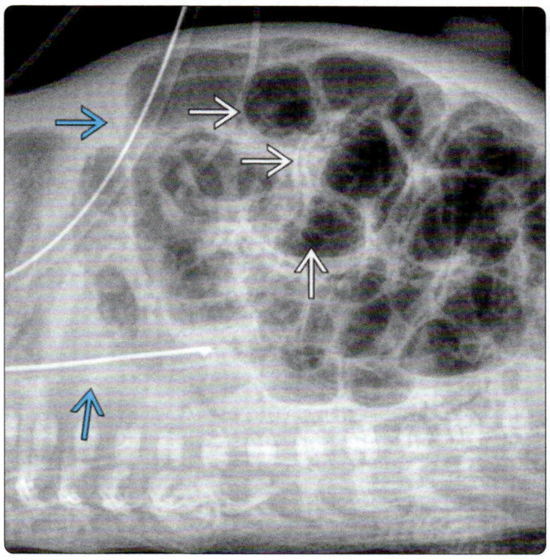

Pseudomembranous Colitis

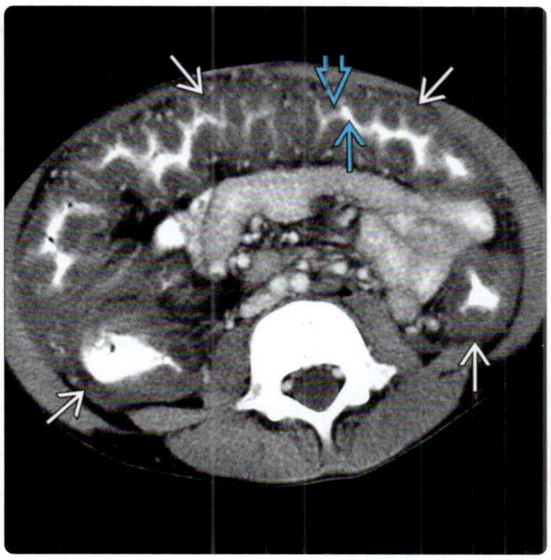

(Left) *Cross-table lateral radiograph of the abdomen in a former 27-week-gestation neonate with necrotizing enterocolitis demonstrates diffuse pneumatosis* ➡ *& branching hepatic lucencies due to portal venous gas* ⇨. **(Right)** *Axial CECT in a 10-year-old child with fever, abdominal pain, & diarrhea depicts pseudomembranous colitis with pancolonic marked wall thickening* ➡. *The alternating bands of hyperdense contrast* ⇨ *between the thickened fluid-density haustra* ⇨ *create the accordion sign.*

Neutropenic Colitis

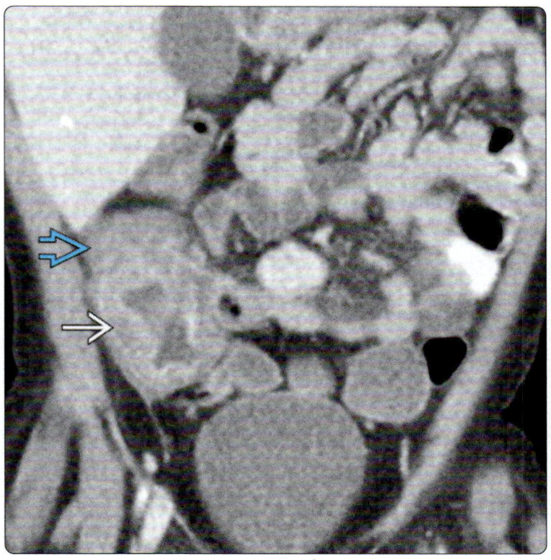

Ischemic Colitis

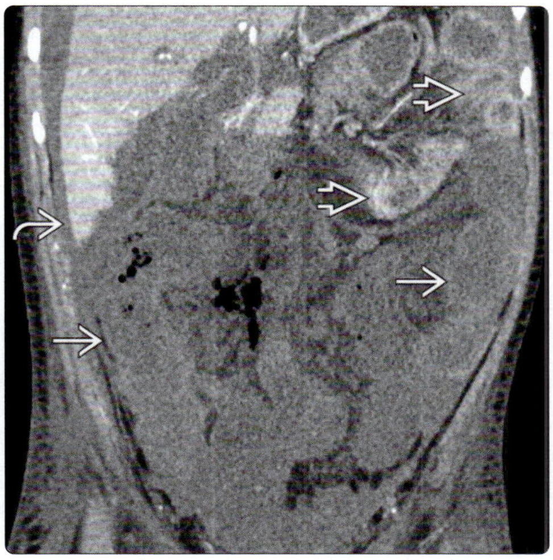

(Left) *Coronal CECT of a 3 year old with acute lymphocytic leukemia, fever, abdominal pain, & neutropenia shows cecal & ascending colon wall thickening* ➡ *& pericolonic stranding* ⇨, *consistent with neutropenic colitis.* **(Right)** *Coronal CECT in an 11 year old with multisystem organ failure demonstrates a lack of enhancement of most of the bowel wall* ➡ *with pericolonic stranding & ascites* ➡. *There are a few enhancing jejunal loops* ➡. *The superior (distal to the jejunal branches) & inferior mesenteric arteries were occluded in this patient.*

Lymphoma (Mimic)

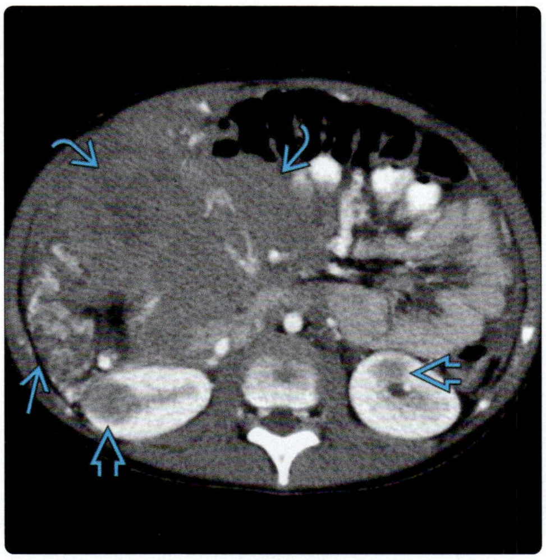

Graft-vs.-Host Disease

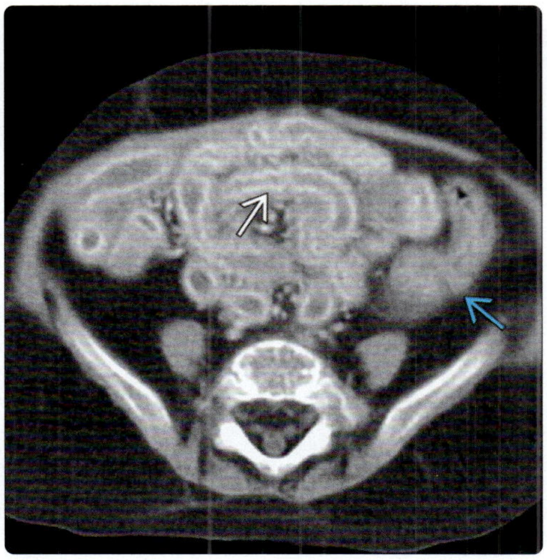

(Left) *Axial CECT in an 11 year old with vomiting shows a large lymphomatous mesenteric mass* ⇨ *encasing vessels + bilateral renal masses* ⇨. *Thickening & heterogeneous enhancement of the colon* ⇨ *may have been from neoplastic involvement or central vascular compression.* **(Right)** *Axial CECT from a 4-year-old bone marrow transplant patient with diarrhea shows small bowel* ➡ *& colonic* ⇨ *wall thickening & featureless mucosal hyperenhancement. UGI showed ribbon-like bowel, typical of GVHD.*

DIFFERENTIAL DIAGNOSIS

Common

- Necrotizing Enterocolitis
- Intraluminal Gas (Mimic)

Less Common

- Bowel Ischemia
- Loss of Mucosal Integrity
- Respiratory Pathologies
- Immunosuppression
- Short-Gut Syndrome

ESSENTIAL INFORMATION

Key Differential Diagnosis Issues

- Clinical history & age are helpful in determining if pneumatosis
  - Indicates severe illness that may require surgical intervention or
  - Is related to other medical/surgical history & will likely follow more benign clinical course
    - Associated peritoneal signs/symptoms favor more critical condition
- Radiographs & CECT are traditional modalities of evaluation
  - Radiographs: Free air & portal venous gas can be seen with benign & urgent etiologies of pneumatosis
  - CECT: Abnormal enhancement, bowel wall thickening, mesenteric stranding, focal dilation, & free fluid may suggest more ominous pathologies
    - CT is not always needed with typical associations & expected clinical findings
  - Ultrasound: Quite helpful in neonates with suspected necrotizing enterocolitis (NEC)

Helpful Clues for Common Diagnoses

- **Necrotizing Enterocolitis**
  - Premature neonate (especially < 1,500 g, < 32 weeks gestation) with bloody stools, feeding intolerance, distended abdomen
  - Ill-appearing patient is at risk of bowel perforation, requiring close monitoring
  - Radiographs/ultrasound: Pneumatosis, portal venous gas, fixed distended bowel loops with ↓ peristalsis, bowel wall thickening or thinning, ↑ or ↓ wall vascularity, pneumoperitoneum, fluid collections
- **Intraluminal Gas (Mimic)**
  - Gas bubbles in intraluminal fluid; will not show curvilinear lucencies within bowel wall
  - Cross-table lateral radiograph can help confirm

Helpful Clues for Less Common Diagnoses

- **Bowel Ischemia**
  - Risk factors: Congenital heart disease, maternal vasoconstrictor use, propensity for thrombosis, obstruction or volvulus, shock
  - CECT: Vascular distribution (often involving watershed areas 1st), bowel wall thinning or thickening, abnormal mucosal enhancement (absent, ↑, or ↓), mesenteric edema, pneumatosis, portal venous gas
- **Loss of Mucosal Integrity**
  - Trauma, obstruction (pyloric stenosis, small bowel stenosis, Hirschsprung), bowel inflammation/infection
- **Respiratory Pathologies**
  - Consider in patients with obstructive pulmonary conditions (asthma, cystic fibrosis) & barotrauma (↑ ventilator pressures)
  - Look for associated pulmonary hyperinflation/lucency, pneumomediastinum, pneumothorax
- **Immunosuppression**
  - History of steroid use, chemotherapy, immunocompromise secondary to medical conditions (HIV, leukemia, bone marrow transplant, solid organ transplantation)
- **Short-Gut Syndrome**
  - Likely secondary to chronic small bowel distension, ↓ lymphoid tissue, & associated infection
  - Commonly related to gastroschisis &/or bowel atresia

Necrotizing Enterocolitis

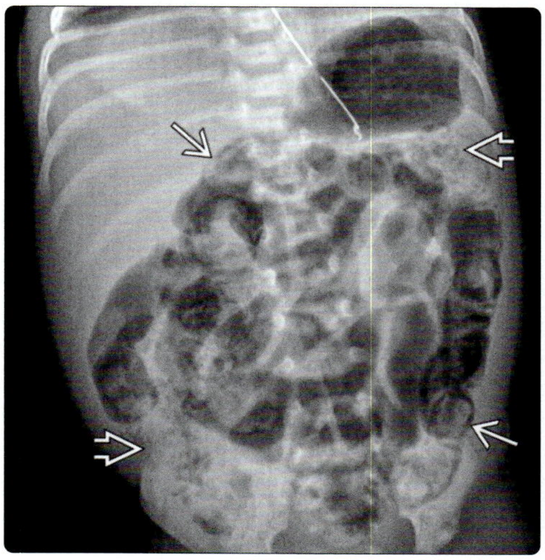

Necrotizing Enterocolitis

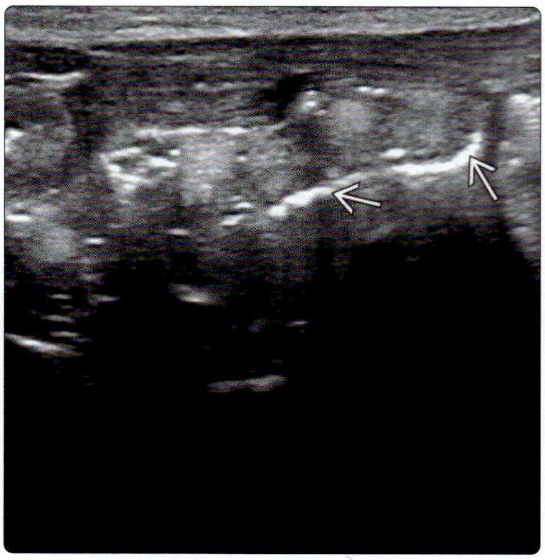

(Left) *AP radiograph in a premature 9 day old with necrotizing enterocolitis shows curvilinear ➡ & bubbly lucencies ➡ along the course of the colon, consistent with pneumatosis.* **(Right)** *Transverse ultrasound from the same patient shows colonic pneumatosis with echogenic intramural foci & associated "dirty" posterior acoustic shadowing at the dependent bowel wall ➡. Ultrasound can also be used to look for bowel wall thickening or thinning, abnormal vascularity, fluid collections, & free air.*

Bowel Ischemia

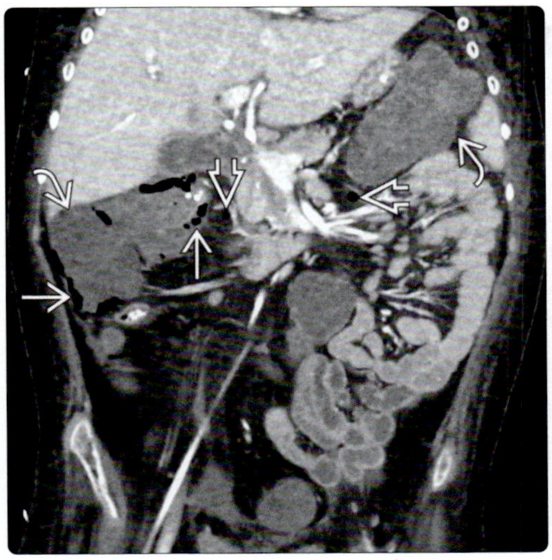

Loss of Mucosal Integrity

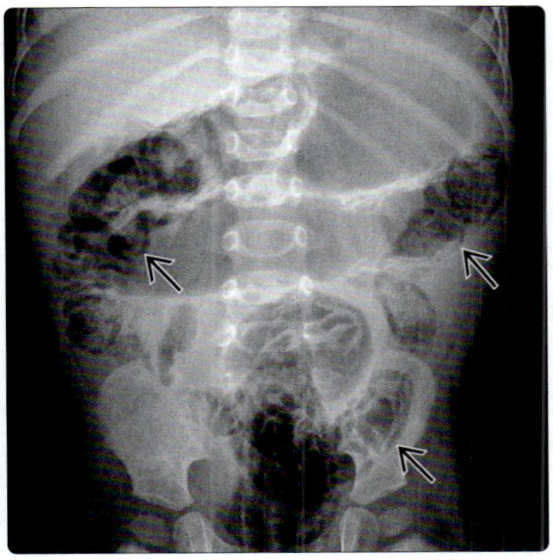

(Left) *Coronal CECT from a 13 year old demonstrates hypoenhancement of the colonic wall with intramural gas, consistent with pneumatosis. Foci of pneumoperitoneum are also present. Ischemic bowel was resected at surgery.* **(Right)** *Frontal radiograph shows pancolonic pneumatosis in this child with a stool culture positive for rotavirus. The child recovered, & the pneumatosis resolved within a week.*

Loss of Mucosal Integrity

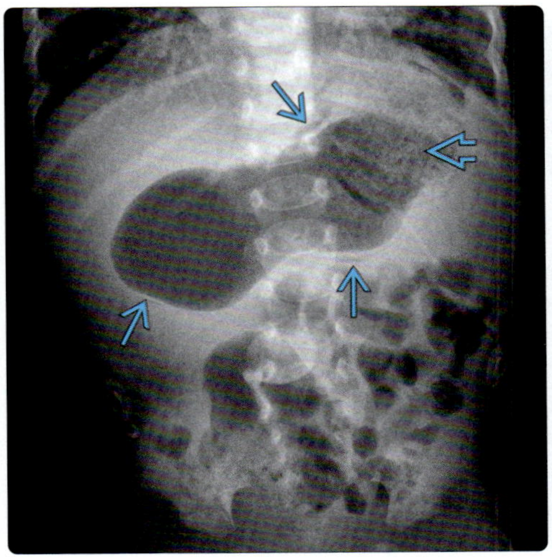

Immunosuppression

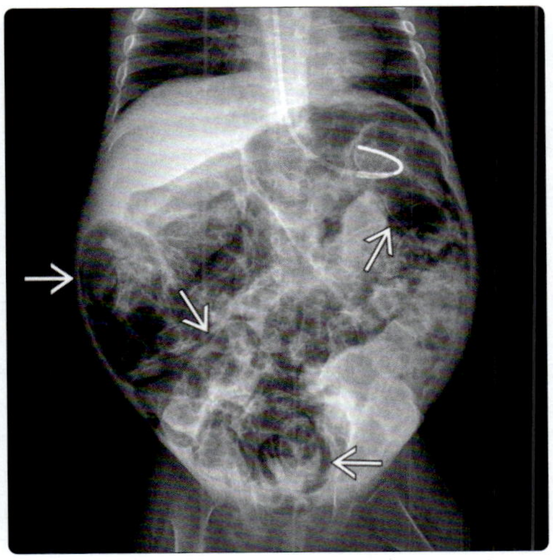

(Left) *Supine frontal radiograph in a 4 week old with vomiting shows curvilinear pneumatosis in the gastric wall. Note the gastric distention in this patient found by ultrasound to have pyloric stenosis. The bubbly lucencies over the proximal stomach could also represent pneumatosis but are more commonly due to retained food.* **(Right)** *Supine frontal radiograph shows extensive pneumatosis in a 2 year old with severe combined immunodeficiency status post bone marrow transplant.*

Immunosuppression

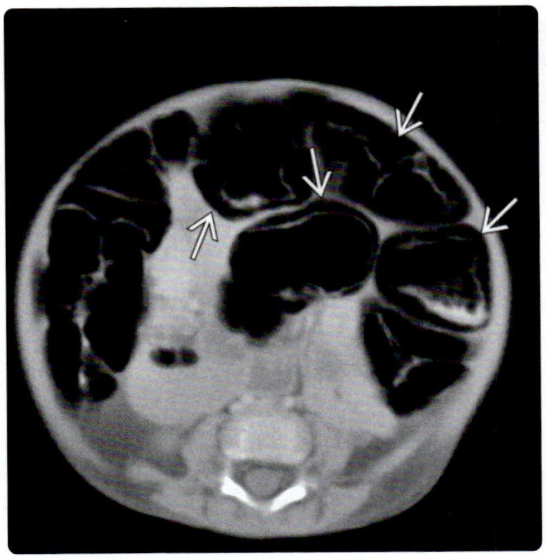

Short-Gut Syndrome

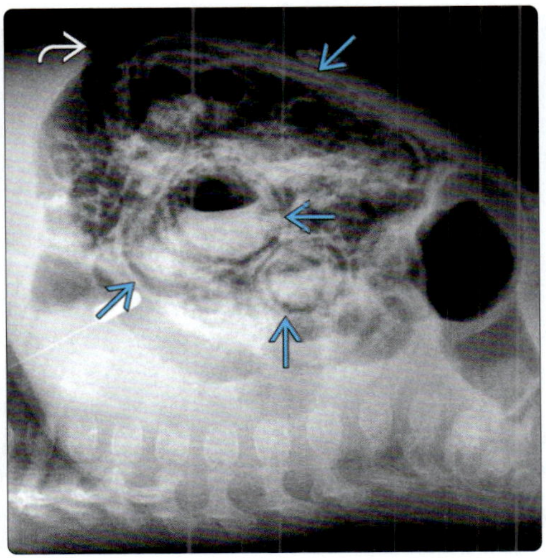

(Left) *Axial CECT from the same patient better depicts the degree of pneumatosis throughout the colon. No wall thickening, abnormal enhancement, or free fluid was seen. The patient was asymptomatic & tolerating feeds with a soft, nontender abdomen. The pneumatosis persisted for months.* **(Right)** *Cross-table lateral radiograph shows extensive curvilinear pneumatosis & a small amount of pneumoperitoneum in this patient with a prior gastroschisis repair.*

DIFFERENTIAL DIAGNOSIS

Common

- Postoperative
- Necrotizing Enterocolitis

Less Common

- Traumatic Bowel Injury
- Dissection From Pneumothorax or Pneumomediastinum
- Obstruction
- Appendicitis
- Iatrogenic
- Infection
- Inflammatory Bowel Disease
- Foreign Body
- Ruptured Pneumatosis

Rare but Important

- Neonatal Gastric/Intestinal Perforation
- Meckel Diverticulitis
- Ischemia
- Lymphoma
- Perforated Peptic Ulcer
- Ehlers-Danlos Syndrome

ESSENTIAL INFORMATION

Key Differential Diagnosis Issues

- Critical to differentiate pneumoperitoneum secondary to gastrointestinal perforation vs. other causes
  - Bowel perforation accounts for 85-95% of cases
- Radiographic signs
  - Triangular, round, or amorphous extraluminal lucency
  - Rigler sign: Air outlining both sides of bowel wall (though directly apposed gas-distended loops can create similar appearance)
  - Upright position: Lucency under right hemidiaphragm
  - Supine position
    - Amorphous lucency: Liver may appear more lucent than heart
    - Visualization of falciform ligament
      - American football sign: Large-volume pneumoperitoneum where air distends flanks & falciform ligament mimics laces on ball
    - Cupola sign: Air outlines central tendon of diaphragm
  - Cross-table lateral: Curvilinear lucency directly underlying ventral abdominal wall, outlining bowel loops or anterior liver margin
  - Left lateral decubitus: Curvilinear lucency between lateral abdominal wall & liver margin
- CT: Much more sensitive than radiographs, particularly with lung windows
- US: Linear echogenic foci underlying anterior peritoneal surface; demonstrate dirty posterior acoustic shadowing
  - Most confidently seen over liver surface

Helpful Clues for Common Diagnoses

- **Postoperative**
  - Common after abdominal surgery
  - Duration of free air is determined by its initial volume & absorption rate
  - Majority resolve within 3 days but may persist for several days more
  - Persistent or ↑ volume should raise suspicion for anastomotic leak
- **Necrotizing Enterocolitis**
  - Prematurity (< 1500 g, < 32-weeks gestation)
  - Presents with bloody stool, feeding intolerance, distended abdomen, bilious aspirates
  - Radiographs & US may show fixed distended bowel loops with ↓ peristalsis, pneumatosis, portal venous gas, bowel wall thickening/thinning, altered vascularity, fluid collections

Helpful Clues for Less Common Diagnoses

- **Traumatic Bowel Injury**
  - Blunt or penetrating trauma
    - Motor vehicle & bicycle accidents are common
      - Relative risk of bowel injury ↑ in patients with seat belt sign
    - Consider child abuse, particularly in infants, if history is inconsistent with injuries or if high-specificity fractures are present
    - Consider sexual assault if rectum is involved
  - CECT: Bowel wall thickening, diffuse or focal abnormal enhancement, mesenteric hematoma/fluid/stranding, & unexplained free fluid all raise concern for bowel injury
    - Look for small foci of extraluminal gas
  - ± other traumatic injuries: Spine, liver, pancreas, brain
- **Dissection From Pneumothorax or Pneumomediastinum**
  - Extension of air from pneumothorax & pneumomediastinum through rents in diaphragm or along vascular planes & normal diaphragmatic openings into peritoneum & retroperitoneum
  - More common in premature patients & patients on mechanical ventilation or CPAP
  - Benign abdominal exam without peritonitis
  - Typically presents after or simultaneous with pneumothorax &/or pneumomediastinum
- **Obstruction**
  - ↑ bowel distention &/or vessel twisting → ischemia/↑ pressure → perforation
  - In neonates, consider atresia, stenosis, midgut volvulus, meconium ileus, Hirschsprung disease
  - In older patients, consider volvulus, adhesions, mass, intussusception, lymphoma, stricture
  - Radiographs: Dilated bowel loops, air fluid levels
  - CECT/US: Twisting, swirling "whirlpool" of mesenteric vessels with volvulus
- **Appendicitis**
  - Pneumoperitoneum is uncommon
  - US/CECT/MR: Dilated appendix with surrounding inflammatory changes; ± appendicolith, complex fluid
- **Iatrogenic**
  - Status post endoscopy, tube/probe placement, peritoneal dialysis, enema
  - Check proper positioning of support devices
- **Infection**
  - Most common cause of nontraumatic colonic perforation
  - ↑ white blood cells, fever
  - CECT/US: Bowel wall thickening, mesenteric stranding

- **Inflammatory Bowel Disease**
  - Crohn disease & ulcerative colitis (UC)
    - Pain, diarrhea, weight loss, bleeding
    - Anemia, leukocytosis, ↑ CRP, ↑ ESR, ↑ fecal calprotectin
    - CECT/US/MR: Bowel wall thickening, hyperemia, adjacent mesenteric stranding
  - Crohn Disease
    - Transmural skip lesions anywhere from mouth to anus; common at terminal ileum
    - Skip lesions, penetrating & stricturing disease, engorged vasa recta, fibrofatty proliferation
  - UC
    - Contiguous proximal extension of inflammation from anus
    - Not transmural (i.e., no penetrating disease); chronic pseudopolyps & loss of haustra
- **Foreign Body**
  - Sharp ingested foreign bodies may perforate bowel
  - Bowel wall may become entrapped between multiple magnets or single magnet + other metallic objects → pressure ulceration, necrosis, & perforation
  - Imaging: Important to look closely at magnets
    - Stacked magnets can appear as single foreign body
    - May have nonradiopaque components
- **Ruptured Pneumatosis**
  - Rupture of subserosal gas-filled cysts without transmural perforation
  - Pneumatosis is characteristic of many serious conditions that can lead to mural perforation: Necrotizing enterocolitis (NEC), obstruction, ischemia
  - Can also occur with benign pneumatosis, as commonly seen with steroids/immunosuppression

Helpful Clues for Rare Diagnoses

- **Neonatal Gastric/Intestinal Perforation**
  - Usually at 2-11 days of life; may be term or preterm
  - Sudden onset of abdominal distension with large volume of pneumoperitoneum (especially with gastric involvement)
- **Meckel Diverticulitis**
  - Remnant of omphalomesenteric duct along antimesenteric border of ileum
  - Diverticulum may obstruct bowel, become inflamed, or cause intestinal bleeding
    - Inflamed Meckel diverticulum may mimic appendicitis; perforation may cause pneumoperitoneum
- **Ischemia**
  - Various etiologies: Volvulus, thrombosis, vasculitis, medications (indomethacin), NEC
  - Imaging: Bowel wall thickening/thinning, abnormal enhancement, absent flow on color Doppler, ↑ lactate
- **Lymphoma**
  - Pneumoperitoneum may be presenting symptom or occur after initiation of chemotherapy
  - Secondary to tumor, obstruction, inflammation, or necrosis
  - Imaging: Marked focal bowel wall thickening; commonly involves terminal ileum
- **Perforated Peptic Ulcer**
  - Risk factors
    - Medications: NSAIDs, steroids, immunosuppressants, antineoplastics
    - Stressors: Shock, sepsis, burns, trauma, intracranial hypertension, surgery
  - Epigastric pain, gastrointestinal bleeding, + *Helicobacter pylori* testing
  - Imaging: Focal bowel inflammation &/or mucosal defect
- **Ehlers-Danlos Syndrome**
  - Connective tissue disorder
  - Spontaneous colonic perforation is seen in type 4

SELECTED REFERENCES

1. Gupta R: Spontaneous pneumoperitoneum in pediatric patients: dilemmas in management. J Indian Assoc Pediatr Surg. 23(3):115-22, 2018
2. Yang T et al: Neonatal gastric perforation: case series and literature review. World J Surg. 42(8):2668-73, 2018
3. Tallant C et al: Spontaneous pneumoperitoneum in pediatric patients: a case series. Int J Surg Case Rep. 22:55-8, 2016
4. Epelman M et al: Necrotizing enterocolitis: review of state-of-the-art imaging findings with pathologic correlation. Radiographics. 27(2):285-305, 2007

Necrotizing Enterocolitis

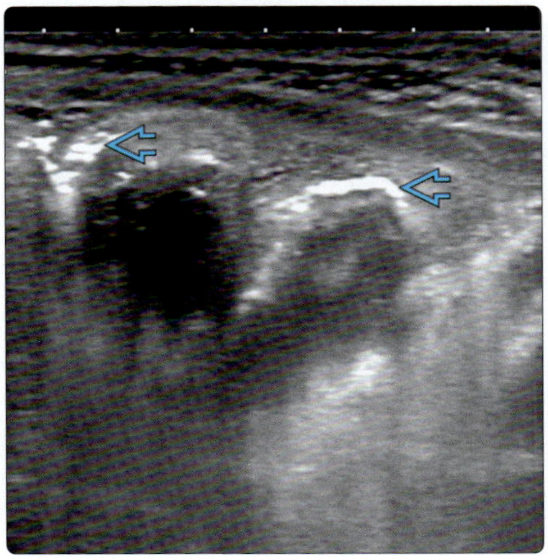

Necrotizing Enterocolitis

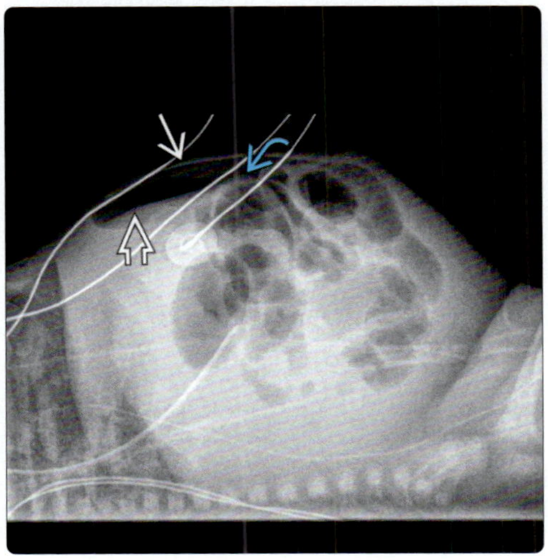

(Left) *Ultrasound from a 1 month old with necrotizing enterocolitis demonstrates intramural echogenic foci ➡ with dirty posterior acoustic shadowing, consistent with pneumatosis. This finding can be difficult to separate from intraluminal air unless it is seen tracking posteriorly around the lumen.* **(Right)** *Cross-table lateral radiograph in the same patient shows pneumoperitoneum with lucency underlying the ventral abdominal wall ➡. Note the delineation of the anterior liver margin ➡ & outer bowel wall ➡.*

(Left) *Supine AP radiograph shows extensive bubbly & curvilinear lucencies of pneumatosis intestinalis ➡ in a neonate. Note the small triangular lucency ⇨ in the right upper quadrant, consistent with a small amount of pneumoperitoneum.* **(Right)** *Axial CECT shows small foci of free air ➡ in a 6 year old that was hit by a car, including a focus adjacent to a jejunal loop in the left upper quadrant ➡. Note the adjacent mesenteric stranding ⇨. A perforated jejunal loop was discovered at surgery.*

Necrotizing Enterocolitis

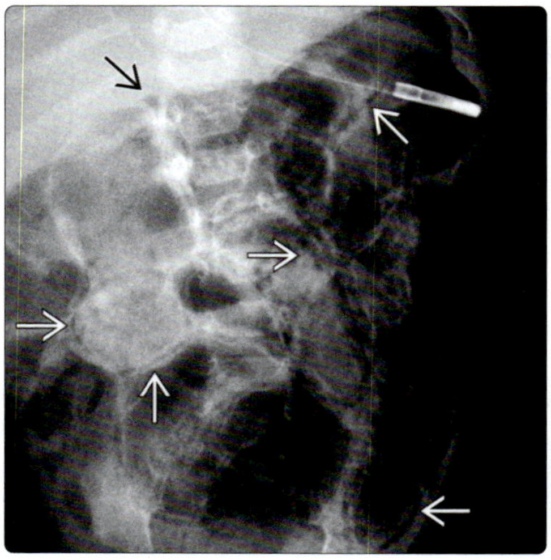

Traumatic Bowel Injury

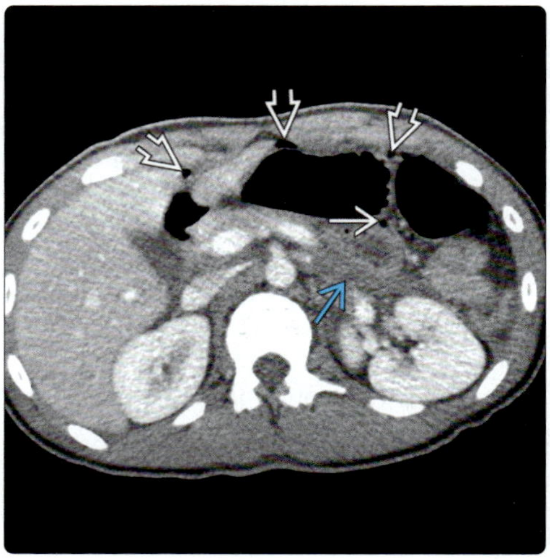

(Left) *AP radiograph shows pneumoperitoneum ➡ in this 2 day old after he developed bilateral pneumothoraces ➡. Note the outline of the falciform ligament ⇨. The abdomen was benign clinically & a small tear was found in the diaphragm.* **(Right)** *Axial CECT from a 16 year old with perforated appendicitis demonstrates an enlarged appendix containing an appendicolith with adjacent inflammatory stranding ➡. Foci of free air are also seen at the right lower quadrant ➡.*

Dissection From Pneumothorax or Pneumomediastinum

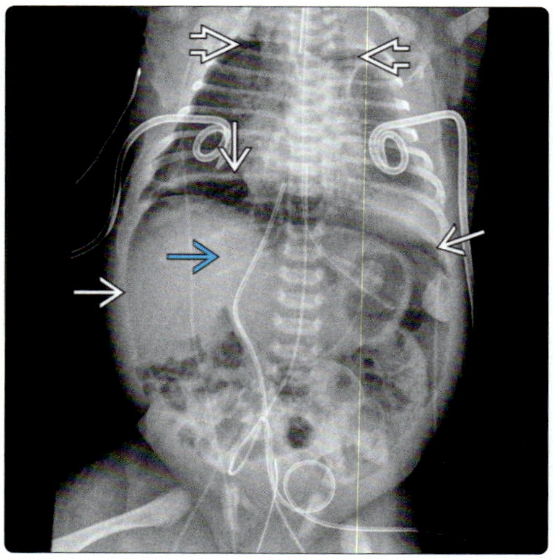

Appendicitis

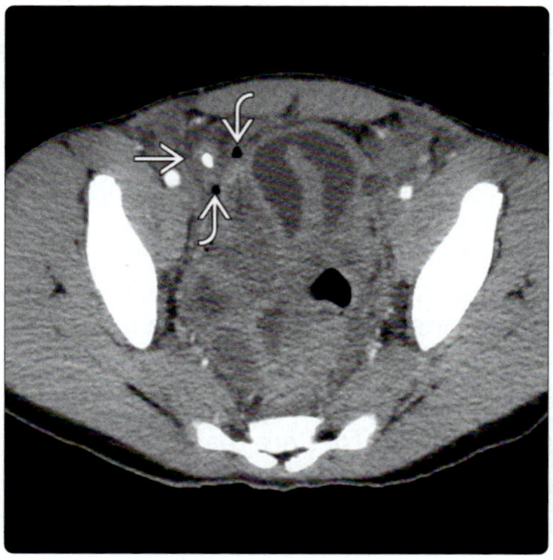

(Left) *Cross-table lateral radiograph shows a large volume of free air ➡ in a 1 year old status post endoscopy. Insufflation of the bowel during endoscopy leads to distended loops with the potential for a large volume of pneumoperitoneum. Note the Rigler signs ➡.* **(Right)** *Axial T2 SSFSE MR in a 12 year old with Crohn disease shows free air ⇨ secondary to a microperforation. The dilated small bowel loops ⇨ were due to strictures that were resected at the exploratory laparotomy that followed this exam.*

Iatrogenic

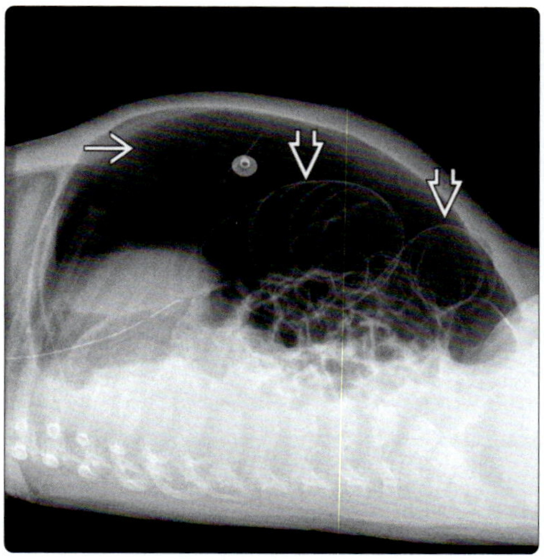

Inflammatory Bowel Disease

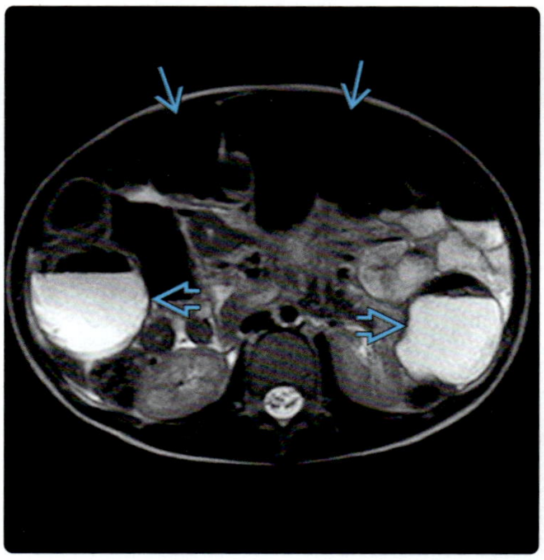

Inflammatory Bowel Disease

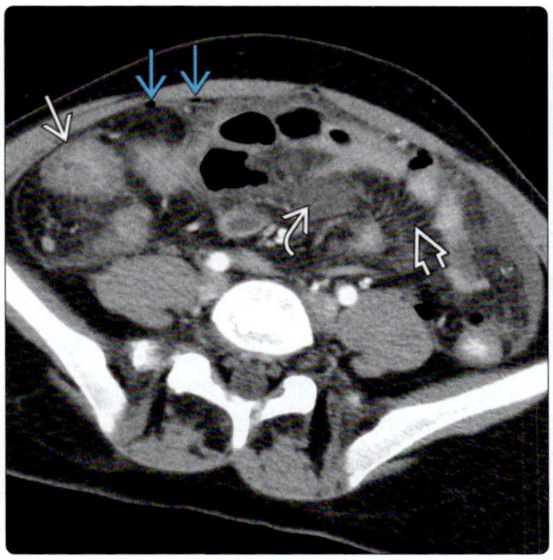

Neonatal Gastric/Intestinal Perforation

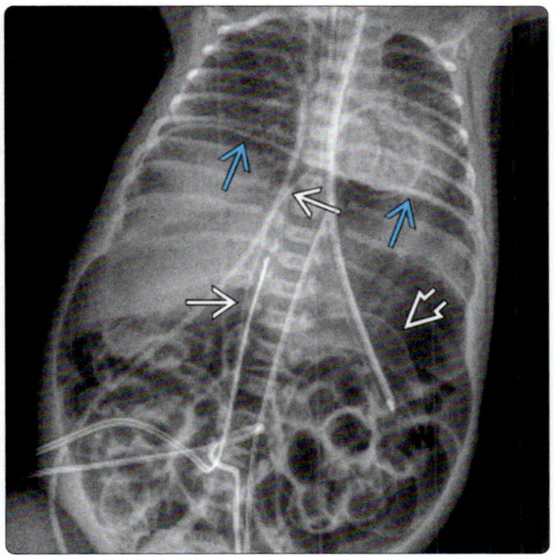

(Left) *Axial CECT shows findings of Crohn disease in a 17 year old with bowel wall thickening ➡, mesenteric fluid ➡, & vascular engorgement ➡. Foci of free air ➡ are also seen, consistent with pneumoperitoneum.* **(Right)** *Supine AP radiograph from a 3 day old with a spontaneous gastric perforation demonstrates a large volume pneumoperitoneum with visualization of the falciform ligament ➡ & inferior surface of the diaphragm ➡ as well as the Rigler sign ➡.*

Meckel Diverticulitis

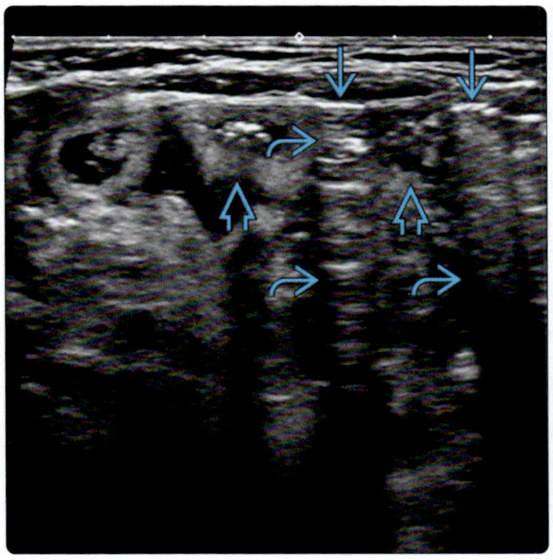

Ischemia

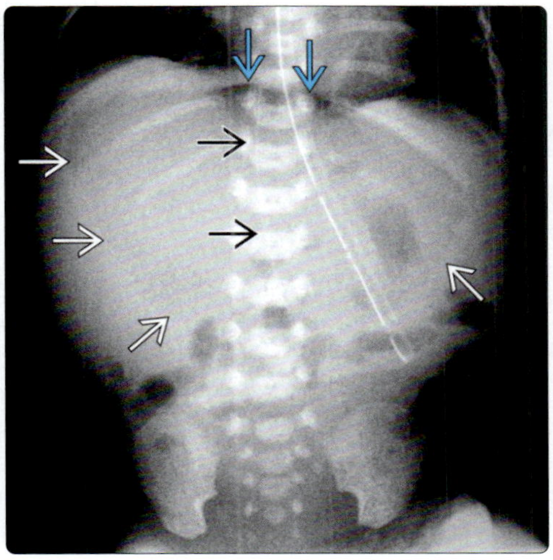

(Left) *Transverse ultrasound of the abdomen in a 4 month old with melena & fussiness shows linear echogenic foci ➡ with dirty posterior acoustic shadowing ➡ along the anterior peritoneum between bowel loops ➡. Radiographs confirmed free air, & a perforated Meckel diverticulum was resected.* **(Right)** *Supine AP radiograph shows free air ➡ in a premature infant treated with indomethacin (which can decrease GI blood flow & lead to perforation). The falciform ligament ➡ is outlined & the cupola sign ➡ is noted.*

Lymphoma

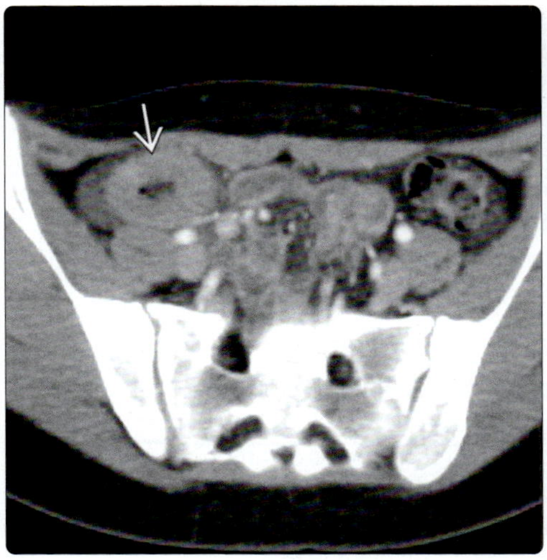

Lymphoma

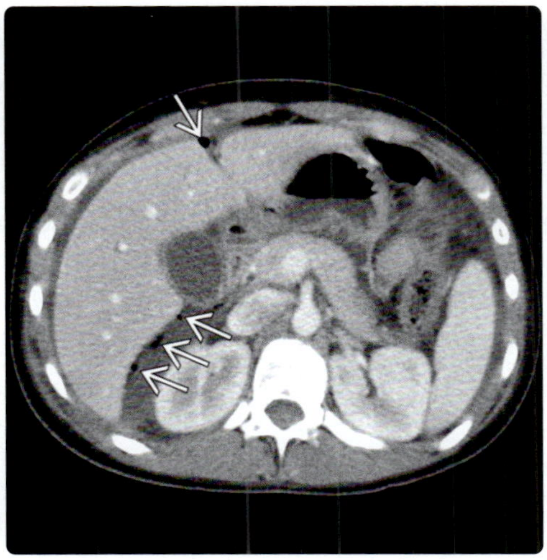

(Left) *Axial CECT from a patient with bowel lymphoma demonstrates focal wall thickening of the terminal ileum ➡.* **(Right)** *Axial CECT from the same patient obtained prior to chemotherapy depicts foci of free air ➡, consistent with perforation. Lymphoma-related perforations can be the presenting symptom of disease or may occur after chemotherapy.*

DIFFERENTIAL DIAGNOSIS

Common

- Lymphatic Malformation
- Reactive Lymphadenopathy
- Abscess

Less Common

- Burkitt Lymphoma
- Neuroblastoma
- Desmoid
- Mesothelial Cyst

Rare but Important

- Inflammatory Myofibroblastic Tumor
- Infantile Hemangioma
- Plexiform Neurofibroma
- Sarcomas
  - Rhabdomyosarcoma
  - Ewing Sarcoma
- Metastases
- Desmoplastic Small Round Cell Tumor
- Castleman Disease
- Tuberculosis

ESSENTIAL INFORMATION

Key Differential Diagnosis Issues

- Mesenteries are specialized peritoneal reflections containing fibrofatty tissue, vessels, & nerves
- Infiltration of mesentery allows lesions to encase bowel

Helpful Clues for Common Diagnoses

- **Lymphatic Malformation**
  - Mass of abnormal lymphatic vessels that do not communicate with normal lymphatics
  - a.k.a. lymphangioma or mesenteric cyst
  - < 5% occur in mesentery
  - Complex, multilocular cystic lesion of variable size
    - Frequently extends across tissue planes
    - Appearance varies depending on cyst size
      - Macrocysts: Cysts of > 1 cm; thin walls with no central enhancement
      - Microcysts: Cysts of < 1 cm; more solid-appearing
    - Cysts have varying degrees of internal complexity
      - Often contain fluid-fluid levels due to hemorrhage
      - Rarely contain fat
    - Relatively compressible cystic components often encase vessels without narrowing them
  - Grow commensurate with patient; may rapidly enlarge due to hemorrhage, infection, or hormonal stimulation
- **Reactive Lymphadenopathy**
  - Benign enlargement from inflammation or infection (e.g., appendicitis, enterocolitis, etc.)
  - Discrete nodes retain normal architecture (i.e., bean shape, central fatty hilum, radiating vasculature)
  - Mesenteric adenitis: Subset of reactive adenopathy without obvious etiology; diagnosis of exclusion
    - Likely secondary to viral inflammation/enteritis
- **Abscess**
  - May be in mesentery or peritoneal space
    - Can extend as continuous or discontinuous collections between leaves of mesentery (interloop abscesses)
  - Discrete walled-off collection(s) of purulent fluid
    - Complex, echogenic debris on US, not layering
      - Swirling with compression
    - Irregular enhancing wall on CECT, ± internal gas
  - Common causes in children: Perforated appendicitis, inflammatory bowel disease, postoperative

Helpful Clues for Less Common Diagnoses

- **Burkitt Lymphoma**
  - Subtype of non-Hodgkin lymphoma
  - Large solitary vs. multiple masses, often bulky
    - Necrosis in large tumors; otherwise homogeneous
      - Ca^{2+} is uncommon prior to treatment
  - Often encases mesenteric vessels
  - Bowel wall can be quite thickened, focally or diffusely
    - Typically narrows lumen, but dilation can occur
  - May have solid organ lesions, peritoneal seeding, & malignant ascites
  - Highly FDG avid
- **Neuroblastoma**
  - Most common extracranial solid malignancy in children
  - Typically originates in paraspinal location
    - Heterogeneous lobulated mass crossing midline, encasing vessels, & invading organs
    - Ca^{2+} in 85-90% by CT
    - Bone & liver metastases are common
  - Commonly spreads from retroperitoneum to mesentery via subperitoneal space
    - Direct invasion by primary mass vs. metastases
- **Desmoid**
  - Benign fibroblastic tumor; can be locally aggressive
  - Increased frequency in familial adenomatous polyposis syndrome; F > M
  - Soft tissue mass of variable size; usually 5-10 cm but can be much larger
    - Hypointense on T1 & T2 MR due to fibrous content
      - T2 hyperintensity with myxoid change
    - Variable enhancement, typically mild or absent
    - Range from circumscribed to spiculated or infiltrative soft tissue masses on CT
      - May be hypodense with myxoid change
    - May encase bowel or vascular structures
    - Often located at mesenteric base near origin of superior mesenteric artery (SMA)
- **Mesothelial Cyst**
  - Accumulation of fluid between mesothelial layers
  - Nonspecific unilocular cyst; very rarely multilocular

Helpful Clues for Rare Diagnoses

- **Inflammatory Myofibroblastic Tumor**
  - Intermediate-grade mesenchymal tumor that is usually benign, but local recurrence is common
  - Most often found in lung, mesentery, & omentum
  - Round or lobulated focal soft tissue mass
    - Circumscribed or ill-defined margins
    - Iso- to hypointense on T1, variable on T2 MR
    - Variable enhancement
      - Large tumors may have areas of necrosis
    - May have central dense Ca^{2+} on CT

- Does not typically encase bowel or vascular structures
- **Infantile Hemangioma**
  - High-flow benign vascular neoplasm, which almost always occurs in skin or subcutaneous tissues
    - Deeper locations, including mesentery, are much more likely with PHACE association
  - Develops in 1st few months of life with rapid growth in 1st year, followed by slow involution over years
  - Doppler: High vessel density with numerous low-resistance arterial waveforms
  - CT: Well-defined, intensely enhancing mass
  - MR: T2 hyperintense with scattered flow voids; avid homogeneous enhancement
- **Plexiform Neurofibroma**
  - Occurs in neurofibromatosis type 1 (NF1)
  - CT: Homogeneously hypoattenuating conglomeration of lobular masses
  - MR: Cross section of individual lesions shows characteristic target sign with T2-hyperintense rim & hypointense center; US can also show target appearance with echogenic center
  - Disproportionate enlargement, increased heterogeneity, SUV > 3.5 on FDG PET raise concern for malignant peripheral nerve sheath tumor (MPNST)
- **Sarcomas**
  - **Rhabdomyosarcoma**
    - Most common sites are head & neck, GU tract
      - Mesenteric disease may represent metastatic involvement or primary site
    - Most commonly seen < 10 years of age
    - Primary: Large heterogeneous mass, variable enhancement, restricted diffusion
    - Metastatic: Carcinomatosis or lymphadenopathy
    - Ca^{2+} is rare; ascites is common
  - **Ewing sarcoma**
    - Rare reports of mesenteric primary
    - May have large cystic components
- **Metastases**
  - Typically due to peritoneal spread of tumor rather than hematogenous spread
    - Ovarian tumors are most common
- **Desmoplastic Small Round Cell Tumor**
  - Rare malignant tumor
  - Far more common in boys (up to 90%)
  - Multiple peritoneal, omental, & serosal masses
    - Often has dominant heterogeneous mass > 10 cm with additional smaller masses; 30% show small Ca^{2+}
    - Diffuse peritoneal thickening, omental caking, & ascites are common
  - Mesenteric adenopathy & extraperitoneal metastatic disease (liver, lung, bone) are common at diagnosis
- **Castleman Disease**
  - Benign lymphoproliferative disorder a.k.a. angiofollicular lymphoid hyperplasia
  - Soft tissue mass ± satellite nodules/lymph nodes
    - Homogeneously hypoechoic on US
    - Ca^{2+} in 10-30%, may appear branching
    - Heterogeneously hyperintense on T2 MR
    - May have central stellate fibrotic scar or necrosis
    - May see peripheral feeding vessels
    - FDG PET uptake is typically lower than lymphoma
    - Characteristic intense enhancement is seen in more common hyaline vascular type
    - Variable enhancement in plasmacytic type
- **Tuberculosis**
  - Peritoneal tuberculosis is uncommon in developed countries
  - Ascites, peritoneal thickening & nodularity, ileocecal thickening, adenopathy, & splenic lesions are typical

SELECTED REFERENCES

1. Morani AC et al: Desmoplastic small round cell tumor: imaging pattern of disease at presentation. AJR Am J Roentgenol. 212(3):W45-54, 2019
2. Dillman JR et al: Imaging of the pediatric peritoneum, mesentery and omentum. Pediatr Radiol. 47(8):987-1000, 2017

Lymphatic Malformation

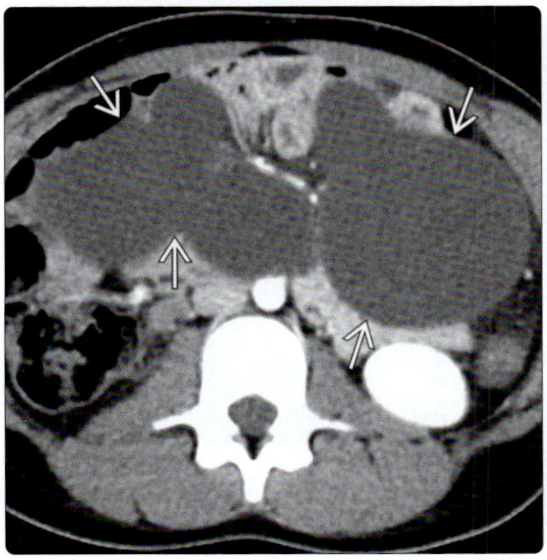

Lymphatic Malformation

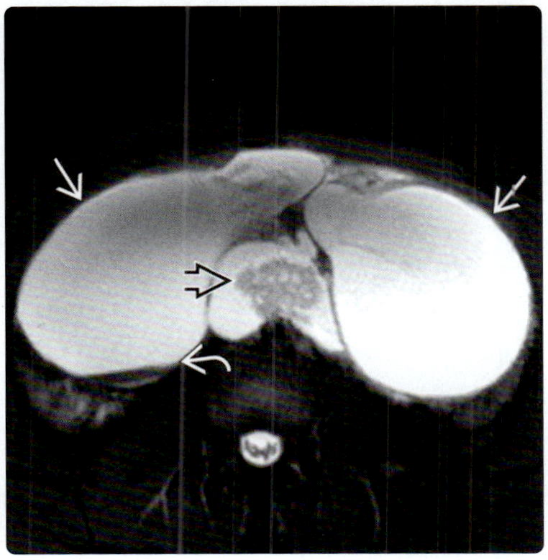

(Left) *Axial CECT in an 11 year old after trauma shows a lobulated fluid-attenuation mesenteric mass ➔ displacing bowel loops anteriorly & posteriorly.* **(Right)** *Axial T2 FS MR in the same patient shows irregular, relatively hypointense material ⇨ & a fluid-fluid level ➔ within different cystic components of the enlarging lesion ➔ due to retracting clot vs. layering blood products, respectively. Note that any nodular enhancement or restricted diffusion (not present in this case) would require more urgent tissue sampling.*

(Left) *Transverse US in the same patient shows the multiloculated mass as predominantly hypoechoic* ➡. *The rounded echogenic debris* ➡ *was avascular, corresponding to the retracting clot seen on MR.* **(Right)** *Coronal CECT in an 11 year old with Crohn disease & abdominal pain shows 2 small abscesses* ➡ *with irregular rim enhancement in the right lower quadrant mesentery due to active inflammation in the terminal ileum* ➡ *(i.e., penetrating disease).*

Lymphatic Malformation

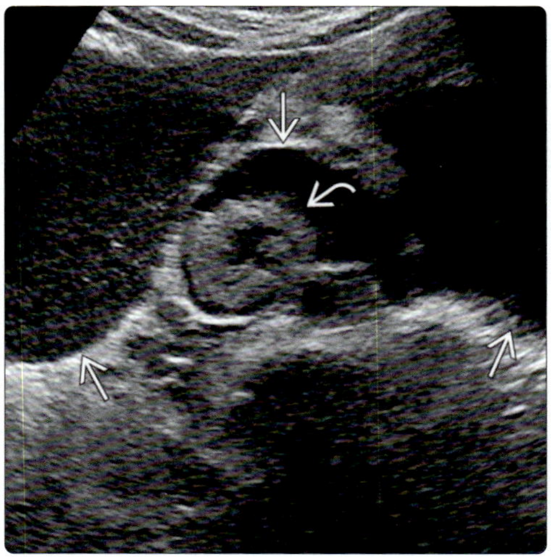

Abscess

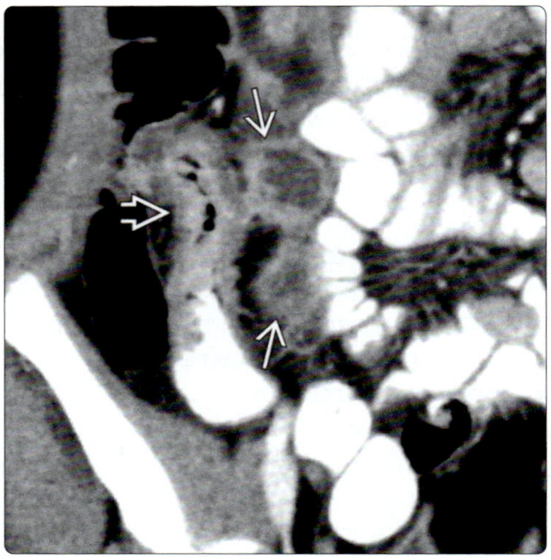

(Left) *Axial CECT in a 4 year old with abdominal pain & diarrhea shows homogeneous hypodense soft tissue masses diffusely involving the mesentery & bowel walls. Luminal narrowing of bowel loops is present at many levels* ➡ *(though involved loops may rarely show dilation). Biopsy confirmed Burkitt lymphoma.* **(Right)** *Coronal PET/CT in the same 4 year old shows intense FDG avidity of the lesions. Though not present in this case, multifocal solid organ lesions also frequently occur with Burkitt lymphoma.*

Burkitt Lymphoma

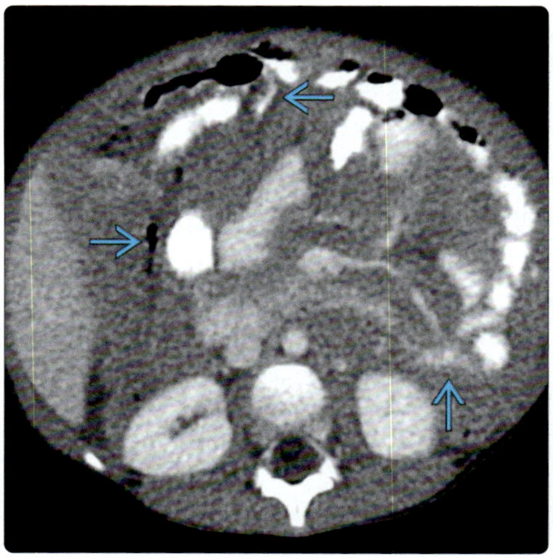

Burkitt Lymphoma

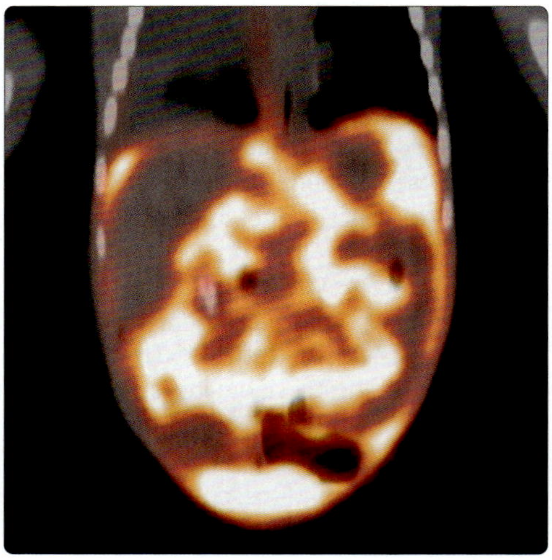

(Left) *Axial CECT in a 2 year old shows lobulated neuroblastoma masses* ➡ *extending from the retroperitoneum into the mesentery with encasement of the SMA* ➡ *& displacement of the aorta* ➡. *Numerous foci of* Ca^{2+} ➡ *are present.* **(Right)** *Axial T2 FS MR shows a desmoid tumor in a 17-year-old girl with familial adenomatous polyposis syndrome. The mass shows characteristic low signal intensity* ➡, *reflecting the fibrous content. These lesions may be well circumscribed or infiltrative.*

Neuroblastoma

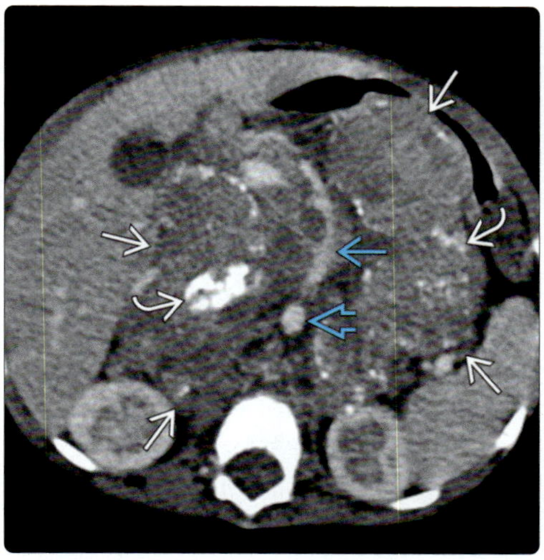

Desmoid

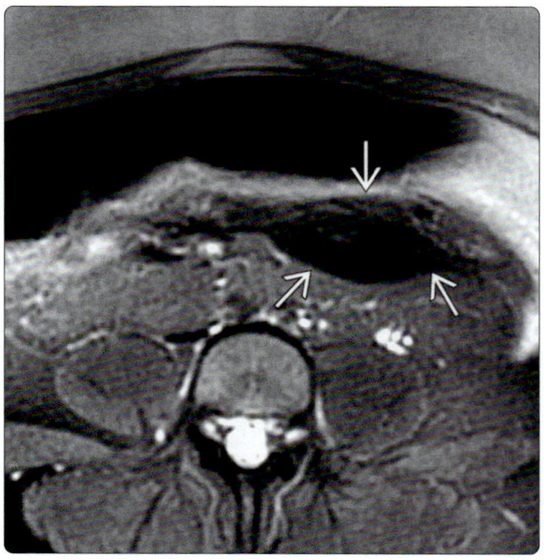

Inflammatory Myofibroblastic Tumor

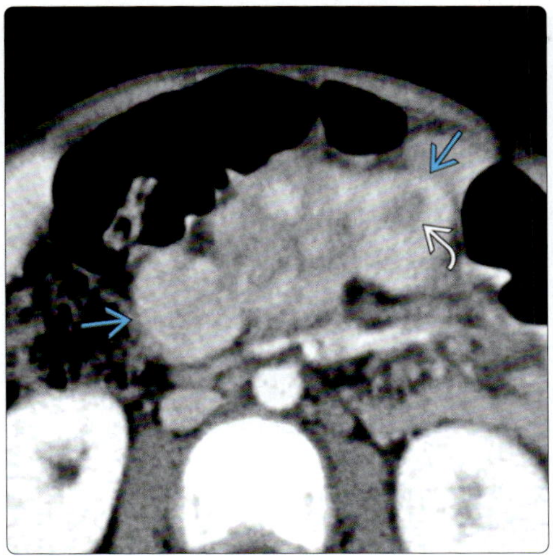

Infantile Hemangioma

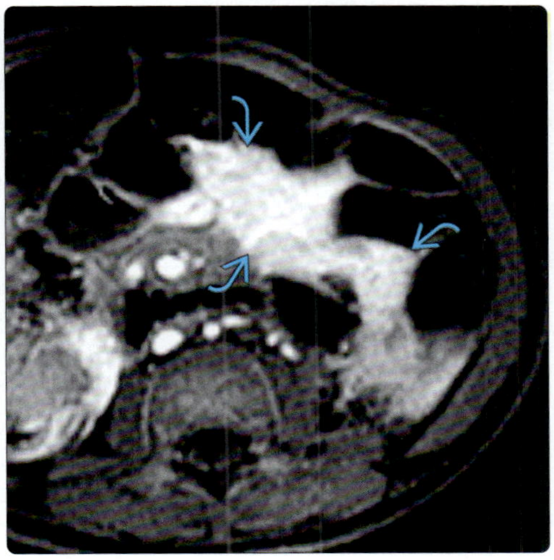

(Left) *Axial CECT shows a lobulated, heterogeneously enhancing mesenteric mass in an 8 year old with fever & abdominal pain, which was found to be an inflammatory myofibroblastic tumor. Note the focus of central necrosis.* **(Right)** *Axial T1 C+ FS MR in a 1 year old with PHACE syndrome shows a large, lobulated infantile hemangioma of the mesentery. There is avid homogeneous enhancement of the lesion. The patient also had hemangiomas in the neck, superior mediastinum, & liver.*

Plexiform Neurofibroma

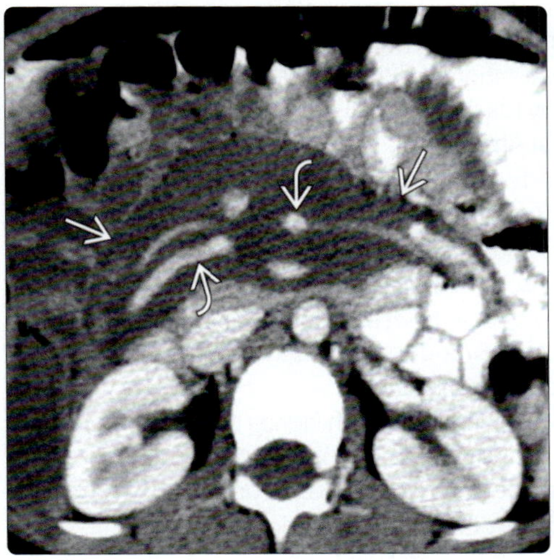

Plexiform Neurofibroma

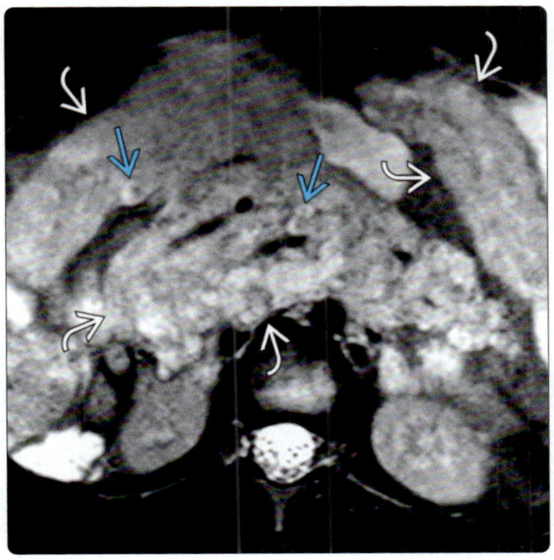

(Left) *Axial CECT performed in a 10 year old after a sports injury shows a large, mesenteric plexiform neurofibroma. Note the homogeneous hypodensity & encasement of mesenteric vessels. The appearance is very similar to a lymphatic malformation.* **(Right)** *Axial T2 FS MR in the same patient shows that the lobulated & infiltrative mass is predominantly hyperintense with individual lobules demonstrating central hypointense signal (the target sign).*

Desmoplastic Small Round Cell Tumor

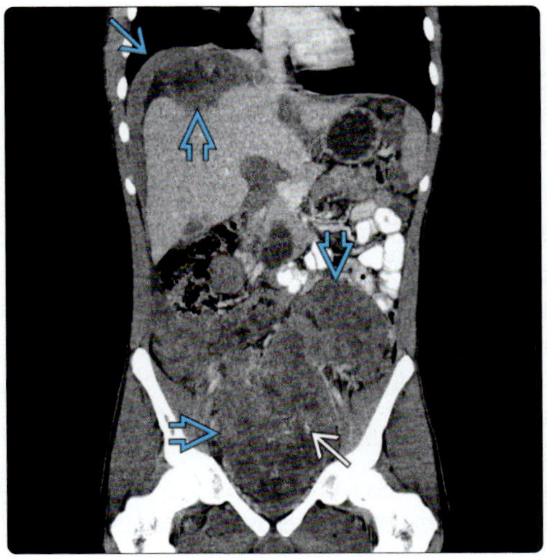

Castleman Disease

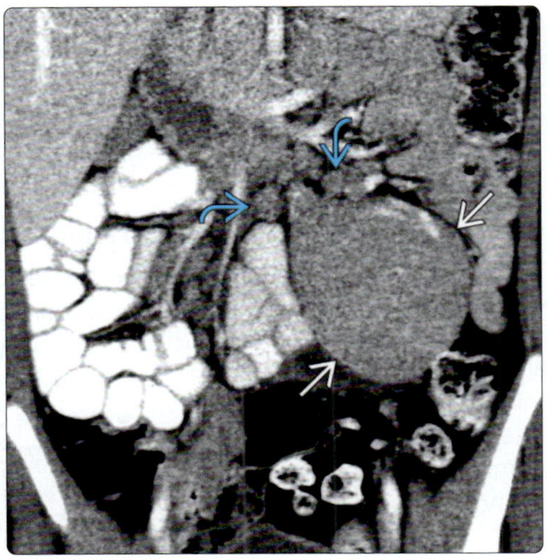

(Left) *Coronal CECT shows multiple mesenteric, omental, & peritoneal masses with diaphragm involvement in this 16 year old with back pain & constipation due to a desmoplastic small round cell tumor. Note the fine Ca^{2+}.* **(Right)** *Coronal CECT shows a solitary mesenteric mass in an 11 year old with anemia, which was found to be the unicentric plasmacytic type of Castleman disease. It lacks the typical hyperenhancement of the hyaline vascular type. There are several small lymph nodes superiorly.*

DIFFERENTIAL DIAGNOSIS

Common

- Ovarian Cyst
- Urinary Bladder
  - Distended Normal Bladder (Mimic)
  - Obstructed Bladder
- Hydronephrosis
- Bowel Obstruction (Mimic)
- Peripancreatic Fluid Collection
- Appendiceal Abscess
- Multicystic Dysplastic Kidney
- Gastrointestinal Duplication Cyst

Less Common

- Splenic Cyst
- Mature Cystic Teratoma
- Lymphatic Malformation
- Hydrometrocolpos
- Choledochal Cyst
- Urachal Cyst
- Peritoneal Inclusion Cyst
- CSF Pseudocyst

Rare but Important

- Cystic Wilms Tumor
- Meconium Pseudocyst
- Multilocular Cystic Renal Tumors
- Mesothelial Cyst
- Tuboovarian Abscess
- Aneurysm

ESSENTIAL INFORMATION

Key Differential Diagnosis Issues

- Organ of origin can be difficult to identify if mass is large
- Patient age & relationship of mass to surrounding structures can focus differential diagnosis

Helpful Clues for Common Diagnoses

- **Ovarian Cyst**
  - Most common in neonates & adolescents
  - ~ 20% of neonatal cysts are > 1 cm
    - Cysts resolve as maternal hormones subside
    - Larger fetal cysts rarely result in torsion & necrosis
  - In adolescents, ovarian cysts are very common
    - Dominant follicle: Can measure up to 3 cm
    - Functional cysts: Can measure up to 3-10 cm
      - Follicular cyst: Normal mature follicle fails to involute; thin wall with anechoic contents
      - Corpus luteal cyst: Dominant follicle after ovulation; may appear thick walled with peripheral hyperemia
      - Hemorrhagic cyst: Uniform internal echoes vs. lace-like retracting clot vs. layering debris, all of which show ↑ through transmission
    - Follow-up of larger cysts shows ↓ in 4-6 weeks
- **Urinary Bladder**
  - **Distended normal bladder (mimic)**
    - May mimic mass; resolves with voiding
  - **Obstructed bladder**
    - Variety of congenital causes, most commonly posterior urethral valves (PUV) in male patients
    - Acquired causes are uncommon & may be mechanical (e.g., mass) or functional (e.g., neurogenic)
- **Hydronephrosis**
  - Many etiologies, including vesicoureteral reflux (VUR), PUV, congenital obstructions at ureteropelvic junction (UPJ) or ureterovesical junction (UVJ), obstructing stone
    - Marked distention of renal pelvis without hydroureter is typical in UPJ obstruction
    - Bilateral hydroureteronephrosis (± renal cystic dysplasia) is typical in male patients with PUV
- **Bowel Obstruction (Mimic)**
  - Many congenital & acquired etiologies
  - Dilated fluid-filled small bowel (SB) loops can mimic cystic mass; must trace loop continuity on US or CT
- **Peripancreatic Fluid Collection**
  - Most common cystic lesion of pediatric pancreas
  - Occurs from recent inflammation &/or trauma
  - Timing (< vs. > 4 weeks) & nature of initial insult (interstitial edema vs. necrosis vs. traumatic duct disruption) determine terminology, natural history, & treatment of fluid collection
    - ↑ organization of fluid & ↓ inflammation with time, typically resulting in well-defined collection
- **Appendiceal Abscess**
  - Due to perforated appendicitis
  - Patients typically have symptoms for > 2 days
  - US shows heterogeneous RLQ/pelvic collection without internal vascularity, ± internal swirling debris
  - CECT shows variable wall thickness & irregularity, ± appendicolith &/or decompressed inflamed appendix
- **Multicystic Dysplastic Kidney**
  - Congenital anomaly in which kidney is entirely replaced by cysts of varying size & has no function
    - Cysts do not connect with renal pelvis
  - Natural history is gradual involution
- **Gastrointestinal Duplication Cyst**
  - Occurs anywhere along GI tract; most common at ileum
    - Adjacent to GI wall; usually spherical or tubular
  - Bowel wall layers (trilaminar or "gut signature") are typically apparent on US
    - Not specific; dilation of hollow viscera (e.g., bladder, vagina, bowel) can have similar appearance
    - Peristalsis increases specificity
  - Can lead to obstruction, bleeding, or intussusception

Helpful Clues for Less Common Diagnoses

- **Splenic Cyst**
  - Congenital or acquired; indistinguishable by imaging
    - Acquired cysts are due to trauma or infection
  - May be simple or mildly complex
- **Mature Cystic Teratoma**
  - a.k.a. dermoid cyst
  - Mixed solid & cystic mass with fat & Ca^{2+}
  - Tip of iceberg: Full extent of mass is obscured by shadowing from superficial echogenic interfaces
  - Dermoid plug: Shadowing echogenic nodule in cyst
  - Dermoid mesh: Echogenic lines & dots due to hair
- **Lymphatic Malformation**
  - Congenital mass of abnormal lymphatic vessels

- Complex, multilocular cystic lesion of variable size
  - Frequently extends across tissue planes
  - Appearance varies depending on cyst size
    - Macrocysts: Cysts of > 1 cm; thin walls with no central enhancement
    - Microcysts: Cysts of < 1 cm; more solid-appearing
  - Cysts have varying degrees of internal complexity
    - Often contain fluid-fluid levels due to hemorrhage
  - Grow commensurate with patient; rapidly enlarge due to hemorrhage, infection, or hormonal stimulation
- **Hydrometrocolpos**
  - Distended fluid- or blood-filled vagina > > > uterus
    - May be due to vaginal septum or imperforate hymen
  - Typically presents in neonates or after onset of puberty
  - Markedly dilated vagina is vertically elongated but round in axial/transverse planes
  - Blood products typically result in bright T1 & intermediate T2 signal intensity, ± layering debris
- **Choledochal Cyst**
  - Cystic or fusiform dilation of biliary tree
  - Todani classification with 5 types: Type 1 (cystic dilation of extrahepatic bile duct) is most common
  - > 60% diagnosed < 10 years of age
  - US most commonly shows dilation of common bile duct > 1 cm in diameter
  - HIDA scan or MR with hepatocellular contrast agent can be used to prove connection to biliary system
  - Long-term risk of cholangiocarcinoma → resection
- **Urachal Cyst**
  - Remnants of embryologic urachus may be found from bladder dome to umbilicus, including cyst, sinus, or diverticulum
  - Cyst above bladder; may be thick walled if infected
- **Peritoneal Inclusion Cyst**
  - Fluid trapped by adhesions of prior surgery or inflammation; often surrounds or displaces ovary
- **CSF Pseudocyst**
  - Localized collection at tip of ventriculoperitoneal shunt
    - Fluid does not track freely around bowel with US compression; typically has lobulated margins

Helpful Clues for Rare Diagnoses

- **Cystic Wilms Tumor**
  - Most common pediatric abdominal neoplasm but typically solid; peak age is 3-4 years
  - Usually heterogeneous solid mass with "claw" of residual renal parenchyma; rarely cystic
    - Look for solid foci with restricted diffusion on MR
- **Meconium Pseudocyst**
  - In utero bowel obstruction → perforation → meconium peritonitis → pseudocyst
  - Wall &/or contents may calcify; wall is typically thick; heterogeneous contents may layer dependently
- **Multilocular Cystic Renal Tumors**
  - Benign spectrum of disease: Cystic nephroma vs. cystic partially differentiated nephroblastoma (CPDN)
  - 2 subtypes are indistinguishable by imaging
    - Classically occurs as well-circumscribed, purely cystic mass with numerous thin septations
    - Herniation into renal pelvis is characteristic
  - Must be differentiated from cystic Wilms tumor
- **Mesothelial Cyst**
  - Accumulation of fluid between mesothelial layers
  - Nonspecific unilocular cyst; very rarely multilocular
- **Tuboovarian Abscess**
  - Fever, cervical tenderness, & vaginal discharge
  - Thick-walled & hyperemic cystic focus along adnexa with surrounding inflammation & free fluid
- **Aneurysm**
  - Etiologies: Posttraumatic (including prior arterial catheterization), infectious, vasculitis, & vasculopathy
  - May see layers of clot in partially thrombosed lumen
  - Doppler is highly sensitive, provides critical component of US interrogation of any cystic lesion
  - CTA/MRA provides better preoperative mapping

SELECTED REFERENCES

1. Dillman JR et al: Imaging of the pediatric peritoneum, mesentery and omentum. Pediatr Radiol. 47(8):987-1000, 2017
2. Ranganath SH et al: Focal cystic abdominal masses in pediatric patients. AJR Am J Roentgenol. 199(1):W1-16, 2012

Ovarian Cyst

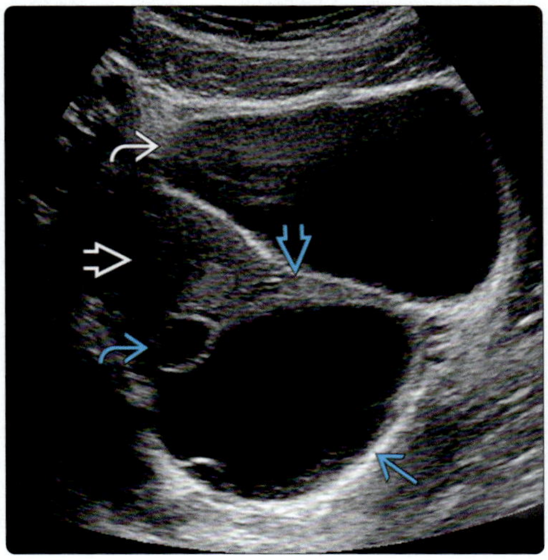

Ovarian Cyst

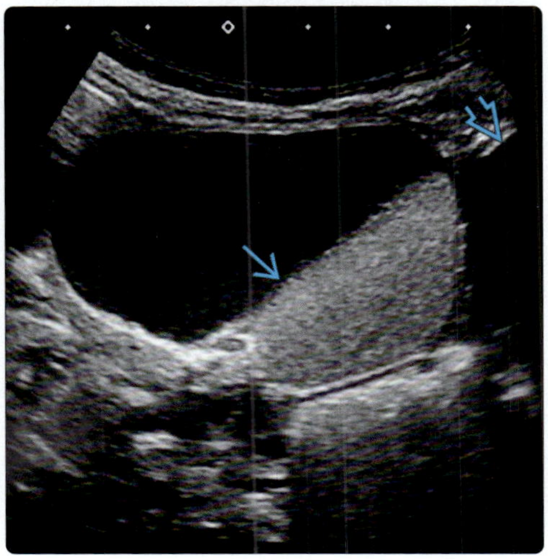

(Left) *Transverse US in a 13 year old with abdominal pain shows a 6-cm simple left ovarian cyst ➡. An adjacent follicle ➡ is noted in the surrounding ovarian parenchyma ➡. The urinary bladder ➡ & uterus ➡ are noted for reference.* **(Right)** *Longitudinal US in a newborn with a prenatally diagnosed cyst shows a fluid-debris level ➡ in a cystic lesion superior to the urinary bladder ➡. No normal left ovary was identified. A "vanishing" ovary due to left in utero torsion was confirmed upon resection.*

(Left) *LPO fluoroscopic VCUG in a 4 day old shows an enlarged irregular bladder with numerous diverticula. Posterior urethral valves (PUV) demarcate the transition from dilated posterior urethra to normal bulbar urethra. There is right grade V vesicoureteral reflux with marked distention of the right ureter & renal collecting system.* **(Right)** *Longitudinal US in the same patient with PUV shows marked right pelvocaliectasis with echogenic parenchyma, suggesting dysplasia due to in utero obstruction.*

Obstructed Bladder

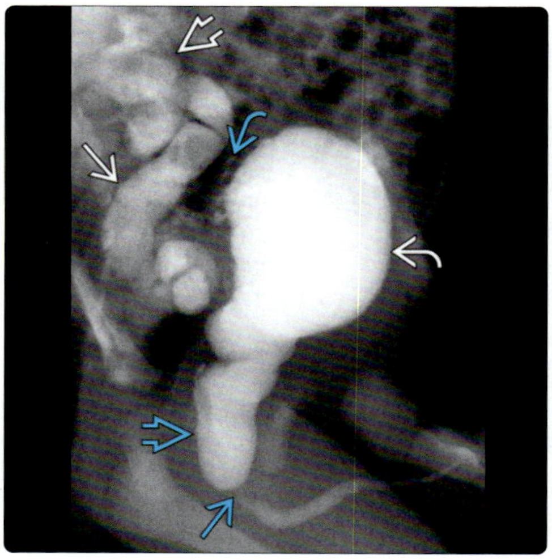

Hydronephrosis

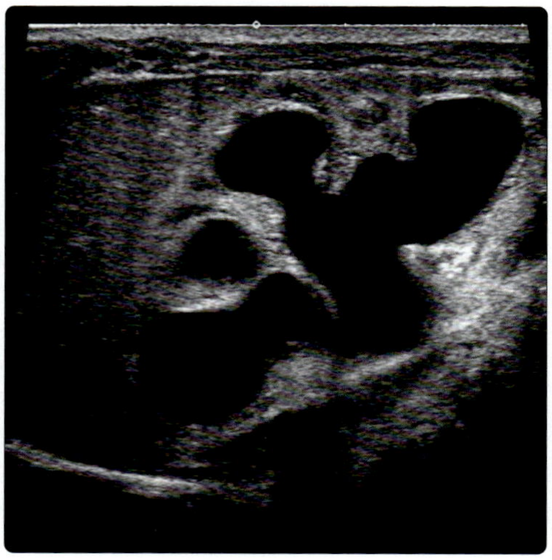

(Left) *Coronal CECT in a 9 year old weeks after an MVA shows multiple dilated fluid-filled small bowel loops due to obstructing strictures from the prior injury. There is mild mass effect on the urinary bladder.* **(Right)** *Axial CECT in a 6 year old 1 month status post pancreatic transection with duct injury shows a well-defined collection in the lesser sac displacing the stomach. This collection had been increasing in size & organization, while the transection, edema, & surrounding inflammatory changes had decreased.*

Bowel Obstruction (Mimic)

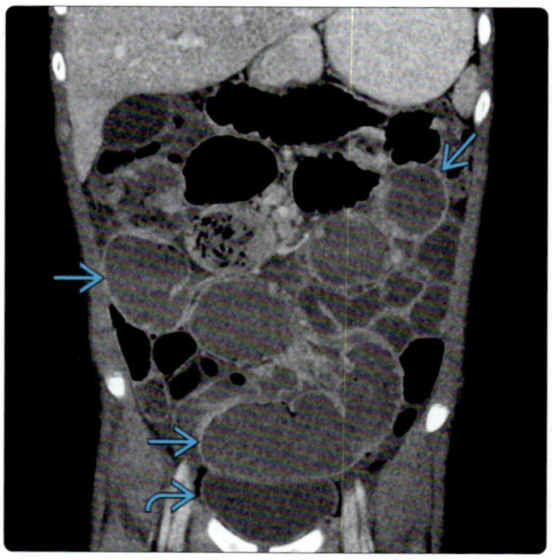

Peripancreatic Fluid Collection

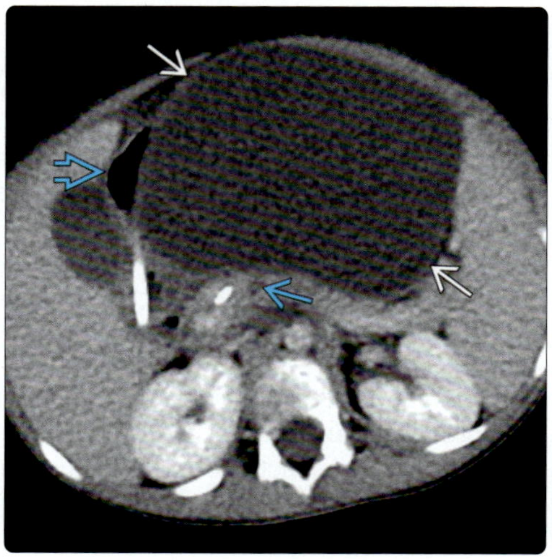

(Left) *Transverse & longitudinal US images in a 3 year old with fever, leukocytosis, & distention show a heterogeneously hypoechoic collection in the pelvis with poorly defined margins.* **(Right)** *Sagittal CECT in the same patient shows a gas- & fluid-containing collection in the pelvis with an irregular, thick, enhancing wall. There is inflammation of the surrounding fat & mass effect on the distended urinary bladder. Pus was found upon transrectal drainage of this abscess due to perforated appendicitis.*

Appendiceal Abscess

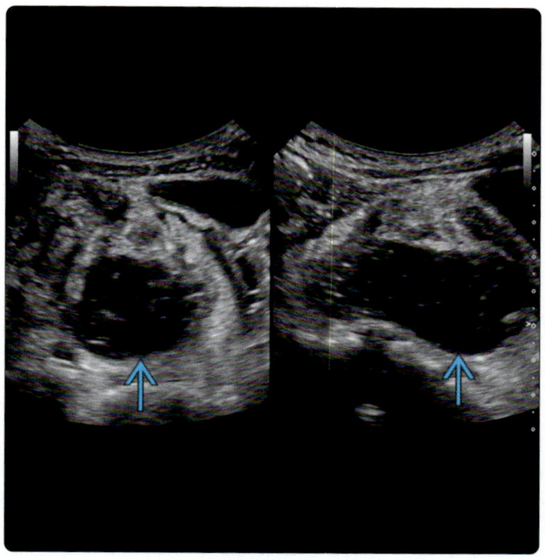

Appendiceal Abscess

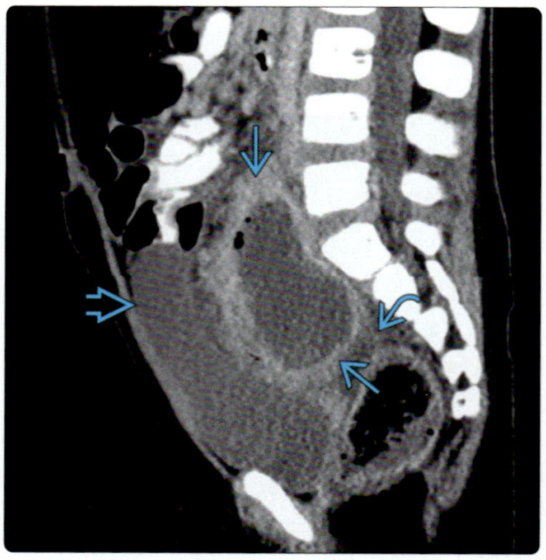

Multicystic Dysplastic Kidney

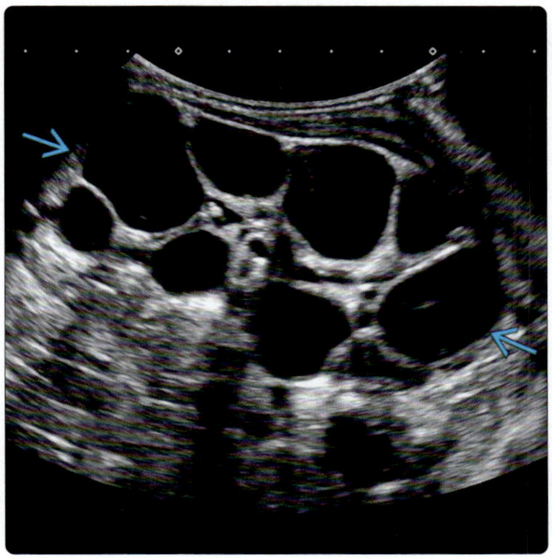

Gastrointestinal Duplication Cyst

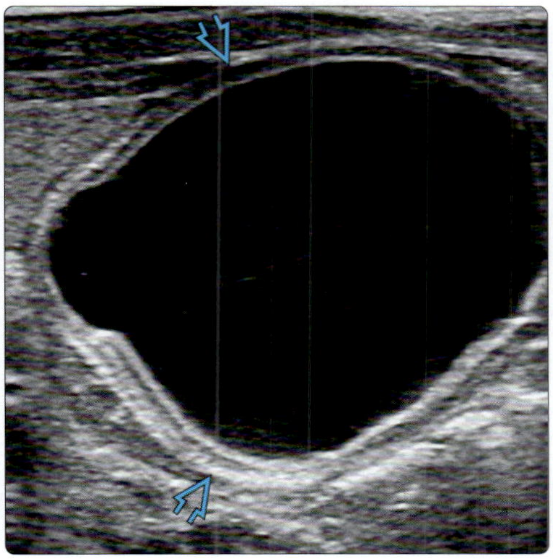

(Left) *Longitudinal US in a 1 month old shows an enlarged 10-cm left kidney that is replaced by numerous cysts & intervening echogenic tissue* → *. There is no detectable normal renal tissue, & no hydronephrosis is seen. Gradual involution would be expected on follow-up imaging.* **(Right)** *Longitudinal US in a 1 month old shows a 5-cm cyst in the right upper quadrant with a well-defined trilaminar "gut signature" wall* → *due to a small bowel duplication cyst. Peristalsis, though rarely seen, would help confirm the diagnosis.*

Splenic Cyst

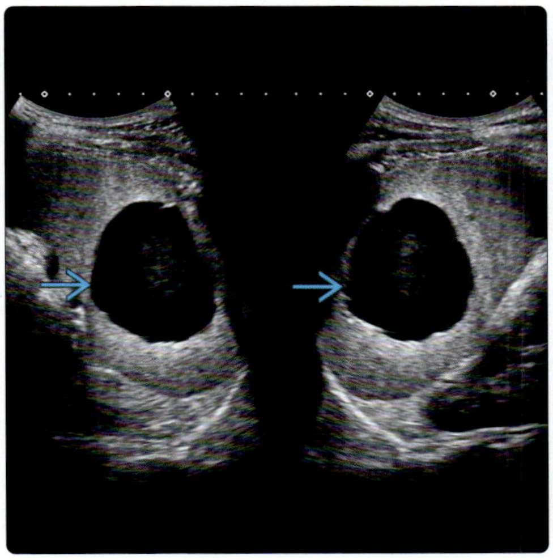

Mature Cystic Teratoma

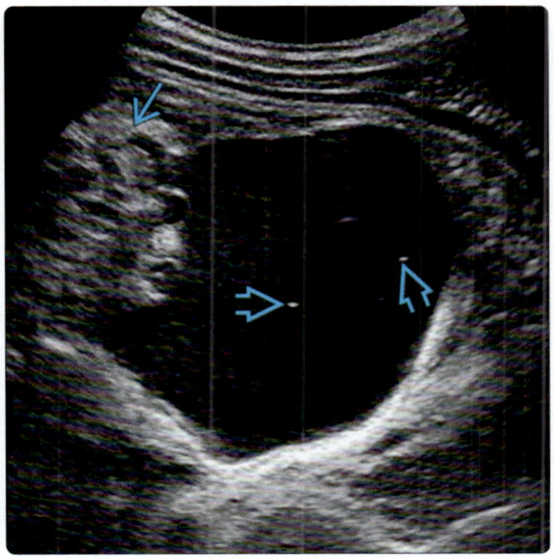

(Left) *Transverse & longitudinal US images in a 17 year old with left upper quadrant pain show a 6-cm lobulated cyst* → *in the spleen. No internal vascularity was seen on color Doppler (not shown). A mesothelial cyst was ultimately proven on biopsy & unroofing procedure.* **(Right)** *Transverse US in a teenage girl with abdominal distention shows a heterogeneous mass with solid* → *& cystic components. Linear & punctate echoes* → *were visualized in the cystic portion due to hair (the dermoid mesh sign).*

Mature Cystic Teratoma

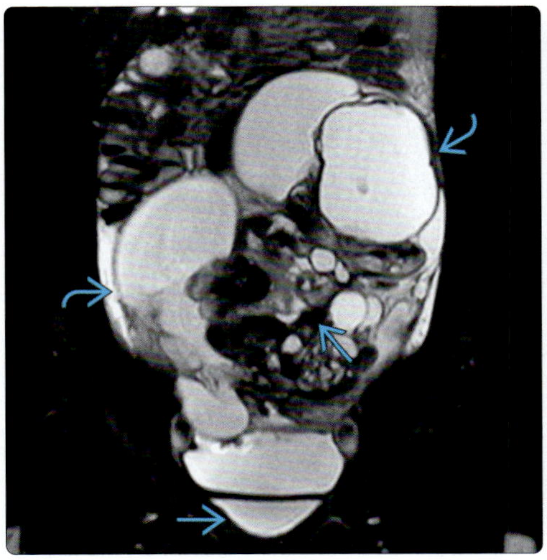

Lymphatic Malformation

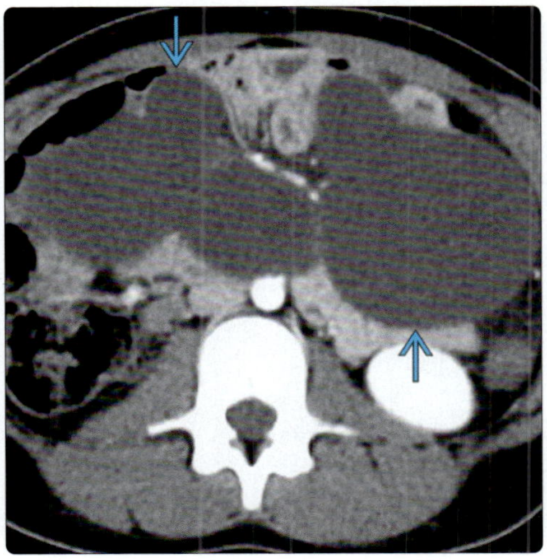

(Left) *Coronal T2 FS MR in the same patient shows a 20-cm lobulated heterogeneous mixed cystic & solid mass* → *extending out of the pelvis & displacing bowel superiorly. The T2 dark foci* → *were T1 bright & T1 FS dark, consistent with fat in this mature cystic teratoma.* **(Right)** *Axial CECT in an 11 year old after trauma shows a lobulated cystic mass with thin walls in the mesenteric leaves* → *separating bowel loops. This lymphatic malformation showed internal blood products on subsequent MR.*

(Left) *Sagittal panoramic US in a 14-year-old girl with flank pain & distention shows an elongated cystic mass in the pelvis posterior to the urinary bladder due to marked distention of the vagina. Note the mildly distended uterus superiorly.* **(Right)** *Coronal T1 MR in the same patient shows marked distention of the vagina by hyperintense blood products. An imperforate hymen was the cause of obstruction in this patient.*

Hydrometrocolpos

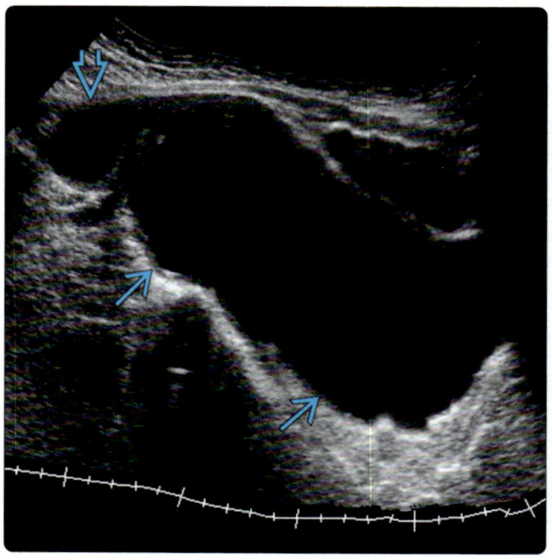

Hydrometrocolpos

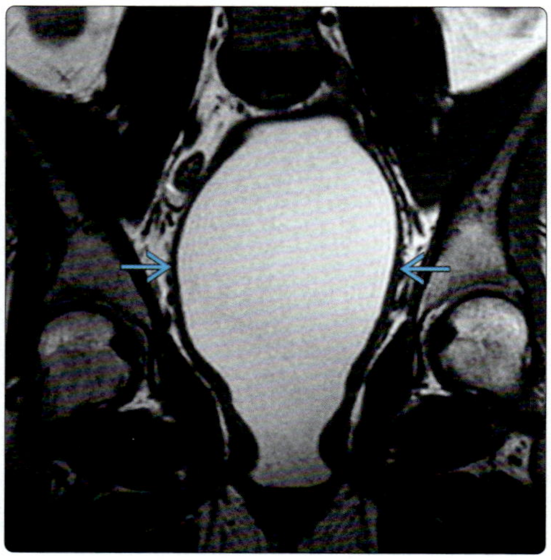

(Left) *Coronal MRCP shows cystic dilation, > 1 cm, of the common bile & hepatic ducts. There is a focal transition to a normal caliber within the midcommon bile duct.* **(Right)** *Frontal ERCP in the same patient shows cystic dilation of the proximal common bile duct & the central intrahepatic ducts. There is a focal tapering of the midcommon bile duct. This is a type 4a choledochal cyst according to the Todani classification.*

Choledochal Cyst

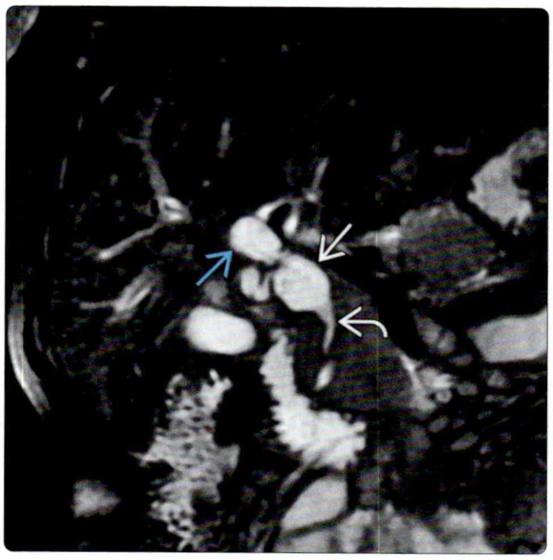

Choledochal Cyst

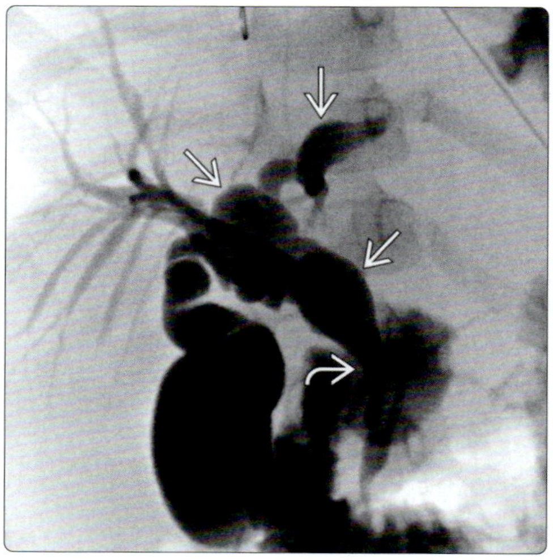

(Left) *Coronal oblique T2 MR in a 13-year-old girl with a history of repaired cloaca shows a fluid collection splaying the bladder & right ovary with multiple thin septations, typical of a peritoneal inclusion cyst.* **(Right)** *Longitudinal US in an 11 year old with shunted hydrocephalus & vomiting shows a localized fluid collection that did not freely communicate with the peritoneal cavity. Note the shunt superiorly in the collection. There are a few mildly dilated bowel loops.*

Peritoneal Inclusion Cyst

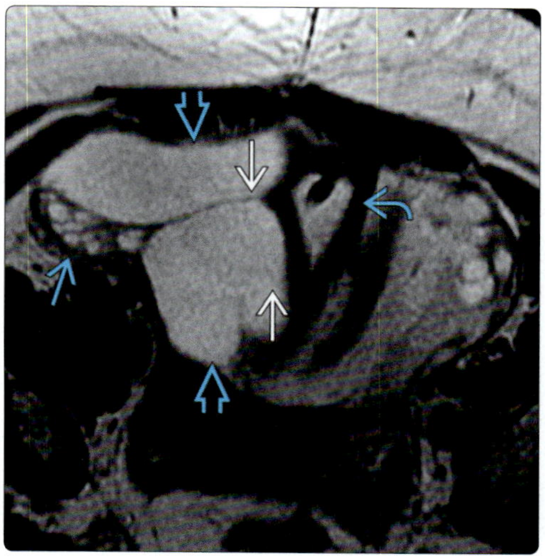

CSF Pseudocyst

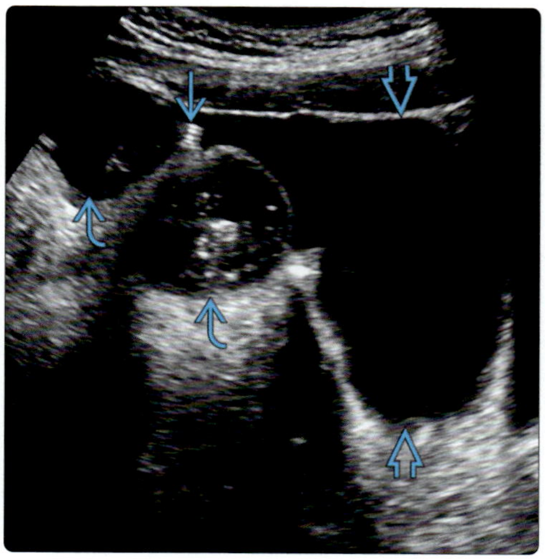

Meconium Pseudocyst

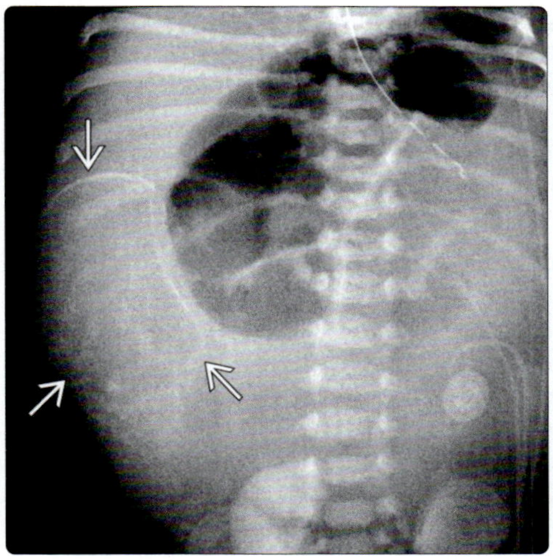

Meconium Pseudocyst

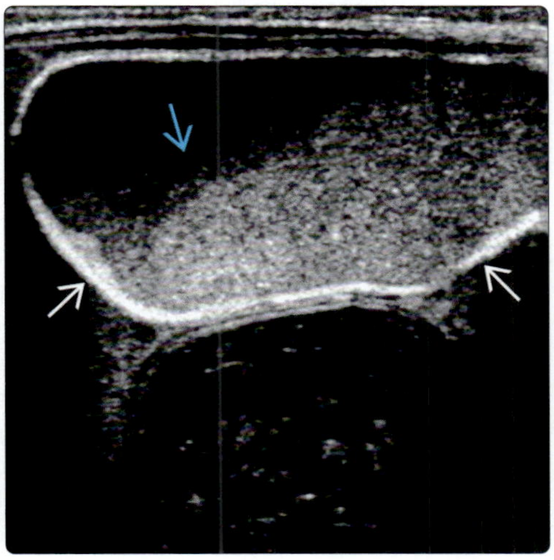

(Left) *AP radiograph shows a partially calcified ovoid mass* ➔ *in the right abdomen of a newborn, displacing dilated bowel to the left. This appearance strongly suggests a meconium pseudocyst with calcified rim due to an in utero distal bowel obstruction with perforation.* **(Right)** *Longitudinal US shows a well-defined cystic abdominal mass in a neonate with a hyperechoic wall* ➔. *Note the layering debris* ➔ *within the mass.*

Multilocular Cystic Renal Tumors

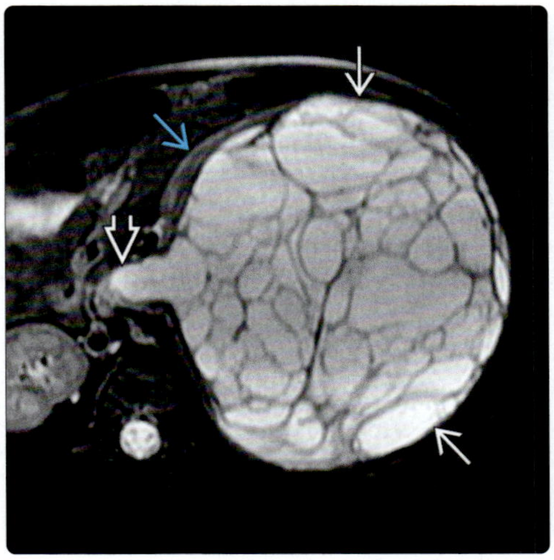

Tuboovarian Abscess

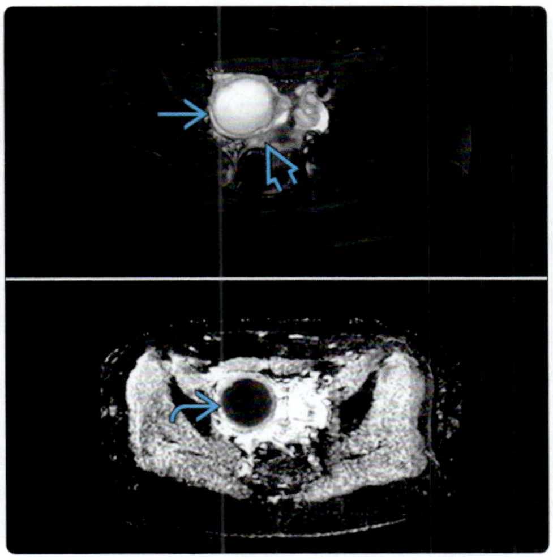

(Left) *Axial T2 FS MR shows a large multiloculated cystic mass* ➔ *with an adjacent "claw" of renal tissue* ➔ *along the margin. The mass extends into the renal pelvis* ➔, *typical of a multilocular cystic renal tumor.* **(Right)** *Axial T2 FS (top) & ADC map (bottom) MR images from a 15 year old with pain demonstrate a round collection with mildly thick, irregular, T2 dark rim* ➔ *& surrounding inflammation* ➔. *There is restricted diffusion centrally* ➔ *due to a tuboovarian abscess.*

Aneurysm

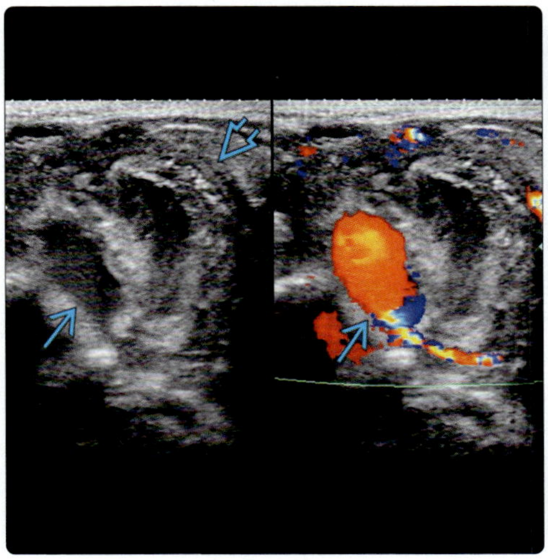

Aneurysm

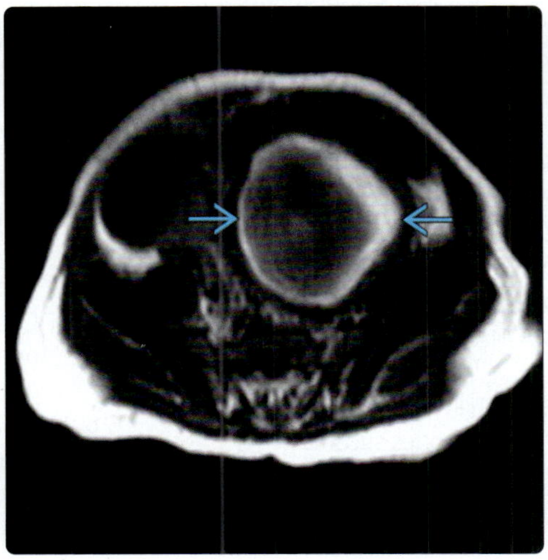

(Left) *Transverse US in a 1 month old shows a heterogeneous 4-cm mass* ➔ *in the left pelvis. Crescentic layers are suggested in the left 1/2 of the mass. The homogeneously hypoechoic ovoid portion* ➔ *filled with pulsatile flow on color Doppler.* **(Right)** *Axial T1 MR in the same patient shows layers of hyperintense signal in the mass due to subacute blood products within a largely thrombosed aneurysm* ➔. *Numerous other aneurysms were found in this infant (who was ultimately diagnosed with polyarteritis nodosa).*

Abdominal Mass in Neonate

DIFFERENTIAL DIAGNOSIS

Common

- Multicystic Dysplastic Kidney
- Obstructed Urinary Bladder
- Hydronephrosis
- Ovarian Cyst
- Adrenal Hemorrhage
- Neuroblastoma
- Gastrointestinal Duplication Cyst
- Sacrococcygeal Teratoma

Less Common

- Mesoblastic Nephroma
- Mesenteric Lymphatic Malformation
- Ovarian Torsion
- Meconium Pseudocyst
- Hepatic Hemangioma
- Bronchopulmonary Sequestration
- Choledochal Cyst

Rare but Important

- Umbilical Venous Catheter Complication
- Hydrocolpos/Hydrometrocolpos
- Hepatoblastoma
- Mesenchymal Hamartoma
- Wilms Tumor

ESSENTIAL INFORMATION

Helpful Clues for Common Diagnoses

- **Multicystic Dysplastic Kidney**
  - Noncommunicating cysts of varying size replace renal parenchyma; no functional tissue remains
    - Involutes over months/years
  - Often has residual intervening echogenic parenchyma
  - May only involve part of kidney if duplicated
  - Contralateral ureteropelvic junction (UPJ) obstruction or vesicoureteral reflux (VUR) in up to 40%
- **Obstructed Urinary Bladder**
  - Variety of congenital causes: Posterior urethral valves, Eagle-Barrett syndrome, obstructing ureterocele, megalourethra, cloaca, megacystis-microcolon-intestinal hypoperistalsis syndrome, mass
- **Hydronephrosis**
  - Many congenital etiologies, including VUR, UPJ obstruction, or ureterovesical junction obstruction
    - Marked distention of renal pelvis without hydroureter is typical in UPJ obstruction
    - Bilateral hydroureteronephrosis (± renal cystic dysplasia) favors bladder outlet obstruction
- **Ovarian Cyst**
  - ~ 20% of neonatal cysts are > 1 cm
    - Cysts resolve as maternal hormones subside
    - Larger fetal cysts rarely result in torsion & necrosis
  - Avascular; variable echogenicity if internal hemorrhage
- **Adrenal Hemorrhage**
  - Heterogeneous avascular suprarenal mass, often with cystic components
  - Involutes over weeks, may develop Ca^{2+}
  - Note that hemorrhage may occur within neuroblastoma
- **Neuroblastoma**
  - Most common malignancy of neonate
  - Origin in paraspinal sympathetic chain ganglia
    - Congenital is most commonly of adrenal origin
  - Often heterogeneous: Mixed cystic & solid lesion, typically hypovascular; Ca^{2+} is common
  - Frequently crosses midline, engulfs vessels, elevates aorta from spine, & invades spinal canal
  - Look for liver, bone, & skin metastases
  - Small congenital lesions may spontaneously regress
- **Gastrointestinal Duplication Cyst**
  - Usually round cystic mass attached to but not communicating with bowel
  - ± trilaminar "gut signature" of wall on US; may rarely show peristalsis
- **Sacrococcygeal Teratoma**
  - Complex presacral solid & cystic mass containing all 3 germ cell layers; fat &/or Ca^{2+} are often present
  - Typically has external/exophytic extension
    - Purely internal forms are more likely to have delayed diagnosis & malignant elements
  - Typically presents prenatally; may lead to fetal hydrops, rupture/hemorrhage, &/or maternal mirror syndrome

Helpful Clues for Less Common Diagnoses

- **Mesoblastic Nephroma**
  - Most common congenital/neonatal renal neoplasm
  - Typically benign hamartomatous tumor
    - Less common cellular subtype is more aggressive
  - May cause prenatal polyhydramnios & premature birth
  - Mass ± hypertension, hypercalcemia in neonates
  - Solid renal mass with heterogeneous enhancement, demonstrating "claw" of splayed residual renal tissue
    - Cystic/necrotic/hemorrhagic foci suggest cellular type
- **Mesenteric Lymphatic Malformation**
  - Complex, multilocular cystic lesion; often transspatial
    - Often have thin internal septations
      - □ Macrocysts: Cysts of > 1 cm; no central enhancement; ± hemorrhage with debris levels
      - □ Microcysts: Cysts of < 1 cm; more solid-appearing
    - Tend to encase vessels without narrowing them
  - Grow with patient; may rapidly enlarge due to hemorrhage, infection, or hormonal stimulation
- **Ovarian Torsion**
  - Imaging appearance is variable in fetus/neonate
    - Complex multiseptated cystic mass; fluid-debris level is highly suggestive if only 1 normal ovary is visualized
      - □ Reflects late findings of hemorrhage & necrosis in clinically silent antenatal torsion
    - Classic appearance of enlarged, edematous ovary with peripheral follicles is less common in neonate
    - ↓ in flow on Doppler US is unreliable
  - May be precipitated by cyst or teratoma
- **Meconium Pseudocyst**
  - Thick-walled cystic mass ± mural Ca^{2+}, internal debris
  - In utero bowel obstruction/ischemia → perforation → meconium peritonitis → pseudocyst
    - ± bowel obstruction related to underlying cause of perforation or subsequent adhesions
- **Hepatic Hemangioma**

- May be congenital hemangioma (CH) or infantile hemangiomas (IHs)
  - Cutaneous hemangiomas in infantile > > congenital
- Highly vascular: Enlarged feeding arteries/draining veins, early peripheral/gradual central enhancement
- CH: Large, solitary mass presenting at birth (or prenatally); does not enlarge postnatally
  - Rapidly involuting CH (RICH) > > noninvoluting CH (NICH)
    - RICH ↓ in size over 3-12 months
  - Moderate to marked internal heterogeneity on US & T2 MR due to internal hemorrhage, fibrosis, &/or Ca^{2+}
    - Central portions do not fully enhance
  - Often have transient coagulopathy; ± heart failure
  - ↑ α-fetoprotein (AFP) levels are likely due to normal neonatal elevations & should trend down
- IHs: Multifocal or diffuse small to moderate masses
  - Develop in 1st few weeks of life, enlarge in 1st year, then involute slowly over years
  - Relatively homogeneous in appearance: Hypoechoic on US, intermediate to high on T2 MR
    - Variable internal vascularity on Doppler US; differs from soft tissue IHs, which are highly vascular
  - Gradually fill in completely on postcontrast imaging
  - Complications are more common with diffuse type
    - Hypothyroidism, liver failure, abdominal compartment syndrome, heart failure

- **Bronchopulmonary Sequestration**
  - Nonfunctioning pulmonary tissue with no tracheobronchial communication
  - 10-15% of extralobar bronchopulmonary sequestrations are intraabdominal
  - Variably echogenic mass near diaphragm
    - Small cysts if components of congenital pulmonary airway malformation are present ("hybrid")
  - Systemic arterial & venous supply
- **Choledochal Cyst**
  - Cystic or fusiform dilation of biliary tree
  - US most commonly shows dilation of common bile duct > 1 cm in diameter
  - HIDA scan or MR imaging with hepatocellular contrast agent can be used to prove connection to biliary system

Helpful Clues for Rare Diagnoses

- **Umbilical Venous Catheter Complication**
  - Often due to malposition in portal system with hypertonic infusion ± laceration
  - Heterogeneous fluid collection in hepatic parenchyma adjacent to vessel currently/previously traversed by umbilical venous catheter
- **Hydrocolpos/Hydrometrocolpos**
  - Distention of vagina > > > uterus, typically by mucus in neonate due to maternal hormonal stimulation
  - Often associated with other GI/GU anomalies
- **Hepatoblastoma**
  - 4% are congenital
  - Large, solid, well-defined liver mass; 80% are solitary
    - May have hemorrhage, necrosis, or Ca^{2+} with heterogeneous enhancement; may invade vessels
  - Persistently high or rising AFP levels
  - Associated with Beckwith-Wiedemann, prematurity, familial adenomatous polyposis, others
- **Mesenchymal Hamartoma**
  - 2nd most common benign hepatic mass of infancy
  - May grow rapidly, leading to compartment syndrome, respiratory distress, rarely heart failure
  - Multiloculated cystic mass in 70%; solid or mixed forms also occur; microcysts may appear solid
  - Reports of spontaneous regression as well as malignant transformation to undifferentiated embryonal sarcoma
- **Wilms Tumor**
  - Typically large, solid, hypoenhancing heterogeneous mass with "claw" of residual renal tissue
    - Cannot differentiate from mesoblastic nephroma by imaging; Wilms is more common > 3 months of age
    - Renal vein/inferior vena cava invasion may occur with Wilms
  - Associated with nephroblastomatosis, Beckwith-Wiedemann, WAGR, Denys-Drash, others

Multicystic Dysplastic Kidney

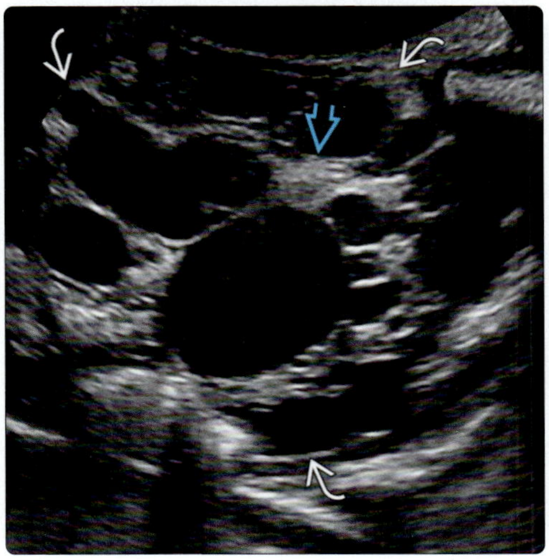

Obstructed Urinary Bladder

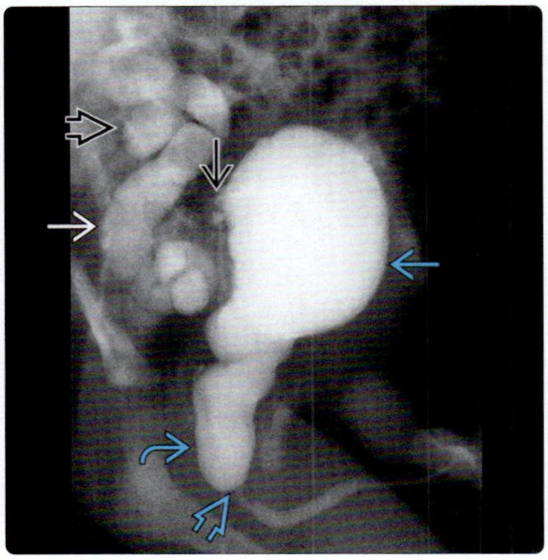

(Left) *Longitudinal US in a 6 day old with suspected prenatal hydronephrosis shows an enlarged left kidney ➔ with numerous noncommunicating cysts of variable size. The intervening dysplastic parenchyma is abnormally echogenic ➔.* **(Right)** *Left posterior oblique fluoroscopic VCUG in a 4 day old shows a dilated urinary bladder ➔ with diverticula ➔. The urethra is dilated ➔ up to the level of posterior urethral valves ➔. Note the grade V vesicoureteral reflux in the dilated ureter ➔ & renal collecting system ➔.*

(Left) *Longitudinal US in a newborn with prenatal hydronephrosis shows dilated calyces connecting with the disproportionately enlarged renal pelvis. No hydroureter was seen. These features are typical of a UPJ obstruction.* **(Right)** *Longitudinal color Doppler US in a newborn girl with a prenatally detected anomaly shows a large pelvic cyst with no internal vascularity but numerous thin internal septations. This lesion gradually regressed over the next 2 months, leaving a normal right ovary.*

Hydronephrosis

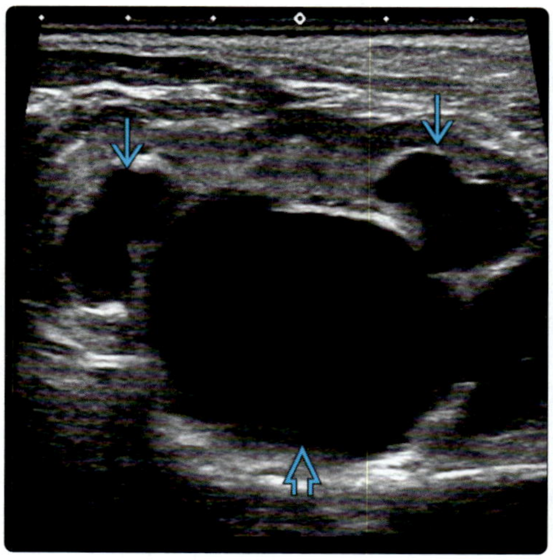

Ovarian Cyst

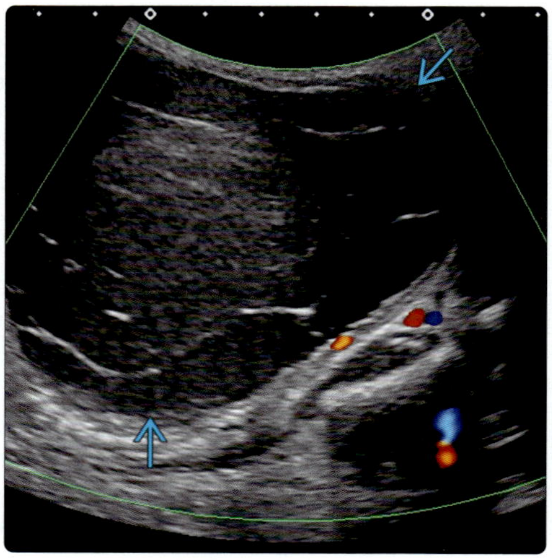

(Left) *Transverse color Doppler US in a 3 day old shows a cystic lesion in the right lower quadrant. The wall demonstrates the trilaminar "gut signature" that suggests (but is not entirely specific for) a GI duplication cyst (ileal, in this case). Note a similar appearance of the urinary bladder wall.* **(Right)** *Longitudinal color Doppler US in a 4 day old shows a heterogeneously hypoechoic & avascular left adrenal lesion. This resolved on follow-up imaging, consistent with adrenal hemorrhage.*

Gastrointestinal Duplication Cyst

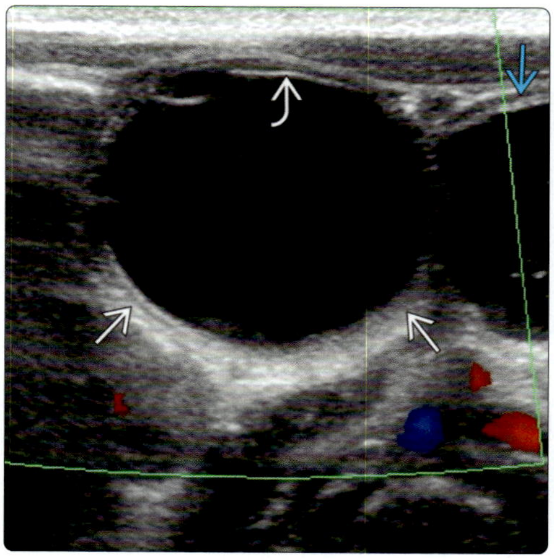

Adrenal Hemorrhage

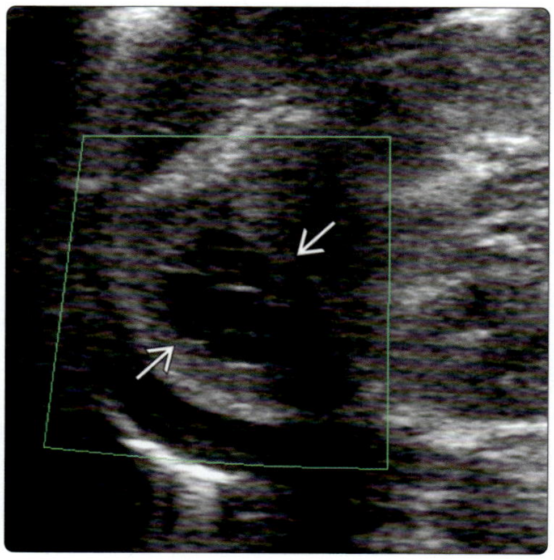

(Left) *Transverse US shows a solid echogenic mass posterior to the spleen & left kidney. A focal Ca^{2+} with posterior acoustic shadowing is a helpful observation in narrowing the differential diagnosis.* **(Right)** *Axial CECT in the same patient shows the mass displacing the left kidney & spleen anteriorly. The mass also demonstrates coarse chunky Ca^{2+}, vessel encasement, & intraspinal extension. The findings are typical of neuroblastoma.*

Neuroblastoma

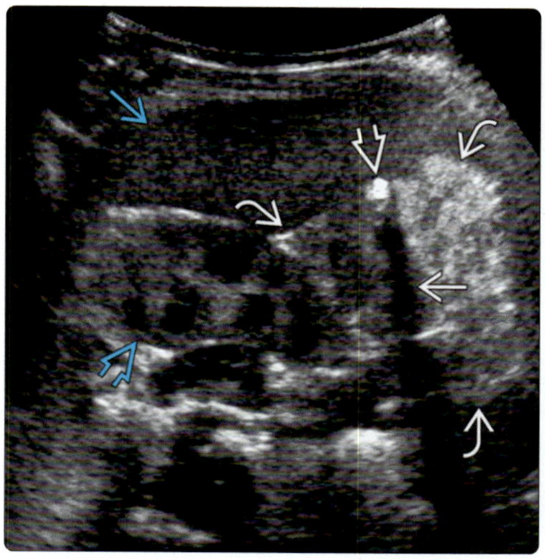

Neuroblastoma

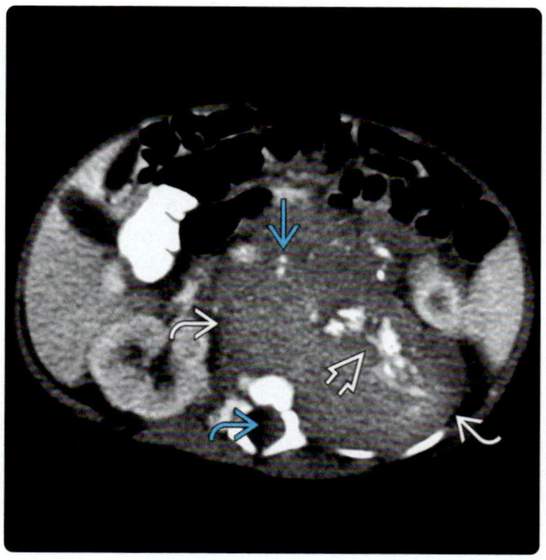

Sacrococcygeal Teratoma

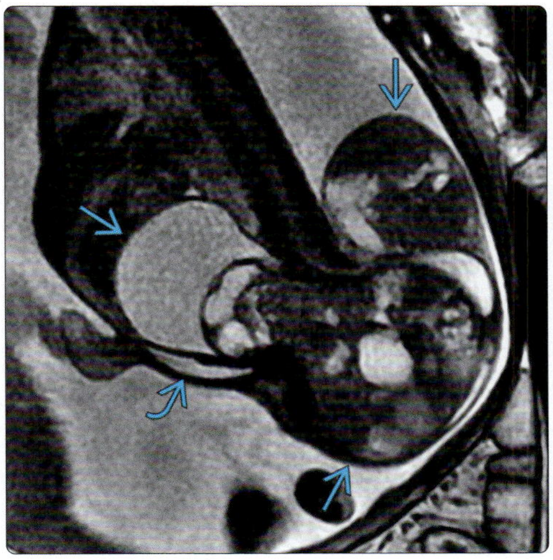

Sacrococcygeal Teratoma

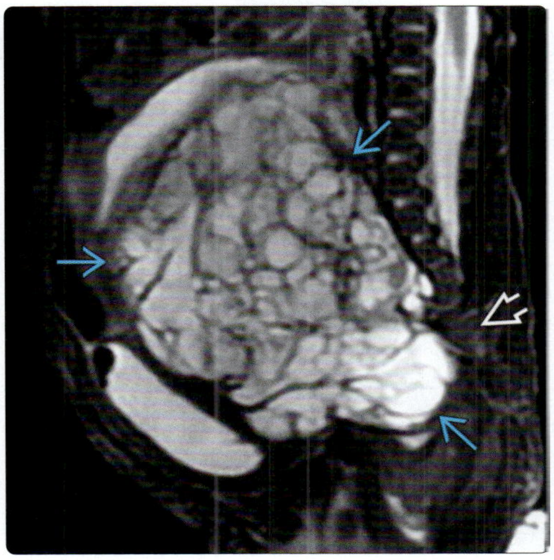

(Left) *Sagittal SSFP MR in a fetus shows a solid & cystic dumbbell-shaped presacral mass extending into the abdomen & pelvis with large exophytic components. The bladder is compressed anteriorly.* **(Right)** *Sagittal STIR MR in the same patient at 2 months of age shows the large residual predominantly cystic intraabdominal portion of the tumor after resection of the exophytic perineal component. The distal sacrum & coccyx have been resected.*

Mesoblastic Nephroma

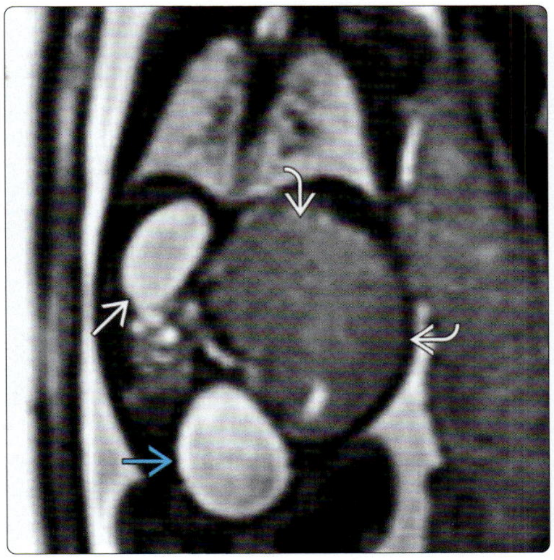

Mesoblastic Nephroma

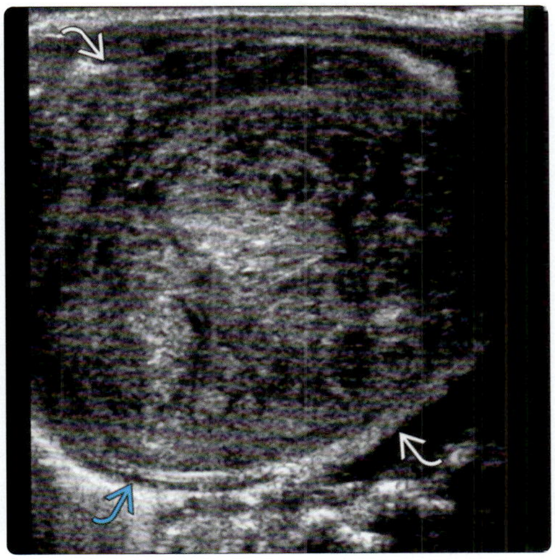

(Left) *Coronal T2 SSFSE MR in a fetus shows a large solid right renal mass due to mesoblastic nephroma, which was resected soon after birth. Note the stomach & bladder.* **(Right)** *Longitudinal US shows the whorled, encapsulated, moderately heterogeneous appearance of the solid mesoblastic nephroma in the same patient. The layered ring sign is evident posteriorly. There are no internal cystic foci, which would favor the more aggressive cellular subtype.*

Mesenteric Lymphatic Malformation

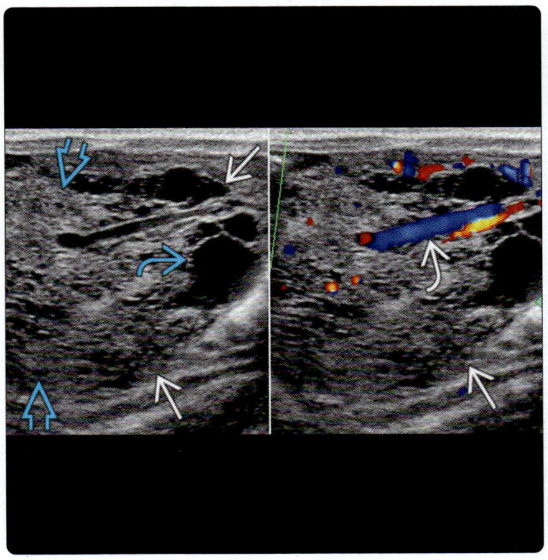

Mesenteric Lymphatic Malformation

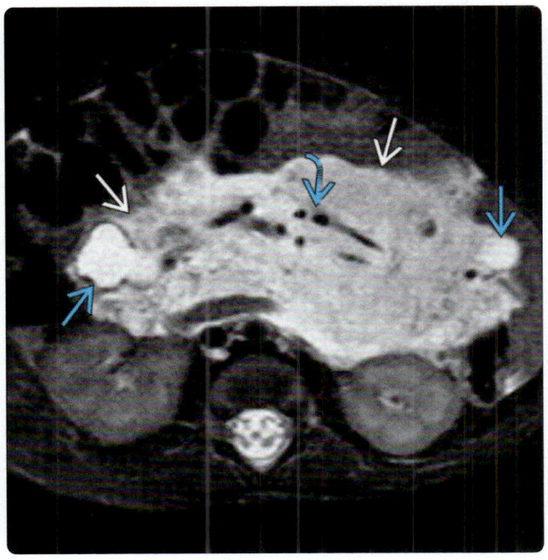

(Left) *Longitudinal US to evaluate a palpable abdominal mass in a 2 week old shows a multicystic mass. This mesenteric lymphatic malformation had both macrocystic & microcystic components. Note that the microcystic components appear nearly solid. Encased vessels course through the mass.* **(Right)** *Axial T2 MR in the same patient shows macrocysts & vascular encasement. Most of the transspatial mass appears microcystic. There was no enhancement on postcontrast imaging (not shown).*

(Left) *Transverse color Doppler US in a newborn girl shows an avascular mass with a central heterogeneously echogenic component* ➔ *within a larger cyst* ↪*, found at surgery to be a chronically torsed left ovary with necrosis. The more echogenic portion represents retracting clot.* **(Right)** *Longitudinal color Doppler US shows an avascular cystic mass* ↪ *with a fluid-debris level* ➔ *in the right lower quadrant of a 9 day old. No normal right ovary was seen. Chronic right ovarian torsion with necrosis was found at surgery.*

Ovarian Torsion

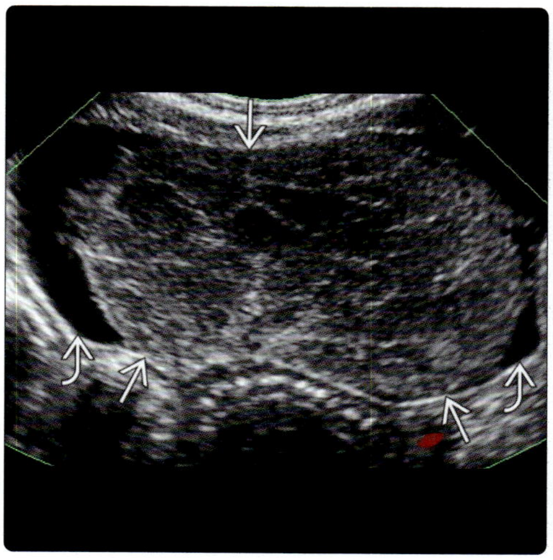

Ovarian Torsion

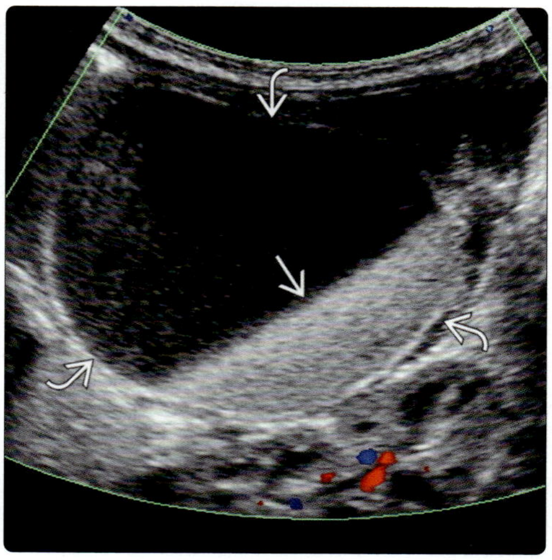

(Left) *AP radiograph shows curvilinear* Ca^{2+} ➔ *in the right lower quadrant of a newborn with a known in utero bowel perforation.* **(Right)** *Subsequent longitudinal US in the same patient demonstrates a complex collection* ↪ *with thick, irregular walls inferior to the liver* ⇨*, consistent with a meconium pseudocyst in the setting of meconium peritonitis from a perforated bowel obstruction.*

Meconium Pseudocyst

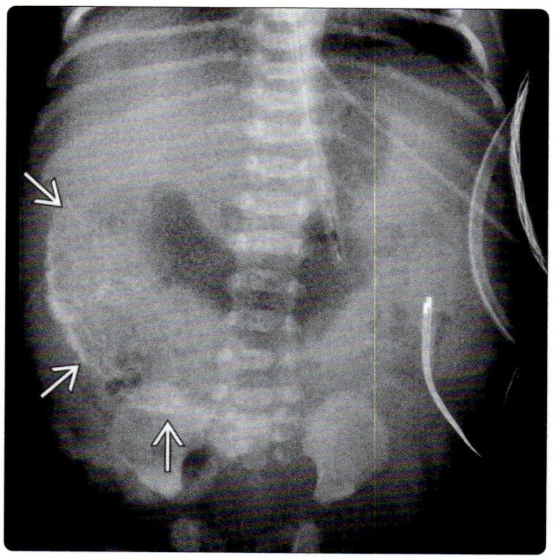

Meconium Pseudocyst

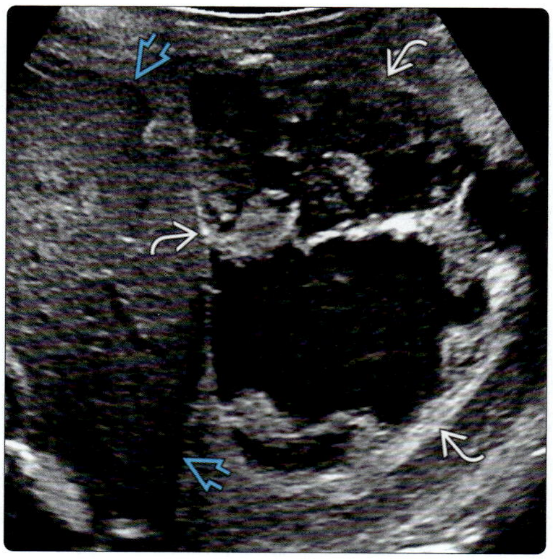

(Left) *Transverse color Doppler US in a newborn shows a large exophytic heterogeneous mass arising from the left lobe of the liver. There is increased peripheral vascularity, typical of a congenital hemangioma. Note that these masses are usually detected prenatally or in the 1st week after delivery.* **(Right)** *Axial SSFSE T2 MR in the same patient shows internal heterogeneity of the mass* ⇨*. The mass regressed to < 1/2 of its size over the next 6 months, typical of a rapidly involuting congenital hemangioma (RICH).*

Hepatic Hemangioma

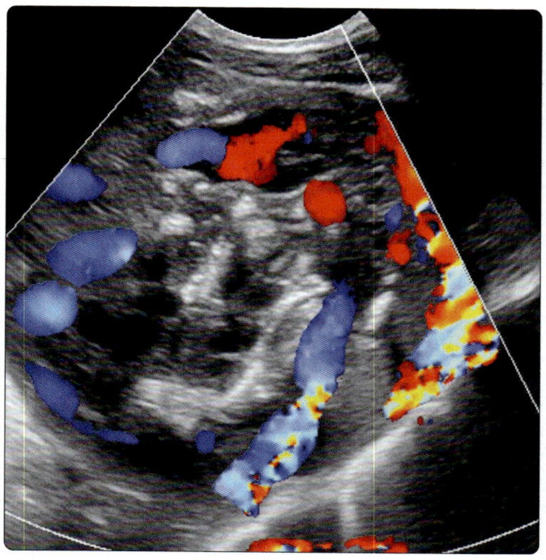

Hepatic Hemangioma

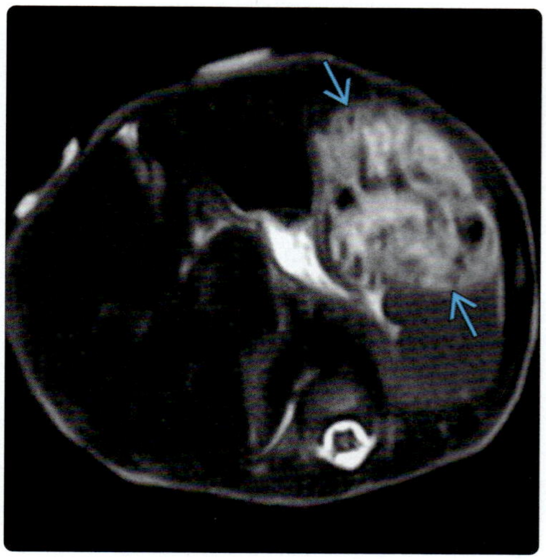

Hepatic Hemangioma

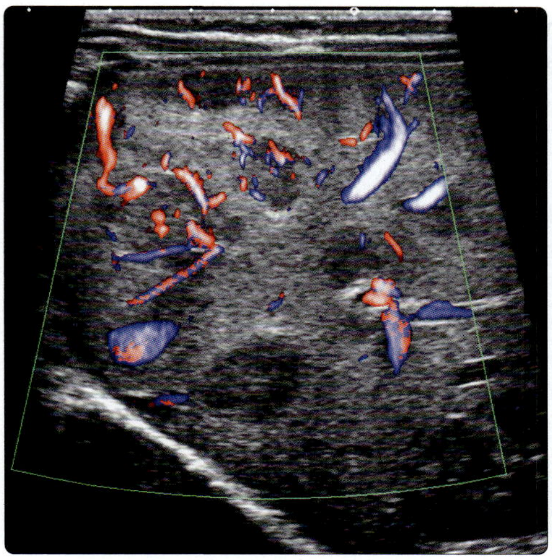

Hepatic Hemangioma

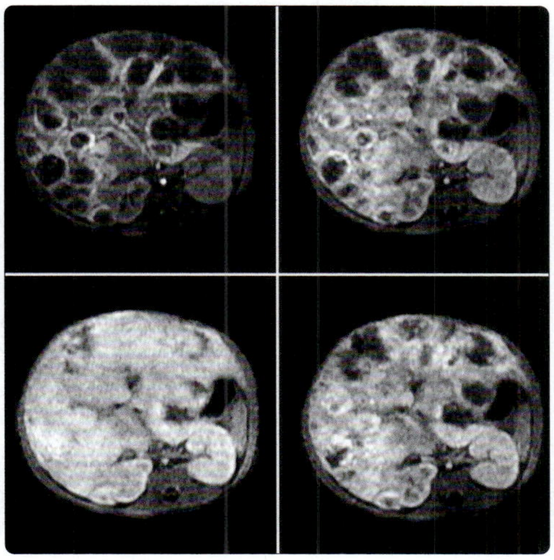

(Left) *Longitudinal color Doppler US in a 4 month old with cutaneous IHs shows scattered, well-circumscribed, round hypoechoic lesions with variable internal vascularity. This appearance is common with hepatic IHs but differs from soft tissue IHs (which always show abundant low-resistance arterial flow in the proliferating phase).* **(Right)** *Dynamic axial T1 C+ FS MR images from early to late (clockwise from the upper left) in a 3 month old with cutaneous IHs show peripheral to central enhancement of the IHs over 2 minutes.*

Bronchopulmonary Sequestration

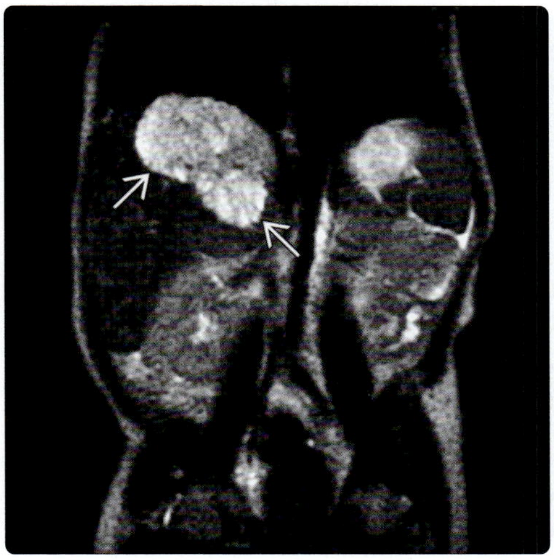

Bronchopulmonary Sequestration

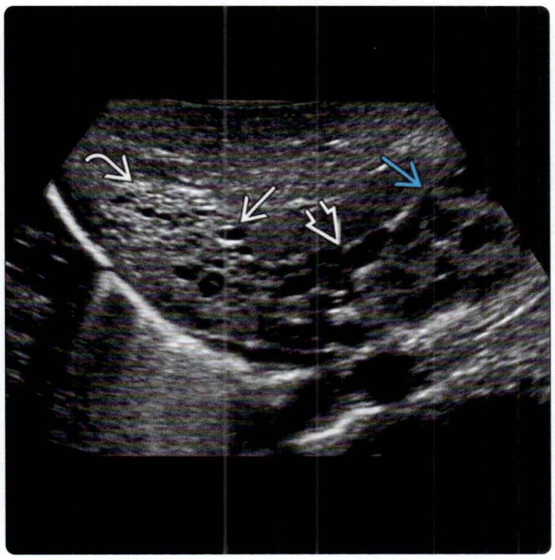

(Left) *Coronal T2 SSFSE MR shows a well-defined multicystic right suprarenal mass along the posterior surface of the liver. This was an infradiaphragmatic bronchopulmonary sequestration.* **(Right)** *Longitudinal US in the same patient shows the heterogeneously echogenic lesion along the posterior margin of the liver. Numerous tiny cysts are seen in the mass. Portions of the normal adrenal gland & kidney are noted.*

Umbilical Venous Catheter Complication

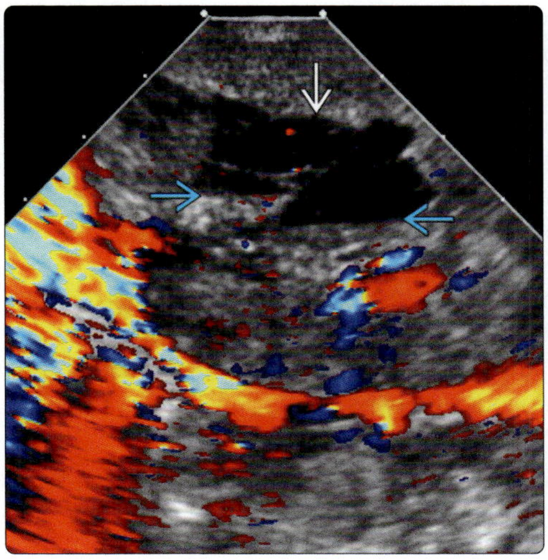

Hepatoblastoma

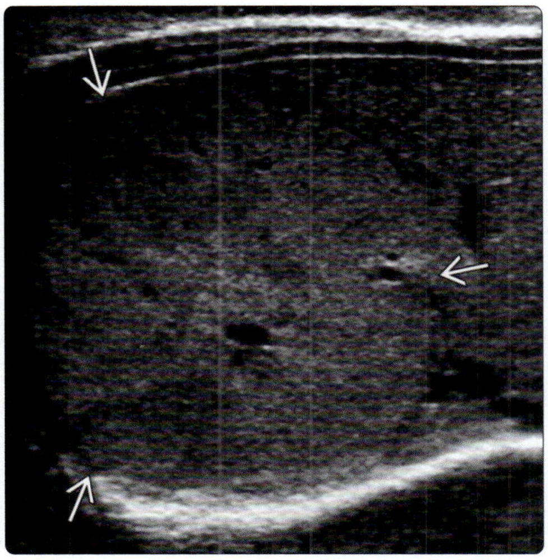

(Left) *Longitudinal color Doppler US in a 2 week old shows a heterogeneous collection in the left hepatic lobe with internal septations, fluid-debris levels, & no internal vascularity. This lesion was due to a UVC extravasation & gradually decreased in size.* **(Right)** *Transverse US shows a well-circumscribed solid mass in the right hepatic lobe on a study performed for pyloric stenosis in a 1 month old. The mass was isolated & hypovascular. The age & appearance are atypical for a hepatic hemangioma.*

DIFFERENTIAL DIAGNOSIS

Common

- Wilms Tumor
- Neuroblastoma

Less Common

- Ovarian Tumors
- Lymphoma
- Hepatic Hemangioma
- Hepatoblastoma
- Rhabdomyosarcoma
- Plexiform Neurofibromas

Rare but Important

- Desmoid/Aggressive Fibromatosis
- Congenital Mesoblastic Nephroma
- Renal Cell Carcinoma
- Angiomyolipoma
- Hepatocellular Carcinoma
- Hepatic Mesenchymal Hamartoma
- Pancreatoblastoma
- Adrenocortical Carcinoma
- Kaposiform Hemangioendothelioma
- Rhabdoid Tumor

ESSENTIAL INFORMATION

Key Differential Diagnosis Issues

- Organ of origin & age help limit differential diagnosis
- Consider mimics of abdominal masses: Splenomegaly, hydronephrosis, abscess, hematoma, ovarian torsion

Helpful Clues for Common Diagnoses

- **Wilms Tumor**
  - Most common pediatric abdominal neoplasm
  - Peak incidence at 3 years; 80% < 5 years
  - May be bilateral (5-10%)
  - Usually presents as abdominal mass ± pain, hematuria
  - Large, heterogeneous, predominantly solid renal mass, typically hypoenhancing; Ca^{2+} in < 20% on CT
    - May invade renal vein, inferior vena cava
  - Associations: WAGR, Denys-Drash, Beckwith-Wiedemann, nephroblastomatosis (persistent metanephric blastema)
- **Neuroblastoma**
  - Malignant tumor of neural crest origin
  - Arises anywhere along sympathetic chain (neck to pelvis)
    - ~ 65% arise in abdomen, most commonly adrenal
  - ~ 30% occur in 1st year of life, > 90% before age 5
  - Usually presents as abdominal mass ± pain, distention
    - May have symptoms attributable to metastatic disease or paraneoplastic effects
    - Urine catecholamines are elevated in 90%
  - Metastases in up to 70% at diagnosis: Bone/marrow, liver, skin
  - Heterogeneously enhancing mass on CECT/MR
    - May be small, round, & well-circumscribed or large, multilobulated, & invasive
    - Often extends across midline & invades adjacent organs: Spine, kidney, pancreas
    - Tends to encase & displace vessels rather than invade
    - Ca^{2+} in ~ 85% on CT
  - I-123 MIBG positive in 90-95%

Helpful Clues for Less Common Diagnoses

- **Ovarian Tumors**
  - Can become very large, filling pelvis/abdomen
  - Teratomas are most common; majority are benign
    - Mixed cystic & solid mass with fat & Ca^{2+}
  - Ovarian malignancies account for 1% of pediatric cancers
    - 75-80% are germ cell tumors
- **Lymphoma**
  - Most cases are > 5 years of age
  - Bulky conglomerations of enlarged lymph nodes that are relatively homogeneous in attenuation
    - May involve any nodal groups
    - Larger masses may become necrotic
    - Rarely contain Ca^{2+} prior to therapy
    - Often encase vessels, efface veins, displace arteries
    - Involvement of bowel & solid organs is common
      - Multifocal round masses of liver, spleen, or kidneys
      - ± lung & bone involvement
- **Hepatic Hemangioma**
  - Congenital hemangiomas: Large focal solitary mass of newborns (discussed elsewhere)
  - Infantile hemangiomas (IHs): Common benign vascular neoplasm
    - Multifocal or diffuse small to moderate masses
    - Develop in 1st few weeks of life, enlarge in 1st year, then involute slowly over years
    - Relatively homogeneous in appearance: Hypoechoic on US, intermediate to high on T2 MR
    - Variable internal vascularity on Doppler US
      - ± enlarged feeding arteries/draining veins
    - Early peripheral enhancement with progressive central filling on dynamic postcontrast imaging
    - ≥ 5 cutaneous IHs ↑ risk of visceral IHs
- **Hepatoblastoma**
  - Most common pediatric liver malignancy
    - Most diagnosed under 18 months of age
  - 90% have increased serum α-fetoprotein (AFP)
  - Large, solid, well-defined liver mass; 80% are solitary
    - Ca^{2+} in 40-55%; ± hemorrhage, necrosis
    - Heterogeneous enhancement; may invade vessels
  - Metastases in 20% at diagnosis: Lung, brain, bone
  - Associations: Low birth weight, Beckwith-Wiedemann, familial adenomatous polyposis, trisomy 18
- **Rhabdomyosarcoma**
  - May be of GU system (bladder, vagina, uterus, prostate) or of soft tissue origin
  - Bimodal age distribution: 2-6 years vs. 14-18 years
  - Heterogeneous solid mass on imaging
- **Plexiform Neurofibroma**
  - Classic cutaneous findings of neurofibromatosis type I (NF1) include café au lait spots & axillary freckling
  - Track along courses of nerves; discrete masses are most common but can diffusely infiltrate hollow viscera
    - Lobulated low-attenuation masses (CT)
    - Classic target sign of individual lobule with T2-hyperintense periphery & hypointense center (MR)

Helpful Clues for Rare Diagnoses

- **Desmoid/Aggressive Fibromatosis**
  - Benign but infiltrative mesenchymal neoplasm
  - Most commonly found in mesentery or abdominal wall
  - Heterogeneous solid mass classically containing low signal intensity components on all MR sequences
  - Associations: Gardner, familial adenomatous polyposis, prior abdominal surgery or trauma
- **Congenital Mesoblastic Nephroma**
  - Most common renal tumor in infants < 3 months of age; 90% diagnosed ≤ 1 year
  - Predominantly solid; cystic/hemorrhagic foci are more suggestive of aggressive cellular subtype
  - Not typical: Ca^{2+}, vascular invasion
- **Renal Cell Carcinoma**
  - Mean age of 9-15 years
  - Typically smaller than Wilms; variable enhancement patterns & likelihood of Ca^{2+} depending on subtype
  - Association: von Hippel-Lindau disease
- **Angiomyolipoma**
  - Benign renal neoplasm, typically multifocal & due to tuberous sclerosis complex (TSC) in children
  - Mean age of 10 years with TSC
  - Intralesional fat is characteristic but solid/vascular components may dominant ("fat poor")
    - Fat components: Hyperechoic (US), hypoattenuating (CT), & following fat signal on all MR sequences
    - Aneurysms are quite uncommon in children
  - Concomitant renal cysts are typical
- **Hepatocellular Carcinoma**
  - 2nd most common pediatric liver malignancy
    - Usually age 10-14 years; rare before age 5
    - ~ 50% have underlying liver disease
  - Elevated AFP in 60-80%
  - May have hemorrhage, necrosis, fat, Ca^{2+}
    - Tumors often large at discovery
    - Arterial enhancement with portal venous phase washout
    - May have capsular enhancement
- **Hepatic Mesenchymal Hamartoma**
  - 2nd most common benign liver mass in children
  - 95% diagnosed < 5 years of age
  - Range from mostly cystic to mostly solid
    - Cysts present in 85% of tumors
    - Variable enhancement of solid components
- **Pancreatoblastoma**
  - Most common in 1st decade of life
  - AFP elevated in up to 55%
  - Usually large, lobulated solitary pancreatic mass
  - Association: Beckwith-Wiedemann
- **Adrenocortical Carcinoma**
  - Median age of 4 years
  - Usually large & hormonally active (virilization, Cushing)
  - Associations: Beckwith-Wiedemann, Li-Fraumeni
- **Kaposiform Hemangioendothelioma**
  - Locally invasive intermediate-grade vascular neoplasm
  - Most occur in infancy; presents as palpable mass, skin discoloration, &/or consumptive coagulopathy (Kasabach-Merritt phenomenon)
  - Lobulated solid mass with intermediate T2 signal intensity ± foci of internal hemorrhage
  - Frequently show poorly defined infiltrative margins with surrounding edema; vigorous enhancement
- **Rhabdoid Tumor**
  - Aggressive renal tumor, 80% diagnosed < 2 years of age
  - Large heterogeneous mass; suggestive features include subcapsular fluid collections, tumor lobulations, & Ca^{2}
  - May have synchronous intracranial masses

SELECTED REFERENCES

1. Chung EM et al: Renal tumors of childhood: radiologic-pathologic correlation part 2. The 2nd decade: from the radiologic pathology archives. Radiographics. 37(5):1538-58, 2017
2. Chung EM et al: Renal tumors of childhood: radiologic-pathologic correlation part 1. The 1st decade: from the radiologic pathology archives. Radiographics. 36(2):499-522, 2016
3. Chung EM et al: From the archives of the AFIP: pediatric liver masses: radiologic-pathologic correlation. Part 2. Malignant tumors. Radiographics. 31(2):483-507, 2011

Wilms Tumor

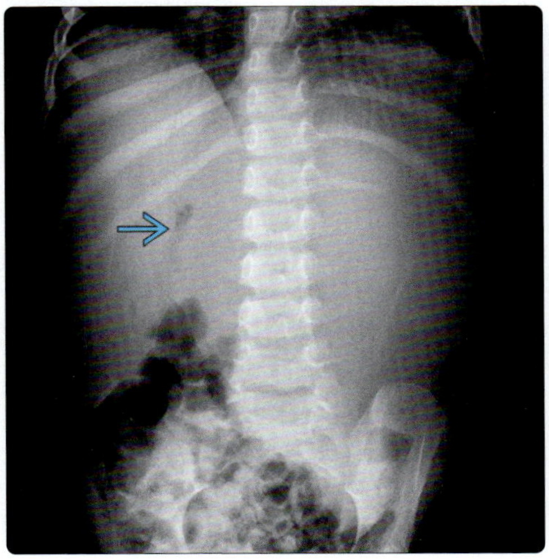

Wilms Tumor

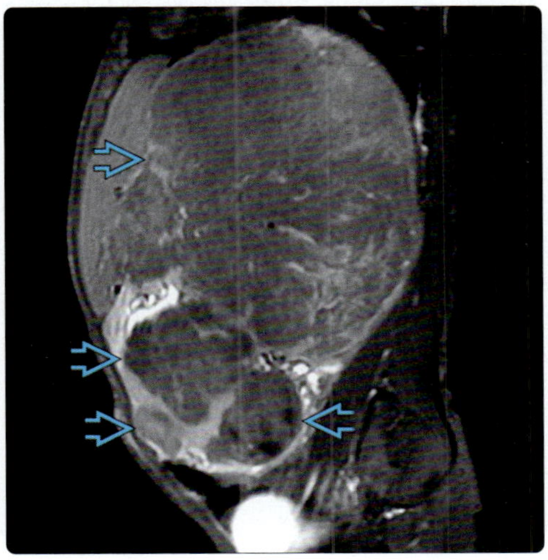

(Left) *AP radiograph in a 4 year old with abdominal distention & a palpable mass shows displacement of the bowel inferiorly by a large left abdominal mass. Note the compressed stomach bubble* ➔ *shifted into the right abdomen.* **(Right)** *Sagittal T1 C+ FS MR in the same patient shows numerous heterogeneously hypoenhancing solid masses* ➔ *of the left kidney due to multifocal Wilms tumor arising from nephroblastomatosis. Both of these entities typically show hypoenhancement relative to the kidney.*

(Left) *Longitudinal color Doppler US in a 6 year old with hematuria shows a hypovascular, round, predominantly solid mass arising at the upper pole of the right kidney.* **(Right)** *Axial T2 FS MR in the same patient shows cystic & solid foci throughout this large, round, right upper pole renal mass. The mass showed restricted diffusion in its solid portions (not shown), consistent with a highly cellular tumor. The patient's age strongly favors a Wilms tumor, confirmed at resection.*

Wilms Tumor

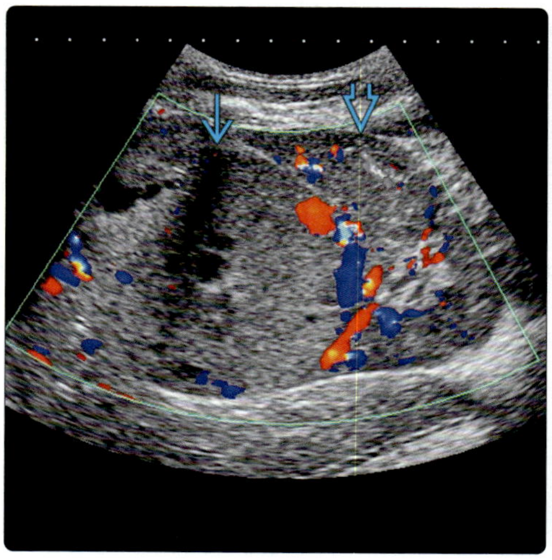

Wilms Tumor

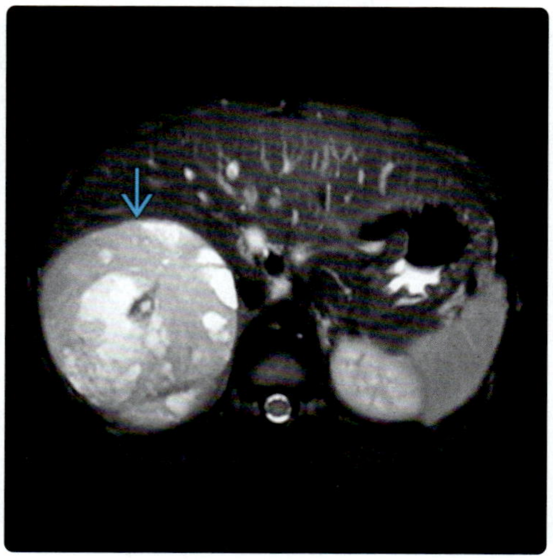

(Left) *AP radiograph in a young child shows a right paraspinal mass with speckled Ca^{2+}, highly concerning for a neuroblastoma.* **(Right)** *Coronal CECT in the same patient shows a lobulated, elongated, partially calcified mass in the right paraspinal region. This mass was not confined to a specific organ. The imaging features are consistent with neuroblastoma, which most commonly arises from the adrenal medulla but can arise anywhere along the sympathetic chain.*

Neuroblastoma

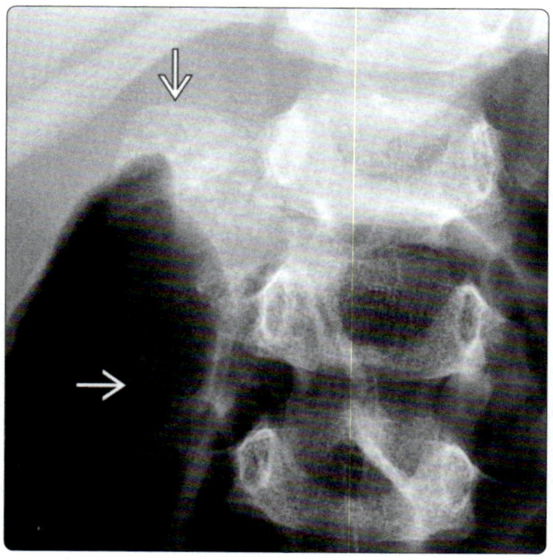

Neuroblastoma

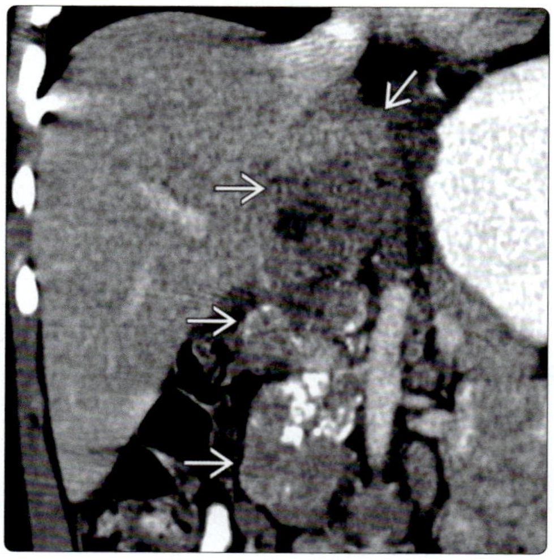

(Left) *Axial CECT in a 3 year old with distention shows a large, round, predominantly fluid-attenuation mass with heterogeneous solid foci containing Ca^{2+} & fat. A right ovarian teratoma was confirmed at resection.* **(Right)** *Coronal CECT in a 10 year old with Burkitt lymphoma shows large retroperitoneal nodal masses displacing bowel & engulfing vessels. Liver metastases & mediastinal nodes are also noted.*

Ovarian Tumors

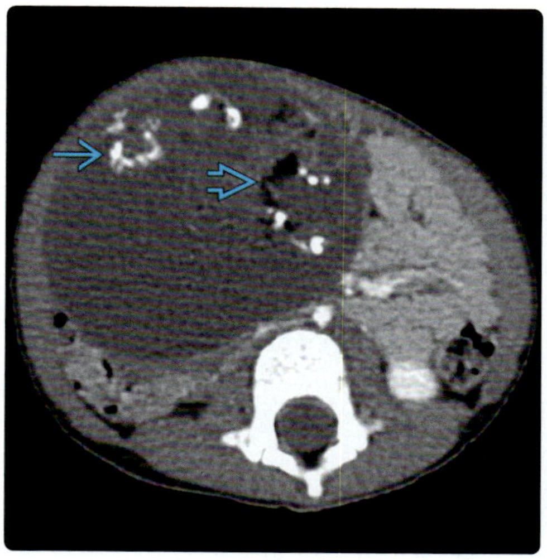

Lymphoma

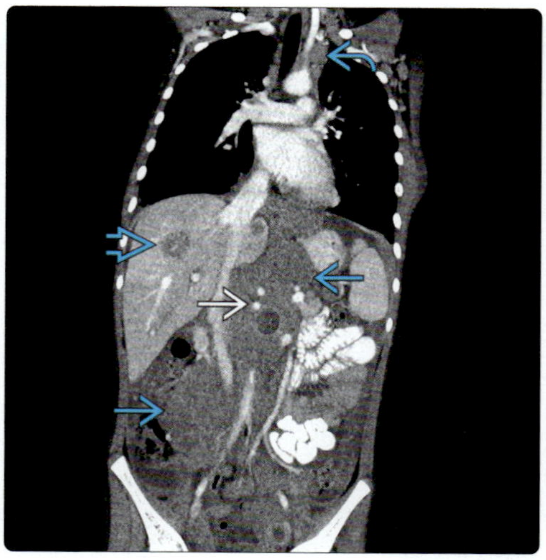

Hepatic Hemangioma

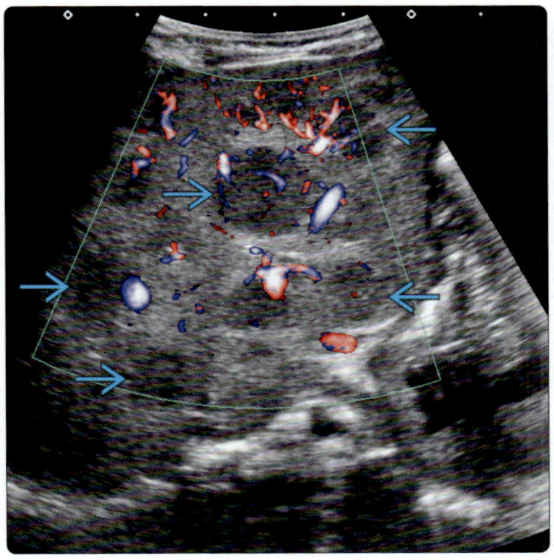

Hepatic Hemangioma

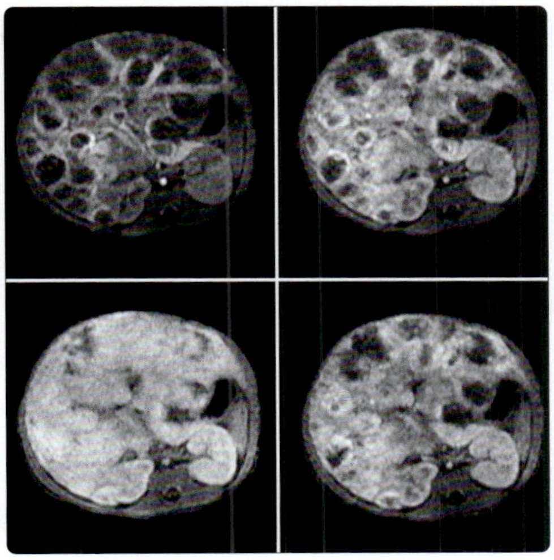

(Left) *Transverse color Doppler US in a 4 month old with > 5 cutaneous infantile hemangiomas (IHs) shows numerous round hypoechoic masses* ⇨ *throughout the liver. Unlike soft tissue IHs (which are uniformly hypervascular in the proliferating phase), hepatic IHs show variable degrees of internal vascularity.* **(Right)** *Dynamic T1 C+ FS MR images (clockwise from the upper left) in a 3 month old with cutaneous IHs show progressive peripheral to central enhancement of the innumerable hepatic IHs.*

Hepatoblastoma

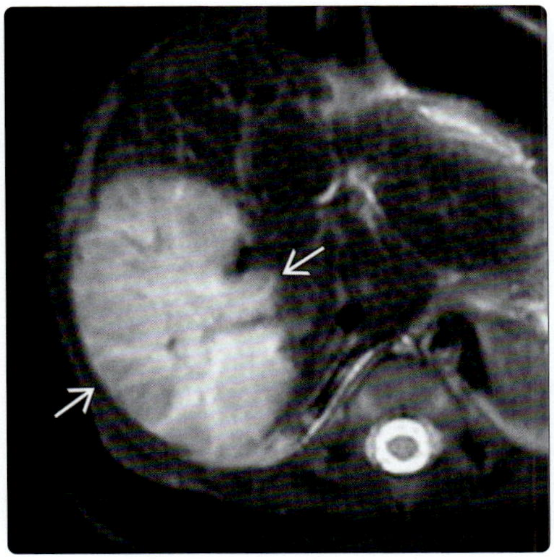

Hepatoblastoma

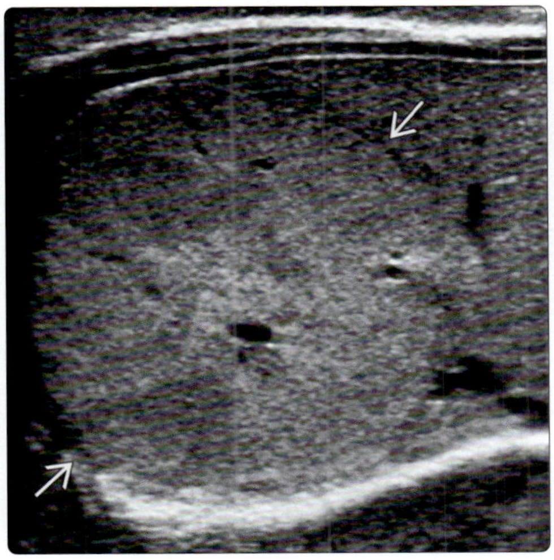

(Left) *Axial T2 MR shows a moderately hyperintense & mildly heterogeneous solid right lobe hepatoblastoma* ➡. **(Right)** *Transverse US shows a well-circumscribed, slightly hyperechoic mass* ➡ *in the right hepatic lobe that was an incidental finding in a 1 month old undergoing US for pyloric stenosis.*

Rhabdomyosarcoma

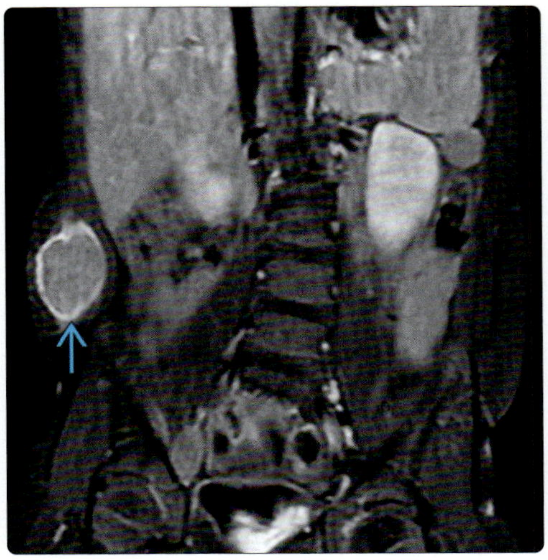

Plexiform Neurofibromas

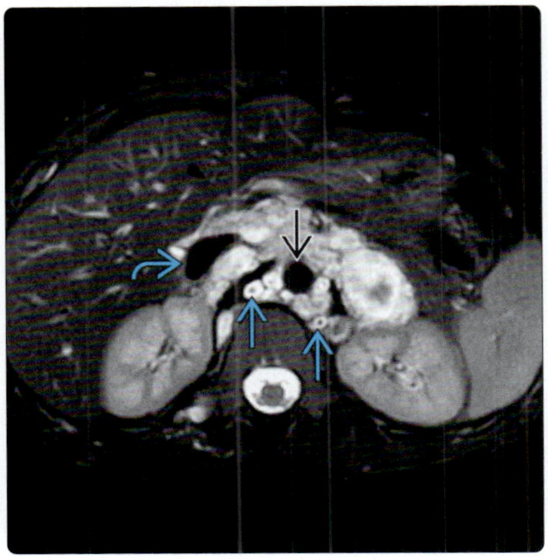

(Left) *Coronal T1 C+ FS MR in a 3 year old with a new right flank mass shows a well-circumscribed, ovoid lesion* ⇨ *with peripheral greater than central enhancement. The mass demonstrated restricted diffusion (not shown), & biopsy confirmed rhabdomyosarcoma.* **(Right)** *Axial T2 FS MR in a 7 year old with neurofibromatosis type I shows a lobulated cluster of hyperintense masses* ⇨ *encasing the aorta* ➡ *& inferior vena cava* ⇨. *The classic target sign is seen in several lesions.*

(Left) *Axial T2 FS MR of an 8 year old with a history of renal transplant & a new firm mass at the incision site shows a heterogeneous lesion → in the muscle with low signal intensity foci. Posttransplant lymphoproliferative disease was an initial clinical consideration, though the MR findings favored a desmoid tumor, which was confirmed with biopsy.* **(Right)** *Axial CECT shows a heterogeneous mass → arising from the right kidney in a young infant due to mesoblastic nephroma.*

Desmoid/Aggressive Fibromatosis

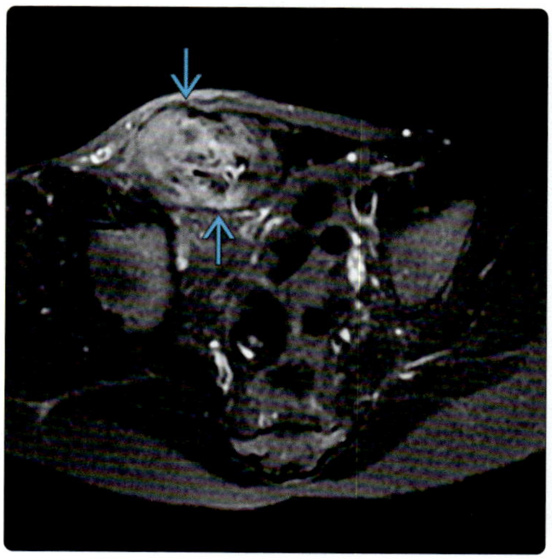

Congenital Mesoblastic Nephroma

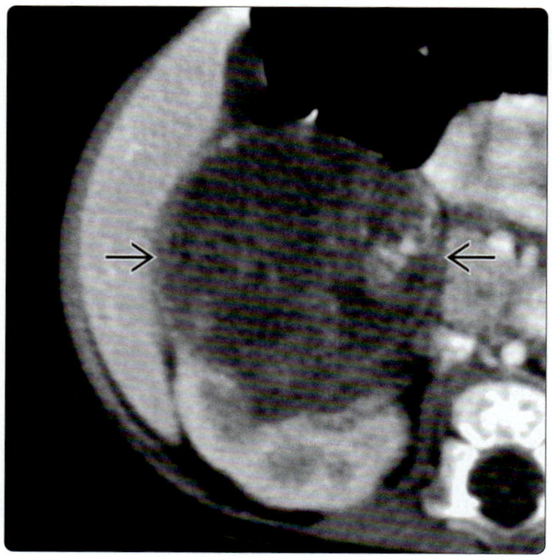

(Left) *Axial T1 C+ FS MR in an 8 year old with an incidentally discovered left renal mass after trauma shows minimal enhancement of a round 3-cm central renal lesion →. Restricted diffusion was seen in the mass (not shown). Resection confirmed renal cell carcinoma.* **(Right)** *Axial T1 MR in a patient with tuberous sclerosis complex shows abundant fat → within a right renal angiomyolipoma*

Renal Cell Carcinoma

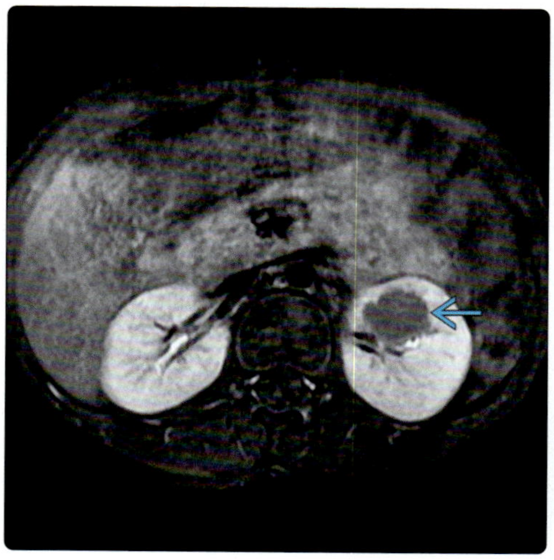

Angiomyolipoma

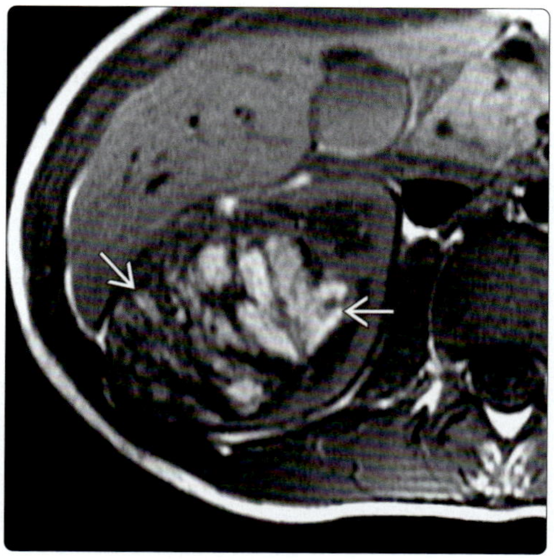

(Left) *Axial T2 FS MR in a 9 year old with cirrhosis secondary to a-1 antitrypsin deficiency shows an enlarging isointense mass → in the right hepatic lobe, found to be hepatocellular carcinoma.* **(Right)** *Axial T2 FS MR in a newborn shows a large & markedly heterogeneous central hepatic mass with enlarged hepatic veins → draped over the lesion. Peripheral enhancement was noted, mimicking a congenital hemangioma. However, a solid mesenchymal hamartoma was found at biopsy.*

Hepatocellular Carcinoma

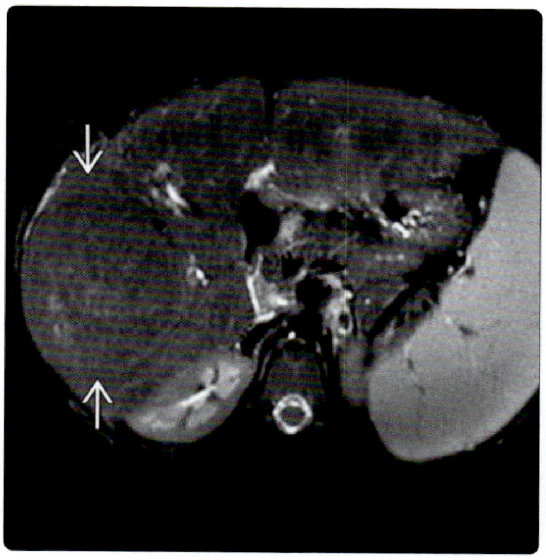

Hepatic Mesenchymal Hamartoma

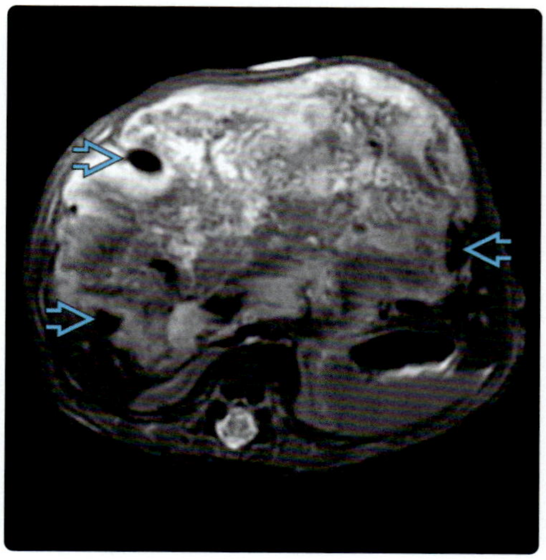

Pancreatoblastoma

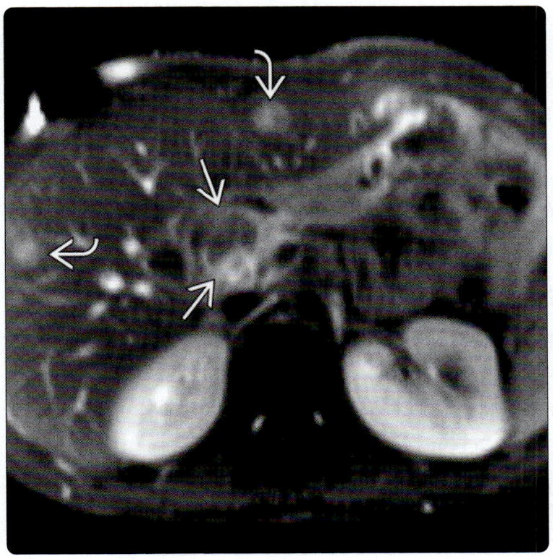

Pancreatoblastoma

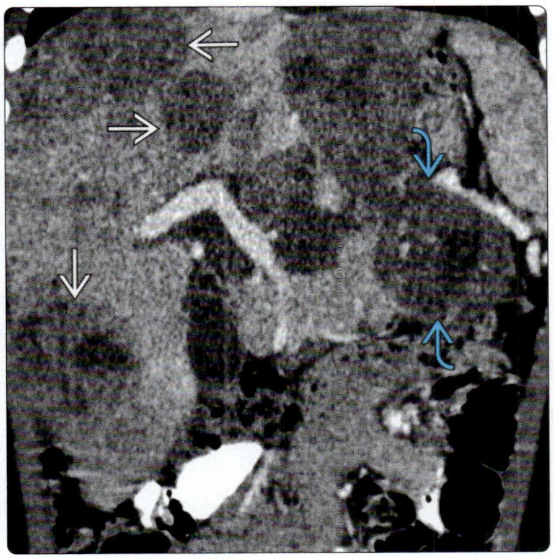

(Left) *Axial T1 C+ FS MR shows a heterogeneously enhancing mass at the superior aspect of the pancreatic head in this 7 year old due to a pancreatoblastoma. The DWI sequence showed restricted diffusion in the mass (not shown). Liver metastases are also seen.* **(Right)** *Coronal CECT shows a heterogeneous mass arising from the tail of the pancreas. There is a "claw" of normal pancreatic tissue splayed along the medial margin of the mass. In addition, there are multiple hepatic metastases.*

Adrenocortical Carcinoma

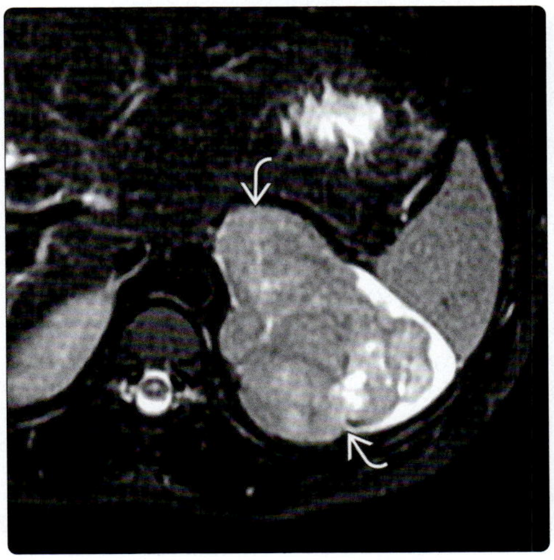

Kaposiform Hemangioendothelioma

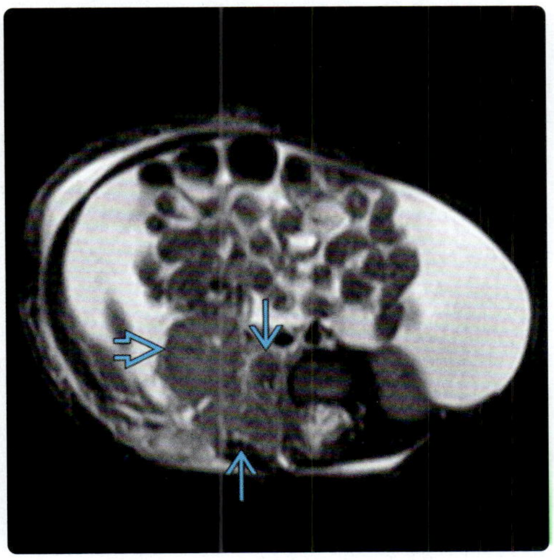

(Left) *Axial T2 FS MR shows a lobulated intermediate signal intensity left suprarenal mass in a 2 year old with virilization & hypertension due to an adrenocortical carcinoma in the setting of Li-Fraumeni syndrome.* **(Right)** *Axial T2 FS MR of a 2 month old with distention & coagulopathy shows an infiltrating intermediate to low signal intensity KHE of the right paraspinal musculature that is inseparable from the right kidney. Note the flank edema & marked ascites.*

Rhabdoid Tumor

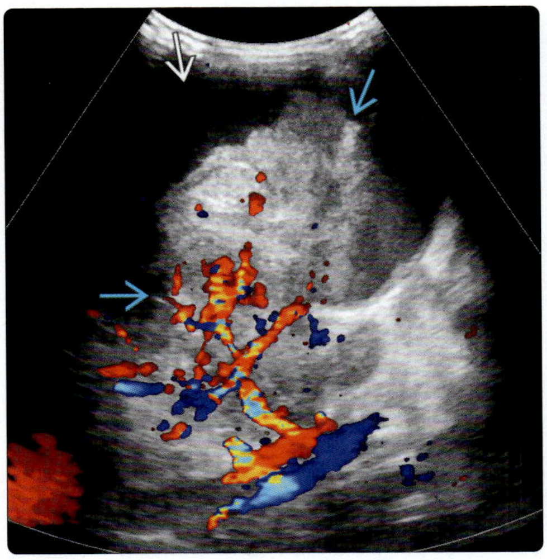

Rhabdoid Tumor

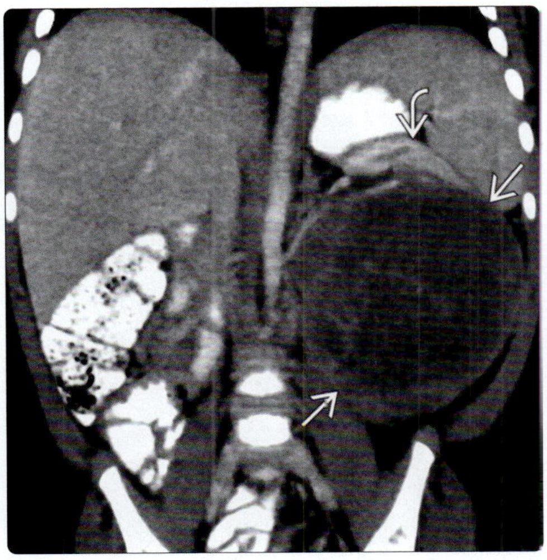

(Left) *Longitudinal color Doppler US in a 1 year old with a large abdominal mass shows a large subcapsular fluid collection overlying a lobulated & highly vascular mass that replaces the left kidney. The patient age & findings favor a malignant rhabdoid tumor.* **(Right)** *Coronal CECT shows a large minimally enhancing left renal rhabdoid tumor involving the renal hilum in this 10 month old. The residual left renal parenchyma is splayed & compressed.*

DIFFERENTIAL DIAGNOSIS

Common

- Middle Aortic Syndrome
- Renal Artery Stenosis

Less Common

- Thromboembolism
- Trauma

Rare but Important

- Abdominal Aortic Aneurysm

ESSENTIAL INFORMATION

Helpful Clues for Common Diagnoses

- **Middle Aortic Syndrome**
  - Segmental narrowing of abdominal aorta with variable involvement of visceral branches (renal > > superior mesenteric > celiac > common iliac arteries)
  - Commonly with hypertension & systolic murmur
  - Causes
    - Idiopathic
    - Genetic: NF1, Williams syndrome, Alagille syndrome
    - Vasculitis: Most commonly Takayasu arteritis; look for active vessel wall inflammation (with thickening, edema, enhancement)
- **Renal Artery Stenosis**
  - Renin-mediated hypertension
  - Most commonly due to fibromuscular dysplasia (FMD) in children
    - Noninflammatory arteriopathy
    - Pediatric fibromuscular dysplasia is histologically distinct from adult-type FMD (consider as separate entity)
    - Commonly also involves mesenteric & carotid arteries; rarely involves abdominal aorta
    - Unlike string-of-beads appearance in adults, renal stenoses in children with FMD are typically more proximal & unifocal or tubular in morphology
  - US for screening
  - CTA or MRA if US positive or moderate clinical suspicion remains; with refractory hypertension, conventional angiography may be required to find intrarenal stenosis
  - Spectral Doppler criteria
    - At stenosis: Elevated peak systolic velocity (> 200 cm/s, > 3.5x peak aortic velocity)
    - Distal to stenosis: Parvus et tardus appearance (delayed systolic upstroke with low resistive index), loss of early systolic compliance peak/reflective-wave complex

Helpful Clues for Less Common Diagnoses

- **Thromboembolism**
  - Neonatal aortic thrombus
    - Most related to umbilical arterial catheter
    - Other risk factors: Cardiopulmonary abnormalities, sepsis, meconium aspiration, extreme prematurity, prothrombotic condition (factor V Leiden mutation)
  - In older children, can be secondary to aortic injury (iatrogenic, trauma, vasculitis)
- **Trauma**
  - Rare; usually in restrained motor vehicle collision passengers
  - May see dissection, intimal tear, periaortic hematoma
  - Almost always have associated bowel & spine injuries

Helpful Clues for Rare Diagnoses

- **Abdominal Aortic Aneurysm**
  - Focal dilation > 3 cm or > 150% of normal aorta
  - Causes
    - Connective tissue disorders: Loeys-Dietz syndrome, vascular Ehlers-Danlos syndrome, Marfan syndrome
    - Other genetic factors: NF1, tuberous sclerosis complex
    - Vasculitis: Takayasu arteritis, Kawasaki disease, polyarteritis nodosa, giant cell arteritis
    - Infection: Bacterial, tuberculosis, fungal
    - Trauma (e.g., umbilical artery catheterization) may lead to pseudoaneurysms
  - Complications: Rupture, dissection, thrombus, intramural hematoma

Middle Aortic Syndrome

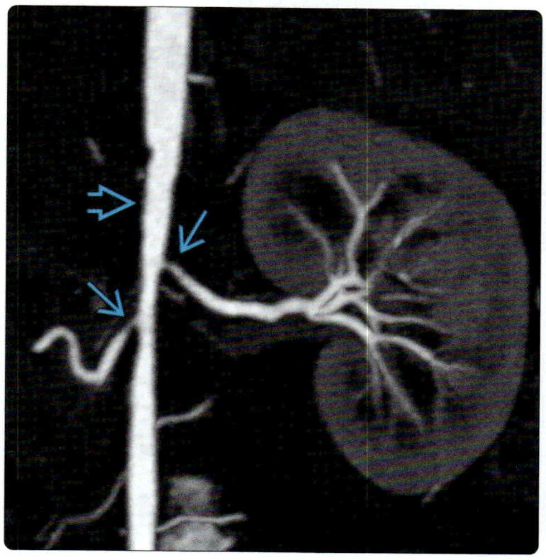

Middle Aortic Syndrome

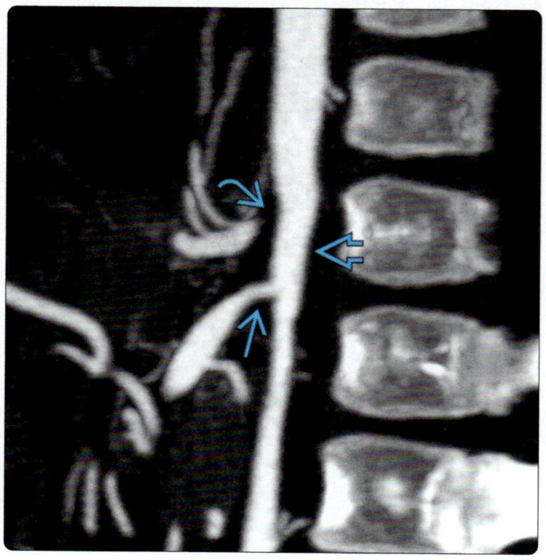

(Left) *Coronal oblique CECT MIP in a 2 year old with neurofibromatosis type 1 (NF1) & hypertension shows irregular segmental tapering of the abdominal aorta ➡, consistent with middle aortic syndrome. There are associated bilateral renal artery stenoses ➡ causing hypertension. This is seen in ~ 1% of NF1 patients.* **(Right)** *Sagittal oblique CECT MIP (same patient) shows irregular narrowing of the abdominal aorta ➡ along with occlusion of the proximal celiac artery ➡ & stenosis of the superior mesenteric artery (SMA) ➡.*

Middle Aortic Syndrome

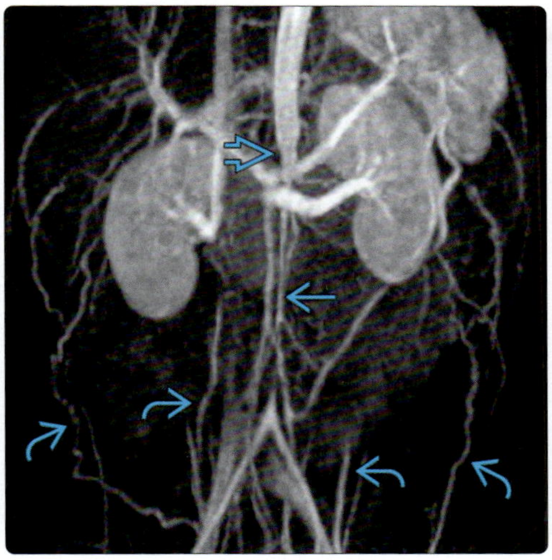

Middle Aortic Syndrome

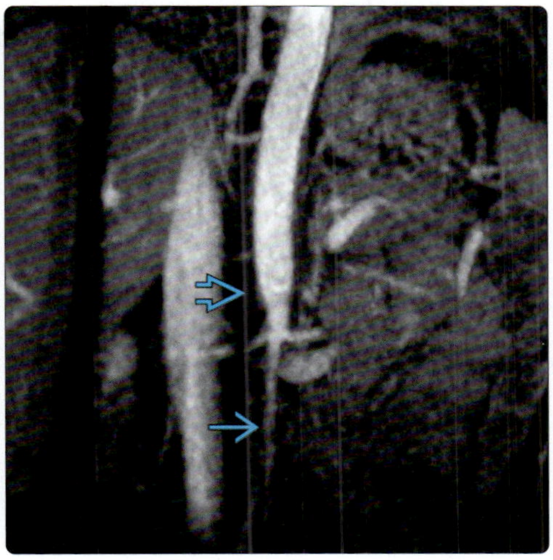

(Left) *Coronal thick-slab MRA MIP in a 14 year old with Takayasu arteritis shows severe narrowing of the perirenal abdominal aorta with a string-like infrarenal aorta. Collaterals bypass the aortic narrowing.* **(Right)** *Thinner slab coronal MRA MIP in the same patient shows the irregular tapering of the abdominal aorta with a string-like infrarenal aorta. Pediatric Takayasu arteritis commonly affects the abdominal aorta & branches (unlike in adults), leading to hypertension in 80% & lower limb claudication in 10-35%.*

Middle Aortic Syndrome

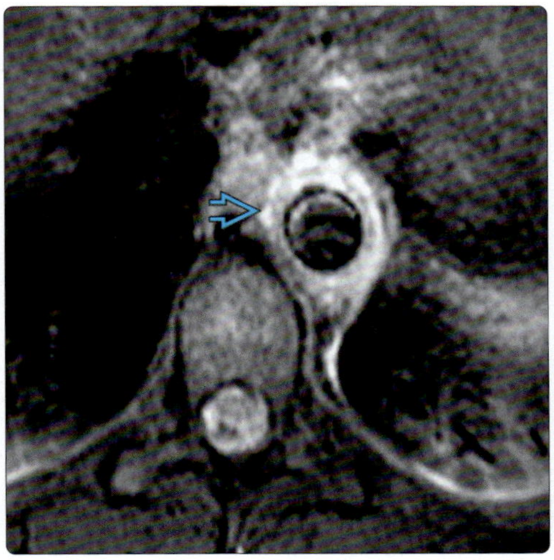

Middle Aortic Syndrome

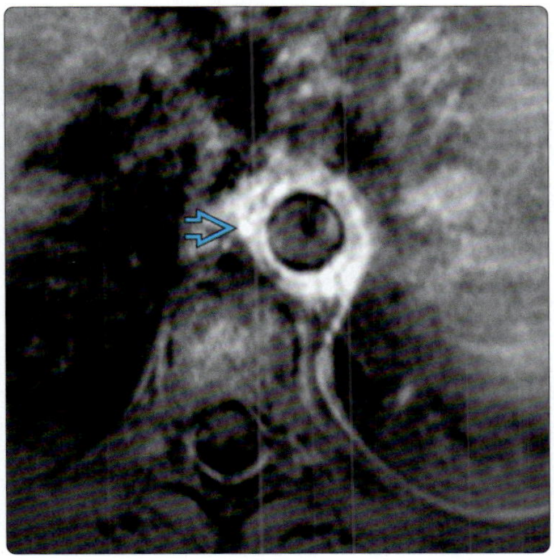

(Left) *Axial STIR MR in the same patient shows wall thickening & edema of the descending thoracic aorta.* **(Right)** *Axial T1 C+ FS MR at the same level shows aortic wall thickening & hyperenhancement. These findings are consistent with active inflammation. MR assessment of active wall inflammation is the most important source of information affecting management, as symptoms & laboratory markers are unreliable for tracking disease activity & therapeutic response.*

Middle Aortic Syndrome

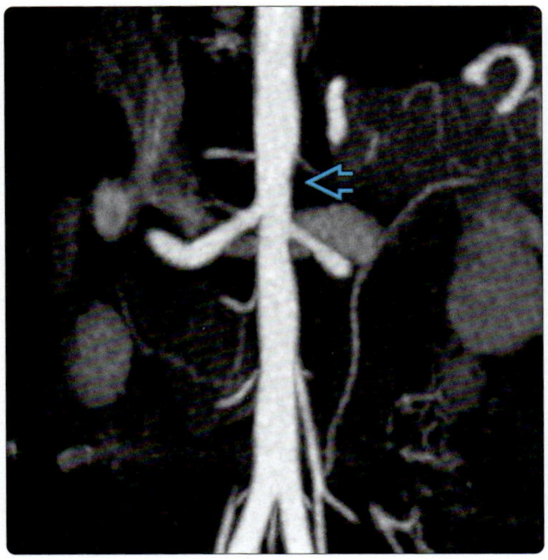

Middle Aortic Syndrome

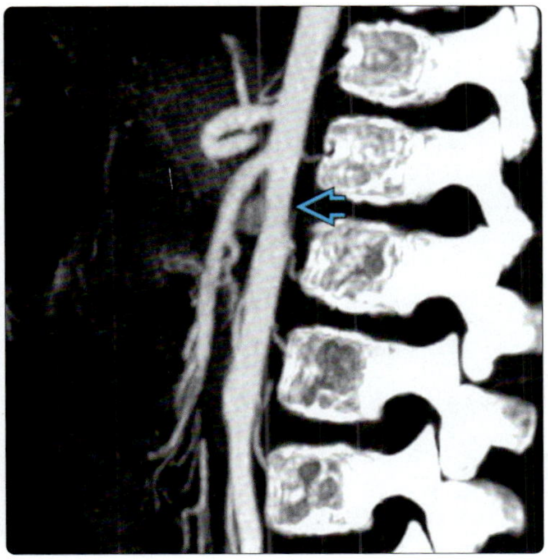

(Left) *Coronal CECT MPR in a 5 year old with Williams syndrome shows mild irregular narrowing of the abdominal aorta, consistent with a mild middle aortic syndrome.* **(Right)** *Sagittal CECT MIP in the same patient again shows mild middle aortic syndrome. Patients with Williams syndrome also characteristically get supravalvular aortic stenosis at the level of the sinotubular junction as well as multiple peripheral pulmonary branch artery stenoses.*

(Left) *Transverse pulsed Doppler US in a 12-year-old girl with hypertensive urgency shows an elevated peak mid right renal artery velocity of 367.9 cm/s, suspicious for renal artery stenosis.* **(Right)** *Transverse color Doppler US in the same patient shows a turbulent poststenotic flow jet distal to the site of elevated renal velocity. Isolated renal artery stenosis in children is most commonly due to fibromuscular dysplasia (FMD).*

Renal Artery Stenosis

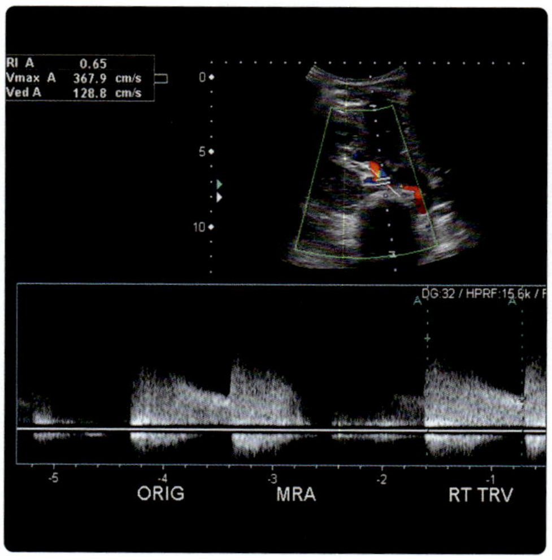

Renal Artery Stenosis

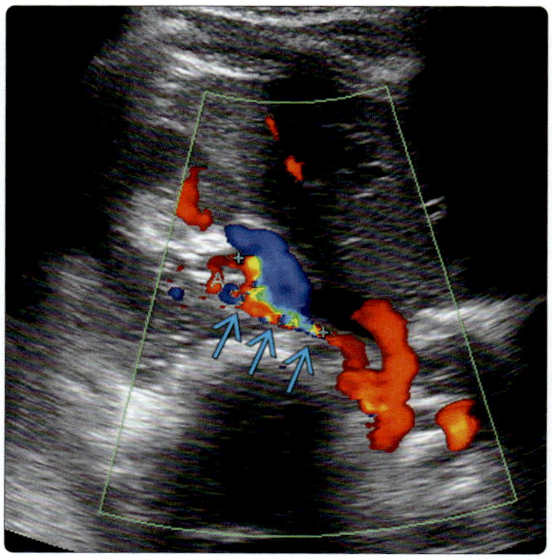

(Left) *Longitudinal pulsed Doppler US in the same patient shows an intrarenal parvus et tardus waveform characterized by a delayed systolic upstroke & a low resistive index.* **(Right)** *Coronal catheter angiogram in the same patient shows bilateral unifocal short-segment stenoses of the mid renal arteries. This appearance is typical of pediatric FMD, which is histologically distinct from adult FMD & should be considered as a separate entity. The primary treatment is with balloon angioplasty.*

Renal Artery Stenosis

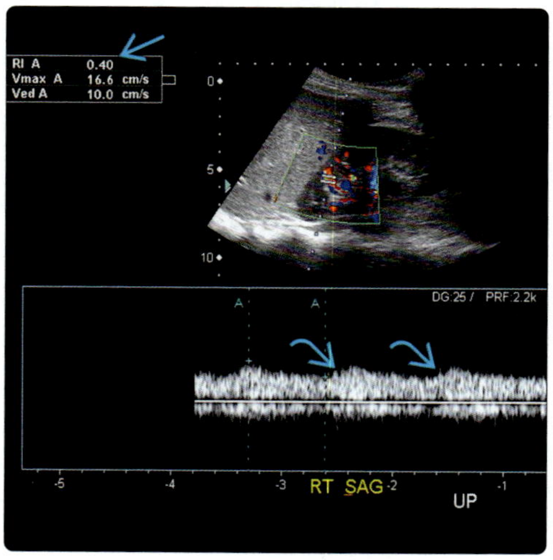

Renal Artery Stenosis

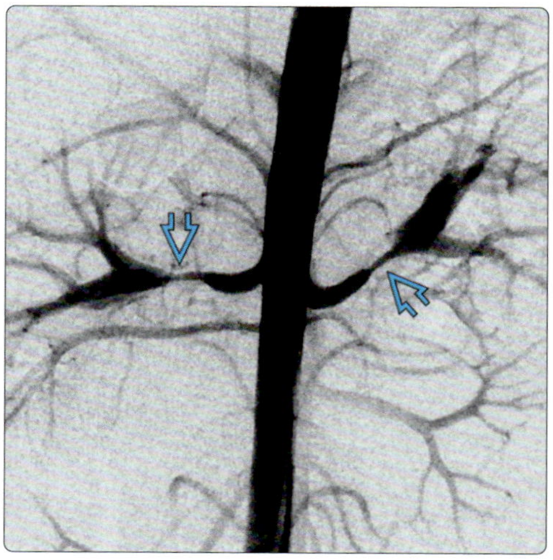

(Left) *Sagittal oblique CECT MIP in a 6 day old with hypernatremia & severe dehydration shows acute occlusive abdominal aortic thrombus below the SMA origin.* **(Right)** *Anterior CECT 3D projection in the same patient shows no opacification of the abdominal aorta below the SMA. The bilateral proximal renal arteries are occluded, supplied retrograde by the phrenic arteries (visualized on the right). The external iliac arteries are supplied by collaterals.*

Thromboembolism

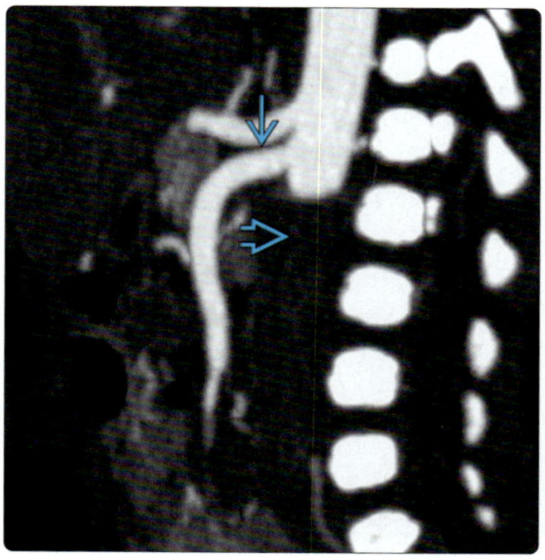

Thromboembolism

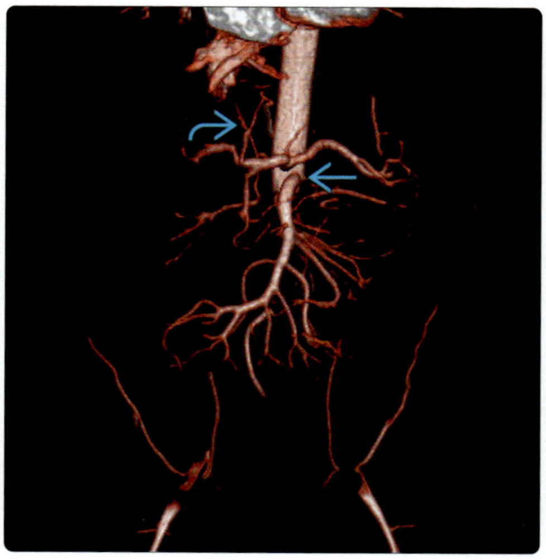

Abdominal Aortic Aneurysm

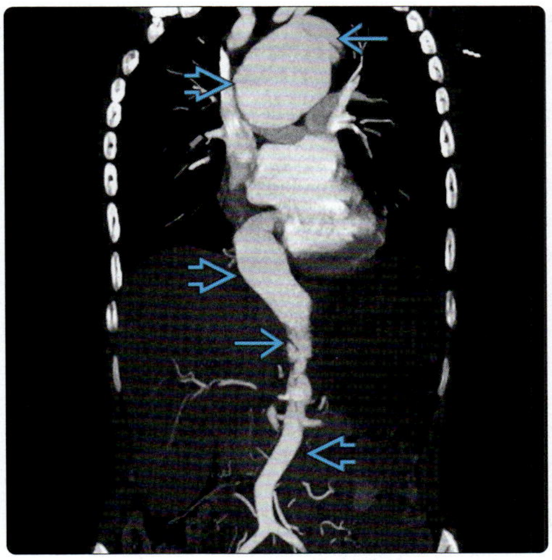

Abdominal Aortic Aneurysm

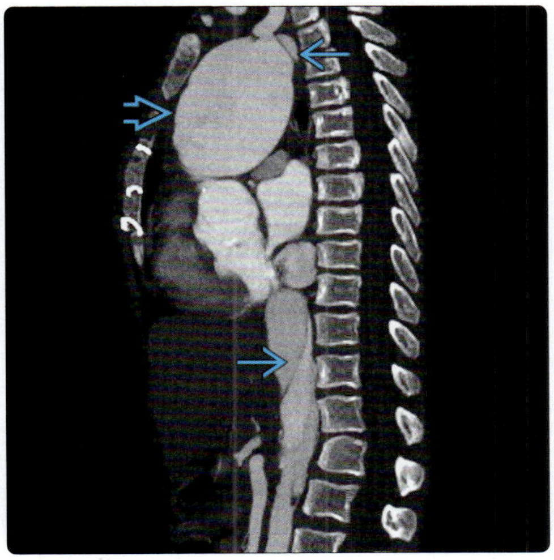

(Left) *Coronal CECT MIP in an 8 year old with Loeys-Dietz syndrome shows a tortuous & dilated aorta ⇨. There is a complication of aortic dissection →.* **(Right)** *Sagittal CECT MIP in the same patient shows the dilated ascending aorta ⇨ with partial visualization of an intimal dissection flap extending from the arch to descending aorta →. Loeys-Dietz syndrome is a craniofacial & vascular connective tissue disorder characterized by arterial aneurysms & tortuosity at a young age with a high risk of dissection or rupture.*

Abdominal Aortic Aneurysm

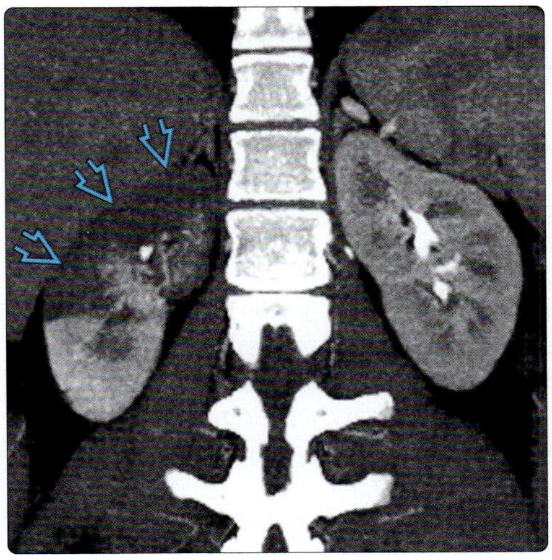

Abdominal Aortic Aneurysm

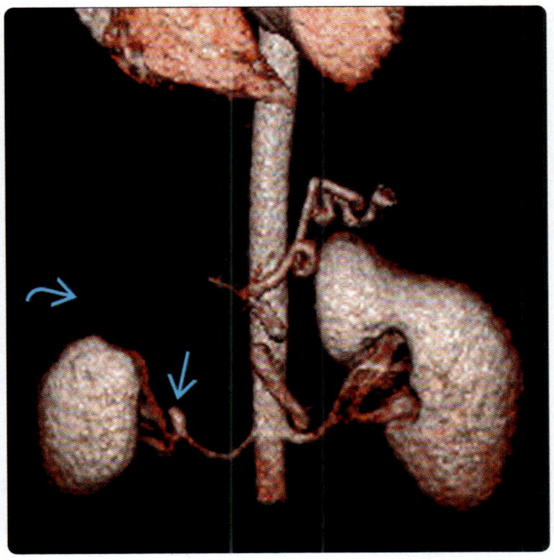

(Left) *Coronal CECT MIP in a 15 year old with vascular Ehlers-Danlos syndrome shows segmental upper pole infarction ⇨ of the right kidney.* **(Right)** *Anterior MRA 3D projection in the same patient shows a small right renal artery aneurysm → that fed a thrombosed upper pole branch artery (not shown), leading to an upper pole infarct ↪. Note that there is also abnormal tortuosity of the splenic artery, which is rare. Vascular Ehlers-Danlos syndrome is characterized by multifocal aneurysms of large & medium-sized vessels.*

Abdominal Aortic Aneurysm

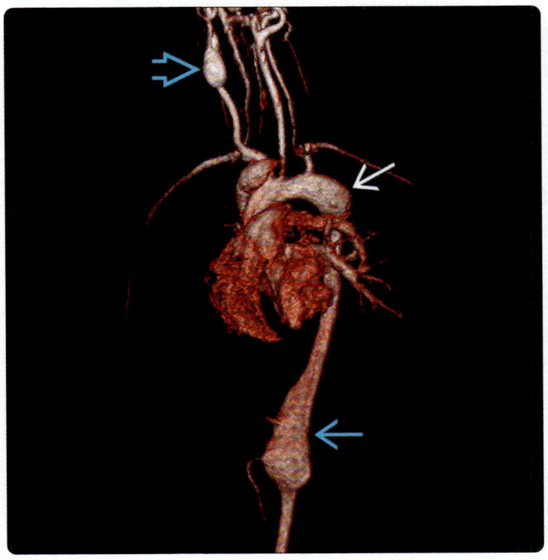

Abdominal Aortic Aneurysm

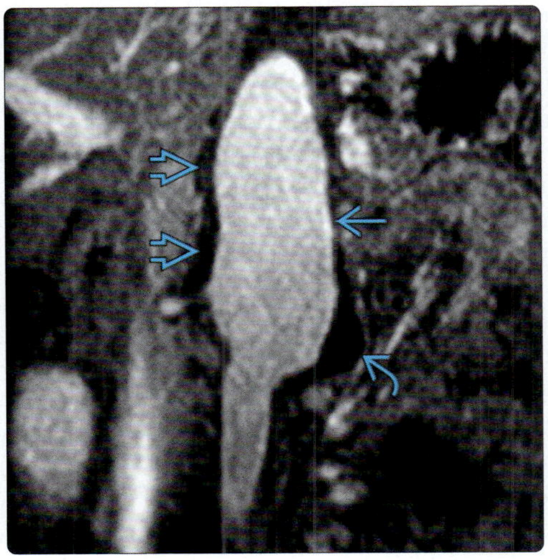

(Left) *Anterior oblique MRA 3D projection in a 12 year old with Takayasu arteritis shows aneurysms of the right common carotid artery ⇨, aortic isthmus ➡, & abdominal aorta →.* **(Right)** *Coronal MRA in the same patient shows the irregular abdominal aortic aneurysm →, wall thickening ⇨, & an irregular crescentic intramural thrombus ↪. While Takayasu arteritis more commonly causes stenoses, a recurrent cycle of intramural inflammation/hemorrhage & healing can lead to aneurysms or dissection.*

DIFFERENTIAL DIAGNOSIS

Common

- Congenital Hemangioma
- Infantile Hemangioma
- Metastases

Less Common

- Hepatoblastoma
- Umbilical Venous Catheter Extravasation
- Mesenchymal Hamartoma
- Congenital Hepatic Cyst
- Choledochal Cyst

Rare but Important

- Abscess
- Cystic Biliary Atresia
- Malignant Rhabdoid Tumor
- Angiosarcoma

ESSENTIAL INFORMATION

Key Differential Diagnosis Issues

- Hepatic tumors are uncommon in perinatal period
  - Much more likely to be benign than malignant
    - Hemangiomas are most common
- Most are identified by antenatal US or neonatal physical
- Skin lesions often occur with neonatal liver pathologies
  - Infantile hemangiomas (IHs), metastatic neuroblastoma, TORCH infections
- Lab tests can help to differentiate masses
  - CBC, α-fetoprotein (AFP), TSH/T4, catecholamines
    - AFP levels are normally elevated in newborns & decrease over 1st few months of life
      - Therefore, neonatal liver mass + elevated initial AFP does not necessarily indicate hepatoblastoma
- Biopsy or resection is often needed for final diagnosis

Helpful Clues for Common Diagnoses

- **Congenital Hemangioma**
  - Solitary focal hypervascular liver mass with shunting
    - **Not** hemangioendothelioma
    - **Not** cavernous hemangioma
  - May present with heart failure & mild coagulopathy
    - True Kasabach-Merritt phenomenon does **not** occur in these liver lesions but is associated with Kaposiform hemangioendothelioma (KHE)
      - KHE: Locally invasive tumor; does not cause focal liver lesions but may infiltrate porta hepatis
  - Should not enlarge after birth (with rare exception of internal hemorrhage) as proliferation is complete; follows 1 of 3 clinical courses
    - Rapidly involuting congenital hemangioma (RICH): 80% volume decrease by age 12 months
    - Noninvoluting congenital hemangioma (NICH): Stable
    - Partially involuting congenital hemangioma (PICH)
  - Imaging: Large, heterogeneous mass (particularly on T2 MR) with increased peripheral vascularity
    - Rapid peripheral enhancement with mild to moderate broadening on dynamic imaging
      - Central areas of nonenhancement (due to fibrosis, Ca^{2+}, necrosis, or hemorrhage) often remain
      - Components may rarely retain hepatocyte-specific contrast media (HSCM) on hepatobiliary phase
    - Intralesional arteriovenous shunting: Enlarged feeding arteries; early enhancement of enlarged draining veins
    - Celiac & hepatic arteries are often enlarged; aorta may taper after celiac takeoff
      - Large vessels are often present on Doppler
  - No medical therapy has yet proven effective; embolization, resection, or transplant may be necessary
- **Infantile Hemangioma**
  - Typically multifocal or diffuse, often in association with cutaneous IHs
  - Not present at birth; typically appear in 1st weeks to months of life, grow rapidly during infancy, & then regress slowly over years
  - Numerous hepatic IHs may lead to heart or liver failure, compartment syndrome, &/or hypothyroidism (due to specific enzyme produced by IHs)
    - Not associated with coagulopathy
  - Imaging: Multiple small to moderate masses of relatively uniform T2-hyperintense signal ± scattered prominent internal flow voids
    - Dynamic imaging shows peripheral to central enhancement with complete fill-in
      - Do not retain HSCM on hepatobiliary phase
    - ± arteriovenous shunting: Enlarged feeding arteries; early enhancement of enlarged draining veins
      - Variable internal/peripheral vascularity on Doppler
    - Celiac & hepatic arteries are often enlarged; aorta may taper after celiac takeoff
  - β-blockers (e.g., propranolol) or steroids are very effective in treating lesions if medical therapy is required
- **Metastases**
  - More common than primary hepatic malignancies
    - Neuroblastoma is most common to cause liver metastases in neonates
    - Leukemia, Wilms tumor, rhabdoid tumor, & others may rarely involve neonatal liver
  - Imaging: Quite variable; may be small to large discrete masses, diffuse infiltration, or combination
    - Lesions are typically hypoenhancing/hypovascular; do not retain HSCM
    - In neuroblastoma, look for suprarenal/paraspinal mass ± Ca^{2+}, as well as marrow & skin/subcutaneous lesions

Helpful Clues for Less Common Diagnoses

- **Hepatoblastoma**
  - Most common primary hepatic malignancy
    - < 5% are congenital
  - Associated with Beckwith-Wiedemann syndrome, familial adenomatous polyposis, extreme prematurity
  - Classically has rising or persistently elevated AFP (vs. normal downward trend in infants)
    - Some subtypes have low/normal levels of AFP
  - Differences compared to typical age range (0.5-3.0 years)
    - Metastases are uncommon but may occur in atypical locations (as fetal circulation bypasses lungs)
    - Tumor rupture can occur during labor/birth
    - Outcomes are similar based on modern treatment
  - Imaging: Large, heterogeneous, hypoenhancing lesion; often restricts diffusion

- Does not retain HSCM on hepatobiliary phase
- ± Ca^{2+}, multifocality, tumor thrombus

- **Umbilical Venous Catheter Extravasation**
  - Often due to malposition in portal system with hypertonic infusion ± laceration
  - May present with acute abdominal distention
  - Imaging: Heterogeneous fluid collection in hepatic parenchyma adjacent to vessel currently/previously traversed by umbilical venous catheter (UVC)
    - Internally avascular; may contain septations & debris
- **Mesenchymal Hamartoma**
  - 2nd most common benign hepatic mass of infancy
    - Typically diagnosed in first 2 years of life
  - May grow rapidly, leading to compartment syndrome, respiratory distress, rarely heart failure
  - AFP may be moderately elevated
  - Imaging: Multiloculated cystic mass in 70%; solid or mixed forms also occur; microcysts may appear solid
    - May rarely mimic hypervascular appearance of congenital hemangioma
    - Solid portions are typically hypoenhancing but may retain HSCM
  - Reports of spontaneous regression as well as malignant transformation to undifferentiated embryonal sarcoma
- **Congenital Hepatic Cyst**
  - Often asymptomatic; may require no intervention
  - Often superficial, just under liver capsule
  - Imaging: Typically simple in appearance without nodularity, wall thickening, or internal vascularity
    - No trilaminar/"gut signature" wall of duplication
    - No connection to biliary system; therefore, will not demonstrate radiotracer activity on HIDA scan or HSCM on hepatobiliary phase MR
- **Choledochal Cyst**
  - Nonobstructive dilation of biliary ducts
    - Todani type I (common bile duct) is most common
  - Presents more commonly with abdominal mass & less commonly with jaundice & pain than in older children
  - Imaging: Fusiform/round dilation of common bile duct, usually > 1 cm in diameter
    - Thin wall, without "gut signature"
    - Continuous with mildly dilated hepatic ducts
      - Will gradually fill with radiotracer on HIDA scan or HSCM on hepatobiliary phase MR
    - Gallbladder is typically normal
  - Treated with excision
    - Malignant degeneration unlikely < 18 years of age

Helpful Clues for Rare Diagnoses

- **Abscess**
  - Usually small & multiple in neonates; solitary in 30%
  - Risks: Prematurity, UVC, sepsis, necrotizing enterocolitis
  - *Staphylococcus aureus*, gram-negative enteric bacteria, & *Candida* are most common organisms
- **Cystic Biliary Atresia**
  - Deficiency or absence of extrahepatic biliary tree; presence of hilar cyst is uncommon form
  - Typically presents in neonatal period with direct hyperbilirubinemia > 2.5 mg/dL
  - Hepatocyte function deteriorates if not treated early
  - Imaging: Cystic form may be confused with choledochal cyst; features favoring biliary atresia include
    - Nondilated intrahepatic ducts
    - Small hilar cyst (typically < 21 mm) without sludge/stones
    - Hypoplastic or absent gallbladder (< 15 mm)
    - Echogenic cord anterior to right portal vein (> 4 mm)
- **Malignant Rhabdoid Tumor**
  - Median age: 8 months; neonatal cases ~ 5%
  - AFP only mildly to moderately elevated; INI1 deficient
  - Imaging: Similar appearance to hepatoblastoma
- **Angiosarcoma**
  - Imaging: Variable appearance, often with dominant mass if lesions are multiple
    - Lesions may be cystic &/or hemorrhagic; enhancement may be early, late, or absent

SELECTED REFERENCES

1. Masand PM: Magnetic resonance imaging features of common focal liver lesions in children. Pediatr Radiol. 48(9):1234-44, 2018

Congenital Hemangioma

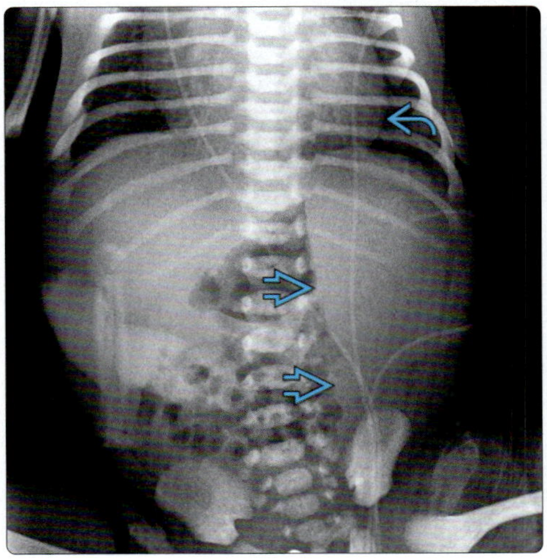

Congenital Hemangioma

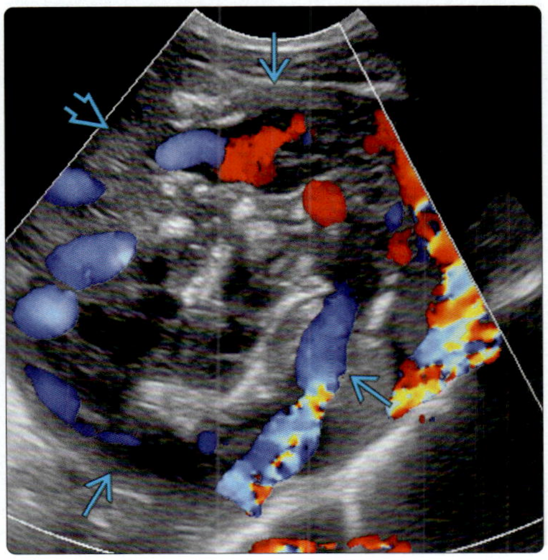

(Left) *Supine AP radiograph in a newborn shows a paucity of bowel gas in the left abdomen ➡. Cardiomegaly ➡ is also present.* **(Right)** *Transverse color Doppler US in the same patient shows a large, exophytic, heterogeneous mass ➡ arising from the left lobe of the liver ➡ with increased peripheral vascularity, typical of a congenital hemangioma (CH). Note that these masses are usually detected prenatally or in the 1st week after delivery.*

(Left) *Coronal arterial-phase CECT in the same patient shows heterogeneous enhancement of the exophytic left hepatic lobe lesion with multiple large vessels seen peripherally. The draining left hepatic vein is enlarged with early enhancement due to shunting in the lesion. The hepatic artery is also enlarged.* **(Right)** *Axial SSFSE T2 MR in the same patient shows internal heterogeneity of the mass. The mass regressed to < 1/2 of its size over the next 6 months, typical of a rapidly involuting CH.*

Congenital Hemangioma

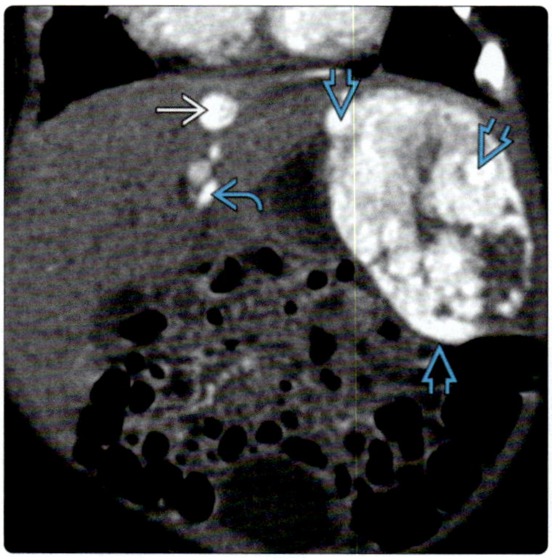

Congenital Hemangioma

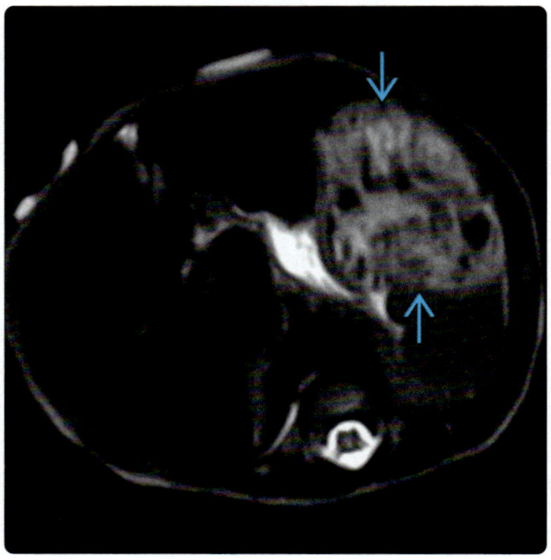

(Left) *Longitudinal color Doppler US in a 4 month old with cutaneous IHs shows scattered, well-circumscribed, round hypoechoic lesions with variable internal vascularity. This appearance is common with hepatic IHs but differs from soft tissue IHs, which always show abundant low-resistance arterial flow in the proliferating phase.* **(Right)** *Transverse color Doppler US in the same patient again shows the hepatic IHs. These lesions typically appear in the 1st few weeks of life, grow rapidly over months, & slowly involute over years.*

Infantile Hemangioma

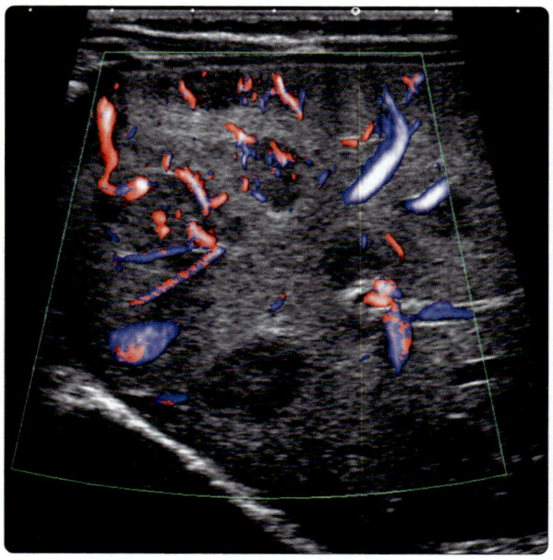

Infantile Hemangioma

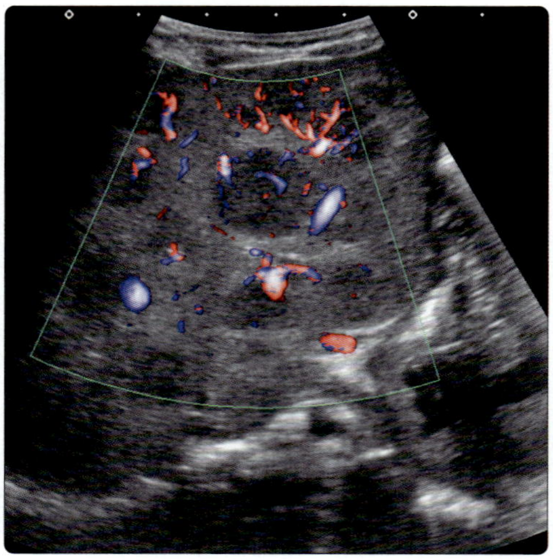

(Left) *Axial T2 MR in a 3 month old with cutaneous IHs, hypothyroidism, & cardiac dysfunction shows numerous round, hyperintense masses replacing most of the liver parenchyma. Only small portions of the liver are spared.* **(Right)** *Axial dynamic T1 C+ FS MR images from early to late (clockwise, from the upper left) in the same patient show peripheral to central enhancement of the IHs over 2 minutes.*

Infantile Hemangioma

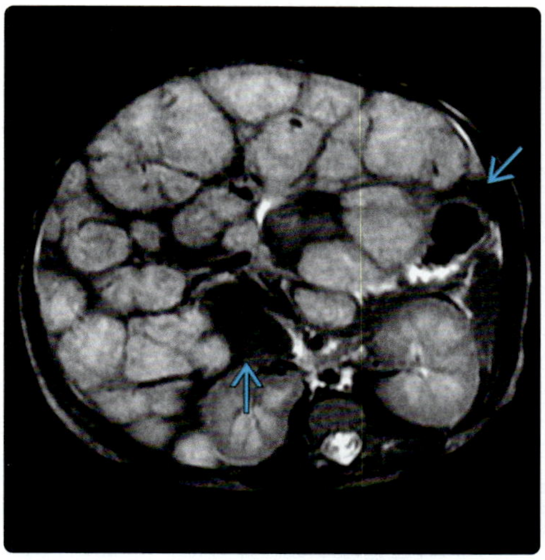

Infantile Hemangioma

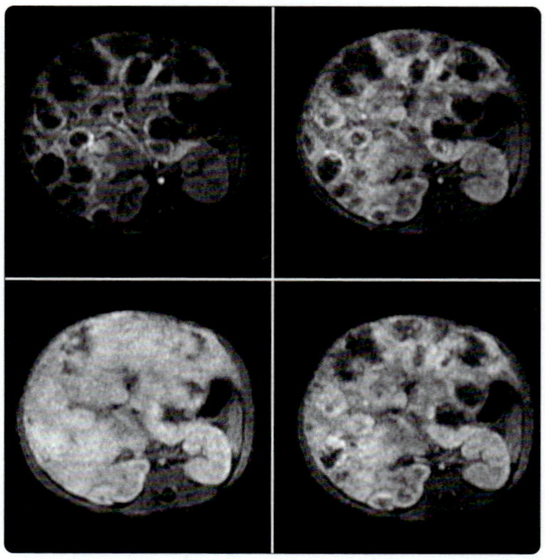

Metastases

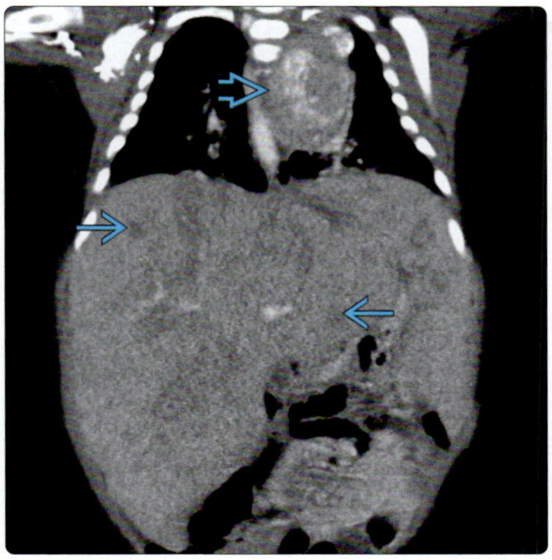

Metastases

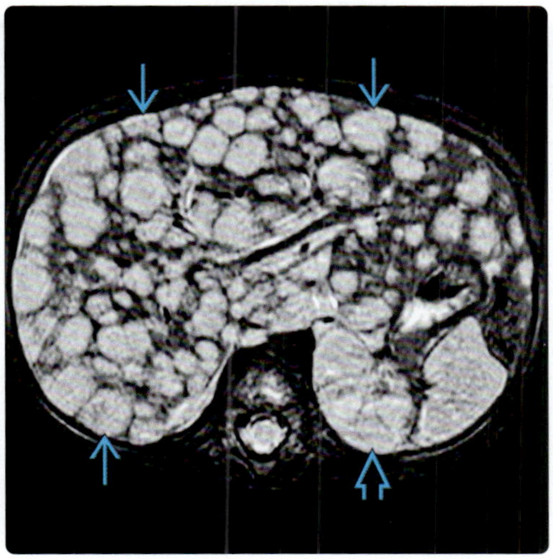

(Left) *Coronal CECT in a 2 month old shows an enlarged & diffusely heterogeneous liver with scattered discrete, hypoenhancing lesions. These findings are secondary to extensive hepatic metastases from the large, partially calcified thoracic neuroblastoma.* **(Right)** *Axial T2 FS MR shows innumerable discrete, hyperintense lesions throughout the liver. The primary neuroblastoma in the left suprarenal fossa is also hyperintense.*

Metastases

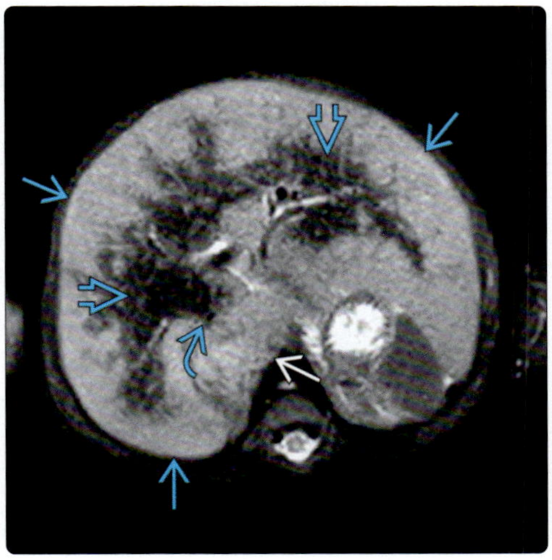

Metastases

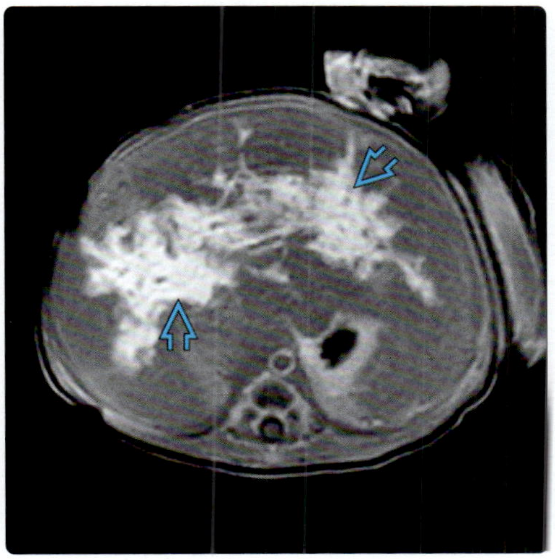

(Left) *Axial T2 FS MR in an 8 day old with hepatomegaly shows a large, confluent rind of hyperintense tissue infiltrating the liver parenchyma. There is sparing of central liver tissue. Note that the IVC is effaced & displaced anteriorly by a similar-appearing suprarenal mass. Neuroblastoma was confirmed at biopsy.* **(Right)** *Axial T1 C+ FS MR with HSCM (in the hepatobiliary phase) shows retention of contrast in the residual central foci of uninvolved liver parenchyma but not the peripheral tumor.*

Hepatoblastoma

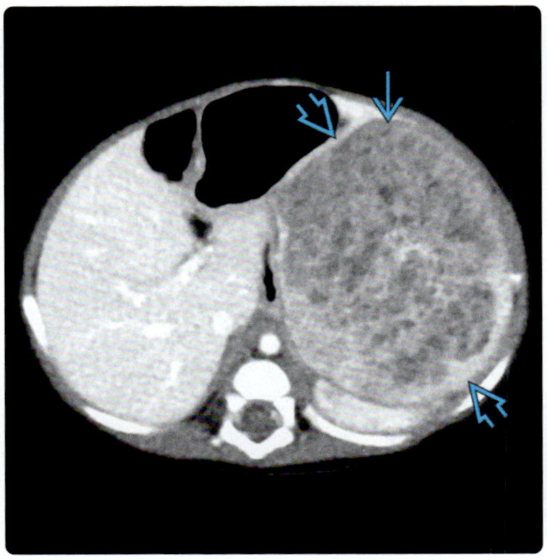

Hepatoblastoma

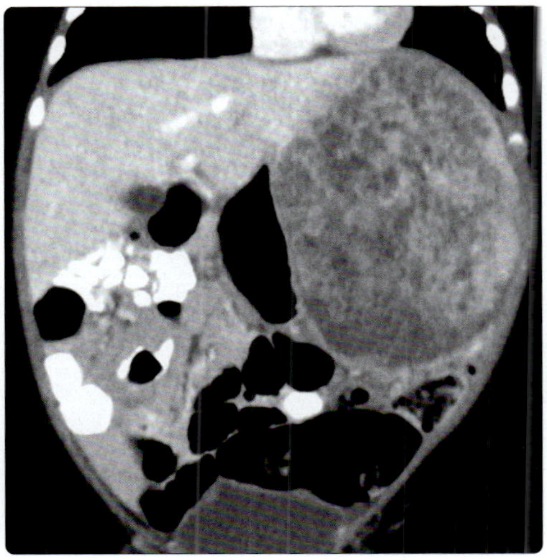

(Left) *Axial CECT in a 2 month old with a palpable left upper quadrant mass shows splaying of the left lobe of the liver by a large mass. As in this case, hepatoblastoma typically shows heterogeneity & hypoenhancement relative to the liver.* **(Right)** *Coronal CECT in the same patient shows the large, exophytic component of the hepatoblastoma filling the left upper abdomen, displacing the stomach medially.*

(Left) *Longitudinal color Doppler US in a 2 week old shows a heterogeneous collection ➔ in the left hepatic lobe with internal septations, fluid-debris levels ➔, & no internal vascularity. This lesion was due to an umbilical venous catheter extravasation & gradually decreased in size.* **(Right)** *Axial T2 FS MR in an 8 month old shows a large, cystic hepatic mass with numerous thin internal septations.*

Umbilical Venous Catheter Extravasation

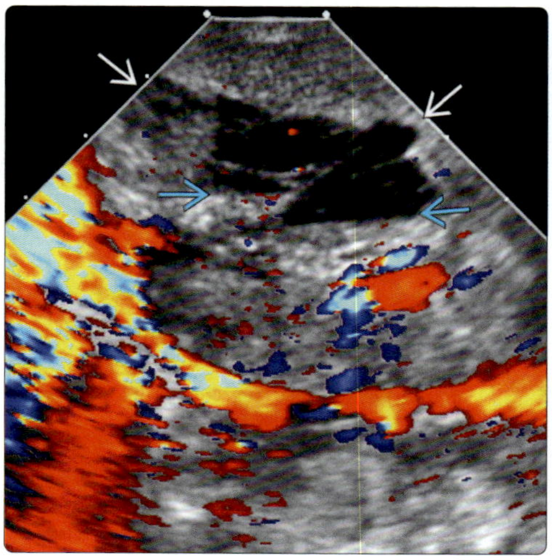

Mesenchymal Hamartoma

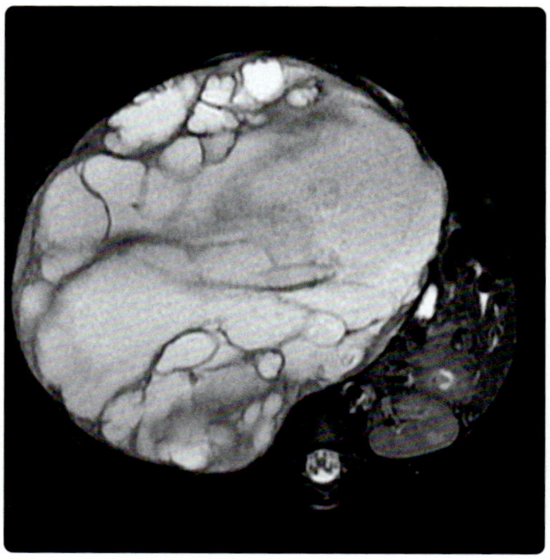

(Left) *Axial T1 C+ FS MR in the same patient shows mild rim & septal enhancement in this congenital mesenchymal hamartoma. Mesenchymal hamartomas are most commonly multicystic but may be solid or mixed.* **(Right)** *Coronal STIR MR shows a large, multicystic & solid mass ➔ of the right hepatic lobe. The cysts vary widely in size in this mesenchymal hamartoma.*

Mesenchymal Hamartoma

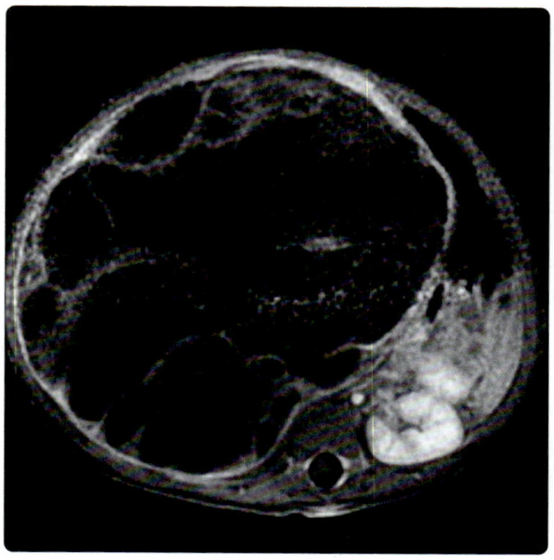

Mesenchymal Hamartoma

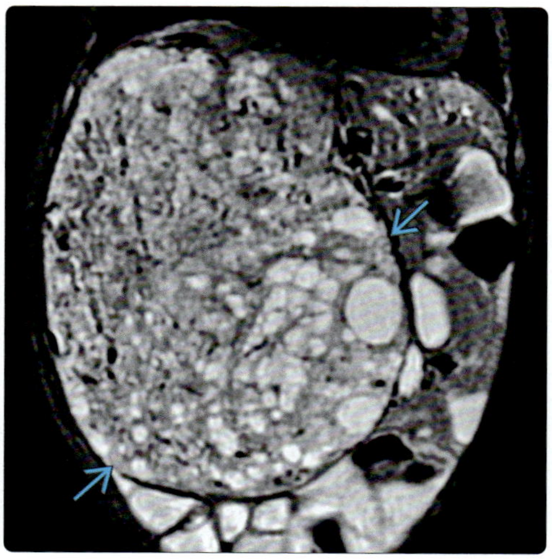

(Left) *Dynamic axial T1 C+ FS MR images (clockwise, from upper left) in a newborn with a prenatally detected mass show a large, heterogeneous hepatic tumor with peripheral to central enhancement, suggestive of a CH. However, biopsy showed a mesenchymal hamartoma. This imaging appearance has rarely been reported with this tumor.* **(Right)** *Coronal T2 SSFSE MR of a 3rd-trimester fetus shows a large, simple-appearing, hyperintense mass ➔ along the inferior edge of the liver.*

Mesenchymal Hamartoma

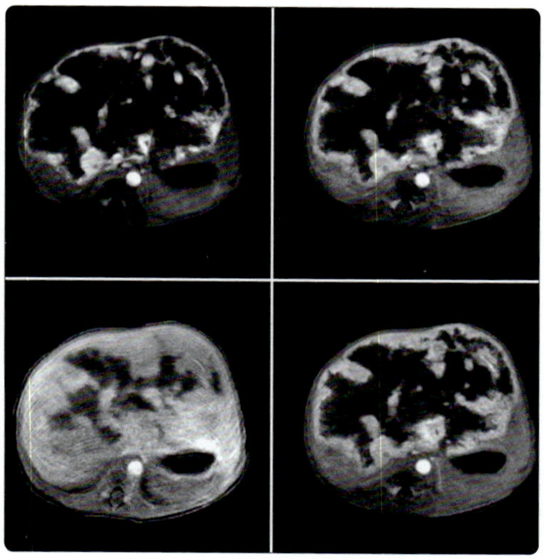

Congenital Hepatic Cyst

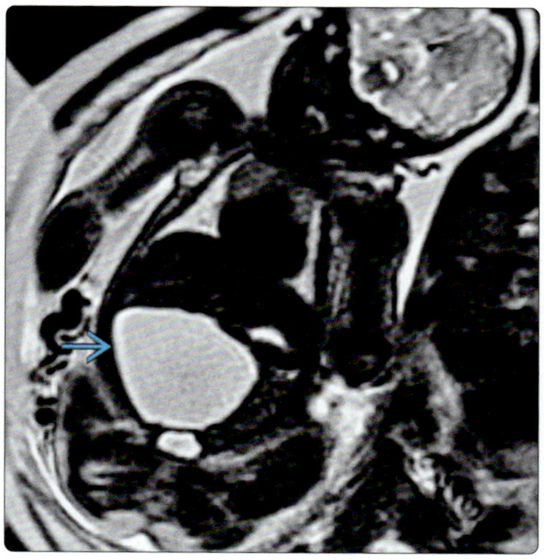

Congenital Hepatic Cyst

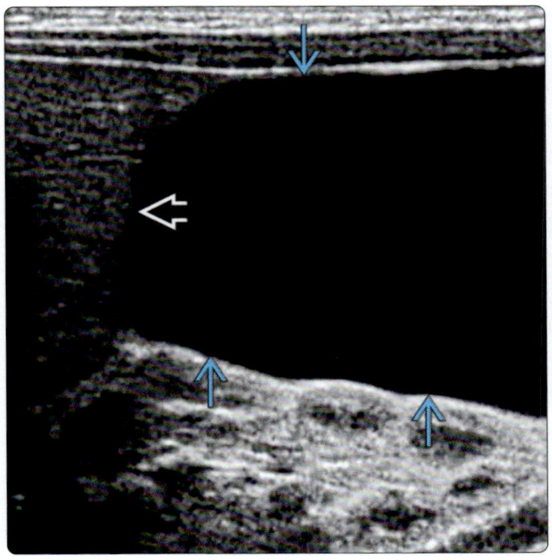

Choledochal Cyst

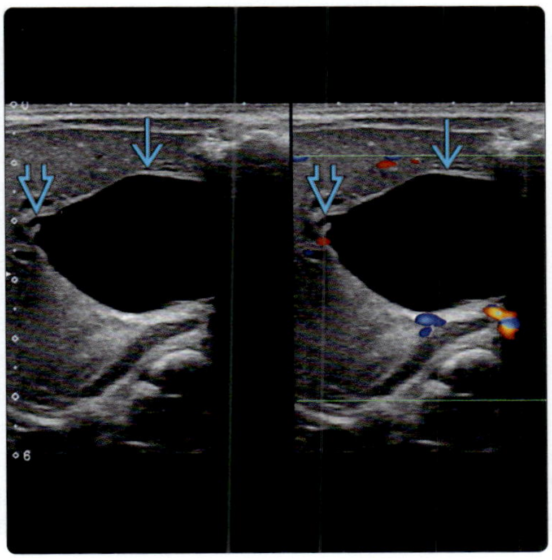

(Left) *Longitudinal US postnatally in the same patient shows a large anechoic lesion arising from the inferior aspect of the liver. This mass has a simple appearance with a thin rim, no septations, & no internal color Doppler flow (not shown). At resection, it was confirmed to be a simple hepatic cyst.* **(Right)** *Longitudinal US images in a 7 day old show an ovoid, cystic mass in the liver hilum with no internal vascularity. The cyst connects to mildly dilated intrahepatic bile ducts.*

Choledochal Cyst

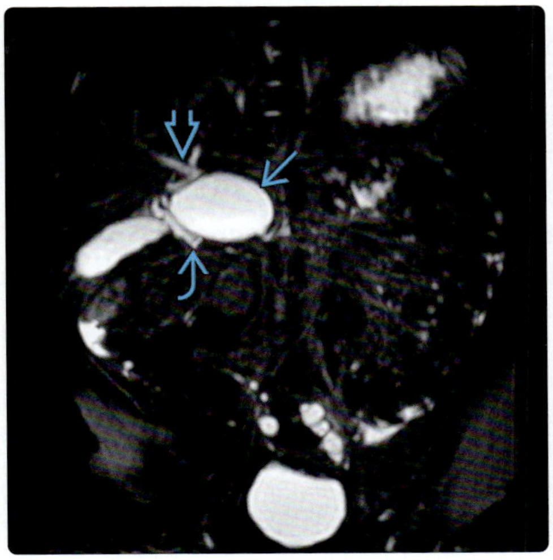

Cystic Biliary Atresia

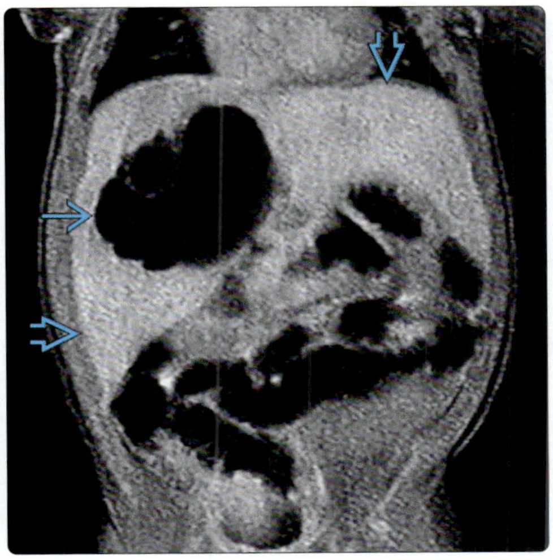

(Left) *Coronal MRCP MIP in the same patient at 5 months of age shows the cyst connecting to the dilated intrahepatic ducts & cystic duct. This type I choledochal cyst was subsequently resected.* **(Right)** *Coronal T1 C+ FS MR (during hepatobiliary phase) in a 3 week old with acholic stools shows a central cystic mass with poor hepatic uptake of HSCM. No gallbladder or common bile duct was seen in this patient with cystic biliary atresia.*

Angiosarcoma

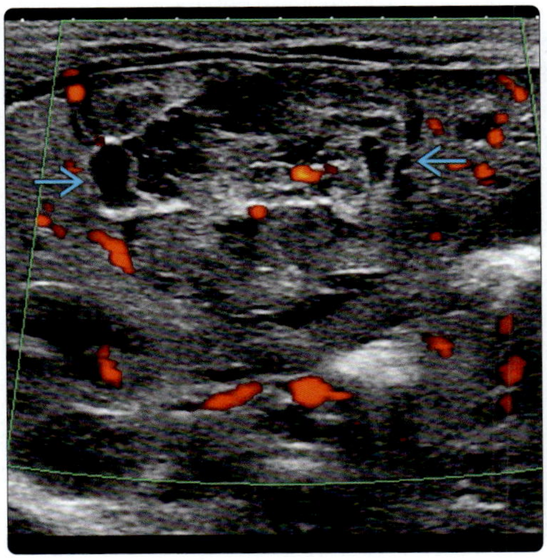

Angiosarcoma

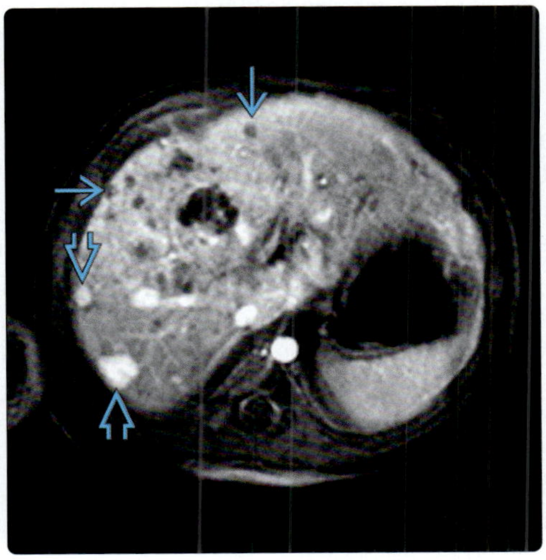

(Left) *Transverse power Doppler US in a 5 day old with numerous hepatic lesions shows a dominant heterogeneous mass with multiple internal septations but little internal vascularity.* **(Right)** *Axial T1 C+ FS MR in the same patient (superior to the dominant mass) shows enhancement of several hepatic lesions during the portal venous phase, though most lesions did not enhance. Many nonenhancing lesions contained low T2 signal fluid levels (not shown) due to blood products.*

DIFFERENTIAL DIAGNOSIS

Common

- Infantile Hemangiomas
- Hepatoblastoma
- Focal Nodular Hyperplasia
- Metastases

Less Common

- Hepatocellular Carcinoma
- Hepatic Adenoma
- Abscess
- Regenerative Nodules
- Mesenchymal Hamartoma

Rare but Important

- Fibrolamellar Hepatocellular Carcinoma
- Undifferentiated Embryonal Sarcoma
- Angiomyolipoma
- Biliary Rhabdomyosarcoma
- Malignant Rhabdoid Tumor

ESSENTIAL INFORMATION

Key Differential Diagnosis Issues

- Differential diagnosis can be focused by age, past medical history, laboratory tests, & imaging features
  - Ultrasound best for screening
  - Dynamic T1 C+ MR particularly useful with hepatocyte-specific contrast media (HSCM) using delayed hepatobiliary phase

Helpful Clues for Common Diagnoses

- **Infantile Hemangiomas**
  - Most common benign hepatic tumor, composed of clusters of plump endothelial cell-lined channels
  - 85% diagnosed in first 6 months but not at birth
    - Proliferating phase: Appear & grow rapidly over 1st few weeks/months of life
    - Involuting phase: Decrease gradually in size over next few months/years
  - Hepatic infantile hemangiomas (IHs) can be single but are more commonly multiple; rarely diffuse (nearly replacing liver)
  - Imaging: Multiple lesions, relatively uniform in size, morphology, & signal characteristics
    - T2 hyperintense ± scattered internal flow voids
    - Rapid enhancement from peripheral to central; do not retain HSCM on delayed hepatocyte phase
    - ± enlarged hepatic artery & veins
    - Doppler ultrasound shows variable degrees of increased internal & peripheral color flow
- **Hepatoblastoma**
  - Most common pediatric hepatic malignancy
  - Median age of 19 months; only 5-10% occur > 4 years
  - 90% have increased serum α-fetoprotein (AFP)
  - Associations: Very low birth weight, Beckwith-Wiedemann, familial adenomatous polyposis
  - Imaging: Solid, large mass; solitary > multifocal
    - Variable heterogeneity; usually have substantial intermediate T2 signal solid components
      - □ Ca^{2+} in 40-55%
    - Usually hypoenhancing on all phases; rarely retain HSCM on hepatobiliary phase
    - ± enhancing tumor thrombus in hepatic & portal veins
    - Solid components often restrict diffusion
  - Distant metastases in 20% at diagnosis
- **Focal Nodular Hyperplasia**
  - Benign hyperplastic nodule composed of hepatocytes & disorganized bile ducts, ± central scar
  - 2 distinct populations
    - Classic solitary lesions (50%): F > > M
    - Multiple lesions: Small, typically in cancer survivors or with preexisting liver disease
  - Imaging: Iso- or slightly T1 hypointense, iso- or slightly T2 hyperintense; hyperenhancing on arterial phase, isointense on portal venous & equilibrium phases, hyperintense on hepatobiliary phase with HSCM
    - Solitary lesions: Relatively larger; T2-hyperintense stellate scar may show delayed enhancement with HSCM or on CECT
    - Multiple lesions: Often subcentimeter with no scar
- **Metastases**
  - More frequent overall than primary hepatic tumors
    - Neuroblastoma, Wilms, & lymphoma most common
  - Imaging: Vary widely in size & morphology
    - Usually hypoenhancing on all phases; do not retain HSCM on hepatobiliary phase
    - Often restrict diffusion due to high cellularity

Helpful Clues for Less Common Diagnoses

- **Hepatocellular Carcinoma**
  - 2nd most common hepatic malignancy in children
  - Rare < 5 years old; patients usually > 10 years old
  - Underlying liver disease (of many different etiologies) is only present in 30-50% of affected children
  - AFP elevated in 70-80%
  - Imaging: Large heterogeneous mass; multifocal in > 50%
    - Variable T1 & T2; restricts diffusion; classic HSCM pattern: Early arterial enhancement with rapid portal venous phase washout & no retention of HSCM
      - □ However, well-differentiated HCC may retain HSCM
    - ± enhancing tumor thrombus in hepatic & portal veins
    - Metastases common: Lymph nodes, lungs, bone
- **Hepatic Adenoma**
  - Benign hepatocellular tumor
  - 4 types: Inflammatory, hepatocyte nuclear factor 1α (HNF1α) inactivated, β-catenin activated, unclassified
    - All can develop hepatocellular carcinoma
    - Lesions > 4 cm at risk for rupture with hemorrhage
  - Predisposing conditions
    - Inflammatory (up to 50%): Obesity, ethanol abuse
    - HNF1α-inactivated (30%): Oral contraceptive use
    - β-catenin activated (10-15%): Glycogen storage disease, familial adenomatous polyposis
  - Imaging
    - Inflammatory: Marked T2 hyperintensity; retain HSCM
    - HNF1α-inactivated: Drop signal on opposed-phase images due to intracellular fat; do not retain HSCM
    - β-catenin activated: Arterial hyperenhancement, retain HSCM
      - □ Highest risk of malignant transformation
    - Unclassified: No specific imaging features

- **Abscess**
  - Associations: Immunodeficiency, systemic infection, abdominal inflammatory processes, & chronic granulomatous disease
    - *Staphylococcus aureus* most common organism
    - Fungal infections (classically *Candida albicans*) & *Bartonella henselae* associated with microabscesses
  - Imaging: Multiple in up to 25% (but 70% in neonates)
    - Microabscesses are typically extensive & subcentimeter, often involving spleen
      - Often hypoechoic on ultrasound, but *Candida* frequently shows central echogenic dot
    - Pyogenic abscesses are larger & more confluent, frequently with enhancing irregular rim
      - Adjacent liver may be T2 hyperintense (edema)
- **Regenerative Nodules**
  - Background liver typically abnormal (cirrhosis, iron deposition, etc.)
    - Predisposing conditions include prior Fontan or Kasai procedures, prior chemotherapy, cholangiopathies, Langerhans cell histiocytosis
  - Imaging: Usually < 2 cm but larger central masses have been reported in cholangiopathies
    - Iso- or hyperintense on T1, variable T2; enhancement typically isointense to liver parenchyma on all phases but arterial hyperenhancement may be seen
- **Mesenchymal Hamartoma**
  - 2nd most common benign hepatic mass of infancy
    - Typically diagnosed in first 2 years of life
  - May grow rapidly, leading to compartment syndrome, respiratory distress, rarely heart failure
  - AFP may be moderately elevated
  - Imaging: Multiloculated large cystic mass in 70%; solid or mixed forms also occur; microcysts may appear solid
    - May rarely mimic hypervascular appearance of congenital hemangioma
    - Solid portions are typically hypoenhancing but may retain HSCM
  - Reports of spontaneous regression as well as malignant transformation to undifferentiated embryonal sarcoma

Helpful Clues for Rare Diagnoses

- **Fibrolamellar Hepatocellular Carcinoma**
  - Occurs in adolescents & young adults
  - AFP is usually not elevated
  - Imaging: Solitary large mass, often with central scar
    - Mass often shows arterial hyperenhancement
    - Scar is low in signal on all MR sequences & shows no enhancement
    - Ca^{2+} is seen in 35-68%
    - Metastatic regional lymph nodes are common
- **Undifferentiated Embryonal Sarcoma**
  - Usually occurs between 5-10 years of age
  - AFP is not elevated
  - Imaging: Large solitary, classically cystic-appearing mass on CECT/MR but solid by ultrasound (due to myxoid content)
    - Low signal fibrous pseudocapsule
    - Often contains foci of hemorrhage
    - May demonstrate enhancing septations & nodules
- **Angiomyolipoma**
  - Associated with tuberous sclerosis
  - Less common than renal angiomyolipoma (AMLs)
  - Imaging: Small lesions with macro- &/or microscopic fat
- **Biliary Rhabdomyosarcoma**
  - Most commonly presents with jaundice < 5 years of age
  - Imaging: Heterogeneous polypoid intraductal mass, most commonly at porta hepatis
    - Upstream biliary ductal dilation is typical
    - Frequent distortion of portal vein
- **Malignant Rhabdoid Tumor**
  - Median age: 8 months; neonatal cases ~ 5%
  - AFP only mildly to moderately elevated; INI1 deficient
  - Imaging: Similar appearance to hepatoblastoma

SELECTED REFERENCES

1. Masand PM: Magnetic resonance imaging features of common focal liver lesions in children. Pediatr Radiol. 48(9):1234-44, 2018
2. Pugmire BS et al: Magnetic resonance imaging of primary pediatric liver tumors. Pediatr Radiol. 46(6):764-77, 2016

Infantile Hemangiomas

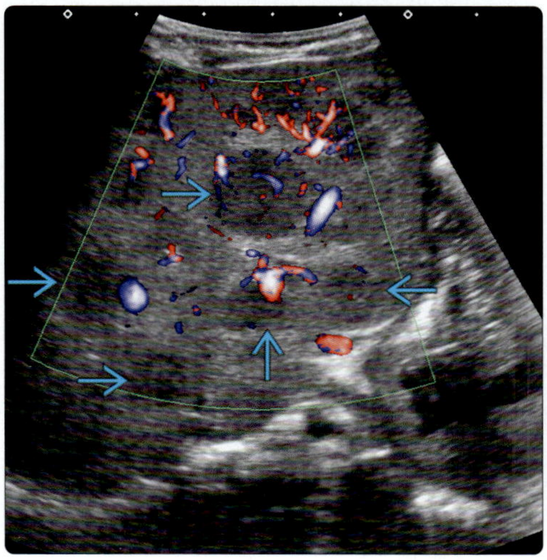

Infantile Hemangiomas

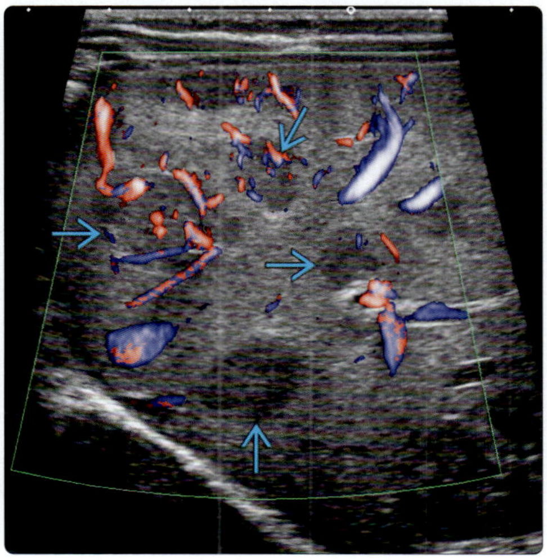

(Left) *Transverse color Doppler ultrasound in a 4 month old with > 5 cutaneous infantile hemangiomas (IHs) shows numerous round hypoechoic masses* ➡ *throughout the liver. Unlike soft tissue IHs (which are uniformly hypervascular in the proliferating phase), hepatic IHs show variable degrees of internal vascularity.* **(Right)** *Longitudinal color Doppler ultrasound in the same patient again demonstrates varying degrees of vascularity in the multifocal IHs* ➡.

(Left) *Axial T2 FS MR in a 3 month old with skin IHs shows innumerable round hyperintense masses nearly completely replacing the liver parenchyma. Only small amounts of normal liver remain ⇨. Patients with this extent of disease may have liver failure, heart failure, compartment syndrome, &/or hypothyroidism.* **(Right)** *Dynamic T1 C+ FS MR images (clockwise, from the upper left) in the same patient show progressive peripheral to central enhancement of the innumerable hepatic lesions, typical of IHs.*

Infantile Hemangiomas

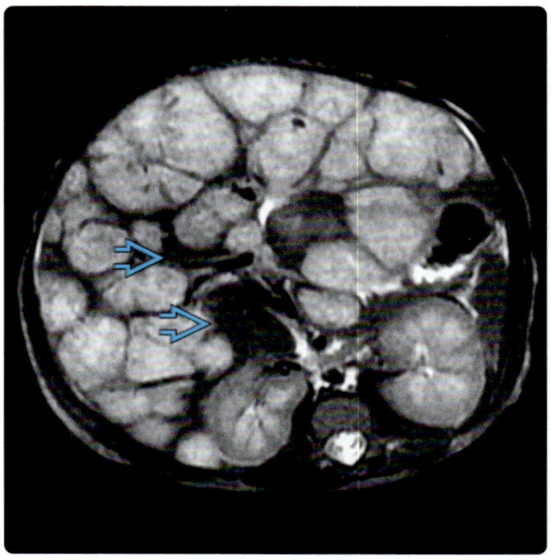

Infantile Hemangiomas

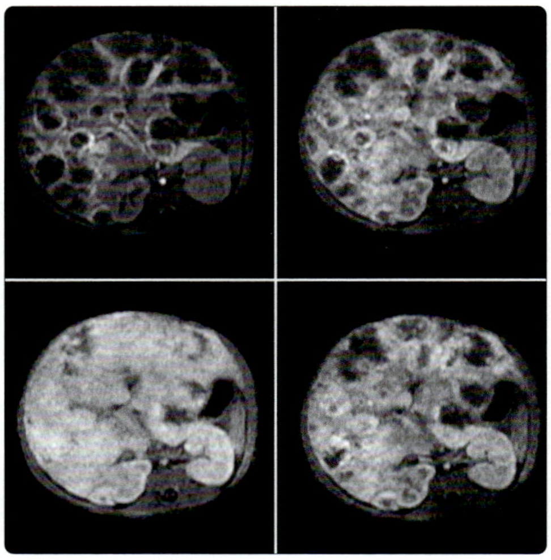

(Left) *Axial T2 FS MR in a 3-year-old patient with hepatoblastoma shows multiple intermediate signal intensity masses ⇨ throughout the liver, some of which are heterogeneous ⇨.* **(Right)** *Axial T1 C+ FS MR images in the same patient, using HSCM, show hypoenhancement & heterogeneity of lesions ⇨ on the equilibrium phase (top) with no retention of contrast ➔ on the hepatobiliary phase (bottom).*

Hepatoblastoma

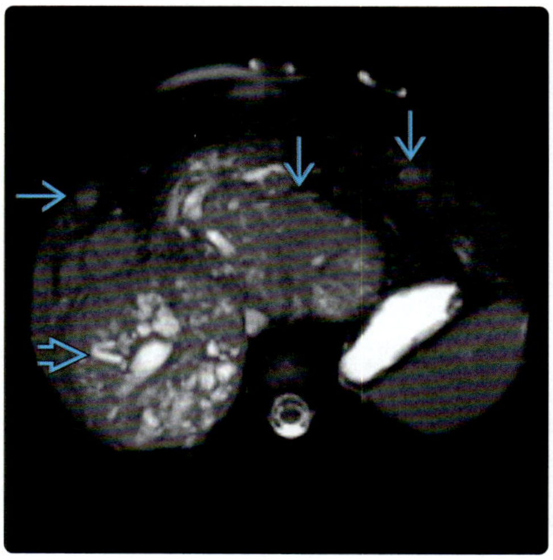

Hepatoblastoma

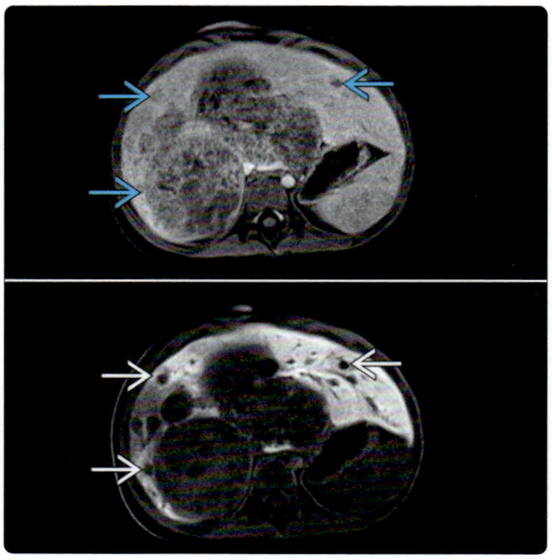

(Left) *Axial DWI MR in the same patient shows restricted diffusion (confirmed on the ADC map, not shown) in all of the foci of hepatoblastoma due to the high cellularity of the lesions.* **(Right)** *Transverse ultrasound in the same patient shows heterogeneous but predominantly increased echogenicity of the hepatoblastoma lesions ⇨ throughout the liver ⇨.*

Hepatoblastoma

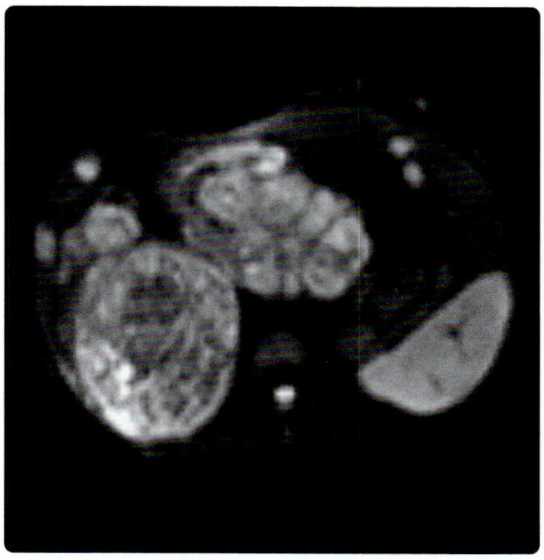

Hepatoblastoma

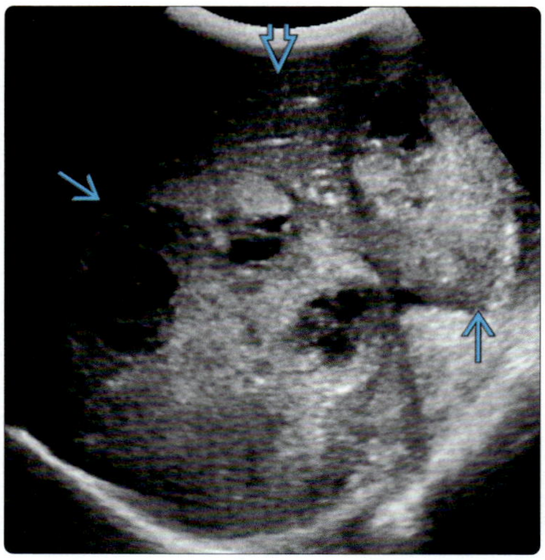

Hepatoblastoma

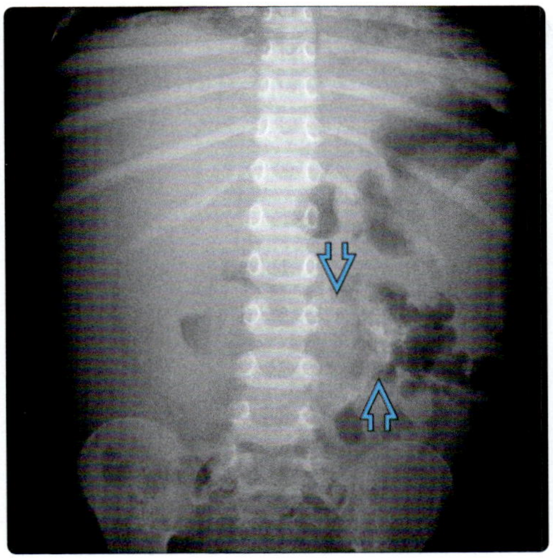

Hepatoblastoma

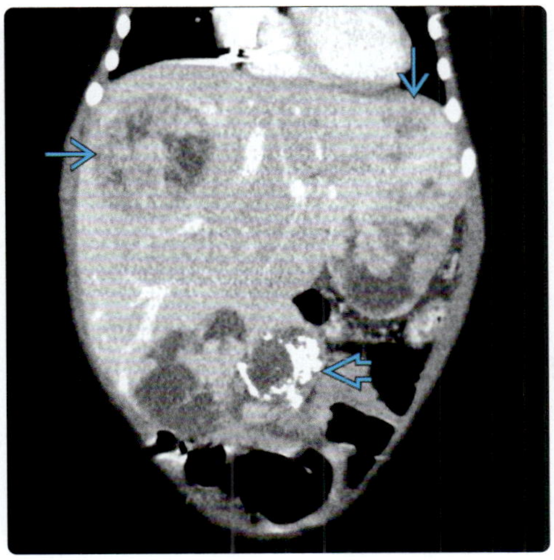

(Left) *Supine frontal radiograph in a 2 year old with hepatomegaly shows displacement of bowel from the right abdomen. There is a partially calcified mass in the medial left abdomen.* **(Right)** *Coronal CECT in the same patient shows multiple heterogeneously enhancing masses in the liver, typical of hepatoblastoma. The more inferomedial lesion is calcified , which is seen in up to 55% of hepatoblastomas.*

Focal Nodular Hyperplasia

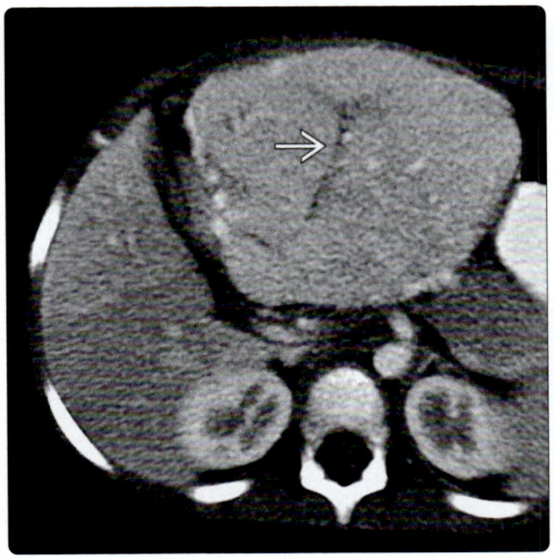

Focal Nodular Hyperplasia

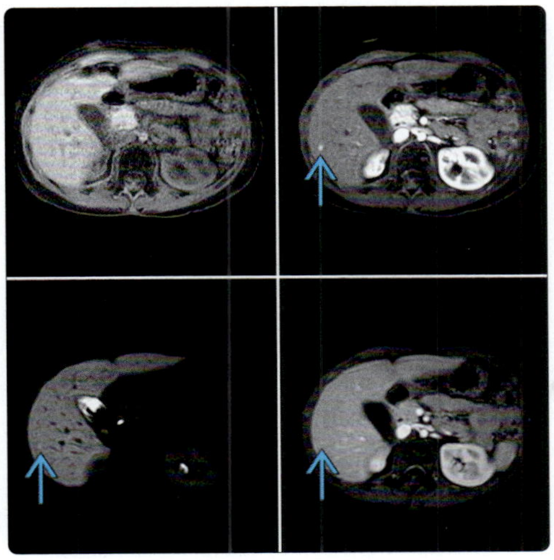

(Left) *Axial CECT shows a slightly hyperenhancing mass of the left hepatic lobe with a central stellate scar . The scar of FNH is classically T2 hyperintense & enhances on MR (not shown).* **(Right)** *Axial T1 FS MR images (clockwise, from the upper left) show a small posterior hepatic lesion in precontrast, arterial phase, portal venous phase, & delayed hepatocyte phase (with HSCM) in an 8 year old with a remote history of neuroblastoma. Many similar lesions were present, typical of FNHs in patients previously treated for malignancy.*

Hepatocellular Carcinoma

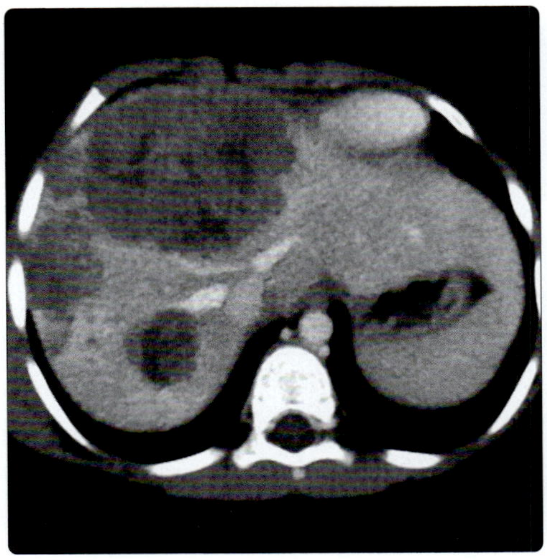

Hepatocellular Carcinoma

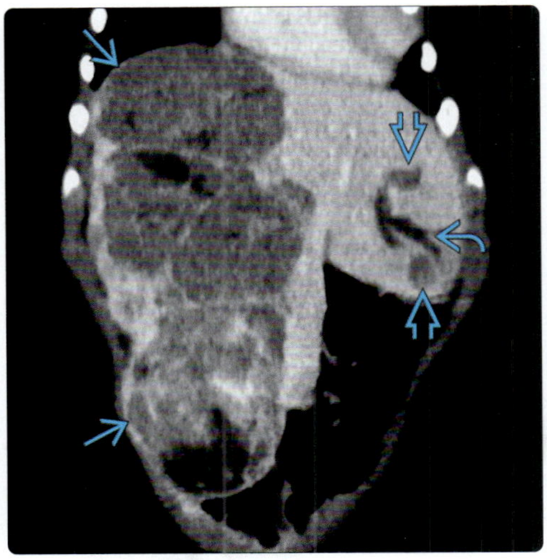

(Left) *Axial CECT in a 6 year old with hepatocellular carcinoma shows multiple hypoenhancing solid masses throughout the liver.* **(Right)** *Coronal CECT in the same patient shows a large multilobulated hypoenhancing tumor throughout the right lobe with multifocal portal venous tumor thrombus in the lateral left lobe. Biliary dilation was also present from central obstruction.*

(Left) *Coronal T1 C+ FS MR MIP in a 16 year old with an Abernethy malformation shows an aberrant connection of the interrupted portal vein* → *to a hepatic vein* ↷. *Biopsy of the hyperenhancing lesions* ⇨ *confirmed inflammatory adenomas.* (Right) *Coronal CECT in the same patient 6 months later shows active arterial extravasation* → *from a large adenoma* ⇨ *with hemoperitoneum* ➡ *& large foci of clotted blood* ↷. *There is profound bowel wall hyperenhancement* ➡ *due to hypoperfusion complex.*

Hepatic Adenoma

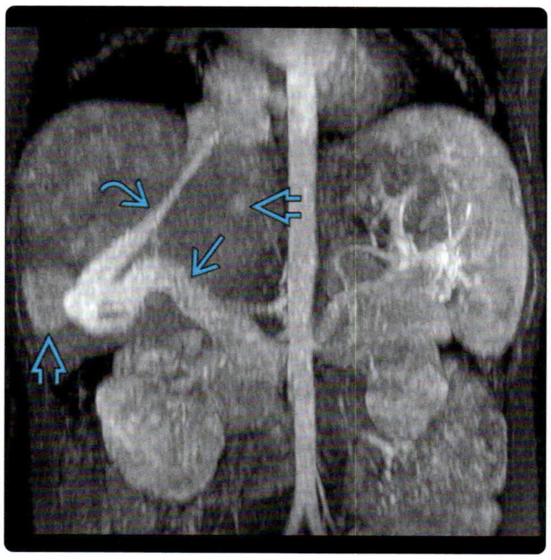

Hepatic Adenoma

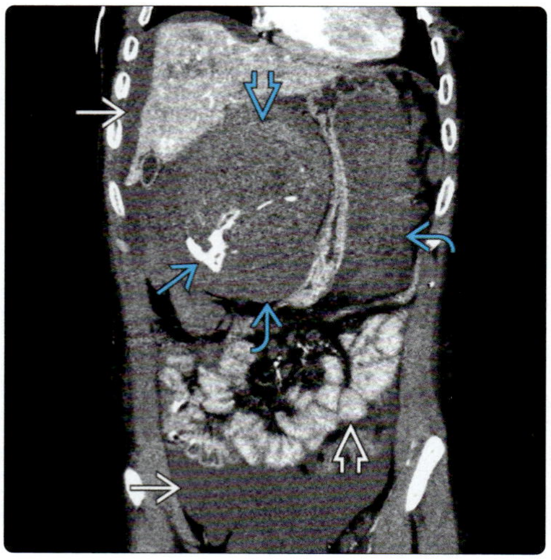

(Left) *Axial T2 FS MR in an 8 month old shows a large predominantly cystic hepatic mass with numerous thin septations* →. *The septations demonstrated enhancement after contrast (not shown). This is the classic appearance for a mesenchymal hamartoma.* (Right) *Axial T1 C+ FS MR in a 21 month old during the portal venous phase shows a relatively homogeneous solid mass, which did not have hyperenhancement on arterial phase, retention of HSCM on hepatobiliary phase, or restricted diffusion.*

Mesenchymal Hamartoma

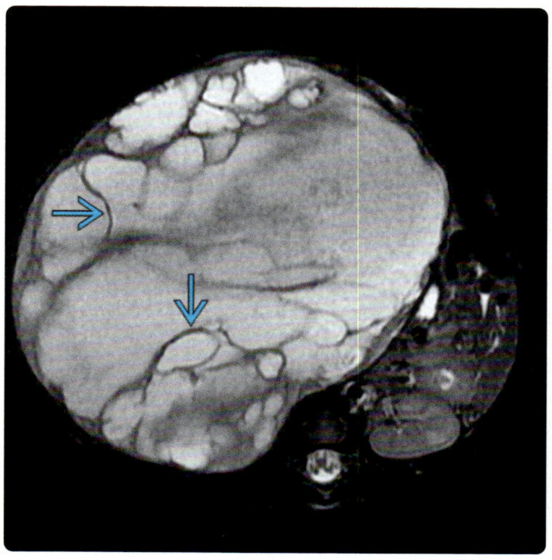

Mesenchymal Hamartoma

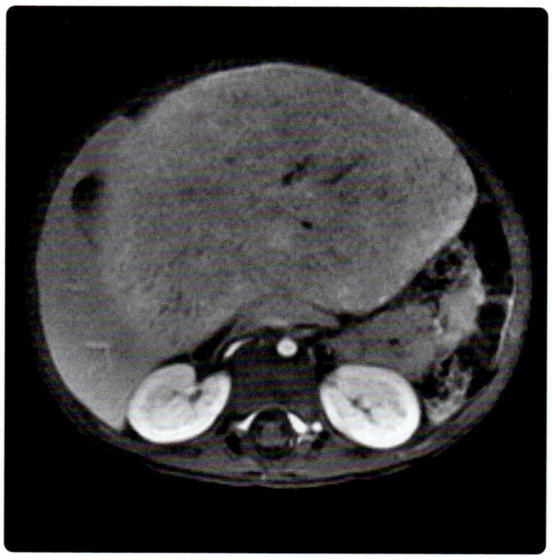

(Left) *Axial T2 FS MR in a 14 year old with a fibrolamellar HCC shows a mildly hyperintense left hepatic mass* ⇨ *with a low signal intensity central scar* →. (Right) *Axial T1 C+ FS MR during the arterial phase in the same patient shows the mass to be slightly hyperenhancing (relative to the liver) except for the nonenhancing scar* →. *The scar & mass were hypoenhancing on all remaining sequences.*

Fibrolamellar Hepatocellular Carcinoma

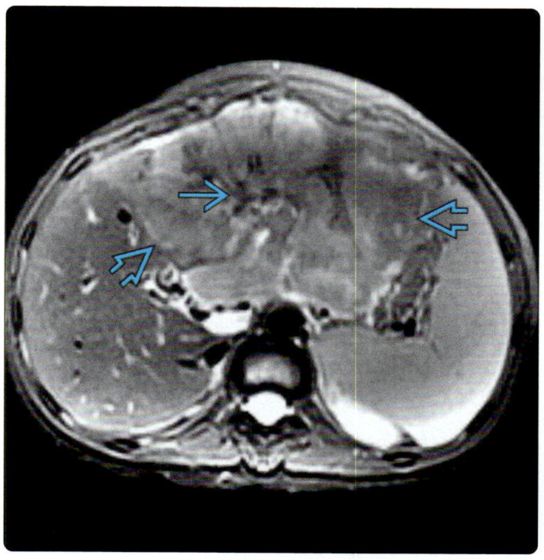

Fibrolamellar Hepatocellular Carcinoma

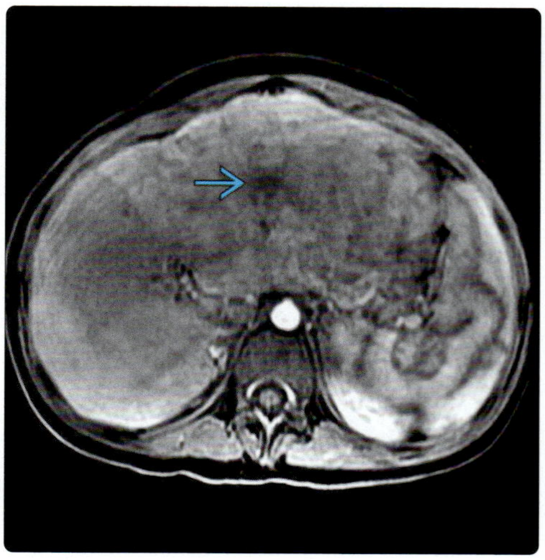

Undifferentiated Embryonal Sarcoma

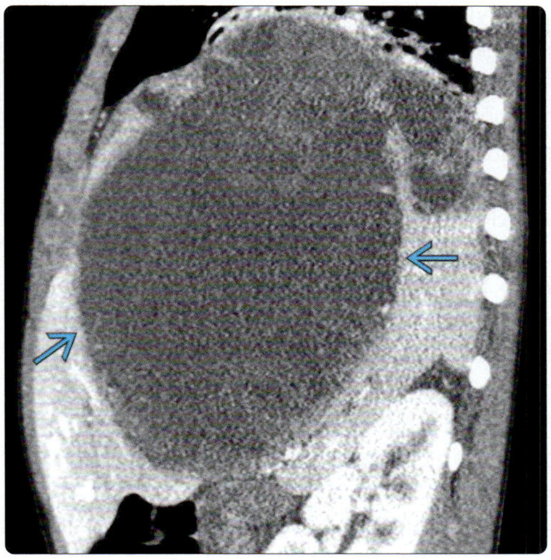

Undifferentiated Embryonal Sarcoma

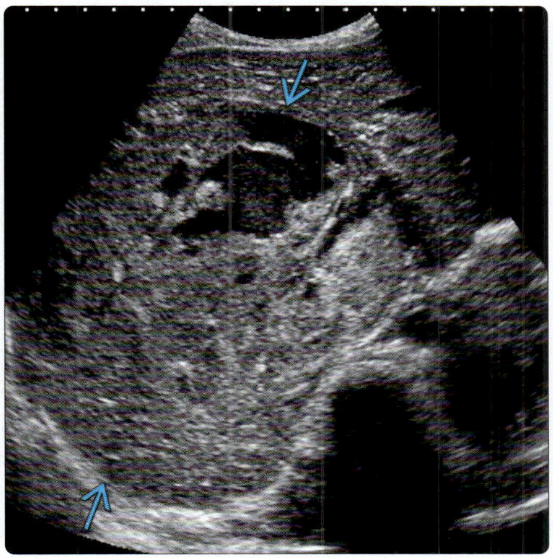

(Left) *Coronal CECT in an 11 year old with right upper quadrant pain shows a large predominantly cystic-appearing mass → centrally in the liver with several satellite lesions.* **(Right)** *Transverse ultrasound in the same patient shows that the mass → is predominantly solid with only small cystic components. The cystic appearance on CECT (& MR, not shown) is typical of undifferentiated embryonal sarcoma (UES) & is due to the myxoid stroma.*

Undifferentiated Embryonal Sarcoma

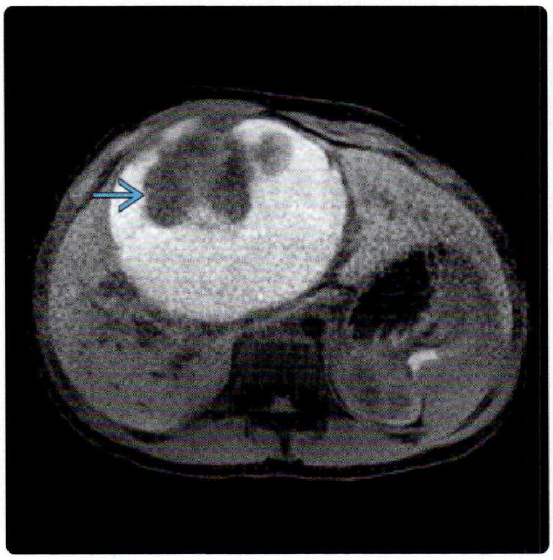

Biliary Rhabdomyosarcoma

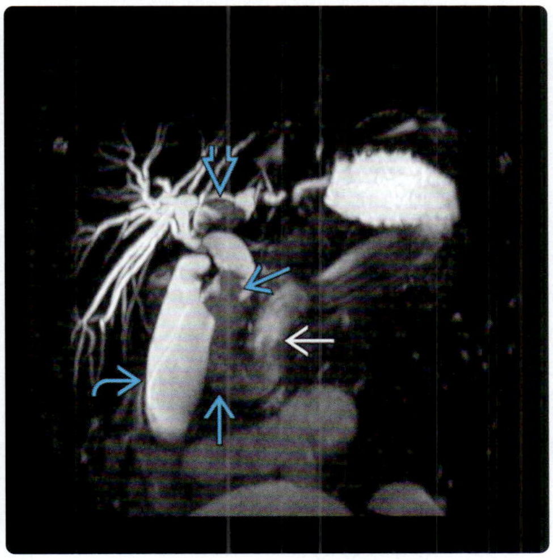

(Left) *Axial T1 FS MR (without contrast) in a patient with UES shows a round mass that is predominantly hyperintense due to internal hemorrhage. The nodular lower signal components → showed no significant enhancement after contrast (not shown).* **(Right)** *Coronal MRCP MIP in a 3 year old shows a lobulated mass filling the common bile duct → & left hepatic duct → with global biliary dilation. The gallbladder → & duodenum ➡ are noted for reference.*

Biliary Rhabdomyosarcoma

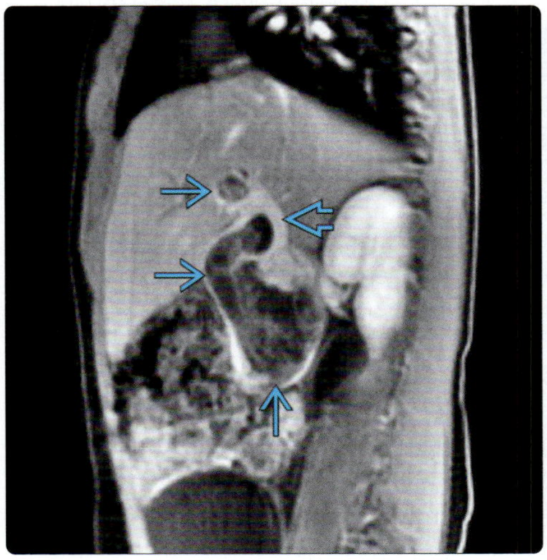

Malignant Rhabdoid Tumor

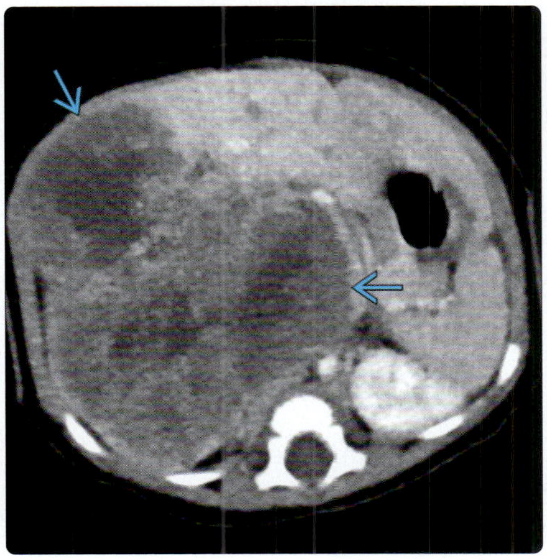

(Left) *Sagittal T1 C+ FS MR in the same patient shows the heterogeneous hypoenhancing mass → in the bile ducts distorting the adjacent portal veins →. Biliary rhabdomyosarcoma was found at surgery.* **(Right)** *Axial CECT in a 3 month old shows a large heterogeneous mass → centered in the right hepatic lobe, most likely a hepatoblastoma in this age. However, the patient's AFP was normal. A malignant rhabdoid tumor was found upon biopsy.*

DIFFERENTIAL DIAGNOSIS

Common

- Infantile Hemangiomas
- Focal Nodular Hyperplasias
- Metastases
  - Neuroblastoma
  - Wilms Tumor
  - Lymphoma

Less Common

- Hepatoblastomas
- Regenerative Nodules
- Hepatic Abscesses
- Adenomas

Rare but Important

- Mesenchymal Hamartomas
- Angiomyolipomas
- Hepatocellular Carcinomas
- Caroli Disease
- Angiosarcomas

ESSENTIAL INFORMATION

Key Differential Diagnosis Issues

- Clinical history is critical
  - Age, skin lesions, preexisting systemic or hepatic disease ± treatment, elevated α-fetoprotein (AFP)
    - Note that neonatal AFP levels are normally elevated & trend down over 1st months of life
- Imaging features often overlap; helpful MR techniques include DWI, in & opposed phase, dynamic & delayed imaging with hepatocyte-specific contrast media (HSCM)

Helpful Clues for Common Diagnoses

- **Infantile Hemangiomas**
  - Most common benign hepatic tumor, composed of clusters of plump endothelial cell-lined channels
  - 85% diagnosed in first 6 months of life but not at birth
    - Proliferating phase: Appear & grow rapidly over 1st few weeks/months of life
    - Involuting phase: Decrease gradually in size over next few months/years
  - Skin infantile hemangiomas (IHs) are present in 50-75% with hepatic IHs
  - Hepatic IHs can be single but are more commonly multiple; rarely diffuse (nearly replacing liver)
  - Diffuse > multifocal can cause
    - Massive hepatomegaly leading to abdominal compartment syndrome & multiorgan failure
    - Liver failure, heart failure
    - Hypothyroidism (due to production of enzymes degrading thyroid hormone)
  - Imaging: Multiple lesions relatively uniform in size, morphology, & signal characteristics
    - T2 hyperintense but not fluid bright, ± scattered internal flow voids
    - Rapid enhancement from peripheral to central; do not retain HSCM on delayed hepatocyte phase
    - ± enlarged hepatic artery & veins
    - Doppler ultrasound shows variable degrees of increased internal & peripheral color flow
- **Focal Nodular Hyperplasias**
  - Benign hyperplastic nodule composed of hepatocytes & disorganized bile ducts, ± central scar
  - 2 distinct populations
    - Classic solitary lesions (50%); F > > M
    - Multiple lesions: Small, typically in cancer survivors or with preexisting liver disease
  - Imaging: Iso- or slightly T1 hypointense, iso- or slightly T2 hyperintense; hyperenhancing on arterial phase, iso- on portal venous & equilibrium phases, hyperintense on delayed hepatobiliary phase with HSCM
    - Solitary lesions: Relatively larger; T2-hyperintense stellate scar may or may not enhance
    - Multiple lesions: Often subcentimeter with no scar
- **Metastases**
  - More frequent overall than primary hepatic tumors
    - Neuroblastoma, Wilms, & lymphoma most common
  - Imaging: Vary widely in size & morphology: May be tiny, innumerable, & diffuse or larger & well circumscribed or even encasing/infiltrating
    - Usually hypoenhancing on all phases; do not retain HSCM on hepatocyte phase
      - ▫ Rarely hyperenhancing on arterial phase
    - Often restrict diffusion due to high cellularity

Helpful Clues for Less Common Diagnoses

- **Hepatoblastomas**
  - Most common pediatric hepatic malignancy
  - Median age of 19 months; only 5-10% occur > 4 years of age; < 5% are congenital
  - 90% have increased serum AFP
  - Associations: Very low birth weight, Beckwith-Wiedemann, familial adenomatous polyposis
  - Imaging: Usually solitary, predominantly solid mass; multifocal lesions usually have 1 dominant mass
    - Variable heterogeneity; usually have substantial intermediate T2 signal components
      - ▫ Ca^{2+} in 40-55%
    - Usually hypoenhancing on all phases; rarely retain HSCM on hepatocyte phase
    - ± enhancing tumor thrombus in hepatic & portal veins
    - Solid components often restrict diffusion
- **Regenerative Nodules**
  - Background liver typically abnormal (cirrhosis, iron deposition, etc.)
    - Predisposing conditions include prior Fontan or Kasai procedures, prior chemotherapy, cholangiopathies, Langerhans cell histiocytosis
  - Imaging: Usually < 2 cm but larger central masses have been reported in cholangiopathies
    - Iso- or hyperintense on T1, variable T2; enhancement typically isointense to liver parenchyma on all phases, but arterial hyperenhancement may be seen
- **Hepatic Abscesses**
  - Associated with immunodeficiency, systemic infection, abdominal inflammatory processes, & chronic granulomatous disease
    - *Staphylococcus aureus* is most common organism

- Fungal infections (classically *Candida albicans*) & *Bartonella henselae* associated with microabscesses
- Risks in neonate include necrotizing enterocolitis & umbilical vein catheterization
- Imaging: Multiple in 20-25% of children & up to 70% in neonates
  - Microabscesses are typically extensive & subcentimeter, often involving spleen
    - Often hypoechoic on ultrasound, but *Candida* frequently shows central echogenic dot
  - Pyogenic abscesses are larger & more confluent, frequently with enhancing, irregular rim
    - Surrounding parenchyma may be T2 hyperintense from edema
  - Ultrasound may be only exam for diagnosis & follow-up in appropriate clinical setting

- **Adenomas**
  - Benign hepatocellular tumor
  - 4 types: Inflammatory, hepatocyte nuclear factor 1α (HNF1α) inactivated, β-catenin activated, unclassified
    - All can develop hepatocellular carcinoma (HCC)
    - Lesions > 4 cm at risk for rupture with hemorrhage
  - Predisposing conditions
    - Inflammatory (up to 50%): Obesity, ethanol abuse
    - HNF1α inactivated (30%): Oral contraceptive use
    - β-catenin activated (10-15%): Glycogen storage disease, familial adenomatous polyposis
  - Imaging
    - Inflammatory: Marked T2 hyperintensity, retention of HSCM
    - HNF1α inactivated: Drop signal on opposed-phase images due to intracellular fat; do not retain HSCM
    - β-catenin activated: Arterial hyperenhancement, retention of HSCM
      - Highest risk of malignant transformation
    - Unclassified: No specific imaging features

Helpful Clues for Rare Diagnoses

- **Mesenchymal Hamartomas**
  - Benign cystic, solid, or mixed mass typically diagnosed in first 2 years of life
  - Imaging: Multiloculated large (usually > 10-cm) solitary cystic mass is classic; rarely multifocal
- **Angiomyolipomas**
  - Associated with tuberous sclerosis
  - Less common than renal angiomyolipomas
  - Imaging: Macro- &/or microscopic fat content
- **Hepatocellular Carcinomas**
  - 2nd most common hepatic malignancy in children
  - Rare < 5 years of age; patients usually > 10 years old
  - Underlying liver disease (of many different etiologies) is only present in 30-50% of affected children
  - AFP elevated in 70-80%
  - Imaging: Disease is multifocal in > 50%
    - Variable T1 & T2; restricts diffusion; classic HSCM pattern: Early arterial enhancement with rapid portal venous phase washout & no retention of HSCM
      - However, well-differentiated HCC may retain HSCM
    - ± enhancing tumor thrombus in hepatic & portal veins
    - Metastases common: Lymph nodes, lungs, bone
- **Caroli Disease**
  - Cystic dilation of intrahepatic bile ducts due to ciliopathy
  - May be associated with autosomal recessive polycystic kidney disease & congenital hepatic fibrosis
  - Patients develop recurrent cholangitis, stones, &/or portal hypertension
  - Imaging: Central dot sign (cross section of dilated bile duct surrounding portal vein radicle) is classic
- **Angiosarcomas**
  - May be solitary or multifocal with dominant mass
  - Imaging: Quite variable due to hemorrhage
    - Solid lesions show variable enhancement

SELECTED REFERENCES

1. Masand PM: Magnetic resonance imaging features of common focal liver lesions in children. Pediatr Radiol. 48(9):1234-44, 2018
2. Trout AT et al: Hepatocyte-specific contrast media: not so simple. Pediatr Radiol. 48(9):1245-55, 2018
3. Pugmire BS et al: Magnetic resonance imaging of primary pediatric liver tumors. Pediatr Radiol. 46(6):764-77, 2016

Infantile Hemangiomas

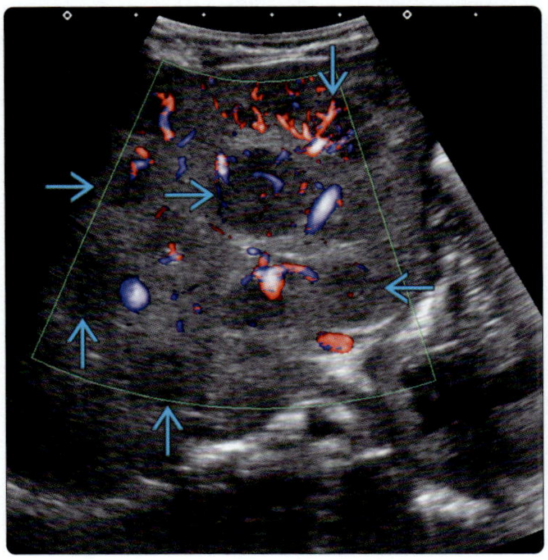

Infantile Hemangiomas

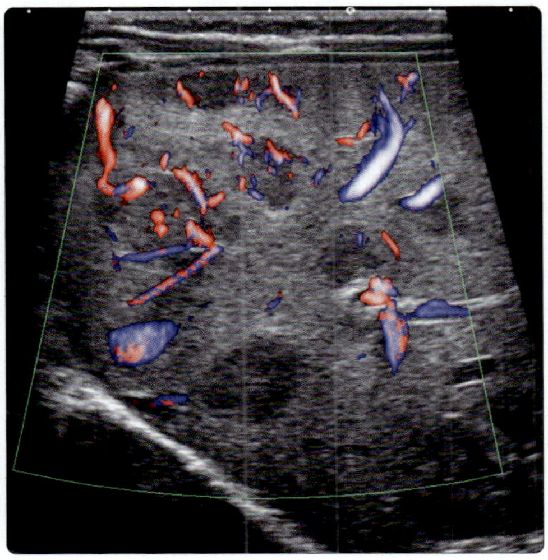

(Left) *Transverse color Doppler ultrasound in a 4 month old with > 5 cutaneous infantile hemangiomas (IHs) shows numerous round, hypoechoic masses* ➡ *throughout the liver. Unlike soft tissue IHs (which are uniformly hypervascular in the proliferating phase), hepatic IHs show variable degrees of internal vascularity.* **(Right)** *Longitudinal color Doppler ultrasound in the same patient again demonstrates varying degrees of vascularity in the multifocal IHs.*

(Left) *AP radiograph in a 3 month old with heart failure & numerous cutaneous IHs shows cardiomegaly & hepatomegaly.* **(Right)** *Axial T2 FS MR in the same patient shows innumerable round, hyperintense (but not fluid-signal-intensity) masses nearly completely replacing the liver parenchyma. Only small amounts of normal liver remain. Patients with this extent of disease may have liver failure, heart failure, compartment syndrome, & hypothyroidism.*

Infantile Hemangiomas

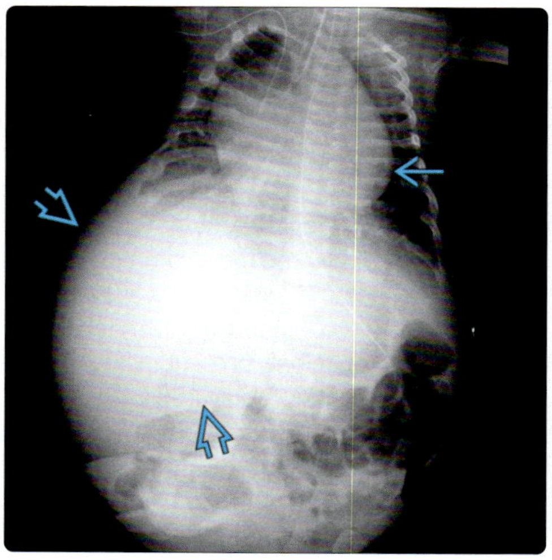

Infantile Hemangiomas

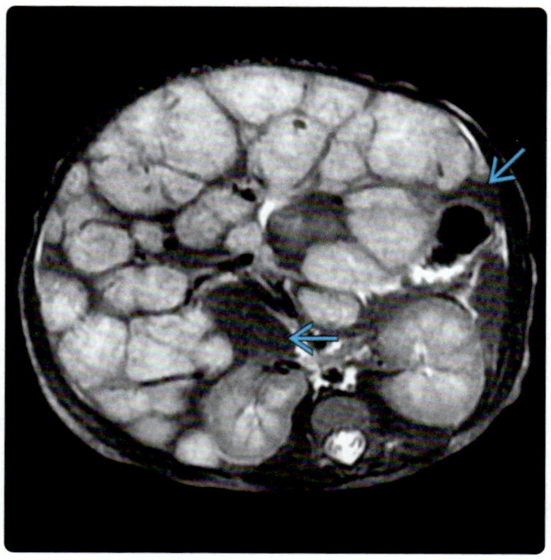

(Left) *Dynamic T1 C+ FS MR images (clockwise from the upper left) in the same patient show progressive peripheral to central enhancement of innumerable hepatic lesions, typical of IHs.* **(Right)** *Axial T1 FS MR images (clockwise from the upper left) show a small posterior hepatic lesion in precontrast, arterial phase, portal venous phase, & delayed hepatocyte phase (with HSCM) in an 8 year old with a remote history of neuroblastoma. Many similar lesions were present, typical of FNHs in patients previously treated for malignancy.*

Infantile Hemangiomas

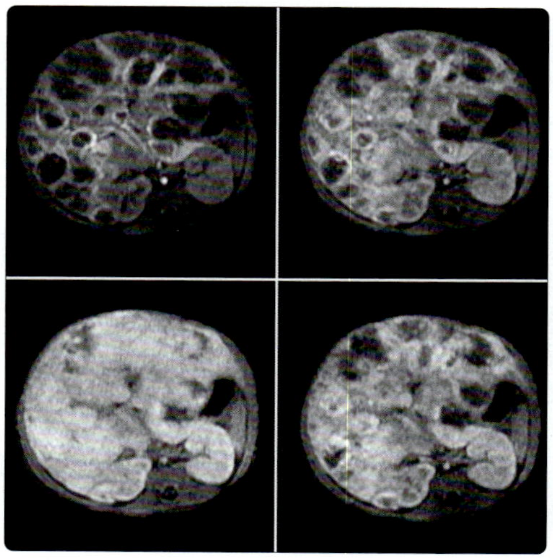

Focal Nodular Hyperplasias

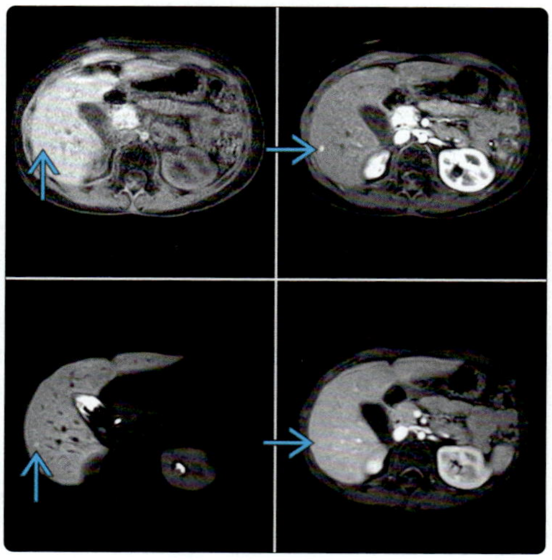

(Left) *Coronal CECT in a 4 month old shows hepatomegaly with a diffusely heterogeneous liver. A few discrete heterogeneous hepatic lesions were also noted. This appearance is due to metastatic neuroblastoma arising in the left adrenal gland.* **(Right)** *Coronal T2 FS MR of a 4 year old with hip pain shows a right suprarenal mass due to neuroblastoma. Multiple subcentimeter metastatic lesions were visualized in the liver, & much of the bone marrow was replaced by tumor.*

Metastases

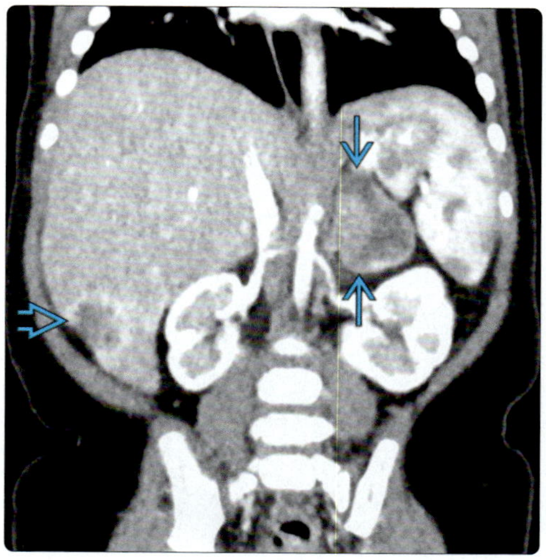

Metastases

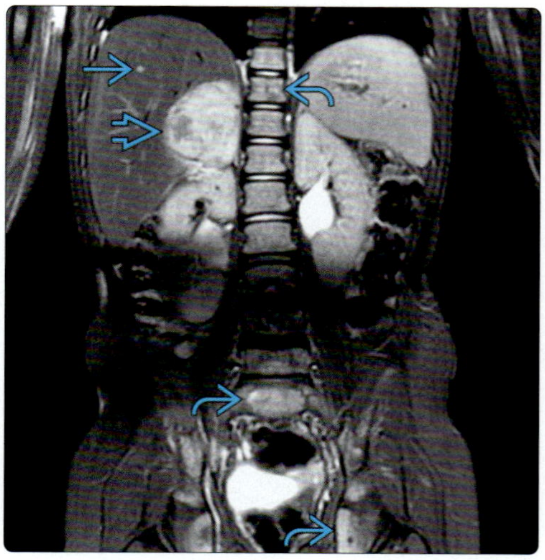

Metastases

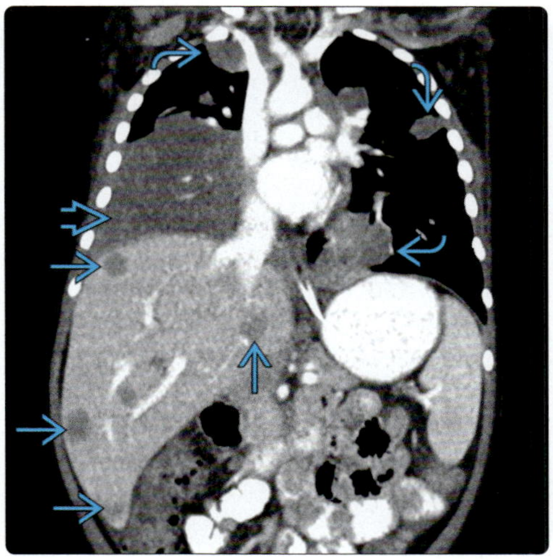

Metastases

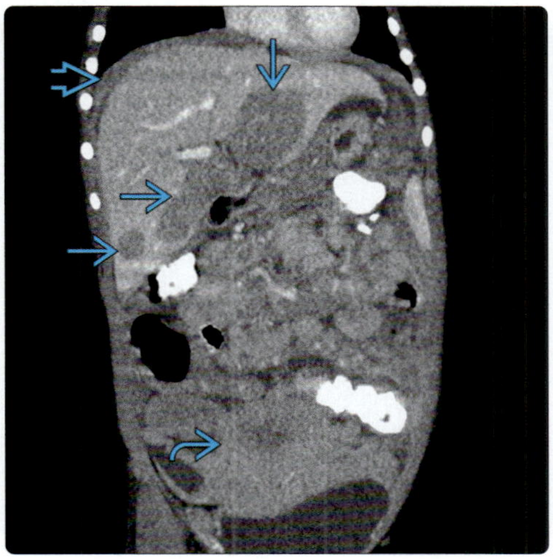

(Left) *Coronal CECT in a 2 year old with respiratory distress shows numerous lung parenchymal lesions, including complete consolidation of the right lower lobe, & multiple well-circumscribed solid liver masses. The patient was ultimately diagnosed with large B-cell lymphoma.* **(Right)** *Coronal CECT in a 7 year old with abdominal distention shows multiple hypodense liver lesions due to Burkitt lymphoma. There is also infiltration of the diaphragm, uterus, mesentery, & segments of bowel.*

Metastases

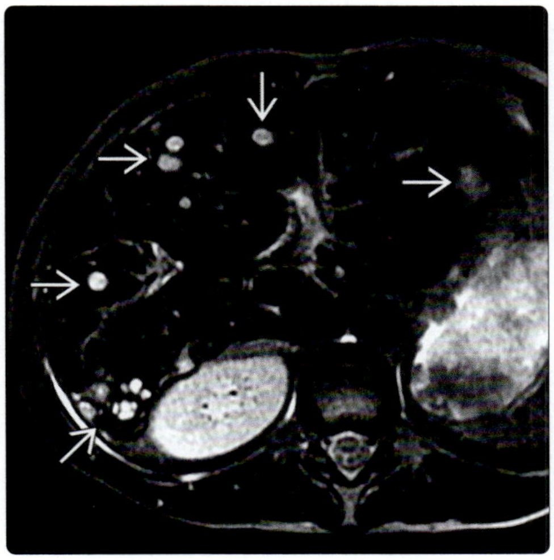

Metastases

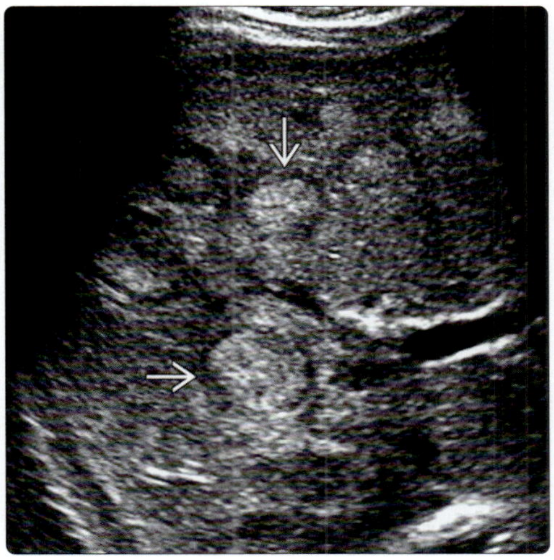

(Left) *Axial T2 FS MR in a patient with a remote history of Wilms tumor shows multiple hyperintense nodules within both lobes of the liver. These metastases demonstrated hypoenhancement after contrast administration.* **(Right)** *Transverse ultrasound shows multiple hyperechoic metastatic lesions in the liver from Wilms tumor. The lesions are well defined with a peripheral hypoechoic rim. Wilms tumor is the 2nd most common tumor to metastasize to the liver in children.*

Hepatoblastomas

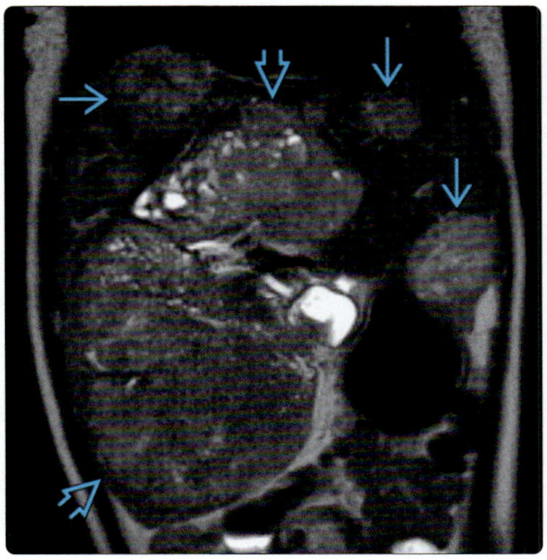

Hepatoblastomas

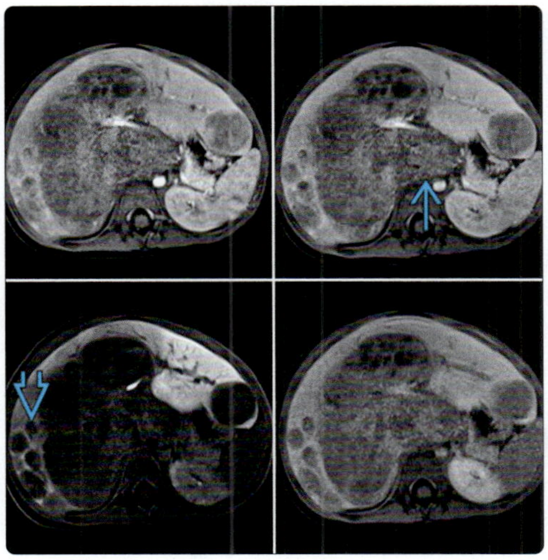

(Left) *Coronal T2 SSFSE MR in a 3 year old with abdominal distention shows numerous solid masses throughout the liver. The dominant mass extends from the medial section into the inferior right lobe.* **(Right)** *Dynamic T1 C+ FS MR images in the same patient (clockwise from upper left) using HSCM show heterogeneous hypoenhancement of the masses on all phases with the satellite lesions best seen on the delayed hepatocyte phase (bottom left). Involvement of the caudate is also seen on these images.*

(Left) *Longitudinal ultrasound in a 2-year-old patient with a palpable mass shows multiple heterogeneous (but predominantly hyperechoic) lesions → in the liver due to hepatoblastoma.* **(Right)** *Axial DWI MR in the same patient with multifocal hepatoblastoma shows restricted diffusion (confirmed on the ADC map, not shown) in the lesions →, typical of a highly cellular tumor.*

Hepatoblastomas

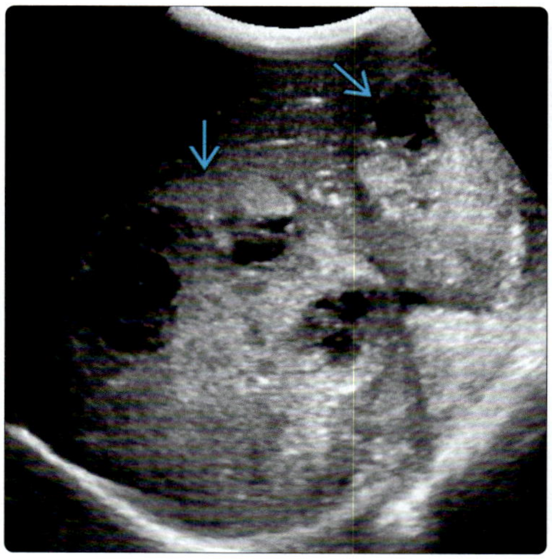

Hepatoblastomas

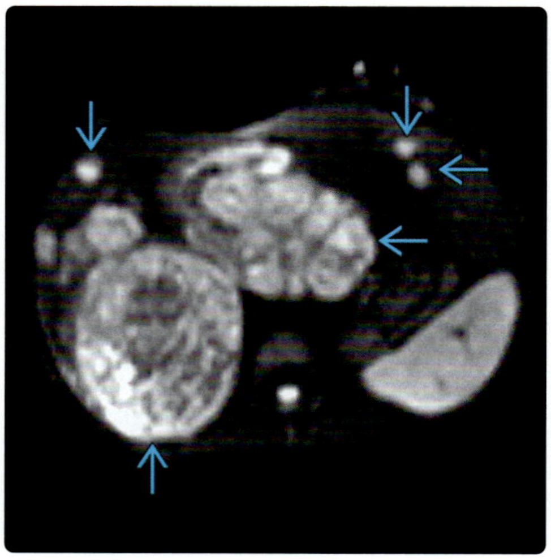

(Left) *Axial T2 FS MR in a 6 year old with a history of a Kasai procedure for biliary atresia shows multiple mildly hypointense, macroscopic regenerative nodules ⇨ centrally in the liver.* **(Right)** *Axial T1 C+ FS MR (in a delayed hepatocyte phase with HSCM) shows isointensity of the central macroscopic nodules ⇨. There are additional tiny, hyperintense lesions → posteriorly, which were not seen on other sequences, likely due to microscopic regenerative nodules or FNH-like lesions.*

Regenerative Nodules

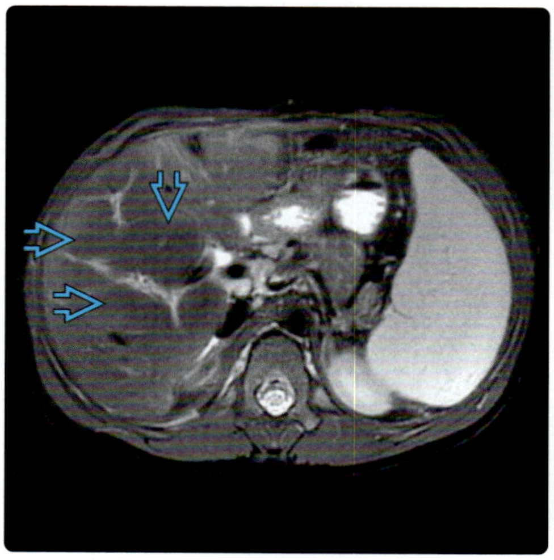

Regenerative Nodules

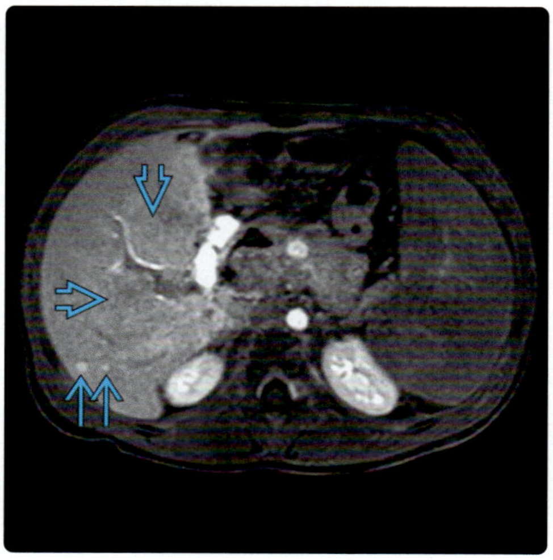

(Left) *Axial CECT in an 8 year old with sickle cell disease status post bone marrow transplant, now with fevers & methicillin-susceptible Staphylococcus aureus (MSSA)-positive blood cultures, shows multiple small, hypodense lesions with irregular wall enhancement →, consistent with abscesses.* **(Right)** *Axial in phase T1 MR in a 4 year old with a history of cryptogenic neonatal liver failure shows multiple hyperintense lesions ➡ throughout the liver parenchyma.*

Hepatic Abscesses

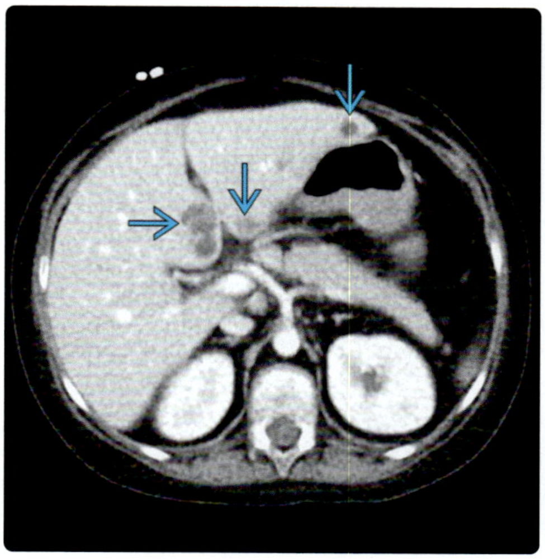

Adenomas

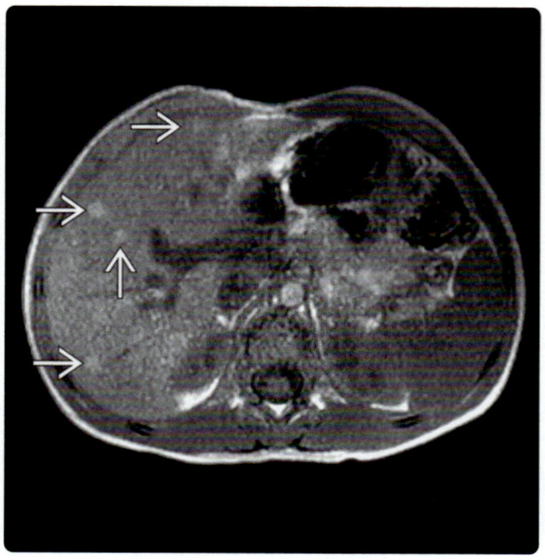

Adenomas

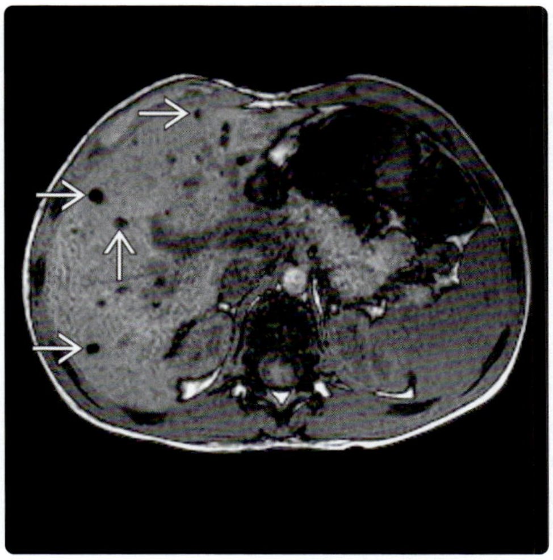

Angiomyolipomas

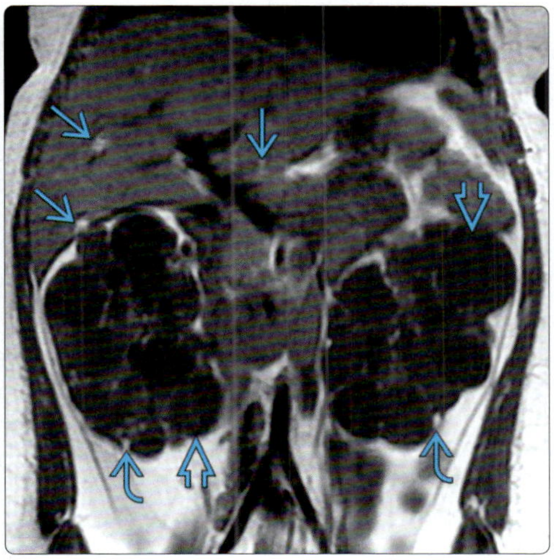

(Left) *Axial opposed-phase T1 MR in the same patient shows signal loss throughout these lesions ➡, consistent with intracellular fat. This finding is characteristic of hepatocyte nuclear factor 1a (HNF1a) inactivated hepatic adenomas.* **(Right)** *Coronal T1 MR in a 14 year old with tuberous sclerosis shows multiple subcentimeter, fat-containing lesions → scattered throughout the liver, typical of angiomyolipomas (AMLs) in this setting. Note the characteristic cysts ⇨ & AMLs ↪ in the kidneys.*

Hepatocellular Carcinomas

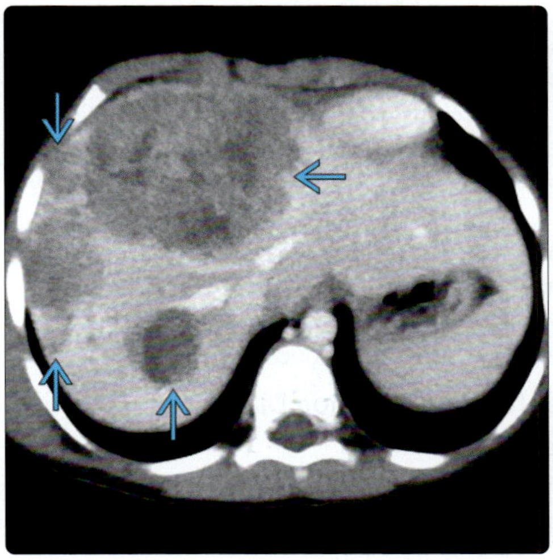

Hepatocellular Carcinomas

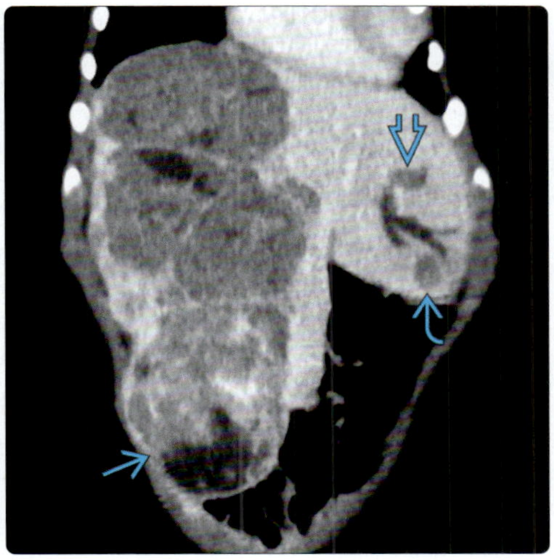

(Left) *Axial CECT in a 6 year old with a palpable right abdominal mass shows multiple heterogeneously hypoenhancing lesions → scattered throughout the liver.* **(Right)** *Coronal CECT in the same patient shows a large, exophytic mass → projecting inferiorly off the right hepatic lobe. Portal venous tumor thrombus ⇨ is seen in the left lobe adjacent to another small mass ↪. A high-grade hepatocellular carcinoma (HCC) was confirmed at biopsy.*

Caroli Disease

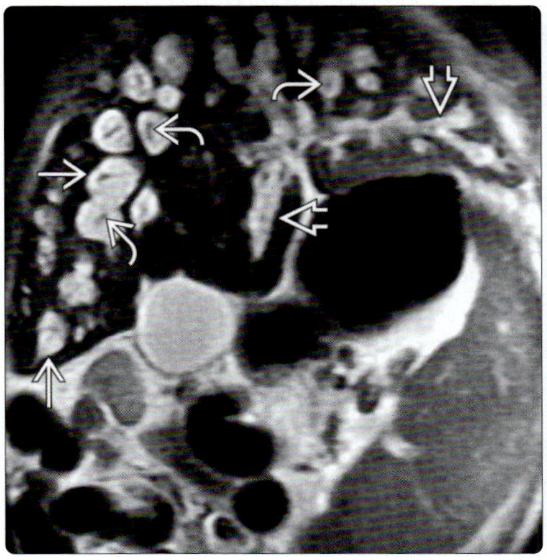

Angiosarcomas

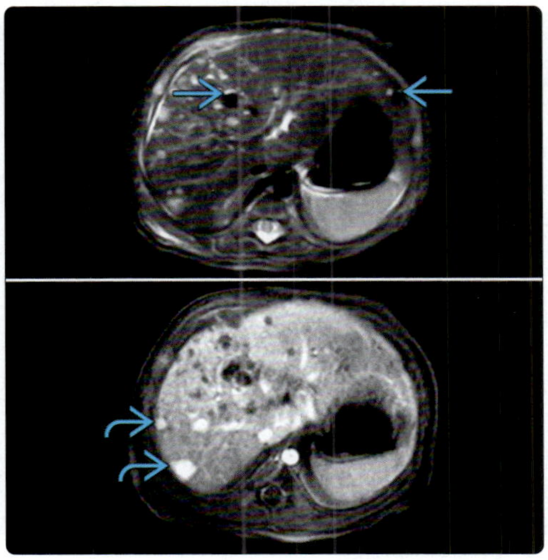

(Left) *Coronal T2 MR shows, in cross section, multiple round, fluid-signal-intensity lesions ➡ with a central hypointense dot ↪. In tangent, these foci are seen to have a contiguous branching pattern ⇨. The findings are typical of Caroli disease.* **(Right)** *Axial T2 FS (top) & T1 C+ FS (bottom) MR images in a newborn with angiosarcoma show numerous hepatic lesions, some of which contain fluid-fluid levels → due to hemorrhage. Other lesions show hyperenhancement ↪. A dominant lesion inferiorly is not shown here.*

DIFFERENTIAL DIAGNOSIS

Common

- Pancreatitis & Complications
- Annular Pancreas
- Solid Pseudopapillary Neoplasm

Less Common

- Metastases
- Pancreatoblastoma
- Neuroendocrine Tumors
- Lymphatic Malformation
- Intrahepatic Splenic Tissue

Rare but Important

- Congenital Pancreatic Cysts
- Congenital Hyperinsulinism of Infancy
- Agenesis of Dorsal Pancreas
- Inflammatory Myofibroblastic Tumor
- Cystadenomas
- Acinar Cell Carcinoma
- Ductal Adenocarcinoma

ESSENTIAL INFORMATION

Key Differential Diagnosis Issues

- Pancreatic tumors are rare in children
  - Account for < 0.2% of pediatric deaths due to malignancy
- DDx for pediatric pancreatic masses is different from DDx in adults
  - Adenocarcinoma is very rare
- Imaging features overlap heavily between different tumors
  - Age, sex, medical history may provide clues
  - Amylase & lipase are quite elevated with inflammation but usually not with tumors
  - Endoscopic ultrasound is often used for biopsy of pancreatic head masses

Helpful Clues for Common Diagnoses

- **Pancreatitis & Complications**
  - Underlying etiologies are more varied than in adult population
    - Accidental & nonaccidental trauma can cause pancreatitis
    - Other causes include infection, medications, hereditary, choledochal cysts, pancreas divisum
  - Imaging: Pancreas can be focally or diffusely enlarged
    - Typically demonstrates surrounding edema &/or fluid
    - Enhancement varies by type of acute pancreatitis
      - Mildly decreased with interstitial edematous subtype
      - Severely decreased in necrotizing subtype
    - Fluid collection nomenclature has therapeutic implications & depends on subtype of acute pancreatitis & timing
      - Acute peripancreatic collection: Nonencapsulated, ≤ 4 weeks from onset of inflammation
      - Pseudocyst: Encapsulated, > 4 weeks from onset
      - Acute necrotic collection: Nonencapsulated collection, ≤ 4 weeks from onset
      - Walled-off necrosis: Encapsulated, > 4 weeks from onset
- **Annular Pancreas**
  - Congenital anomaly in which pancreatic tissue surrounds mid 2nd duodenum (D2)
  - May be asymptomatic or present as
    - Neonate with duodenal obstruction
      - Associated anomalies include duodenal stenosis or atresia, Down syndrome, tracheoesophageal fistula, congenital heart disease
    - Older child/adult with pain, pancreatitis
  - Imaging: Tissue that is isodense (CT)/isointense (MR) to pancreas encircles duodenum, extending more laterally than normal pancreatic head
    - Abrupt caliber change of D2 is typical at this level, appearing more round & narrow on axial plane
    - Can rarely create double-bubble bowel gas pattern in neonate, though distal gas may be present
- **Solid Pseudopapillary Neoplasm**
  - Most common primary pediatric tumor of pancreas
    - Demonstrates low malignant potential
  - Typically occurs in adolescent girls & young women
  - Presents with abdominal pain, nausea/vomiting, weight loss, &/or mass
  - Imaging: Well-circumscribed solid or mixed solid & cystic mass, typically in pancreatic head or tail, often > 5 cm
    - Hypoenhancement is typical, may appear cystic on CECT
    - Enhancing fibrous capsule & internal hemorrhage are common; Ca^{2+} in up to 1/3 of cases
  - Excellent outcomes with resection; metastases rare
    - Males may have worse prognosis

Helpful Clues for Less Common Diagnoses

- **Metastases**
  - Lymphoma is most common, typically of Burkitt or large cell subtypes
    - May rarely occur as primary
  - Neuroblastoma is also common, though local invasion accounts for some cases
  - Sarcomas may also spread to (or rarely arise primarily in) pancreas
  - Imaging: Focal hypoenhancing parenchymal lesions vs. complete infiltration/replacement, ± adjacent nodal involvement & masses of other organs
    - MR: Diffusion restriction may increase conspicuity
- **Pancreatoblastoma**
  - Most common in 1st decade of life; mean age: 4 years
  - M:F ratio = 2:1
  - Most commonly presents as asymptomatic mass
  - α-fetoprotein is elevated in up to 55%
  - Can be associated with Beckwith-Wiedemann syndrome
  - Imaging: Usually large, solitary, hypoenhancing mass
    - Well defined with lobulated margins; may be poorly defined with higher grades
    - May be difficult to identify organ of origin
      - ~ 50% arise from pancreatic head
    - May extend beyond pancreas, typically with mass effect rather than invasion
      - May encase vessels
    - ± hemorrhage, cysts, Ca^{2+}

- Metastases to liver & lymph nodes occur in up to 35% of patients
- **Neuroendocrine Tumors**
  - a.k.a. islet cell tumors
  - Account for 20% of pediatric pancreatic malignancies
  - May be functioning or nonfunctioning
    - Functioning tumors produce symptoms related to hormonal release & typically present earlier with smaller tumors
  - Associated with von Hippel-Lindau (VHL) disease & multiple endocrine neoplasia (MEN) type 1
  - Insulinomas are most common in children; most are sporadic
  - Imaging: Classically hypervascular/hyperenhancing
    - Insulinomas are usually in body or tail of pancreas
    - Gastrinomas are usually in pancreatic head
- **Lymphatic Malformation**
  - Congenital errors of lymphatic vessel development
  - Result in conglomerations of macro- & microcystic masses infiltrating multiple compartments
  - Rarely limited to pancreas
  - Imaging: Fluid attenuation/signal intensity mass extending across tissue planes & infiltrating pancreas
    - Multiple thin septations between larger cysts; cysts may contain fluid-fluid levels from hemorrhage
    - More confluent microcysts may show enhancement
- **Intrahepatic Splenic Tissue**
  - Imaging: Focal, round tissue in pancreatic tail; follows splenic characteristics on all modalities/sequences
    - DWI MR is particularly helpful

Helpful Clues for Rare Diagnoses

- **Congenital Pancreatic Cysts**
  - Usually asymptomatic; can be solitary or multiple
  - Multiple cysts associated with syndromes: VHL, Beckwith-Wiedemann, autosomal dominant polycystic kidney disease
- **Congenital Hyperinsulinism of Infancy**
  - a.k.a. nesidioblastosis
  - Hyperfunctioning B cells → hyperinsulinemia → refractory hypoglycemia in neonates/infants
    - Diffuse vs. focal types
  - Imaging: Pancreas is diffusely enlarged without focal mass
    - ^{18}F-DOPA PET useful in detection/characterization
- **Agenesis of Dorsal Pancreas**
  - a.k.a. congenitally short pancreas
  - Associated with polysplenia
  - Risk of diabetes mellitus, as most islet cells are in pancreatic tail
  - Imaging: Pancreas appears rounded & short, may mimic mass
- **Inflammatory Myofibroblastic Tumor**
  - Adolescent females are affected most commonly
  - Imaging: May have necrosis, Ca^{2+}
    - Solid portions enhance similar to pancreas on CECT
- **Cystadenomas**
  - Imaging
    - Serous: Numerous cysts, central scar, & Ca^{2+}
      - Increased risk in vHL
    - Mucinous: Multiloculated mass with large cysts
- **Acinar Cell Carcinoma**
  - Imaging: Necrosis & Ca^{2+} are common
- **Ductal Adenocarcinoma**
  - Extremely rare < 40 years of age
  - Most pediatric cases have familial predisposition
  - Imaging: Hypoenhancing mass, often small
    - Metastases are common in children

SELECTED REFERENCES

1. Bohl CE et al: FDG-PET CT in the evaluation of primary and secondary pancreatic malignancies. Pediatr Blood Cancer. 65(10):e27115, 2018
2. Ozcan HN et al: Imaging features of primary malignant pancreatic tumors in children. AJR Am J Roentgenol. 203(3):662-7, 2014
3. Shet NS et al: Imaging of pediatric pancreatic neoplasms with radiologic-histopathologic correlation. AJR Am J Roentgenol. 202(6):1337-48, 2014
4. Ahmed TS et al: Imaging features of pancreatic tumors in children: 13-year experience at a pediatric tertiary hospital. Pediatr Radiol. 43(11):1435-43, 2013
5. van den Akker M et al: Malignant pancreatic tumors in children: a single-institution series. J Pediatr Surg. 47(4):681-7, 2012

Pancreatitis & Complications

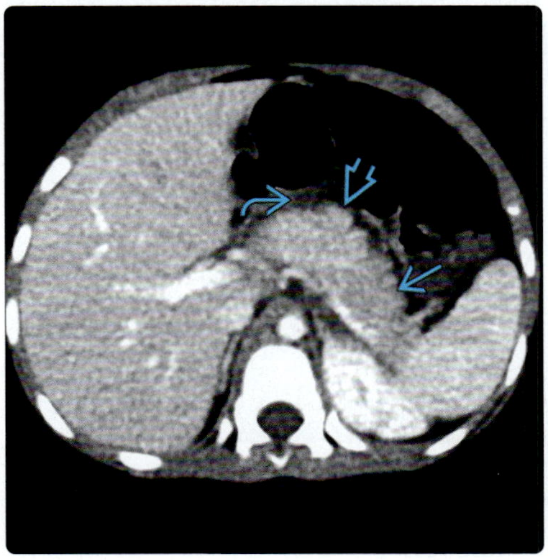

Pancreatitis & Complications

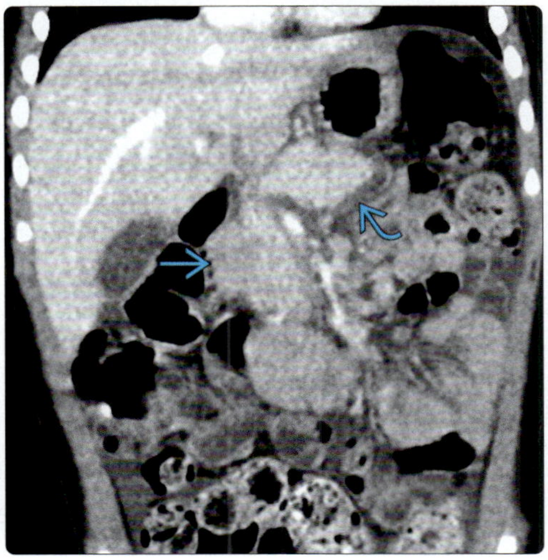

(Left) *Axial CECT in a 3 year old with pain & leukocytosis shows mild generalized enlargement of the pancreas ⇨ with patchy regions of slightly decreased enhancement → & mild surrounding edema ↗. Viral pancreatitis was ultimately confirmed.* **(Right)** *Coronal CECT in the same patient shows pancreatic head enlargement with patchy foci of slightly decreased enhancement → & surrounding edema ↗, consistent with acute interstitial edematous pancreatitis.*

(Left) *Axial CECT in a patient involved in a motor vehicle accident shows a linear hypodense band in the tail of the pancreas with surrounding peripancreatic edema. Isolated pancreatic injury (in this case, pancreatic transection) is more common in children than adults. Pancreatic ductal injury must be considered with this appearance.* **(Right)** *Axial CECT in the same patient 8 days later shows the development of a bilobed acute peripancreatic collection with an enhancing wall at the site of transection.*

Pancreatitis & Complications

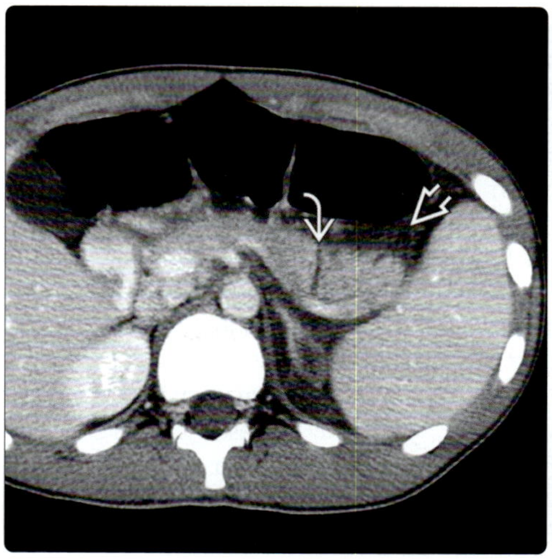

Pancreatitis & Complications

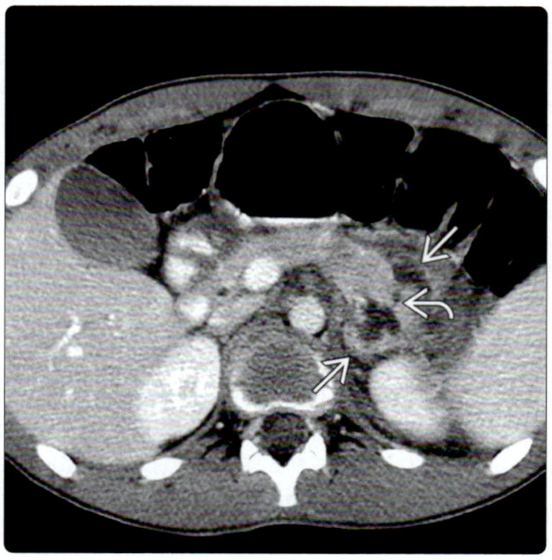

(Left) *Axial CECT shows a markedly abnormal pancreas that is diffusely edematous & poorly enhancing. Only a small portion of the pancreas enhances normally. There is moderate peripancreatic fluid. The findings are typical of necrotizing pancreatitis.* **(Right)** *Axial CECT in the same patient 8 days later shows an irregular, rim-enhancing collection of fluid & necrotic tissue replacing & extending from the pancreas, consistent with an acute necrotic collection.*

Pancreatitis & Complications

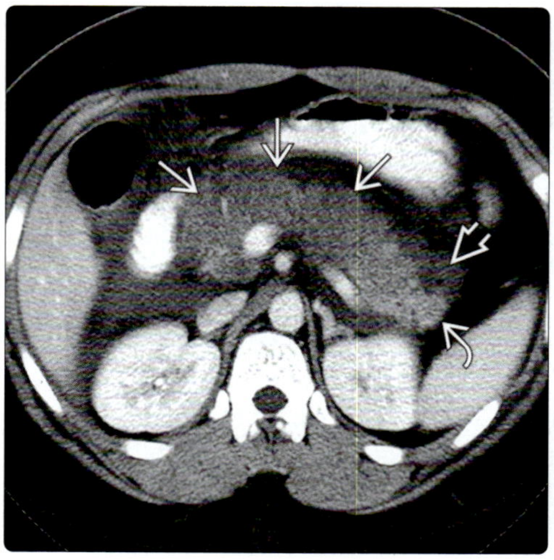

Pancreatitis & Complications

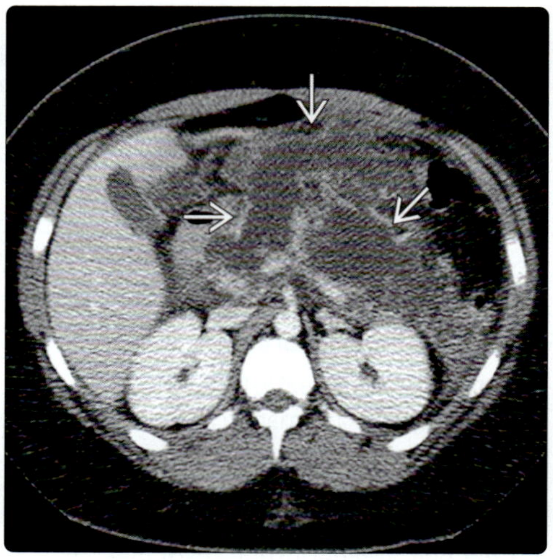

(Left) *Axial CECT in a 9 year old with cerebral palsy shows necrotizing pancreatitis with an onset of ~ 2 weeks prior. There is a heterogeneous acute necrotic collection replacing portions of the pancreatic neck & body. Mild dilation of the pancreatic duct is noted with poor enhancement of the adjacent parenchyma. There is also surrounding inflammatory change.* **(Right)** *Axial T1 C+ FS MR in the same patient several weeks later shows mass-like regions of walled-off necrosis (as > 4 weeks have passed).*

Pancreatitis & Complications

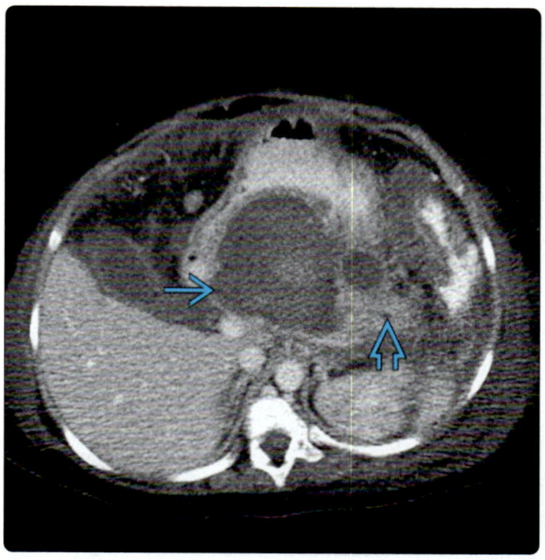

Pancreatitis & Complications

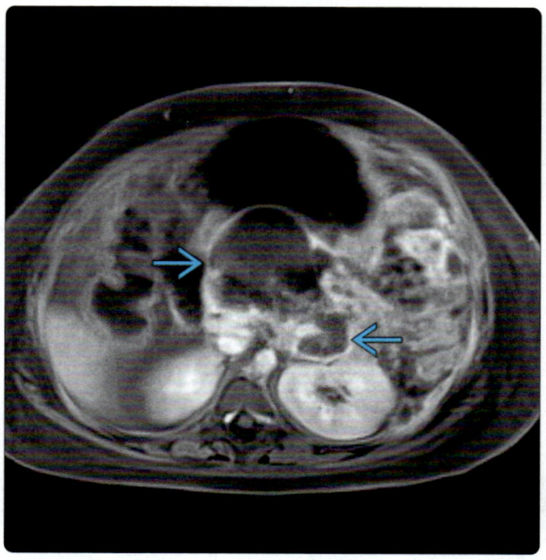

Annular Pancreas

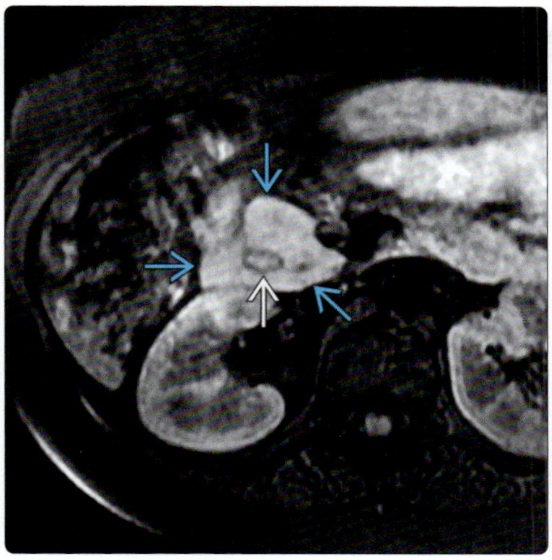

Annular Pancreas

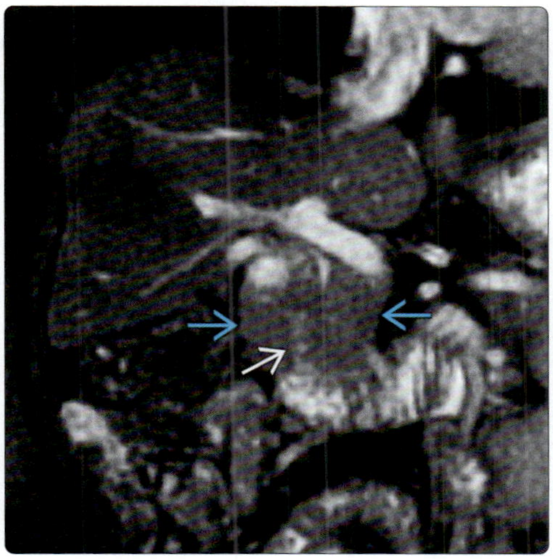

(Left) *Axial T1 FS MR shows a hypointense "lesion" in the head of the pancreas with a central area of increased signal due to the 2nd duodenum being encased by an annular pancreas. Note the continuity of the otherwise normal T1-hyperintense pancreatic tissue around the narrowed duodenum.* **(Right)** *Coronal SSFP MR in the same patient shows a narrowed hyperintense 2nd duodenum passing through the hypointense pancreas .*

Solid Pseudopapillary Neoplasm

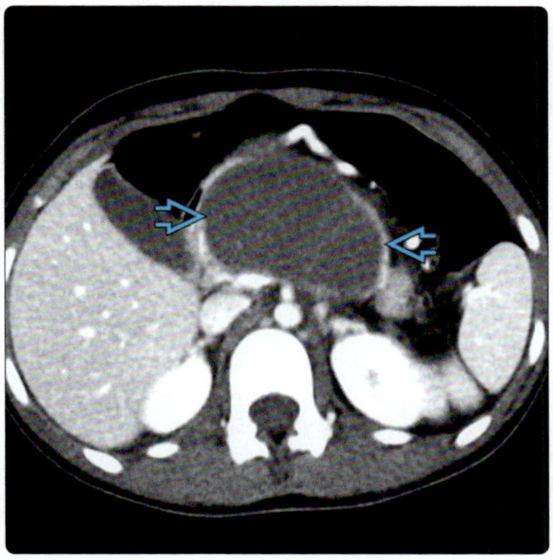

Solid Pseudopapillary Neoplasm

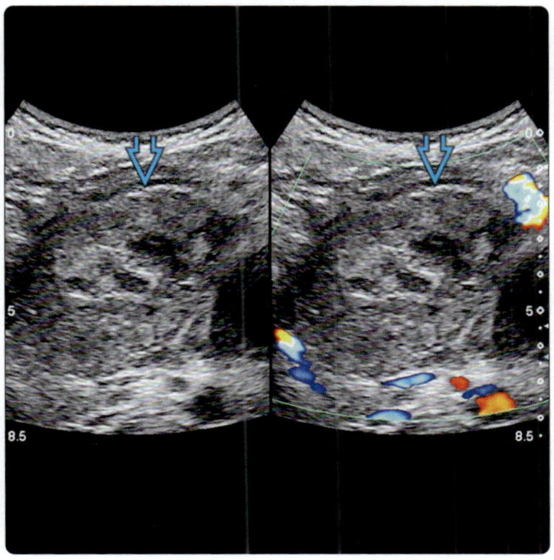

(Left) *Axial CECT in a 13-year-old girl with epigastric pain shows a well-circumscribed, ovoid, fluid-attenuation, 6-cm mass in the pancreatic neck with subtle internal heterogeneity. No Ca^{2+} was seen.* **(Right)** *Transverse grayscale & color Doppler ultrasound images in the same patient show a heterogeneous relatively avascular mass with probable cystic & solid foci in the pancreatic neck.*

Solid Pseudopapillary Neoplasm

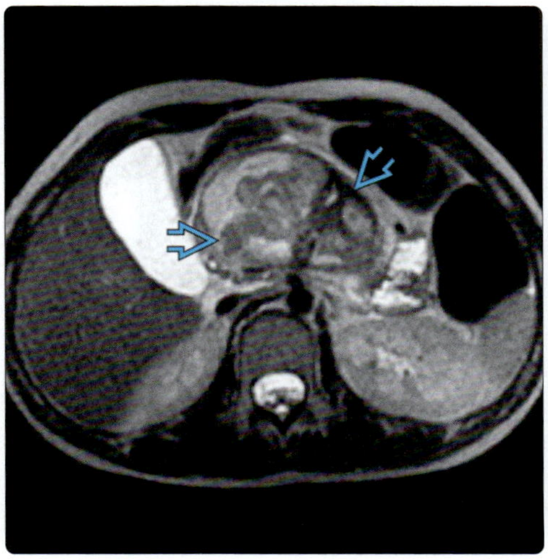

Solid Pseudopapillary Neoplasm

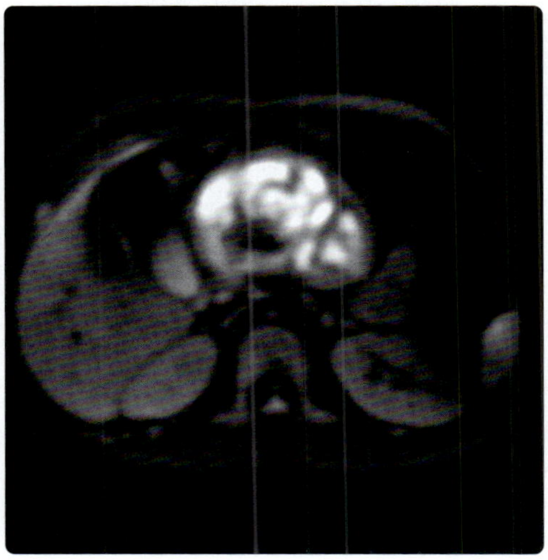

(Left) *Axial T2 MR in the same patient shows marked internal heterogeneity of the lesion with multiple foci of intermediate to low signal intensity throughout the mass, likely due to hemorrhage.* **(Right)** *Axial DWI MR in the same patient shows multiple foci of restricted diffusion in the lesion. Large regions of tumor necrosis & hemorrhage were found upon resection of this solid pseudopapillary neoplasm.*

(Left) *Axial CECT in a 5 year old with Burkitt lymphoma shows confluent hypoenhancing tissue replacing the pancreas & encasing the splenic artery & celiac axis. Also note the multiple lymphomatous masses in the right kidney.* **(Right)** *Axial T2 FS MR in a 7 year old with a left adrenal neuroblastoma shows complete replacement of the pancreas by lobulated solid masses. The splenic vein, portal vein, & inferior aspect of the primary tumor are noted.*

Metastases

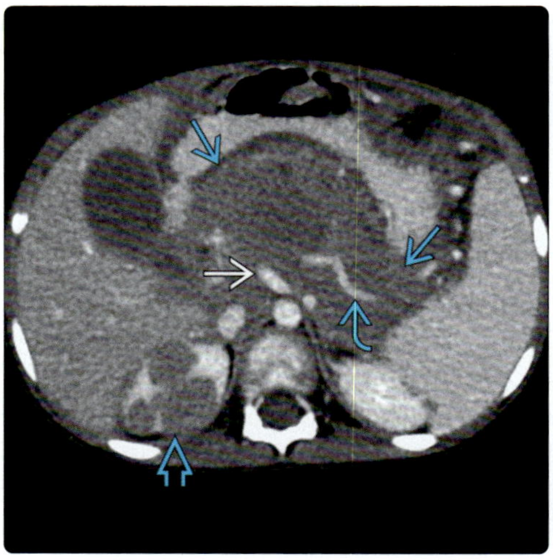

Metastases

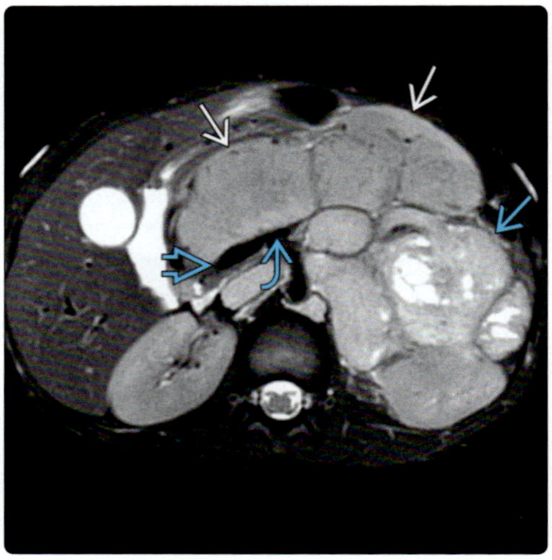

(Left) *Coronal T2 SSFSE FS MR in an 8-year-old boy shows a heterogeneous lobulated mixed solid & cystic mass arising from & extending beyond the pancreatic head & neck. Biopsy confirmed a pancreatoblastoma.* **(Right)** *Axial CECT in a 6-year-old boy shows a large lobulated mass arising from the pancreatic head & neck & extending anteriorly, displacing the stomach. Most pancreatoblastomas arise from the pancreatic head.*

Pancreatoblastoma

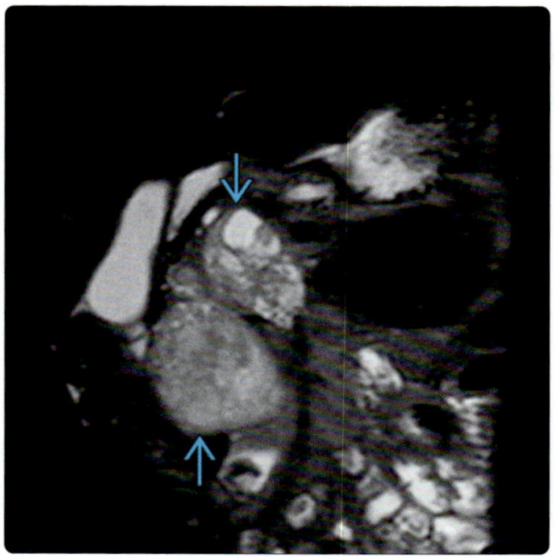

Pancreatoblastoma

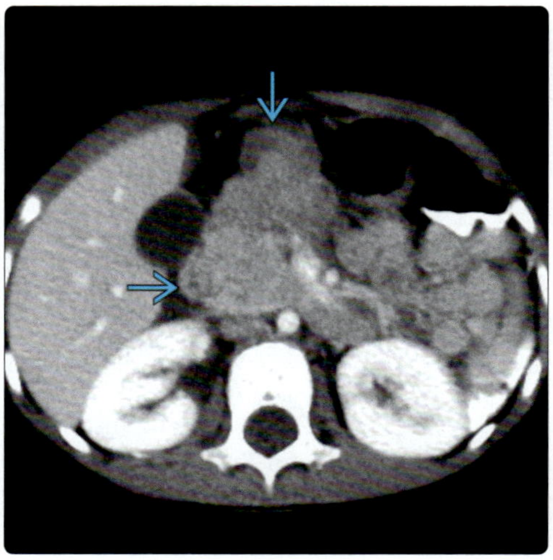

(Left) *Axial CECT in a 15 year old with von Hippel-Lindau syndrome shows a hyperenhancing mass in the tail of an otherwise normal-appearing pancreas. Resection confirmed a well-differentiated endocrine tumor.* **(Right)** *Axial DWI MR in a 34 year old with hepatitis C shows a small round focus of restricted diffusion in the pancreatic tail. This focus was isointense to the spleen on all sequences, consistent with intrapancreatic accessory splenic tissue.*

Neuroendocrine Tumors

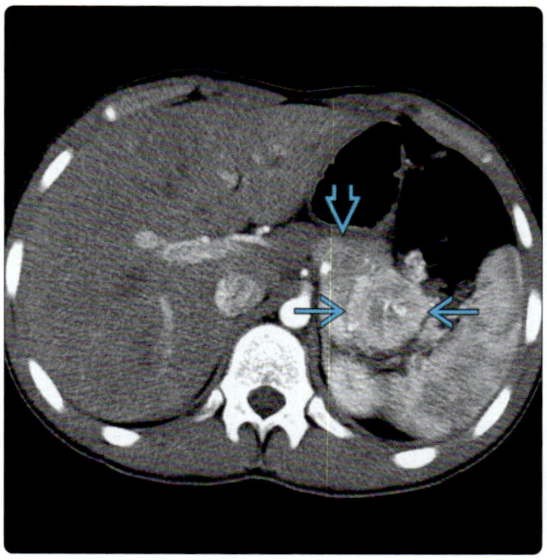

Intrahepatic Splenic Tissue

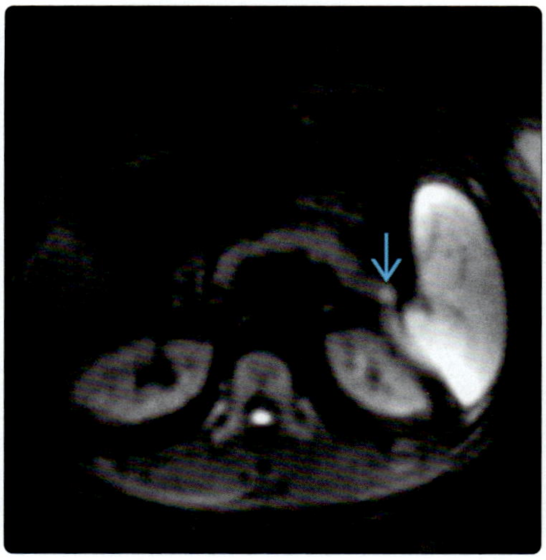

Congenital Pancreatic Cysts

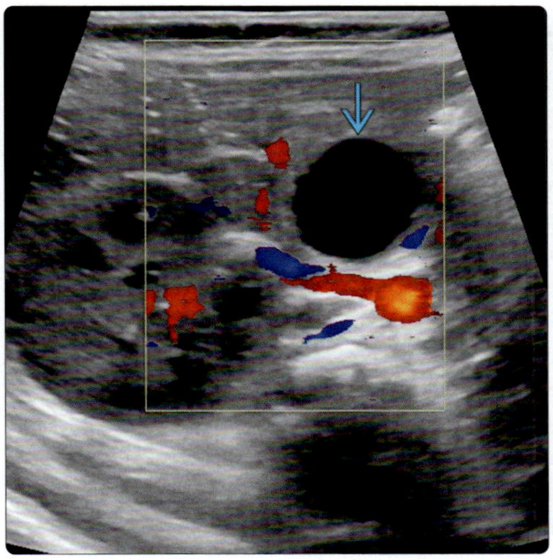

Congenital Pancreatic Cysts

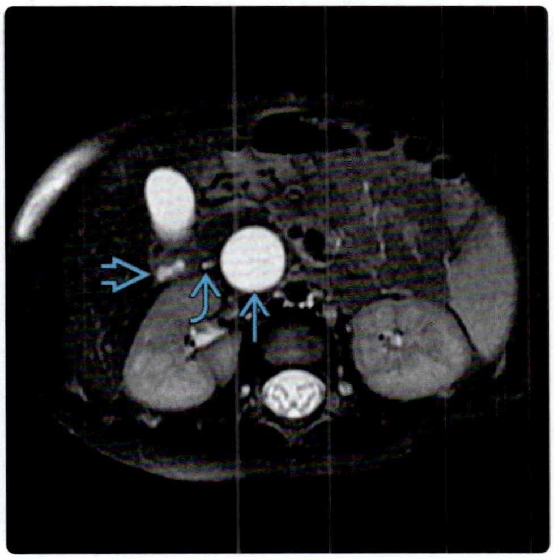

(Left) *Color Doppler ultrasound in a 3 month old with a history of a prenatally detected right upper quadrant cystic lesion shows a round, anechoic, thin-walled avascular cyst ➡ of the pancreatic head & uncinate process.* **(Right)** *Axial T2 FS MR in the same patient shows homogeneous fluid signal intensity of the cyst ➡ along the posterior aspect of the pancreas, separate from the common bile duct ➡ & duodenum ➡. Surgery confirmed a benign epithelial cyst, & a cyst duodenostomy was performed.*

Agenesis of Dorsal Pancreas

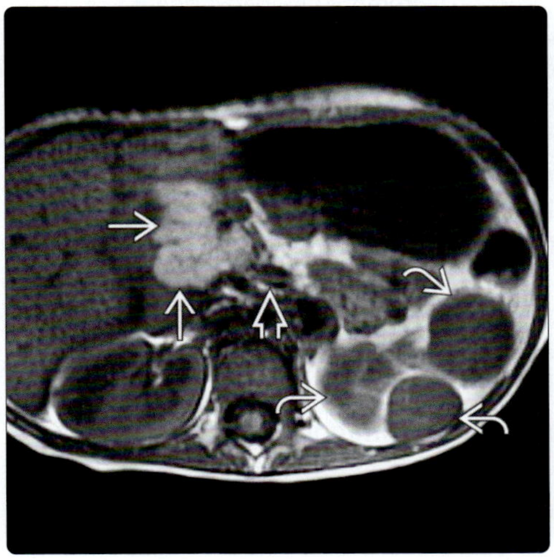

Inflammatory Myofibroblastic Tumor

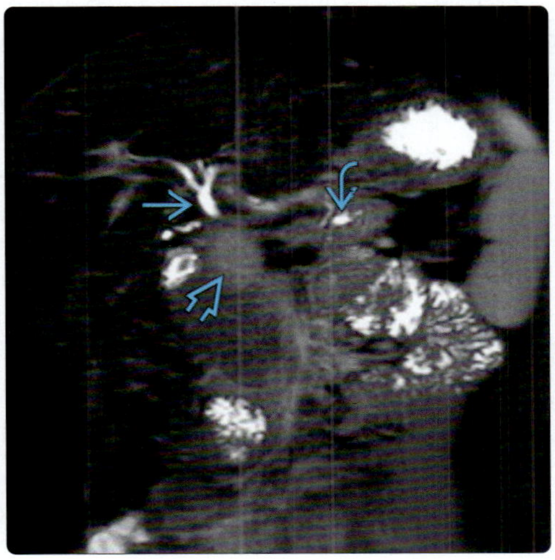

(Left) *Axial T1 MR shows a relatively hyperintense pancreas ➡ with an abnormal morphology. The pancreas does not extend to the left of the mesenteric vessels ➡. Multiple spleens are present ➡, which is a common association with dorsal agenesis.* **(Right)** *Coronal T2 SSFSE FS MR in a 17 year old with jaundice shows a slightly hyperintense mass ➡ in the pancreatic neck. There is associated biliary ➡ & pancreatic ➡ ductal dilation.*

Inflammatory Myofibroblastic Tumor

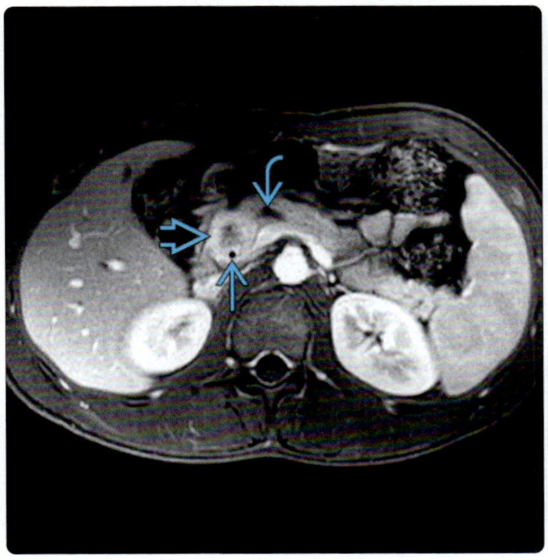

Ductal Adenocarcinoma

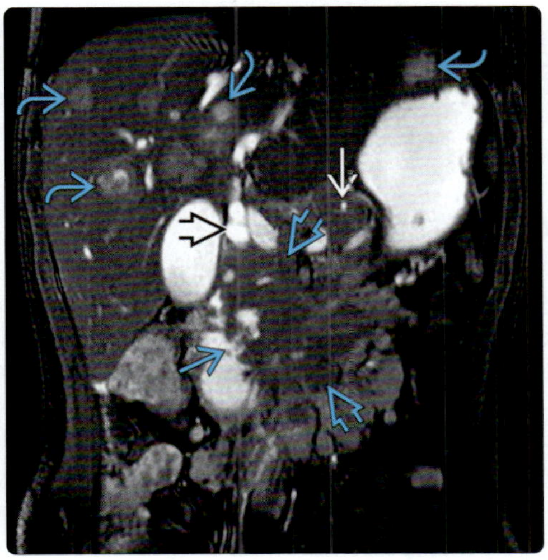

(Left) *Axial T1 C+ FS MR in the same patient shows peripheral enhancement of the pancreatic neck mass ➡. There is a stent in the encased common bile duct ➡. Dilation of the pancreatic duct ➡ is also visible.* **(Right)** *Coronal SSFP MR in a 13 year old with weight loss & pain shows a large, heterogeneous, irregular lesion of the pancreatic head ➡ with ulceration of the duodenal wall ➡, dilation of the biliary ➡ & pancreatic ➡ ducts, & numerous hepatic metastases ➡ from ductal adenocarcinoma.*

DIFFERENTIAL DIAGNOSIS

Common

- Perfusion Artifact (Mimic)
- Trauma
- Granulomatous Disease
- Cleft (Mimic)

Less Common

- Infarction
- Lymphoma
- Epithelial Cyst
- Pseudocyst
- Infection/Abscess
- Posttransplant Lymphoproliferative Disease

Rare but Important

- Hamartoma
- Vascular Malformations
  - Lymphatic Malformation
    - Isolated
    - Generalized Lymphatic Anomaly
    - Kaposiform Lymphangiomatosis
  - Venous Malformation
- Vascular Neoplasms
  - Congenital Hemangioma
  - Littoral Cell Angioma/Hemangioma
  - Hemangioendothelioma
  - Angiosarcoma
- Metastases

ESSENTIAL INFORMATION

Key Differential Diagnosis Issues

- Beyond lymphoma & leukemia, malignancy in pediatric spleen is extremely rare
- Important clinical considerations
  - Immunocompromised state
  - Recent or remote trauma
  - Sickle cell disease or other hemoglobinopathy
  - Coagulopathy
  - Known malignancy
- Important lesion imaging considerations
  - Cystic vs. solid
  - Solitary vs. multiple
  - Lesions in other organs

Helpful Clues for Common Diagnoses

- **Perfusion Artifact (Mimic)**
  - Transient & predictable: Seen during arterial phase of CECT or MR, resolving on venous phases
  - Classic appearance is archiform zebra-stripe enhancement
    - Focal & diffuse heterogeneity are less common
  - Ultrasound helpful if lesions are still suspected
- **Trauma**
  - Splenic injury is more common with splenomegaly (as seen with infectious mononucleosis, etc.)
  - May include hematoma, laceration, fracture, or rupture
    - Laceration: Irregular linear/branching fluid attenuation foci
    - Fracture: Laceration extending from one surface to another
    - Rupture: Multiple fractures with discontinuous fragments
    - Hematoma: Collection in or adjacent to spleen
    - Surrounding free fluid usually present with splenic injury, 0-30 HU on CT
      - May have hematocrit level with layering cells causing increased density dependently (particularly in pelvis)
      - Higher attenuation (40-80 HU) focal collection may represent clotted blood adjacent to injured organ (sentinel clot sign)
    - Active bleeding (extravasation) & pseudoaneurysm
      - Foci of high attenuation (isoattenuating to vascular contrast) that do not conform to normal vessel size, morphology, or course
- **Granulomatous Disease**
  - Active disease (uncommonly imaged) may have splenomegaly with scattered hypoechoic/hypoattenuating lesions
  - Remote infection (commonly imaged incidentally) usually has normal-sized spleen with scattered calcified (echogenic/hyperattenuating) foci
  - Etiologies largely depend on region/country
    - Common: Histoplasmosis, tuberculosis
    - Less common: Cat-scratch disease, sarcoid, Wegener
- **Cleft (Mimic)**
  - Congenital variant in contour
  - Smooth, thin linear/curvilinear focus of decreased attenuation extending from 1 splenic surface into parenchyma
  - No surrounding fluid

Helpful Clues for Less Common Diagnoses

- **Infarction**
  - Secondary to occlusion of noncommunicating end arteries
  - Commonly seen in children with hemoglobinopathies, such as sickle cell disease, & some malignancies
  - Variable appearance, depending on stage
    - Early: Ill-defined mottled changes in attenuation/echogenicity
    - Late: Well-defined peripheral hypoechoic/hypoattenuating wedge-shaped foci with parenchymal volume loss
      - Islands of preserved splenic tissue: Hypoechoic round lesions scattered throughout echogenic parenchyma
      - Chronic global infarction: Small, calcified spleen
  - May also resolve completely or evolve into acquired cyst
- **Lymphoma**
  - Hodgkin or non-Hodgkin types
  - Focal lesions vs. diffuse involvement
    - May be round, geographic, or poorly defined
  - Typically hypoattenuating/hypoechoic
  - Look for lymphadenopathy & other visceral lesions
    - Kidneys, liver, bowel, pleura, lung
- **Epithelial Cyst**
  - Epidermoid vs. mesothelial cyst
  - May be simple or mildly complex

- **Pseudocyst**
  - Lacks epithelial lining
  - Typically results from prior trauma, infarct, or infection
  - Differentiation by imaging from epithelial cyst is not reliable
- **Infection & Abscess**
  - Fungal & bacterial infections occur most frequently in immunocompromised patients
  - Fungal abscesses are typically small & hypoechoic/hypoattenuating; echogenic centers are characteristic
    - Look for lesions in other organs
  - Limb or neck adenopathy in healthy patient with small splenic lesions may suggest cat-scratch disease
  - Hydatid abscesses are rare
- **Posttransplant Lymphoproliferative Disease**
  - Spectrum of disease, ranging from benign to malignant
  - Most commonly due to Epstein-Barr virus (EBV) infection
  - Highest risk with small bowel transplant
  - Similar imaging appearance to lymphoma
  - Look for nodal conglomerations & multifocal visceral masses
    - Kidneys, liver, lung, bowel, CNS
    - Spleen involved in ~ 20% of cases

Helpful Clues for Rare Diagnoses

- **Hamartoma**
  - Benign mixture of normal splenic elements
  - Can be seen in tuberous sclerosis patients with hamartomas in other organs
  - Nonspecific solid mass
- **Vascular Malformations**
  - **Lymphatic malformation:** May take 1 of 2 forms
    - Isolated splenic/perisplenic macrocystic mass
      - Multilobulated fluid-filled lesion with thin septations
      - May contain debris or fluid-fluid levels
    - Numerous tiny cysts < 1-2 cm
      - Look for cystic bone lesions & pleural involvement with generalized lymphatic anomaly (GLA) or Kaposiform lymphangiomatosis
  - **Venous malformation**
    - More correct histologic term for cavernous hemangioma
    - Delayed centripetal enhancement typical
    - Multiple lesions are often associated venous malformations at other soft tissue & visceral sites
      - Blue rubber bleb nevus syndrome: Numerous, often punctate, lesions found in gastrointestinal tract, leading to bleeding
- **Vascular Neoplasms**
  - **Congenital hemangioma**: Variable vascularity ± Ca^{2+}; may present with heart failure &/or coagulopathy
  - **Littoral cell angioma/hemangioma**: Nonspecific imaging; often found incidentally upon resection of enlarged spleen
  - **Kaposiform hemangioendothelioma**: Most commonly manifests as poorly defined infiltrative retroperitoneal mass in infants with severe coagulopathy
    - May rarely occur as multiple splenic lesions
  - **Angiosarcoma**: Variable appearance, usually not hypervascular
- **Metastases**
  - Extremely rare
  - Variable imaging appearance
  - Look for metastases in other viscera

SELECTED REFERENCES

1. Lee HJ et al: Cross-sectional imaging of splenic lesions: radiographics fundamentals | Online Presentation. Radiographics. 38(2):435-36, 2018
2. Hodge MG et al: Splenic cysts in the pediatric population: a report of 21 cases with review of the literature. Fetal Pediatr Pathol. 31(2):54-62, 2012
3. Hilmes MA et al: The pediatric spleen. Semin Ultrasound CT MR. 28(1):3-11, 2007

Perfusion Artifact (Mimic)

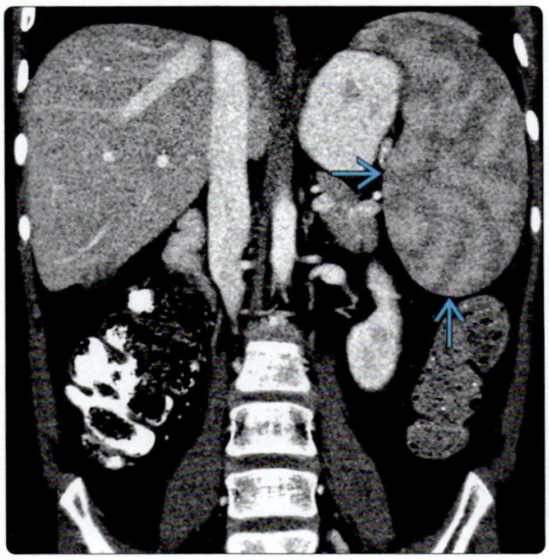

Perfusion Artifact (Mimic)

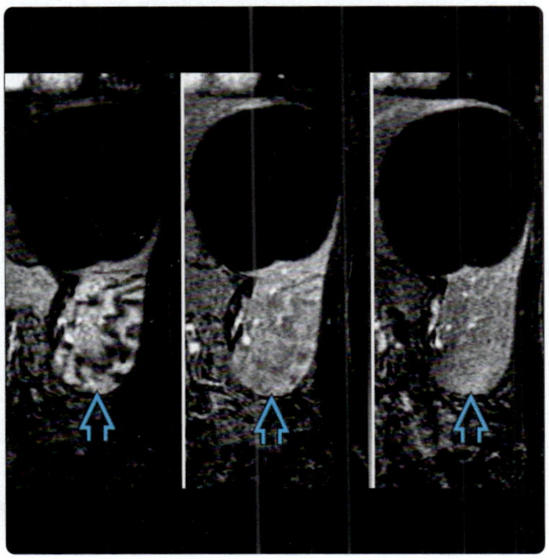

(Left) *Coronal CECT shows heterogeneous stripes of low attenuation in the spleen ➡, a common transient finding seen during arterial-phase imaging.* **(Right)** *Subtracted dynamic T1 C+ FS MR images of an epithelial cyst in the splenic upper pole of a 15 year old show no internal enhancement of the lesion. Note the normal progression in the postcontrast appearance of the spleen ➡ from early arterial (left) to late venous (right) phases.*

Perfusion Artifact (Mimic)

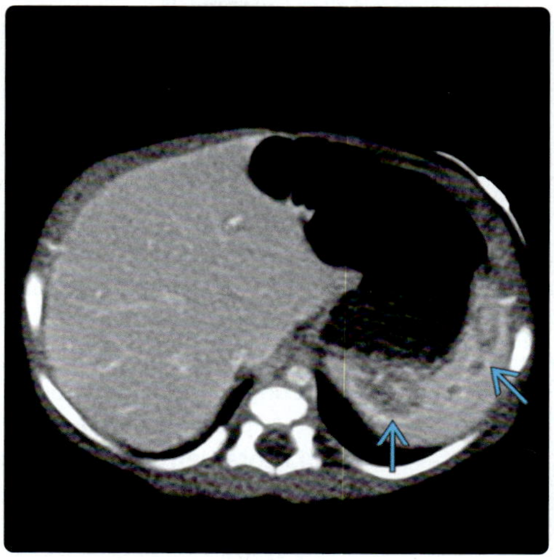

Perfusion Artifact (Mimic)

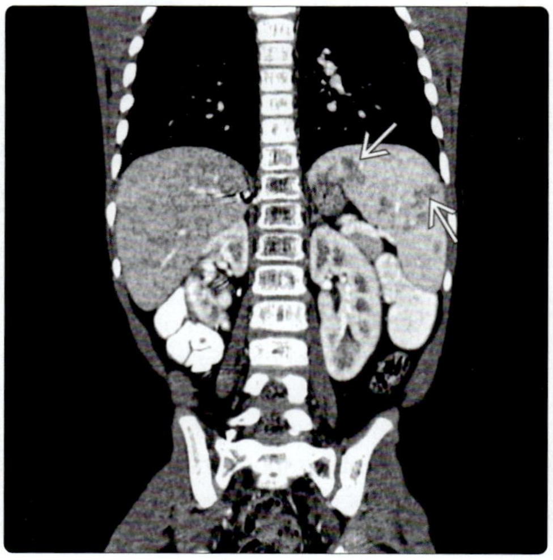

(Left) *Axial CECT shows multiple foci of heterogeneous enhancement in the spleen that proved to be transient perfusion artifacts. The spleen was normal on a follow-up ultrasound.* **(Right)** *Coronal CECT shows multiple foci of heterogeneously decreased enhancement of the spleen that resolved on portal venous-phase imaging.*

Trauma

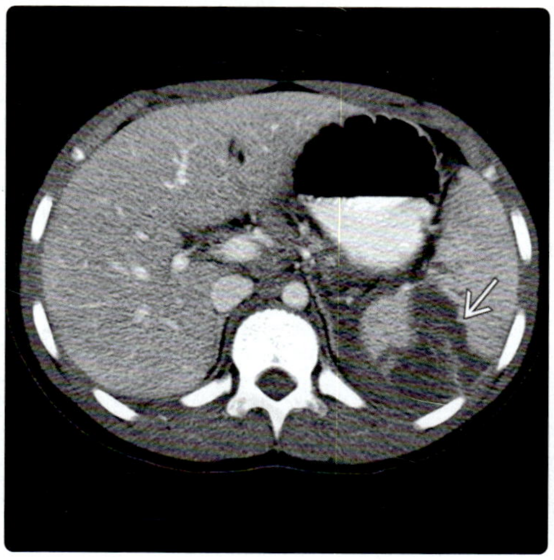

Trauma

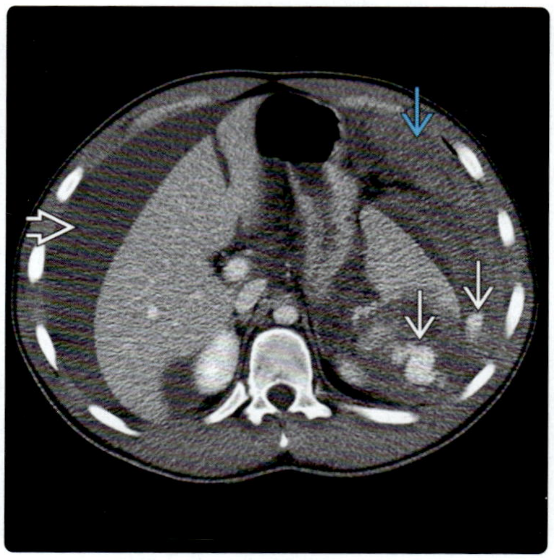

(Left) *Axial CECT shows a splenic fracture in a 9 year old with splenomegaly from infectious mononucleosis. There was no active contrast extravasation.* **(Right)** *Axial CECT shows a traumatic laceration of the spleen with active contrast extravasation & a large volume of hemoperitoneum in this 16 year old who suffered a football-related injury. Note the relatively dense sentinel clot adjacent to the site of injury.*

Granulomatous Disease

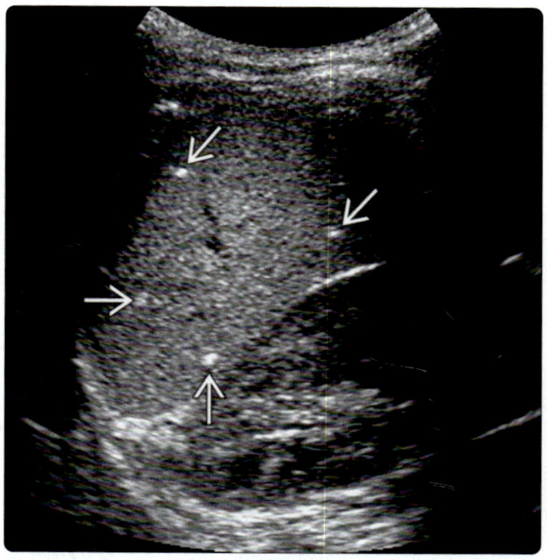

Granulomatous Disease

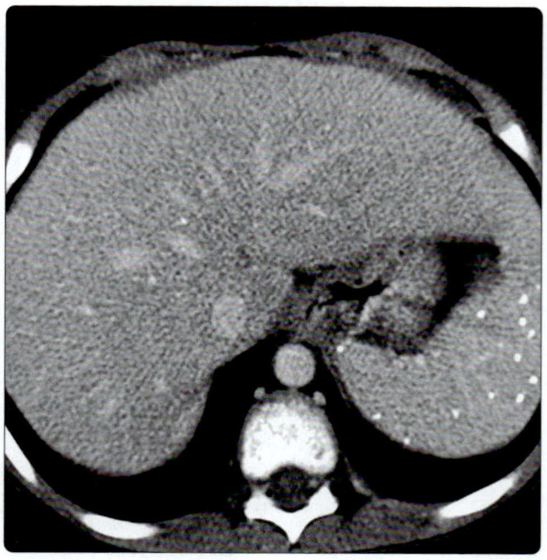

(Left) *Longitudinal US shows scattered punctate echogenic foci in an otherwise normal-appearing spleen, consistent with calcifications due to prior granulomatous disease.* **(Right)** *Axial CECT in a 12-year-old patient shows multiple punctate calcified foci scattered throughout the spleen, consistent with prior granulomatous disease.*

Granulomatous Disease

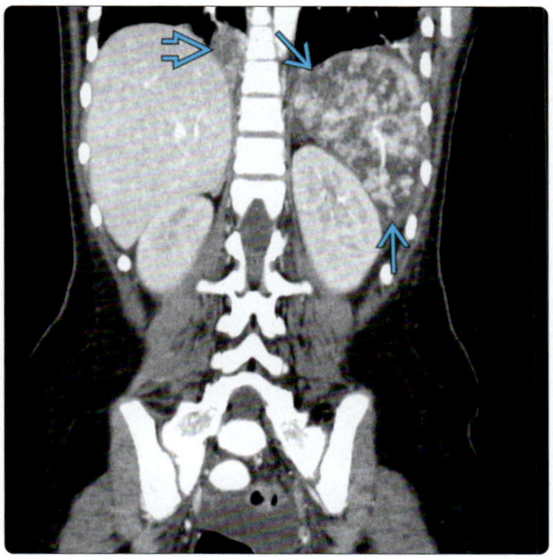

Infarction

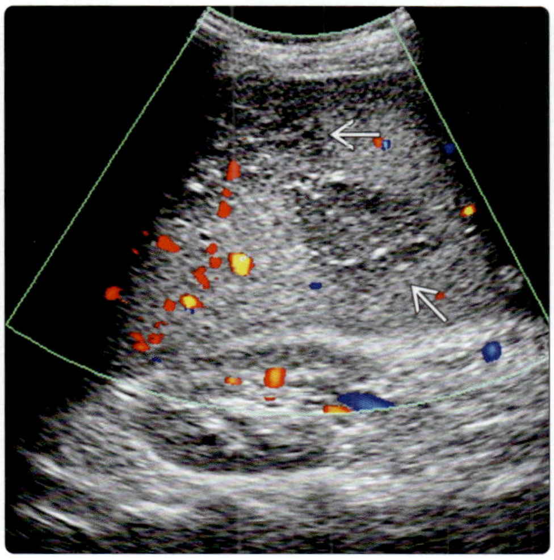

(Left) *Coronal CECT in a 13 year old with proteinuria & leukocytosis shows a markedly heterogeneous spleen ⇨ with nodules of preserved parenchyma intermixed with patchy foci of nonenhancement. Note lung disease ⇨; patient diagnosed with Wegener granulomatosis.* **(Right)** *Longitudinal color Doppler US in a patient with splenomegaly shows wedge-shaped peripheral foci ➡ of heterogeneously ↓ echogenicity & flow relative to the adjacent splenic parenchyma, consistent with splenic infarcts.*

Infarction

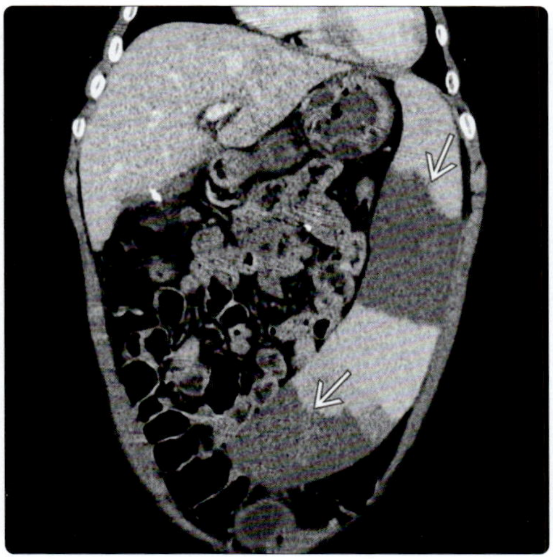

Infarction

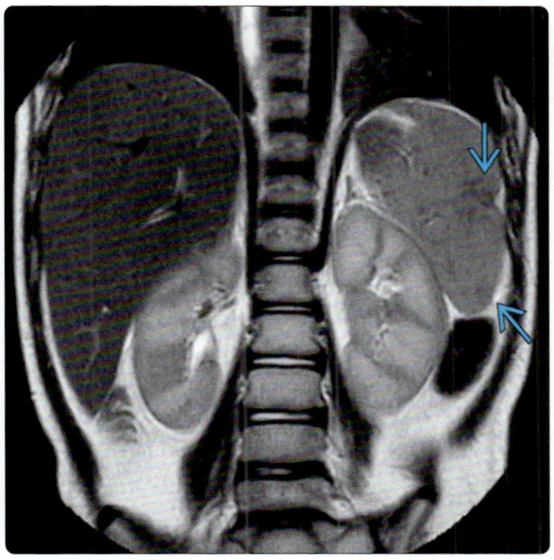

(Left) *Coronal CECT in a 9-year-old liver transplant recipient shows splenomegaly with well-demarcated regions of decreased enhancement ➡, consistent with infarcts.* **(Right)** *Coronal T2 MR in a 5 year old with a history of a heart transplant & pancreatitis shows peripheral foci of decreased signal intensity with capsular retraction →, consistent with chronic infarcts.*

Infarction

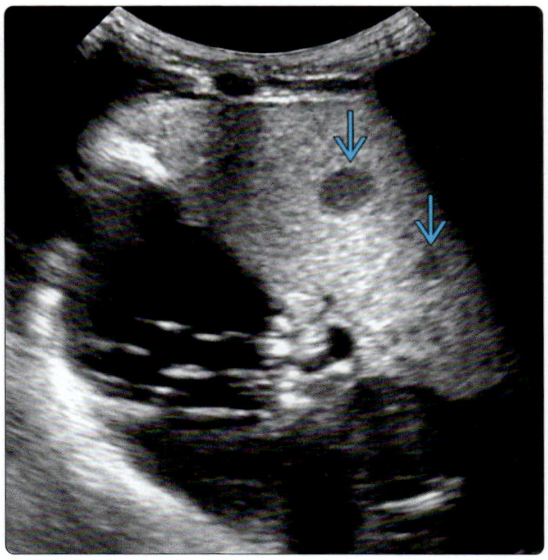

Lymphoma

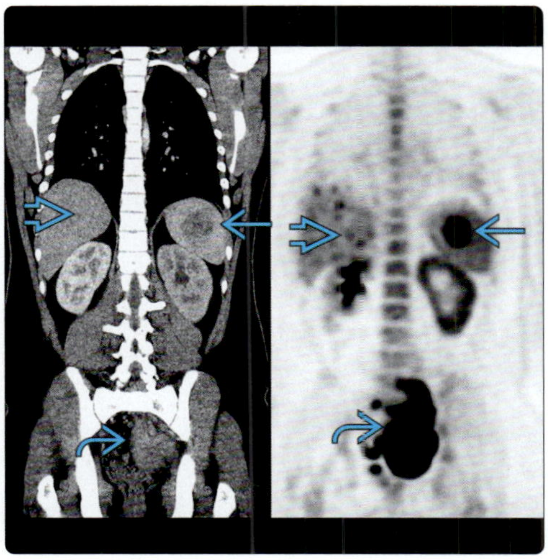

(Left) *Transverse US in a 12 year old with sickle cell disease shows a mildly enlarged echogenic spleen with multiple well-circumscribed foci of decreased echogenicity →. These pseudolesions were due to preserved islands of functional splenic tissue surrounded by extensive evolving splenic infarctions.* **(Right)** *Coronal CECT (left) & PET (right) images in a 16 year old show hypermetabolic hypoattenuating lesions in the spleen →, pelvis ↷, & liver ⇨. Biopsy showed a large B-cell lymphoma.*

(Left) *Upright radiograph in a 13 year old with upper abdominal pain & fullness shows a left upper quadrant mass (presumed to be splenomegaly) displacing the stomach & bowel.* **(Right)** *Longitudinal ultrasound of the same patient show a rind (or "claw") of splenic tissue along the margin of a large left upper quadrant cyst. The cyst shows moderate internal echoes, which swirled in real time. The left kidney is displaced inferiorly by the cyst. Resection confirmed an epithelial cyst.*

Epithelial Cyst

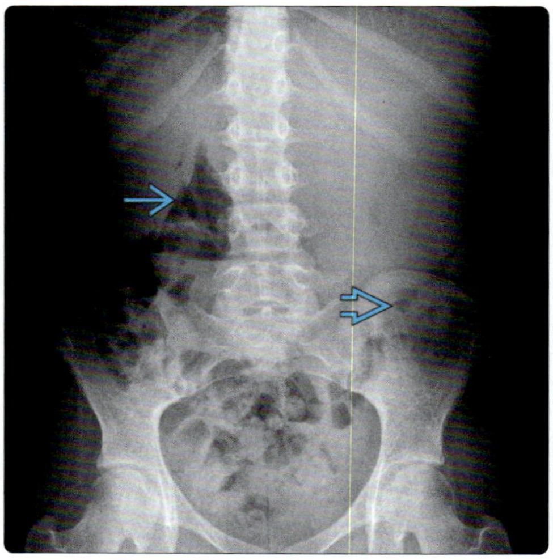

Epithelial Cyst

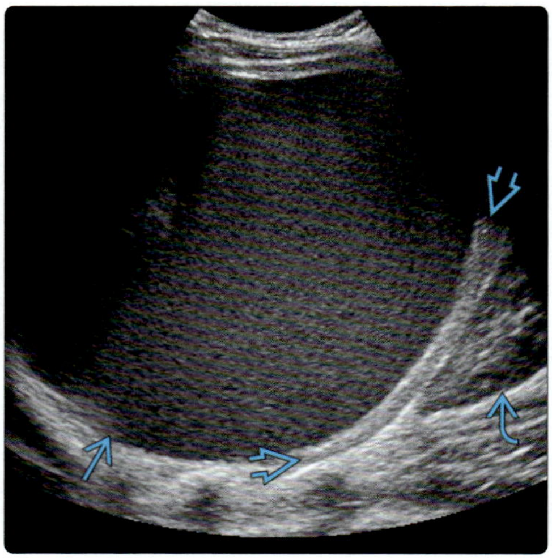

(Left) *Coronal T2 FS MR shows 2 discrete mildly lobulated high signal intensity cysts in the spleen. Resection confirmed the mesothelial type of epithelial cysts.* **(Right)** *Axial T1 FS MR in a 12 year old with left upper quadrant fullness shows a large well-circumscribed homogeneously hyperintense cyst originating from the spleen. The T1 shortening was due to high protein content/blood products. Resection confirmed a pseudocyst, likely posttraumatic.*

Epithelial Cyst

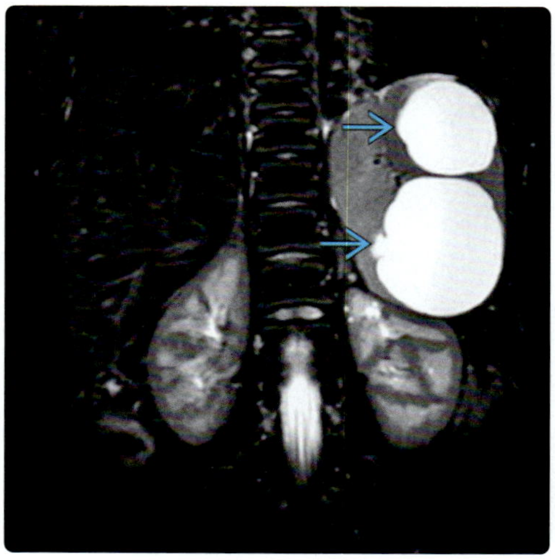

Pseudocyst

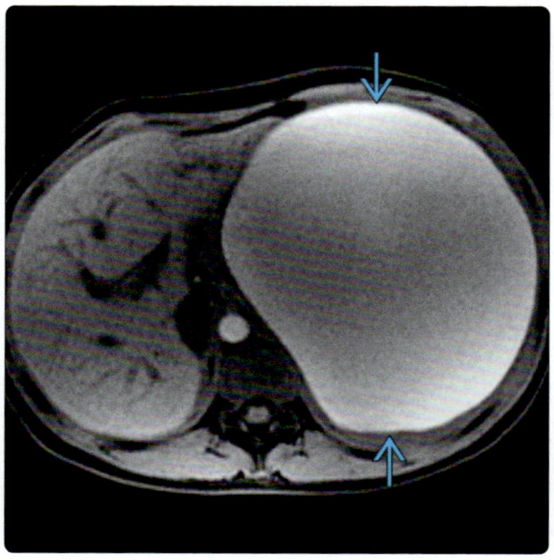

(Left) *Longitudinal ultrasound of the spleen in a 7 month old with leukemia & fungemia shows a round hypoechoic subcentimeter lesion. Numerous such lesions were present & decreased with appropriate therapy, consistent with microabscesses. Many of the liver lesions demonstrated a typical echogenic center (not shown).* **(Right)** *Axial CECT in the same patient shows hypoenhancing lesions of the spleen & liver, typical of microabscesses.*

Infection/Abscess

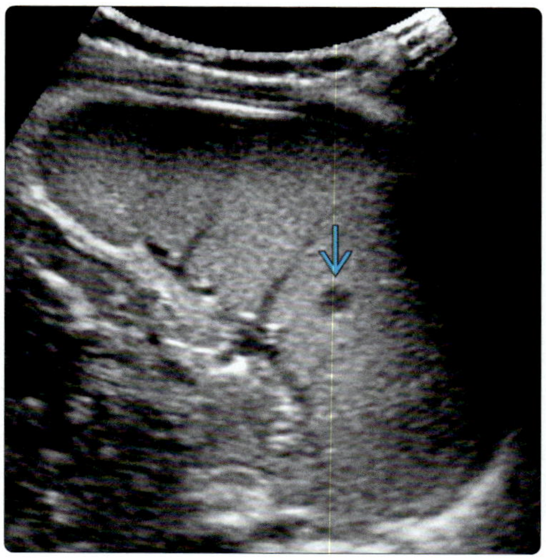

Infection/Abscess

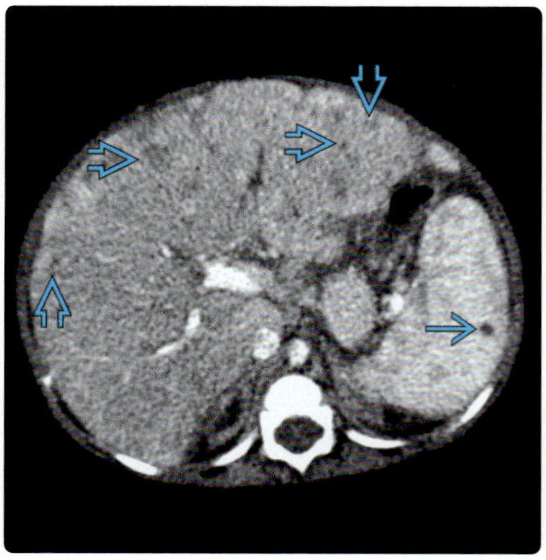

Posttransplant Lymphoproliferative Disease

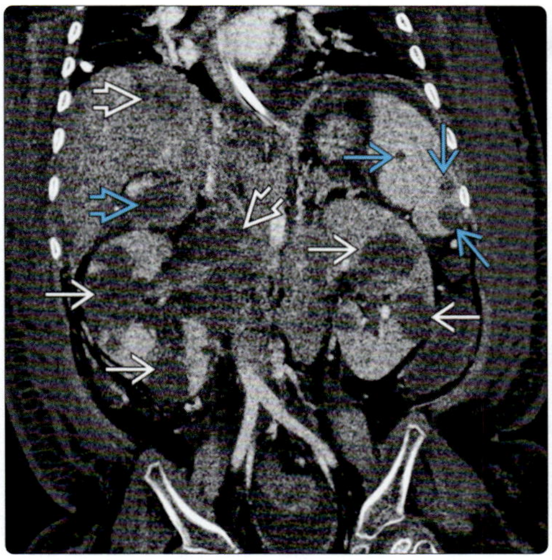

Posttransplant Lymphoproliferative Disease

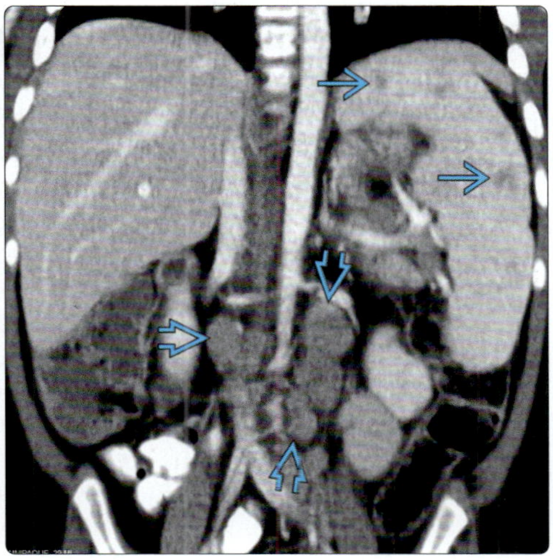

(Left) *Coronal CECT in a 2-year-old liver transplant patient shows multiple hypodense masses within the spleen. Note the adenopathy as well as additional masses in the liver & kidneys. Biopsy demonstrated posttransplant lymphoproliferative disease.* **(Right)** *Coronal CECT in a 4-year-old heart transplant patient with posttransplant lymphoproliferative disease shows multiple hypoattenuating splenic lesions as well as retroperitoneal adenopathy.*

Hamartoma

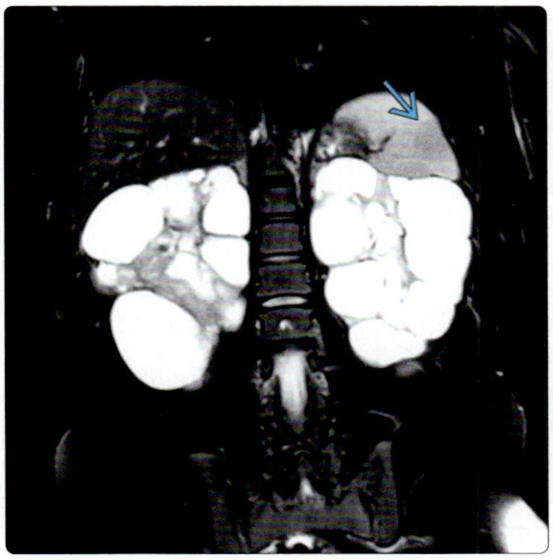

Hamartoma

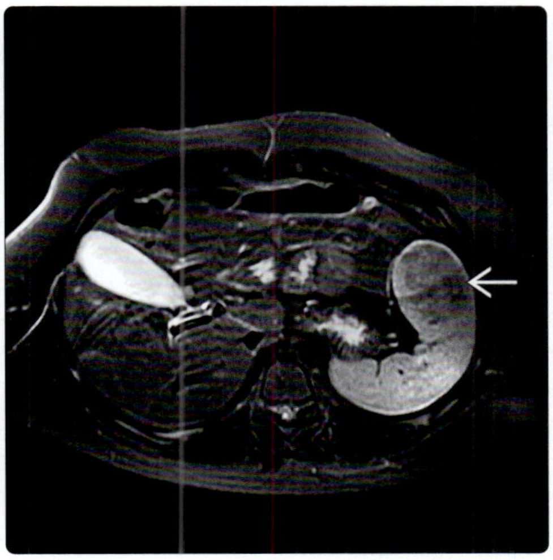

(Left) *Coronal T2 FS MR in an 11 year old with tuberous sclerosis complex (TSC) & autosomal dominant polycystic kidney disease shows a round, well-circumscribed hypointense splenic lesion, consistent with a hamartoma in the setting of TSC.* **(Right)** *Axial T2 FS MR in a 15 year old with TSC shows a hypointense splenic mass that was stable over years, presumed to be a splenic hamartoma.*

Lymphatic Malformation

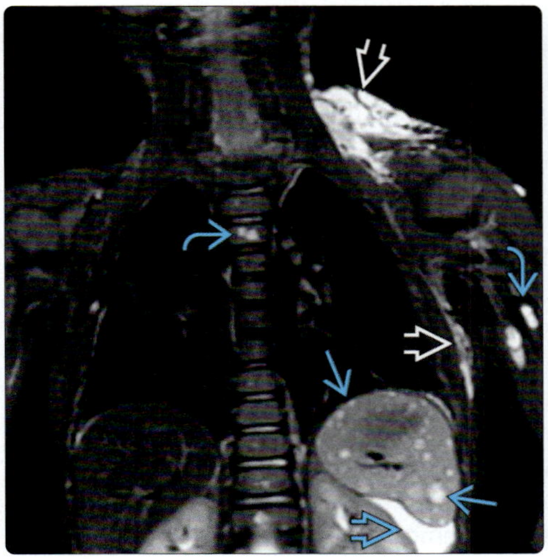

Hemangioendothelioma

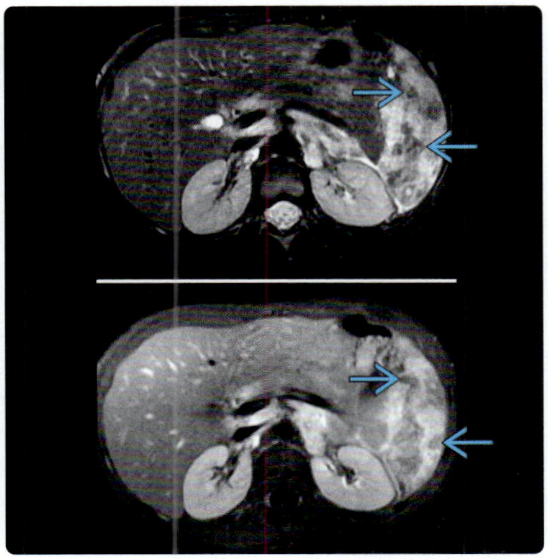

(Left) *Coronal STIR MR of a 1 year old with a chest wall lymphatic malformation shows cystic lesions in the spleen, bones, & peritoneum, consistent with generalized lymphatic anomaly.* **(Right)** *Axial T2 FS (top) & T1 C+ FS MR (bottom) images in a 6 year old with coagulopathy show hypointense splenic lesions. Splenectomy revealed Kaposiform hemangioendothelioma, which more commonly presents in infants as an infiltrative retroperitoneal or extremity mass.*

DIFFERENTIAL DIAGNOSIS

Common

- Appendicolith
- Nephrolithiasis
- Splenic & Hepatic Granulomas
- Ovarian Teratoma
- Neuroblastoma
- Remote Adrenal Hemorrhage

Less Common

- Cholelithiasis
- Hepatoblastoma
- Meconium Peritonitis
- Chronic Pancreatitis

Rare but Important

- Intestinal Calcifications

ESSENTIAL INFORMATION

Key Differential Diagnosis Issues

- Age of patient: Newborn, toddler, adolescent, etc.
- Location of Ca^{2+}: In solid organ, hollow organ, mass, or peritoneal cavity
- Morphology of Ca^{2+}: Coarse, punctate, or curvilinear

Helpful Clues for Common Diagnoses

- **Appendicolith**
  - May be present ± acute appendicitis
  - Usually in right lower abdomen/pelvis; may be in right upper abdomen with retrocecal appendix
  - Radiographs: Round or oval calcific density
    - Seen in 10-15% of acute appendicitis cases
  - US: Echogenic focus with posterior shadowing in appendix
  - CT: Hyperdense Ca^{2+} in appendix
  - Findings supporting acute appendicitis on imaging
    - Noncompressible, fluid-filled appendix
    - Increased echogenicity/induration of adjacent fat
    - Appendix diameter > 6 mm on US (less reliable on CT)
    - ± thickened, irregular wall; enhancement & vascularity are variable
    - ± dilated bowel in right lower abdomen
    - Abscess &/or extraluminal appendicolith (perforation)
- **Nephrolithiasis**
  - Increasing incidence of nephrolithiasis in children
  - Presents with pain, hematuria, &/or infection
  - Up to 84% have underlying metabolic abnormality: Hypercalciuria & hypocitraturia are most common
    - GU tract abnormalities, genetic factors, inflammatory bowel disease, cystic fibrosis, myelomeningocele, & cerebral palsy have increased stone formation
  - Calcium-based stones are most common in children
    - Calcium oxalate in 40-60%
  - Radiographs: Punctate or coarse Ca^{2+} that projects over renal shadow, ureteral course, or bladder
  - US: Echogenic foci with posterior shadowing
    - Color Doppler may be used to look for twinkling artifact or comet tail artifact posterior to small renal or ureterovesical junction stones
    - May see pelvocaliectasis with obstructing, nonvisualized ureteral calculus
      - Absence of ipsilateral ureteral jet in bladder on color Doppler may also suggest obstructing stone
  - CT: Hyperdense calculi in urinary tract
- **Splenic & Hepatic Granulomas**
  - Typically incidental sequelae of prior infection (most commonly fungal or tuberculous)
  - Radiographs: Multiple, punctate, round or ovoid Ca^{2+} projecting over spleen &/or liver
  - US: Multiple punctate echogenic foci that may or may not have posterior acoustic shadowing
  - CT: Multiple, punctate, round or ovoid densities within liver or spleen; may also see in lung bases & mediastinal/hilar lymph nodes
- **Ovarian Teratoma**
  - Germ cell tumor containing all 3 germ layers
    - May have intralesional hair, fat, Ca^{2+}
  - Vast majority in abdomen & pelvis arise from ovary
    - Benign mature teratoma (a.k.a. dermoid cyst) is most common pediatric ovarian neoplasm
  - May be bilateral in up to 15% of cases
  - Radiographs: Punctate or coarse Ca^{2+} projecting over pelvis; may be shaped like tooth
    - ± mass effect on adjacent structures
  - US: Heterogeneous, cystic & solid mass
    - Ca^{2+} are echogenic with posterior shadowing
    - May contain fat-fluid levels
    - Tip of iceberg sign: Full extent of mass is obscured by shadowing from superficial echogenic interfaces
    - Dermoid plug sign: Shadowing echogenic nodule in lumen of cyst
    - Dermoid mesh sign: Thin echogenic "lines & dots" due to hair in cyst
    - Ovarian torsion may be complication
  - CT: Mixed cystic & solid mass; fat & Ca^{2+} are diagnostic
- **Neuroblastoma**
  - Can arise anywhere along sympathetic chain from skull base to pelvis; 70% originate in retroperitoneum
  - Median age at diagnosis: 15-22 months
  - Abdominal mass is most common presentation
  - Radiographs: Paraspinal soft tissue mass
    - 30% will have visible Ca^{2+}
    - ± displacement of bowel loops, widening of paraspinal stripe, local osseous changes (i.e., erosions), hepatomegaly (from metastases)
    - ± lucent permeative bone metastases
  - US/CT/MR: Mass may be round & well circumscribed or large, multilobulated, & invasive
    - Heterogeneous due to necrosis &/or hemorrhage
    - Ca^{2+} in up to 85% by CT
    - Larger masses frequently cross midline, encase vessels, & invade spine, kidney, pancreas, or bowel
    - Metastasis are most common to liver & bone
  - MIBG: Uptake in 90-95% of patients
- **Remote Adrenal Hemorrhage**
  - Adrenal hemorrhage most commonly occurs secondary to stress in perinatal period
  - May be bilateral

- US: Hemorrhage initially appears as heterogeneous, avascular suprarenal mass
  - Clot gradually lyses, becoming smaller & more hypoechoic over weeks
  - Eventually resolves with minimal residua, ± Ca^{2+}
    - Should not see any associated mass
- Radiographs: Suprarenal Ca^{2+} (coarse, irregular, or adreniform) may be seen after weeks/months
  - If morphology, extent, or size leave any question to nature of Ca^{2+}, obtain further imaging to exclude neuroblastoma

Helpful Clues for Less Common Diagnoses

- **Cholelithiasis**
  - Risk factors
    - Neonate/infant: Sepsis, diuretics, total parenteral nutrition
    - Child/adolescent: Hemolytic anemia (i.e., sickle cell disease), cystic fibrosis, small bowel disorders
  - Radiographs: ~ 30% of gallstones are detectable
    - Look for Ca^{2+} along inferior hepatic margin
  - US: Highly sensitive & specific
    - Gallstones are echogenic with posterior shadowing
    - Mobile, unless impacted
    - Look for biliary ductal dilation due to choledocholithiasis
    - Look for signs of acute cholecystitis: Gallbladder wall thickening, pericholecystic fluid, surrounding hyperemia, sonographic Murphy sign
  - MRCP: Filling defects in gallbladder or bile ducts; may be subtle
- **Hepatoblastoma**
  - Most common pediatric liver malignancy
  - Median age of 19 months
  - Elevated α-fetoprotein levels in 90%
  - Radiographs: Large mass/hepatomegaly in upper abdomen, displacing bowel
  - US/CT/MR: Large, heterogeneous mass within or extending exophytically from liver; may be multifocal
    - Typically hypovascular/hypoenhancing relative to liver
    - ~ 50% have coarse Ca^{2+}
    - Often invades hepatic or portal veins
- **Meconium Peritonitis**
  - Sterile chemical reaction resulting from bowel perforation in utero
  - Radiographs: Ca^{2+} may be focal or scattered throughout peritoneal cavity, including visceral surfaces
    - Ca^{2+} may be punctate, coarse, or curvilinear
    - May see numerous dilated bowel loops of distal obstruction or paucity of gas
    - Pseudocyst: Walled-off collection of meconium & fluid; Ca^{2+} of wall is common; typically displaces bowel
    - Free air may be seen if perforation has not sealed
  - US: Hyperechoic punctate/curvilinear foci ± shadowing
    - May extend along hepatic surface & into scrotum
    - ± simple or complex ascites &/or bowel dilation
    - Pseudocyst: Cystic, heterogeneous mass with thick, irregular, partially calcified wall
- **Chronic Pancreatitis**
  - Up to 30% of children with acute pancreatitis will progress to recurrent & then chronic pancreatitis
  - Risk factors not as clear as in adults (alcohol, gallstones)
    - Genetic/metabolic (including cystic fibrosis) & structural biliary anomalies most common in children
  - Radiographs: Ca^{2+} scattered over region of pancreas
  - US/CT/MR: Pancreatic parenchymal volume loss with ductal dilation & scattered Ca^{2+}

Helpful Clues for Rare Diagnoses

- **Intestinal Calcifications**
  - In newborn, typically seen with distal bowel obstruction
    - Anorectal malformation: Ca^{2+} due to mixing of meconium & urine in utero due to rectourinary fistula
    - Multiple intestinal atresias: May be due to stasis
    - Hirschsprung disease (rare)
  - Radiographs: Variable appearance; scattered, small, & punctate vs. extensive
    - Some degree of bowel dilation is typically present

Appendicolith

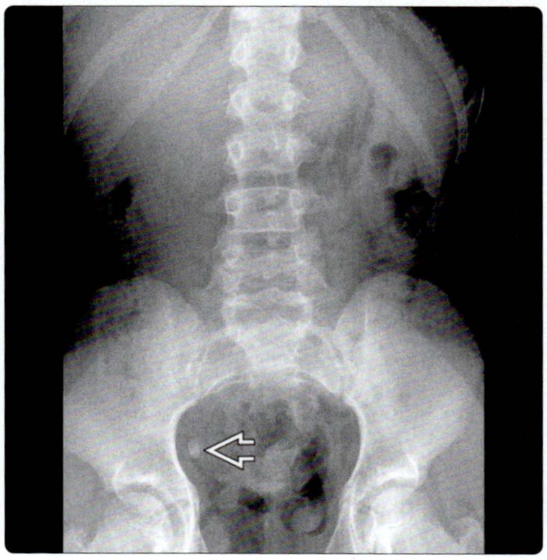

Appendicolith

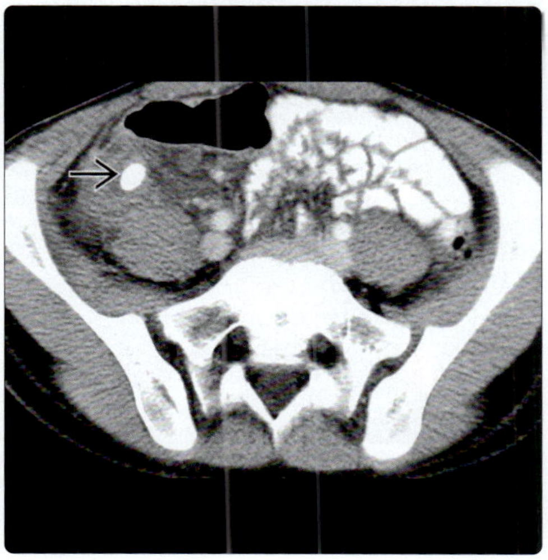

(Left) *Frontal radiograph demonstrates an ovoid Ca^{2+} in the right lower pelvis ⇨. The Ca^{2+} could be located in the appendix, in an ovary, or in a mass. Appendicoliths are identified on conventional radiographs in 10-15% of patients. This patient had a positive McBurney sign.* **(Right)** *Axial CECT demonstrates an extraluminal appendicolith ➙ due to perforated appendicitis. Note the surrounding inflammatory change. Any appendicolith must be removed at surgery as it can serve as a nidus for recurrent infections if it is retained.*

(Left) *Oblique US in a patient with right lower quadrant pain shows an echogenic appendicolith with posterior shadowing. The appendix is dilated & fluid-filled with increased echogenicity & thickening of the adjacent fat.* **(Right)** *Frontal radiograph shows 2 rounded Ca^{2+} projecting over the left renal shadow. An upright or decubitus view can help to show that the Ca^{2+} remain over the kidney.*

Appendicolith

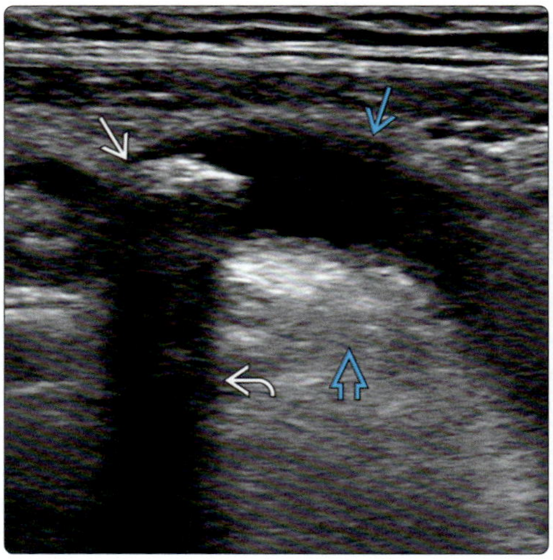

Nephrolithiasis

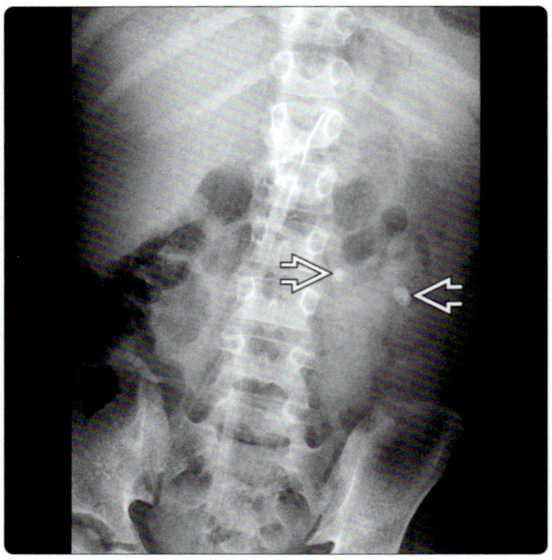

(Left) *Longitudinal US shows an echogenic, shadowing renal stone. The associated hydronephrosis of the kidney suggests that there is an obstructing stone distally in the collecting system.* **(Right)** *Transverse US demonstrates an echogenic stone lodged at the right ureterovesical junction. Twinkling artifact on Doppler can help find such stones. Doppler is also useful to confirm obstruction with absence of an ipsilateral ureteral jet.*

Nephrolithiasis

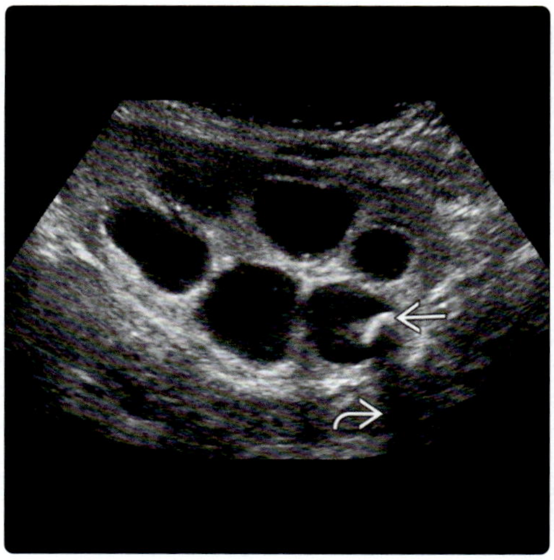

Nephrolithiasis

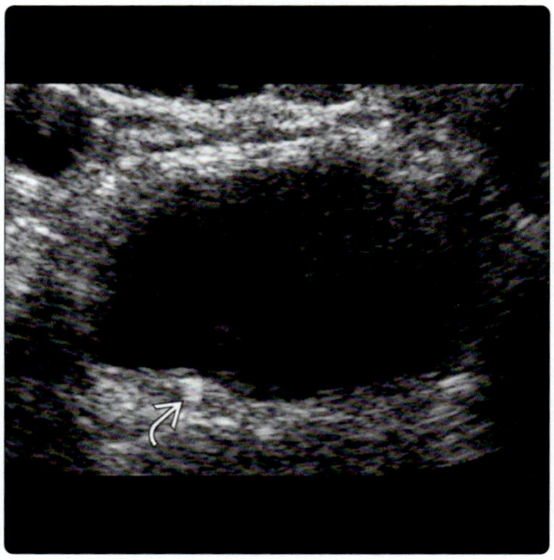

(Left) *Longitudinal color Doppler US in the upper pole of the right kidney in an 11 year old with nephrolithiasis shows twinkling artifact associated with an echogenic calculus.* **(Right)** *Coronal NECT MIP in an 11 year old with Menkes syndrome shows a 12-mm calculus in the upper pole of the right kidney, punctate calculi in the left kidney, & multiple calculi in the distal right ureter.*

Nephrolithiasis

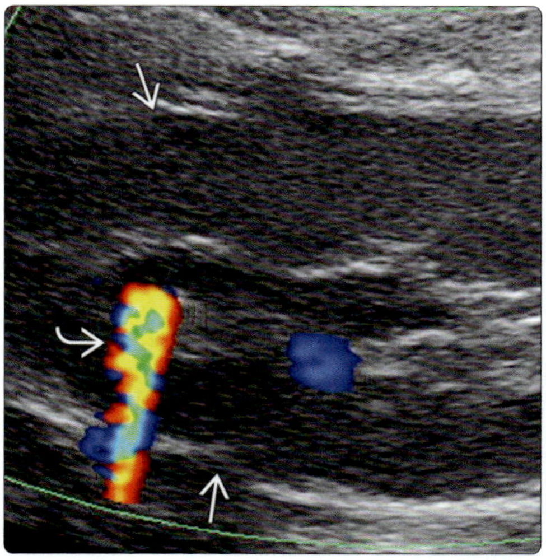

Nephrolithiasis

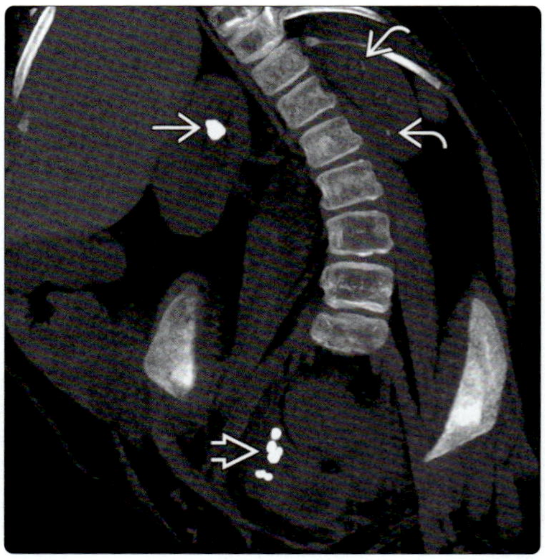

Splenic & Hepatic Granulomas

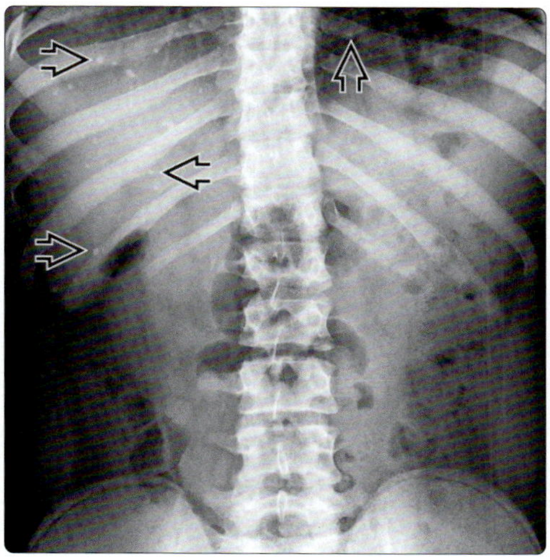

Splenic & Hepatic Granulomas

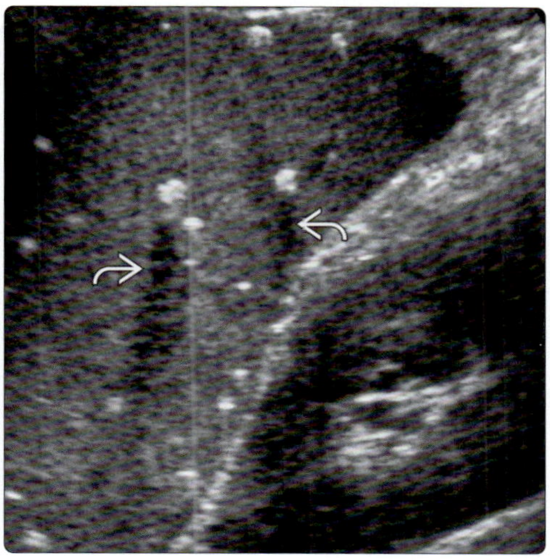

(Left) *Frontal radiograph shows numerous punctate Ca^{2+} projecting over the liver. The number & distribution of Ca^{2+}, in conjunction with the lack of hepatomegaly or bulging mass, help to narrow the differential diagnosis.* **(Right)** *Longitudinal US demonstrates numerous scattered echogenic foci throughout the liver. Only a minority of these echogenic foci demonstrate posterior acoustic shadowing.*

Ovarian Teratoma

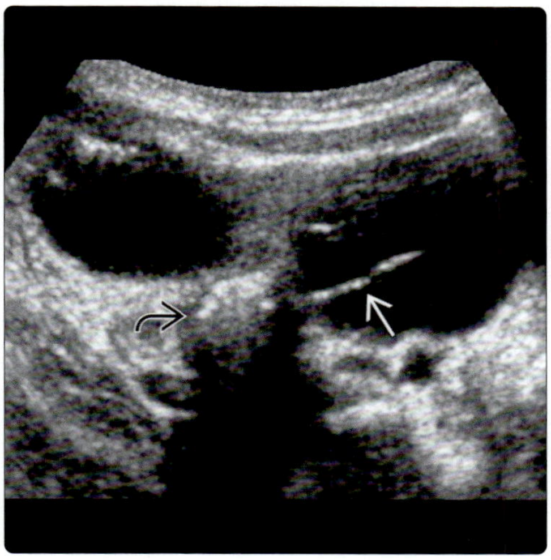

Ovarian Teratoma

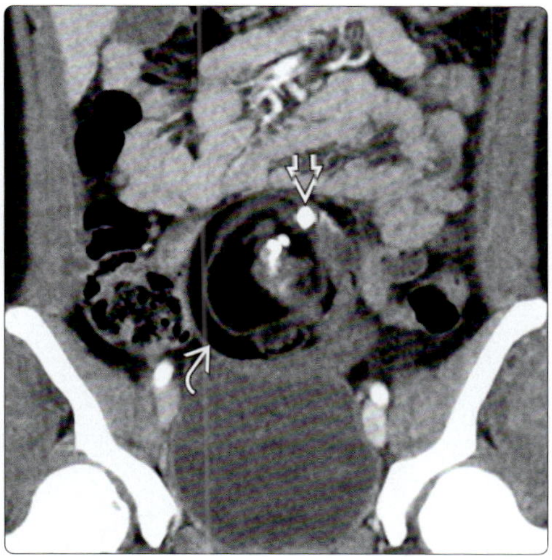

(Left) *Transverse US demonstrates a mixed cystic & solid lesion in the left adnexa. There are numerous shadowing Ca^{2+} associated with this mass. The linear echogenicities likely represent hair ("dermoid mesh").* **(Right)** *Coronal CECT shows a complex mass containing both fat & Ca^{2+} in this 11-year-old girl undergoing CT for trauma. This was a mature teratoma at excision.*

Ovarian Teratoma

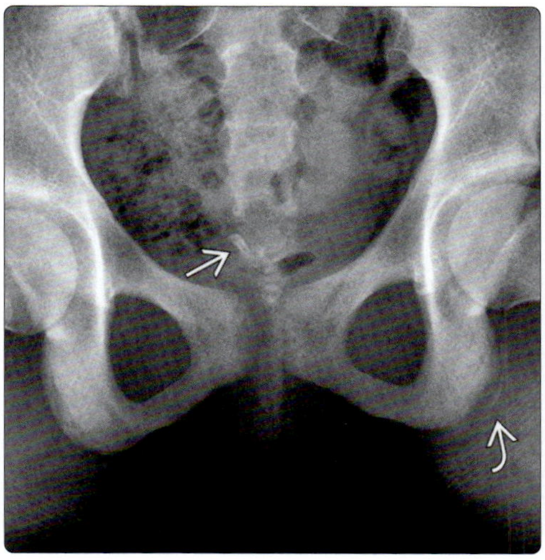

Ovarian Teratoma

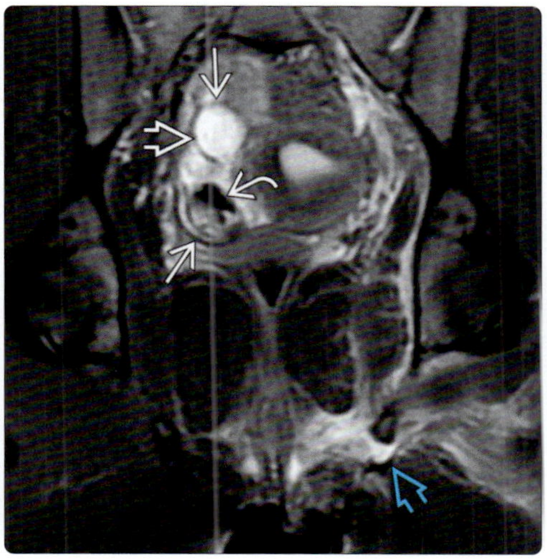

(Left) *AP radiograph in a 13 year old with a cheerleading injury shows a left ischial avulsion fracture. However, tooth-like Ca^{2+} are also seen projecting over the lower pelvis.* **(Right)** *Coronal T2 FS MR in the same patient shows a right ovarian mass containing cystic components & hypointense fat. Ca^{2+} is better demonstrated on radiography, CT, & US as compared to MR. The left ischial avulsion injury is again seen.*

(**Left**) *Frontal radiograph shows a tight cluster of punctate & coarse Ca^{2+} to the right of the spine in a patient with neuroblastoma. No adjacent bony erosion or lucent lesion is identified.* (**Right**) *Axial CECT demonstrates curvilinear Ca^{2+} associated with a solid mass in a right paraspinal location. No intraspinal extension was identified. The inferior vena cava is partially encased by the mass.*

Neuroblastoma

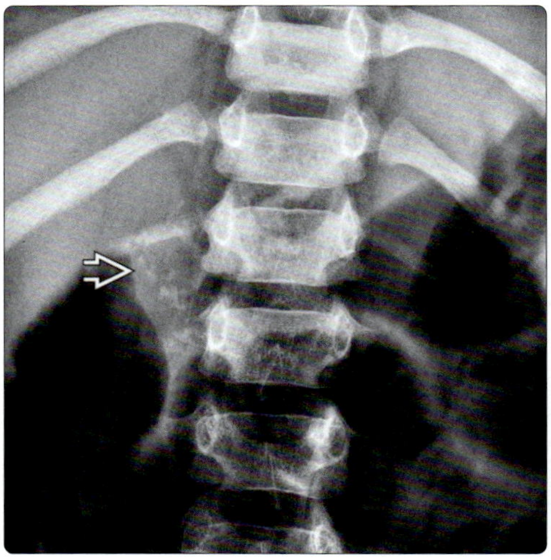

Neuroblastoma

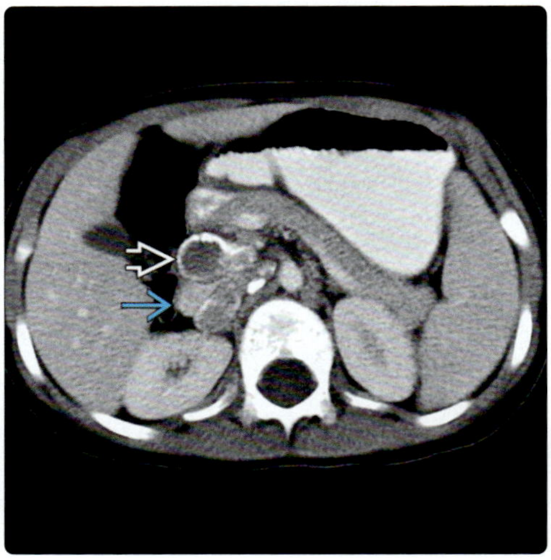

(**Left**) *AP radiograph shows incidental Ca^{2+} in the right paraspinal region of this 1 year old. The differential diagnosis includes remote adrenal hemorrhage, neuroblastoma, & hepatoblastoma.* (**Right**) *Longitudinal US in the same patient shows shadowing echogenic Ca^{2+} in an otherwise normal adrenal gland just superior to the right kidney. No suprarenal mass is identified.*

Remote Adrenal Hemorrhage

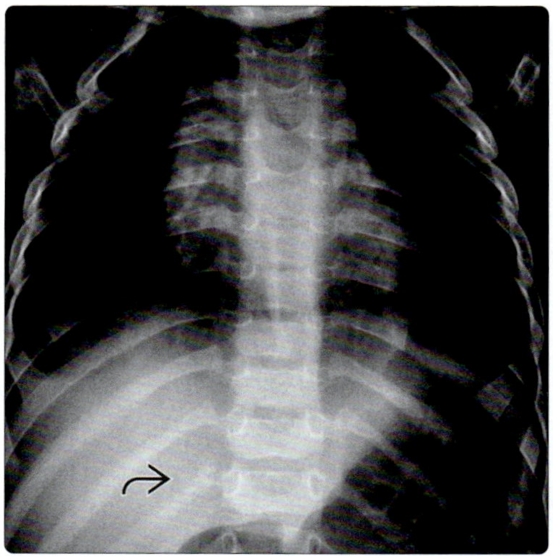

Remote Adrenal Hemorrhage

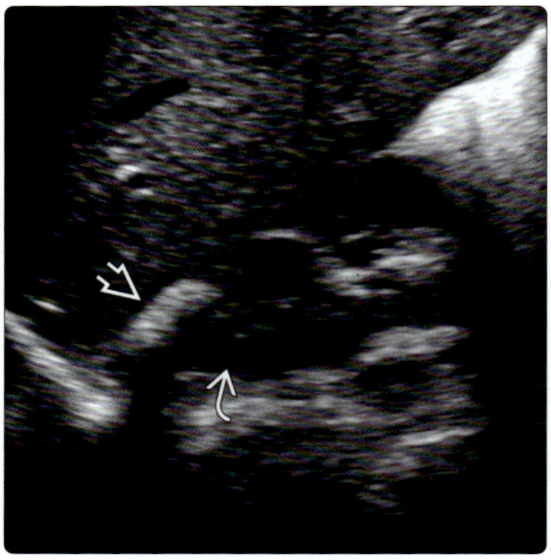

(**Left**) *Transverse US shows an echogenic focus with posterior shadowing dependently within the gallbladder lumen of a 12 year old with chronic right upper quadrant pain. There was no gallbladder wall thickening or pericholecystic fluid to suggest acute cholecystitis.* (**Right**) *Transverse US in a 16 year old with right upper quadrant pain & vomiting shows a shadowing echogenic focus in the gallbladder lumen, consistent with cholelithiasis. The wall thickening may represent acute cholecystitis.*

Cholelithiasis

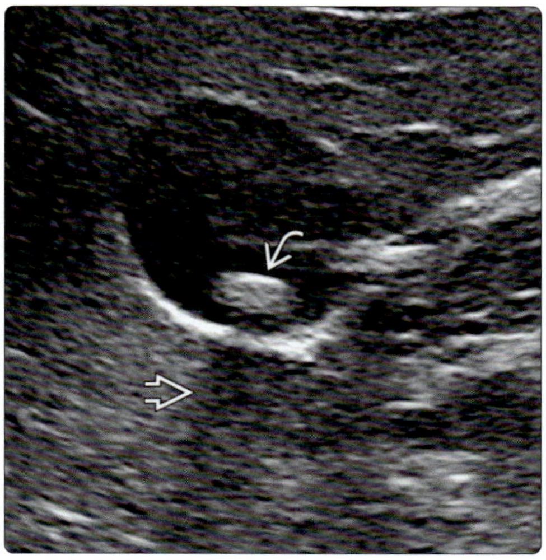

Cholelithiasis

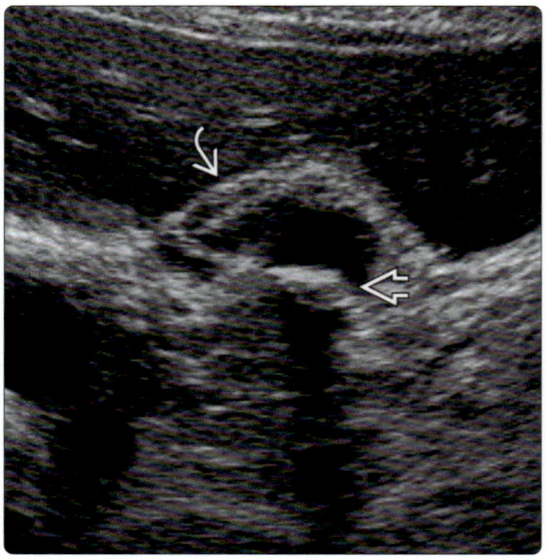

Hepatoblastoma

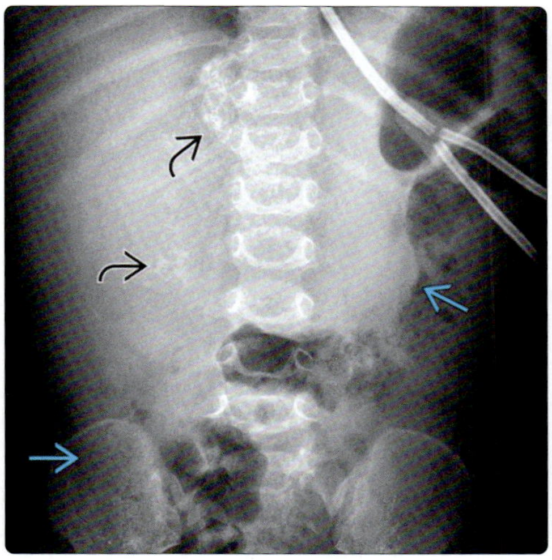

Hepatoblastoma

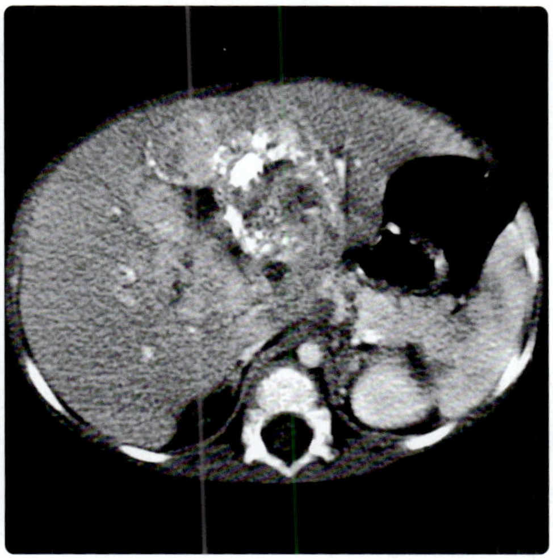

(Left) *Frontal radiograph shows clusters of coarse Ca^{2+} projecting over the upper abdomen. Note the mass effect on adjacent bowel. With the high paraspinal concentration of Ca^{2+}, both neuroblastoma & hepatoblastoma should be considered.* **(Right)** *Axial CECT in the same patient shows numerous coarse Ca^{2+} associated with a heterogeneous left hepatic mass.*

Meconium Peritonitis

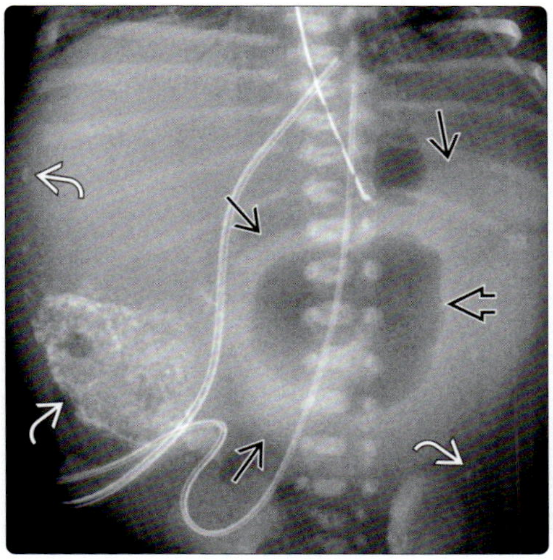

Chronic Pancreatitis

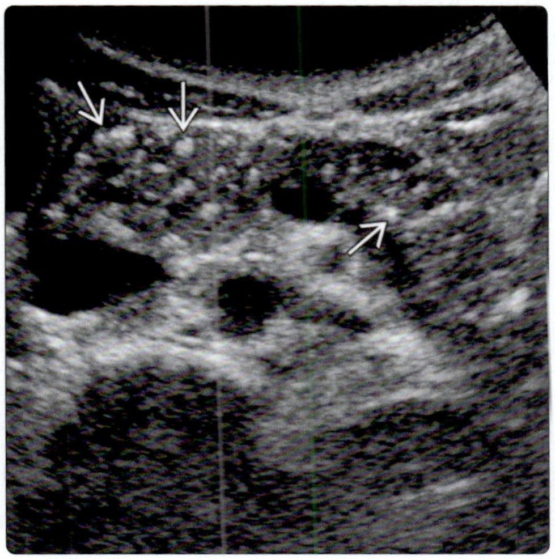

(Left) *Frontal radiograph in a newborn shows peritoneal Ca^{2+} reflective of meconium peritonitis. The vague ovoid hyperdensity in the central abdomen corresponds to contrast within a meconium pseudocyst ,which was seen to communicate with the colon on a contrast enema. Gas is also present within the pseudocyst.* **(Right)** *Transverse US shows numerous echogenic foci scattered throughout the pancreatic parenchyma, corresponding to Ca^{2+} in this 14 year old with chronic pancreatitis.*

Chronic Pancreatitis

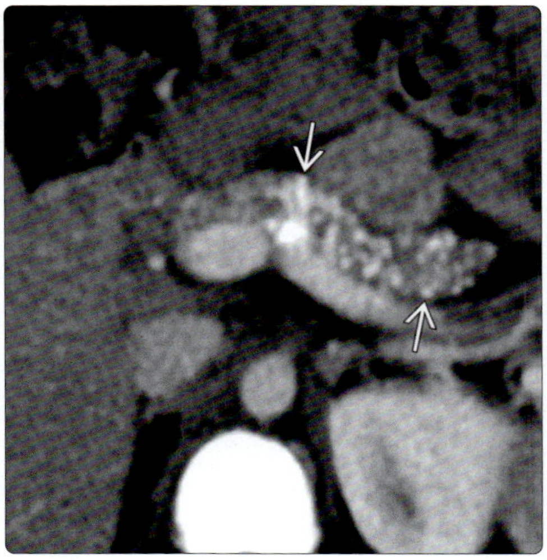

Intestinal Calcifications

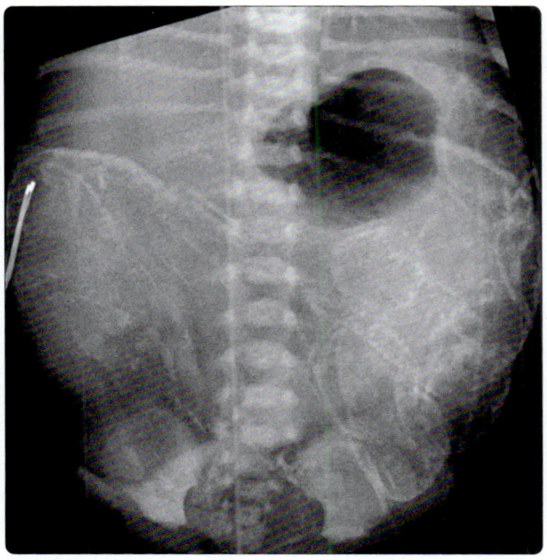

(Left) *Axial CECT shows multiple Ca^{2+} throughout the pancreatic body & tail of this 14 year old with cystic fibrosis & chronic pancreatitis.* **(Right)** *Frontal radiograph in a newborn with a prenatally detected bowel obstruction shows extensive intestinal Ca^{2+} with a paucity of bowel gas. Fluoroscopic & surgical investigations showed multiple intestinal atresias, including pyloric atresia. The patient was ultimately diagnosed with hereditary multiple intestinal atresias after showing the typical immunodeficiencies.*

DIFFERENTIAL DIAGNOSIS

Common
- Coins
- Artifact (Mimic)

Less Common
- Button Battery
- Magnets
- Sharp Objects (Nails, Pins, Tacks, Needles)
- Bullets

Rare but Important
- Lead-Containing Foreign Body

ESSENTIAL INFORMATION

Key Differential Diagnosis Issues
- Shape & pattern of density
- Location & migration
- History

Helpful Clues for Common Diagnoses
- **Coins**
  - Disc-shaped & typically homogeneous without lucent halo or step-off
  - Measurements cannot determine coin type
  - Most common sites of impaction: Upper esophagus at thoracic inlet, midesophagus at aortic arch, lower esophageal sphincter
- **Artifact (Mimic)**
  - Metallic density external to patient
  - Orthogonal/tangential views assist localization

Helpful Clues for Less Common Diagnoses
- **Button Battery**
  - Disc-shaped but with step-off/beveled edge on lateral view, halo or double density on AP view
    - 2 directly apposed coins of different sizes may mimic this appearance
  - Smaller negative pole is more likely site of severe injury
  - Tissue edema leads to tracheal displacement/narrowing
  - Risk of complications higher with: Prolonged esophageal contact, size ≥ 20 mm, < 5 years old, multiple batteries
    - Esophageal perforation, esophageal stricture, aortoenteric fistula, tracheoesophageal fistula
    - May see mediastinal widening &/or gas
  - Emergent removal required for esophageal location
  - ± CTA to look for aortic/vascular injury
- **Magnets**
  - Variable shapes: Rod, disc, sphere/ball bearing
  - Stacked magnets may simulate single foreign body
  - Potential for bowel ulceration, perforation, fistulae
  - Evaluate for gap between closely apposed magnets &/or adjacent metallic objects, failure of magnet(s) to move on sequential radiographs, dilated bowel, free air
- **Sharp Objects (Nails, Pins, Tacks, Needles)**
  - Linear metallic density
  - Serial radiographs to look for progression if asymptomatic & object lies beyond ligament of Treitz for < 3 days or if object is short with blunt end & lies in stomach
  - Esophageal location prompts urgent removal
  - Evaluate for pneumomediastinum, retropharyngeal gas, pneumoperitoneum
- **Bullet**
  - Appearance depends on construction, velocity, impacted tissue
    - Full metal jacket often remains in 1 piece
    - Semijacketed, hollow-point, nonjacketed, & soft-point bullets deform/fragment on impact
    - Shotgun pellets "buck/birdshot" are round
  - Identify entry & exit sites: Bone bevels in direction of travel; conical fragment distribution with apex at entry
  - May rarely enter artery & embolize

Helpful Clues for Rare Diagnoses
- **Lead-Containing Foreign Body**
  - No distinguishing radiographic features
  - Elevated blood lead levels within 90 minutes; higher absorption in stomach due to gastric acid

Coins

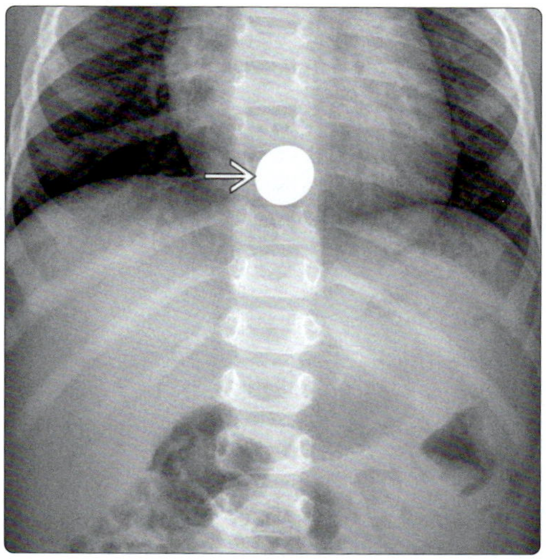

Button Battery

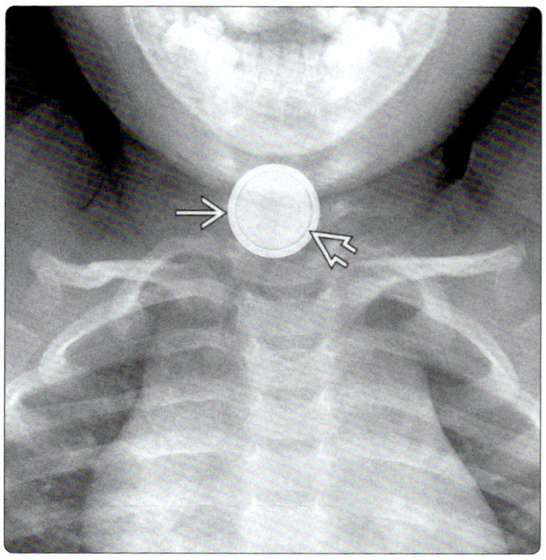

(Left) *Frontal radiograph of a 2 year old with emesis shows a metallic disc ➡, consistent with a coin, projecting over the distal esophagus. Note the homogeneous density of the object. A dime was removed at endoscopy.* **(Right)** *Frontal radiograph of a 1 year old with acute cough, gagging, & emesis but no witnessed ingestion shows a disc-shaped foreign body ➡ with a concentric lucent halo ➡ (or "double density") in the proximal esophagus, consistent with a button battery.*

Button Battery

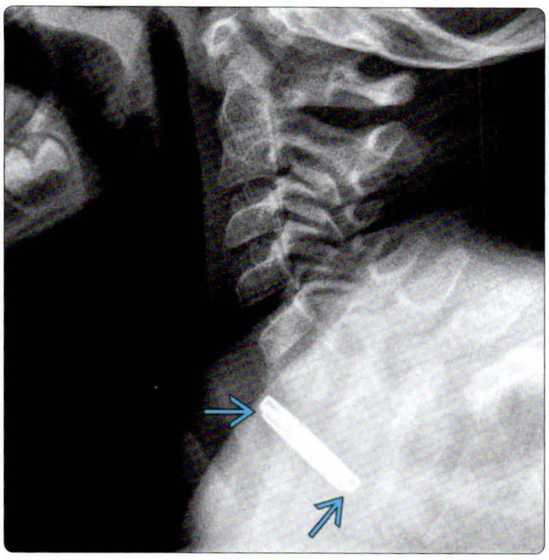

Magnets

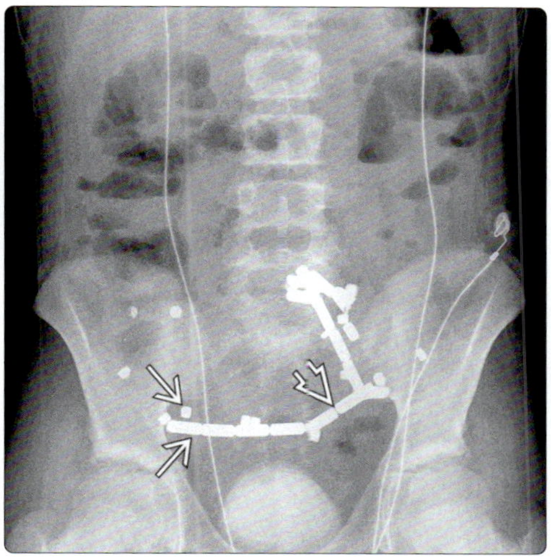

(Left) *Lateral radiograph in a 3 year old shows a button battery in the cervical esophagus. Note the typical step-off/beveled edge* ⇨ *at the margins of the battery (which help distinguish it from a coin). Emergent removal by endoscopy is required.* **(Right)** *Frontal upright view in a 12 year old with abdominal pain & emesis shows multiple rod-shaped metallic foreign bodies* ➡ *in the lower abdomen. Small gaps between the magnets represent entrapped intervening bowel* ➡*. Small bowel perforations & fistulae were noted at surgery.*

Sharp Objects (Nails, Pins, Tacks, Needles)

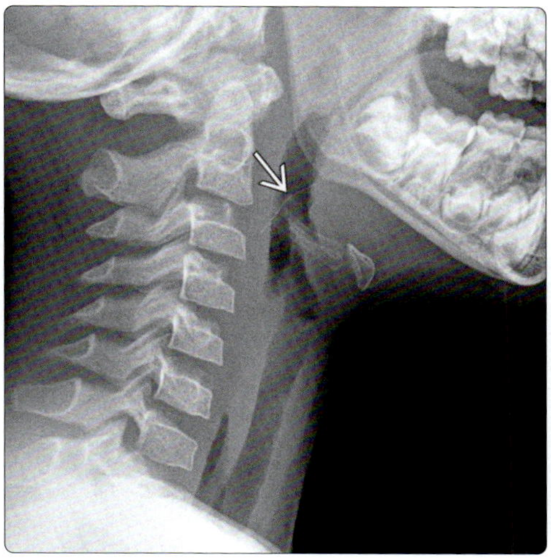

Sharp Objects (Nails, Pins, Tacks, Needles)

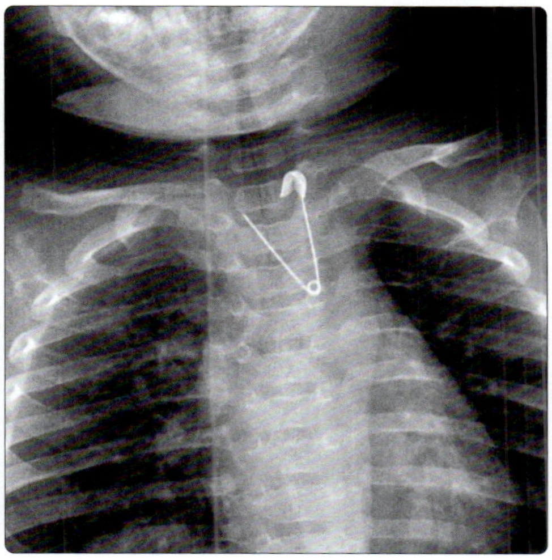

(Left) *Lateral radiograph of the neck obtained in a patient complaining of pain with swallowing demonstrates a linear metallic density in the hypopharynx* ➡*. Upon removal, this object was found to be a metal bristle from a BBQ grill cleaning brush.* **(Right)** *Frontal radiograph obtained after a witnessed ingestion of an open safety pin by an infant demonstrates the foreign body projecting over the upper esophagus. There is no evidence of pneumomediastinum or pneumothorax.*

Bullets

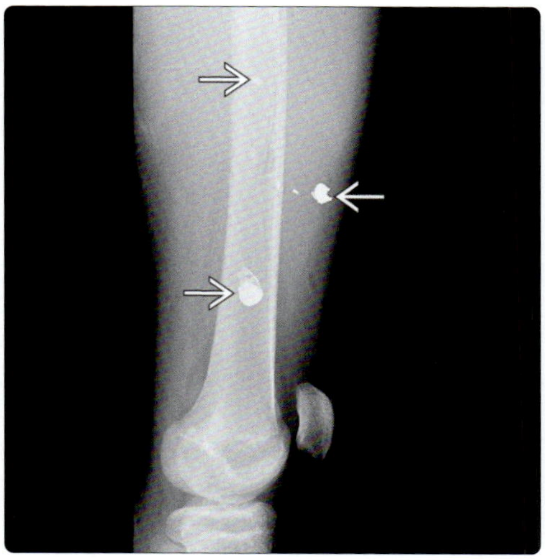

Bullets

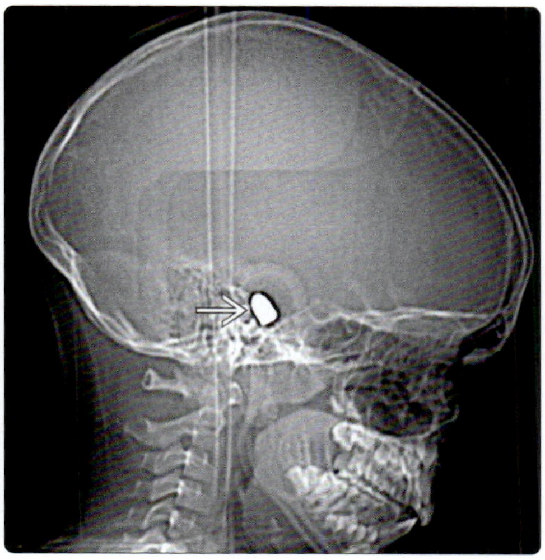

(Left) *Cross-table lateral radiograph of the leg demonstrates multiple irregular bullet fragments* ➡ *in the soft tissues & medullary cavity of the femur.* **(Right)** *Scout image from a CT of an 8-year-old boy with a gunshot injury to the head depicts a bullet* ➡ *with minimal fragmentation or deformation in the right temporal region.*

SECTION 4

Genitourinary

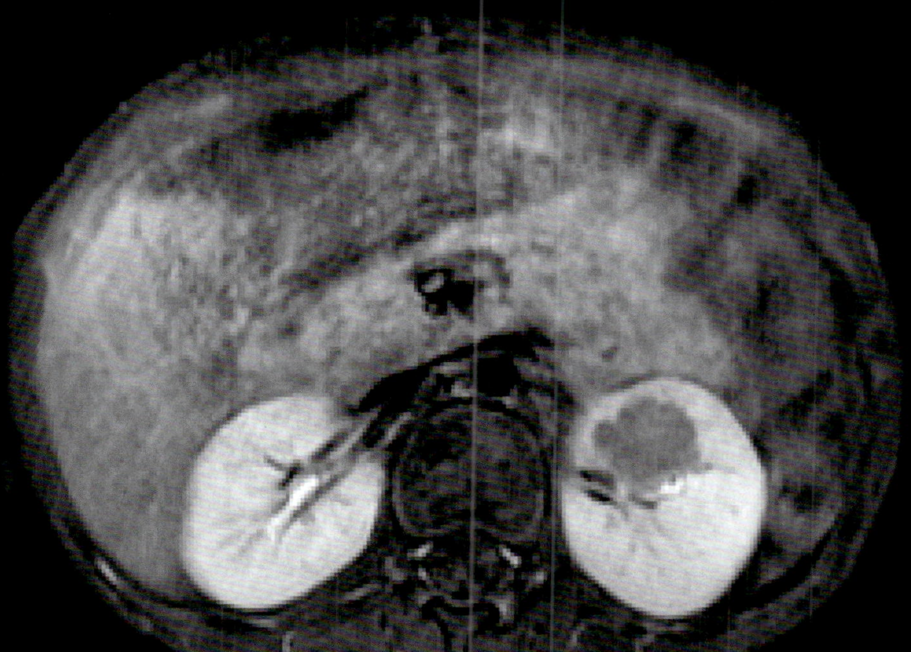

DIFFERENTIAL DIAGNOSIS

Common

- Lymphoma
- Neuroblastoma

Less Common

- Abscess
- Lymphatic Malformation
- Metastases
- Retroperitoneal Hematoma
- Duodenal Hematoma
- Plexiform Neurofibroma
- Ganglioneuroma

Rare but Important

- Paraganglioma
- Teratoma
- Lipoblastoma
- Kaposiform Hemangioendothelioma
- Inflammatory Myofibroblastic Tumor
- Castleman Disease
- Desmoplastic Small Round Cell Tumor

ESSENTIAL INFORMATION

Key Differential Diagnosis Issues

- Most solid retroperitoneal masses are malignant
  - Lesions clearly arising from solid organs (e.g., kidney, pancreas) are discussed separately
- US is useful screening modality; CECT or MR is typically required to define extent & further characterize lesion

Helpful Clues for Common Diagnoses

- **Lymphoma**
  - Most cases are > 5 years of age
    - Non-Hodgkin lymphoma is more common than Hodgkin lymphoma in children < 10 years old
    - Burkitt & diffuse large B-cell lymphoma are most common types to affect retroperitoneum
  - Imaging: Bulky conglomerations of enlarged lymph nodes that are relatively homogeneous in attenuation
    - May involve any nodal groups
    - Larger masses may become necrotic
    - Rarely contain Ca^{2+} prior to therapy
    - Often encase vessels, efface veins, displace arteries
    - Involvement of bowel & solid organs is common
      - Multifocal round masses of liver, spleen, or kidneys
      - ± lung & bone involvement
- **Neuroblastoma**
  - > 90% of patients diagnosed before age 5
    - Median age is 15-22 months
  - Can arise anywhere along sympathetic chain
    - ~ 70% originate in retroperitoneum: 35% in adrenal medulla, 30-35% in extraadrenal paraspinal ganglia
  - Abdominal mass is most common presentation
    - Wide variety of presentations due to metastases (e.g., limp, orbital swelling) > > paraneoplastic phenomena
      - Metastases to bone/marrow, liver, &/or skin are common at diagnosis (~ 50%)
  - Mass may be round & well circumscribed or large, multilobulated, & invasive; Ca^{2+} in ~ 85%
    - Larger masses frequently cross midline, encase vessels, & invade spine, kidney, pancreas, or bowel
  - MIBG uptake in 90-95% of patients

Helpful Clues for Less Common Diagnoses

- **Abscess**
  - Can be due to perforated appendicitis, Crohn disease, prior surgery, or osteomyelitis
  - Walled-off fluid collection ± internal gas
  - Enhancing rim typically has irregular margins of variable thickness (CECT/MR)
    - May show peripheral low T2 MR signal intensity & central restricted diffusion
  - Internal swirling contents upon compression with US transducer
  - Consider tuberculosis if vertebral osteomyelitis extends to retroperitoneal soft tissues
- **Lymphatic Malformation**
  - a.k.a. lymphangioma
  - Mass of abnormal lymphatic vessels that do not communicate with normal lymphatics
  - Complex, multilocular cystic lesion of variable size
  - Frequently extends across tissue planes
  - Appearance varies depending on cyst size
    - Macrocysts: > 1 cm; thin walls, no central enhancement
    - Microcysts: < 1 cm; more solid appearing
  - Cysts have varying degrees of internal complexity
    - Often contain fluid-fluid levels due to hemorrhage
    - Rarely contain fat
  - Relatively compressible cystic components often encase vessels without narrowing them
  - Grow commensurate with patient; may rapidly enlarge due to hemorrhage, infection, or hormonal stimulation
- **Metastases**
  - Testicular metastases are most common
    - Spread to retroperitoneal lymph nodes
- **Retroperitoneal Hematoma**
  - Seen with trauma, bleeding disorder, or anticoagulation
  - Time from hemorrhage to imaging dictates appearance
- **Duodenal Hematoma**
  - Typically occurs with trauma: Accidental (e.g., handlebar injury), nonaccidental (i.e., child abuse), or iatrogenic (e.g., EGD with biopsy)
  - May be intraluminal (expanding but obstructing lumen) or intramural (effacing lumen)
  - Most commonly occurs at 2nd/3rd duodenum
  - Volume of paraduodenal hematoma is variable
  - Associated with pancreatic injuries
- **Plexiform Neurofibroma**
  - Classic cutaneous findings of neurofibromatosis type 1 (NF1) include café au lait spots & axillary freckling
  - Discrete masses are most common but can diffusely infiltrate hollow viscera
    - Track along courses of nerves
    - Lobulated low attenuation masses (CT)
    - Classic target sign of individual lobule with T2-hyperintense periphery & hypointense center (MR)
  - Can compress spinal cord & vessels

- Focal discordant growth, cystic change, peripheral enhancement, & PET SUV > 3.5 suggest malignancy
- **Ganglioneuroma**
  - Differentiated benign neuroblastic tumor of older children
  - Well-defined paraspinal mass; Ca^{2+} in 10-25%

Helpful Clues for Rare Diagnoses

- **Paraganglioma**
  - ~ 30% of all pediatric pheochromocytomas are extraadrenal, 85% of which are retroperitoneal
    - Organ of Zuckerkandl is most common site of origin
  - Most common in 2nd-3rd decade of life
  - Associated with von Hippel-Lindau, MEN type 2, & NF1
  - 20-50% are malignant
    - Most commonly metastasize to bone, liver, & lungs
  - Often presents with hypertension
  - Intermediate to high T2 signal intensity
  - MIBG uptake is typical
- **Teratoma**
  - Heterogeneous mixed solid & cystic mass containing all 3 germ cell layers; foci of fat & Ca^{2+} are quite common
  - Mature, benign >> immature > malignant forms
- **Lipoblastoma**
  - Most common in children under age 3
  - Heterogeneous fatty mass, often large
    - Fat in soft tissue mass in young child is not specific but confers benignity
- **Kaposiform Hemangioendothelioma**
  - Locally invasive intermediate grade vascula neoplasm
  - Most occur in infancy
  - Typically presents as palpable mass, skin discoloration, &/or coagulopathy
    - Consumptive coagulopathy may be severe (true Kasabach-Merritt phenomenon)
  - Lobulated solid mass with intermediate T2 signal intensity ± foci of internal hemorrhage
  - Frequently show poorly defined infiltrative margins with surrounding edema
  - Vigorous enhancement; ± prominent vessels, more commonly along base than in lesion
  - ± regional adenopathy; no distant metastases
- **Inflammatory Myofibroblastic Tumor**
  - Intermediate-grade mesenchymal tumor that is usually benign, but local recurrence is common
  - Round or lobulated focal soft tissue mass; circumscribed or ill-defined margins
  - May have central dense Ca^{2+} on CT
  - Iso- to hypointense on T1, variable on T2 MR; variable enhancement
  - Does not typically encase bowel or vascular structures
- **Castleman Disease**
  - Benign lymphoproliferative disorder, a.k.a. angiofollicular lymphoid hyperplasia
  - Soft tissue mass ± satellite nodules/lymph nodes
  - Ca^{2+} in 10-30%, may appear branching
  - Heterogeneously hyperintense on T2 MR; may have central stellate fibrotic scar or necrosis
  - Characteristic intense enhancement is seen in more common hyaline vascular type
    - Variable enhancement in plasmacytic type
  - FDG PET uptake is typically lower than lymphoma
- **Desmoplastic Small Round Cell Tumor**
  - Rare malignant tumor, far more common in boys
  - Typically shows multifocal peritoneal masses with ascites; 30% show small Ca^{2+}
    - ~ 50% have retroperitoneal involvement

SELECTED REFERENCES

1. Morani AC et al: Desmoplastic small round cell tumor: imaging pattern of disease at presentation. AJR Am J Roentgenol. 212(3):W45-54, 2019
2. Chen AM et al: A review of neuroblastoma image-defined risk factors on magnetic resonance imaging. Pediatr Radiol. 48(9):1337-47, 2018
3. Sakamoto S et al: A large retroperitoneal lipoblastoma: a case report and literature review. Medicine (Baltimore). 97(40):e12711, 2018

Lymphoma

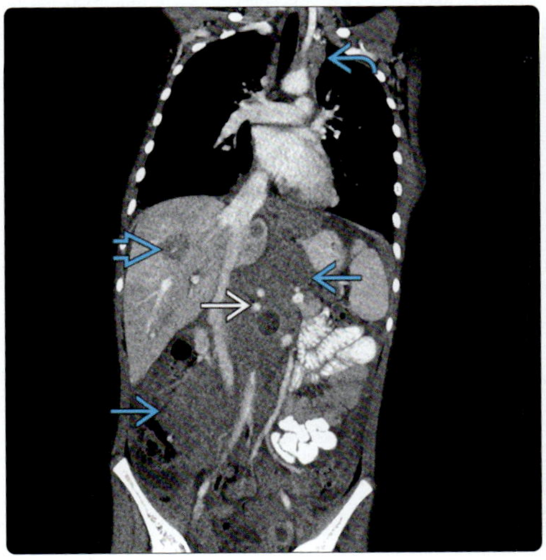

Lymphoma

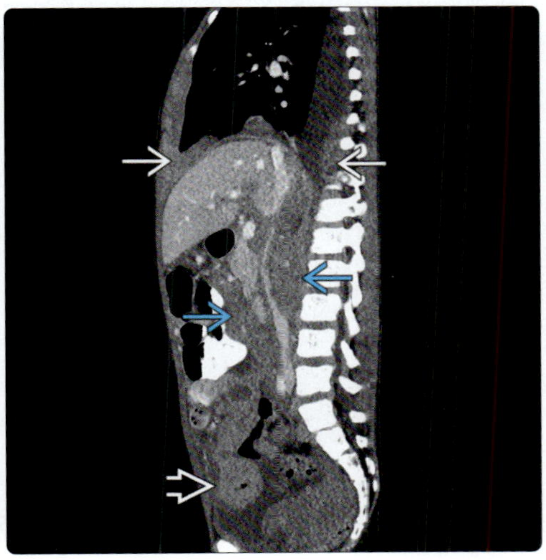

(Left) *Coronal CECT in a 10 year old with Burkitt lymphoma shows large retroperitoneal nodal masses ⇨ displacing bowel & engulfing vessels ➡. Liver metastases ⇨ & mediastinal nodes ⇨ are also noted.* **(Right)** *Sagittal CECT in the same patient shows pleural masses ➡ (with effusion) as well as large retroperitoneal masses ⇨. Foci of bowel involvement ➡ are also noted, typical of lymphoma.*

(Left) *Transverse color Doppler US in an 18 month old with a palpable abdominal mass shows displacement of the left kidney by a large lobulated relatively hypovascular solid mass.* **(Right)** *Axial T2 FS MR in the same patient shows the large retroperitoneal mass encasing the aorta & displacing the left kidney. Diffusion restriction was seen throughout the mass due to high cellularity (not shown). The findings & age are typical for neuroblastoma.*

Neuroblastoma

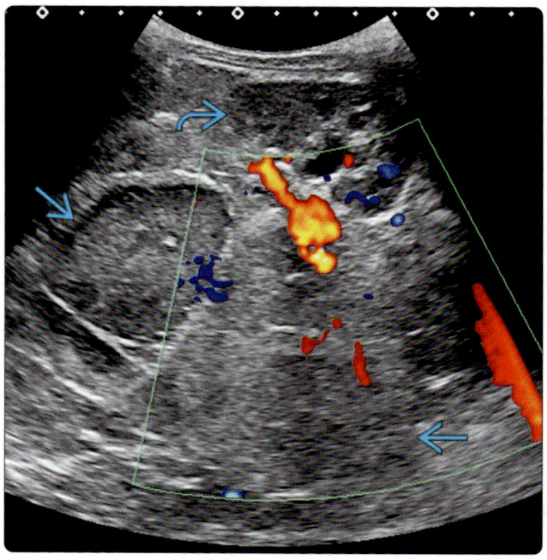

Neuroblastoma

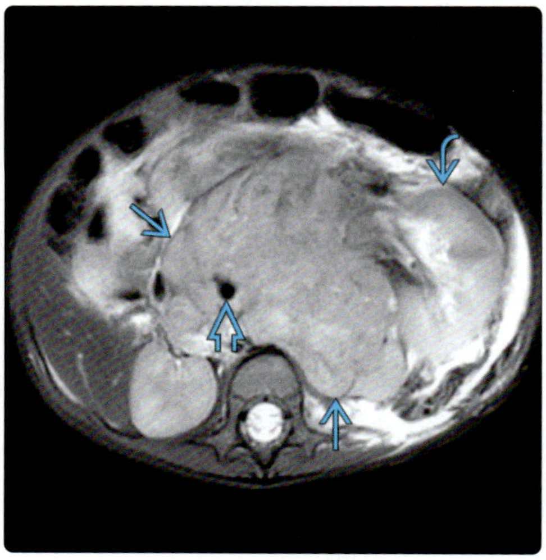

(Left) *Axial CECT in a 4 year old with abdominal distention shows a large multilobulated soft tissue mass of the retroperitoneum lifting & encasing the aorta & inferior vena cava (IVC) & invading the spinal canal. Note the Ca^{2+} in this typical neuroblastoma.* **(Right)** *Anterior & posterior MIBG images in the same patient show intense uptake of the primary tumor as well as numerous sites of bony metastatic disease. (Note that the bones should not be visualized on an MIBG scan.)*

Neuroblastoma

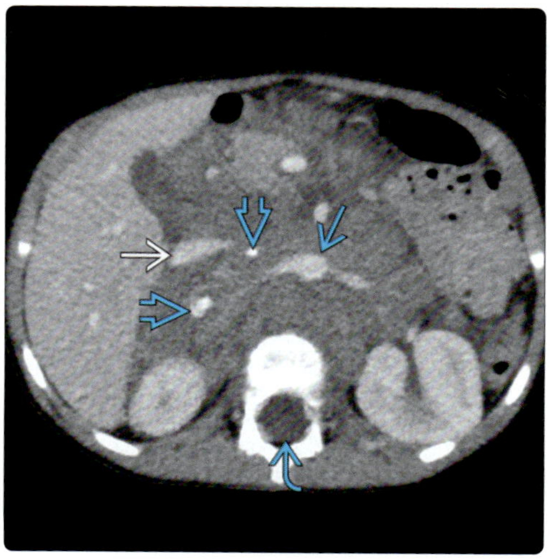

Neuroblastoma

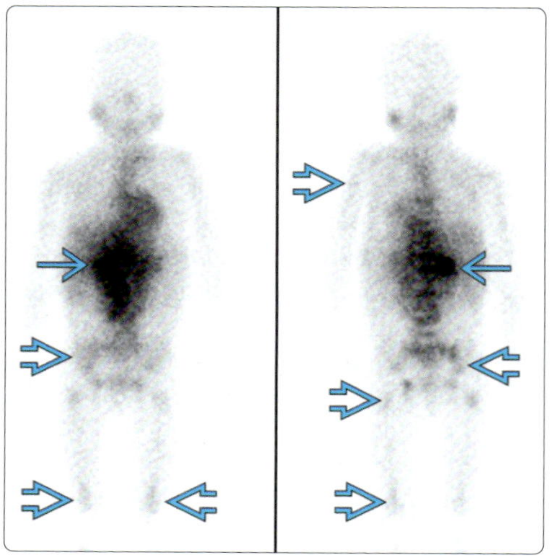

(Left) *Axial CECT in a 17 year old with Crohn disease & new pain shows irregular wall enhancement of a fluid collection in the right psoas muscle. The source of this intramuscular abscess is penetrating disease of the inflamed terminal ileum.* **(Right)** *Axial T2 FS (top) & T1 C+ FS (bottom) MR images in a patient with prior retrocecal appendicitis show a fluid collection with a T2-hypointense rim & irregular enhancing margins, typical of abscess.*

Abscess

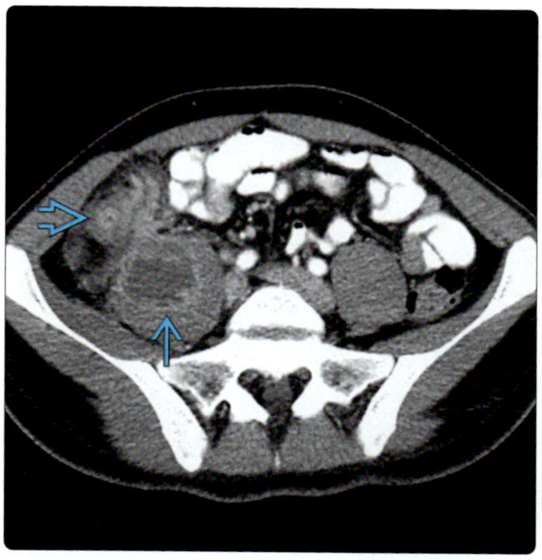

Abscess

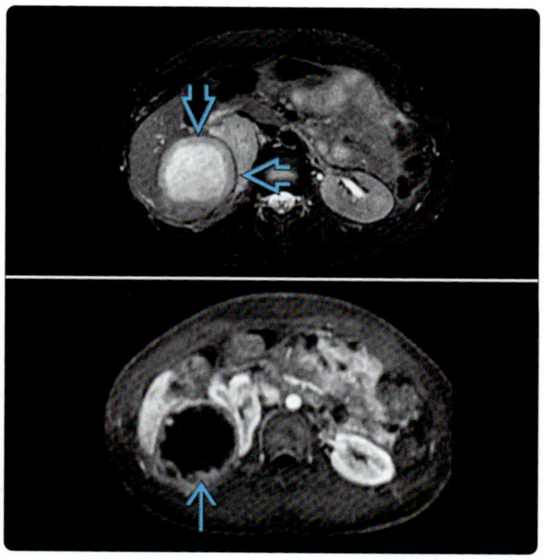

Abscess

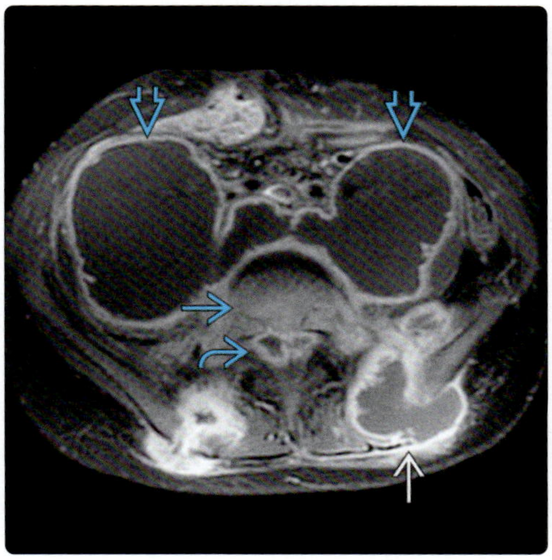

Lymphatic Malformation

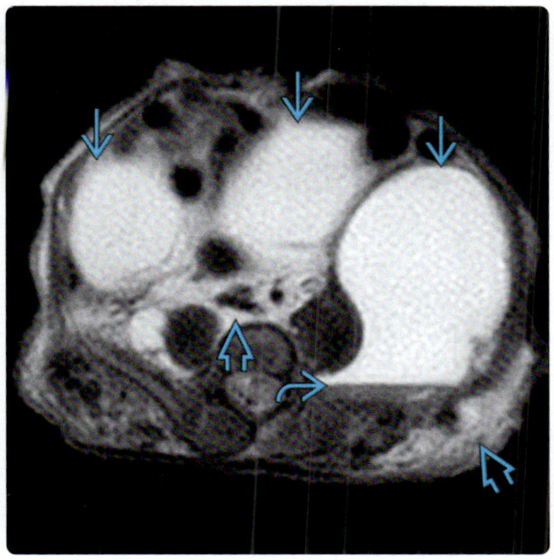

(Left) *Axial T1 C+ FS MR in a girl with tuberculosis shows large retroperitoneal abscesses ⇒ emanating from a vertebral infection →. Also note the epidural ↗ & posterior paraspinal ➡ abscesses.* **(Right)** *Axial T2 FS MR in a newborn shows numerous large thin-walled cysts → displacing the bowel anteriorly. A fluid-fluid level ↗ (due to blood products) is seen in one cyst. The findings are typical of a macrocystic lymphatic malformation. More poorly defined microcystic disease is seen in the left flank & paraspinal regions ⇒.*

Metastases

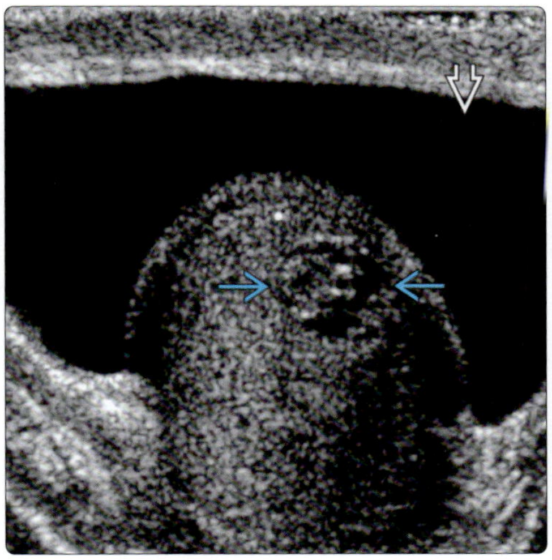

Metastases

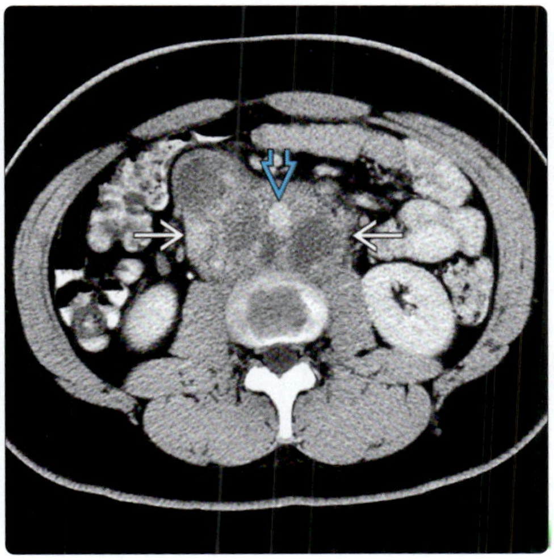

(Left) *Transverse US in a teenager with scrotal swelling shows a heterogeneous mass → of the testis with a moderate hydrocele ➡.* **(Right)** *Axial CECT in the same patient shows a conglomerate nodal mass ➡ surrounding the aorta ⇒ at the level of the kidneys due to retroperitoneal metastases from the testicular germ cell tumor. Many of the lymph nodes appear necrotic.*

Metastases

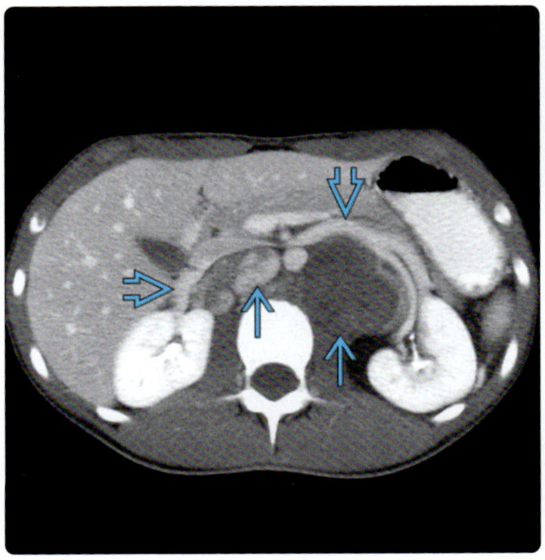

Retroperitoneal Hematoma

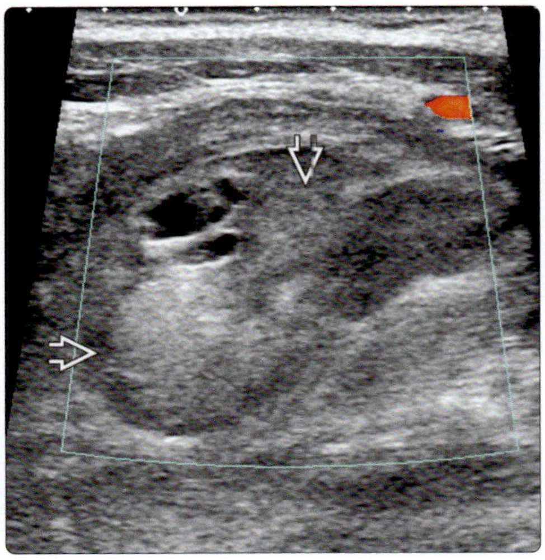

(Left) *Axial CECT in a 16-year-old boy shows multiple lobulated masses of variable enhancement → displacing renal veins anteriorly ⇒. These metastatic nodal masses were due to a paratesticular rhabdomyosarcoma.* **(Right)** *Longitudinal color Doppler US in an anticoagulated 16 year old with new right flank pain shows a nondescript avascular mass ➡ expanding iliopsoas musculature due to hematoma. Patient had history of antiphospholipid antibody syndrome & was being treated for arterial clot.*

(Left) *Axial CTA in the same patient shows intramuscular hemorrhage expanding the right iliopsoas musculature. Note that the hematoma is similar in attenuation to the muscle on this arterial phase study.* **(Right)** *Axial CECT in a 5 year old status post EGD & biopsy shows a homogeneous hematoma expanding the duodenum. Hemorrhage tracks into the anterior pararenal space & peritoneal cavity. Note the featureless ribbon-like appearance of the hyperenhancing bowel wall, typical of graft-vs.-host disease.*

Retroperitoneal Hematoma

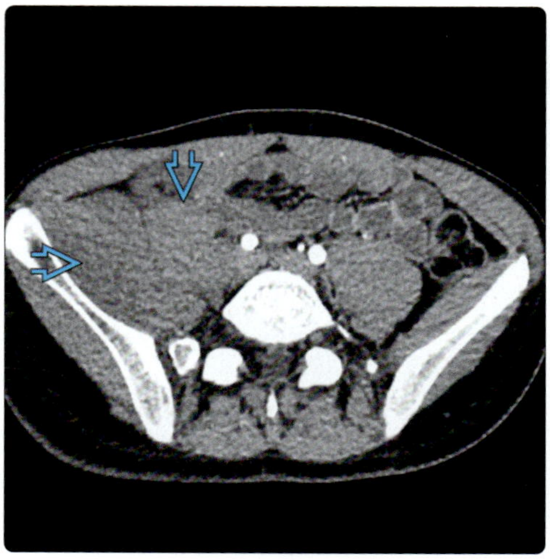

Duodenal Hematoma

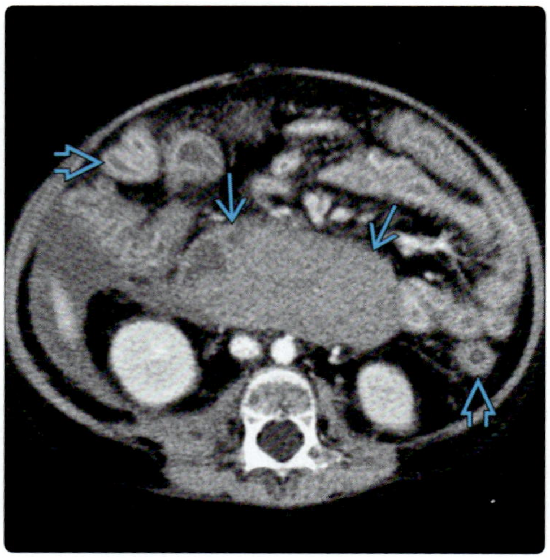

(Left) *Oblique US of the upper abdomen shows a C-shaped hypoechoic focus. No vascular flow was seen on color Doppler imaging (not shown), & no peristalsis was observed real-time.* **(Right)** *Lateral upper GI image shows a filling defect expanding the 1st portion of the duodenum. Contrast did not easily pass beyond this filling defect, which was secondary to a hematoma. Pediatric patients with duodenal hematoma will typically have a history of a recent biopsy or other trauma (e.g., handlebar injury or child abuse).*

Duodenal Hematoma

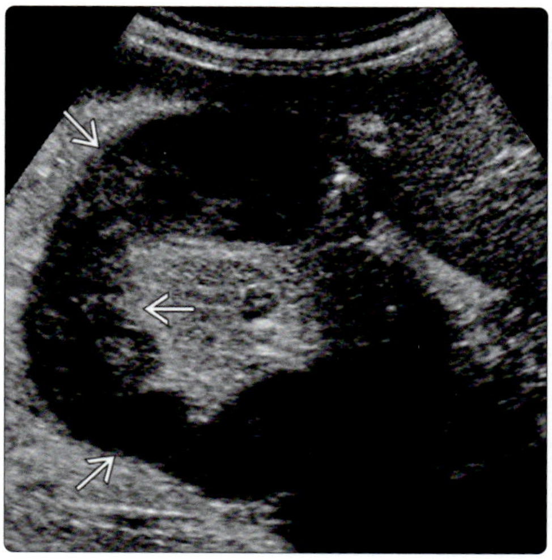

Duodenal Hematoma

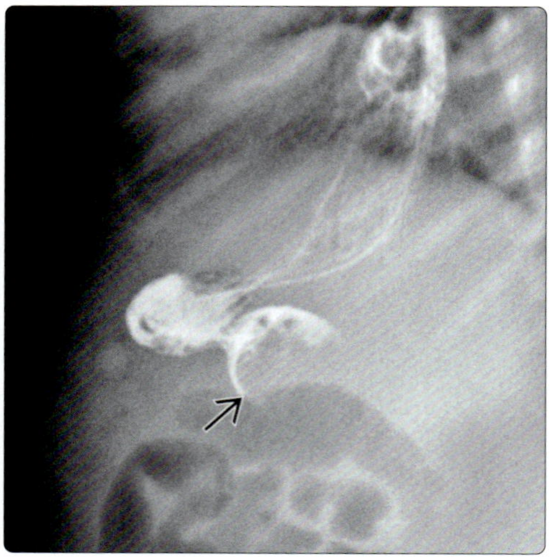

(Left) *Axial T2 FS MR in a 6 year old with NF1 shows numerous lobulated hyperintense lesions of the retroperitoneum elevating the aorta & IVC. Some lesions show a classic target appearance of plexiform neurofibromas with a hypointense center.* **(Right)** *Axial T1 C+ FS MR in the same patient shows variable enhancement of the lesions, some showing a target-like appearance. A suspected MPNST shows heterogeneous enhancement.*

Plexiform Neurofibroma

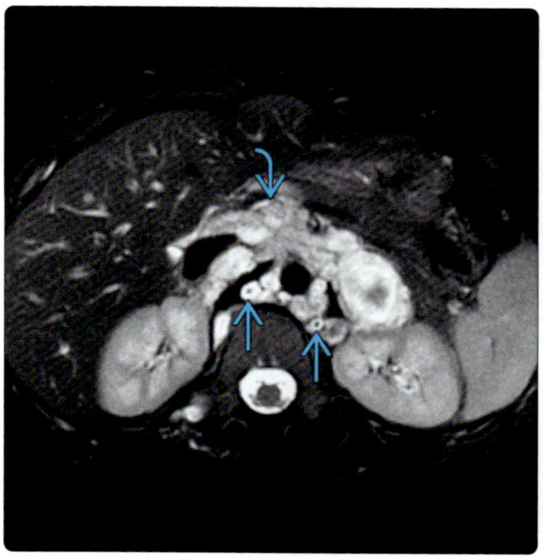

Plexiform Neurofibroma

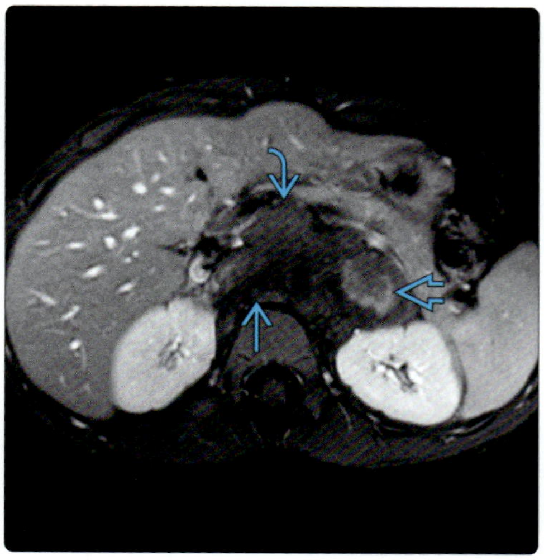

Teratoma

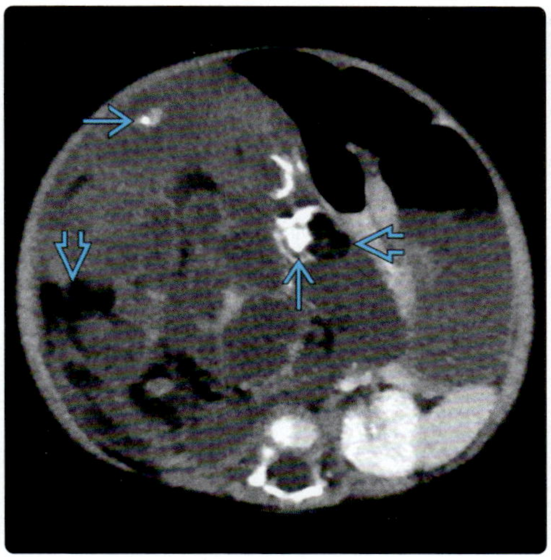

Teratoma

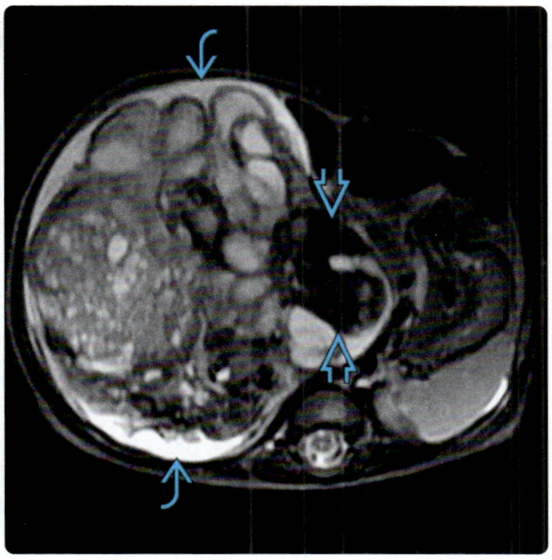

(Left) *Axial CECT in a 4 month old with abdominal distention shows a large heterogeneous mass of the retroperitoneum displacing bowel anteriorly & medially. Numerous foci of fat & Ca^{2+} are seen in the mass, typical of a teratoma.* **(Right)** *Axial T2 FS MR in the same patient shows the large mixed solid & cystic teratoma of the retroperitoneum. The components of fat & Ca^{2+} are more difficult to separate on this sequence.*

Kaposiform Hemangioendothelioma

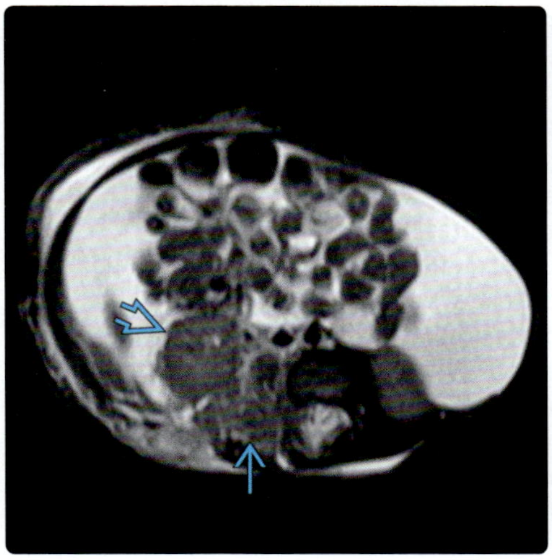

Kaposiform Hemangioendothelioma

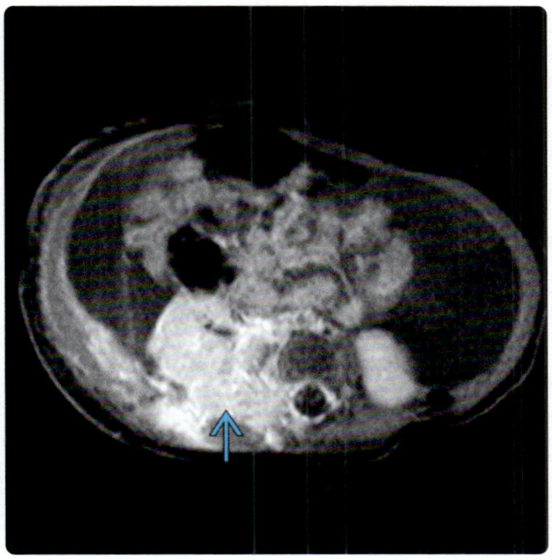

(Left) *Axial T2 FS MR of a 2 month old with abdominal distention & profound coagulopathy shows a poorly defined, infiltrating, intermediate-to-low-signal intensity mass of the right paraspinal musculature & perinephric fat that is inseparable from the right kidney. Note the right flank edema & marked ascites.* **(Right)** *Axial T1 C+ FS MR in the same patient shows vigorous enhancement of the poorly defined paraspinal lesion, typical of a Kaposiform hemangioendothelioma.*

Castleman Disease

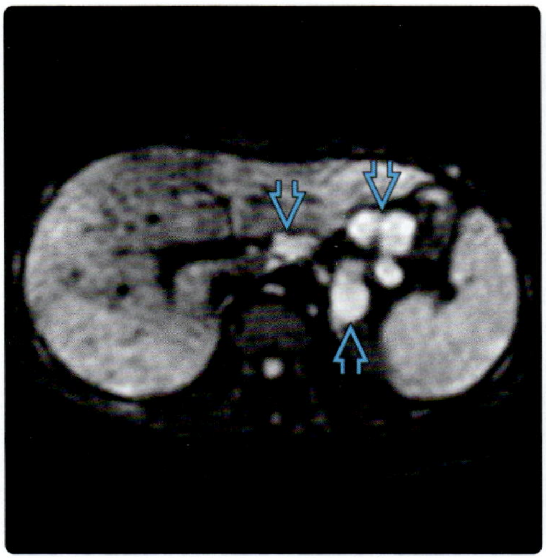

Desmoplastic Small Round Cell Tumor

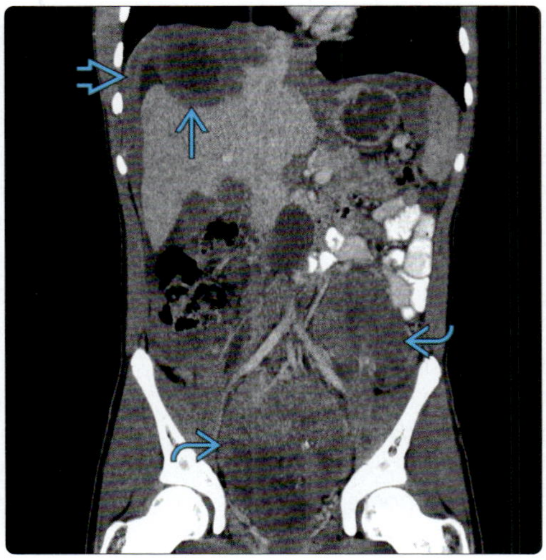

(Left) *Axial DWI MR in a 17 year old with fever, anemia, & elevated sedimentation rate shows multiple enlarged lymph nodes of the peritoneum & retroperitoneum due to Castleman disease.* **(Right)** *Coronal CECT in a 16-year-old boy shows solid, mildly heterogeneous soft tissue masses in the pelvis with ascites, right hemidiaphragm thickening, & a necrotic perihepatic mass. Peritoneal spread of a desmoplastic small round cell tumor was found at surgery.*

DIFFERENTIAL DIAGNOSIS

Common

- Normal Adrenal Hypertrophy of Neonate
- Neuroblastoma
- Adrenal Hemorrhage

Less Common

- Bronchopulmonary Sequestration
- Ganglioneuroma
- Ganglioneuroblastoma

Rare but Important

- Adrenocortical Carcinoma
- Adrenal Adenoma
- Congenital Adrenal Hyperplasia
- Pheochromocytoma
- Wolman Disease

ESSENTIAL INFORMATION

Key Differential Diagnosis Issues

- Pediatric adrenal neoplasms are usually malignant
- DDx for suprarenal mass in fetus or neonate
  - Adrenal hemorrhage, neuroblastoma, pulmonary sequestration
    - Urine/blood will usually show elevated catecholamines in neuroblastic tumors

Helpful Clues for Common Diagnoses

- **Normal Adrenal Hypertrophy of Neonate**
  - At birth, normal adrenal is 10-20x larger than adult gland relative to body weight
    - ~ 1/3 size of neonatal kidney
    - Normal limb thickness < 4 mm
  - Gland decreases in size over first 2 weeks
  - Thick hypoechoic outer layer & echogenic core on US
- **Neuroblastoma**
  - Malignant tumor of primitive neural crest cells
  - Most common solid pediatric extracranial malignancy
    - 2nd most common abdominal neoplasm after Wilms
  - Can arise anywhere along sympathetic chain (neck to pelvis); ~ 65% originate in abdomen
    - 2/3 of these arise in adrenal medulla
  - > 90% of patients are diagnosed at < 5 years of age
    - Median age at diagnosis is 15-22 months
    - Patients < 18 months of age have better prognosis
  - Wide variety of metastatic & paraneoplastic presentations
    - Abdominal mass, pain, or distention remain most common
  - Most common congenital malignancy
    - More commonly adrenal in origin (90%)
    - Metastases to liver, bone marrow, & skin are often present at diagnosis (50%)
    - > 90% survival if congenital; may spontaneously regress
  - Heterogeneously enhancing mass on CECT/MR
    - May be round & well circumscribed or large, multilobulated, & invasive
      - □ Often extends across midline & invades adjacent organs: Spine, kidney, pancreas
    - Ca^{2+} is present in ~ 85% of tumors (by CT)
    - Tends to encase & displace vessels
      - □ Often lifts aorta off of spine
  - 50-70% have metastases at diagnosis
    - Most common to lymph nodes, liver, & bone/marrow
      - □ Hepatic metastases can be diffuse or nodular
  - I-123 MIBG uptake in 90-95% of patients
- **Adrenal Hemorrhage**
  - Most commonly seen in neonates or trauma
    - Most common neonatal suprarenal mass
  - Multiple causes, including perinatal stress &/or hypoxia, trauma, sepsis, coagulopathies, renal vein thrombosis, & Henoch-Schönlein purpura
  - Bilateral in 10%; when unilateral R > L
  - Can be asymptomatic or life threatening
  - US: Avascular mass expanding adrenal gland
    - Acute: Echogenic
    - Subacute: Heterogeneous as it liquefies & contracts
    - Chronic/remote: Normal size ± Ca^{2+} or cyst
  - CECT/MR: Nonenhancing mass enlarging, splaying, or compressing enhancing gland
    - Acute: More dense than simple fluid (CT); variable intensity on MR
    - Subacute: Hypodense (CT); may layer (T2) or bloom (T2*) on MR
    - Chronic/remote: Ca^{2+}
    - CT usually only performed in setting of trauma
      - □ Active extravasation rarely seen
      - □ Look for other abdominal & thoracic injuries
  - Radiographs: May see Ca^{2+} of remote hemorrhage
    - Coarse, irregular, adreniform
    - If any uncertainty, evaluate with US to exclude mass (as bilateral Ca^{2+} may simulate neuroblastoma crossing midline)
  - Short-term (3- to 4-week) follow-up US in neonate to confirm expected evolution of hemorrhage
    - Urine & blood will be negative for excess catecholamines

Helpful Clues for Less Common Diagnoses

- **Bronchopulmonary Sequestration**
  - Congenital anomaly, more commonly in thorax
    - May be prenatally diagnosed in 2nd trimester
  - Nonfunctioning pulmonary tissue
    - No connection to tracheobronchial tree
    - Systemic arterial supply
  - Intralobar: Bronchopulmonary sequestration (BPS) shares pleura with normal lung
  - Extralobar: BPS has separate pleura from normal lung
    - Intraabdominal in 10-15%; may be suprarenal
    - Typically has systemic venous drainage
    - May rarely torse & infarct
  - US: Homogeneously or heterogeneously echogenic
    - Hybrid lesion (with CPAM) may have small cysts
    - Feeding vessel may be visible on prenatal Doppler/MR or postnatal CTA/MRA
- **Ganglioneuroma**
  - Well-differentiated benign neural crest cell tumor

- Neuroblastoma or ganglioneuroblastoma can mature to ganglioneuroma
- Median age at diagnosis is 7 years
- Most common in mediastinum, retroperitoneum, & adrenal gland
- Typically homogeneous on US & CT
  - May have small Ca^{2+} (50%)

- **Ganglioneuroblastoma**
  - Intermediate-grade tumor between ganglioneuroma & neuroblastoma
  - Seen in similar locations as neuroblastoma
  - Has malignant potential

Helpful Clues for Rare Diagnoses

- **Adrenocortical Carcinoma**
  - Median age of 4 years
  - Most are hormonally active
    - Virilization, Cushing syndrome
  - Associated with Beckwith-Wiedemann & Li-Fraumeni syndromes
  - Tumors are usually large at presentation
  - Difficult to differentiate from adenoma in children
    - More common in adrenocortical carcinoma (ACC): Hemorrhage, necrosis, Ca^{2+}, size > 5 cm, invasion of inferior vena cava, & metastases
  - Imaging & age can be similar to neuroblastoma
    - ACC has clinical findings of hormonal stimulation
- **Adrenal Adenoma**
  - Less common (by 2-9x) than ACC in children
  - Most are hormonally active in children
    - Cushing syndrome, precocious puberty, virilization, hypertension
  - Unlike adults, diagnostic criteria are not established
    - Almost always < 8 cm (mean of 4.4 cm in one study) but may still be heterogeneous
    - Do not reliably have high lipid content
- **Congenital Adrenal Hyperplasia**
  - Inborn error of metabolism
    - Defective cortisol & aldosterone synthesis → excess stimulation & hyperplasia of adrenal cortex
  - Typical neonatal presentations
    - Virilization in female patients
    - Salt wasting in male patients
  - Characteristic US appearance
    - Enlarged with cerebriform or wrinkled contour
      - Normal corticomedullary differentiation
      - ≥ 20-mm length, ≥ 4-mm limb thickness
- **Pheochromocytoma**
  - 10-20% of pheochromocytomas occur in children
    - Mean age of 11 years
  - Presents with sustained hypertension, palpitations, sweating, headaches, blurred vision, flushing
  - ~ 40% hereditary vs. 10% in adults
    - von Hippel-Lindau, multiple endocrine neoplasia type 2, neurofibromatosis type 1, familial paraganglioma syndromes
    - More likely to be multifocal
  - 50-85% arise in adrenal medulla
  - Bilateral in 19-38%
  - Variably hyperintense on T2 MR
  - Intense enhancement on CECT/MR imaging
  - Larger tumors may have cystic or hemorrhagic areas
  - I-123 MIBG uptake
  - Less commonly malignant in children
- **Wolman Disease**
  - Rare disorder of lipid metabolism
    - Due to lysosomal acid lipase deficiency
  - Hepatosplenomegaly, jaundice, vomiting, developmental delay
  - Results in enlarged calcified adrenal glands
  - Classically fatal in 1st year of life; stem cell transplant & new enzyme replacements may improve outcomes

SELECTED REFERENCES

1. Swift CC et al: Updates in diagnosis, management, and treatment of neuroblastoma. Radiographics. 38(2):566-80, 2018
2. Sargar KM et al: Imaging of nonmalignant adrenal lesions in children. Radiographics. 37(6):1648-64, 2017
3. Flynt KA et al: Pediatric adrenocortical neoplasms: can imaging reliably discriminate adenomas from carcinomas? Pediatr Radiol. 45(8):1160-8, 2015

Normal Adrenal Hypertrophy of Neonate

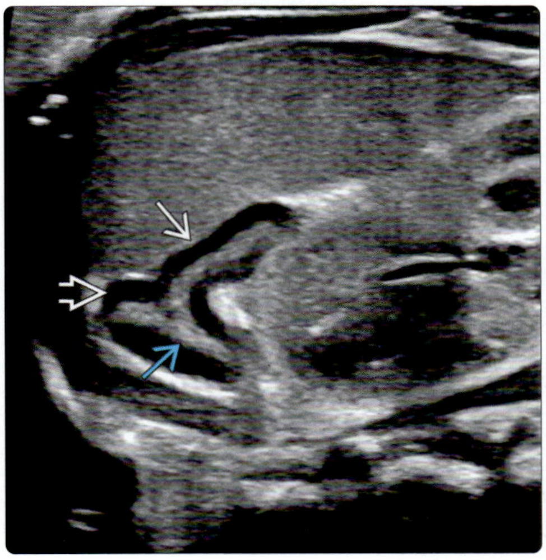

Normal Adrenal Hypertrophy of Neonate

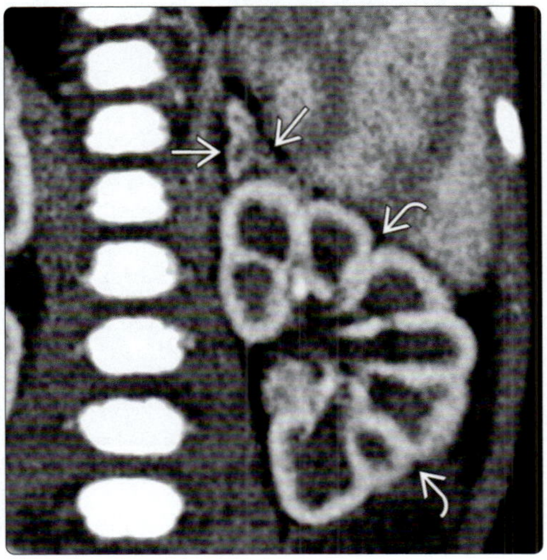

(Left) *Longitudinal ultrasound in a 1-day-old infant demonstrates normal neonatal adrenal hypertrophy ➡ with a hypoechoic cortex ➡ & echogenic medulla ➡. The normal neonatal adrenal gland may be up to 1/3 of the length of the kidney. The normal λ or inverted Y shape is maintained.* **(Right)** *Coronal CECT shows a prominent left adrenal gland ➡ with an enhancing cortex & hypodense core. There is fetal lobation of the left kidney ➡.*

(Left) *AP radiograph in a 3 year old with neuroblastoma demonstrates lobulated, mass-like suprarenal Ca^{2+} bilaterally with inferior extension over the paraspinal soft tissues.* **(Right)** *Axial CECT in the same patient demonstrates a large, heterogeneous mass arising from the right adrenal gland with multifocal coarse Ca^{2+}. Up to 90% of neuroblastomas will have Ca^{2+} by CT.*

Neuroblastoma

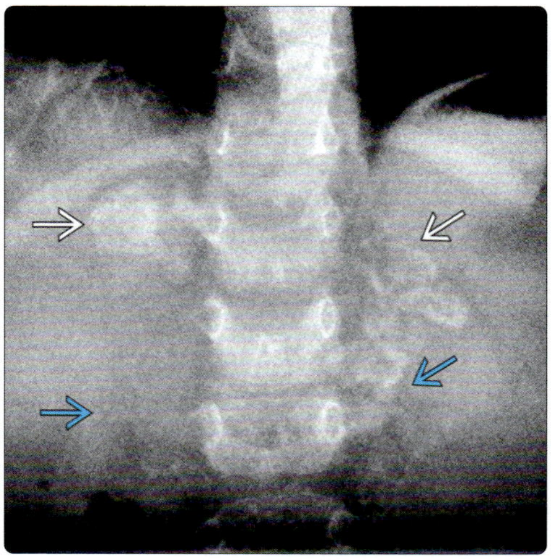

Neuroblastoma

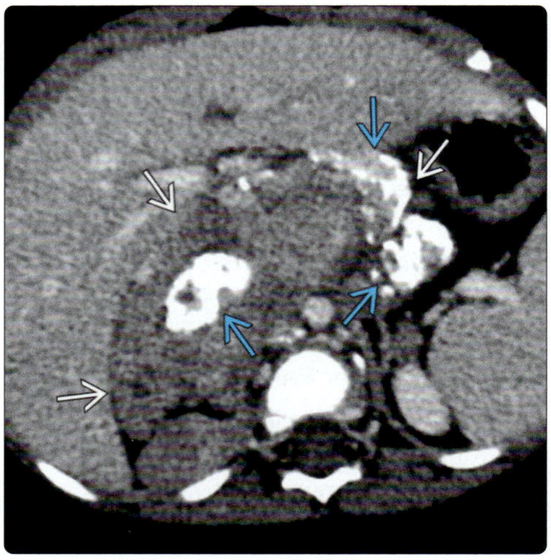

(Left) *Sagittal SSFSE T2 MR of a fetus shows a heterogeneous left suprarenal mass displacing the kidney inferiorly. The differential diagnosis for a suprarenal mass in a fetus is neuroblastoma, adrenal hemorrhage, & bronchopulmonary sequestration (BPS).* **(Right)** *Longitudinal ultrasound in the same patient after birth shows a large, heterogeneously hyperechoic suprarenal mass. The mass still displaces the kidney inferiorly.*

Neuroblastoma

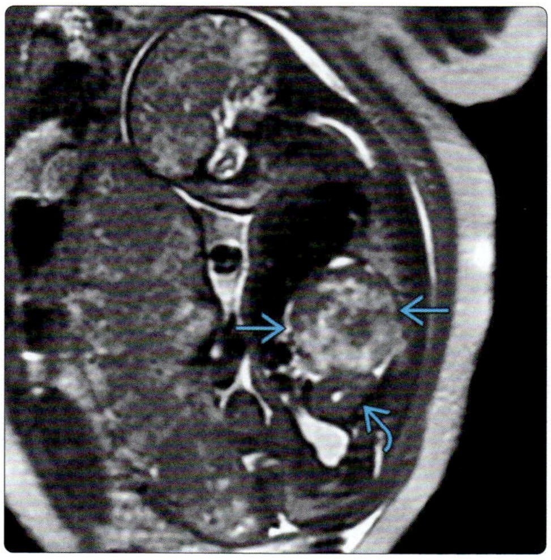

Neuroblastoma

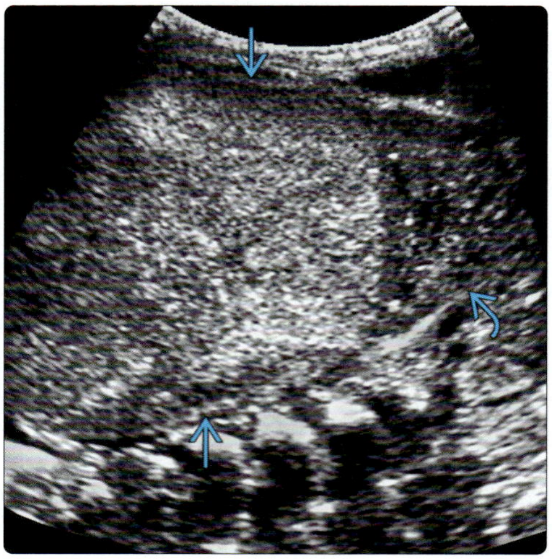

(Left) *Coronal T2 MR in the same patient shows a large, heterogeneous mass displacing the left kidney inferiorly. Neuroblastoma is the most common malignancy in the 1st month of life.* **(Right)** *Coronal PET in the same patient shows FDG uptake in the periphery of the large suprarenal mass. Note the considerable uptake in the brown fat in the upper thorax. Congenital neuroblastoma has a relatively good prognosis & is almost always adrenal in origin.*

Neuroblastoma

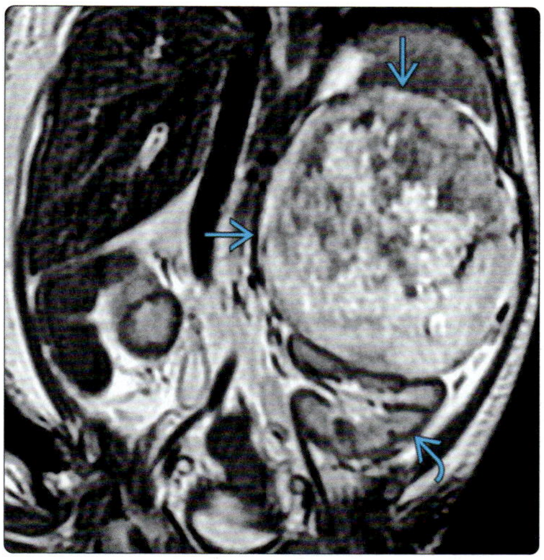

Neuroblastoma

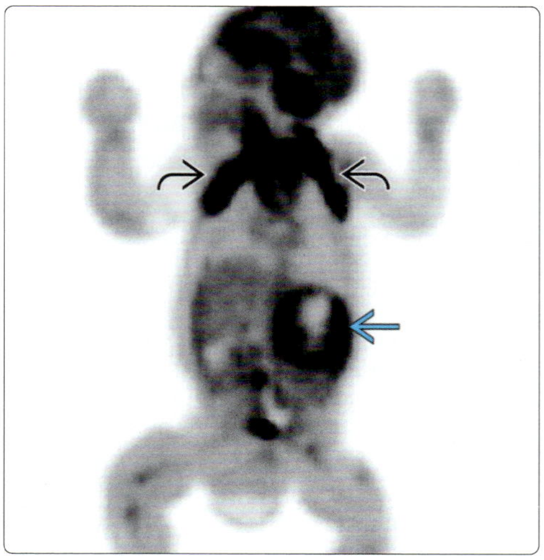

Adrenal Hemorrhage

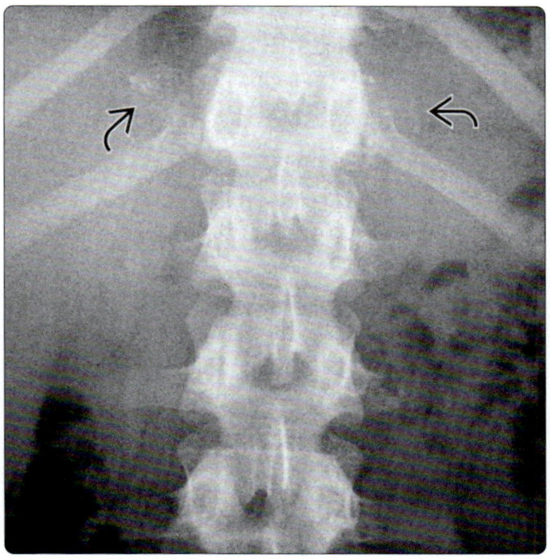

Adrenal Hemorrhage

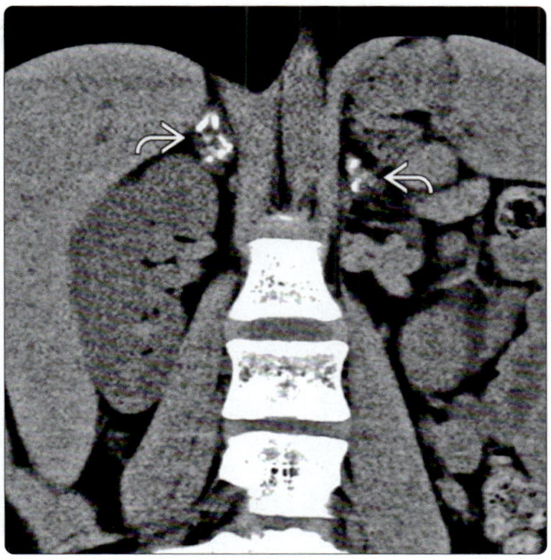

(Left) *AP radiograph shows faint Ca^{2+} in the suprarenal regions bilaterally. Suprarenal Ca^{2+} are most commonly due to neuroblastoma or sequela of adrenal hemorrhage. US or limited CT can be used to distinguish between these causes.* **(Right)** *Coronal NECT shows bilateral adrenal Ca^{2+} without a mass. Specifically, the adrenal glands maintain their adeniform shapes. Note that adrenal hemorrhage is bilateral in 10% of patients.*

Adrenal Hemorrhage

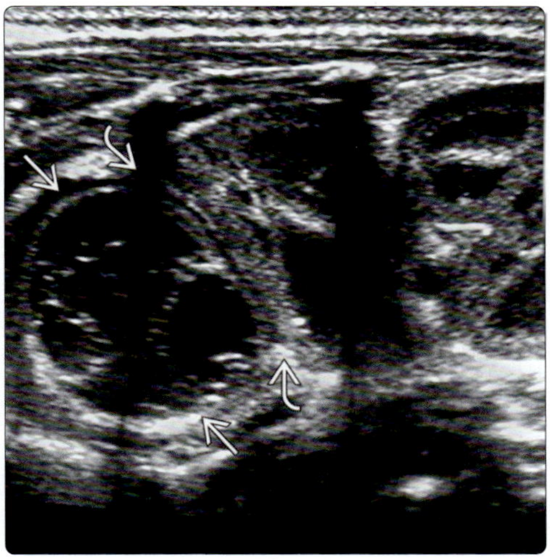

Adrenal Hemorrhage

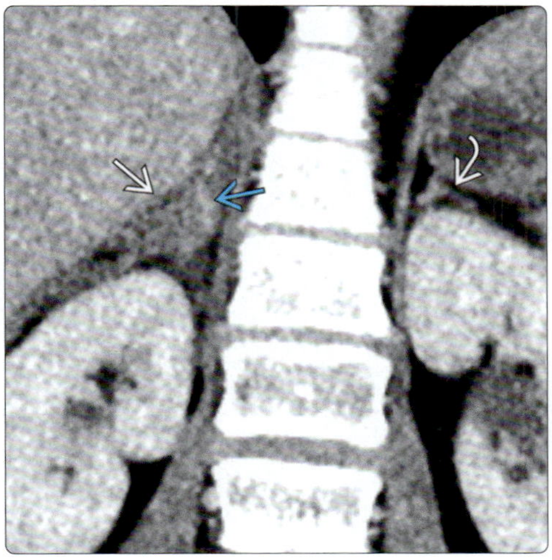

(Left) *Longitudinal ultrasound shows a hypoechoic suprarenal mass with an echogenic rim & internal septations. No internal vascularity was seen on Doppler. The mass distorts the upper pole of the kidney.* **(Right)** *Coronal CECT in a 13 year old in an ATV accident demonstrates ill-defined enlargement of the right adrenal gland, consistent with adrenal hemorrhage. Note the internal hyperdensity. The patient also had a right renal laceration (not shown). The left adrenal gland is normal.*

Bronchopulmonary Sequestration

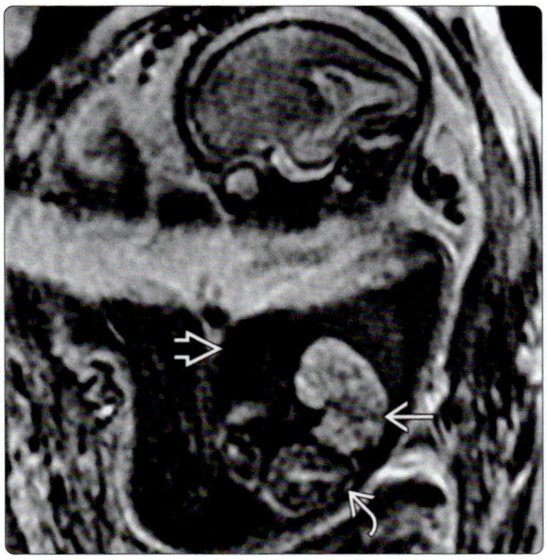

Bronchopulmonary Sequestration

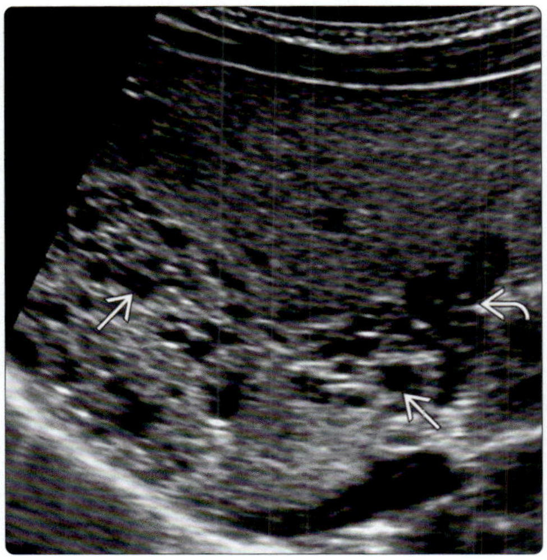

(Left) *Sagittal SSFSE T2 MR of a fetus shows a nonspecific, hyperintense, bilobed right suprarenal mass. The mass deforms the adjacent liver & kidney. Extralobar pulmonary sequestration is intraabdominal in 10-15% of patients.* **(Right)** *Longitudinal ultrasound (after delivery) in the same patient shows an echogenic right suprarenal mass with small anechoic foci. The normal adrenal gland is distinct from the mass. Resection confirmed a BPS.*

(Left) *Axial CECT shows a small, hypodense lesion of the left adrenal gland →. Ganglioneuromas are composed of ganglion cells & schwannian stroma & can arise independently or represent maturation of neuroblastoma or ganglioneuroblastoma.* **(Right)** *Coronal T2 MR shows a linear, hyperintense lesion in the left suprarenal region ↶. Ganglioneuromas present later in life than neuroblastomas with a median age of 7 years at diagnosis.*

Ganglioneuroma

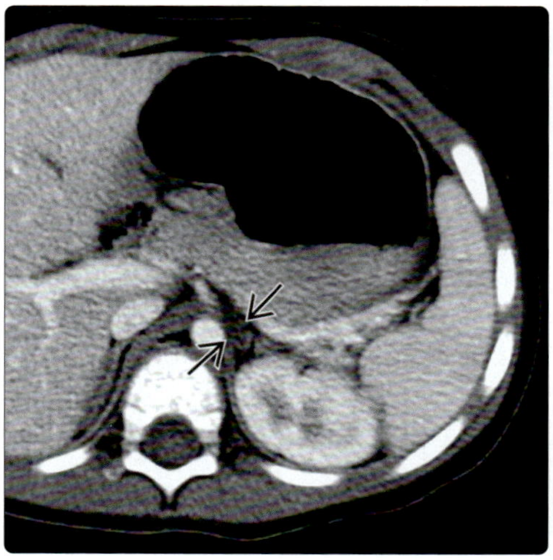

Ganglioneuroma

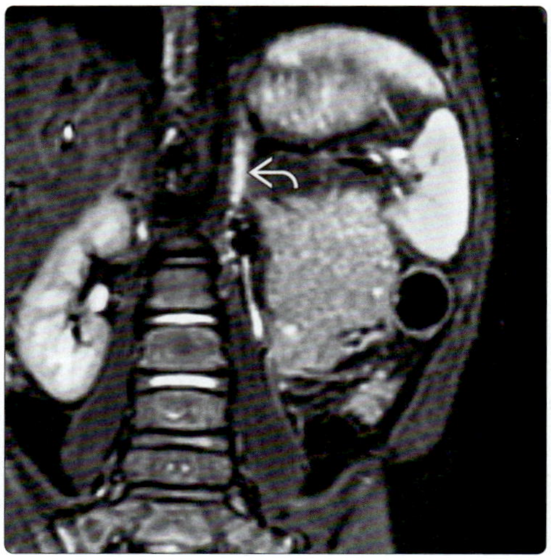

(Left) *Coronal CECT shows a large, heterogeneous mass ➡ surrounding the left renal artery →. Ganglioneuroblastoma has malignant potential & is an intermediate-grade tumor between neuroblastoma & ganglioneuroma.* **(Right)** *MIBG scintigraphy in the anterior & posterior projection shows uptake in the left suprarenal mass → & at the site of injection ↷ in the right shoulder. Ganglioneuroblastoma occurs at the same locations as neuroblastoma.*

Ganglioneuroblastoma

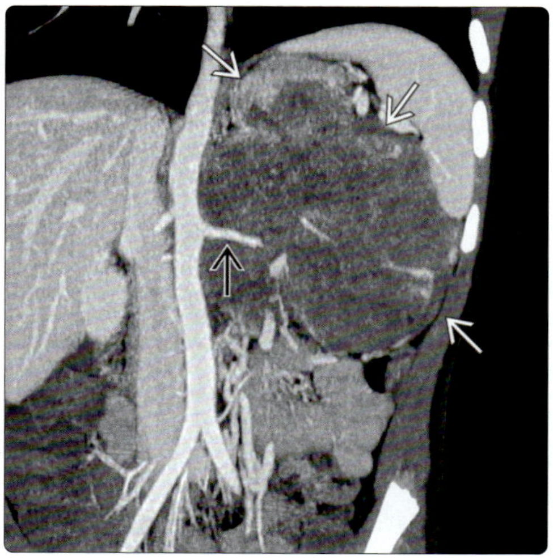

Ganglioneuroblastoma

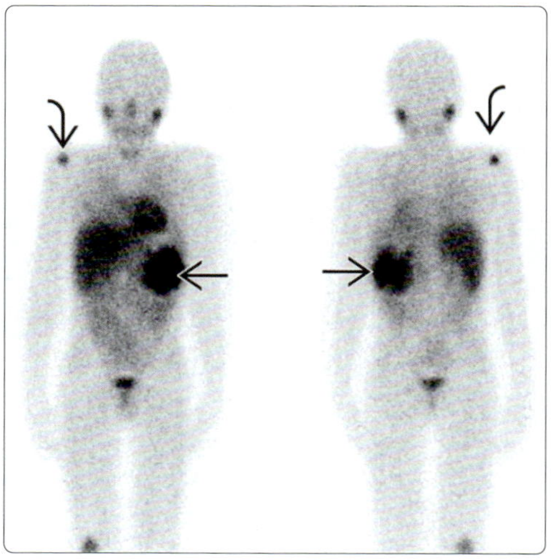

(Left) *Coronal T2 FS MR demonstrates a heterogeneous left suprarenal mass ➡ in a 2-year-old girl who presented with virilization & hypertension. While the age & imaging are most typical of neuroblastoma, the hormonal findings strongly suggest adrenal cortical carcinoma, confirmed at biopsy.* **(Right)** *PET/CT in the same patient demonstrates avid FDG uptake in the mass ➡. This patient was found to have Li-Fraumeni syndrome. ACC is also associated with Beckwith-Wiedemann syndrome.*

Adrenocortical Carcinoma

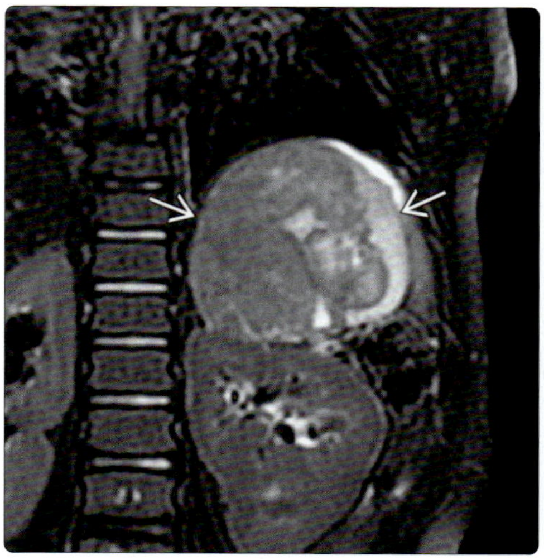

Adrenocortical Carcinoma

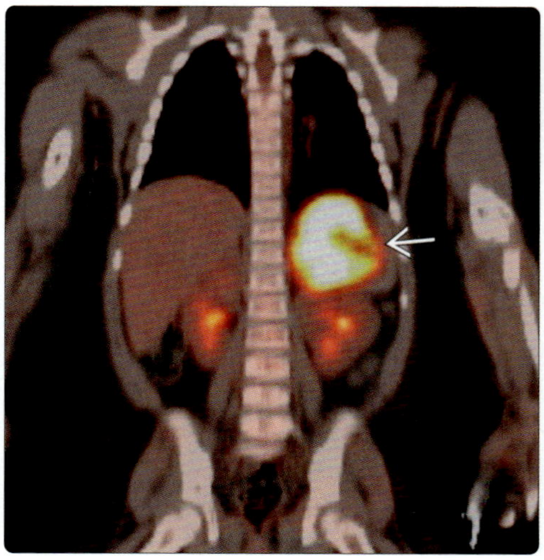

Adrenal Adenoma

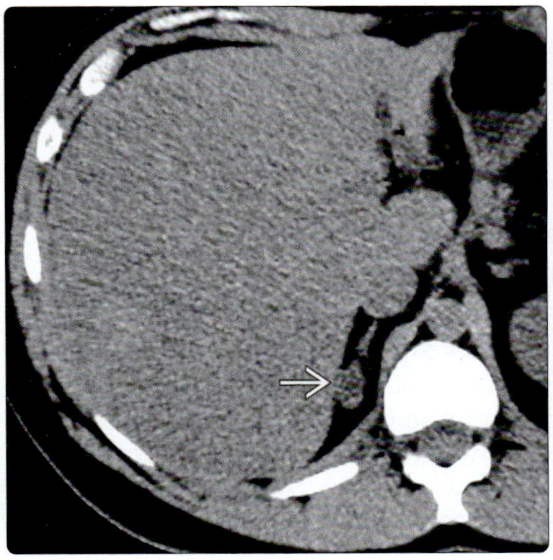

Adrenal Adenoma

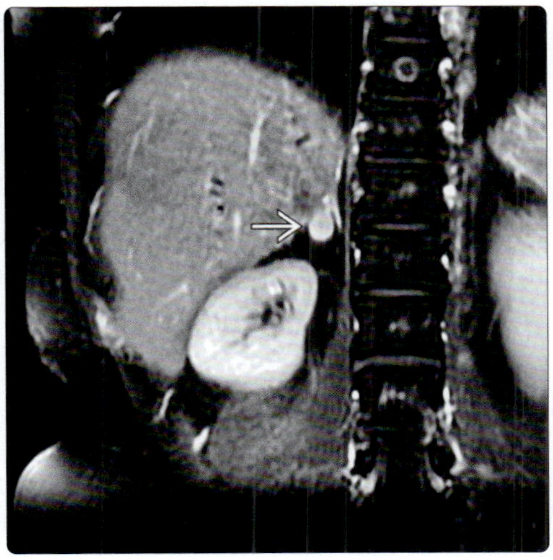

(Left) *Axial NECT shows a slightly hypodense mass* ➔ *arising from the right adrenal gland. This mass was stable in size over several years. Adrenal adenomas are rare in children & much less common than ACC (though the latter tends to be larger & more heterogeneous).* **(Right)** *Coronal T1 C+ FS MR shows an enhancing nodule* ➔ *arising from the lateral arm of the right adrenal gland. Adrenal adenomas are often hormonally active in children. Cushing syndrome is the most frequent presentation.*

Adrenal Adenoma

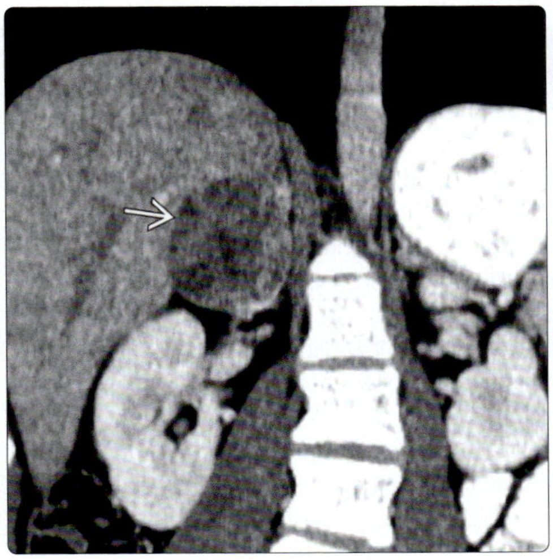

Congenital Adrenal Hyperplasia

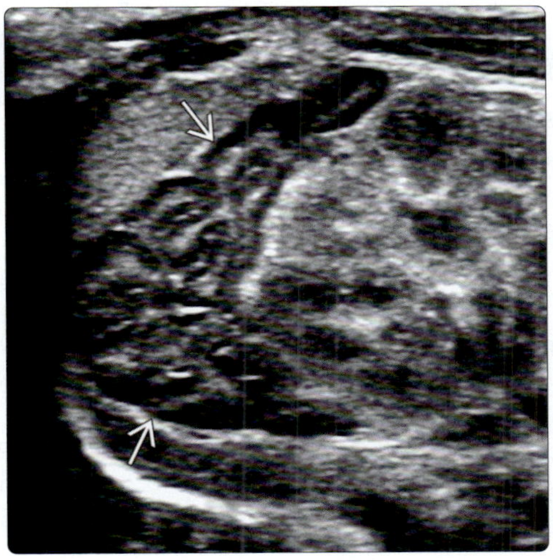

(Left) *Coronal CECT shows a heterogeneous right adrenal mass* ➔ *that measured ~ 5 cm & had grown from a prior study, concerning for malignancy. Differentiation of these entities can be difficult, but this was found to be an adenoma.* **(Right)** *Longitudinal ultrasound in a newborn with ambiguous genitalia shows an enlarged adrenal* ➔ *with the "cerebriform" contour of congenital adrenal hyperplasia. Contrast this with the normal neonatal adrenal, which has a thicker, more hypoechoic cortex & λ shape.*

Pheochromocytoma

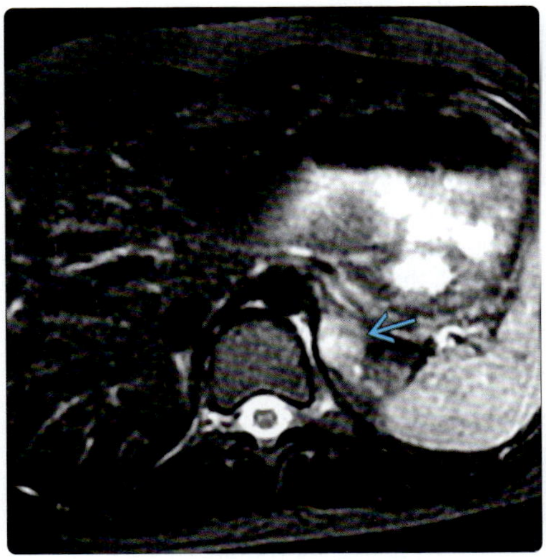

Pheochromocytoma

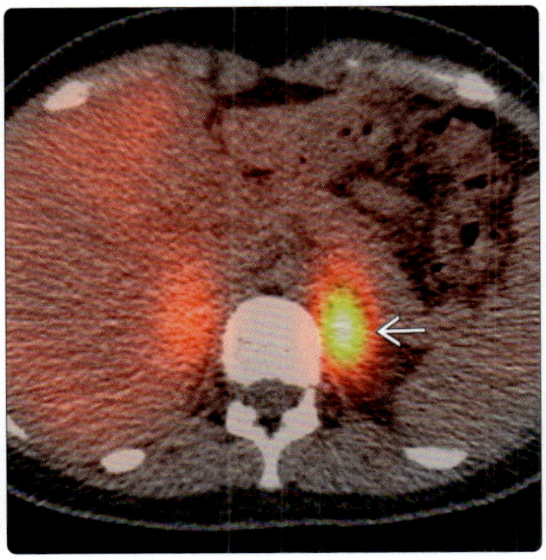

(Left) *Axial T2 FS MR shows a left adrenal nodule* ➔ *in a 16-year-old girl with MEN2A syndrome & elevated plasma metanephrine screening. Pheochromocytoma is often T2 hyperintense.* **(Right)** *Fused axial I-123 MIBG SPECT/CT in the same patient demonstrates intense MIBG uptake* ➔ *in the mass. MEN2A syndrome is also associated with medullary thyroid carcinoma & parathyroid hyperplasia. MIBG can be particularly useful when looking for extraadrenal pheochromocytoma (paraganglioma).*

DIFFERENTIAL DIAGNOSIS

Common

- Pyelonephritis/Abscess
- Wilms Tumor

Less Common

- Congenital Mesoblastic Nephroma
- Renal Cell Carcinoma
- Clear Cell Sarcoma
- Lymphoma
- Nephroblastomatosis
- Angiomyolipoma

Rare but Important

- Rhabdoid Tumor
- Xanthogranulomatous Pyelonephritis
- Renal Medullary Carcinoma
- Metanephric Tumors
- Primitive Neuroectodermal Tumor
- Desmoplastic Small Round Cell Tumor
- Ossifying Renal Tumor of Infancy

ESSENTIAL INFORMATION

Key Differential Diagnosis Issues

- Age is quite helpful, as many imaging features overlap
- Signs/symptoms for solid renal masses are nonspecific: Incidental palpable mass, pain, hematuria, hypertension
- On imaging, "claw" of residual renal parenchyma splayed along tumor margin helps confirm renal origin

Helpful Clues for Common Diagnoses

- **Pyelonephritis/Abscess**
  - Signs/symptoms/labs typically (but not always) include: Fever, flank pain, cloudy urine, leukocytosis
  - Predisposing factors: Vesicoureteral reflux, urinary tract obstruction or anomalies, septic emboli
  - Imaging: Depends on presence of complications
    - Pyelonephritis: Wedge-shaped or sharply demarcated focus/foci of edema/corticomedullary loss/↓ perfusion/delayed enhancement with swelling & perinephric stranding
      - Typically occurs at renal poles
    - Abscess: Heterogeneous necrotic-appearing collection with septa, irregular wall, diminished surrounding enhancement
- **Wilms Tumor**
  - Most common primary childhood renal tumor (> 90%)
  - Age of presentation peaks at 3-4 years; 80% < 5 years
    - Earlier peak for bilateral Wilms at 15 months
  - Associations: Cryptorchidism, hypospadias, sporadic aniridia, & hemihypertrophy
    - WAGR syndrome: **W**ilms, **a**niridia, **G**U anomalies, mental **r**etardation
    - Drash syndrome: Male pseudohermaphroditism, glomerulonephritis
    - Beckwith-Wiedemann syndrome: Omphalocele, macroglossia, organomegaly
  - Imaging: Large, well-circumscribed heterogeneous solid mass, frequently with cystic components; Ca^{2+} in up to 15%; fat is rarely seen
    - Typically hypoenhancing (CT/MR) with intermediate to high T2 & restricted diffusion (MR)
    - Look for capsular rupture with surrounding fluid
    - Up to 10% invade renal vein; ± inferior vena cava (IVC) (& even right atrial) tumor thrombus
    - Multifocal (unilateral or bilateral) hypoenhancing masses suggest underlying nephrogenic rests
    - Metastases: Lungs & regional lymph nodes > liver

Helpful Clues for Less Common Diagnoses

- **Congenital Mesoblastic Nephroma**
  - Most common solid renal tumor in neonates
  - Majority present < 3 months of age; 90% by age 1 year
  - Imaging: May demonstrate polyhydramnios in utero
    - Classic subtype: Homogeneous benign solid mass; ± surrounding hyperechoic/hypoechoic (US) rings with ↑ Doppler flow
    - Cellular subtype: Larger more aggressive tumors with heterogeneity from necrosis/hemorrhage/cysts
      - May show local & distant spread; prone to rupture on resection
- **Renal Cell Carcinoma**
  - 2nd most common pediatric renal malignancy
    - More common than Wilms in 2nd decade of life
  - Reported in ages 6 months to adulthood
  - Imaging
    - Translocation renal cell carcinoma (RCC): Up to 50% of pediatric RCCs
      - Heterogeneous, often with rim Ca^{2+} & nodal spread
    - Clear cell RCC: Associated with von Hippel Lindau (VHL) syndrome
      - Heterogeneous with solid portions showing enhancement similar to renal cortex
      - Look for bilateral tumors + other VHL features: Renal cysts, pancreatic cysts & tumors, spine hemangioblastomas
    - Papillary RCC: Homogeneously hypoenhancing, ± Ca^{2+}
    - Metastases in up to 20% at diagnosis
- **Clear Cell Sarcoma**
  - 2nd most common renal malignancy under age 10 years of age; mean: 3 years of age
  - Imaging: Similar features of mass to Wilms tumor
    - Metastasizes in up to 18% at presentation: Bones, lymph nodes, brain, liver, & lung
      - Bone is uncommon site of spread for Wilms tumor
- **Lymphoma**
  - Primary involvement of kidney is rare
  - Imaging: Multiple hypoenhancing masses (CT/MR); hypoechoic with ↑ through transmission (US)
    - Solitary lesions are uncommon
    - Look for adjacent adenopathy & other visceral lesions (e.g., liver, spleen, bowel, lung/pleura)
- **Nephroblastomatosis**
  - Nephrogenic rests normally persist to 36-weeks gestational age; rests are seen in 1% of infants
  - Give rise to 30-40% of Wilms tumors
  - Found in 99% of bilateral Wilms tumors
  - Imaging: Focal lobular homogeneously hypoenhancing (CT/MR) & hypoechoic (US) masses along cortex or in parenchyma; may create confluent rind of abnormal tissue around distorted kidney

- Increasing size & heterogeneity suggest Wilms tumor
- **Angiomyolipoma**
  - Benign lesions; almost always multifocal & occurring with tuberous sclerosis complex (TSC) in children
  - Mean age of 10 years in TSC
  - Imaging: Intralesional fat is characteristic but solid/vascular components may dominant (fat poor)
    - Fat components: Hyperechoic (US), hypoattenuating (CT), & following fat signal on all MR sequences
      - Opposed-phase MR shows signal drop in fat-poor lesions & "India ink" artifact at margin of angiomyolipoma & renal parenchyma
    - Lesions > 4 cm: ↑ risk of hemorrhage
    - Renal cysts are also common
    - Rare epithelioid subtype is locally invasive & may metastasize in adult population

Helpful Clues for Rare Diagnoses

- **Rhabdoid Tumor**
  - Aggressive tumor with poor prognosis
  - Mean age: 11 months; 80% before 2 years of age
  - 15% have synchronous intracranial neoplasms (atypical teratoid-rhabdoid tumor & others)
  - Imaging: Similar to Wilms; suggestive features of rhabdoid tumors include subcapsular fluid collections, tumor lobulations, & Ca^{2+}
    - Renal vein/IVC extension may occur
    - Metastases are common
- **Xanthogranulomatous Pyelonephritis**
  - Chronic inflammation with obstruction & parenchymal destruction/fibrosis
  - Imaging
    - Diffuse type: Enlarged kidney with loss of corticomedullary differentiation, collecting system dilation, & calculi (often staghorn)
    - Focal type: Cystic/hypoenhancing mass of 1 pole; difficult to distinguish from mass or abscess
    - Perinephric extension may be seen with either type
- **Renal Medullary Carcinoma**
  - Adolescent with sickle cell trait or hemoglobin SC, not hemoglobin SS
  - Mean age of ~ 15 years
    - Under 25 years, M > F (3:1)
  - Extremely aggressive with poor prognosis
  - Imaging: Central, infiltrative, poorly defined necrotic tumor causing caliectasis
    - May mimic renal abscess
    - Enlargement of kidney with preserved renal shape
    - Lymph nodes & perinephric fat are often involved
    - Lymphangitic lung metastases are common
- **Metanephric Tumors**
  - Spectrum of benign tumors
    - Adenomas: Most common; typically occur in adults
    - Adenofibromas: Mean age of 7 years
    - Stromal tumors: Mean age of 2 years
  - Imaging: Well circumscribed, hyperechoic (US), hyperattenuating (NECT), hypoenhancing (CECT or MR), T2 hypointense; foci of Ca^{2+} or hemorrhage are common
- **Primitive Neuroectodermal Tumor**
  - Mean age of 24-27 years
  - Imaging: Often large & poorly defined; variable T2 (MR)
    - May extend into IVC
    - Metastatic disease in up to 50%
- **Desmoplastic Small Round Cell Tumor**
  - Usually occurs as extensive primary peritoneal disease
  - Renal cases: Typically < 20 years of age
  - M > > F (3-5:1)
  - Imaging: Variable
- **Ossifying Renal Tumor of Infancy**
  - Benign extremely uncommon lesion; M > F
  - Imaging: Ca^{2+} 2- to 3-cm mass, may mimic staghorn calculus

SELECTED REFERENCES

1. Chung EM et al: Renal tumors of childhood: radiologic-pathologic correlation part 2. The 2nd decade: from the radiologic pathology archives. Radiographics. 37(5):1538-58, 2017
2. Chung EM et al: Renal tumors of childhood: radiologic-pathologic correlation part 1. The 1st decade: from the radiologic pathology archives. Radiographics. 35(2):499-522, 2016

Pyelonephritis/Abscess

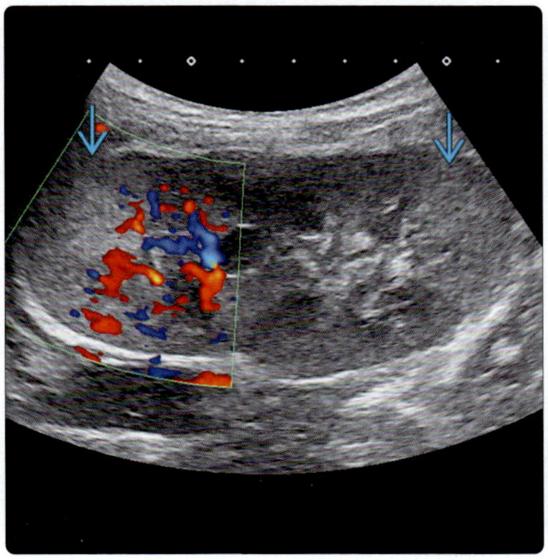

Pyelonephritis/Abscess

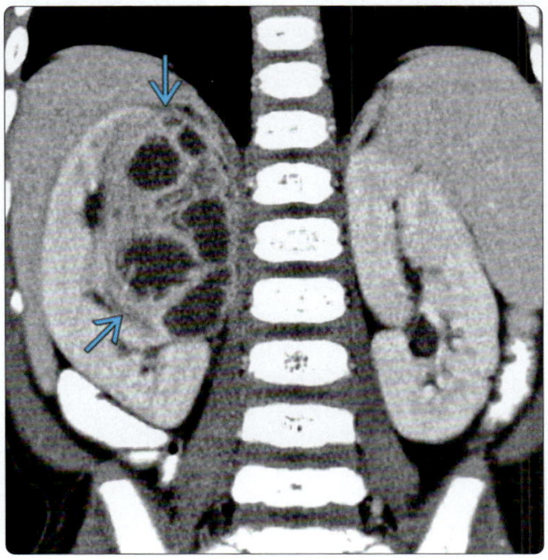

(Left) *Longitudinal color Doppler US in a 7 year old with vomiting, pain, & an Enterococcus urinary tract infection shows an enlarged right kidney with upper & lower pole wedge-shaped foci of increased echogenicity ➔ but decreased vascularity. The findings are typical of pyelonephritis.* **(Right)** *Coronal CECT in a 7 year old with fever shows a complex mass ➔ in the right kidney with fluid-density foci separated by thick, irregular septations due to an abscess. US had shown a less well-defined & more solid appearance to the lesion.*

(Left) *Axial CECT in a 12 year old with fever, pain, & vomiting shows a round fluid-attenuation focus ➔ of the renal parenchyma with a thick irregular wall. Note the adjacent soft tissue stranding ➯.* **(Right)** *Coronal CECT in the same patient shows a round fluid-attenuation focus of the left renal upper pole with an irregular rim & surrounding decreased parenchymal enhancement ➔. There was an adjacent gas & fluid-containing collection ➯ of the spleen with a poorly defined wall. These abscesses were due to septic emboli.*

Pyelonephritis/Abscess

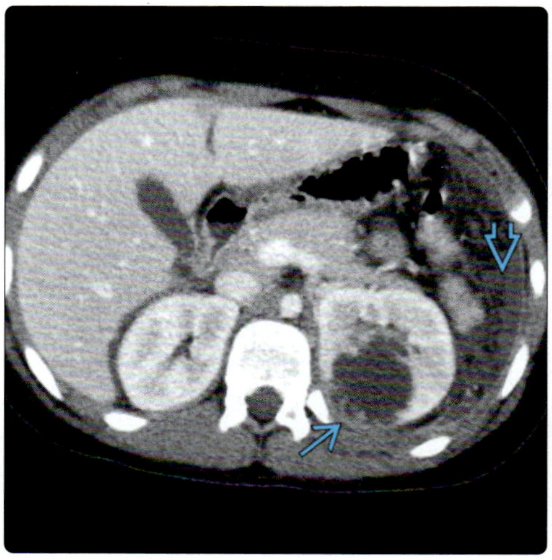

Pyelonephritis/Abscess

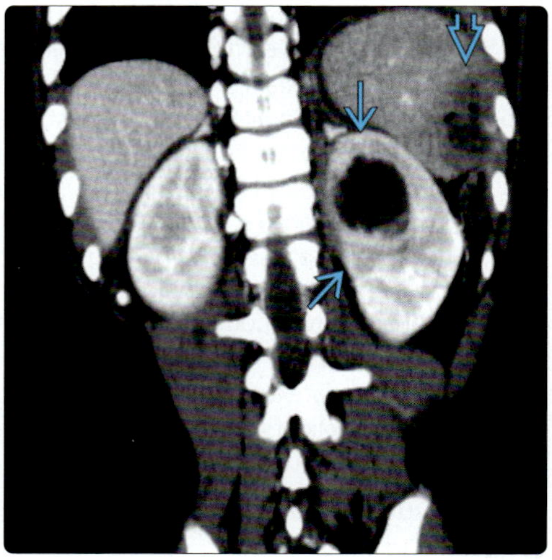

(Left) *AP radiograph in a 4 year old with abdominal distention & a palpable mass shows displacement of the bowel inferiorly by a large left abdominal mass. Note the compressed stomach bubble ➔ shifted into the right abdomen.* **(Right)** *Sagittal T1 C+ FS MR in the same patient shows numerous heterogeneously hypoenhancing solid masses ➯ of the left kidney due to multifocal Wilms tumor arising from nephroblastomatosis. Both of these entities typically show hypoenhancement relative to the kidney.*

Wilms Tumor

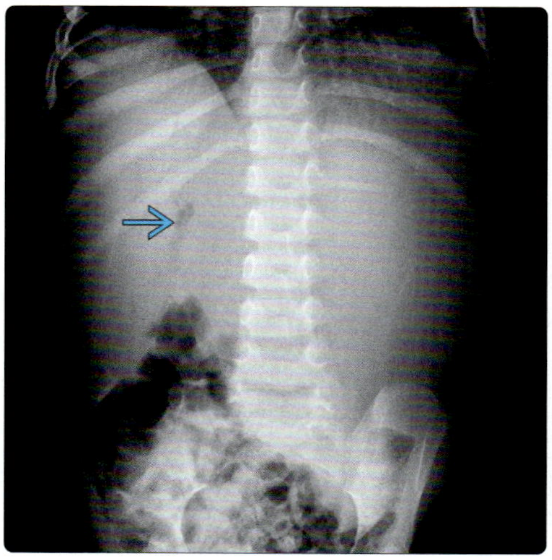

Wilms Tumor

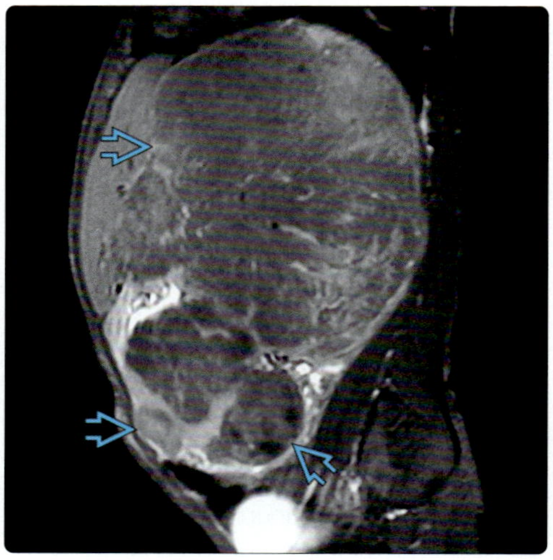

(Left) *Longitudinal color Doppler US in a 6 year old with hematuria shows a hypovascular, round, predominantly solid mass ➔ arising at the upper pole of the right kidney ➯.* **(Right)** *Axial T2 FS MR in the same patient shows cystic & solid foci throughout this large, round right upper pole renal mass ➔. The mass showed restricted diffusion in its solid portions (not shown), consistent with a highly cellular tumor. The patient's age strongly favors a Wilms tumor, confirmed at resection.*

Wilms Tumor

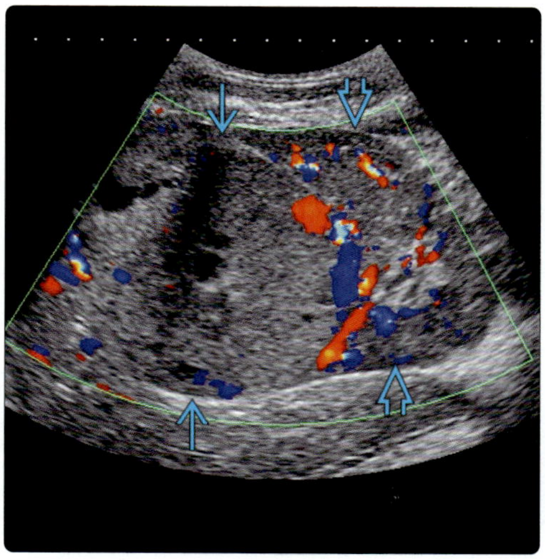

Wilms Tumor

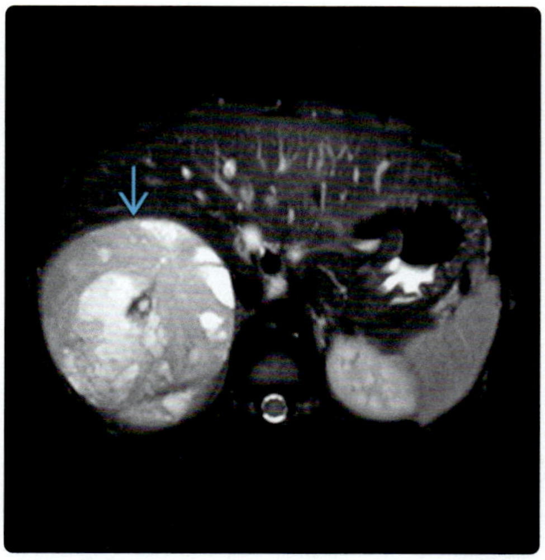

Wilms Tumor

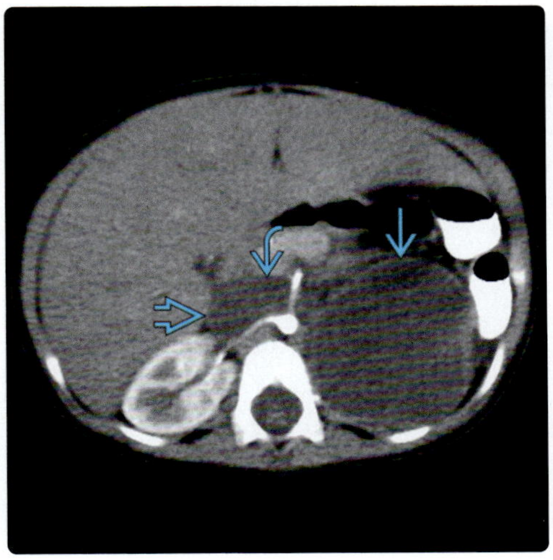

Wilms Tumor

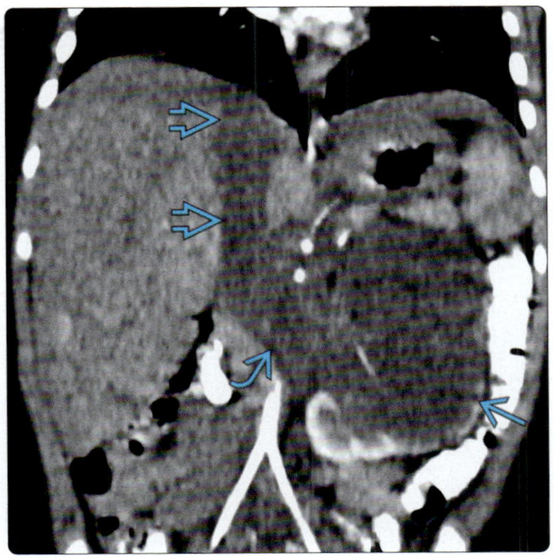

(Left) *Axial CECT in a 2 year old with a hypoenhancing left upper pole Wilms tumor ➡ shows a large tumor thrombus expanding the left renal vein ➡ & inferior vena cava (IVC) ➡. No other renal lesions were identified.* **(Right)** *Coronal CECT in the same patient shows the large hypoenhancing left renal tumor ➡ extending through the left renal vein ➡ into the IVC ➡. A large contiguous tumor thrombus was also present in the right atrium (not shown).*

Wilms Tumor

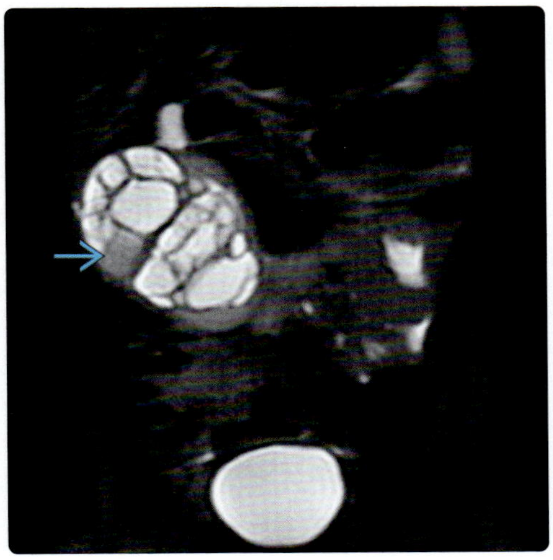

Congenital Mesoblastic Nephroma

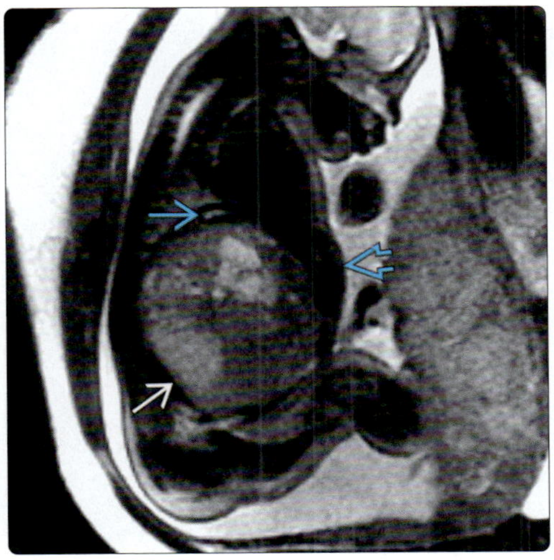

(Left) *Coronal T2 FS MR in a 1 year old shows a predominantly cystic Wilms tumor of the right kidney with a single solid nodule ➡. Wilms tumors often have cystic foci but are rarely predominantly cystic.* **(Right)** *Sagittal SSFSE T2 MR in a 37-weeks-gestation fetus shows a heterogeneous solid & cystic renal mass ➡ displacing the stomach ➡ & liver ➡, suggesting a mesoblastic nephroma (which is the most common renal tumor in neonates).*

Congenital Mesoblastic Nephroma

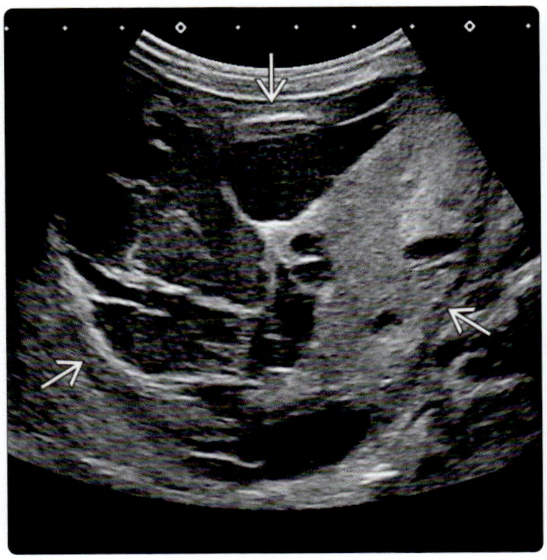

Renal Cell Carcinoma

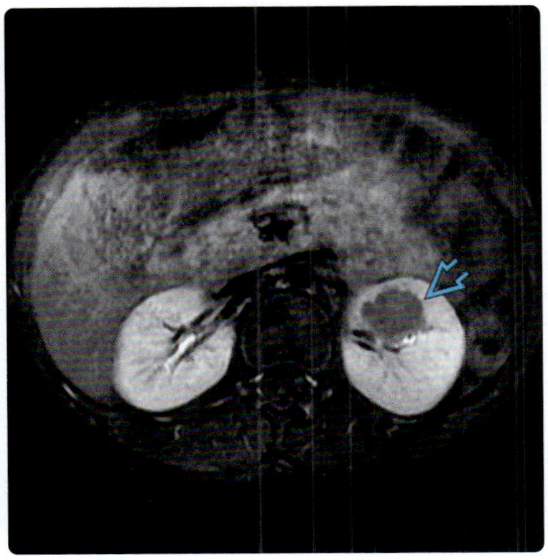

(Left) *Longitudinal US in the same patient after delivery shows a cystic & solid mass ➡ replacing the left kidney. A cellular subtype of mesoblastic nephroma was confirmed upon resection. Cystic foci are common in the cellular subtype of this tumor.* **(Right)** *Axial T1 C+ FS MR in a previously healthy 7 year old with hematuria after trauma shows a mildly lobular hypoenhancing mass ➡ of the anterior interpolar kidney. Other sequences confirmed a solid lesion with restricted diffusion. Resection revealed a papillary renal cell carcinoma.*

Renal Cell Carcinoma

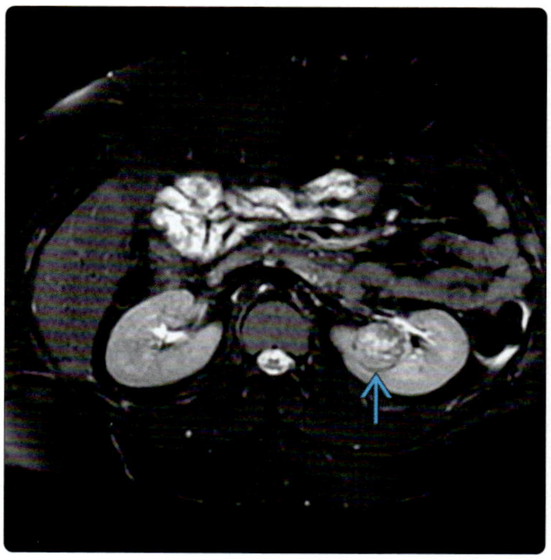

Clear Cell Sarcoma

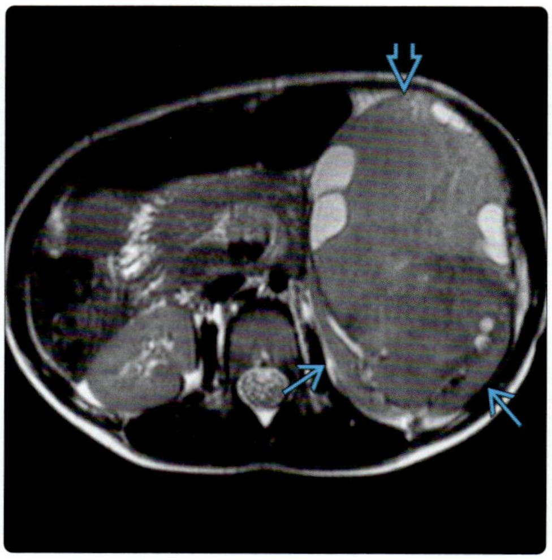

(Left) *Axial T2 FS MR in a 14 year old with von Hippel Lindau (vHL) syndrome shows a heterogeneous mass* → *in the medial left kidney. Resection confirmed a clear cell subtype of renal cell carcinoma (which is typical for pediatric vHL patients).* **(Right)** *Axial T2 MR in a 4 year old with a left upper quadrant mass shows a predominantly solid mass* ⇨ *with scattered cystic foci arising from the left kidney* →*.*

Clear Cell Sarcoma

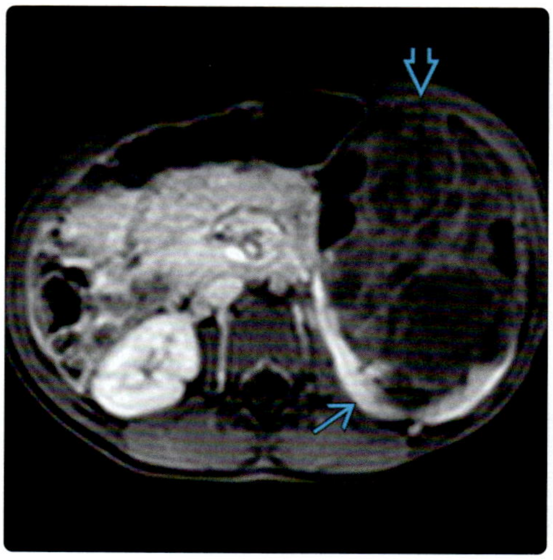

Nephroblastomatosis

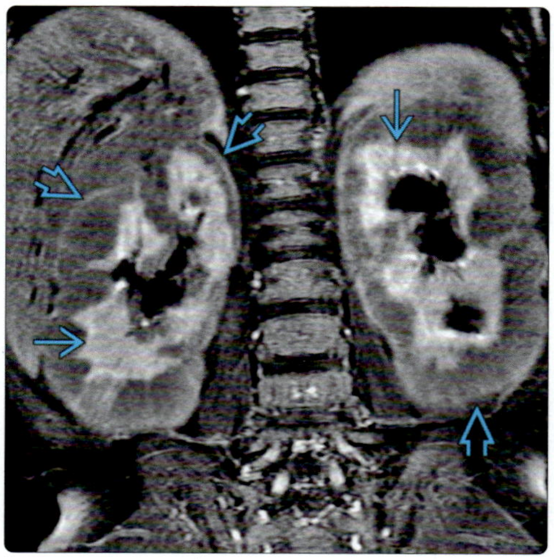

(Left) *Axial T1 C+ FS MR in the same patient shows only mild heterogeneous enhancement of this predominantly solid mass* ⇨ *arising from the left kidney* →*. A clear cell sarcoma was found at biopsy. No bone metastases were identified on nuclear scans.* **(Right)** *Coronal T1 C+ FS MR shows encasement of enhancing (but distorted) renal tissue* → *by a lobular rind of hypoenhancing perilobar nephroblastomatosis* ⇨ *bilaterally. No larger, focal, heterogeneous mass was identified to suggest degeneration to a Wilms tumor at this time.*

Angiomyolipoma

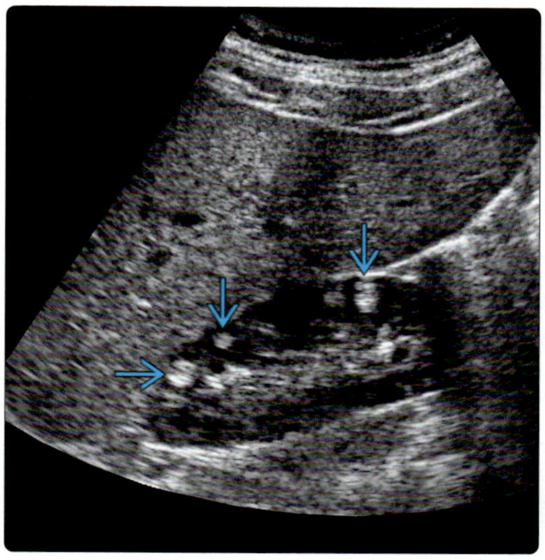

Angiomyolipoma

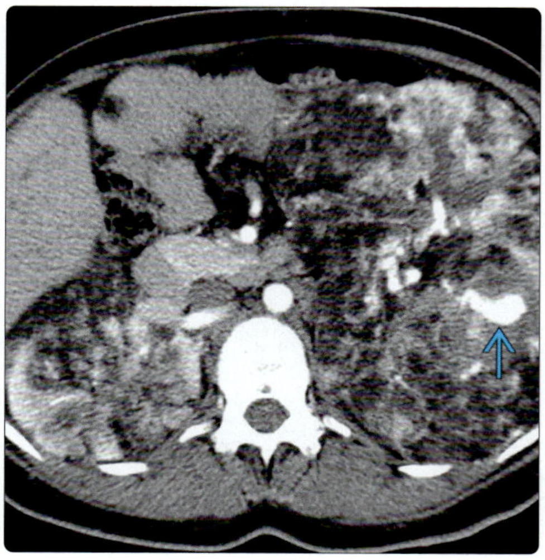

(Left) *Longitudinal US shows multiple small echogenic renal cortical foci* → *without posterior acoustic shadowing in a child with a history of tuberous sclerosis complex (TSC). This is the typical US appearance of small angiomyolipomas. No renal cysts were seen.* **(Right)** *Axial CECT in a teenager with TSC shows extensive fatty renal masses bilaterally, replacing virtually all normal renal parenchyma. An aneurysm* → *was found in a larger mass on the left & was ultimately embolized.*

Rhabdoid Tumor

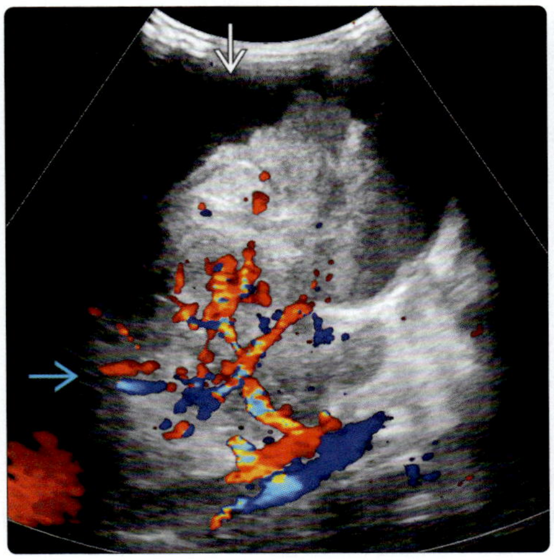

Rhabdoid Tumor

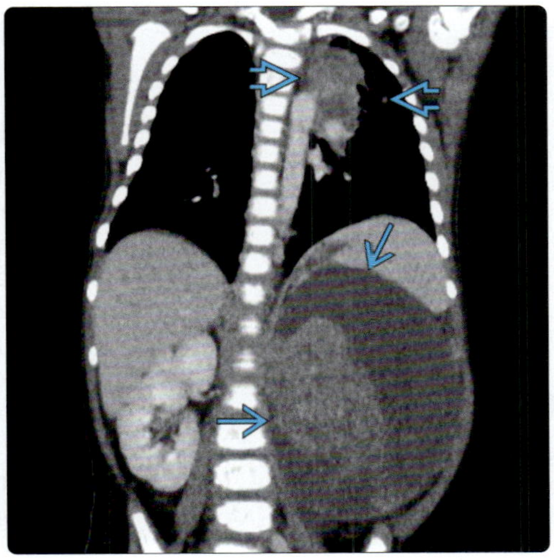

(Left) *Longitudinal color Doppler US in a 1 year old with a large abdominal mass shows a large subcapsular fluid collection overlying a lobulated & highly vascular mass replacing the left kidney. The patient age & findings favor a malignant rhabdoid tumor.* **(Right)** *Coronal CECT in the same patient shows a cystic & solid mass replacing the left kidney. Multiple lung metastases were present in this patient with a renal rhabdoid tumor, but no intracranial lesions were found.*

Renal Medullary Carcinoma

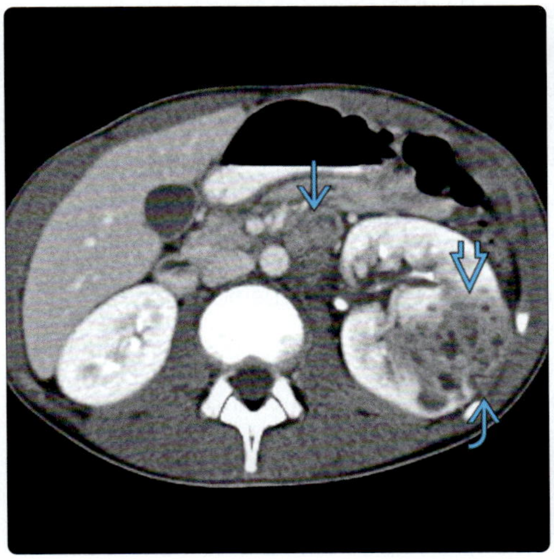

Renal Medullary Carcinoma

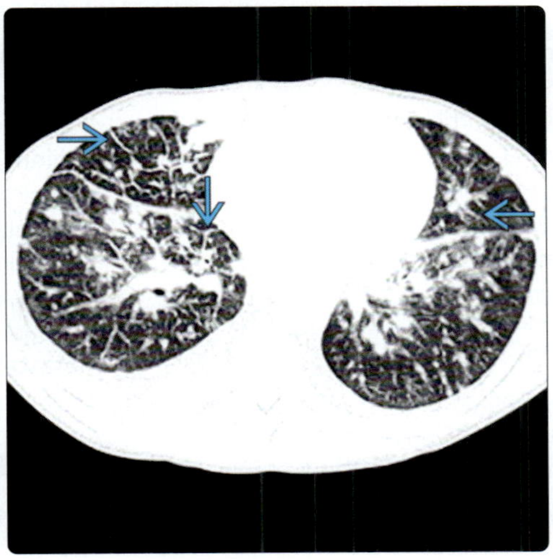

(Left) *Axial CECT in a teenager with flank pain & sickle cell trait shows a heterogeneous, poorly defined infiltrative mass of the left kidney with extracapsular extension & enlarged adjacent lymph nodes. A renal medullary carcinoma (RMC) was ultimately confirmed.* **(Right)** *Axial CECT of the lungs in the same patient shows extensive interlobular septal thickening intermixed with regions of ground-glass opacity. Lymphangitic spread of tumor is common in patients with RMC.*

Primitive Neuroectodermal Tumor

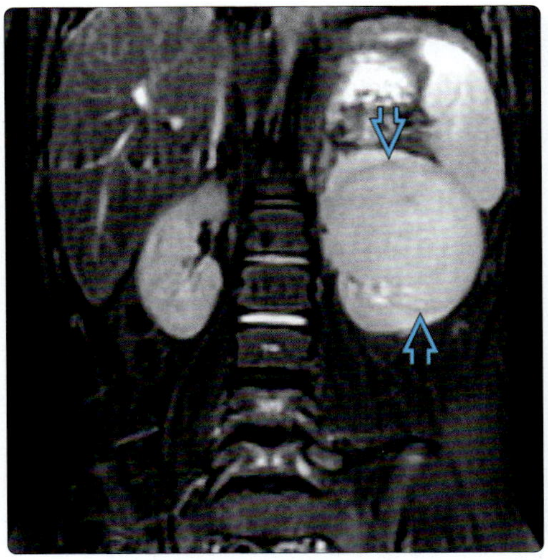

Primitive Neuroectodermal Tumor

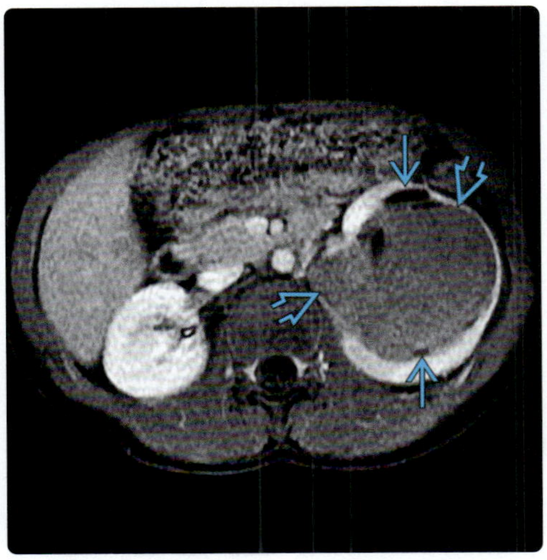

(Left) *Coronal T2 FS MR in a 7 year old shows a solid, round, intermediate-signal-intensity mass of the central left kidney. A renal primitive neuroectodermal tumor was found upon resection.* **(Right)** *Axial T1 C+ FS MR in the same patient shows only mild enhancement of the solid central left renal mass that splays the obstructed dilated calyces. Adjacent subcentimeter lymph nodes were positive for tumor in this patient.*

DIFFERENTIAL DIAGNOSIS

Common

- Pyelonephritis (Mimic)

Less Common

- Nephroblastomatosis
- Lymphoma

Rare but Important

- Wilms Tumors
- Angiomyolipomas
- Metastases

ESSENTIAL INFORMATION

Key Differential Diagnosis Issues

- Major determinants
  - Age
    - < 5 years: More likely nephroblastomatosis ± multifocal Wilms
    - > 5 years: Lymphoma more likely
  - Morphology
    - Discrete, bulging, &/or exophytic masses: Wilms, angiomyolipomas
    - Vague renal enlargement (particularly by ultrasound): Pyelonephritis, lymphoma, nephroblastomatosis
      - These may also lead to discrete masses
  - Involvement of other viscera
    - Bowel, spleen, lymph nodes, pleura: Lymphoma
    - Lymph nodes, renal vein/inferior vena cava: Wilms
    - Liver & lung in both
  - Underlying syndrome
    - Tuberous sclerosis (TS): Angiomyolipomas
    - Beckwith-Wiedemann, WAGR, Denys-Drash, others: Nephroblastomatosis ± multifocal Wilms

Helpful Clues for Common Diagnoses

- **Pyelonephritis (Mimic)**
  - Typically occurs with febrile urinary tract infection & costovertebral angle tenderness, but not always
  - Wedge-shaped peripheral foci of decreased perfusion/enhancement & increased echogenicity
    - Single or multifocal, unilateral or bilateral
  - Some lesions may develop multicystic mass (abscess) with irregular thick rim & surrounding inflammation

Helpful Clues for Less Common Diagnoses

- **Nephroblastomatosis**
  - Discrete homogeneous masses of persistent primitive metanephric blastema within or around kidneys; may form plaque of tissue encasing kidneys
  - Best seen as uniform hypoenhancing masses surrounding/distorting normally enhancing renal parenchyma on CECT or MR
  - Disproportionately large & heterogeneous masses suggest transformation to Wilms (solitary or multifocal)
- **Lymphoma**
  - Numerous typically homogeneous solid round or irregular hypoenhancing masses
  - Multiple nodal groups are typically involved at diagnosis ± spleen, bowel, liver, lungs/pleura

Helpful Clues for Rare Diagnoses

- **Wilms Tumors**
  - Large, heterogeneous solid renal mass in young child
  - Multifocality occurs in setting of nephroblastomatosis
- **Angiomyolipomas**
  - Typically occurs in TS with numerous renal cysts
  - Usually contain macroscopic fat but may be fat poor by imaging
    - In-/out-of-phase MR may help demonstrate fat not visible on other sequences
- **Metastases**
  - Quite uncommon outside of lymphoma

SELECTED REFERENCES

1. Chung EM et al: Renal tumors of childhood: radiologic-pathologic correlation part 2. The 2nd decade: from the radiologic pathology archives. Radiographics. 37(5):1538-58, 2017
2. Chung EM et al: Renal tumors of childhood: radiologic-pathologic correlation part 1. The 1st decade: from the radiologic pathology archives. Radiographics. 36(2):499-522, 2016

Pyelonephritis (Mimic)

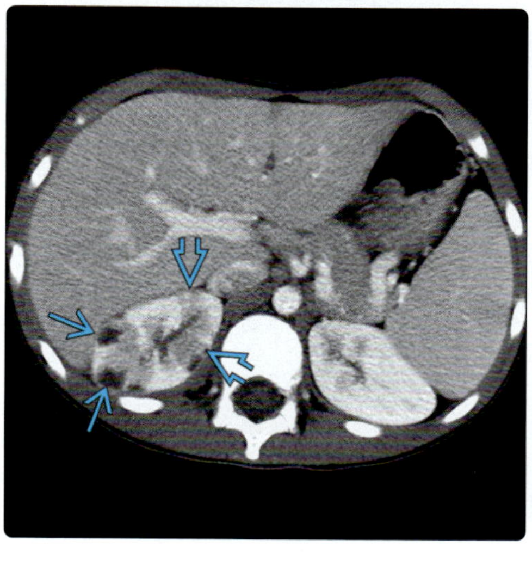

Pyelonephritis (Mimic)

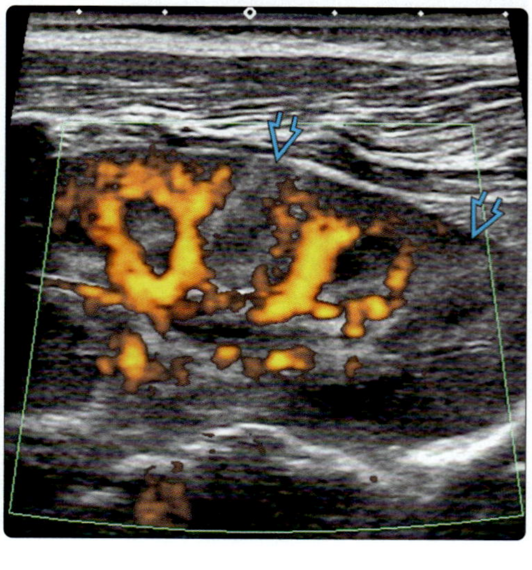

(Left) *Axial CECT in a 12 year old with right flank pain & fever shows multifocal wedge-shaped regions of diminished enhancement ➡ in the right kidney, some of which contain cystic-appearing foci →. The urinalysis confirmed pyelonephritis.* **(Right)** *Longitudinal power Doppler ultrasound in a 4 year old with fever & infected urine shows several regions of increased cortical echogenicity & decreased perfusion ➡, typical of pyelonephritis.*

Nephroblastomatosis

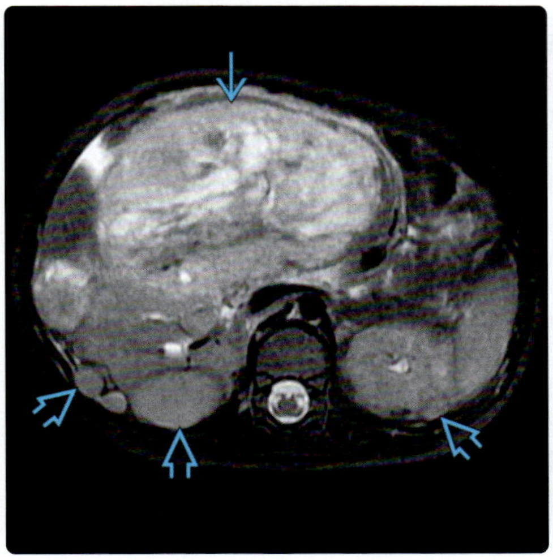

Nephroblastomatosis

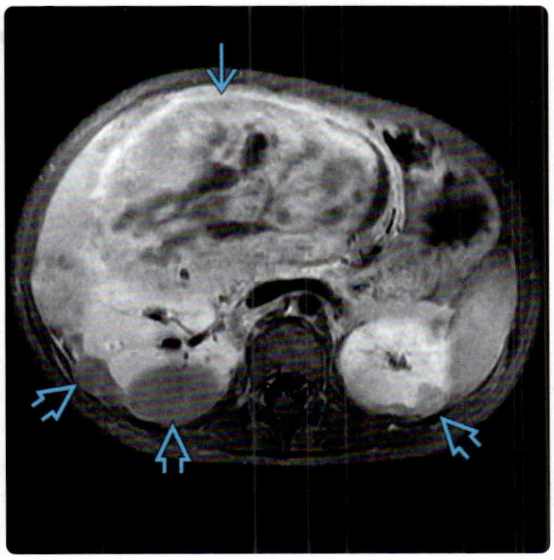

(Left) *Axial T2 FS MR in a 3 year old with an abdominal mass shows numerous ovoid lesions of largely homogeneous intermediate signal intensity along the renal cortex bilaterally, typical of nephroblastomatosis. There is a larger heterogeneous Wilms tumor arising from the anterior right kidney.* **(Right)** *Axial T1 C+ FS MR in the same child shows uniform hypoenhancement of the foci of nephroblastomatosis. However, the Wilms tumor shows heterogeneous enhancement.*

Nephroblastomatosis

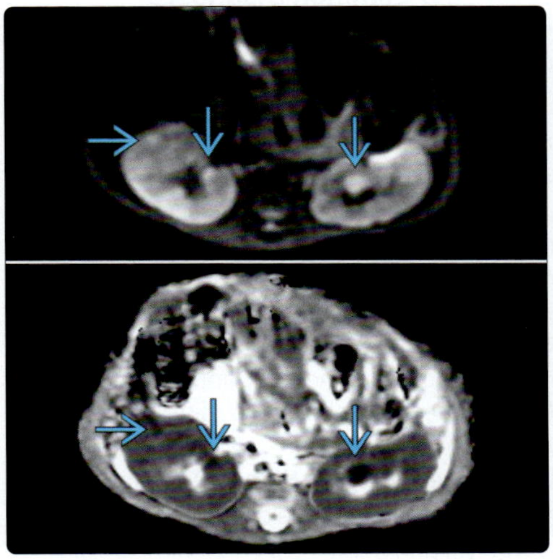

Lymphoma

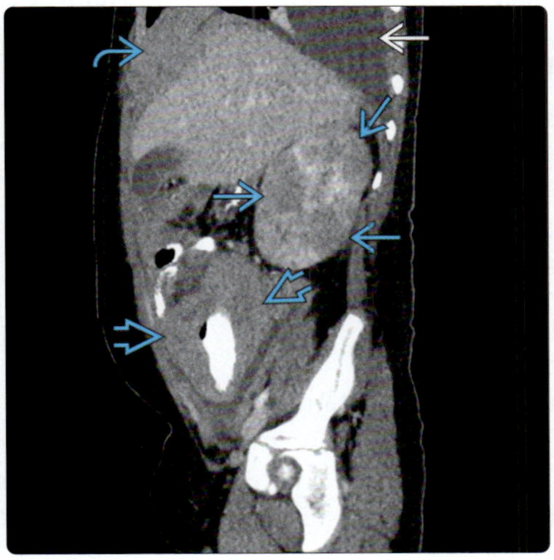

(Left) *Axial DWI (top) & ADC (bottom) MR images in a 24 day old with hepatomegaly show restricted diffusion within numerous small round hypoenhancing (not shown) renal lesions, typical of nephroblastomatosis. This patient was ultimately determined to have Beckwith-Wiedemann syndrome.* **(Right)** *Sagittal CECT in an 8 year old with abdominal pain shows multifocal hypoenhancing masses in the right kidney. There is also bowel wall, & diaphragmatic, & pleural disease in this patient with Burkitt lymphoma.*

Angiomyolipomas

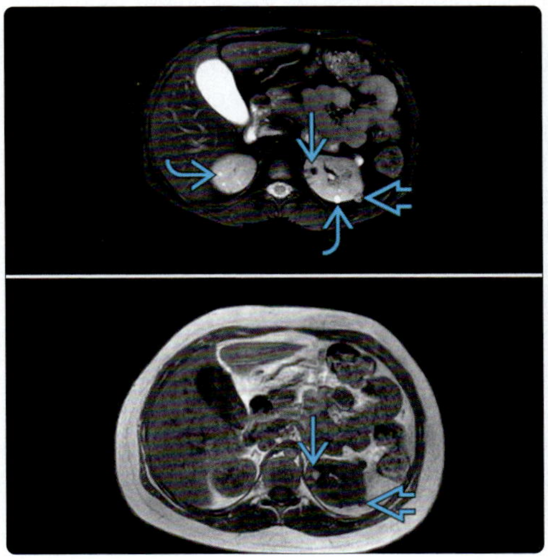

Metastases

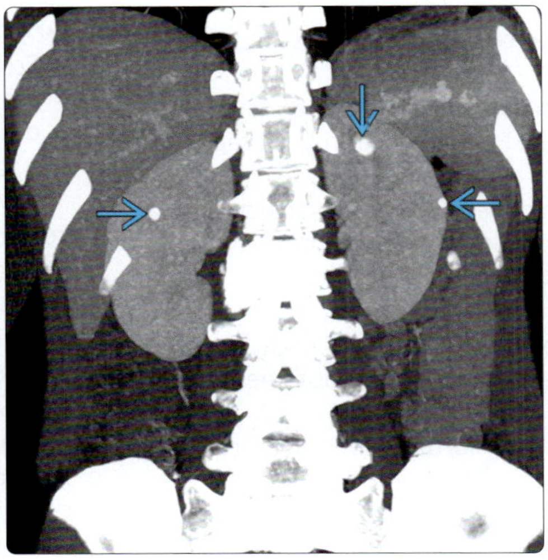

(Left) *Axial T2 FS (top) & in-phase T1 (bottom) MR images in a 9 year old with tuberous sclerosis show bilateral renal lesions, including cysts. A typical angiomyolipoma (AML) follows fat signal intensity on both sequences, though a fat-poor AML shows intermediate signal intensity.* **(Right)** *Coronal CECT MIP image in an 18 year old with a humeral osteosarcoma demonstrates multiple calcified lesions in the the bilateral kidneys, confirmed to be metastases.*

DIFFERENTIAL DIAGNOSIS

Common

- Simple Renal Cyst
- Calyceal Diverticulum
- Cystic Renal Dysplasia
- Multicystic Dysplastic Kidney
- Ureteropelvic Duplications (Mimic)

Less Common

- Abscess
- Autosomal Recessive Polycystic Kidney Disease
- Autosomal Dominant Polycystic Kidney Disease
- Tuberous Sclerosis Complex

Rare but Important

- Medullary Cystic Kidney Disease Complex
- von Hippel-Lindau
- Acquired Cystic Kidney Disease
- Congenital Mesoblastic Nephroma
- Wilms Tumor
- Multilocular Cystic Renal Tumors

ESSENTIAL INFORMATION

Key Differential Diagnosis Issues

- Number & size of cysts, bilaterality, & appearance of background renal parenchyma help direct differential
  - Scattered, relatively small simple cysts (micro- vs. macrocysts) vs. single large cystic/multicystic renal mass
  - Normal vs. abnormal kidney otherwise (size, echogenicity, additional lesions)
  - Unilateral vs. bilateral process
- In utero severe bilateral renal diseases → ↓ fetal urine production → oligohydramnios → pulmonary hypoplasia → ↓ survival

Helpful Clues for Common Diagnoses

- **Simple Renal Cyst**
  - Imaging: Smooth, well-circumscribed, round lesion with thin imperceptible wall & no internal complexity (i.e., nodularity, septation, vascularity, or Ca^{2+})
    - Posterior acoustic enhancement on US; does not enhance on CT or MR
    - Complexity requiring further work-up: Wall thickness > 1 mm, nodularity or soft tissue, vascularity, > 4 septa, septa > 1 mm thick
  - ~ 8% risk of autosomal dominant (AD) polycystic kidney disease for incidental pediatric renal cysts; more likely if larger (22 vs. 13 mm), growing, or multiple
- **Calyceal Diverticulum**
  - Urine-filled eventration of calyx into renal parenchyma, connected by narrow channel; typically unifocal; mean size of ~ 1 cm
  - Imaging: Smooth, round to ovoid, thin walled; abuts calyx
    - May contain stones or debris; delayed filling by contrast is diagnostic
- **Cystic Renal Dysplasia**
  - Abnormal renal development due to chronic injury
  - Most commonly secondary to in utero bladder outlet obstruction, such as posterior urethral valves
  - Imaging: Diffusely ↑ parenchymal echogenicity with scattered cysts, most commonly small & peripheral; may be unilateral or bilateral
- **Multicystic Dysplastic Kidney**
  - Congenital anomaly of nonfunctioning tissue; considered as most common & severe subtype of cystic dysplasia
  - Typically unilateral; bilateral is usually fatal
  - Imaging: Noncommunicating cysts of varying size replace renal parenchyma; no functional tissue remains
    - Often has residual intervening echogenic parenchyma
    - Lacks uptake on nuclear medicine renal scan
    - Involutes over months/years
    - May only involve part of kidney if duplicated
  - Contralateral ureteropelvic junction obstruction or vesicoureteral reflux (VUR) in up to 40%
- **Ureteropelvic Duplications (Mimic)**
  - Upper pole of completely duplicated system tends to obstruct due to ectopic ureteral insertion or ureterocele
    - May result in hydronephrosis &/or cystic dysplasia
  - Lower pole has high incidence of VUR

Helpful Clues for Less Common Diagnoses

- **Abscess**
  - Signs/symptoms/labs typically (but not always) include fever, flank pain, cloudy urine, leukocytosis
  - Predisposing factors: VUR, urinary tract obstruction or anomalies, septic emboli
  - Imaging: Depends on presence of complications
    - Pyelonephritis: Wedge-shaped or sharply demarcated focus/foci of edema/corticomedullary loss/↓ perfusion/delayed enhancement with swelling & perinephric stranding (typically occurs at renal poles)
    - Abscess: Heterogeneous necrotic-appearing collection with septa, irregular wall, diminished surrounding enhancement
- **Autosomal Recessive Polycystic Kidney Disease**
  - Most common inherited infantile cystic renal disease
  - Ciliopathy with varying degrees of congenital hepatic fibrosis & Caroli disease
  - Imaging: Bilateral, enlarged microcystic kidneys with ↓ corticomedullary differentiation & ↓ amniotic fluid index (AFI)
    - Ectatic collecting ducts create innumerable radiating linear hypoechoic foci & may ↑ medullary echogenicity (due to more interfaces)
    - ± scattered macrocysts; may bulge flanks & displace bowel centrally
- **Autosomal Dominant Polycystic Kidney Disease**
  - Ciliopathy, which rarely manifests in childhood
    - Typically found when screening family members or during routine in utero US; may present with hypertension in child
  - 5-15% are sporadic mutations
  - 50% have renal cysts in 1st decade, 72% in 2nd
  - Manifestations during lifetime: Renal cysts (100%), liver cysts (50%), pancreatic cysts (9%), cardiac valvular disease (26%), cerebral aneurysms (5-10%)
  - Imaging: Small simple cysts (of cortex & medulla) early, unilateral or bilateral; gradual ↑ in size, number, & complexity of cysts, ultimately causing renal enlargement

- Prenatal: Normal to mildly enlarged kidneys with preserved or accentuated corticomedullary differentiation, scattered cysts, & normal AFI
  - May rarely present with appearance of autosomal recessive polycystic kidney disease in setting of homozygous *PKD* mutations: Bilateral marked renal enlargement with diffusely ↑ echogenicity, scattered tiny cysts, & anhydramnios
- **Tuberous Sclerosis Complex**
  - Neurocutaneous syndrome: Hamartomatosis
  - AD inheritance; 66% with sporadic mutation
  - Classic clinical triad (only present in ~ 33%): Adenoma sebaceum, seizures, & intellectual disability
  - Imaging: Bilateral cysts of varying size
    - Look for additional fatty renal lesions (angiomyolipomas): May be small; less common than cysts in children
    - Other commonly affected organs: Brain, heart, lung, bones, skin

Helpful Clues for Rare Diagnoses

- **Medullary Cystic Disease Complex**
  - Ciliopathies with many genetic mutations, traditionally classified as nephronophthisis or medullary cystic disease
  - Imaging: Kidneys are normal in size or small with poor corticomedullary differentiation & small cysts
    - Medullary cystic disease: Cysts are clustered in medulla with relative cortical sparing
    - Nephronophthisis: Corticomedullary cysts, associated with various syndromes (Joubert, Meckel-Gruber, Bardet-Biedl, Jeune)
- **von Hippel-Lindau**
  - AD neurocutaneous syndrome of cysts & tumors
  - Imaging: Renal cysts & renal cell carcinoma (RCC), pheochromocytoma, CNS hemangioblastomas, pancreatic cysts & neoplasms
- **Acquired Cystic Kidney Disease**
  - Classically develops in native kidneys while on dialysis, but may be seen in chronic renal disease prior to dialysis or after transplant
    - Cysts ↑ with length of time on dialysis
  - Defined by ≥ 3 cysts in each kidney (adults) &/or new renal cysts (children) in vulnerable populations; affects ~ 22-46% of at-risk population
  - Develop at mean of ~ 50 months after initiating dialysis
  - Imaging: Small kidneys with small cysts; ↑ risk of RCC (0-8% in pediatric acquired cystic kidney disease patients)
- **Congenital Mesoblastic Nephroma**
  - Most common solid renal tumor in neonates
  - Majority present < 3 months of age; 90% by age 1 year
  - Imaging: May demonstrate polyhydramnios in utero
    - Classic subtype: Homogeneous benign solid mass; ± surrounding hyperechoic/hypoechoic (US) rings with ↑ Doppler flow
    - Cellular subtype: Larger, more aggressive tumors with heterogeneity from necrosis/hemorrhage/cysts
- **Wilms Tumor**
  - Most common pediatric renal malignancy but rarely predominantly cystic
  - Age of presentation peaks at 3-4 years; 80% < 5 years
    - Earlier peak for bilateral Wilms at 15 months
  - Numerous associations
  - Imaging: Large, well-circumscribed heterogeneous solid mass, frequently with some cystic/necrotic components; Ca^{2+} in up to 15%
    - Typically hypoenhancing (CT/MR) with intermediate to high T2 & restricted diffusion (MR)
    - Up to 10% invade renal vein; ± inferior vena cava (& even right atrial) tumor thrombus
    - Multifocal (unilateral or bilateral) hypoenhancing masses suggest underlying nephrogenic rests
- **Multilocular Cystic Renal Tumors**
  - Benign spectrum of disease: Cystic nephroma vs. cystic partially differentiated nephroblastoma (CPDN)
  - Associated with *DICER1* tumor predisposition syndrome
  - Imaging: 2 subtypes are indistinguishable
    - Classically occurs as well-circumscribed, purely cystic mass with numerous thin septations; no nodular or solid components (should raise concern for Wilms)
    - Herniation into renal pelvis is characteristic

Simple Renal Cyst

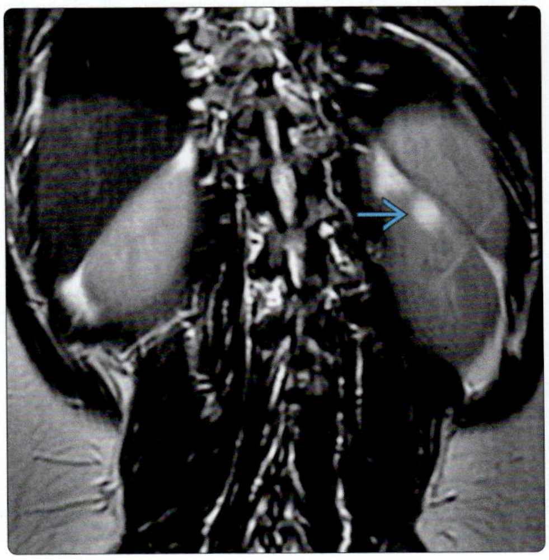

Simple Renal Cyst

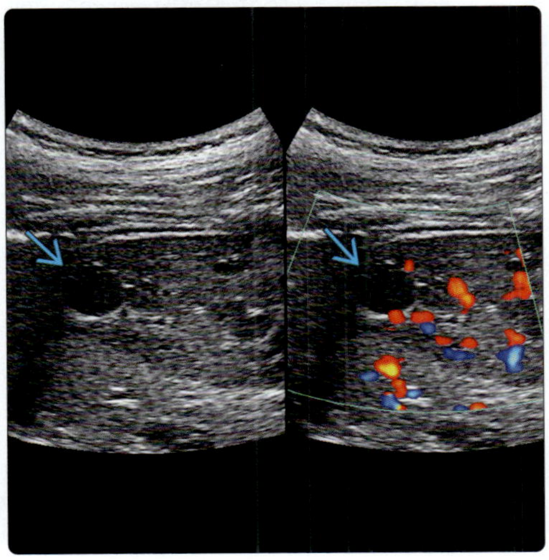

(Left) *Coronal T2 spine MR of a 12 year old with worsening scoliosis shows an incidental cystic lesion of the left renal upper pole ➡. Due to the technique of this spine exam & the motion artifact with volume averaging, the lesion could not be fully characterized.* **(Right)** *Longitudinal grayscale & color Doppler US images in the same patient show the cyst to be well defined, round, & anechoic with an imperceptible wall, posterior acoustic enhancement, & no internal vascularity ➡, typical of a simple cyst.*

(Left) *Longitudinal US in a patient shows a well-defined cyst with smooth walls & ↑ through transmission in the right renal upper pole.* **(Right)** *Longitudinal US shows a large cyst in the upper pole of the right kidney in a 17 year old with intermittent hematuria & flank pain. Note the dependently layering echogenic material.*

Simple Renal Cyst

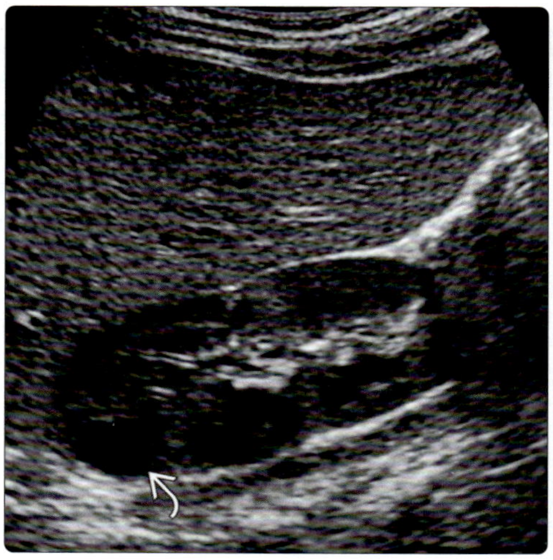

Calyceal Diverticulum

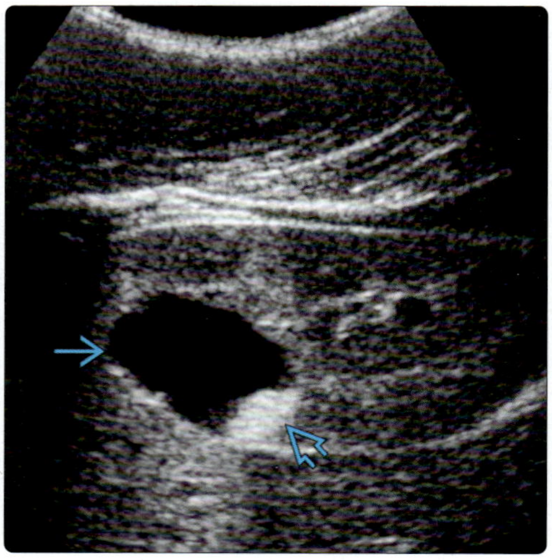

(Left) *Axial NECT in the same patient shows Ca^{2+} layering dependently within the cyst of the right renal upper pole.* **(Right)** *Frontal IVP in the same patient shows contrast filling the right upper pole cystic lesion as contrast is being excreted by the kidneys, typical of a calyceal diverticulum. This focus has a narrow neck connecting it to the central calyces.*

Calyceal Diverticulum

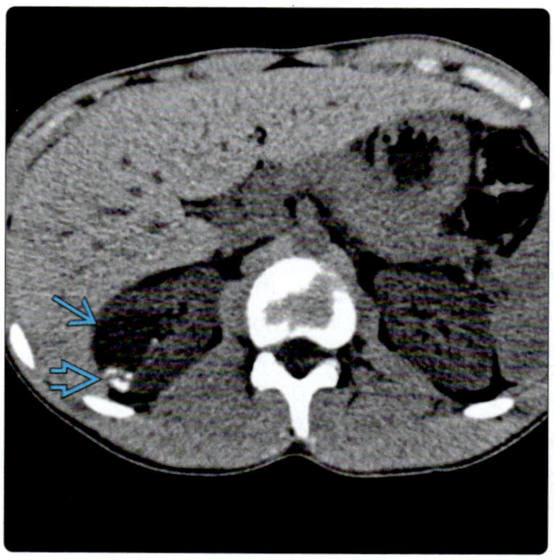

Calyceal Diverticulum

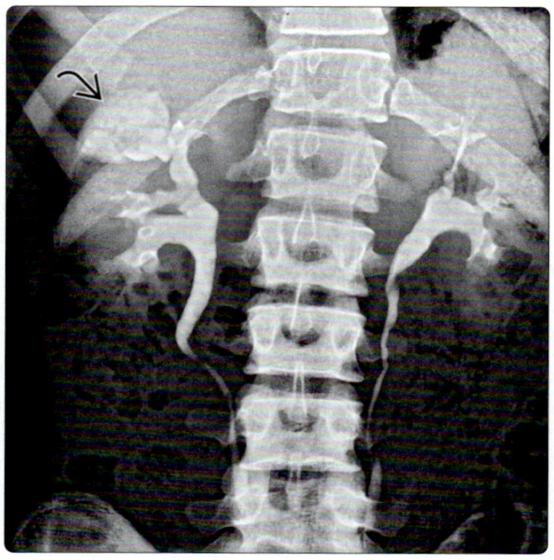

(Left) *Sagittal SSFP MR MIP of a 32-week fetus with anhydramnios shows a bladder outlet obstruction with dilated posterior urethra, hydroureter, & numerous tiny cortical cysts (which were present bilaterally). Posterior urethral valves (PUV) were confirmed after delivery.* **(Right)** *Longitudinal US in a newborn with PUV shows diffusely echogenic left renal parenchyma with numerous tiny cortical cyst, typical of cystic renal dysplasia from chronic in utero obstruction. There is mild pelvocaliectasis.*

Cystic Renal Dysplasia

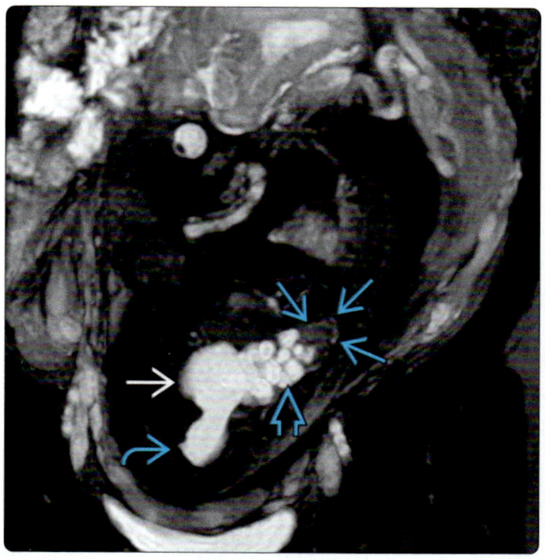

Cystic Renal Dysplasia

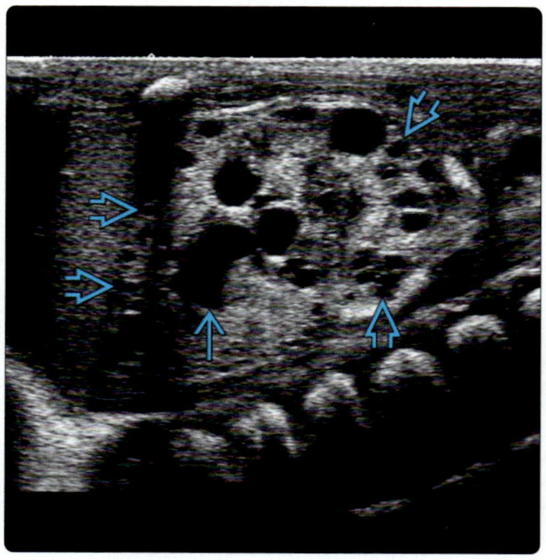

Multicystic Dysplastic Kidney

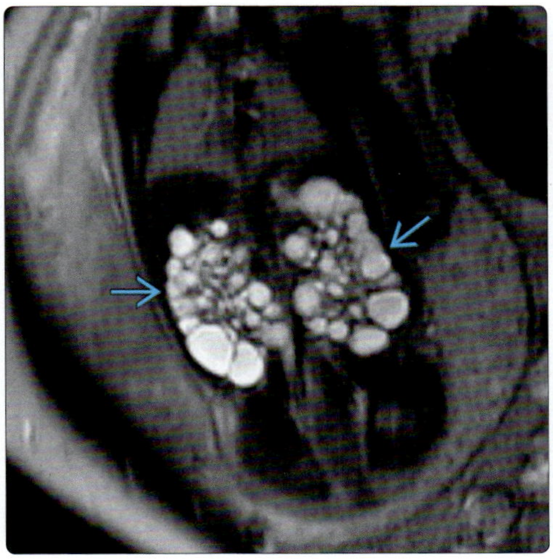

Multicystic Dysplastic Kidney

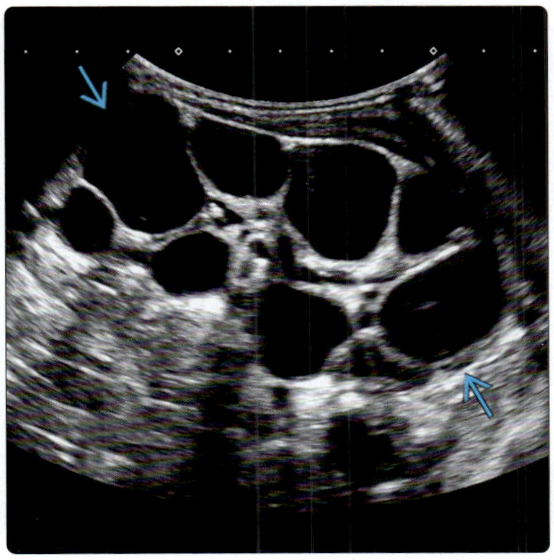

(Left) *Coronal T2 MR SSFSE in a 32-week fetus with anhydramnios shows replacement of both kidneys → by innumerable cysts of varying size, typical of multicystic dysplastic kidney (MCDK). No bladder is seen, as there is no functional renal tissue.* **(Right)** *Longitudinal US in newborn with normal right kidney demonstrates left renal enlargement → (10 cm) by numerous noncommunicating cysts of varying size & interspersed echogenic tissue. No normal left renal tissue is seen, typical of MCDK. There is no hydronephrosis.*

Multicystic Dysplastic Kidney

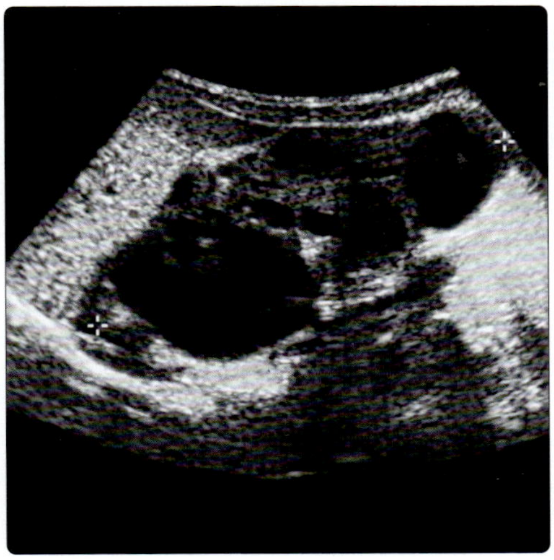

Multicystic Dysplastic Kidney

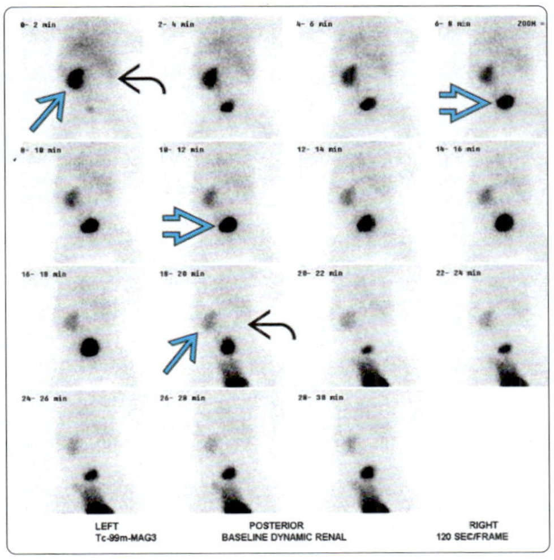

(Left) *Longitudinal US shows an enlarged but reniform collection of cysts & echogenic soft tissue (denoted by calipers) in the right renal fossa of a newborn.* **(Right)** *Posterior Tc-99m MAG3 nuclear medicine renal scan in the same patient shows no functional right renal tissue →, consistent with MCDK. The left kidney → shows normal uptake & excretion, accounting for the bladder filling with excreted radiotracer →.*

Ureteropelvic Duplications (Mimic)

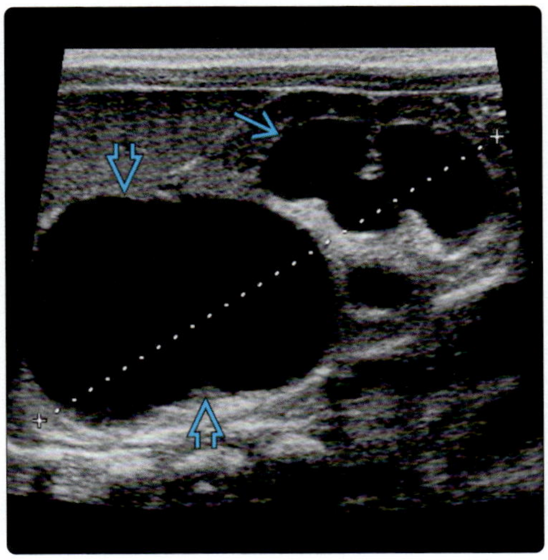

Abscess

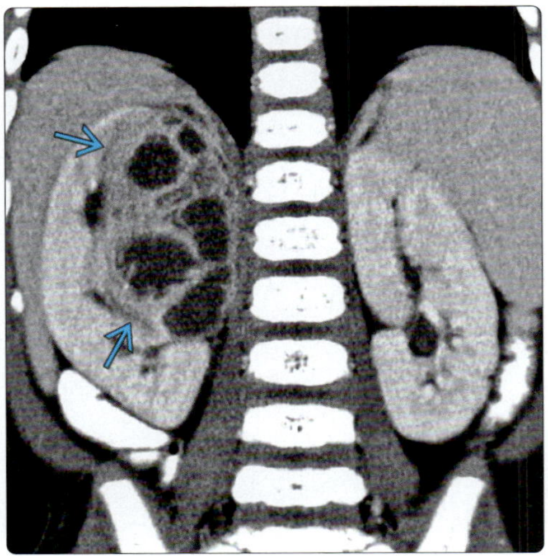

(Left) *Longitudinal US in a newborn shows a large "cyst" → in the upper pole of the left kidney with a severely thinned cortex. There is also marked caliectasis in the lower pole →. US of the bladder (not shown) revealed an obstructing ureterocele from the left upper pole moiety, & a subsequent VCUG confirmed vesicoureteral reflux into the lower pole moiety.* **(Right)** *Coronal CECT in a 7 year old with fever shows a complex mass → in the right kidney with fluid density foci separated by thick, irregular septations due to an abscess.*

(Left) *AP radiograph in a newborn with respiratory distress & a distended abdomen shows bulging flanks & central displacement of bowel loops. The lungs are poorly aerated in this anuric infant.* **(Right)** *Transverse US through the lower abdomen in the same newborn shows that both kidneys are dramatically enlarged, touching in the midline ➡. The ↑ medullary echogenicity ↪ is due to the higher concentration of dilated tubules (creating interfaces) at these levels.*

Autosomal Recessive Polycystic Kidney Disease

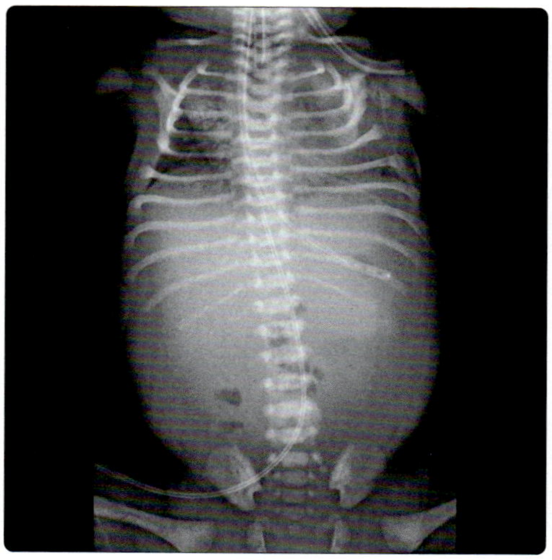

Autosomal Recessive Polycystic Kidney Disease

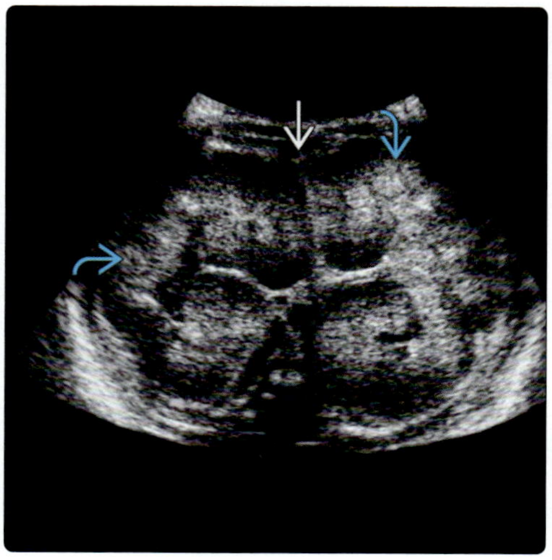

(Left) *Longitudinal US with a high-frequency linear transducer in the same newborn shows the radiating dilated tubules with innumerable tiny cysts. Scattered macrocysts may rarely be seen as well.* **(Right)** *Longitudinal color Doppler US in a 17 year old with hypertension shows multiple simple cysts → scattered throughout the right kidney with mild splaying of the adjacent vessels. Genetic testing confirmed autosomal dominant polycystic kidney disease (ADPKD).*

Autosomal Recessive Polycystic Kidney Disease

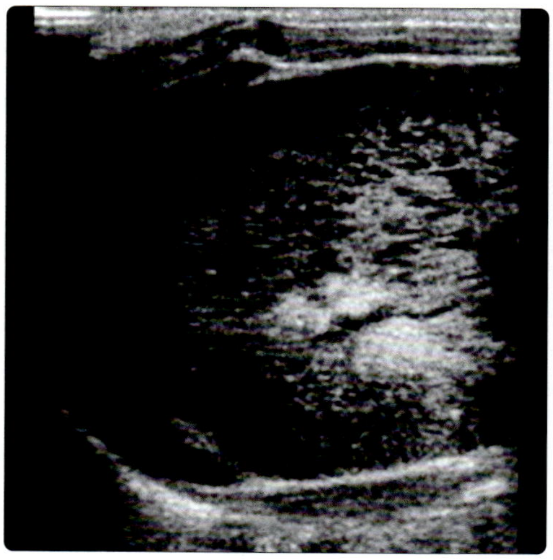

Autosomal Dominant Polycystic Kidney Disease

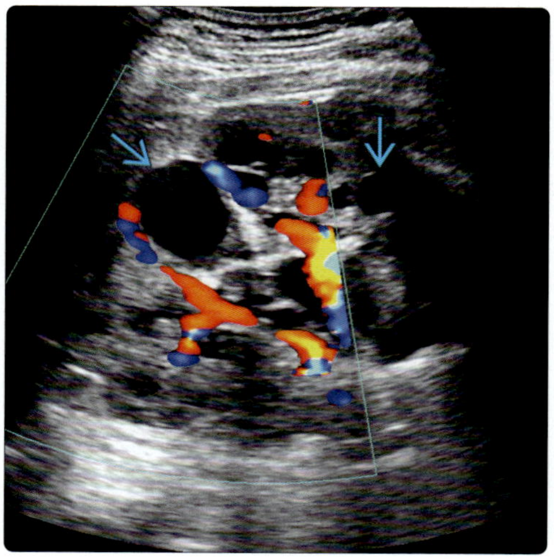

(Left) *Axial SSFSE T2 MR in a 31-week fetus with anhydramnios shows massive enlargement of the kidneys → with diffusely hyperintense parenchyma due to a rare phenotype of ADPKD, typically with homozygous mutations of the PKD1 gene.* **(Right)** *Coronal oblique SSFP MR of the same fetus shows the massively enlarged & hyperintense right kidney →. Note the numerous tiny cysts in the normal-sized maternal kidney ⇨; the mother tested positive for a PKD1 mutation, confirming ADPKD for her.*

Autosomal Dominant Polycystic Kidney Disease

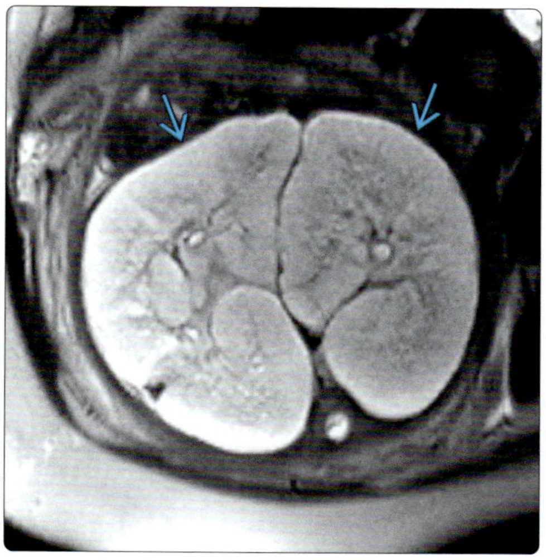

Autosomal Dominant Polycystic Kidney Disease

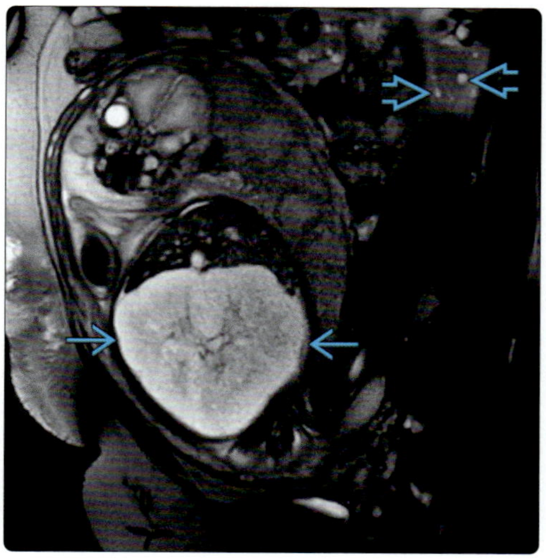

Tuberous Sclerosis Complex

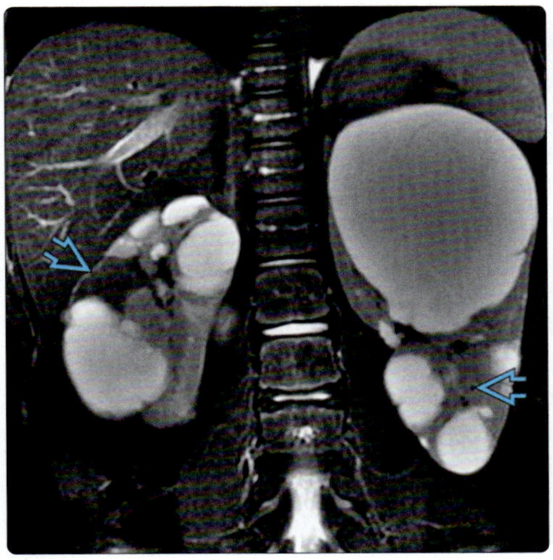

Tuberous Sclerosis Complex

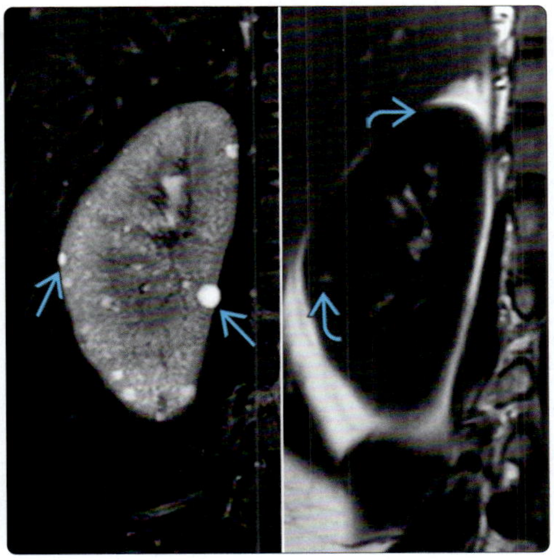

(Left) *Coronal T2 FS MR in a 10 year old with tuberous sclerosis complex (TSC) shows numerous cysts of varying size throughout both kidneys. A fat-poor angiomyolipoma (with no T1 shortening, not shown) was also present in the right kidney.* **(Right)** *Coronal T2 FS (left) & T1 (right) MR images in an 8 year old with TSC show scattered subcentimeter macroscopic cysts among innumerable tiny parenchymal cysts. A few small, fat-containing angiomyolipomas are also noted.*

Medullary Cystic Kidney Disease Complex

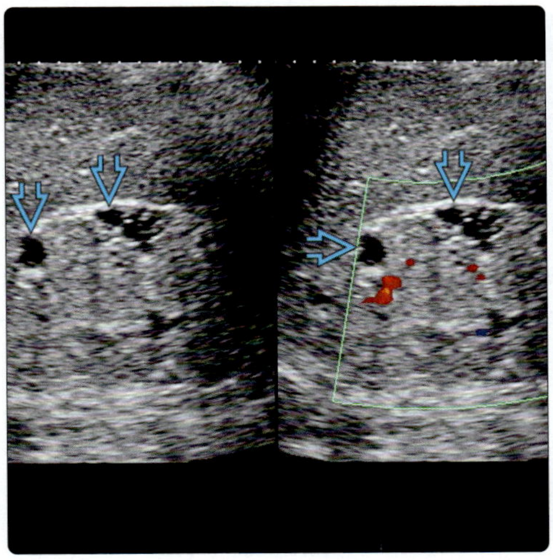

Congenital Mesoblastic Nephroma

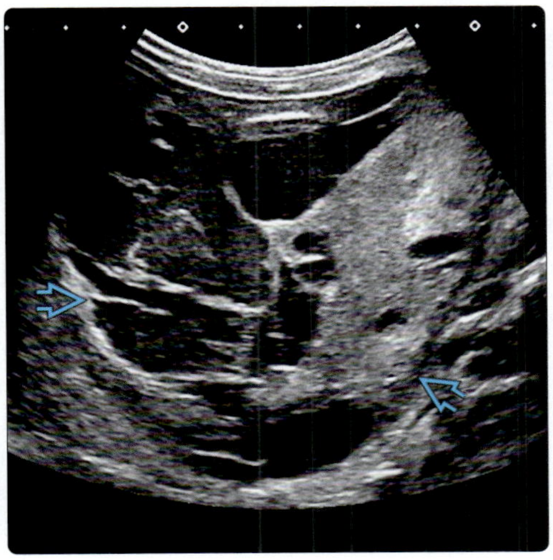

(Left) *Longitudinal grayscale & color Doppler US images in a child with Joubert syndrome & deteriorating kidney function show loss of normal renal corticomedullary differentiation with scattered cortical cysts. The left kidney had a similar appearance (not shown).* **(Right)** *Longitudinal US in a newborn shows a cystic & solid mass replacing the left kidney. A cellular subtype of congenital mesoblastic nephroma was confirmed upon resection.*

Wilms Tumor

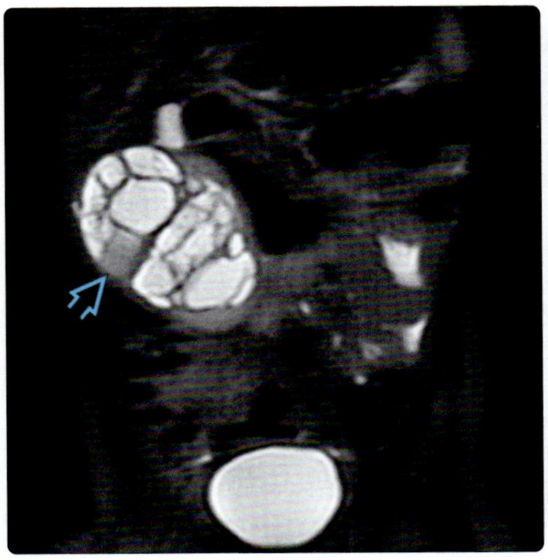

Multilocular Cystic Renal Tumors

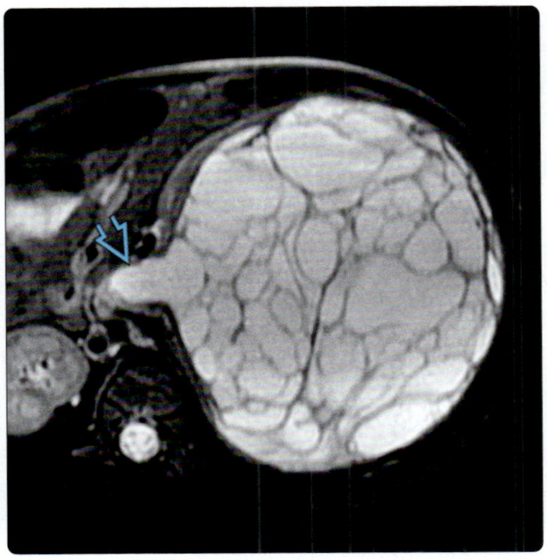

(Left) *Coronal T2 FS MR in a 1 year old shows a predominantly cystic Wilms tumor of the right kidney with a single solid nodule (which restricted diffusion, not shown). Wilms tumors often have cystic foci but are rarely predominantly cystic.* **(Right)** *Axial T2 FS MR in a toddler shows a mass composed entirely of thin-walled cysts replacing most of the left kidney. Note the herniation of the mass into the left renal pelvis, which is typical of these benign tumors.*

DIFFERENTIAL DIAGNOSIS

Common

- Vesicoureteral Reflux
- Posterior Urethral Valves
- Neurogenic Bladder

Less Common

- Primary Megaureter
- Crossed Fused Ectopia
- Horseshoe Kidney
- Ureterocele
- Megacystis-Megaureter
- Bladder Mass
- Extrinsic Pelvic Neoplasm
- Bilateral Ureteropelvic Junction Obstructions

Rare but Important

- Cloacal Malformation
- Eagle-Barrett Syndrome (Prune Belly)
- Anterior Urethral Valves
- Congenital Megalourethra
- Megacystis-Microcolon-Intestinal Hypoperistalsis
- Urethral Duplication
- Megacalycosis

ESSENTIAL INFORMATION

Key Differential Diagnosis Issues

- Pelvocaliectasis (renal collecting system dilation of any cause) & hydronephrosis (which implies obstruction as cause of dilation) are often used interchangeably
- Some underlying diagnoses may lead to unilateral or bilateral renal collecting system dilation
- Dilation may also be due to > 1 cause, & some etiologies are poorly understood/indistinct
- Mechanical or functional bladder outlet obstructions (BOO) often lead to vesicoureteral reflux (VUR)
  - Longstanding obstructions &/or VUR can lead to chronic renal damage ± stones & urinary tract infections (UTI)
  - Severe in utero obstructions may lead to ↓ fetal micturition → ↓ amniotic fluid → ↓ lung development (pulmonary hypoplasia) → ↓ survival
- However, prenatally detected urinary tract dilation (typically mild) is transient or physiologic in 50-70% of cases

Helpful Clues for Common Diagnoses

- **Vesicoureteral Reflux**
  - Retrograde flow of urine from bladder toward kidneys
  - Graded by fluoroscopic VCUG from I (mild) to V (severe)
    - NM cystogram is more sensitive for VUR but lacks other anatomic detail of GU tract
    - US may be normal or only show urothelial thickening
  - May be isolated or secondary to distal obstruction
  - Most common in children < 2 years of age
    - Most cases are mild & discovered during work-up of febrile UTI; 80% outgrow VUR by puberty
  - Complications: Recurrent pyelonephritis & renal scarring that may lead to renal insufficiency & hypertension
- **Posterior Urethral Valves**
  - Most common congenital BOO; occurs only in male patients
  - Persistent or prominent plicae colliculi in urethra cause variable degree of obstruction
  - Complete obstruction in fetus leads to
    - Oligo-/anhydramnios → pulmonary hypoplasia
    - Bladder dysfunction
    - Chronic hydroureteronephrosis → cystic renal dysplasia → renal failure
  - Mild obstruction may go undetected for several years
    - Presents late with renal failure, bladder dysfunction
  - Typically detected prenatally with large, thick-walled bladder & "keyhole" dilated posterior urethra
    - ± marked uni- vs. bilateral hydroureteronephrosis
    - ± echogenic kidneys with numerous cortical cysts
  - Bladder may be decompressed prior to postnatal US
  - Fluoroscopic VCUG shows thin valve tissue at transition from dilated posterior to bulbar urethra
    - Irregular bladder with trabeculation & diverticula
    - Varying degrees of VUR
- **Neurogenic Bladder**
  - Malfunctioning bladder from any neurologic disorder
  - Upper tract is compromised by poor bladder emptying, ↑ bladder pressures, VUR, & infection
  - Early: Highly compliant, poorly emptying bladder
  - Gradually develops muscular hypertrophy with ↓ compliance & capacity
  - Late: Low capacity, noncompliant, noncontractile
  - Imaging shows bladder wall trabeculation, VUR, diverticula, ↓ capacity, & poor emptying

Helpful Clues for Less Common Diagnoses

- **Primary Megaureter**
  - Focal concentric narrowing of extravesical distal ureter anywhere from 0.5-4.0 cm in length
    - Distal segment is adynamic/aperistaltic due to abnormal innervation or abnormal musculature
    - Ureter dilates above this narrowed distal segment
  - Results in variable combinations of VUR & obstruction
    - VUR: Ipsilateral in 5%, contralateral in 10%
- **Crossed Fused Ectopia**
  - Upper kidney is orthotopic; other kidney is on wrong side & in low position
  - Lower pole of orthotopic kidney is fused to upper pole of ectopic kidney (which typically has different long axis compared to orthotopic kidney)
  - Ureter from lower kidney crosses to contralateral trigone
  - Associated with aberrant & accessory vessels
  - ↑ risk of VUR & ureteropelvic junction (UPJ) obstruction; pelvocaliectasis may be diffuse or segmental
- **Horseshoe Kidney**
  - Lower poles of kidneys are fused in midline; variable volume of functional renal tissue at "isthmus" that connects kidneys (& lies between inferior mesenteric artery & aorta)
  - Upper poles are lower than usual
  - Aberrant & accessory vessels & ureters are common
  - ↑ risk of VUR & UPJ obstruction; pelvocaliectasis may be diffuse or segmental
  - ↑ risk of Wilms tumor
- **Ureterocele**
  - Congenital cystic dilation of distal submucosal ureter

- Possible insertions: Orthotopic at trigone (simple) vs. ectopic insertion anywhere else, typically medial & distal
- Kidney being drained may have single collecting system (typically orthotopic) or duplex (typically ectopic)
- US shows thin-walled, cystic-appearing lesion protruding into urinary bladder from ureterovesical junction; associated renal collecting system & ureter are typically dilated
- Fluoroscopic VCUG shows round filling defect on early bladder-filling images; may evert later
  - Depending on size, ureterocele may constantly or intermittently block bladder outlet

- **Megacystis-Megaureter**
  - Large, thin-walled, smooth bladder due to constant recycling of refluxed urine
  - Not neurogenic: Bladder contracts normally but never empties completely due to drainage of dilated ureters
  - Bladder capacity & function typically normalize when VUR is corrected
- **Bladder Mass**
  - Obstructs at ureterovesical junction or bladder outlet
  - Intrinsic neoplastic or inflammatory lesion
    - Numerous etiologies, generally indistinguishable by imaging: Rhabdomyosarcoma (RMS), inflammatory pseudotumor, eosinophilic cystitis, hemorrhagic cystitis, neurofibromas, fibroepithelial polyp
    - Nonmobile, varying degrees of internal vascularity
  - Other intraluminal considerations: Hematoma, stone, & fungal balls; will be mobile & avascular
- **Extrinsic Pelvic Neoplasm**
  - RMS (of prostate, vagina, or soft tissues), neuroblastoma, sacrococcygeal teratoma, lymphoma, ovarian mass
- **Bilateral Ureteropelvic Junction Obstructions**
  - UPJ is most common congenital urinary obstruction
  - Bilateral in up to 30%
  - Focal narrowing at junction of renal pelvis & ureter
    - Renal pelvis is often disproportionately dilated relative to calyces; ureter is not dilated
  - Obstruction may be intrinsic or extrinsic
    - Intrinsic: Abnormal smooth muscle orientation, fibrosis &/or abnormal innervation
    - Extrinsic: Crossing vessels, adenopathy, or mass
    - Presentation: Most found by prenatal US; may have recurrent UTI, flank pain, hematuria, vomiting

Helpful Clues for Rare Diagnoses

- **Cloacal Malformation**
  - Anorectal malformation with common channel/single orifice of GI & GU tracts in female patients
  - Associated with various GU anomalies
  - Hydrocolpos can obstruct bladder outlet
- **Eagle-Barrett Syndrome (Prune Belly)**
  - Classic triad: Absent/hypoplastic abdominal wall muscles, cryptorchidism, patulous urinary tract (including various urethral anomalies)
  - Affects male patients almost exclusively (95-97%)
- **Anterior Urethral Valves**
  - Similar tissue as in posterior urethral valves (PUV) but in anterior urethra (at variable locations, with variable degrees of obstruction)
- **Congenital Megalourethra**
  - Similar to PUV but anterior penile urethra is dilated
    - Enlarged fluid-filled anterior urethra/penis result in tubular fluid-filled mobile structure at genitals
  - May be secondary to deficient corpus spongiosum or cavernosum tissue vs. anterior urethral valves
- **Megacystis-Microcolon-Intestinal Hypoperistalsis**
  - Autosomal recessive disorder, typically affects female patients
  - Functional bowel & urinary bladder obstructions resulting in marked abdominal distention
  - Malrotation of midgut is typical
- **Urethral Duplication**
  - May obstruct, leading to hydroureteronephrosis
- **Megacalycosis**
  - Congenital anomaly of nonobstructive calyceal dilation due to hypoplastic renal pyramids

Vesicoureteral Reflux

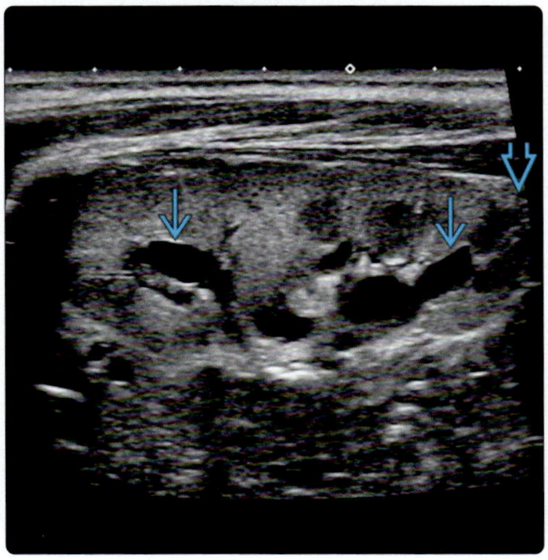

Vesicoureteral Reflux

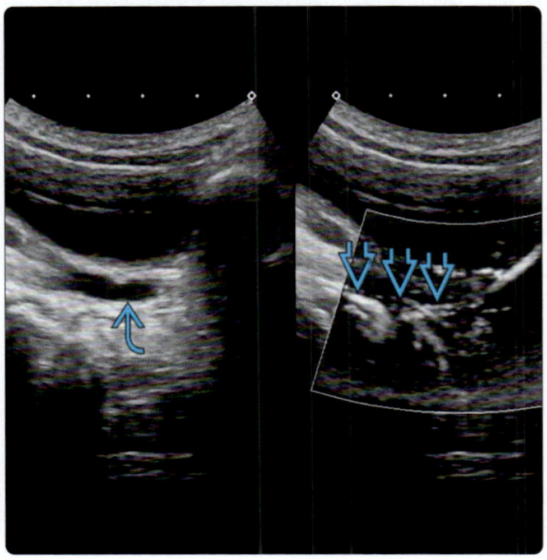

(Left) *Longitudinal US of the left kidney in a 1-year-old girl with a history of 2 febrile urinary tract infections shows mild left pelvocaliectasis with thinning of the lower pole parenchyma. The right kidney showed a similar appearance without scarring.* **(Right)** *Longitudinal US in the same patient shows dilation of the distal left ureter. Doppler maximized for slow flow showed intermittent retrograde flow of urine into the left ureter on real-time scanning, consistent with vesicoureteral reflux (VUR).*

(Left) *Posterior Tc-99m DTPA nuclear medicine cystogram in the same patient shows left ➙ worse than right ➙ VUR.* **(Right)** *Sagittal SSFSE T2 MR shows marked dilation & wall thickening of the urinary bladder ➙ in a male fetus at 21-weeks gestation. Note the dilation of the posterior urethra ➙ & oligohydramnios ➙.*

Vesicoureteral Reflux

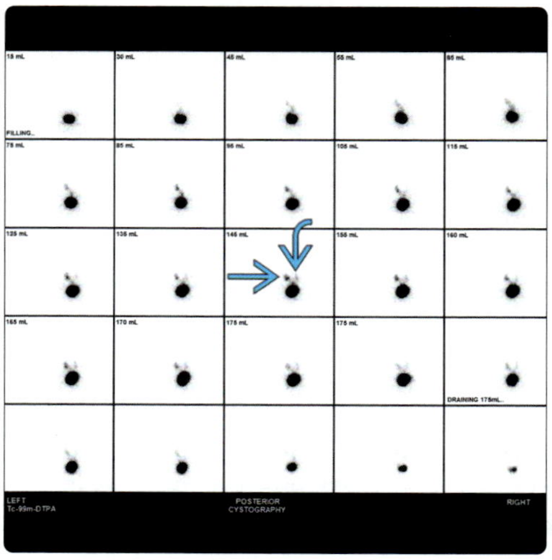

Posterior Urethral Valves

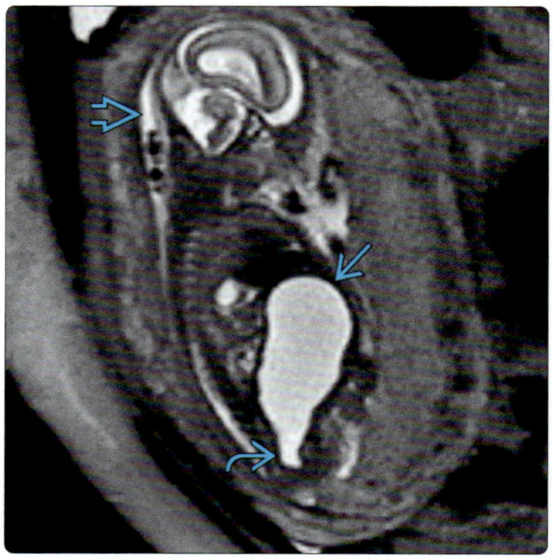

(Left) *Axial SSFSE T2 MR in the same fetus shows bilateral hydronephrosis ➙ in addition to the urinary bladder dilation & wall thickening ➙.* **(Right)** *Longitudinal postnatal US in the same patient shows diffusely echogenic left renal parenchyma with numerous tiny cortical cysts ➙, typical of cystic renal dysplasia from chronic in utero obstruction. There is mild pelvocaliectasis ➙. The right kidney (not shown) demonstrated more severe dilation with echogenic parenchyma but no cortical cysts.*

Posterior Urethral Valves

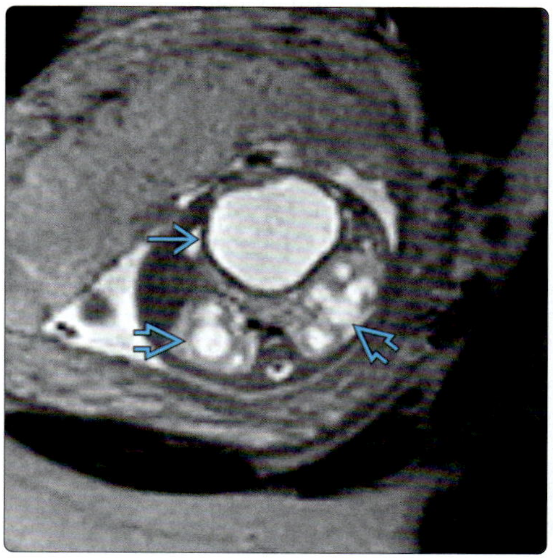

Posterior Urethral Valves

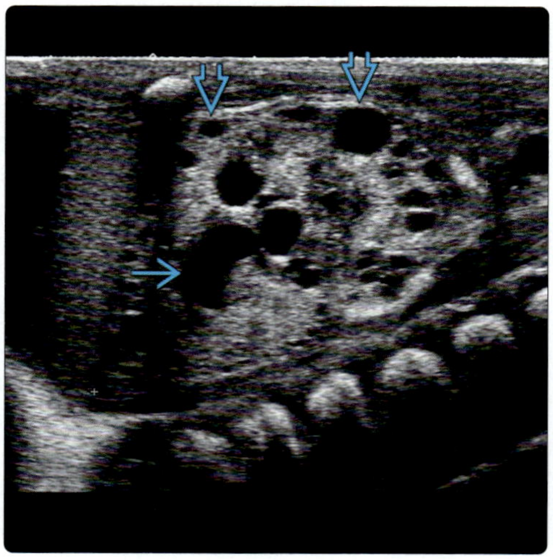

(Left) *LPO fluoroscopic VCUG in a 4 day old with a prenatally detected bladder outlet obstruction shows a dilated bladder ➙ with diverticula ➙. There is marked dilation of the posterior urethra ➙ with valve tissue ➙ seen at the junction with the bulbar urethra. Grade V VUR ➙ is noted.* **(Right)** *Supine fluoroscopic VCUG in a 6 month old with a history of myelomeningocele (MMC) & neurogenic bladder shows bilateral grade V VUR ➙. A ventriculoperitoneal shunt is coiled in the abdomen.*

Posterior Urethral Valves

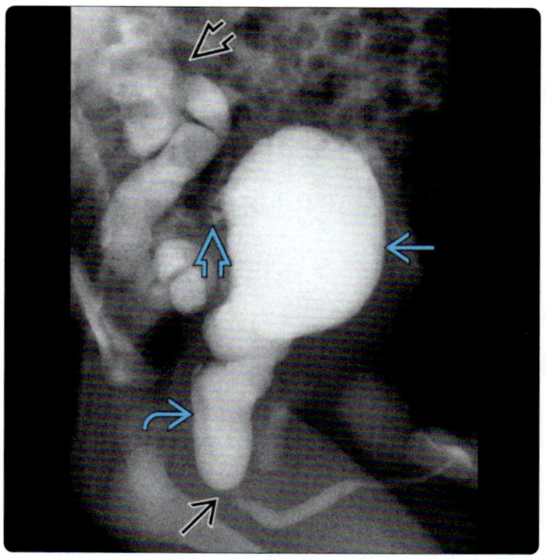

Neurogenic Bladder

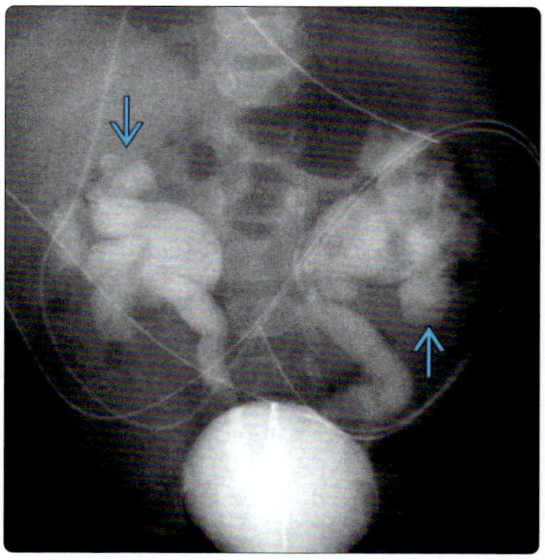

Neurogenic Bladder

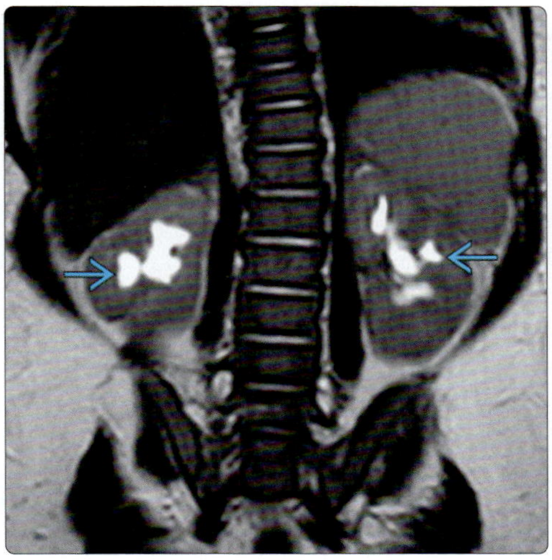

Primary Megaureter

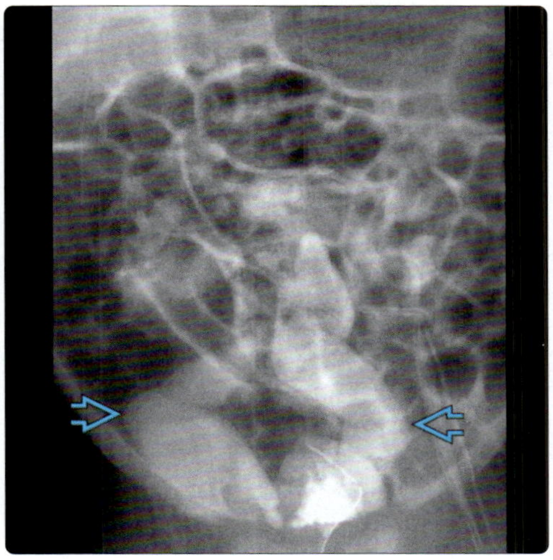

(Left) *Coronal T2 MR of the spine in the same patient with a repaired MMC (not shown) demonstrates bilateral pelvocaliectasis .* **(Right)** *Supine frontal fluoroscopic VCUG in a 10 day old shows bilateral grade V VUR with massive ureteral dilation . This post-void image (& images from a 2nd fill & void) showed no significant change in ureteral opacification, suggesting an obstructing component to these refluxing megaureters.*

Crossed Fused Ectopia

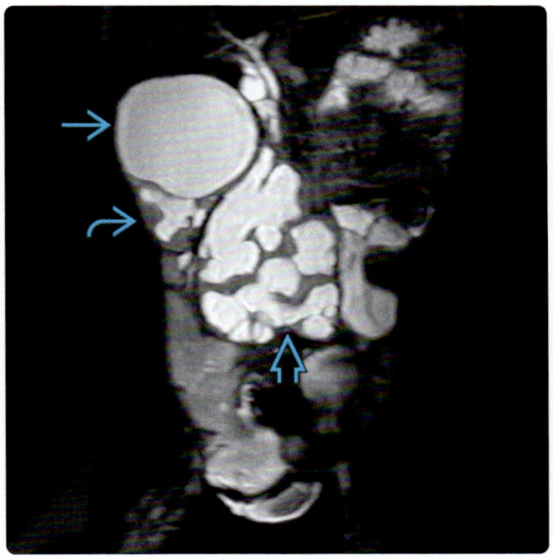

Crossed Fused Ectopia

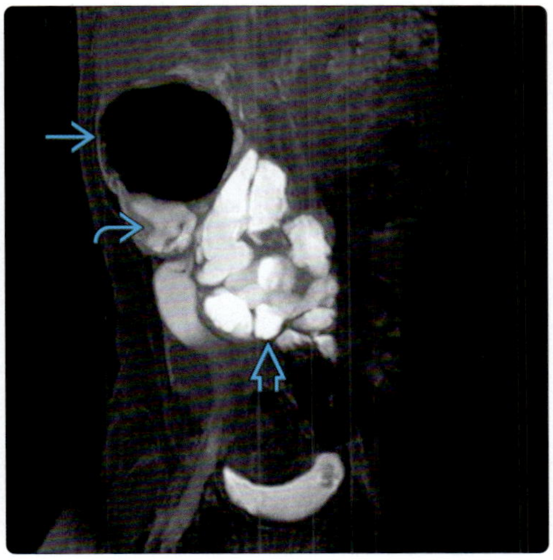

(Left) *Coronal MR urogram MIP in a 5-year-old girl with bilateral ureteral reimplantations for a right obstructed ureterocele & left ectopic ureter shows cross-fused ectopia with left kidney fused to right lower pole . Moderate to severe dilation is seen in all moieties, most pronounced at right upper pole .* **(Right)** *Delayed coronal T1 C+ FS MR MIP in the same patient shows contrast filling left & right lower moieties but not the right upper pole due to a concomitant ureteropelvic junction (UPJ) obstruction.*

Horseshoe Kidney

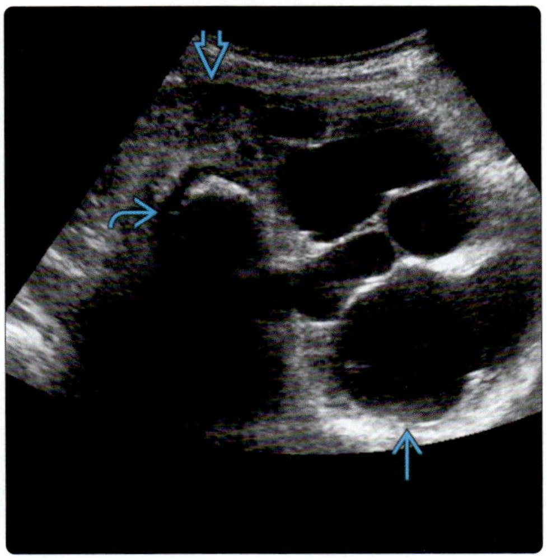

Horseshoe Kidney

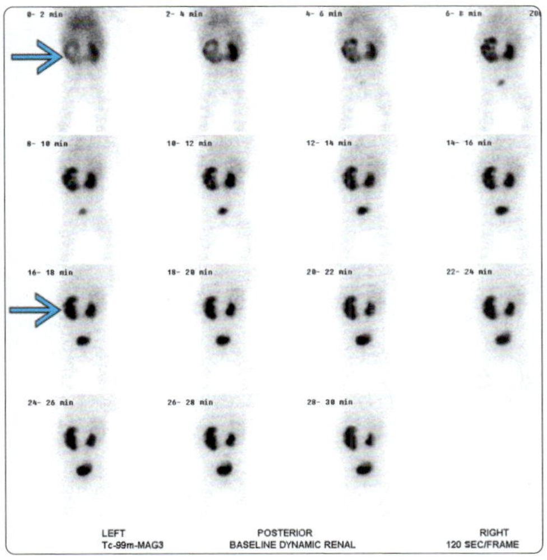

(Left) *Transverse US in the midline abdomen shows marked pelvocaliectasis of renal tissue crossing the midline in this patient with horseshoe kidney. Note the isthmus of renal tissue overlying the spine .* **(Right)** *Posterior nuclear medicine renal scan in the same patient shows bilateral prominence of the intrarenal collecting systems, worse on the left . The long axis of each moiety is abnormal, with the lower poles directed medially. Dilation, stasis, & stones are common complications of horseshoe kidney.*

(Left) *Coronal oblique SSFP MR in a 30-weeks gestation fetus shows marked dilation of the left upper pole moiety in a duplicated system. Also note the hydroureter draining this moiety.* **(Right)** *Coronal oblique SSFP MR in the same fetus shows that the ureter of the left upper pole moiety terminates in a ureterocele that is obstructing the urinary bladder & causing right hydroureteronephrosis.*

Ureterocele

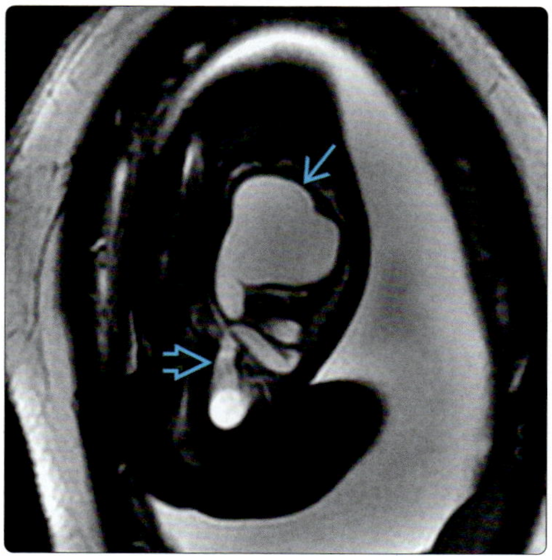

Ureterocele

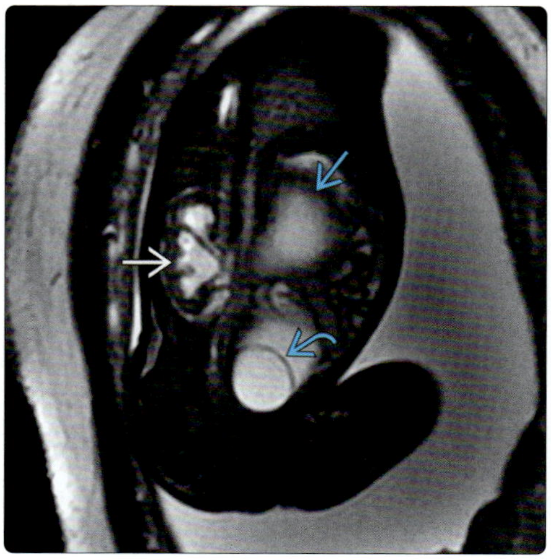

(Left) *RPO fluoroscopic VCUG shows bilateral, high-grade VUR but a thin-walled, smooth bladder, characteristic of megacystis megaureter. Refluxed urine constantly refills the bladder (which is not a neurogenic bladder) in this scenario.* **(Right)** *Oblique fluoroscopic VCUG shows a lobulated filling defect at the bladder base in this child with hematuria. Subsequent biopsy showed a botryoid rhabdomyosarcoma. These intrinsic tumors may cause bladder outlet obstruction, as can extrinsic pelvic tumors.*

Megacystis-Megaureter

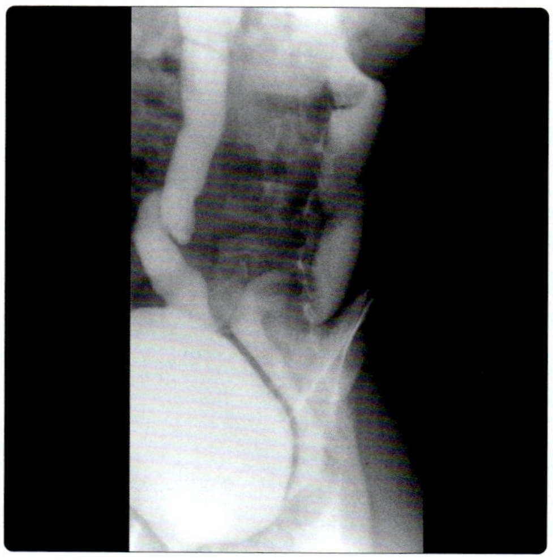

Bladder Mass

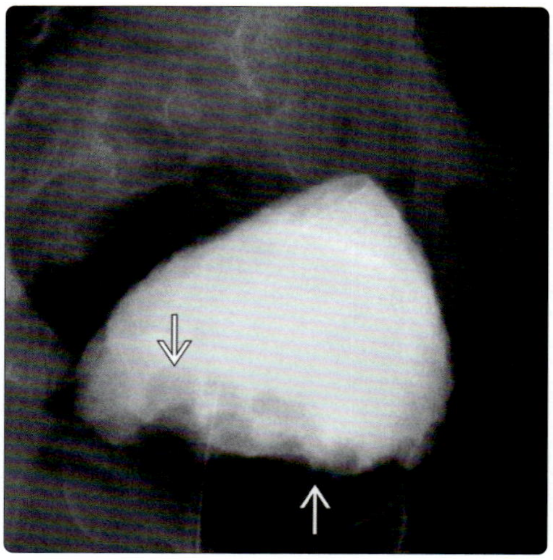

(Left) *Coronal SSFSE T2 MR in a newborn shows a large, predominantly solid presacral mass with external protrusion. This sacrococcygeal teratoma was causing bladder outlet obstruction (not shown), leading to bilateral hydronephrosis.* **(Right)** *Coronal CECT in a 7 year old with back pain, constipation, & urinary retention shows a large, solid mass in the pelvis with scattered* Ca^{2+}*. This neuroblastoma caused bladder outlet obstruction with bilateral hydronephrosis.*

Extrinsic Pelvic Neoplasm

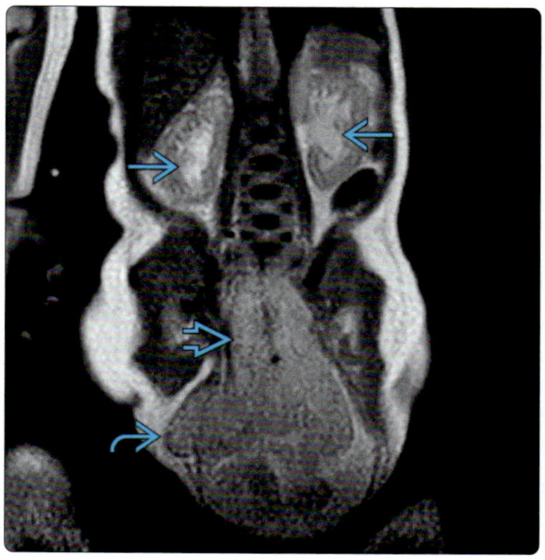

Extrinsic Pelvic Neoplasm

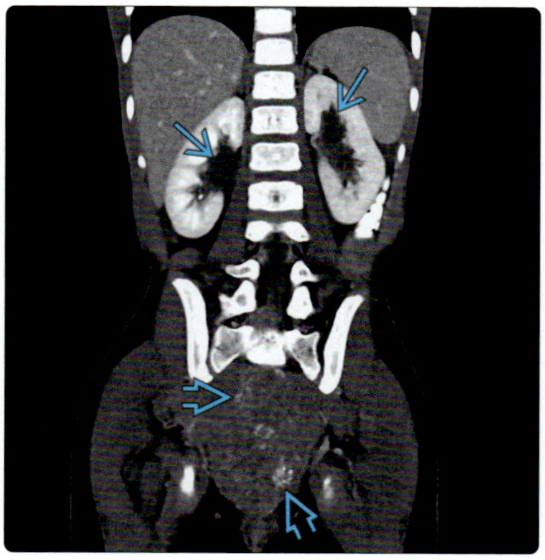

Bilateral Ureteropelvic Junction Obstructions

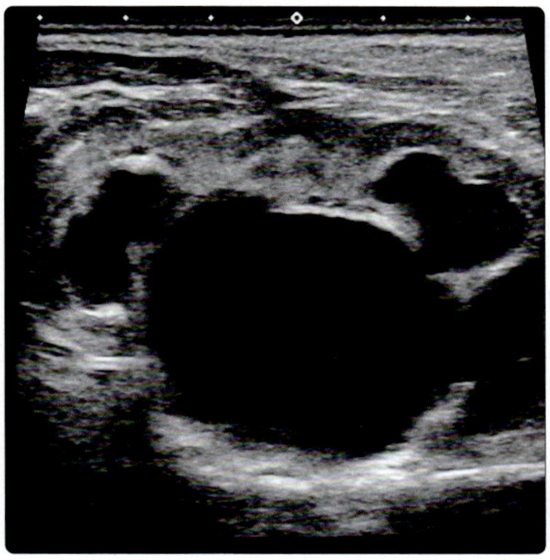

Bilateral Ureteropelvic Junction Obstructions

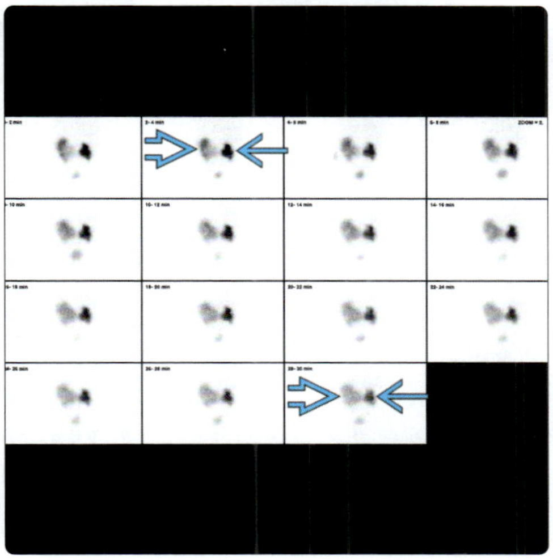

(Left) *Longitudinal US in a newborn shows severe pelvocaliectasis. Other images showed disproportionate dilation of the renal pelvis but no ureterectasis, typical of a UPJ obstruction. Less pronounced but similar findings were also seen on the right (not shown).* **(Right)** *Posterior diuretic renogram in the same patient after Lasix administration shows dilation & impaired drainage of the left → > right → systems.*

Bilateral Ureteropelvic Junction Obstructions

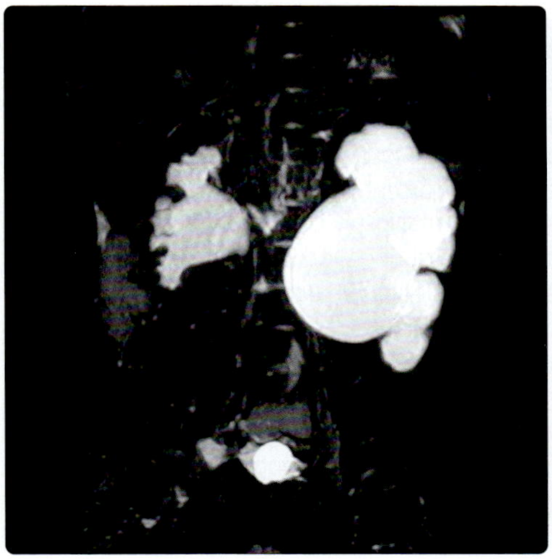

Bilateral Ureteropelvic Junction Obstructions

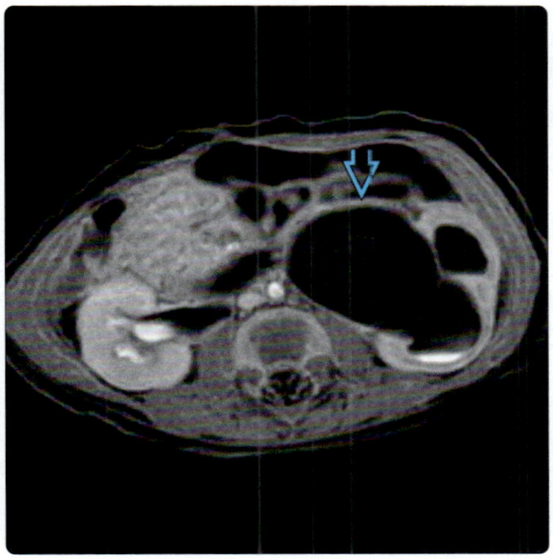

(Left) *Coronal MR urogram MIP in the same patient at 8 months of age shows bilateral UPJ obstructions, left worse than right. No ureteral dilation is seen.* **(Right)** *Delayed axial T1 C+ FS MR in the same patient shows excretion of contrast into the right > left collecting systems, but no ureteral contrast was visualized. The ballooning of the left renal pelvis → is quite typical in severe UPJ obstructions. Bilateral pyeloplasties were subsequently performed in this patient.*

Eagle-Barrett Syndrome (Prune Belly)

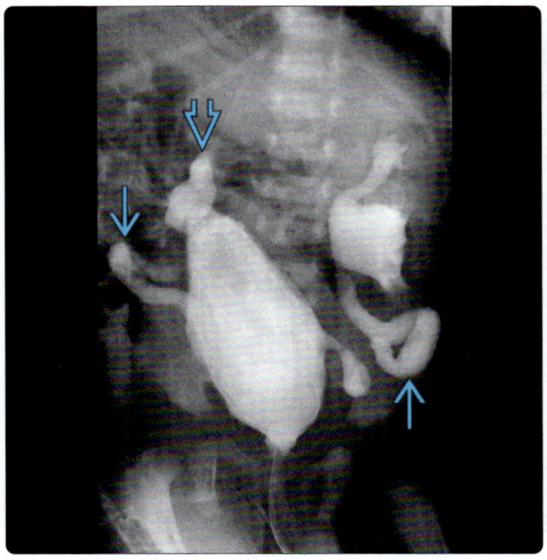

Congenital Megalourethra

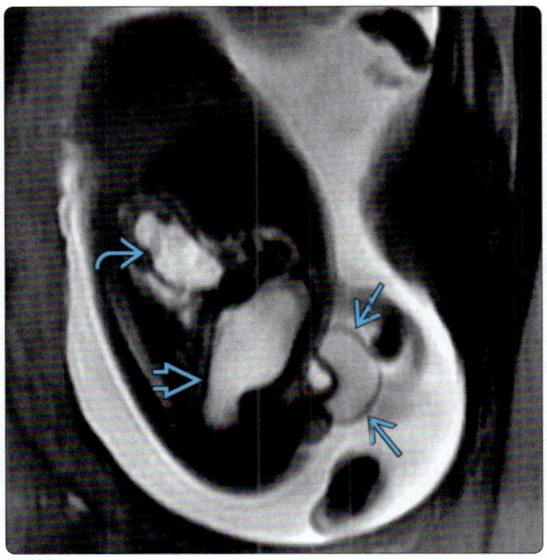

(Left) *Supine frontal fluoroscopic VCUG shows bilateral VUR with markedly tortuous ureters → given their relatively mild dilation. There is a vertically oriented bladder with a urachal remnant → in this male newborn with a flaccid anterior abdominal wall.* **(Right)** *Sagittal SSFP MR in a 23-weeks-gestation male fetus shows a dilated, fluid-filled anterior urethra expanding the penis →. Note the distended bladder → & dilated renal collecting system →. However, the amniotic fluid is normal.*

DIFFERENTIAL DIAGNOSIS

Common

- Ureteropelvic Junction Obstruction
- Vesicoureteral Reflux
- Ureterovesical Junction Obstruction
  - Primary Megaureter
  - Other Intrinsic Causes
  - Other Extrinsic Causes
- Urolithiasis (Stones)

Less Common

- Multicystic Dysplastic Kidney (Mimic)
- Congenital Bladder Outlet Obstruction
  - Posterior Urethral Valves
  - Others
- Ureterocele

Rare but Important

- Bladder Mass
- Iatrogenic
- Ureteral Fibroepithelial Polyp

ESSENTIAL INFORMATION

Key Differential Diagnosis Issues

- Prenatal urinary tract dilation is transient/physiologic in 50-70% of cases
- However, severe in utero obstructions can lead to
  - Chronic renal damage
  - ↓ fetal micturition → ↓ amniotic fluid → ↓ lung development (pulmonary hypoplasia) → ↓ survival
- Determining extent of dilation helps narrow differential
  - Dilated calyces & disproportionately enlarged renal pelvis without ureterectasis suggest ureteropelvic junction (UPJ) obstruction
  - Dilation from top to bottom points to problems at ureterovesical junction (UVJ) or bladder outlet
  - Midureteral transitions to normal caliber are unusual; if present, consider
    - Urolithiasis
    - Aberrant anatomy: Crossing vessel
    - Stricture: Postsurgical or radiation related
    - Compression by adjacent mass
    - Ureteral mass or polyp (very uncommon)
- Imaging modalities
  - US & nuclear medicine (NM) diuretic renography are mainstays for determining degree of obstruction, associated scarring/renal growth/renal function, & superimposed infection
  - Fluoroscopic VCUG primarily evaluates for vesicoureteral reflux (VUR) but also demonstrates bladder & urethral anatomy
  - MR urography may be used in complex cases
  - Cystoscopy & retrograde ureterography further evaluate bladder masses & ureteral/collecting system obstructions

Helpful Clues for Common Diagnoses

- **Ureteropelvic Junction Obstruction**
  - Most common cause of urinary tract dilation from obstruction in children
  - Focal narrowing at junction of renal pelvis & ureter
    - Renal pelvis is often disproportionately dilated relative to calyces; ureter is not dilated
  - Degree of UPJ obstruction
    - Varies from mild to severely obstructed
    - May change with age & hydration state
  - Obstruction may be intrinsic or extrinsic
    - Intrinsic: Abnormal smooth muscle orientation, fibrosis, &/or abnormal innervation
    - Extrinsic: Crossing vessels, adenopathy, or mass
  - Presentation: Most found by prenatal US
    - May have recurrent UTI, intermittent flank pain, hematuria, vomiting
    - Older children often have crossing vessel as etiology
- **Vesicoureteral Reflux**
  - Retrograde flow of urine from bladder toward kidney
  - Graded by fluoroscopic VCUG from 1 (mild, with only ureteral extension of contrast) to 5 (severe, resulting in marked dilation & tortuosity of ureter with severely blunted renal calyces)
    - NM cystogram is more sensitive for VUR but lacks other anatomic detail of GU tract
    - US may be normal or only show urothelial thickening
  - Most common in children < 2 years of age
    - Most cases are mild
    - 80% of children outgrow VUR by puberty
  - Complications: Recurrent pyelonephritis & renal scarring that may lead to renal insufficiency & hypertension
  - Usually discovered during work-up of febrile UTI
- **Ureterovesical Junction Obstruction**
  - **Primary megaureter**
    - Focal concentric narrowing of extravesical distal ureter, anywhere from 0.5-4.0 cm in length
      - Distal segment is adynamic/aperistaltic due to abnormal innervation or abnormal musculature
      - Ureter dilates above this narrowed distal segment
    - VUR: Ipsilateral in 5%, contralateral in 10%
  - **Other intrinsic causes**
    - Stricture, fibrosis, aberrant anatomy
  - **Other extrinsic causes**
    - Compressed distal ureter due to bladder wall hypertrophy, mass, adenopathy, etc.
- **Urolithiasis (Stones)**
  - Much less common in children than adults
  - Degree of obstruction varies with stone size & location
  - US shows round/elongated echogenic focus anywhere in urinary tract (though bowel gas obscures much of ureter)
    - Twinkling artifact: Artifactual color Doppler signal in or posterior to stone
    - ± acoustic shadowing posterior to stone
    - ± loss of ureteral jet in urinary bladder
    - ± hydroureteronephrosis, renal enlargement
  - NECT is highly sensitive for calcified stones

Helpful Clues for Less Common Diagnoses

- **Multicystic Dysplastic Kidney (Mimic)**
  - Noncommunicating cysts of varying size replace renal parenchyma; no functional tissue remains
    - Involutes over months/years

- Often has residual intervening echogenic parenchyma
- May only involve part of kidney if duplicated
- Contralateral UPJ obstruction or VUR in up to 40%

- **Congenital Bladder Outlet Obstruction**
  - Often causes dilated bladder & bilateral hydroureteronephrosis
  - **Posterior urethral valves**
    - Most common form of bladder outlet obstruction; occurs only in male patients
    - Persistent tissue just distal to verumontanum obstructs posterior urethra
    - Complete obstruction in fetus leads to
      - Oligo-/anhydramnios → pulmonary hypoplasia
      - Bladder dysfunction
      - Chronic hydroureteronephrosis → cystic renal dysplasia → renal failure
    - Mild obstruction may go undetected for several years
      - Can present late with renal failure, bladder dysfunction
    - Unilateral VUR or urinoma (from UVJ or calyceal rupture) may protect contralateral kidney
      - Better long-term prognosis
    - Typically detected prenatally with large, thick-walled bladder & "keyhole" dilated posterior urethra
      - ± marked uni- vs. bilateral hydroureteronephrosis
      - ± echogenic kidneys with numerous cortical cysts
    - Bladder may have been decompressed prior to postnatal US
    - Fluoroscopic VCUG shows thin valve tissue at transition from dilated posterior to bulbar urethra
      - Irregular bladder with trabeculation & diverticula
      - Varying degrees of VUR
  - **Others**
    - Numerous etiologies: Eagle-Barrett syndrome, obstructing ureterocele, urethral atresia, megalourethra, cloaca, megacystis-microcolon-intestinal hypoperistalsis syndrome
- **Ureterocele**
  - Congenital cystic dilation of distal submucosal ureter
  - Location: Intra- or extravesical
  - Possible insertions: Orthotopic at trigone (simple) vs. ectopic insertion anywhere else, typically medial & distal
  - Kidney being drained may be single collecting system (typically simple, intravesical variety of ureterocele) or duplex (typically ectopic)
  - US shows thin-walled cystic-appearing lesion protruding into urinary bladder from UVJ, ± ureteral jet in bladder
  - Fluoroscopic VCUG shows round filling defect on early bladder-filling images; may evert later

Helpful Clues for Rare Diagnoses

- **Bladder Mass**
  - Intrinsic neoplasm or inflammatory lesion
    - Numerous etiologies, generally indistinguishable by imaging. Rhabdomyosarcoma (RMS), inflammatory pseudotumor, eosinophilic cystitis, hemorrhagic cystitis, neurofibromas
    - Nonmobile, varying degrees of internal vascularity
  - Extrinsic neoplasm may also cause obstruction
    - Prostatic or vaginal RMS, neuroblastoma, sacrococcygeal teratoma, etc.
  - Other intraluminal considerations: Hematoma, stone, & fungal balls; will be mobile & avascular
- **Iatrogenic**
  - Potential complications with recent surgery/procedure
    - VUR status post ureterocele incision
    - Deflux complications
    - Ureteral reimplantation
    - Stent malposition or blockage
    - Ureteral ligation during pelvic surgery
- **Ureteral Fibroepithelial Polyp**
  - Benign fibrovascular polyp
  - Small, well-circumscribed pedunculated mass ± internal vascularity
  - May be seen at bladder neck or in ureter

SELECTED REFERENCES

1. Morin CE et al: Use of MR urography in pediatric patients. Curr Urol Rep. 19(11):93, 2018
2. Phelps AS et al: Urinary tract dilation illustrations. Pediatr Radiol. 47(9):1214-5, 2017

Ureteropelvic Junction Obstruction

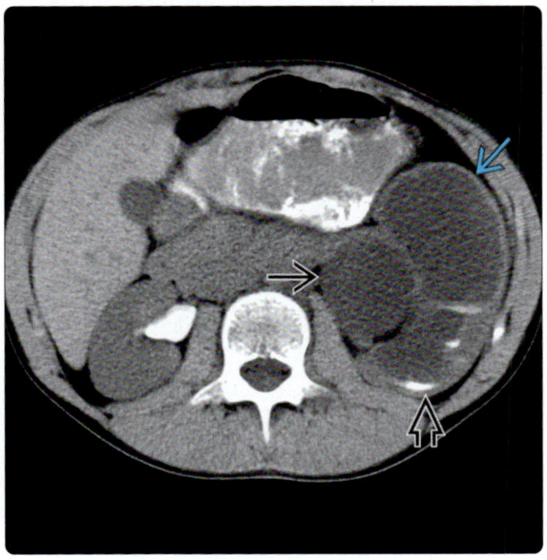

Ureteropelvic Junction Obstruction

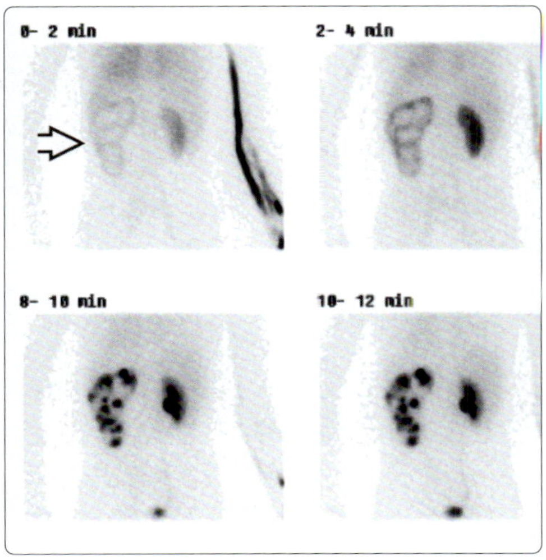

(Left) *Delayed axial CECT shows marked dilation of the left renal pelvis ➡ & calyces with minimal contrast layering in the calyces ➡. There is marked thinning of the left renal parenchyma ➡. Excreted contrast is seen in the nondilated right renal pelvis with none in the left.* **(Right)** *Posterior nuclear medicine Tc-99m renogram in the same patient shows delayed uptake & excretion of the enlarged, hydronephrotic left kidney ➡. The right kidney is normal.*

(Left) *Posterior nuclear medicine renogram in the same patient following diuretic challenge shows gradual filling of the dilated left renal pelvis but no visualization of the left ureter. The right kidney drains rapidly & is only faintly seen.* (Right) *Diuretic renography time-activity curves in the same patient show prompt drainage with decreasing counts in the normal right kidney but a flat curve with no washout in the left kidney typical of a left ureteropelvic junction obstruction.*

Ureteropelvic Junction Obstruction

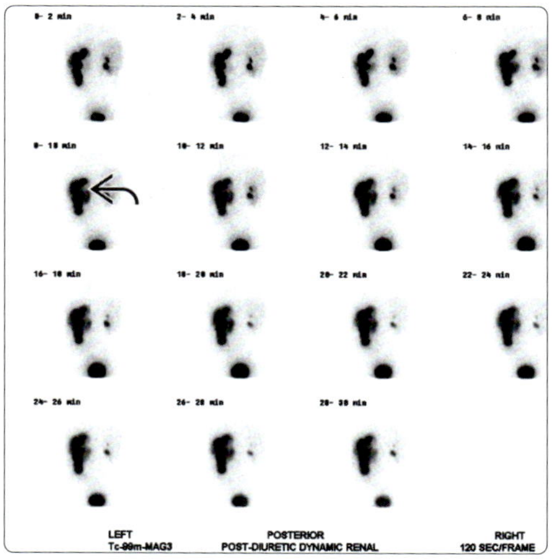

Ureteropelvic Junction Obstruction

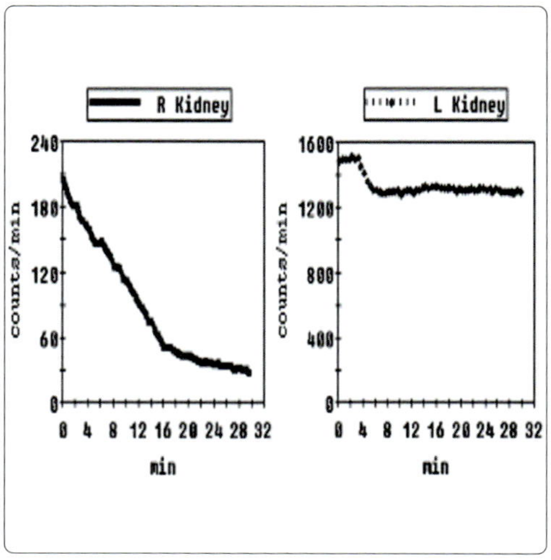

(Left) *Supine frontal fluoroscopic VCUG in an infant shows grade V vesicoureteral reflux (VUR) into the left ureter & renal collecting system.* (Right) *Coronal MR urogram MIP in a 2 month old shows marked dilation of the left ureter & renal collecting system. The dilated ureter did not clearly connect to the urinary bladder on other views. No orifice was visualized at cystoscopy. A pinpoint ureterovesical junction (UVJ) opening was found upon pathologic examination, consistent with a congenital UVJ obstruction.*

Vesicoureteral Reflux

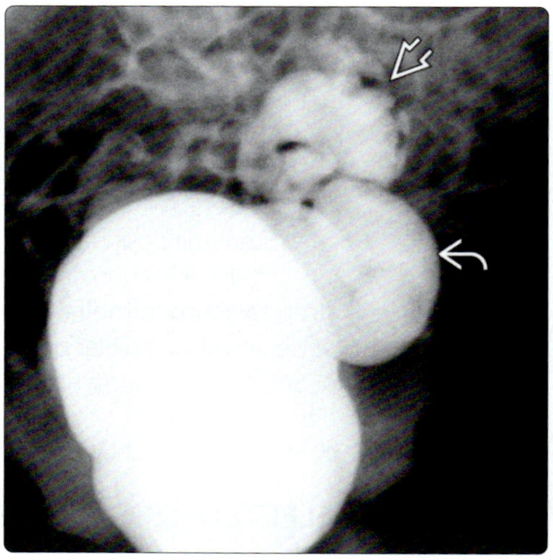

Ureterovesical Junction Obstruction

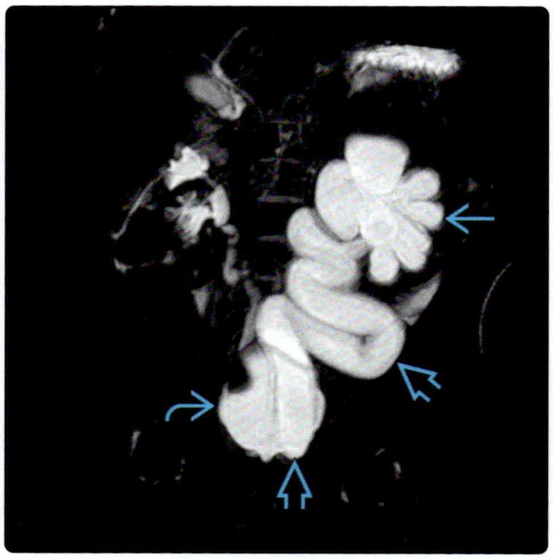

(Left) *RPO fluoroscopic VCUG shows a normal-caliber male urethra & VUR into the dilated left ureter. Note the short segment of the narrowed distal ureter in this patient with a refluxing primary megaureter.* (Right) *Posterior diuretic renography shows poor drainage from the dilated left kidney & ureter in the same patient, who has a refluxing & partially obstructed megaureter. The normal right kidney is not seen at the end of the exam.*

Primary Megaureter

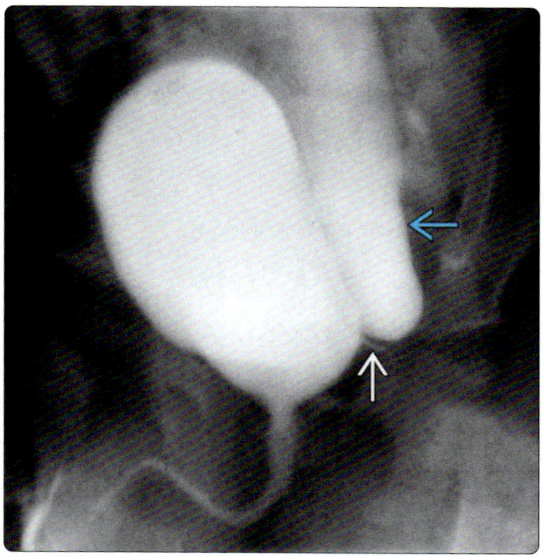

Primary Megaureter

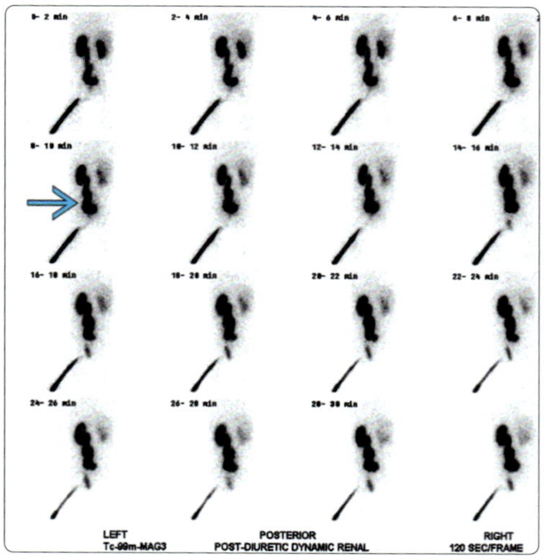

Urolithiasis (Stones)

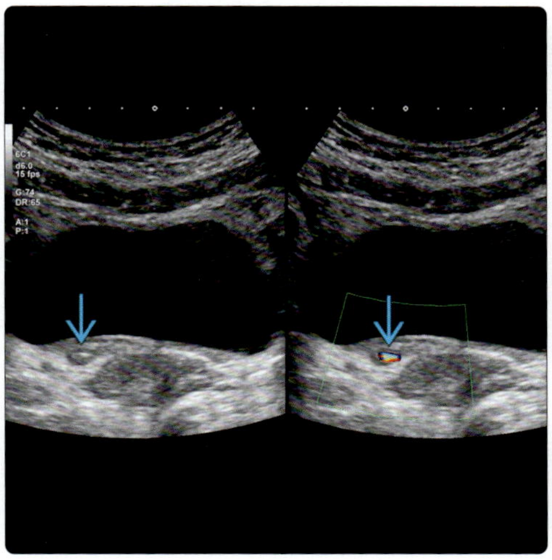

Urolithiasis (Stones)

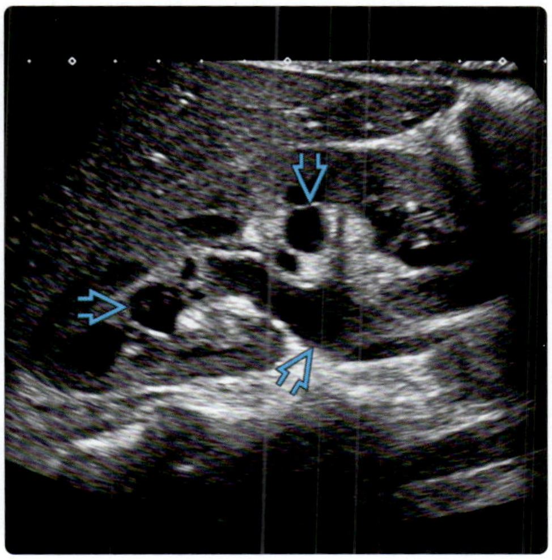

(Left) *Transverse grayscale & color Doppler US in a 14 year old with right flank pain & hematuria show a 4-mm echogenic focus with twinkling artifact (but no posterior acoustic shadowing) in the distal right ureter. No right ureteral jet was seen, & the distal right ureter was mildly dilated (not shown), typical of an obstructing stone.* **(Right)** *Longitudinal US in the same patient shows mild right hydronephrosis secondary to the distal right ureteral stone.*

Urolithiasis (Stones)

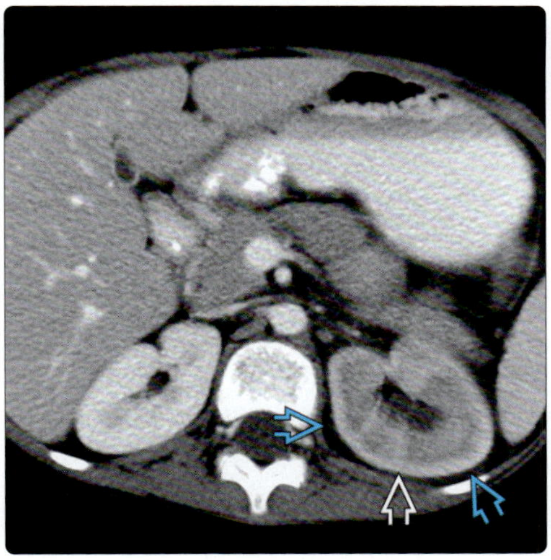

Urolithiasis (Stones)

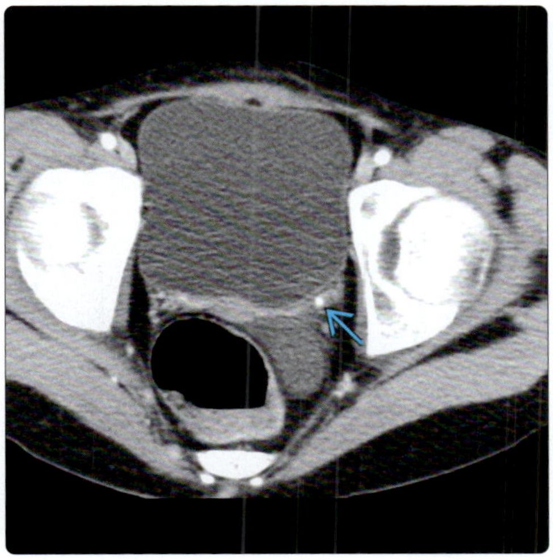

(Left) *Axial CECT shows delayed enhancement of the left kidney in this 9-year-old girl with acute left flank pain. The left kidney is mildly swollen with slight dilation of the left renal collecting system & mild edema of the surrounding fat.* **(Right)** *Axial CECT shows a calcific density in the left distal ureter of the same patient, consistent with a partially obstructing distal ureteral calculus. Additional imaging in this patient failed to show any other stones.*

Urolithiasis (Stones)

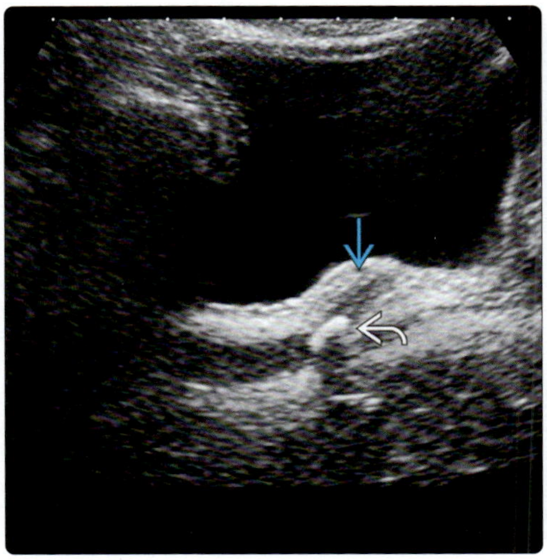

Multicystic Dysplastic Kidney (Mimic)

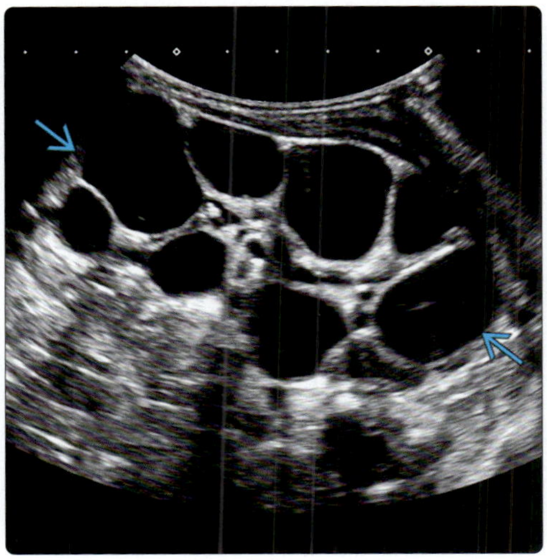

(Left) *Longitudinal US shows an echogenic, shadowing calculus in a teenager with hematuria & pain. Note the edema in the ureter distal to the stone. A ureteral jet could not be demonstrated.* **(Right)** *Longitudinal US in a newborn shows that the left kidney is enlarged (10 cm) & entirely replaced with cysts of varying size with interspersed echogenic tissue. No normal left renal tissue is identified, typical of MCDK. Note that the cysts do not communicate, & there is no renal pelvis dilation to suggest hydronephrosis.*

(Left) *Oblique sagittal SSFSE T2 MR in a 16-week male fetus shows dilation of the posterior urethra & urinary bladder, suggesting posterior urethral valves (PUVs). There is marked left hydronephrosis. The amniotic fluid is currently normal.* **(Right)** *LPO fluoroscopic VCUG in the same patient 4 days after birth shows PUVs at the junction of the dilated posterior urethra & normal bulbar urethra. There is grade V VUR into a dilated left ureter & displaced duplicated left lower pole renal collecting system.*

Posterior Urethral Valves

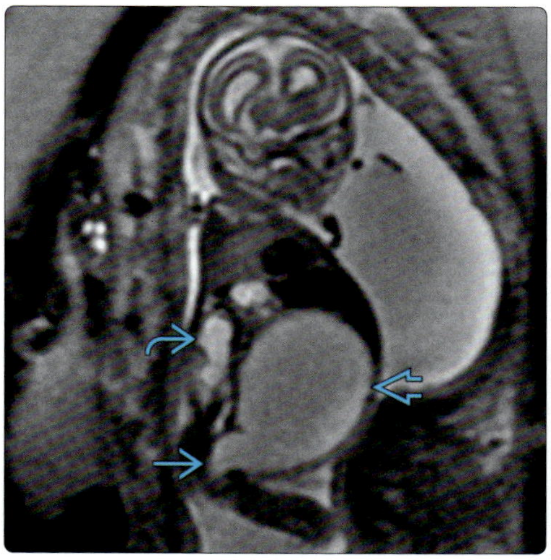

Posterior Urethral Valves

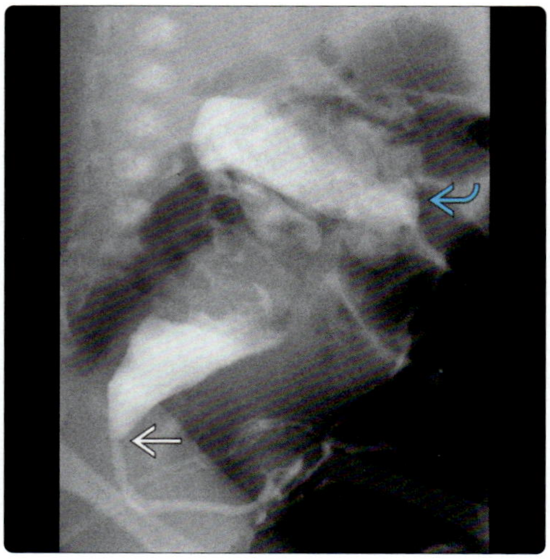

(Left) *LPO fluoroscopic VCUG shows high-grade VUR into the right ureter & renal collecting system in this newborn with a prenatal diagnosis of bladder outlet obstruction & unilateral hydroureteronephrosis. Note the dilation of the posterior urethra.* **(Right)** *Longitudinal US shows a round, thin-walled, cystic lesion within the urinary bladder protruding from the left UVJ. The distal left ureter is dilated but peristalsed vigorously on real-time imaging.*

Posterior Urethral Valves

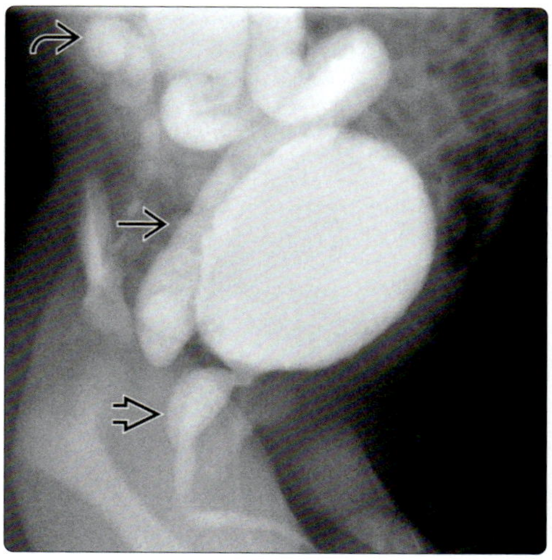

Ureterocele

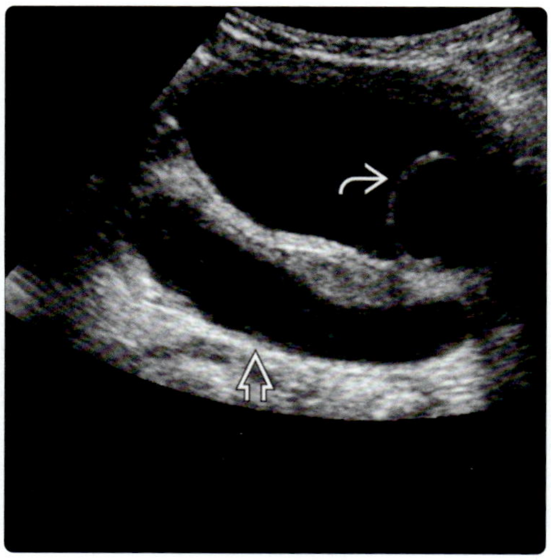

(Left) *Posterior nuclear medicine renal scan shows left-sided hydroureteronephrosis & a filling defect in the left bladder base representing the obstructed ureterocele.* **(Right)** *Longitudinal oblique color Doppler US in a 20-month-old male patient with hematuria shows blood vessels branching within a round bladder mass, excluding a clot or fungus ball. No flow is seen in the distal left ureter.*

Ureterocele

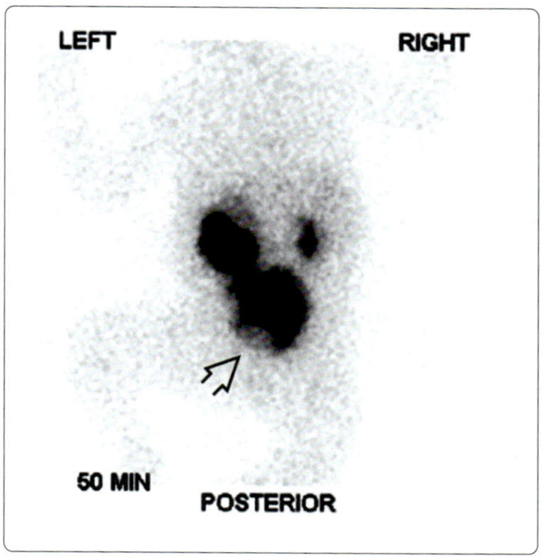

Bladder Mass

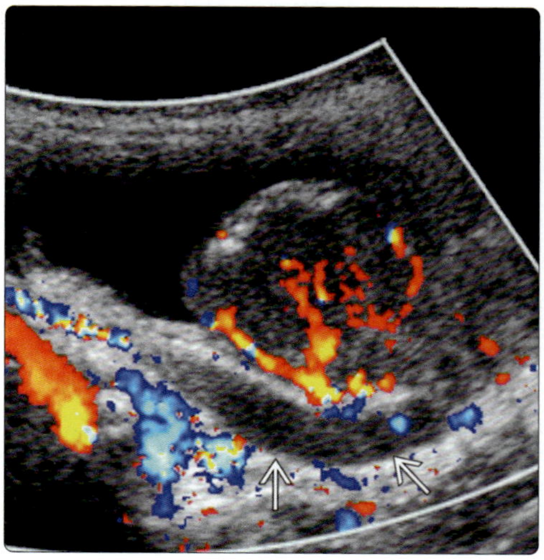

Bladder Mass

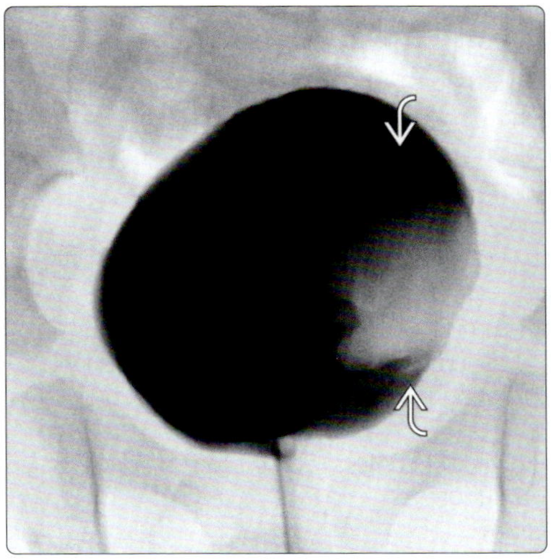

Bladder Mass

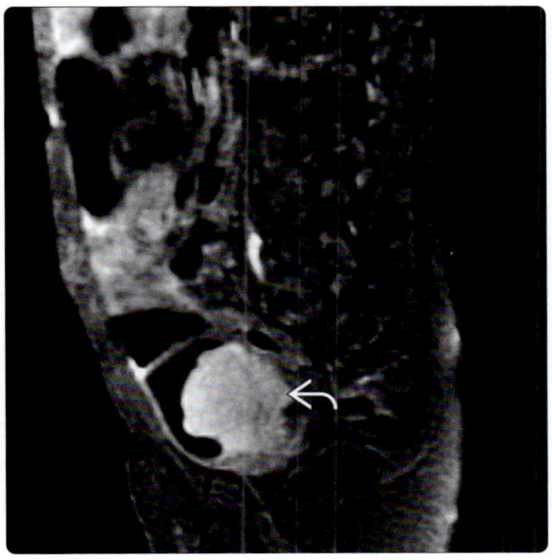

(Left) *Supine fluoroscopic VCUG in the same patient shows a lobulated filling defect in the left side of the bladder. It was difficult to know from either the US or VCUG if the mass had extended beyond the bladder wall into the surrounding pelvic tissues.* **(Right)** *Sagittal T1 C+ FS MR in the same patient shows the enhancing lobulated mass in the bladder base. The mass was resected & pathologically proven to be an inflammatory myofibroblastic tumor (benign).*

Iatrogenic

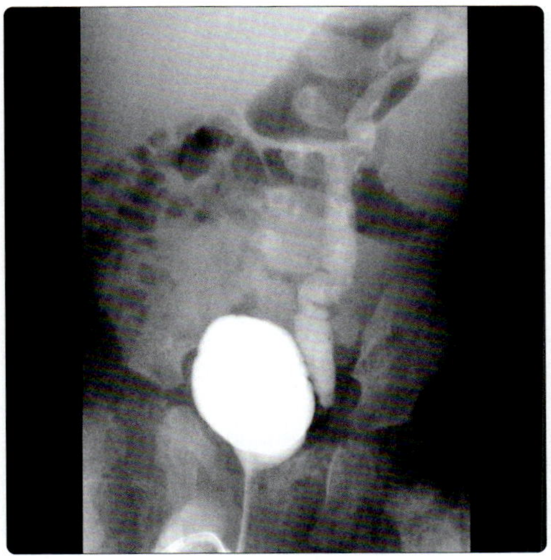

Iatrogenic

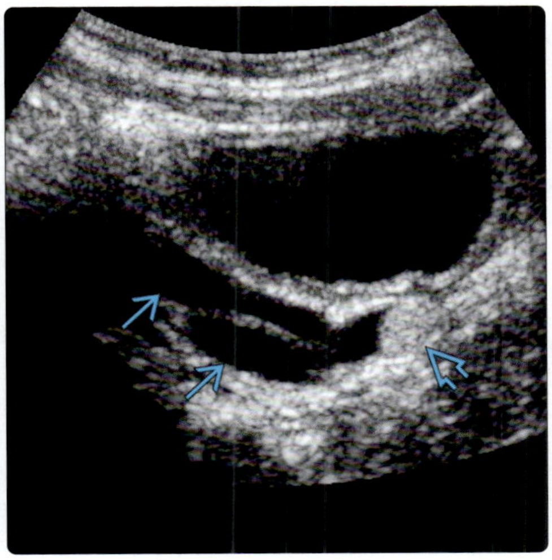

(Left) *Supine frontal fluoroscopic VCUG shows new reflux into a left ureter in a patient who recently had a large left-sided obstructed ureterocele incised through a cystoscope. VUR after ureterocele incision is fairly common.* **(Right)** *Longitudinal oblique US shows dilated ureters joining above the bladder. There is an echogenic mound of Deflux material just outside the bladder wall. This Y-shaped ureter was not dilated prior to the Deflux procedure.*

Ureteral Fibroepithelial Polyp

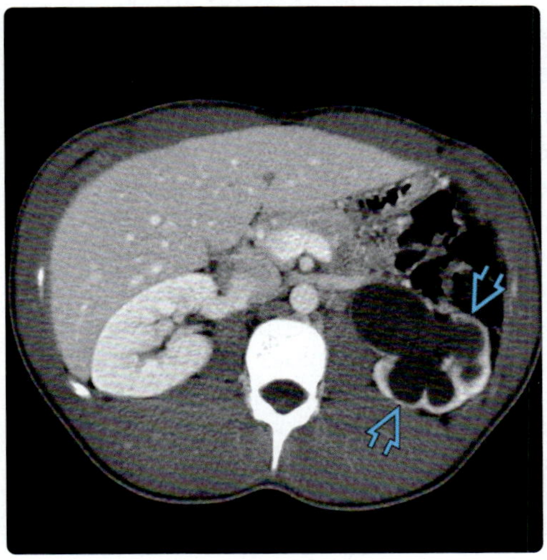

Ureteral Fibroepithelial Polyp

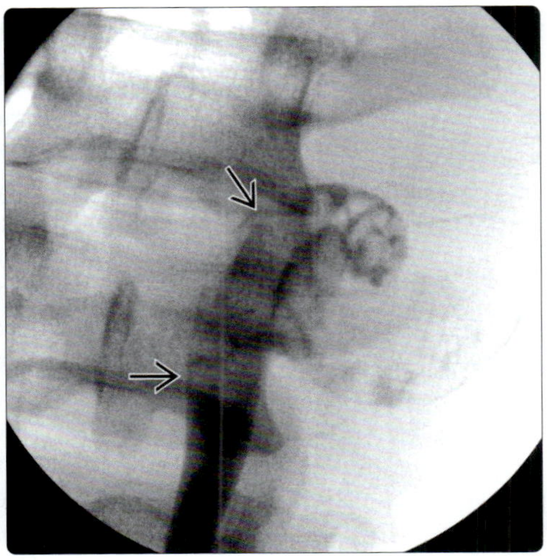

(Left) *Axial CECT shows marked hydronephrosis of the left kidney with global cortical thinning in this 17 year old with chronic intermittent hematuria & flank pain. Images more inferiorly showed soft tissue in the dilated ureter, initially thought to be a hematoma.* **(Right)** *Supine fluoroscopic retrograde pyelogram performed in the operating room shows a tubular filling defect in the proximal ureter. There was a normal-caliber ureter distally (not shown). Biopsy of the intraluminal lesion showed a fibroepithelial polyp.*

DIFFERENTIAL DIAGNOSIS

Common

- Ovarian Cyst
- Paraovarian Cyst
- Peritoneal Inclusion Cyst
- Ovarian Neoplasm
- Ovarian Torsion
- Pelvic Abscess

Less Common

- Hydrometrocolpos/Hematometrocolpos
- Lower Urinary Tract Anomalies
- Renal Ectopia & Fusion
- Sacrococcygeal Teratoma
- Neuroblastoma
- Burkitt Lymphoma
- Enteric Cyst
- Ewing Sarcoma
- Rhabdomyosarcoma

Rare but Important

- Anterior Sacral Meningocele
- Ectopic Pregnancy

ESSENTIAL INFORMATION

Key Differential Diagnosis Issues

- Sex & age of patient
- Any ovarian mass (especially > 5 cm) predisposes to & may coexist with ovarian torsion

Helpful Clues for Common Diagnoses

- **Ovarian Cyst**
  - Simple cyst: Anechoic, > 3 cm
  - Hemorrhagic cyst: Avascular; may appear solid, have lacy reticular echoes, fluid-debris levels, or contracting clot
- **Paraovarian Cyst**
  - Wolffian duct remnant
  - Separate from ovary
  - Anechoic, thin walled; 95% are unilocular
  - Variable size, mean of 4 cm
  - Appearance/size will not change with time
- **Peritoneal Inclusion Cyst**
  - Peritoneal fluid trapped by adhesions
    - History of surgery or inflammation
  - Irregular unilocular or multilocular cystic lesion, often surrounding or displacing ovary
- **Ovarian Neoplasm**
  - Germ cell tumors
    - Teratoma: Mixed cystic & solid mass with fat & Ca^{2+}
      - Benign mature teratoma (a.k.a. dermoid cyst) is most common pediatric ovarian neoplasm
      - Immature teratoma is not reliably differentiated on imaging; generally has greater solid component
      - Tip of iceberg sign: Full extent of mass is obscured by shadowing from superficial echogenic interfaces
      - Dermoid plug sign: Shadowing echogenic nodule in lumen of cyst
      - Dermoid mesh sign: Thin echogenic "lines & dots" due to hair in cyst
      - May see fat-fluid interface
    - Dysgerminoma, yolk sac tumor, embryonal cell carcinoma, choriocarcinoma: Heterogeneous solid & cystic masses
  - Epithelial cell tumors
    - Cystadenoma > > cystadenocarcinoma
    - Predominantly cystic appearance
    - Thick & irregular walls & septations suggest malignancy
    - Serous contents appear more homogeneous
    - Mucinous contents show varying density
  - Stromal cell tumors
    - Granulosa cell tumor: Large solid mass with variable cystic component; may cause isosexual precocious puberty
    - Sertoli-Leydig cell tumors: Cystic, solid, or mixed; may cause virilization
- **Ovarian Torsion**
  - Twisting of vascular pedicle of ovary &/or fallopian tube
  - Marked asymmetry in ovarian volumes
    - > 100 mL highly suggestive
    - Median volume 12x normal side
  - May be displaced to midline or contralateral pelvis
  - Appearance varies with chronicity
    - Enlarged, rounded ovary
    - Hypoechoic or heterogeneous
    - Peripheral mildly enlarged follicles may be seen
  - Ovarian morphology is important
    - Normal Doppler flow does not exclude ovarian torsion
  - Underlying cyst or mass is common
- **Pelvic Abscess**
  - Consider perforated appendicitis, Crohn disease, tuboovarian abscess
  - Complex cystic mass with thick enhancing rim, adjacent free fluid, & inflammation
  - May see reactive or secondary findings
    - Bowel wall thickening
    - Ileus or bowel obstruction
    - Ureteropelvocaliectasis
  - Abscess secondary to bowel pathology is more likely to contain gas than tuboovarian abscess

Helpful Clues for Less Common Diagnoses

- **Hydrometrocolpos/Hematometrocolpos**
  - Dilation of vagina ± uterus with fluid or blood
    - May see nondilated or mildly dilated uterus arising from dome of collection (as vaginal walls are much more distensible)
  - Bimodal age presentation: Infancy, peripubertal
  - Causes range from simple imperforate hymen to complex müllerian duct anomalies
  - Cystic pelvic mass in cloacal malformation most commonly corresponds to hydrocolpos
- **Lower Urinary Tract Anomalies**
  - Bladder outlet obstruction: Posterior urethral valves, cloaca, obstructing mass
    - Also consider urinary retention: Neurogenic bladder, infection, constipation
  - Bladder diverticulum: Thin-walled, fluid-filled structure, continuity with bladder wall, M > F
  - Ureterocele: Cystic intravesical mass on US

- Ureteral dilation: Tubular fluid-filled structures; tortuous & redundant when severe
- **Renal Ectopia & Fusion**
  - Varying degrees of ectopia & fusion configurations
    - Frequently have multiple vessels & ureters
  - Horseshoe kidney: Fused at lower poles, lie lower than normal kidneys
  - Crossed fused renal ectopia: Kidney fused to lower pole of contralateral kidney
  - Pelvic kidney: Parenchyma may otherwise appear normal
  - Ptotic or mobile kidney may only be in pelvis when standing
- **Sacrococcygeal Teratoma**
  - Congenital heterogeneous mixed cystic/solid presacral mass ± Ca^{2+}, fat
  - Ranges from large & exophytic to entirely internal
- **Neuroblastoma**
  - Arises from neural crest cells in sympathetic chain; 2-3% in pelvis
  - Typical CT/US/MR findings
    - Heterogeneous soft tissue mass with Ca^{2+}, necrosis, hemorrhage
    - Metastases typically to liver, bones, & skin (younger ages)
  - 95% diagnosed before age 7 years
- **Burkitt Lymphoma**
  - Homogeneous soft tissue masses involving solid organs or bowel, especially ileocecal region
  - Clinically causes obstruction or intussusception
  - Can grow rapidly with very acute presentation
  - Mean age of 8 years, M > > F
- **Enteric Cyst**
  - Enteric duplication cyst (ileum >> rectum), tailgut cyst (presacral/retrorectal)
  - Round or tubular fluid-filled structure
  - Hypoechoic on US, low attenuation on CT
    - May see bowel wall layers on US
- **Ewing Sarcoma**
  - Pelvic & lumbosacral origins are common
  - Bone: Permeative destruction, often with expansile component; may involve entire bone
  - Soft tissues: Large heterogeneous mass is typical
- **Rhabdomyosarcoma**
  - Genitourinary system is 2nd most common site of origin after head & neck
    - Bladder, vagina, uterus, or prostate
    - May also arise from other pelvic soft tissues
  - Heterogeneous solid mass
  - Bimodal age distribution: 2-6 years, 14-18 years

Helpful Clues for Rare Diagnoses

- **Anterior Sacral Meningocele**
  - Usually purely cystic in appearance
  - Osseous defects on radiographs: Sacral deficiency, scimitar sacrum
  - May be asymptomatic or present with urinary or bowel symptoms
  - Associations: Anorectal malformations, neurofibromatosis type 1 (NF1), Marfan syndrome
- **Ectopic Pregnancy**
  - Heterogeneous ring-like adnexal mass with positive pregnancy test
    - 95% in fallopian tube, separate from ovary
    - Ring of fire color Doppler appearance, also seen with corpus luteum cyst
    - ± hemoperitoneum
  - No intrauterine pregnancy
    - Pseudosac in uterus in 10-20%
  - Correlate findings with quantitative hCG

SELECTED REFERENCES

1. Paltiel HJ et al: US of the pediatric female pelvis. Radiology. 270(3):644-57, 2014
2. Anthony EY et al: Adnexal masses in female pediatric patients. AJR Am J Roentgenol. 198(5):W426-31, 2012
3. Moyle PL et al: Nonovarian cystic lesions of the pelvis. Radiographics. 30(4):921-33, 2010
4. Kocaoglu M et al: Pediatric presacral masses. Radiographics. 26(3):833-57, 2006

Ovarian Cyst

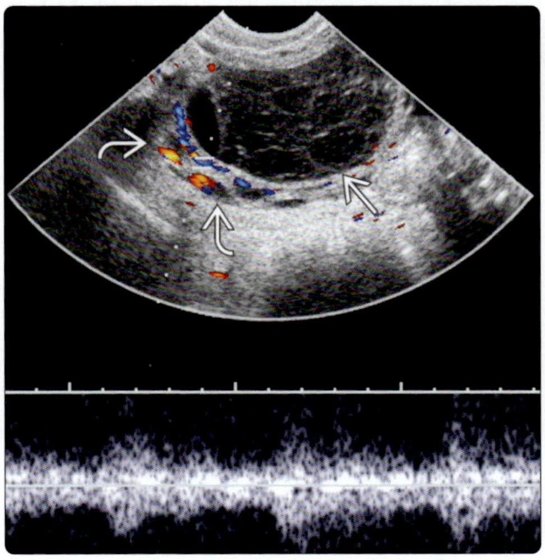

Ovarian Cyst

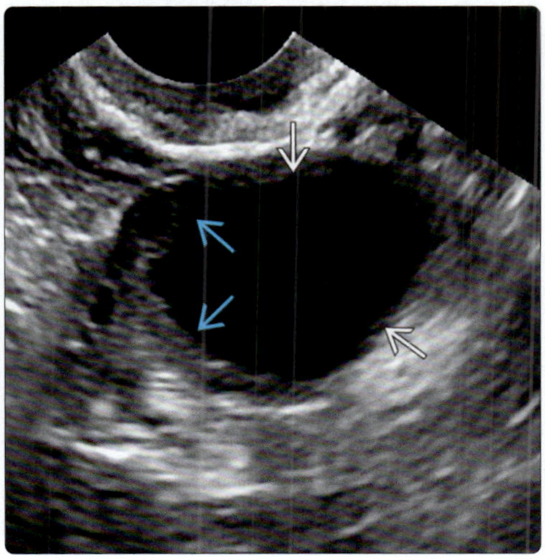

(Left) *Longitudinal US shows a circumscribed, hypoechoic, ovoid pelvic mass ➡ with no internal vascularity. The internal reticular echoes are typical of a hemorrhagic ovarian cyst. There is a crescent of normal ovarian tissue with internal vascularity stretched along its edge ➡.* **(Right)** *Transverse US shows a 3-cm anechoic lesion ➡ in the right ovary in a 15 year old with pain. The lesion was also avascular (not shown), consistent with a simple cyst. A thin rim of ovarian tissue ➡ confirms its origin.*

(Left) *Longitudinal US shows a small anechoic structure* ➔ *adjacent to but separate from the normal right ovary* → *in this 13 year old with pain. It was unchanged on a pelvic US 2 years later, consistent with a paraovarian cyst.* **(Right)** *Axial T2 FS MR shows a fluid collection* ➔ *surrounding the right ovary* ↗, *consistent with a peritoneal inclusion cyst in this 12-year-old girl who had a history of multiple abdominal surgeries. The septations* → *are typically thin.*

Paraovarian Cyst

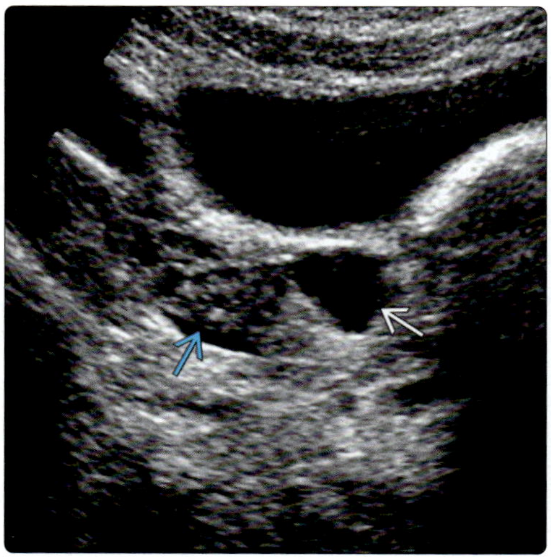

Peritoneal Inclusion Cyst

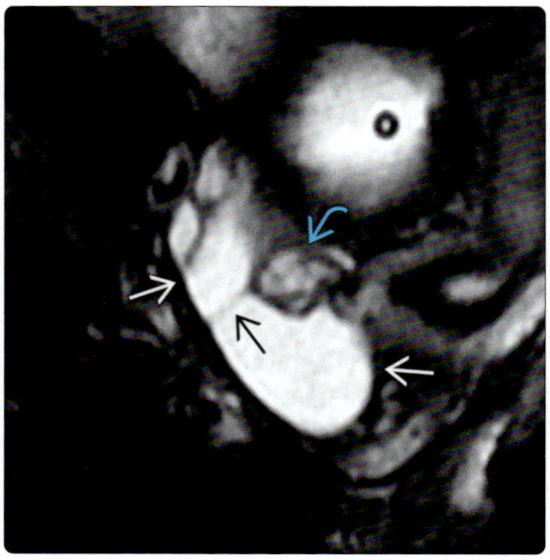

(Left) *Axial CECT shows an ovoid pelvic lesion in the left adnexal region. Note the classic components of this mature teratoma: Predominantly cystic* ⇒, *low-attenuation fat* ➔, *& Ca^{2+}* →. **(Right)** *Axial CECT shows a large complex mass* ➔ *arising from the pelvis in this 3-year-old girl. Low-attenuation areas represent cysts & necrosis in this juvenile granulosa cell tumor. Premature breast development was also seen, indicating a hormonally active tumor.*

Ovarian Neoplasm

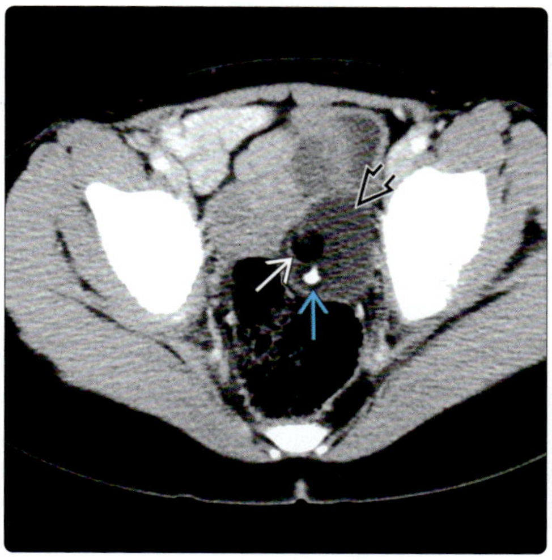

Ovarian Neoplasm

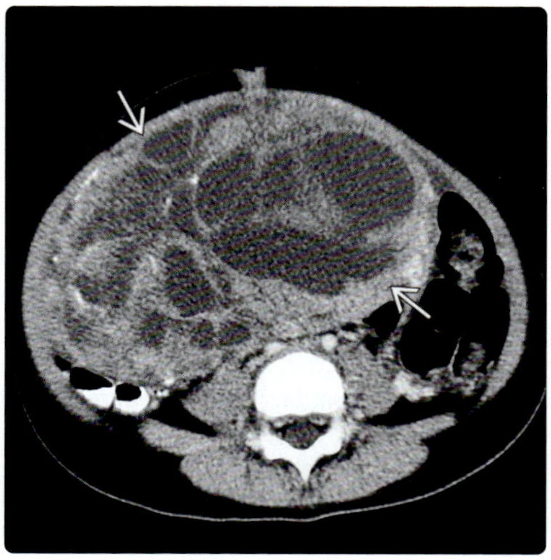

(Left) *Transverse US in this 16 year old with acute pelvic pain & vomiting shows an enlarged left ovary* ➔ *containing a hemorrhagic cyst* →. *The ovarian parenchyma was heterogeneously hypoechoic & blood flow was diminished. Ovarian volumes were 86 mL on the left & 13 mL on the right.* **(Right)** *Axial CECT in a 3 year old shows a fluid & gas* → *collection* ➔ *with a thick irregular wall secondary to perforated appendicitis, the most common cause of abdominopelvic abscesses in children.*

Ovarian Torsion

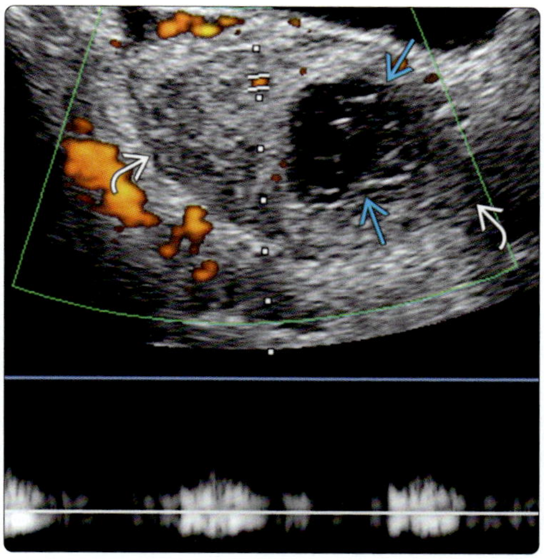

Pelvic Abscess

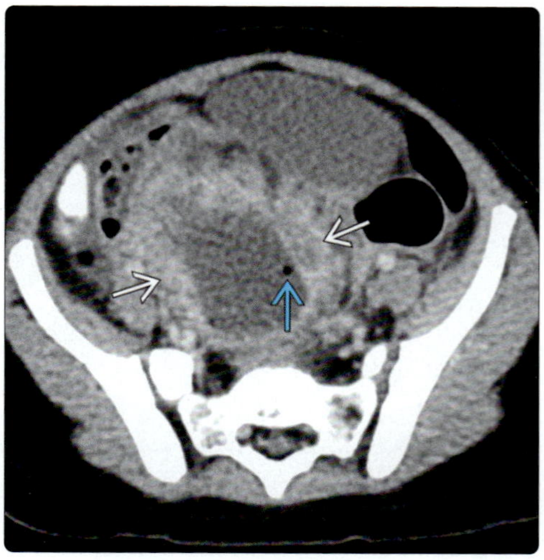

Hydrometrocolpos/Hematometrocolpos

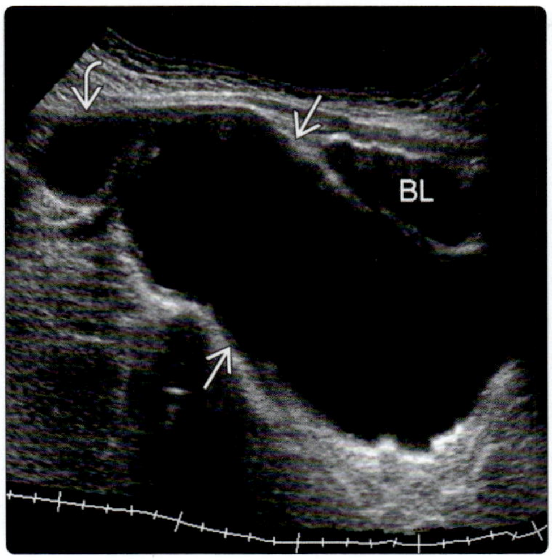

Hydrometrocolpos/Hematometrocolpos

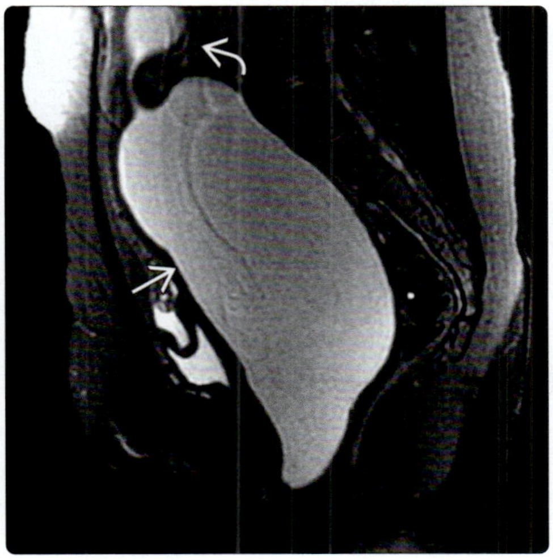

(Left) *Longitudinal US in a 14-year-old girl with flank pain & a palpable mass demonstrates a distended, fluid-filled vagina & uterus. This was an isolated finding, but coexistent renal anomalies are common.* **(Right)** *Sagittal T2 FS MR in the same patient demonstrates the distended vagina & uterus. This patient was found to have an imperforate hymen. The contents were also hyperintense on T1 (not shown), consistent with blood products.*

Lower Urinary Tract Anomalies

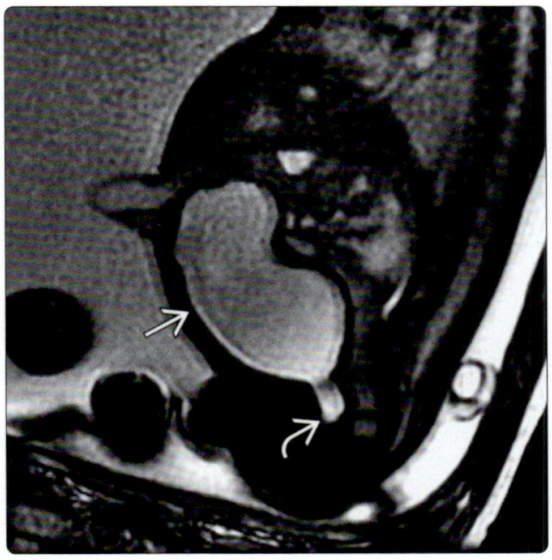

Renal Ectopia & Fusion

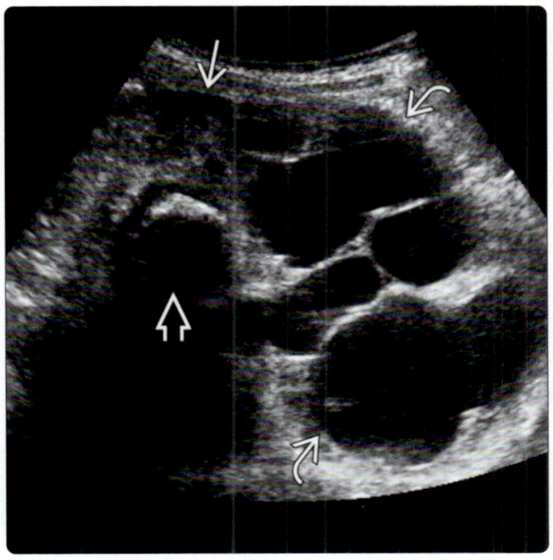

(Left) *Sagittal SSFP MR of a male fetus shows a dilated bladder & posterior urethra, typical of posterior urethral valves resulting in bladder outlet obstruction. There was also bilateral hydroureteronephrosis (not shown).* **(Right)** *Transverse US in this 2 year old shows a pelvic horseshoe kidney with a hydronephrotic left moiety. The isthmus of the horseshoe kidney extends across midline anterior to the spine. This location increases the risk of traumatic injury.*

Sacrococcygeal Teratoma

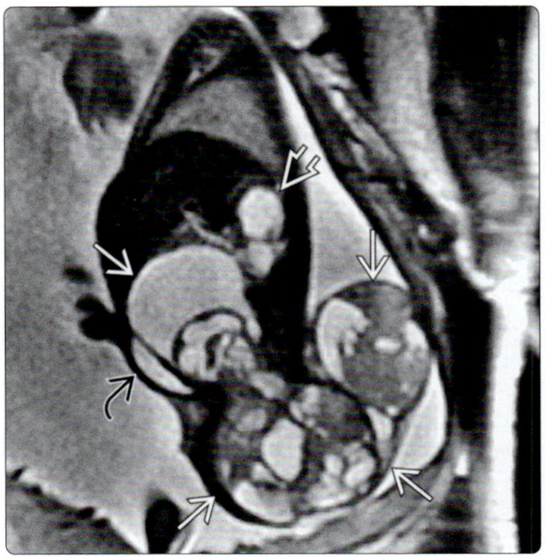

Sacrococcygeal Teratoma

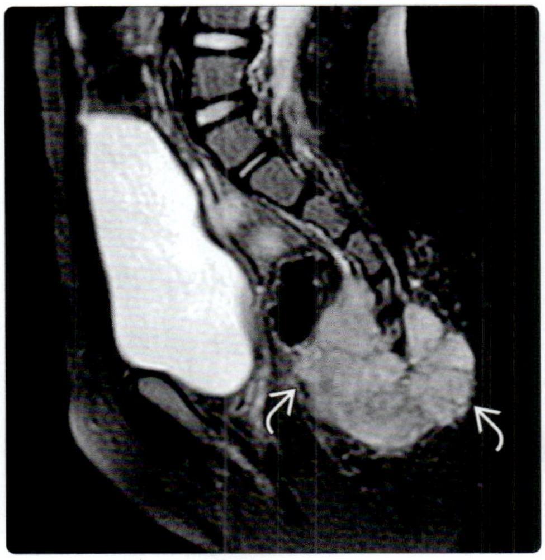

(Left) *Sagittal T2 MR of a fetus demonstrates a very large mixed cystic & solid mass with exophytic & intrapelvic components, consistent with a sacrococcygeal teratoma. The bladder is compressed anteriorly & there is hydronephrosis.* **(Right)** *Sagittal T2 FS MR shows a lobular high signal intensity mass encircling the coccyx. This purely internal sacrococcygeal teratoma was discovered not by physical exam but by a renal/bladder US after a urinary tract infection.*

(Left) *Transverse US shows a heterogeneous pelvic mass with scattered flecks of* Ca^{2+}*, some demonstrating subtle posterior acoustic shadowing. This lesion was very low in the pelvis, a less common location for neuroblastoma.* **(Right)** *Axial CECT shows the same lesion, though the mass now appears only mildly heterogeneous. Note the* Ca^{2+} *& extension into the sacral neural foramen & spinal canal.*

Neuroblastoma

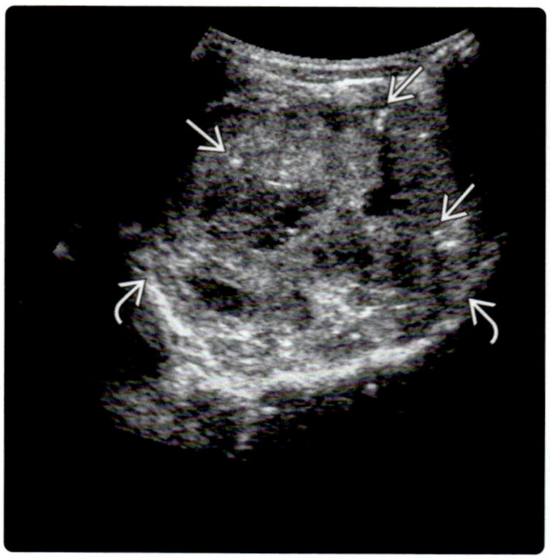

Neuroblastoma

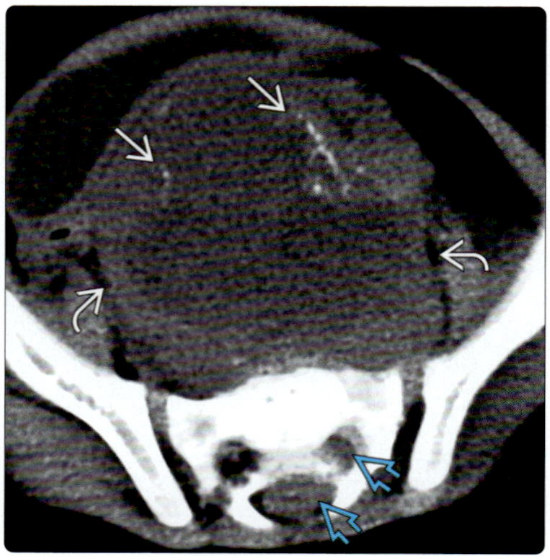

(Left) *Axial CECT shows a homogeneous soft tissue mass deep in the pelvis in a patient who presented after 5 days of abdominal pain & distension. The mass displaces the bladder anteriorly.* **(Right)** *Axial T2 FS MR from the same patient shows a homogeneous soft tissue mass of Burkitt lymphoma encircling the rectum & causing obstruction. Note the urethra anteriorly.*

Burkitt Lymphoma

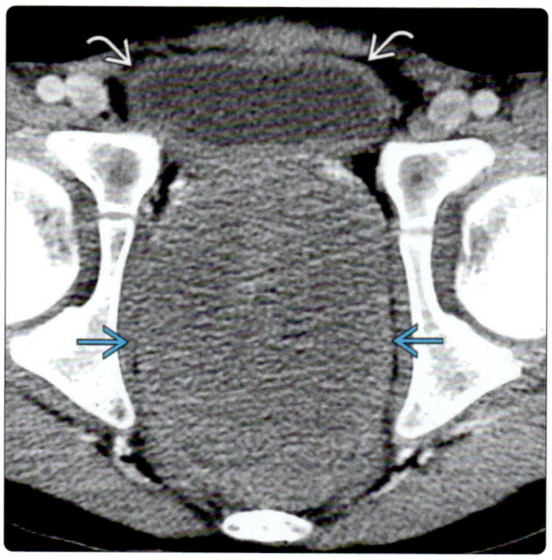

Burkitt Lymphoma

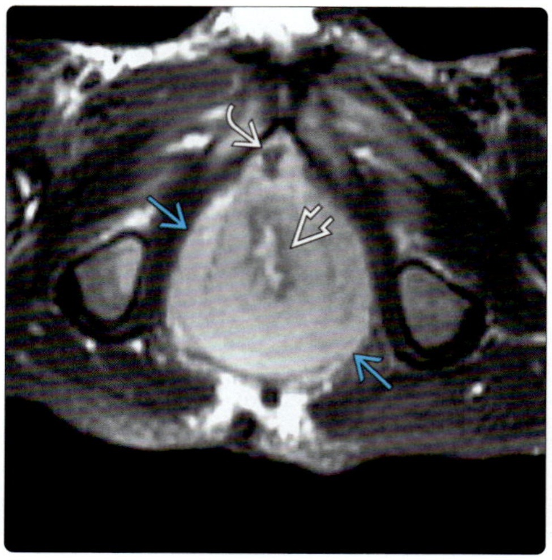

(Left) *Coronal oblique T2 FS MR of the pelvis in a 12-year-old girl being evaluated for perirectal abscess shows a lobulated hyperintense retrorectal mass. This lesion was found to be a tailgut cyst with inflammation & focal fistula formation on pathology.* **(Right)** *Transverse US shows a cystic pelvic lesion with posterior acoustic enhancement. The wall lacks the characteristic "gut signature" that is often suggestive of a duplication cyst. This was an ileal duplication cyst.*

Enteric Cyst

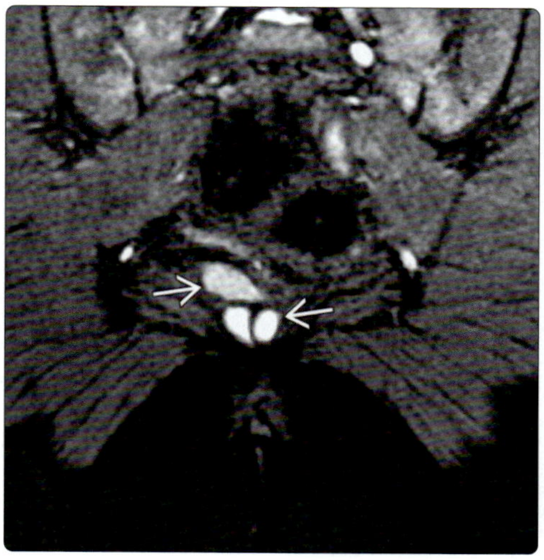

Enteric Cyst

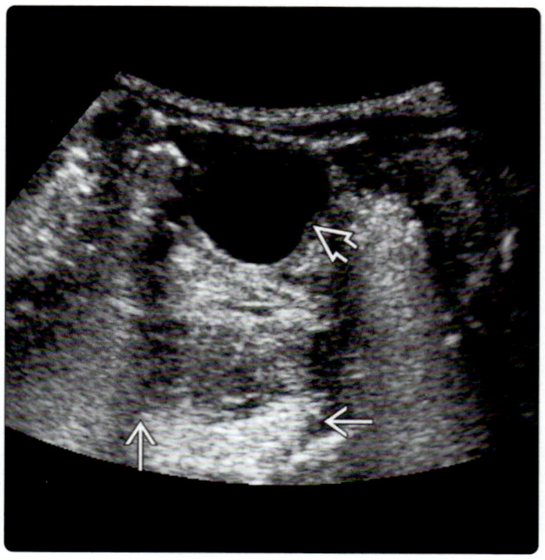

Ewing Sarcoma

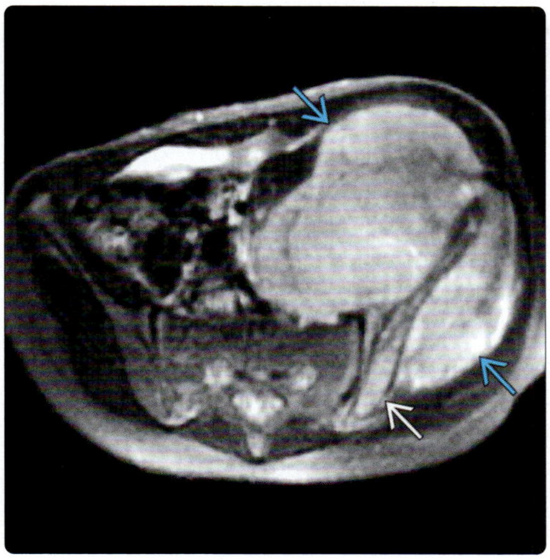

Ewing Sarcoma

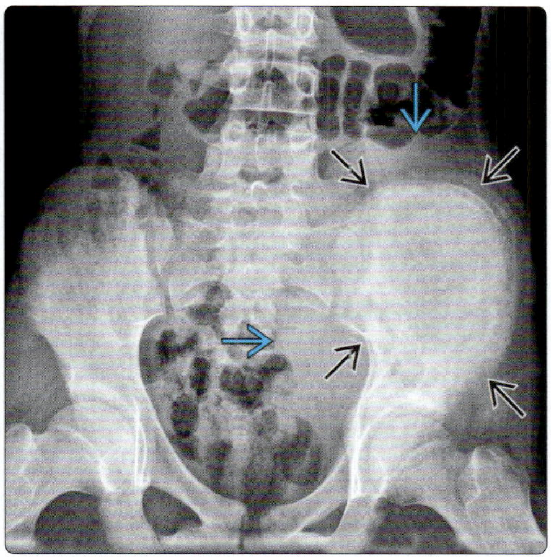

(Left) *Axial T2 MR shows a bulky high signal intensity mass ⇨ arising from the left iliac wing in this child with metastatic Ewing sarcoma who initially presented with a 5-month history of intermittent hip pain. Note also the marrow signal abnormality of the iliac bone ⇨.* **(Right)** *AP radiograph in the same patient shows expansion, permeation, sclerosis, & periosteal reaction of the left iliac bone ⇨ with an associated large soft tissue mass ⇨ due to Ewing sarcoma.*

Rhabdomyosarcoma

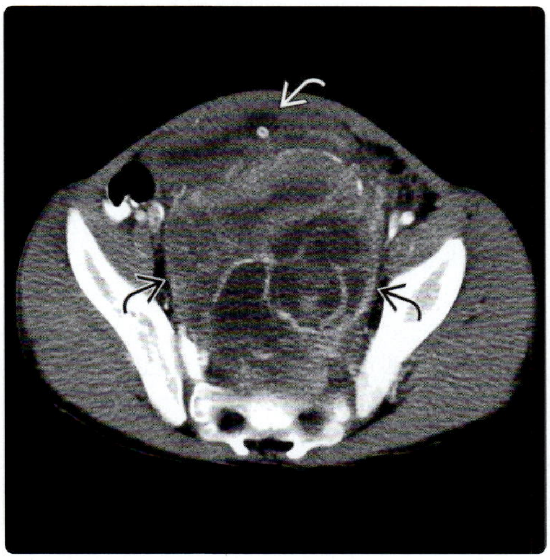

Anterior Sacral Meningocele

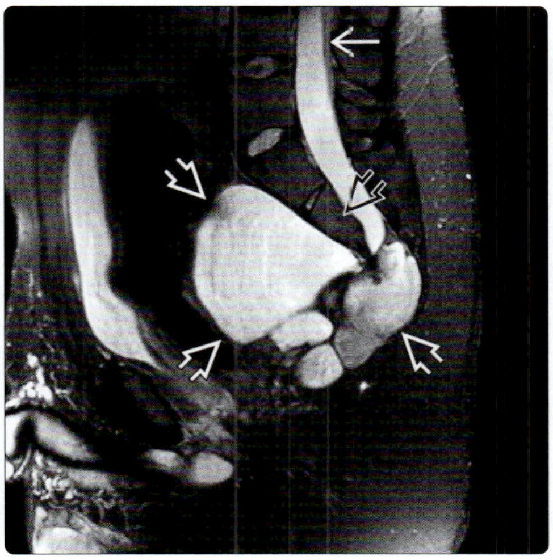

(Left) *Axial CECT shows a circumscribed, heterogeneous pelvic mass ⇨, without Ca^{2+}, found to emanate from the prostate. The urinary bladder is displaced superiorly & anteriorly ⇨, containing a Foley catheter.* **(Right)** *Sagittal T2 FS MR shows a lobular, cystic lesion ⇨ anterior & inferior to an abnormally truncated sacrum ⇨. Note the tethered nerve roots clinging to the posterior spinal canal ⇨.*

Anterior Sacral Meningocele

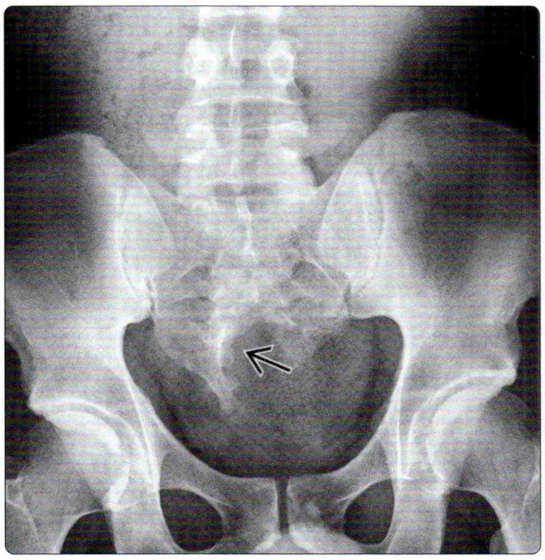

Ectopic Pregnancy

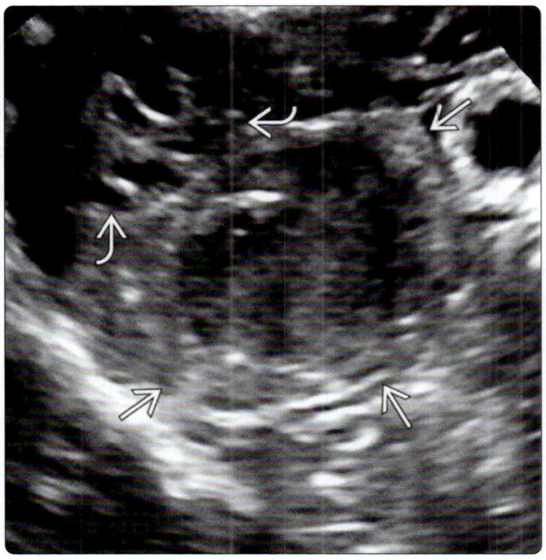

(Left) *Frontal radiograph in the same patient shows an abnormally curved scimitar sacrum ⇨. The 3 findings of a scimitar sacrum, any presacral mass, & an anorectal malformation comprise the Currarino triad.* **(Right)** *Transverse US shows a heterogeneous right adnexal mass ⇨ in an adolescent with right lower quadrant pain & a positive urine pregnancy test. The mass was intraoperatively confirmed to be a tubal ectopic pregnancy. The normal right ovary lies immediately adjacent ⇨.*

DIFFERENTIAL DIAGNOSIS

Common

- Functional Ovarian Cysts
- Hemorrhagic Cyst
- Ovarian Torsion
- Mature Teratoma
- Polycystic Ovary Syndrome

Less Common

- Tuboovarian Abscess
- Ectopic Pregnancy
- Dysgerminoma
- Mixed Germ Cell Tumor
- Yolk Sac Tumor
- Sertoli-Leydig Cell Tumor
- Epithelial Tumors

Rare but Important

- Small Cell Carcinoma, Hypercalcemic Type
- Ovarian Fibroma
- Juvenile Granulosa Cell Tumor

ESSENTIAL INFORMATION

Key Differential Diagnosis Issues

- Pediatric ovarian masses can be
  - Functional/nonneoplastic
  - Neoplastic: Benign > malignant (10-20%)
- Findings suggestive of malignancy
  - Predominantly solid
  - Large or growing mass
  - Hormonally active
  - Positive serum tumor markers (AFP, β-hCG, LDH, CA-125)
  - Invasion or metastases
  - Peritoneal fluid & implants
- Any ovarian mass predisposes to ovarian torsion

Helpful Clues for Common Diagnoses

- **Functional Ovarian Cysts**
  - Most common pediatric ovarian "mass"
    - Seen most commonly in neonatal period & again in peripubertal/postpubertal girls
  - Imaging: Round/ovoid, well circumscribed, anechoic, thin walled, avascular
  - Cysts > 3 cm should be reimaged in 6-8 weeks
    - > 90% will resolve spontaneously
    - < 3 cm is considered physiologic
    - Adult-centric guidelines on incidental ovarian cysts are not applicable to pediatric patients with pain
  - Fetal ovarian cysts
    - Stimulated by maternal & fetal gonadotropins
    - May be displaced into abdomen & palpable
    - Usually regress in 3-4 months, up to 1 year
  - Corpus luteal cyst
    - Residua of dominant follicle after ovulation
    - Typically < 3 cm
    - Thicker, irregular, hypervascular wall
- **Hemorrhagic Cyst**
  - Avascular complex cyst containing debris
  - Imaging: Contents are variable in appearance, including homogeneously echogenic, lacy reticular echoes, fluid-debris level, &/or contracting echogenic clot
  - Should regress/involute in 6-8 weeks
    - > 5 cm are less likely to spontaneously regress
- **Ovarian Torsion**
  - Twisting of ovary, fallopian tube, or both → ischemia
  - Bimodal distribution: < 1 year & ~ 12 years
    - ~ 10% neonatal, ~ 50% 9-14 years
  - Imaging: Unilateral enlarged ovary, > 5-12x contralateral volume; stromal edema → peripheral follicles
    - ± parenchymal hemorrhage
      - ▫ May appear as midline "pelvic mass" with visualization of only 1 normal ovary
    - Free pelvic fluid/blood
    - Normal Doppler exam does not exclude torsion with concerning grayscale appearance & clinical findings
  - 51-84% of pediatric ovarian torsion is associated with underlying lesion
    - More likely if mass > 5 cm
  - Treatment: Urgent surgical detorsion, conservation of ovarian tissue
    - Length of symptoms does not predict viability
- **Mature Teratoma**
  - Benign germ cell tumor, containing all 3 layers
    - Hair, fat, & teeth may be seen on imaging
  - Most common pediatric ovarian neoplasm
  - Imaging: Typical appearance is mixed cystic & solid mass with areas of fat & Ca^{2+}
    - In general, cystic > solid components
    - Ultrasound signs
      - ▫ Tip of iceberg: Full extent of mass obscured by shadowing superficial interfaces
      - ▫ Dermoid plug: Floating echogenic nodule
      - ▫ Dermoid mesh: Echogenic lines & dots (due to hair) surrounded by fluid
    - Immature teratoma is not reliably differentiated, but generally solid > cystic components
  - Bilateral in up to 15-25%
- **Polycystic Ovary Syndrome**
  - Ovulatory dysfunction, hyperandrogenism, polycystic ovaries, insulin resistance
  - Imaging: Ultrasound findings are supportive but not diagnostic in absence of clinical findings
    - ≥ 25 follicles/ovary with ultrasound transducer ≥ 8 MHz
      - ▫ Peripheral, uniform size, string of pearls appearance
    - Ovarian volume ≥ 10 mL
    - Normal morphology does not exclude diagnosis

Helpful Clues for Less Common Diagnoses

- **Tuboovarian Abscess**
  - Fever, cervical tenderness, & vaginal discharge
  - Imaging: Complex solid & cystic adnexal mass
    - Thick-walled & hyperemic cystic regions
    - Surrounding inflammation & free fluid
    - Internal gas is rare → consider bowel pathology
    - CT or MR may be necessary to exclude appendiceal abscess
  - Generally treated medically, not surgically

- **Ectopic Pregnancy**
  - Imaging: Heterogeneous, sometimes ring-like adnexal mass with positive pregnancy test
    - Decidual reaction/fluid in uterus with no true intrauterine gestational sac
    - May see gestational sac in adnexa in minority of cases
      - Usually on same side as corpus luteum
    - Ring of fire appearance is nonspecific
      - Corpus luteum is far more common than ovarian ectopic
    - ± hemoperitoneum
  - Correlate findings with quantitative β-hCG level
  - Ovarian ectopic is rare; 90-95% are tubal
- **Dysgerminoma**
  - Analogous to testicular seminoma
  - 5% secrete β-hCG
  - Imaging: Multilobulated solid mass, enhancing septa
    - May have areas of necrosis, hemorrhage, Ca^{2+}
    - Septa hypointense on T2 MR imaging
    - 10-15% bilateral
  - 15% recur but are retreated with good prognosis
  - Association with gonadal dysgenesis, Turner syndrome
- **Mixed Germ Cell Tumors**
  - Contain > 1 type of germ cell tumor
    - Teratoma, dysgerminoma, & yolk sac tumor are most common elements
    - Embryonal carcinoma & nongestational choriocarcinoma are extremely rare germ cell tumors
      - May occur as pure or mixed tumor
- **Yolk Sac Tumor**
  - May secrete α-fetoprotein (AFP)
  - Imaging: Large heterogeneous enhancing solid > cystic mass ± areas of necrosis, hemorrhage
  - Hematogenous & peritoneal metastases are common
    - May have ascites
- **Sertoli-Leydig Cell Tumor**
  - Sex cord-stromal tumor
  - May cause virilization (30%)
  - Recurrence & malignant behavior are seen with poorly differentiated subtypes
  - Imaging: Predominantly solid mass with some cystic components; occasionally predominantly cystic
- **Epithelial Tumors**
  - 15-20% of pediatric ovarian tumors
  - Imaging
    - Benign cystadenoma is most common in children
      - Uni- or multilocular cystic thin-walled mass
      - Serous versus mucinous
    - Borderline epithelial tumor
      - Papillary projections in cystic lesion
    - Malignant epithelial tumor
      - Large complex mass with thick irregular walls

Helpful Clues for Rare Diagnoses

- **Small Cell Carcinoma, Hypercalcemic Type**
  - Aggressive malignancy
  - Mean age: 24 years
  - Paraneoplastic hypercalcemia in > 60%
  - Imaging: Nonspecific, heterogeneous mass
- **Ovarian Fibroma**
  - Imaging: Homogeneous or heterogeneous solid mass
    - Often have Ca^{2+}
    - Low signal on T1 & T2 MR due to fibrous content
  - Meigs syndrome with ascites & pleural effusion
- **Juvenile Granulosa Cell Tumor**
  - Granulosa cell tumor may be juvenile or adult type
    - 5% are juvenile type
  - Often secrete estrogen causing precocious puberty
    - May also cause endometrial thickening on ultrasound
  - Imaging: Mixed solid & cystic mass
    - May have sponge-like appearance

SELECTED REFERENCES

1. Heo SH et al: Review of ovarian tumors in children and adolescents: radiologic-pathologic correlation. Radiographics. 34(7):2039-55, 2014
2. Anthony EY et al: Adnexal masses in female pediatric patients. AJR Am J Roentgenol. 198(5):W426-31, 2012

Functional Ovarian Cysts

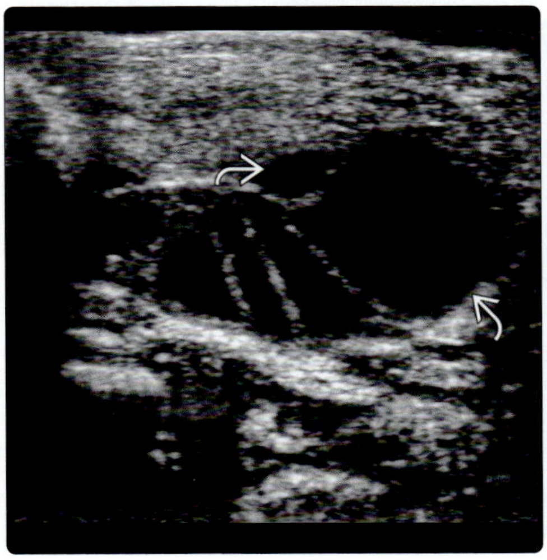

Functional Ovarian Cysts

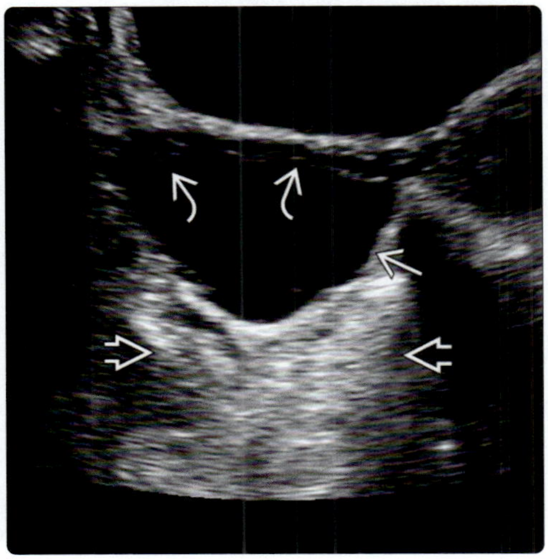

(Left) *Longitudinal ultrasound shows several small, functional, physiologic cysts ➡ in a newborn girl. Ovarian cysts are common in newborns due to the influence of maternal hormones.* **(Right)** *Transverse ultrasound shows a simple right ovarian cyst ➡ in a 15 year old. The cyst is anechoic with posterior acoustic enhancement ➡ & a claw sign of ovarian tissue ➡ splayed along the cyst margin. This cyst measured > 5 cm, which increases the risk of superimposed ovarian torsion.*

(Left) *Transvaginal ultrasound shows a complex cystic lesion* ➡ *with reticular lace-like internal echoes in the left ovary of an adolescent girl. Note the crescent of normal-appearing ovarian tissue* ➡ *along the deep margin of the lesion.* **(Right)** *Transvaginal ultrasound in the same patient shows abundant color Doppler flow around the lesion with no significant internal flow. The findings are most typical of a hemorrhagic cyst in this age.*

Hemorrhagic Cyst

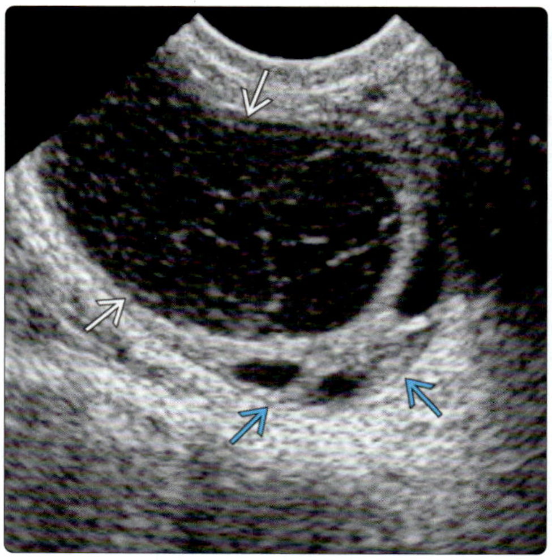

Hemorrhagic Cyst

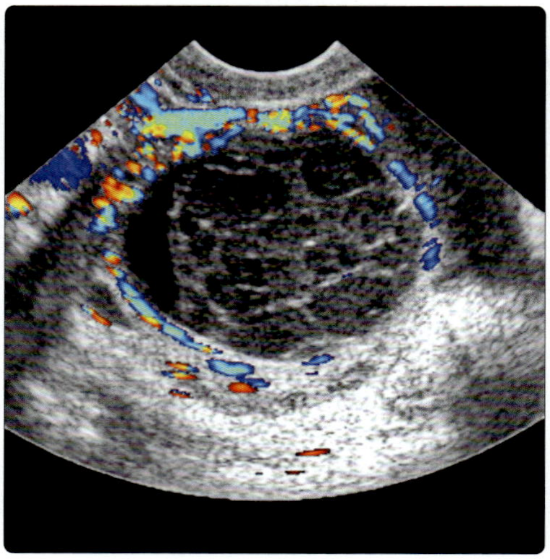

(Left) *Longitudinal ultrasound in a 6 year old presenting with right lower quadrant pain shows an enlarged hypoechoic right ovary (calipers) with peripheral follicles* ➡*. This appearance was noted during an evaluation for appendicitis.* **(Right)** *Transverse color Doppler ultrasound in the same patient shows asymmetry in size of the right* ➡ *& left* ➡ *ovaries. No vascular flow was able to be demonstrated in the right ovary. Reactive free fluid is also present* ➡*. Right ovarian torsion was confirmed intraoperatively.*

Ovarian Torsion

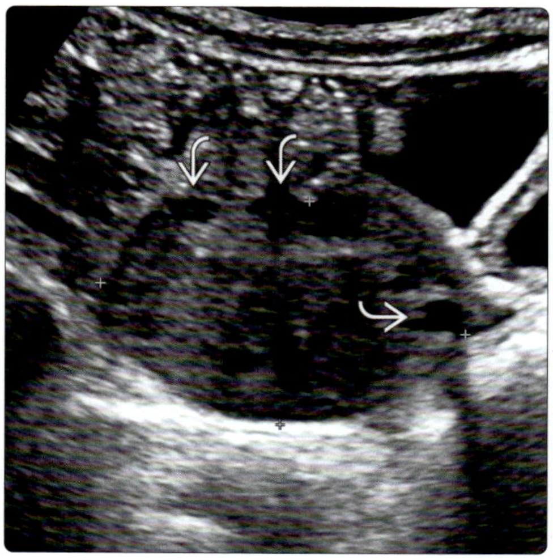

Ovarian Torsion

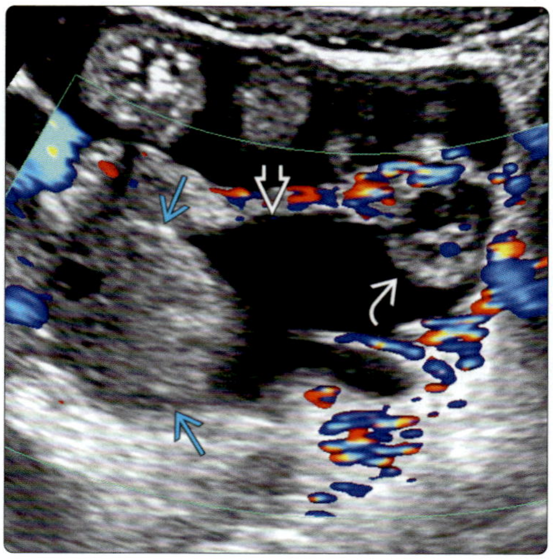

(Left) *Transverse ultrasound shows a large complex right adnexal lesion* ➡ *in an 11-year-old girl with right lower quadrant pain. This mass was predominantly cystic with heterogeneous nodular components* ➡*. Multiple "line & dot" echoes* ➡ *corresponded to hair seen intraoperatively in this mature teratoma (the dermoid mesh sign).* **(Right)** *Axial T2 FS (left) & T1 (right) MR images in the same patient demonstrate the cystic* ➡ *& solid* ➡ *components of the mass, including T1-hyperintense fat* ➡*.*

Mature Teratoma

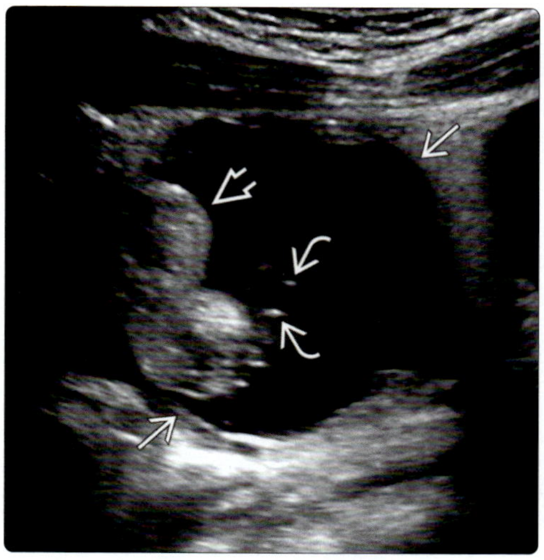

Mature Teratoma

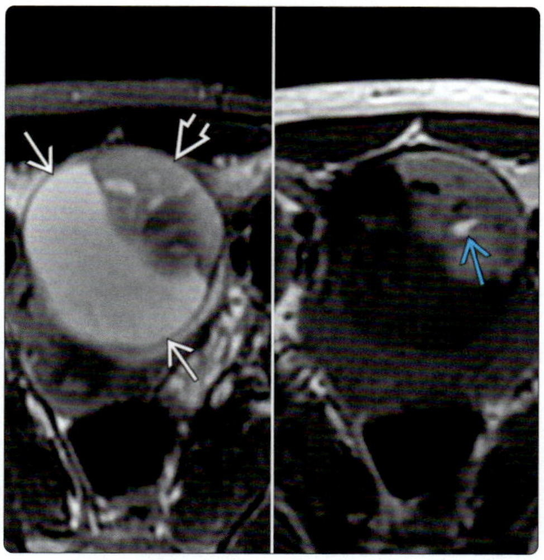

Polycystic Ovary Syndrome

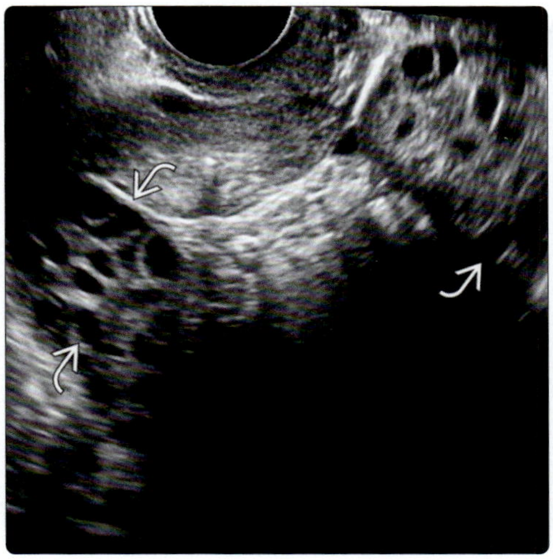

Tuboovarian Abscess

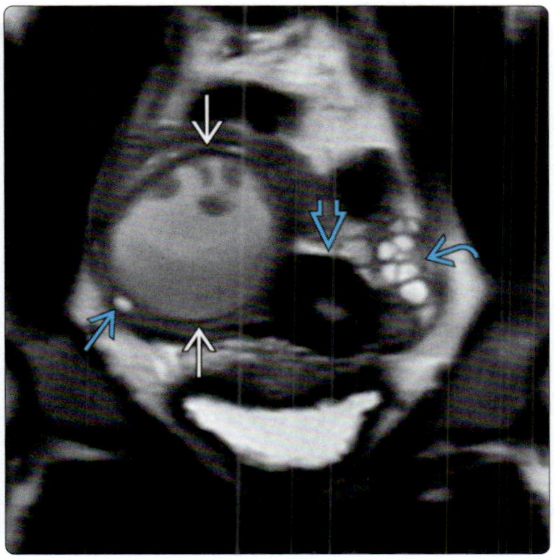

(Left) *Transvaginal ultrasound in this 17 year old with clinical & laboratory findings of polycystic ovary syndrome demonstrates bilaterally enlarged ovaries ➡ with numerous small follicles, supportive of the clinical diagnosis.* **(Right)** *Coronal T2 MR in a 14 year old demonstrates a complex right adnexal lesion with a low-signal rim ➡. There was also internal diffusion restriction (not shown). Note the peripheral right ovarian follicles ➡ & normal left ovary ➡ & uterus ➡. Purulent fluid was drained intraoperatively.*

Tuboovarian Abscess

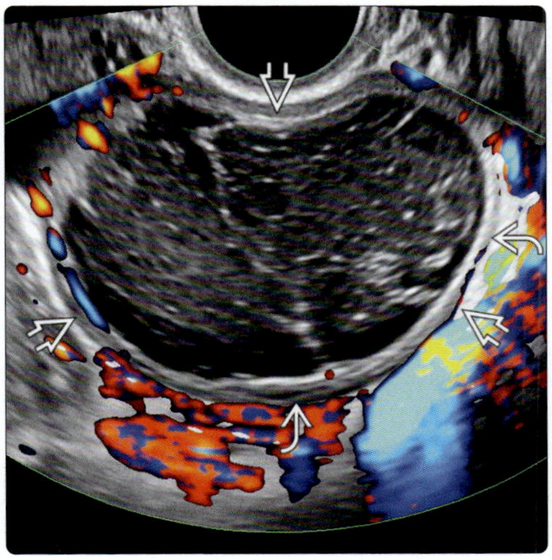

Ectopic Pregnancy

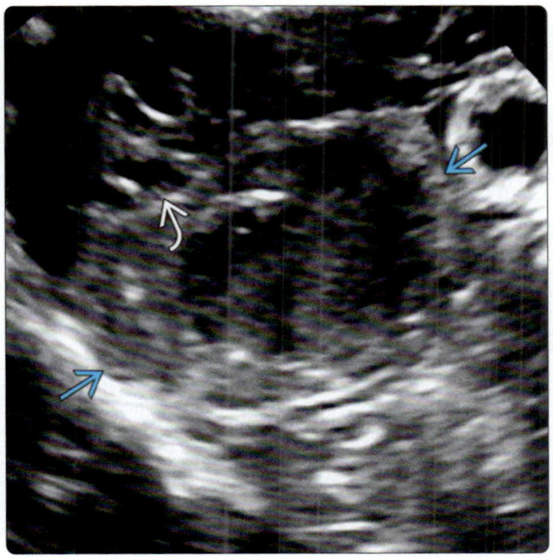

(Left) *Transvaginal color Doppler ultrasound in an 18 year old with pelvic inflammatory disease shows a heterogeneously hypoechoic left tuboovarian abscess ➡ with a thick wall ➡ & surrounding hyperemia.* **(Right)** *Transverse ultrasound shows a heterogeneous right adnexal mass ➡ in an adolescent with right lower quadrant pain & a positive pregnancy test, found to be an ectopic pregnancy. The right ovary ➡ is immediately adjacent. Ovarian ectopic pregnancy is rare. As in this case, 90-95% are tubal.*

Ectopic Pregnancy

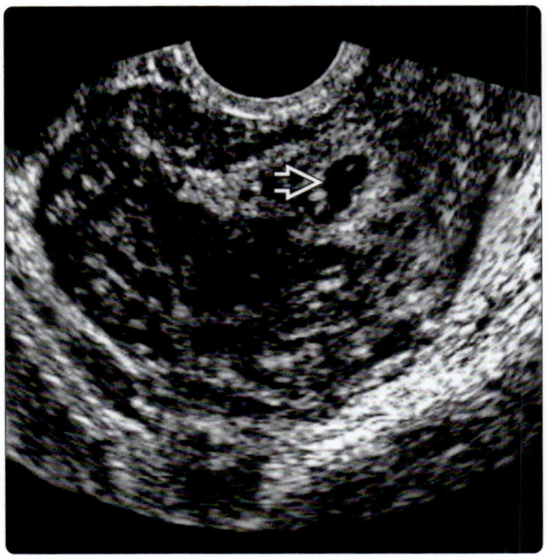

Ectopic Pregnancy

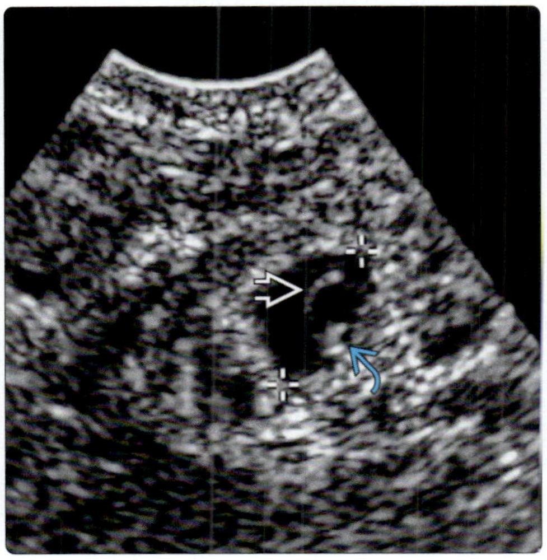

(Left) *Transvaginal ultrasound shows an enlarged & heterogeneous right adnexal mass containing a small cystic region ➡ in this adolescent with vaginal bleeding, pelvic pain, & a positive pregnancy test.* **(Right)** *Higher magnification ultrasound in the same patient shows the gestational sac (calipers). A tiny fetal pole ➡ & yolk sac ➡ are visible in this case of right adnexal ectopic pregnancy.*

(Left) *Transverse color Doppler ultrasound in a 10 year old with intermittent abdominal pain shows a solid right adnexal mass* ➔ *with internal vascular flow. Tumor markers (LDH & β-hCG) were elevated.* **(Right)** *Axial T2 FS MR in the same patient demonstrates a lobulated, solid mass* ➔ *with hypointense septa* ⇨ *found to be a right ovarian dysgerminoma. This patient's karyotype was normal, & there were no findings of ovarian dysgenesis.*

Dysgerminoma

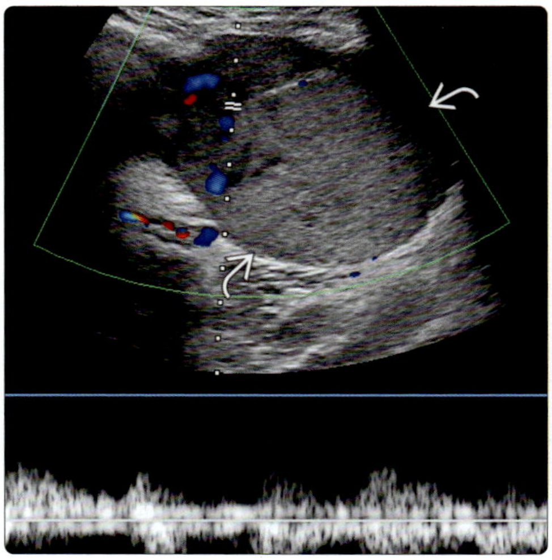

Dysgerminoma

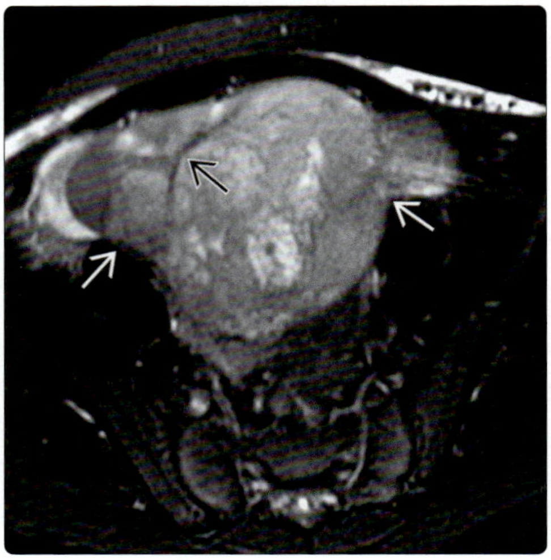

(Left) *Coronal CECT shows a predominantly solid ovarian mass* ➔ *in an 8-year-old girl with an elevated AFP due to a malignant mixed germ cell tumor with yolk sac tumor & dysgerminoma components. Note also the ascites* ➔ *& lymph node metastases* ⇨*. Embryonal carcinoma & choriocarcinoma may also occur as part of a mixed germ cell tumor.* **(Right)** *Extended field-of-view ultrasound was needed to show the extent of a large yolk sac tumor* ➔ *arising in the pelvis in a 14-year-old girl.*

Mixed Germ Cell Tumor

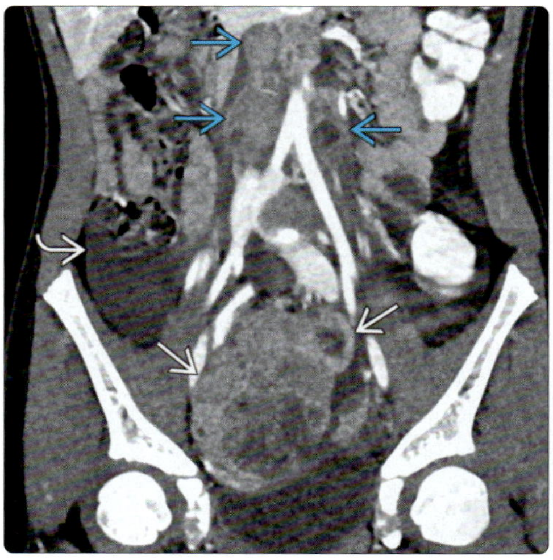

Yolk Sac Tumor

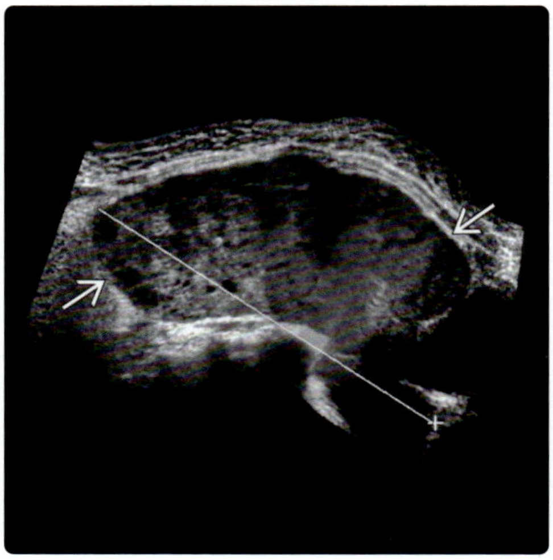

(Left) *Longitudinal ultrasound shows a very large solid & cystic mass* ➔ *extending up from the pelvis (anterior to the right kidney) in this 9 year old with vomiting & a palpable mass.* **(Right)** *Coronal CECT in the same patient shows linear areas of enhancement* ➔ *in the large mass with a relatively well-defined capsule. This patient had a right salpingo-ophorectomy & received chemotherapy for this Sertoli-Leydig cell tumor.*

Sertoli-Leydig Cell Tumor

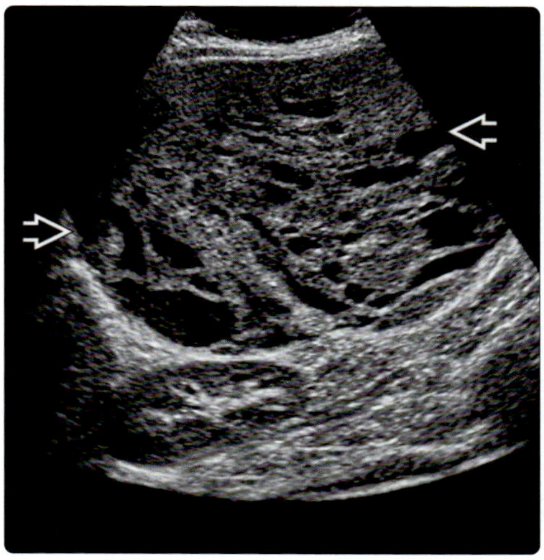

Sertoli-Leydig Cell Tumor

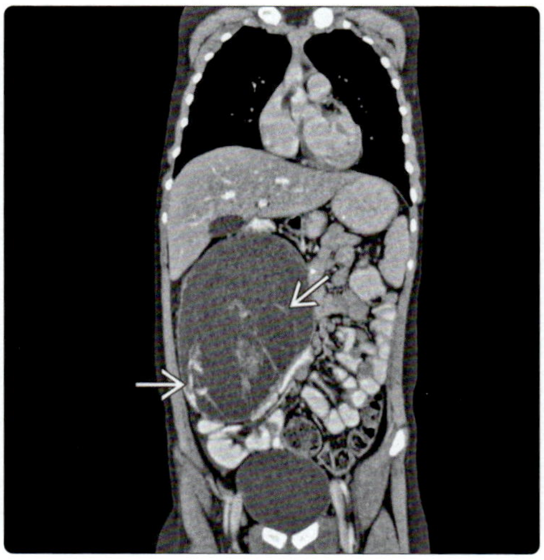

Epithelial Tumors

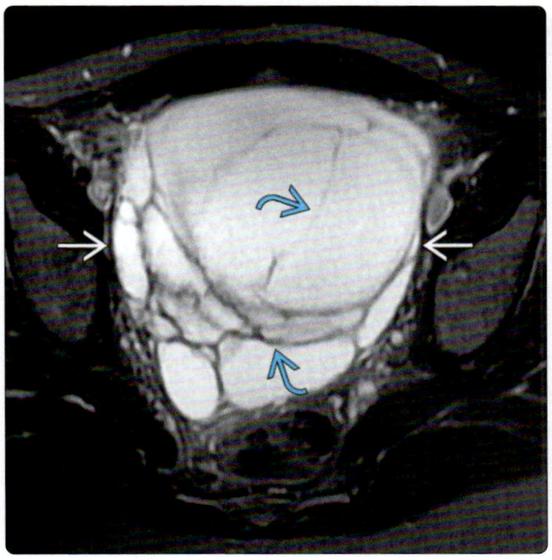

Epithelial Tumors

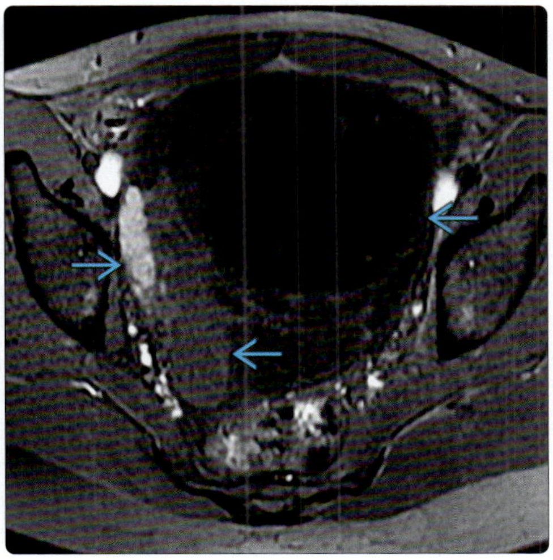

(Left) *Axial T2 FS MR shows a multilocular cystic-appearing mass ➡ in a 17-year-old girl. The mass has internal septations ⇨ amidst hyperintense contents.* **(Right)** *Axial T1 FS MR in the same patient demonstrates variable signal intensities of the cysts ⇨, reflecting various mucinous contents in this mucinous cystadenoma. There were no borderline or malignant features on pathology.*

Small Cell Carcinoma, Hypercalcemic Type

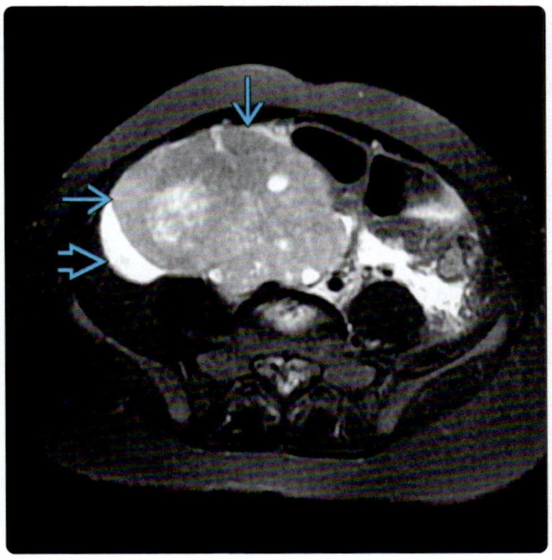

Small Cell Carcinoma, Hypercalcemic Type

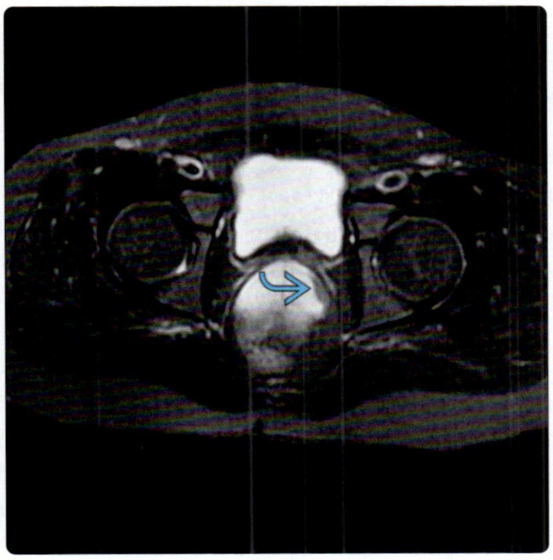

(Left) *Axial T2 FS MR in an 8-year-old girl with lower abdominal pain shows a heterogeneous predominantly solid ovarian mass ⇨, found to be a small cell carcinoma at surgery. Note the ascites ⇨.* **(Right)** *Axial T2 FS MR in the same patient shows a solid nodule ⇨ along the peritoneal lining in the rectouterine pouch. Both this nodule & the primary tumor demonstrated restricted diffusion (not shown) due to high cellularity. The findings are consistent with peritoneal metastases.*

Ovarian Fibroma

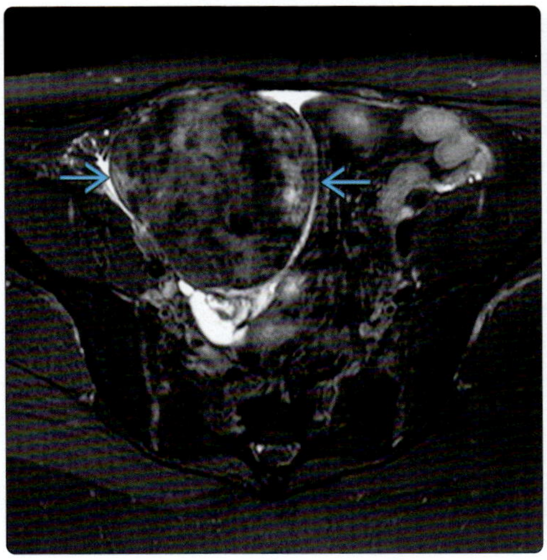

Juvenile Granulosa Cell Tumor

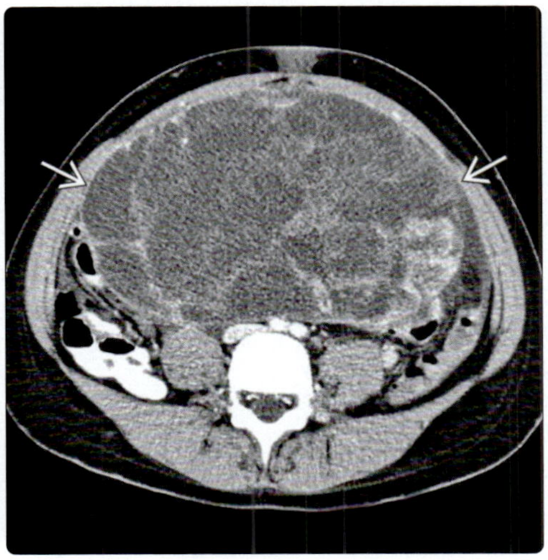

(Left) *Axial T2 FS MR in a young adult girl with a history of an anorectal malformation shows a heterogeneously hypointense mass ⇨ of the right ovary that proved to be a fibroma upon resection.* **(Right)** *Axial CECT shows a large, heterogeneously enhancing mixed solid & cystic mass ➡ extending out of the pelvis in this 12-year-old girl. A juvenile granulosa cell tumor was found at surgery.*

DIFFERENTIAL DIAGNOSIS

Common

- Hydrocele
- Inguinal-Scrotal Hernia
- Varicocele
- Torsion of Testicular Appendage
- Epididymitis/Epididymoorchitis
- Testicular Torsion
- Spermatocele/Epididymal Cyst

Less Common

- Testicular Rupture/Hematoma
- Testicular Tumors
- Paratesticular Rhabdomyosarcoma
- Epidermoid Cyst
- Tubular Ectasia

Rare but Important

- Henoch-Schönlein Purpura
- Meconium Peritonitis
- Scrotal Pneumatosis
- Adrenal Rests

ESSENTIAL INFORMATION

Key Differential Diagnosis Issues

- Begin by determining structural origin of scrotal mass
  - Testicle, epididymis, tunica albuginea or vaginalis, spermatic cord, fat & connective tissues, etc.
- Next, determine character of mass
  - Solid tissue, fluid or cyst, vascular, peristalsing, or combination
- Finally, confirm normal blood flow in testicle
  - Testicular ischemia can be complication of paratesticular masses
  - Alternatively, twisted spermatic cord of torsion can mimic mass

Helpful Clues for Common Diagnoses

- **Hydrocele**
  - Most common pediatric scrotal "mass"
    - Congenital: Patent processus vaginalis
    - Acquired: Trauma, infection, torsion, neoplasm, etc.
  - Fluid within tunica vaginalis surrounds testicle except for "bare area"
    - Should not displace or compress testicle
  - Important to define extent
    - Limited to scrotum
    - Limited to spermatic cord/inguinal canal
    - Freely communicating with peritoneal cavity
    - Contained but bulging into peritoneal cavity
  - Debris &/or septations may be present with infection (pyocele), trauma (hematocele), or chronicity
    - Uniform, tiny, low-level mobile echoes are typically of no significance
- **Inguinal-Scrotal Hernia**
  - Typically heterogeneous, mixed soft tissue mass
    - May contain echogenic peritoneal fat &/or bowel
  - Look for hernia neck pointing to inguinal canal or frank communication with peritoneal cavity
    - May spontaneously reduce during or prior to study; confirmation may require specific maneuvers (i.e., upright position & Valsalva)
  - Peristalsis may be diminished/absent when bowel is incarcerated
  - Testicle may be displaced to bottom of scrotal sac
    - Confirm normal blood flow in testis
- **Varicocele**
  - Dilated veins of pampiniform plexus > 2-3 mm, increasing with Valsalva
    - Typically isolated to spermatic cord; may involve testis
  - L side > > R; may be bilateral
    - Isolated right-sided varicocele should prompt evaluation for retroperitoneal mass
  - May result in chronic testicular atrophy
    - Most common correctable cause of male infertility
- **Torsion of Testicular Appendage**
  - Twisting of testicular or epididymal appendage
  - Small avascular mass adjacent to testis or between testis & epididymis
    - Variable echogenicity, depending on duration of symptoms; typically hypoechoic acutely
    - Surrounding hyperemia
  - Associated hydrocele is common
  - May mimic epididymitis but is more common in prepubertal males
- **Epididymitis/Epididymoorchitis**
  - Enlarged, hypoechoic, & often heterogeneous epididymis
  - Marked hyperemia of epididymis (± testis) on Doppler
  - Associated hydrocele is common
- **Testicular Torsion**
  - Twisted spermatic cord → venous congestion & ischemia
    - May see "knot" of twist just above testicle
  - Appearance of testicle depends on duration
    - Acute: Enlarged with absent flow
    - Subacute/Chronic: May appear heterogeneous
  - Doppler hypoperfusion is key to diagnosis
    - Always compare to asymptomatic side
    - Incomplete/intermittent torsion may have normal flow; spontaneous detorsion may appear hyperemic
  - Lie of testicle is often abnormal
  - May have reactive hydrocele
  - Surgical emergency
    - Testicular salvage rate drops with symptom duration
- **Spermatocele/Epididymal Cyst**
  - Both result from dilated epididymal tubule
  - Identical imaging appearance
    - Anechoic cystic lesion ± internal septations
  - Spermatocele
    - Contains spermatozoa & sediment
    - Most often in epididymal head
  - Epididymal cyst
    - Contains clear serous fluid
    - Found anywhere in epididymis

Helpful Clues for Less Common Diagnoses

- **Testicular Rupture/Hematoma**
  - Appearance depends on severity, acuity, & type of injury
  - Parenchymal hematoma: Avascular mass

- Conservative treatment
- Follow-up (to exclude underlying testicular neoplasm) shows interval ↓ in size
  - Rupture: Irregular testicular contour with interruption of echogenic tunica albuginea
    - Generally treated as surgical emergency
  - Confirm normal testicular perfusion (i.e., no torsion)
  - Extratesticular hematoma (hematocele) is treated nonsurgically
- **Testicular Tumors**
  - Bimodal age peaks
    - < 2 years old & late adolescence
  - General imaging appearance
    - Hypoechoic; may have cystic or necrotic foci or Ca^{2+}
    - Usually hypervascular relative to testicle
    - Reactive hydrocele in 15-20%
  - Germ cell variety (60-77%)
    - Yolk sac tumor: Elevated α-fetoprotein
    - Teratoma: Benign in prepubertal patients; malignant in postpubertal
      - May contain echogenic calcific or fatty elements
    - Choriocarcinoma: Malignant with early hematogenous metastases, ↑ β-HCG
    - Mixed: Variable behavior
    - Seminomas: Rare in children
  - Sertoli cell & Leydig cell tumors
    - Gonadal stromal tumors
    - Hormonally active: Gynecomastia, precocious puberty
    - Typically appear as small hypoechoic mass
  - Juvenile granulosa cell tumors
    - 27% of all neonatal testicular tumors; benign
    - Appearance resembles ovarian follicles
  - Gonadoblastoma: Patients with disorders of sexual development
  - Leukemia/lymphoma
    - Solitary, multifocal, or diffusely infiltrating hypoechoic lesion; often hypervascular; may be bilateral
    - "Sanctuary organ" for leukemia recurrence
  - Metastases: Neuroblastoma, Wilms tumor, etc.
- **Paratesticular Rhabdomyosarcoma**
  - Malignant tumor outside of testicle; may be quite large & heterogeneous with variable vascularity
  - 70% have retroperitoneal nodal spread at diagnosis
- **Epidermoid Cyst**
  - Benign intratesticular avascular mass
  - Concentric rings of keratin give onion skin appearance
  - Characteristic appearance → testicle-sparing surgery
- **Tubular Ectasia**
  - Dilation of rete testis
  - Variably sized avascular cysts or tubules
  - Radiate from mediastinum testis

Helpful Clues for Rare Diagnoses

- **Henoch-Schönlein Purpura**
  - Small vessel vasculitis leading to bowel edema/hemorrhage, rash, arthritis, nephritis
  - Scrotal involvement in up to 15%
    - Scrotal skin thickening, enlarged epididymis, hydrocele; testes usually appear normal
    - Cellulitis, insect bite, & allergic reaction can also have this appearance
- **Meconium Peritonitis**
  - Sequela of in utero bowel perforation
  - Ca^{2+} & fluid extend into scrotum ("meconium orchitis")
- **Scrotal Pneumatosis**
  - Abnormal gas extends from peritoneum or perineum
  - Look for bowel perforation, pneumatosis, adjacent soft tissue infection
- **Adrenal Rests**
  - Adolescents with congenital adrenal hyperplasia
  - Symmetric bilateral hypoechoic hypervascular masses, typically lobulated & infiltrating mediastinum testis

SELECTED REFERENCES

1. Alkhori NA et al: Pediatric scrotal ultrasound: review and update. Pediatr Radiol. 47(9):1125-33, 2017
2. Basta AM et al: Scrotal swelling in the neonate. J Ultrasound Med. 34(3):495-505, 2015
3. Delaney LR et al: Ultrasound of the pediatric scrotum. Semin Ultrasound CT MR. 34(3):248-56, 2013

Hydrocele

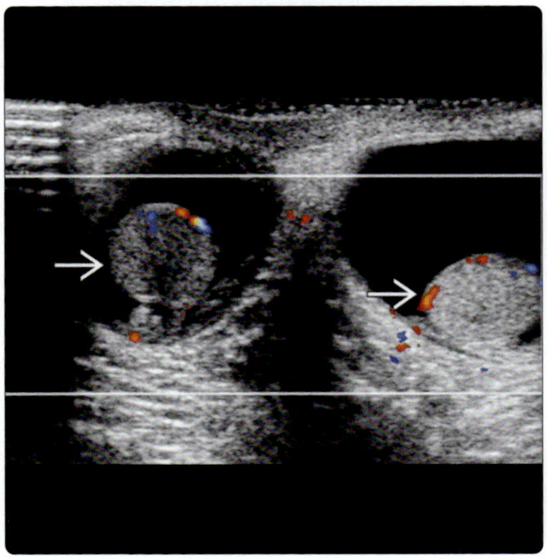

Inguinal-Scrotal Hernia

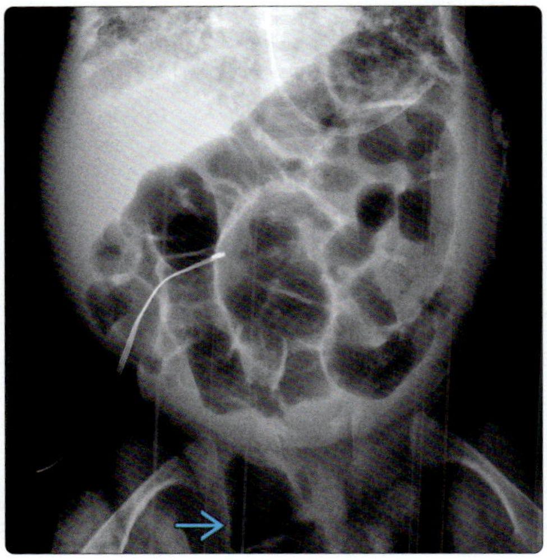

(Left) *Transverse color Doppler ultrasound shows normal perfusion of both testes ➔, which are both nearly surrounded by anechoic fluid. This infant had large bilateral hydroceles, causing scrotal enlargement. Note that both testes are normally fixed to the scrotal wall & not completely surrounded by fluid (which would suggest a bell clapper deformity).* **(Right)** *Frontal radiograph in a neonate with scrotal swelling shows gas-filled bowel herniated through the inguinal canal into the right scrotum ➔.*

(Left) *Longitudinal ultrasound with extended field of view shows bowel & fat* → *extending through the right inguinal canal into the scrotum in this child with scrotal fullness. The testicle* ↷ *is displaced inferiorly. Normal bowel will show continued peristalsis & blood flow without thickening.* **(Right)** *Longitudinal ultrasound shows herniation of echogenic fat* ➡ *from the peritoneal cavity into the right inguinal canal & superior scrotum. The right testicle* ⇨ *is normal.*

Inguinal-Scrotal Hernia

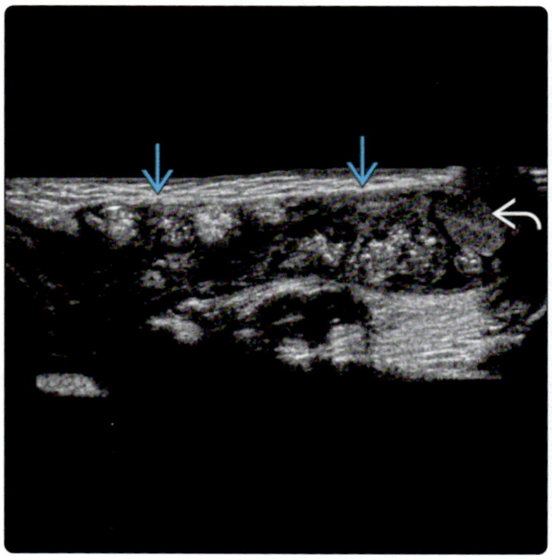

Inguinal-Scrotal Hernia

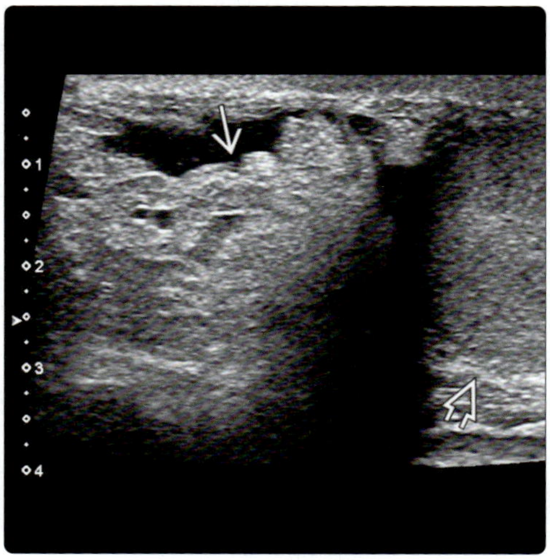

(Left) *Transverse ultrasound shows a normal testicle* ➡ *adjacent to serpiginous anechoic tubular foci* ↷*, typical of a varicocele. Varicoceles enlarge during Valsalva & show flow on color Doppler. They occasionally involve the testis. Over time, the ipsilateral testicle may decrease in volume.* **(Right)** *Longitudinal color Doppler ultrasound of the left inguinal canal during a Valsalva maneuver demonstrates prominent color flow in an isolated left varicocele.*

Varicocele

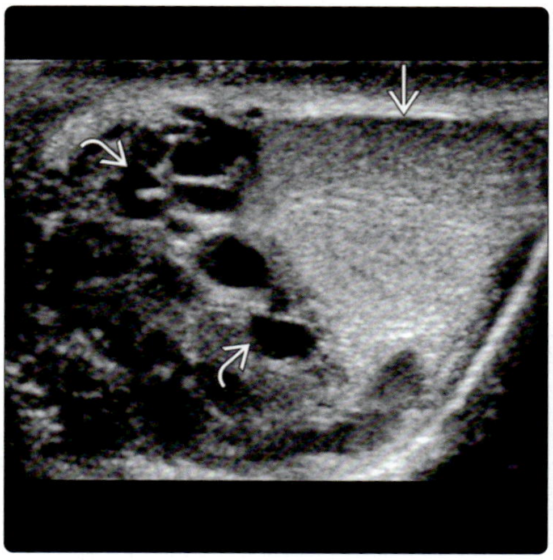

Varicocele

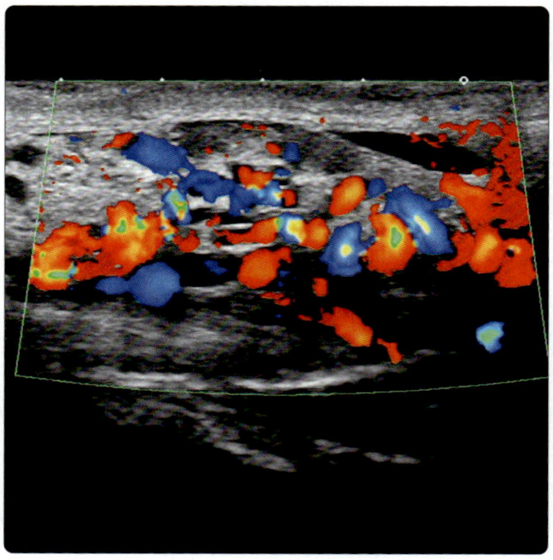

(Left) *Longitudinal grayscale & color Doppler ultrasound in a 9-year-old boy with acute scrotal pain demonstrates an avascular heterogeneously hypoechoic mass* ➡ *at the superior pole of the testis* ⇨ *with surrounding hyperemia, typical of a torsed appendage.* **(Right)** *Transverse color Doppler ultrasound shows absence of flow in a hyperechoic nodule* ➡ *adjacent to a hyperemic epididymis* ⇨ *in a teenager with pain for days. The torsed appendage becomes hyperechoic with time, gradually decreasing in size.*

Torsion of Testicular Appendage

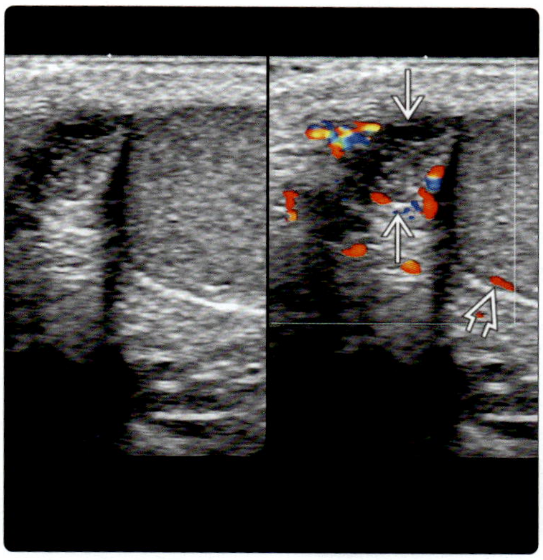

Torsion of Testicular Appendage

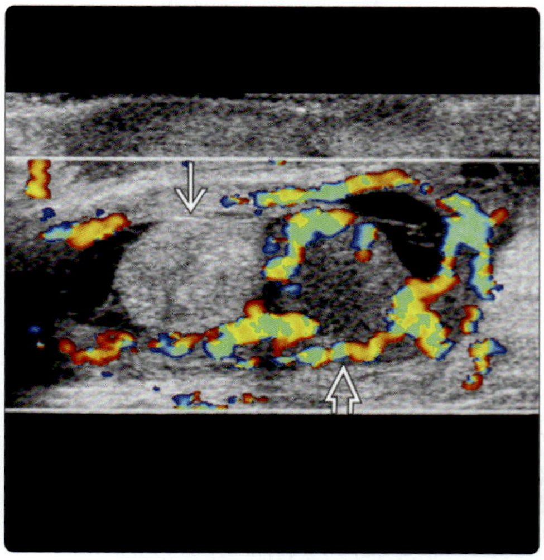

Epididymitis/Epididymoorchitis

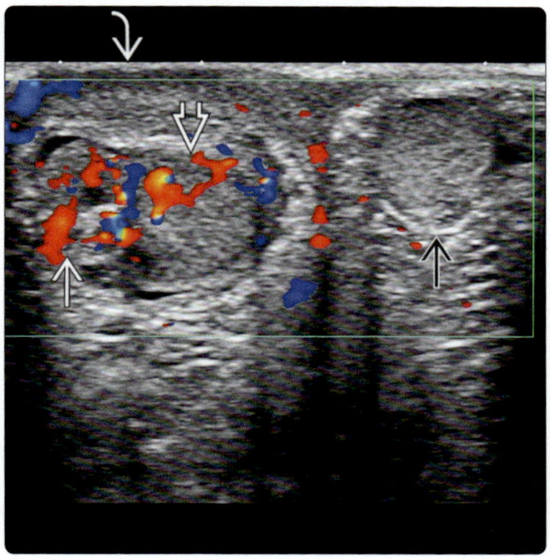

Epididymitis/Epididymoorchitis

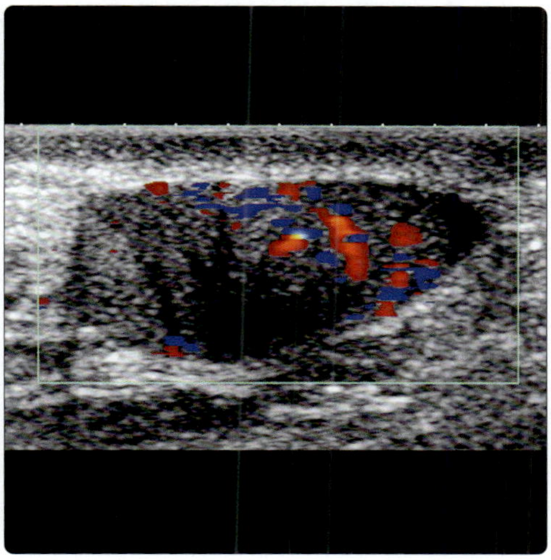

(Left) *Transverse ultrasound in a 4-year-old boy with right epididymoorchitis demonstrates enlargement & hyperemia of the right epididymis → as well as hyperemia of the right testis →. There is overlying scrotal wall edema →. The left testis → is normal.* **(Right)** *Longitudinal color Doppler ultrasound shows hyperemia in an inflamed, relatively hypoechoic epididymis, consistent with epididymitis. The testicles (not shown) were normal bilaterally.*

Testicular Torsion

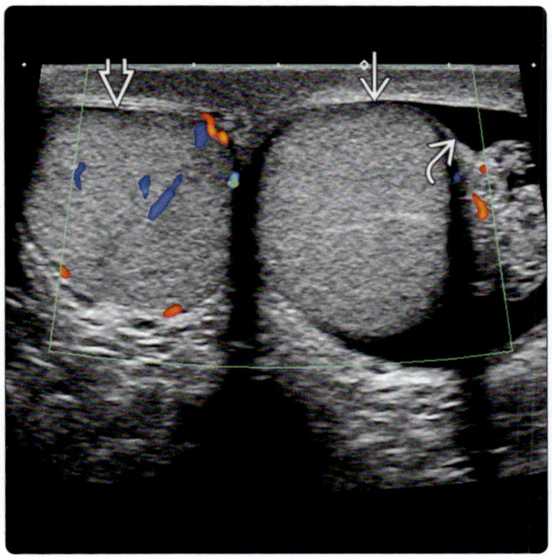

Testicular Torsion

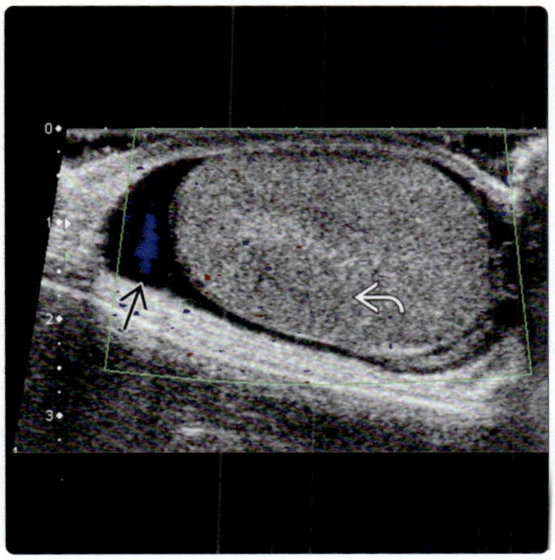

(Left) *Transverse color Doppler ultrasound demonstrates mild enlargement of the left testicle → with absent blood flow. The normal right testicle → with normal blood flow provides internal comparison. Reactive hydrocele → is also seen.* **(Right)** *Longitudinal color Doppler ultrasound shows a small hydrocele → surrounding a torsed left testicle. There is mild prominence of the rete testis → radiating out from the mediastinum testis, reflecting swelling/edema.*

Spermatocele/Epididymal Cyst

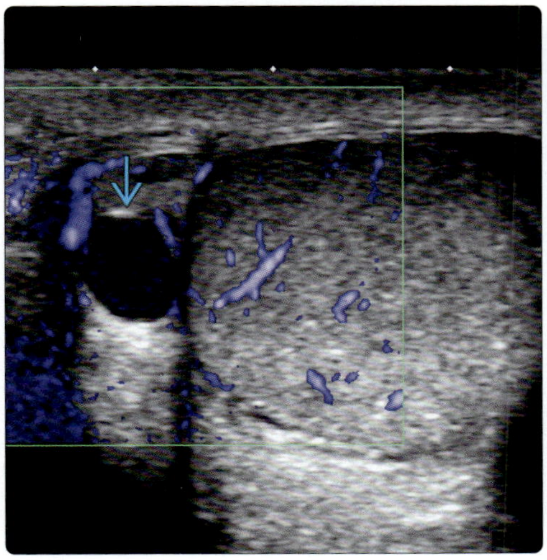

Testicular Rupture/Hematoma

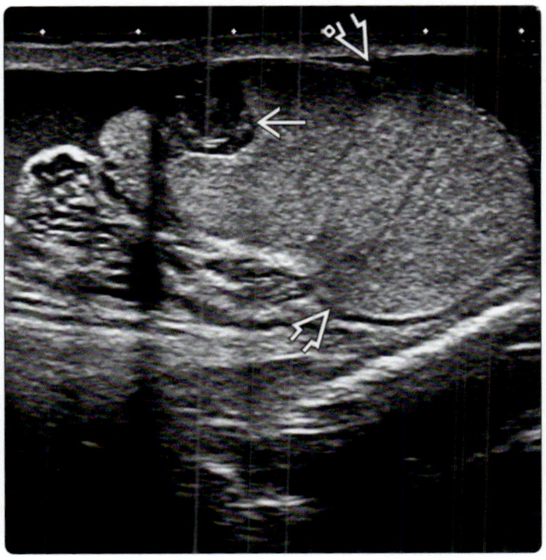

(Left) *Longitudinal color Doppler ultrasound in a 13-year-old boy with pain shows a well-circumscribed, avascular, thin-walled, anechoic, 6-mm cyst → in the epididymal head, likely an epididymal cyst.* **(Right)** *Longitudinal ultrasound in a teenager with a direct blow to the scrotum demonstrates a heterogeneously hypoechoic intratesticular hematoma →, which was avascular on color Doppler evaluation. The abnormal testicular contour & interruption of the echogenic tunica are consistent with testicular rupture →.*

(Left) *Transverse ultrasound shows a heterogeneous predominantly hypoechoic mass in the right testicle with an echogenic shadowing focus, suggesting Ca2+.* **(Right)** *Longitudinal ultrasound shows the same mass in a perpendicular plane. The mass appears heterogeneous but relatively well circumscribed with a focus of Ca2+. It was subsequently removed & found to be a testicular teratoma.*

Testicular Tumors

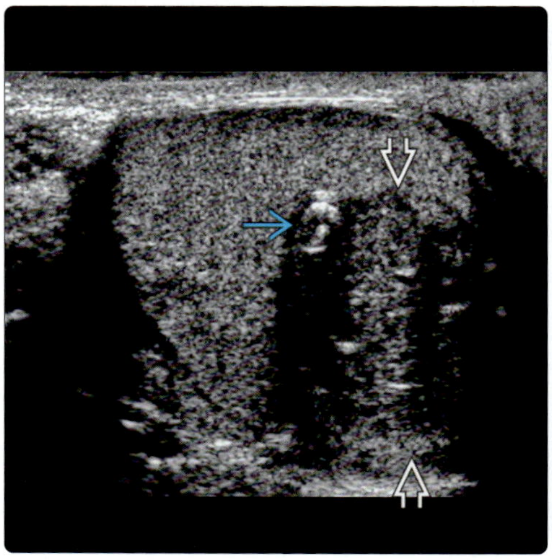

Testicular Tumors

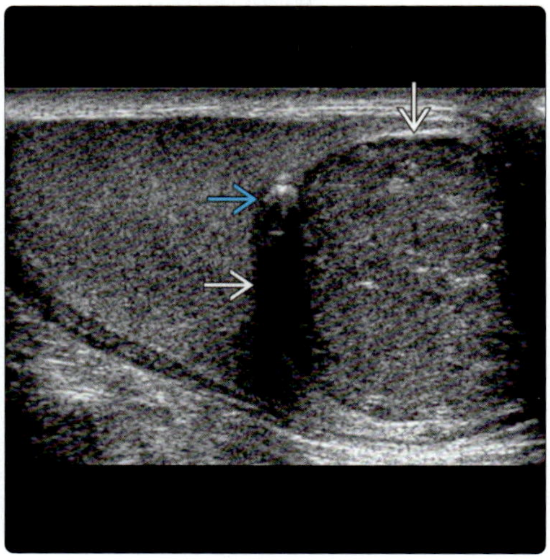

(Left) *Extended field-of-view ultrasound shows complete replacement of the left testicle with a heterogeneous mass. There is a large complex hydrocele in this 17-year-old boy who reported that his left scrotum had been enlarged for months.* **(Right)** *Axial CECT in the same patient shows bulky periaortic adenopathy, ascites, & delayed left nephrogram from hydronephrosis. The findings are most consistent with a metastatic testicular tumor, though lymphoma & infection were also considered.*

Testicular Tumors

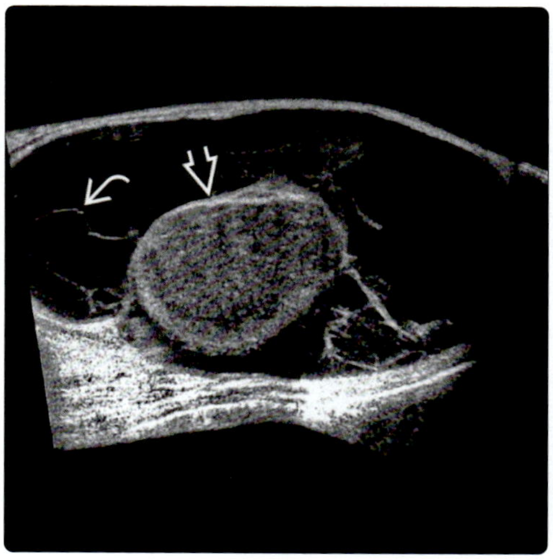

Testicular Tumors

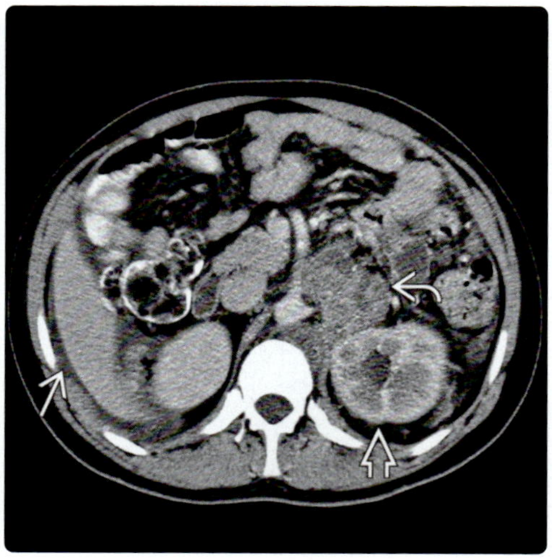

(Left) *Axial CECT shows numerous lung metastases in the same teenage boy, consistent with a metastatic testicular tumor. The tumor was later shown to be a germ cell tumor.* **(Right)** *Transverse ultrasound shows massive enlargement & subtle heterogeneity of the right testis in a child with relapsed acute lymphocytic leukemia. The left testis is normal. Note that bilateral involvement is common & often symmetric. Disorganized & increased vascularity may also be seen with testicular involvement.*

Testicular Tumors

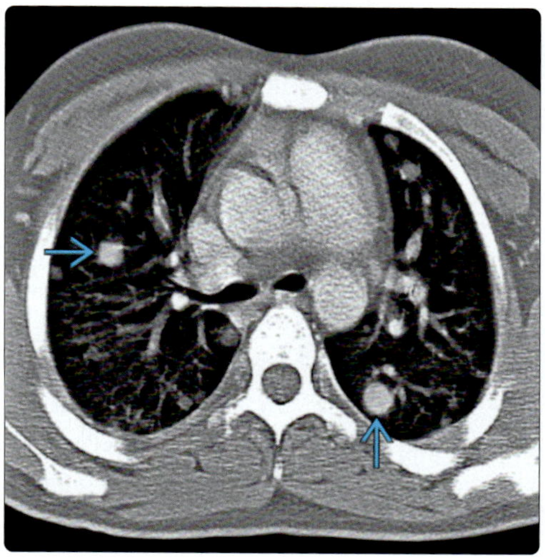

Testicular Tumors

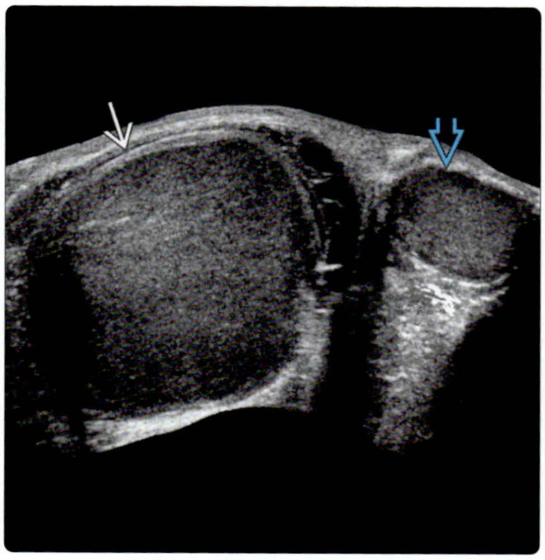

Paratesticular Rhabdomyosarcoma

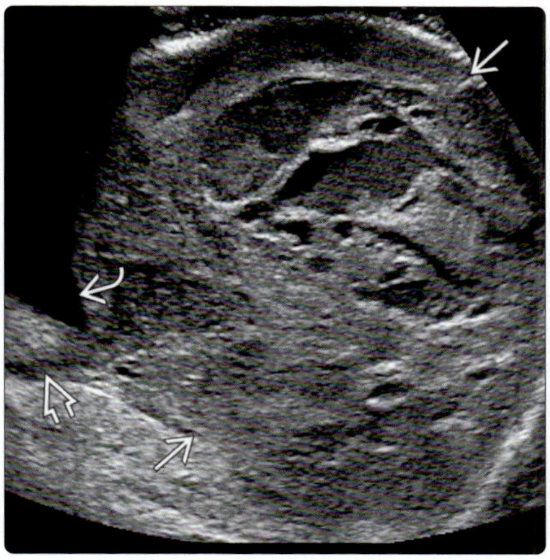

Epidermoid Cyst

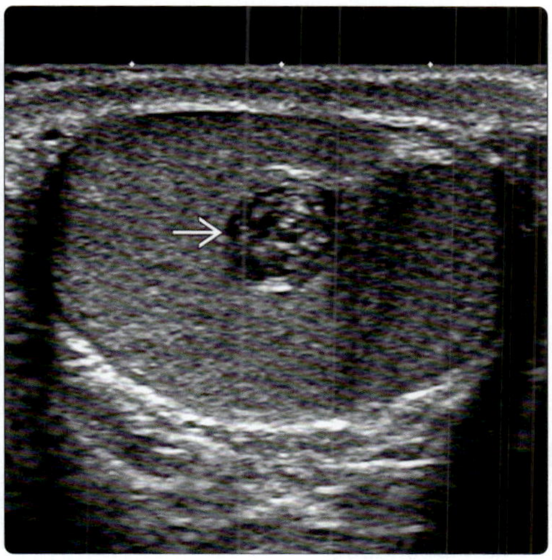

(Left) *Longitudinal ultrasound of the right scrotum in a 16-year-old boy with a painless scrotal mass for several months demonstrates a large heterogeneous extratesticular mass ➡. The separate right testis ➡ is partially visualized, compressed by the mass & associated hydrocele ➡.* **(Right)** *Longitudinal ultrasound of the left testicle in a 15-year-old boy demonstrates the characteristic lamellated appearance of an epidermoid cyst ➡. The mass was avascular on color Doppler ultrasound.*

Tubular Ectasia

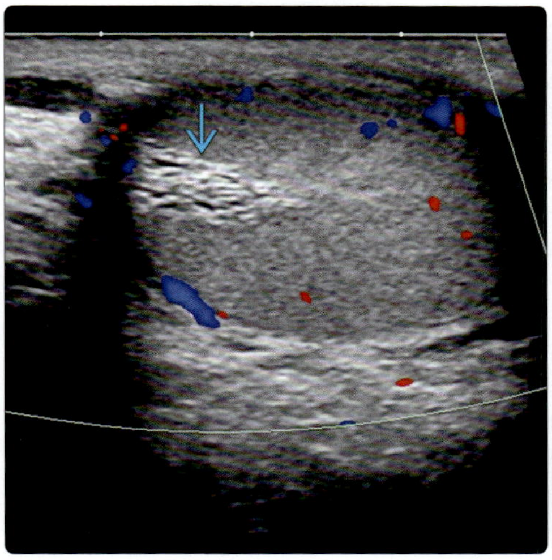

Henoch-Schönlein Purpura

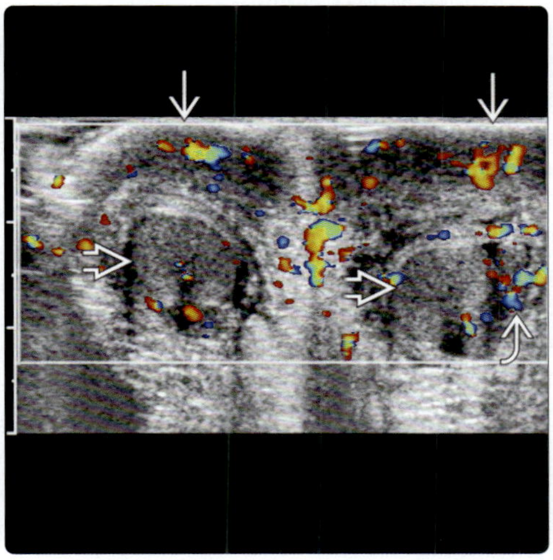

(Left) *Transverse color Doppler ultrasound in a 13 year old shows tubular ectasia of the rete testis ➡ in the echogenic mediastinum testis. The surrounding parenchyma is normal, & there is no internal vascularity to suggest tumor.* **(Right)** *Transverse color Doppler ultrasound shows scrotal wall thickening & hyperemia ➡ as well as left epididymal enlargement & hyperemia ➡. The testicles ➡ are normal in this patient with Henoch-Schönlein purpura. Note that cellulitis, allergic reaction, & insect bite could all have this appearance.*

Meconium Peritonitis

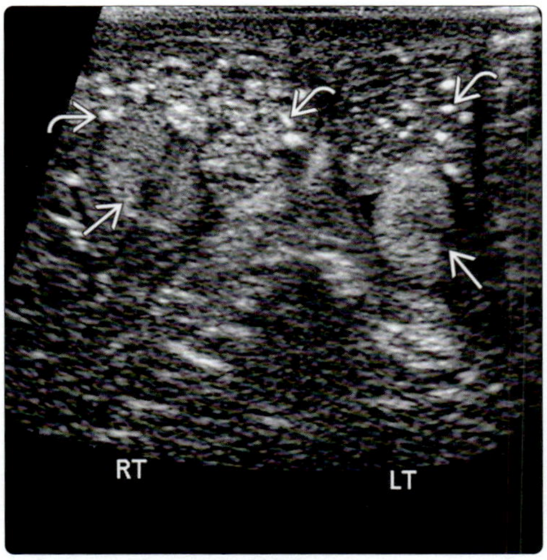

Adrenal Rests

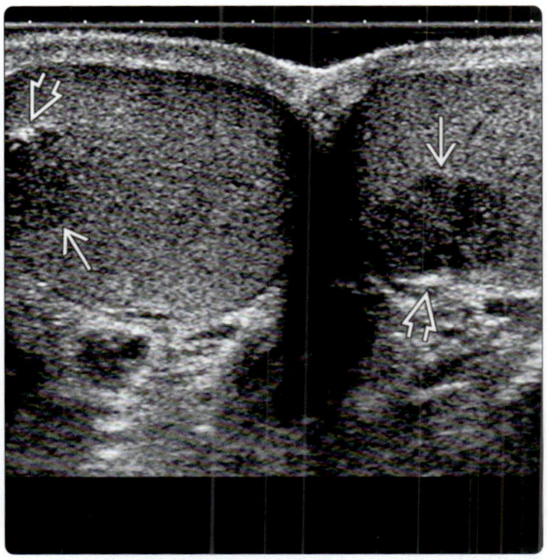

(Left) *Transverse ultrasound shows numerous echogenic foci ➡ surrounding normal testicles ➡ in this infant with a history of in utero bowel perforation & meconium peritonitis. Extension through a patent processus vaginalis may result in "meconium orchitis."* **(Right)** *Transverse ultrasound in a 17-year-old boy with congenital adrenal hyperplasia demonstrates bilateral hypoechoic testicular masses ➡, consistent with adrenal rests. These are typically found in the echogenic mediastinum ➡ & are usually hypervascular.*

DIFFERENTIAL DIAGNOSIS

Common

- Torsion of Testicular/Epididymal Appendage
- Epididymitis/Epididymoorchitis
- Testicular Torsion
- Inguinal Hernia
- Varicocele
- Urinary Tract Calculus

Less Common

- Testicular Trauma
- Henoch-Schönlein Purpura
- Testicular Neoplasm

ESSENTIAL INFORMATION

Helpful Clues for Common Diagnoses

- **Torsion of Testicular/Epididymal Appendage**
  - More common in prepubertal males
  - May involve appendix testis or appendix epididymis
  - Small, round, avascular mass in epididymis or along surface of testis
    - Acute: Hypoechoic with scattered echogenic dots & septa (salt & pepper); > 5-6 mm overall size
    - Subacute-chronic: ↓ size, ↑ echogenicity; adjacent hyperemia/hydrocele mimics epididymitis
- **Epididymitis/Epididymoorchitis**
  - More common in postpubertal males
  - Epididymis/testis is often enlarged, hypoechoic/heterogeneous, hypervascular
  - Reactive hydrocele is often present
  - If recurrent, consider congenital anomaly (e.g., ectopic insertion of ureter), especially in prepubertal patient
- **Testicular Torsion**
  - Appearance depends on duration
    - Acute: Absent parenchymal flow; ± abnormal lie, hydrocele, surrounding hyperemia
      - Absent (or even just diminished) internal vascularity compared to painless testis is key feature
      - ± hyperemia with spontaneous detorsion
    - Subacute/chronic: Heterogeneous parenchyma
  - Twisting of spermatic cord ("knot") directly above testis
- **Inguinal Hernia**
  - Bowel in scrotum usually peristalsis, though not always
  - Hernia contents may only be echogenic mesenteric fat
  - Can cause ↓ testicular flow in infants
- **Varicocele**
  - Dilated veins > 2-3 mm, ↑ with Valsalva
  - Usually left sided, occasionally bilateral
    - Isolated right sided should prompt evaluation for retroperitoneal mass
- **Urinary Tract Calculus**
  - Referred pain; ± hematuria
  - Look for echogenic focus (with twinkling artifact ± posterior shadowing) at ureterovesical junction or in ureter; ± hydroureteronephrosis, absent ureteral jet

Helpful Clues for Less Common Diagnoses

- **Testicular Trauma**
  - Rupture: Disruption of echogenic tunica albuginea; irregular contour to parenchymal margin
  - Fracture: Linear hypoechoic disruption of testicular parenchyma
  - Hematoma: Heterogeneous avascular lesion within testis
    - Follow-up to exclude underlying mass
- **Henoch-Schönlein Purpura**
  - Scrotal involvement in up to 15%
  - Scrotal skin thickening with hyperemia, enlarged epididymis, hydrocele
    - Similar scrotal wall thickening may also be seen with allergic reaction, insect bite, or cellulitis
  - Testes usually appear normal
- **Testicular Neoplasm**
  - Usually painless; may delay diagnosis when presenting with pain
  - Variable echogenicity & vascularity
    - May be small & focal or replace entire testis
  - Primary: Germ cell tumors, stromal tumors
  - Metastases: Leukemia, lymphoma

Torsion of Testicular/Epididymal Appendage

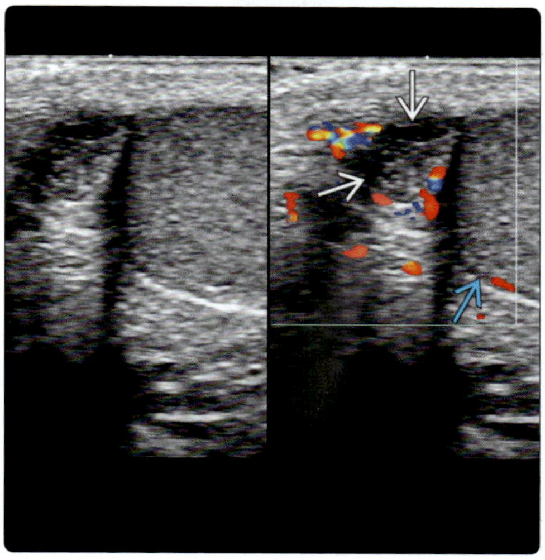

Epididymitis/Epididymoorchitis

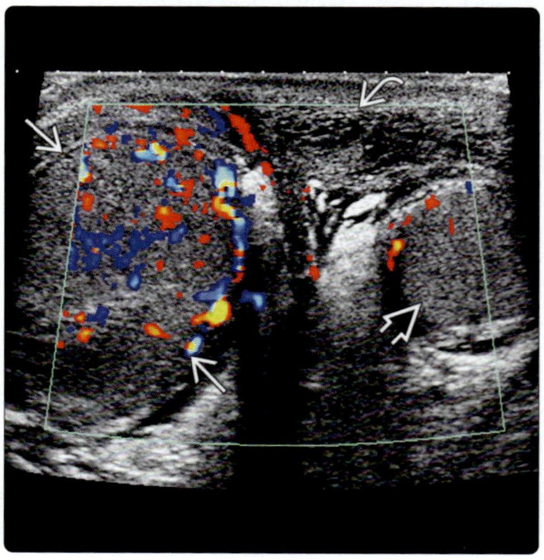

(Left) *Longitudinal color Doppler US of the scrotum in a 9 year old with acute scrotal pain demonstrates an avascular hypoechoic nodule ➡ adjacent to the superior pole of the testis ⇨. Note surrounding hyperemia.* **(Right)** *Transverse color Doppler US shows an enlarged, painful right testis ➡ with diffuse scrotal wall thickening ➡ & hyperemia. The left testis is normal ➡. Isolated orchitis is uncommon; the epididymis (not shown) is typically enlarged, heterogeneous, & hyperemic as well (or in isolation).*

Testicular Torsion

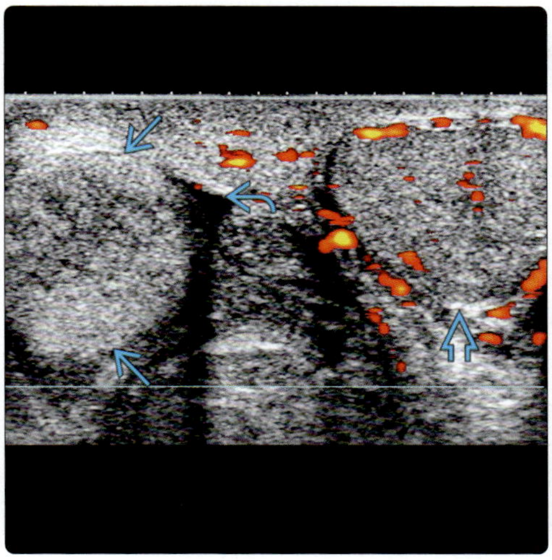

Inguinal Hernia

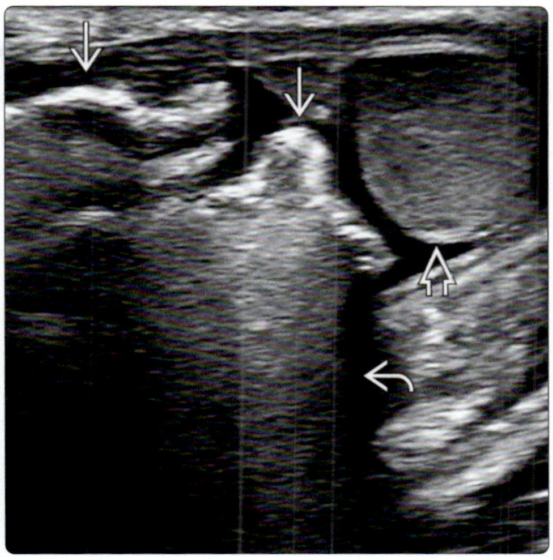

(Left) *Transverse power Doppler US shows no blood flow in an acutely torsed right testis, which is mildly heterogeneous in echotexture compared with the normal left testis. Note the small hydrocele.* **(Right)** *Longitudinal US demonstrates bowel loops extending through the inguinal canal into the upper scrotum. Echogenic gas within the bowel loops results in dirty posterior acoustic shadowing. The normal right testis lies in the inferior scrotum.*

Varicocele

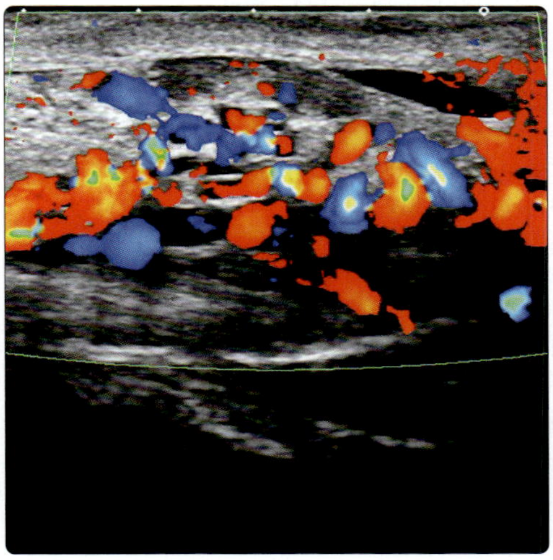

Testicular Trauma

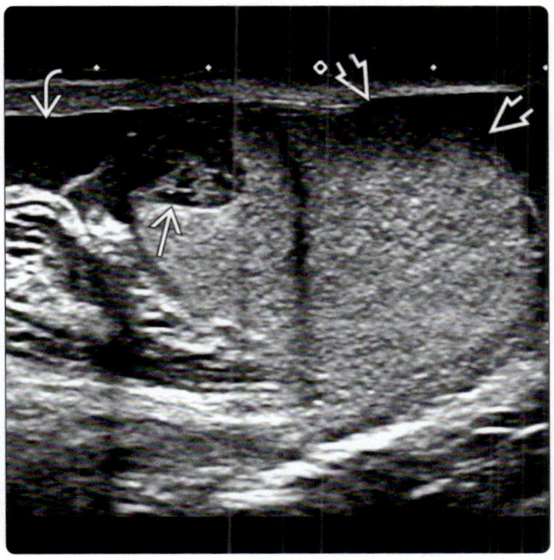

(Left) *Longitudinal color Doppler US of the left inguinal canal demonstrates prominent color flow within the dilated veins of a varicocele during a Valsalva maneuver.* **(Right)** *Longitudinal US of the scrotum in an adolescent with sports-related scrotal trauma demonstrates a heterogeneously hypoechoic testicular hematoma & surrounding hematocele. Abnormal contour of the testis with loss of the overlying echogenic tunica albuginea is consistent with testicular rupture.*

Henoch-Schönlein Purpura

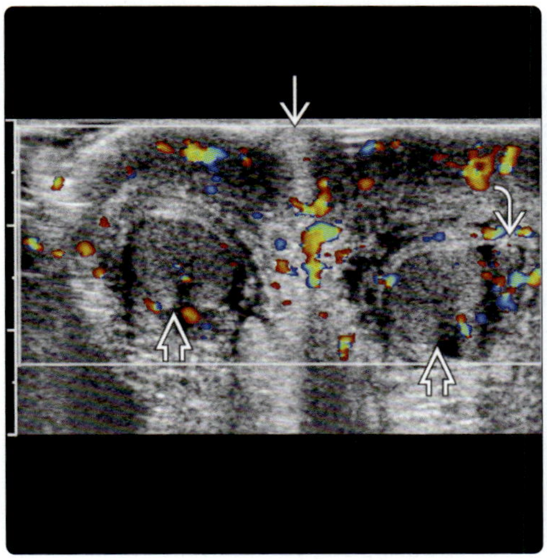

Testicular Neoplasm

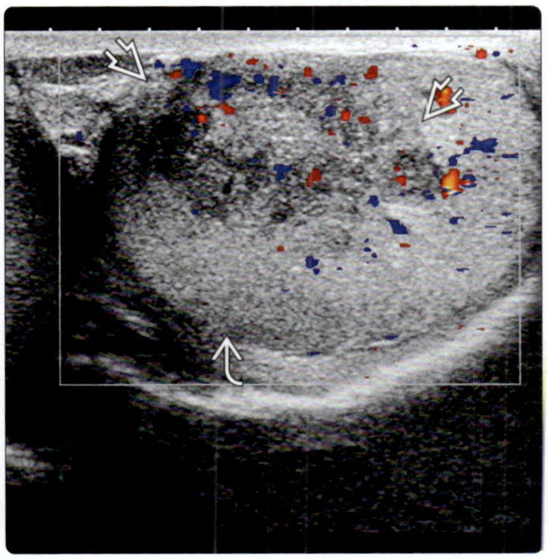

(Left) *Transverse color Doppler US shows scrotal wall thickening & hyperemia as well as left epididymal enlargement & hyperemia. The testes are normal in this patient with Henoch-Schönlein purpura.* **(Right)** *Longitudinal color Doppler US shows a heterogeneous & mildly hypervascular lesion within the left testis, proven to be an embryonal carcinoma. Primary testicular neoplasms usually present as palpable masses rather than scrotal pain (unless an infarction, hemorrhage, or hydrocele develops).*

DIFFERENTIAL DIAGNOSIS

Common

- Ureterocele
- Antireflux Intervention at Ureterovesical Junction
- Cystitis

Less Common

- Calculus
- Hematoma
- Rhabdomyosarcoma
- Fibroepithelial Polyp
- Urothelial Neoplasms
  - Papillary Urothelial Neoplasm of Low Malignant Potential
  - Urothelial Papilloma
  - Urothelial Carcinoma

Rare but Important

- Foreign Body
- Inflammatory Myofibroblastic Tumor
- Fungus Ball
- Neurofibroma
- Metanephric Adenoma

ESSENTIAL INFORMATION

Key Differential Diagnosis Issues

- Clinical considerations
  - Typical symptoms include
    - Difficulty voiding
    - Dysuria
    - Urgency
    - Frequency
    - Hematuria
- Imaging considerations
  - Modalities
    - Ultrasound (with full bladder) may be only imaging necessary prior to cystoscopy & biopsy
    - Fluoroscopic voiding cystourethrogram (VCUG) may pick up
      - Ureteroceles & associated vesicoureteral reflux (VUR) in duplicated systems or bladder neck obstruction
      - Prolapse of polyps into urethra on voiding
    - MR may be useful in some tumors to assess local invasion & adenopathy
  - Characteristics of intrinsic masses
    - Solid vs. cystic
    - Fixed vs. mobile
    - Infiltrative vs. pedunculated
    - Presence or absence of internal vascularity
    - Relationship to urethra & ureterovesical junction
  - Also consider extrinsic compression or invasion/infiltration of bladder by adjacent masses
    - Rhabdomyosarcoma of prostate or vagina
    - Hydrometrocolpos
    - Burkitt lymphoma
    - Vascular malformation
- **Take home point**
  - Most fixed solid bladder masses will not be distinguishable by imaging, necessitating cystoscopy & biopsy/excision

Helpful Clues for Common Diagnoses

- **Ureterocele**
  - Smooth, round, thin-walled cystic dilation of distal ureter protruding from ureterovesical junction into bladder
    - Depending on degree of obstruction, may visualize
      - Ureteral jet from ureterocele on color Doppler
      - Ureteral & collecting system dilation
  - After puncture (to relieve obstruction), decompressed ureterocele will appear smaller & more thick walled or solid
- **Antireflux Intervention at Ureterovesical Junction**
  - Various bulking agents (e.g., Deflux) may be injected into ureterovesical junction to decrease VUR
    - Typically leaves round, smooth, homogeneous, avascular mass
      - Mass may calcify over time
  - Ureteral reimplantation may cause focal round or longitudinal distortion of bladder wall
- **Cystitis**
  - Mild generalized wall thickening is commonly seen with routine urinary tract infections
  - Various forms of cystitis, particularly chronic, may cause more focal mass-like thickening ± hyperemia
    - Hemorrhagic cystitis: Classically seen in setting of chemotherapy or stem cell transplant
    - Eosinophilic cystitis: May have atopy
    - Cystitis cystica
    - Cystitis glandularis
    - Polypoid cystitis

Helpful Clues for Less Common Diagnoses

- **Calculus**
  - Uncommon in children without predisposing history of chronic bladder dysfunction
    - Stasis & recurrent infections
      - Neurogenic bladder
      - Bladder augmentation
    - Lack of animal proteins
  - Typically mobile & highly echogenic with twinkling artifact on color Doppler; ± posterior acoustic shadowing
- **Hematoma**
  - Hematuria typically present
  - Layered appearance of round avascular mass is characteristic, decreasing over days with bladder irrigations
- **Rhabdomyosarcoma**
  - Most common bladder malignancy in children
  - Bimodal age distribution: < 2 years old vs. adolescence
  - Sporadic vs. genetic predisposition syndromes
    - Neurofibromatosis type I
    - Li-Fraumeni syndrome
    - Multiple endocrine neoplasia type (MEN) 2A
  - Typical embryonal subtype large & solid with variable internal vascularity/enhancement
    - Botryoid subtype may appear like grapes with clusters of thin-walled cysts
  - Up to 20% have metastases at diagnosis

- **Fibroepithelial Polyp**
  - a.k.a. fibrovascular polyp
  - Typically small, well-circumscribed pedunculated mass ± internal vascularity at bladder neck
  - May prolapse into urethra
- **Urothelial Neoplasms**
  - **Papillary urothelial neoplasm of low malignant potential**
    - Typically 1-2 cm
    - 35% recurrence rate after resection
  - **Urothelial papilloma**
    - May have frond-like appearance
  - **Urothelial carcinoma**
    - More common in adolescents
    - Most are solitary & low grade
    - Predisposing conditions include
      - Prior bladder augmentation
      - Costello syndrome

Helpful Clues for Rare Diagnoses

- **Foreign Body**
  - Variable appearance depending on composition; look for
    - Straight margins or angles
    - Repeating patterns of echogenicity
    - Posterior acoustic shadowing or enhanced transmission
    - Unusual mobility
  - History of urethral insertion may not be provided
- **Inflammatory Myofibroblastic Tumor**
  - Spindle cell neoplasm with low malignant potential
  - Solid tumor similar to rhabdomyosarcoma in appearance
    - ± necrosis, Ca^{2+}, delayed enhancement
- **Fungus Ball**
  - Avascular mobile focus
    - May rarely obstruct urinary tract
  - Classically due to *Candida* species infections in premature neonates
- **Neurofibroma**
  - Plexiform or diffuse type may be localized or infiltrating
  - Plexiform lesions in cross section typically have characteristic target appearance on MR
    - Fluid-sensitive sequences: Central round intermediate signal surrounded by rim of high signal
    - Post contrast: Central enhancement
  - Conglomerations of lesions often tubular & infiltrating with bag-of-worms-like appearance
- **Metanephric Adenoma**
  - Metaplasia, often in setting of prior trauma, inflammation, or procedure
    - 10% found in renal transplant patients

SELECTED REFERENCES

1. Mohseny AB et al: Late-onset sepsis due to urinary tract infection in very preterm neonates is not uncommon. Eur J Pediatr. 177(1):33-8, 2018
2. Shelmerdine SC et al: Pearls and pitfalls in diagnosing pediatric urinary bladder masses. Radiographics. 37(6):1872-91, 2017
3. Soliman NA et al: Endemic bladder calculi in children. Pediatr Nephrol. 32(9):1489-99, 2017
4. Arena S et al: Bladder mass in newborn: case report and review of literature. Urology. 86(5):1004-7, 2015
5. Huppmann AR et al: Polyps and masses of the pediatric urinary bladder: a 21-year pathology review. Pediatr Dev Pathol. 14(6):438-44, 2011
6. Shah RU et al: Imaging of pediatric pelvic neoplasms. Radiol Clin North Am. 49(4):729-48, v, 2011
7. Young RH: Tumor-like lesions of the urinary bladder. Mod Pathol. 22 Suppl 2:S37-52, 2009
8. Netto JM et al: Pediatric inflammatory bladder tumors: myofibroblastic and eosinophilic subtypes. J Urol. 162(4):1424-9, 1999

Ureterocele

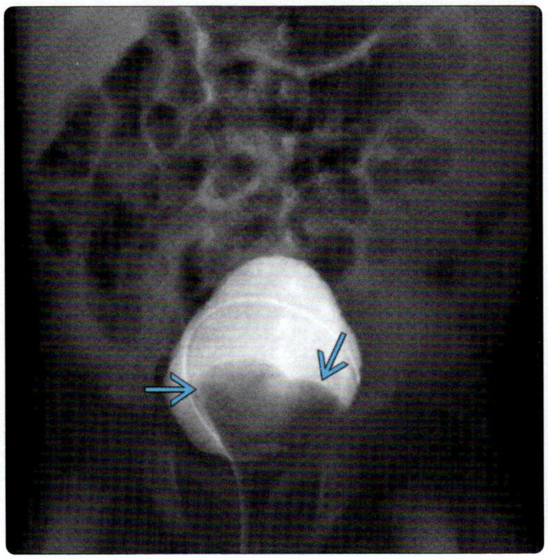

Ureterocele

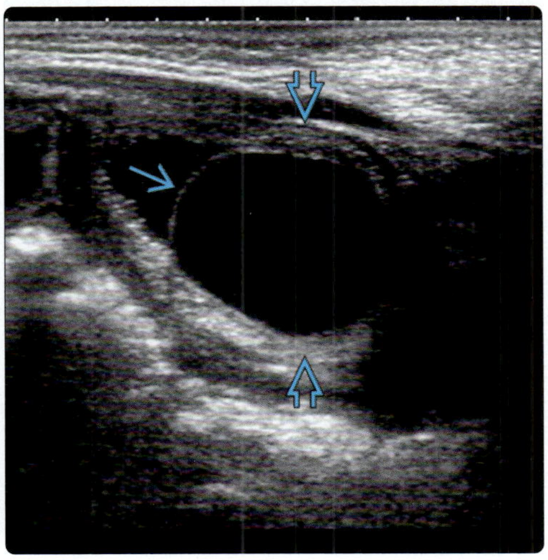

(Left) *Fluoroscopic VCUG image in a neonate with prenatally detected hydronephrosis shows a smooth, mildly lobulated filling defect* ➡ *in the otherwise contrast-filled urinary bladder.* **(Right)** *Longitudinal ultrasound in the same patient shows the thin-walled urine-filled ureterocele* ➡ *in the bladder base* ⇨. *This ectopic ureterocele was associated with an obstructed upper pole moiety of the left kidney.*

(Left) *Transverse color Doppler ultrasound of the urinary bladder in a 5 year old status post bilateral ureterovesical junction (UVJ) is shown. Deflux injections show prominent round intramural mounds of the bulking agent ➡. A ureteral jet emanates from the left UVJ orifice.* **(Right)** *Transverse color Doppler ultrasound in a 5 year old on chemotherapy for neuroblastoma who presented with new hematuria shows lobular posterior bladder wall thickening & hyperemia due to hemorrhagic cystitis.*

Antireflux Intervention at Ureterovesical Junction

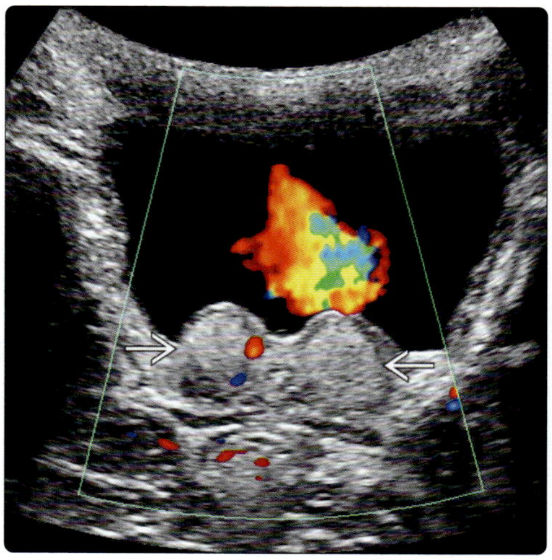

Cystitis

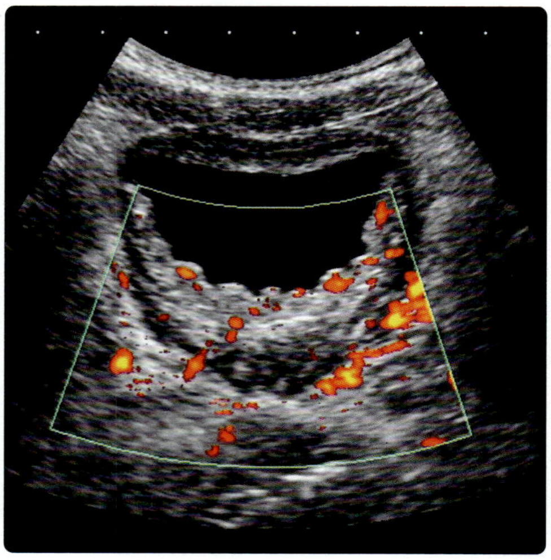

(Left) *Transverse ultrasound in a 2 year old shows 2 round echogenic foci ➡ with posterior acoustic shadowing ⇨. These foci were mobile with changes in patient position, consistent with bladder calculi.* **(Right)** *Transverse color Doppler ultrasound in a 3 year old with pre-B-cell acute lymphoblastic lymphoma (ALL) & hematuria shows a large intravesical avascular mass with layered echogenicity ⇨, typical of a bladder clot.*

Calculus

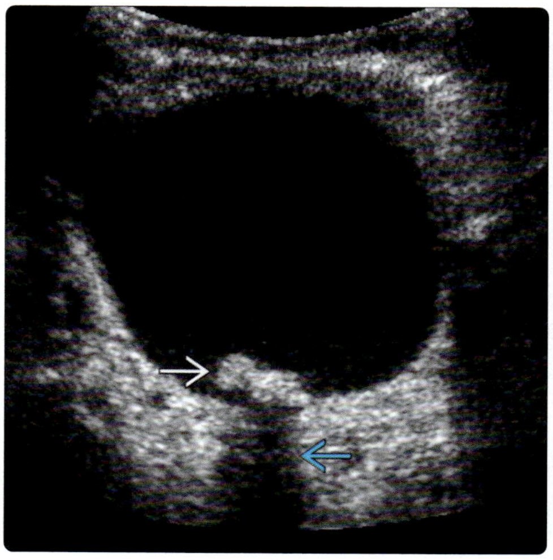

Hematoma

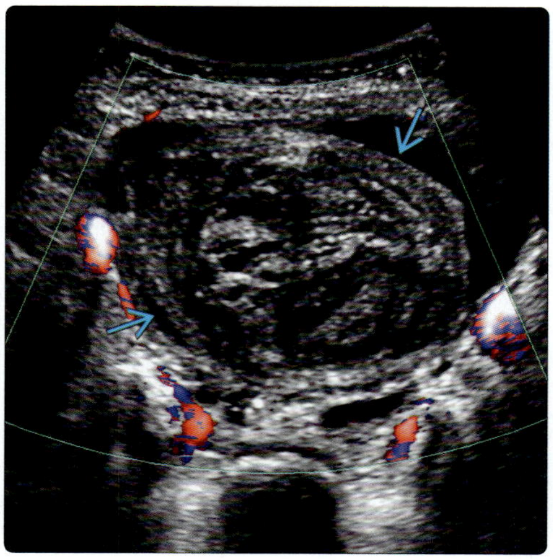

(Left) *Longitudinal color Doppler ultrasound of the bladder in a 3-month-old boy shows a solid mass ⇨ with mild internal vascularity in the bladder base ➡. A prostatic rhabdomyosarcoma was found upon further imaging.* **(Right)** *Transverse color Doppler ultrasound in a 12 year old with a tumor predisposition syndrome shows a nonspecific polypoid bladder mass ⇨ with internal vascularity. Resection confirmed a papillary urothelial neoplasm of low malignant potential.*

Rhabdomyosarcoma

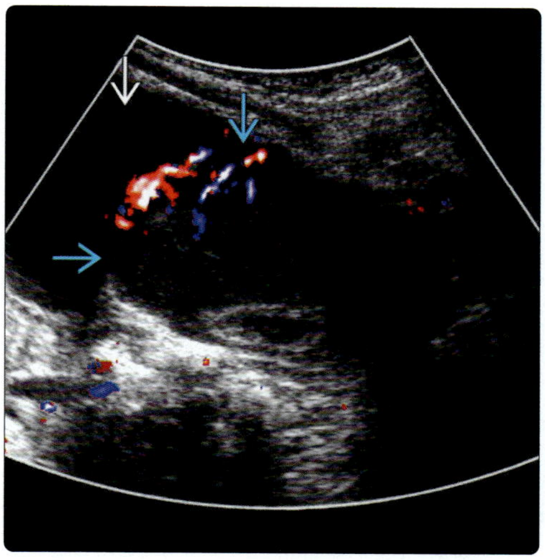

Urothelial Neoplasms

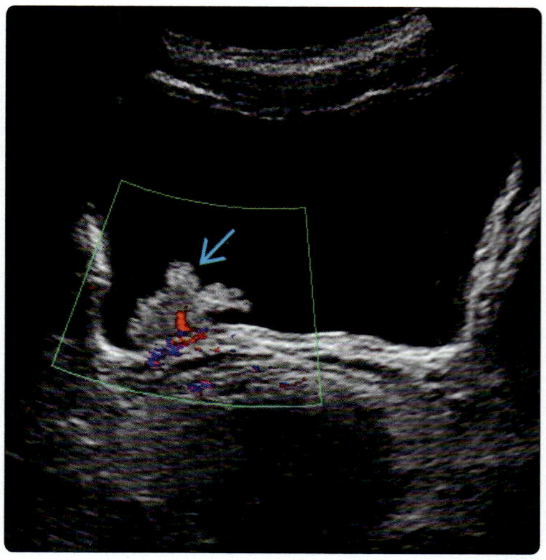

Urothelial Carcinoma

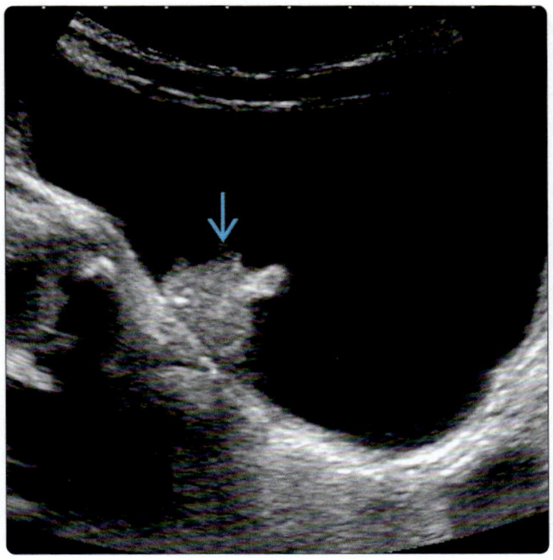

Foreign Body

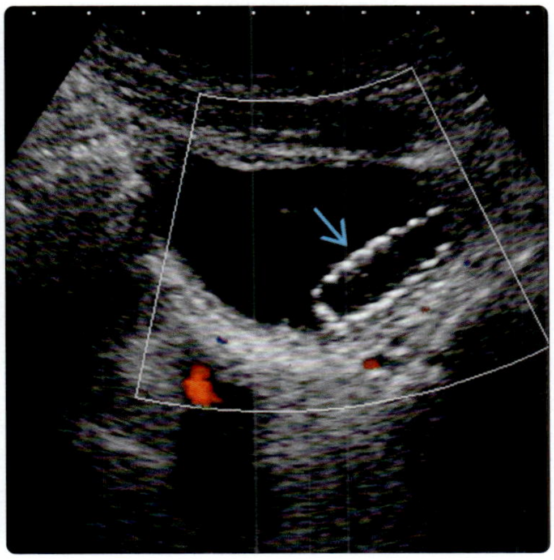

(Left) *Longitudinal ultrasound in a 5 year old with hematuria shows a solid nonmobile polypoid mass in the bladder. Resection showed a high-grade urothelial neoplasm.* **(Right)** *Longitudinal color Doppler ultrasound in a 13-year-old boy who had inserted a fishing lure into his urethra shows a cylindrical foreign body with echogenic striations in the bladder.*

Inflammatory Myofibroblastic Tumor

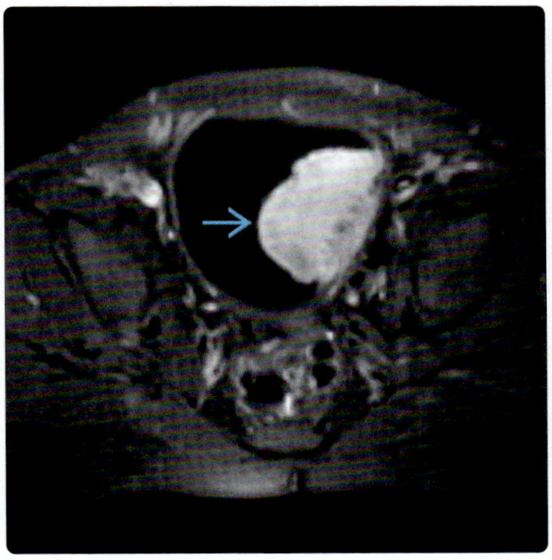

Inflammatory Myofibroblastic Tumor

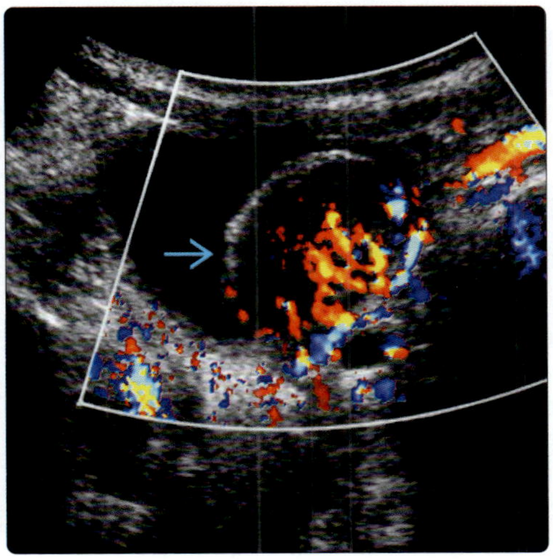

(Left) *Axial T1 C+ FS MR in the same patient shows diffuse enhancement of the mass . Biopsy confirmed an inflammatory myofibroblastic tumor.* **(Right)** *Transverse color Doppler ultrasound in a 2 year old shows a solid ovoid mass attached to the left lateral bladder wall. There is notable hyperemia in the base of the lesion.*

Fungus Ball

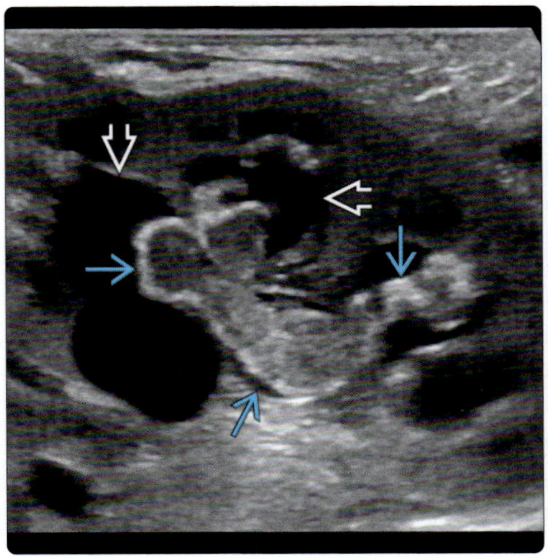

Neurofibroma

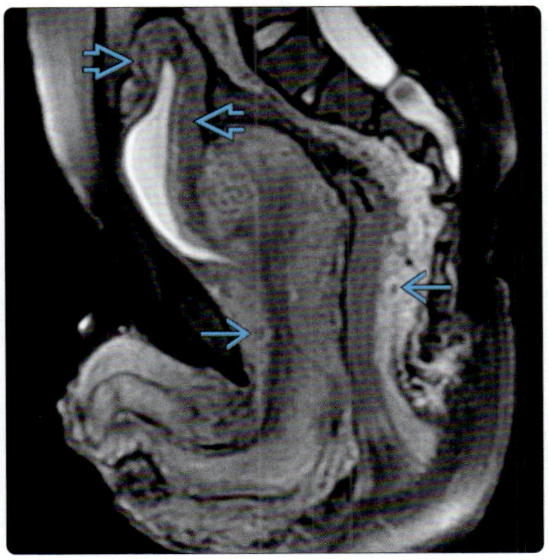

(Left) *Longitudinal US of a kidney in a premature neonate with candiduria shows lobulated echogenic material obstructing renal collecting system , consistent with fungus balls. Only irregular debris was seen in the urinary bladder. (Courtesy L. Linscott, MD.)* **(Right)** *Sagittal T2 FS MR in a patient with neurofibromatosis type 1 shows large plexiform neurofibromas infiltrating the penis, prostate, & bladder wall . Several pelvic components show the classic lesional cross section of a target appearance .*

DIFFERENTIAL DIAGNOSIS

Common

- Normal Male Urethra
- Normal Female Urethra
- Posterior Urethral Valves
- Prostatic Utricle
- Bladder Sphincter Dyssynergia

Less Common

- Cowper Duct Syringocele
- Ejaculatory Duct Reflux
- Prostatic Reflux
- Reflux Into Ectopic Ureter
- Urethral Trauma
- Urethral Stricture
- Anorectal Malformation
- Prune Belly Syndrome
- Lacuna Magna

Rare but Important

- Anterior Urethral Valve
- Urethral Polyp
- Congenital Megalourethra
- Urethral Duplication
- Congenital Urethroperineal Fistula

ESSENTIAL INFORMATION

Helpful Clues for Common Diagnoses

- **Normal Male Urethra**
  - Divided into prostatic, membranous, bulbous, & penile
    - Prostatic
      - Longitudinal filling defect along posterior wall: Urethral crest/verumontanum (site of ejaculatory duct & prostatic utricle openings)
      - Focal anterior indentation: Intermuscular incisura
      - Normal circumferential urethral folds extending distally from verumontanum: Plicae colliculi; do not cause bladder outlet obstruction
    - Membranous: Short segment coursing through external sphincter/urogenital diaphragm
    - Bulbous: Proximal segment of anterior urethra
      - Paired Cowper ducts run along ventral urethra from Cowper glands in external sphincter to orifices at distal bulbous urethra
    - Penile: Beyond suspensory ligament
- **Normal Female Urethra**
  - Relatively short, smooth tubular or conical passage
  - May see indentations (from proximal to distal) at bladder neck, incisura, & urogenital diaphragm/external sphincter
  - Vaginal reflux of urine occurs in up to 60% normally
- **Posterior Urethral Valves**
  - Membrane/diaphragm obstructing distal posterior urethra near external sphincter; may be complete or have central perforation
  - Most common cause of bladder outlet obstruction; occurs in male patients only
  - Spectrum of presentations
    - Complete obstruction in fetus
      - Oligo-/anhydramnios → pulmonary hypoplasia
      - Chronic hydroureteronephrosis → cystic renal dysplasia → renal failure
      - Bladder dysfunction
    - Lesser degrees of obstruction may go undetected for years, presenting as voiding dysfunction & renal failure
  - US: Bladder wall thickening, elongation, irregularity, or diverticula; may be decompressed by catheter
    - Hydroureteronephrosis ± echogenic kidneys with variably sized peripheral cysts (cystic renal dysplasia)
  - VCUG: Dilated posterior urethra with abrupt transition to normal or narrow caliber anterior urethra near membranous segment
    - Discrete thin valve tissue may not be visible
    - Thick bladder wall with irregular morphology; ± diverticula, urachal remnant
    - ± vesicoureteral reflux (VUR), intrarenal reflux
- **Prostatic Utricle**
  - Normal blind-ending pouch/diverticulum arising from posterior wall of posterior prostatic urethra
    - Müllerian duct remnant; may be termed müllerian duct cyst if it lacks communication with urethra
  - Typically small; may be incidentally visualized
  - Enlargement may be seen with hypospadias, sexual differentiation disorders, & prune belly syndrome (PBS)
    - Larger size correlates with more severe hypospadias
    - May be seen after repair of imperforate anus
      - Posterior urethral diverticulum vs. residual rectourethral fistula
  - VCUG: Appears as posterior urethral diverticulum
    - Optimally imaged during voiding in steep obliquity
  - US, CT, or MR: May be incidentally noted when performed for other indication
- **Bladder Sphincter Dyssynergia**
  - Disruption of CNS regulation of micturition → lack of bladder & urethral sphincter coordination
    - During bladder detrusor contraction, urethral sphincter fails to relax
    - Most common pediatric CNS associations: Myelomeningocele, tethered cord, spinal cord injury
  - VCUG: Dilation of posterior urethra to closed urethral sphincter (spinning top appearance in females)

Helpful Clues for Less Common Diagnoses

- **Cowper Duct Syringocele**
  - Cystic dilation at end of Cowper duct
  - Frequently asymptomatic; can present as urinary infection, hematuria, dysuria, obstructive symptoms
  - VCUG: May only demonstrate mild mass effect of unopacified cyst on bulbous urethra at orifice of duct
    - Larger patulous defect → contrast filling of distal Cowper duct
      - May occur with distal urethral obstruction or rupture of retention cyst
- **Ejaculatory Duct Reflux**
  - Associated with neurogenic bladder
    - Bladder-sphincter dyssynergia, anorectal malformation
  - May lead to recurrent epididymitis
- **Prostatic Reflux**
  - Associated with variable degrees of urethral obstruction

- VCUG: Poorly defined, cloud-like ↓ density surrounding prostatic urethra
- **Reflux Into Ectopic Ureter**
  - Ectopic ureter may be associated with
    - Single system, predominantly in males
      - Inserts above external sphincter in males
    - Upper pole of duplex kidney, usually in females
      - May insert below sphincter in females
- **Urethral Trauma**
  - Anterior urethra: Often due to straddle-type injury
  - Posterior: Higher association pelvic fractures from MVA
  - Classification of urethral injuries
    - Type 1: Intact but stretched
    - Type 2: Disrupted above external sphincter
    - Type 3 (most common): Tear at urogenital diaphragm
    - Type 4: Involves bladder neck
    - Type 5: Anterior urethral injury
- **Urethral Stricture**
  - Variable locations & lengths, depending on etiology: Trauma, infection, postsurgical (hypospadias, epispadias)
  - Sexually transmitted infection causing urethritis may take years to develop stricture, often in bulbous urethra
- **Anorectal Malformation**
  - Most variations of anorectal malformation (ARM) will have outlet of abnormal distal colon; many will involve urinary tract
    - Males: Fistula from distal rectal pouch to perineum, urethra (50%), or bladder neck
    - Females: Cloacal malformation (common channel draining rectum, vagina, & urethra), rectoperineal fistula, or rectovestibular fistula
  - Most ARMs require initial diverting colostomy with delayed definitive repair
- **Prune Belly Syndrome**
  - a.k.a. Eagle-Barrett syndrome
  - Classic triad in male patient: Cryptorchidism, deficiency of abdominal wall musculature, urinary tract anomalies; rarely seen in females with other genital anomalies
  - Smooth dilated bladder with severely dilated & tortuous ureters; no mechanical obstruction
  - Associated urethral anomalies: Dilated prostatic urethra (especially posterior wall, due to hypoplastic prostate), diffusely or focally enlarged penile urethra
    - Rarely atretic urethra or posterior urethral valves (PUV)
  - Amniotic fluid is typically normal in utero
- **Lacuna Magna**
  - Dorsal diverticulum at roof of fossa navicularis
  - Often asymptomatic; may result in dysuria, end-void gross hematuria, or hematospermia

Helpful Clues for Rare Diagnoses

- **Anterior Urethral Valve**
  - Most are caused by anterior urethral diverticulum
  - Diverticulum expands into urethral lumen during voiding, occluding urethral flow
  - Variable obstruction, mild to severe
- **Urethral Polyp**
  - Symptoms of obstruction or hematuria
  - Usually solitary, pedunculated, urothelial-lined benign mass from verumontanum
  - Mildly mobile filling defect in prostatic urethra, ± internal vascularity
- **Congenital Megalourethra**
  - Nonobstructive urethral dilation; overlap of genitourinary anomalies with PBS
  - Deficiency of corpus spongiosum & cavernosa
    - Scaphoid type: Focally abnormal spongiosum
    - Fusiform: Abnormal spongiosum & cavernosa
- **Urethral Duplication**
  - Complete vs. incomplete
  - Typically in sagittal plane with 2 meatal openings
    - Ventral urethra is typically functional
    - Y-type: Functional urethra opens on perineum
  - Often incidentally discovered; may be associated with other genitourinary anomalies
- **Congenital Urethroperineal Fistula**
  - Fistula from posterior urethra to perineum is minimally functional, unlike Y-type duplication

Normal Male Urethra

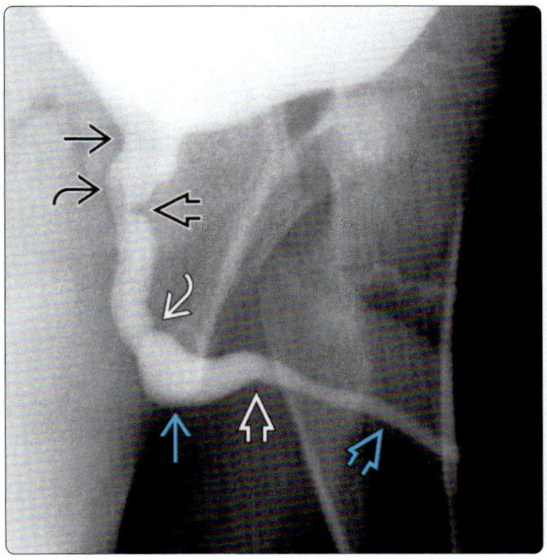

Normal Male Urethra

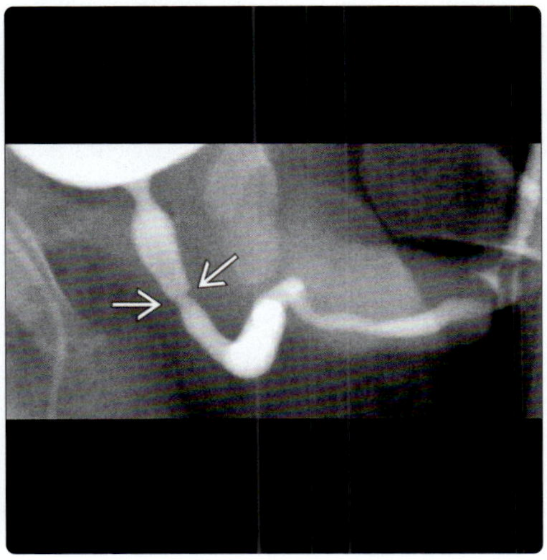

(Left) *Oblique VCUG shows the features of a normal male urethra, including the bladder neck ➔, intermuscular incisura ➔, verumontanum ➔, external urethral sphincter (membranous urethra) ➔, & suspensory ligament of penis ➔ at the junction of the bulbous ➔ & penile ➔ urethra.* **(Right)** *Oblique VCUG in a 1-week-old boy shows prominent plicae colliculae ➔, which can mimic subtle posterior urethral valves (PUV). Secondary signs of bladder outlet obstruction were not present.*

(Left) *Frontal VCUG in an 8-year-old girl with a history of urinary tract infections demonstrates the typical normal appearance of a mildly cone-shaped, smooth-walled female urethra ⇒. No vaginal reflux is present on this image.* **(Right)** *Oblique VCUG of a normal female urethra shows the bladder neck ⇒, external urethral sphincter ➡, external urethral meatus ➡, & incidental vaginal reflux ➡. The spinning top appearance of the urethra ⇒ is normal in some cases but can be seen with bladder sphincter dyssynergia.*

Normal Female Urethra

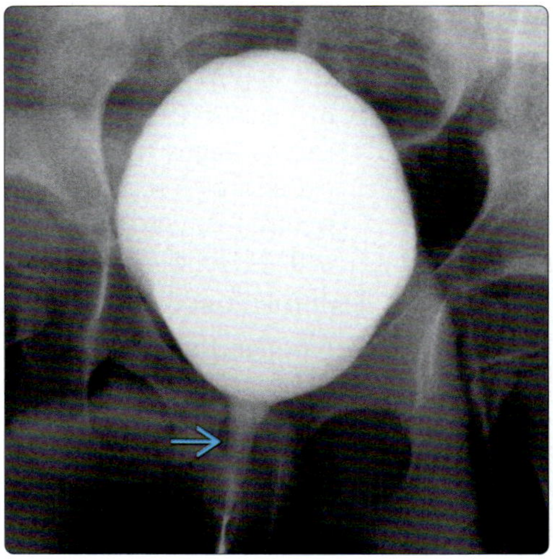

Normal Female Urethra

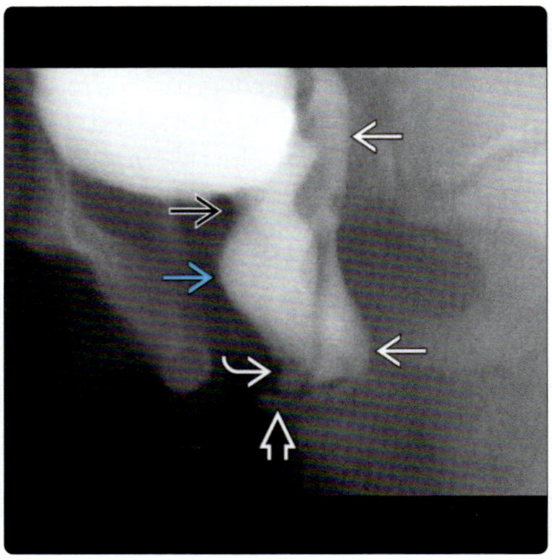

(Left) *Sagittal T2 SSFSE MR in a 21-week fetus shows a dilated, thick-walled urinary bladder ⇒ with a dilated posterior urethra ⇒. Note the oligohydramnios ⇒ & small chest. The accompanying hydroureteronephrosis is not shown on this image.* **(Right)** *Oblique VCUG in a 2-day-old boy shows a dilated posterior urethra ⇒ with abrupt transition to a narrow anterior urethra ⇒ at the level of PUV ⇒. The trabeculated urinary bladder ➡ has almost completely emptied. Note the right grade 5 vesicoureteral reflux (VUR) ➡.*

Posterior Urethral Valves

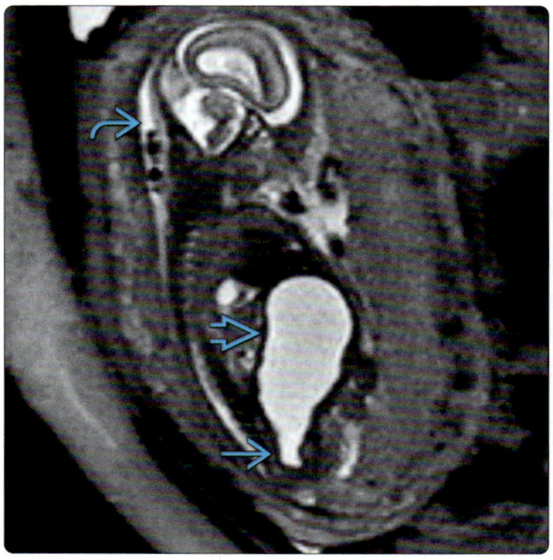

Posterior Urethral Valves

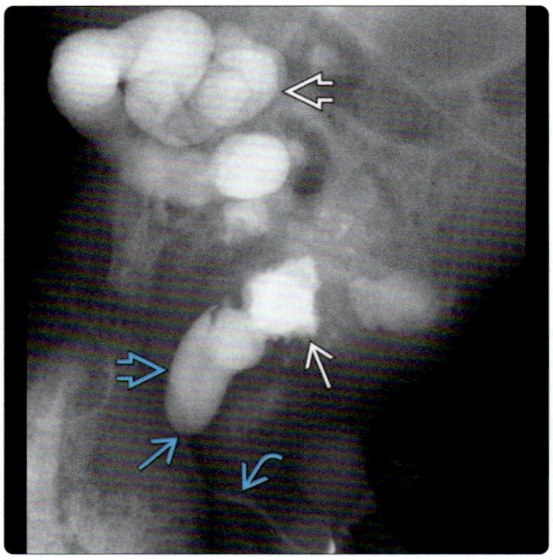

(Left) *Oblique VCUG shows minor PUV ⇒ & an incidental lacuna magna ⇒.* **(Right)** *Longitudinal US of the perineum in the same patient (oriented similar to the VCUG) shows the anechoic dilated posterior urethra ⇒ just below the bladder neck ⇒. Varying degrees of posterior urethral dilation may occur, depending on the severity of the obstruction.*

Posterior Urethral Valves

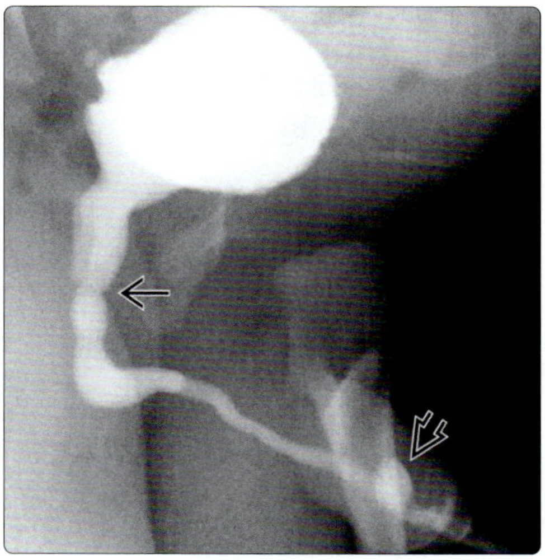

Posterior Urethral Valves

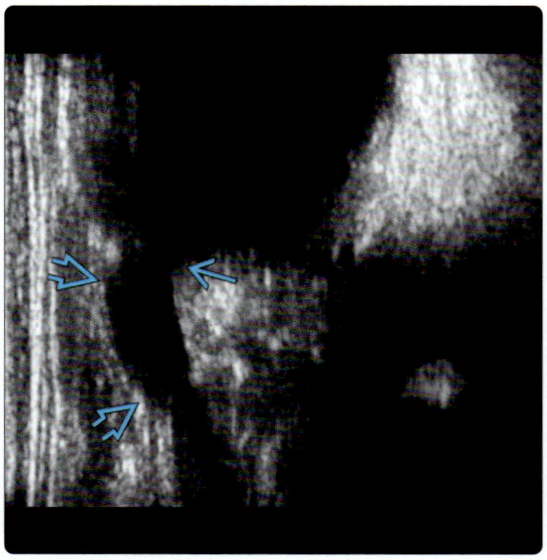

Prostatic Utricle

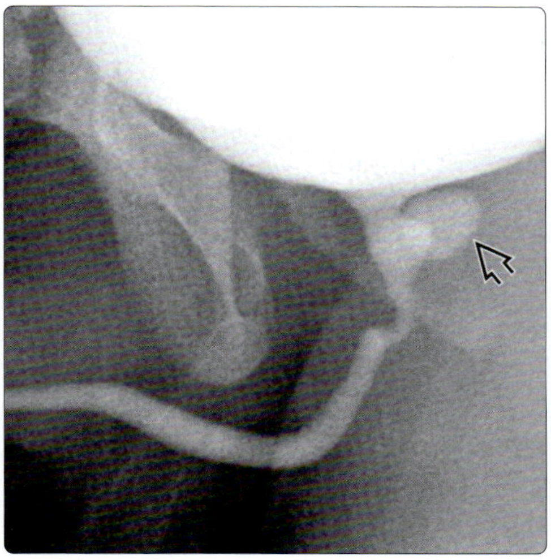

Bladder Sphincter Dyssynergia

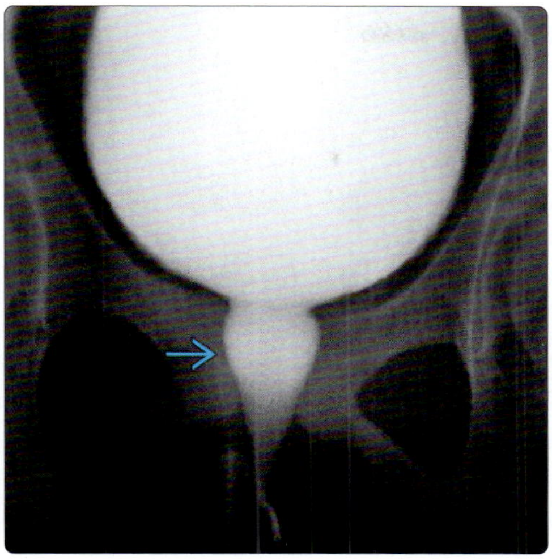

(Left) *Oblique VCUG in a 2-year-old boy shows a contrast-filled diverticulum arising from the posterior prostatic urethra, consistent with a utricle in this patient, who also had a history of hypospadias.* **(Right)** *Frontal VCUG in a young girl with day & night wetting & a history of a tethered spinal cord shows a spinning top appearance of the urethra during intermittent "start-stop" voiding, which can be seen in bladder sphincter dyssynergia.*

Cowper Duct Syringocele

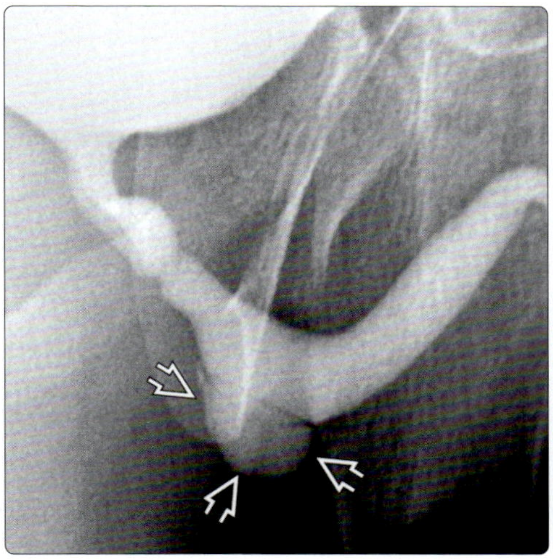

Ejaculatory Duct Reflux

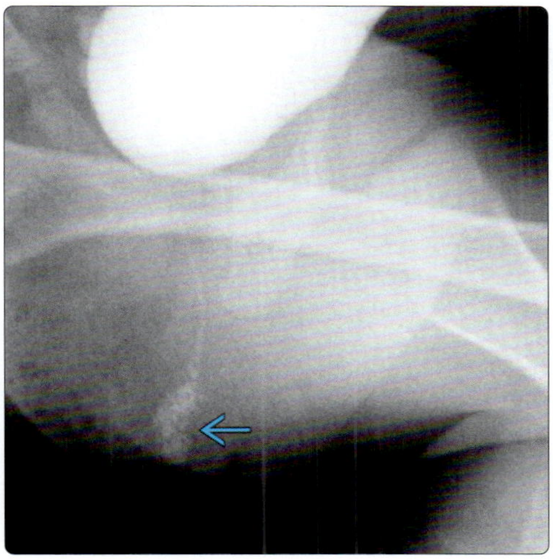

(Left) *Oblique VCUG shows an outpouching of contrast toward the undersurface of the bulbous urethra, characteristic of a Cowper duct syringocele.* **(Right)** *Lateral VCUG in a patient with an anorectal malformation shows contrast extending along the ejaculatory duct to the epididymis. Recurrent epididymitis can occur in such patients.*

Reflux Into Ectopic Ureter

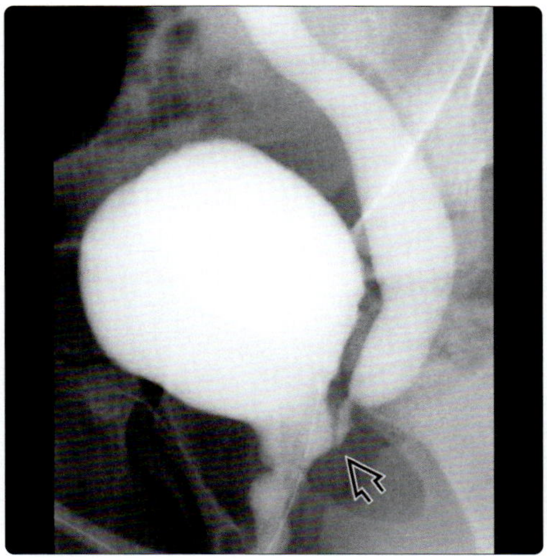

Urethral Trauma

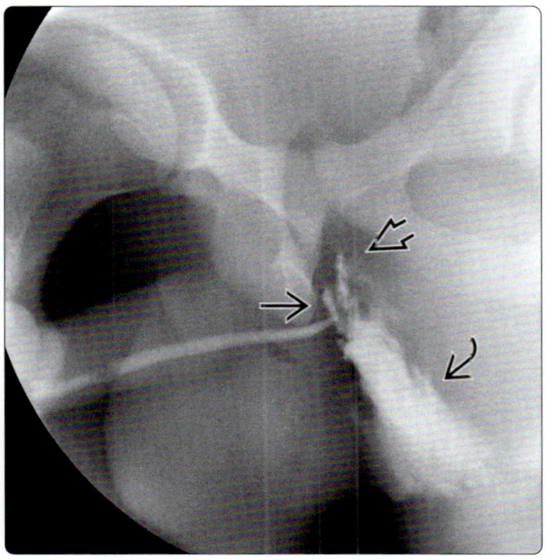

(Left) *Oblique VCUG in a male patient shows ectopic insertion of the left ureter into the prostatic urethra. In males, an ectopic ureter is more likely to be associated with a single renal collecting system rather than a duplicated system.* **(Right)** *Oblique retrograde urethrogram shows contrast extravasation at the level of the urogenital diaphragm & extending toward the perineum & scrotum.*

Urethral Stricture

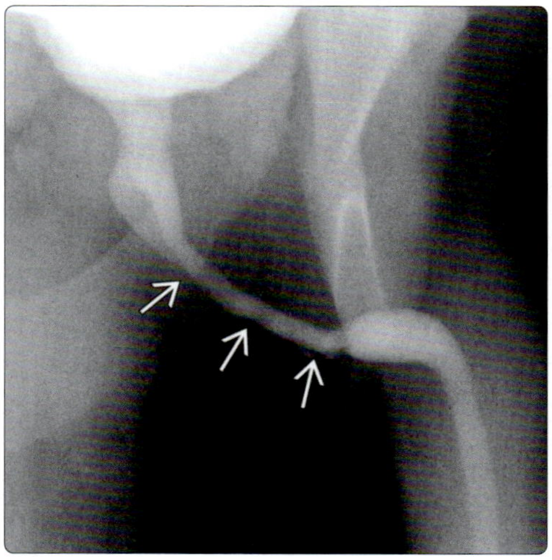

Urethral Stricture

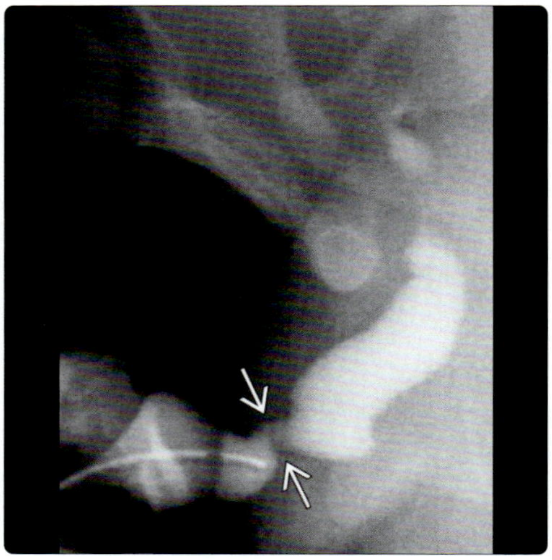

(Left) *Oblique VCUG shows long-segment narrowing of the bulbous urethra in this adolescent boy, who had a urethral swab positive for gonorrhea.* **(Right)** *Oblique retrograde urethrogram shows an anterior urethral stricture in this patient treated for hypospadias as an infant. A VCUG could not be performed because the catheter would not pass through the stricture.*

Anorectal Malformation

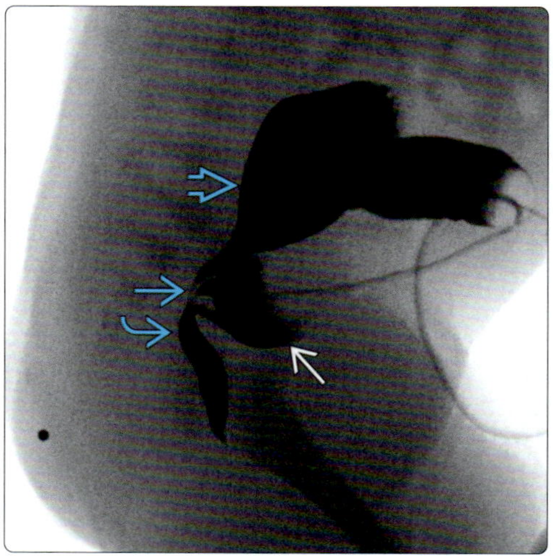

Anorectal Malformation

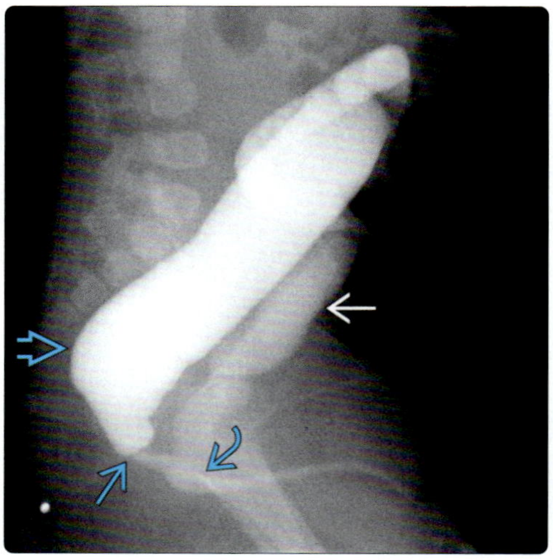

(Left) *Lateral view of distal colostogram in a 3 month old with anorectal malformation post colostomy shows a fistula from rectum to prostatic urethra (i.e., rectoprostatic fistula) with reflux into urinary bladder. Metallic marker lies at expected level of anus.* **(Right)** *Lateral view of distal colostogram in a 4 month old with anorectal malformation post colostomy shows a fistula from rectum to bulbous urethra (i.e., rectobulbar fistula) with reflux into urinary bladder. Metallic marker lies at expected level of anus.*

Prune Belly Syndrome

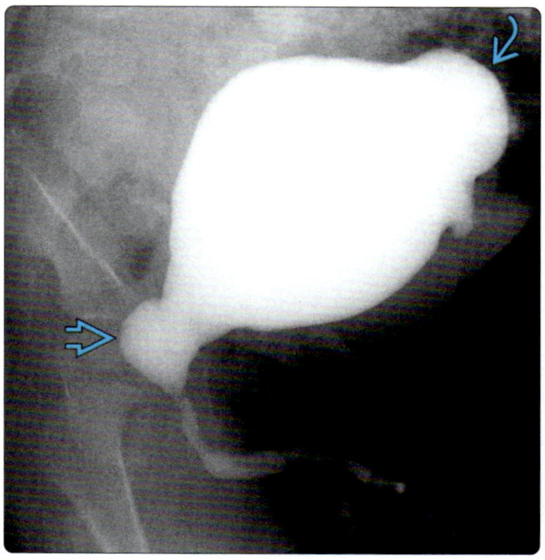

Prune Belly Syndrome

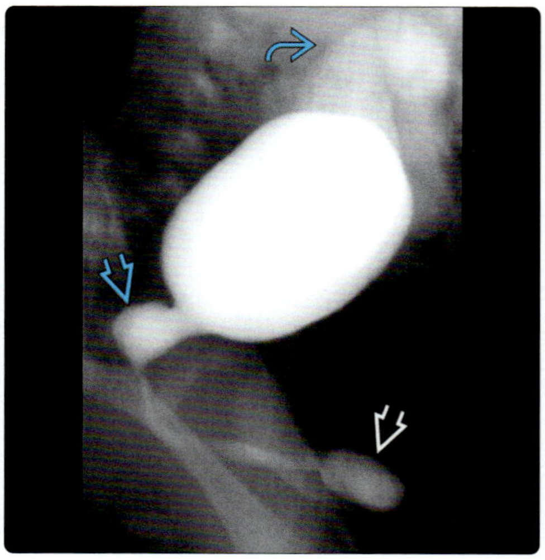

(Left) *Oblique VCUG in a 13 month old with prune belly syndrome (PBS) shows a dilated prostatic urethra (with characteristic bulging posterior wall). The bulging focus at the bladder dome suggests a urachal diverticulum.* **(Right)** *Oblique VCUG in a patient with PBS shows a dilated prostatic urethra (with bulging posterior wall), distal scaphoid megalourethra, & a urachal remnant.*

Urethral Polyp

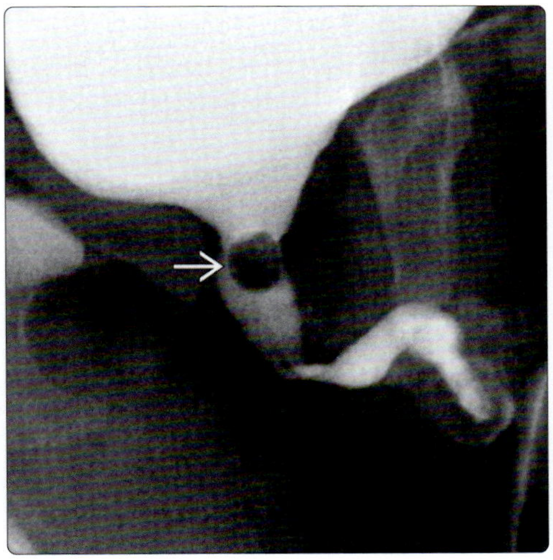

Congenital Megalourethra

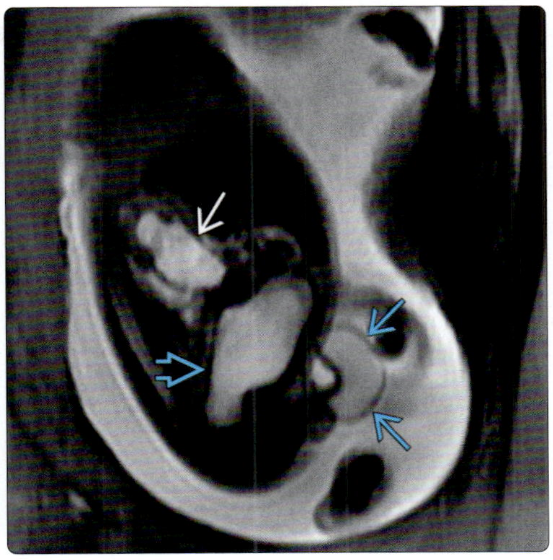

(Left) *Oblique VCUG shows a round filling defect ➡ within the posterior urethra that intermittently prolapses between the bladder neck & posterior urethra during filling & voiding.* **(Right)** *Sagittal MR urogram of the same fetus shows the congenital megalourethra ⇨, dilated urinary bladder ⇨, & hydroureteronephrosis ➡. The amniotic fluid is normal.*

Congenital Megalourethra

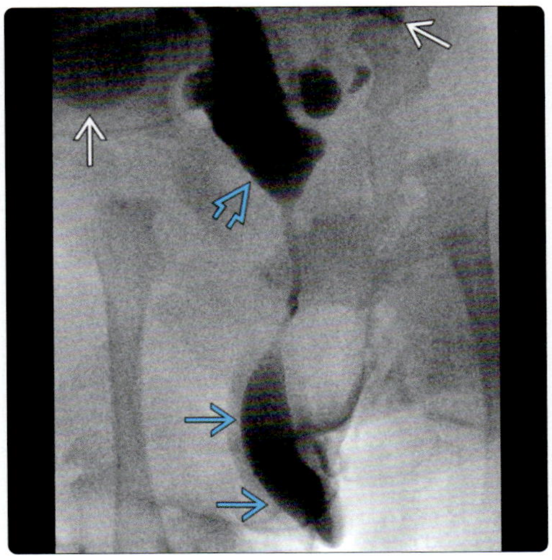

Congenital Megalourethra

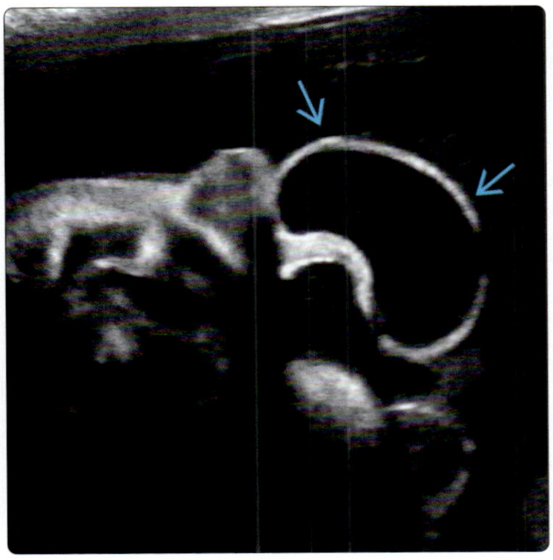

(Left) *VCUG in the same patient at 5 months old shows dilated anterior urethra ⇨. Urinary bladder is elongated ⇨ with multiple diverticula. Bilateral grade 5 VUR ➡ was noted. While this child also had cryptorchidism, the typical abdominal wall features of PBS were not present.* **(Right)** *US in a 23-week fetus with a dilated bladder & bilateral hydroureter (not shown) demonstrates a large, mobile, tubular, fluid-filled structure ⇨ between the lower extremities, suggesting an enlarged phallus with a fusiform megalourethra.*

Urethral Duplication

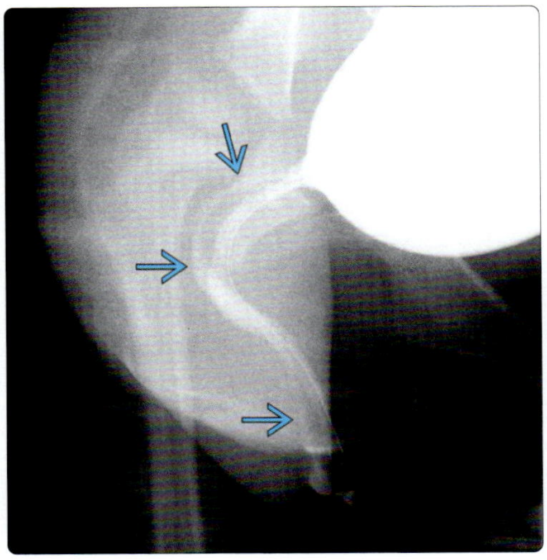

Urethral Duplication

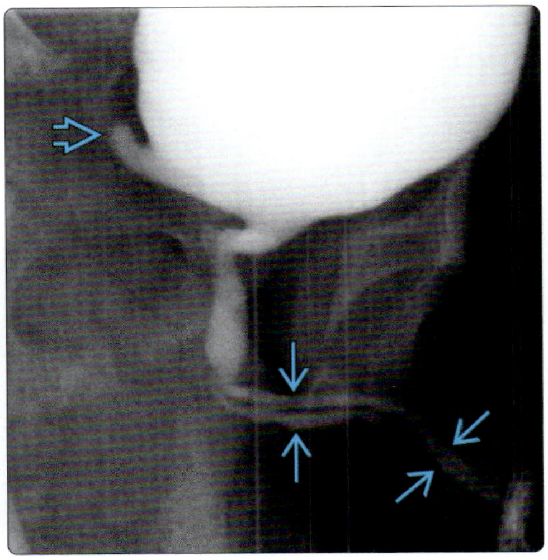

(Left) *Oblique VCUG in a 2-year-old boy with multiple congenital anomalies shows a complete duplication of the urethra ⇨.* **(Right)** *Oblique VCUG in a 3 year old with a history of anorectal malformation shows duplication of the anterior urethra ⇨ as well as a bladder diverticulum ⇨.*

SECTION 5

Musculoskeletal

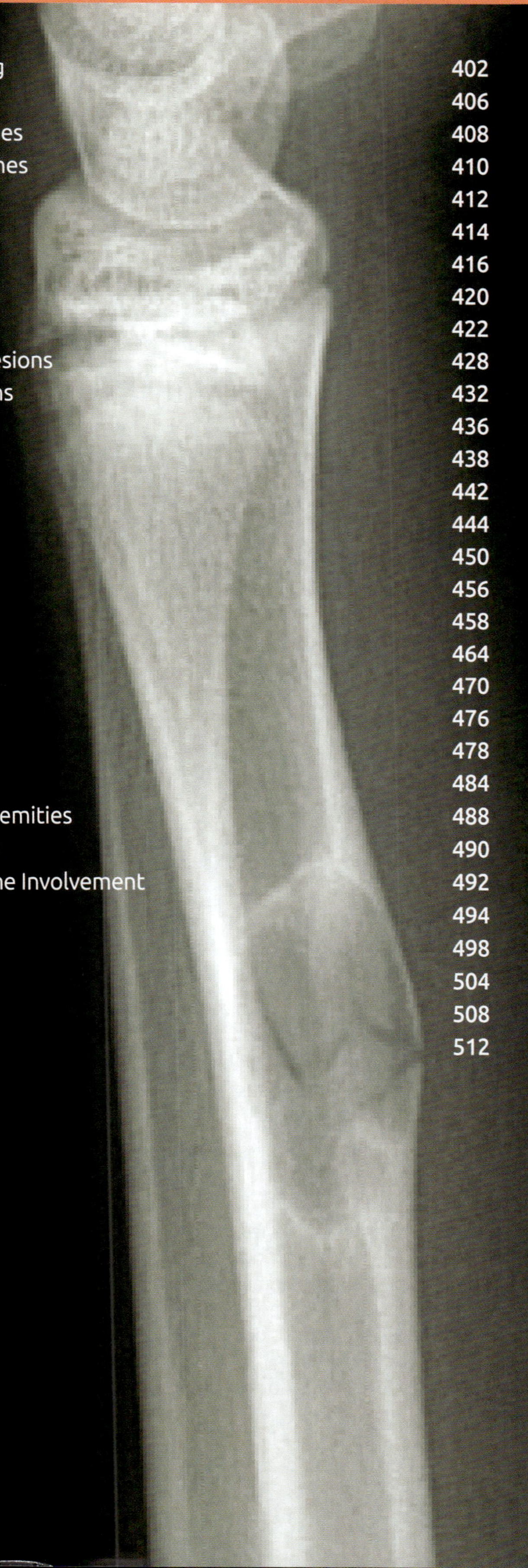

DIFFERENTIAL DIAGNOSIS

Common

- Developmental Irregular Ossification
- Osteomyelitis & Septic Arthritis
- Avascular Necrosis
- Osteochondroses

Less Common

- Osteochondritis Dissecans
- Juvenile Idiopathic Arthritis
- Rickets
- Hypothyroidism
- Fetal Alcohol Syndrome

Rare but Important

- Epiphyseal Dysplasias
- Pseudoachondroplasia
- Chondrodysplasia Punctata
- Trevor-Fairbank Disease (Dysplasia Epiphysealis Hemimelica)
- Thermal Injury or Frostbite
- Complications of Warfarin (Coumadin)

ESSENTIAL INFORMATION

Key Differential Diagnosis Issues

- May be able to separate into irregular vs. stippled epiphyses
  - Differential diagnosis for irregular epiphyses
    - Developmental irregular ossification
    - Avascular necrosis
    - Osteomyelitis & septic arthritis
    - Osteochondrosis
    - Juvenile idiopathic arthritis
    - Rickets
    - Trevor-Fairbank disease
    - Epiphyseal dysplasias
  - Differential diagnoses for stippled epiphyses
    - Hypothyroidism
    - Warfarin embryopathy
    - Chondrodysplasia punctata
    - Fetal alcohol syndrome
    - Epiphyseal dysplasias
  - Some entities such as epiphyseal dysplasias may have stippled &/or irregular epiphyses

Helpful Clues for Common Diagnoses

- **Developmental Irregular Ossification**
  - Multiple &/or irregular growth centers are **normal** at many locations in pediatric skeleton
    - Upper extremity: Trochlea, pisiform
    - Lower extremity: Femoral condyles, tibial tubercle, medial malleolus, calcaneal apophysis, cuneiforms
  - Knowing common sites of developmental irregular ossification prevents mistaking these for pathology [e.g., avascular necrosis, osteochondritis dissecans (OCD), dysplasia]
  - MR: Normal ossification centers do not have abnormal edema/fluid signal
    - Cartilage precursors may show increased fluid signal prior to ossification at some locations
- **Osteomyelitis & Septic Arthritis**
  - Epiphyseal involvement: May be primary site in infants vs. spread from metaphysis or joint in any child
  - Typically have signs/symptoms of infection
  - May show sclerosis, irregularity, or destruction of involved epiphysis, particularly from chronic infection or sequela of septic arthritis
- **Avascular Necrosis**
  - Osteonecrosis of epiphysis → subchondral sclerosis → irregularity & subchondral collapse
    - Prior to significant flattening, may see fragments at site of necrosis
  - Etiologies in children: Acute lymphoblastic leukemia, steroids, sickle cell disease, trauma, vasculitis
- **Osteochondroses**
  - Collection of poorly understood "disorders" of immature skeleton
  - Many entities reflect symptomatic growth disturbances with elements of idiopathic osteonecrosis &/or chronic repetitive overuse injury
  - Symptoms range from asymptomatic → pain → growth disturbances
  - Outcomes range from resolution of self-limited process to permanent deformity
  - Many cause temporary epiphyseal/apophyseal irregularity
    - Capitellum: Panner disease, OCD
    - Femoral head
      - Legg-Calvé-Perthes (LCP): Symptomatic & may lead to permanent deformity
      - Meyer dysplasia: Irregular/delayed ossification of femoral epiphysis (unilateral or bilateral), which typically normalizes without treatment
    - Medial tibia: Blount disease
    - Tibial tubercle: Osgood-Schlatter disease
    - Calcaneal apophysis: Sever disease
    - Tarsal navicular: Köhler disease
    - 2nd or 3rd metatarsal head: Freiberg disease

Helpful Clues for Less Common Diagnoses

- **Osteochondritis Dissecans**
  - Sometimes classified with osteochondroses but more often classified as distinct entity
  - Etiology: Chronic repetitive overuse injury to secondary growth center of involved epiphyses
  - Radiographs: Focal area of subchondral lucency & sclerosis; may lead to intraarticular loose bodies
  - MR: Bone marrow edema, loss of secondary epiphyseal growth plate, & thickening of unossified epiphyseal cartilage distinguish from developmental irregular ossification
    - MR is also useful in distinguishing stable from unstable OCD lesions
  - Most common sites
    - Knee (femoral condyles >> patella > trochlea)
    - Elbow (capitellum > trochlea)
    - Ankle (talar dome)
- **Juvenile Idiopathic Arthritis**
  - Synovial inflammatory disease of unknown cause
  - < 16 years old & symptoms > 6 weeks in duration
  - Early: Joint effusion/synovitis

- Late: Joint space narrowing, erosions
- **Rickets**
  - Metaphyseal cupping & fraying with loss of metaphyseal zone of provisional calcification (ZPC)
  - Loss of ZPC of secondary epiphyseal ossification centers results in irregular epiphyseal margins
- **Hypothyroidism**
  - Infant: Stippled epiphyses
  - Toddler: Severe delay in skeletal maturation
    - Fragmentation of femoral capital epiphysis
- **Fetal Alcohol Syndrome**
  - Stippled epiphyses
  - Typically involves lower but not upper extremities

Helpful Clues for Rare Diagnoses

- **Epiphyseal Dysplasias**
  - Multiple epiphyseal dysplasia (MED)
    - Abnormal endochondral ossification of epiphyses/physes
      - Autosomal dominant & recessive forms
    - Often presents in late childhood/adolescence
    - Small, irregular, fragmented epiphyses ± flattening
    - Most pronounced in lower extremities (especially femoral heads)
    - Can mimic LCP; other epiphyseal involvement can suggest MED
  - Spondyloepiphyseal dysplasia (SED)
    - Group of skeletal dysplasias primarily involving vertebrae & proximal epiphyseal centers
      - Platyspondyly + abnormal epiphyses
    - Congenita (evident at birth) & tarda (presents at 5-10 years) forms
  - Both MED & SED have been described with irregular &/or stippled epiphyses
  - Many other skeletal dysplasias can cause variable amounts of epiphyseal irregularity
    - Typically associated with diffuse skeletal findings
- **Pseudoachondroplasia**
  - Heterogeneous inherited skeletal dysplasia with short stature
  - Vertebrae: Mild platyspondyly (early) → normalize (later)
  - Miniepiphyses in hips, hands/feet
  - Irregular carpal/tarsal bones
  - Irregular, splayed metaphyses
- **Chondrodysplasia Punctata**
  - Stippled epiphyses
  - Nonrhizomelic type: Conradi Hünermann
    - Nonlethal & autosomal dominant
  - Rhizomelic type: Lethal autosomal recessive
    - Multiple other abnormalities
- **Trevor-Fairbank Disease (Dysplasia Epiphysealis Hemimelica)**
  - Developmental abnormality with osteochondroma-like mass(es) arising from epiphysis or apophysis
  - Appears as irregularly ossified exophytic lesion projecting off epiphysis or as lobulations superimposed on epiphyses
    - May appear as discontinuous intraarticular fragments in early childhood
  - Lower limb (knee, ankle, hip) is most frequently affected
  - May be polyarticular; typically monomelic
- **Thermal Injury & Frostbite**
  - Epiphyses are at risk for vascular injury with vasoconstriction from cold temperature
  - May become dense & fragmented
  - Early fusion results in short phalanges
  - Thumb is generally not involved (as often folded into palm in cold temperatures)
- **Complications of Warfarin (Coumadin)**
  - Maternal ingestion during early pregnancy → stippled epiphyses
  - Hypoplastic nose, eye malformations, mental retardation

SELECTED REFERENCES

1. Jaimes C et al: MR imaging of normal epiphyseal development and common epiphyseal disorders. Radiographics. 34(2):449-71, 2014
2. Lachman R. Taybi & Lachman's Radiology of Syndromes, Metabolic Disorders & Skeletal Dysplasias, 5e. Philadelphia: Mosby, 2006

Developmental Irregular Ossification

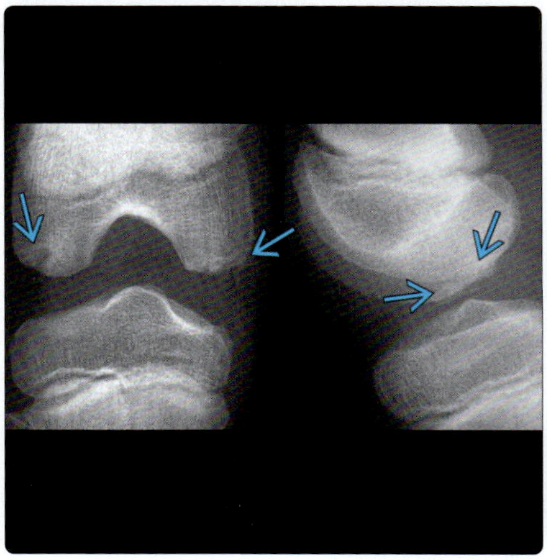

Developmental Irregular Ossification

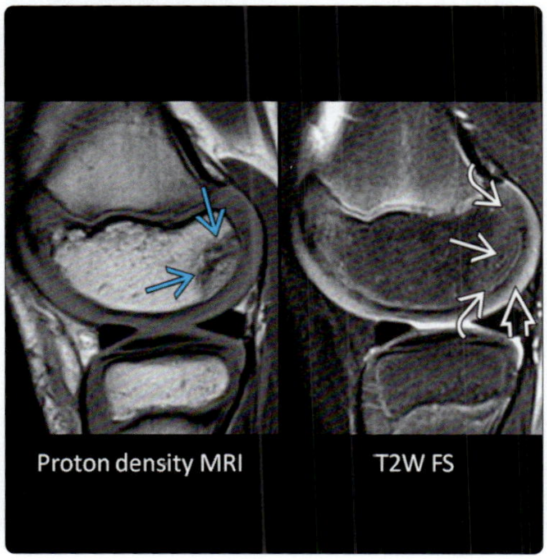

(Left) *Tunnel & lateral knee radiographs of an 8-year-old boy show irregularity of the femoral condyles ➔. Juvenile osteochondritis dissecans (OCD) can have a similar appearance. If symptoms are concerning for OCD, MR can be performed.* **(Right)** *Sagittal PD MR in the same child shows irregular ossification ➔. The T2 FS MR shows no underlying marrow edema ➨, a normal secondary physis ➨ (the physis of the epiphysis), & normal overlying cartilage ➨ in this area. These MR findings distinguish irregular ossification from OCD.*

(Left) *Frontal radiograph in a 15-year-old boy with a history of left hip septic arthritis & proximal femoral osteomyelitis shows irregularity of the left femoral head with secondary osteoarthritis. Ischemia & destruction of the femoral head are feared complications of hip septic arthritis & are more likely if treatment is delayed.* **(Right)** *AP radiograph in a 9-year-old girl with sickle cell disease & bilateral hip pain shows sclerosis & lucency of the bilateral femoral heads with flattening & irregularity of the left femoral head →.*

Osteomyelitis & Septic Arthritis

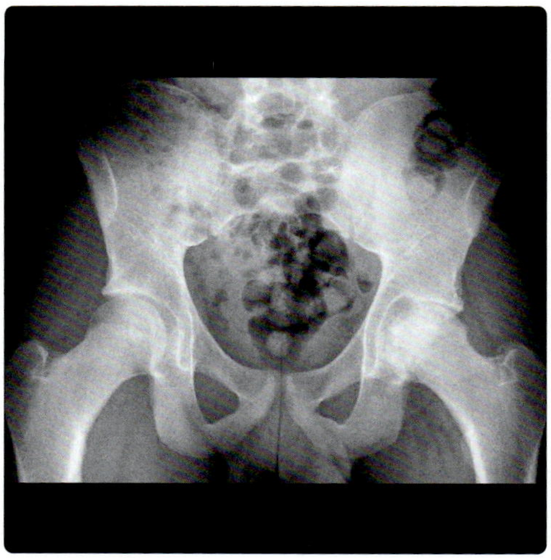

Avascular Necrosis

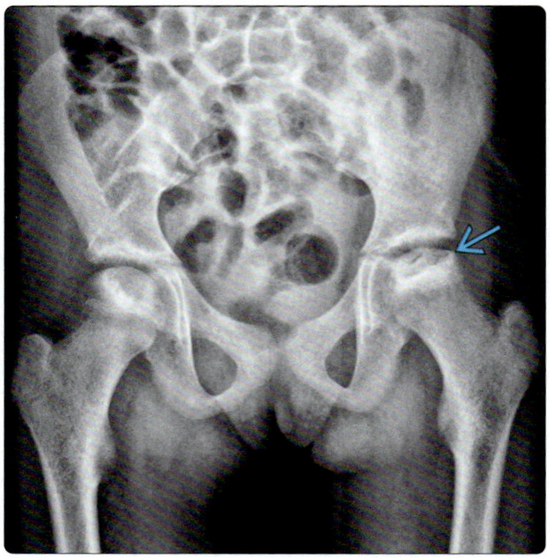

(Left) *Initial frontal radiograph (left) of the left hip in a patient with Legg-Calvé-Perthes (LCP) disease shows an irregular, fragmented, & flattened femoral head →. Two years later (right), there is extrusion of the femoral head laterally →. LCP is idiopathic osteonecrosis of the femoral head.* **(Right)** *PA radiograph shows irregularity of the carpals & radial epiphysis in a patient with JIA due to erosions & overgrowth. The ankylosis at the carpometacarpal joints → is also typical of longstanding disease.*

Osteochondroses

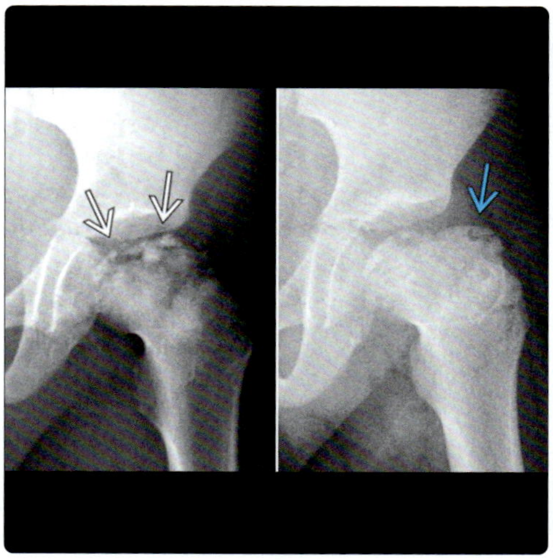

Juvenile Idiopathic Arthritis

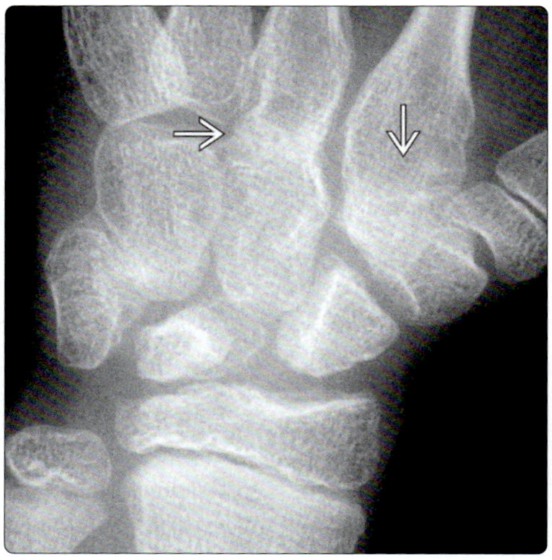

(Left) *AP radiograph shows cupping & fraying of the proximal femoral metaphysis → with loss of the zone of provisional calcification. Also note that the epiphysis has slipped →. The femoral head irregularity is due to a similar (though less pronounced) effect on endochondral bone formation at this secondary ossification center.* **(Right)** *AP radiograph in an infant shows stippled epiphyses → at the femoral head & greater trochanter. Hypothyroidism is one of several entities that may present with stippled epiphyses.*

Rickets

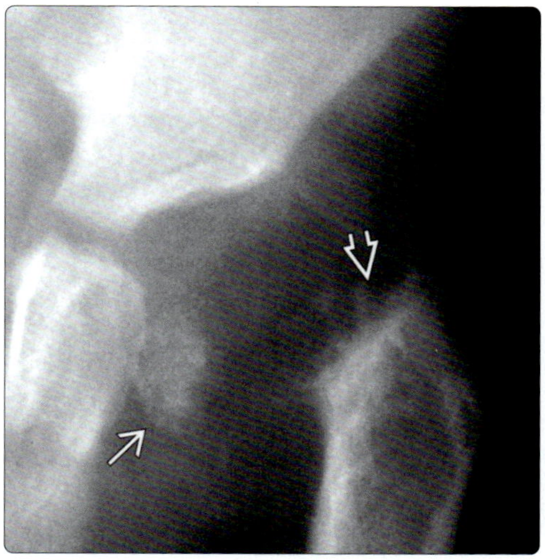

Hypothyroidism

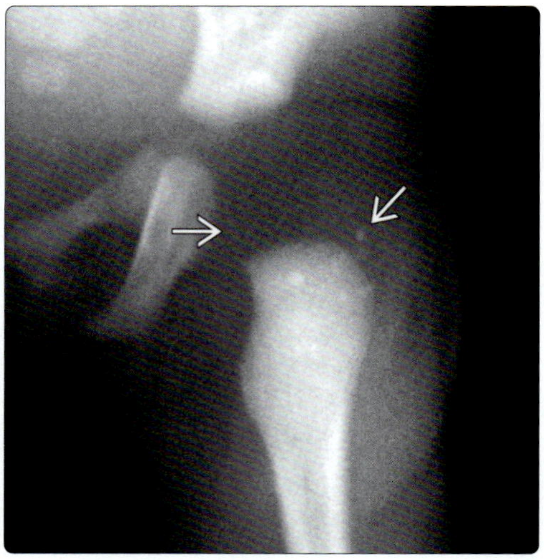

Epiphyseal Dysplasias

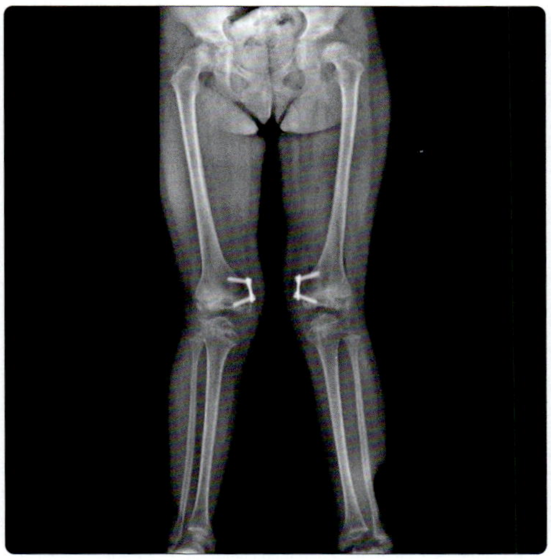

Epiphyseal Dysplasias

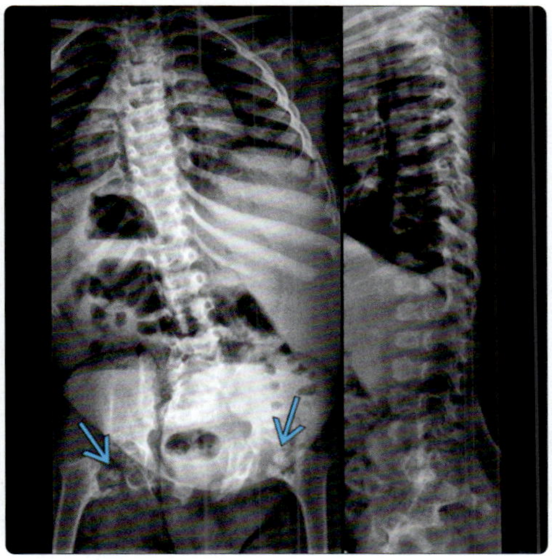

(Left) *Frontal radiograph of the lower extremities in a 10 year old with multiple epiphyseal dysplasia shows hypoplasia & irregularity of all visible epiphyses. Medial distal femoral epiphysiodeses were performed to treat genu valgum.* **(Right)** *Frontal & lateral spine radiographs in a 4-year-old boy with spondyloepiphyseal dysplasia show hypoplastic & markedly irregular femoral heads →. There are bilateral coxa vara deformities. Vertebral abnormalities are also present throughout the spine.*

Chondrodysplasia Punctata

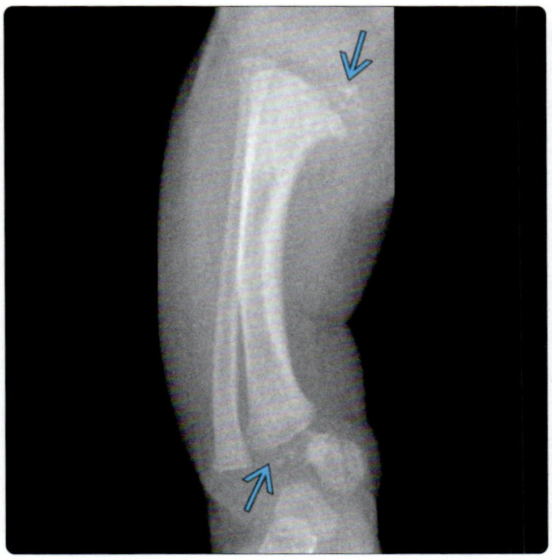

Chondrodysplasia Punctata

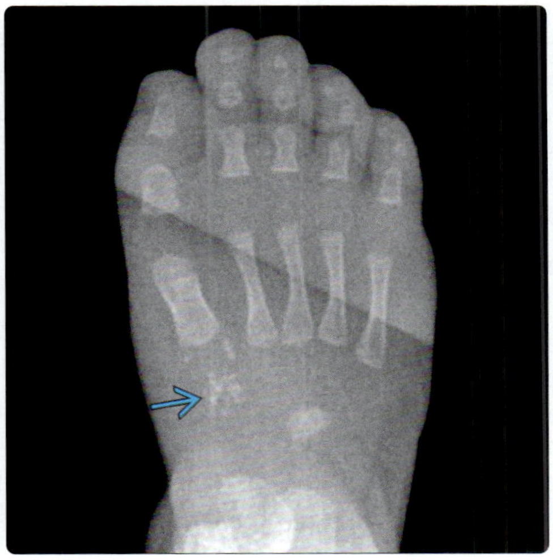

(Left) *Frontal radiograph of the right leg in an infant shows punctate Ca^{2+} of the proximal & distal tibial epiphyses →, which have a stippled appearance.* **(Right)** *Frontal radiograph of the right foot in the same infant shows punctate Ca^{2+} → at the ossification center of the medial cuneiform, which is an epiphyseal equivalent. Similar finding were also present in the contralateral extremity (not shown).*

Trevor-Fairbank Disease (Dysplasia Epiphysealis Hemimelica)

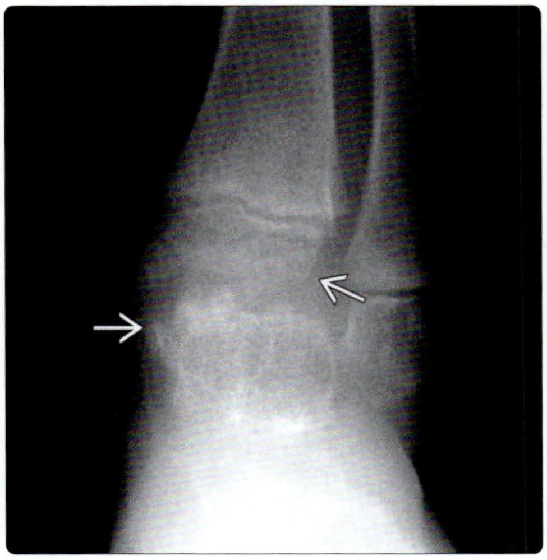

Complications of Warfarin (Coumadin)

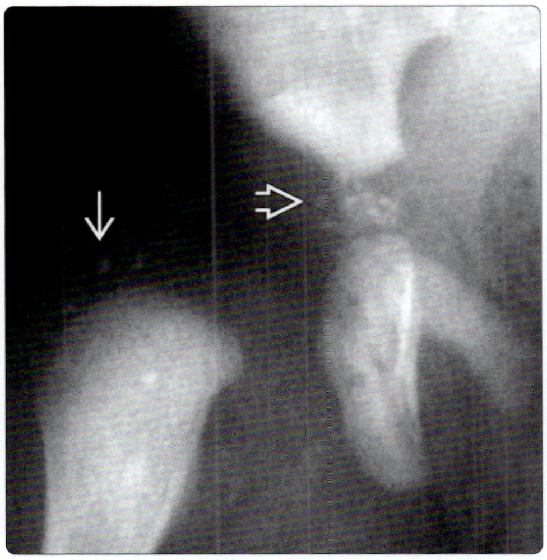

(Left) *AP radiograph shows irregularity of the epiphyses of the tibiotalar joint → due to epiphyseal osteochondroma-like lesions, termed Trevor-Fairbank disease.* **(Right)** *AP radiograph shows stippling of the unossified femoral head & greater trochanter → as well as the triradiate cartilage of the acetabulum →. This infant's mother had been given warfarin during pregnancy; stippled epiphyses are one of the manifestations of warfarin embryopathy.*

DIFFERENTIAL DIAGNOSIS

Common

- Fracture
- Septic Arthritis

Less Common

- Hemarthrosis (Recurrent)
- Juvenile Idiopathic Arthritis
- Avascular Necrosis
- Mimics (Blount Disease & Turner Syndrome)

Rare but Important

- Skeletal Dysplasias

ESSENTIAL INFORMATION

Key Differential Diagnosis Issues

- In skeletally immature patients, prolonged joint hyperemia leads to
  - Overgrowth (ballooning) of epiphysis; early physeal fusion with limb shortening
- Classic DDx for childhood epiphyseal overgrowth due to hyperemia: Juvenile idiopathic arthritis (JIA) & hemophilia
  - In modern era, earlier diagnosis & improved treatments rarely lead to classic late changes of JIA & hemophilia
- However, any cause of hyperemia may lead to overgrowth; other causes include healing between displaced fragments & dysplasias

Helpful Clues for Common Diagnoses

- **Fracture**
  - Epiphyseal or metaphyseal fractures
    - Fracture healing → hyperemia → overgrowth
    - Healing between separated fragments may also lead to chronic enlargement
  - Look for residual findings of healing/posttraumatic deformity
- **Septic Arthritis**
  - Effusion, synovitis → cartilage loss, erosions, ± avascular necrosis (AVN)
    - Often leads to small or destroyed femoral head
  - Atypical infections (e.g., TB or fungal) more often lead to overgrowth vs. typical pyogenic infections
    - More indolent, allowing chronic hyperemia

Helpful Clues for Less Common Diagnoses

- **Hemarthrosis (Recurrent)**
  - Recurrent hemarthrosis → chronic inflammation → overgrowth
  - Dense effusion & hemosiderin deposition
    - Look for blooming of hemosiderin on T2* GRE MR
  - Eventually → cartilage loss, degenerative joint disease
  - Etiologies: Hemophilia or intraarticular vascular anomalies (typically venous malformations)
    - Venous malformation: Phleboliths (radiographs or US), discrete or clustered serpentine venous channels (US or MR)
- **Juvenile Idiopathic Arthritis**
  - Chronic synovitis → chronic inflammation → overgrowth
  - Knee > elbow > ankle
  - Associated findings: Marginal erosions, cartilage loss, ankylosis (late)
- **Avascular Necrosis**
  - AVN of femoral head from various causes may lead to epiphysis enlargement during reparative phase
    - Such as coxa magna in Legg-Calvé-Perthes
- **Mimics (Blount Disease & Turner Syndrome)**
  - Both can cause changes to medial tibial condyle with relative overgrowth of medial femoral condyle
    - Femoral epiphyseal overgrowth is secondary

Helpful Clues for Rare Diagnoses

- **Skeletal Dysplasias**
  - Various dysplasias can cause epiphyseal enlargement (megaepiphyses)
    - Includes epiphyseal, spondyloepiphyseal, spondylo-megaepiphyseal-metaphyseal, metaphyseal chondro- & Kniest dysplasias
  - Irregularity/fragmentation of epiphyses & metaphyses may be present
  - Associated with other diffuse skeletal findings

Fracture

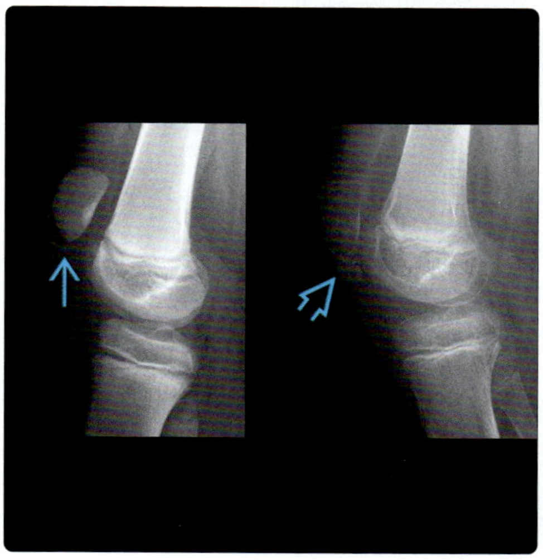

Septic Arthritis

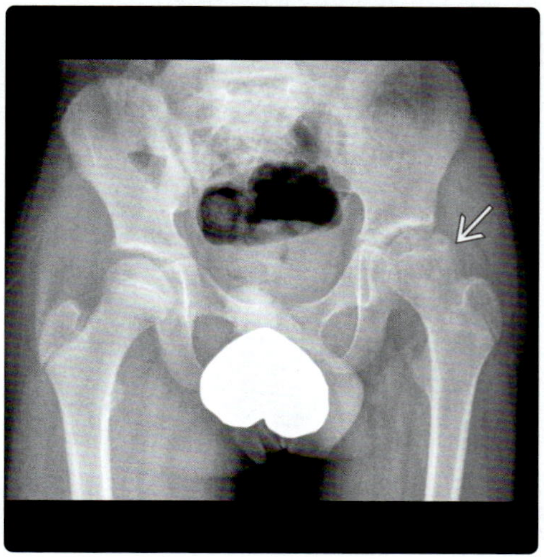

(Left) *Lateral radiograph in a 10 year old (left) initially shows an inferior pole patellar sleeve avulsion fracture ⇒. Follow-up image 3 months later (right) shows progressive ossification of the displaced growth cartilage ⇒ with bridging bone extending to the residual inferior pole, creating an elongated patella.* **(Right)** *AP radiograph shows an enlarged left femoral head & neck ➡ in a 12 year old with a history of a septic joint treated 9 months earlier. The hyperemia from this process resulted in femoral head overgrowth in this child.*

Hemarthrosis (Recurrent)

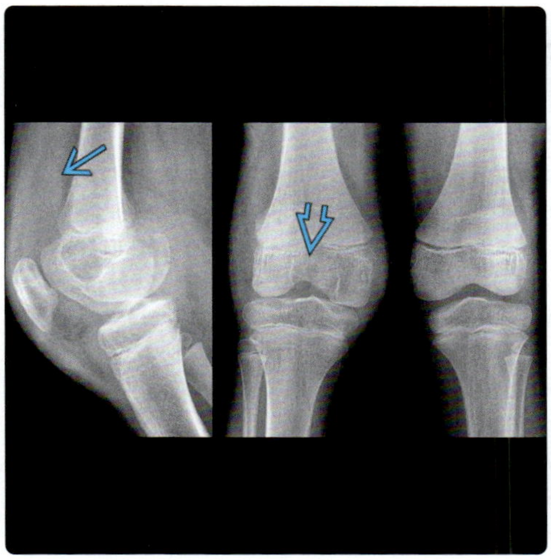

Hemarthrosis (Recurrent)

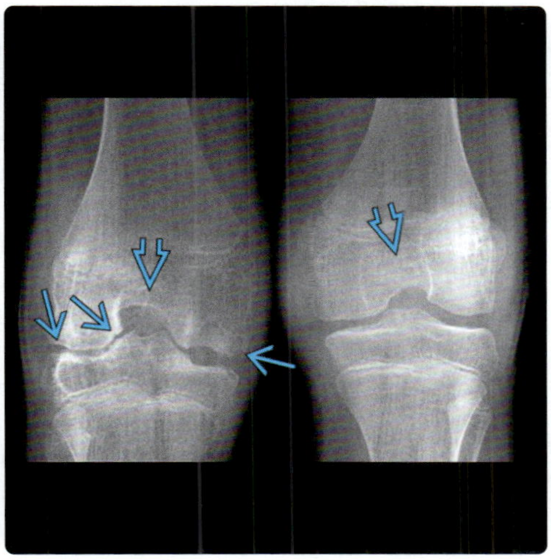

(Left) *Radiographs in an 8-year-old boy with hemophilia show a large right joint effusion* ➡. *The frontal views of both knees show enlargement of the femoral epiphyses, worse on the right than the left, & widening of the right intercondylar notch* ⇨. **(Right)** *Frontal knee radiographs in the same child 2 years later show progression of the femoral epiphyseal overgrowth & widening of the intercondylar notches* ⇨. *Also note the condylar irregularity* ➡ *due to erosions & degenerative changes.*

Juvenile Idiopathic Arthritis

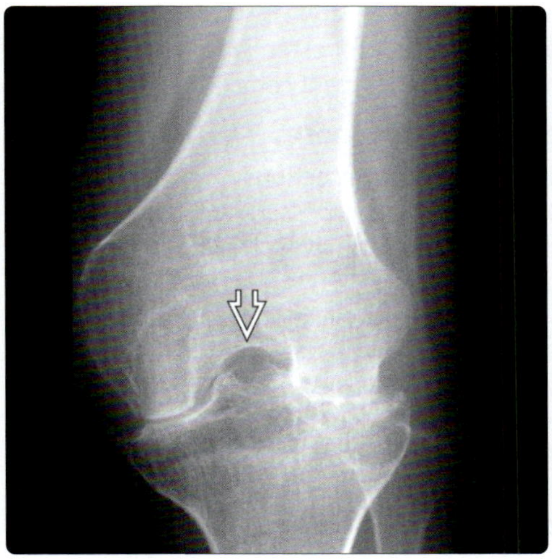

Mimics (Blount Disease & Turner Syndrome)

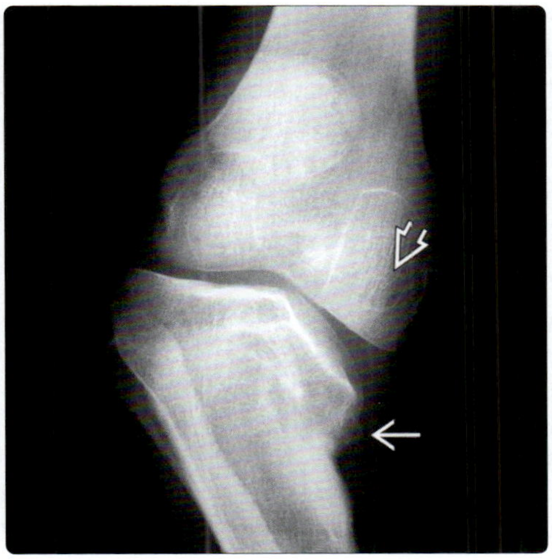

(Left) *AP radiograph shows significant enlargement (overgrowth) of the femoral epiphysis relative to the diaphysis. There are severe erosions & widening of the intercondylar notch* ⇨ *in this patient with juvenile idiopathic arthritis.* **(Right)** *AP radiograph shows collapse of the medial tibial metaphysis* ➡ *in this patient with Blount disease. There is compensatory overgrowth of the medial femoral condyle* ⇨. *Also note the associated varus deformity.*

Skeletal Dysplasias

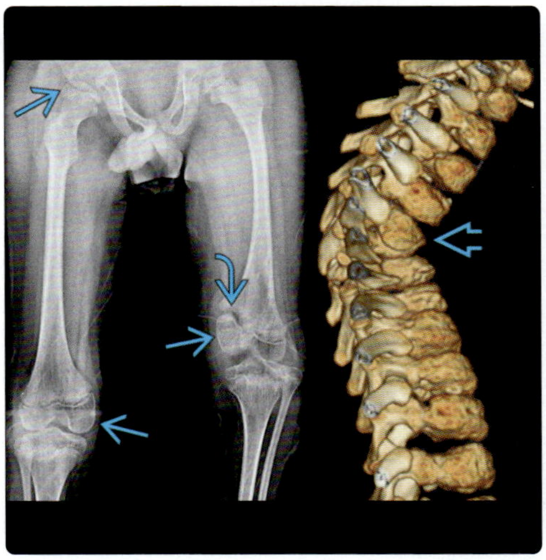

Skeletal Dysplasias

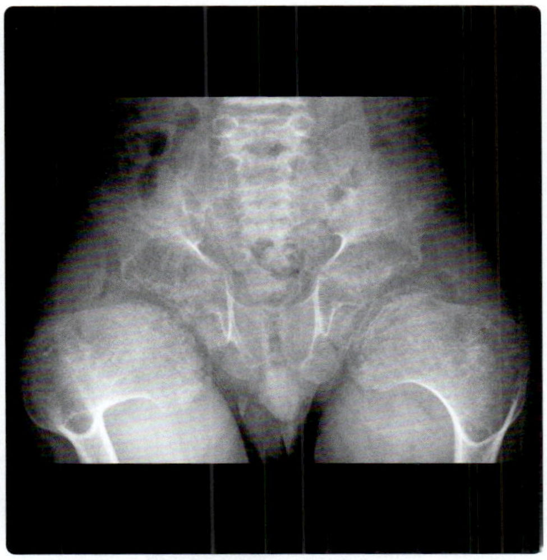

(Left) *AP radiographs in a child with spondylo-megaepiphyseal dysplasia show enlargement of multiple epiphyses* ➡ & *metaphyseal irregularity* ↷. *3D bone CT of the spine shows diffuse irregularity of vertebrae, hypoplasia of vertebral bodies, & severe kyphosis* ⇨. **(Right)** *AP radiograph in a 10-year-old boy with Kniest dysplasia shows severe bilateral coxa magna with overgrowth of the femoral heads & necks. Multiple other skeletal deformities indicate that this is part of a systemic skeletal dysplasia.*

Dense Metaphyseal Bands and Lines

DIFFERENTIAL DIAGNOSIS

Common

- Physiologic Dense Metaphyseal Bands
- Growth Arrest Lines
- Trauma

Less Common

- Heavy Metal (Lead) or Chemical Ingestion
- Rickets
- Malignancy
- Radiation
- Medications

Rare but Important

- Congenital Transplacental Infections
- Scurvy
- Skeletal Dysplasias
- Osteopetrosis

ESSENTIAL INFORMATION

Key Differential Diagnosis Issues

- Most conspicuous at sites of rapid growth (e.g., knee, wrist)
- Orientation of metaphyseal bands: Transverse vs. vertical
- Some entities have alternating lucent & sclerotic bands
- Sites of Involvement
  - Diffuse: Lead ingestion, medication
  - Localized: Trauma, radiation

Helpful Clues for Common Diagnoses

- **Physiologic Dense Metaphyseal Bands**
  - Occur mainly at 2-6 years of age
  - Formed at zone of provisional calcification (ZPC)
  - ~ density & width of adjacent cortex
  - Typically do not involve fibula (vs. lead poisoning)
- **Growth Arrest Lines**
  - Usually attributed to slowed growth during stress
  - Move away from physis in parallel fashion when stress ceases & growth resumes
- **Trauma**
  - Subacute/healing fractures develop marginal sclerosis
  - Stress injury of bone causes transverse band of sclerosis
    - Often does not traverse entire bone width
  - Repetitive growth plate microtrauma leads to physeal elongation with metaphyseal irregularity ± sclerosis

Helpful Clues for Less Common Diagnoses

- **Heavy Metal (Lead) or Chemical Ingestion**
  - Lead poisoning most common (usually < 2 years of age)
  - Typically involves all metaphyses (including fibula)
  - Bands may be more dense & thick than cortex
  - Radiograph abdomen for lead paint chip ingestion
- **Rickets**
  - Metaphyseal irregularity, cupping, fraying
  - May develop sclerotic bands with healing
- **Malignancy**
  - Metastases (e.g., neuroblastoma): Lucent or sclerotic
  - Leukemia: Lucent bands may become dense with healing
  - ± permeative lesions, aggressive periosteal reaction
- **Radiation**
  - Regional bands & osteoporosis
- **Medications**
  - Bisphosphonate therapy for osteogenesis imperfecta
  - Fluoride & vitamin D treatment complications

Helpful Clues for Rare Diagnoses

- **Congenital Transplacental Infections**
  - **TORCHS**: **T**oxoplasmosis, **r**ubella, **C**MV, **H**SV, **s**yphilis
  - Alternating lucent/sclerotic vertical bands ("celery stalk")
- **Scurvy**
  - Alternating dense band (Frankel line) & lucent band (Trümmerfeld zone)
- **Skeletal Dysplasias**
  - Some have sclerotic or alternating lucent/sclerotic bands (e.g., metaphyseal dysplasias)
  - Typically have more diffuse skeletal abnormalities
- **Osteopetrosis**
  - Group of disorders with increased bone density
    - Actually fragile with increased risk for fractures
  - Diffuse or metaphyseal sclerosis, "bone-in-bone"

Physiologic Dense Metaphyseal Bands

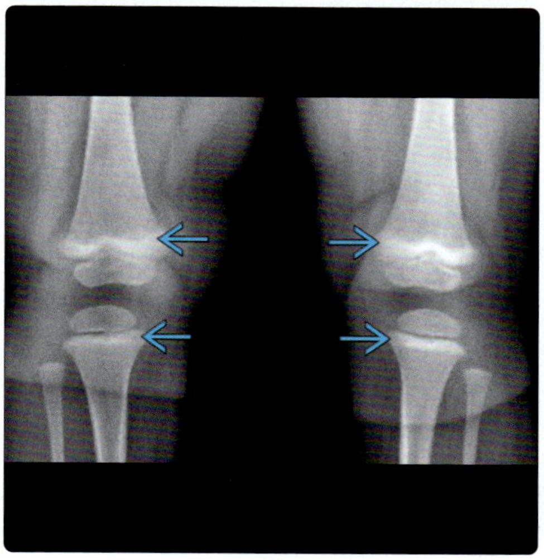

Trauma

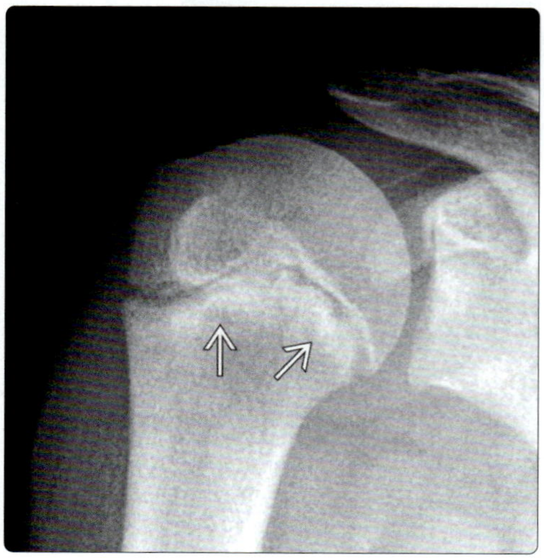

(Left) *Frontal radiographs in an asymptomatic 2-year-old girl to evaluate lower extremity alignment show dense transverse metaphyseal bands* ⇨ *in the femurs & tibiae but not the fibulae, typical of physiologic dense bands.* **(Right)** *External rotation radiograph shows irregularity & sclerosis of the metaphysis* ➡ *in this baseball pitcher with a chronic repetitive injury (a.k.a., Little Leaguer's shoulder).*

Heavy Metal (Lead) or Chemical Ingestion

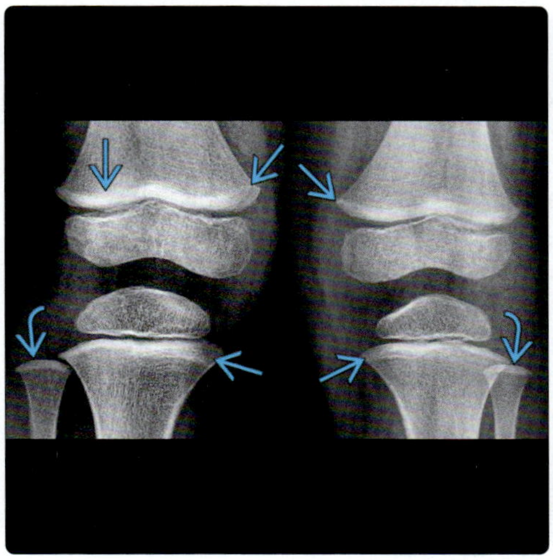

Rickets

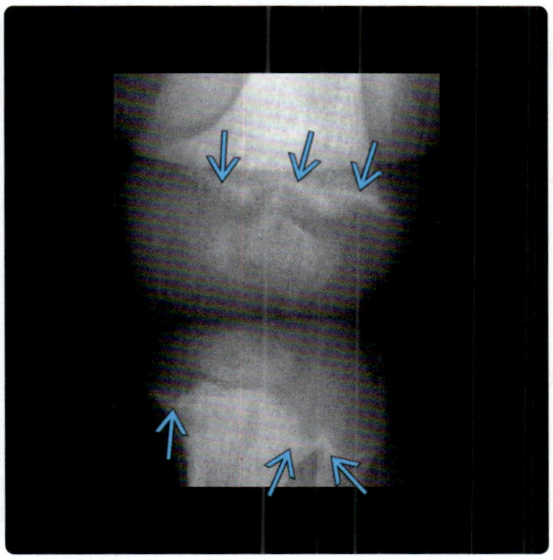

(Left) *Frontal radiographs in a 3-year-old girl with dense metaphyseal bands from lead paint chip ingestion show that the dense bands are present in not only the femurs & tibias but also the fibulae.* **(Right)** *Frontal radiograph of the knee in a child with rickets shortly after the initiation of treatment shows the classic metaphyseal cupping/fraying of rickets as well as foci of transverse linear sclerosis from early recovery of the zones of provisional calcification (ZPC).*

Medications

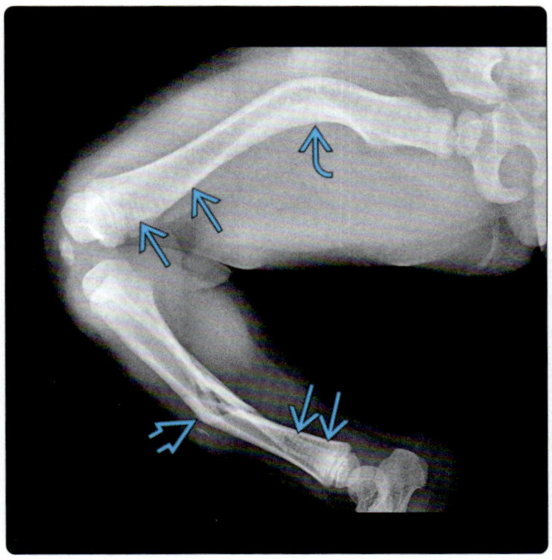

Scurvy

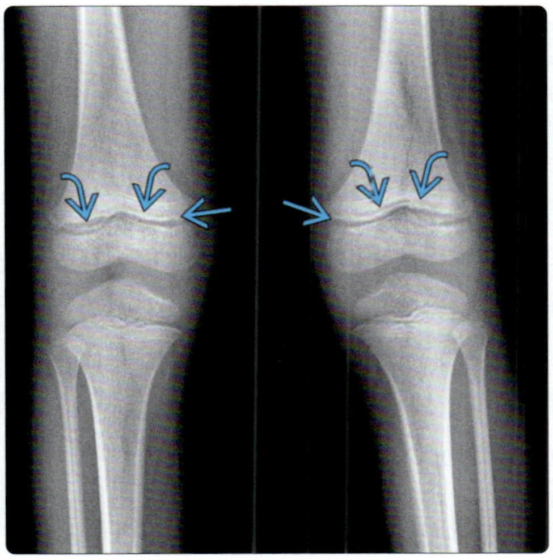

(Left) *Lateral radiograph of right lower extremity in child with osteogenesis imperfecta shows bowing of femur from malunion of a prior fracture & acute fractures of tibia & fibula. Multiple thin dense transverse bands parallel to the distal femoral & tibial metaphyses are from bisphosphonate treatments.* **(Right)** *Radiographs of a boy with bilateral lower extremity pain show alternating dense transverse metaphyseal bands (Frankel lines) & adjacent metaphyseal lucent bands (Trümmerfeld zones) from scurvy.*

Scurvy

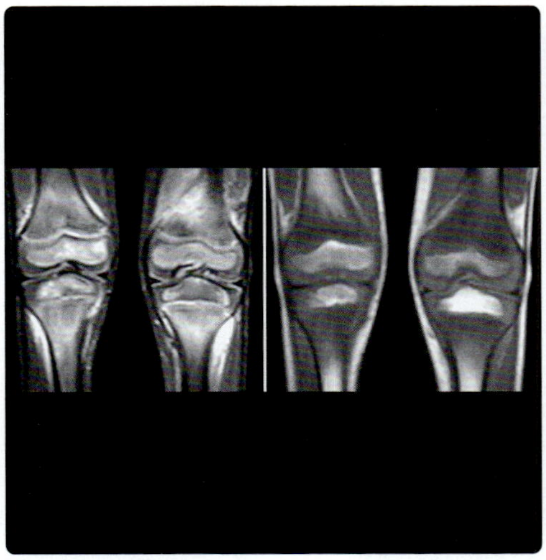

Osteopetrosis

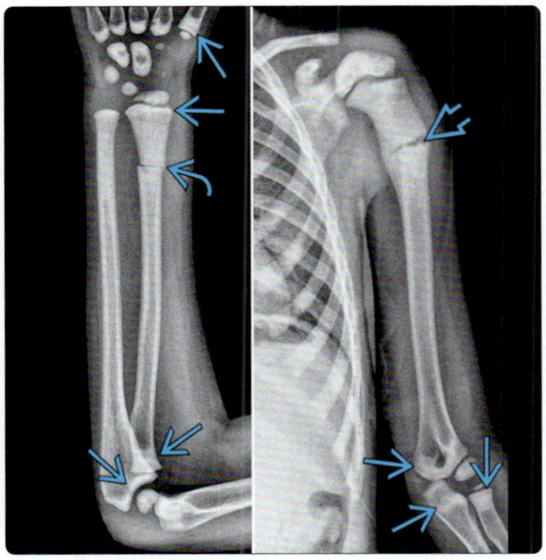

(Left) *Coronal STIR (left) & T1 (right) MR images of both knees in the same boy show nonspecific edema-like signal of the distal femurs & proximal tibiae. This child was found to have scurvy & responded to oral vitamin C treatment.* **(Right)** *Frontal radiographs in a 6-year-old boy after minor trauma show acute distal radial & healing proximal humeral fractures. The bones are diffusely dense with prominent metaphyseal sclerosis due to autosomal dominant osteopetrosis.*

DIFFERENTIAL DIAGNOSIS

Common

- Osteoporosis/Systemic Stress
- Trauma

Less Common

- Hyperemia of Inflammation
- Rickets
- Leukemia/Metastases
- Radiation

Rare but Important

- Congenital Transplacental Infection
- Scurvy
- Hypophosphatasia
- Skeletal Dysplasias
- Infantile Myofibromatosis

ESSENTIAL INFORMATION

Key Differential Diagnosis Issues

- Orientation of band relative to physis
  - Transverse: Parallel (e.g., leukemia, systemic stress)
  - Vertical: Perpendicular (e.g., congenital infections)
- Presence of zone of provisional calcification (ZPC)
  - Disrupted (e.g., rickets, repetitive trauma)
  - Intact (e.g., leukemia, osteoporosis/systemic stress)
- Location
  - Diffuse (e.g., systemic stress, rickets, leukemia)
  - Regional (e.g., trauma, radiation)
- Some entities have alternating lucent & sclerotic bands
- Transverse metaphyseal lucent bands in child (i.e., not neonate) without other cause: **Must consider leukemia**

Helpful Clues for Common Diagnoses

- **Osteoporosis/Systemic Stress**
  - Diffuse (e.g., systemic stress) or localized (e.g., disuse)
    - Changes of birth/neonatal stress: < 6 weeks of life
- **Trauma**
  - Lucency of acute fracture or delayed disuse/hyperemia

Helpful Clues for Less Common Diagnoses

- **Hyperemia of Inflammation**
  - Localized ↑ blood flow (e.g., juvenile idiopathic arthritis)
- **Rickets**
  - Metaphyseal osteolysis, cupping, fraying
  - Loss of normal ZPC with physeal widening (elongation)
  - Healing may show transverse lucent & sclerotic bands
- **Leukemia/Metastases**
  - Leukemic lines: Transverse lucent bands
    - Attributed to multiple causes (e.g., systemic stress, fractures, leukemic infiltrates, & others)
  - Metastases (most commonly neuroblastoma) can appear similar to leukemia ± focal aggressive lesions
  - Either may have extensive marrow replacement on MR
- **Radiation**
  - Regional osteoporosis; ± growth arrest, osteochondromas

Helpful Clues for Rare Diagnoses

- **Congenital Transplacental Infection**
  - **TORCHS: T**oxoplasmosis, **r**ubella, **C**MV, **H**SV, **s**yphilis
    - Viral: Lucent/sclerotic vertical striations ("celery stalk")
    - Syphilis: Lucent transverse metaphyseal bands, metaphyseal irregularity/destruction
- **Scurvy**
  - Vitamin C deficiency
  - Alternating dense transverse metaphyseal band (Frankel line) & adjacent lucent band (Trümmerfeld zone)
- **Hypophosphatasia**
  - Metaphyseal osteolysis, cupping, fraying (like rickets)
    - Portions of growth plate often spared
  - Lucent vertical extensions into metaphysis from physis
  - Bowdler spurs (classically in fibulae)
- **Skeletal Dysplasias**
  - ± lucencies, alternating bands/striations (e.g., spondyloepimetaphyseal dysplasias, enchondromatosis)
- **Infantile Myofibromatosis**
  - Relatively symmetric bubbly lucent lesions of metadiaphyses in multiple long bones
  - ± sclerotic bone lesions, visceral lesions

Osteoporosis/Systemic Stress

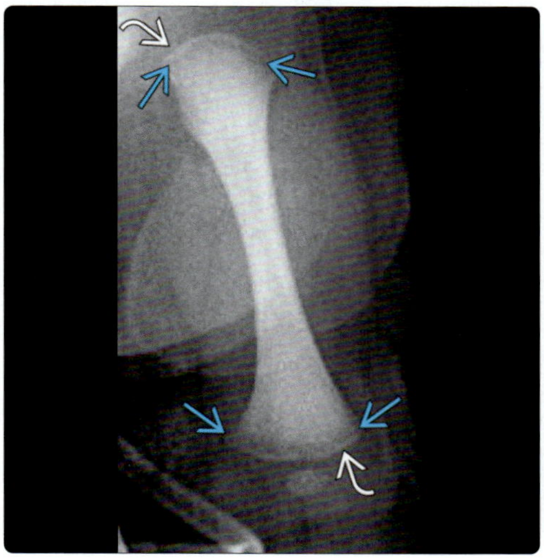

Trauma

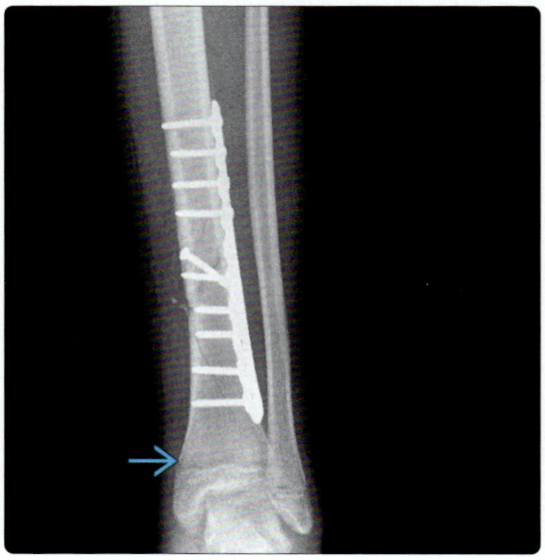

(Left) *Frontal radiograph of the left femur of a 4 week old with tetralogy of Fallot & a wound infection shows transverse lucent bands* ➡ *in the proximal & distal femoral metaphyses. Note that the thin sclerotic zones of provisional calcifications (ZPC) are intact* ➡. **(Right)** *Frontal radiograph shows a transverse lucent metaphyseal band* ➡ *in the distal tibia due to disuse osteoporosis following immobilization after open reduction & internal fixation (ORIF) of a diaphyseal fracture.*

Rickets

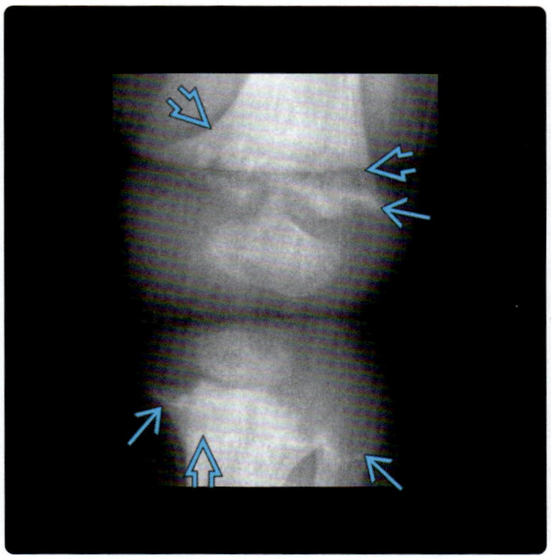

Leukemia/Metastases

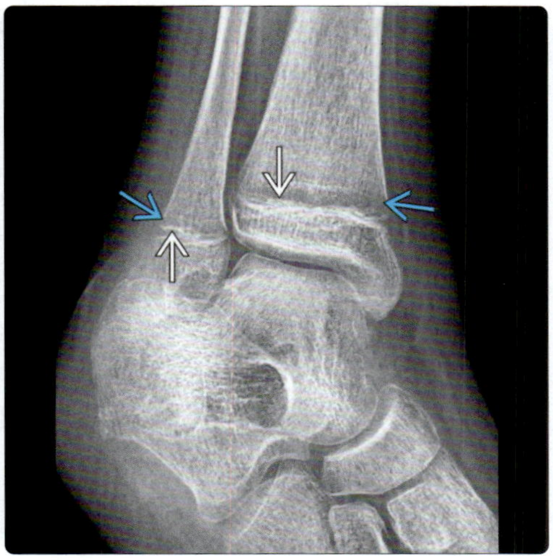

(Left) *AP knee radiograph in a child with rickets shortly after the initiation of treatment shows metaphyseal cupping & fraying. The foci of transverse sclerosis are from early recovery of the initially lost ZPCs with adjacent transverse lucencies.* **(Right)** *Oblique radiograph of the right ankle in a 12-year-old girl with leukemia shows transverse metaphyseal lucent bands in the distal right tibia & fibula. The adjacent ZPCs are intact. Leukemic lines have been attributed to the stress of the disease &/ or leukemic infiltrates.*

Congenital Transplacental Infection

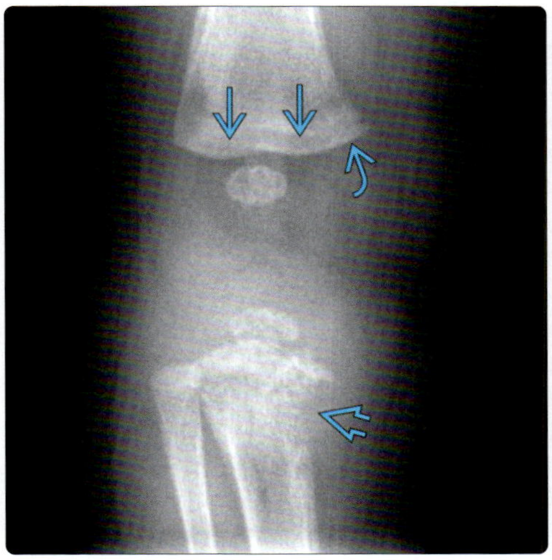

Scurvy

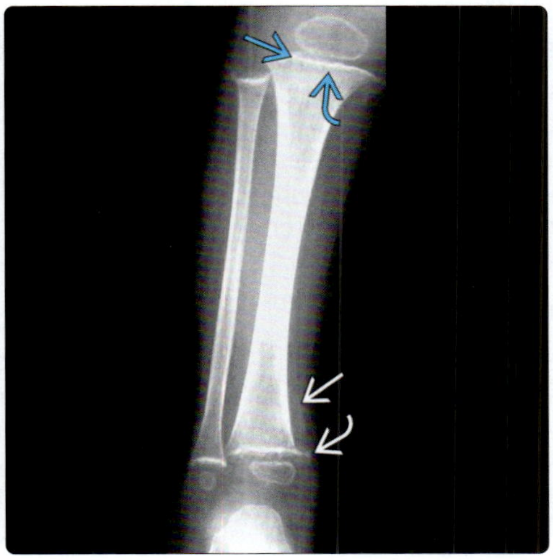

(Left) *AP radiograph shows findings of congenital syphilis with metaphyseal osteitis, which appears as lucent bands (note the intact ZPC). The tibia shows a Wimberger corner sign with localized medial proximal tibial destruction.* **(Right)** *AP radiograph in a child with scurvy shows a metaphyseal fracture with wide periosteal reaction related to subperiosteal hemorrhage. Also note the transverse sclerotic band (Frankel line) & lucent band (Trümmerfeld zone).*

Hypophosphatasia

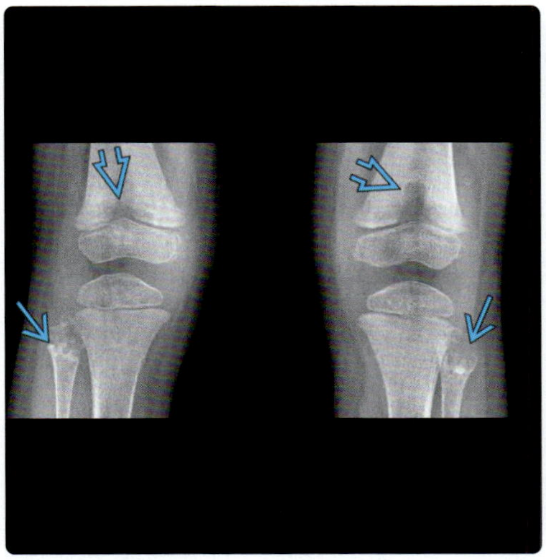

Skeletal Dysplasias

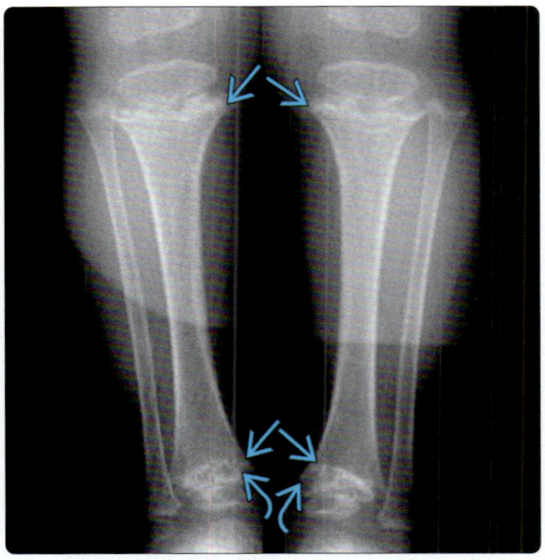

(Left) *Frontal radiograph of both knees in a 3-year old-girl shows metaphyseal cupping & irregularity in the bilateral proximal fibulae. Additionally, there are focal vertical lucencies extending into the metaphyses from the physes in the distal femurs, also due to hypophosphatasia.* **(Right)** *Frontal radiograph in a 2 year old with spondyloepimetaphyseal dysplasia shows irregular metaphyses of the proximal & distal tibiae & fibulae with transverse sclerotic & lucent bands.*

Metaphyseal Fraying/Irregularity

DIFFERENTIAL DIAGNOSIS

Common

- Chronic Physeal Stress Injuries
- Physeal Fractures
- Osteomyelitis

Less Common

- Metaphyseal Corner Fracture
- Rickets
- Chronic Recurrent Multifocal Osteomyelitis
- Leukemia

Rare but Important

- Skeletal Dysplasias
- Neuropathic Disease
- Hypophosphatasia
- Copper Deficiency, Infantile
- Scurvy
- Congenital syphilis

ESSENTIAL INFORMATION

Key Differential Diagnosis Issues

- Age, history, & extent (i.e., systemic vs. isolated/multisite involvement) limit differential
  - Systemic: Metabolic disorders, skeletal dysplasias
  - Isolated/multisite: Chronic physeal stress, fractures (accidental or nonaccidental), osteomyelitis, chronic recurrent multifocal osteomyelitis

Helpful Clues for Common Diagnoses

- **Chronic Physeal Stress Injuries**
  - Sport/situation & site specific
    - Throwers: Proximal humerus, medial epicondyle
    - Gymnasts: Distal radius; runners: distal femur
- **Physeal Fractures**
  - Look for displacement of epiphysis
- **Osteomyelitis**
  - Focal metaphyseal osteoporosis & destruction
  - Soft tissue edema seen much earlier than bone changes

Helpful Clues for Less Common Diagnoses

- **Metaphyseal Corner Fracture**
  - Infantile injuries of child abuse, often asymmetric
- **Rickets**
  - Diffuse metaphyseal cupping & fraying with loss of dense periphyseal zones of provisional calcification (ZPC), most pronounced at sites of rapid growth
  - ± osteoporosis, delayed skeletal maturation, bowing
- **Chronic Recurrent Multifocal Osteomyelitis**
  - Multifocal nonpyogenic inflammatory bone lesions; most common at long bone metaphyses
- **Leukemia**
  - Typically lucent metaphyseal bands with intact ZPC

Helpful Clues for Rare Diagnoses

- **Skeletal Dysplasias**
  - Many cause metaphyseal irregularity (e.g., metaphyseal chondrodysplasias, spondyloepimetaphyseal dysplasias)
  - Associated with diffuse skeletal findings
- **Neuropathic Disease**
  - Exaggerated changes, including extensive fragmentation, layered periosteal reaction, ± joint debris
- **Hypophosphatasia**
  - Distinct lucent extensions into metaphysis from physis
  - ± osteoporosis, craniosynostosis, bowing, fractures, diaphyseal Bowdler spurs
- **Copper Deficiency, Infantile**
  - Metaphyseal cupping, ↑ density of ZPC, spurs of medial distal femurs; hypotonia, anemia, pallor
- **Scurvy**
  - Osteoporosis, thin cortices, "field of rubble" metaphyseal heterogeneity, persistent/dense ZPC
  - Bleeding tendency
- **Congenital Syphilis**
  - Range of metaphyseal findings: Lucent bands, irregularity (serrated, sawtooth), destructive lesions
  - Wimberger corner sign: Focal proximal medial tibial metaphyseal concavity/irregularity distal to physis
  - ± hepatosplenomegaly, adenopathy, rash

(Left) *Frontal radiographs of both shoulders in a left hand dominant Little League pitcher with left shoulder pain show mild "widening" (lengthening) of the proximal left humeral physis with associated mild metaphyseal irregularity* ➜. **(Right)** *Frontal radiograph (left) & gradient-echo MR (right) images of the right knee in a 14-year-old soccer player with chronic pain show "widening" (lengthening) of the lateral aspect of the distal femoral growth plate* ➜ *with associated mild metaphyseal irregularity* ➜. *These findings resolved with rest.*

Chronic Physeal Stress Injuries

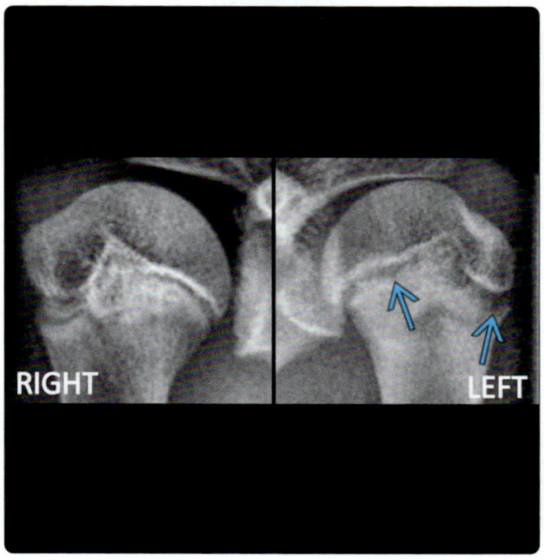

Chronic Physeal Stress Injuries

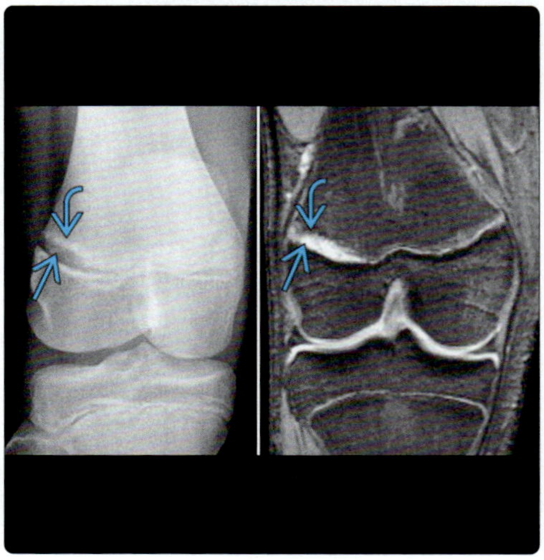

Physeal Fractures

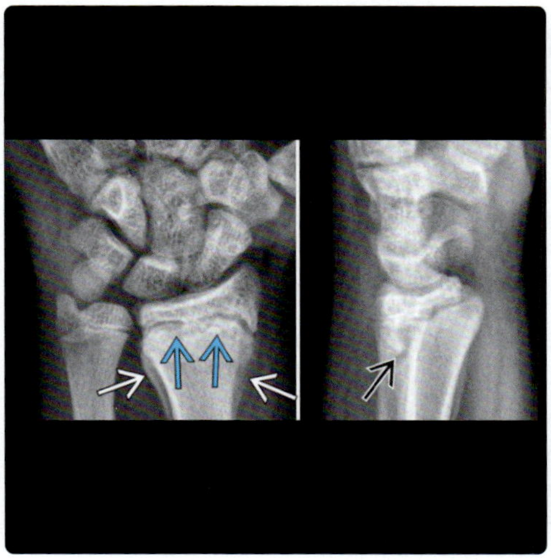

Osteomyelitis

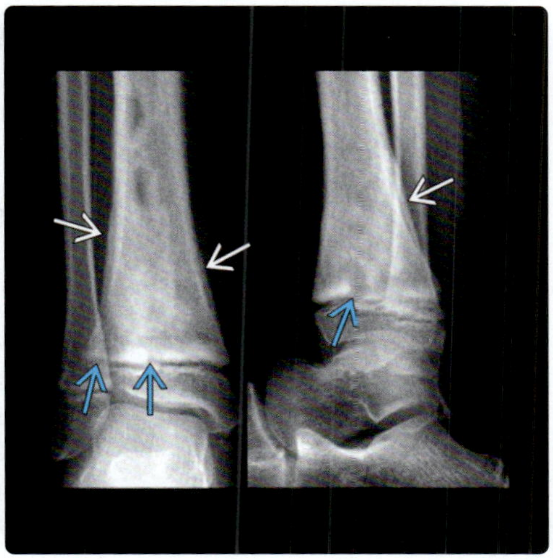

(Left) *Frontal & lateral wrist radiographs in a 13-year-old boy show distal radial metaphyseal irregularity* ⇨ *& periosteal reaction* ➡*. The healing Salter-Harris II fracture* ⇨ *extends through the distal radial metaphysis & physis. There is mild dorsal displacement of the distal fracture fragment.* **(Right)** *Frontal & lateral radiographs of the ankle in a 10 year old with subacute to chronic osteomyelitis show tibial metaphyseal irregularities* ⇨ *with proximal extension of medullary sclerosis & lucency + periosteal reaction* ➡*.*

Metaphyseal Corner Fracture

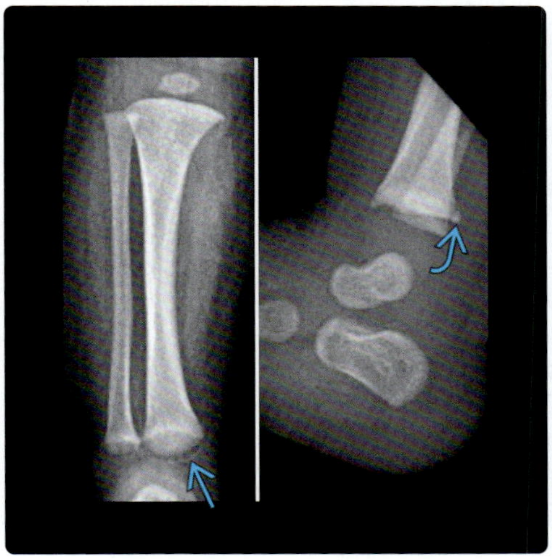

Rickets

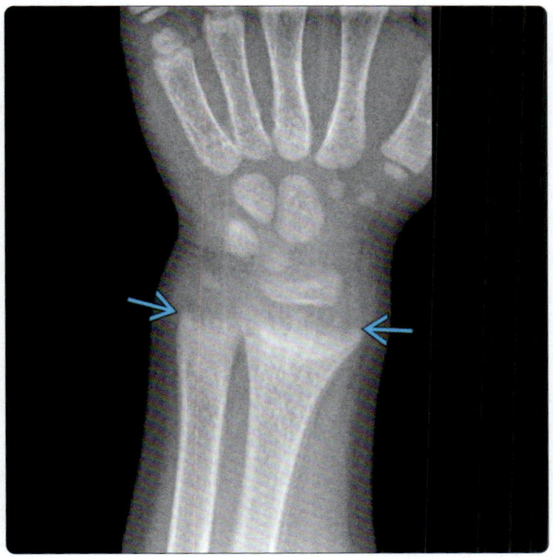

(Left) *Frontal radiograph of the right leg (left) from a skeletal survey in a 2-month-old girl with bruising shows a bucket-handle fracture of the distal tibial metaphysis* ⇨*. When seen on the lateral view (right), this has a classic metaphyseal corner fracture appearance* ⇨*.* **(Right)** *Frontal radiograph of the wrist in a 2 year old with rickets shows cupping & fraying* ⇨ *of the distal radial & ulnar metaphyses with loss of the normal dense periphyseal zones of provisional calcification.*

Chronic Recurrent Multifocal Osteomyelitis

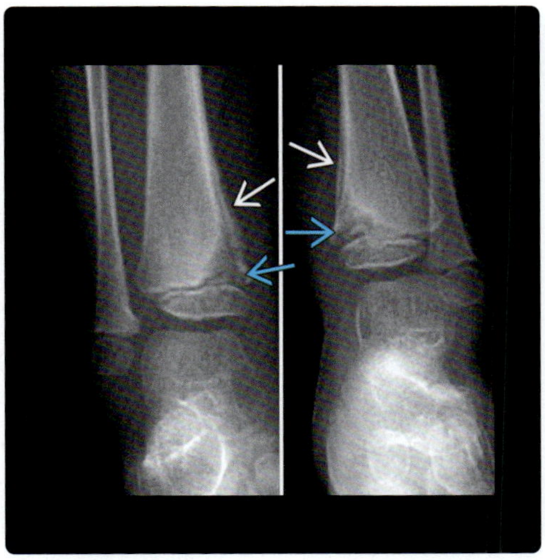

Skeletal Dysplasias

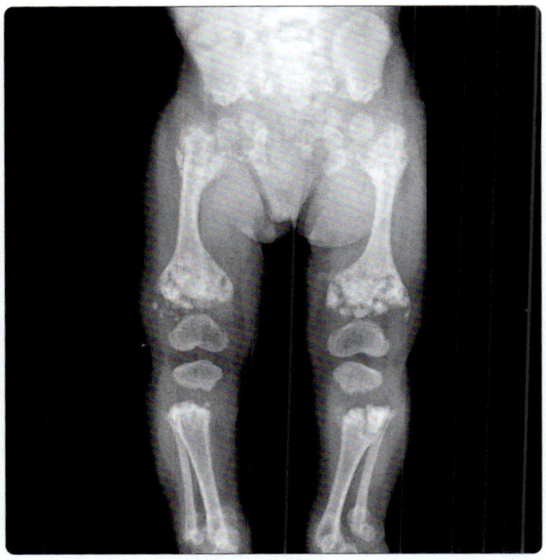

(Left) *Frontal radiographs in a 4-year-old girl with bilateral ankle pain show lucent lesions & irregularities in both distal tibias* ⇨ *with associated periosteal reaction* ➡*. This child also had a lesion in the right clavicle (not shown), which is another commonly affected area.* **(Right)** *Radiographs in a 4-year-old boy with Jansen-type metaphyseal chondrodysplasia show marked irregularity & expansion of the metaphyses. By contrast, the epiphyses are enlarged but relatively normal in shape, which is typical of this disorder.*

DIFFERENTIAL DIAGNOSIS

Common

- Normal Variant
- Rickets
- Repetitive Stress
- Healing Fracture (Mimic)

Less Common

- Renal Osteodystrophy
- Chronic Recurrent Multifocal Osteomyelitis
- Skeletal Dysplasias

Rare but Important

- Scurvy
- Hypophosphatasia
- Therapy-Induced Infarction

ESSENTIAL INFORMATION

Key Differential Diagnosis Issues

- Number of physes involved: All, one, random, or bilateral/symmetric at specific locations
- Extent of involvement at individual physis: Uniform/diffuse, heterogeneous, or focal
- Zone of provisional Ca^{2+} (ZPC): Normal, thin, dense line at junction of ossified metaphysis & lucent growth cartilage
    - Classic causes of "lucent metaphyseal bands" (such as leukemia) generally leave ZPC intact
    - True interruption of endochondral ossification results in abnormal ZPC (e.g., absent, interrupted, or widened)
- Metabolic disorders (e.g., rickets, renal osteodystrophy) can lead to overgrowth of disorganized cartilage
    - Diffuse but most noticeable at sites of rapid growth (e.g., distal radius/ulna, distal femur, proximal tibia)

Helpful Clues for Common Diagnoses

- **Normal Variant**
    - Minimal cupping & irregularity; symmetric
    - Distal ulna is most common
- **Rickets**
    - Cupping, fraying, splaying, & loss of normal ZPC with widening of physis; all growth plates are affected
- **Repetitive Stress**
    - Focal or uniform metaphyseal changes with loss of ZPC & physeal widening; often bilateral at same location (depending on type of athletic activity)
        - Gymnast wrist, Little League shoulder, etc.
    - Relative sparing of adjacent bones bearing less weight
- **Healing Metaphyseal Fracture (Mimic)**
    - Corner fractures ("classic metaphyseal lesion") of child abuse or Salter-Harris II/IV fractures

Helpful Clues for Less Common Diagnoses

- **Renal Osteodystrophy**
    - Combination of rickets & hyperparathyroidism
- **Chronic Recurrent Multifocal Osteomyelitis (CRMO)**
    - Periphyseal lesions, often symmetric: Lucent, bubbly, or destructive; epiphyseal & metaphyseal marrow edema with relative physeal sparing
        - No soft tissue abscess
    - Look for pelvis, spine, & clavicle involvement
- **Skeletal Dysplasias**
    - Many cause metaphyseal cupping (e.g., achondroplasia, metaphyseal chondrodysplasia)
    - Variable in appearance by dysplasia, but typically diffuse ± additional skeletal findings

Helpful Clues for Rare Diagnoses

- **Scurvy**
    - Thickened ZPC with subjacent lucencies ± metaphyseal fractures, spurring, cupping
    - ± subperiosteal hemorrhage
- **Hypophosphatasia**
    - Variable severity & age of presentation
    - Distinct lucent extensions into metaphysis from physis; may be relatively random across physis
    - Coarse trabecula, Bowdler spurs in fibulae > ulnae
- **Therapy-Induced Infarction**
    - Periphyseal marrow infarct may focally disrupt endochondral ossification

Normal Variant

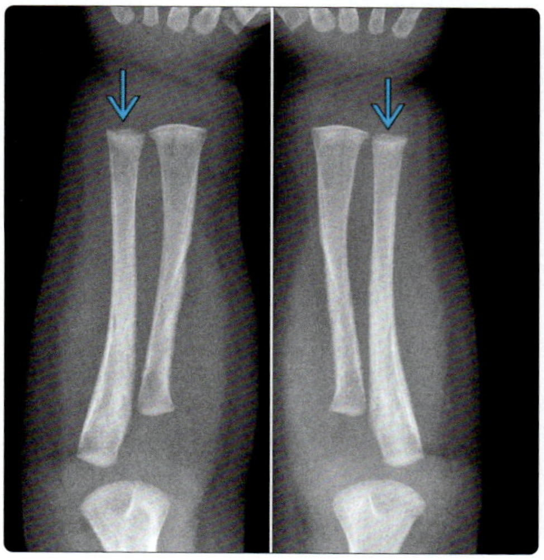

Rickets

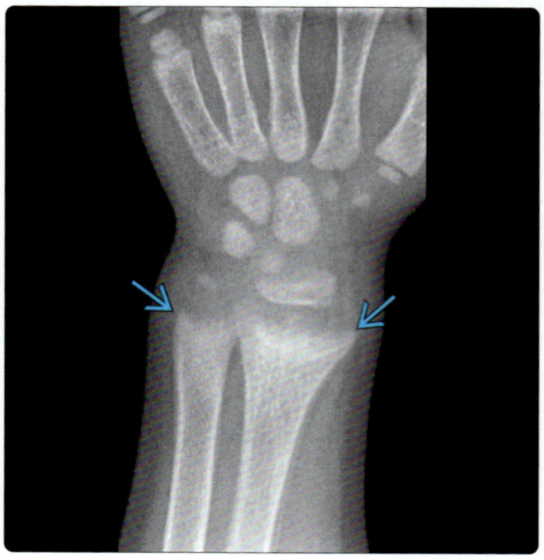

(Left) *AP radiographs of a 2 month old with traumatic brain injury show symmetric cupping of the ulnar metaphyses bilaterally* → *, a normal variant commonly seen in infants.* **(Right)** *PA radiograph of the wrist in a 2 year old with rickets shows classic "cupping, fraying, & splaying"* → *of the distal radial & ulnar metaphyses with loss of the normal zones of provisional* Ca^{2+} *(ZPC). These findings were symmetric at the wrists & knees.*

Metaphyseal Cupping

Repetitive Stress

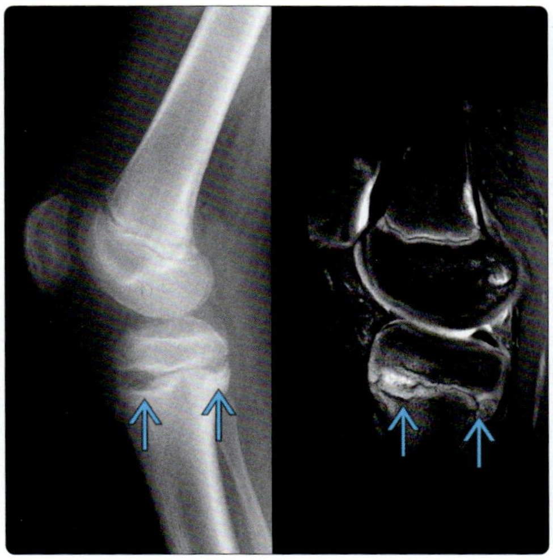

Healing Fracture (Mimic)

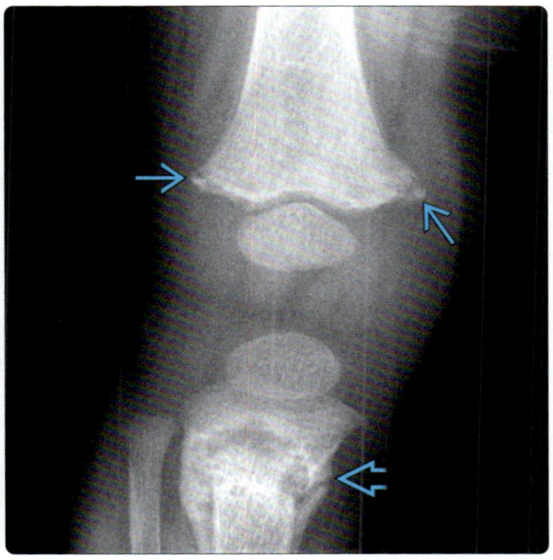

(Left) *Lateral radiograph (left) & sagittal T2 FS MR (right) show foci of physeal widening* → *due to repetitive stress injuries. The appearance was seen only at the bilateral proximal tibiae.* **(Right)** *AP knee radiograph in a 7 month old with bruising shows splaying, fraying, & accentuated cupping of the femoral metaphysis (which has an intact ZPC) due to a healing metaphyseal corner/bucket handle fracture* → *of child abuse. An additional healing tibial diaphyseal fracture* ⇨ *is noted. The other visible metaphyses appear normal.*

Skeletal Dysplasias

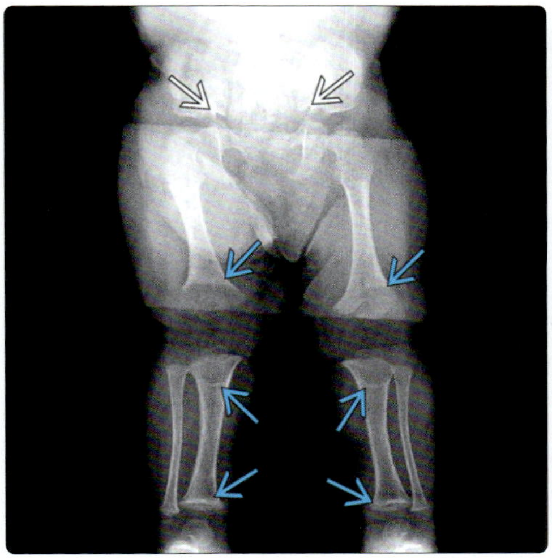

Skeletal Dysplasias

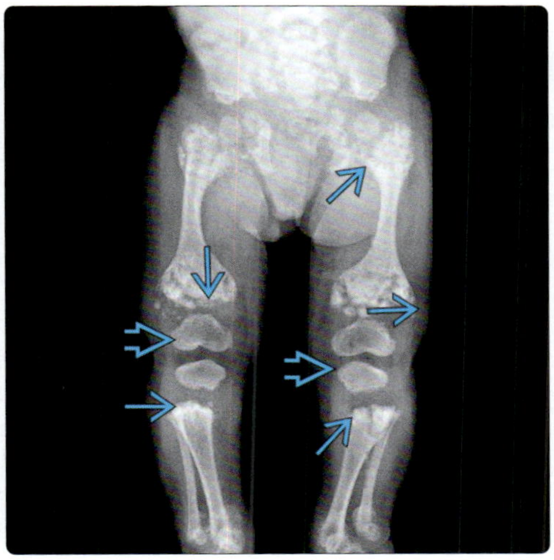

(Left) *Frontal radiograph of the lower extremities in a 2 year old shows cupping of the metaphyses* →*. There is also long bone shortening, small iliac wings with rounded iliac crests, horizontal acetabula, & narrowed sacrosciatic notches* ➡*, typical of achondroplasia.* **(Right)** *Frontal radiograph in a 4 year old with Jansen type metaphyseal chondrodysplasia shows marked irregularity & cupping of the metaphyses diffusely* → *with widened physes & elongated epiphyses* ⇨*.*

Scurvy

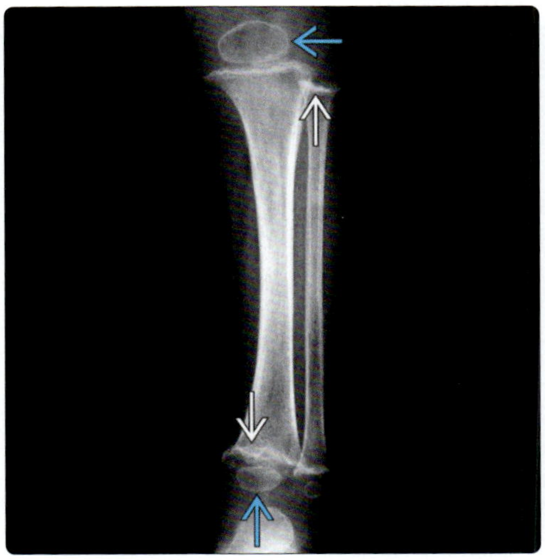

Hypophosphatasia

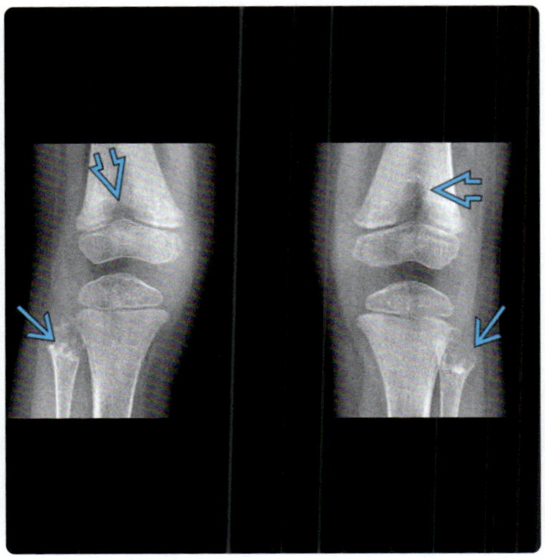

(Left) *Frontal radiograph shows signs of scurvy, including osteoporosis & dense lines at the metaphyses & epiphyses* →*. Mild metaphyseal cupping* ➡ *is also present in multiple locations.* **(Right)** *Frontal radiograph in a 3 year old shows metaphyseal cupping & irregularity in the proximal fibulae* →*. Additional focal lucencies were seen extending into the metaphyses from the physes in the distal femurs* ⇨*. The pattern of physeal/metaphyseal involvement can be relatively random in hypophosphatasia.*

DIFFERENTIAL DIAGNOSIS

Common

- Physeal Fracture (Salter-Harris)
- Chronic Repetitive Physeal Injury
- Apophyseal Avulsion/Apophysitis

Less Common

- Osteomyelitis (Pyogenic)
- Chronic Recurrent Multifocal Osteomyelitis
- Rickets
- Leukemia (Mimic)
- Renal Osteodystrophy
- Osteochondroses

Rare but Important

- Hypophosphatasia
- Mucopolysaccharidoses
- Chronic Physeal Fractures of Myelodysplasia
- Scurvy
- Skeletal Dysplasias
- Copper Deficiency

ESSENTIAL INFORMATION

Key Differential Diagnosis Issues

- Key clinical information: Acuity of symptom onset
  - Chronic repetitive injuries may appear similar to acute
- Key imaging features
  - Extension of lucency from physis into metaphysis, either focal or uniform across metaphysis
    - Loss of radiodense zone of provisional calcification (ZPC) at junction of lucent cartilaginous growth plate & new metaphyseal bone
    - Metaphyseal-physeal interface, usually well-defined & mildly undulating, becomes irregular/poorly defined
    - Lucencies may be due to unossified cartilage vs. loss of formed bone at site of pathology
    - Differs from lucent metaphyseal bands of systemic stress, leukemia, etc. where ZPC often remains intact
  - Traditionally termed physeal widening, though this process occurs with (not against) long axis of bone (i.e., lengthening may be better term)
    - Epiphysiolysis is incorrect
  - **Localized**: Involvement of single or several adjacent physes
    - Physeal fractures & chronic repetitive injuries, osteomyelitis, slipped capital femoral epiphysis (SCFE), Legg-Calvé-Perthes disease (LCP)
  - **Generalized**: Involvement of all (or most) physes, implying systemic process; often have other associated findings
    - Metabolic & nutritional causes
    - Endocrine disorders
    - Skeletal dysplasias & syndromes

Helpful Clues for Common Diagnoses

- **Physeal Fracture (Salter-Harris)**
  - Fracture plane courses through physis
    - Usually also extends through metaphysis (Salter-Harris type II)
      - ◻ Metaphyseal fragment or displacement of epiphysis may be most conspicuous feature
    - Less commonly extends into epiphysis (Salter-Harris type III) or both (Salter-Harris type IV)
    - Salter-Harris type I (SCFE) is uncommon
      - ◻ SCFE is likely due to minor trauma superimposed on chronic stress of weight bearing
      - ◻ Typically, femoral head slips posterior & medial
      - ◻ Bilateral in 18-80% (need not be synchronous)
      - ◻ Age: Girls 8-15 years; boys 10-17 years
  - ZPC is largely intact
  - Soft tissue swelling & appropriate history are evident
- **Chronic Repetitive Physeal Injury**
  - Chronic repetitive overuse → injury of metaphyseal blood supply → localized disruption of endochondral ossification → physeal widening & metaphyseal irregularity
  - May result in growth arrest with angular deformities (e.g., genu varum or valgum) if not treated with rest
  - Characteristic involvement of specific growth plates with certain activities/sports
    - Little League pitchers: Proximal humerus (Little Leaguer shoulder)
    - Gymnasts: Distal radius (gymnast wrist)
    - Running sports: Distal femur & proximal tibia
- **Apophysis Avulsion/Apophysitis**
  - Growth plate of apophysis = physeal equivalent
    - Cartilage remains "weak link" in skeletally immature teenagers with increasing muscle bulk
      - ◻ Osteocartilaginous avulsion is more likely than musculotendinous injury
  - Can be wide/irregular from chronic overuse (apophysitis) vs. acute avulsion injury
    - Acute often comes with clear history of "pop" & sudden onset of pain during classic activity
  - Common sites: Medial humeral epicondyle, anterior superior & inferior iliac spines, ischial tuberosity, lesser trochanter, tibial tubercle

Helpful Clues for Less Common Diagnoses

- **Osteomyelitis (Pyogenic)**
  - Most commonly occurs in metaphysis of children
  - May spread to physis with apparent widening
    - Physeal involvement can later lead to premature physeal closure (bone bridge formation)
  - Typically diagnosed by MR imaging before radiographic bone changes occur
    - Poorly defined marrow abnormality centered at metaphysis with periosteal & soft tissue changes (± fluid collections)
- **Chronic Recurrent Multifocal Osteomyelitis**
  - Noninfectious inflammatory process
  - Cystic lucencies within periphyseal metaphysis
  - MR: Marrow & soft tissue edema without fluid collections; often bilateral & relatively symmetric
- **Rickets**
  - Failure to mineralize cartilage/osteoid at physis
    - Due to ↓ in calcium or phosphorous
    - Most commonly from vitamin D deficiency
    - Can also be due to renal defects (i.e., renal rickets)
  - Radiographs

- Metaphyseal osteolysis, cupping, fraying
    - Loss of ZPC with widening of physis
    - ↓ bone density, smudged trabeculae
    - Generalized bowing of long bones
- **Leukemia (Mimic)**
    - Metaphyseal lucent bands ± permeative cortical destruction, aggressive periosteal reaction, osteoporosis, fractures
    - ZPC typically remains intact
- **Renal Osteodystrophy**
    - Combined findings of rickets & hyperparathyroidism
        - Signs of hyperparathyroidism
            - Subperiosteal resorption
            - Subchondral resorption with collapse
            - Cystic "brown tumors"
- **Osteochondroses**
    - Symptomatic growth disturbance of epiphysis secondary to repetitive microtrauma &/or avascular necrosis
    - Frequently results in fragmentation, sclerosis, & abnormal morphology of epiphysis/metaphysis or equivalent
        - LCP (femoral head) may also have metaphyseal abnormalities
        - Blount disease primarily affects medial tibial metaphysis (but medial epiphysis is also abnormal)

Helpful Clues for Rare Diagnoses

- **Hypophosphatasia**
    - Distinct lucent extensions into metaphysis from physis
    - Most growth plates/metaphyses are affected but to variable degrees
        - Often asymmetric; also nonuniform at single physis
    - Osteoporosis
- **Mucopolysaccharidoses**
    - Heterogeneous group of lysosomal storage diseases
    - Dysostosis multiplex (DM): Constellation of bone dysplasia features seen variably in MPS
    - Delay in epiphyseal ossification may mimic apparent widening of physis
    - Spine: Anteriorly beaked vertebral bodies associated with kyphosis
    - Pelvis: Ilia taper inferiorly, steep acetabular roofs
    - Oar-shaped ribs & diaphyseal widening of long bones
- **Chronic Physeal Fractures of Myelodysplasia**
    - Patients with decreased sensation (e.g., myelomeningocele, chronic insensitivity to pain) develop recurrent fracture/refracture pattern with incomplete healing between episodes
        - Results in aggressive layered periosteal reaction
    - Often have background osteoporosis, gracile long bones, muscle wasting
    - May have adjacent neuropathic joint
- **Scurvy**
    - Vitamin C deficiency → ↑ bleeding, ↓ collagen synthesis
    - Osteoporosis with thin cortices, dense ZPC (white line of Frankel), metaphyseal lucencies (Trümmerfeld zone), & sclerotic rim of epiphysis (Wimberger sign)
    - Metaphyseal corner spur/fracture
    - Diaphyseal periosteal lifting/reaction due to subperiosteal hemorrhage
- **Skeletal Dysplasias**
    - Many have true or apparent physeal widening
        - e.g., metaphyseal, spondylometaphyseal & metaphyseal chondrodysplasias
    - Metaphyses are flared & irregular with apparent physeal widening
- **Copper Deficiency**
    - Etiologies: Nutritional (including TPN), malabsorption, & congenital
        - Menkes: Rare X-linked recessive disorder that disrupts copper absorption
            - Metaphyseal irregularity, cupping, & spurs with increased density
            - Tortuous intracranial arteries, Wormian bones

SELECTED REFERENCES

1. Nguyen JC et al: Imaging of pediatric growth plate disturbances. Radiographics. 37(6):1791-812, 2017
2. Laor T et al: Physeal widening in the knee due to stress injury in child athletes. AJR Am J Roentgenol. 186(5):1260-4, 2006

Physeal Fracture (Salter-Harris)

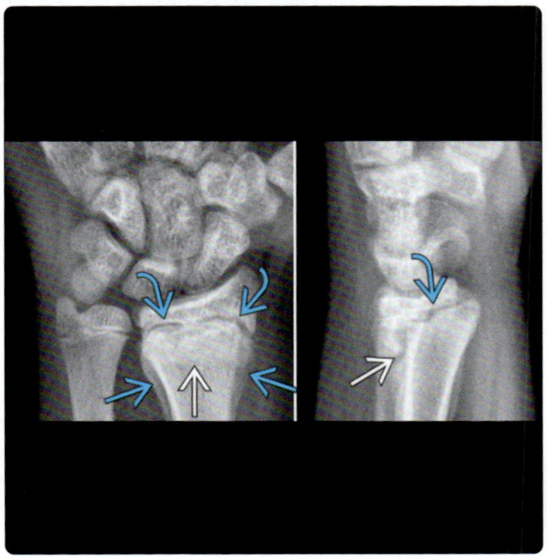

Physeal Fracture (Salter-Harris)

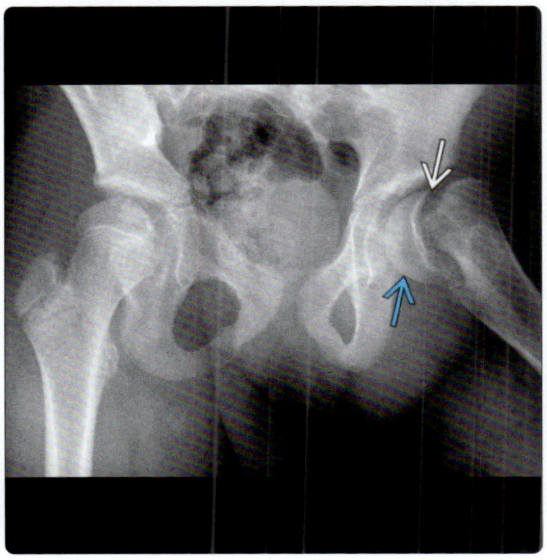

(Left) *Frontal & lateral wrist radiographs in a 13-year-old boy show distal radial metaphyseal irregularity & periosteal reaction. The healing Salter-Harris II fracture extends through the distal radial physis, which is widened.* **(Right)** *AP radiograph in a 10-year-old girl with left hip pain shows widening of the left proximal femoral physis due to severe displacement (slip) of the capital femoral epiphysis medially.*

(Left) *Frontal radiographs of both shoulders in a left-hand-dominant Little League pitcher with left shoulder pain show mild widening of the proximal left humeral physis with associated mild metaphyseal irregularity.* **(Right)** *Frontal radiograph & gradient-echo MR images of the right knee in a 14-year-old soccer player with chronic pain show widening of the lateral aspect of the distal femoral growth plate with associated mild metaphyseal irregularity. These findings resolved with rest.*

Chronic Repetitive Physeal Injury

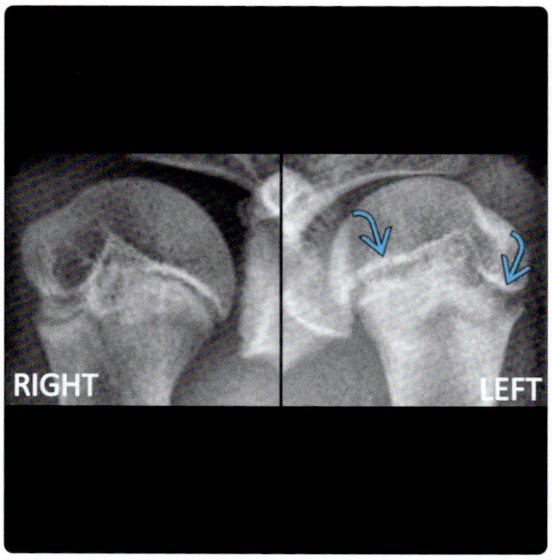

Chronic Repetitive Physeal Injury

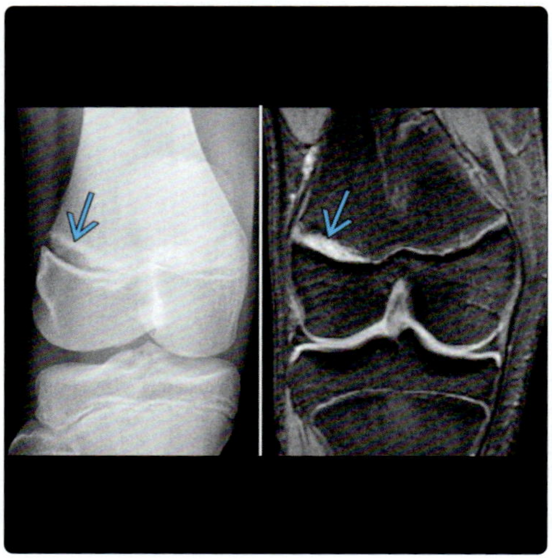

(Left) *AP radiographs in a 15-year-old right-handed Little League pitcher show an avulsion fracture of the inferior right medial epicondyle with widening of the growth plate. Note the normal left medial epicondyle.* **(Right)** *Oblique radiograph & sagittal T2 FS MR images in a 10 year old with L > R ankle pain show a lobulated periphyseal lucent/hyperintense lesion of the metaphysis with similar signal abnormality in the epiphysis. The findings are typical for CRMO & are frequently bilateral.*

Apophyseal Avulsion/Apophysitis

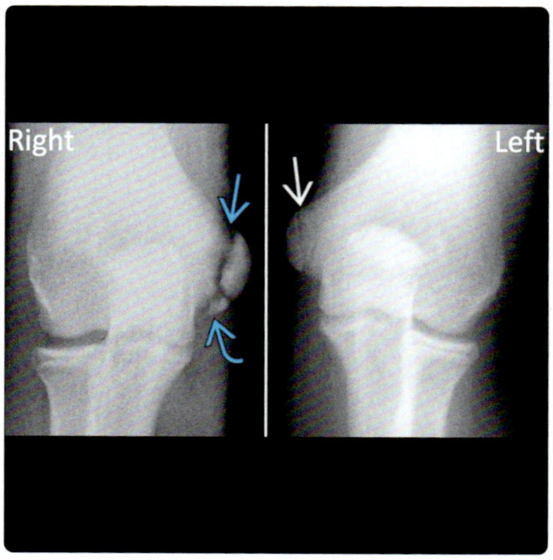

Chronic Recurrent Multifocal Osteomyelitis

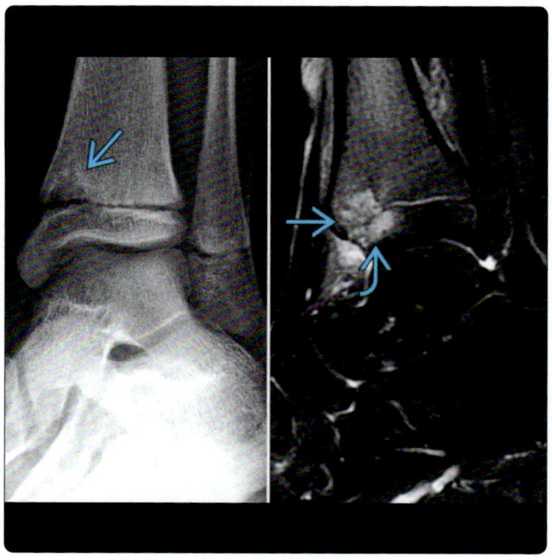

(Left) *PA radiograph in a 2 year old with rickets shows cupping & fraying of the distal radial & ulnar metaphyses, loss of the ZPC, & widening of the radial & ulnar physes.* **(Right)** *AP radiographs in a 9 year old with bilateral knee pain for 2 months show lucent bands throughout the visible metaphyses. These are more irregular at the proximal left tibia where there is also periosteal reaction. The radiodense ZPCs bordering the cartilaginous growth plates are largely intact. Leukemia was ultimately diagnosed.*

Rickets

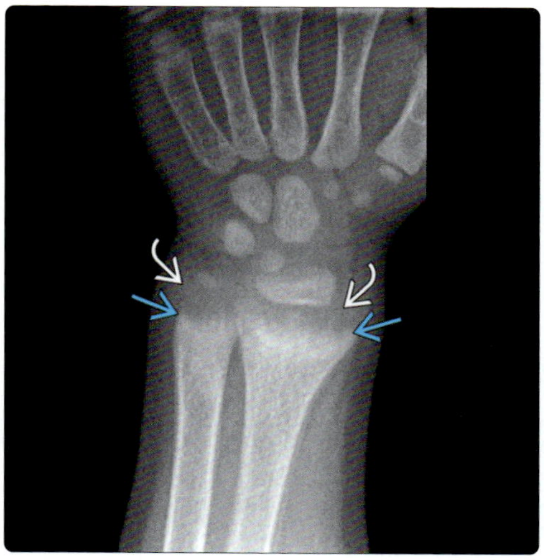

Leukemia (Mimic)

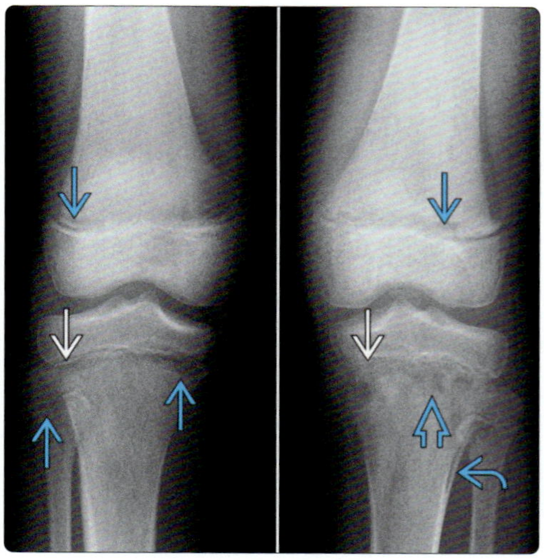

Renal Osteodystrophy

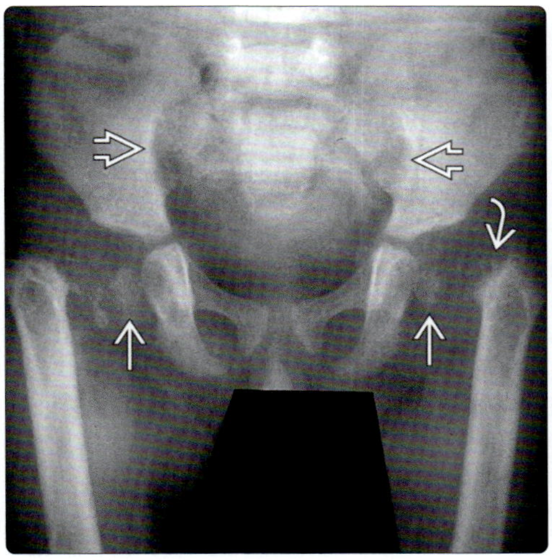

Hypophosphatasia

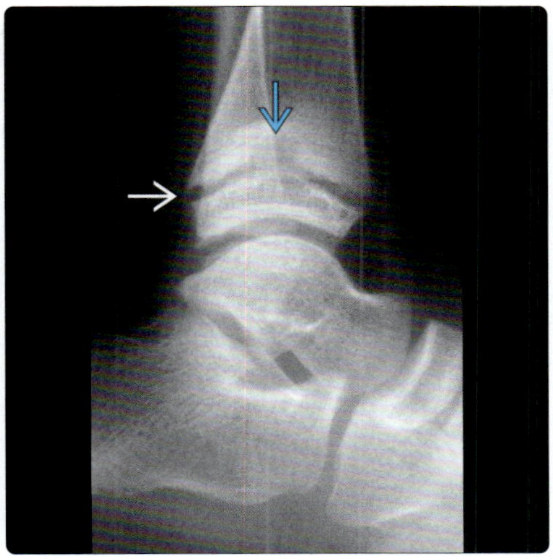

(Left) *AP radiograph shows severe renal osteodystrophy, apparent in the hips as rickets, with loss of the ZPCs ➡ & slip of the capital epiphyses ➡. There are also findings of hyperparathyroidism with widened sacroiliac joints ➡ due to subchondral resorption & "smudged" trabecula.* **(Right)** *Lateral radiograph shows widening of the tibial physis ➡. Also note the more focal lucency extending from the physis into the metaphysis ➡ due to unossified cartilage in hypophosphatasia.*

Mucopolysaccharidoses

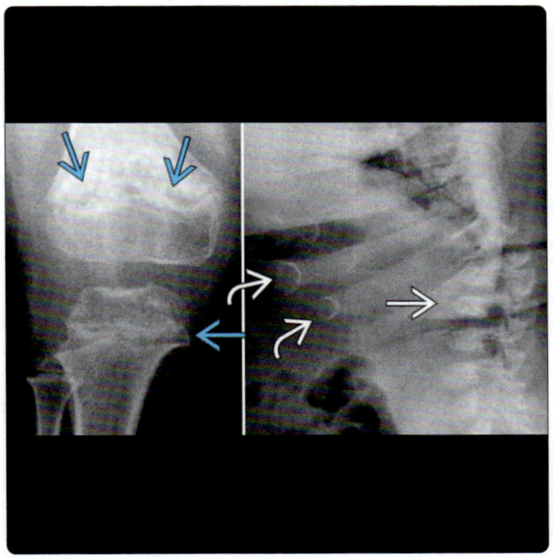

Chronic Physeal Fractures of Myelodysplasia

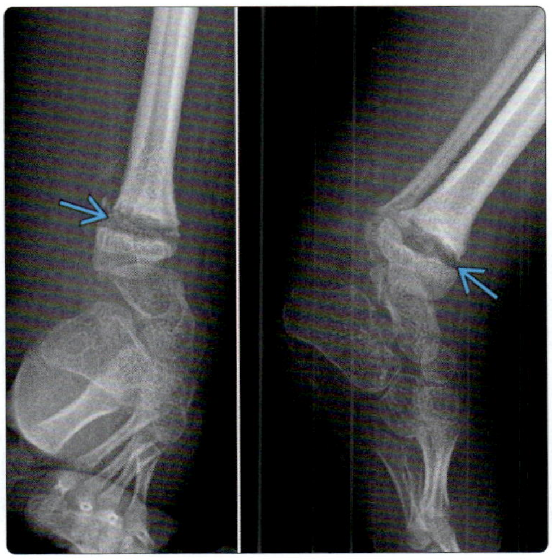

(Left) *Radiographs in a 12-year-old girl with Morquio syndrome show widening of distal femoral & proximal tibial physes ➡ as well as anterior vertebral beaking ➡ & oar-shaped (proximally narrowed & distally expanded) ribs ➡.* **(Right)** *Radiographs in a 7 year old with myelomeningocele show chronic changes of neuromuscular disease, including osteoporosis, gracile long bones, & muscle wasting. Note the wide physis ➡ of the tibia due to recurrent fractures with incomplete healing.*

Scurvy

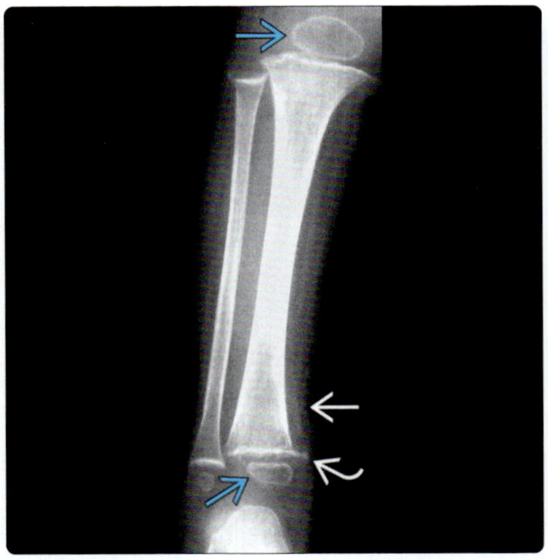

Skeletal Dysplasias

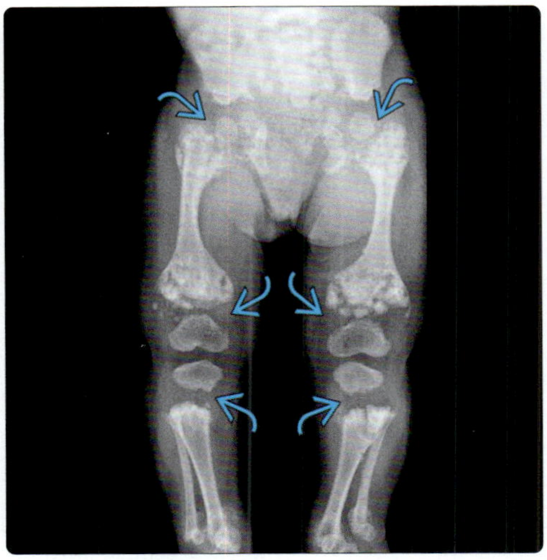

(Left) *AP radiograph shows findings of scurvy with a metaphyseal fracture/spur ➡. Note the wide periosteal reaction ➡ related to subperiosteal hemorrhage as well as the relatively dense epiphyseal margins ➡.* **(Right)** *AP radiographs in a 4-year-old boy with Jansen-type metaphyseal chondrodysplasia show marked irregularity & expansion of the metaphyses. By contrast, the epiphyses are enlarged but relatively normal in shape, which is typical of this disorder. There is also widening (lengthening) of the physes ➡.*

Physeal Bridge/Growth Arrest

DIFFERENTIAL DIAGNOSIS

Common

- Fracture

Less Common

- Infection
- Iatrogenic (Surgical)
- Osteochondroses
- Advanced Bone Age
- Juvenile Idiopathic Arthritis
- Chronic Recurrent Multifocal Osteomyelitis
- Focal Periphyseal Edema Zone (Mimic)

Rare but Important

- Tumors
- Radiation-Induced Growth Deformities
- Thermal Injury

ESSENTIAL INFORMATION

Key Differential Diagnosis Issues

- History & distribution of physes involved limits differential
- Common mechanisms
  - Physeal injury → transphyseal vessels → bone deposition
  - Hyperemia → early closure
- Bridge may restrict growth regardless of cause
  - Central bone bridge → longitudinal growth restriction
  - Peripheral bone bridge → angular deformity
- Bridges are diagnosed based on direct & indirect findings
  - Direct: Visualization of bone bridge interrupting physis
  - Indirect: Newly narrowed or indistinct physis as compared to prior exam &/or adjacent or contralateral bone, obliquely oriented growth recovery line in adjacent metaphysis (sloping toward bridge), new angular deformity or relative shortening of affected bone

Helpful Clues for Common Diagnoses

- **Fracture**
  - Analyze physis on follow-up of Salter-Harris (SH) injuries
    - Bridges are more common in lower extremity

Helpful Clues for Less Common Diagnoses

- **Infection**
  - Osteomyelitis of metaphyses may involve physis
  - Hyperemia of septic arthritis & osteomyelitis may also lead to bridge without direct physeal involvement
- **Iatrogenic (Surgical)**
  - Epiphysiodesis: Intentional surgical closure of physis by screws, staples, or drilling
    - Treatment for angular & limb length deformities
- **Osteochondroses**
  - Collection of poorly understood "disorders" related to avascular necrosis, repetitive stress, or normal variation
  - Blount & Legg-Calvé-Perthes can result in physeal bridge
- **Advanced Bone Age**
  - Precocious puberty, congenital adrenal hyperplasia, etc.
  - All growth centers uniformly affected
- **Juvenile Idiopathic Arthritis**
  - Chronic hyperemia from synovitis at involved joints may lead to osteoporosis, erosions, joint space loss, epiphyseal overgrowth, physeal closure
- **Chronic Recurrent Multifocal Osteomyelitis**
  - Multifocal nonpyogenic inflammatory bone lesions
  - Commonly metaphyseal but can involve physis
- **Focal Periphyseal Edema Zone (Mimic)**
  - Periphyseal edema seen in adolescents
  - Likely related to early physiologic physeal closure
  - Associated with pain; no intervention required

Helpful Clues for Rare Diagnoses

- **Tumors**
  - Any lesion that breaches physis can lead to bridge
  - Hereditary multiple exostoses & enchondromatosis can lead to short bones due to displaced growth cartilage
- **Radiation-Induced Growth Deformities**
  - Vasculitis from radiation may lead to early fusion in distribution of radiation field
  - ± avascular necrosis & osteochondromas
- **Thermal Injury**
  - Typical history of burns or frostbite

Fracture

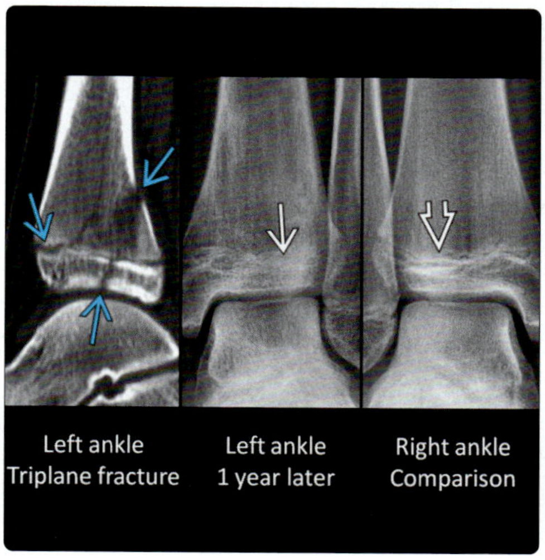

Fracture

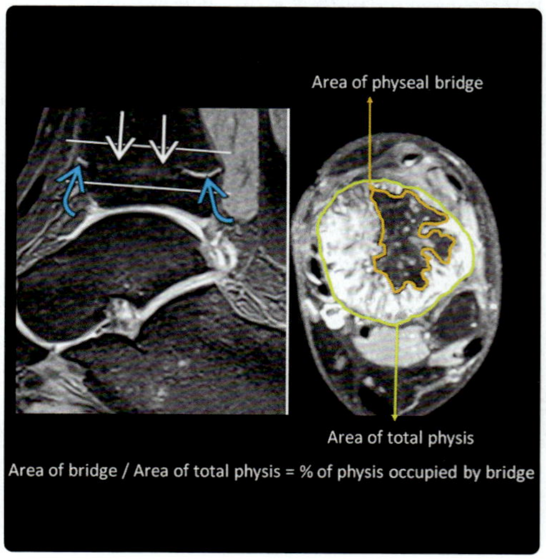

(Left) *Sagittal bone CT in a 13-year-old boy shows a left tibial triplane fracture ⇨. Follow-up frontal radiographs show poor definition of the left tibial physis centrally ➡ due to a bone bridge. Note the normal distal right tibial physis ➡, which remains open.* **(Right)** *Sagittal 3D FSPGR MR (left) in the same patient shows a dark osseous bridge ➡ interrupting the bright cartilaginous physis ⇨. Axial MIP through the physis (right) allows area measurements of the bridge (outlined in orange) & total physis (outlined in yellow).*

Infection

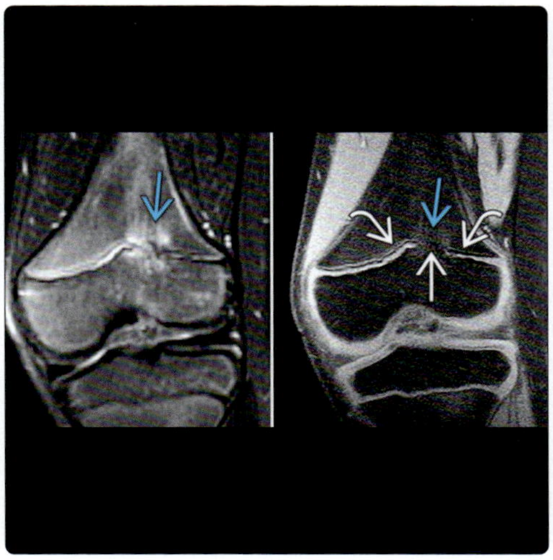

Iatrogenic (Surgical)

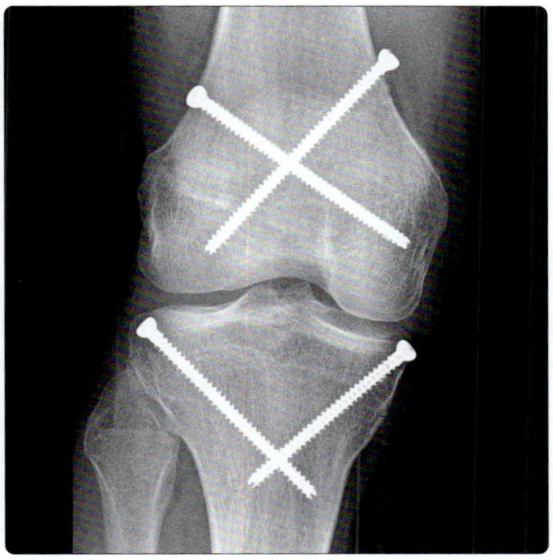

(Left) *Coronal T2 FS (left) & GRE (right) MR images in a 9-year-old boy with a history of distal right femoral osteomyelitis show loss of the normal central physis with adjacent marrow edema* →*. The GRE image confirms an osseous bridge* → *extending across the bright physeal cartilage* →*.* **(Right)** *Frontal radiograph in a 13-year-old boy shows that transphyseal screws were placed across the distal femoral & proximal tibial physes to induce early closure (in order to treat a leg length discrepancy in this patient).*

Osteochondroses

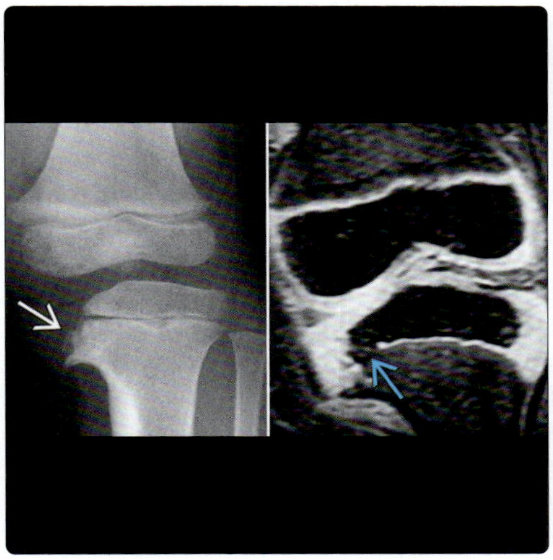

Juvenile Idiopathic Arthritis

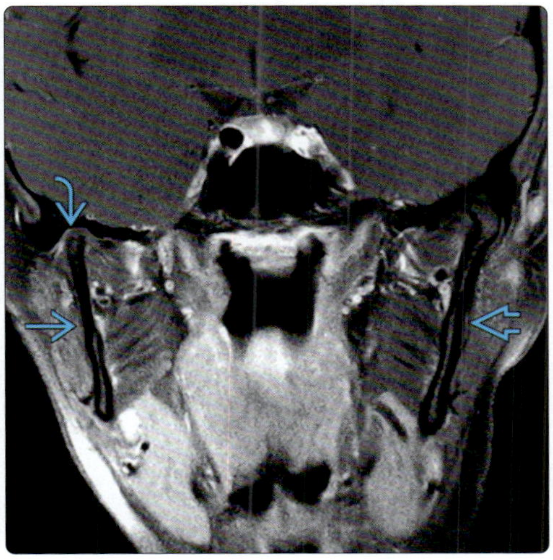

(Left) *AP radiograph (left) shows downsloping, beaking, & irregularity of the medial tibial metaphysis (Blount disease)* →*. Follow-up coronal GRE MR (right) shows an osseous bridge* → *crossing the medial tibial physis.* **(Right)** *Coronal T1 C+ FS MR of the temporomandibular joints in an 18 year old with juvenile idiopathic arthritis shows a shortened right mandibular ramus* → *relative to the left* →*. This is likely due to chronic erosive disease & premature growth plate closure at the right condyle* →*.*

Focal Periphyseal Edema Zone (Mimic)

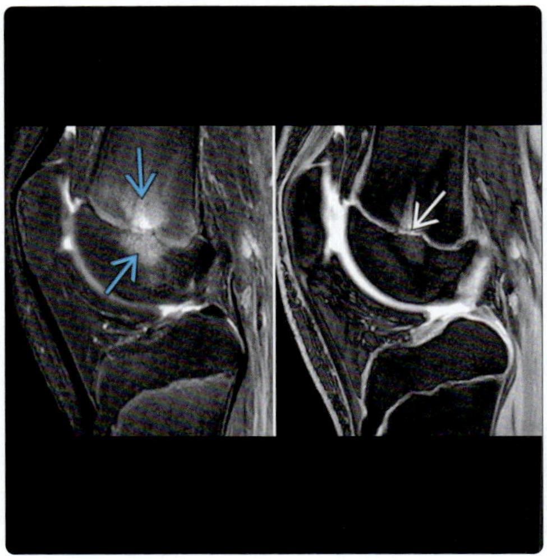

Thermal Injury

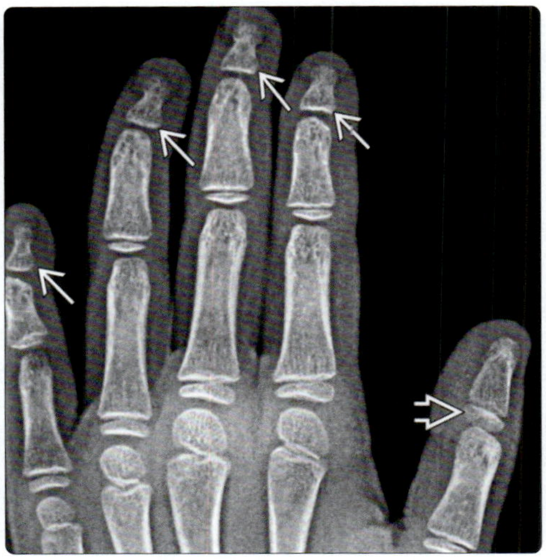

(Left) *Sagittal T2 FS (left) & GRE (right) MR images of the knee in a 13-year-old girl show foci of periphyseal edema* →*. The GRE image shows that the physis is normal* →*. Focal periphyseal edema zones are seen in adolescents nearing physeal closure & should not be confused with a bone bridge.* **(Right)** *PA radiograph shows premature closure of the physes at the 2nd-5th distal phalanges* →*, resulting in short digits. This is due to vascular damage from frostbite. Note the normal physis & distal phalanx of the thumb* →*.*

DIFFERENTIAL DIAGNOSIS

Common

- Fibroxanthoma

Less Common

- Simple Bone Cyst
- Aneurysmal Bone Cyst
- Fibrous Dysplasia
- Langerhans Cell Histiocytosis
- Enchondroma
- Primary Sarcoma or Metastatic Disease

Rare but Important

- Osteoblastoma
- Chondroblastoma
- Chondromyxoid Fibroma
- Osteofibrous Dysplasia/Adamantinoma
- Giant Cell Tumor

ESSENTIAL INFORMATION

Helpful Clues for Common Diagnoses

- **Fibroxanthoma**
  - Encompasses fibrous cortical defect (FCD) & nonossifying fibroma (NOF)
    - FCD: < 2-3 cm, within cortex
    - NOF: > 2-3 cm, extends into medullary cavity
  - Developmental defect, usually discovered as incidental finding on radiograph or MR
  - Age: 2-20 years
  - M:F = 2:1; 30-40% of all children
  - Typically affects metadiaphyseal region of long bones, most commonly around knee
    - Femur (38%), tibia (43%), fibula (8%), humerus (5%)
  - Radiographs: Eccentric, bubbly, multiloculated, subcortical, lucent lesion with sclerotic border
    - Often has scalloped margin
    - Cortex may be mildly expanded or appear absent
    - Lacks periosteal reaction unless fracture (or, less commonly, infection) is superimposed
    - Gradual ossification/regression of lesions
  - MR: Low to intermediate T1/T2 intensity with hypointense (sclerotic) rim; typically enhances
  - Usually asymptomatic, requiring no treatment
    - Involvement of > 50% diameter of weight-bearing bone increases risk of pathologic fracture
    - Curettage & bone grafting to prevent fracture
  - Jaffe-Campanacci syndrome
    - Café-au-lait lesions, intellectual disability, hypogonadism, ocular & cardiovascular abnormalities
    - Associated with multiple fibroxanthomas

Helpful Clues for Less Common Diagnoses

- **Simple Bone Cyst**
  - a.k.a. solitary bone cyst, unicameral bone cyst (UBC)
  - Age: 10-20 years; ~ 2/3 present with pathologic fracture
  - Proximal humerus & femur in up to 80-90%
  - Radiographs: Central, metaphyseal, well-defined, lucent lesion; lacks periosteal reaction without fracture
    - Generally lacks significant septations or expansion
    - Fallen-fragment sign is pathognomonic
      - □ Pathologic fracture fragment falls dependently within fluid of lesion
  - MR: May contain fluid-fluid level if traumatized; no solid enhancing component
- **Aneurysmal Bone Cyst**
  - Etiology unknown, possibly due to venous obstruction or arteriovenous fistula vs. reparative process
  - Lesion contains thin-walled, blood-filled cystic cavities
  - Age: 10-30 years; rare ≤ 5 years
  - Primary (1°) or secondary (2°)
    - 1°: No recognized preexisting lesion
    - 2°: Arising in preexisting lesion
      - □ Benign lesions: Giant cell tumor, chondroblastoma, fibrous dysplasia, osteoblastoma, chondromyxoid fibroma, fibroxanthoma
      - □ Malignant lesions: Osteosarcoma (e.g., telangiectatic variant), chondrosarcoma
  - Typically metaphyseal, most commonly around knee
  - Tubular long bones (70-80%), leg (29%), pelvis (5-10%), clavicle & ribs (5%), spinal posterior elements (16%)
  - Radiographs: Multicystic eccentric expansile lesion
    - Periosteal reaction
    - Cortex often severely thinned, rarely disrupted
  - MR: Characteristic fluid-fluid levels within cavities of differing signal intensity
    - Hypointense rim surrounds lesion
    - Mural & septal enhancement is typical without significant solid components
- **Fibrous Dysplasia**
  - Age: 5-20 years
  - Radiographs: Monostotic or polyostotic expansile lesion with endosteal scalloping
    - Typically lucent to ground glass (i.e., smudged/frosted) matrix
    - Less commonly: Mixed lucent & sclerotic
    - No periostitis unless pathologic fracture
  - MR: Variable, but active lesions are T2 hyperintense with enhancement
  - CT: May be helpful to confirm characteristic matrix if radiographs & MR are unclear
  - McCune-Albright: Precocious puberty, café-au-lait spots, & polyostotic fibrous dysplasia
- **Langerhans Cell Histiocytosis**
  - Benign neoplasm of atypical Langerhans cells
  - Age: 50% < 10 years
  - Single system unifocal or multifocal disease vs. multisystem disease
    - Involvement: Bones (80-90%) > skin (50%) > viscera
    - Skull (50%), axial skeleton (25%), long bones (15%)
  - Radiographs: Lytic, sharply demarcated lesion without sclerotic margin, unless healing
    - Axial skeleton
      - □ "Punched-out" skull lesions ± "beveled edge"; spiculated periosteal reaction & permeation are atypical
      - □ Classic cause of vertebra plana
    - Appendicular skeleton
      - □ Nonaggressive to aggressive appearance; expansion is rare

- One of classic "flat bone" lesions
- MR: Bone defect typically is filled with enhancing soft tissue, but large soft tissue mass is not typical
  - May have disproportionate surrounding marrow edema compared to overlying soft tissues
- **Enchondroma**
  - Age: 15-40 years
  - Most common: Small tubular hand/foot bones & ribs
    - Typically central diaphysis in long bones
  - Radiographs: Well-defined lucent lesion with endosteal scalloping, marginal sclerosis
    - ± chondroid matrix: Dots, arcs, or rings of Ca^{2+}
    - ± mild expansile remodeling of bone
  - Enchondromatoses: Conditions with multiple enchondromas
    - Ollier disease: May be unilateral with lucent metaphyseal streaks & eccentric surface lesions
    - Maffucci syndrome: Multiple enchondromas + slow-flow vascular anomalies
      - Phleboliths in soft tissues on radiographs
- **Primary Bone Sarcoma or Metastatic Disease**
  - Radiographs: Typically have more aggressive appearance with wide zone of transition, permeation, & periosteal reaction (i.e., interruption, layering, spiculation, etc.)
    - 2° ABC may create bubbly appearance

Helpful Clues for Rare Diagnoses

- **Osteoblastoma**
  - Benign osseous lesion with osteoid production
  - Related to osteoid osteoma (OO): Osteoblastoma > 1.5 cm vs. OO < 1.5 cm
  - Age: 10-20 years old
  - Spine (40%), long bones (30%), hands & feet (15%), skull & face (15%)
    - May present with painful scoliosis
  - Radiographs: Lytic, expansile lesion with sclerotic margin, variable central Ca^{2+}
  - MR: Inflammatory change can mimic infection or trauma
- **Chondroblastoma**
  - Benign bone tumor with immature cartilage cells
  - Peak: 15-20 years; range: 3-85 years
  - Majority arise in epiphysis or equivalent
  - Most commonly around knee & proximal humerus
    - Long bones (80%), hands & feet (10%)
  - Radiographs: Well-defined, lucent lesion; sclerotic border
    - Calcified chondroid matrix in 50%
      - Better visualized on CT
  - MR: Heterogeneous with low-signal rim; adjacent marrow/periosteal/soft tissue edema, reactive joint effusion
- **Chondromyxoid Fibroma**
  - Eccentric, lucent with sclerotic margin
  - Male predominance; chondromyxoid fibromas present with pain
  - Treatment: Curettage, recurrence in 25%
- **Osteofibrous Dysplasia/Adamantinoma**
  - Osteofibrous dysplasia (OFD): Fibroosseous lesion primarily affecting tibia in children
    - Usually eccentrically involves anterior tibial diaphysis/metadiaphysis
    - Radiographs: Lucent & sclerotic; solitary or multifocal
      - Can synchronously involve fibula
    - May lead to fracture & pseudoarthrosis
  - Adamantinoma: Similar but is low-grade malignancy
    - Radiographs: Can be identical to OFD but typically occurs in older children
      - Worrisome features include periosteal reaction, permeative destruction, & soft tissue extension
- **Giant Cell Tumor**
  - Usually occurs after growth plate closure
  - Long bones (75-90%), around knee (50%)
  - Radiographs: Metaepiphyseal/epiphyseal, extending to subarticular bone; eccentric & lytic lesion with nonsclerotic margin ± periosteal reaction
  - Pathologic fracture (30%)

Fibroxanthoma

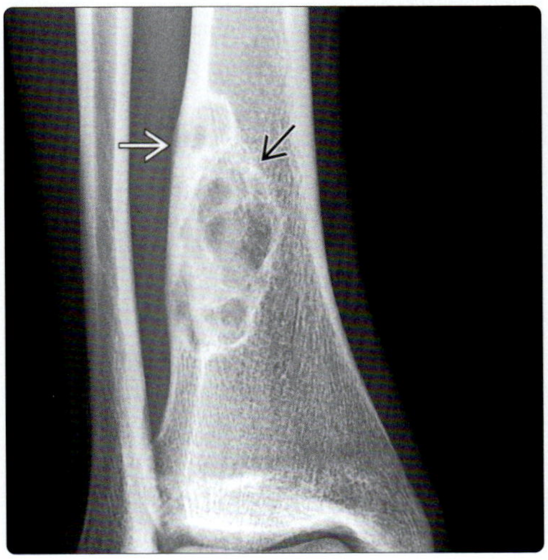

Fibroxanthoma

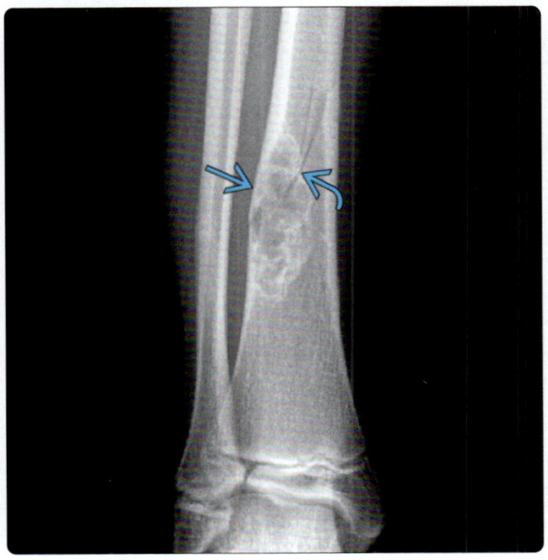

(Left) *AP radiograph shows a bubbly, eccentric, lucent lesion ➔ with a scalloped sclerotic margin in the distal tibial diaphysis. Note the cortical margin thinning ➔ & mild expansion by the nonossifying fibroma (fibroxanthoma).* **(Right)** *AP radiograph in a 13 year old with leg pain after a minor injury shows a pathologic fracture ➔ through a fibroxanthoma ➔ of the distal tibial diaphysis. Fibroxanthomas that involve > 50% of the diameter of the bone are at increased risk for pathologic fractures.*

(Left) *AP radiographs of the ankle were obtained in a boy at 11 (left) & 14 (right) years of age. The initial radiographs show a fibroxanthoma* ➙ *that has nearly resolved on the follow-up study.* (Right) *AP radiograph (left) shows a pathologic fracture* ➙ *through a distal left tibial fibroxanthoma* ➙*. The 2nd radiograph (right) was obtained after curettage & bone grafting of the lesion. Fibroxanthomas are considered "do-not-touch" lesions but may be treated after (or to prevent) a pathologic fracture.*

Fibroxanthoma

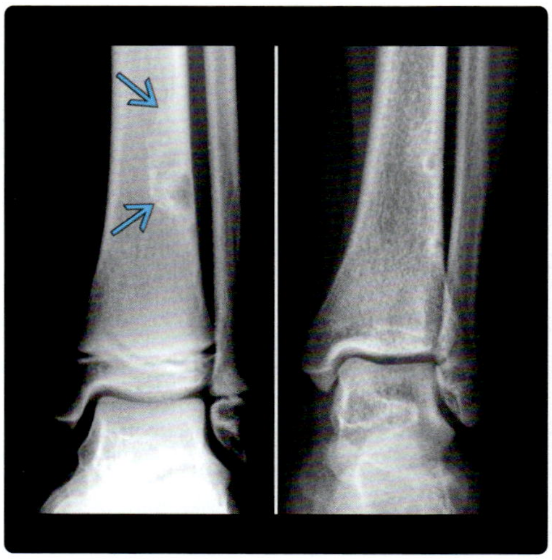

Fibroxanthoma

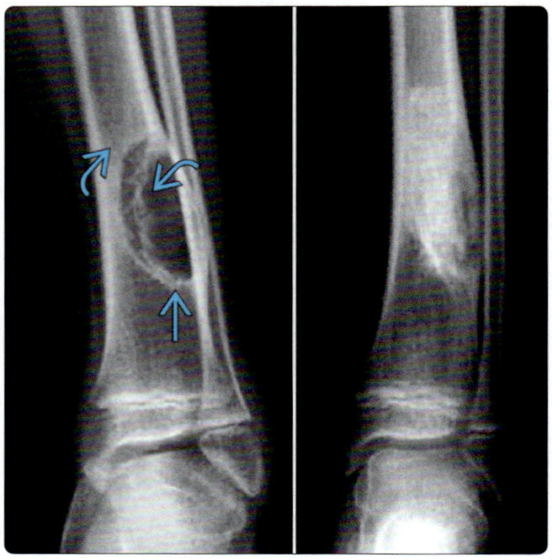

(Left) *AP radiographs in a 10-year-old girl with Jaffe-Campanacci syndrome show multiple fibroxanthomas in the bilateral tibiae* ➙*. Callus formation* ➙ *along the distal left tibial lesion is due to a healing pathologic fracture.* (Right) *Lateral radiograph shows a well-circumscribed lucent calcaneal lesion* ➙ *that was confirmed by MR to be a simple bone cyst. Simple bone cysts should be differentiated from a normal region of triangular lucency that frequently occurs in the anterior calcaneus between the major trabecular groups.*

Fibroxanthoma

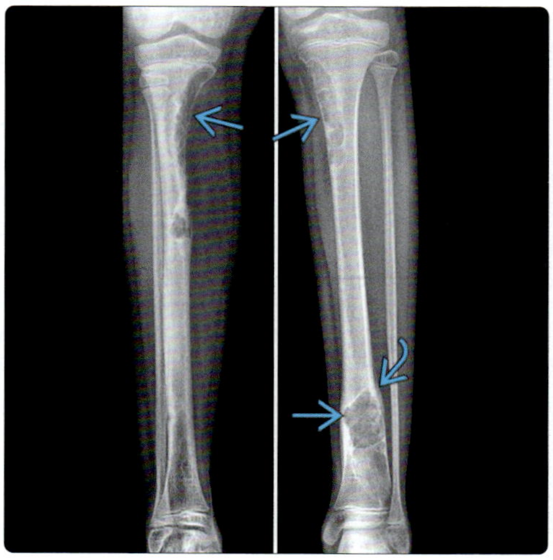

Simple Bone Cyst

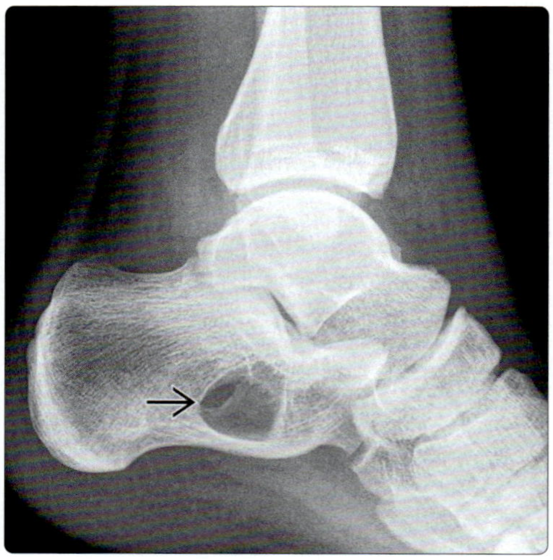

(Left) *Scapular Y lateral view in a 10-year-old girl with left arm pain after a minor injury shows a pathologic fracture* ➙ *across a nonaggressive-appearing lucent lesion in the proximal left humeral diaphysis* ➙*. There is a fallen fragment of bone within the dependent portion of the lesion* ➙*.* (Right) *PA & lateral radiographs in a 10 year old with right distal forearm pain & swelling show a well-circumscribed expansile lytic lesion* ➙ *in the distal radius. Thin septations are seen in the lesion* ➙*, & there is associated periosteal reaction* ➙*.*

Simple Bone Cyst

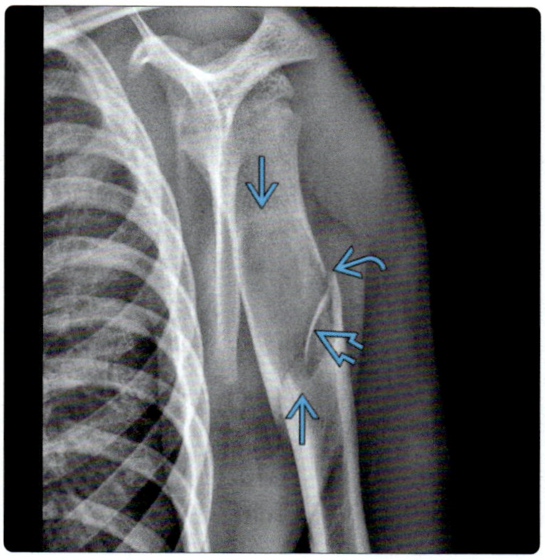

Aneurysmal Bone Cyst

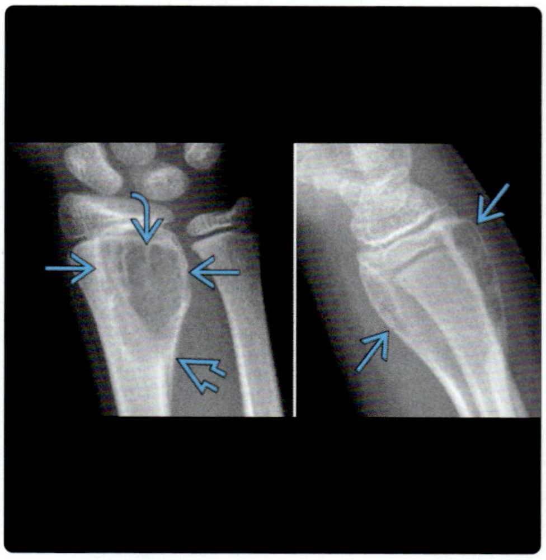

Aneurysmal Bone Cyst

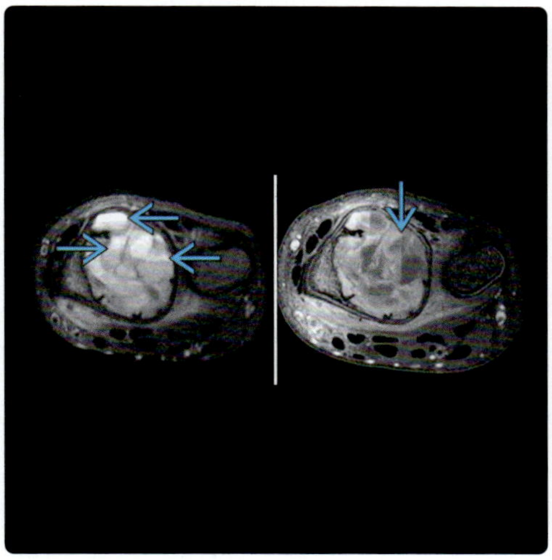

Aneurysmal Bone Cyst

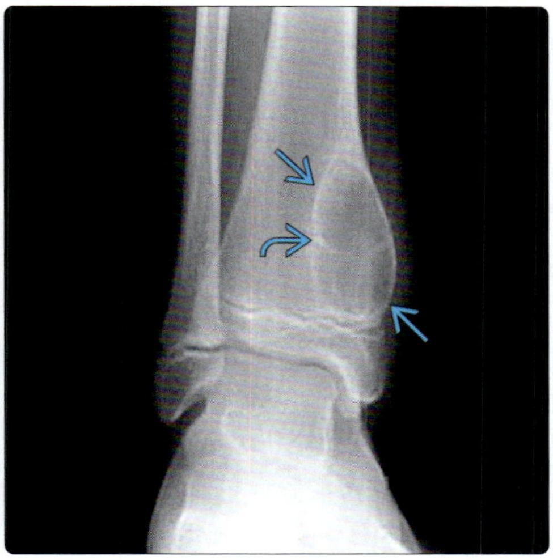

(Left) *Axial T2 FS (left) & T1 C+ FS (right) MR images in the same patient show multiple internal fluid-fluid levels (that shifted in orientation due to a change in wrist position during the scan). There is peripheral & septal enhancement on the postcontrast image, typical of an aneurysmal bone cyst (ABC).* **(Right)** *Frontal radiograph in a 13-year-old boy with distal leg swelling & pain shows a well-defined, expansile lytic lesion in the distal tibia that contains thin septations.*

Aneurysmal Bone Cyst

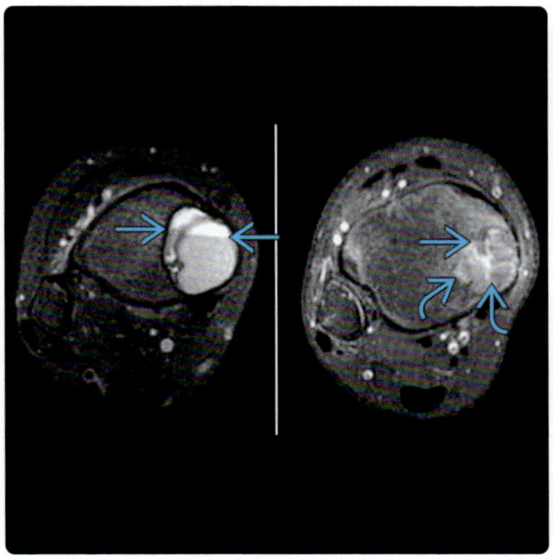

Fibrous Dysplasia

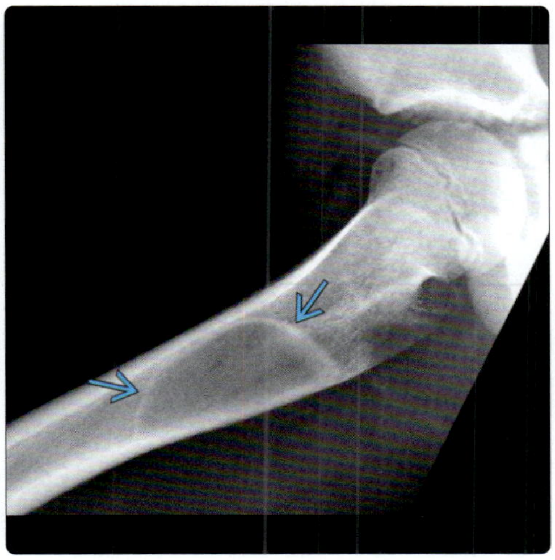

(Left) *Axial T2 FS (left) & T1 C+ FS (right) MR images in the same patient show multiple fluid-fluid levels in the lesion. The postcontrast image shows mild peripheral & septal enhancement, typical of ABCs.* **(Right)** *Lateral radiograph of the proximal right femur in a 10-year-old boy with right hip pain shows a well-defined lytic lesion with a sclerotic margin & a subtle ground-glass matrix, typical of fibrous dysplasia.*

Langerhans Cell Histiocytosis

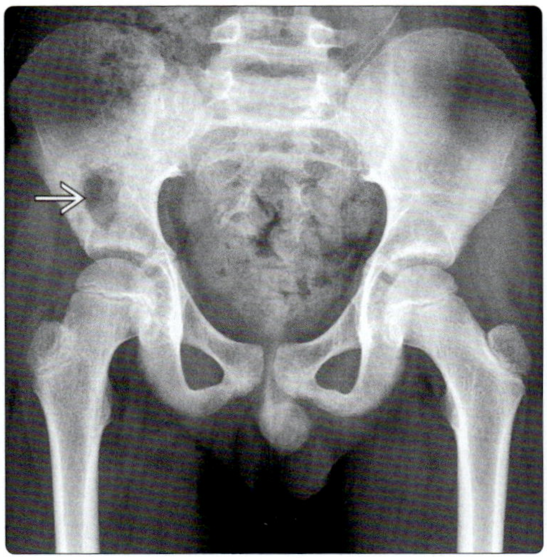

Langerhans Cell Histiocytosis

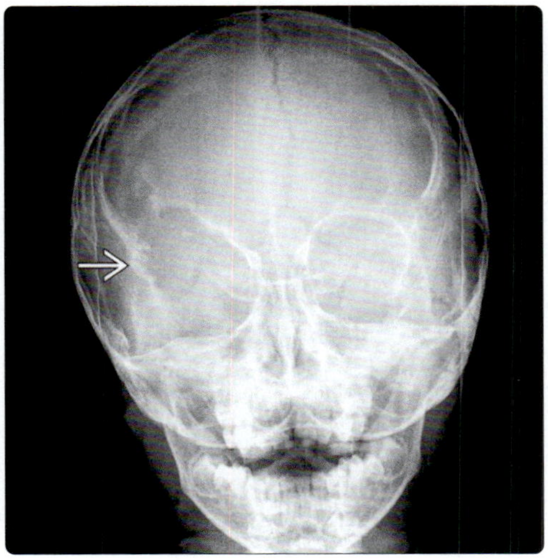

(Left) *AP radiograph shows a geographic, well-defined, lucent lesion without a sclerotic margin in the right iliac bone. This patient had a known history of Langerhans cell histiocytosis (LCH).* **(Right)** *AP radiograph of the skull in the same patient shows destruction of the right lateral orbital wall. LCH is a classic "flat bone lesion," & solitary lesions (i.e., single-system unifocal disease) are 3-5x more common than multifocal bone lesions.*

(Left) *Townes skull radiograph in a 2 year old with LCH shows innumerable geographic lytic lesions, none of which clearly shows the classically described beveled edge appearance.* **(Right)** *Radiographs of the proximal humeri (top) & femurs (bottom) in the same child show lytic lesions in the metadiaphyses with frank cortical destruction. Also note the lytic lesions in the bilateral femoral heads.*

Langerhans Cell Histiocytosis

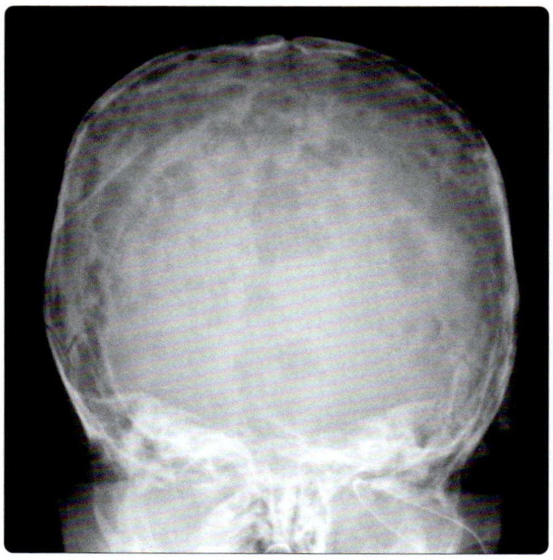

Langerhans Cell Histiocytosis

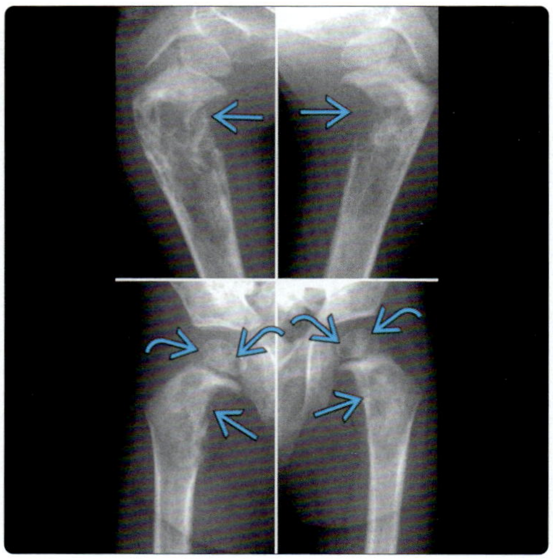

(Left) *PA radiograph of the index finger in a child with pain after minor trauma shows a pathologic fracture across a well-defined bubbly lucent lesion in the proximal phalanx. The internal matrix shows subtle arcs/rings of Ca^{2+}, typical of enchondromas. Also note the typical endosteal scalloping.* **(Right)** *AP radiograph in a 15 year old with knee pain shows a lytic lesion with a wide zone of transition & aggressive periosteal reaction in the distal femoral metaphysis medially.*

Enchondroma

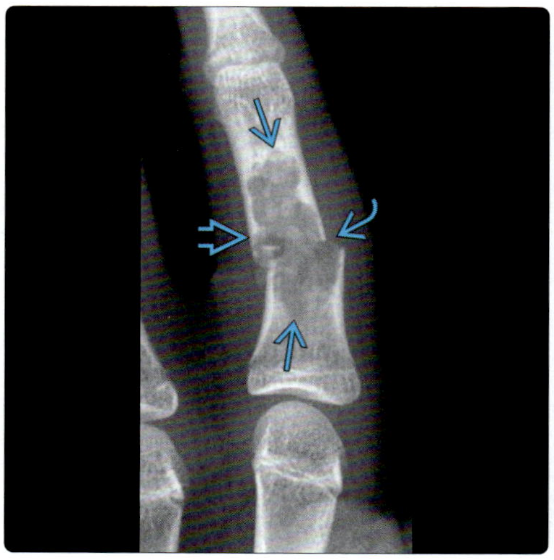

Primary Sarcoma or Metastatic Disease

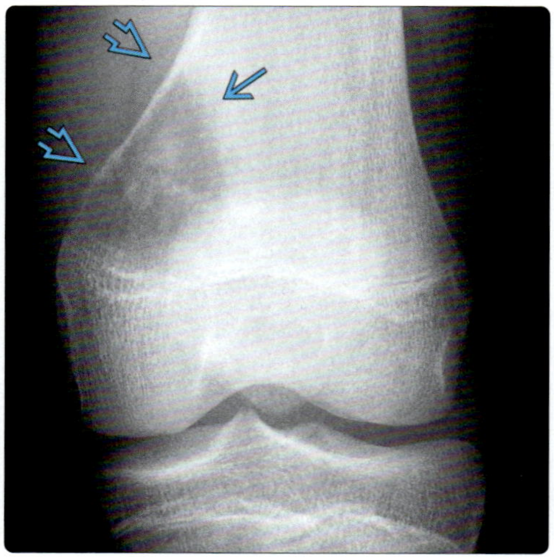

(Left) *Axial T2 FS MR in the same patient shows a few scattered fluid-fluid levels in this telangiectatic osteosarcoma. Note the cortical permeation & periosteal elevation by the tumor.* **(Right)** *Oblique radiograph (left) & coronal bone CT (right) in a child with chest wall pain shows a lucent, expansile lesion in the left 7th rib. Internal Ca^{2+} can be seen on both studies. Biopsy confirmed osteoblastoma.*

Primary Sarcoma or Metastatic Disease

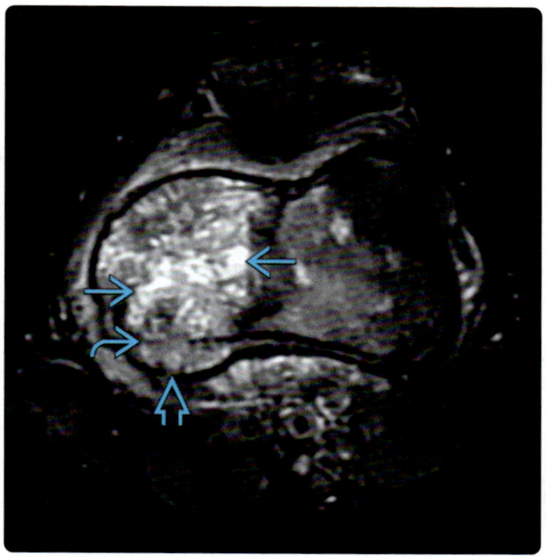

Osteoblastoma

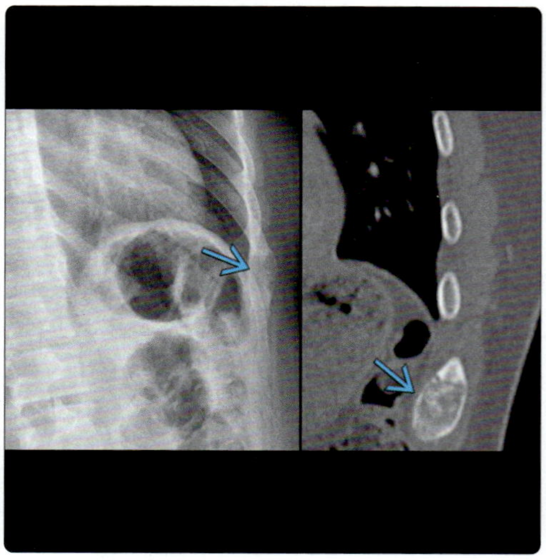

Chondroblastoma | **Chondroblastoma**

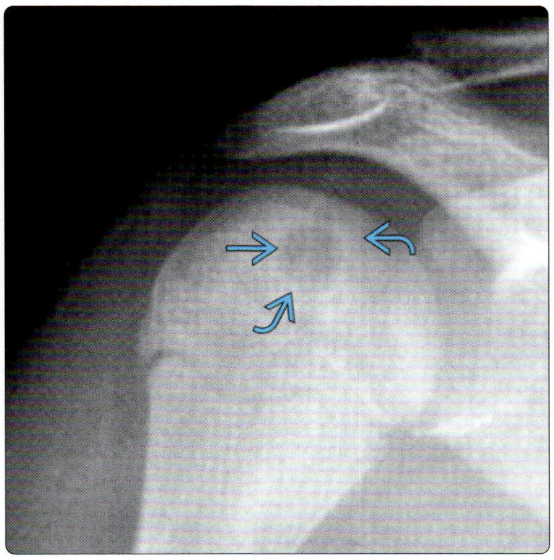

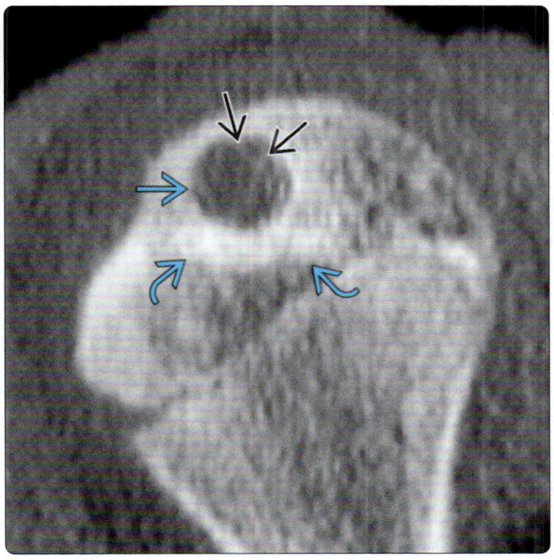

(Left) *Internal rotation radiograph in a 10-year-old boy with right shoulder pain shows a well-defined lytic lesion* → *in the right humeral epiphysis. A subtle surrounding rim of sclerosis* ↷ *is noted.* **(Right)** *Sagittal reformatted image from an NECT in the same child shows the lytic lesion* → *in the humeral epiphysis. The internal matrix of the lesion, which contains subtle arcs & rings of* Ca^{2+} ➜, *is typical of cartilage tumors. The adjacent sclerosis* ↷ *& internal matrix are better seen on this CT than on the radiographs.*

Chondromyxoid Fibroma | **Chondromyxoid Fibroma**

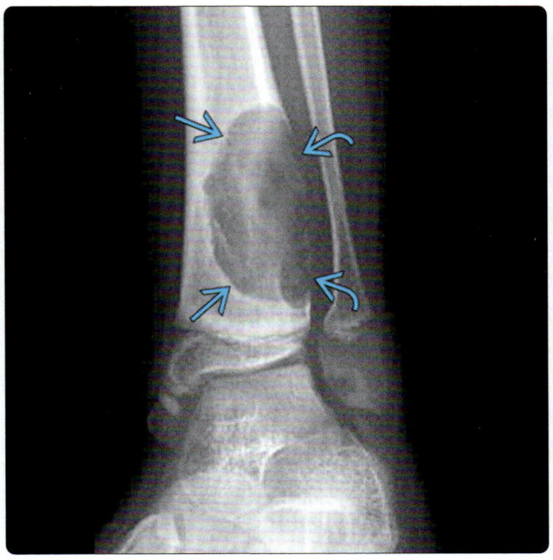

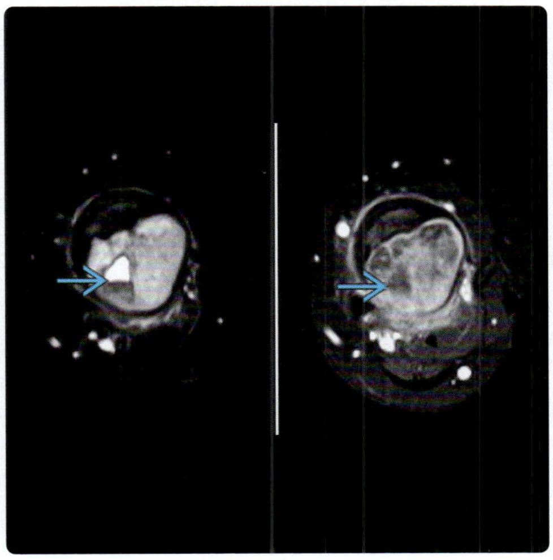

(Left) *Oblique radiograph in a 7-year-old boy with a well-circumscribed lytic lesion in the distal left tibia* → *shows thinning & destruction of the lateral tibial cortex* ↷. **(Right)** *Axial T2 FS (left) & T1 C+ FS (right) MR images in the same child show a focal cystic area that contains a fluid-fluid level* →, *suggesting a secondary ABC. On the postcontrast images, the majority of the lesion enhanced. Pathology showed a chondromyxoid fibroma with a small secondary ABC.*

Osteofibrous Dysplasia/Adamantinoma | **Giant Cell Tumor**

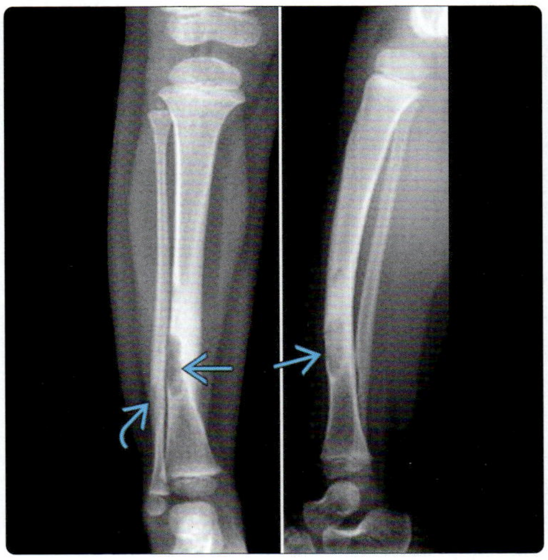

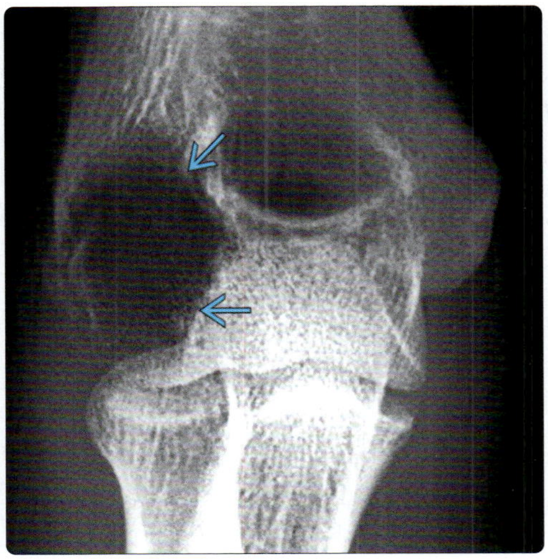

(Left) *Frontal & lateral radiographs of the right leg in a 2-year old girl with osteofibrous dysplasia show a tibial lesion with lytic* → *& sclerotic components. There is associated anterior tibial bowing. A more subtle lesion is also present in the distal fibula* ↷. **(Right)** *AP radiograph shows a lytic lesion* → *within the distal lateral humerus. Note closed growth plates & extension of the lesion to the articular surface. Although benign, giant cell tumors have a tendency for bone destruction & local recurrence with rare metastasis.*

DIFFERENTIAL DIAGNOSIS

Common

- Fibroxanthomas

Less Common

- Enchondromas
- Osteochondromas
- Fibrous Dysplasia, Polyostotic
- Langerhans Cell Histiocytosis

Rare but Important

- Generalized Lymphatic Anomaly
- Brown Tumors
- Trevor-Fairbank Disease
- Infantile Myofibromatosis
- Osteopoikilosis & Osteopathia Striata
- Melorheostosis

ESSENTIAL INFORMATION

Key Differential Diagnosis Issues

- Many of these lesions can be solitary or multiple
    - Numerous lesions may indicate syndromic association
        - e.g., Jaffe-Campanacci, Maffucci
- Imaging of nonaggressive bone lesions in children
    - Radiographs classically show
        - Narrow zone of transition (well defined)
        - Absent or nonaggressive periosteal reaction
            - Smooth, solid, &/or continuous
        - ± expansile remodeling
    - Multifocal, nonaggressive bone lesions in children may have pathognomonic radiographic appearance
        - Fibroxanthomas, osteochondromas, & enchondromas
            - These typically do **not** need further investigation
            - Advanced imaging (e.g., MR) can be used to assess for complications or preoperative planning
    - Assessment of entire skeleton (via skeletal survey, whole-body MR, &/or nuclear medicine imaging) can determine
        - Extent of disease
        - Most easily biopsied lesion (if diagnosis is unclear)
        - Response to therapy

Helpful Clues for Common Diagnoses

- **Fibroxanthomas**
    - Developmental defect, usually discovered incidentally
    - Encompasses fibrous cortical defect (FCD) & nonossifying fibroma (NOF)
        - FCD: < 2-3 cm, within cortex
        - NOF: > 2-3 cm, extends into medullary cavity
    - Age: 2-20 years
    - M:F = 2:1; 30-40% of all children
    - Typically at metadiaphyseal region of long bones, most commonly around knee
    - Radiographs: Eccentric, bubbly, multiloculated, subcortical, lucent lesion with sclerotic border
        - Often has scalloped margin
        - Cortex may be mildly expanded or appear absent
        - Lacks periosteal reaction unless fracture (or, less commonly, infection) is superimposed
        - Gradual ossification/regression of lesions
    - MR: Variable T2 signal intensity & enhancement with hypointense (sclerotic) rim
    - Usually asymptomatic, requiring no treatment
        - Involvement of > 50% diameter of weight-bearing bone increases risk of pathologic fracture
        - Curettage & bone grafting to prevent fracture
    - Fibroxanthomas are often multiple
        - Consider Jaffe-Campanacci syndrome if widespread
            - Café au lait lesions, intellectual disability, hypogonadism, ocular & cardiovascular anomalies

Helpful Clues for Less Common Diagnoses

- **Enchondromas**
    - Thought to be due to displaced rests of physeal cartilage
    - Most commonly affect small tubular bones of hands & feet + ribs
        - Typically central in location, especially in long bones
    - Radiographs: Well-defined lucent lesion with endosteal scalloping & marginal sclerosis
        - ± chondroid matrix: Dots, arcs, or rings of Ca^{2+}
        - ± mild expansile remodeling of bone
    - Enchondromatoses: Conditions with multiple enchondromas
        - Typical medullary lesions plus
            - Intracortical & periosteal (juxtacortical) chondromas, which may mimic osteochondromas
            - Linear metaphyseal/diaphyseal columns of cartilage extending from physes
        - Ollier disease: May be unilateral with lucent metaphyseal streaks & eccentric surface lesions
        - Maffucci syndrome: Multiple enchondromas + soft tissue slow-flow vascular anomalies
            - Phleboliths in soft tissues are due to venous malformation-like spindle cell hemangiomas
            - Predisposition to multiple malignancies
    - Multiple enchondromas are common in hand phalanges without enchondromatosis
- **Osteochondromas**
    - Common benign bone lesion arising from displaced physeal cartilage
    - Most common in long bone metaphyses (70%); less common in ribs, scapula, pelvis
    - Pedunculated or sessile with cortical & medullary continuity to parent bone
        - Multiple hereditary exostoses (MHE) can mimic dysplasia
    - Cartilage cap thickness is variable during childhood
    - Malignant degeneration is very rare in childhood
        - Growth after skeletal maturity or pain raises concern for malignant degeneration
            - Increased risk in patients with MHE
            - Pain is more commonly due to exostosis fracture or irritation of overlying soft tissues ± bursa
        - Other complications include: Angular deformities, neurovascular impingement
- **Fibrous Dysplasia, Polyostotic**
    - Age: 5-20 years
    - Radiographs: Monostotic or polyostotic expansile lesion with endosteal scalloping

- Typically lucent to ground-glass (i.e., smudged/frosted) matrix
- No periostitis unless pathologic fracture
- Less commonly: Mixed lucent & sclerotic

- MR: Variable; active lesions are T2 bright with enhancement
- CT: May be helpful to confirm characteristic matrix if radiographs & MR are unclear
- McCune-Albright: Precocious puberty, café au lait spots, & polyostotic fibrous dysplasia
- Mazabraud: Polyostotic FD with intramuscular myxoma; rare

- **Langerhans Cell Histiocytosis**
  - Benign neoplasm of atypical Langerhans cells
  - Age: 50% < 10 years
  - Single-system, unifocal or multifocal disease vs. multisystem disease
    - Involvement: Bones (80-90%) > skin (50%) > viscera
    - Skull (50%), axial skeleton (25%), long bones (15%)
  - Radiographs: Lytic, sharply demarcated lesion without sclerotic margin (unless healing)
    - Axial skeleton
      - "Punched-out" skull lesions ± "beveled edge"; spiculated periosteal reaction & permeation is not typical
      - Classic cause of vertebra plana
    - Appendicular skeleton
      - Nonaggressive to aggressive appearance; expansion is rare
      - One of classic "flat bone" lesions
  - MR: Bone defect is typically filled with enhancing soft tissue, but large soft tissue mass is not typical
    - May have disproportionate surrounding marrow edema compared to overlying soft tissues

Helpful Clues for Rare Diagnoses

- **Generalized Lymphatic Anomaly**
  - Often called "lymphangiomatosis" of bone
  - Numerous cystic lesions of all bones; may be expansile
  - Some bone lesions will show increased fat deposition
  - Splenic & pleural involvement frequent, ± discrete macrocystic soft tissue lymphatic malformations (LM)
  - Gorham-Stout: Destruction of adjacent bones at one location from microcystic LM
- **Brown Tumors**
  - Can occur in 1° or 2° hyperparathyroidism (HPTH) with renal osteocystrophy
  - Nonaggressive expansile lucent lesions
    - Geographic nonsclerotic margins; no cortical destruction, periosteal reaction, or matrix
    - Look for systemic changes of HPTH, including classic sites of bone resorption & tendon/ligament rupture
- **Trevor-Fairbank Disease**
  - a.k.a. dysplasia epiphysealis hemimelica, Trevor disease
  - Intraarticular osteochondroma-like lesion arising from epiphysis or epiphyseal equivalent
  - In young children with much unossified cartilage, these lesions may mimic
    - Accessory ossification centers
    - Loose intraarticular bodies
  - Can be monoarticular or involve 1 side of multiple joints of extremity (unilateral)
- **Infantile Myofibromatosis**
  - Relatively symmetric distribution of well-defined metaphyseal/metadiaphyseal lucent lesions
  - May show expansion &/or frank cortical lysis
  - Involved bones may have bizarre morphology
- **Osteopoikilosis & Osteopathia Striata**
  - Asymptomatic disorders of endochondral ossification
  - Osteopoikilosis: Multiple enostoses; may be associated with dermatofibrosis lenticularis disseminata
  - Osteopathia striata: Sclerotic striations
- **Melorheostosis**
  - Abnormal endochondral & intramembranous ossification
  - Cortical & medullary hyperostosis of 1 or more adjacent bones: Dripping candle wax appearance
  - Can be associated with joint contractures, muscular atrophy, & skin changes

Fibroxanthomas

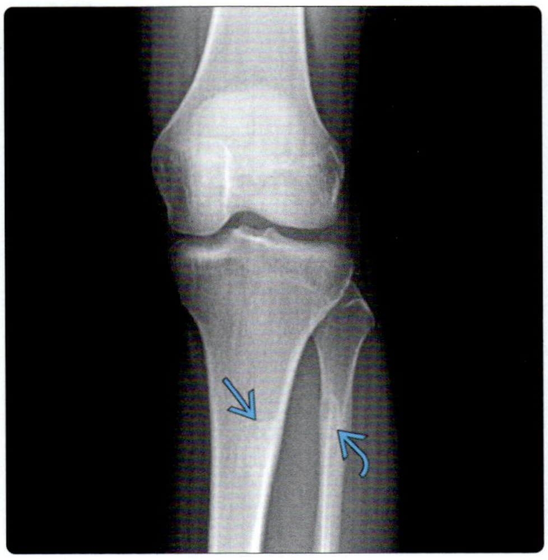

Fibroxanthomas

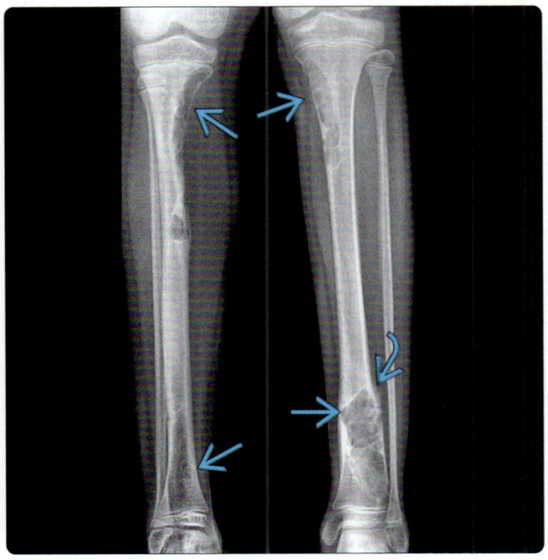

(Left) *AP radiograph in a 16-year-old girl with left knee pain shows fibroxanthomas in the proximal tibia → & proximal fibula →. The majority of fibroxanthomas are detected incidentally, as in this patient. They may be multiple without syndromic association.* **(Right)** *AP radiograph in a 10-year-old girl with Jaffe-Campanacci syndrome shows multiple fibroxanthomas in the bilateral tibiae →. Periosteal reaction → along the distal left tibial lesion is due to a healing pathologic fracture.*

(**Left**) *Oblique radiograph shows multiple lucent lesions in the hand ➔, predominantly central & diaphyseal in location, with associated endosteal scalloping. Faint cartilage matrix can be seen within some of the lesions, though this is not always the case. Several lesions are eccentric & expansile.* (**Right**) *Lateral radiograph shows linear lucent striations → extending into the femoral diaphysis from the physis. An eccentric surface enchondroma is also seen in the fibula ⇨. The findings are typical of enchondromatosis.*

Enchondromas

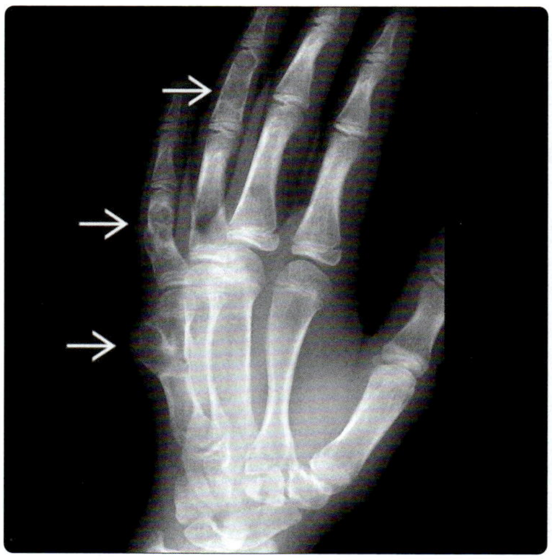

Enchondromas

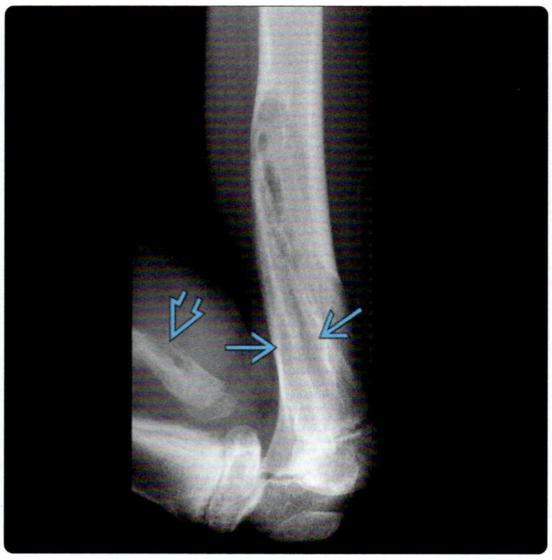

(**Left**) *AP radiograph in a 13-year-old boy with multiple hereditary exostoses shows sessile & pedunculated osteochondromas arising from the distal femurs, proximal tibiae, & proximal fibulae.* (**Right**) *Axial T2 FS MR images at different levels of the left knee in the same child show multiple osteochondromas extending off the distal femur & proximal tibia, most of which have small, bright cartilaginous caps →. These lesions are deforming the normal femoral & tibial morphologies.*

Osteochondromas

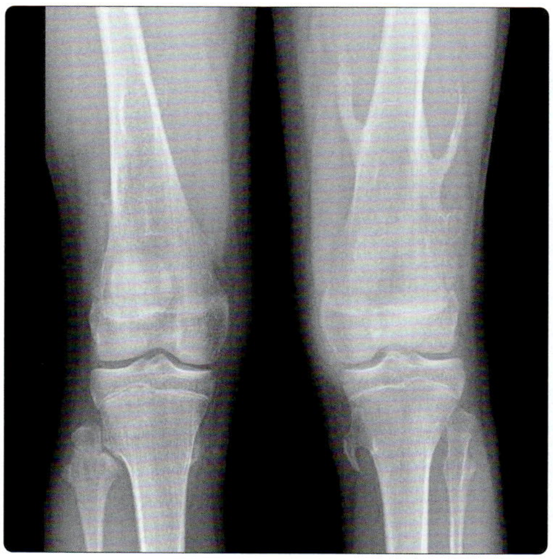

Osteochondromas

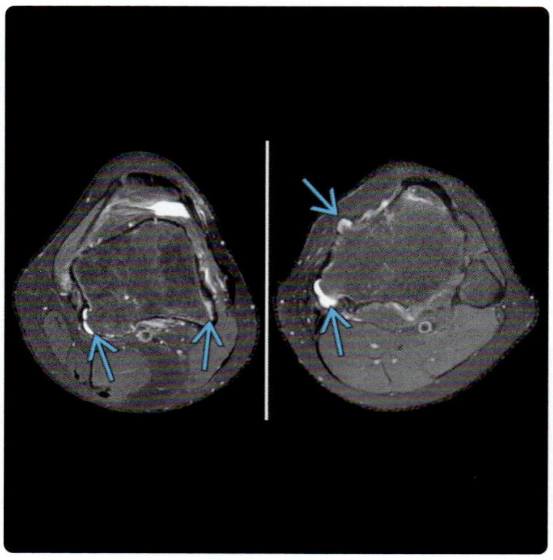

(**Left**) *AP radiographs of the lower legs in a 12 year old with polyostotic fibrous dysplasia show multiple mildly expansile fibular → & tibial ⇨ diaphyseal lesions with a classic ground-glass matrix.* (**Right**) *AP radiograph in a 2-year-old girl with left hip pain shows a nonaggressive-appearing lucent lesion → in the intertrochanteric left proximal femur.*

Fibrous Dysplasia, Polyostotic

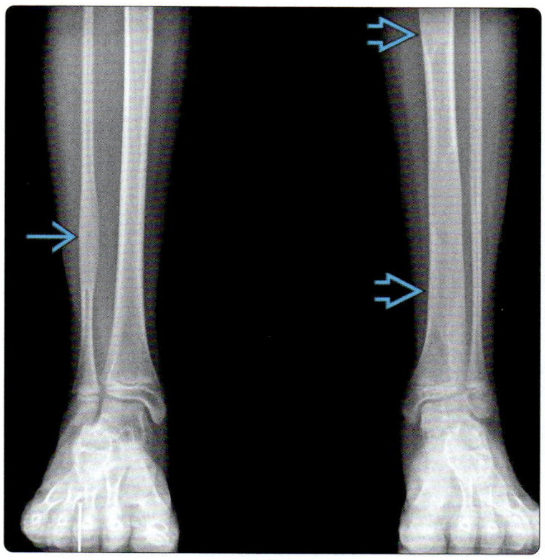

Langerhans Cell Histiocytosis

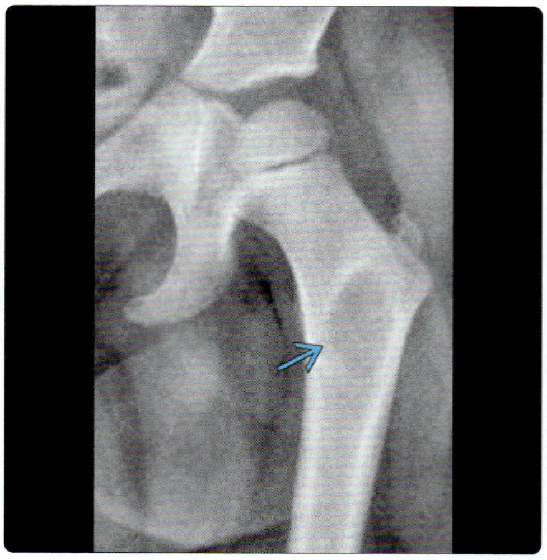

Langerhans Cell Histiocytosis

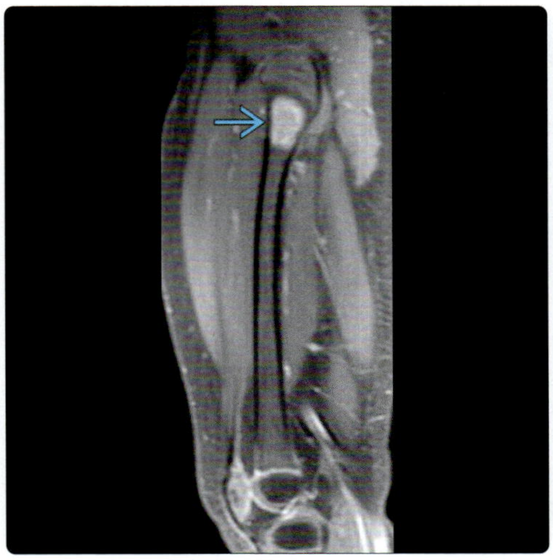

Generalized Lymphatic Anomaly

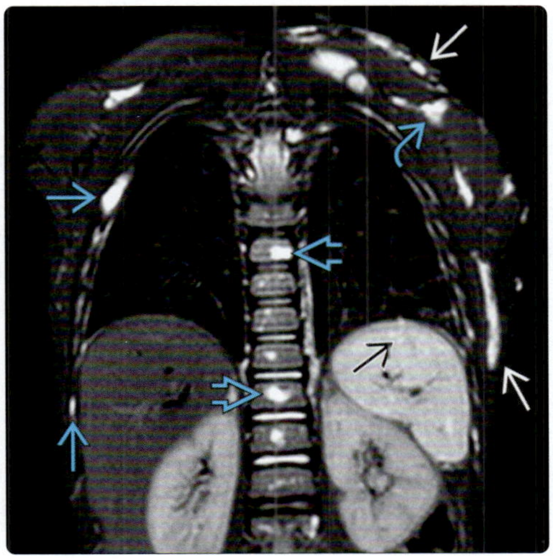

(Left) *Sagittal T1 C+ FS MR from the same child shows moderate homogeneous enhancement of the well-defined lesion* → *in proximal femur. LCH bone lesions can range in appearance from nonaggressive, as in this child, to aggressive with frank cortical destruction.* **(Right)** *Coronal STIR MR in a 4 year old with generalized lymphatic anomaly shows multiple cystic-appearing lesions of vertebrae* ⇨*, ribs* →*, & left scapula* ↗*. Additional lesions are seen in soft tissues* ➡ *& spleen* ⇨*.*

Brown Tumors

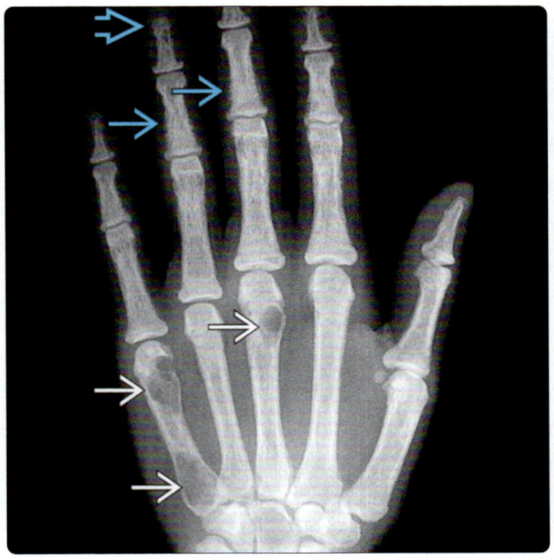

Trevor-Fairbank Disease

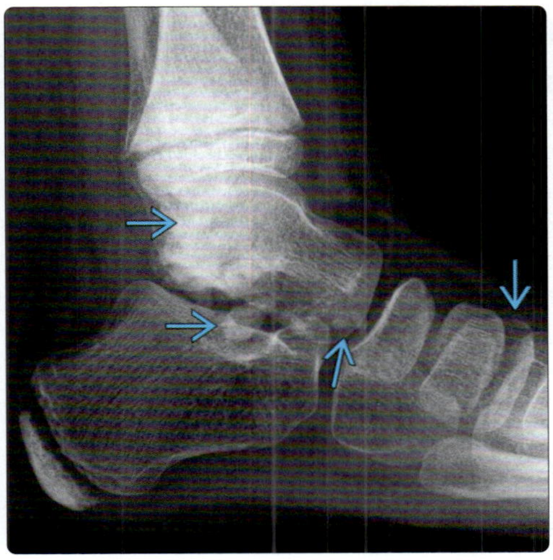

(Left) *PA radiograph shows findings of renal osteodystrophy & secondary hyperparathyroidism in a teenager with end-stage renal disease. There is subperiosteal* → *& tuft* ⇨ *resorption of the phalanges with multiple lucent lesions* ➡ *due to brown tumors.* **(Right)** *Lateral radiograph in a 7 year old with ankle pain shows numerous small ossific bodies* → *about the ankle. These bony foci were due to incompletely ossified exostoses arising from epiphyseal equivalent bones of the hindfoot & midfoot as well as the fibular epiphysis.*

Osteopoikilosis & Osteopathia Striata

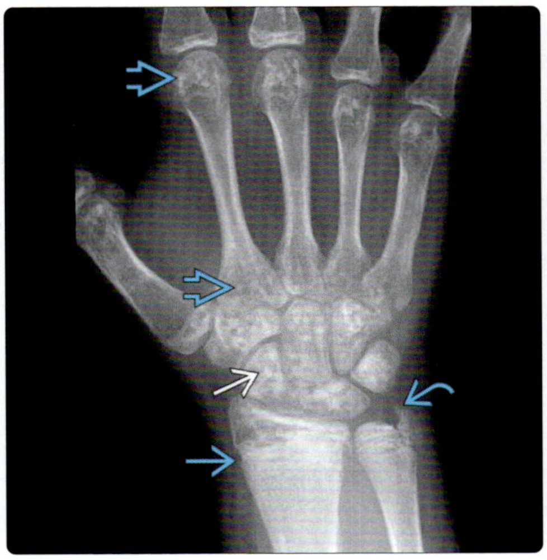

Melorheostosis

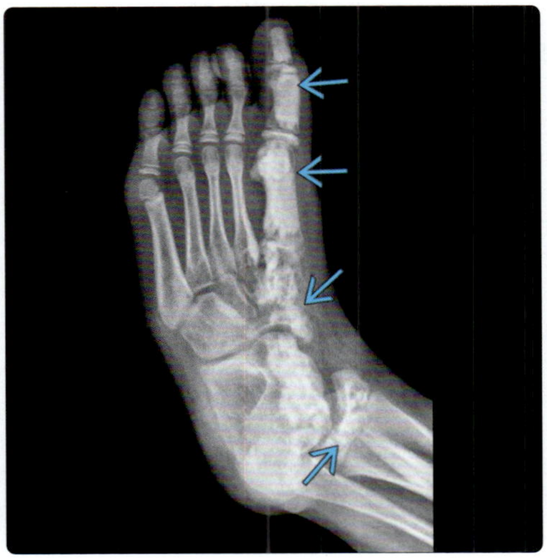

(Left) *PA radiograph of the wrist in a 16 year old following distal radial* → *& ulnar styloid* ↗ *fractures shows multiple enostoses (bone islands) throughout the carpals* ➡ *& metacarpals* ⇨*. These were found incidentally due to the fractures.* **(Right)** *Oblique foot radiograph in a 12 year old shows geographic sclerotic lesions* → *of the 1st digit, medial tarsals, & distal tibia. Melorheostosis often follows a sclerotome distribution, giving a dripping candle wax appearance of adjacent bones.*

DIFFERENTIAL DIAGNOSIS

Common

- Neuroblastoma
- Leukemia
- Osteomyelitis (Pyogenic)

Less Common

- Chronic Recurrent Multifocal Osteomyelitis
- Langerhans Cell Histiocytosis
- Rhabdomyosarcoma
- Ewing Sarcoma
- Lymphoma
- Osteosarcoma

Rare but Important

- Retinoblastoma
- Medulloblastoma
- Clear Cell Sarcoma of Kidney
- Infantile Myofibromatosis
- Congenital Syphilis

ESSENTIAL INFORMATION

Key Differential Diagnosis Issues

- Imaging of aggressive bone lesions in children
  - Radiographs: Wide zone of transition (ill defined), aggressive periosteal reaction (e.g., lamellated, spiculated, interrupted), cortical destruction
    - Extensive marrow lesions may be subtle/occult
  - MR: May be confluent & extensive or discrete, well-circumscribed lesions with sharp interfaces against normal fatty marrow
    - T1 is best for defining margins of tumor
    - Majority of lesions are T2 bright; T2 dark lesions are typically seen with sclerosis
    - Enhancement variable; extensive marrow lesions may show superimposed foci of necrosis/infarction
    - ± periosteal reaction, soft tissue mass
  - Skeletal survey, whole-body MR, &/or nuclear medicine imaging (i.e., bone scan or PET/CT) can help determine
    - Extent/staging of disease
    - Most easily biopsied lesion
    - Response to therapy
  - While some imaging features may suggest specific entity, biopsy is almost always required
    - Metastatic bone disease is common cause for multifocal aggressive bone lesions (though lung metastases are more frequent with MSK sarcomas)
    - Generally looks similar regardless of specific primary
      - Most lesions are lytic; can be sclerotic or mixed
      - Some malignancies favor sclerotic over lytic
- In children, residual red marrow & red marrow reconversion must be distinguished from pathologic marrow infiltration
  - Red marrow will have normal radiographs but can mimic multifocal marrow replacement on MR
  - Keys to diagnosing red marrow
    - Iso- to mildly hyperintense on T1 MR compared to skeletal muscle & intervertebral discs
    - In long bones, often flame-shaped in metaphyses
    - Drops signal on opposed-phase MR

Helpful Clues for Common Diagnoses

- **Neuroblastoma**
  - Malignant tumor of sympathetic chain neural crest
    - Primary tumor: Adrenal > extraadrenal retroperitoneum > posterior mediastinum
  - Most common pediatric cause of bone metastases
    - Up to 60% have skeletal metastases
      - Can present with pain & limp
    - Liver metastases are also common
  - Median age of 15-17 months at diagnosis
- **Leukemia**
  - Often has diffuse skeletal involvement & may initially present with bone pain
  - Spectrum of radiographic findings: Normal, diffuse osteoporosis, lucent metaphyseal bands (leukemic lines), periosteal reaction , bone destruction, sclerosis, pathologic fracture, chloroma
- **Osteomyelitis (Pyogenic)**
  - Can be multifocal, particularly in children with septicemia
  - Early radiographs can be normal but can progress to aggressive-appearing in lesions ~ 2 weeks
  - MR (as compared to neoplasms)
    - Margins less well-defined against normal marrow fat
    - Soft tissue edema & fluid collections are more likely

Helpful Clues for Less Common Diagnoses

- **Chronic Recurrent Multifocal Osteomyelitis**
  - Multifocal nonpyogenic inflammatory bone lesions with relapsing/remitting course
  - Associated with other inflammatory conditions (e.g., psoriasis, inflammatory bowel disease)
  - Typically involves periphyseal regions
  - Most common sites: Tibia, femur, spine, pelvis, clavicle
    - Multiple sites over course of disease in ~ 80%
      - Can be bilateral & relatively symmetric
    - Medial clavicular involvement suggests chronic recurrent multifocal osteomyelitis
  - Radiographs: Features may be mixed at presentation
    - Acute: Lytic lesion (usually in metaphysis near physis)
    - Late: Progressive adjacent sclerosis
    - Recurrence: New lytic areas or periosteal reaction
  - MR: Enhancement of lesion & surrounding marrow
    - ± soft tissue & periosteal edema (but no abscess)
    - ± reactive adjacent joint effusion/synovitis
- **Langerhans Cell Histiocytosis**
  - Benign neoplasm of atypical Langerhans cells
  - Axial skeleton
    - Well-defined lytic skull lesions without sclerotic rim are characteristic ("punched-out")
    - Classic cause of vertebra plana
  - Appendicular skeleton
    - Aggressive features > nonaggressive
  - Sensitivity of screening studies for suspected Langerhans cell histiocytosis: PET > skeletal survey > bone scan
- **Rhabdomyosarcoma**
  - Most common soft tissue sarcoma in children
- **Ewing Sarcoma**
  - Ewing sarcoma (ES) family of tumors
    - Aggressive small round blue cell tumors

– Includes: Osseous ES, extraosseous (soft tissue) ES, & Askin tumor (extraskeletal ES of chest)
- **Lymphoma**
  - Bone involvement can be secondary or primary
    - Primary lymphoma of bone is rare
  - Variable appearance
    - Typically lucent, permeative lesions
      - ± areas of sclerosis, periosteal reaction
    - Can be radiographically occult despite extensive marrow involvement
    - MR tends to show aggressive marrow lesions without significant extraosseous extension
      - May demonstrate geographic foci of decreased medullary enhancement in tumor
- **Osteosarcoma**
  - Most common malignant primary bone tumor in children
  - Bone metastases may be blastic

Helpful Clues for Rare Diagnoses

- **Retinoblastoma**
  - Malignant primary retinal neoplasm of young children
  - May have blastic bone metastases
- **Medulloblastoma**
  - Malignant posterior fossa tumor
  - May have blastic bone metastases
- **Clear Cell Sarcoma of Kidney**
  - Rare malignant renal tumor in young children
  - Metastases: Lymph nodes, bone, lung
- **Infantile Myofibromatosis**
  - Solitary or multifocal soft tissue mass(es) in infant, often distorting adjacent bone
  - Multifocal bone lesions are rare but classically lucent, well-defined, & relatively symmetric in metaphyses
- **Congenital Syphilis**
  - Lucent metaphyseal bands are typical
  - Wimberger corner sign: Lytic proximal medial tibial lesion

SELECTED REFERENCES

1. Smets AM et al: Whole-body magnetic resonance imaging for detection of skeletal metastases in children and young people with primary solid tumors - systematic review. Pediatr Radiol. 48(2):241-52, 2018

Neuroblastoma

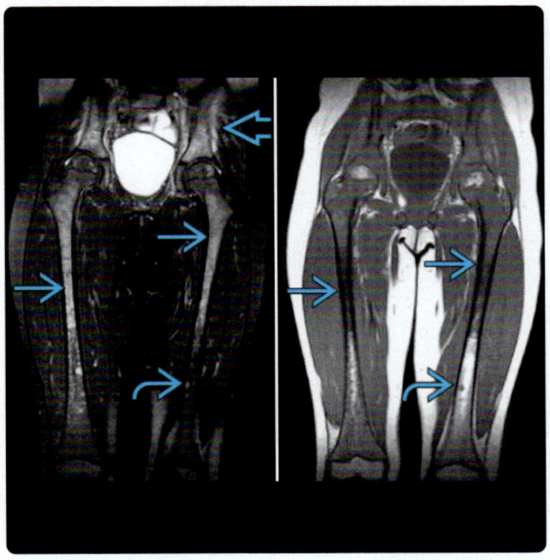

Neuroblastoma

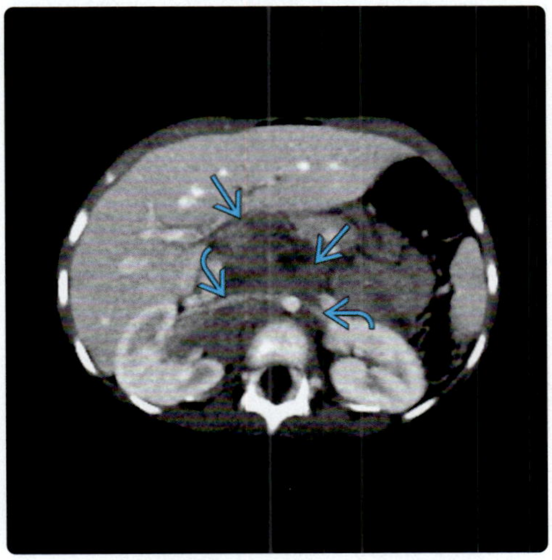

(Left) *Coronal T2 FS (left) & T1 (right) MR images in a 4 year old with left hip pain & limping show widespread bony metastases. Some lesions are extensive & confluent ➔, some are small & well defined ➔, & some show periosteal edema ➔.* **(Right)** *Axial CECT of the abdomen in the same patient shows a midline lobulated mass ➔ encasing the aorta & renal arteries ➔, typical of neuroblastoma in a young child.*

Leukemia

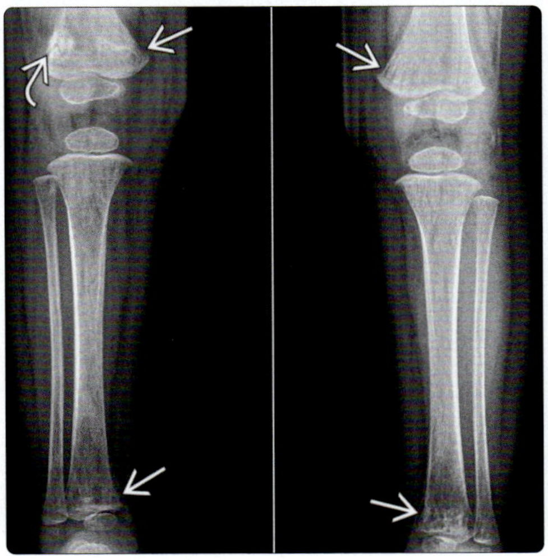

Osteomyelitis (Pyogenic)

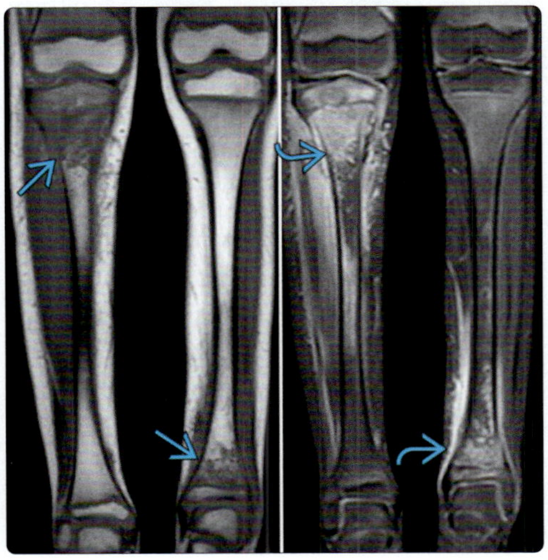

(Left) *AP radiographs of the legs show poorly defined lucent & sclerotic lesions ➔ within the bilateral distal femoral, distal tibial, & distal fibular metaphyses with a pathologic fracture in the right femur ➔.* **(Right)** *Coronal T1 (left) & STIR (right) MR images in a 6 year old with leg pain & limping show poorly defined areas of low signal ➔ & high signal ➔, respectively, in the distal left tibia & proximal right tibia. There is adjacent periosteal edema in both regions. The findings are typical of pyogenic osteomyelitis.*

(Left) *AP radiograph (top) in a 4-year-old girl with right clavicle & bilateral ankle pain shows expansion & permeation of the right medial clavicle →. On coronal STIR MR (bottom), there is increased signal within & periosteal reaction along the right clavicle → with adjacent soft tissue inflammation →.* **(Right)** *Frontal radiographs of both ankles in the same child with chronic recurrent multifocal osteomyelitis show lucent lesions in the bilateral distal tibial metaphyses with cortical thinning & layered periosteal reaction →.*

Chronic Recurrent Multifocal Osteomyelitis

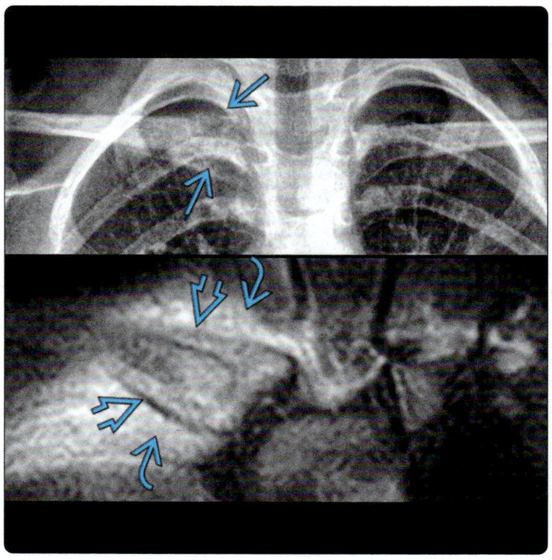

Chronic Recurrent Multifocal Osteomyelitis

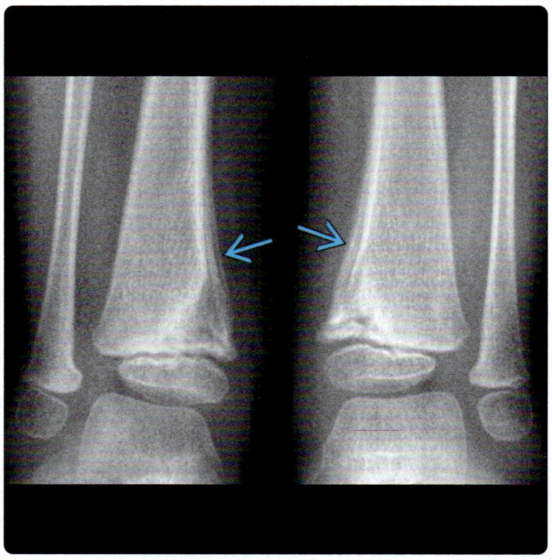

(Left) *Radiographs of the proximal humeri (top) & femurs (bottom) in a 2 year old presenting with a limp show lytic lesions in the bilateral proximal humeral & femoral metadiaphyses with frank cortical destruction →, typical of LCH. Also note the lytic lesions in the bilateral femoral heads →.* **(Right)** *Radiographs of the thoracic spine & skull in the same child show innumerable lytic lesions. Also note the thoracic vertebra plana deformity →. While not specific, LCH is the classic cause of pediatric vertebra plana.*

Langerhans Cell Histiocytosis

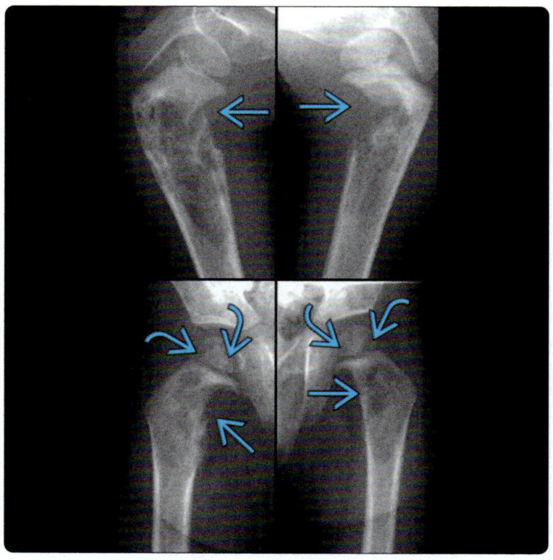

Langerhans Cell Histiocytosis

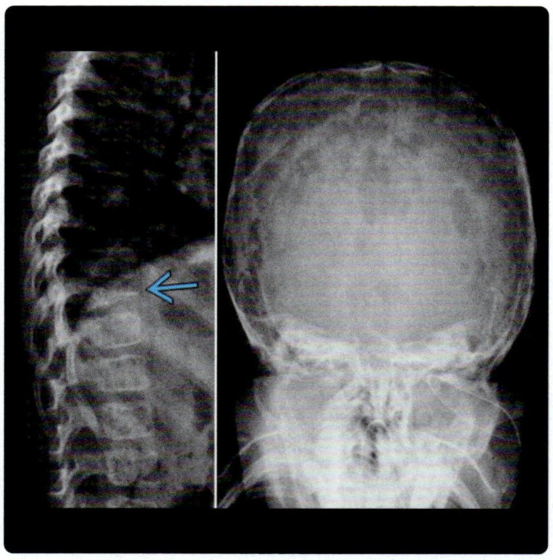

(Left) *Coronal NECT of the chest in a 12 year old with metastatic rhabdomyosarcoma shows multiple lytic lesions throughout the vertebral bodies, in the right 9th rib →, & in the right scapula →. Note the compression deformity of the 10th vertebral body → from a pathologic fracture.* **(Right)** *Axial NECT shows diffuse mixed lytic & sclerotic metastases → within the iliac wings & sacrum from Ewing sarcoma.*

Rhabdomyosarcoma

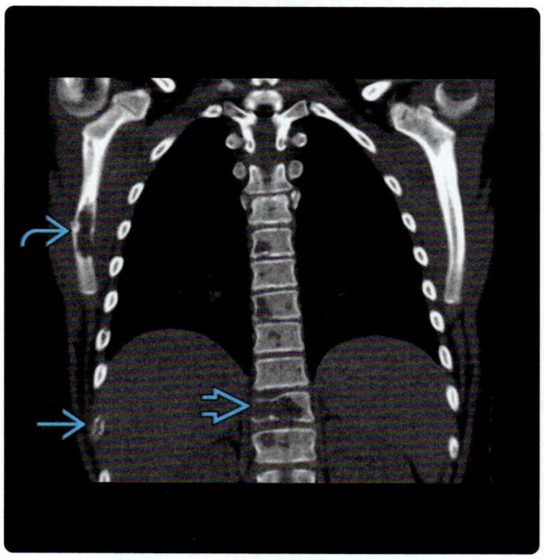

Ewing Sarcoma

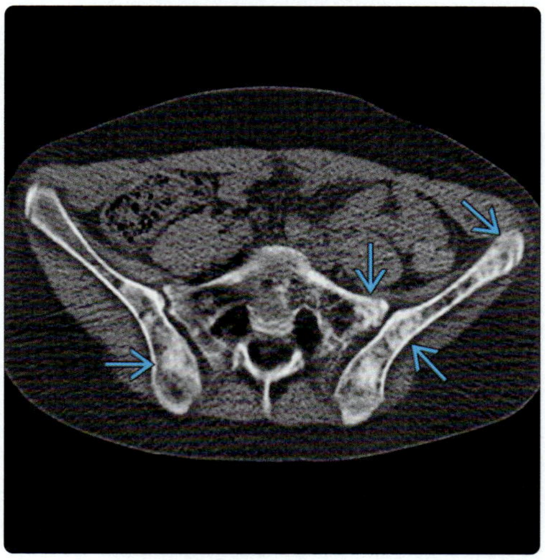

Lymphoma

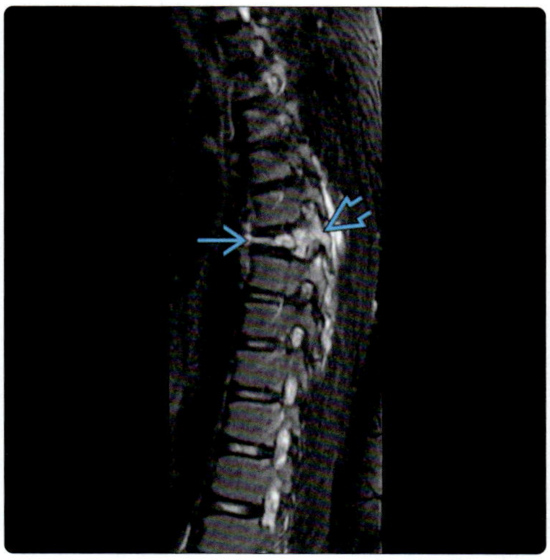

Lymphoma

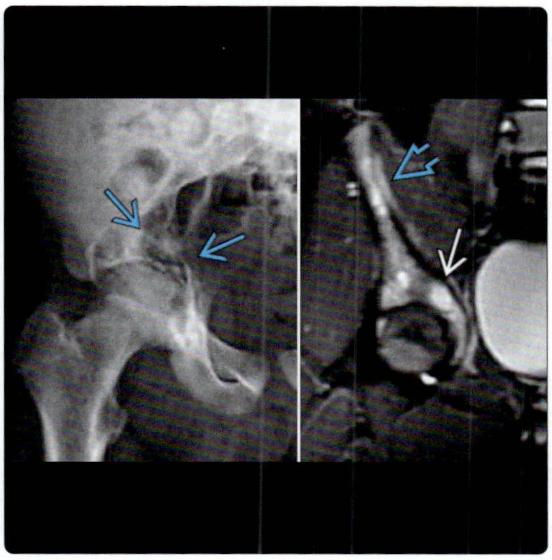

(Left) *Sagittal STIR MR of the thoracic spine in a 14 year old with back pain shows T5 vertebra plana. Also note the diffusely increased signal intensity throughout the T5 vertebra, including the posterior elements.* **(Right)** *Radiograph (left) of the right hip in the same patient shows an aggressive lesion in the right acetabulum. Coronal STIR MR (right) shows the acetabular lesion & an additional lesion in the right ilium. LCH was suspected, but biopsy showed lymphoma.*

Osteosarcoma

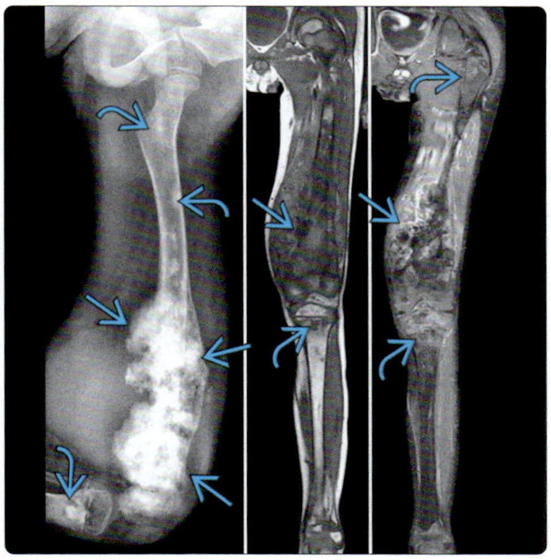

Retinoblastoma

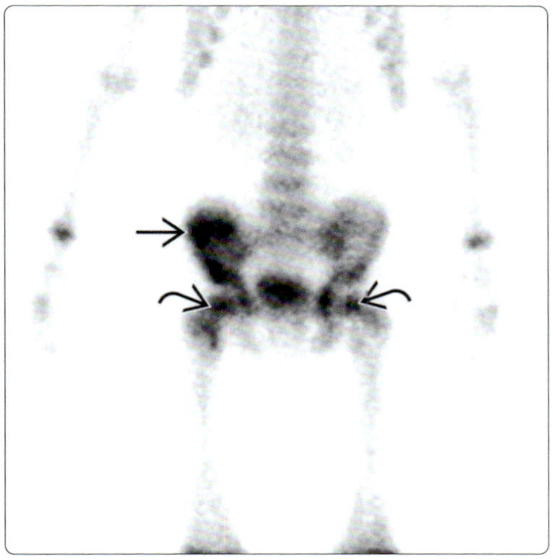

(Left) *Right femur radiograph (left), T1 MR (middle), & T1 C+ FS MR (right) images in a 5 year old presenting with right femur pain show a distal femoral osteosarcoma. Metastatic lesions are seen in the femur & tibia.* **(Right)** *Anterior nuclear medicine bone scan in a child with retinoblastoma shows increased radiopharmaceutical uptake within metastatic disease in the right iliac wing & bilateral proximal femurs.*

Infantile Myofibromatosis

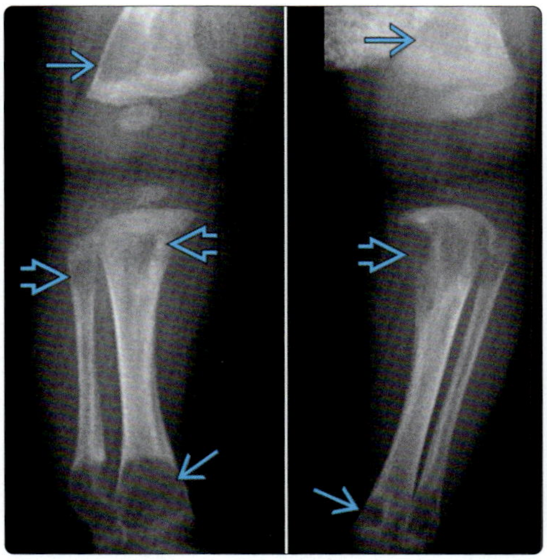

Congenital Syphilis

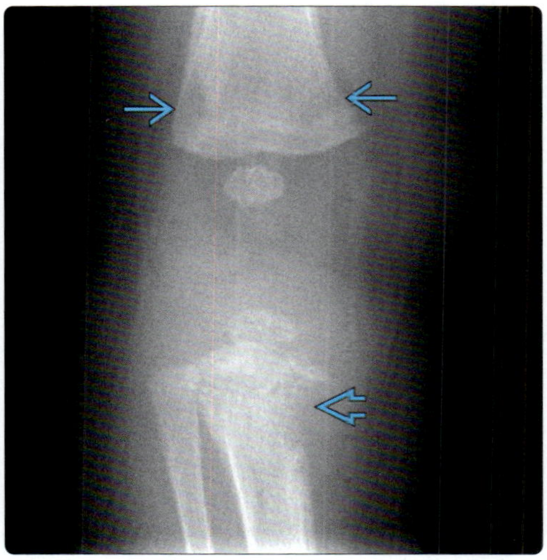

(Left) *AP radiographs of lower legs in a 2 month old show lucent lesions in all metadiaphyses. Some lesions show indolent features of expansion & narrow zones of transition, while others show cortical destruction with wide zones of transition. Biopsy confirmed infantile myofibromatosis.* **(Right)** *AP knee radiograph in a patient with congenital syphilis (CS) shows multiple lucent metaphyseal lesions. The proximal tibial lesion shows permeation & medial cortical destruction, typical of the Wimberger corner sign in CS.*

DIFFERENTIAL DIAGNOSIS

Common

- Physiologic Red Marrow (Mimic)
- Red Marrow Reconversion
- Neoplastic Marrow Replacement

Less Common

- Chemotherapy/Radiation Therapy
- Iron Overload Syndromes

Rare but Important

- Gaucher Disease
- Serous Atrophy of Bone Marrow
- Osteopetrosis

ESSENTIAL INFORMATION

Helpful Clues for Common Diagnoses

- **Physiologic Red Marrow (Mimic)**
  - Conversion of hematopoietic red to fatty yellow marrow begins shortly after birth & follows predictable pattern
    - Appendicular before axial skeleton
    - Distal before proximal extremities
    - Epiphyses → central diaphysis → metaphyses
      - Metaphyseal red marrow often persists in adults
      - Typically flame-shaped or poorly defined
  - Spin-echo-based T1 MR (best marrow sequence)
    - Iso- or slightly ↑ vs. muscle & intervertebral discs
  - Fluid-sensitive MR sequences (T2 FS or STIR)
    - Typically iso- or slightly ↑ vs. muscle
- **Red Marrow Reconversion**
  - Occurs in reverse order from initial conversion
  - Typically due to increased hematopoietic demand
    - Sickle cell disease & chronic anemias, high altitude
  - Drops signal on opposed-phase vs. in-phase MR
- **Neoplastic Marrow Replacement**
  - Leukemia, lymphoma, metastases (e.g., neuroblastoma)
  - Diffuse confluent or multifocal well-defined marrow lesions ± cortical destruction, periosteal reaction
  - Iso- to ↓ vs. skeletal muscle & intervertebral discs on T1, usually ↑ on T2 FS/STIR MR
  - No drop of signal intensity on opposed-phase MR

Helpful Clues for Less Common Diagnoses

- **Chemotherapy/Radiation Therapy**
  - Chemotherapy
    - Early: Edema (↓ T1 & ↑ T2 FS/STIR)
    - Later: Fatty conversion (↑ T1 & ↓ T2 FS/STIR)
    - Recovery: Regeneration of hematopoietic cells
      - Foci of ↓ T1 & ↑ T2 FS
    - May also lead to iron overload pattern
  - Granulocyte colony stimulating factor (GCSF) → exaggerated diffuse reconversion
  - Radiation therapy: Time & dose dependent
    - Early post radiation: Edema (↓ T1 & ↑ T2 FS)
    - Subacute: Hemorrhage (focal ↑ T1 & ↓ T2 FS)
    - Late: Fatty transformation in port distribution
- **Iron Overload Syndromes**
  - Typically due to transfusion therapy for hereditary anemias; may also be seen with chemotherapy
  - Leads to iron deposition in reticuloendothelial system
    - Liver, spleen, & bone marrow
  - Decreased signal intensity on all pulse sequences

Helpful Clues for Rare Diagnoses

- **Gaucher Disease**
  - Glucosylceramide accumulates in reticuloendothelium
  - Distribution & signal similar to marrow reconversion
  - Other findings typically present: Endosteal scalloping, Erlenmeyer flask deformities (undertubulation), bone infarcts, hepatosplenomegaly
- **Serous Atrophy of Bone Marrow**
  - Typically in patients with severe weight loss & anemia
  - Causes: Severe malnutrition (e.g., anorexia nervosa), malabsorption, malignancies, chronic conditions
  - Marrow & subcutaneous fat: ↓ T1 & ↑ T2 FS
- **Osteopetrosis**
  - Diffuse sclerosis on radiographs; ↓ T1 & T2 on MR

Physiologic Red Marrow (Mimic)

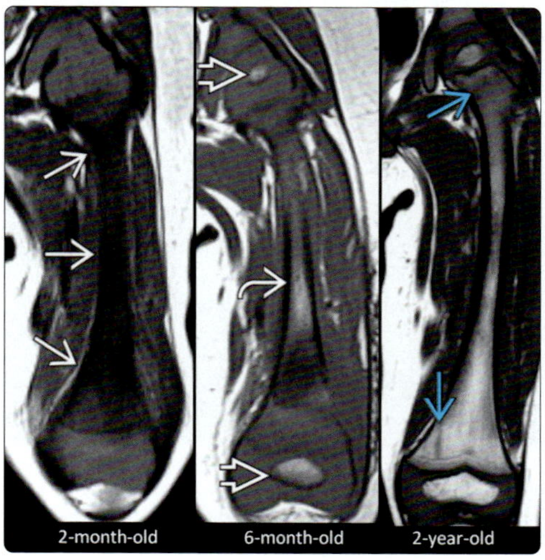

Physiologic Red Marrow (Mimic)

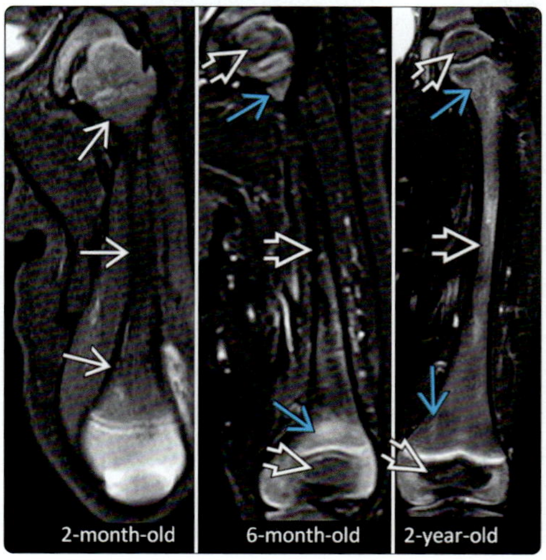

(Left) *Coronal T1 MR images in children of various ages show normal femur marrow patterns. Initially, there is diffuse low-signal red (cellular) marrow. Yellow marrow appears first in the epiphyses & central diaphysis, later progressing to the metaphyses. However, metaphyseal red marrow persists.* **(Right)** *Corresponding coronal STIR MR images show low signal intensity early. Later, epiphyseal & diaphyseal yellow marrow is of lower signal intensity than metaphyseal red marrow.*

Red Marrow Reconversion

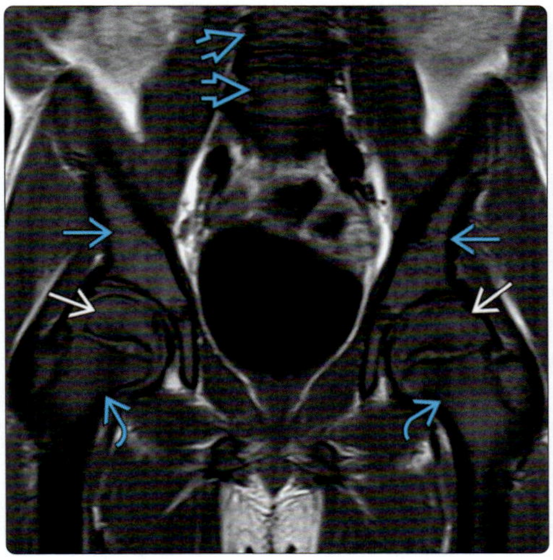

Red Marrow Reconversion

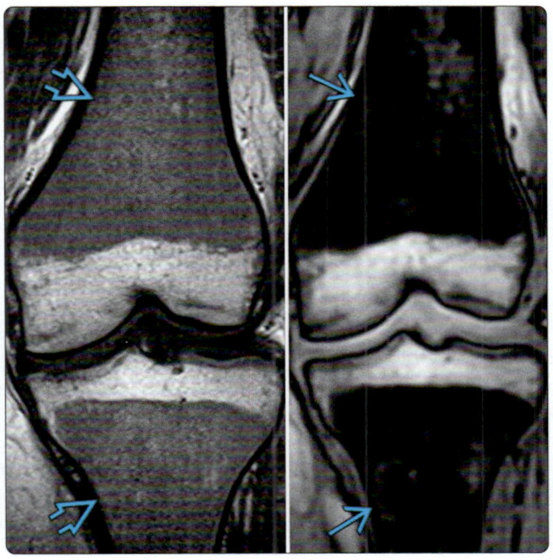

(Left) *Coronal T1 MR in a 7 year old with chronic anemia from sickle cell disease shows an increased volume of intermediate-signal red marrow throughout the pelvis, vertebral bodies, & proximal femurs, including the epiphyses.* **(Right)** *Coronal T1 in- (left) & opposed- (right) phase MR images in a child with sickle cell disease show red marrow in the metadiaphyses that drops signal on the opposed-phase image because of persistent microscopic fat (whereas neoplastic cells would not show signal drop).*

Neoplastic Marrow Replacement

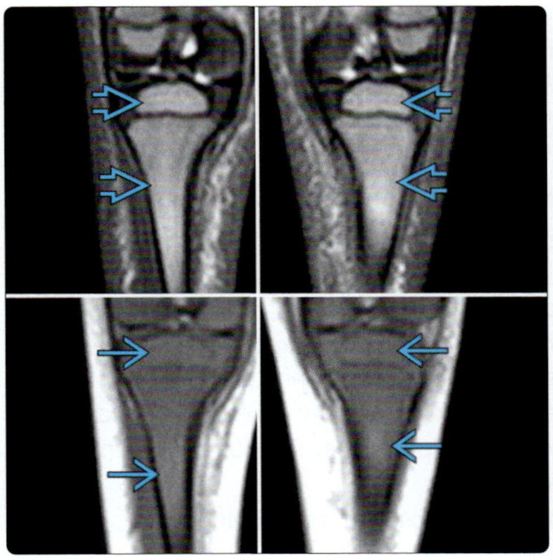

Chemotherapy/Radiation Therapy

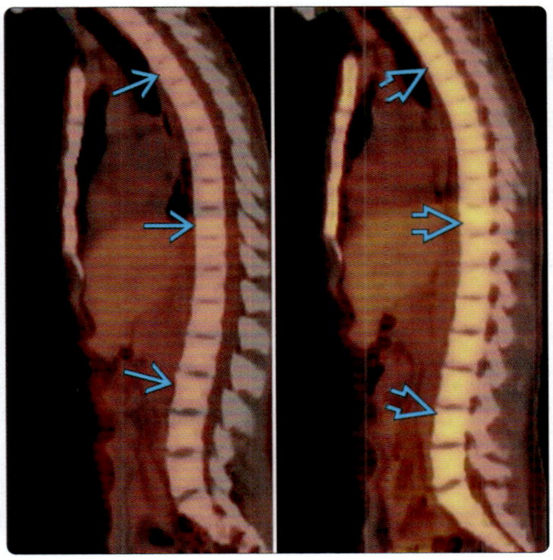

(Left) *Coronal STIR (top) & T1 (bottom) MR images of the legs in a girl with leukemia show diffusely increased STIR & decreased T1 signal intensity.* **(Right)** *Sagittal FDG PET/CT images show therapy-related changes in spinal marrow in a 17 year old on chemotherapy. The left image (pretreatment) shows normal low-level metabolic activity in the vertebral bodies. After chemotherapy & granulocyte-colony stimulating factor (right), there is diffusely increased low-level metabolic activity in the spine due to red marrow stimulation.*

Iron Overload Syndromes

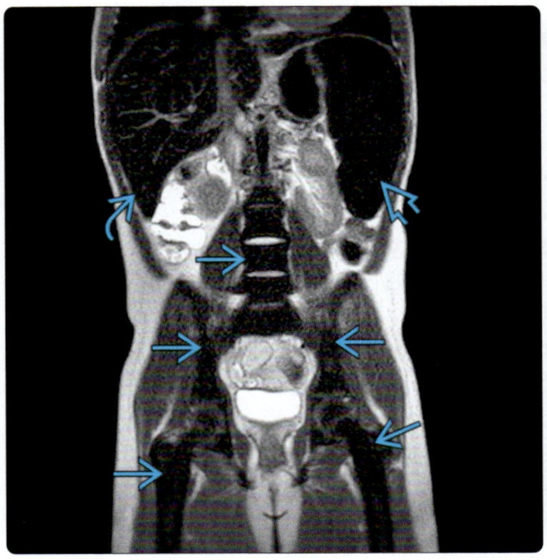

Gaucher Disease

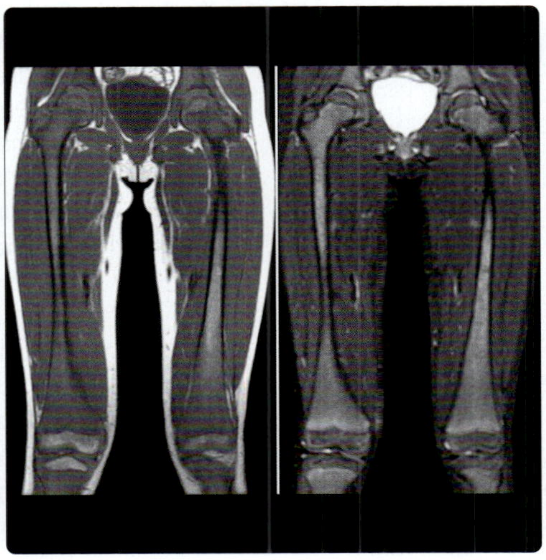

(Left) *Coronal T2 MR in a 14 year old with sickle cell disease shows diffuse low signal intensity throughout the bone marrow secondary to iron deposition. Also note the low signal in the liver & spleen.* **(Right)** *Coronal T1 (left) & STIR (right) MR images in a 6 year old with Gaucher disease show diffusely abnormal marrow of the femurs with intermediate to low T1 & intermediate to high STIR signal intensity. This appearance is due to abnormal marrow accumulation of glucosylceramide.*

Diaphyseal Lesion

DIFFERENTIAL DIAGNOSIS

Common

- Osteoid Osteoma
- Fibrous Dysplasia
- Osteomyelitis (Pyogenic)

Less Common

- Bone Infarcts
- Metastases
- Ewing Sarcoma
- Langerhans Cell Histiocytosis
- Chronic Recurrent Multifocal Osteomyelitis
- Leukemia
- Lymphoma
- Osteosarcoma
- Enchondroma

Rare but Important

- Vascular Anomaly
- Osteofibrous Dysplasia/Adamantinoma
- Chondrosarcoma

ESSENTIAL INFORMATION

Key Differential Diagnosis Issues

- Majority of pediatric bone lesions are found in metaphyses
  - Nonaggressive-appearing lesions (e.g., fibroxanthoma, enchondroma)
    - May start in metaphysis but migrate away from physis as child grows
    - Typically remain in metadiaphyseal region
  - Aggressive-appearing lesions
    - Some preferentially arise in metaphysis (e.g., osteosarcoma, osteomyelitis) & less commonly arise in diaphysis
    - Others preferentially arise in diaphysis (e.g., Ewing sarcoma) & less commonly arise in metaphysis
    - Obtain joint-to-joint long bone MR imaging to look for skip metastases
- Many diaphyseal lesion considerations are small round blue cell tumors
  - Can be indistinguishable from one another
    - Ewing sarcoma
    - Langerhans cell histiocytosis
    - Leukemia
    - Metastases
    - Osteomyelitis & chronic recurrent multifocal osteomyelitis (CRMO)
    - Lymphoma
  - Note that each of these lesions may be polyostotic

Helpful Clues for Common Diagnoses

- **Osteoid Osteoma**
  - Benign neoplasm with nidus of osteoid (< 2 cm)
  - Pain at night relieved by NSAIDs
  - Various types: Cortical (most common), medullary, endosteal, & subperiosteal
    - Diaphyseal lesions are typically cortical
  - Imaging: Cortical thickening ± lucent nidus
    - Surrounding marrow & soft tissue edema is common on MR
      - □ Dynamic T1 C+ FS images show early nidus enhancement
- **Fibrous Dysplasia**
  - Mono- or polyostotic benign fibroosseous lesion
  - Imaging: Expansile lesion(s) with endosteal scalloping
    - Typically lucent to ground-glass (i.e., smudged/frosted) matrix
      - □ Less commonly: Mixed lucent & sclerotic
    - Typically without periosteal reaction unless pathologic fracture occurs
    - MR: Variable, but active lesions are T2 hyperintense with enhancement
      - □ Margins are typically sharp on MR
- **Osteomyelitis (Pyogenic)**
  - Imaging: Pediatric patients typically present prior to bone changes on radiographs
    - Soft tissue swelling is most common early finding; aggressive-appearing bone lesions require ~ 2 weeks
    - MR (as compared to neoplasms)
      - □ Margins are less well-defined against normal marrow fat (especially on T1)
      - □ Soft tissue edema & fluid collections are more likely
    - Subacute/chronic/healing infections (± pathologic fracture): Abnormal radiographs are more likely

Helpful Clues for Less Common Diagnoses

- **Bone Infarcts**
  - Early bone infarcts (particularly dactylitis) present with radiographic periosteal reaction
    - Poorly defined marrow & periosteal edema are frequent on MR; can mimic infection
  - Subacute/chronic infarcts show mixed lucency/sclerosis
    - MR shows well-defined, serpiginous double line sign
- **Metastases**
  - Neuroblastoma is most common etiology
  - Usually polyostotic in children
  - Metaphysis > diaphysis
  - May be diffusely infiltrating with mild periosteal reaction & mottling of bone vs. more focal destructive lesions
- **Ewing Sarcoma**
  - Predilection for long bone diaphysis & flat bones of patients 5-25 years of age
  - Permeative with aggressive periosteal reaction ± mild expansion; MR often shows large soft tissue mass
  - May present with osseous metastases
- **Langerhans Cell Histiocytosis**
  - Benign neoplasm of atypical Langerhans cells
  - Axial skeleton
    - Well-defined lytic skull lesions without sclerotic rim ("punched-out")
    - Classic cause of vertebra plana
  - Appendicular skeleton
    - Aggressive features > nonaggressive
    - Can involve diaphysis, metaphysis, or epiphysis
  - Whole-body imaging to evaluate extent
    - MR, PET, or skeletal survey
- **Chronic Recurrent Multifocal Osteomyelitis**
  - Multifocal nonpyogenic inflammatory bone lesions with relapsing/remitting course

- Associated with other inflammatory conditions (e.g., psoriasis, inflammatory bowel disease)
- Typically periphyseal regions but can involve diaphysis
- Most common sites: Tibia, femur, spine, pelvis, clavicle
  - Multiple sites over course of disease in ~ 80% cases
    - Can be bilateral & relatively symmetric
  - Medial clavicular involvement suggests CRMO
- Radiographic features may be mixed at presentation
  - Acute: Lytic lesion (usually in metaphysis near physis)
  - Late: Progressive adjacent sclerosis
  - Recurrence: New lytic areas or periosteal reaction
- MR: Enhancement of lesion & surrounding marrow
  - ± soft tissue & periosteal edema (but no abscess)
  - ± reactive adjacent joint effusion/synovitis

- **Leukemia**
  - Usually polyostotic
  - Often has diffuse skeletal involvement & may initially present with bone pain
  - Spectrum of radiographic findings: Normal, diffuse osteoporosis, lucent metaphyseal bands ("leukemic lines"), periosteal reaction, bone destruction, sclerosis, pathologic fracture, chloroma
  - MR may show diffuse marrow replacement vs. multifocal lesions
- **Lymphoma**
  - 50% are polyostotic at presentation
  - Metaphyseal are more common than diaphyseal lesions
  - Bone involvement can be secondary or primary
    - Primary lymphoma of bone is rare
  - Variable appearance
    - Typically lucent, permeative lesions
      - ± areas of sclerosis, periosteal reaction
    - Can be radiographically occult despite extensive marrow involvement
    - MR tends to show aggressive marrow lesions without significant extraosseous extension
      - May demonstrate geographic foci of decreased medullary enhancement in tumor
- **Osteosarcoma**
  - Most common primary bone malignancy in children
    - Typically metaphyseal, less commonly diaphyseal
  - Wide zone of transition with aggressive periosteal reaction; often has osteoid matrix
- **Enchondroma**
  - Benign bubbly lucent lesion of diaphysis that is most common in bones of hand
  - Endosteal scalloping, mild expansile remodeling, & chondroid matrix are typical
  - MR shows classic cartilage matrix: Lobules of high T2 signal tumor with thin low-signal septations & peripheral nodular septal enhancement

Helpful Clues for Rare Diagnoses

- **Vascular Anomaly**
  - Congenital vascular malformations more commonly involve bone than vascular neoplasms
    - High flow: Arteriovenous malformation
    - Low flow: Venous or lymphatic malformation
  - May be focal & well-circumscribed lucent lesions vs. diffusely infiltrating with expansion
- **Osteofibrous Dysplasia/Adamantinoma**
  - Osteofibrous dysplasia (OFD): Fibroosseous lesion primarily affecting tibia in children
    - Usually eccentrically involves anterior tibial diaphysis/metadiaphysis
    - Lucent & sclerotic; solitary or multifocal
      - Can synchronously involve fibula
    - May lead to fracture & pseudoarthrosis
  - Adamantinoma: Similar, but is low-grade malignancy
    - Can be identical to OFD on imaging but typically occurs in older children
      - Worrisome features include periosteal reaction, permeative destruction, & soft tissue extension
- **Chondrosarcoma**
  - Considered if chondroid matrix is present in aggressive diaphyseal lesion of teenager

SELECTED REFERENCES

1. Raissaki M et al: Multifocal bone and bone marrow lesions in children - MRI findings. Pediatr Radiol. 47(3):342-60, 2017

Osteoid Osteoma

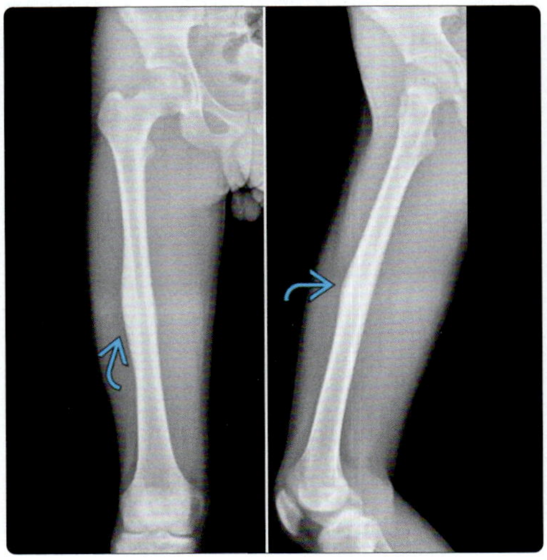

Fibrous Dysplasia

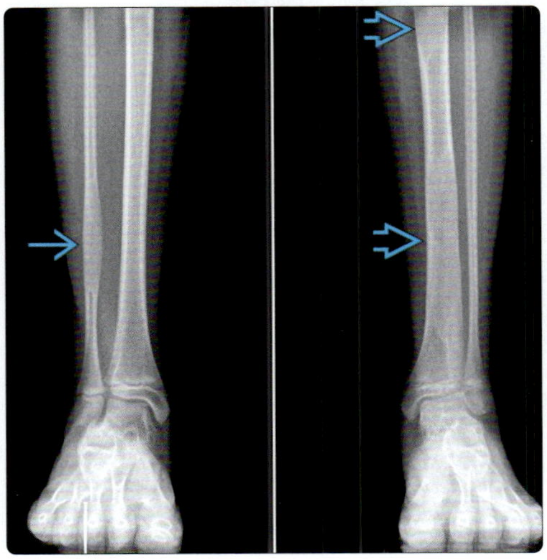

(Left) *AP & lateral radiographs in a 15-year-old boy with right thigh pain show focal mature cortical thickening* ➔ *of the anterolateral mid right femoral diaphysis. MR imaging (not shown) confirmed a central nidus, & the child's symptoms resolved with radiofrequency ablation.* **(Right)** *AP radiographs in a 12 year old with fibrous dysplasia show classic radiographic features in the right fibula* ➔ *& left tibia* ➔*, including well-defined, mildly expansile central diaphyseal lesions with a smudged or ground-glass matrix.*

(Left) *Coronal T1 C+ FS MR in an 8 month old with swelling & fever shows extensive tibial osteomyelitis with patchy decreased marrow enhancement → due to necrosis &/or pus. A small subperiosteal abscess → is noted. The initial radiographs were normal except for soft tissue edema.* **(Right)** *AP & lateral radiographs in the same patient 6 weeks later show somewhat aggressive changes of the tibia with patchy regions of lucency & sclerosis, solid but interrupted periosteal reaction, & a pathologic fracture.*

Osteomyelitis (Pyogenic)

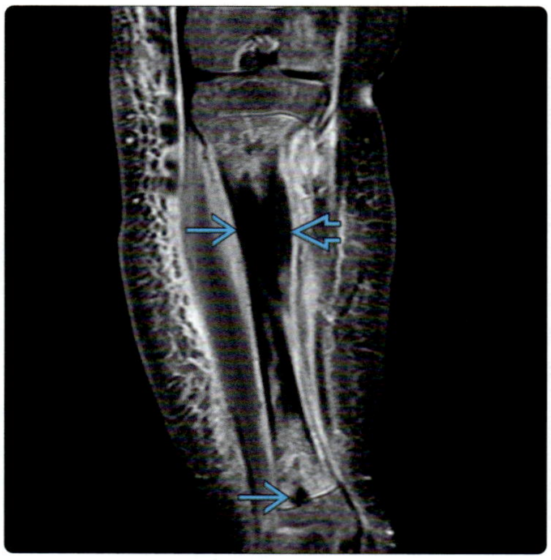

Osteomyelitis (Pyogenic)

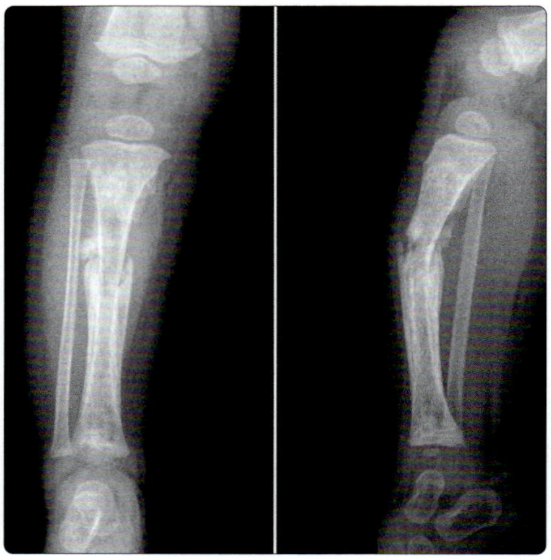

(Left) *Coronal T2 FS & T1 MR images in a child with known SCD & right thigh pain show 2 stages of femur infarcts. The more cranial lesion → has a sharply defined double line sign (bright inner & dark outer lines) of subacute/chronic infarcts. A more acute inferior lesion → has adjacent marrow & periosteal edema →.* **(Right)** *AP & lateral radiographs in a 6-year-old boy with a distal femoral osteosarcoma → show sclerotic skip metastases in the proximal femoral diaphysis →. Note a proximal tibial metastasis →.*

Bone Infarcts

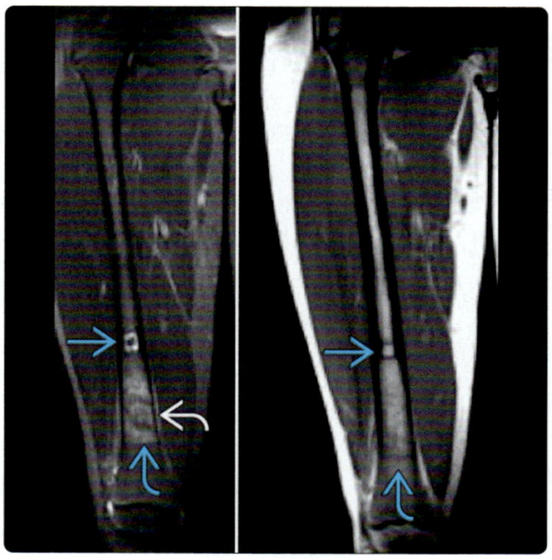

Metastases

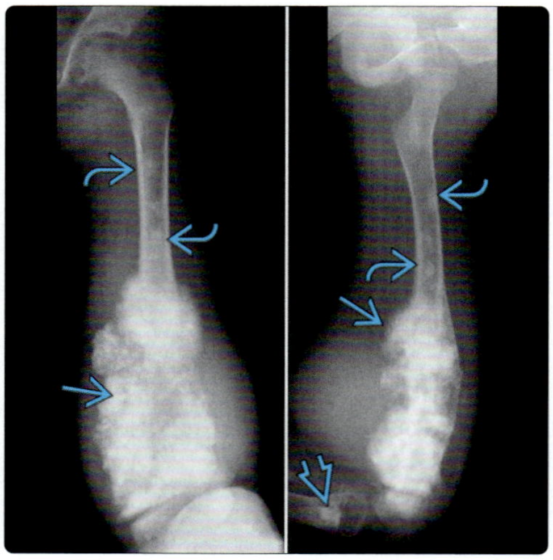

(Left) *Frontal & lateral radiographs of the right femur in a 13 year old with right knee pain show a permeative lesion in the proximal to mid femoral diaphysis → with aggressive periosteal reaction.* **(Right)** *Coronal STIR & T1 C+ FS MR images in the same child show the extent of the intraosseous → & overlying soft tissue → components. Note that the intraosseous margins of bone tumors are actually best defined on T1 imaging without contrast or fat suppression (not shown).*

Ewing Sarcoma

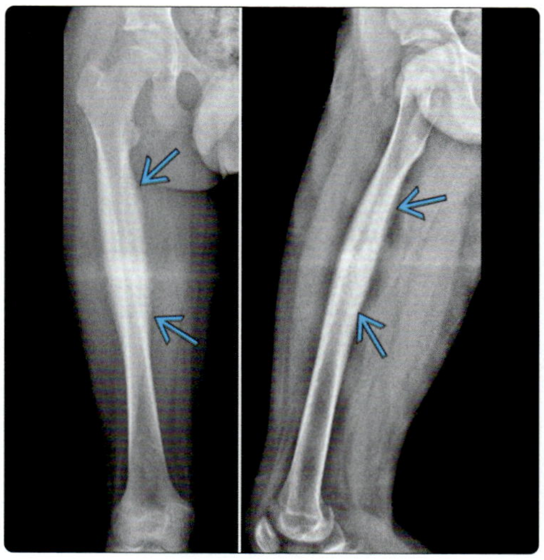

Ewing Sarcoma

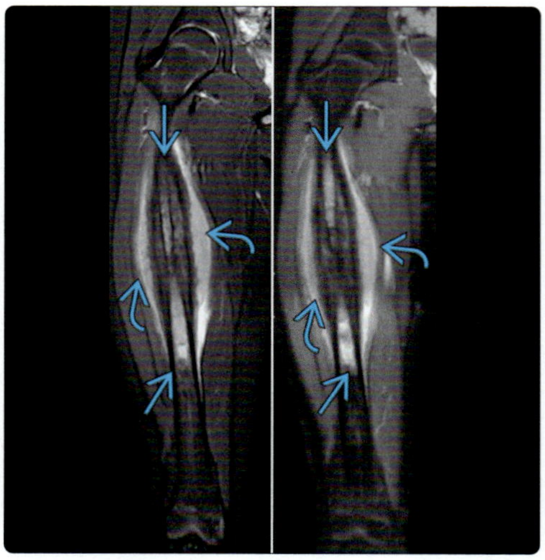

Langerhans Cell Histiocytosis

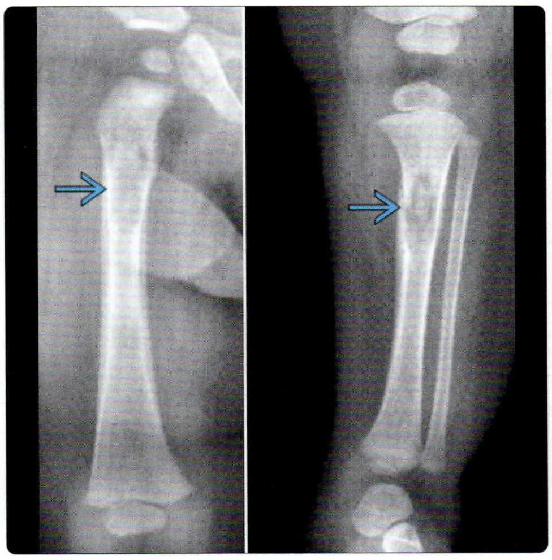

Enchondroma

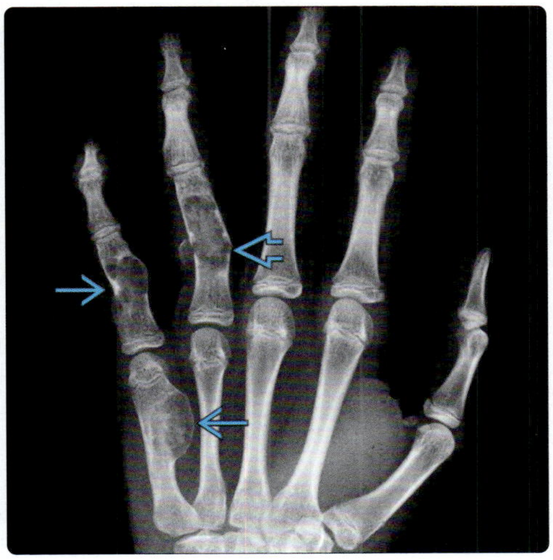

(Left) *AP radiographs in a 6 month old with Langerhans cell histiocytosis (LCH) show focal lytic lesions in the proximal right femoral & left tibial diaphyses.* **(Right)** *PA radiograph of the hand in a 12 year old shows a pathologic fracture through one of several bubbly lucent diaphyseal lesions. Expansile remodeling, endosteal scalloping, & chondroid matrix are noted, all typical of enchondromas.*

Vascular Anomaly

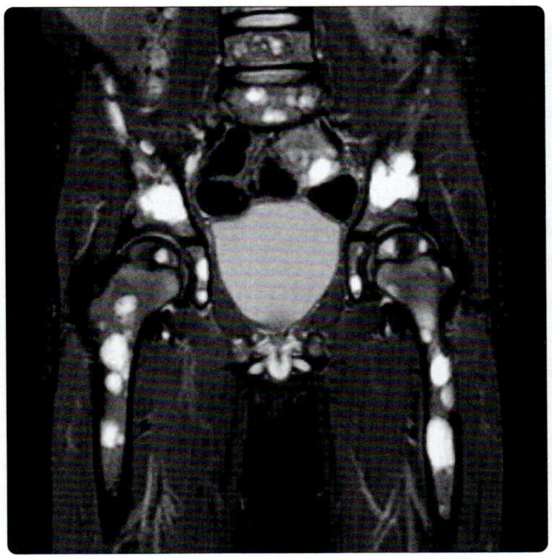

Osteofibrous Dysplasia/Adamantinoma

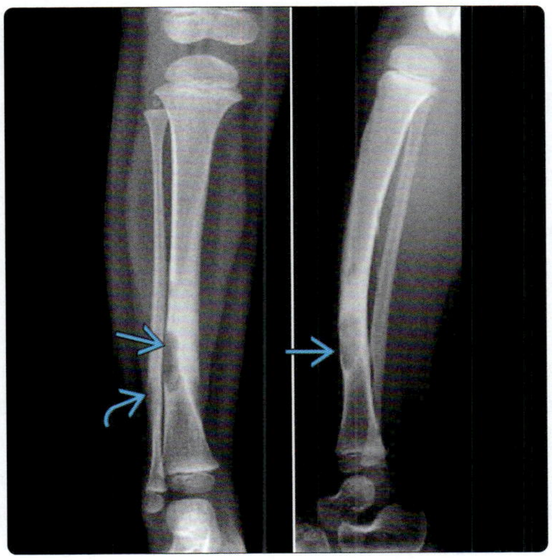

(Left) *Coronal STIR MR in a 6 year old with generalized lymphatic anomaly (GLA) shows typical bubbly cystic lesions of the bones that can be mildly expansile. GLA patients often have splenic lesions & pleural disease as well.* **(Right)** *Frontal & lateral radiographs of the right leg in a 2-year-old girl with osteofibrous dysplasia (OFD) show a distal tibial diaphyseal lesion with lucent & sclerotic components. There is associated anterior tibial bowing. A more subtle lesion is also present in the distal fibula.*

Chondrosarcoma

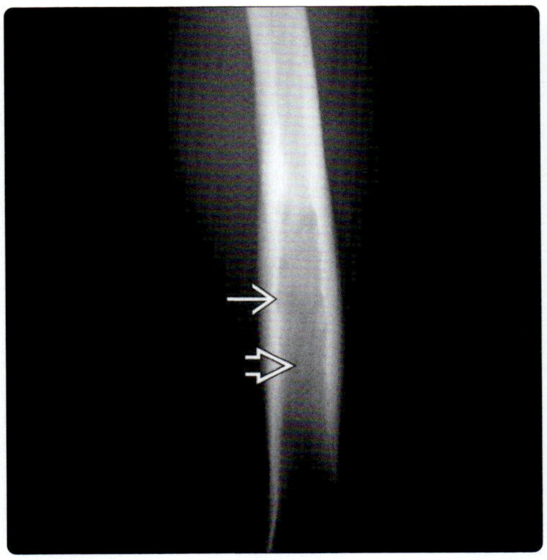

Chondrosarcoma

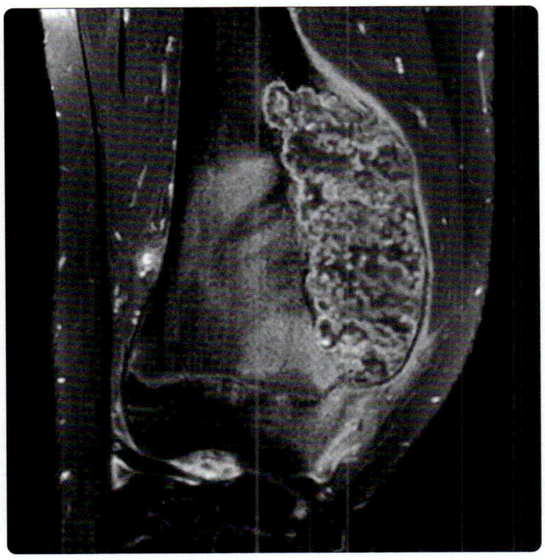

(Left) *Lateral radiograph in a 17 year old shows mild expansion of the femoral diaphysis by a lucent lesion with endosteal scalloping. Subtle internal matrix proved to be chondroid in nature.* **(Right)** *Coronal T1 C+ FS MR in a 15 year old with pain shows a femoral surface metadiaphyseal lesion with mixed aggressive & nonaggressive features. The lobulated & nodular septal enhancement is typical of tumor cartilage. Pathology showed a low-grade chondrosarcoma.*

DIFFERENTIAL DIAGNOSIS

Common

- Enostosis (Bone Island)
- Ossifying Fibroxanthoma
- Healing Fracture
- Chronic Recurrent Multifocal Osteomyelitis

Less Common

- Osteomyelitis
- Osteoid Osteoma
- Osteosarcoma
- Osteonecrosis
- Enchondroma
- Fibrous Dysplasia

Rare but Important

- Metastases
- Lymphoma
- Osteoma
- Ewing Sarcoma
- Osteopoikilosis & Osteopathia Striata
- Melorheostosis

ESSENTIAL INFORMATION

Helpful Clues for Common Diagnoses

- **Enostosis (Bone Island)**
    - Focus of cortical bone within trabecular bone
    - Typically < 1-cm, ovoid, intramedullary focus ± spiculation
- **Ossifying Fibroxanthoma**
    - Encompasses fibrous cortical defect [(FCD), < 3 cm] & nonossifying fibroma [(NOF), > 3 cm]
    - Eccentric bubbly lucent lesion with sclerotic border, typically metadiaphyseal; gradually ossifies
- **Healing Fracture**
    - Sclerosis along margins of fracture & callus
- **Chronic Recurrent Multifocal Osteomyelitis**
    - May cause lytic or sclerotic lesions without abscesses

Helpful Clues for Less Common Diagnoses

- **Osteomyelitis**
    - Chronic osteomyelitis can be sclerotic or mixed lucent/sclerotic ± expansion & intraosseous abscesses
- **Osteoid Osteoma**
    - Benign neoplasm with nidus of osteoid (< 2 cm)
    - Pain at night relieved by NSAIDs
    - Cortical thickening ± lucent nidus
- **Osteosarcoma**
    - Most common malignant primary bone tumor in children
    - Aggressive lesion with variable mix of lysis & sclerosis, usually in long bone metaphysis
        - Cloud-like osteoid often extends beyond bone
- **Osteonecrosis**
    - Focal serpentine or vague sclerosis
    - Often bilateral in predisposing conditions (e.g., sickle cell disease, leukemia treated with steroids)
- **Enchondroma**
    - Typically central lucent diaphyseal lesion with endosteal scalloping, often in digits
    - ± chondroid matrix (punctate, arcs, rings of Ca^{2+})
- **Fibrous Dysplasia**
    - Mixed lucent & sclerotic vs. classic ground-glass matrix

Helpful Clues for Rare Diagnoses

- **Metastases**
    - Lytic > sclerotic; usually multifocal
    - May be well defined or more aggressive
- **Lymphoma**
    - May be sclerotic & involve large portion of single bone
- **Osteoma**
    - Benign & bone forming, primarily in paranasal sinuses
- **Ewing Sarcoma**
    - More commonly permeative diaphysial/flat bone lesion
- **Osteopoikilosis & Osteopathia Striata**
    - Osteopoikilosis: Multiple enostoses
    - Osteopathia striata: Sclerotic striations
- **Melorheostosis**
    - Dripping candle wax appearance

Enostosis (Bone Island)

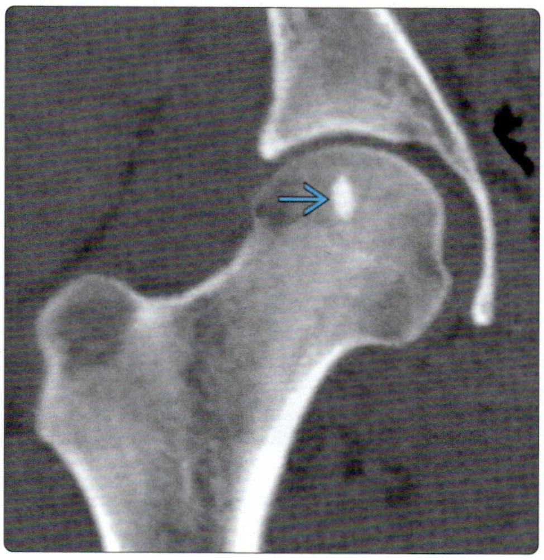

Ossifying Fibroxanthoma

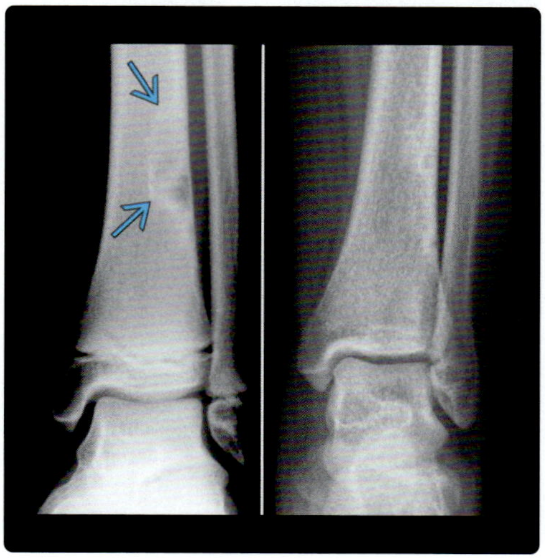

(Left) *Coronal reformatted abdominal/pelvic CECT from a girl with abdominal pain shows an incidental ovid sclerotic lesion in the femoral head* →. **(Right)** *Frontal radiographs of the ankle were obtained in a boy at 11 (left) & 14 (right) years of age. The initial radiographs show a nonaggressive eccentric mixed lucent & sclerotic lesion in the distal tibial diaphysis with a sclerotic margin* →. *The follow-up study shows near resolution of the lesion.*

Osteoid Osteoma

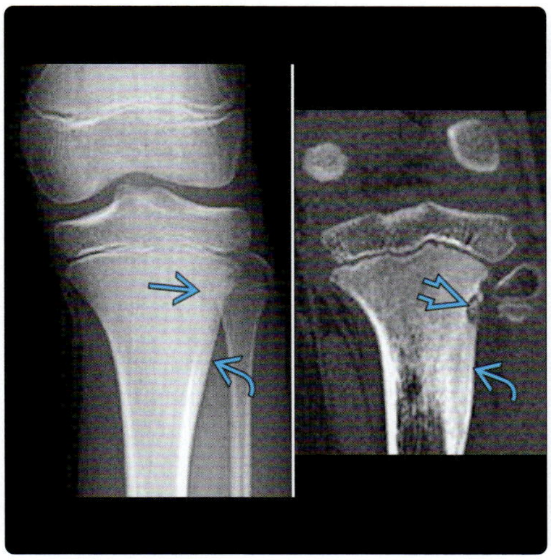

Osteosarcoma

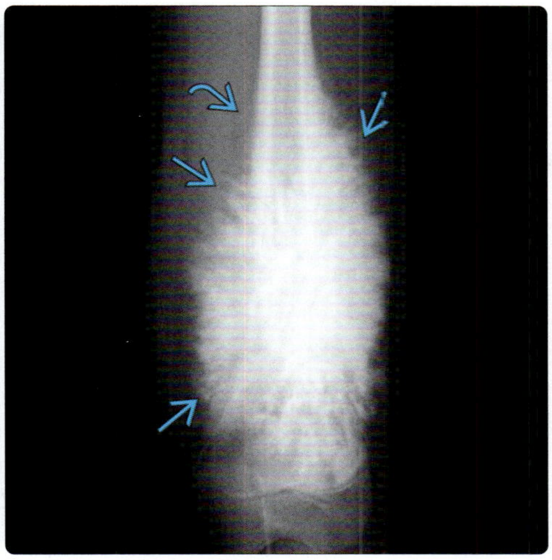

(Left) *Frontal radiograph (left) & coronal NECT (right) images of the proximal left tibia in a child with knee pain show an osteoid osteoma. The nidus of the lesion is subtle on the radiograph, but the adjacent cortical thickening is well seen on both studies. The CT shows central* Ca^{2+} *within the nidus.* **(Right)** *AP radiograph in a 12-year-old boy with left knee pain shows a poorly defined (wide zone of transition) tumor in the distal femur with a cloud-like osseous matrix & aggressive periosteal reaction (both sunburst & interrupted).*

Metastases

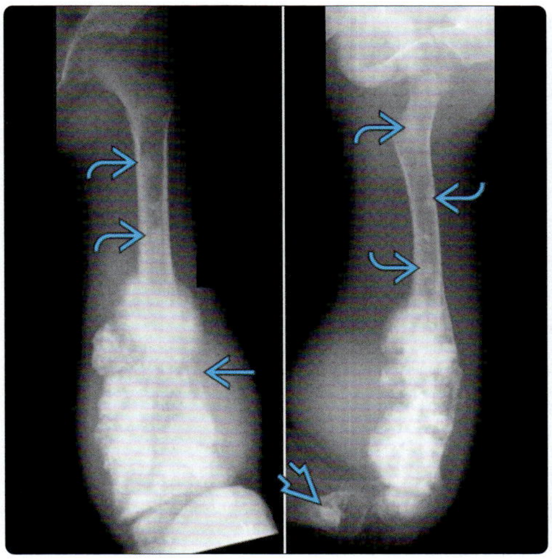

Ewing Sarcoma

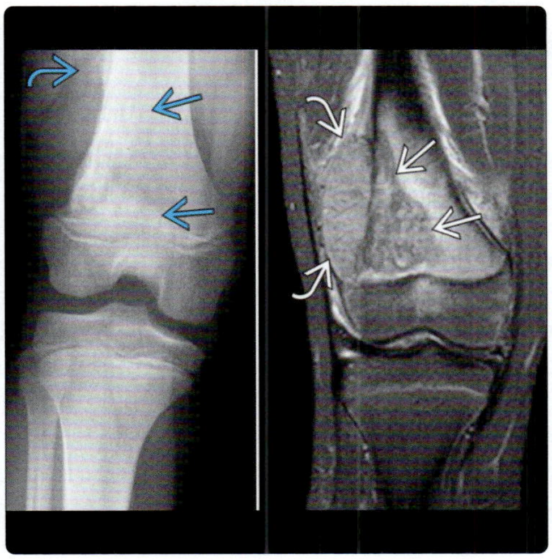

(Left) *AP (left) & lateral (right) radiographs in a 6-year-old boy with a distal femoral osteosarcoma show multiple sclerotic skip metastases in the proximal femur & proximal tibia.* **(Right)** *AP radiograph (left) in a 10-year-old girl with right knee swelling shows a subtle sclerotic lesion in the distal femoral metaphysis with aggressive periosteal reaction. The coronal T2 FS MR (right) shows the intraosseous portion of the tumor & a soft tissue component in this atypical Ewing sarcoma.*

Osteopoikilosis & Osteopathia Striata

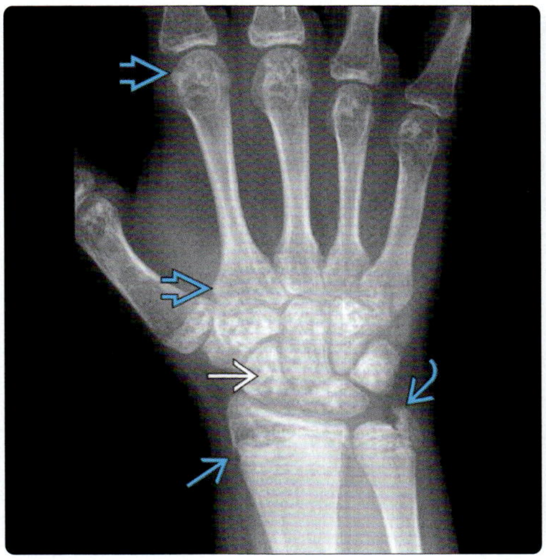

Melorheostosis

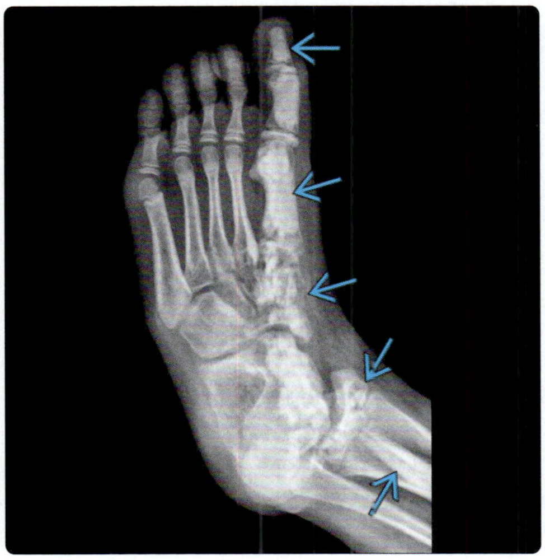

(Left) *PA radiograph of the wrist in a 16 year old following distal radial & ulnar styloid fractures shows multiple enostoses (bone islands) throughout the carpal bones of the wrist & within the metacarpals. These were found incidentally due to the fractures.* **(Right)** *Oblique foot radiograph in a 12-year-old boy shows geographic sclerotic lesions of the 1st digit, medial tarsals, & distal tibia. Melorheostosis often follows a sclerotome distribution, giving a dripping candle wax appearance of adjacent bones.*

DIFFERENTIAL DIAGNOSIS

Common

- Transient Synovitis
- Septic Arthritis
- Osteomyelitis
- Slipped Capital Femoral Epiphysis
- Legg-Calvé-Perthes
- Trauma

Less Common

- Juvenile Idiopathic Arthritis
- Chronic Recurrent Multifocal Osteomyelitis
- Osteonecrosis
- Femoral Acetabular Impingement & Labral Tears
- Osteoid Osteoma
- Other Bone Tumors

Rare but Important

- Idiopathic Chondrolysis

ESSENTIAL INFORMATION

Key Differential Diagnosis Issues

- Age & history are helpful in narrowing differential diagnosis
- Imaging considerations
  - Radiographs are not sensitive for hip joint effusion or early marrow abnormalities
  - Ultrasound is very sensitive for hip joint effusions but cannot distinguish infected from sterile fluid
  - CT provides excellent cortical bone detail but limited soft tissue & marrow evaluation
  - MR is most sensitive for pediatric musculoskeletal pathologies but requires anesthesia for young children
  - Nuclear medicine now has limited roles in work-ups of musculoskeletal pain

Helpful Clues for Common Diagnoses

- **Transient Synovitis**
  - a.k.a. irritable hip, toxic synovitis
  - Age: 18 months to 10 years; peak: 4-7 years old
  - Typically follows recent upper respiratory infection
  - Hip, thigh, or knee pain with limp ± mild fever
  - May have mildly ↑ ESR & WBC
  - Radiographs: Typically normal ± signs of joint effusion
  - Ultrasound: Effusion ± synovial thickening, hyperemia
  - Treatment is supportive (rest + NSAIDs)
  - Symptoms typically last 7-10 days with 17% recurrence
- **Septic Arthritis**
  - Microbial joint infection; *Staphylococcus aureus* is most common
  - Peak age: 2-3 years old
  - Important to diagnose early to avoid destruction of joint
    - Delay in treatment ≥ 4 days → poorer outcomes
  - Fever, pain, swelling, limp or non-weight bearing
  - Radiographs: Typically normal early ± signs of effusion
  - Ultrasound: Effusion ± synovial thickening, hyperemia
    - Fluid can appear simple to complex
    - Cannot predict if fluid is sterile vs. infected
      - Correlate with clinical & laboratory Kocher criteria
  - MR: Joint effusion ± synovial thickening, hyperemia
    - Adjacent marrow & soft tissue edema make septic arthritis more likely than transient synovitis
    - Also detects osteomyelitis & soft tissue abscesses
  - Treatment: Surgical drainage, intravenous (IV) antibiotics
- **Osteomyelitis**
  - Microbial infection of bone; *S. aureus* is most common
  - Important to evaluate SI joints & lower spine when imaging hips, as pain may be referred
  - Radiographs: May take 10-14 days to depict bony changes of osteomyelitis
    - Earlier: Soft tissue swelling ± signs of hip effusion
    - Later: Periosteal reaction & lytic lesions
  - MR: Detects early marrow & soft tissue abnormalities
  - MR & ultrasound: Can detect associated joint effusions + subperiosteal & soft tissue abscesses
  - Treatment: Antibiotics, debridement, abscess drainage
- **Slipped Capital Femoral Epiphysis**
  - Salter-Harris type I proximal femoral fracture
  - Age: 10-15 years old
  - Predispositions: Obesity & endocrine disorders
  - Bilateral (18-36%): Contralateral within 18-24 months
  - Radiographs
    - Widened/elongated femoral physis, often appearing smoother than undulating normal side
    - Medial/posterior displacement of femoral head (best seen on frog leg lateral view)
    - Klein line drawn along lateral femoral neck normally intersects femoral head on AP view
      - Slipped femoral head often lies medial to Klein line
  - MR: Can detect preslip prior to radiographic findings
- **Legg-Calvé-Perthes**
  - Osteonecrosis of femoral head of unknown etiology
  - Age: 3-12 years old; peak: 6-8 years old
  - Bilateral (10-20%)
  - Radiographs
    - Flattening, fragmentation, & sclerosis of femoral head
    - May be normal in early stages
  - MR: More sensitive than radiographs for early stages
    - Postcontrast subtracted images yield earliest detection of decreased perfusion
  - Prognosis depends on containment of femoral head
- **Trauma**
  - Ranges from minor muscular injuries to apophyseal avulsions to hip dislocations & pelvic fractures
  - May be due to acute injury or repetitive stress
  - Radiographs: Often show fractures & dislocations
  - CT & MR: Can detect radiographically occult fractures
    - CT: Important to characterize complex pelvic fractures
    - MR: Can also evaluate cartilage & labral injuries

Helpful Clues for Less Common Diagnoses

- **Juvenile Idiopathic Arthritis**
  - Synovial inflammatory disease of unknown cause
  - < 16 years old & symptoms > 6 weeks in duration
  - Stiff, swollen, painful joint with decreased motion
  - US: Joint effusion, synovial thickening, & hyperemia
  - MR: Effusion, synovial thickening & hyperenhancement, ± erosions, ± rice bodies
  - Late: Joint space narrowing & ankylosis
- **Chronic Recurrent Multifocal Osteomyelitis**

- Multifocal nonpyogenic inflammatory bone lesions
- Relapsing/remitting course
- Associated with other conditions (e.g., juvenile idiopathic arthritis)
- Radiographs
  - Acute: Lytic lesion (usually in metaphysis near physis)
  - Late: Progressive adjacent sclerosis
- MR: Edema/enhancement of lesion & adjacent marrow
  - ± soft tissue & periosteal inflammation but no abscess
  - ± reactive adjacent joint effusion/synovitis

- **Osteonecrosis**
  - Most commonly in anterolateral weight-bearing portion of femoral head
  - Etiologies: Acute lymphoblastic leukemia, steroids, sickle cell disease, trauma, vasculitis, others
  - Radiographs: Flattening, sclerosis, fragmentation of femoral head ± subchondral fracture
    - Radiograph may be normal early
  - MR: Earlier diagnosis than radiographs with abnormal signal intensity & decreased femoral head perfusion
    - Subacute/chronic: T2 double line sign
      - High-signal-intensity inner line = granulation tissue
      - Low-signal-intensity outer line = sclerotic bone
- **Femoral Acetabular Impingement & Labral Tears**
  - Pathologic contact (impingement) of femur & acetabulum during hip motion
  - Divided into 2 morphologic types
    - Cam type: Aspherical femoral head, abnormal femoral head/neck junction
    - Pincer type: Focal or general acetabular overcoverage
  - Can be primary or secondary
    - Secondary femoral acetabular impingement (FAI) may result from various pediatric hip diseases [e.g., slipped capital femoral epiphysis (SCFE), Legg-Calvé-Perthes (LCP), dysplasias] or their treatments (e.g., pelvic osteotomies)
      - SCFE & LCP → cam-type FAI → labral tears
  - Labral pathology can also be secondary to untreated developmental hip dysplasia (DDH)
    - Secondary to lateral uncovering of femoral head → chronic labral stress (rather than FAI)
    - Pelvic osteotomies treating DDH → pincer-type FAI
  - Radiographs show features of cam & pincer types of FAI but are not specific (as patients may be asymptomatic)
  - MR arthrography used to evaluate labrum & cartilage
- **Osteoid Osteoma**
  - Benign osteoblastic neoplasm composed of osteoid & woven bone in fibrovascular stroma, < 2-cm nidus
  - Age: Peak: 10-20 years old
  - Pain at night relieved by NSAIDs
  - Various types: Cortical (most common), medullary, endosteal, & subperiosteal
  - Radiographs show cortical thickening ± lucent nidus
    - Intramedullary & intraarticular osteoid osteoma (OO) less frequently show cortical thickening
  - CT & MR can both show OO & may be complimentary in evaluating atypical OO
  - Dynamic postcontrast MR shows increased specificity
    - Early nidus enhancement with later partial washout
    - Adjacent marrow edema enhances later than nidus
- **Other Bone Tumors**
  - Primary of pelvis (e.g., Ewing sarcoma), proximal femur (e.g., chondroblastoma), or marrow (e.g., leukemia)
  - Metastatic disease: Most commonly neuroblastoma
  - ± pathologic fracture

Helpful Clues for Rare Diagnoses

- **Idiopathic Chondrolysis**
  - Increased pressure of unknown cause → femoral & acetabular cartilage destruction
  - Preadolescent/adolescent with hip pain, stiffness, & limp
  - Radiographs: Concentric joint space narrowing + osteoporosis (late findings)
  - MR: Rectangular increased T2 signal & enhancement in central femoral head + ill-defined edema in acetabulum
    - ± mild synovial hypertrophy, minimal effusion

Transient Synovitis

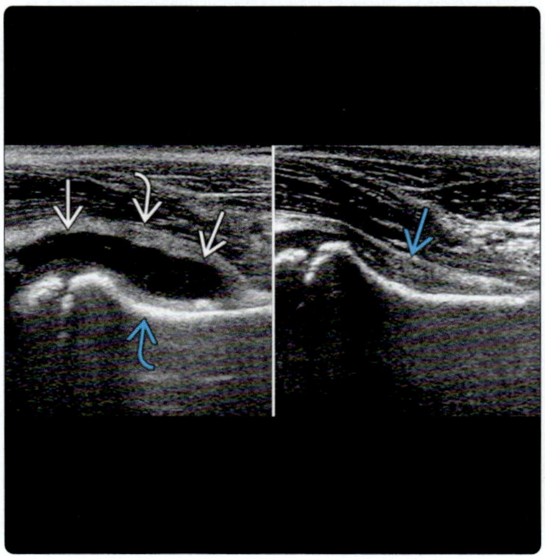

Septic Arthritis

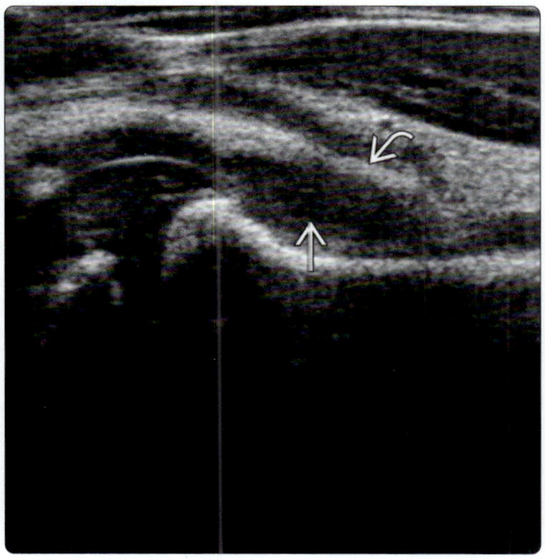

(Left) *Anterior approach longitudinal ultrasound of the left hip at the level of the femoral neck ➡ shows a widened anechoic joint space ➡ with a convex outer margin, consistent with a hip effusion. Note the echogenic synovial thickening ➡ along the capsule. The normal right hip ➡ shows no significant fluid.* **(Right)** *Anterior approach longitudinal ultrasound of the hip shows complex joint fluid ➡ with convex bowing ➡ of the joint capsule. One cannot predict if the fluid is infected or not based on ultrasound.*

(Left) *Axial T1 C+ FS MR in a patient with right hip pain & normal radiographs (not shown) shows abnormal increased enhancement of the ischium & adjacent musculature secondary to osteomyelitis. A small abscess extends from the ischiopubic synchondrosis.* **(Right)** *Coronal T1 C+ FS MR in a 13 year old with ischiopubic osteomyelitis shows heterogeneous osseous enhancement with extension of an abscess into the obturator externus muscle.*

Osteomyelitis

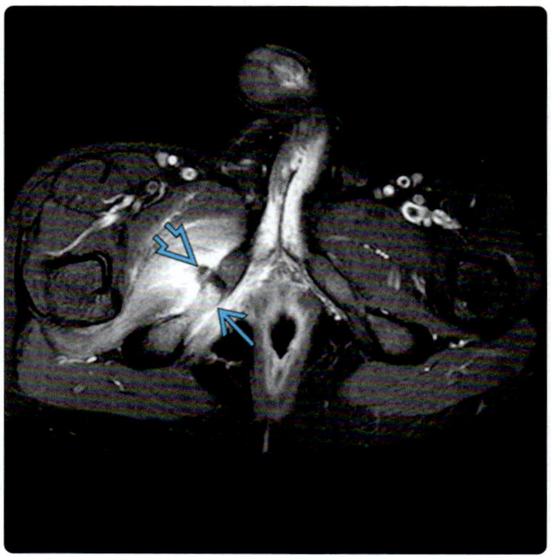

Osteomyelitis

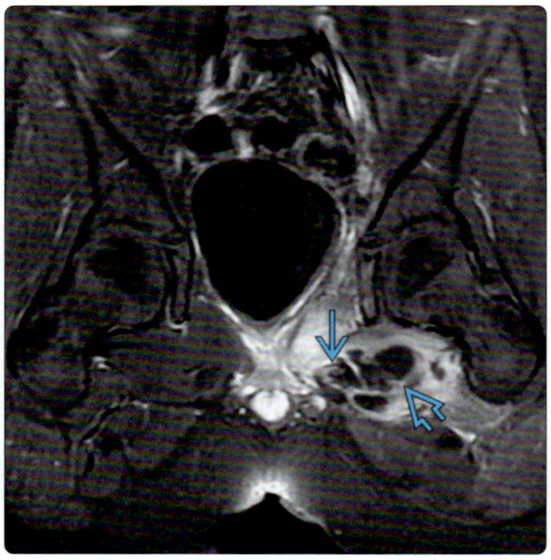

(Left) *AP radiograph in a 10-year-old girl with left hip pain shows that the left subcapital femoral physis appears more lucent, wide, & curved as compared to the right.* **(Right)** *Frog leg lateral view of the hips in the same patient shows posteromedial slippage of the left femoral head relative to the femoral neck, consistent with a slipped capital femoral epiphysis (SCFE). There is a normal femoral head-neck relationship on the right.*

Slipped Capital Femoral Epiphysis

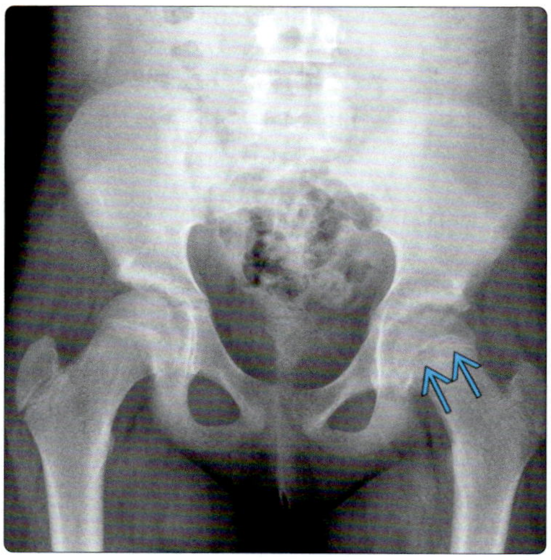

Slipped Capital Femoral Epiphysis

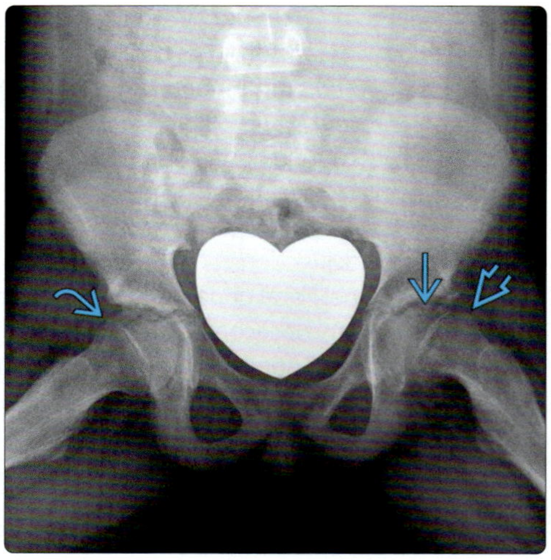

(Left) *AP radiograph in a 7 year old with left hip pain shows a typical appearance of Legg-Calvé-Perthes disease, including flattening, fragmentation, & mixed sclerosis & lucency of the left femoral head.* **(Right)** *Subtracted T1 C+ FS MR in the same patient shows a large central region of left femoral head nonenhancement (i.e., necrosis) with surrounding hyperenhancement (due to reperfusion &/or reactive edema). There is normal enhancement of the right femoral head.*

Legg-Calvé-Perthes

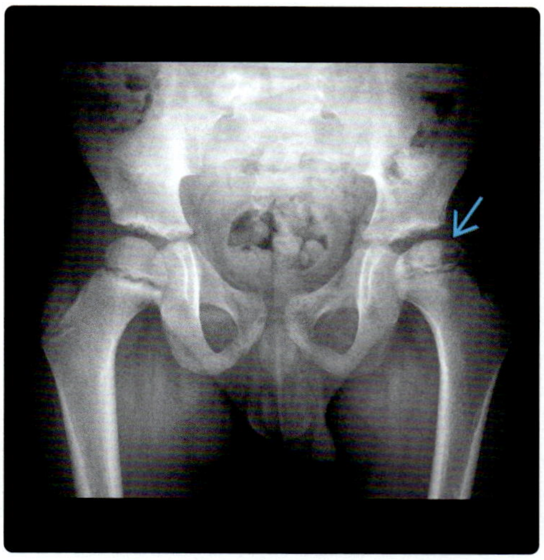

Legg-Calvé-Perthes

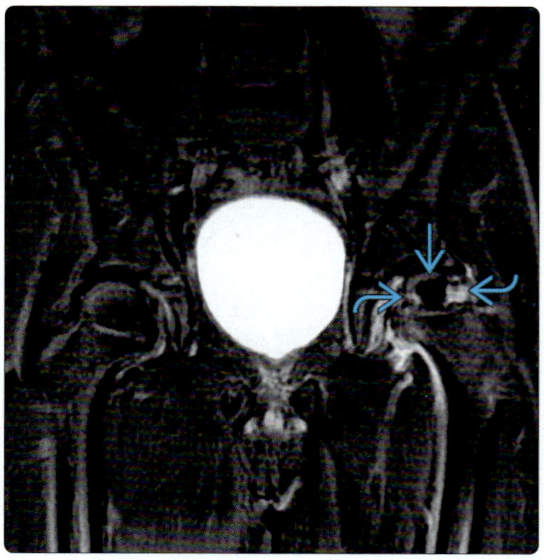

Trauma

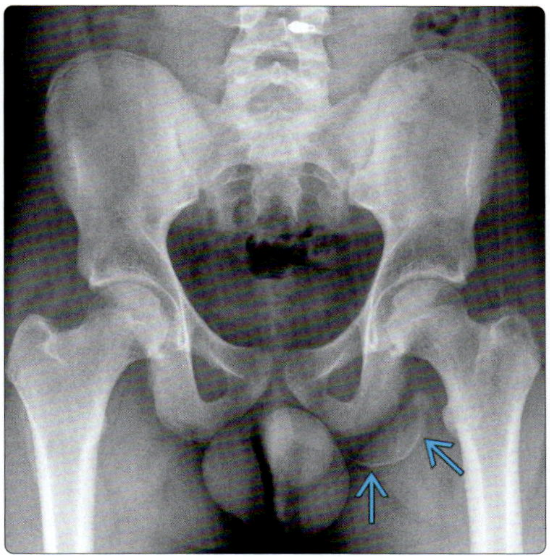

Trauma

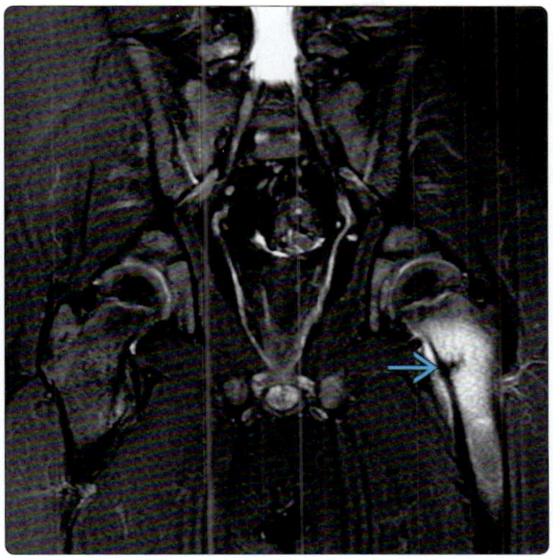

(Left) *AP radiograph in a 13-year-old boy with the sudden sensation of a "pop" & left hip pain while running shows a displaced avulsion fracture of the left ischial tuberosity apophysis.* **(Right)** *Coronal T2 FS MR in a 4 year old with left hip pain & normal radiographs shows a linear focus of low signal intensity extending perpendicular to the medial femoral neck cortex with surrounding marrow & soft tissue edema, typical of a stress fracture. Progressive sclerosis was seen at this level on follow-up radiographs.*

Trauma

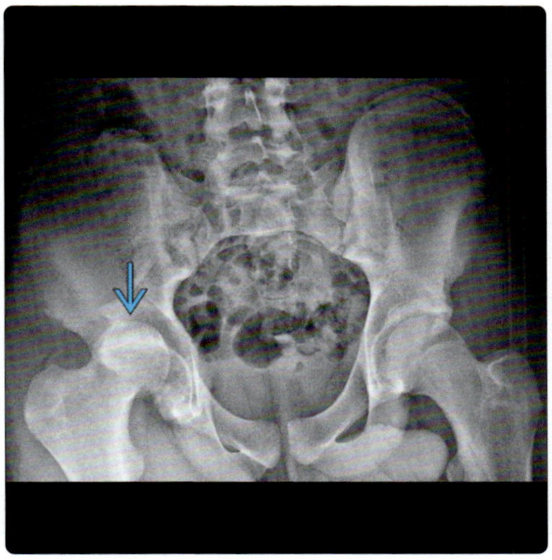

Trauma

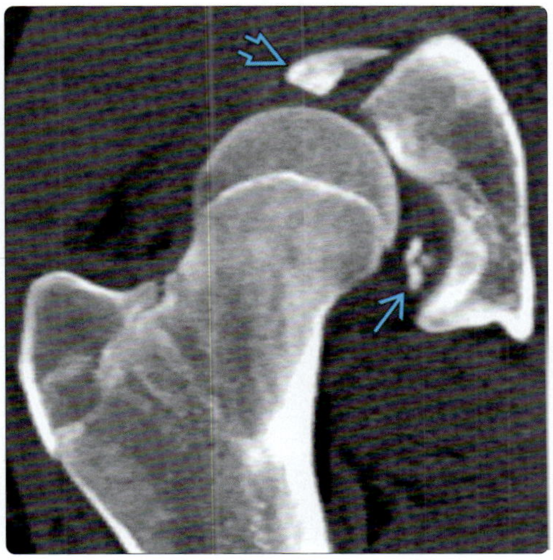

(Left) *AP pelvic radiograph from a 16-year-old boy after trauma shows a posterior superior dislocation of the right femoral head.* **(Right)** *Coronal oblique reformatted NECT in the same patient after femoral head reduction shows a fracture fragment of the posterior wall of the acetabulum + incarcerated intraarticular bone fragments within the right hip joint.*

Juvenile Idiopathic Arthritis

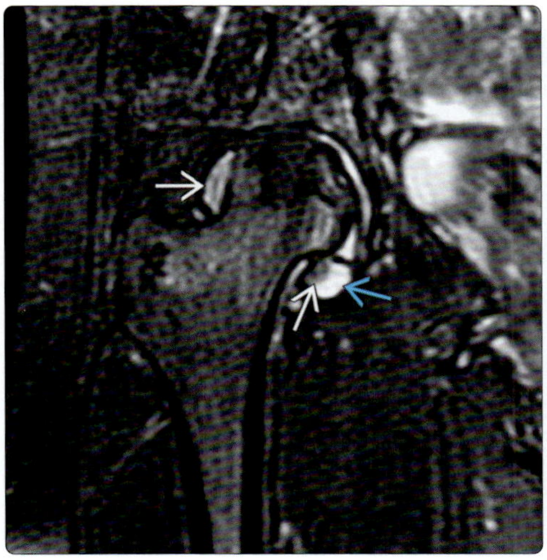

Juvenile Idiopathic Arthritis

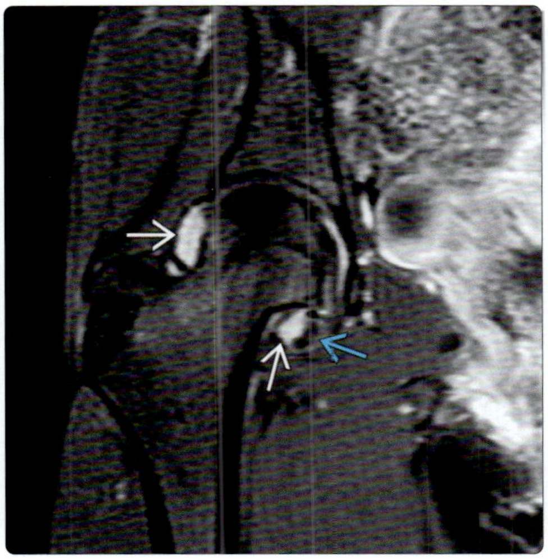

(Left) *Coronal T2 FS MR shows distention of the right hip joint with intermediate signal intensity synovium & high signal intensity fluid. Comparison with early postcontrast images is helpful to confirm active synovitis. Joint space narrowing, especially superolaterally, had progressed when compared to prior studies (not shown).* **(Right)** *Coronal T1 C+ FS MR in the same child confirms regions of abnormally thickened, enhancing synovium as well as nonenhancing fluid.*

(Left) *Axial T2 FS MR in a 5-year-old girl with bilateral hip pain shows poorly defined increased signal intensity in the right iliac bone → & adjacent soft tissues ↗.* **(Right)** *Coronal STIR MR from the same patient shows poorly defined hyperintense signal in the intertrochanteric left femur → & greater trochanter ↗ surrounding the physis. Biopsy of the right iliac lesion showed no organisms & was consistent with chronic recurrent multifocal osteomyelitis (CRMO).*

Chronic Recurrent Multifocal Osteomyelitis

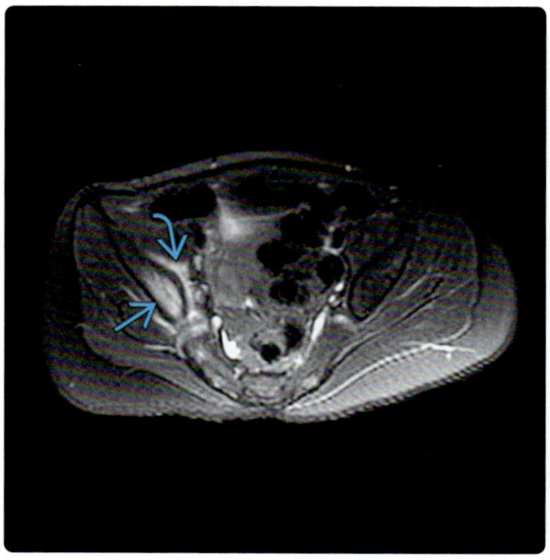

Chronic Recurrent Multifocal Osteomyelitis

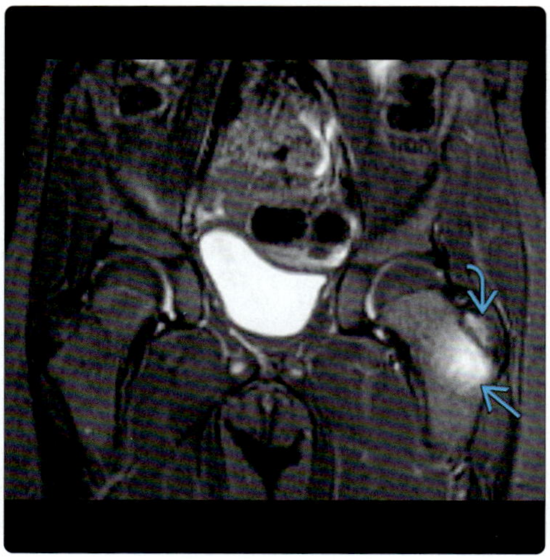

(Left) *AP radiograph in a child with hip pain shows sclerosis & flattening of the right femoral head ➔. Note the large, metaphyseal, cyst-like lucency ➔, a common finding in skeletally immature patients with femoral head osteonecrosis. This child had a predisposing history of acute lymphoblastic leukemia & steroid therapy.* **(Right)** *Coronal T1 MR in a patient with osteonecrosis shows typical serpentine hypointense bands ➔ surrounding hyperintense foci.*

Osteonecrosis

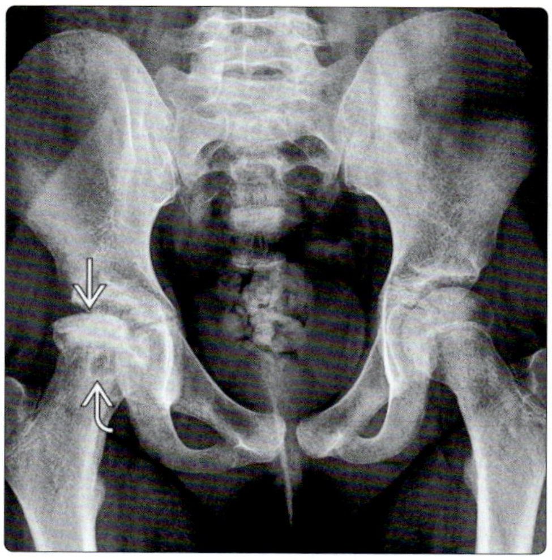

Osteonecrosis

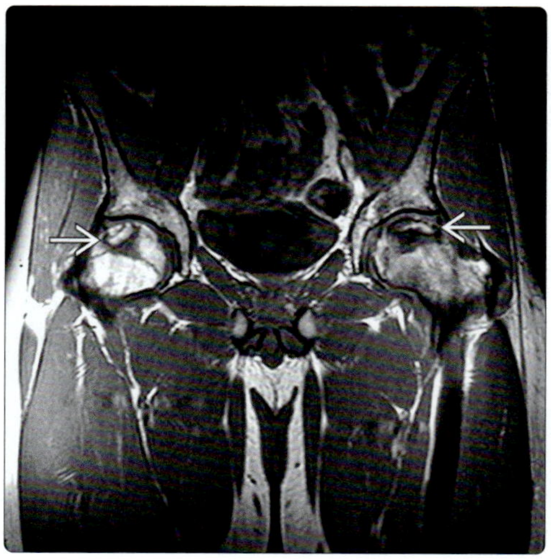

(Left) *Frontal radiograph in a 16-year-old boy with right hip pain & a remote history of SCFE shows right coxa vara & a large cam-type deformity at the right femoral head-neck junction → due to the prior SCFE.* **(Right)** *Coronal proton density MR in the same patient shows the large cam-type deformity → from the prior SCFE with irregularity & attenuation of the labrum ↗ from chronic tearing. Note that a number of pediatric hip disorders can cause chronic morphologic changes leading to secondary femoral acetabular impingement (FAI).*

Femoral Acetabular Impingement & Labral Tears

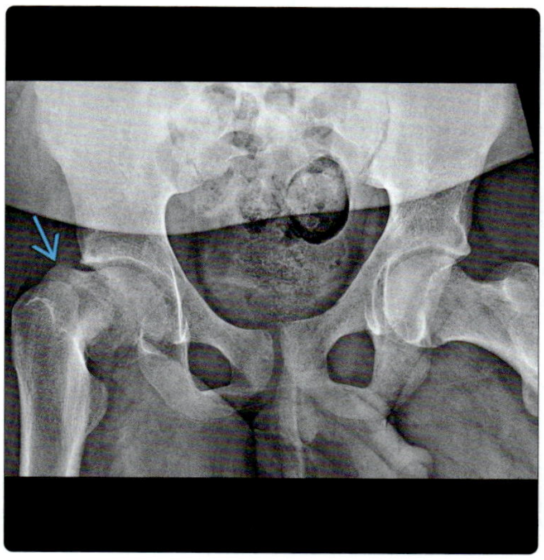

Femoral Acetabular Impingement & Labral Tears

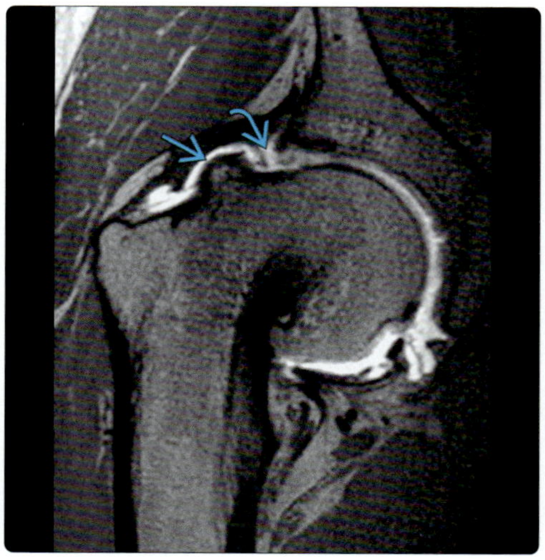

Osteoid Osteoma

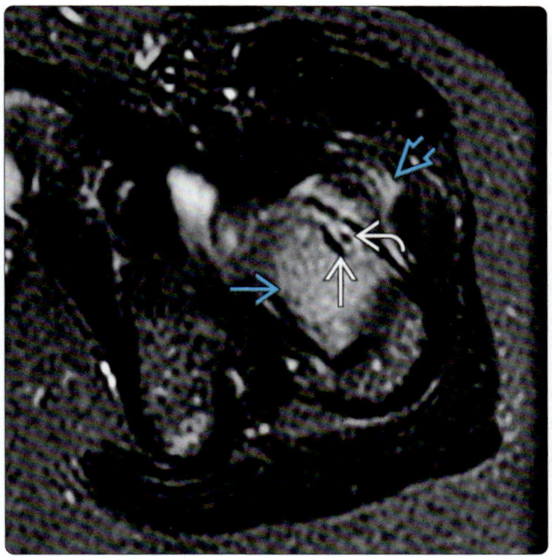

Osteoid Osteoma

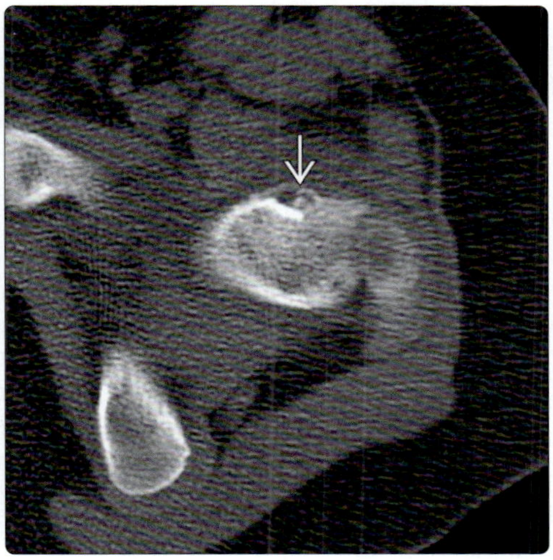

(Left) *Axial T2 FS MR of the left hip shows a cortically based lesion within the anterior femoral neck. There is a central hypointense focus with edema of the adjacent marrow & soft tissues, typical of an osteoid osteoma.* **(Right)** *Axial NECT in the same patient shows a tiny sclerotic focus within a radiolucent nidus (characteristic of an osteoid osteoma) along the anterior left femoral neck.*

Other Bone Tumors

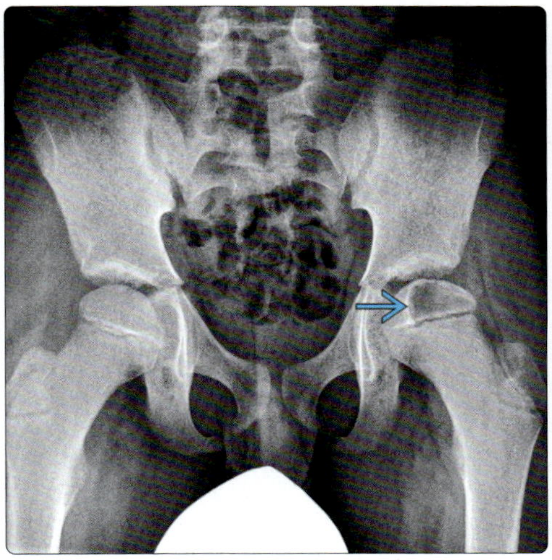

Other Bone Tumors

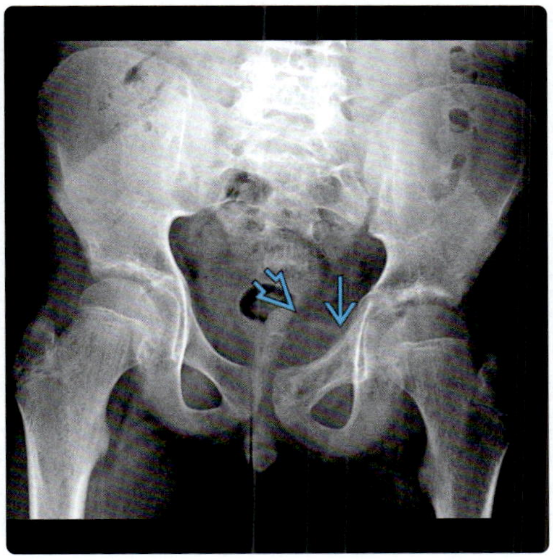

(Left) *AP radiograph shows a lucent lesion in the left femoral head. The lesion was biopsied & proven to be a chondroblastoma. Chondroblastomas typically occur in epiphyses (or equivalent bones) & often incite a local inflammatory response.* **(Right)** *AP radiograph in a 10-year-old boy with left hip pain shows expansion & mottling of the left superior pubic ramus with associated periosteal reaction. There is an associated soft tissue mass.*

Other Bone Tumors

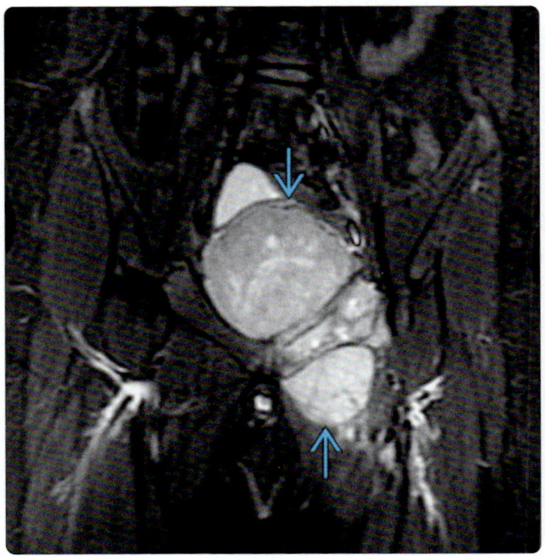

Idiopathic Chondrolysis

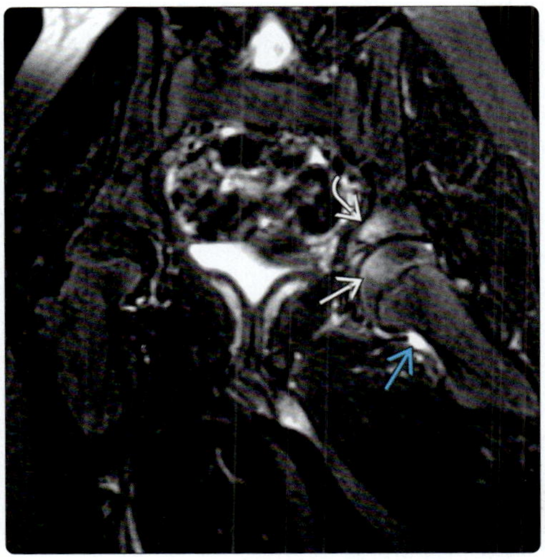

(Left) *Coronal T2 FS MR in the same child shows a tumor in the left superior pubic ramus with large soft tissue components extending superiorly & inferiorly. Pathology confirmed a Ewing sarcoma. Large soft tissue masses are often seen with this malignancy, particularly in the pelvis.* **(Right)** *Coronal T2 FS MR shows a rectangular-shaped area of edema in the central left femoral head. There is also mild edema within the adjacent acetabulum. Note minimal synovial thickening &/or joint fluid.*

DIFFERENTIAL DIAGNOSIS

Common

- Developmental Irregular Ossification
- Developmental Dysplasia of Hip

Less Common

- Legg-Calvé-Perthes Disease
- Avascular Necrosis
- Septic Arthritis
- Juvenile Idiopathic Arthritis
- Slipped Capital Femoral Epiphysis

Rare but Important

- Meyer Dysplasia
- Idiopathic Chondrolysis
- Epiphyseal Bone Tumors & Tumor-Like Conditions
- Epiphyseal Dysplasias
- Proximal Focal Femoral Deficiency

ESSENTIAL INFORMATION

Key Differential Diagnosis Issues

- Age & clinical presentation are key
- Associated findings (e.g., other bones involved, shallow acetabulum) limit differential
- Must exclude infection in child with hip pain & joint fluid, ± femoral head destruction

Helpful Clues for Common Diagnoses

- **Developmental Irregular Ossification**
  - Femoral head ossification center appears between 3-6 months of age
  - Mild irregularity at margins is common
  - Rarely, more pronounced developmental irregularity is seen at superior central aspect
    - Lack of symptoms + normalization on follow-up radiographs distinguishes from Legg-Calvé-Perthes disease (LCP) & other etiologies
    - MR of normal hip will not show marrow edema or joint effusion
- **Developmental Dysplasia of Hip**
  - Spectrum of abnormalities of acetabulum/femoral head
  - Typically diagnosed in infancy
  - Untreated developmental dysplasia of hip (DDH)
    - Displaced femoral head → abnormal hip development
    - Femoral head
      - Early: Subluxed/dislocated + decreased ossification
      - Late: Coxa magna & degenerative changes
    - Concomitant shallow acetabulum
      - Helps differentiate early DDH from some entities
      - Pseudoacetabulum may ultimately form
  - Avascular necrosis (AVN) can complicate DDH treatment

Helpful Clues for Less Common Diagnoses

- **Legg-Calvé-Perthes Disease**
  - AVN of femoral head of unknown etiology
  - Age: 3-14 years; peak: 5-6 years; bilateral in 10-20%
  - Stages
    - Initial/necrosis: Initial ischemia & osteonecrosis
    - Fragmentation: Necrotic bone is resorbed, ± metaphyseal cysts (cartilage), ± collapse
    - Reossification/remodeling: New bone formation
  - Radiographs
    - May be normal in early LCP
    - Flattening, sclerosis, fragmentation of femoral head ± subchondral fracture (best seen on frog-leg view)
  - Bone scintigraphy: Earlier diagnosis than radiographs with decreased or absent perfusion
  - MR: Earlier diagnosis than radiographs with abnormal signal intensity + decreased femoral head perfusion
  - Prognosis depends on femoral head containment
    - Femoral head grows laterally (extrusion of femoral head) with widening of medial joint space → incongruence of femoral head & acetabulum
    - Point of maximum weight bearing shifts laterally → labral degeneration → osteoarthritis in later life
- **Avascular Necrosis**
  - Etiologies: Acute lymphoblastic leukemia, steroids, sickle cell disease, trauma, vasculitis, others
  - Most commonly located in anterolateral weight-bearing portion of femoral head but can occur anywhere
  - Important to detect & treat prior to subchondral fracture → subchondral collapse
  - Radiographs: Flattening, sclerosis, fragmentation of femoral head ± subchondral fracture
    - Radiograph may be normal in early AVN
  - Bone scintigraphy: More sensitive than radiographs
    - Early photopenia; late shows increased uptake (revascularization)
  - MR: Earlier diagnosis than radiographs with abnormal signal intensity & decreased femoral head perfusion
    - T2: Pathognomonic "double-line" sign in subacute/chronic stages
- **Septic Arthritis**
  - *Staphylococcus aureus* is most common
  - Early diagnosis & treatment to prevent joint destruction
    - Ultrasound: Detects effusion (but cannot distinguish infected vs. aseptic fluid)
      - Correlate with clinical & laboratory Kocher criteria
    - Complications: Erosions, osteomyelitis, osteonecrosis, soft tissue abscesses; cartilage destruction → degenerative joint disease
- **Juvenile Idiopathic Arthritis**
  - Synovial inflammatory disease of unknown cause
  - < 16 years old & symptoms > 6 weeks in duration
  - Early: Joint effusion/synovitis
  - Late: Joint space narrowing, erosions
- **Slipped Capital Femoral Epiphysis**
  - Salter-Harris I fracture of subcapital femoral physis
  - Femoral head slips medial/posterior
  - Bilateral in 18-80%
    - Contralateral slipped capital femoral epiphysis occurs within 18 months
  - Age: Girls 8-15 years; boys 10-17 years
  - Predisposing conditions: Obesity, growth spurt, endocrine deficiencies, Down syndrome, renal rickets
  - Radiographs
    - Early: Normal or wide & smooth physis
      - MR may be useful to diagnose "preslip"
    - AP view shows medial component of slip

- Frog-leg view is much more sensitive for posterior direction (which usually predominates)
- Complications
  - Chondrolysis (10%)
  - AVN (1%): Increased risk in open reduction & fixation or if pins extend across superolateral femoral head ossification center
  - Pin penetration into joint

Helpful Clues for Rare Diagnoses

- **Meyer Dysplasia**
  - Poorly understood femoral head dysostosis
  - Age: 2-4 years; boys > girls; bilateral in 60%
  - Radiographs: Irregular ossification/fragmentation of femoral head(s)
  - Asymptomatic; if symptomatic, consider LCP
- **Idiopathic Chondrolysis**
  - Increased pressure of unknown cause → femoral & acetabular cartilage destruction
  - Presents with stiffness, limp, & hip pain in adolescent or preadolescent
  - Radiographs: Findings late with concentric joint space narrowing + osteoporosis
  - MR: Rectangular increased T2 signal & enhancement in central femoral head + ill-defined edema in acetabulum
    - ± mild synovial hypertrophy, minimal effusion
- **Epiphyseal Bone Tumors & Tumor-Like Conditions**
  - Chondroblastoma
    - Benign bone tumor with immature cartilage cells
    - Majority arise in epiphysis or equivalent
    - Peak age: 15-20 years; range: 3-85 years
    - Imaging
      - Calcified chondroid matrix in 50%
      - Well-defined, lucent lesion with sclerotic border
      - MR: Heterogeneous, low-signal rim, adjacent marrow/periosteal edema, reactive joint effusion
  - Langerhans cell histiocytosis
    - Disease of unknown etiology characterized by proliferation of atypical Langerhans cells
    - Varied osseous lesions, classically focal & lytic
    - Can involve epiphyses (including femoral head)
  - Giant cell tumor
    - Locally aggressive tumor of proliferating mononuclear cells + multinucleated giant cells
    - Occurs almost exclusively after physeal closure
    - Lytic lesion originates in metaphysis → epiphysis → subarticular bone
- **Epiphyseal Dysplasias**
  - Multiple epiphyseal dysplasia
    - Abnormal endochondral ossification of epiphyses/physes
    - Autosomal dominant & recessive forms
    - Often presents in late childhood/adolescence
    - Small, irregular, fragmented epiphyses ± flattening
      - Most pronounced in lower extremities (especially femoral heads)
  - Spondyloepiphyseal dysplasia
    - Group of skeletal dysplasias primarily involving vertebrae & proximal epiphyseal centers
      - Platyspondyly + abnormal epiphyses
    - Congenita (evident at birth) & tarda (presents at 5-10 years) forms
- **Proximal Focal Femoral Deficiency**
  - Rare congenital anomaly with failure of normal development of proximal femur
  - Range of dysplasia of proximal femur & acetabulum
  - MR is better than radiographs for early assessment due to visualization of unossified structures

SELECTED REFERENCES

1. Atweh LA et al: Multimodality imaging of developmental dysplasia of hip. Pediatr Radiol. 43 Suppl 1:S166-71, 2013
2. Jarrett DY et al: Imaging SCFE: diagnosis, treatment and complications. Pediatr Radiol. 43 Suppl 1:S71-82, 2013
3. Biko DM et al: Proximal focal femoral deficiency: evaluation by MR imaging. Pediatr Radiol. 42(1):50-6, 2012
4. Dimeglio A et al: Imaging in Legg-Calvé-Perthes disease. Orthop Clin North Am. 42(3):297-302, v, 2011
5. Dillman JR et al: MRI of Legg-Calve-Perthes disease. AJR Am J Roentgenol. 193(5):1394-407, 2009

Developmental Irregular Ossification

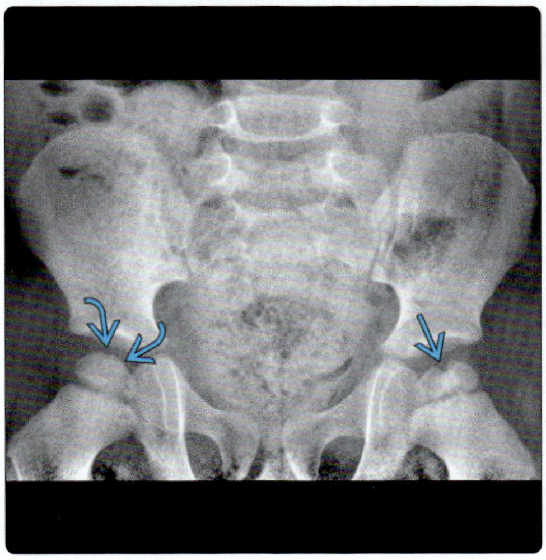

Developmental Irregular Ossification

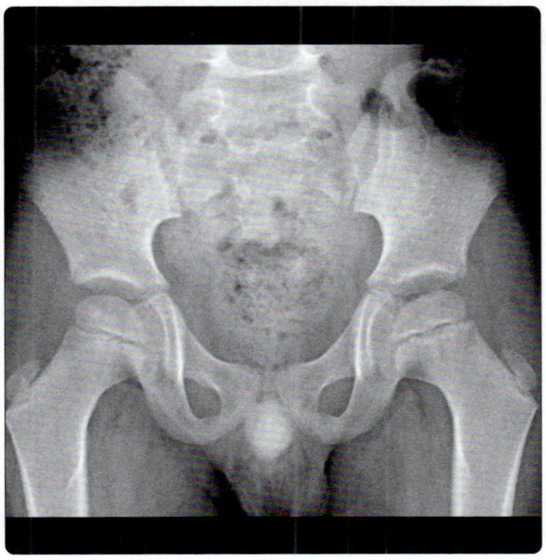

(Left) *AP radiograph in a 3-year-old boy with abdominal pain shows minimal irregularity of the right femoral head* ➔ *& more pronounced central irregularity of the left femoral head with a prominent cleft* ➔*. The child had no hip pain.* **(Right)** *AP radiograph of the pelvis in the same child 2 years later shows resolution of the previously seen cleft in the left femoral head & only minimal residual irregular ossification of the femoral epiphyses. This child never developed any signs or symptoms of hip pathology.*

Developmental Dysplasia of Hip

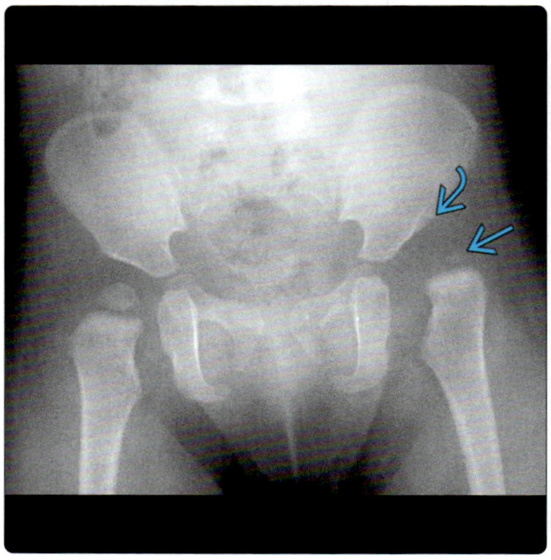

Developmental Dysplasia of Hip

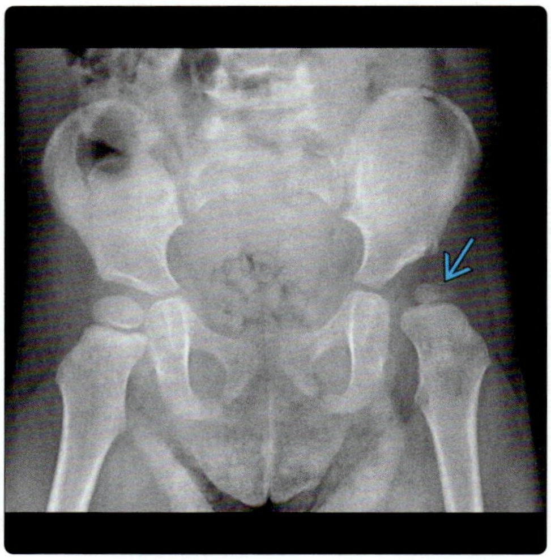

(Left) *AP radiograph in a 1-year-old girl with undiagnosed left hip dysplasia shows a shallow left acetabulum. There is marked superolateral subluxation of the left femoral head with only a small ossification center.* **(Right)** *Follow-up radiograph in the same child after spica casting shows progressive ossification of the left femoral head, though it remains small. Mild irregularity is likely due to avascular necrosis (AVN), a complication that may occur with excessive hip abduction during casting.*

Developmental Dysplasia of Hip

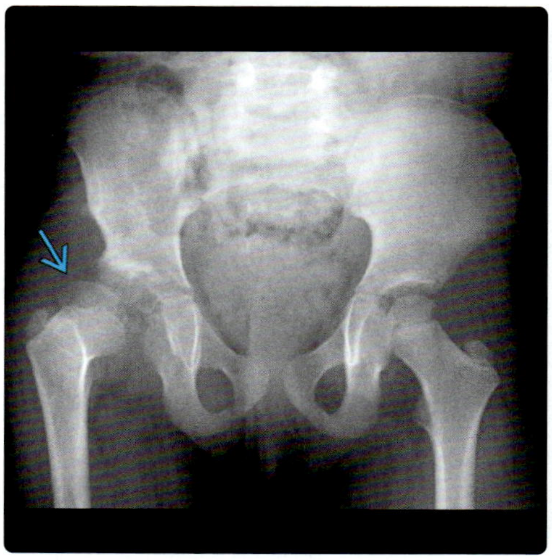

Developmental Dysplasia of Hip

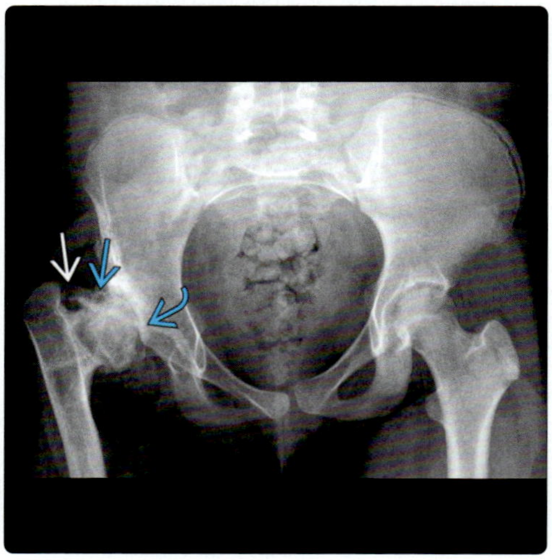

(Left) *AP radiograph in a 6 year old with a delayed diagnosis of right developmental hip dysplasia shows a shallow right acetabulum despite prior pelvic osteotomies. There is coxa magna & lateral subluxation of the right femoral head.* **(Right)** *A follow-up radiograph 6 years later shows pseudoacetabulum formation & joint degeneration with loss of the joint space, osteophyte formation, & subchondral cystic changes. The right coxa vara is from a prior osteotomy.*

Legg-Calvé-Perthes Disease

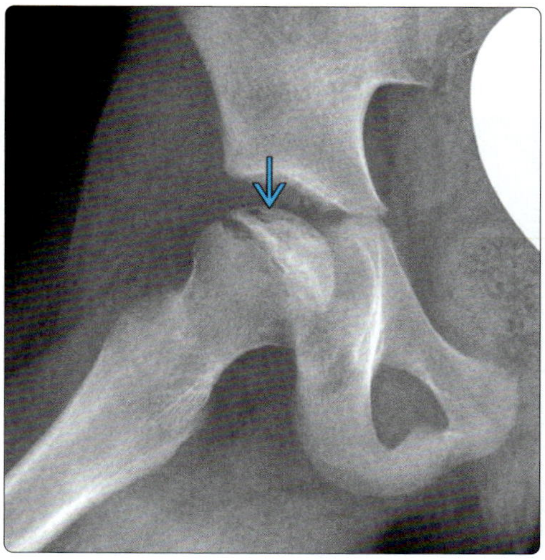

Legg-Calvé-Perthes Disease

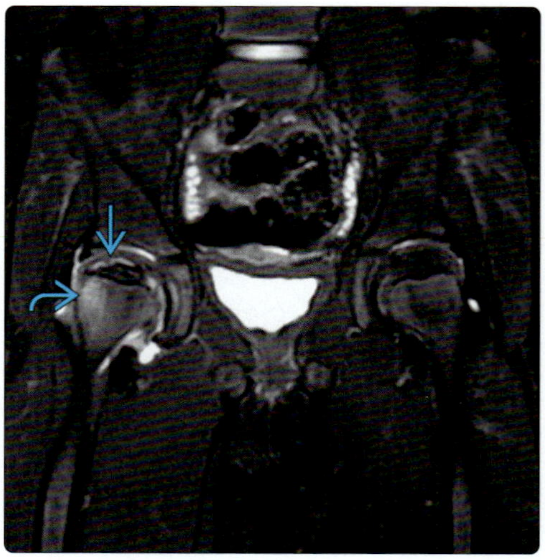

(Left) *Frog-leg lateral radiograph in an 8 year old with right hip pain shows sclerosis & flattening of the right femoral head, typical of Legg-Calvé-Perthes (LCP) disease. Note the lucent subchondral fracture, which is typically better visualized on this view.* **(Right)** *Coronal T2 FS MR of the same patient with LCP disease shows the subchondral fracture as a curvilinear hyperintense focus. Note the abnormal right femoral head morphology, femoral neck marrow edema, & joint effusion.*

Legg-Calvé-Perthes Disease

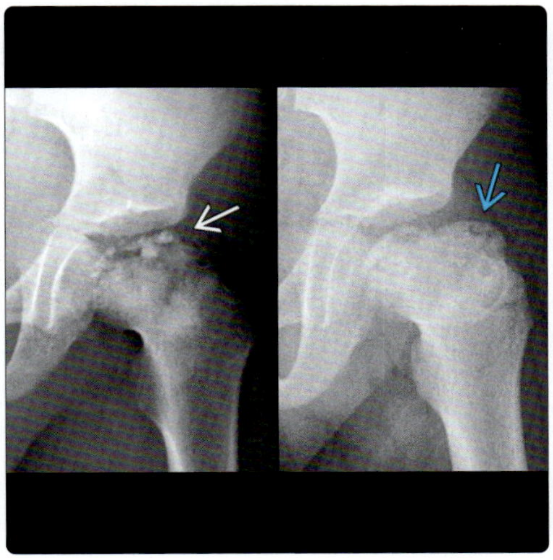

Avascular Necrosis

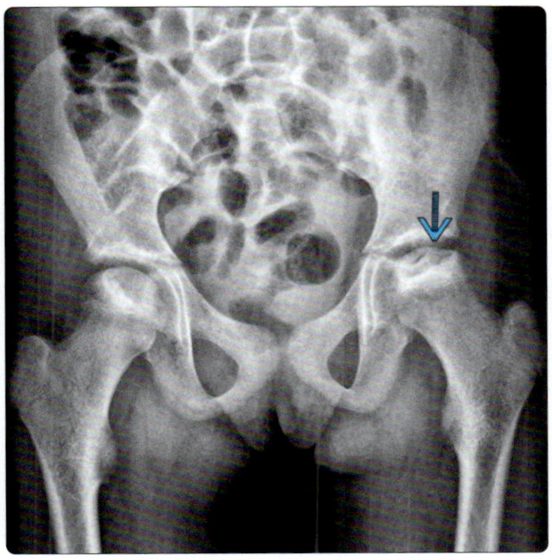

(Left) *Initial frontal radiograph (left image) of the left hip in a patient with LCP disease shows a fragmented & flattened femoral head ➡ with widening of the femoral neck. Two years later (right image), there is extrusion of the femoral head laterally ➡. Note the increasing ossification of the femoral head.* **(Right)** *AP radiograph in a 9-year-old girl with sickle cell disease & bilateral hip pain shows sclerosis & lucency of the bilateral femoral heads with flattening & irregularity of the left femoral head ➡.*

Avascular Necrosis

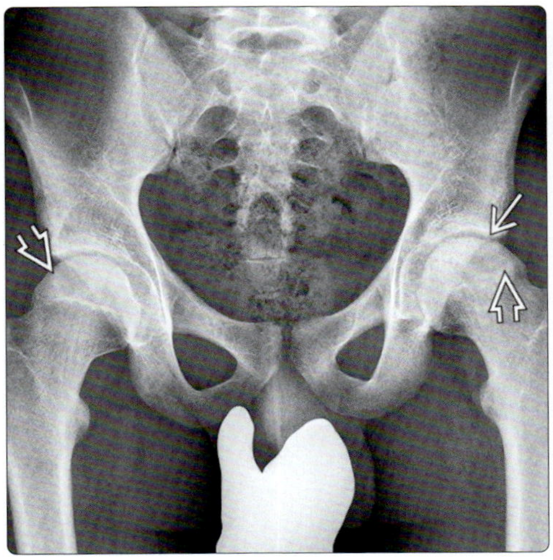

Avascular Necrosis

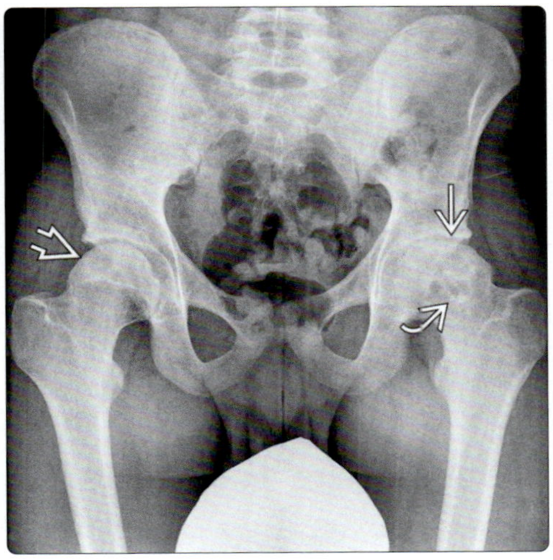

(Left) *AP radiograph shows mild left femoral head irregularity ➡ with patchy areas of increased sclerosis in both femoral heads ➡. This child had a history of dermatomyositis treated with steroid therapy.* **(Right)** *AP radiograph in the same patient 1 year later shows increasing deformity of the left femoral head ➡ with a stable appearance of the right ➡. Note the development of cystic-appearing lucencies in the left femoral neck ➡.*

Septic Arthritis

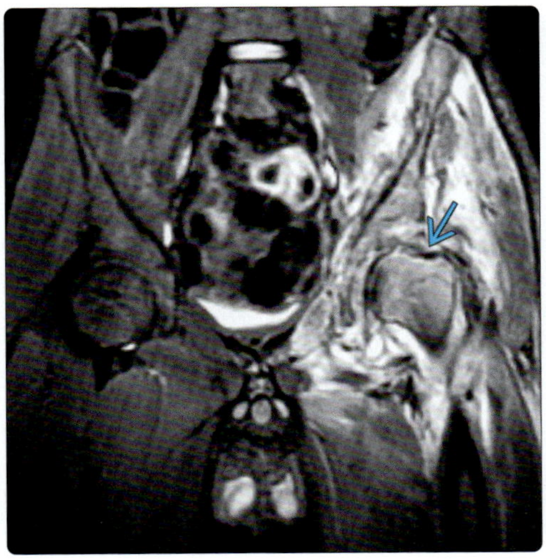

Septic Arthritis

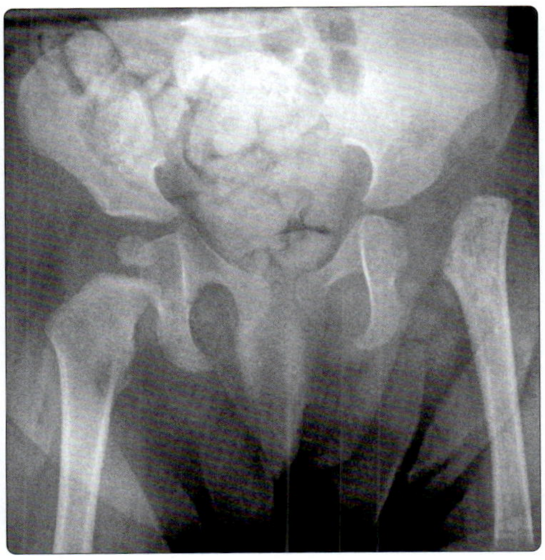

(Left) *Coronal STIR MR in a 15 year old diagnosed 1 month prior with left hip septic arthritis shows loss of the normal articular cartilage with femoral head erosions ➡. The extensive abnormal marrow & soft tissue signal intensity was due to concomitant osteomyelitis & soft tissue abscesses.* **(Right)** *AP radiograph in an 18 month old with a history of neonatal left hip septic arthritis shows sequelae of joint destruction with loss of a normal left femoral head ossification center & associated dysplasia of the acetabulum.*

(Left) *Coronal T1 C+ FS MR shows joint space narrowing with loss of articular cartilage along both sides of the bilateral hip joints. Subchondral foci of enhancement in both femoral heads are due to inflammation/erosions &/or mechanical degeneration with edema.* **(Right)** *Frontal pelvic radiograph in a 10-year-old girl with left hip pain shows marked widening of the left proximal femoral physis due to severe displacement of the capital femoral epiphysis medially.*

Juvenile Idiopathic Arthritis

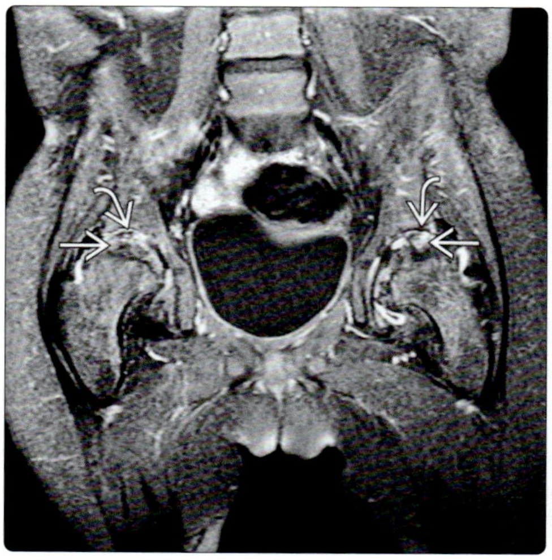

Slipped Capital Femoral Epiphysis

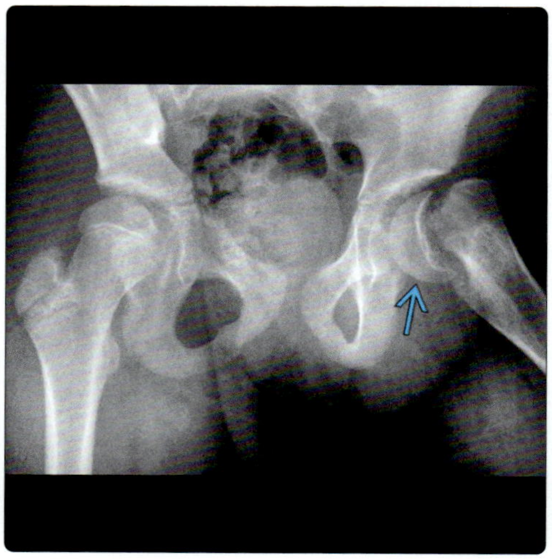

(Left) *Initial (left) & 3-month follow-up (right) postoperative radiographs in the same patient with slipped capital femoral epiphysis (SCFE) show the development of irregularity, sclerosis, & collapse of the femoral head. These findings are consistent with AVN, a known complication of SCFE &/or treatment.* **(Right)** *Frontal radiograph in a 2 year old presenting with a traumatic right femur fracture shows small, fragmented femoral epiphyses. This was an incidental finding with no history of hip pain.*

Slipped Capital Femoral Epiphysis

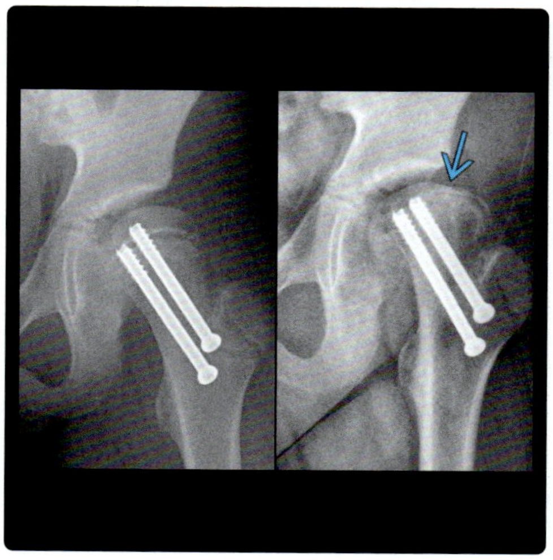

Meyer Dysplasia

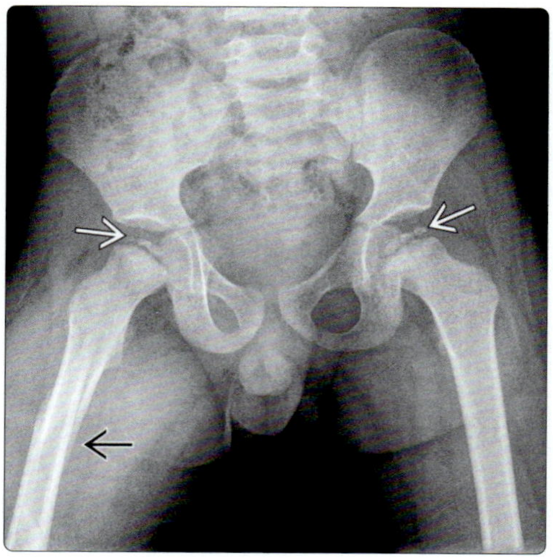

(Left) *Coronal T2 FS MR in a patient with left hip pain shows a rectangular-shaped focus of hyperintense signal within the central left femoral head. Note also that mild hyperintense signal is present within the adjacent acetabulum.* **(Right)** *AP radiograph in the same patient 4 years later shows irregularity of both femoral heads, joint space narrowing, & osteophyte formation. This patient had developed chondrolysis of the right hip in the interval.*

Idiopathic Chondrolysis

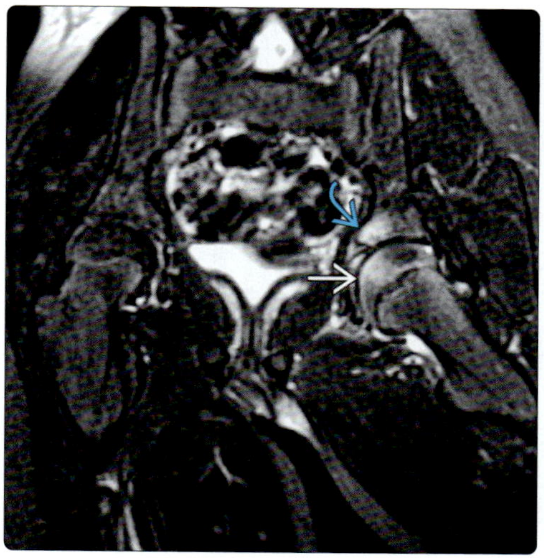

Idiopathic Chondrolysis

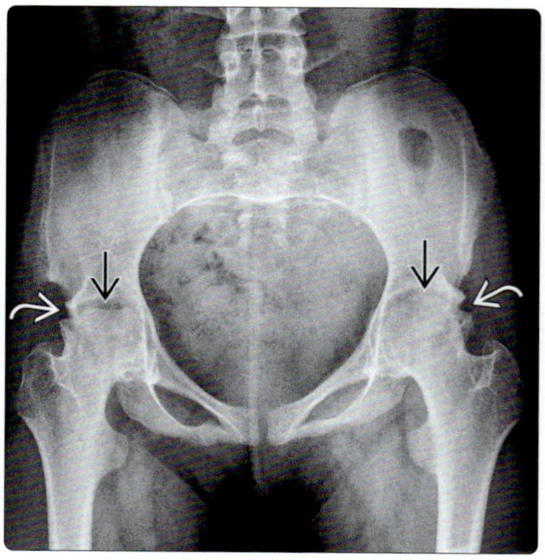

Epiphyseal Bone Tumors & Tumor-Like Conditions

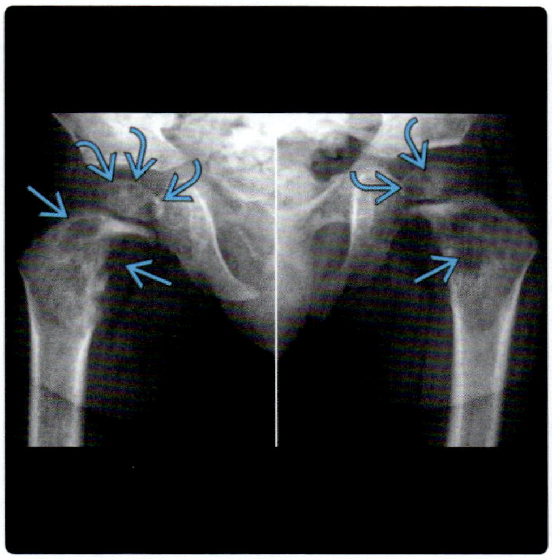

Epiphyseal Bone Tumors & Tumor-Like Conditions

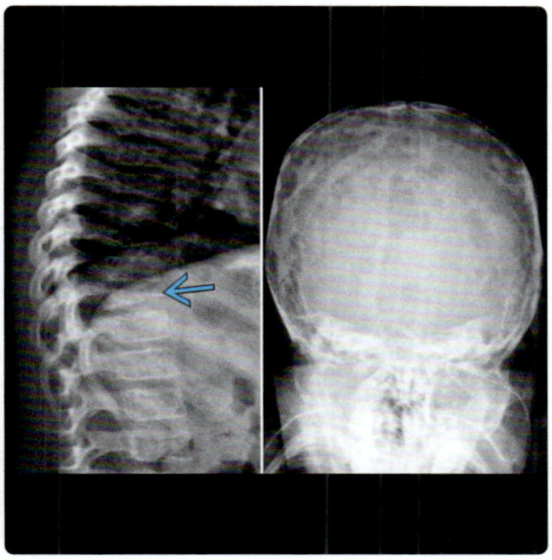

(Left) *Frontal radiographs of both hips in a 2 year old who presented with a limp show lucent lesions within both femoral heads* →*. Additionally, there are lucent lesions within both proximal femoral metaphyses* →*. The child was eventually diagnosed with Langerhans cell histiocytosis.* **(Right)** *Radiographs of the thoracic spine & skull in the same child show innumerable lytic lesions. Also note the vertebra plana deformity of a thoracic vertebra* →*, which is often seen in Langerhans cell histiocytosis.*

Epiphyseal Bone Tumors & Tumor-Like Conditions

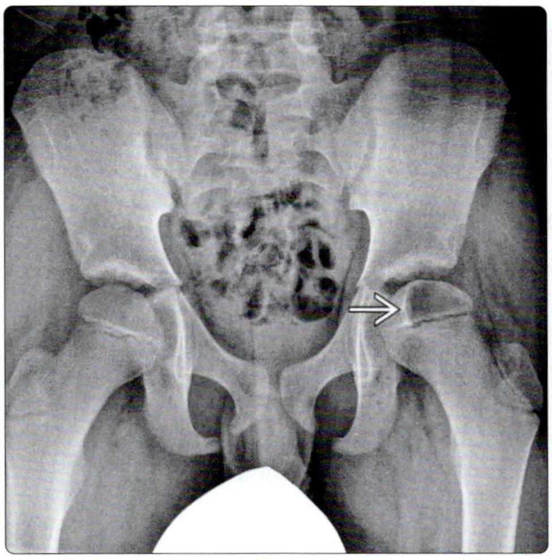

Epiphyseal Dysplasias

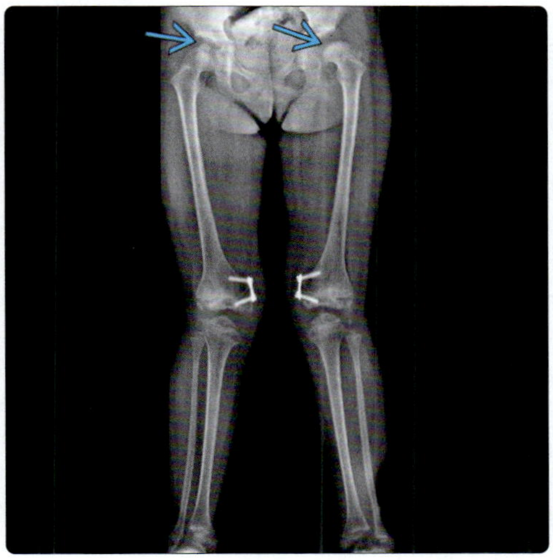

(Left) *Frontal radiograph shows a well-defined lytic lesion with a sclerotic margin within the left femoral head* → *+ mild femoral head flattening. A chondroblastoma was diagnosed by pathology.* **(Right)** *Frontal radiograph of the lower extremities in a 10 year old with multiple epiphyseal dysplasia shows hypoplastic & irregular femoral heads* →*. There is also irregularity of the remaining visualized epiphyses. Medial distal femoral epiphysiodeses were performed to treat genu valgum.*

Epiphyseal Dysplasias

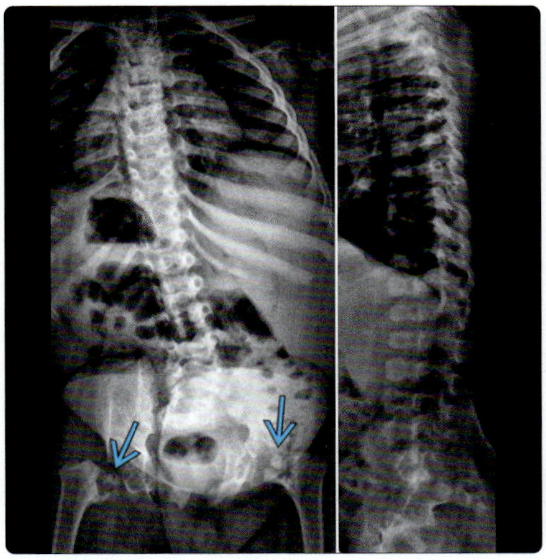

Proximal Focal Femoral Deficiency

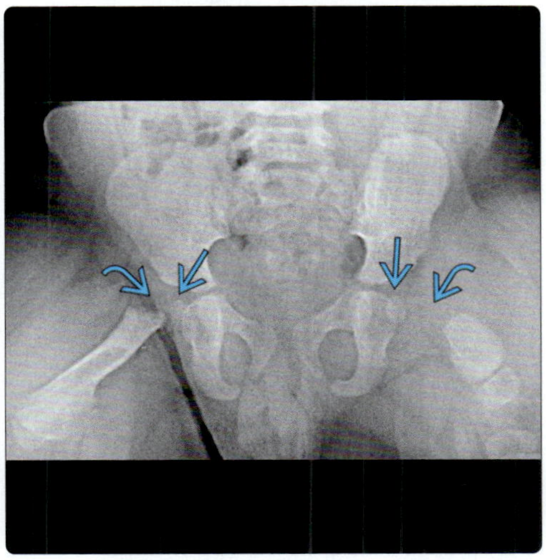

(Left) *Frontal & lateral spine radiographs in a 4-year-old boy with spondyloepiphyseal dysplasia show hypoplastic & markedly irregular femoral heads* →*. There are bilateral coxa vara deformities. Vertebral abnormalities are also present throughout the spine.* **(Right)** *Frontal radiograph of the pelvis in a 1 year old with lower extremity deformities shows small femoral heads* → *with deficiencies of the proximal femoral shafts* → *& shortening of the bilateral femurs.*

DIFFERENTIAL DIAGNOSIS

Common

- Legg-Calvé-Perthes
- Slipped Capital Femoral Epiphysis
- Developmental Dysplasia of Hip
- Septic Hip

Less Common

- Hip/Femur Trauma
- Juvenile Idiopathic Arthritis

Rare but Important

- Skeletal Dysplasias
- Transient Synovitis

ESSENTIAL INFORMATION

Key Differential Diagnosis Issues

- Coxa magna: Overgrowth of femoral head & neck
  - Exact definitions in medical literature vary; generally considered as widening/broadening
- Causation thought to be: Various insults → hyperemia → cartilage hyperplasia & hypertrophy → overgrowth of developing femoral head/neck
- History & associated findings are key to differentiating causes of coxa magna
- Degree of associated acetabular dysplasia largely depends on primary site of pathology & age of hip pathology onset (as earlier pathology impacts hip development earlier)

Helpful Clues for Common Diagnoses

- **Legg-Calvé-Perthes (LCP)**
  - Idiopathic avascular necrosis of femoral head in child
  - Peak age: 5-7 years
  - Fragmentation & flattening of head leads to coxa magna deformity
  - Hint (for LCP as cause): Femoral head remains centered on neck; acetabulum is relatively normal but femoral head is markedly abnormal
- **Slipped Capital Femoral Epiphysis (SCFE)**
  - Femoral head slips posterior & medial to metaphysis
    - Slipped femoral head appears short/broad on short/broad neck
  - Peak age: 11-14 years
  - Hint (for SCFE as cause): Femoral head posterior/medial on neck; acetabulum normal
- **Developmental Dysplasia of Hip (DDH)**
  - Abnormal position of femoral head relative to acetabulum during & beyond infancy → abnormal growth of both femoral head & acetabulum
  - Untreated severe DDH → femoral head & neck are broad & short
  - Hint (for DDH as cause): Shallow acetabulum on earliest images
    - May not be present after pelvic osteotomy
- **Septic Hip**
  - Microbial infection of joint → osteocartilaginous destruction & avascular necrosis
    - **Or** hyperemia → overgrowth of femoral head & neck

Helpful Clues for Less Common Diagnoses

- **Hip/Femur Trauma**
  - Resorption &/or impaction of neck or malalignment → coxa magna
- **Juvenile Idiopathic Arthritis**
  - Chronic inflammation → hyperemia → overgrowth of femoral head/neck

Helpful Clues for Rare Diagnoses

- **Skeletal Dysplasias**
  - Many can cause coxa magna
    - Will have systemic osseous deformities
  - Hint (due to dysplasia): Systemic features involving pelvis & other bones
- **Transient Synovitis**
  - Idiopathic inflammation of hip joint in children
  - Very common diagnosis but typically self-limited & without sequela
    - Rare reports of transient synovitis → coxa magna

Legg-Calvé-Perthes

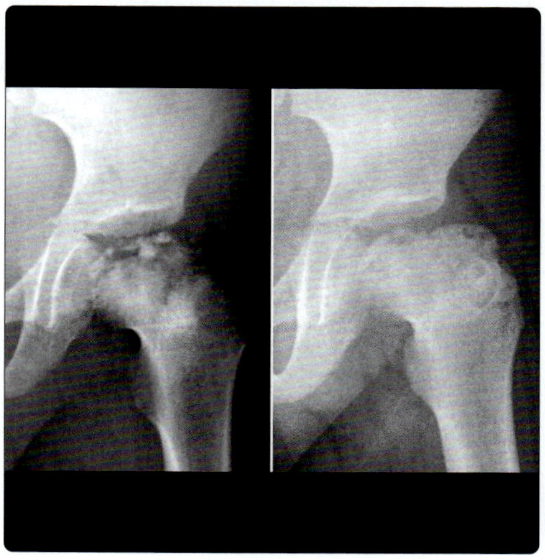

Legg-Calvé-Perthes

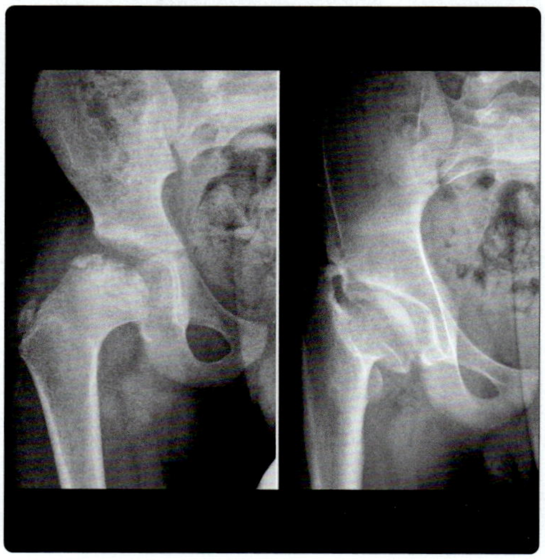

(Left) *Initial AP radiograph (left) of the hip in a patient with Legg-Calvé-Perthes (LCP) shows a fragmented & flattened left femoral head. Two years later (right), there is coxa magna with continued flattening & fragmentation. The acetabulum is only mildly dysplastic.* **(Right)** *Initial AP radiograph in a 6 year old (left) shows fragmentation & flattening of the right femoral head. Eight years later (right), after pelvic & femoral osteotomies, there is severe shortening & broadening of the femoral head & neck.*

Slipped Capital Femoral Epiphysis

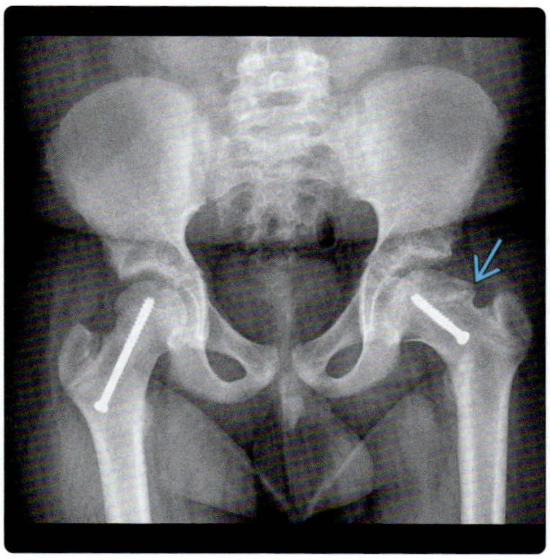

Developmental Dysplasia of Hip

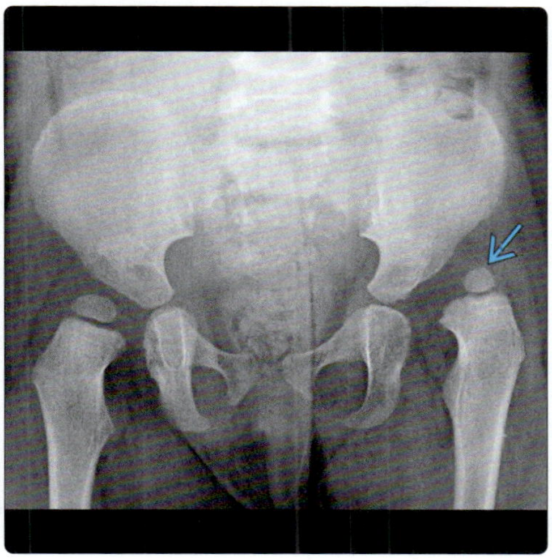

(Left) *AP radiograph in a 12 year old boy with bilateral SCFE treated with transphyseal screws shows that the left hip was complicated by avascular necrosis, which led to coxa magna. Also note the Cam-type deformity at the left femoral head & neck junction →.* **(Right)** *AP radiograph of the pelvis in 1-year-old girl shows shallow acetabula bilaterally. There is lateral subluxation of the right femoral head & superolateral dislocation of the left femoral head →, which is less developed than the right.*

Developmental Dysplasia of Hip

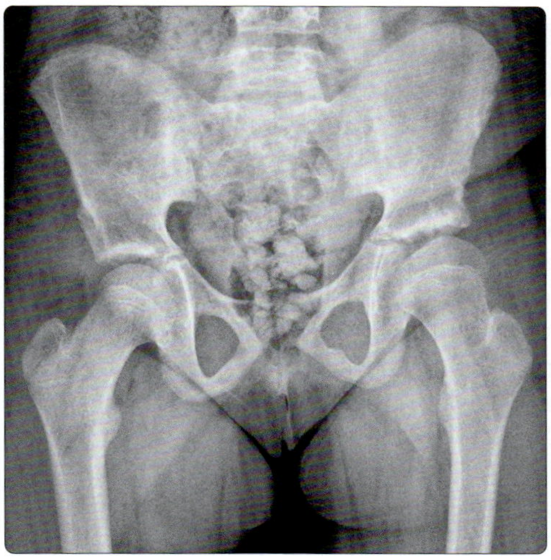

Septic Hip

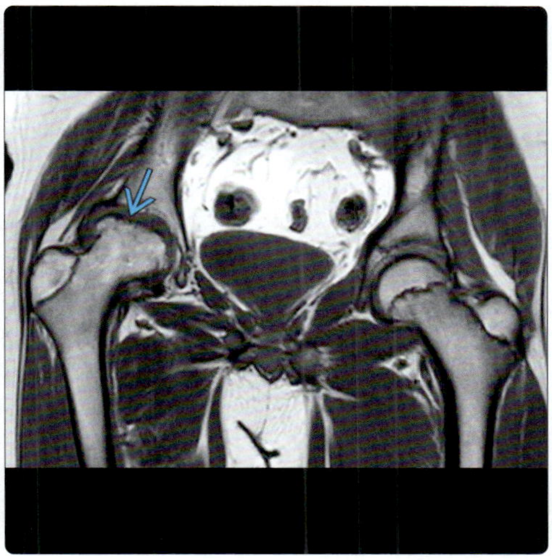

(Left) *AP radiograph in the same girl at 10 years of age (after spica casting & bilateral pelvic osteotomies) shows coxa magna of the left proximal femur (which was the more affected side previously). The acetabula are not shallow due to the prior realignment osteotomies.* **(Right)** *Coronal T1 MR of the pelvis in a 14 year old with a history of chronic right hip pain & a remote history of right hip septic arthritis shows right coxa magna with associated irregularity & flattening of the right femoral head →.*

Septic Hip

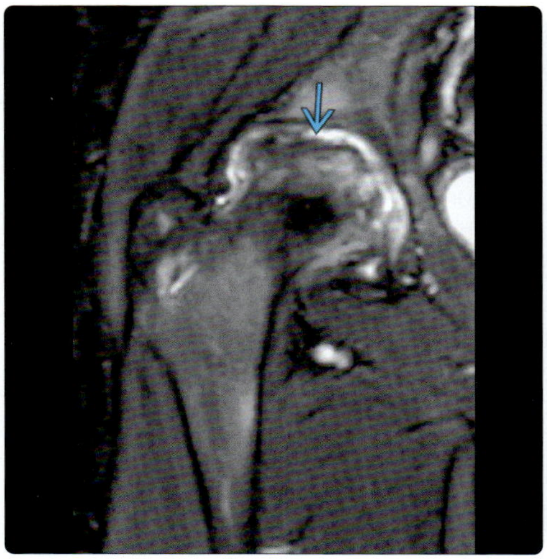

Skeletal Dysplasias

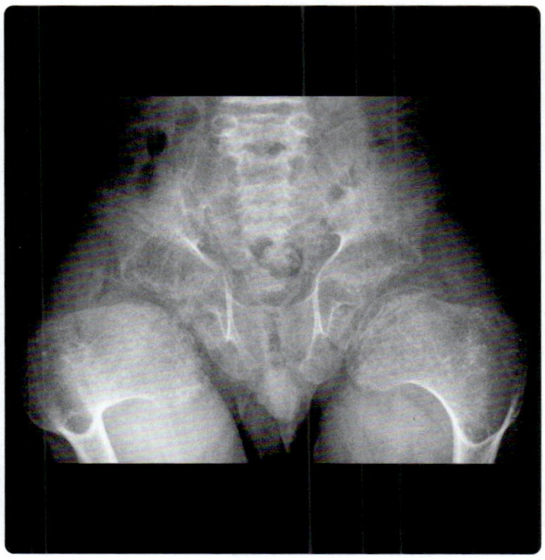

(Left) *Coronal T2 FS MR in the same child shows articular cartilage loss → & subchondral bone marrow edema.* **(Right)** *AP radiograph in a 10-year-old boy with Kniest dysplasia shows severe bilateral coxa magna with overgrowth of the femoral heads & necks. Multiple other skeletal deformities indicate that this is part of a systemic skeletal dysplasia.*

DIFFERENTIAL DIAGNOSIS

Common

- Trauma
- Septic Arthritis
- Transient Synovitis
- Juvenile Idiopathic Arthritis
- Normal Cartilage in Young Child (Mimic)

Less Common

- Osteonecrosis/Infarct
- Synovial Venous Malformation
- Pigmented Villonodular Synovitis
- Hemophilic Arthropathy
- Periarticular/Intraarticular Bone Tumor
- Intraarticular Loose Body

Rare but Important

- Marrow Infiltrating Processes
- Synovial Sarcoma (Mimic)
- Synovial Osteochondromatosis
- Idiopathic Chondrolysis
- Lyme Disease
- Vasculitis

ESSENTIAL INFORMATION

Key Differential Diagnosis Issues

- Clinical features to consider
  - Age
  - Timing of onset + duration of symptoms
  - Number & location of joints involved
  - Degree of functional limitation
  - Presence or absence of
    - Injury
    - Fever
    - Elevated inflammatory markers
    - Previously established medical condition
- Modality considerations
  - Radiographs
    - Excellent evaluation of cortical bone
    - Cannot differentiate fluid from abnormal synovium
    - Will miss effusions in some joints (e.g., hips, shoulders)
    - Will not show early sequelae of arthritis
  - Ultrasound
    - Excellent depiction of fluid in joints
      - Certain joints need specific views
      - Fluid may be confused with hypoechoic synovium & unossified cartilage (both of which do not compress & may show internal vascularity)
  - MR
    - Best depiction of entire joint + marrow & soft tissues
    - Most etiologies show simple fluid ± regions of enhancing synovium > 2 mm thick
      - IV contrast improves conspicuity of synovitis (though it may be visible on T2-weighted images)
      - T2* GRE increases sensitivity for blood products
- Take home points
  - Many pathologies result in joint effusions ± synovitis
  - Imaging generally cannot distinguish infected from sterile fluid

Helpful Clues for Common Diagnoses

- **Trauma**
  - Exceedingly common in children
    - Event of injury may not be recognized in very young
  - Look for subtle fractures
  - MR is typically reserved for suspected soft tissue injuries
    - Reveals reactive fluid vs. layering hemarthrosis or lipohemarthrosis
    - Mild synovitis is often present with subacute or recurrent trauma
- **Septic Arthritis**
  - New onset of swelling, redness, & warmth, usually without trauma history & typically isolated to 1 joint
  - Presence of increased number of Kocher criteria increases specificity for infection: Fever > 38.5°C, non-weight-bearing, WBC > 12,000, ESR ≥ 40 mm/hour; some include CRP > 20 mg/L
    - Joint aspiration is required with any suspicion
  - Synovial thickening is typically mild unless infection is chronic/indolent
  - Presence of marrow & soft tissue edema on MR increases likelihood of joint infection over transient synovitis
    - Diminished enhancement of periarticular marrow may occur in tight joints (due to ischemia)
  - Urgent joint washout & IV antibiotics are required due to risk of rapid joint destruction
- **Transient Synovitis**
  - Typically 3-8 years of age
  - Hip is affected most commonly
  - More commonly bilateral than septic arthritis
  - Ultrasound is frequently used to detect hip fluid
    - Cannot distinguish infected from sterile fluid regardless of complexity, volume, or synovitis
    - Presence of fluid must be coupled with absence of Kocher criteria to exclude need for joint aspiration
  - Surrounding soft tissues are normal on MR
- **Juvenile Idiopathic Arthritis**
  - Pain for ≥ 6 weeks, usually indolent
  - Age < 16 years
  - Radiographs are most specific in chronic disease
    - Epiphyseal (or equivalent) overgrowth, erosions, joint space loss (rarely leading to ankylosis)
  - MR is best for early changes
    - Mild to moderate synovial thickening (> 2 mm) throughout joint
    - Rice bodies (tiny, uniform, T2-hypointense foci) in joint strongly suggest diagnosis
    - ± foci of marrow edema, osteocartilaginous erosions
- **Normal Cartilage in Young Child (Mimic)**
  - Unossified cartilage of epiphyses & epiphyseal equivalents at joints can mimic fluid on radiographs & ultrasound
    - Knowing expected adult shapes of bones & visualizing cartilage margins flush with metaphyseal cortex can be helpful
    - Sonography demonstrates tiny, round, echogenic fibrovascular channels throughout noncompressible unossified cartilage

Helpful Clues for Less Common Diagnoses

- **Osteonecrosis/Infarct**
  - Legg-Calvé-Perthes is most common pediatric form
    - Radiographs show femoral head sclerosis, lucency, fragmentation, broadening
    - MR shows heterogeneous marrow
      - Patchy increased fluid signal intensity of marrow acutely with diminished enhancement
      - Decreased T1 & T2 signal intensity chronically suggests sclerosis with nonenhancement of necrosis; hyperenhancement suggests reperfusion
      - Classic double line sign may be seen chronically
  - Otherwise uncommon in children without predisposition
    - Sickle cell disease
    - Leukemia with steroid treatment
    - Infection in tight joint
- **Synovial Venous Malformation**
  - Lobulated masses ± tubular foci about joint on MR, extending into synovium
    - Mass protrudes into effusion from joint capsule
    - Fluid-fluid levels & low-signal thrombi in mass
    - Enhancement typically patchy & gradual
  - Synovium blooms on T2* GRE due to hemosiderin
- **Pigmented Villonodular Synovitis**
  - Frond-like protrusions extend into synovium with variable enhancement; may have more focal mass
  - Synovium blooms on T2* GRE due to hemosiderin
- **Hemophilic Arthropathy**
  - Diagnosis of hemophilia is typically known
  - Synovium blooms on T2* GRE due to hemosiderin
- **Periarticular/Intraarticular Bone Tumor**
  - Certain bone tumors (such as osteoid osteoma & chondroblastoma) are known to incite marked inflammatory reaction of surrounding tissues
  - Intraarticular extension of other tumors also results in joint effusion &/or synovitis
- **Intraarticular Loose Body**
  - Unstable osteochondral lesions, particularly those with loose/free fragments, may irritate joint
    - Check classic locations for donor site (medial talar dome, capitellum, medial femoral condyle)
    - MR shows typical signal of cartilage ± bone fragment
  - Penetrating injuries may rarely lead to retained intraarticular foreign bodies

Helpful Clues for Rare Diagnoses

- **Marrow Infiltrating Processes**
  - Look for extensive marrow signal abnormalities on MR
    - Loss of T1-bright yellow marrow, increase of fluid content on T2 FS or STIR
  - Most commonly due to leukemia or metastatic neuroblastoma in children
- **Synovial Sarcoma (Mimic)**
  - Often occurs near joint, rarely in joint
    - Does not originate from synovium
  - Can begin as small, lobulated, cyst-like mass
- **Synovial Osteochondromatosis**
  - Appearance of intraarticular bodies varies by content
    - Cartilage, calcification, &/or fatty marrow of ossification
- **Idiopathic Chondrolysis**
  - Rare hip disorder in preadolescents where increased intracapsular pressure leads to cartilage loss
  - Vertical column of T2-hyperintense MR signal & enhancement centrally within femoral head
- **Lyme Disease**
  - Characteristic rash + history of tick bite helpful
- **Vasculitis**
  - Systemic clues (lung, renal, or CNS involvement) helpful

SELECTED REFERENCES

1. Dimitriou C et al: Imaging of juvenile idiopathic arthritis. Radiol Clin North Am. 55(5):1071-83, 2017
2. Nguyen JC et al: US evaluation of juvenile idiopathic arthritis and osteoarticular infection. Radiographics. 37(4):1181-201, 2017
3. Kim HK et al: MR findings of synovial disease in children and young adults: Part 2. Pediatr Radiol. 41(4):512-24, 2011
4. Kim HK et al: MR findings of synovial disease in children and young adults: Part 1. Pediatr Radiol. 41(4):495-511; quiz 545-6, 2011

Trauma

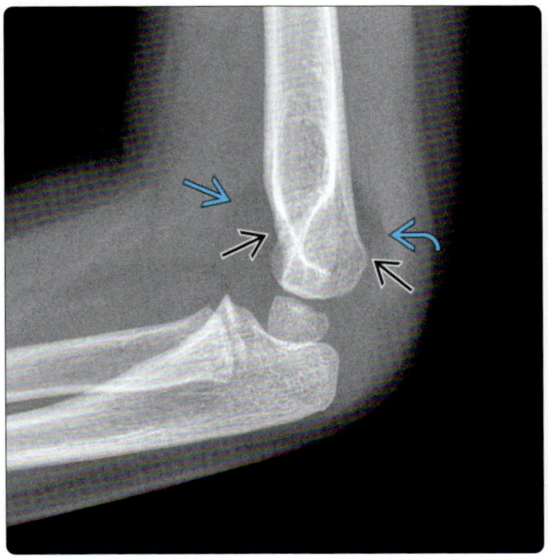

Trauma

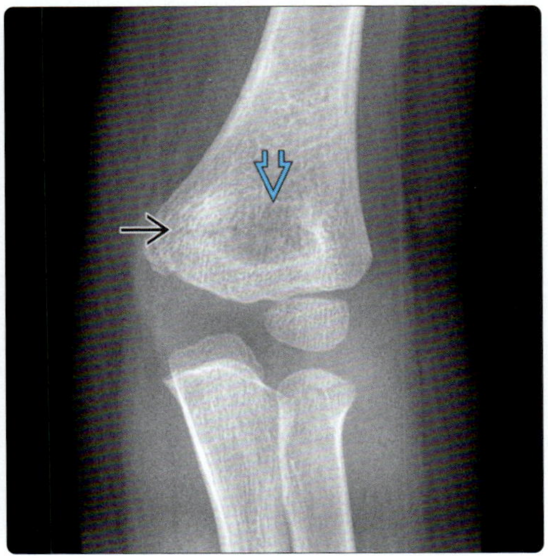

(Left) *Lateral radiograph in a 4 year old after a fall shows displacement of the anterior ➡ & posterior ➡ fat pads, consistent with an elbow joint effusion after trauma. The location & morphology of cortical disruption ➡ are typical of a nondisplaced supracondylar fracture.* **(Right)** *AP radiograph in the same patient confirms the supracondylar fracture line ➡ traversing the level of the coronoid & olecranon fossae ➡.*

(Left) *Lateral knee radiograph in a 13-year-old girl with pain after being kicked shows moderate distention of the suprapatellar pouch, most commonly due to a traumatic effusion/hemarthrosis.* (Right) *Sunrise view of the knee in the same patient shows lateral subluxation of the patella with avulsion of a small bone fragment from the medial pole at the site of the medial patellofemoral ligament attachment, consistent with a transient patellar dislocation.*

Trauma

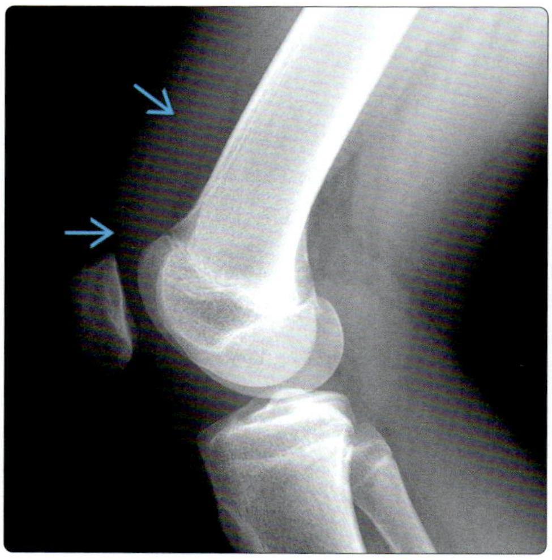

Trauma

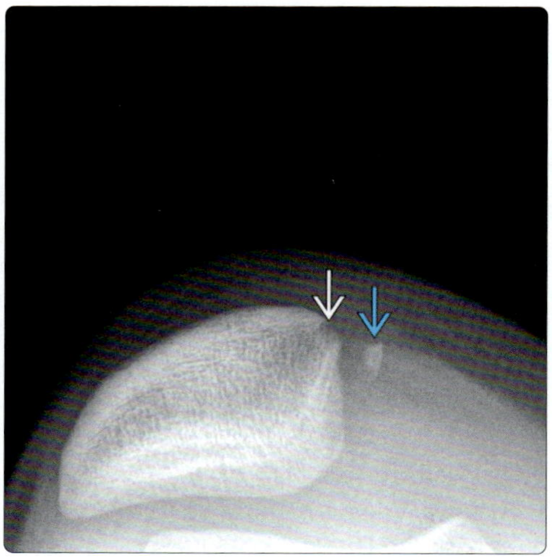

(Left) *Lateral radiograph in a 13-year-old boy after an injury shows a Salter-Harris II fracture of the distal tibia. There is a moderate joint effusion.* (Right) *Posterior transverse ultrasound of the right shoulder in a 9 month old with fever shows fluid distending the joint capsule around the hypoechoic unossified humeral head & echogenic labrum. Note the ossified portions of the glenoid & humeral head.*

Trauma

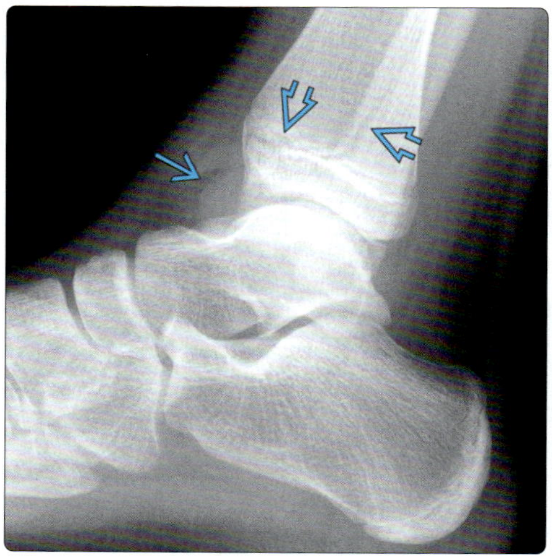

Septic Arthritis

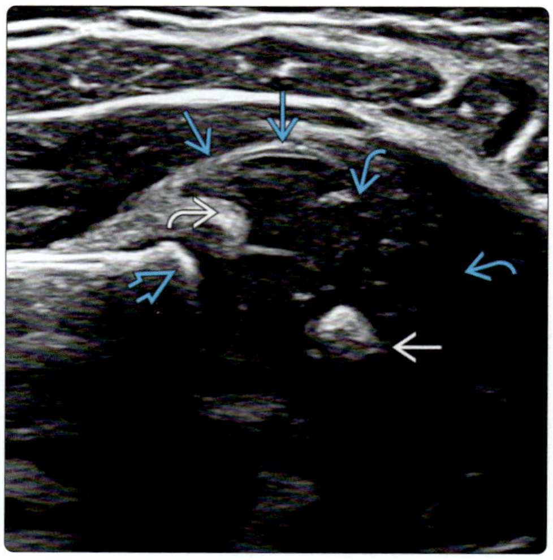

(Left) *Axial T2 FS MR in the same patient shows the effusion & synovitis of the glenohumeral joint. Note the edema in the partially ossified humeral head & the overlying soft tissues. Septic arthritis was confirmed upon drainage.* (Right) *AP radiograph in a 2-year-old boy with hip pain shows symmetric positions of the femoral heads with normal gluteal fat pads. However, hip joint effusions are often occult on radiographs.*

Septic Arthritis

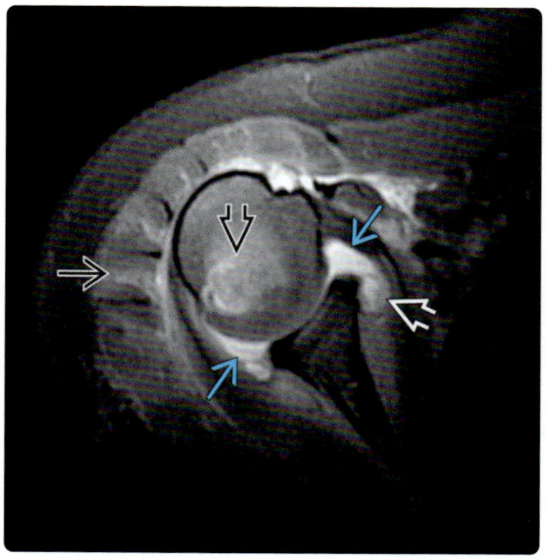

Transient Synovitis

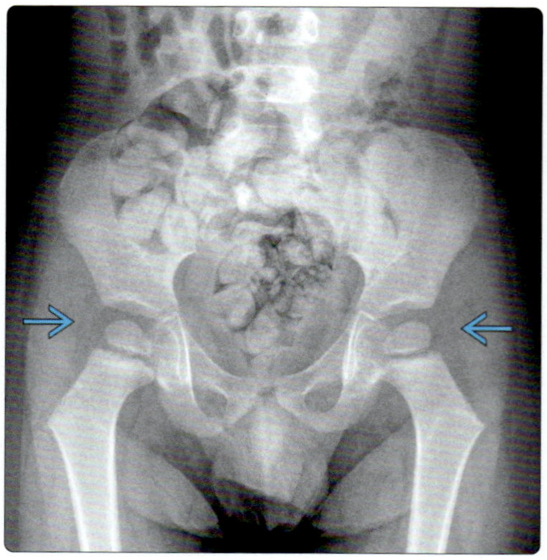

Transient Synovitis

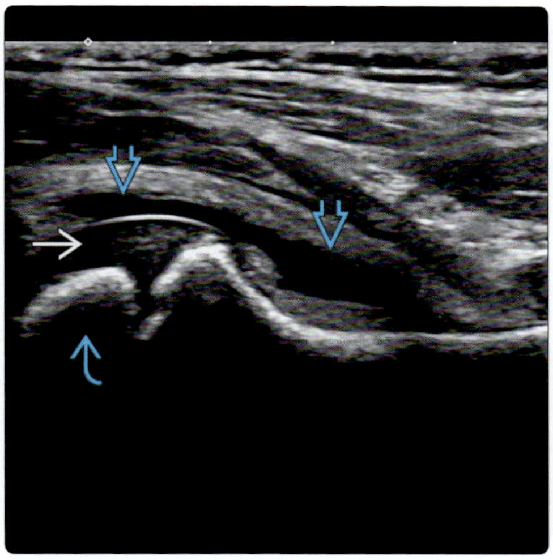

Juvenile Idiopathic Arthritis

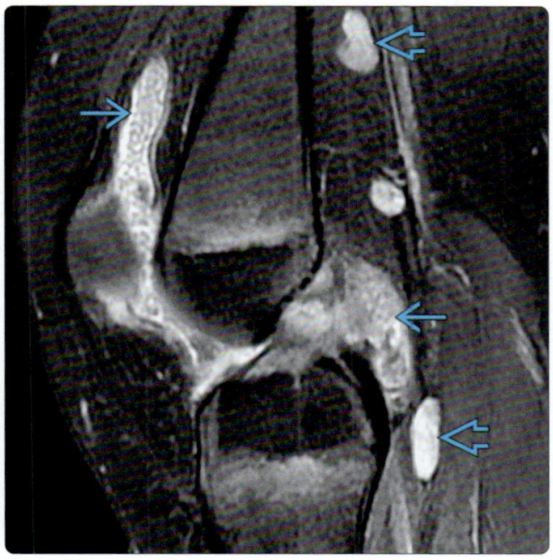

(Left) *Sagittal ultrasound in the same patient shows a moderate effusion ⇨ of the left hip joint. Note the hypoechoic appearance of the unossified cartilage ➡ surrounding the femoral head ossification center ⇨.* **(Right)** *Sagittal T2 FS MR in a 12-year-old girl with systemic juvenile idiopathic arthritis (JIA) shows distention of the knee joint by fluid & numerous tiny hypointense bodies ⇨ that are uniform in size. These rice bodies & popliteal adenopathy ⇨ are common in JIA.*

Juvenile Idiopathic Arthritis

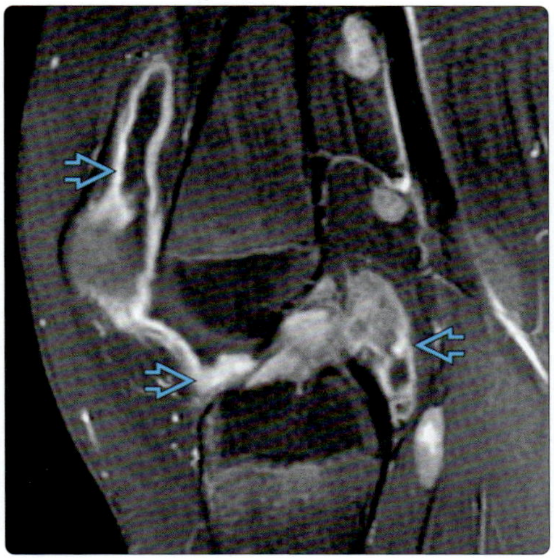

Normal Cartilage in Young Child (Mimic)

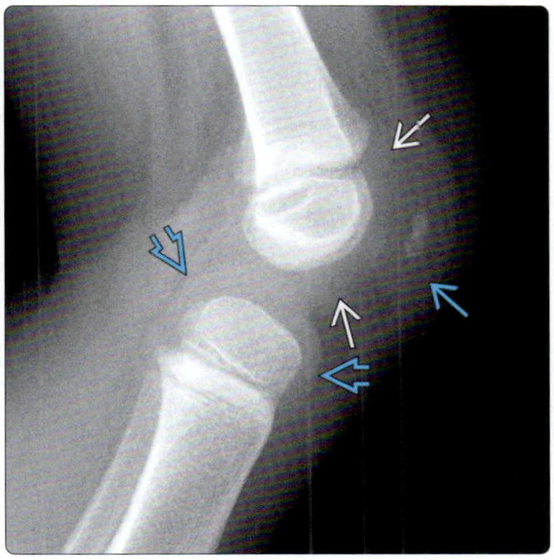

(Left) *Sagittal T1 C+ FS MR in the same patient shows abnormally thickened, enhancing synovium ⇨ throughout the joint.* **(Right)** *Lateral radiograph of a normal knee in a 3 year old with pain shows soft tissue (fluid) attenuation by the unossified epiphyseal cartilages about the knee, including the distal femur ➡, proximal tibia ⇨, & patella ⇨. These cartilages can mimic abnormal fluid collections in young children.*

Osteonecrosis/Infarct

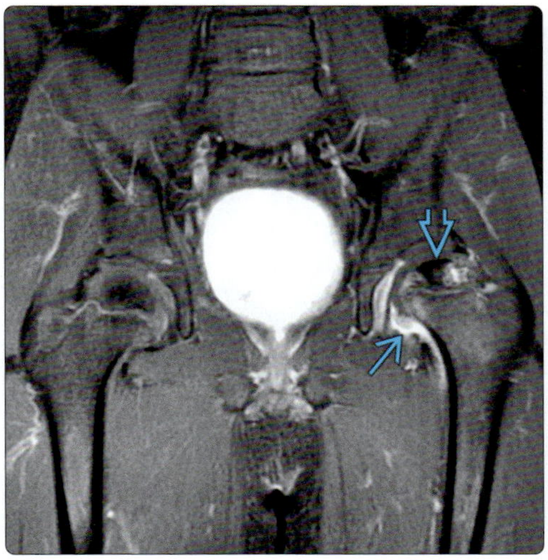

Osteonecrosis/Infarct

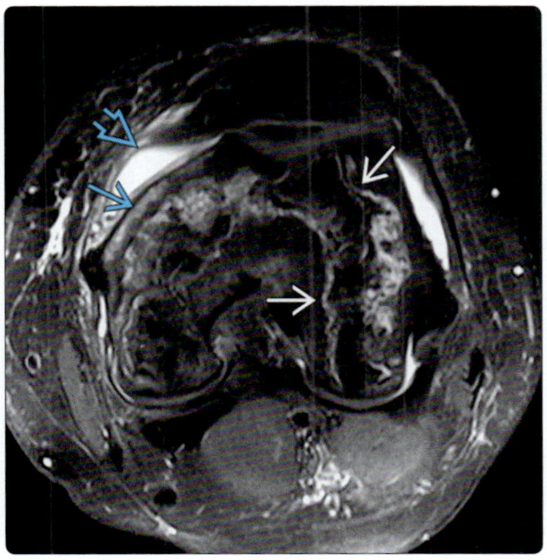

(Left) *Coronal T1 C+ FS MR in a 7-year-old girl with known Legg-Calvé-Perthes disease shows a mildly flattened femoral head with central hypoenhancement ⇨ that is surrounded by peripheral hyperenhancement & synovitis ⇨.* **(Right)** *Axial T2 FS MR in a 16 year old shows the classic double line sign of chronic bone infarcts ➡. However, there is more focal, poorly defined edema ⇨ medially due to a superimposed acute or subacute infarct that resulted in the joint effusion ⇨.*

(Left) *Sagittal T2 FS MR in a 7 year old with a venous malformation shows the lesion protruding into the suprapatellar pouch with inferior extensions along the Hoffa fat & ACL. Note the characteristic fluid-fluid levels & thrombi within the mass.* **(Right)** *Sagittal T2* GRE MR of the same knee shows "blooming" of the hemosiderin lining the synovium. The blood products & associated enzymes of recurrent hemarthrosis can lead to accelerated joint degeneration.*

Synovial Venous Malformation

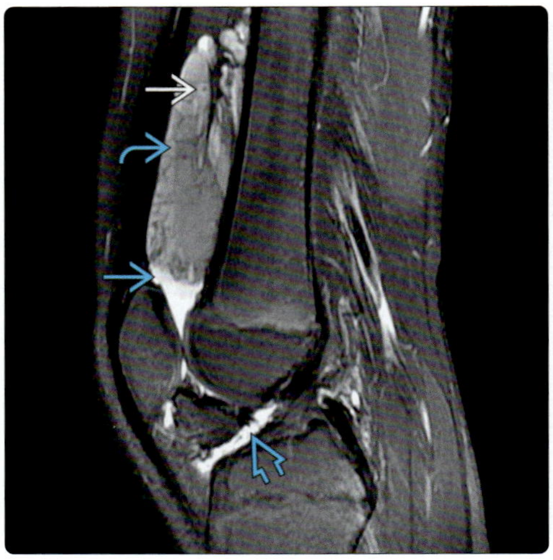

Synovial Venous Malformation

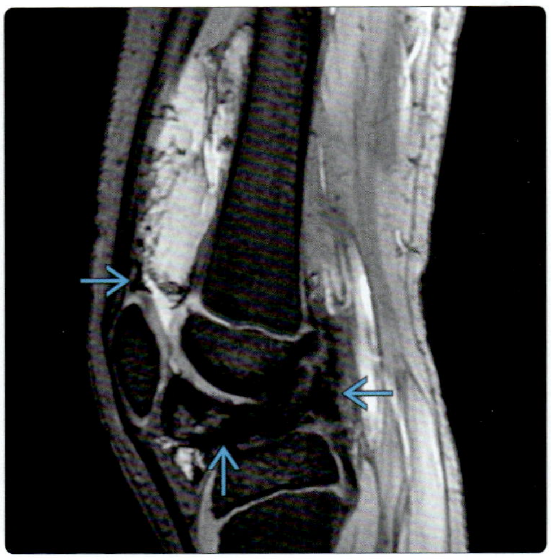

(Left) *Sagittal T2 FS MR in a 14 year old with hemophilia A shows an elbow joint effusion with low signal intensity hemosiderin lining the synovium. Aggressive factor replacement regimens have decreased the frequency of recurrent hemarthroses.* **(Right)** *Coronal T2 FS MR in a 16 year old with hip pain shows the target appearance of an osteoid osteoma nidus in the superolateral acetabulum. There is edema of the adjacent marrow plus a joint effusion.*

Hemophilic Arthropathy

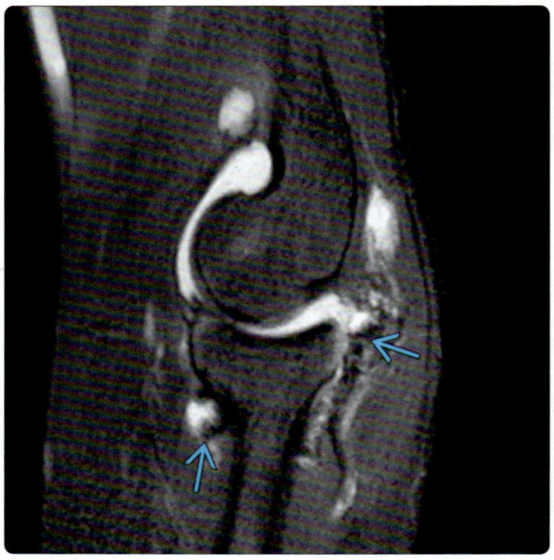

Periarticular/Intraarticular Bone Tumor

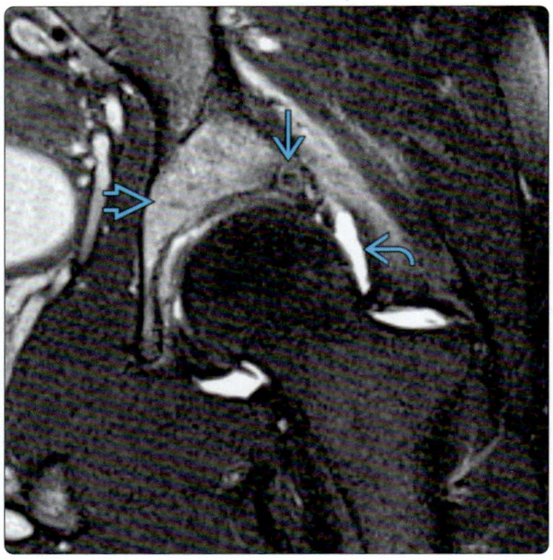

(Left) *Sagittal T2 FS MR in a 13-year-old girl shows a heterogeneously hypointense lesion in the posterior tibial epiphysis & metaphysis. There is marked surrounding marrow & soft tissue edema as well as a joint effusion. These findings are all typical of a chondroblastoma.* **(Right)** *Sagittal T2 FS MR of the right elbow in a 14 year old shows a detached osteochondral fragment in the posterior joint. There is loss of cartilage & bone at the anterior capitellum, which is a typical site for osteochondritis dissecans.*

Periarticular/Intraarticular Bone Tumor

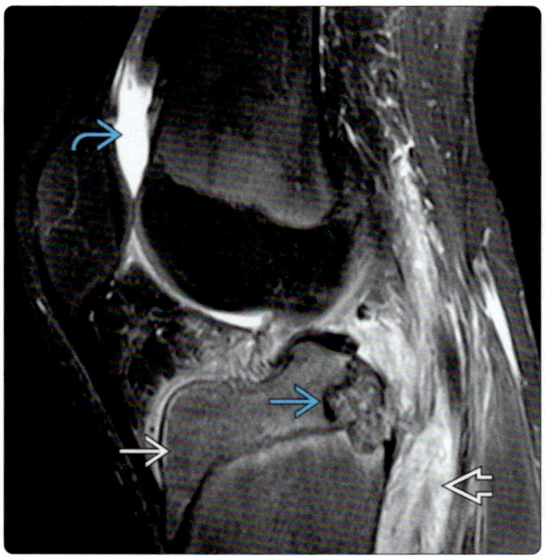

Intraarticular Loose Body

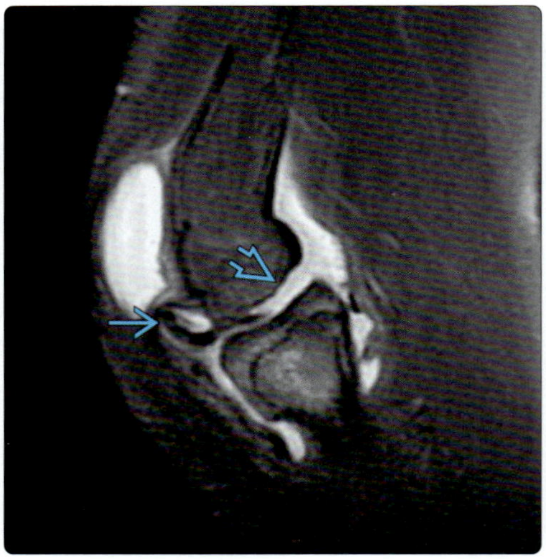

Marrow Infiltrating Processes

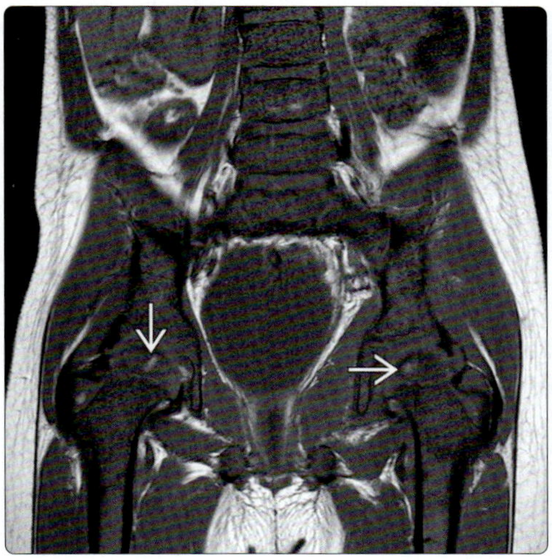

Marrow Infiltrating Processes

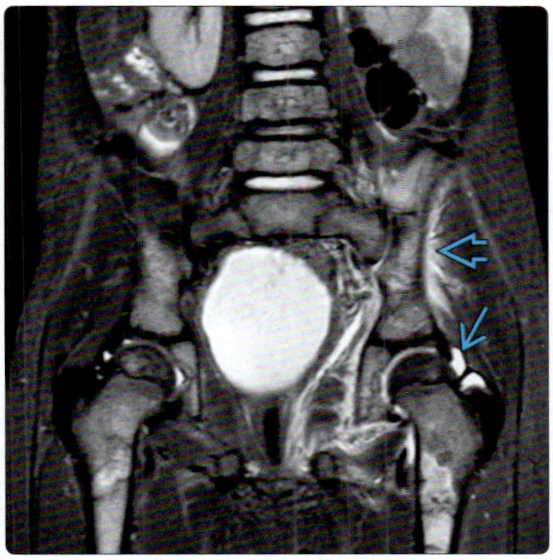

(Left) *Coronal T1 MR in a 3-year-old boy with left hip pain, malaise, & anemia shows diffuse replacement of fatty marrow with minimal residual T1-bright fat in the femoral heads. In young children, this appearance is most commonly seen with leukemia or metastatic neuroblastoma.* **(Right)** *Coronal STIR MR in the same patient shows abnormally bright signal of the marrow diffusely. There is periosteal & soft tissue edema as well as a joint effusion on the left. Metastatic neuroblastoma was ultimately diagnosed.*

Synovial Sarcoma (Mimic)

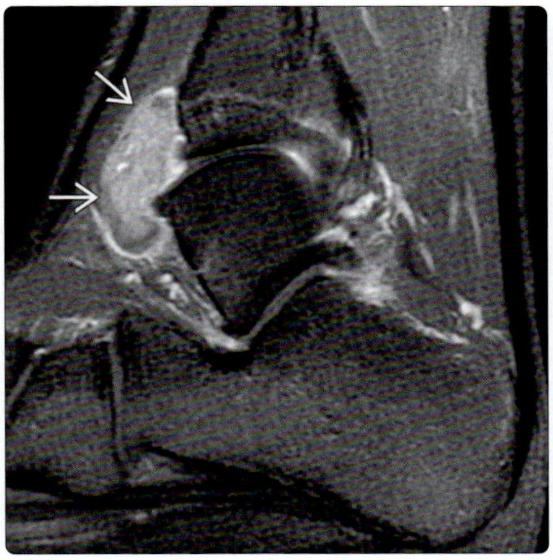

Synovial Osteochondromatosis

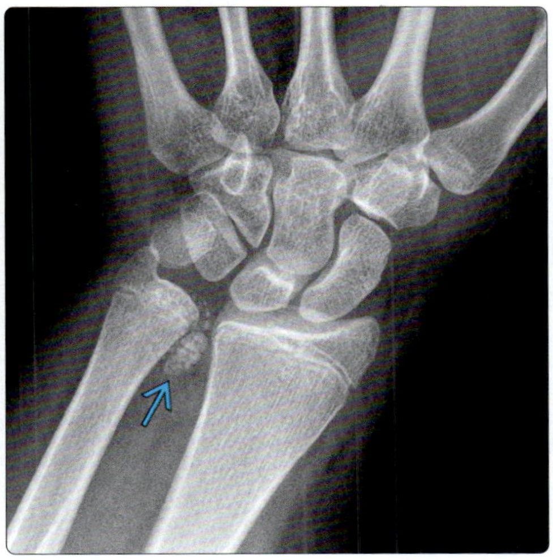

(Left) *Sagittal T1 C+ FS MR in a 15-year-old boy shows a moderately enhancing, solid mass along the anterior tibiotalar articulation. Synovial sarcoma was found on biopsy. These lesions more commonly occur near a joint rather than in a joint.* **(Right)** *PA radiograph of the wrist in a 12-year-old girl shows numerous tiny, calcified bodies in the distal radioulnar joint. Synovial osteochondromatosis was confirmed on a subsequent MR.*

Idiopathic Chondrolysis

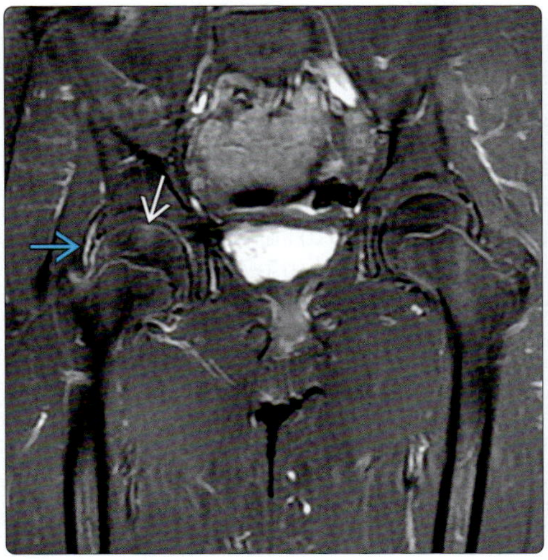

Vasculitis

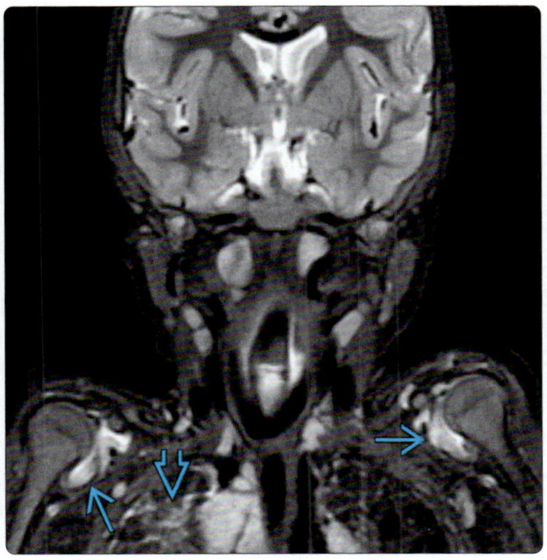

(Left) *Coronal T1 C+ FS MR in a 9-year-old girl with right hip pain demonstrates mild synovitis & a central column of increased femoral head enhancement, typical of idiopathic chondrolysis.* **(Right)** *Coronal STIR MR in a 4-year-old girl with ANCA vasculitis & multifocal joint swelling shows synovitis of the bilateral glenohumeral joints. Her associated lung disease was better detailed on CT.*

DIFFERENTIAL DIAGNOSIS

Common

- Septic Arthritis
- Juvenile Idiopathic Arthritis
- Trauma

Less Common

- Developmental Dysplasia of Hip
- Legg-Calvé-Perthes
- Other Avascular Necrosis
- Venous Malformation

Rare but Important

- Lyme Disease
- Pigmented Villonodular Synovitis
- Hemophilia
- Osteoid Osteoma
- Malignancy
- Neuropathic Joint
- Synovial Osteochondromatosis
- Tuberculous Arthropathy
- Vasculitis
- Trevor-Fairbank Disease
- Epiphyseal Dysplasia (Mimic)
- Multicentric Carpal-Tarsal Osteolysis (Mimic)
- Gorham-Stout Disease (Mimic)

ESSENTIAL INFORMATION

Key Differential Diagnosis Issues

- Imaging features overlap between many articular diseases
  - Acute: Variable degrees of T2-hyperintense joint fluid; synovial thickening (> 2 mm) along joint capsule, often slightly hypointense to fluid on T2; ± adjacent marrow abnormalities
    - Active synovitis is best demonstrated on early postcontrast MR images
  - Chronic: Cartilage loss, erosions, subchondral cysts, osteophytes
    - Longstanding hyperemia may lead to epiphyseal overgrowth &/or early growth plate closure
    - Changes of repetitive mechanical dysfunction & associated degeneration may be difficult to discern from ongoing primary disease
- Some imaging clues narrow differential: Ca^{2+}, hemosiderin, loose bodies
- Prior studies may provide insight into underlying disorders
- Clinical history is helpful, including age of onset, duration of symptoms, number of joints involved, involvement of other organ systems, & laboratory markers
  - Imaging alone does not exclude infected joint fluid
- Detection & treatment of active disease early will lessen &/or prevent chronic debilitating joint disease

Helpful Clues for Common Diagnoses

- **Septic Arthritis**
  - Bacterial infection of joint; usually monostotic with rapid onset of symptoms
  - Requires urgent confirmation & joint washout
  - Kocher criteria ↑ specificity in acute setting: Fever > 38.5°C (101.3°F), non-weight-bearing, WBC > 12,000 cells/mm³, ESR > 40 mm/hour; some add CRP > 20 mg/L
  - Acute imaging: Size of effusion is variable; synovitis is typically mild to moderate
    - Adjacent marrow & soft tissue edema & ↓ epiphyseal enhancement on MR ↑ likelihood of infection
    - Bulky synovium should raise other considerations [such as juvenile idiopathic arthritis (JIA), focal pigmented villonodular synovitis (PVNS), tumor, indolent infection]
  - Chronic imaging (if not rapidly treated in acute setting): Joint destruction (particularly at tight joints like hip)
- **Juvenile Idiopathic Arthritis**
  - > 6 weeks of symptoms
  - < 16 years of age at onset
  - Classified into 7 types
    - Systemic (Still disease): Recurring daily fever, rash, hepatomegaly, serositis, lymphadenopathy
    - Oligoarticular: < 5 joints affected in first 6 months of disease; large joints primarily affected
    - Polyarticular: > 5 joints affected in first 6 months
      - □ Rheumatoid factor (RF) positive
      - □ RF negative
    - Psoriatic: Characteristic rash, dactylitis, nail pitting
    - Enthesitis related: Includes ankylosing spondylitis & inflammatory bowel disease-related arthritis
    - Undifferentiated
  - Acute imaging: Nonspecific synovitis & effusion
    - Rice bodies (innumerable small uniform T2-hypointense bodies throughout joint fluid due to necrotic synovium) in child strongly suggest JIA
    - Periosteal reaction may suggest adjacent tenosynovitis
  - Chronic imaging: Erosions, cartilage loss, epiphyseal overgrowth, meniscal hypoplasia, widened intercondylar notch, ankylosis in carpals & cervical spine
- **Trauma**
  - Mild synovial reaction is common with traumatic episode
  - Single hemarthrosis does not typically incite long-term synovitis & rebleeding
  - However, chronic mechanical dysfunction from prior &/or repetitive injuries may lead to joint degeneration

Helpful Clues for Less Common Diagnoses

- **Developmental Dysplasia of Hip**
  - Chronic poor coverage of femoral head by deficient acetabulum ultimately leads to labral hypertrophy with degeneration & tearing & early osteoarthrosis
- **Legg-Calvé-Perthes**
  - Idiopathic avascular necrosis (AVN) of femoral head with typical onset in 1st decade of life (peak: 5-7 years of age)
  - M:F = 4-5:1
  - Early changes of sclerosis, fragmentation, &/or subchondral fracture on radiographs; ↓ perfusion of femoral head, often with effusion & synovitis, on postcontrast MR imaging
  - Chronic changes of coxa magna & coxa plana with lateral femoral head extrusion leading to long-term mechanical dysfunction, labral tearing, & osteoarthrosis
- **Other Avascular Necrosis**

- Sickle cell disease, leukemia with steroid treatment, etc.
- Patchy sclerosis & or serpentine infarcts of medullary cavities; gradual subchondral fracture, collapse
- Acutely may have more poorly defined marrow edema with periosteal reaction on MR

- **Venous Malformation**
  - Congenital but may not present until trauma, infection, or hormonal stimulation leads to rapid growth of lesions
  - Tubular & lobular masses of abnormal venous channels
    - ± phleboliths, fluid-fluid levels, gradual patchy enhancement
  - May involve synovium, leading to recurrent hemarthrosis with accelerated joint degeneration

Helpful Clues for Rare Diagnoses

- **Lyme Disease**
  - History of tick bite & characteristic rash may be absent
- **Pigmented Villonodular Synovitis**
  - Monoarticular; may be focal (mass-like) or, more commonly, diffuse (with frond-like extensions of proliferative synovium intermixed with hemosiderin)
- **Hemophilia**
  - Effusion may be dense; leads to chronic hemosiderin deposition & friable synovium prone to rebleeding
  - Chronic change less frequently seen due to aggressive factor replacement regimens & joint washouts
- **Osteoid Osteoma**
  - Benign osteoblastic lesion inciting marked inflammation of surrounding tissues
  - Lucent nidus with surrounding sclerosis &/or edema
- **Malignancy**
  - Marrow infiltrating lesions (e.g., leukemia, metastatic neuroblastoma) may lead to reactive effusion & synovitis, particularly with superimposed AVN or infection
  - Focal neoplasms may directly invade joint
- **Neuropathic Joint**
  - May be seen in children with myelomeningocele or congenital insensitivity to pain
  - ↓ sensation leads to chronic abnormal mechanics with joint debris, destruction
  - Osteoporosis, gracile long bones, muscle wasting
  - May have repetitive physeal fractures with aggressive-appearing periosteal reaction
- **Synovial Osteochondromatosis**
  - Benign neoplastic transformation of synovium leads to variably sized intraarticular bodies containing cartilage, Ca^{2+}, &/or fatty marrow
- **Tuberculous Arthropathy**
  - Marked synovial proliferation with joint subluxation, destruction, soft tissue abscesses
- **Vasculitis**
  - Other organ systems typically involved
- **Trevor-Fairbank Disease**
  - a.k.a. dysplasia epiphysealis hemimelica
  - Irregular-appearing epiphyses (& equivalents) due to articular surface osteochondroma-like lesions
  - Early on, appears as numerous accessory ossification centers &/or intraarticular Ca^{2+}
  - May lead to osteoarthrosis without treatment
- **Epiphyseal Dysplasias (Mimic)**
  - Typically symmetric abnormal appearance of epiphyseal ossification centers diffusely
  - ± spine involvement
- **Multicentric Carpal-Tarsal Osteolysis (Mimic)**
  - Poorly understood autosomal dominant disorder not responsive to typical rheumatologic treatments
  - ± nephropathy
- **Gorham-Stout Disease (Mimic)**
  - Progressive osteolysis of multiple contiguous bones due to infiltrating microcystic lymphatic malformation

SELECTED REFERENCES

1. Hemke R et al: Imaging of the knee in juvenile idiopathic arthritis. Pediatr Radiol. 48(6):818-27, 2018
2. Dimitriou C et al: Imaging of juvenile idiopathic arthritis. Radiol Clin North Am. 55(5):1071-83, 2017
3. Kraus C et al: Imaging of juvenile hip conditions predisposing to premature osteoarthritis: pediatric imaging. Radiographics. 37(7):2204-05, 2017
4. Kim HK et al: MR findings of synovial disease in children and young adults: part 2. Pediatr Radiol. 41(4):512-24, 2011
5. Kim HK et al: MR findings of synovial disease in children and young adults: part 1. Pediatr Radiol. 41(4):495-511; quiz 545-6, 2011

Septic Arthritis

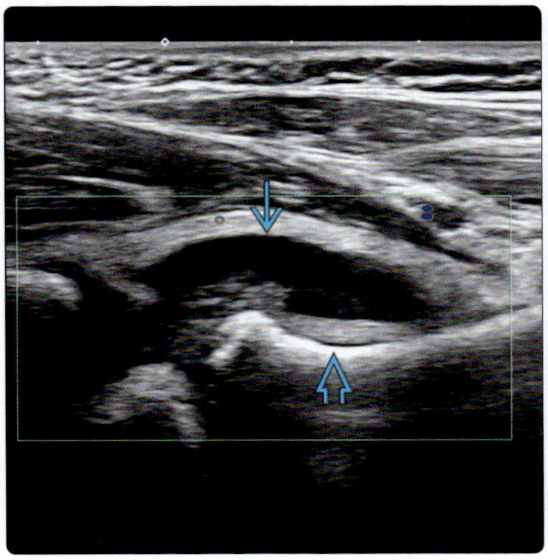

Septic Arthritis

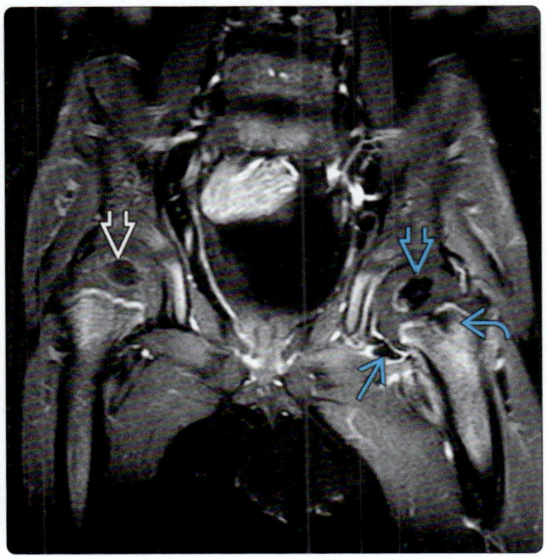

(Left) *Anterior ultrasound of the left hip in a 17 month old with fever, refusal to bear weight, & elevated inflammatory markers shows distention of the joint capsule by a large effusion* ➔ *at the level of the femoral neck* ➔. **(Right)** *Coronal T1 C+ FS MR in the same patient shows decreased perfusion of the left femoral head* ➔ *& neck* ➔ *compared to the right* ➔, *consistent with ischemia &/or osteomyelitis in the setting of a joint effusion* ➔. *Purulent joint fluid positive for Streptococcus pneumoniae was found at surgery.*

(Left) *Coronal T2* GRE MR in a 17-month-old patient with a history of neonatal left hip septic arthritis shows complete destruction of the left femoral head & acetabular cartilage due to the prior infection. The right hip is normal for this age.* **(Right)** *Sagittal T2 FS MR in an 11 year old with oligoarticular juvenile idiopathic arthritis (JIA) shows a small amount of joint fluid but pronounced synovial proliferation that is less hyperintense than fluid.*

Septic Arthritis

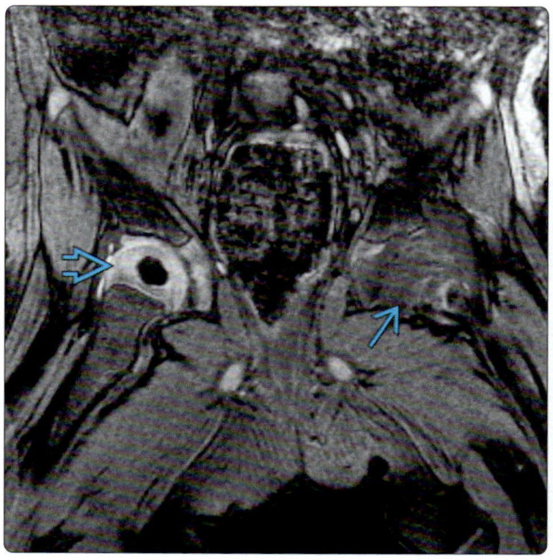

Juvenile Idiopathic Arthritis

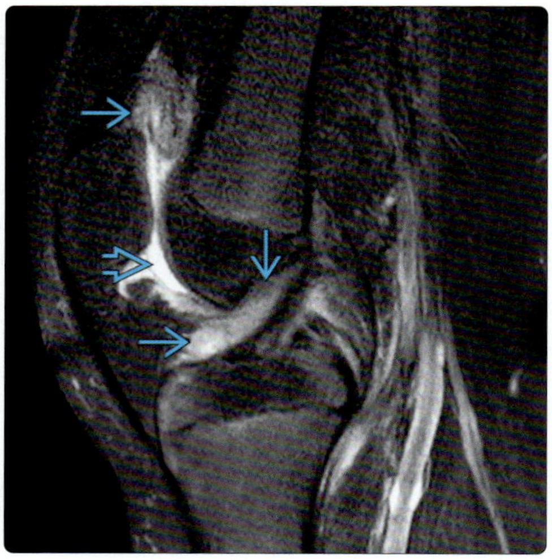

(Left) *Axial T1 C+ FS MR in a 9 year old with hip & back pain shows L > R sacroiliitis plus enthesitis at the right anterior superior iliac spine. There is wall thickening & mural stratification of the terminal ileum, suggesting Crohn disease. The findings likely represent enthesitis-related JIA.* **(Right)** *Coronal T1 C+ FS MR in a 12-year-old patient with longstanding rheumatoid-factor-negative polyarticular JIA shows marked synovitis of all wrist compartments with numerous bone erosions, marrow edema, & joint space loss.*

Juvenile Idiopathic Arthritis

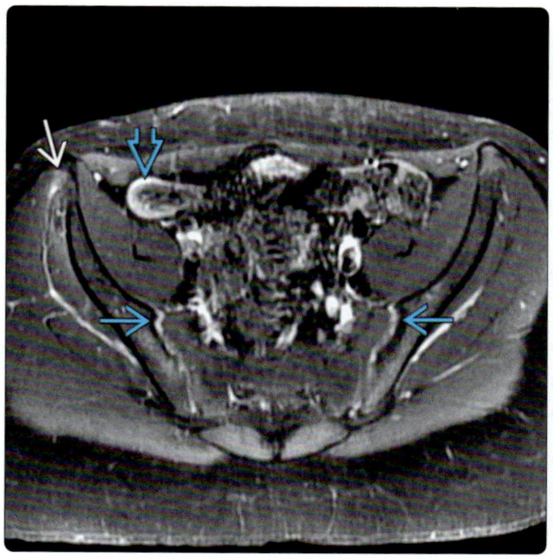

Juvenile Idiopathic Arthritis

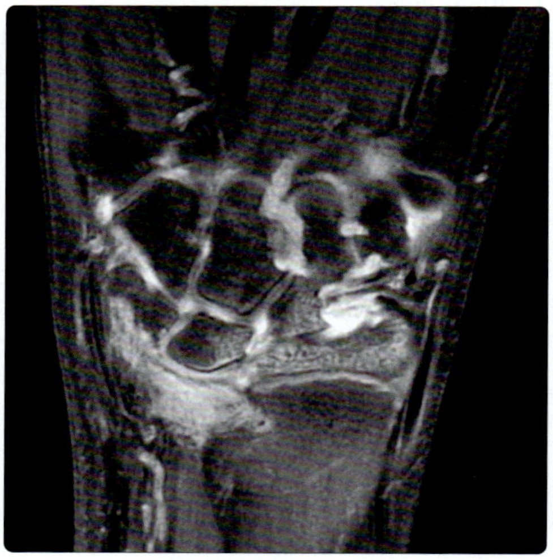

(Left) *AP radiograph in a 9-year-old patient with rheumatoid-factor-negative polyarticular JIA shows epiphyseal overgrowth, joint space loss, & focal erosions at the tibiotalar joint.* **(Right)** *Axial 3D T2* GRE MR arthrogram in a teenager with recurrent shoulder dislocations due to seizures shows large Hill-Sachs & osseous Bankart lesions of the glenohumeral joint. There is moderate hemosiderin-laden synovitis throughout the joint capsule.*

Juvenile Idiopathic Arthritis

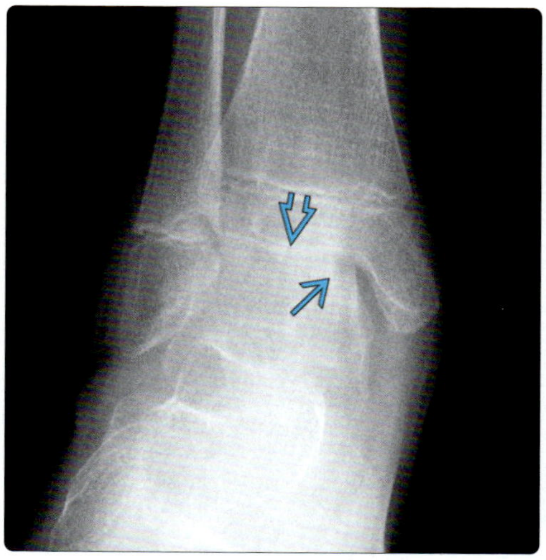

Trauma

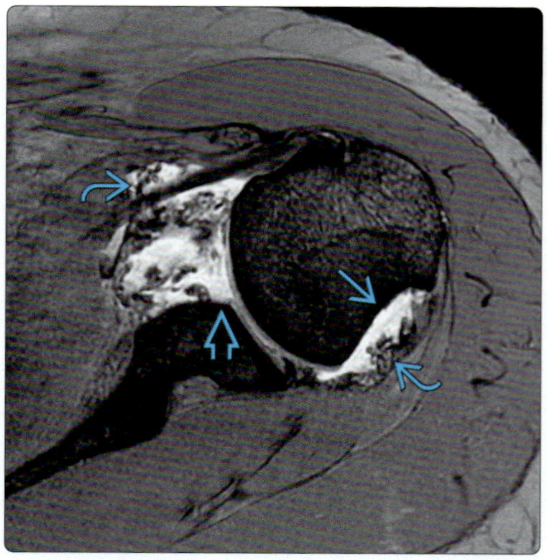

Developmental Dysplasia of Hip

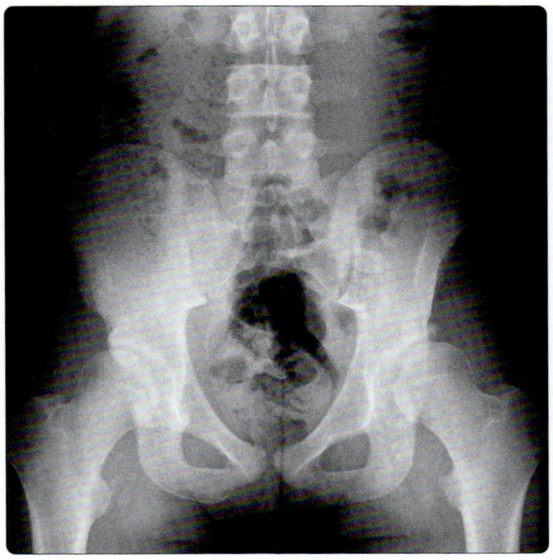

Developmental Dysplasia of Hip

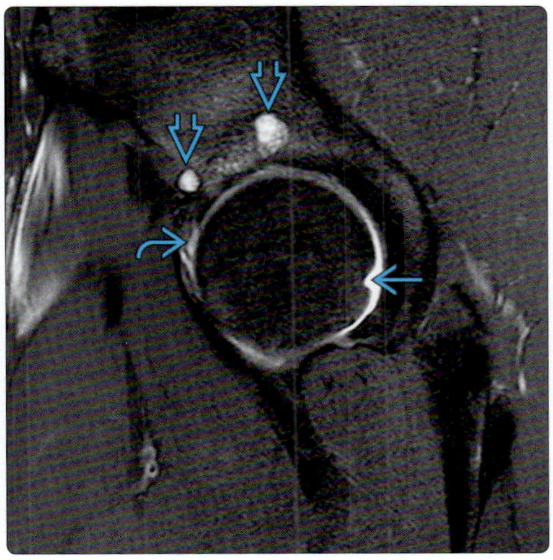

(Left) *AP radiograph in a 16 year old with left hip pain & bilateral hip dysplasia shows (left worse than right) shallow & steep acetabula with uncovering of the femoral heads.* **(Right)** *Sagittal T2 FS MR in the same patient shows degenerative changes of the left hip with generalized cartilage thinning, focal osteochondral loss →, subchondral cystic change →, & a complex labral tear →.*

Legg-Calvé-Perthes

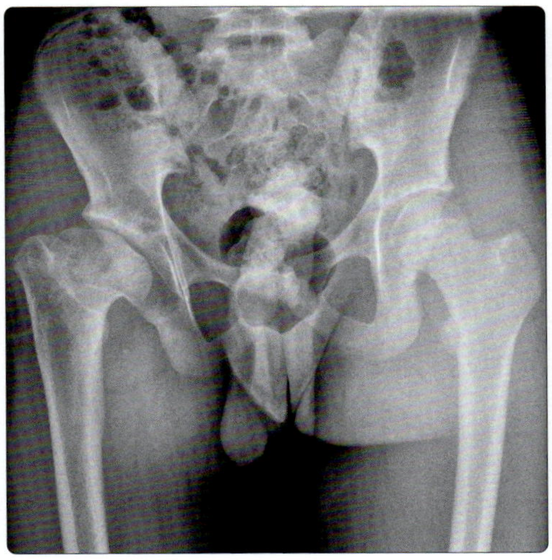

Legg-Calvé-Perthes

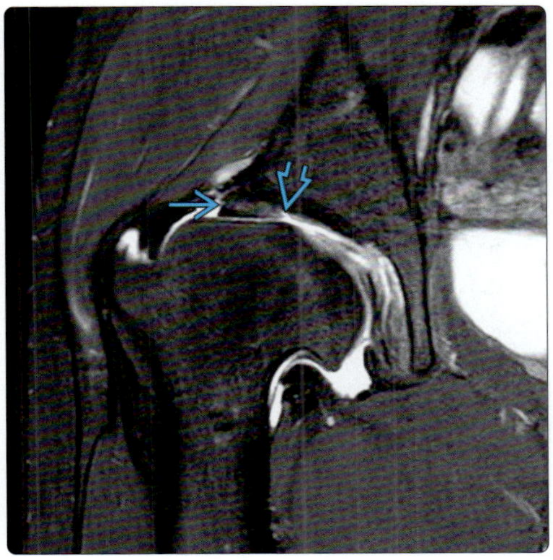

(Left) *AP radiograph of the hips in a 14 year old with chronic changes of right Legg-Calvé-Perthes disease shows right coxa plana (flat), coxa magna (broad), coxa vara (decreased angle), coxa brevis (short), & extrusion (lateral uncovering) of the femoral head & neck with a dysplastic acetabulum.* **(Right)** *Coronal T2 FS MR arthrogram in the same patient shows chronic labral degeneration & tearing → with cartilage loss of the femoral head & acetabulum →.*

Other Avascular Necrosis

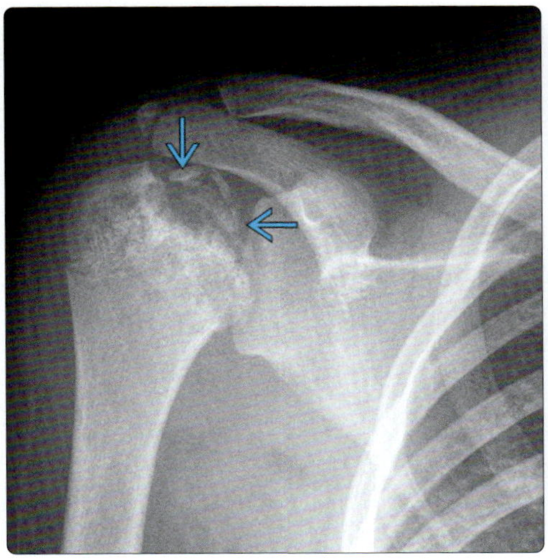

Other Avascular Necrosis

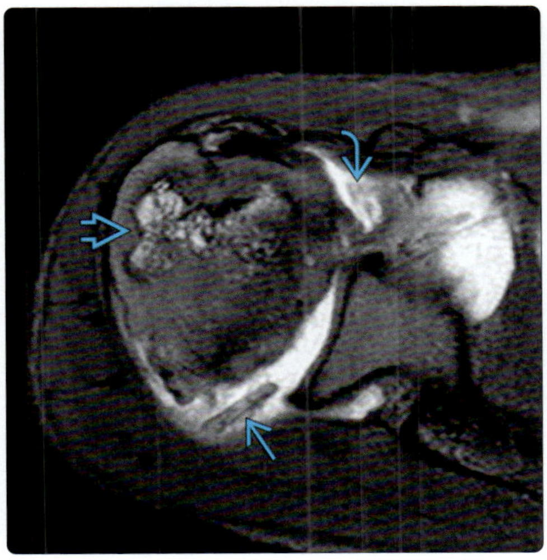

(Left) *External rotation radiograph in a patient with hemoglobin SS (sickle cell disease) & shoulder pain shows fragmentation → & subchondral collapse of the humeral head.* **(Right)** *Axial T2 FS MR in the same patient shows chronic bone infarction → in the irregular humeral head. Proliferative synovium → as well as bone & cartilage fragments → are visualized within the glenohumeral joint.*

(Left) *Sagittal T2 FS MR in a 5 year old with an extensive lower extremity venous malformation → shows intraarticular extension with malformation surrounding the cruciate ligaments →. Intraosseous lesions &/or erosions are seen in the intercondylar roof →, & a small joint effusion is present →.* **(Right)** *Sagittal T2* GRE MR in the same patient shows "blooming" of hemosiderin → along the synovium due to recurrent hemarthrosis. This will lead to accelerated joint degeneration without intervention.*

Venous Malformation

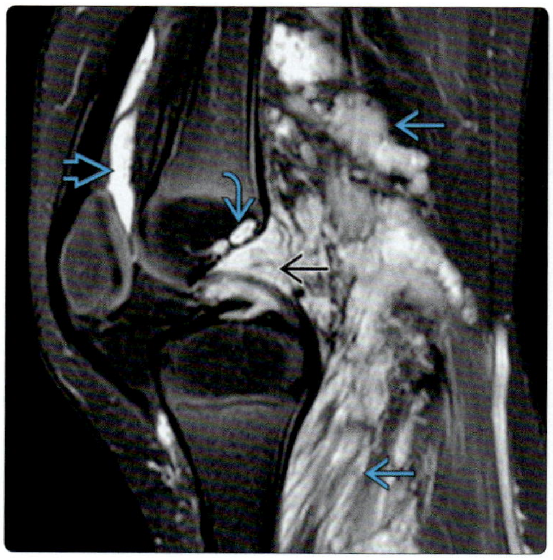

Venous Malformation

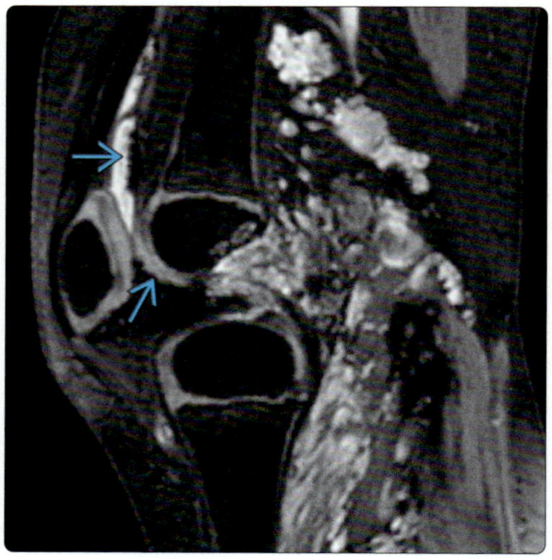

(Left) *Sagittal T1 C+ FS MR in an 18 year old with a history of a characteristic rash & recurrent knee swelling shows a large joint effusion with synovitis →. Titers for Lyme disease antibodies were positive.* **(Right)** *Sagittal T2 FS MR in a 16 year old with a recent knee injury shows a mild joint effusion with heterogeneous frond-like proliferation of the synovium →. No significant internal derangement was otherwise identified.*

Lyme Disease

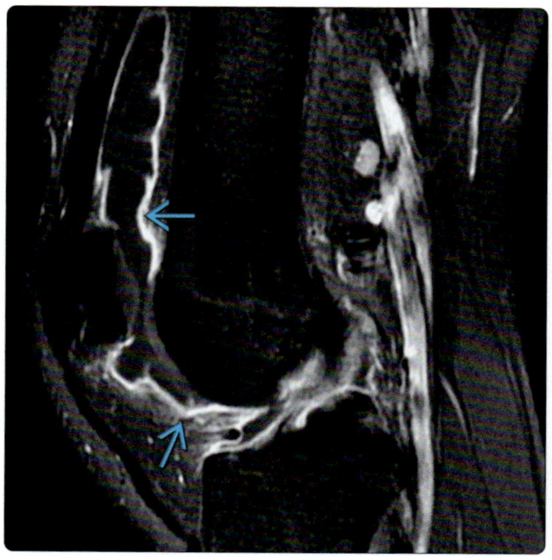

Pigmented Villonodular Synovitis

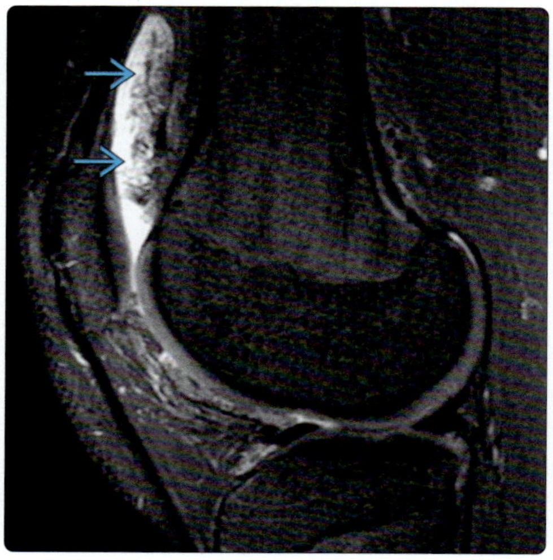

(Left) *Sagittal T2* GRE MR in the same patient demonstrates "blooming" → (exaggerated signal loss) of the hemosiderin-stained synovium, typical of accumulated blood products. Biopsy confirmed pigmented villonodular synovitis, & a synovectomy was performed to prevent further bleeding & synovitis leading to joint degeneration.* **(Right)** *Coronal bone CT in a 16 year old with hip pain shows the calcified center of a lucent osteoid osteoma nidus →. There is mild surrounding sclerosis.*

Pigmented Villonodular Synovitis

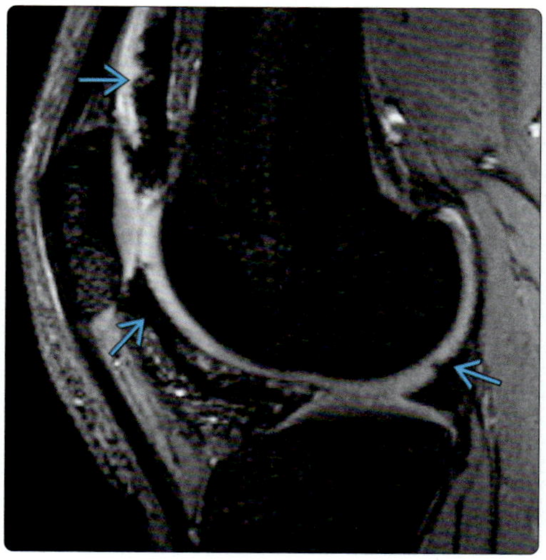

Osteoid Osteoma

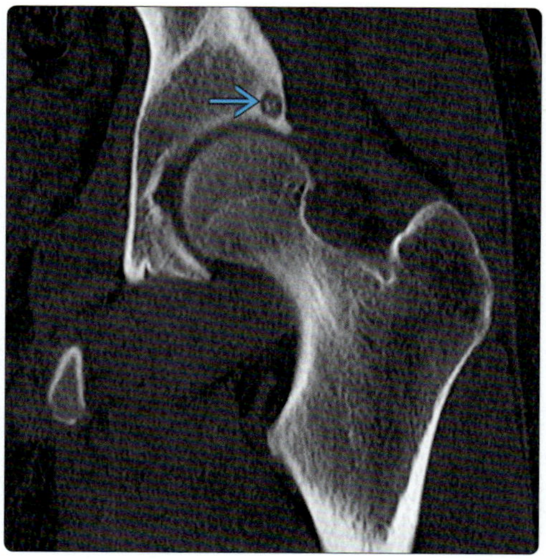

Osteoid Osteoma

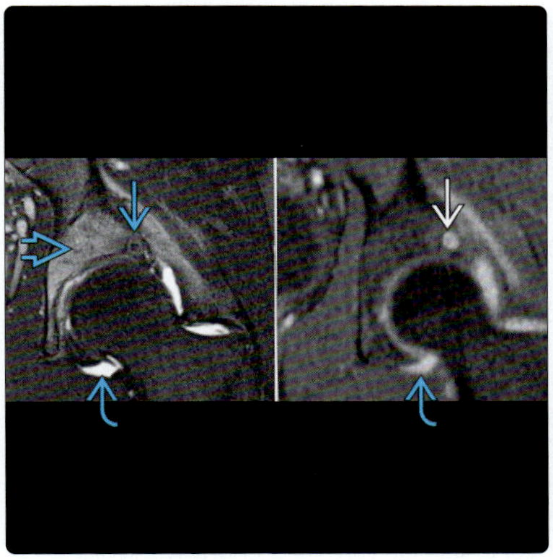

Synovial Osteochondromatosis

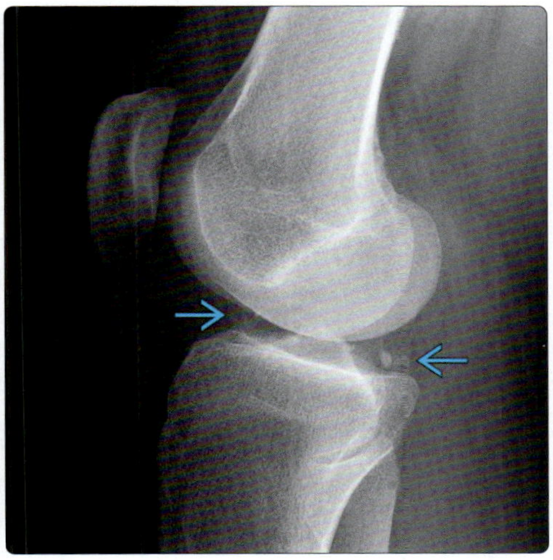

(Left) *Coronal T2 FS (left) & early dynamic T1 C+ FS (right) MR images in the same patient show low signal intensity → & early enhancement ➡ of the osteoid osteoma nidus. Note adjacent marrow edema → & joint effusion/synovitis →. The marrow edema demonstrated typical delayed enhancement (not shown).* **(Right)** *Lateral radiograph of the knee in a 15 year old with chronic pain shows numerous calcified bodies → in the joint. These bodies were removed, & a synovectomy was performed to prevent recurrence leading to joint degeneration.*

Tuberculous Arthropathy

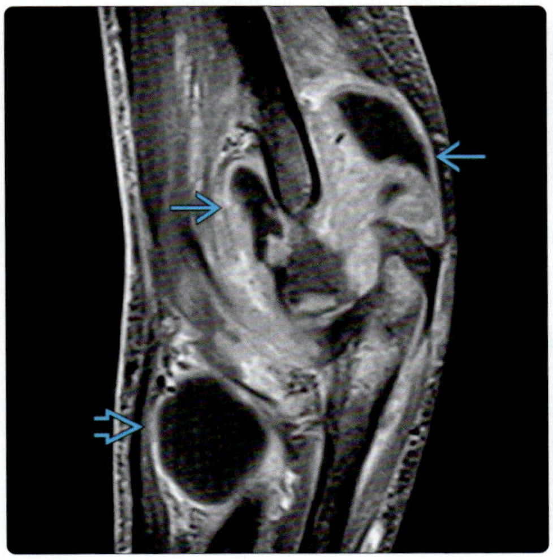

Trevor-Fairbank Disease

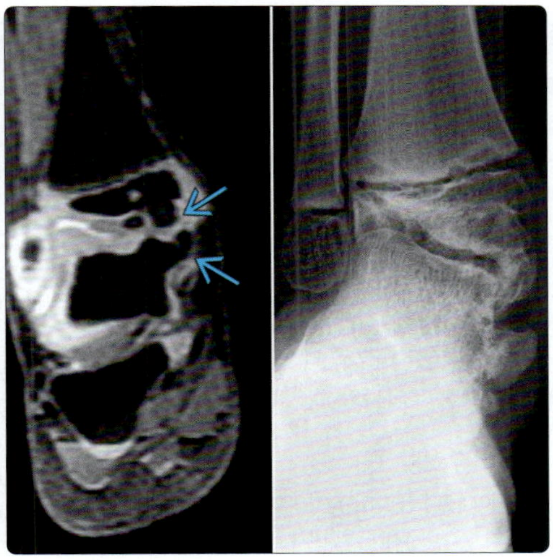

(Left) *Sagittal T1 C+ FS MR in an immunosuppressed adolescent shows massive synovial proliferation & fluid in the elbow joint → due to tuberculosis. Abscesses extend into the soft tissues →.* **(Right)** *Coronal T2* GRE MR in a 3 year old with shows abutting osteocartilaginous excrescences → arising from the medial tibial plafond & talar dome. AP radiograph 3 years later shows worsening valgus alignment.*

Epiphyseal Dysplasia (Mimic)

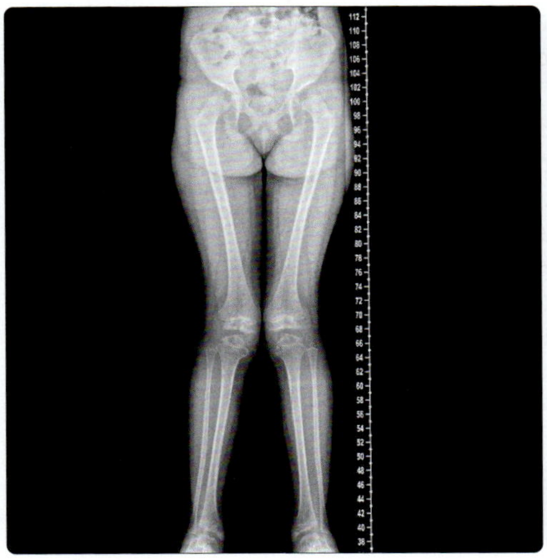

Multicentric Carpal-Tarsal Osteolysis (Mimic)

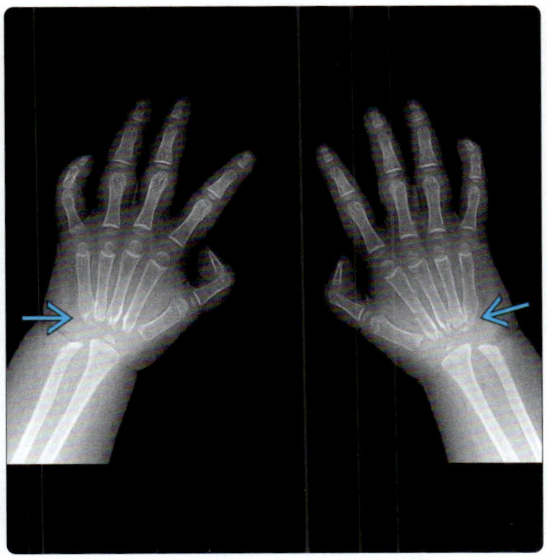

(Left) *AP limb length radiograph shows symmetric hypoplasia & irregularity of all visible epiphyseal ossification centers due to spondyloepiphyseal dysplasia.* **(Right)** *PA radiograph of the wrists in a 3 year old with pain & swelling shows typical findings of carpal-tarsal osteolysis with loss of the carpal ossification centers, proximal tapering of the metacarpal bases →, & tapered distal ulnas.*

DIFFERENTIAL DIAGNOSIS

Common

- Supracondylar Fracture
- Lateral Condylar Fracture
- Medial Epicondyle Avulsion
- Radial Neck Fracture
- Traumatic Effusion Without Fracture

Less Common

- Olecranon Fracture
- Monteggia Fracture-Dislocation
- Complete Elbow Dislocation
- Osteochondritis Dissecans (Mimic)
- Juvenile Idiopathic Arthritis (Mimic)
- Septic Arthritis (Mimic)

Rare but Important

- Distal Humeral Epiphyseal Separation
- Capitellar Shear Injury
- Panner Disease (Mimic)

ESSENTIAL INFORMATION

Key Differential Diagnosis Issues

- Developmental order of ossification center appearances at elbow: **C**apitellum, **r**adial head, medial (**i**nternal) epicondyle, **t**rochlea, **o**lecranon, lateral (**e**xternal) epicondyle (**CRITOE**)
  - Most important point (for acute trauma): Trochlear ossification center appears after medial epicondyle
    - If bone fragment projects over region of trochlea without visible medial epicondyle in normal location, suspect avulsed medial epicondyle in joint
- Alignment: Normal vs. trauma
  - Anterior humeral line
    - Lateral view: Line drawn along anterior humerus should pass through middle 1/3 of capitellum
    - Classic teaching: If capitellum lies posterior to this line, supracondylar fracture should be suspected
    - In isolation, this "rule" is not sensitive or specific
      - Not all supracondylar fractures will have enough displacement to fail this test
      - Other less common fractures may fail this test
      - Also, distal humerus has mild curvature normally; therefore, length/position of anterior line affects its relationship to capitellum
  - Radiocapitellar line
    - Any view: Line drawn from center of proximal radial shaft classically bisects capitellar ossification center
      - Eccentric ossification of capitellum in younger patients may create mild offset on AP view
    - When abnormal, radial head dislocation is likely
      - Markedly displaced lateral condylar fracture would also disrupt relationship
- Fat pads overlie joint capsule at distal humerus
  - Anterior: Mildly visualized in normal elbows
    - Elevation (sail sign) implies joint effusion or synovitis
    - With trauma, must exclude occult fracture (typically by immobilization & follow-up in 10-14 days to assess for healing changes)
  - Posterior: Not normally visualized; therefore, its visualization is more sensitive for occult fractures
  - Fat pad displacement requires intact joint capsule
    - Disruption (leading to joint fluid leak) is more likely with marked displacement or true dislocation
  - Some fractures (such as medial epicondyle) may be extraarticular & lack joint effusion

Helpful Clues for Common Diagnoses

- **Supracondylar Fracture**
  - ~ 50-70% of elbow fractures in children
  - Age: 3-10 years
  - Fracture line courses horizontally through distal humerus at level of coronoid & olecranon fossae
    - May rarely have additional intercondylar component of distal extension in sagittal plane to articular surface, termed T-fracture
  - Degrees of displacement are quite variable; distal fragment generally translates posteriorly with volar angulation of fracture apex
    - Severe displacement can mimic dislocation (but radiocapitellar alignment is maintained)
- **Lateral Condylar Fracture**
  - ~ 20% of elbow fractures in children
  - Age: 4-10 years
  - Distal humeral metaphyseal fracture parallels lateral portion of physis, typically entering middle portion of physis
    - Fracture then typically extends distally into unossified cartilage between capitellum & trochlea as Salter-Harris (SH) IV injury
      - This component is radiographically occult but may be inferred with more severe displacement
      - Distal fracture component less commonly continues medially through physis as SH II
  - Oblique views are often helpful in detection & assessment of displacement
    - Displacement ranges from minimal to marked rotation of metaphyseal fragment (& capitellum) out of alignment with radius
    - ≥ 2 mm of displacement typically requires open surgical reduction & pinning
- **Medial Epicondyle Avulsion**
  - ~ 15% of elbow fractures in children
  - Age: 8-15 years
  - Entirety or portion of medial epicondyle ossification center avulsed by ulnar collateral ligament (UCL)
    - May become displaced & trapped in elbow joint, simulating trochlear ossification center
  - 50% associated with elbow dislocations
  - Unreliable fat pad sign: Fracture tends to be extracapsular in location in children > 2 years old
- **Radial Neck Fracture**
  - 4-17% of pediatric elbow fractures
  - Average age of 10 years
  - Focal angulation of metaphyseal cortex at lateral margin of radial neck, particularly on AP view
    - Typically SH II type injury with variable degrees of radial head angulation & translation
  - May occur in conjunction with olecranon fracture
- **Traumatic Effusion Without Fracture**

- Reactive vs. hemarthrosis from occult fracture
  - Likelihood of occult fracture when only joint effusion is seen on initial radiographs varies in literature (from 54% to > 90%)

Helpful Clues for Less Common Diagnoses

- **Olecranon Fracture**
  - ~ 4-7% of pediatric elbow fractures
  - Typically occurs in base with intraarticular extension
    - Avulsion of apophysis is uncommon except in osteogenesis imperfecta
  - Often occurs in association with radial neck fractures
- **Monteggia Fracture-Dislocation**
  - Radial head dislocation in conjunction with proximal ulnar fracture
  - Isolated radial head dislocation is uncommon in children: Look for variations of ulnar injuries (including plastic deformation) or more distal ulnar injury
  - Radial head subluxation (nursemaid elbow) is often reduced before or during radiographs
- **Complete Elbow Dislocation**
  - 3-5% of pediatric elbow injuries
  - Uncommon in 1st decade of life; peaks at 12-13 years
  - Radius & ulna no longer articulate with capitellum & trochlea, respectively; usually translate posterior & lateral
  - Medial epicondyle avulsion & intraarticular displacement are common; must exclude postreduction incarceration
  - Other fractures may also occur
- **Osteochondritis Dissecans (Mimic)**
  - a.k.a. osteochondral lesion
  - Typically adolescent boys (11-15 years old)
    - Due to repetitive valgus stress & impaction
  - Subchondral ovoid/lobulated lucency of anterior capitellum, ± surrounding sclerosis
  - Loose body may displace into humeral fossae
- **Juvenile Idiopathic Arthritis (Mimic)**
  - Begins < 16 years old, symptoms > 6 weeks
  - Synovitis, effusion ± rice bodies, erosions; epiphyseal overgrowth & ankylosis less commonly
- **Septic Arthritis (Mimic)**
  - *Staphylococcus aureus* is most common pathogen, typically from hematogenous seeding
  - Fever, arthralgia, & joint swelling are typical
  - Nonspecific effusion & soft tissue swelling are initial radiographic manifestations

Helpful Clues for Rare Diagnoses

- **Distal Humeral Epiphyseal Separation**
  - a.k.a. transphyseal fracture
  - Usually < 3 years of age
  - High association with child abuse or birth trauma
  - Fracture plane through distal humeral physis ± small metaphyseal component
  - Medial & posterior translation of radius & ulna
    - Displaced capitellum remains aligned with radius, though young age may limit capitellar visualization
      - Displaced humeral epiphyseal cartilage must be inferred radiographically by age & position of radius & ulna
      - Cartilage may be visualized with ultrasound, MR, or conventional arthrography
- **Capitellar Shear Injury**
  - Adolescents
  - Coronal fracture plane at variable capitellar depth; may be subtle radiographically
  - ± radial head/neck fractures
- **Panner Disease (Mimic)**
  - Irregular ossification of capitellum, possibly due to avascular necrosis
  - Typically involves dominant arm of boys 5-12 years old
  - Entire capitellum is often abnormal in appearance by radiographs or MR imaging, but fragmentation with loose bodies is not typical

SELECTED REFERENCES

1. Little KJ: Elbow fractures and dislocations. Orthop Clin North Am. 45(3):327-40, 2014
2. Iyer RS et al: Pediatric bone imaging: imaging elbow trauma in children–a review of acute and chronic injuries. AJR Am J Roentgenol. 198(5):1053-68, 2012

Supracondylar Fracture

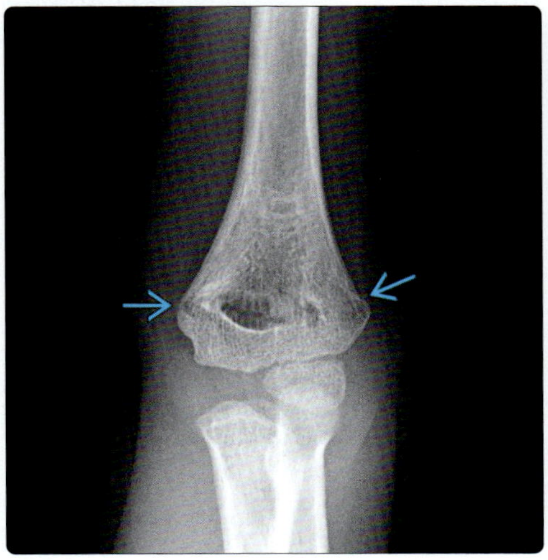

Supracondylar Fracture

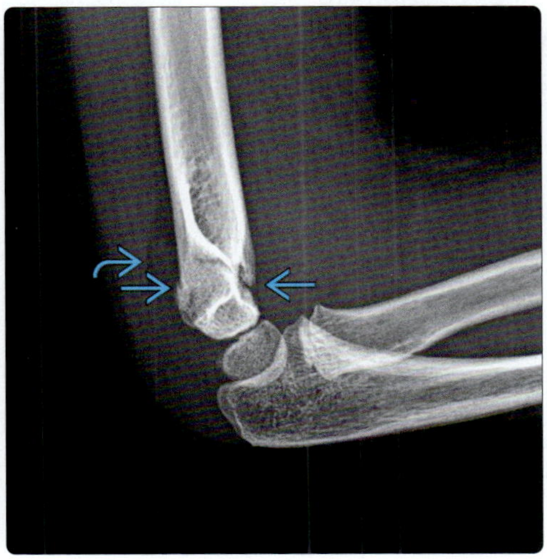

(Left) *AP radiograph in a 5 year old shows the classic location of a supracondylar fracture traversing the distal humerus at the level of the coronoid & olecranon fossae.* **(Right)** *Lateral radiograph in the same patient shows the fracture traversing the "waist of the hourglass" (at the coronoid & olecranon fossae of the humerus). Note the displacement of the posterior fat pad due to the associated joint effusion.*

(Left) *AP radiograph shows a supracondylar fracture with posterior translation & rotation of the distal humeral fracture fragments. This does not represent a true elbow dislocation as the radial & capitellar alignment is maintained.* **(Right)** *Lateral radiograph in the same patient shows marked posterior translation of the distal humeral fracture fragment. The elbow articulations remain intact.*

Supracondylar Fracture

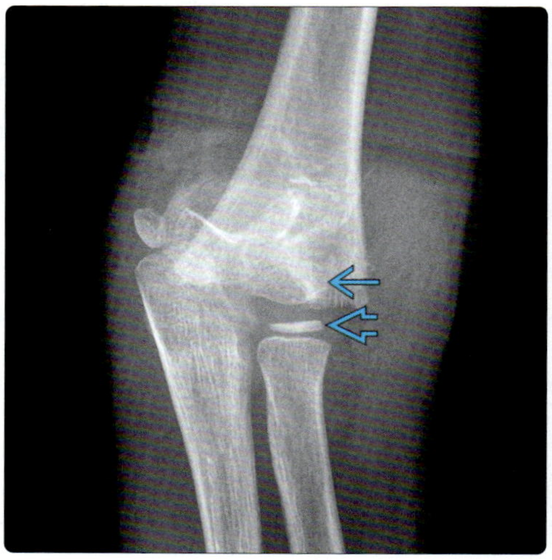

Supracondylar Fracture

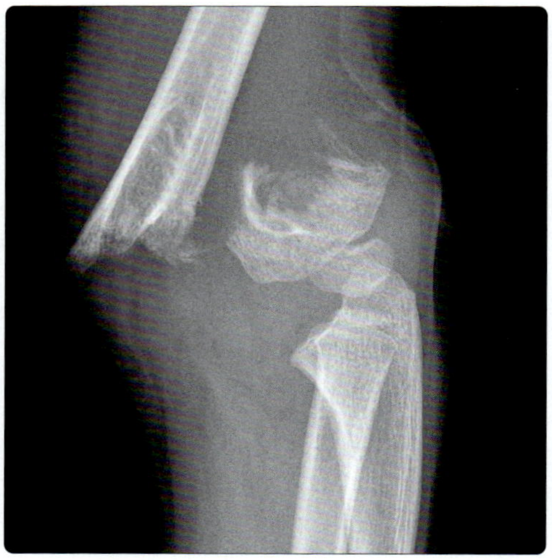

(Left) *AP radiograph in a 3 year old shows a minimally displaced lateral condylar fracture of the distal humerus with overlying soft tissue swelling. The posterior component of the fracture extends more proximally in the humerus. The distal component of the fracture typically extends across the physis into the unossified humeral epiphyseal cartilage.* **(Right)** *Lateral radiograph in the same patient shows the typical oblique extension of a lateral condylar fracture in the posterior aspect of the distal humeral metaphysis.*

Lateral Condylar Fracture

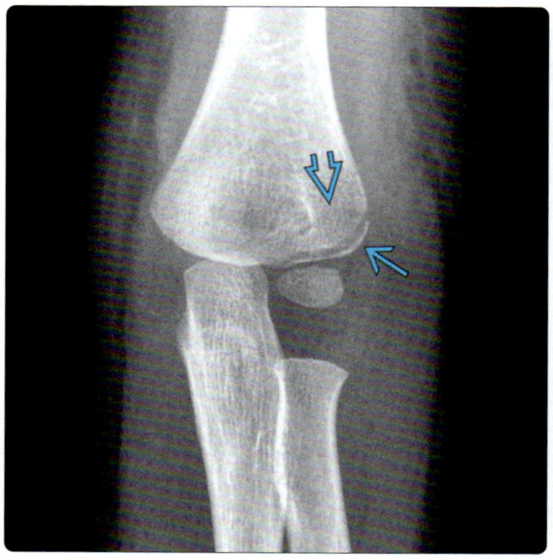

Lateral Condylar Fracture

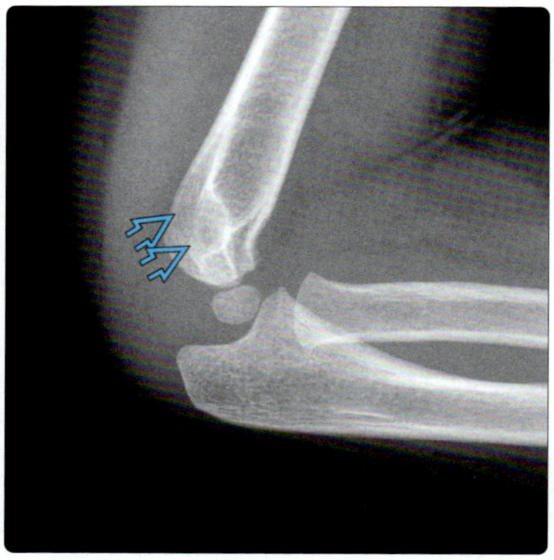

(Left) *AP radiograph in a 5 year old shows lateral translation & medial rotation of a large lateral condylar fracture fragment, including a metaphyseal sliver & the capitellar ossification center. This is consistent with the Salter-Harris IV fracture plane extending distally through the unossified cartilage to the articular surface medial to the capitellum.* **(Right)** *Lateral radiograph in the same patient shows the anterior displacement of the lateral condylar fragment with dissociation of the capitellum from the radial head.*

Lateral Condylar Fracture

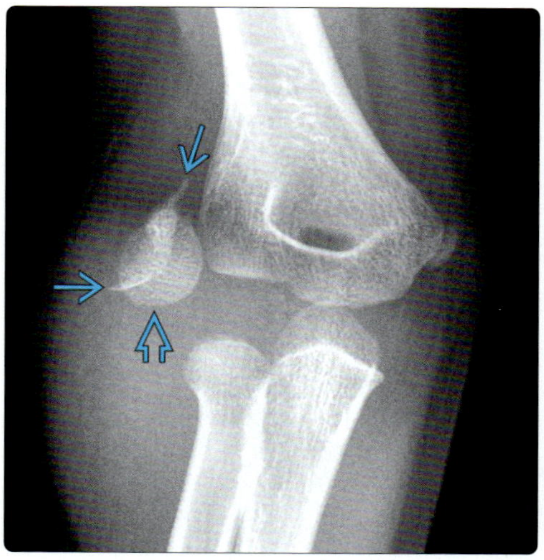

Lateral Condylar Fracture

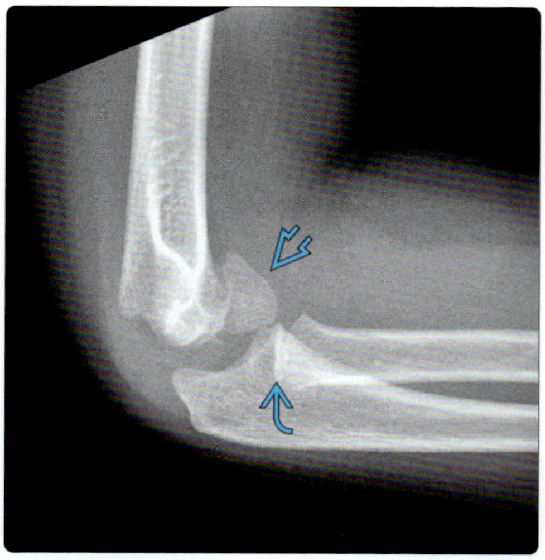

Medial Epicondyle Avulsion

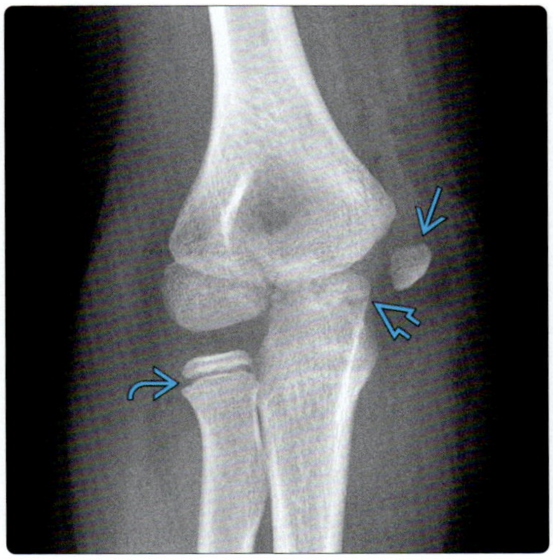

Medial Epicondyle Avulsion

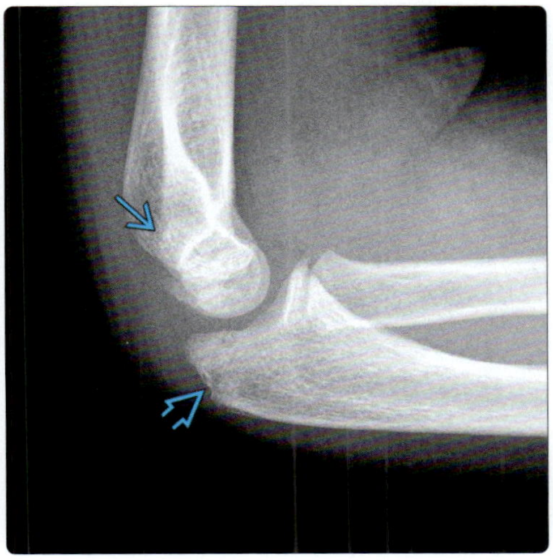

(Left) *AP radiograph in a 9 year old shows distraction & medial translation of the medial epicondyle ossification center from the humerus. An additional intraarticular olecranon fracture is noted. The mild step-off of the lateral radial metaphysis is normal on this view.* **(Right)** *Lateral radiograph in the same patient shows mild anterior displacement of the medial epicondyle ossification center, which usually sits more posteriorly along the humerus. The olecranon fracture is again noted.*

Medial Epicondyle Avulsion

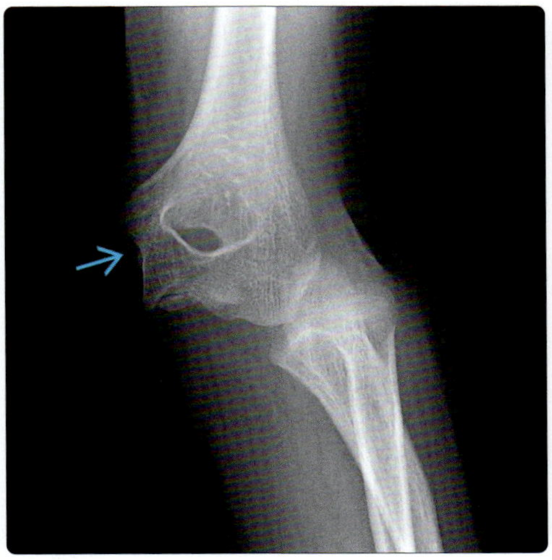

Medial Epicondyle Avulsion

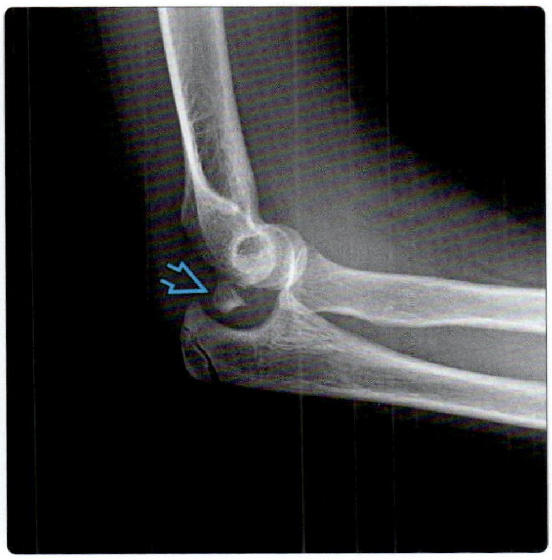

(Left) *AP radiograph in an 11 year old shows lateral dislocation of the radius & ulna. Only a tiny fragment of the medial epicondyle ossification center remains in its expected location.* **(Right)** *Lateral radiograph in the same patient shows posterior dislocation of the ulna relative to the humerus with a large portion of the medial epicondyle ossification center displaced between these articular surfaces.*

Radial Neck Fracture

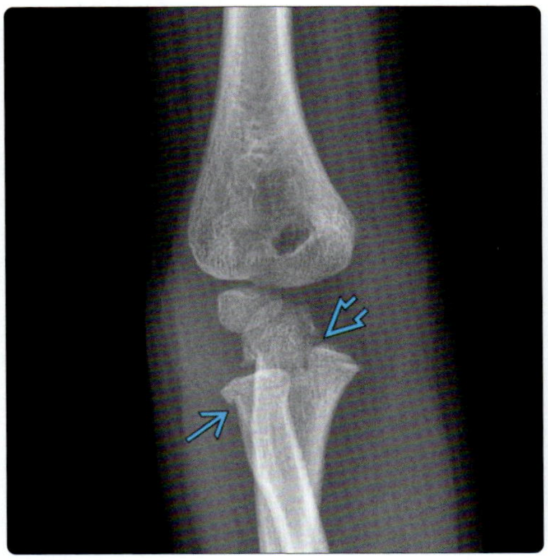

Radial Neck Fracture

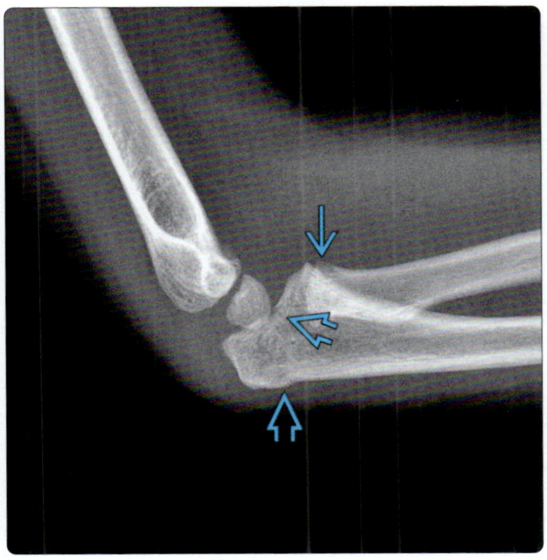

(Left) *AP radiograph in a 4 year old after a fall shows a Salter-Harris II fracture of the radial neck. There is an accompanying intraarticular fracture of the ulnar olecranon. These fractures often occur together but may each occur in isolation (with the radial neck being more common).* **(Right)** *Lateral radiograph in the same patient clearly shows the olecranon fracture while the radial neck fracture is more subtle (as is often the case on the lateral view).*

(Left) *AP radiograph in an 8 year old shows a complex fracture of the olecranon as well as a lateral condylar fracture.* (Right) *Lateral radiograph in the same patient shows a coronoid fracture as part of the complex olecranon fracture. The posterior component of the lateral condylar fracture is also visible in the distal humerus. "Satisfaction of search" errors must be remembered at the elbow as > 1 fracture may be present, potentially altering management considerations.*

Olecranon Fracture

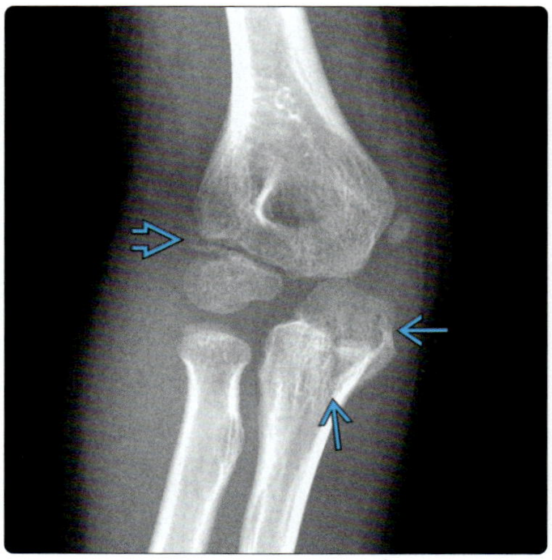

Olecranon Fracture

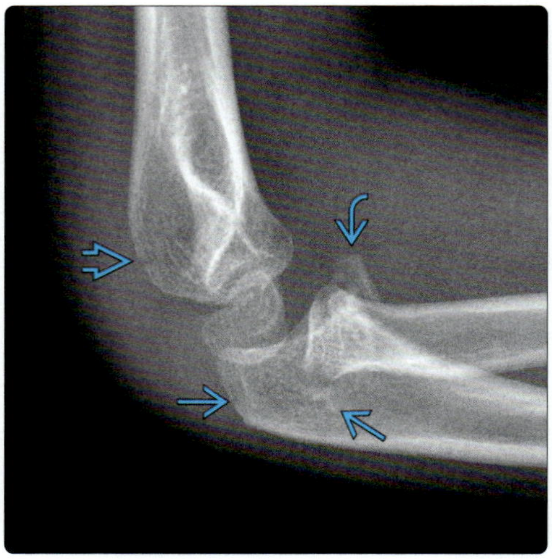

(Left) *AP radiograph in a 3 year old shows dislocation of the radius from the capitellum. The ulna appears normal on this view.* (Right) *Lateral radiograph in the same patient shows the volar dislocation of the radius from the capitellum as well as a fracture of the proximal 1/3 of the ulna, consistent with a Monteggia fracture-dislocation. As isolated radial head dislocations are uncommon in children, the entire forearm may need to be imaged to find the ulnar fracture.*

Monteggia Fracture-Dislocation

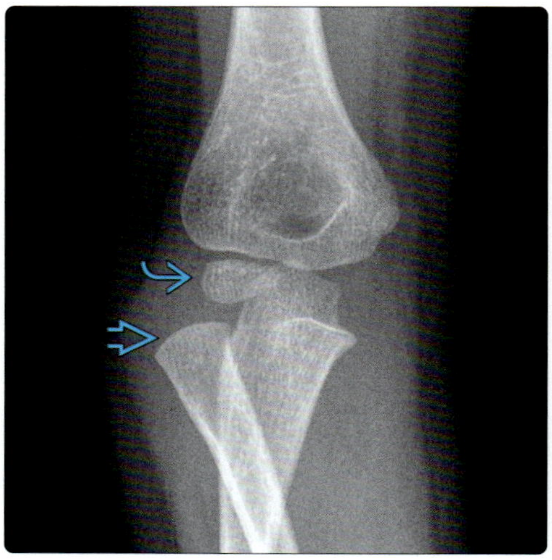

Monteggia Fracture-Dislocation

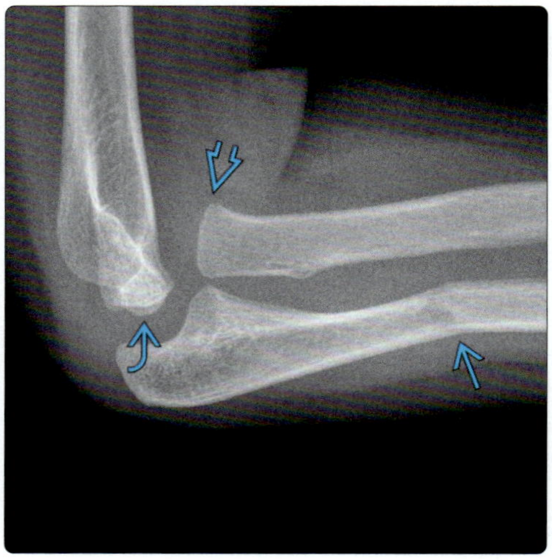

(Left) *AP radiograph in a 13 year old with elbow pain shows an irregular lucency of the subchondral capitellum.* (Right) *Coronal T2 FS MR in the same patient shows an osteochondritis dissecans (OCD) of the capitellum with cartilage fissuring, a finding concerning for fragment instability. Only edema is seen deep to the OCD lesion without a true fluid cleft or cystic change (which are additional findings that can suggest instability).*

Osteochondritis Dissecans (Mimic)

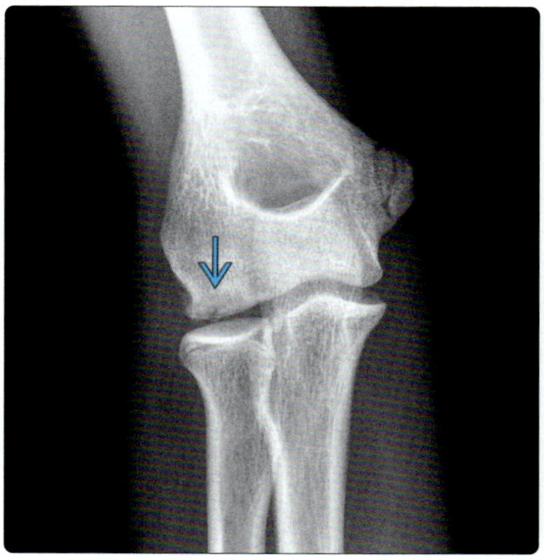

Osteochondritis Dissecans (Mimic)

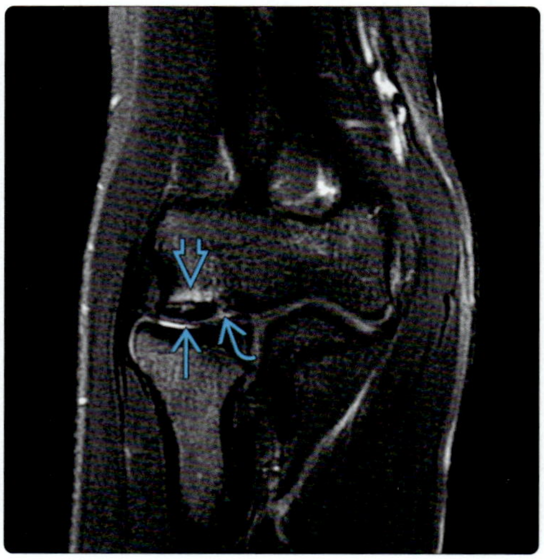

Septic Arthritis (Mimic)

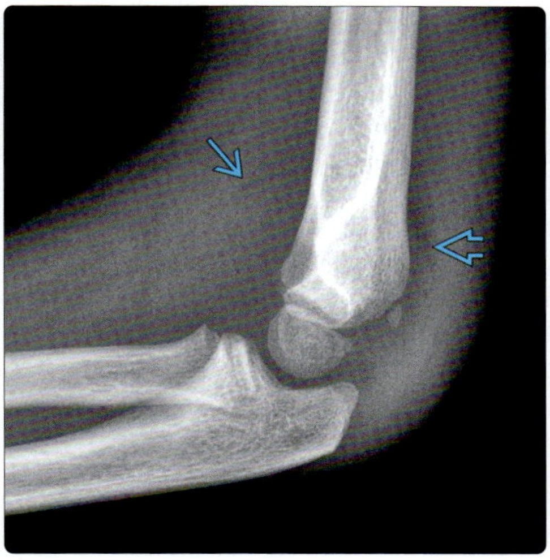

Septic Arthritis (Mimic)

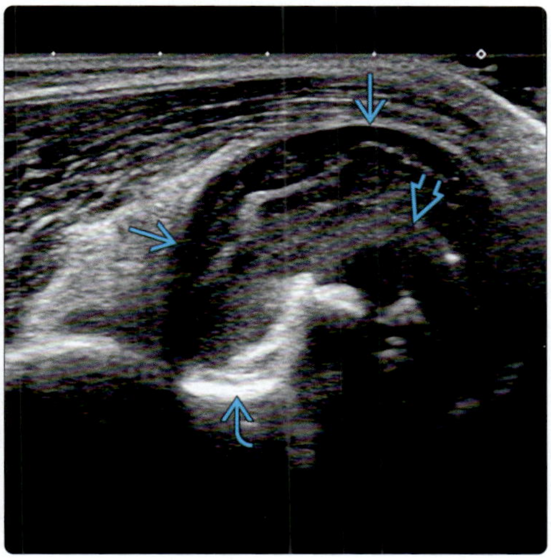

(Left) *Lateral radiograph in a 5 year old with elbow swelling, pain, & elevated inflammatory markers shows displacement of the anterior ➙ & posterior ➙ fat pads, consistent with joint effusion &/or synovitis.* **(Right)** *Anterior longitudinal ultrasound of the elbow in the same patient shows a large complex joint effusion ➙ at the level of the partially ossified humeral capitellar cartilage ➙ & coronoid fossa ➙. Purulent material was found upon needle sampling, leading to an arthrotomy & irrigation for septic arthritis.*

Distal Humeral Epiphyseal Separation

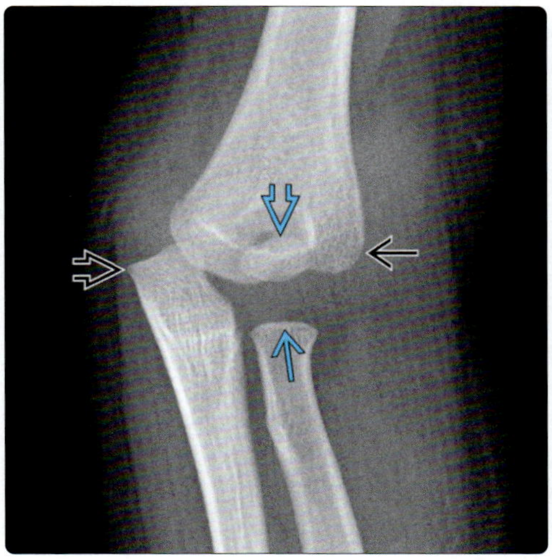

Distal Humeral Epiphyseal Separation

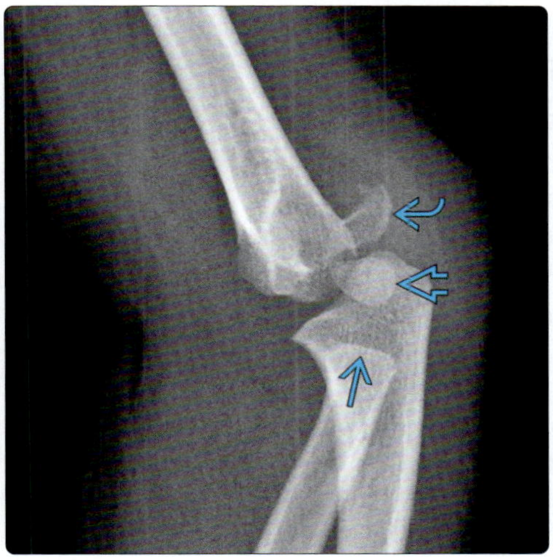

(Left) *AP radiograph in a 3 year old after a fall shows medial translation of the capitellum ➙, radius ➙, & ulna ➙ relative to the humeral metaphysis ➙. However, the radiocapitellar alignment is maintained.* **(Right)** *Lateral radiograph in the same patient shows posterior translation of the radius ➙ & capitellum ➙ as well as a lateral condylar fragment ➙. This configuration is typical of a distal humeral epiphyseal separation, up to 50% of which are due to child abuse.*

Capitellar Shear Injury

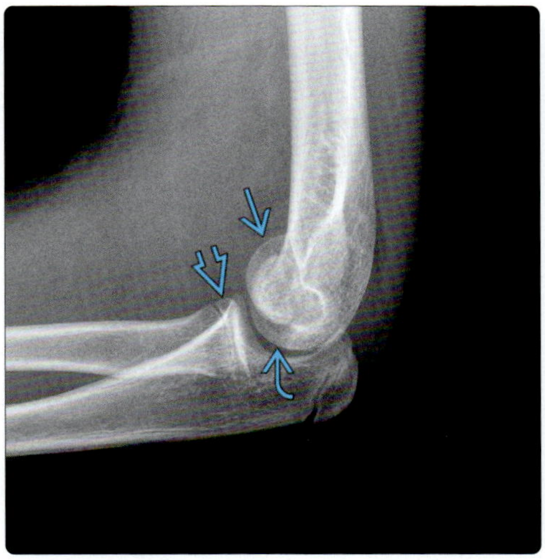

Capitellar Shear Injury

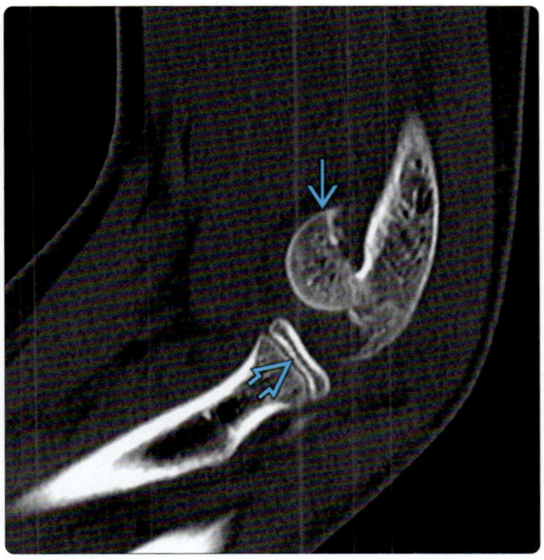

(Left) *Lateral radiograph in a 14 year old shows proximal displacement of the capitellum ➙ relative to the radial head ➙ & trochlear ➙ ossification centers.* **(Right)** *Sagittal bone CT in the same patient confirms a shear fracture through the base of the capitellum with dissociation of the proximally translated capitellar ossification center ➙ from the radial head ➙. While not seen in this case, radial head/neck fractures may also be present with these types of capitellar injuries.*

Radial Dysplasia/Aplasia

DIFFERENTIAL DIAGNOSIS

Common

- VACTERL Association
- Thrombocytopenia-Absent Radius Syndrome
- Fanconi Anemia
- Holt-Oram Syndrome

Less Common

- Trisomies 18 & 13
- Klippel-Feil Syndrome
- Congenital Radial Head Dislocation
- Radioulnar Synostosis
- Amniotic Band Syndrome
- Poland Syndrome

Rare but Important

- Mesomelic Dysplasia Group
- Teratogens
- Cornelia de Lange Syndrome
- Oculo-Auriculo-Vertebral Dysplasia
- Nail Patella Disease (Fong)

ESSENTIAL INFORMATION

Key Differential Diagnosis Issues

- Radial longitudinal deficiency (a.k.a. radial club hand)
- Spectrum of radial hypoplasia → aplasia
  - Associated: Ulnar hypoplasia; dysplasia/absence of scaphoid, trapezium, thumb metacarpal & phalanges

Helpful Clues for Diagnoses

- **VACTERL Association**
  - ≥ 3: **V**ertebral, **a**nal, **c**ardiac, **t**racheo**e**sophageal, anomalies, **r**enal, **l**imb (especially radial ray)
- **Thrombocytopenia-Absent Radius Syndrome**
  - Absent radius (typically bilateral); thumb present
  - Thrombocytopenia presenting at/near birth
- **Fanconi Anemia**
  - Hypoplastic → absent radius, scaphoid, trapezium; thumb may be absent, hypoplastic, or supernumerary
  - Absent, hypoplastic, or supernumerary
  - Pancytopenia: Usually appears by 5-10 years of age
- **Holt-Oram Syndrome**
  - a.k.a: Heart-hand or cardiac-limb syndrome
  - Radius: Hypoplastic → absent
  - Carpal bones: Absent, fused, &/or delayed ossification
  - Thumb: Absent, hypoplastic, triphalangeal, or bifid
  - Cardiac anomalies (most commonly atrial septal defect/ventricular septal defect)
- **Trisomy 18 & 13**
  - Multiple anomalies found on prenatal US
- **Klippel-Feil Syndrome**
  - Segmentation failure of ≥ 2 cervical vertebrae
  - ± Sprengel deformity, omovertebral bone
- **Congenital Radial Head Dislocation**
  - Dome-shaped radial head + hypoplastic capitellum
- **Radioulnar Synostosis**
  - Congenital fusion of proximal radius & ulna
  - Radial head dysplastic & dorsally dislocated
- **Amniotic Band Syndrome**
  - Extremity constriction → fracture → amputation
  - Bizarre patterns of limb, body wall, & face involvement
- **Poland Syndrome**
  - Unilateral absence of pectoralis musculature
  - ± shortened radius/ulna, symbrachydactyly
- **Mesomelic Dysplasia Group**
  - Symmetric shortening of mid limb segment
  - Dyschondrosteosis is most common
- **Teratogens**
  - Fetal thalidomide, varicella, & valproic acid exposure
- **Cornelia de Lange Syndrome**
  - ± severe deformities: Microbrachycephaly, phocomelia
  - Intellectual disability, small stature, long philtrum
  - Synophrys (continuous eyebrow across midline)
- **Oculo-Auriculo-Vertebral Dysplasia**
  - Facial, vertebral, rib, & limb anomalies
- **Nail Patella Disease (Fong)**
  - Nail dysplasia, patella hypoplasia/aplasia, iliac horns
  - Hypoplastic radial head + subluxation/dislocation

VACTERL Association

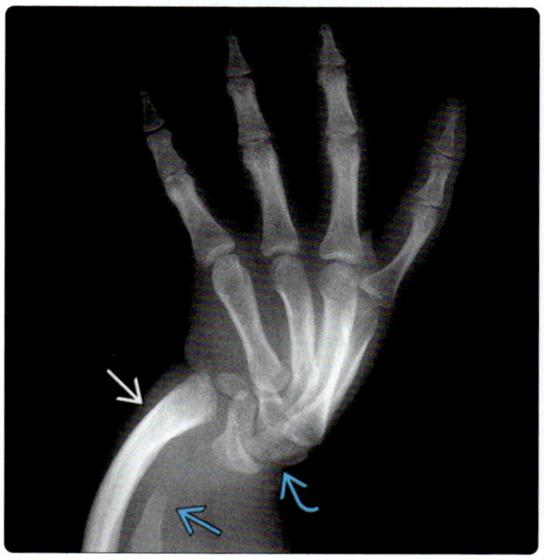

Thrombocytopenia-Absent Radius Syndrome

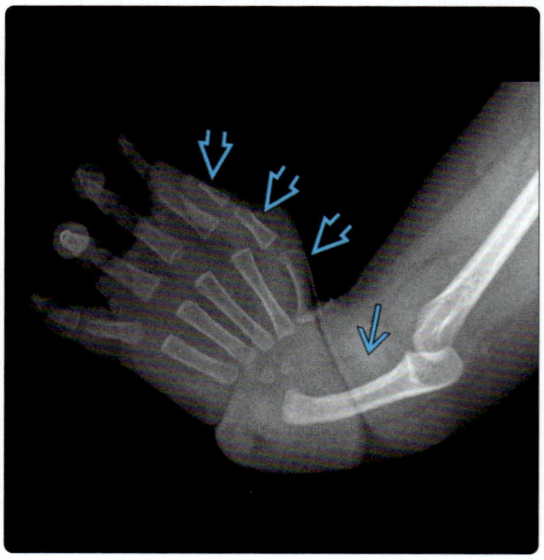

(Left) *PA radiograph shows a hypoplastic radius ➞, an absent thumb, a short curved ulna ➞, & carpal bone fusions ➞. The findings were bilateral, & the patient had other typical VACTERL anomalies.* **(Right)** *Frontal radiograph in a 1 year old with thrombocytopenia-absent radius (TAR) syndrome shows complete absence of the radius ➞, which was bilateral. The right thumb is present ➞, which differs from other disorders associated with an absent radius.*

Fanconi Anemia

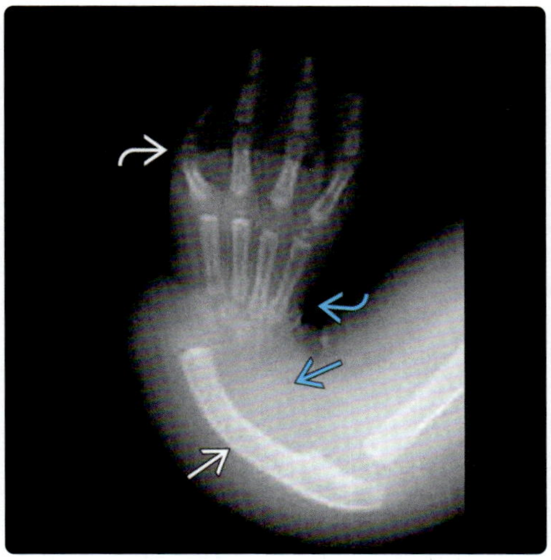

Holt-Oram Syndrome

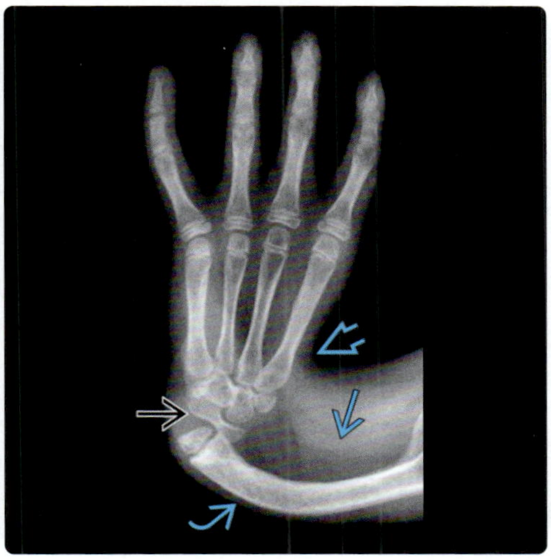

(Left) *Frontal radiograph in a patient with Fanconi anemia shows absence of the radius & thumb. The ulna is bowed, & there is clinodactyly of the 5th digit.* **(Right)** *Frontal radiograph in a 12 year old with Holt-Oram syndrome shows that the radius & thumb are completely absent. The ulna is bowed, & there is fusion of the carpal bones. Holt-Oram is associated with cardiac deformities, most commonly an atrial septal defect or a ventricular septal defect.*

Congenital Radial Head Dislocation

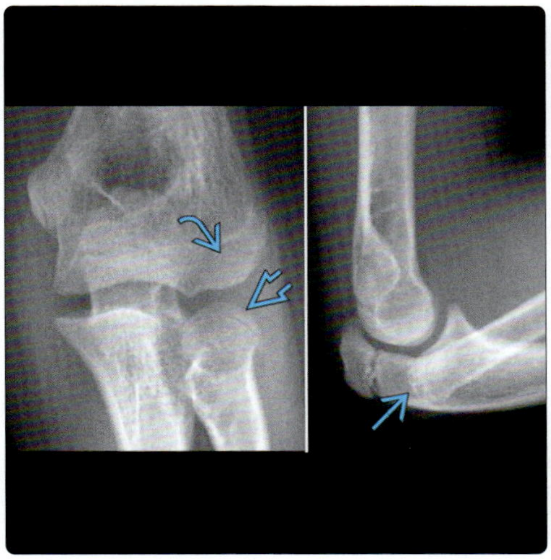

Radioulnar Synostosis

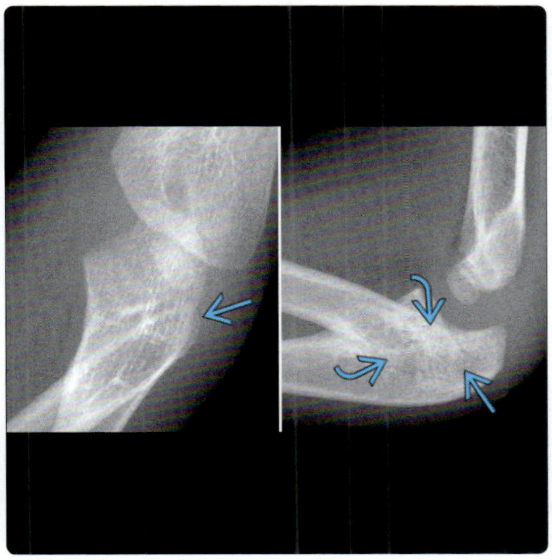

(Left) *Radiographs in a 10 year old with a left elbow injury show a dome-shaped radial head, which is dorsally dislocated. Also note the hypoplastic capitellum. These findings distinguish this entity from a traumatic dislocation.* **(Right)** *Radiographs in a 4 year old with decreased pronation/supination of the forearm show a dysplastic appearance of the radial head, which is dorsally & laterally dislocated. There is also osseous fusion of the proximal radius & ulna.*

Amniotic Band Syndrome

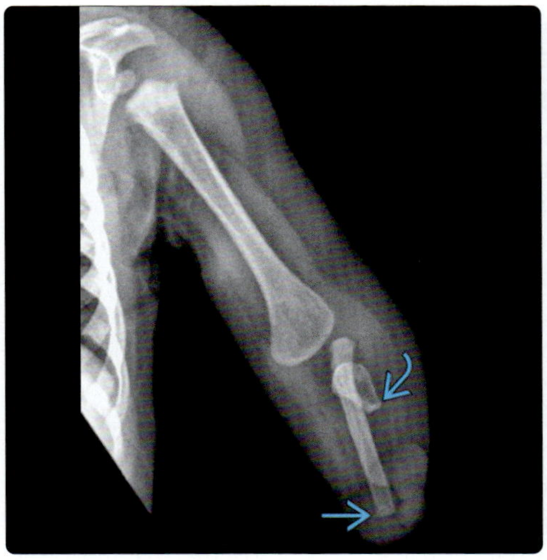

Cornelia de Lange Syndrome

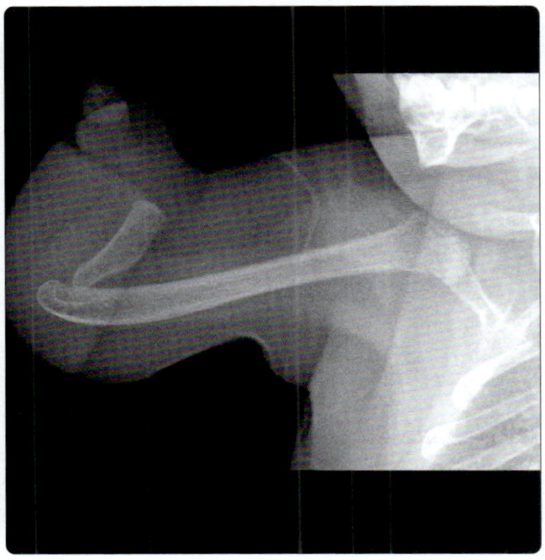

(Left) *AP radiograph in a 10-month-old girl with amniotic band syndrome shows amputation of the left forearm at the distal radius & proximal ulna.* **(Right)** *Lateral radiograph in a 15 month old with Cornelia de Lange syndrome shows a common upper extremity deformity of this disorder with severe deficiency of the bones of the forearm, wrist, & hand. This anomaly was present bilaterally.*

DIFFERENTIAL DIAGNOSIS

Common

- Physiologic Bowing
- Blount Disease
- Injury

Less Common

- Congenital/Infantile Tibial Bowing
- Metabolic Bone Disease
- Fibrous Dysplasia

Rare but Important

- Skeletal Dysplasias
- Osteogenesis Imperfecta
- Osteofibrous Dysplasia/Adamantinoma

ESSENTIAL INFORMATION

Key Differential Diagnosis Issues

- Extent: Isolated or generalized bowing
- Location: Bowing at knee vs. localized to leg or femur
  - Genu varum or genu valgum: Lower extremity bowing centered at knee
    - Varus alignment
      - Apex of curve points away from midline
      - Extremity distal to apex deviates toward midline
    - Valgus alignment
      - Apex of curve points toward midline
      - Extremity distal to apex deviates away from midline
  - Tibial bowing
    - Infantile/congenital tibial bowing characterized by direction of apex
    - Localized tibial bowing in child is rarely from osteofibrous dysplasia (OFD) or adamantinoma
  - Femoral bowing: Less common & typically associated with diffuse osseous abnormalities, such as skeletal dysplasia, osteogenesis Imperfecta (OI)
- Cause: Physiologic vs. pathologic
  - Physiologic genu varum normal in infant
    - As child begins walking, typically decreases & becomes valgus
    - Genu varum is abnormal in child > 2 years of age

Helpful Clues for Common Diagnoses

- **Physiologic Bowing**
  - Developmental changes of lower extremity alignment centered at knee occur during childhood
  - Normal progression from genu varum → valgum
    - 0-1 year of age: Normal ~ 10-17° varus
    - 1-2 years: Normal ~ 0-10° varus
    - 3-4 years: Normal ~ 0-10° valgus
    - 4-13 years: Normal ~ 6° valgus
  - Exaggerated physiologic bowing (varus)
    - More common in early walkers, overweight, & African American children
    - Prominent, mildly beaked medial proximal tibial/distal femoral metaphyses
      - Tibial metaphysis is also mildly depressed
      - Should not be fragmented (as in Blount disease)
    - Thickening of medial tibial & femoral cortices
    - Metaphyseal-diaphyseal angle (MDA): Angle between proximal tibial metaphysis & line perpendicular to long axis of tibial diaphysis
      - Physiologic bowing is typically ≤ 11°
      - Blount disease is typically > 11°
      - However, there is overlap: 8-11° is considered borderline & warrants clinical + radiographic follow-up
    - Exaggerated physiologic varus typically resolves without treatment
- **Blount Disease**
  - Developmental disorder with disrupted endochondral ossification of medial proximal tibial physis
  - Thought to result from abnormal stress on proximal medial tibial physis
  - Diagnosed by progressive bowing on clinical exam + characteristic radiographic changes
  - Infantile type: 1-3 years, bilateral in 60-80%
    - Must differentiate from physiologic bowing
  - Adolescent type: 8-14 years, more commonly unilateral
  - Predisposed: Early walkers, obese children, & African Americans
  - Medial tibial metaphysis is depressed, fragmented, ± physeal bridge of proximal medial tibia, genu varum
  - MDA in Blount disease is typically > 11°
  - Enlarged epiphyseal cartilage & medial meniscus on MR
- **Injury**
  - Growth plate injury
    - Various insults to growth plate can lead to physeal bridge
      - If peripheral, may lead to angular deformity
    - Possible causes: Fracture, infection, medications (retinoids), radiation
  - Overuse injury
    - Chronic repetitive overuse can injure metaphyseal blood supply
    - Localized disruption of endochondral ossification can lead to varus/valgus angulation depending upon area of growth plate involvement
  - Fracture malunion
    - Less common in children due to greater remodeling

Helpful Clues for Less Common Diagnoses

- **Congenital/Infantile Tibial Bowing**
  - Typically unilateral congenital or infantile diaphyseal deformity
  - 3 classic patterns characterized by direction of apex
    - Posteromedial
      - Typically physiologic
      - Secondary to intrauterine positioning
      - ± associated calcaneovalgus foot deformity
    - Anteromedial
      - Associated with fibular hemimelia (range of fibular abnormalities from hypoplastic to absent)
    - Anterolateral
      - High association with neurofibromatosis type 1
      - Bowing is typically at junction of mid to distal 1/3 of tibia
      - Often with narrowing, sclerosis, or cystic change at apex
      - May develop fracture & pseudarthrosis

- **Metabolic Bone Disease**
  - Various etiologies can cause bowing
  - Rickets: Classic childhood metabolic bone disease
    - Failure to mineralize cartilage/osteoid at physis
      - Due to decreased calcium or phosphorous
      - Most commonly from vitamin D deficiency
    - Loss of zone of provisional calcification (ZPC) with metaphyseal osteolysis, cupping, & fraying
      - Most pronounced at sites of rapid growth: Distal femur, proximal tibia, distal radius
    - Generalized bowing
- **Fibrous Dysplasia**
  - Replacement of portions of medullary cavity with fibrous stroma & dysplastic trabecular
  - Long bone medullary space widening, endosteal scalloping, coarse or obliterated trabeculation
    - Classically ground-glass (think "frosted" or "smudged" glass) fibrous matrix
      - May have more lytic or sclerotic areas
  - Monostotic (~ 80%) or polyostotic (~ 20%)
    - Polyostotic tends to be unilateral
    - Polyostotic may have syndromic association
      - McCune-Albright, Mazabraud syndromes

Helpful Clues for Rare Diagnoses

- **Skeletal Dysplasia**
  - Many skeletal dysplasias can present with bending of long bones, genu varum, or genu valgum
  - Achondroplasia
    - Most common form of short limb dwarfism
    - Generalized bowing
    - Short, thick long bones with metaphyseal cupping & flaring; short, broad phalanges
    - Short rectangular iliac bones, narrow sacrosciatic notches, flat acetabular roof
    - Bullet-shaped vertebral bodies with posterior scalloping, progressive narrowing of interpediculate distances inferiorly in lumbar spine
  - Campomelic dysplasia
    - Often fatal in infancy
    - Anterolateral bowing of lower > upper extremities
    - Bowed femur with short bowed tibia
    - Large skull with small face, hypoplastic scapula, narrow pelvis, dislocated hips, bell-shaped chest
- **Osteogenesis Imperfecta**
  - Group of clinically heterogeneous genetic disorders caused by type I collagen abnormalities
  - Increased bone fragility → frequent fractures → malunion & bowing
    - Higher likelihood of subsequent fractures
  - Treatment: Bisphosphonates, physical therapy, orthopedic surgery
    - Bisphosphonates → sclerotic metaphyseal bands paralleling growth plates
- **Osteofibrous Dysplasia/Adamantinoma**
  - OFD
    - Fibroosseous lesion primarily affecting tibia in children
      - Usually tibial diaphysis &/or metadiaphysis
      - Can synchronously involve fibula
    - May present with painless anterior bowing
    - Fracture & pseudoarthrosis can also occur
    - Usually eccentrically involves anterior tibia
    - Lucent & sclerotic, solitary or multifocal
  - Adamantinoma
    - Similar to OFD but is low-grade malignancy
    - More common in older patients than OFD
    - Differentiated form can be seen in children & can be radiographically identical to OFD
    - Worrisome features include periosteal reaction, permeative destruction, & soft tissue extension

SELECTED REFERENCES

1. Lachman R. Taybi and Lachman's Radiology of Syndromes, Metabolic Disorders and Skeletal Dysplasias. 5th ed. Philadelphia: Mosby, 2006
2. Cheema JI et al: Radiographic characteristics of lower-extremity bowing in children. Radiographics. 23(4):871-80, 2003

Physiologic Bowing

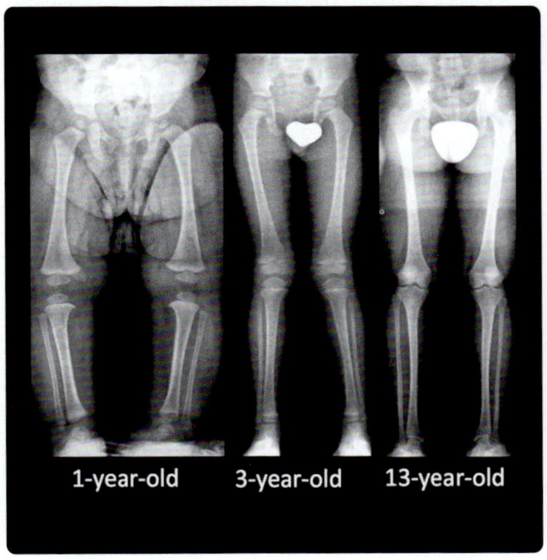

Physiologic Bowing

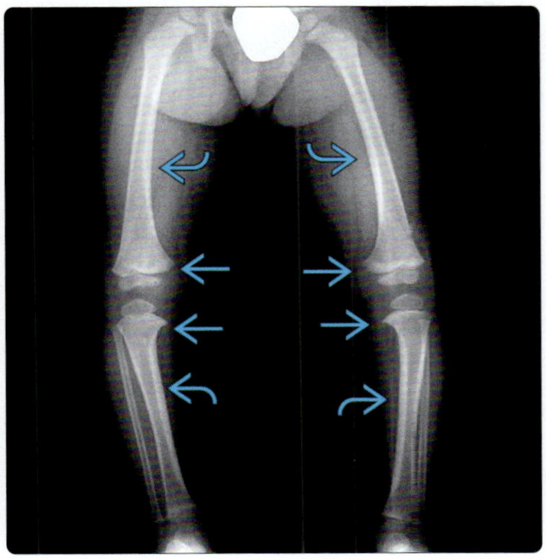

(Left) *Lower extremity radiographs show the normal changes in alignment with age. There is normal genu varum at 1 year. After children begin walking, this transitions to genu valgum (3 years old) & then decreases after 4 years to the minimal valgus/near neutral alignment of adolescents.* **(Right)** *AP radiograph in a 23 month old shows genu varum (or > 10° at this age). The knee medial metaphyses are beaked ➔ with mild downsloping of the tibial metaphyses. Also note the medial cortical thickening ➔.*

Physiologic Bowing

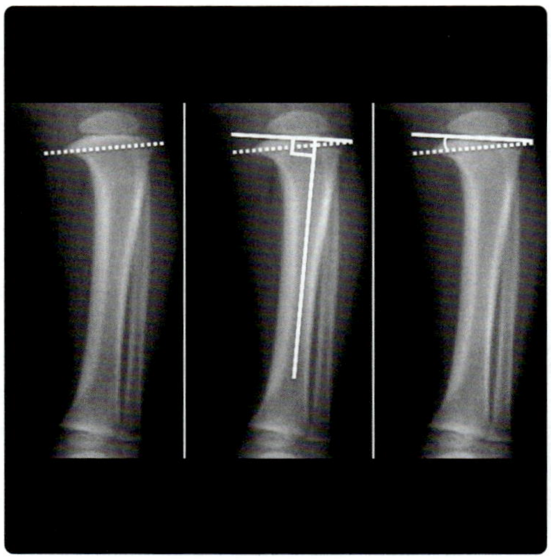

Physiologic Bowing

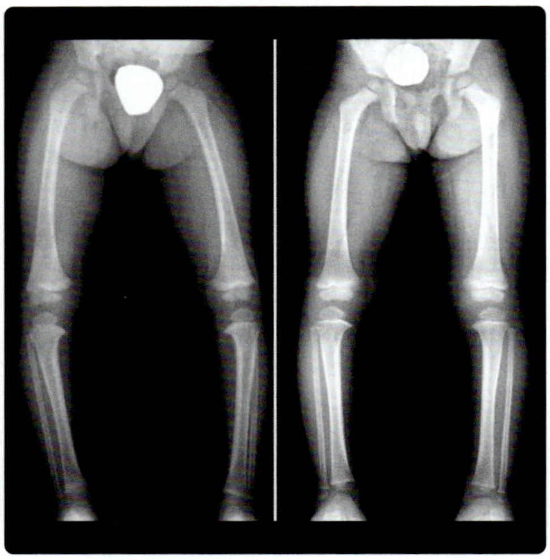

(Left) *Radiographs show measurement of the metaphyseal-diaphyseal angle (MDA). The metaphyseal line (dashed line) connects the corners of the proximal tibial metaphysis. A 2nd line is drawn perpendicular to the long axis of the tibia (solid line). The angle between these lines (far right) is the MDA. In this patient, the MDA was borderline at 10°.* **(Right)** *Initial (left) & follow-up (right) radiographs in the same patient show improvement of the genu varum, confirming that this was exaggerated physiologic bowing.*

Blount Disease

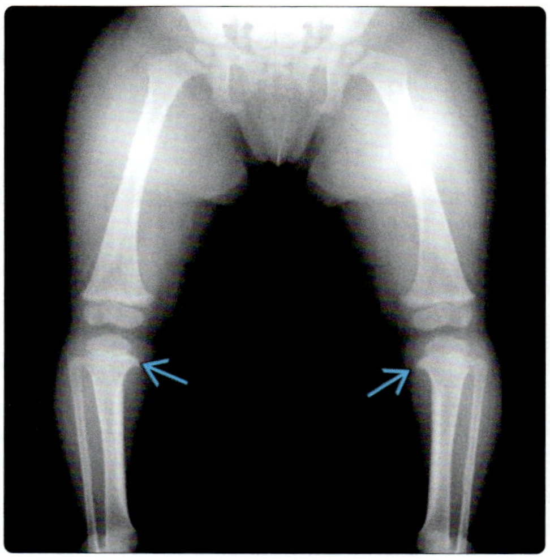

Blount Disease

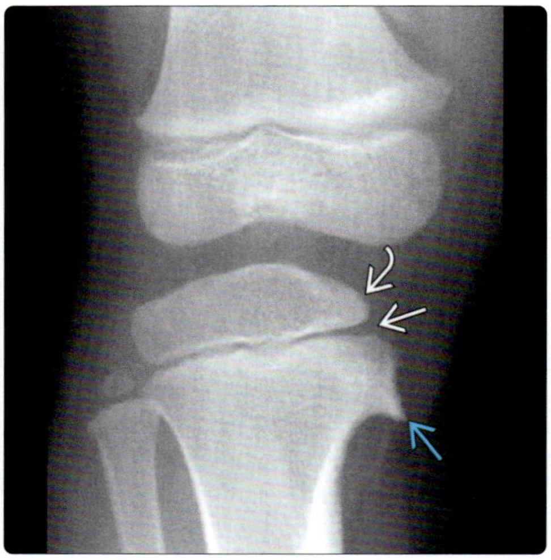

(Left) *Frontal radiograph in a 15-month-old girl shows genu varum with beaked proximal medial tibial metaphyses ➔. This girl's MDA angles measured 12°.* **(Right)** *Follow-up frontal radiograph of the right knee in the same girl 1 year later shows a beaked & markedly downsloped proximal medial tibial metaphysis ➔, underdeveloped adjacent epiphysis ➔, & widened adjacent physis ➔. Similar findings developed in the contralateral knee (not shown).*

Blount Disease

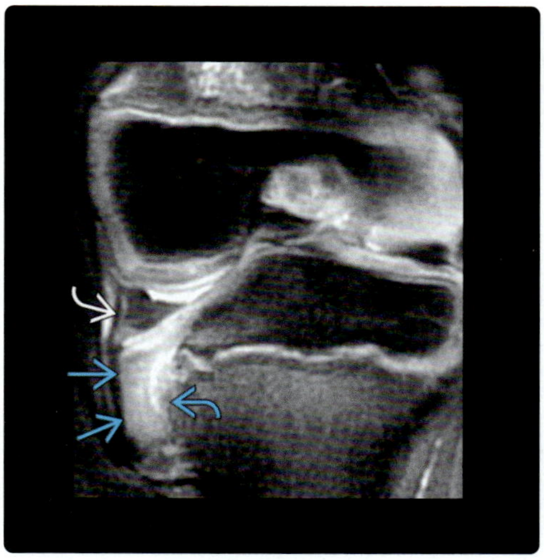

Blount Disease

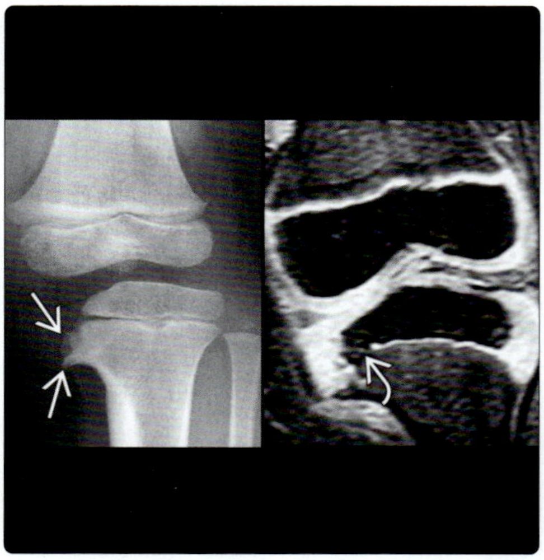

(Left) *Coronal T2 FS MR of the left knee in a child with Blount disease shows medial proximal tibial downsloping ➔ & thickening of the unossified epiphyseal cartilage ➔ in this area. Also note the thickening of the medial meniscus ➔.* **(Right)** *AP radiograph (left) shows downsloping, beaking, & irregularity of the medial tibial metaphysis ➔ (Blount disease). Coronal GRE MR (right) shows abnormal ossification of the medial tibial epiphysis & metaphysis with an osseous bridge ➔ crossing the tibial physis.*

Injury

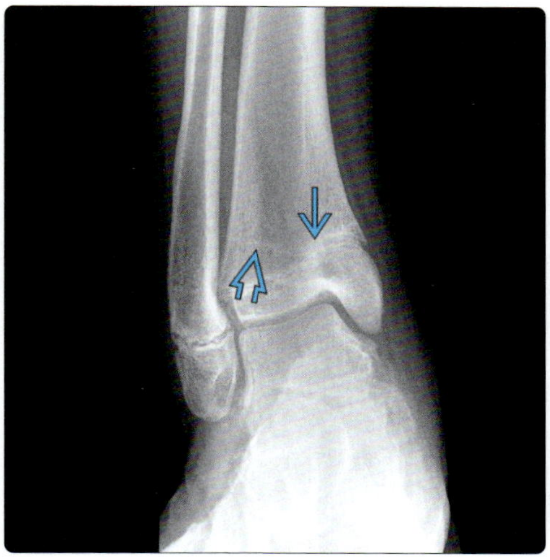

Congenital/Infantile Tibial Bowing

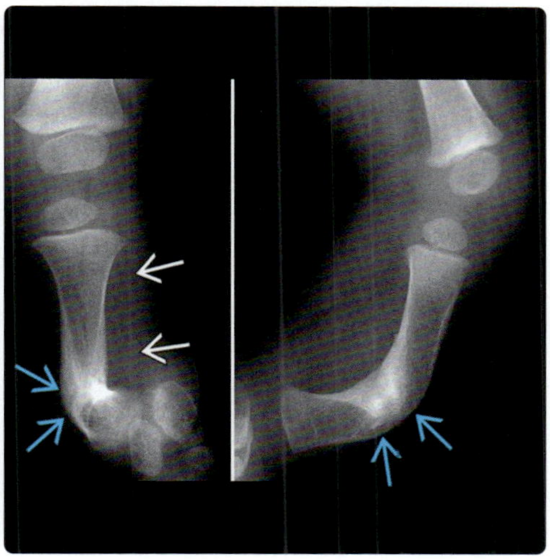

(Left) *Standing AP radiograph of the ankle in an 11 year old 3 years after distal tibial & fibular physeal fractures shows varus alignment of the ankle due to a medial tibial bone bridge ⇨. Note the growth arrest line ⇨ that is sloped medially toward the bridge.* **(Right)** *Frontal (left) & lateral (right) radiographs in an 8 month old with fibular hemimelia show anteromedial tibial bowing ⇨ associated with absence of the fibula ➡.*

Congenital/Infantile Tibial Bowing

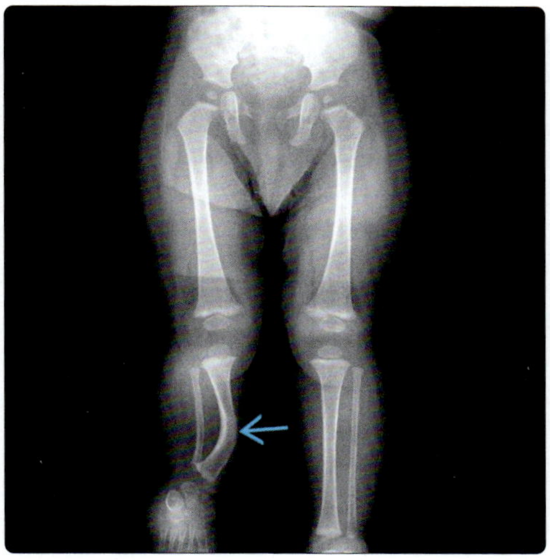

Congenital/Infantile Tibial Bowing

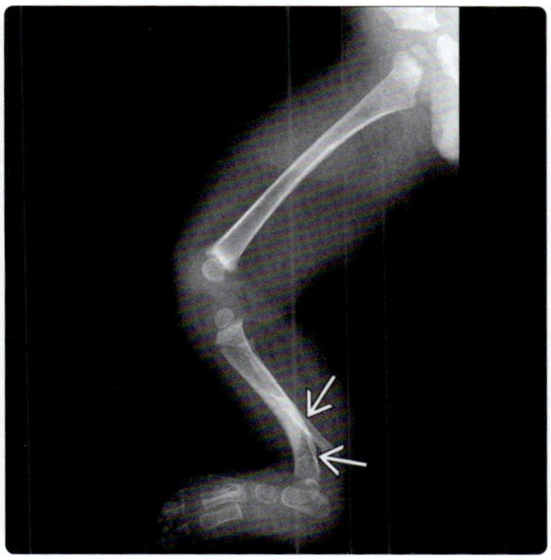

(Left) *Frontal radiograph of the lower extremities in a 1 year old shows medial tibial bowing on the right ⇨. There is shortening of the right tibia & fibula with an associated limb length discrepancy.* **(Right)** *Lateral radiograph in the same child shows posterior bowing of the tibia ➡. An associated calcaneovalgus deformity is suggested, though weight-bearing radiographs are required to adequately assess disorders of foot alignment.*

Congenital/Infantile Tibial Bowing

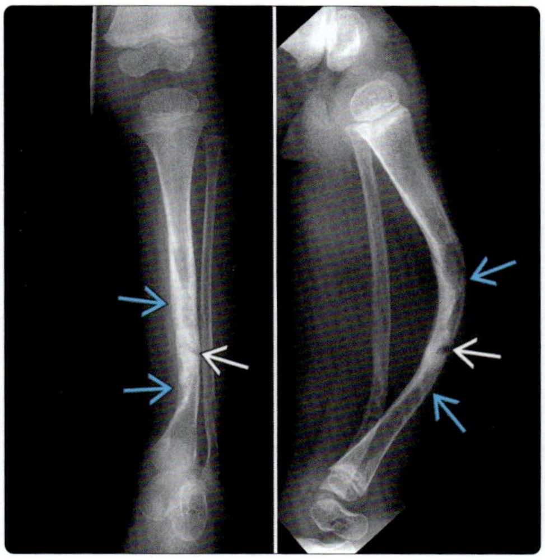

Congenital/Infantile Tibial Bowing

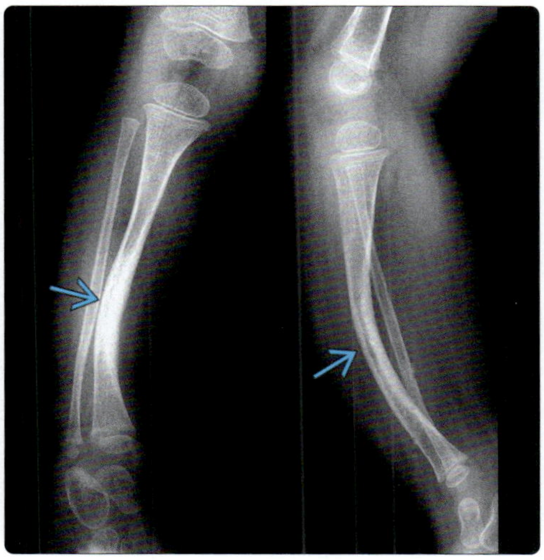

(Left) *Frontal & lateral radiographs in a 2-year-old boy with neurofibromatosis type 1 show anterolateral bowing of the midtibial diaphysis ⇨ with associated increased sclerosis & cortical thickening. There is a developing fracture ➡, which ultimately progressed to a pseudarthrosis.* **(Right)** *AP & lateral radiographs of the lower leg in a 1 year old with neurofibromatosis type 1 show anterolateral tibial bowing ⇨ with associated cortical thickening. No fracture or pseudarthrosis is present at this time.*

(**Left**) *AP radiograph shows the typical findings of rickets, including loss of the dense zones of provisional calcification (ZPCs) with metaphyseal flaring, cupping, & fragmentation + growth plate widening/lengthening ➡. Note the more prominent focal bowing at the ankles.* (**Right**) *AP radiograph in the same patient a few years later shows residual bowing of the distal tibia & fibula ➡ with thickening of the distal medial tibial cortices. The previous changes of rickets have largely resolved with intact ZPCs now visible ⇨.*

Metabolic Bone Disease

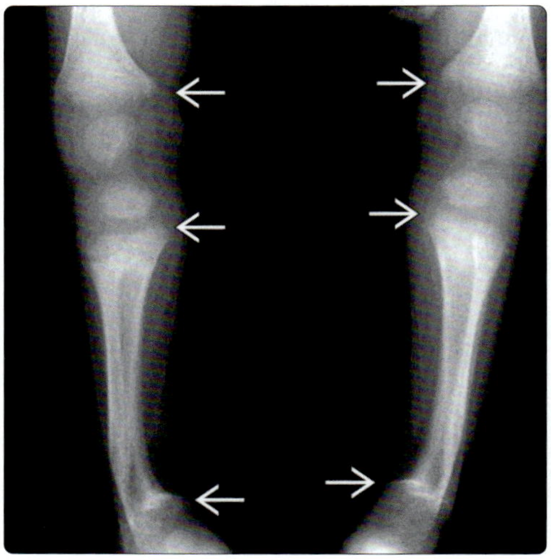

Metabolic Bone Disease

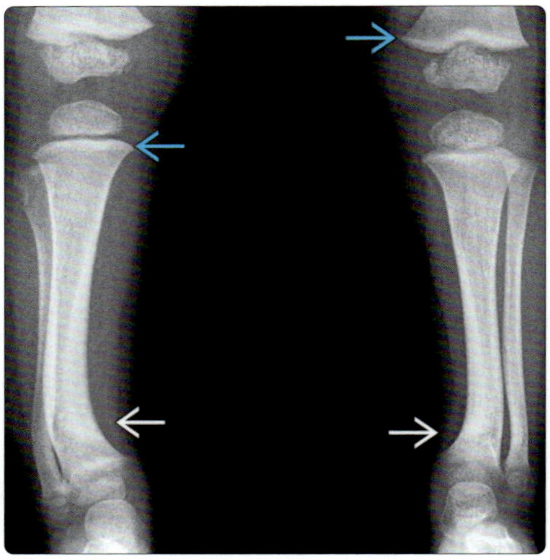

(**Left**) *AP radiograph of the lower extremities shows cupped, frayed metaphyses ⇨ & lower extremity bowing in a child with rickets.* (**Right**) *Right hip radiograph in a girl with McCune-Albright syndrome shows irregular widening of the medullary cavity & loss of normal trabeculation (which is replaced by the ground-glass matrix of fibrous dysplasia in the proximal femur & pelvis). Also note the severe coxa vara (shepherd's crook) deformity ⇨ of the proximal femur + bowing from a healing pathologic fracture of the mid femur ⇨.*

Metabolic Bone Disease

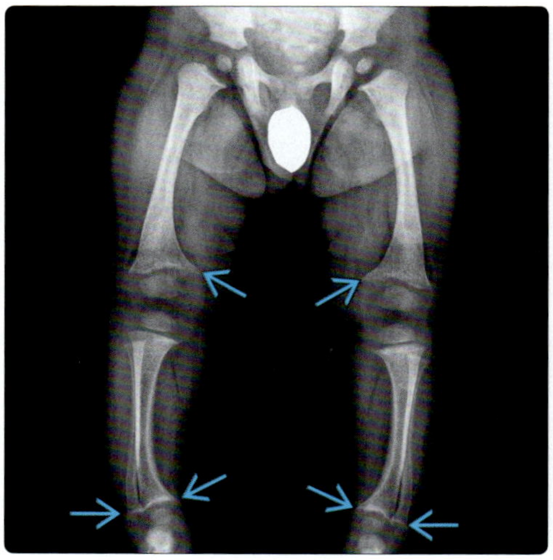

Fibrous Dysplasia

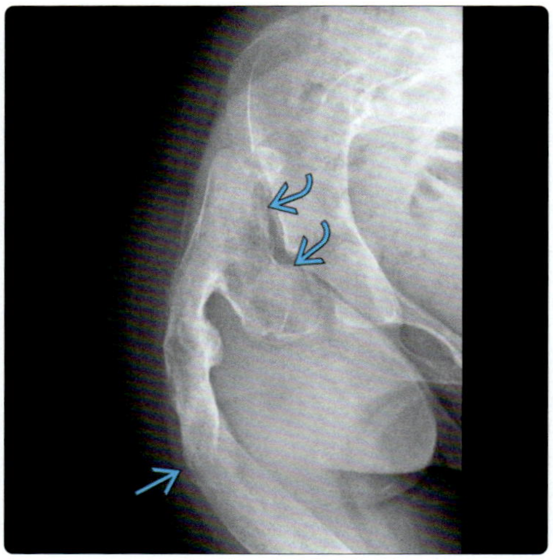

(**Left**) *Frontal radiograph of the lower extremities in a 4-year-old boy with achondroplasia shows bilateral genu varum. Other findings of achondroplasia include cone (chevron)-shaped distal femoral/proximal tibial metaphyses/epiphyses ⇨, small squared iliac wings, rounded iliac crests, horizontal acetabular roofs ➡, & relatively long fibulae.* (**Right**) *AP radiograph in a boy with campomelic dysplasia shows lateral bowing of the proximal femurs. Note the mild medial bowing of the right tibia & short bilateral fibulae.*

Skeletal Dysplasias

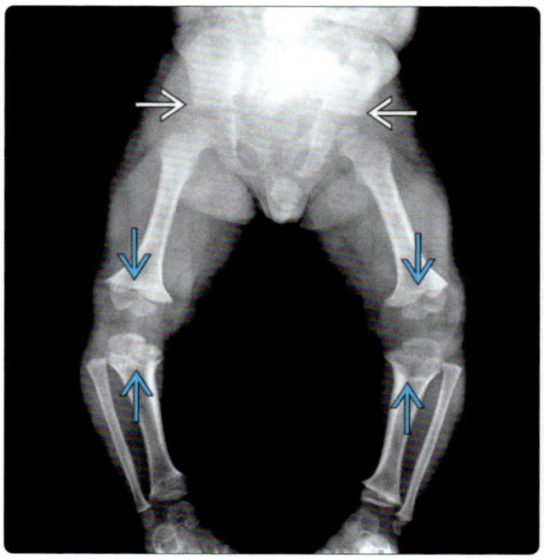

Skeletal Dysplasias

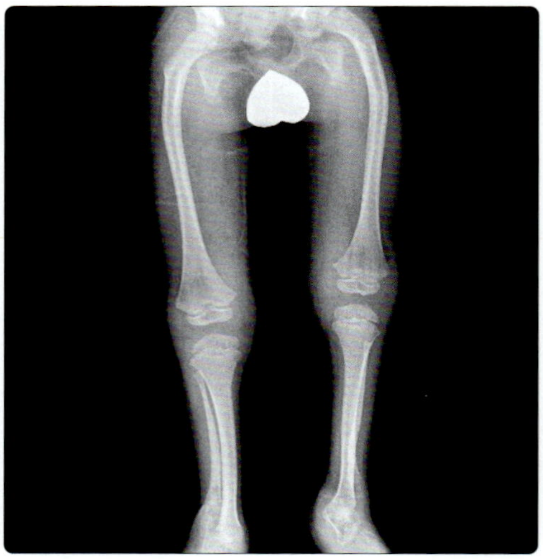

Osteogenesis Imperfecta

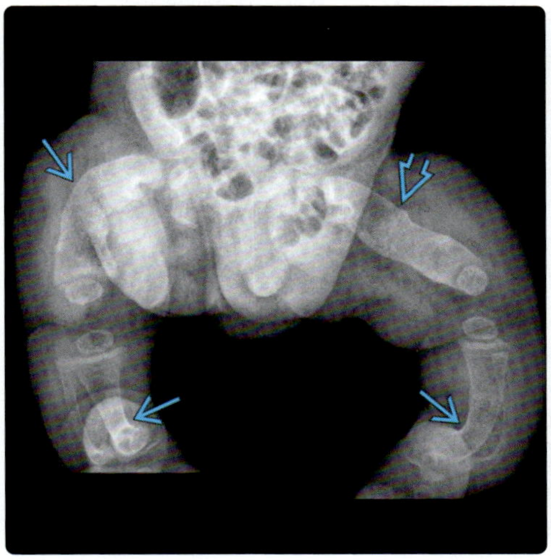

Osteogenesis Imperfecta

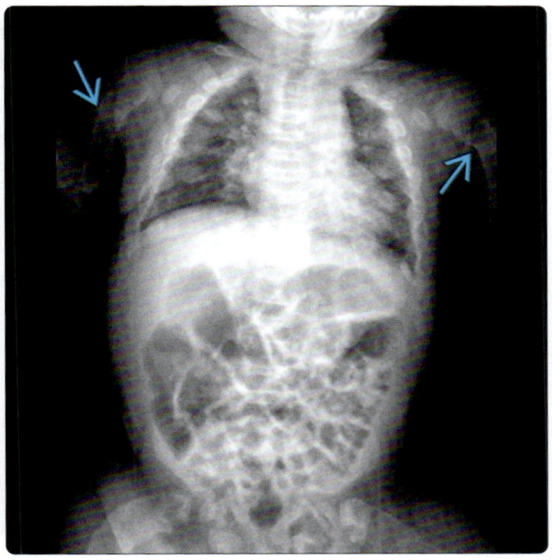

(Left) *Frontal radiograph of the lower extremities in a 4 month old who was born with multiple fractures shows diffuse osseous abnormalities, including osteoporosis, short long bones with irregular diaphyseal widening →, & bowing of the right femur & both tibiae/fibulae →.* **(Right)** *Frontal radiograph of the chest & abdomen in the same patient shows bilateral healing humeral fractures → & a beaded appearance of the bilateral ribs due to innumerable healing rib fractures.*

Osteogenesis Imperfecta

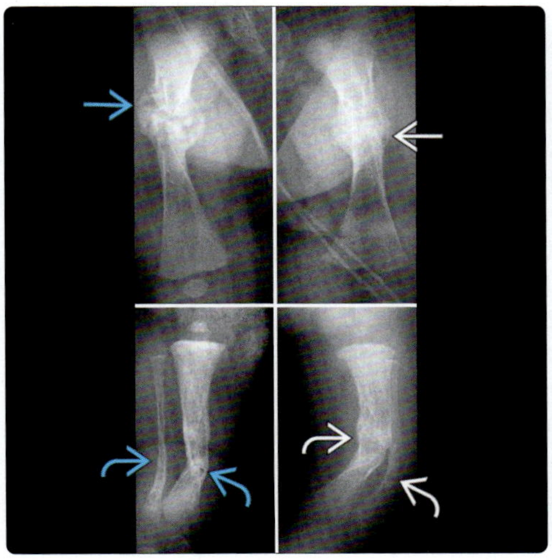

Osteogenesis Imperfecta

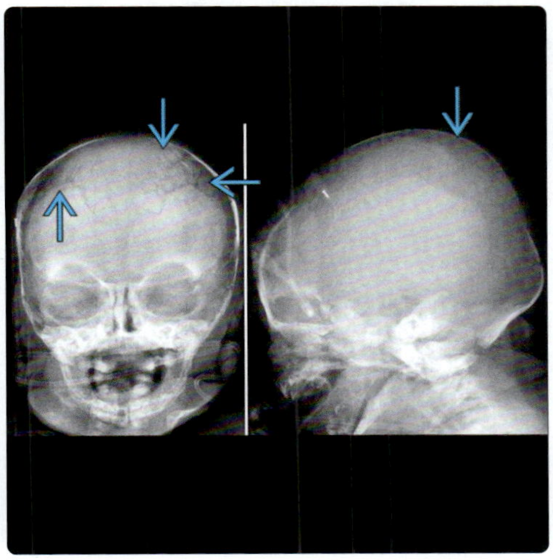

(Left) *Frontal radiographs of both lower extremities in a 1-day-old girl show healing fractures of the right → & left → femurs. Bowing deformities of both the right → & left → tibiae/fibulae (secondary to healing fractures) are also noted.* **(Right)** *Skull radiographs in the same girl show multiple (> 10) wormian bones → throughout the skull. This girl also had bilateral rib & upper extremity fractures (not shown) & was subsequently diagnosed with type III osteogenesis imperfecta.*

Osteofibrous Dysplasia/Adamantinoma

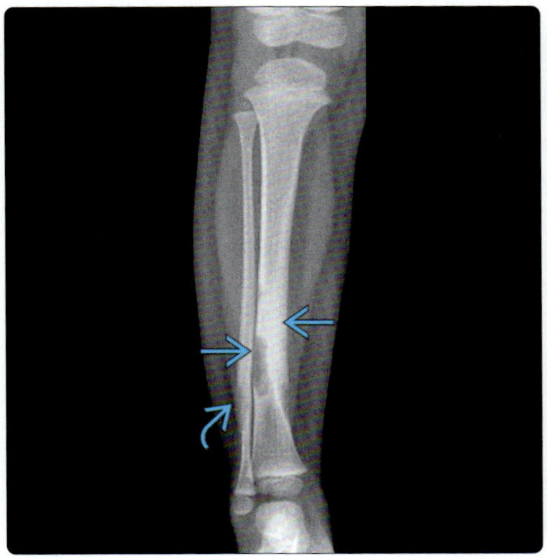

Osteofibrous Dysplasia/Adamantinoma

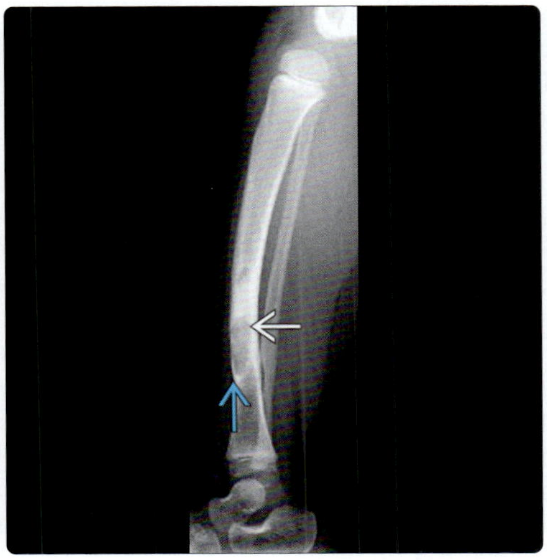

(Left) *Frontal radiograph of the right leg in a 2-year-old girl shows a sclerotic & lytic lesion → of the distal right tibial diaphysis associated with mild lateral tibial bowing. A more subtle lesion is also present in the distal fibula →.* **(Right)** *Lateral radiograph in the same girl shows that the sclerotic & lytic tibial lesion involves the anterior cortex → & is associated with mild anterior bowing & a pathologic fracture →. Biopsy showed osteofibrous dysplasia.*

DIFFERENTIAL DIAGNOSIS

Common

- Metatarsus Adductus
- Pes Planovalgus
- Club Foot (Talipes Equinovarus)
- Tarsal Coalition
- Hallux Valgus

Less Common

- Congenital Vertical Talus
- Oblique Talus
- Pes Cavus/Neuromuscular Disorders (Mimic)
-

Rare but Important

- Polydactyly
- Skewfoot
- Delta Phalanx (Bracket Epiphysis)
- Ectrodactyly (Split Hand/Split Foot Malformation)

ESSENTIAL INFORMATION

Key Differential Diagnosis Issues

- Foot alignment should only be assessed on weight-bearing/simulated weight-bearing radiographs
- Most congenital foot deformities can be diagnosed by evaluating 3 relationships
  - Hindfoot equinus or calcaneus
    - On lateral radiograph, normal angle between long axes of calcaneus & tibia ranges from 60-90°
    - Hindfoot equinus: Tibiocalcaneal angle > 90° (excessive plantarflexion of calcaneus)
    - Hindfoot calcaneus: Tibiocalcaneal angle < 60° (excessive dorsiflexion of calcaneus)
  - Hindfoot varus or valgus
    - On lateral radiograph, normal angle between long axes of talus & calcaneus ranges between 30-45° (Kite angle or lateral talocalcaneal angle)
    - On AP radiograph, normal angle between long axes of talus & calcaneus ranges between 30-45°
    - Varus hindfoot: ↓ talocalcaneal angle (i.e., bones nearly parallel), < 30° on lateral, < 30° on AP
    - Valgus hindfoot: ↑ talocalcaneal angle (i.e., bones diverge), > 45° on lateral, > 45° on AP
  - Forefoot varus or valgus
    - On lateral radiograph, metatarsals (MTs) are normally moderately superimposed, with 5th in plantar-most position; angle of inclination of MTs gradually ↑ from 5° for 5th to 20° for 1st
    - On AP radiograph, MTs normally show moderate convergence of bases
    - Varus forefoot: Inversion & supination; on lateral, ↓ superimposition of MTs (ladder-like) with 5th MT in plantar-most position; on AP, ↑ overlap of MT bases
    - Valgus forefoot: Eversion & pronation; on lateral, ↑ superimposition of MTs with 1st MT in plantar-most position; on AP, ↓ convergence of MT bases
- **Hint**: Most congenital foot deformities match type of hindfoot & forefoot deformities
  - Varus hindfoot with varus forefoot
  - Valgus hindfoot with valgus forefoot
- **Hint**: If hindfoot & forefoot deformities are unmatched (i.e., varus hindfoot & valgus forefoot or valgus hindfoot & varus forefoot), is usually due to spastic foot

Helpful Clues for Common Diagnoses

- **Metatarsus Adductus**
  - Most common structural foot abnormality of infants
  - Adduction of MTs; normal hindfoot
  - Rarely imaged, since it is flexible & typically self-correcting
- **Pes Planovalgus**
  - Common (4% of population)
  - Flexible; non-weight-bearing radiographs are normal
  - Abnormalities on weight-bearing radiographs
    - Hindfoot valgus, **no** equinus
- **Club Foot (Talipes Equinovarus)**
  - Fixed structural abnormalities
    - Plantarflexion of calcaneus relative to tibia (equinus)
    - Hindfoot varus
    - Forefoot adduction (varus)
  - Incidence of 1:1,000 births
  - M > F (2-3:1)
  - Treatment is primarily conservative with manipulation & casting; selective use of surgery
- **Tarsal Coalition**
  - Usually secondary to congenital lack of segmentation of bones of hindfoot
  - Symptoms begin in late 1st or 2nd decade
  - Painful flatfoot: Persistent or intermittent spasm of peroneal muscles
  - 25-50% bilaterality
  - Most commonly calcaneonavicular or talocalcaneal
    - Others (e.g., cubonavicular, talonavicular, calcaneocuboid) are less common
  - Secondary signs
    - Talar beak: Due to excessive motion at talonavicular joint because of rigid subtalar joint
    - C-sign: Continuous C-shaped line (on lateral radiograph in talocalcaneal coalition) formed by superior outline of talar dome & inferior outline of sustentaculum tali posteriorly
    - Ball & socket tibiotalar joint: Conversion of this hinge joint to rounded articulation; due to extensive subtalar coalition
  - Calcaneonavicular coalition
    - Anterior process of calcaneus extends & broadens at union with navicular
    - Directly visualized on oblique foot radiograph
  - Talocalcaneal coalition
    - Generally at mid subtalar joint & not well visualized on standard foot radiographs
      - Harris-Beath (posterior tangential) view of foot: Sole of foot flat on detector with beam angled ~ 45° toward heel
      - Best radiographic view for subtalar coalition
    - Rarely involves posterior &/or anterior subtalar facets
  - CT or MR allows for best evaluation
  - Both feet should be imaged due to high incidence of bilateral tarsal coalitions
- **Hallux Valgus**

- May be idiopathic or secondary to other alignment disorder
- Girls > boys
- Intermetatarsal (1st & 2nd) angle > 10°; 1st MT-proximal phalanx angle > 15-20°

Helpful Clues for Less Common Diagnoses

- **Congenital Vertical Talus**
  - Rigid flatfoot
  - Isolated or part of syndrome/disorder (frequently associated with myelomeningocele)
  - Constant structural abnormalities
    - Hindfoot equinus
    - Hindfoot valgus
    - Plantar flexed talus with talonavicular dissociation
    - Forefoot valgus
  - Plantar flexion lateral radiograph used to evaluate if talonavicular dissociation persists
    - If long axis of talus remains inferior to navicular = congenital vertical talus (vs. oblique talus)
    - Talonavicular alignment can only be assessed radiographically once navicular ossifies (~ 2-5 years)
      - US or MR can be used prior to navicular ossification
    - Some use talar-1st MT alignment as surrogate on radiographs for talonavicular alignment prior to navicular ossification
      - Long axis of talus should be oriented along or above long axis of 1st MT
- **Oblique Talus**
  - Inferior orientation of talus, less severe than vertical talus
  - Talonavicular subluxation reduces with plantar flexion
    - Assessed on radiographs after ossification of navicular
    - Can be assessed on US prior to navicular ossification
- **Pes Cavus/Neuromuscular Disorders (Mimics)**
  - Multiple etiologies; not strictly congenital
    - Upper motor neuron lesions (Friedrich ataxia)
    - Lower motor neuron lesions (poliomyelitis)
    - Cerebral palsy, vascular ischemia, Charcot-Marie-Tooth
  - Spastic abnormalities, often with mismatch of hindfoot & forefoot abnormalities (varus-valgus)
  - Soft tissues show muscle atrophy

Helpful Clues for Rare Diagnoses

- **Polydactyly**
  - Extra digits
  - Preaxial (tibial side), post axial (fibular side), or mesoaxial (central)
  - Can be associated with syndactyly (either soft tissue or osseous fusion of digits)
  - Extra digit can range from small skin tag → digit with hypoplastic bones → fully developed extra digit
- **Skewfoot**
  - Hindfoot valgus, navicular laterally subluxed, MTs adducted
  - Compared to metatarsus adductus, there is fixed forefoot varus & hindfoot valgus
- **Delta Phalanx (Bracket Epiphysis)**
  - a.k.a. longitudinally bracketed epiphysis
  - C-shaped epiphysis along medial side of MT from proximal to distal aspect
  - Results in curved 1st MT
  - Clinical appearance is similar to metatarsus adductus, but deformity is rigid
- **Ectrodactyly (Split Hand/Split Foot Malformation)**
  - Deep, central, V-shaped cleft in feet (& hands)
  - Soft tissue & osseous syndactyly + aplasia & hypoplasia of residual phalanges/MTs
  - Associated with numerous gene mutations & syndromes

SELECTED REFERENCES

1. Miron MC et al: Ultrasound evaluation of foot deformities in infants. Pediatr Radiol. 46(2):193-209; quiz 190-2, 2016
2. Chu A: Managing pediatric foot and ankle deformity. Foot Ankle Clin. 20(4):xiii-xiv, 2015
3. Thapa MM et al: Radiographic assessment of pediatric foot alignment: review. AJR Am J Roentgenol. 194(6 Suppl):S51-8, 2010

Metatarsus Adductus

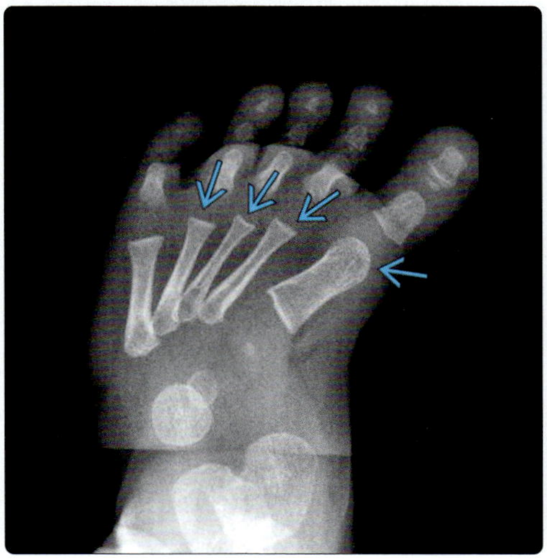

Metatarsus Adductus

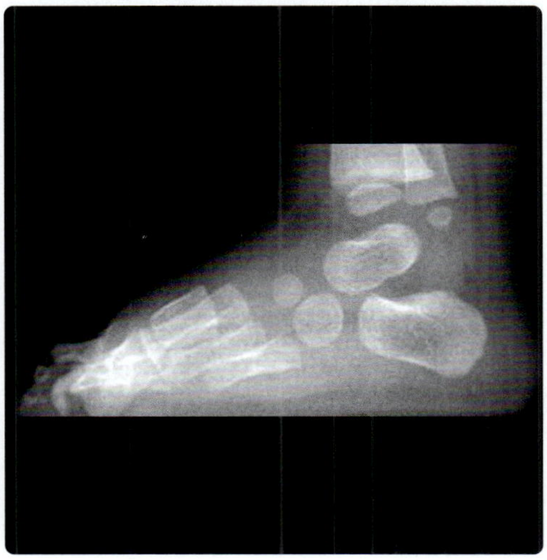

(Left) *AP weight-bearing radiograph of the left foot in a 1-year-old girl shows medial deviation of the metatarsals ⇒ with overlap of their bases. Note that the 1st metatarsal is more deviated than the 5th, & the midfoot & hindfoot are normal. These findings are typical in metatarsus adductus.* **(Right)** *Lateral weight-bearing radiograph of the same foot confirms normal alignment of the midfoot & hindfoot. There were similar findings in this patient's other foot (not shown); both were corrected without surgical intervention.*

(Left) *AP radiograph in a 7 year old shows that the long axis of the talus → is oriented medial to the long axis of the 1st metatarsal ➡ (due to hindfoot valgus).* **(Right)** *Lateral radiograph shows that the long axis of the talus (solid line) is oriented inferior to the long axis of the 1st metatarsal (dashed line). This lateral talar-1st metatarsal angle (Meary's angle) should be 0° ± 4°. If the talus is > 4° inferior to the 1st metatarsal, the foot is considered planus; if it is > 4° above it, the foot is considered cavus.*

Pes Planovalgus

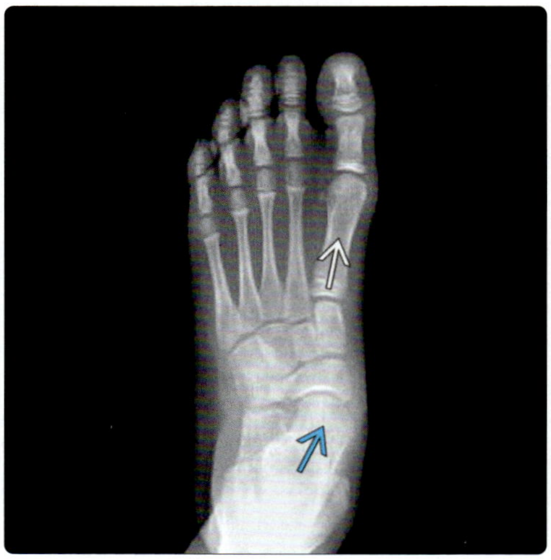

Pes Planovalgus

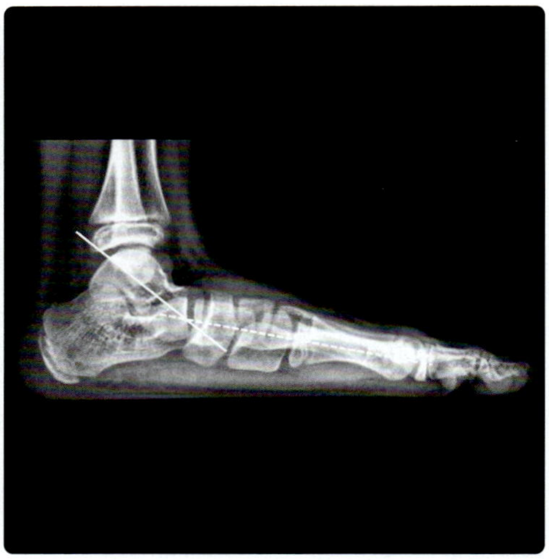

(Left) *AP radiograph of both feet in an 8-year-old boy shows bilateral hindfoot valgus with the long axes of both tali → oriented medial to the long axes of the 1st metatarsals ➡.* **(Right)** *Lateral radiographs of the left foot (top) & right foot (bottom) in the same child show hindfoot valgus with inferior orientation of the long axis of each talus →. Note that the navicular → is not dissociated from the talar head in either foot. There is also pes planus with loss of each longitudinal arch.*

Pes Planovalgus

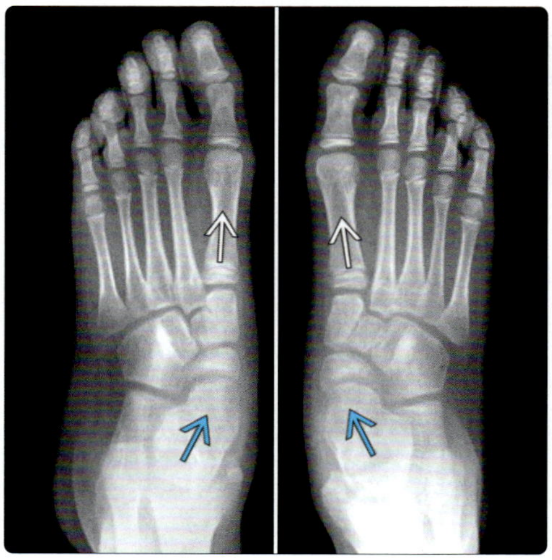

Pes Planovalgus

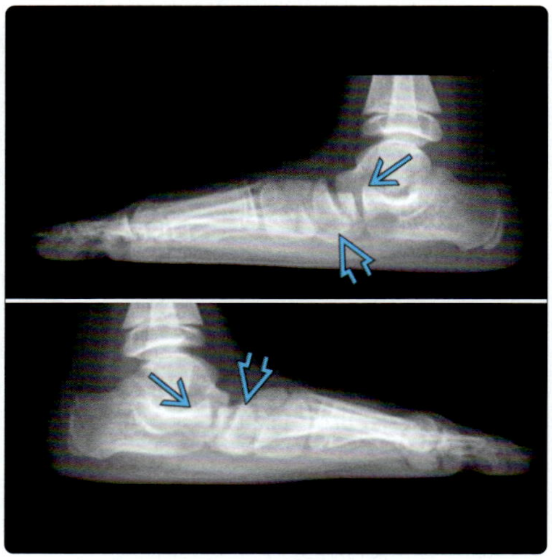

(Left) *AP simulated weight-bearing radiograph in a 1 year old shows the typical features of club foot, including hindfoot varus (with a lateral orientation of the talus → & a reduced angle between the long axes of the talus & calcaneus →).* **(Right)** *Lateral simulated weight-bearing radiograph in the same child shows that the calcaneus → is directed inferiorly. There is a decreased angle between the long axes of the talus → & that of the calcaneus. There is also a parallel configuration of the metatarsals ➡.*

Club Foot (Talipes Equinovarus)

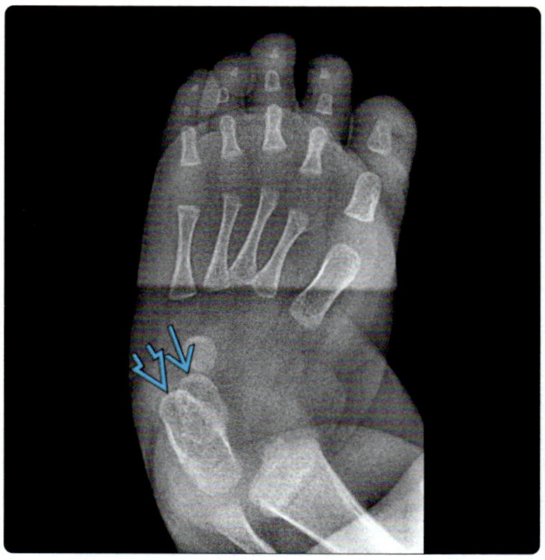

Club Foot (Talipes Equinovarus)

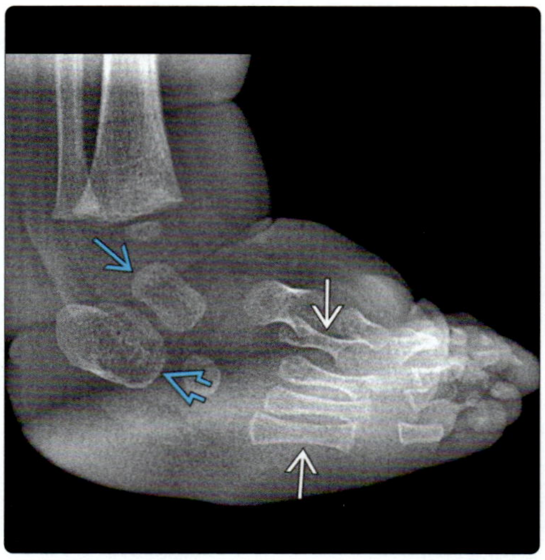

Tarsal Coalition

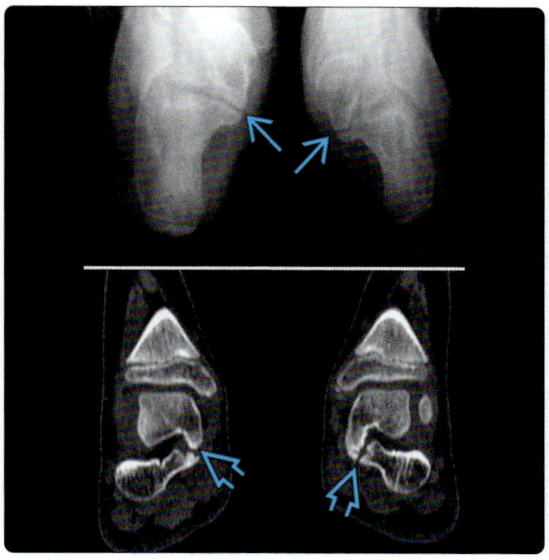

Congenital Vertical Talus

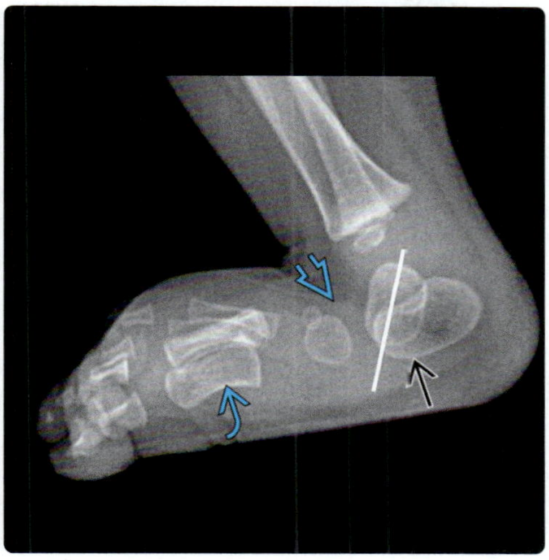

(Left) *Harris-Beath radiograph of both feet shows medial downsloping & narrowing of bilateral middle subtalar articulations. Coronal NECT better demonstrates bilateral fibrocartilaginous coalitions.* **(Right)** *Lateral simulated weight-bearing radiograph shows the long axis of the talus (white line) is oriented inferior to the expected location of the unossified navicular. Some use the long axis of the 1st metatarsal as a surrogate for normal talar orientation prior to navicular ossification. Note calcaneal equinus.*

Congenital Vertical Talus

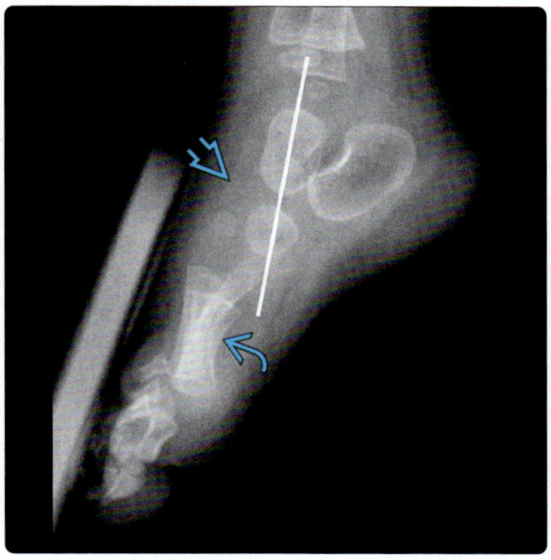

Skewfoot

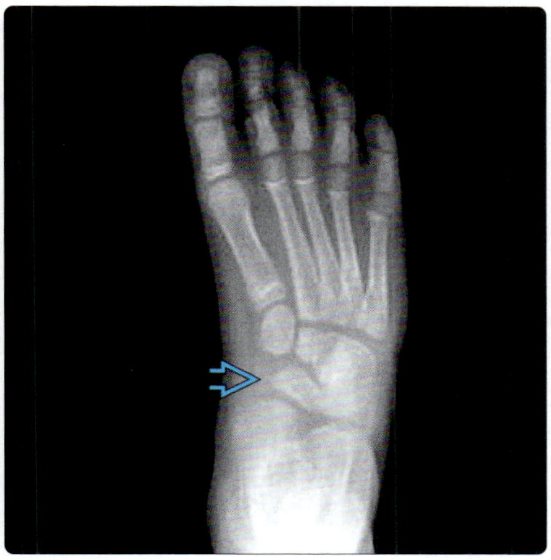

(Left) *Plantar flexion radiograph of the same foot shows that the talar orientation (white line) remains inferior to the unossified navicular & long axis of the 1st metatarsal.* **(Right)** *AP foot radiograph in a 6-year-old girl shows hindfoot valgus, lateral subluxation of the navicular, & metatarsus adductus.*

Delta Phalanx (Bracket Epiphysis)

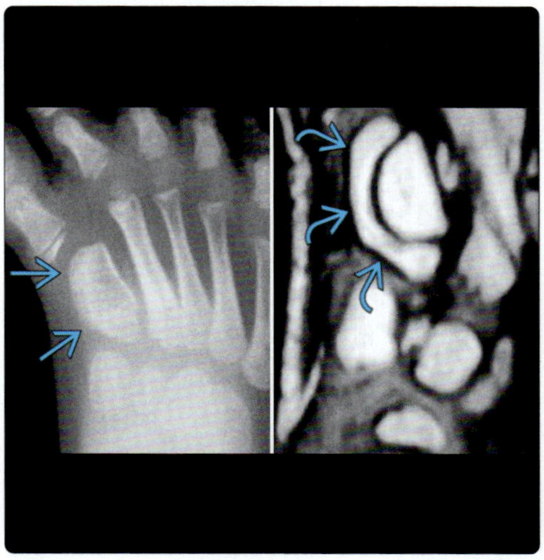

Ectrodactyly (Split Hand/Split Foot Malformation)

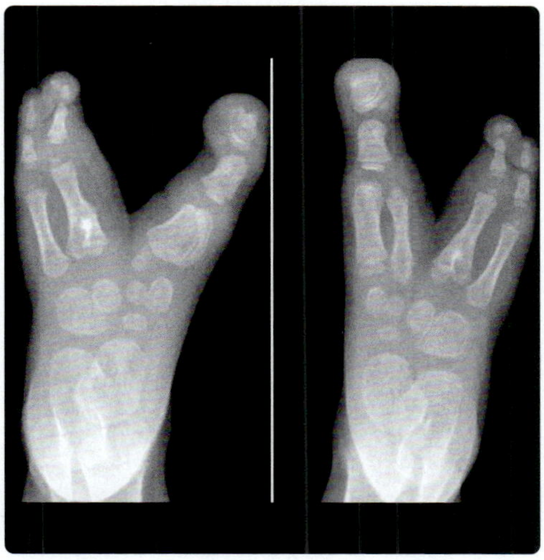

(Left) *Frontal radiograph (left image) of the right foot shows a short, broad 1st metatarsal with a curved medial margin. This causes medial deviation of the metatarsals. T1 MR (right image) show that the 1st metatarsal epiphysis extends along the entire medial aspect of the shaft from proximal to distal.* **(Right)** *AP radiographs in a 3-year-old girl with bilateral ectrodactyly shows deep, central, V-shaped clefts in both feet with soft tissue & osseous syndactyly. This child also had bilateral hand deformities (not shown).*

DIFFERENTIAL DIAGNOSIS

Common

- Achondroplasia
  - Hypochondroplasia
- Pseudoachondroplasia
- Thanatophoric Dysplasia
- Mesomelic Dysplasias
- Multiple Epiphyseal Dysplasia

Less Common

- Osteogenesis Imperfecta
- Campomelic Dysplasia
- Asphyxiating Thoracic Dysplasia (Jeune Syndrome)
- Chondrodysplasia Punctata
- Chondroectodermal Dysplasia (Ellis-van Creveld)

Rare but Important

- Achondrogenesis
- Spondyloepiphyseal Dysplasia
- Kniest Dysplasia
- Short Rib Polydactyly Syndrome

ESSENTIAL INFORMATION

Definitions of Limb Shortening

- Rhizomelia: Relative proximal (humeri, femurs) shortening
- Mesomelia: Relative middle (forearm/leg) shortening
- Acromelia: Relative shortening of bones of hands/feet
- Micromelia: Generalized shortening

Helpful Clues for Diagnoses

- **Achondroplasia**
  - Rhizomelic long bone shortening
  - Limbs: Short, thick tubular bones with flared metaphyses
  - Pelvis: Rounded ilia, horizontal acetabula
  - Vertebrae: Posterior scalloping, short pedicles + ↓ interpediculate distance inferiorly
  - **Hypochondroplasia**: Milder variant
- **Pseudoachondroplasia**
  - Vertebrae: Mild platyspondyly (early) → normalize (later)
  - Limbs: Miniepiphyses in hips, hands/feet; irregular carpal/tarsal bones; irregular, splayed metaphyses
- **Thanatophoric Dysplasia**
  - Most common lethal dysplasia
  - Micromelia, severe platyspondyly, short ribs
- **Mesomelic Dysplasias**
  - Group of dysplasias with mesomelic shortening
  - Dyschondrosteosis (most common type): Madelung deformity + variable tibial/fibular shortening
- **Multiple Epiphyseal Dysplasia**
  - Small, irregular epiphyses
- **Osteogenesis Imperfecta**
  - Generalized osteoporosis + fractures → short stature
- **Campomelic Dysplasia**
  - Spine: Hypoplasia, ↓ ossification of cervical vertebrae
  - Thorax: Short ribs & hypoplastic scapulae
  - Limbs: Bowed femurs, hypoplastic tibiae/fibulae
- **Asphyxiating Thoracic Dysplasia (Jeune Syndrome)**
  - Short horizontal ribs, normal spine
  - Limbs: Micromelia; cone-shaped epiphyses in hands; irregular/flared metaphyses
- **Chondrodysplasia Punctata**
  - Rhizomelic type: Rhizomelia + stippled epiphyses
- **Chondroectodermal Dysplasia (Ellis-van Creveld)**
  - Short, heavy tubular bones (including ribs), polydactyly
- **Achondrogenesis**
  - Short tubular & long bones, minimal/absent ossification of vertebral bodies
- **Spondyloepiphyseal Dysplasia**
  - Platyspondyly + abnormal epiphyses
- **Kniest Dysplasia**
  - Progressive bone abnormalities from infancy
  - Vertebrae: Coronal clefts (early) → platyspondyly
  - Limbs: Short, dumbbell-shaped (splayed epiphyses & metaphyses); irregular epiphyses → megaepiphyses
- **Short Rib Polydactyly Syndrome**
  - Vertebrae: Platyspondyly with irregular vertebrae
  - Thorax: Very short ribs
  - Limbs: Micromelia, metaphyseal spurs, polydactyly

Achondroplasia

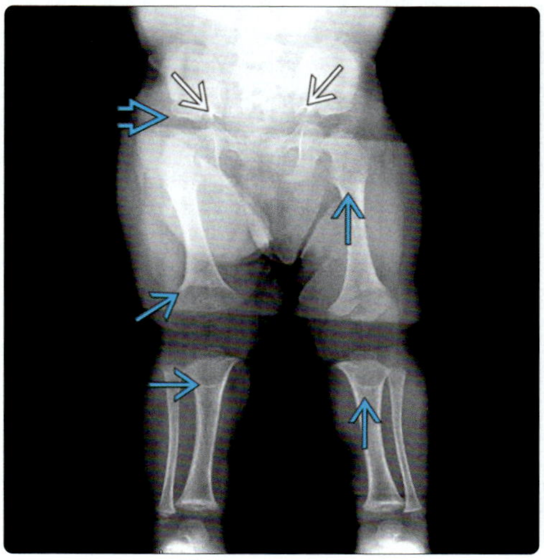

Achondroplasia

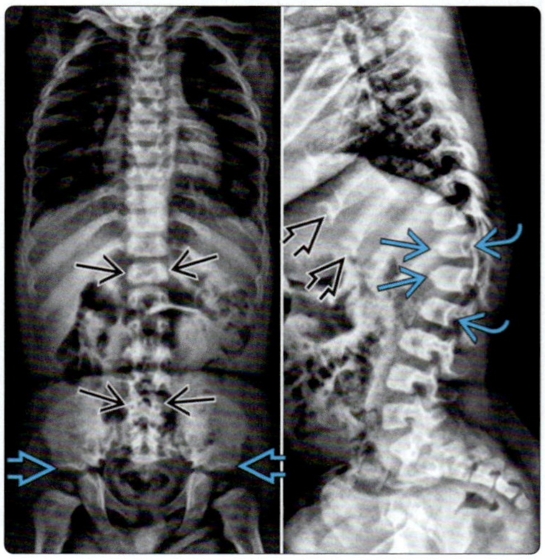

(Left) *Frontal radiograph of the lower extremities in a 2-year-old girl shows flaring of the metaphyses ➔, long bone shortening, small rounded iliac crests, horizontal acetabula ➔, & narrowed sacrosciatic notches ➔.* **(Right)** *Spine radiographs in a 2-year-old boy show central anterior beaking of the vertebral bodies ➔. Note also the posterior vertebral body scalloping ➔, short pedicles, inferior narrowing of the interpedicular distances ➔, flared anterior ribs ➔, squared iliac bones, & horizontal acetabula ➔.*

Thanatophoric Dysplasia

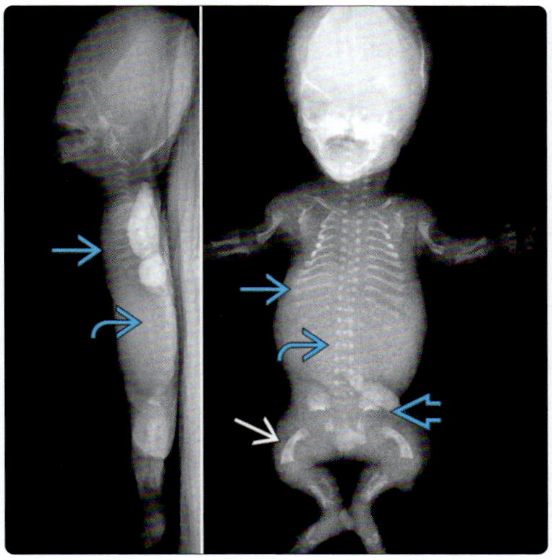

Asphyxiating Thoracic Dysplasia (Jeune Syndrome)

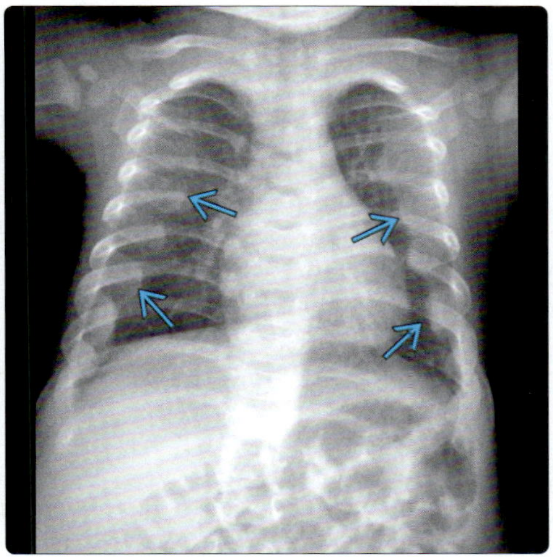

(Left) *Radiographs of a deceased 22-week fetus show multiple characteristic features of type I thanatophoric dysplasia, including very short ribs* →, *platyspondyly* →, *horizontal acetabula* →, *& "French telephone receiver" femurs* →. **(Right)** *Frontal radiograph of the chest in a 6 month old with asphyxiating thoracic dysplasia shows a small, bell-shaped thoracic cage. Note the horizontal orientation of the ribs, which are short with bulbous ends* →.

Chondroectodermal Dysplasia (Ellis-van Creveld)

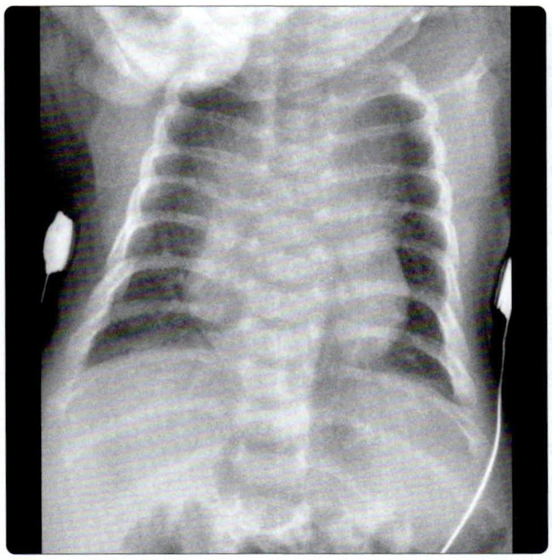

Chondroectodermal Dysplasia (Ellis-van Creveld)

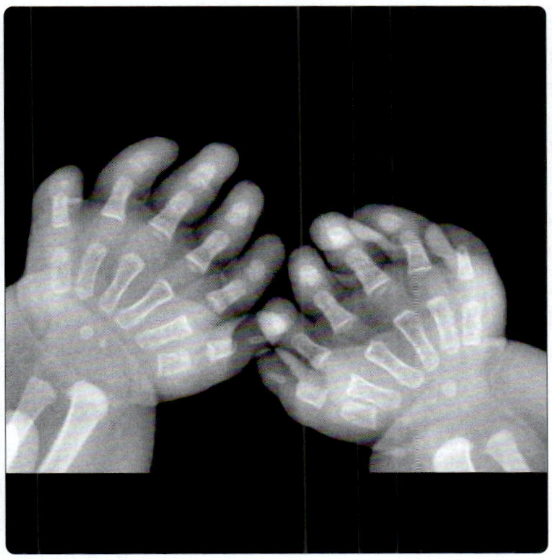

(Left) *Frontal radiograph in a 1 year old with chondroectodermal dysplasia shows short ribs.* **(Right)** *PA hand radiographs in the same child show bilateral postaxial polydactyly with 6 fingers on each hand. Polydactyly (including hands & feet) is usually seen in chondroectodermal dysplasia & can help limit the differential diagnosis in children with short stature & short ribs.*

Spondyloepiphyseal Dysplasia

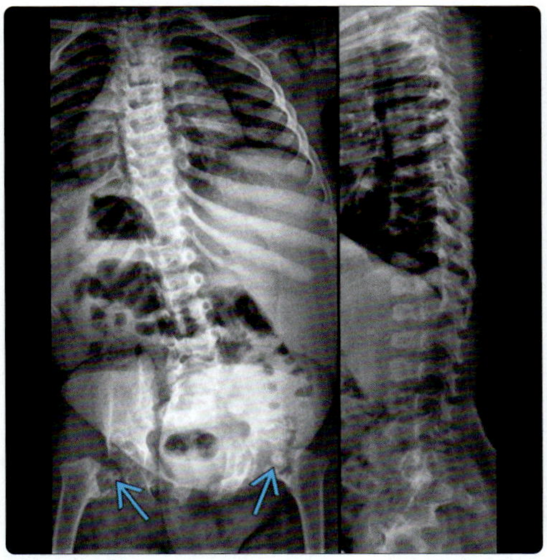

Kniest Dysplasia

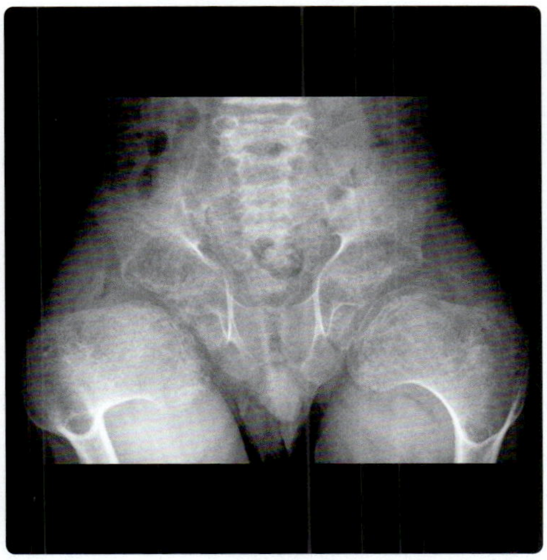

(Left) *Frontal & lateral spine radiographs in a 4-year-old boy with spondyloepiphyseal dysplasia show hypoplastic & markedly irregular femoral heads* → *with bilateral coxa vara deformities. Vertebral abnormalities are also present throughout the spine.* **(Right)** *AP radiograph in a 10-year-old boy with Kniest dysplasia shows severe bilateral coxa magna with overgrowth of the femoral heads & necks. Note the widening & lucency of pelvic bones about each acetabulum.*

DIFFERENTIAL DIAGNOSIS

Common

- Achondroplasia

Less Common

- Pseudoachondroplasia
- Thanatophoric Dysplasia

Rare but Important

- Osteogenesis Imperfecta Type II
- Asphyxiating Thoracic Dysplasia (Jeune Syndrome)
- Hypophosphatasia
- Campomelic Dysplasia
- Achondrogenesis
- Cleidocranial Dysplasia
- Chondroectodermal Dysplasia (Ellis-van Creveld)
- Otopalatodigital Syndrome
- Short Rib-Polydactyly Syndrome

ESSENTIAL INFORMATION

Key Differential Diagnosis Issues

- Severity of rib shortening correlates with degree of pulmonary hypoplasia & survivability

Helpful Clues for Diagnoses

- **Achondroplasia**
  - Short trunk with short, wide ribs
  - Short, thick tubular bones with flared metaphyses
  - Classic vertebral findings include
    - Bullet-shaped or "beaked" vertebral bodies
    - Posterior vertebral body scalloping
    - Narrowed lumbar interpediculate distances
    - Short pedicles
    - Accentuated lumbosacral lordosis
    - Craniocervical junction stenosis
- **Pseudoachondroplasia**
  - Short limbs & short trunk
  - Splayed, fragmented, irregular metaphyses
  - Normal vertebrae at birth → diffuse platyspondyly by 2-4 years
- **Thanatophoric Dysplasia**
  - Most common lethal bone dysplasia (1:10,000 births)
  - Short ribs with cupped costochondral junctions
  - Long trunk with narrow chest
  - Platyspondyly
  - "French telephone receiver" femurs
- **Osteogenesis Imperfecta Type II**
  - Multiple in utero/perinatal fractures
  - Short, poorly mineralized "crumpled" bones with short "beaded" ribs
- **Asphyxiating Thoracic Dysplasia (Jeune Syndrome)**
  - Small, bell-shaped thoracic cage
  - Horizontal, short ribs with bulbous ends
  - Normal spine
- **Hypophosphatasia**
  - Poor, irregular ossification of skeleton
- **Campomelic Dysplasia**
  - Bell-shaped thorax
  - 11 pairs of shortened ribs
  - Hypoplastic cervical vertebrae & scapulae
- **Achondrogenesis**
  - Short tubular & long bones
  - Minimal (if any) mineralization of vertebral bodies
- **Cleidocranial Dysplasia**
  - Cone-shaped chest with mildly shortened, downward-sloping ribs
  - Hypoplastic or absent clavicles
  - Hypoplastic central portions of pubic rami
- **Chondroectodermal Dysplasia (Ellis-van Creveld)**
  - Short, heavy tubular bones (including ribs)
  - Polydactyly
- **Otopalatodigital Syndrome**
  - Ribs are short, wavy, & angled
  - Long bones show increased density & bowing
- **Short Rib-Polydactyly Syndrome**
  - Extremely short, horizontal ribs
  - Polydactyly

Achondroplasia

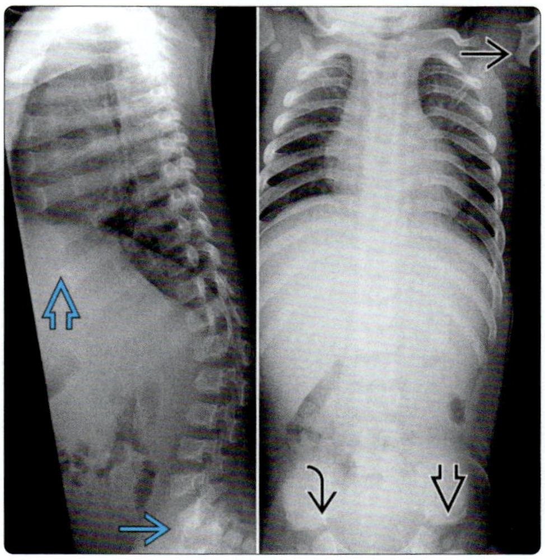

Thanatophoric Dysplasia

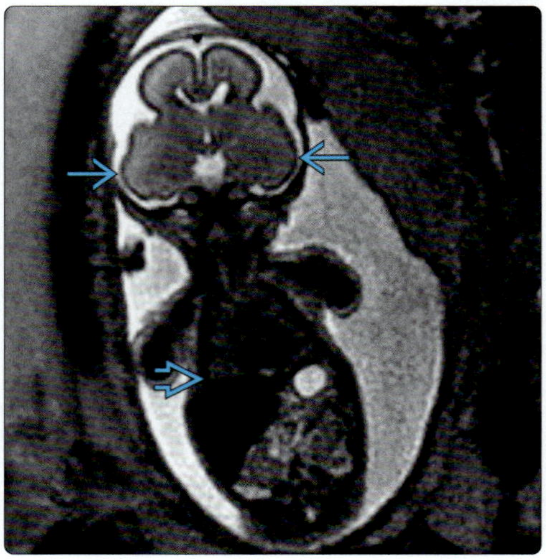

(Left) *Radiographs in a 16 month old with achondroplasia show numerous typical features, including mildly shortened flared ribs ⇒, lumbosacral lordosis →, flared metaphyses →, horizontal acetabula ⇒, & narrowed sacrosciatic notches ⇒.* **(Right)** *Coronal SSFSE T2 MR of a 23-week fetus with short limbs shows a small chest ⇒ (with lung volumes confirming hypoplasia). Note the overgrowth & abnormal sulcation of the temporal lobes →, a finding most commonly reported in thanatophoric dysplasia.*

Thanatophoric Dysplasia

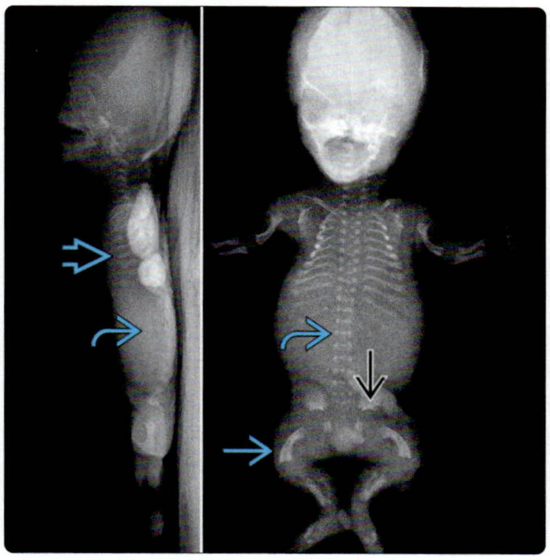

Osteogenesis Imperfecta Type II

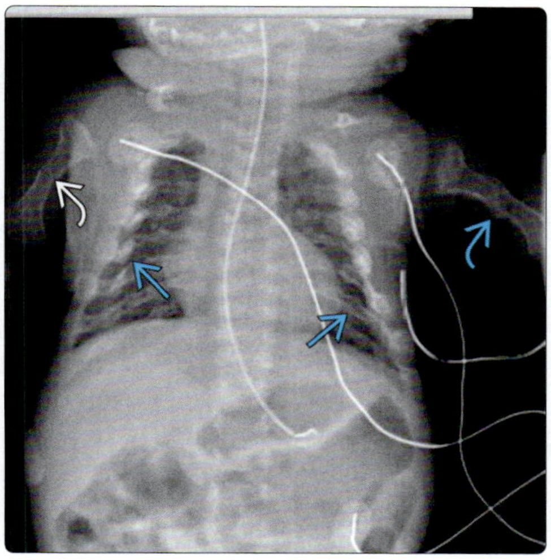

(Left) *Radiographs of a deceased 22-week fetus show multiple characteristic features of thanatophoric dysplasia, including very short ribs, platyspondyly, flat acetabula, & "French telephone receiver" femurs.* **(Right)** *Frontal radiograph of the chest in a newborn with osteogenesis imperfecta type II shows a narrow thorax & a beaded appearance of the ribs from multiple in utero/perinatal fractures. There is also an acute fracture of the right humerus & a healing fracture of the left humerus.*

Asphyxiating Thoracic Dysplasia (Jeune Syndrome)

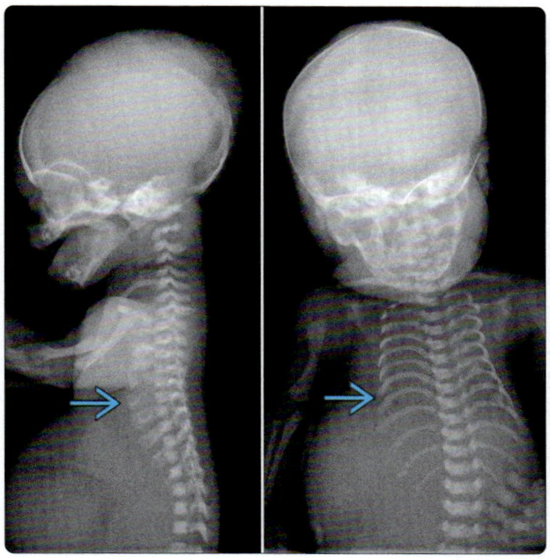

Achondrogenesis

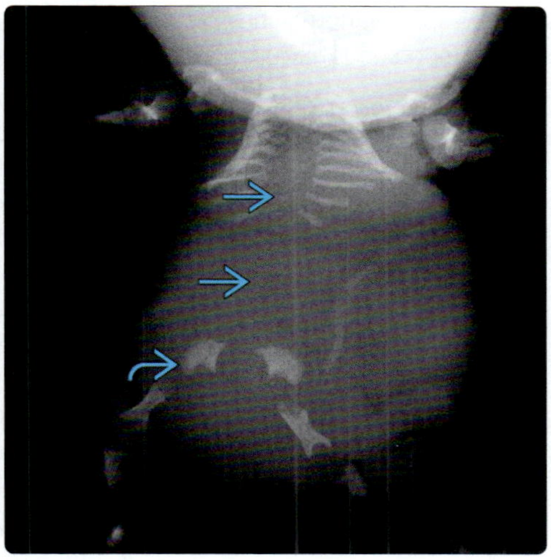

(Left) *Radiographs in a stillborn 35-week fetus show typical findings of Jeune syndrome, including very short horizontal ribs with bulbous ends, short long bones, & a normal spine.* **(Right)** *AP radiograph in a deceased 31-week fetus shows very short ribs & long bones, deformed iliac bones, & characteristic near-complete absence of vertebral body ossification.*

Chondroectodermal Dysplasia (Ellis-van Creveld)

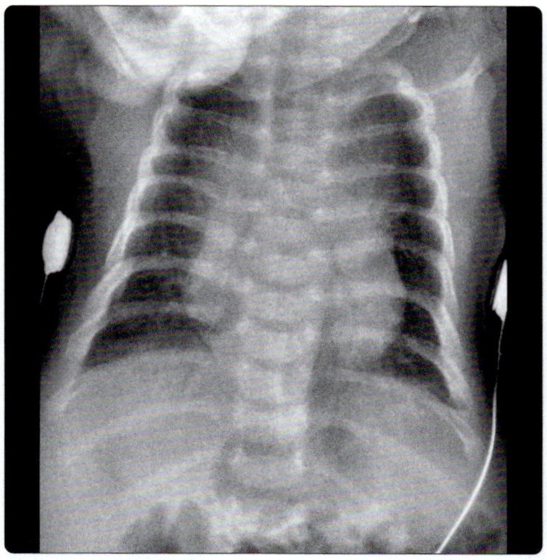

Chondroectodermal Dysplasia (Ellis-van Creveld)

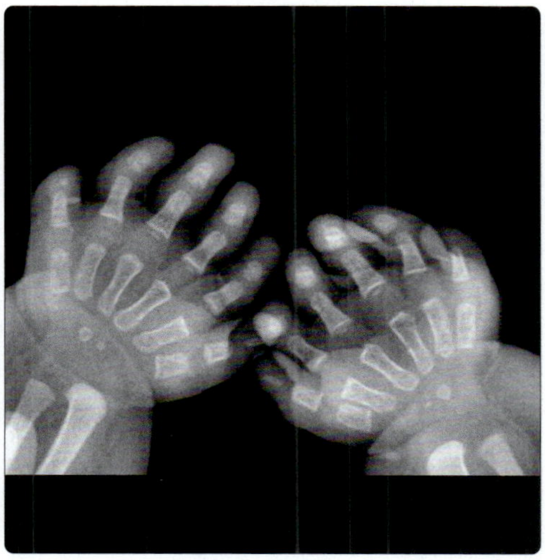

(Left) *AP radiograph in a 1 year old with chondroectodermal dysplasia shows mildly short ribs.* **(Right)** *PA hand radiographs in the same child show bilateral postaxial polydactyly with 6 fingers. Polydactyly is usually seen in chondroectodermal dysplasia (also at the feet) & can help limit the differential diagnosis in children with nonlethal skeletal dysplasias that include short ribs.*

Skeletal Dysplasia With Major Spine Involvement

DIFFERENTIAL DIAGNOSIS

Common

- Achondroplasia
- Pseudoachondroplasia
- Thanatophoric Dysplasia

Less Common

- Spondyloepiphyseal Dysplasia
- Osteogenesis Imperfecta
- Mucopolysaccharidoses

Rare but Important

- Achondrogenesis
- Campomelic Dysplasia
- Short Rib Polydactyly Syndrome Type I
- Diastrophic Dysplasia
- Metatropic Dysplasia

ESSENTIAL INFORMATION

Key Differential Diagnosis Issues

- Many disorders have short stature & spine abnormalities
- Vertebral shape + other osseous & nonosseous features help limit differential

Helpful Clues for Diagnoses

- **Achondroplasia**
  - Most common nonlethal skeletal dysplasia
  - Bullet-shaped vertebral bodies with posterior scalloping & short pedicles
  - Decreasing interpediculate distances from L1 → L5
  - Accentuated lumbosacral lordosis
  - Craniocervical junction stenosis
  - Numerous other characteristic skeletal findings
- **Pseudoachondroplasia**
  - Mild platyspondyly + anterior tongue seen by 2-4 years
  - Vertebrae normalize later
- **Thanatophoric Dysplasia**
  - Most common lethal skeletal dysplasia
  - Severe platyspondyly
  - Long narrow trunk with severely shortened ribs
  - "French telephone receiver" femurs
- **Spondyloepiphyseal Dysplasia**
  - Ovoid or pear-shaped vertebrae in infancy
  - Central, anterior vertebral body beak
  - Odontoid hypoplasia
  - Delayed ossification of epiphyses, ultimately appearing irregular or hypoplastic
- **Osteogenesis Imperfecta**
  - Generalized osteoporosis + fractures → short stature
  - Spine: Kyphoscoliosis, biconcave or flattened vertebral bodies (platyspondyly), compression fractures
- **Mucopolysaccharidoses**
  - Heterogeneous group of lysosomal storage diseases
  - Variable platyspondyly + anterior vertebral beaking
    - Morquio: Central, anterior beak with hypoplastic dens
    - Hurler/Hunter: Anteroinferior beak
- **Achondrogenesis**
  - Short ribs, short limbs
  - Absent or minimal vertebral body ossification diffusely
- **Campomelic Dysplasia**
  - Hypoplastic cervical vertebrae
  - Nonossified thoracic pedicles
  - Hypoplastic scapulae
- **Short Rib Polydactyly Syndrome Type I**
  - Very short ribs
  - Diffuse platyspondyly with irregular vertebrae
  - Spiked distal femurs
- **Diastrophic Dysplasia**
  - Cervical kyphosis, scoliosis, ± narrowed spinal canal
  - "Hitchhiker thumb"
- **Kniest Dysplasia**
  - Platyspondyly with narrow interpediculate distance
  - Coronal vertebral body clefts in infants
  - Dumbbell femurs
  - Epiphyses are small/dysplastic early, enlarged late
- **Metatropic Dysplasia**
  - Severe platyspondyly at birth

Achondroplasia

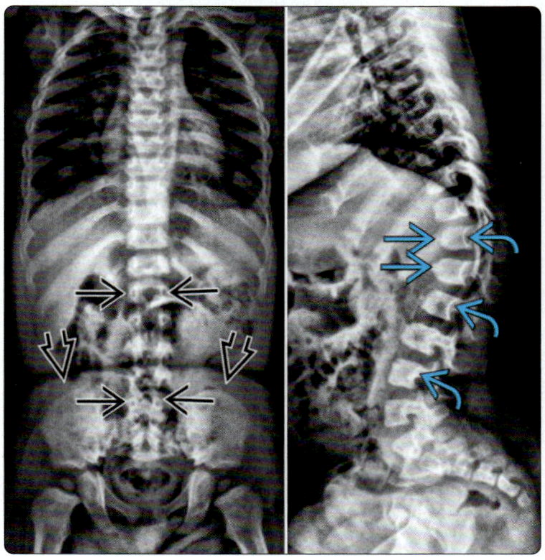

Pseudoachondroplasia

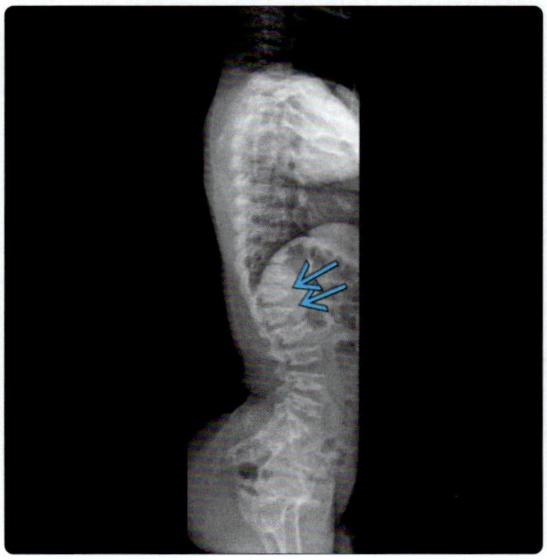

(Left) *Frontal & lateral radiographs in a 2 year old with achondroplasia show central anterior vertebral body beaking ➔. Other characteristic findings include posterior vertebral body scalloping ➔, short pedicles, inferior narrowing of the interpedicular distances ➔, flared anterior ribs, squared iliac bones ➔, & horizontal acetabula.* **(Right)** *Lateral radiograph in a 17-year-old boy with pseudoachondroplasia shows mild platyspondyly & anterior vertebral body beaking ➔.*

Thanatophoric Dysplasia

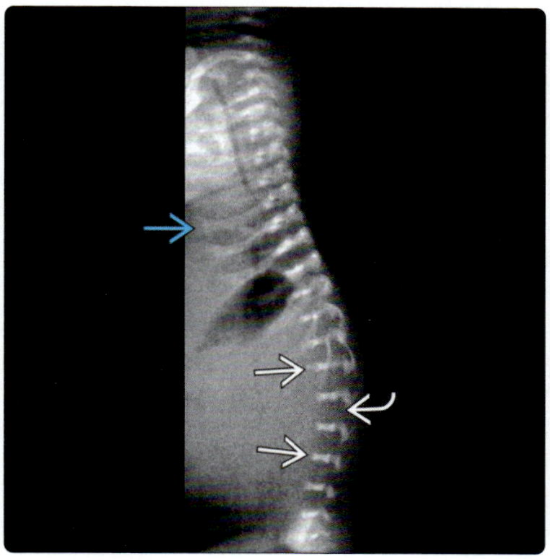

Spondyloepiphyseal Dysplasia

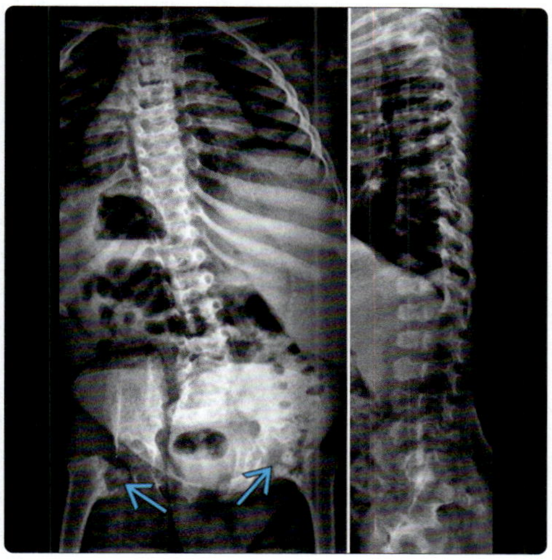

(Left) *Lateral radiograph shows classic platyspondyly → with widened intervertebral disk spaces →. Thus, the normal truncal length is maintained despite the flat vertebral bodies. Note the severely shortened ribs →. This is a lethal dysplasia.* **(Right)** *Frontal & lateral radiographs in a 4 year old with SED show hypoplastic & irregular femoral heads → with bilateral coxa vara deformities. Vertebral abnormalities (with irregularity & mild platyspondyly) are also present throughout.*

Osteogenesis Imperfecta

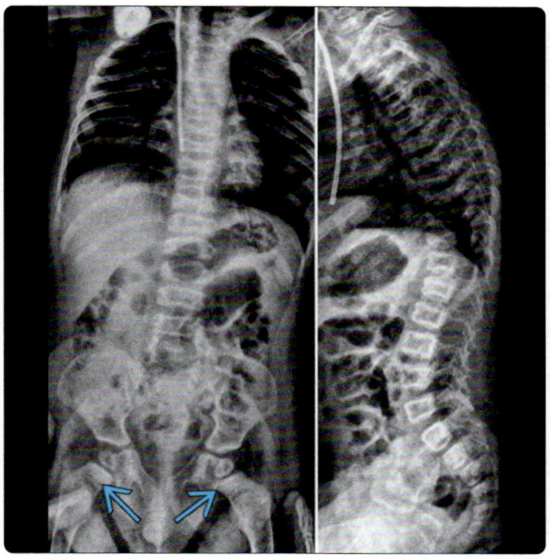

Mucopolysaccharidoses

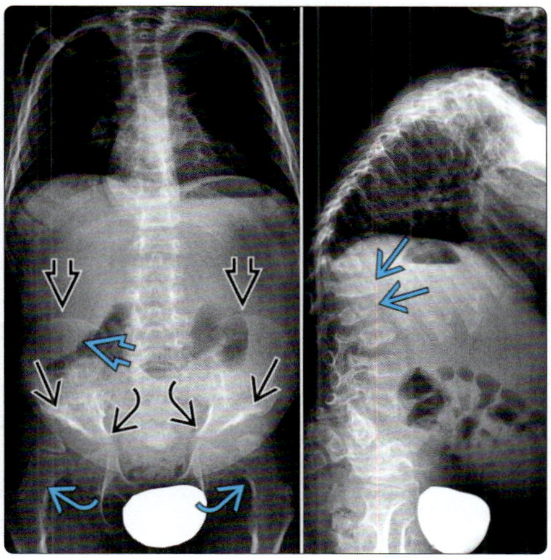

(Left) *Frontal & lateral radiographs in a 1 year old with OI show height loss of multiple thoracic vertebral bodies from compression fractures. Also note the sclerotic metaphyseal bands → paralleling growth plates from bisphosphonate treatments.* **(Right)** *AP & lateral radiographs in a 6 year old with MPS type IV show thoracolumbar kyphosis, small irregular vertebrae, beaked vertebrae →, broad ribs, hepatomegaly →, coxa valga →, dysplastic acetabula →, & rounded iliac wings → with inferiorly tapered ilia →.*

Mucopolysaccharidoses

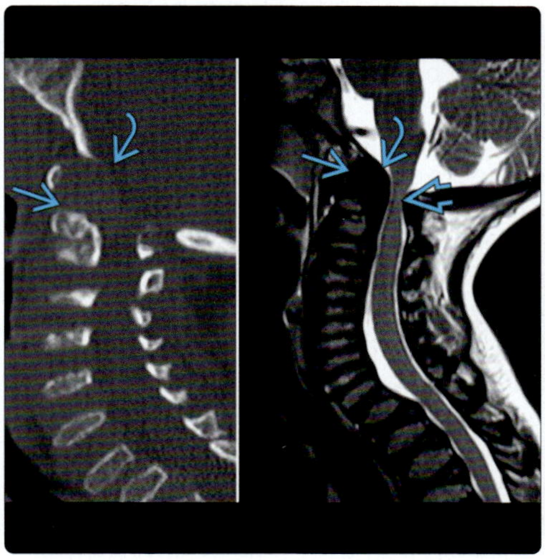

Achondrogenesis

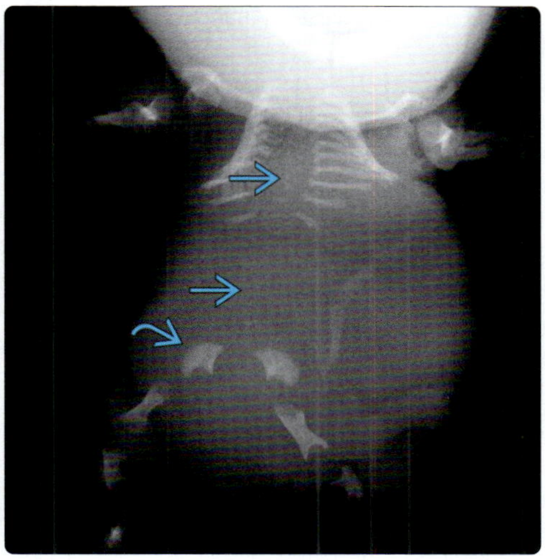

(Left) *Sagittal cervical spine CT (left) & T2 MR (right) in the same patient show a hypoplastic odontoid → with ligamentous infiltration →. There is narrowing of the craniocervical junction → with cord compression.* **(Right)** *AP radiograph in a deceased 31-week fetus shows very short ribs & long bones, deformed iliac bones →, & characteristic near-complete absence of vertebral body ossification → due to achondrogenesis.*

DIFFERENTIAL DIAGNOSIS

Common

- Isolated Vascular Malformations
  - Venous Malformation
  - Lymphatic Malformation
  - Arteriovenous Malformation
- Neurofibromatosis Type I

Less Common

- Hyperemia
  - Juvenile Idiopathic Arthritis
  - Hemophilia
  - Fracture
  - Infection
- Beckwith-Wiedemann Syndrome
- Klippel-Trenaunay Syndrome
- Fibrous Dysplasia
- Enchondromatosis

Rare but Important

- PTEN Hamartoma Tumor Syndrome
- Parkes-Weber Syndrome
- CLOVES Syndrome
- Proteus Syndrome
- Macrodystrophia Lipomatosa

ESSENTIAL INFORMATION

Key Differential Diagnosis Issues

- Identify tissue(s) involved: Fat, muscle, bone, vessels
- Vascular malformations
  - May cause enlargement of focally involved area
  - Several syndromes have extensive vascular malformations + limb overgrowth; some have ↑ risk of other tumors
- Hyperemia from any cause in developing joint can lead to osseous overgrowth

Helpful Clues for Common Diagnoses

- **Isolated Vascular Malformations**
  - Congenital soft tissue masses of abnormal vessels that grow commensurate with patient
    - May rapidly enlarge with trauma, infection, or hormonal stimulation
    - Characteristic cutaneous stigmata may be present
    - Can be focal or quite extensive & infiltrative
  - **Venous malformation**
    - Low-flow lesion with clusters of abnormal veins
      - Numerous thin septations are present throughout lobulated fluid-signal-intensity lesions; frequently contain fluid-fluid levels due to stagnant blood
      - Shows gradual patchy enhancement
      - Intramuscular components are often oriented with long axis of muscle
      - Phleboliths are common
      - Variable amounts of fatty stroma
      - Often soft & compressible
    - Osseous changes are variable
      - Overgrowth secondary to hyperemia
      - Periosteal new bone, cortical thickening, pressure erosions, intraosseous lesions
  - **Lymphatic malformation**
    - Low-flow lesion with numerous cystic spaces of abnormal lymphatics
      - Macrocysts (> 1 cm): Thin, enhancing septations & variable amounts of debris (± fluid-fluid levels); no central enhancement
      - Microcysts (< 1 cm): Can be more solid-appearing
    - Frequently involve face, neck, chest wall, mediastinum, & axilla
    - Localized osseous involvement is uncommon; multifocal bone involvement is seen in systemic forms
  - **Arteriovenous malformation**
    - High-flow lesion with enlarged arteries & veins
      - Variably sized clusters/tangles of flow voids on MR
      - Variable amounts of abnormal soft tissue in mass
    - Intraosseous extension may be seen
- **Neurofibromatosis Type I**
  - Overgrowth is mainly from plexiform neurofibromas
    - Lobulated lesions show target sign in cross section on T2 MR with ↑ peripheral & ↓ central signal intensity
    - Can be quite extensive & infiltrative
    - May be bilateral but are often asymmetric
    - Involved digits may not be contiguous
  - Cutaneous changes: Café au lait spots, axillary & inguinal freckling
  - Other disease manifestations
    - Mesodermal dysplasia: Bowing & pseudoarthrosis of tibia, subperiosteal hemorrhage
    - Optic glioma, Lisch nodule (iris nevi)

Helpful Clues for Less Common Diagnoses

- **Hyperemia**
  - In skeletally immature patients, prolonged joint hyperemia may lead to overgrowth of epiphysis
    - Classic differential: Juvenile idiopathic arthritis (JIA) & hemophilia
      - Knee: Enlarged epiphyses, wide intercondylar notch
      - ± erosions, cartilage loss, osteoarthrosis, & ankylosis
      - Intrarticular hemarthrosis in hemophilia, venous malformation, or pigmented villonodular synovitis will show blooming of susceptibility artifact on T2* GRE MR
    - Earlier diagnosis & improved treatments prevent these classic late changes in JIA & hemophilia
  - Any cause of chronic hyperemia may lead to overgrowth
    - Fracture: Epiphyseal or metaphyseal fractures → hyperemia → overgrowth
      - Healing between separated fragments may also lead to chronic enlargement
      - Fractures may lead to shortening by physeal bridge
    - Infection: Osteomyelitis &/or septic arthritis
      - Osteomyelitis is often periphyseal with hyperemia
      - Septic arthritis: Especially if chronic/indolent; look for cartilage loss, erosions
  - Note that hyperemia can lead to premature growth plate closure → shortening
- **Beckwith-Wiedemann Syndrome**
  - Macrosomia, hemihyperplasia, macroglossia; ± ventral wall defects & neonatal hypoglycemia

- Tumor predisposition: Wilms, hepatoblastoma, others
- Hemihyperplasia or hemihypertrophy also occurs with other congenital syndromes
- **Klippel-Trenaunay Syndrome**
  - Affected limb (≥ 2 present for phenotypic diagnosis)
    - Capillary malformations (port-wine stain)
    - Venous &/or lymphatic malformations
    - Bone &/or soft tissue overgrowth
  - Overgrowth ranges from macrodactyly to hemihypertrophy; lower extremity > upper extremity
  - Large lateral embryonic/primitive vein(s); hypoplastic deep venous system
  - No high-flow vascular anomaly
- **Fibrous Dysplasia**
  - Monostotic vs. polyostotic process
    - Multifocal lesions are often unilateral in extremities
    - Common involvement of facial bones & skull base
  - May be bubbly or sclerotic; classic lesion shows ground-glass matrix ("frosted glass" or "smudged glass")
  - Frequently expansile ± characteristic deformities of specific bones (e.g., "shepherd's crook" femur)
- **Enchondromatosis**
  - Typical medullary lesions +
    - Intracortical & periosteal (juxtacortical) chondromas, which may mimic osteochondromas
    - Linear metaphyseal/diaphyseal columns of cartilage extending from physes
  - Ollier disease: Multiple enchondromas, often unilateral
  - Maffucci syndrome: Multiple enchondromas (often very expansile) + soft tissue slow-flow vascular anomalies
    - Phleboliths in soft tissues due to venous malformation-like spindle cell hemangiomas
    - Predisposition to numerous malignancies

Helpful Clues for Rare Diagnoses

- **PTEN Hamartoma Tumor Syndromes**
  - Include: Cowden & Bannayan-Riley-Ruvalcaba syndromes
  - Various soft tissue hamartomatous growths, often containing fat, myxoid tissue, & vessels
  - May have high- or low-flow lesions
  - Frequently have macrocephaly & penile freckling
- **Parkes-Weber Syndrome**
  - Affected limb shows
    - Overgrowth of soft tissue &/or bone
    - Capillary malformations (port-wine stain)
    - Mix of low- & high-flow lesions
      - Has arteriovenous malformations (AVMs)/arteriovenous fistulas, which can lead to ulcerations or high-output cardiac failure
- **CLOVES Syndrome**
  - **C**ongenital **l**ipomatous **o**vergrowth, **v**ascular anomalies, **e**pidermal nevi, **s**coliosis/skeletal/spinal anomalies
  - Thoracic/trunk lipomatous overgrowth
  - Lymphatic, venous, & capillary malformations ± AVMs
    - High-flow spinal/paraspinal malformations may lead to myelopathy
  - Linear epidermal nevi
  - ↑ incidence of Wilms tumor
- **Proteus Syndrome**
  - Normal at birth but develop severe deformities
  - Craniofacial dysmorphism
  - Asymmetric soft tissue/fatty limb overgrowth
  - Epidermal lesions/nevi
  - Abnormal CNS development &/or intellectual disability
  - Vascular anomalies (low flow)
- **Macrodystrophia Lipomatosa**
  - Unilateral; 1 or more contiguous digits
    - 2nd & 3rd digits most common
    - Most severe involvement along distal digit
    - Volar surface > dorsal surface, creating dorsal bowing
  - Overgrowth of soft tissue (especially fat) & bone
  - Neural enlargement

SELECTED REFERENCES

1. Bertino F et al: Congenital limb overgrowth syndromes associated with vascular anomalies. Radiographics. 39(2):491-515, 2019
2. Edmondson AC et al: Overgrowth syndromes. J Pediatr Genet. 4(3):136-43, 2015

Venous Malformation

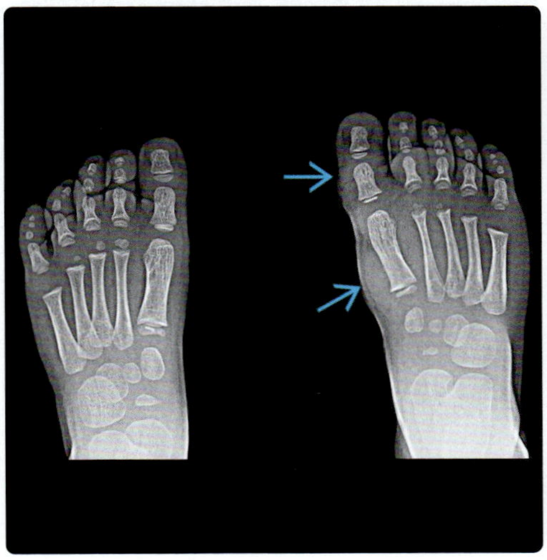

Venous Malformation

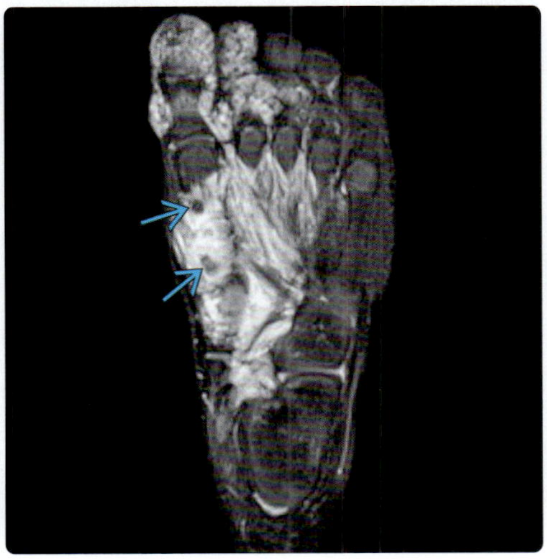

(Left) *AP radiographs in a 2-year-old girl with left foot enlargement show medial soft tissue swelling ➔ as compared to the normal contralateral foot. The bones appear normal.* **(Right)** *Long-axis STIR MR of the left foot in the same girl shows an infiltrating high signal intensity lesion in the subcutaneous fat & musculature of the medial foot. The lesion enhanced diffusely (not shown), except for low-signal-intensity thrombi ➔.*

(Left) *Frontal DSA of the hand in a 9 year old with chronic swelling & pain of the middle finger shows a tangle of abnormal arteries & veins in the affected digit. Note the early venous visualization secondary to shunting.* **(Right)** *Coronal STIR MR of a 15-year-old girl with neurofibromatosis type 1 (NF1) shows extensive plexiform neurofibromas (PNs) with massive disfiguring enlargement of both thighs, left > right. The right femoral head is noted for orientation.*

Arteriovenous Malformation

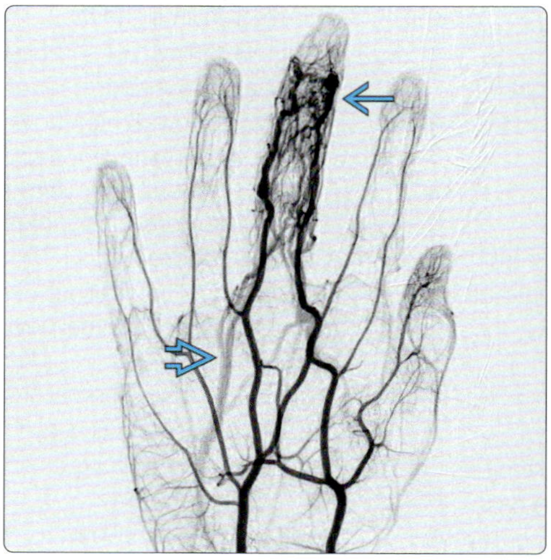

Neurofibromatosis Type I

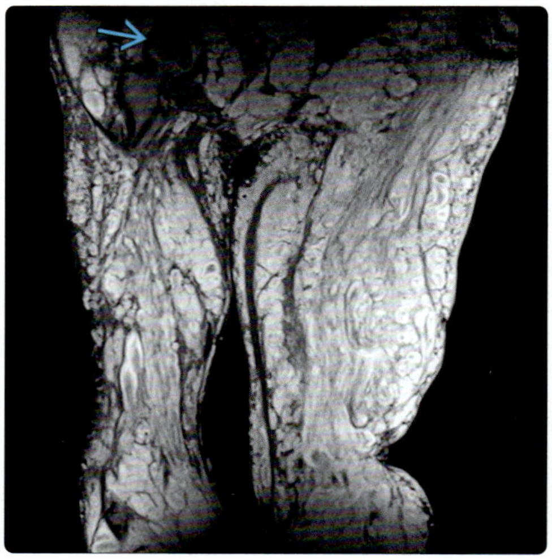

(Left) *Axial T2 FS MR image in the same girl with NF1 shows extensive PNs throughout both thighs. The lobulated, infiltrative masses are predominantly high in signal intensity with many showing a target sign of low signal intensity centrally, classic for PNs.* **(Right)** *AP radiograph in an 8-year-old boy with prior left femoral pyogenic osteomyelitis shows residual heterogeneity of the distal left femoral metaphysis. This child ultimately had a 2-cm leg length discrepancy from left femoral overgrowth (note the pelvic tilt).*

Neurofibromatosis Type I

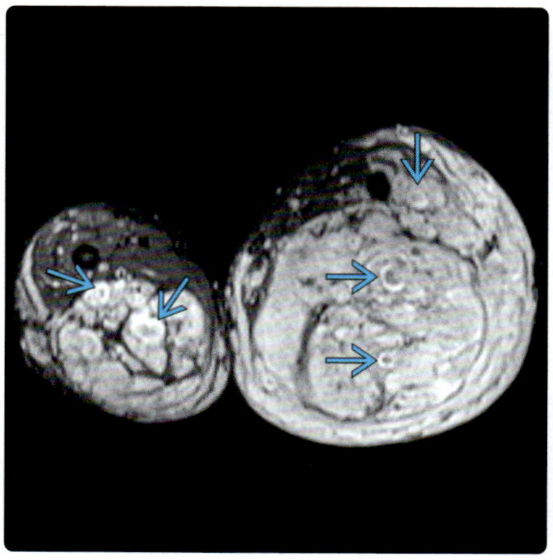

Hyperemia

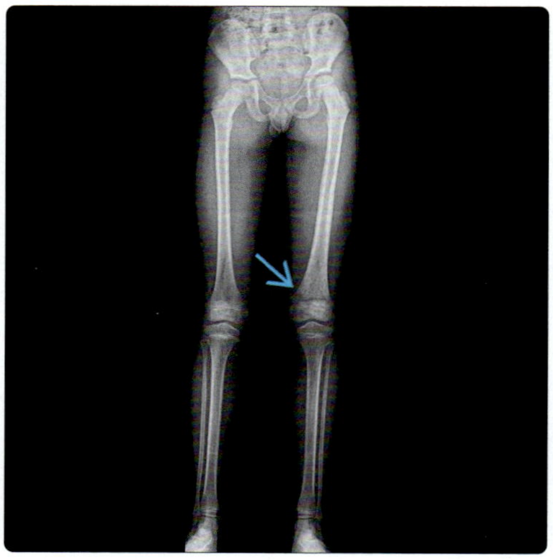

(Left) *AP radiograph in a 1 year old with Klippel-Trenaunay syndrome shows marked enlargement of the right lower extremity. The overgrowth is predominantly of the soft tissues, but there is overgrowth of the right femur & tibia as well. The lack of pelvic tilt is due to a 2-cm lift under the left foot.* **(Right)** *Coronal STIR MR in the same girl shows diffuse infiltration of the subcutaneous fat of the right lower extremity by high-signal-intensity lesions of a mixed venous & lymphatic malformation.*

Klippel-Trenaunay Syndrome

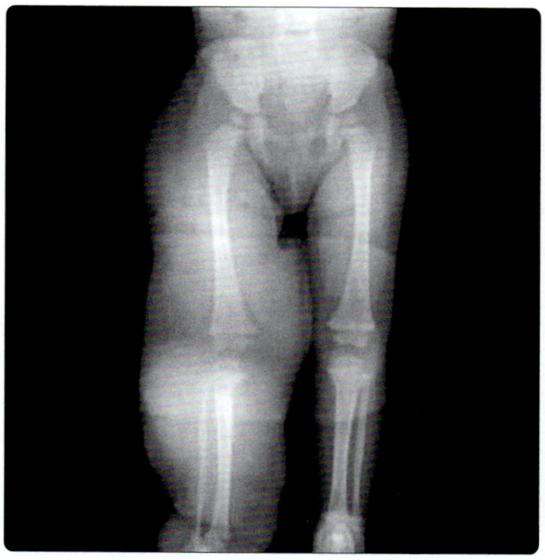

Klippel-Trenaunay Syndrome

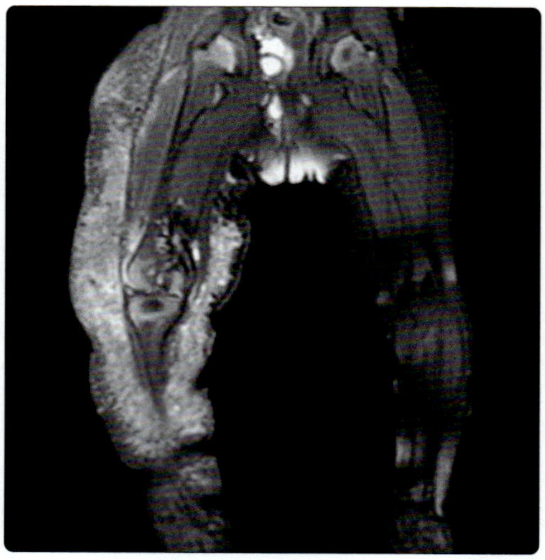

Fibrous Dysplasia

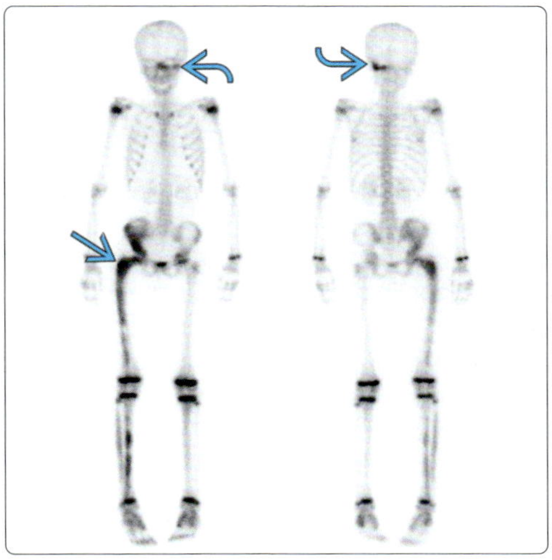

Fibrous Dysplasia

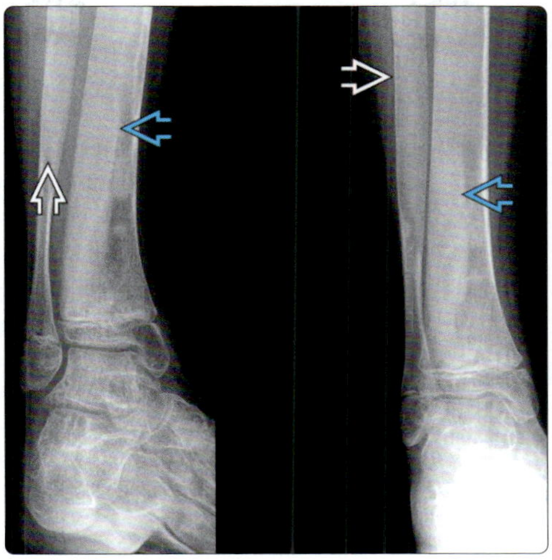

(Left) *Anterior & posterior nuclear medicine bone scans show patchy foci of increased radiotracer uptake throughout the right lower extremity & the left skull base ➡. Note the "shepherd's crook" deformity of the right femur ➡ as well as the limb overgrowth.* **(Right)** *Oblique (left) & AP (right) radiographs of the right ankle in the same patient with polyostotic fibrous dysplasia show characteristic expansile lesions with ground-glass matrix in the tibia ➡ & fibula ➡.*

Enchondromatosis

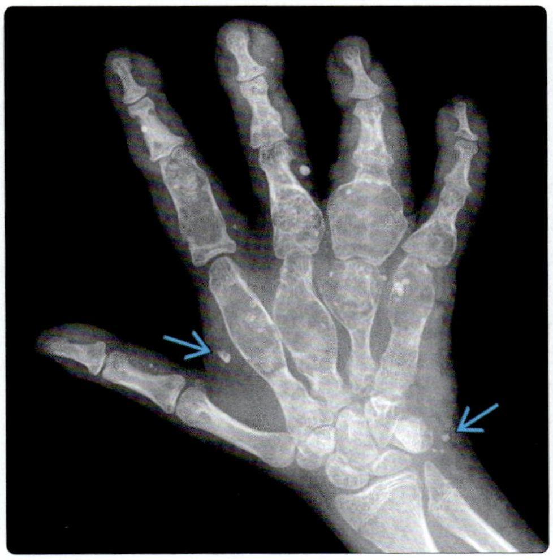

CLOVES Syndrome

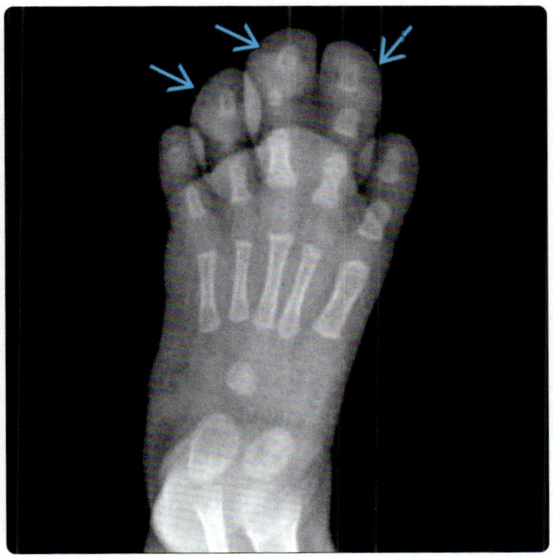

(Left) *PA radiograph of the right hand shows numerous central expansile lucent lesions of the metacarpals & phalanges with endosteal scalloping & chondroid matrix, typical of enchondromas. Soft tissue lobulations & phleboliths ➡ are secondary to venous malformation-like lesions in Maffucci syndrome.* **(Right)** *AP radiograph in a 2 month old with CLOVES syndrome shows soft tissue & osseous overgrowth of the 2nd-4th toes ➡.*

CLOVES Syndrome

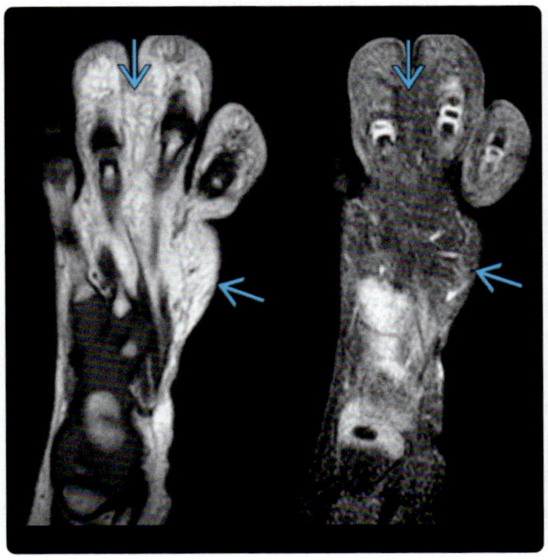

Macrodystrophia Lipomatosa

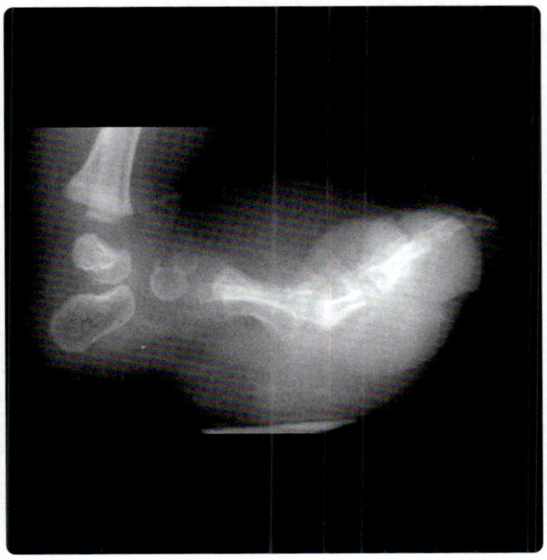

(Left) *Long-axis T1 MR images without (left) & with (right) FS of the right foot in the same child show that the soft tissue overgrowth ➡ follows fat signal intensity on both pulse sequences. This child also had an area of thoracic lipomatous overgrowth with an overlying linear epidermal nevus, characteristic of CLOVES.* **(Right)** *Lateral radiograph shows a normal hindfoot & midfoot with giantism of both the soft tissues & osseous structures of the forefoot in this patient with macrodystrophia lipomatosa.*

DIFFERENTIAL DIAGNOSIS

Common

- Lymphadenopathy
- Abscess
- Dermoid
- Pilomatrixoma
- Ganglion Cyst
- Baker Cyst
- Vascular Malformations
  - Venous Malformation
  - Lymphatic Malformation
  - Arteriovenous Malformation
- Infantile Hemangioma

Less Common

- Hematoma
- Fat Injury
- Granuloma Annulare
- Rhabdomyosarcoma
- Plexiform Neurofibroma
- Muscle Hernia
- Lipoma

Rare but Important

- Synovial Sarcoma
- Myositis Ossificans
- Fibromatosis
- Infantile Myofibroma
- Nodular Fasciitis
- Extraosseous Ewing Sarcoma
- Infantile Fibrosarcoma
- Malignant Peripheral Nerve Sheath Tumor
- Kaposiform Hemangioendothelioma
- Lipoblastoma
- Extrarenal Rhabdoid Tumor

ESSENTIAL INFORMATION

Key Differential Diagnosis Issues

- Critical clinical factors: Patient age, duration & location of lesion, associated symptoms, & firmness on palpation
- Bottom line: Most round to ovoid solid masses will require tissue sampling due to ↑ likelihood of malignancy

Helpful Clues for Common Diagnoses

- **Lymphadenopathy**
  - Locations suggesting lymph nodes: Inguinal, axillary, epitrochlear, posterior auricular, etc.
  - Infectious/inflammatory
    - Reactive: Preserved nodal architecture, ± hyperemia
    - Necrotic: Surrounding cellulitis, heterogeneity with foci of ↓ echogenicity & vascularity
  - Neoplastic: Greater ovoid enlargement of multiple groups with effacement of fatty hilum, variable internal vascularity, no surrounding inflammation
- **Abscess**
  - May originate in nodes vs. myositis/osteomyelitis
  - Irregular enhancing wall, often T2 hypointense
  - Central restricted diffusion with no internal vascularity
  - Swirling internal debris on US with compression
- **Dermoid**
  - Small round to ovoid lesion with no internal vascularity
    - Larger lesions may show mobile internal debris
  - Classically overlies calvarial suture & results in subjacent outer table concavity (i.e., remodeling)
  - May also be seen over spine or sternum
- **Pilomatrixoma**
  - Round, well-circumscribed benign neoplasm of hair follicle in subcutaneous fat
  - Hypoechoic ± internal Ca^{2+}, may show peripheral hyperemia & ↑ echogenicity of surrounding fat
- **Ganglion Cyst**
  - Lobulated homogeneous fluid signal intensity mass ± thin septations & peripheral enhancement
    - Have low threshold for giving contrast on MR as synovial sarcoma can mimic ganglion
  - Communicates with joint space or tendon sheath
- **Baker Cyst**
  - Elongated cyst in popliteal fossa
  - Tail extends between gastrocnemius medial head & semimembranosus toward joint
  - Minimal internal complexity without vascularity
  - Rupture may incite surrounding inflammation
- **Vascular Malformations**
  - Present from birth; grow commensurate with patient but may rapidly enlarge with infection, trauma, or hormonal stimulation; often extend across tissue planes
  - **Venous malformation**: Low flow with slow gradual enhancement; clusters of abnormal T2-hyperintense venous channels; phleboliths are diagnostic in pediatric mass; ± fluid-fluid levels from stagnant blood products
  - **Lymphatic malformation**: Low flow with thin rim enhancement; may be infiltrating & more solid-appearing (microcystic) vs. multiple macrocysts (> 1 cm); ± fluid-fluid levels
  - **Arteriovenous malformation**: High flow; numerous flow voids in mass; variable soft tissue components
- **Infantile Hemangioma**
  - Benign vascular neoplasm; not present at birth, grows rapidly in 1st weeks-months, slowly involutes over years
  - Soft, lobular, ovoid/elongated subcutaneous mass of mixed echogenicity in infant
  - Highly vascular (> 5 vessels/cm^2) on Doppler with low-resistance arterial flow
  - Strawberry-/cherry-red skin discoloration if superficial vs. bluish color in deeper hemangiomas

Helpful Clues for Less Common Diagnoses

- **Hematoma**
  - History of trauma (accidental, nonaccidental, or iatrogenic), anticoagulation, or bleeding disorder
  - Variable internal echogenicity/signal intensity depending on age of blood products; may layer with fluid-fluid levels
- **Fat Injury**
  - Most commonly follows trauma at bony protuberances
  - Classic subacute/chronic appearance of impaction/shear injury (a.k.a. Morel-Lavallée lesion): Elongated collection at junction of subcutaneous fat & fascia with angular margins & internal fat debris
    - More heterogeneous with surrounding edema early
  - May evolve to stellate or linear focus without mass

- **Granuloma Annulare**
  - Painless inflammatory lesion, often self-limited, occurring most commonly from ages 2-5 years
  - Most common in pretibial/infrapatellar locations
  - Poorly defined or mildly nodular subcutaneous mass abutting periosteum or fascia; can be multifocal
  - Variable enhancement & T2 heterogeneity
- **Rhabdomyosarcoma**
  - Most common soft tissue sarcoma in children
  - Often well-circumscribed solid & firm soft tissue mass without surrounding edema
  - Variable internal vascularity but most commonly hypovascular/hypoenhancing; restricts on DWI MR
- **Plexiform Neurofibroma**
  - Occurs in neurofibromatosis type 1 (NF1)
  - Lobulated ↑ T2 signal intensity masses with central low intensity (target sign)
  - Follow courses of nerves; may be extensive
- **Muscle Hernia**
  - Typically small; most common in lower leg
  - Dynamic US is quite helpful → distal flexion/extension (or other maneuver) may show muscle protruding/retracting through defect in echogenic fascia
  - MR may appear normal if hernia is reduced during scan
- **Lipoma**
  - Soft, nearly completely fatty mass; minimal thin septa
  - May simply appear as thickened subcutaneous fat
    - Intramuscular lipomas may appear more complex with interspersed muscle fibers & poor definition

Helpful Clues for Rare Diagnoses

- **Synovial Sarcoma**
  - Typically 15-35 years old
  - Ca^{2+} in ~ 30%; often near joint, rarely in joint
  - Often small & well circumscribed; may appear cystic
- **Myositis Ossificans**
  - Intense muscle edema surrounding heterogeneous mass
  - Peripheral Ca^{2+} develops in weeks; seen on nuclear bone scan, CT, US (& possibly MR) before radiographs
  - Trauma history is often lacking (~ 30-40%)
- **Fibromatosis**
  - Benign but locally aggressive infiltrating mass, often with substantial sheet-like regions of ↓ T2 signal intensity
- **Infantile Myofibroma**
  - Heterogeneous well-circumscribed vs. infiltrating mass; ± Ca^{2+}, bizarre remodeling of adjacent bone
  - May have rim, heterogeneous, or uniform enhancement
  - ± multifocal relatively symmetric metadiaphyseal lytic bone lesions, visceral lesions
- **Nodular Fasciitis**
  - Benign lesion with rapid growth & intense enhancement, typically along fascial planes
- **Extraosseous Ewing Sarcoma**
  - Typically well-circumscribed solid & firm soft tissue mass without surrounding edema; may be cystic
- **Infantile Fibrosarcoma**
  - Often large solid & cystic mass, may be hypervascular
- **Malignant Peripheral Nerve Sheath Tumor**
  - Consider malignant degeneration of plexiform neurofibroma (PNF) in NF1 with rapid growth, cystic change, & ↑ SUV on PET
- **Kaposiform Hemangioendothelioma**
  - Most are diagnosed in infants
  - May present as palpable mass &/or consumptive coagulopathy (Kasabach-Merritt phenomenon)
  - Intermediate T2 signal nodules with infiltrative margins & surrounding edema, intense enhancement
- **Lipoblastoma**
  - Benign fatty mass, primarily < 3 years old
  - Heterogeneous mix of fat & myxoid tissue
- **Extrarenal Rhabdoid Tumor**
  - Aggressive malignancy of young children

SELECTED REFERENCES

1. Caro-Domínguez P et al: Imaging appearances of soft-tissue tumors of the pediatric foot: review of a 15-year experience at a tertiary pediatric hospital. Pediatr Radiol. 47(12):1555-71, 2017
2. Johnson CM et al: Clinical and sonographic features of pediatric soft-tissue vascular anomalies part 2: vascular malformations. Pediatr Radiol. 47(9):1196-1208, 2017

Lymphadenopathy

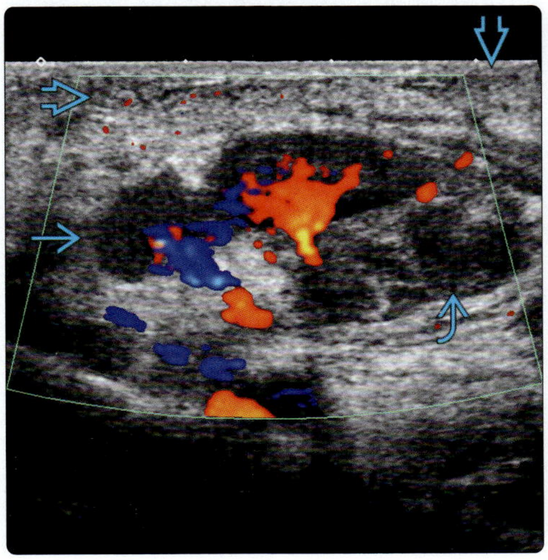

Lymphadenopathy

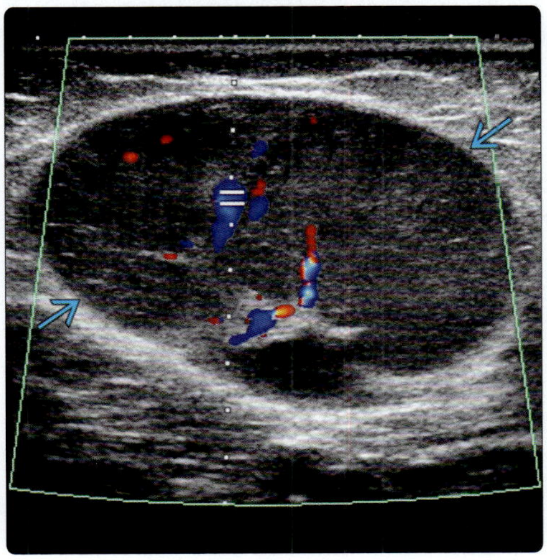

(Left) *Longitudinal color Doppler US in a 2 year old with inguinal swelling shows an enlarged heterogeneous lymph node ➡ with fatty hilum & radiating vessels. Foci of decreased echogenicity & vascularity suggest necrosis ➡. There is overlying fat induration ➡. The findings suggest infectious adenitis & cellulitis.* **(Right)** *Longitudinal color Doppler US shows mass-like enlargement of an inguinal node ➡ in a 13 year old due to lymphoma. The vascularity & fatty hilum are effaced, & the overlying soft tissues are normal.*

(Left) *Longitudinal color Doppler US in a 13 year old with increasing inguinal pain & swelling for 2 months shows a predominantly cystic mass ⇨ with irregular walls & a vascularized peripheral nodule →.* **(Right)** *Sagittal T2 FS (left) & T1 C+ FS (right) MR images in the same patient show a large inguinal fluid collection with enhancing rim & nodule → as well as surrounding edema ↷. The location suggests a nodal abscess, & cat-scratch disease was confirmed by serum titers.*

Abscess

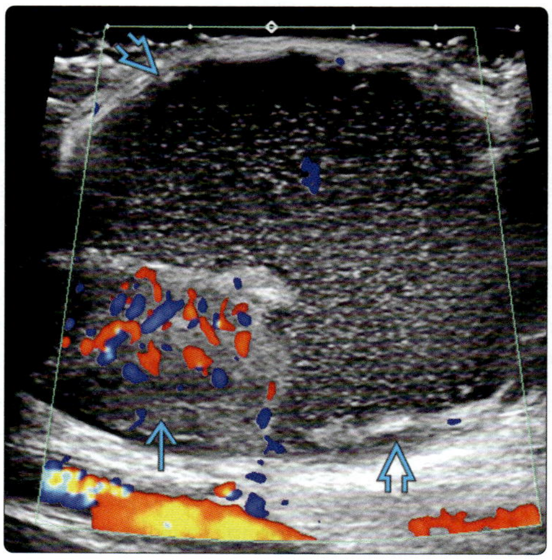

Abscess

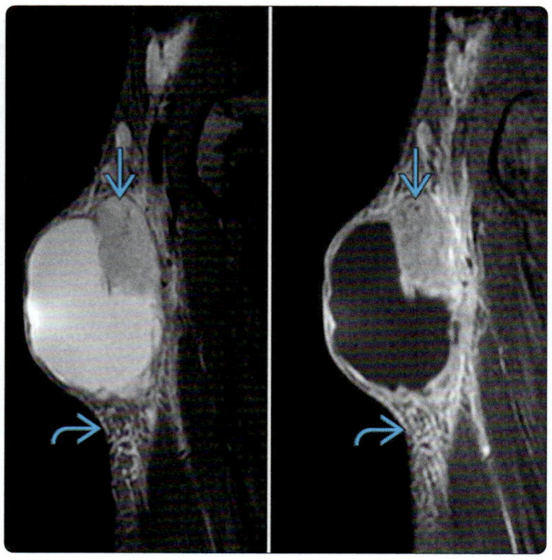

(Left) *Coronal color Doppler US in a 2 month old with a firm scalp nodule shows a 5-mm ovoid hypoechoic mass ⇨ overlying the sagittal suture & superior sagittal sinus →. Dermoids often abut a suture & may remodel the outer calvarium.* **(Right)** *Transverse color Doppler US of the chest wall in a 13 year old with a bump for 1 month shows a round, well-circumscribed, hypoechoic mass in the subcutaneous fat with increased through transmission & peripheral vascularity. Resection confirmed a pilomatrixoma.*

Dermoid

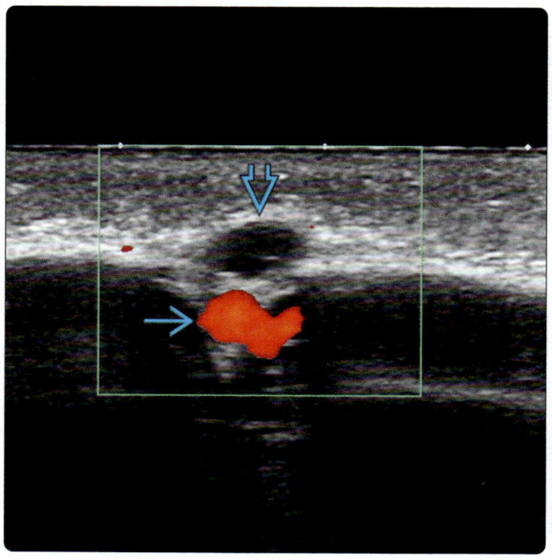

Pilomatrixoma

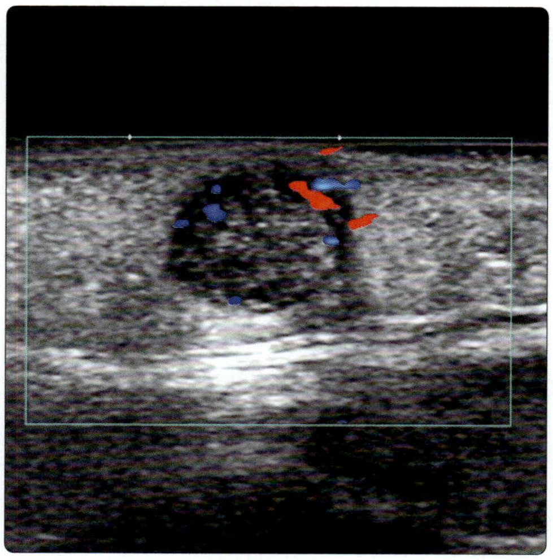

(Left) *Longitudinal US of the lateral knee in an 11 year old with a soft mass shows a lobulated cystic lesion → that measured 4 cm in length & demonstrated no internal vascularity on Doppler (not shown). Note the subjacent fibular head ⇨.* **(Right)** *Coronal T2 FS MR images in the same patient show a lobulated cystic mass with thin septations insinuating along adjacent tendons & ligaments, originating from the tibiofibular articulation ⇨ (which is a common site for a ganglion).*

Ganglion Cyst

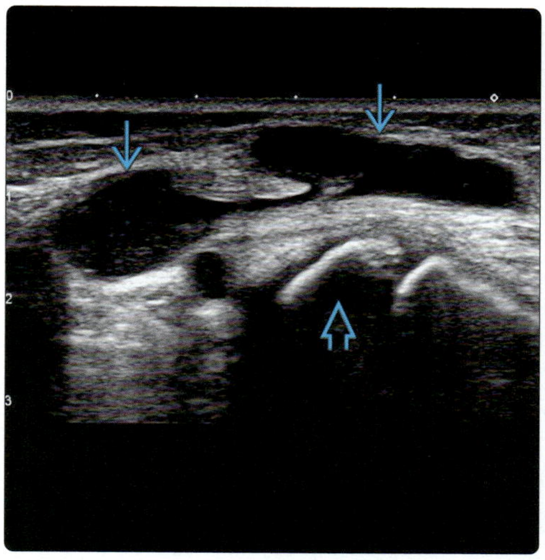

Ganglion Cyst

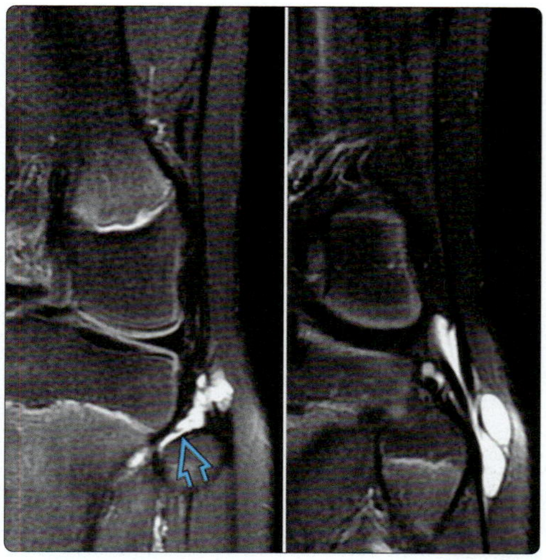

Venous Malformation

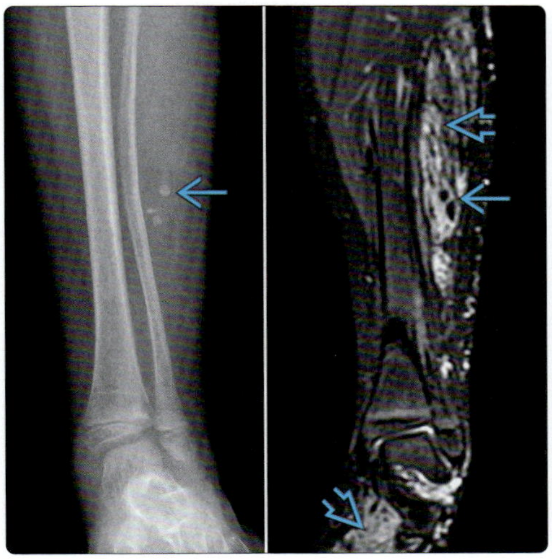

Venous Malformation

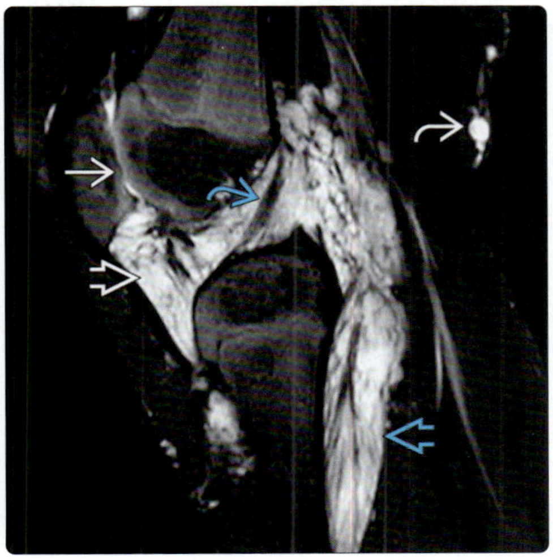

(Left) *Frontal radiographic (left) & coronal STIR MR (right) images show phleboliths* ⇨ *in an extensive lower leg venous malformation* ⇨. **(Right)** *Sagittal T2 FS MR shows intramuscular* ⇨ *& intraarticular* ➡ *venous malformations with discrete superficial aberrant veins* ➡. *The synovial involvement (demonstrated along the ACL* ⇨*) has led to prior hemarthrosis & early cartilage degeneration* ➡.

Lymphatic Malformation

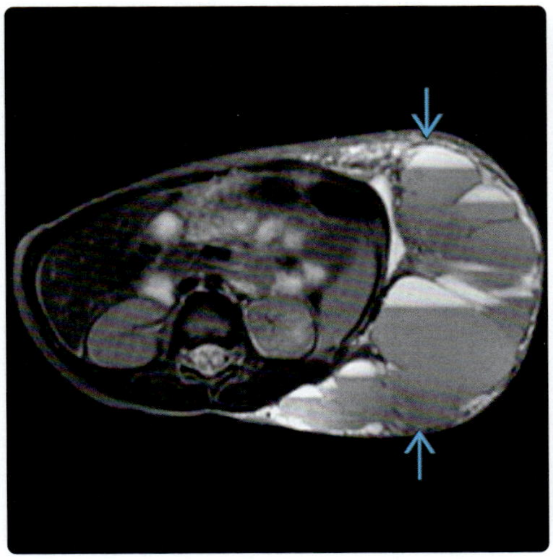

Arteriovenous Malformation

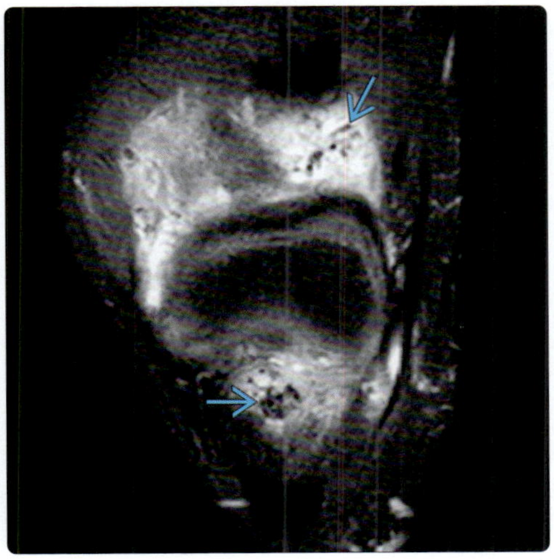

(Left) *Axial T2 FS MR in a 3 year old with a lymphatic malformation of the flank shows numerous thin-walled cysts* ⇨ *containing fluid levels due to internal hemorrhage. The mass had rapidly expanded after minor trauma.* **(Right)** *Coronal T2 FS MR in a 5 year old with a longstanding mass & worsening knee pain shows clusters of small flow voids* ⇨ *(due to high-flow vessels) within an otherwise solid-appearing, poorly defined lesion at the patella.*

Arteriovenous Malformation

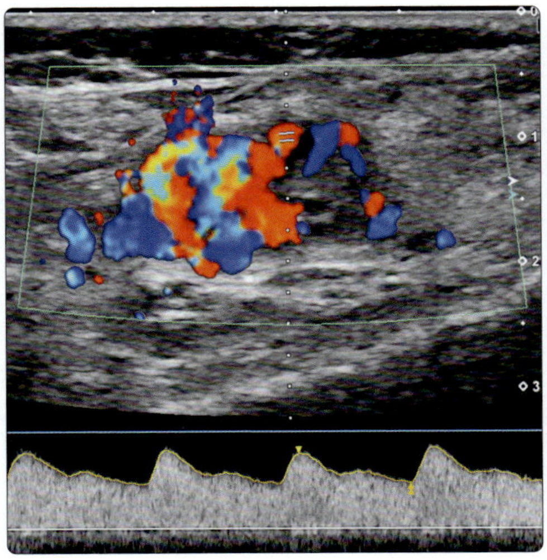

Infantile Hemangioma

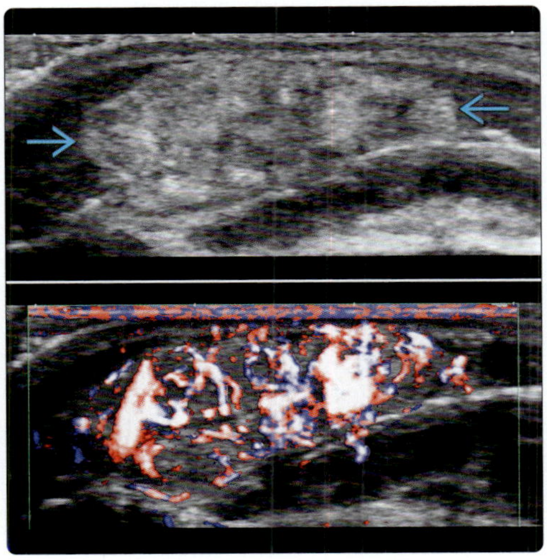

(Left) *Longitudinal spectral Doppler US in the same patient shows abnormally low-resistance arteries within this cluster of vessels, typical of an arteriovenous malformation.* **(Right)** *Transverse grayscale & color Doppler US images in a 1 month old show an ovoid mass* ⇨ *of the subcutaneous fat. The mass is heterogeneously hyperechoic with a high vessel density on Doppler. Spectral tracings showed low-resistance arterial waveforms in much of the mass, consistent with infantile hemangioma.*

(Left) *Axial T2 FS MR in a 16 year old after an injury shows an elongated collection with angular margins in the subcutaneous fat. A small globule of fat is seen in the lesion, which is typical of fat-shearing injuries.* **(Right)** *Sagittal STIR (left) & T1 C+ FS (right) MR images in a 3 year old with a painless mass show a poorly circumscribed heterogeneous lesion of the subcutaneous fat overlying the patellar tendon. The presentation, age, location, & imaging are typical of subcutaneous granuloma annulare.*

Fat Injury

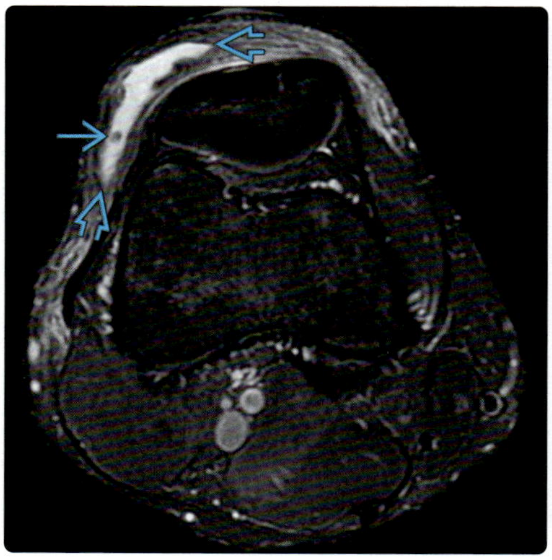

Granuloma Annulare

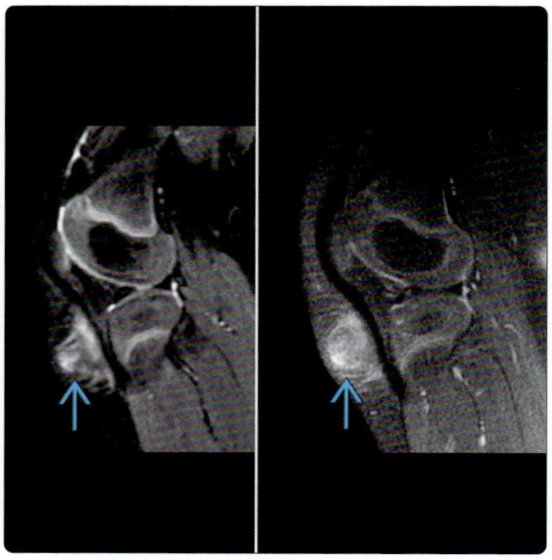

(Left) *Axial (to the foot) T2 FS (left) & T1 C+ FS (right) MR images in a 3 year old with a painless firm mass show a lobulated but well-circumscribed mass of the foot extending between the metatarsals. The mass appears cystic by T2 with mild enhancement. DWI (not shown) confirmed restricted diffusion in the lesion.* **(Right)** *Axial T2 FS MR in a 16 year old with a palpable mass shows a small, ovoid, well-circumscribed but heterogeneous lesion within the vastus musculature.*

Rhabdomyosarcoma

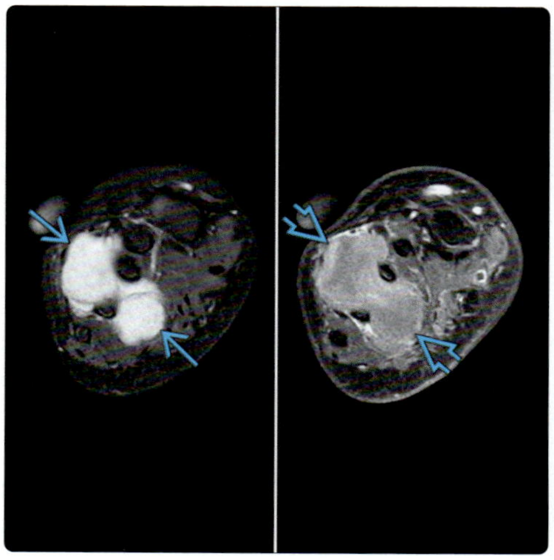

Synovial Sarcoma

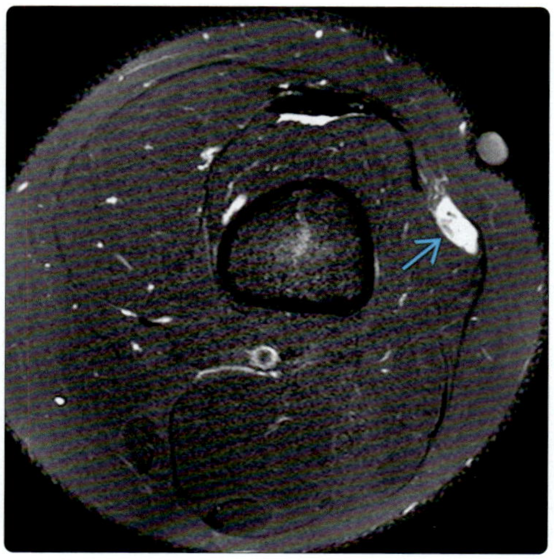

(Left) *Frontal radiograph in the same patient shows small irregular Ca^{2+} within the lesion. Excision confirmed a synovial sarcoma. Synovial sarcomas often occur near a joint & calcify in up to 30% of cases.* **(Right)** *Sagittal T2 FS MR in a 17 year old with a firm lower leg mass shows an elongated intramuscular lesion with well-defined hypointense & hyperintense foci, typical of many desmoid tumors.*

Synovial Sarcoma

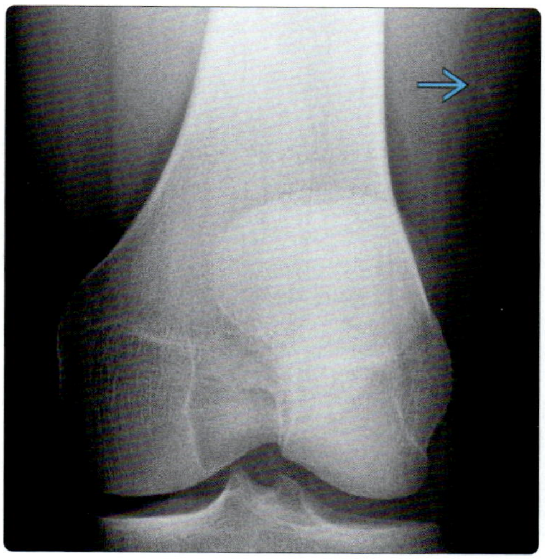

Fibromatosis

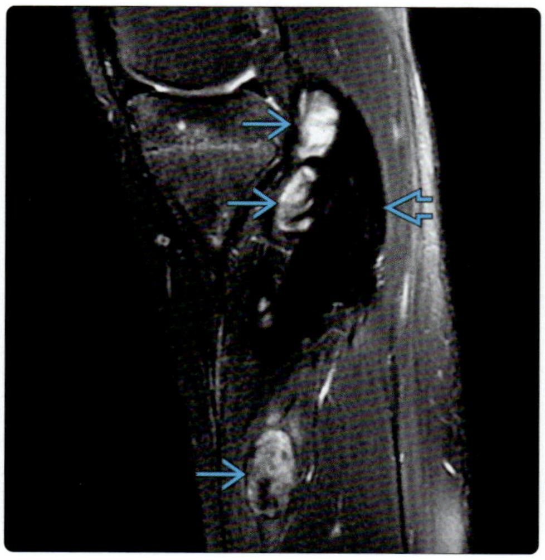

Infantile Myofibroma

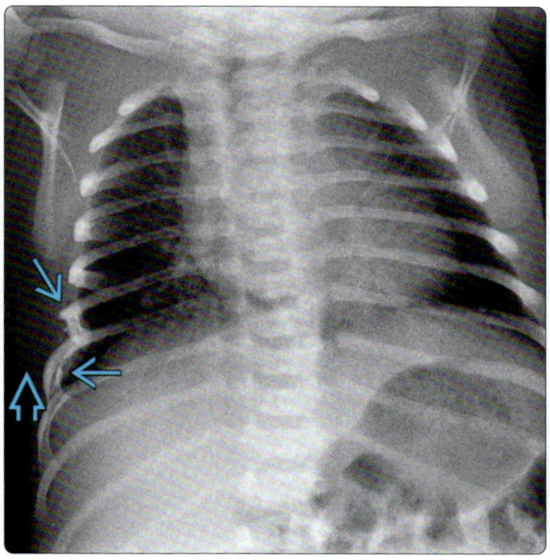

Infantile Myofibroma

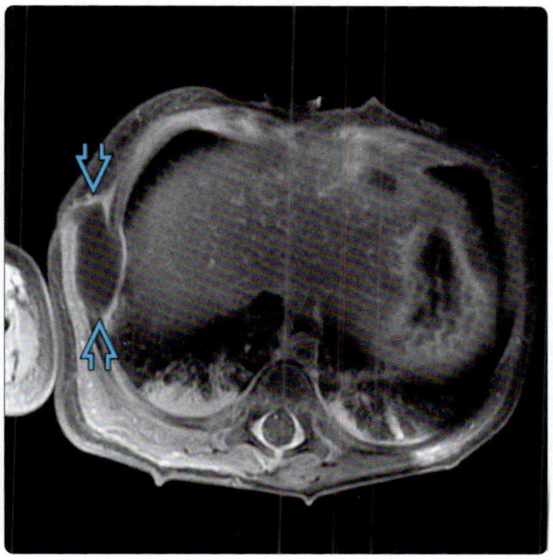

(Left) *AP radiograph in a newborn with a firm chest wall mass → shows irregular distortion of multiple subjacent ribs →.* **(Right)** *Axial T1 C+ FS MR in the same newborn shows only rim enhancement of the firm lesion →. A target pattern of enhancement has been described with infantile myofibromas but is not sensitive or specific. An abscess could have a similar enhancement pattern, though surrounding inflammation would be expected.*

Infantile Fibrosarcoma

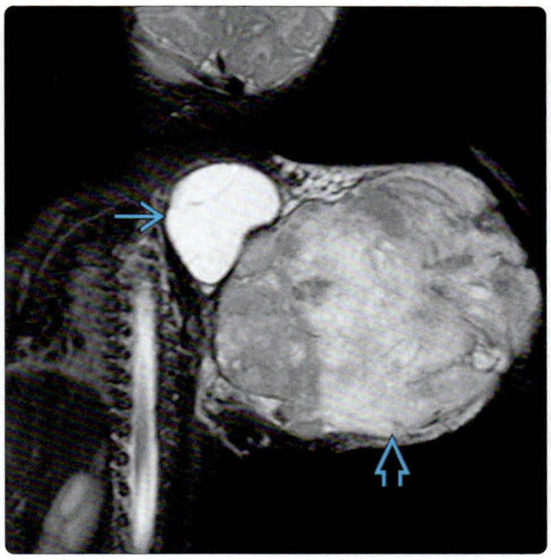

Malignant Peripheral Nerve Sheath Tumor

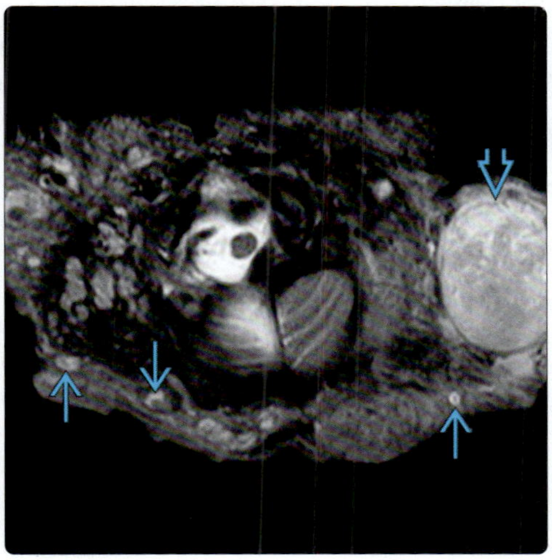

(Left) *Coronal STIR MR in a 2 month old with a rapidly growing mass shows a large heterogeneous solid → & cystic → lesion of the left back. Biopsy confirmed an infantile fibrosarcoma.* **(Right)** *Axial STIR MR in a 16 year old with NF1 shows extensive plexiform neurofibromas, many of which demonstrate the classic target sign →. A rapidly growing heterogeneous lesion → of the left neck showed increasing SUV on PET studies (up to 4.5) & was resected, confirming an MPNST.*

Lipoblastoma

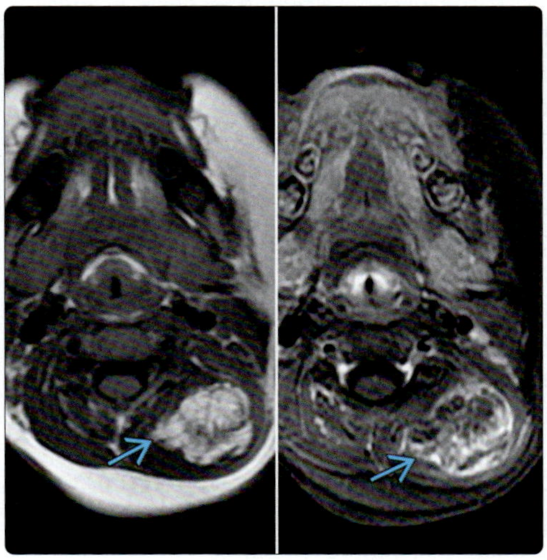

Extrarenal Rhabdoid Tumor

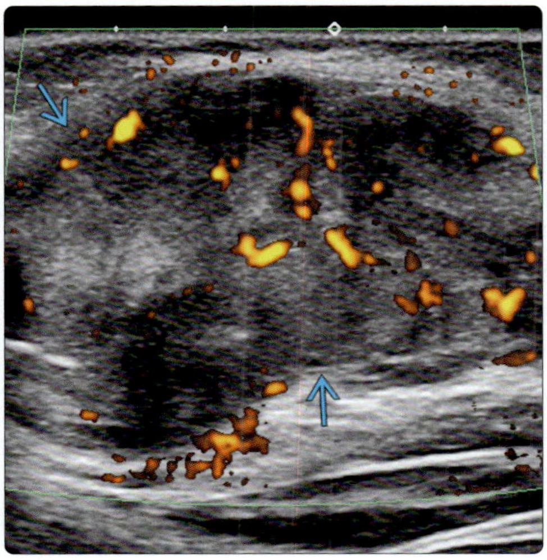

(Left) *Axial T1 (left) & T1 C+ FS (right) MR images in an 11 month old show a predominantly fatty but heterogeneous mass → of the paraspinal muscles, found to be a lipoblastoma on resection.* **(Right)** *Longitudinal color Doppler US in a 3 year old with an extrarenal rhabdoid tumor shows a well-circumscribed ovoid solid mass → with moderate internal vascularity. This sonographic appearance is highly concerning for malignancy.*

Soft Tissue Calcifications

DIFFERENTIAL DIAGNOSIS

Common

- Venous Malformation
- Heterotopic Ossification

Less Common

- Myositis Ossificans
- Pilomatrixoma
- Injection Granuloma
- Juvenile Dermatomyositis
- Synovial Sarcoma
- Iatrogenic

Rare but Important

- Hypercalcemia
- Tumoral Calcinosis
- Infantile Myofibroma
- Parasitic
- Trevor-Fairbank Disease (Mimic)
- Osteosarcoma
- Synovial Osteochondromatosis (Mimic)
- Chondrodysplasia Punctata (Mimic)
- Fibrodysplasia Ossificans Progressiva

ESSENTIAL INFORMATION

Helpful Clues for Common Diagnoses

- **Venous Malformation**
  - Congenital low-flow vascular anomaly
  - Grows proportional to child but may rapidly enlarge or become painful with thrombosis, trauma, infection, or hormonal stimulation (such as puberty)
  - Generally soft & compressible except for thrombi
    - MR: Clusters of abnormal T2-hyperintense venous channels
      - ± fluid-fluid levels from stagnant blood products
      - Gradual patchy enhancement is typical
    - Radiographs/US: Phleboliths are diagnostic in pediatric mass
- **Heterotopic Ossification**
  - Lamellar bone formation in soft tissues where bone does not exist
  - Frequently occurs after musculoskeletal trauma or surgery, burns, or neurologic injury
  - Occurs adjacent to large joints typically 1-4 months (up to 18 months) following injury
  - Alkaline phosphatase is commonly elevated up to 3.5x normal with peak ~ 12 weeks following injury

Helpful Clues for Less Common Diagnoses

- **Myositis Ossificans**
  - Subtype of heterotopic ossification, typically due to trauma
    - Prior single injury vs. repetitive trauma; history is lacking in ~ 30-40%
  - Early on, MR shows intense muscle edema surrounding focal heterogeneous mass
  - Peripheral Ca^{2+} develops in weeks; seen on nuclear bone scan, CT, US (& possibly MR) before radiographs (which may take 4-6 weeks)
  - Once mature, MR shows fatty marrow signal in calcified mass with no surrounding edema
- **Pilomatrixoma**
  - Round, well-circumscribed, benign neoplasm of hair follicle in subcutaneous fat
  - US: Hypoechoic ± internal Ca^{2+}, may show peripheral hyperemia & ↑ echogenicity of surrounding fat
- **Injection Granuloma**
  - Small heterogeneous foci in typical locations of injections (e.g., subcutaneous fat of upper arm, buttocks, thighs)
- **Juvenile Dermatomyositis**
  - Collagen vascular disease with proximal muscle weakness ± tenderness, easy fatigue
  - Characteristic skin changes: Heliotrope eyelid rash & Gottron papules
  - Soft tissue Ca^{2+} in 30-70%; develops months to years after disease onset, usually periarticular
    - Typically elbows, knees, digits, & extremities
  - Juvenile dermatomyositis (JDM) diagnosis is classically made by characteristic skin rash + 3 of following
    - Symmetric proximal muscle weakness
    - ↑ muscle enzymes in serum
    - Characteristic electromyography
    - Characteristic changes on muscle biopsy
  - Diagnosis confirmation now more commonly employs characteristic MR findings & autoantibody profiles
- **Synovial Sarcoma**
  - Typically 15-35 years old
  - Ca^{2+} in ~ 30%; often near joint, rarely in joint
  - Often small & well circumscribed; may appear cystic
    - Have low threshold for administering intravenous (IV) contrast for cyst that could be ganglion, etc.
- **Iatrogenic**
  - Surgically placed bone graft may displace from initial position, especially by fluid collection
  - IV calcium administrations may infiltrate soft tissues

Helpful Clues for Rare Diagnoses

- **Hypercalcemia**
  - a.k.a. "metastatic Ca^{2+}"
  - Any process that causes ↑ calcium-phosphate product may lead to precipitation of calcium in soft tissue
    - Secondary hyperparathyroidism, hypervitaminosis D, sarcoidosis, milk-alkali syndrome
    - Subcutaneous fat necrosis: Perinatal/maternal stress → panniculitis with erythematous subcutaneous nodule(s) → necrotic cells release calcium → hypercalcemia → calcium deposition in kidneys, skin, heart, etc.
      - Typically in term infants, often with therapeutic cooling for hypoxic-ischemic encephalopathy
- **Tumoral Calcinosis**
  - Periarticular Ca^{2+} along extensor surfaces (hip, elbow, shoulder, foot, wrist)
    - Seen primarily in first 2 decades of life
  - Classically due to familial renal disorder resulting in hyperphosphatemia; may be idiopathic
- **Infantile Myofibroma**
  - Heterogeneous, well-circumscribed vs. infiltrating mass; ± Ca^{2+}, bizarre remodeling of adjacent bone
  - May have rim, heterogeneous, or uniform enhancement

- ± multifocal relatively symmetric metadiaphyseal lytic bone lesions, visceral lesions
- **Parasitic**
  - Cysticercosis: "Rice grain" Ca^{2+}
    - Caused by pork tapeworm (*Taenia solium*) found worldwide
  - Dracunculiasis: Crescentic Ca^{2+}
    - a.k.a. guinea worm disease
    - Most commonly seen in Africa
  - Others: Loiasis, hydatid disease, trichinosis
- **Trevor-Fairbank Disease (Mimic)**
  - a.k.a. dysplasia epiphysealis hemimelica
  - Epiphyseal (or equivalent) osteochondromas
  - Multiple bones of single extremity are often involved on either medial or lateral side
  - Lower extremity (particularly foot/ankle) is much more commonly affected than upper
  - Mechanical symptoms & limb deformity are common
  - Classic appearance in infants/toddlers: "Too many ossicles" along 1 side of multiple adjacent joints
  - MR/US: Confirms cartilaginous continuity of radiographic "accessory ossification centers" with underlying bones in very young patients
- **Osteosarcoma**
  - Conventional intramedullary or surface osteosarcomas frequently extend beyond bone & produce tumor osteoid bulging into soft tissues
  - Extraskeletal osteosarcoma typically occurs in much older population
- **Synovial Osteochondromatosis (Mimic)**
  - Depending on joint involved & initial views obtained, ossified intraarticular bodies may mimic soft tissue Ca^{2+}
- **Chondrodysplasia Punctata (Mimic)**
  - Diverse group of skeletal dysplasias featuring stippled epiphyses
- **Fibrodysplasia Ossificans Progressiva**
  - Progressive debilitating bridging ossification of soft tissues between bones
    - Typically truncal distribution, particularly of neck & back
  - Starts with edema of fascia & ligaments, leads to mature bone formation over months
  - Associated with great toe & thumb anomalies

SELECTED REFERENCES

1. Meyers C et al: Heterotopic ossification: a comprehensive review. JBMR Plus. 3(4):e10172, 2019
2. Del Pozzo-Magaña BR et al: Subcutaneous fat necrosis of the newborn: a 20-year retrospective study. Pediatr Dermatol. 33(6):e353-5, 2016
3. Sargar KM et al: Pediatric fibroblastic and myofibroblastic tumors: a pictorial review. Radiographics. 36(4):1195-214, 2016
4. Cherian EV et al: Iatrogenic calcinosis cutis in a neonate. BMJ Case Rep. 2013, 2013
5. Dabadie A et al: A rare case of a calcified glomus tumour in the thigh of an adolescent. Pediatr Radiol. 43(8):1045-8, 2013

Venous Malformation

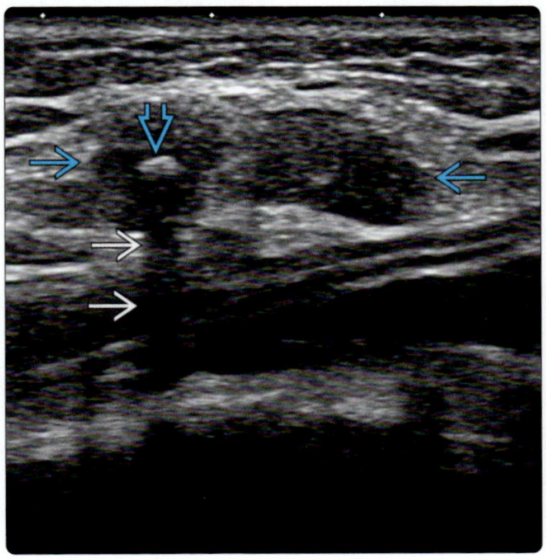

Venous Malformation

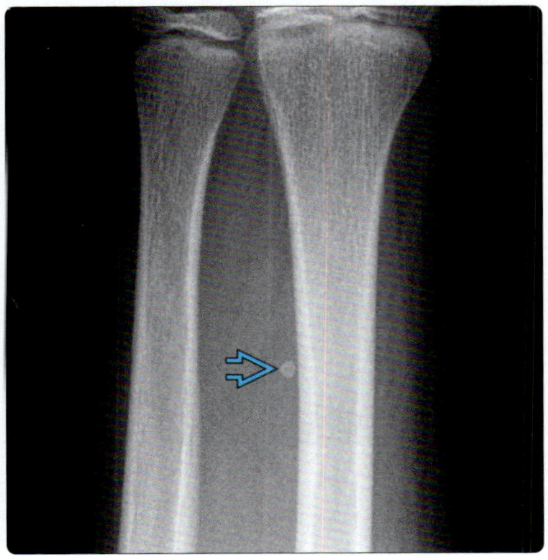

(Left) *Longitudinal US in a 12 year old reporting a palpable lump for 2 years shows a lobular hypoechoic mass ➡ in the subcutaneous fat of the forearm. A round echogenic focus ➡ in the lesion demonstrates posterior acoustic shadowing ➡, suggesting Ca^{2+} (possibly a phlebolith).* **(Right)** *AP radiograph in the same patient shows that the Ca^{2+} ➡ is round, well defined, & has a lucent center, consistent with a phlebolith. This confirms the mass to be a venous malformation.*

(Left) *AP radiograph in a 15 year old with bilateral hip pain shows exuberant ossification extending from the right anterior inferior iliac spine into the rectus femoris muscle due to prior trauma. The patient also has vigorous bone formation at a site of remote ischial tuberosity avulsion.* **(Right)** *AP radiograph shows heterotopic ossification along the diaphysis of the left femur distal to a surgical plate that transfixes a femoral neck fracture.*

Heterotopic Ossification

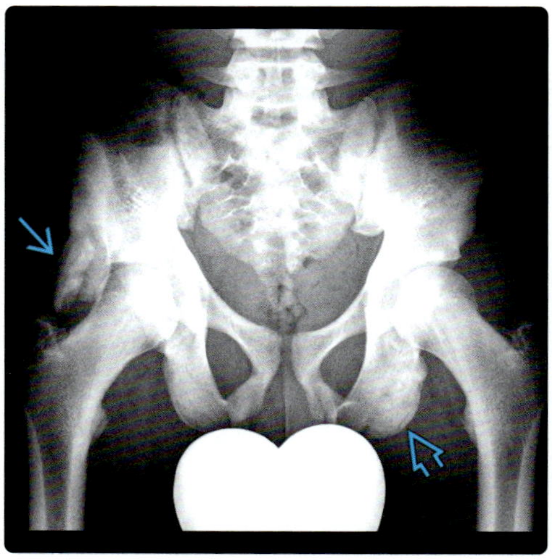

Heterotopic Ossification

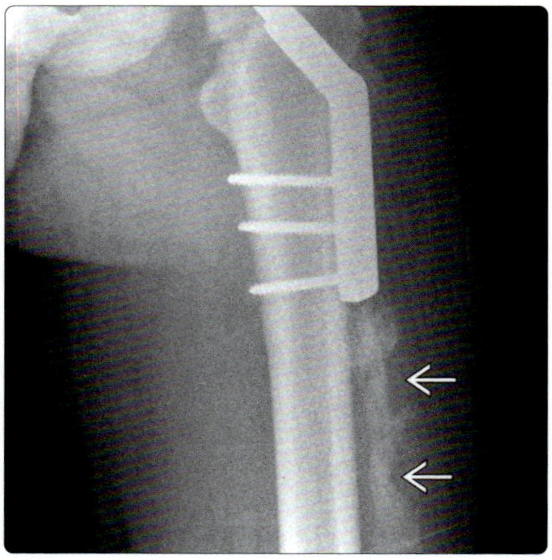

(Left) *Axial bone CT in a 4 year old with a hard mass noted months after trauma shows a peripherally calcified intramuscular mass, typical of myositis ossificans.* **(Right)** *Coronal STIR MR in the same patient 3 months prior to the CT shows marked edema of the masseter muscle surrounding a heterogeneously low signal intensity, round mass inferiorly. There was no Ca^{2+} in the mass by radiographs at this time.*

Myositis Ossificans

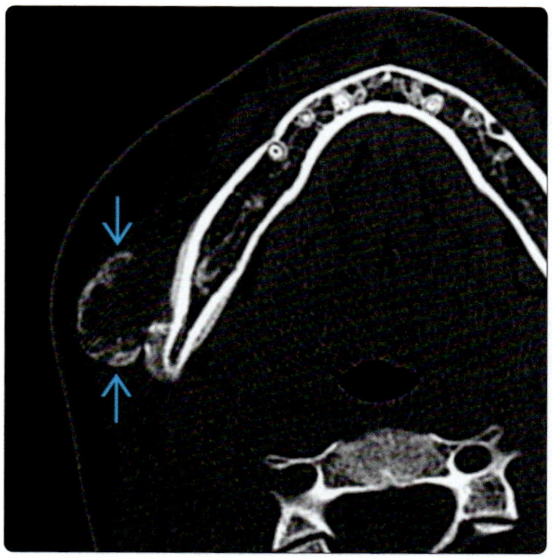

Myositis Ossificans

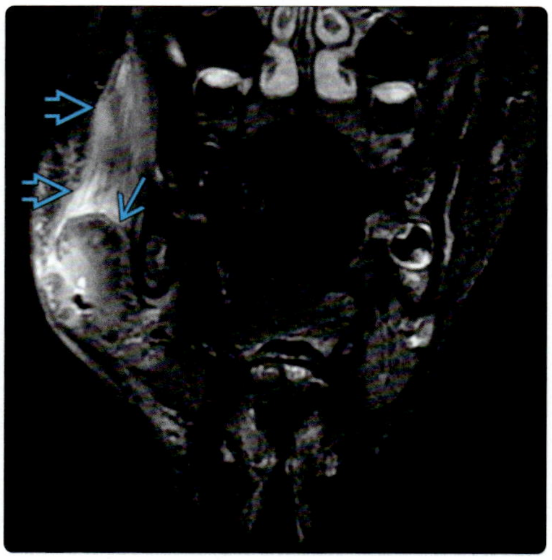

(Left) *Transverse US in a 12 year old with a scalp mass shows a well-circumscribed, ovoid hypoechoic mass of the subcutaneous fat. Numerous tiny punctate echogenic foci are seen in the lesion. There is mild increased echogenicity of the surrounding soft tissues. This is a common appearance for a pilomatrixoma.* **(Right)** *AP radiograph shows extensive periarticular Ca^{2+} around the knee in this child with juvenile dermatomyositis (JDM). Soft tissue Ca^{2+} develop in 25-50% of these patients.*

Pilomatrixoma

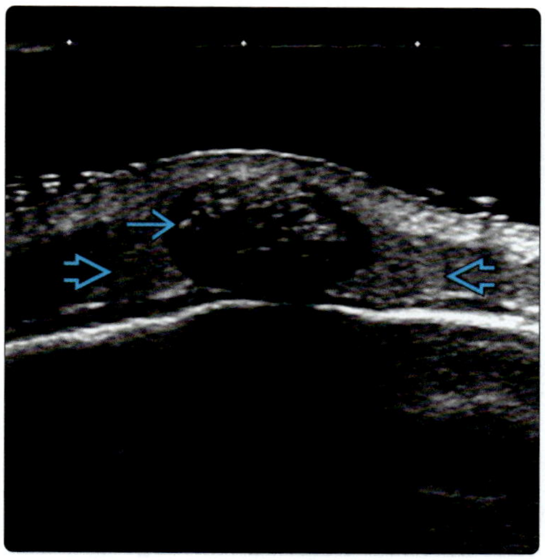

Juvenile Dermatomyositis

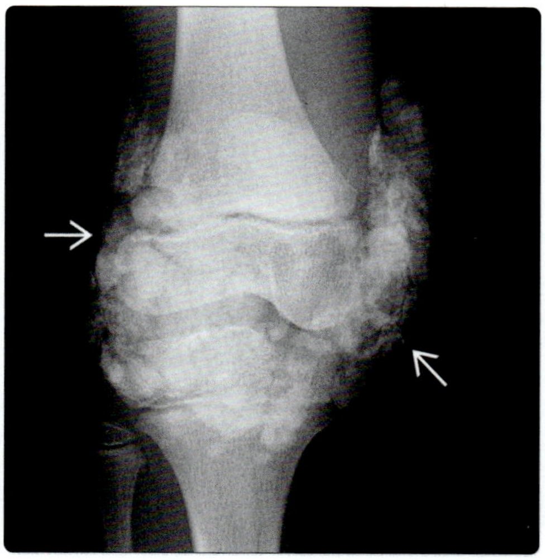

Synovial Sarcoma

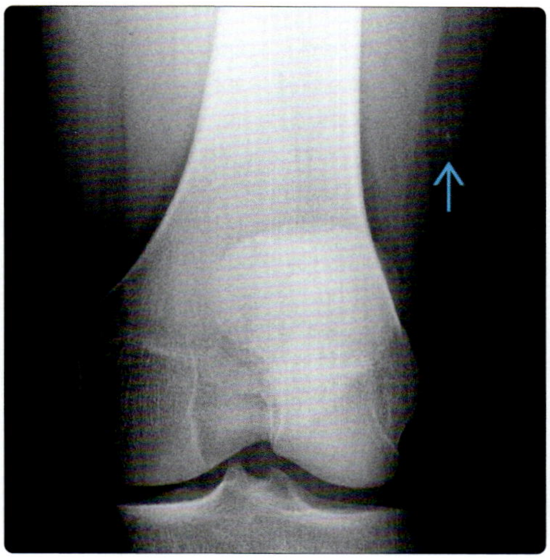

Synovial Sarcoma

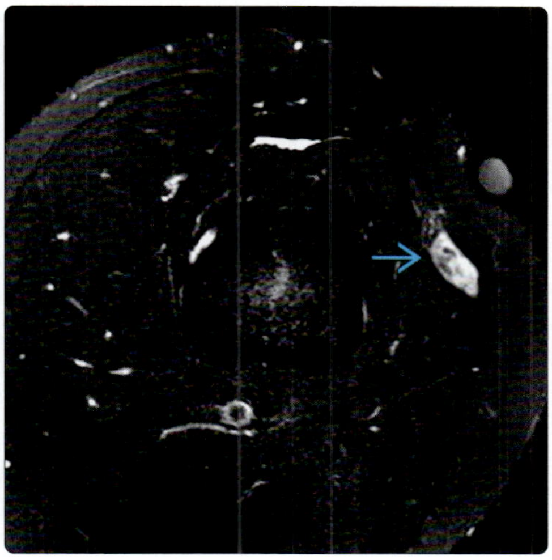

(Left) *AP radiograph in a 15 year old with a small firm thigh mass shows a cluster of punctate* Ca^{2+} *in the lateral soft tissues just proximal to the knee.* **(Right)** *Axial T2 FS MR in the same patient shows a small, well-circumscribed, mildly heterogeneous mass of the distal vastus lateralis muscle just deep to the fascia. Excision showed a synovial sarcoma. While they can be large, synovial sarcomas are notorious for being small, well circumscribed, & cystic-appearing at presentation.*

Tumoral Calcinosis

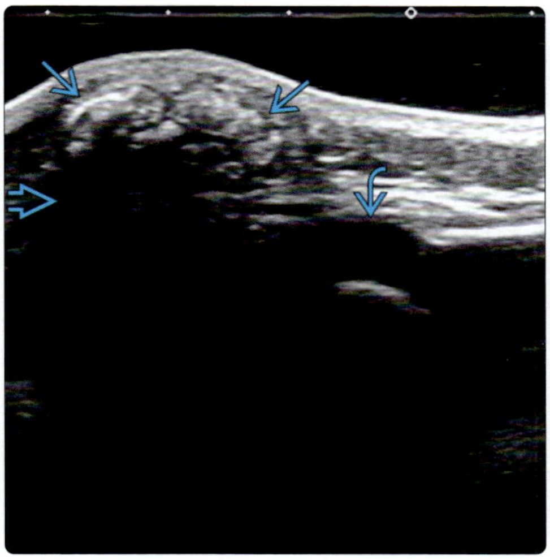

Tumoral Calcinosis

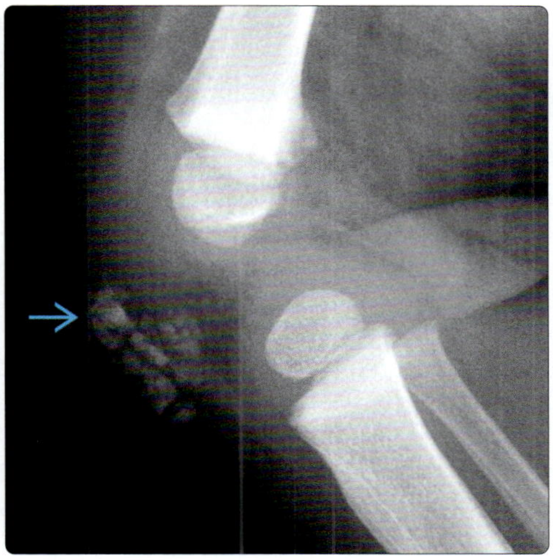

(Left) *Longitudinal US in a 1 year old with a firm infrapatellar mass shows a heterogeneously hyperechoic lesion with posterior acoustic shadowing, suggesting heavy* Ca^{2+}*. The partially ossified tibial epiphysis is noted for reference.* **(Right)** *Lateral radiograph in the same patient confirms amorphous cloud-like* Ca^{2+} *in the mass. Excision of the mass, in conjunction with serum & urine laboratory investigations, proved this to be idiopathic tumoral calcinosis.*

Infantile Myofibroma

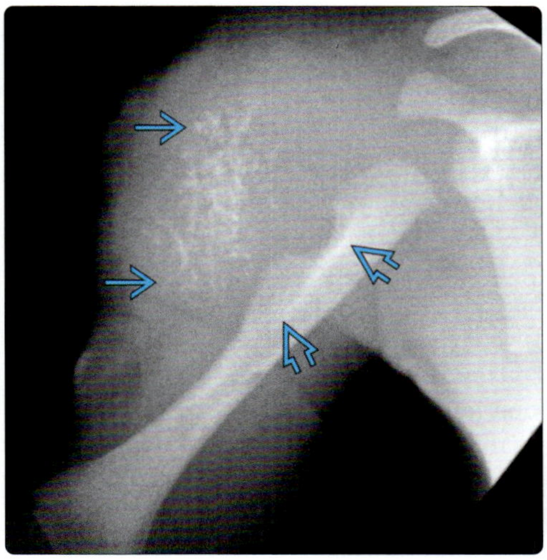

Infantile Myofibroma

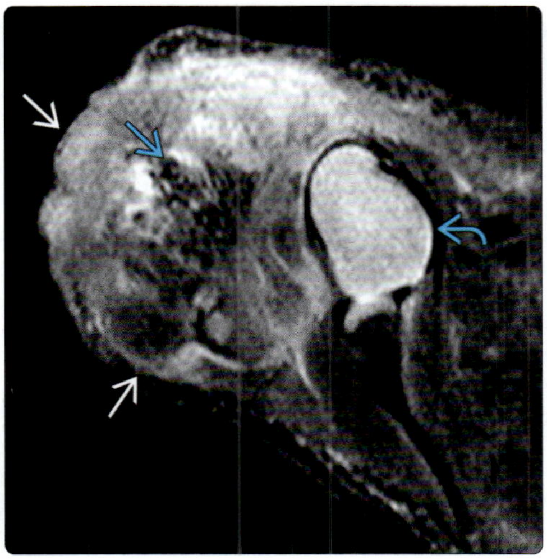

(Left) *AP radiograph in a 1 day old shows a large heterogeneous mass of the upper right arm containing numerous fine* Ca^{2+}*. There is unusual remodeling of the underlying humerus. The age & imaging features strongly suggest an infantile myofibroma.* **(Right)** *Axial STIR MR in the same patient shows marked heterogeneity of the mass with the low-signal foci corresponding to* Ca^{2+} *& fibrous tissue. The unossified humeral head is noted for reference. An infantile myofibroma was proven by biopsy.*

DIFFERENTIAL DIAGNOSIS

Common

- Physiologic
- Child Abuse

Less Common

- Chronic Recurrent Multifocal Osteomyelitis
- Prostaglandins
- Multifocal Malignancy
- Multifocal Osteomyelitis (Infectious)
- Langerhans Cell Histiocytosis
- Juvenile Idiopathic Arthritis
- Sickle Cell Dactylitis
- Osteogenesis Imperfecta
- Chemotherapy

Rare but Important

- Renal Osteodystrophy (Mimic)
- Scurvy
- Caffey Disease
- Hypervitaminosis A
- Hypertrophic Osteoarthropathy

ESSENTIAL INFORMATION

Key Differential Diagnosis Issues

- Periostitis: Generalized term for periosteal reaction (but incorrectly implies inflammation in all cases); often used when no focal lesion is visible radiographically
  - Monostotic: Common with numerous pathologies
  - Polyostotic: Much less common
    - Patient age, distribution/extent, degree of symmetry, & aggressive vs. nonaggressive features help limit differential
    - 1st appearance before 6 months of age: Physiologic (peaks at 6 months), prostaglandin-induced, congenital osteomyelitis, Caffey disease
- **Hint:** Consider abuse with unexplained multifocal periosteal reaction in young children (particularly if asymmetric)

Helpful Clues for Common Diagnoses

- **Physiologic**
  - Periosteal new bone along long bone diaphyses
    - Smooth, solid, mild; usually bilateral & symmetric
    - Humeri, femurs, tibiae
  - Likely secondary to rapid bone growth
  - Not seen before 1 month of age; peaks at 6 months
- **Child Abuse**
  - Always consider when periosteal reaction is seen in infants, particularly if multifocal & asymmetric
  - Often due to metaphyseal corner fracture
    - Fracture causes subperiosteal bleeding & lifting of periosteum
  - May occur without fracture (due to loose periosteum & twisting injuries)

Helpful Clues for Less Common Diagnoses

- **Chronic Recurrent Multifocal Osteomyelitis**
  - Multifocal nonpyogenic inflammatory bone lesions with relapsing/remitting course
  - Associated with other inflammatory conditions (e.g., psoriasis, inflammatory bowel disease)
  - Typically involves periphyseal regions
  - Most common sites: Tibia, femur, spine, pelvis, clavicle
    - Multiple sites over course of disease in ~ 80%
    - Can be bilateral & relatively symmetric
    - Medial clavicular involvement suggests chronic recurrent multifocal osteomyelitis
  - Radiographs: Features may be mixed at presentation
    - Acute: Lytic lesion (usually in metaphysis near physis)
    - Late: Progressive adjacent sclerosis
    - Recurrence: New lytic areas or periosteal reaction
  - MR: Enhancement of lesion & surrounding marrow
    - ± soft tissue & periosteal edema (but no abscess)
    - ± reactive adjacent joint effusion/synovitis
- **Prostaglandins**
  - Used to maintain patent ductus arteriosus in infants with congenital heart disease
  - Similar to physiologic appearance but worse
    - Symmetric involvement of extremity long bones, ribs, clavicles, & scapulae; rarely involves mandible
  - Typically develops after ≥ 40 days of treatment
  - After stopping prostaglandins, periosteal reaction is incorporated into bone over 6-12 months
- **Multifocal Malignancy**
  - Bone metastases
    - Primary bone tumor, soft tissue sarcomas, & other tumors (e.g., neuroblastoma, medulloblastoma)
  - Leukemia: More typically presents with lucent metaphyseal bands or diffuse osteoporosis
    - Periostitis is rare manifestation
- **Multifocal Osteomyelitis (Infectious)**
  - Congenital infections
    - TORCH/TORCHES infections
      - **To**xoplasmosis, **r**ubella, **c**ytomegalovirus, **he**rpes, **s**yphilis
      - "O" sometimes used for other: Varicella-zoster virus, Zika virus, Parvovirus B19
  - Multifocal osteomyelitis later in childhood
    - Hematogenous spread (metaphyseal)
  - Tuberculosis (TB) involvement in hands: Dactylitis termed spina ventosa
- **Langerhans Cell Histiocytosis**
  - Benign neoplasm of atypical Langerhans cells
  - Axial skeleton
    - Well-defined lytic skull lesions without sclerotic rim ("punched-out")
    - Classic cause of vertebra plana
  - Appendicular skeleton
    - Aggressive features > nonaggressive
    - Periosteal reaction variable; may be absent
- **Juvenile Idiopathic Arthritis**
  - 1st osseous manifestation may be periostitis of hand or foot phalanges
    - Typically secondary to adjacent tenosynovitis
  - Later, joints will be involved
  - Differential includes: Sickle cell & TB dactylitis
- **Sickle Cell Dactylitis**
  - Generally young children (< 7 years of age)

- Cold temperature → vasoconstriction of terminal vessels in phalanges → sludging of sickled red blood cells → bone infarct
- Bone infarct may initially elicit periostitis; eventually has mixed lytic & sclerotic appearance

- **Osteogenesis Imperfecta**
  - Group of clinically heterogeneous genetic disorders caused by type I collagen abnormalities
  - Increased bone fragility → frequent fractures → malunion & bowing
  - Numerous in utero or perinatal fractures of short, poorly mineralized bones (most severe form, type II)
  - Other types: Multiple fractures in thin, overtubulated long bones + vertebral fractures + osteoporosis
- **Chemotherapy**
  - Some chemotherapeutics may rarely cause periosteal reaction (e.g., methotrexate)
  - Retinoids
    - Used to treat severe acne; also used in some chemotherapeutic regimens (e.g., neuroblastoma)
    - May cause variety of musculoskeletal changes: Hyperostosis, syndesmophytes, premature physeal closure
    - Periosteal reaction is less common
  - Differential diagnosis includes osteomyelitis & bone infarcts in oncology patients

Helpful Clues for Rare Diagnoses

- **Renal Osteodystrophy (Mimic)**
  - Severe subperiosteal resorption, especially at proximal humeral, tibial, or femoral metaphyses or at radial aspects of middle phalanges; may mimic fluffy periostitis
    - Watch for underlying abnormal bone density, signs of rickets with widening physes of loss of normal zones of provisional calcification (ZPC)
  - Severe renal osteodystrophy may result in bone accretion when effective treatment is initiated; mimics periosteal reaction
- **Scurvy**
  - Hypovitaminosis C → ↓ collagen synthesis
  - Thickened sclerotic ZPC, a.k.a. white line of Frankel
    - Sclerotic but brittle; therefore fractures may develop in this zone
  - Lucent/demineralized area deep to sclerotic ZPC is called scurvy or Trümmerfeld zone
    - Demineralized zone also prone to fractures
  - Subperiosteal hemorrhage (especially with corner fracture) → subperiosteal new bone formation covering enlarged subperiosteal space
  - Wimberger ring sign: Dense ZPC outlining secondary ossification centers
  - Usually occurs at 6 months to 2 years of age
- **Caffey Disease**
  - a.k.a. infantile cortical hyperostosis
  - Rare disease, manifests at birth
  - Painful periostitis of long bones
  - Involvement of clavicle & mandible is suggestive of diagnosis in infants
  - Self-limited; spontaneously resolves over first 2 years of life
- **Hypervitaminosis A**
  - Excessive intake of vitamin A results in pain with periosteal reaction
    - Subtle at first but may become dense & thick
  - Continued use of excessive vitamin A may lead to coned epiphyses
- **Hypertrophic Osteoarthropathy**
  - Lung disease (e.g., cystic fibrosis) may elicit hypertrophic osteoarthropathy, just as in adults
  - Periosteal reaction with pain, referred to joints

SELECTED REFERENCES

1. Raissaki M et al: Multifocal bone and bone marrow lesions in children - MRI findings. Pediatr Radiol. 47(3):342-60, 2017
2. Sidhu HS et al: Imaging features of therapeutic drug-induced musculoskeletal abnormalities. Radiographics. 32(1):105-27, 2012
3. Dwek JR: The periosteum: what is it, where is it, and what mimics it in its absence? Skeletal Radiol. 39(4):319-23, 2010
4. Lachman R. Taybi & Lachman's Radiology of Syndromes, Metabolic Disorders & Skeletal Dysplasias, 5e. Philadelphia: Mosby, 2006

Physiologic

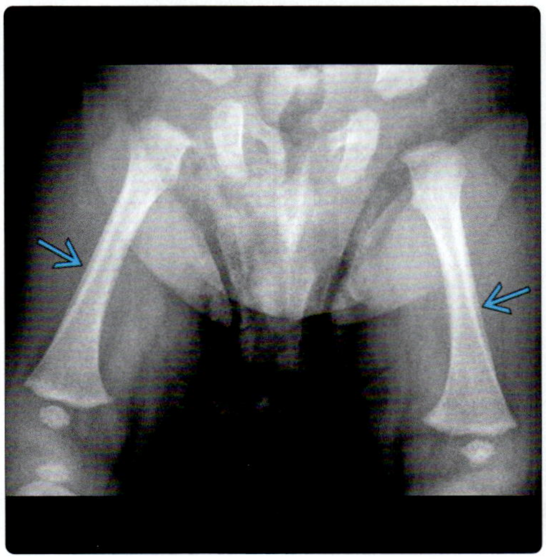

Child Abuse

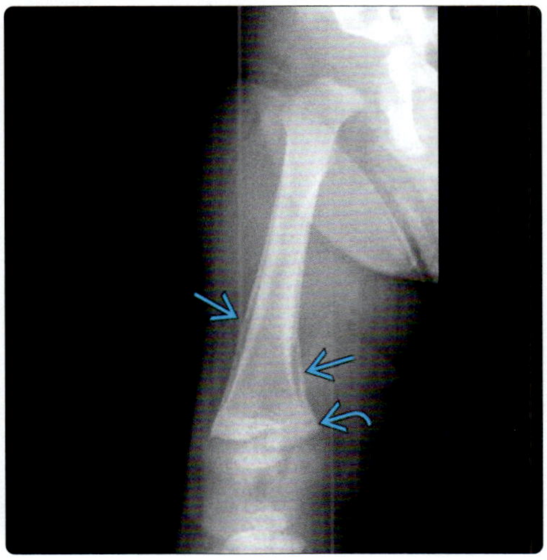

(Left) *AP radiograph in a 3-month-old boy shows smooth, solid, & symmetric physiologic periosteal reaction along the femoral diaphyses ➙. This entity is not seen before 1 month of age & peaks at 6 months. The femurs, tibiae, & humeri are classic sites of involvement.* **(Right)** *AP radiograph in a 2-month-old boy who had a skeletal survey performed for a suspicion of nonaccidental injury shows more focal & slightly bulging periosteal reaction along the distal femur ➙ due to a healing metaphyseal fracture ➙.*

(Left) *Oblique radiograph of the left forearm in the same child shows a healing radial fracture → with mature callus →. This child also had multiple healing posterior rib fractures (not shown). These findings are consistent with nonaccidental trauma.* **(Right)** *AP radiograph in a 3 month old with subdural hematomas (not shown) reveals numerous healing rib fractures → & a healing right clavicle fracture →. The constellation of findings is highly suggestive of child abuse.*

Child Abuse

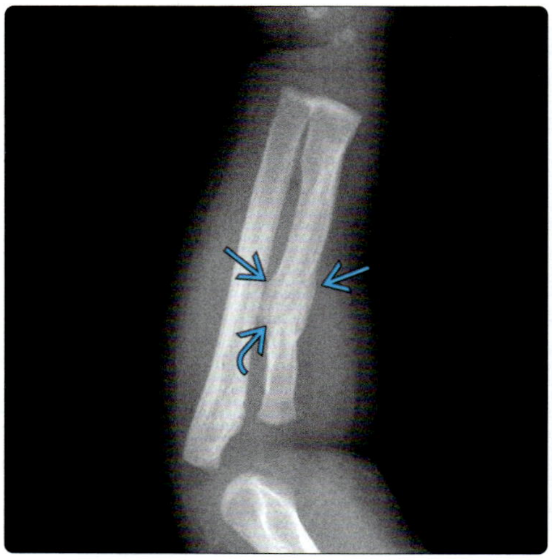

Child Abuse

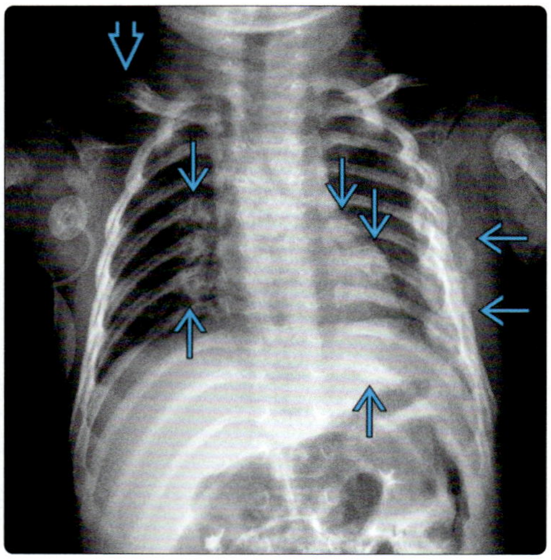

(Left) *AP radiograph (top) in a 4-year-old girl with right clavicle & bilateral ankle pain shows expansion & permeation of the right medial clavicle → with periosteal reaction. On the coronal STIR MR (bottom), there is increased signal within & periosteal reaction along the right clavicle → with adjacent soft tissue inflammation →.* **(Right)** *Frontal radiographs of both ankles in the same child with CRMO show lucent lesions in the bilateral distal tibial metaphyses with cortical thinning & layered periosteal reaction →.*

Chronic Recurrent Multifocal Osteomyelitis

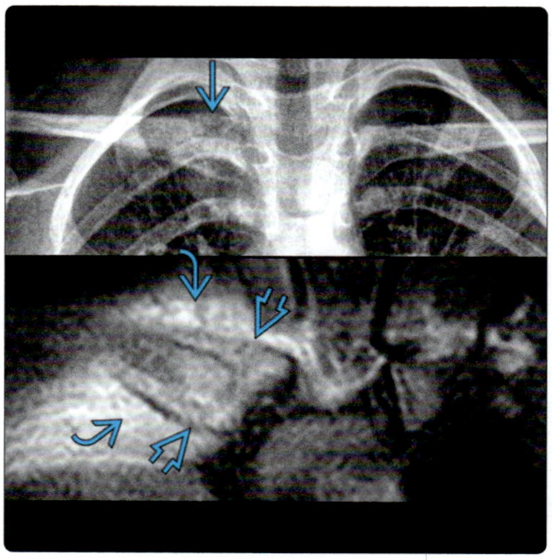

Chronic Recurrent Multifocal Osteomyelitis

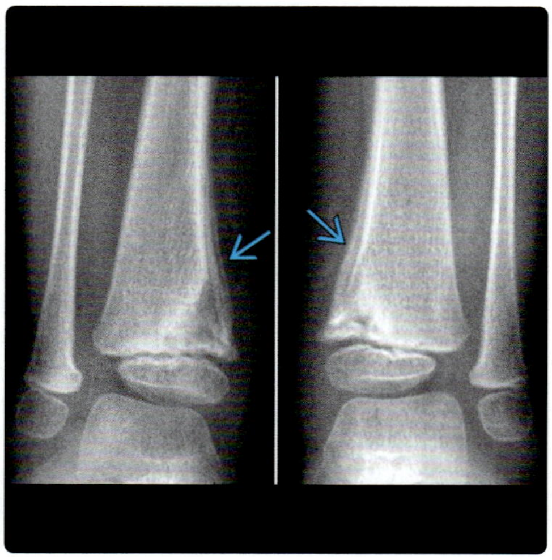

(Left) *Lateral right femur (left) & left lower leg (right) radiographs show multifocal interrupted periosteal reaction → with metaphyseal lucent bands → & a pathologic fracture →. Bone marrow aspiration revealed acute myelogenous leukemia in this toddler with fever & anemia.* **(Right)** *Coronal CECT in an infant with metastatic neuroblastoma shows a characteristic pattern of aggressive periosteal reaction where radiating perpendicular spicules of new bone → project into associated soft tissue masses →.*

Multifocal Malignancy

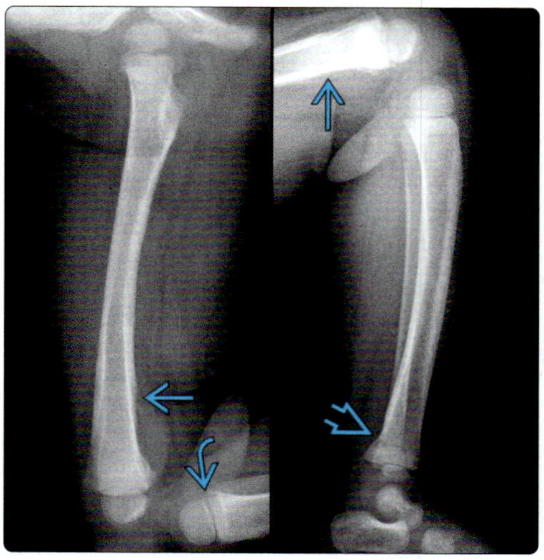

Multifocal Malignancy

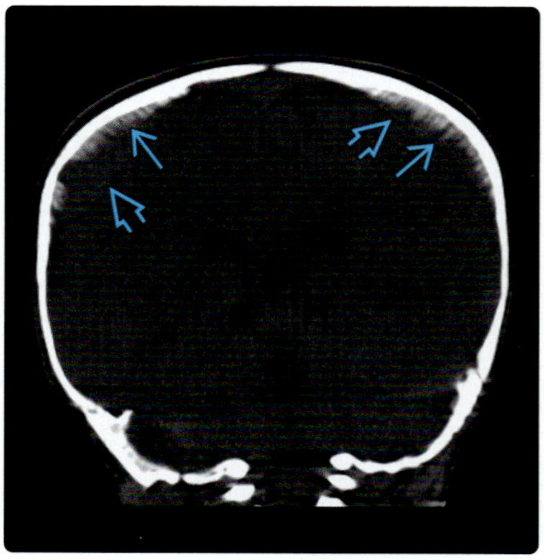

Multifocal Osteomyelitis (Infectious)

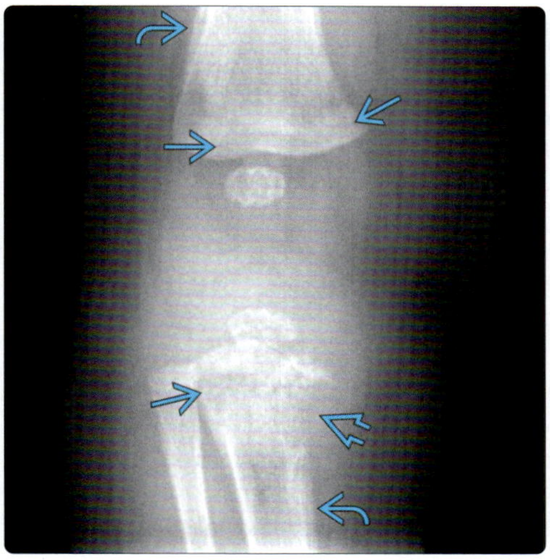

Juvenile Idiopathic Arthritis

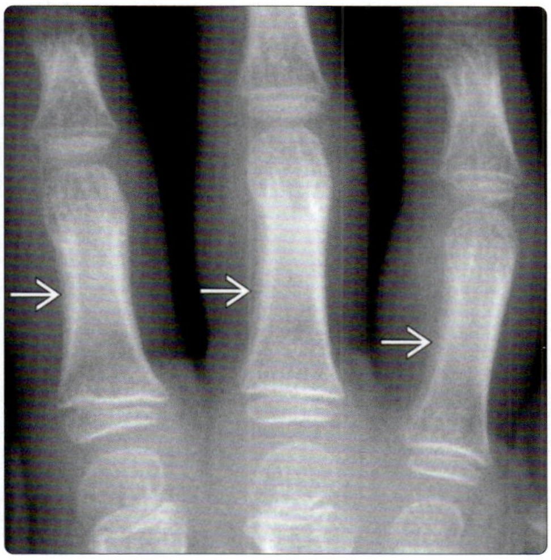

(Left) *AP radiograph of the right knee in an infant shows metaphyseal lucencies & a destructive proximal tibial lesion medially, typical of the Wimberger corner sign in congenital syphilis. There is adjacent periosteal reaction. These findings were bilateral.* **(Right)** *PA radiograph in a patient with juvenile idiopathic arthritis demonstrates phalangeal periosteal reaction, typically due to nearby tenosynovitis. Sickle cell dactylitis is also in the differential diagnosis for this appearance.*

Sickle Cell Dactylitis

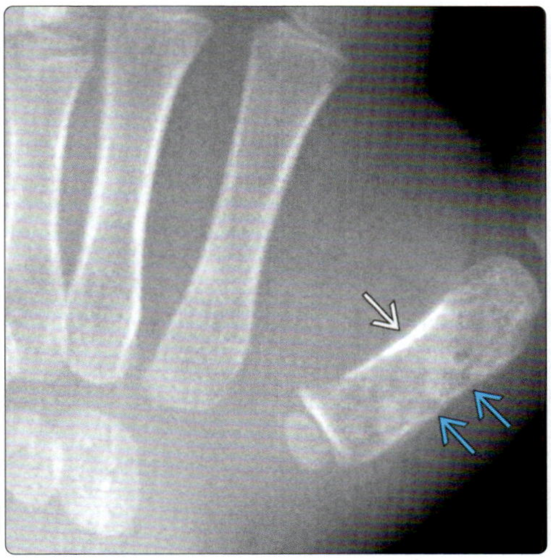

Renal Osteodystrophy (Mimic)

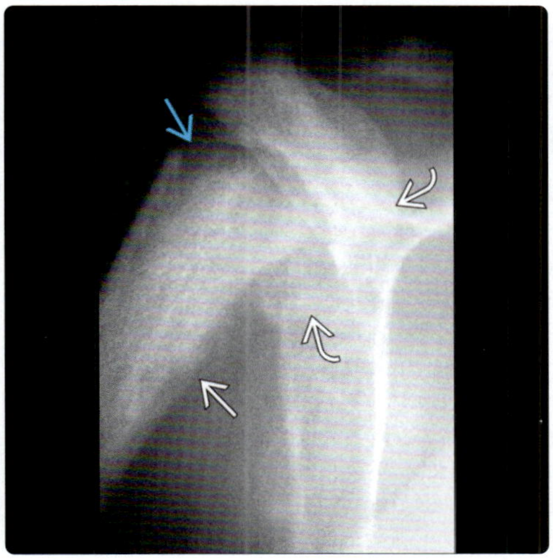

(Left) *PA radiograph shows subtle periosteal reaction & underlying bone permeation/mottling in this child with sickle cell disease who developed recent hand pain. This appearance is due to a bone infarct.* **(Right)** *Oblique radiograph shows what might be mistaken for fluffy periostitis along the proximal humerus, but this patient has aggressive subperiosteal resorption due to renal disease. Also note the cupped, frayed metaphysis & slipped humeral epiphysis secondary to renal rickets.*

Scurvy

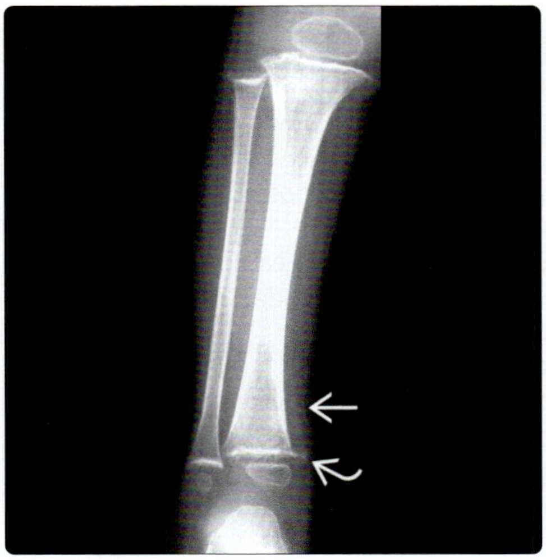

Caffey Disease

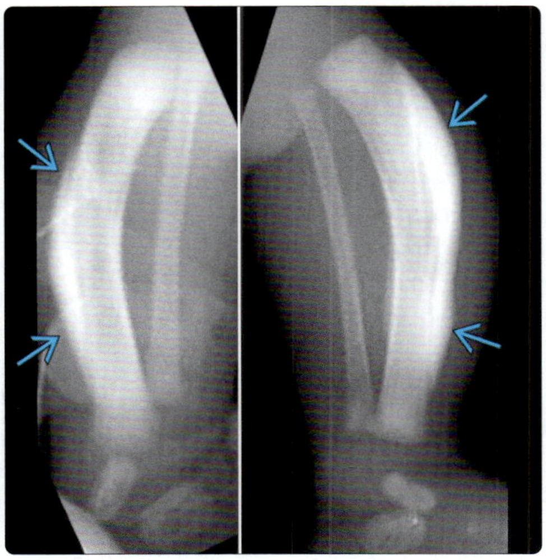

(Left) *AP radiograph shows dense metaphyseal lines of Frankel plus a metaphyseal corner irregularity in this patient with scurvy. Subperiosteal hemorrhage can also lead to periosteal bone formation in such patients.* **(Right)** *Lateral radiographs of both lower legs in a 3-week-old girl with Caffey disease show dense cortical thickening of the anterior aspects of both tibiae. Caffey disease typically manifests at birth & spontaneously resolves over the first 2 years of life.*

DIFFERENTIAL DIAGNOSIS

Common

- Child Abuse
- Accidental Trauma
- Birth Trauma
- Benign Enlargement of Subarachnoid Spaces
- Periosteal Reaction of Other Causes
- Normal Anatomic Variants
- Wormian Bones & Accessory Sutures
- Artifacts
- Osteomyelitis

Less Common

- Rickets
- Leukemia
- CPR-Related Rib Fractures

Rare but Important

- Osteogenesis Imperfecta
- Congenital Syphilis
- Scurvy
- Menkes Syndrome
- Skeletal Dysplasias

ESSENTIAL INFORMATION

Key Differential Diagnosis Issues

- Any injury inconsistent with reported mechanism or stage of development should raise suspicion for child abuse
- Associated clinical, laboratory, & imaging findings
  - Injuries of varying age, bruising in nonmobile infant, patterned bruises or burns, & retinal hemorrhages should raise suspicion for child abuse
  - Laboratory results, genetic testing, & constellation of imaging findings may identify or exclude underlying metabolic & genetic diseases that can mimic abuse

Helpful Clues for Common Diagnoses

- **Child Abuse**
  - Majority of deaths occur in children < 3 years old
    - Infants ≤ 1 year old are at greatest risk of abuse
  - May present with no history to explain injury or with mechanism inconsistent with injury or stage of development
  - Physical exam findings may include: Retinal hemorrhages, patterned bruising or burns, injuries of varying age, palpable callus or crepitus at rib fractures
  - Fractures with high specificity for child abuse
    - Classic metaphyseal lesion (a.k.a. metaphyseal corner fracture or bucket handle fracture)
    - Posterior rib fractures
    - Scapular fracture
    - Spinous process fracture
    - Sternal fracture
  - Abusive head trauma
    - Leading cause of fatal head injuries & serious/fatal traumatic brain injury in children < 2 years old
    - Most common findings: Subdural hemorrhage (SDH), hypoxic-ischemic injury, skull fractures
      - Complex skull fractures are significantly associated with intracranial injury & positive skeletal survey
- **Accidental Trauma**
  - History & mechanism are consistent with injury & stage of development
  - May be difficult to distinguish fractures with low or moderate specificity for abuse as accidental
- **Birth Trauma**
  - Correlate appearance of fracture relative to delivery date as well as other factors: Mode of delivery, degree of difficulty, use of vacuum or forceps, need for resuscitation
  - Clavicle is most common obstetric-related fracture
  - Oblique/spiral diaphyseal long bone fractures can be seen
  - Can have fractures of metaphysis & epiphysis identical to those of abuse, though very rare
  - Small birth-related subdural hematomas are common, resolve in 4-6 weeks, & do not rebleed
- **Benign Enlargement of Subarachnoid Spaces**
  - Common cause of macrocephaly in infants; typically resolves by 24 months
    - Normal neurological development or mild delay
    - Family history of macrocephaly is often present
  - ↑ frontal/temporal subarachnoid spaces (SAS), ± mild ventriculomegaly
    - Veins are seen crossing SAS
    - No evidence of ↑ intracranial pressure or mass effect
  - Echogenicity & MR signal follow CSF
    - Tiny subdural collections are seen in < 6%
      - Anything other than tiny, simple-appearing collection should trigger child abuse work-up
- **Periosteal Reaction of Other Causes**
  - Physiologic
    - Seen in infants 1-6 months of age
    - Smooth, thin (< 2 mm), diaphyseal, & symmetric
      - Typically involves femurs, tibiae, & humeri
    - No callus formation on follow-up
  - Drug related: Prostaglandin E1 used to maintain patency of ductus arteriosus
- **Normal Anatomic Variants**
  - Variations of normal anatomy & development can mimic fractures of child abuse
  - Ossification centers
    - Well corticated
    - No callus formation on follow-up
  - Metaphyseal step-off & spur
    - Step-off: Junction of subperiosteal bone collar & cortex
    - Spur: Extension of subperiosteal bone collar
    - Unlike fracture, no lucency undercuts subperiosteal bone collar
  - Rib fusion
  - Congenital pseudarthrosis of clavicle or ribs
    - Smooth margins, may appear hypoplastic
- **Wormian Bones & Accessory Sutures**
  - Intrasutural wormian bones & accessory sutures may be mistaken for skull fractures
    - Multiple wormian bones are associated with various syndromes, including osteogenesis imperfecta
  - Assess for typical location of common types: Interparietal bone, mendosal suture

- No overlying soft tissue injury or intracranial injury
- **Artifacts**
  - Sternal ossification centers overlap posterior ribs on oblique projections, simulating fractures
  - Normal clavicle contour may simulate fracture
- **Osteomyelitis**
  - ↑ inflammatory markers
  - Periosteal reaction, focal osteoporosis, osseous destruction, abscess

Helpful Clues for Less Common Diagnoses

- **Rickets**
  - Metaphyseal cupping, fraying, & splaying with loss of dense zone of provisional Ca^{2+} (ZPC)
  - History, clinical, & laboratory findings should support metabolic bone disease
  - Important points about fractures in rickets
    - Rickets does not cause high-specificity fractures seen with child abuse
    - Fractures seen in rickets typically occur in older mobile infants
    - Fractures due to rickets do not occur without osseous changes of rickets
- **Leukemia**
  - Metaphyseal lucent bands, osteoporosis
  - ± cortical permeation, periosteal reaction, soft tissue mass, pathologic fractures
    - No classic metaphyseal lesions
  - Abnormal CBC, hepatosplenomegaly, bruising/petechiae
- **CPR-Related Rib Fractures**
  - Correlate with history
  - Very rare, typically anterior even with new 2-handed CPR technique

Helpful Clues for Rare Diagnoses

- **Osteogenesis Imperfecta**
  - Disorder of genes controlling collagen synthesis
  - Numerous types, varying in severity of osteoporosis & number of fractures
  - Wormian bones are often present
  - Sclera may be blue or gray in many types
- **Congenital Syphilis**
  - Positive serology
  - Lucent &/or destructive changes at metaphyses, including Wimberger sign at proximal & medial tibial metadiaphyses
    - Pathologic fractures may mimic child abuse
  - ± hepatosplenomegaly, adenopathy, rash
- **Scurvy**
  - Hypovitaminosis C → impaired collagen synthesis, ↑ bleeding, osteoporosis
  - Severe cortical thinning, irregular metaphyseal lucencies with horizontal spurs, dense ZPC
- **Menkes Syndrome**
  - X-linked recessive defect in copper absorption
    - ↓ serum copper & ceruloplasmin
  - Osteoporosis, wormian bones, metaphyseal spurs/irregularity, long bone fractures
  - Thin & coarse "kinky" hair, seizures, hypotonia, vascular tortuosity, bladder diverticula
- **Skeletal Dysplasias**
  - Extensive symmetric metaphyseal abnormalities that will not change on follow-up radiographs
    - Metaphyseal chondrodysplasia, Schmid type
      - Enlarged femoral heads, coxa vara, femoral bowing
    - Spondylometaphyseal dysplasia, Sutcliffe/corner fracture type
      - Severe coxa vara, Blount-like changes of proximal tibiae, odontoid hypoplasia

SELECTED REFERENCES

1. Choudhary AK et al: Consensus statement on abusive head trauma in infants and young children. Pediatr Radiol. 48(8):1048-65, 2018
2. Servaes S et al: The etiology and significance of fractures in infants and young children: a critical multidisciplinary review. Pediatr Radiol. 46(5):591-600, 2016
3. Kleinman PK. Diagnostic Imaging of Child Abuse. 3rd ed. Cambridge, United Kingdom New York: Cambridge University Press, 2015.

Child Abuse

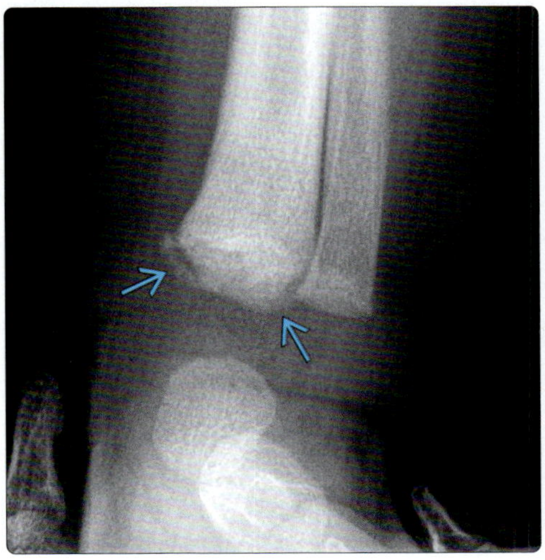

Child Abuse

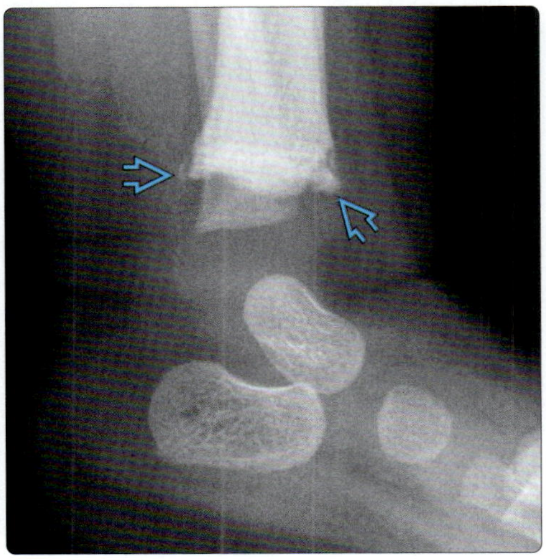

(Left) *AP radiograph of the left ankle in a 5 month old with bruising shows a bucket handle appearance ⇨ of a classic metaphyseal lesion from child abuse.* **(Right)** *Lateral radiograph in the same patient shows the same injury of the left tibia at a tangential view, appearing as metaphyseal corner fractures ⇨. Note the lucency undercutting the fragments. This patient also had numerous rib fractures.*

Child Abuse

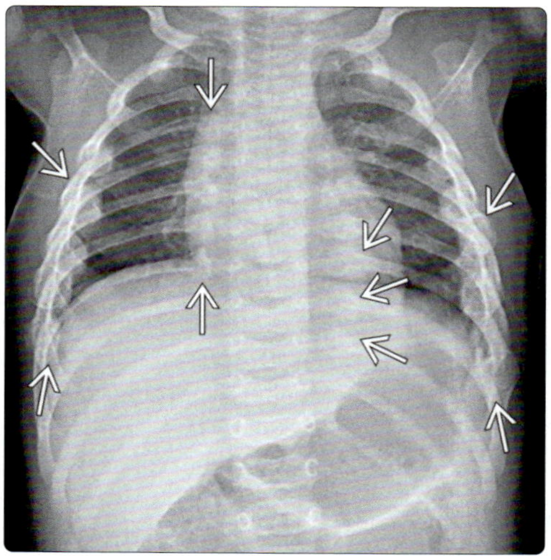

Child Abuse

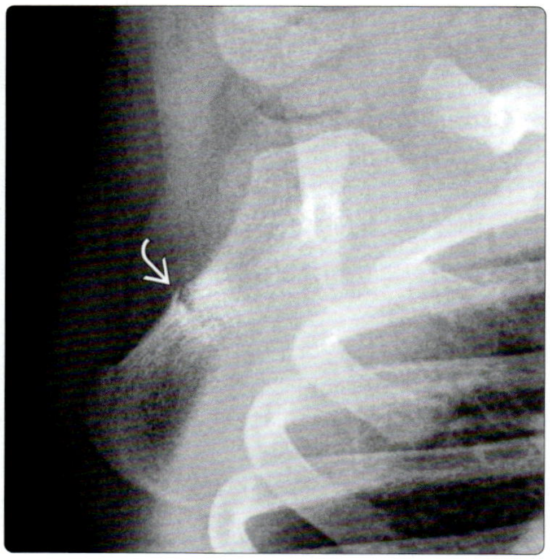

(Left) *AP radiograph of a 12 week old demonstrates multiple healing posterior & lateral rib fractures bilaterally . The reported history of a recent fall was inconsistent with these injuries (which are highly specific for child abuse).* **(Right)** *AP radiograph shows a fracture through the lateral margin of the right scapula in this 2 year old who presented with unexplained bruising. Scapular injuries are highly specific for child abuse, as they require a great deal of force. A sibling was also discovered to have long bone fractures.*

Child Abuse

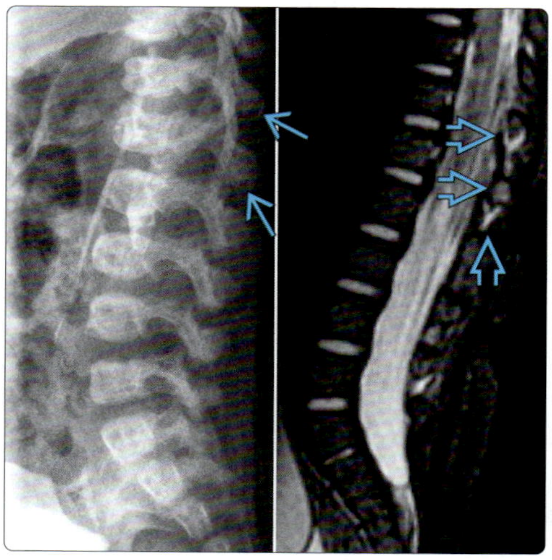

Child Abuse

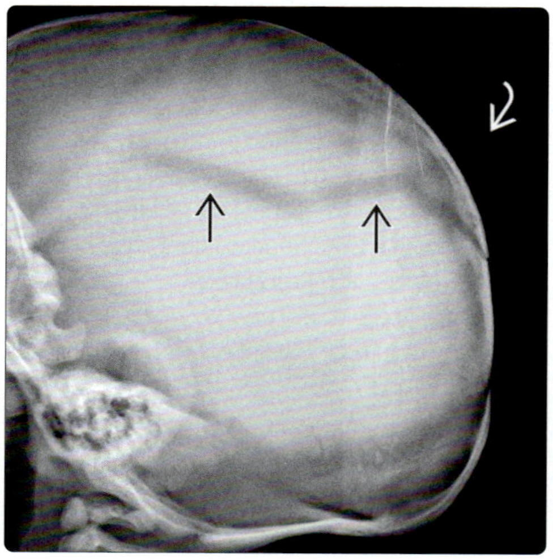

(Left) *Lateral radiographic (left) & STIR MR (right) images in an 8 month old with petechia show osseous fragmentation of the spinous processes with corresponding marrow edema & soft tissue injury due to abuse.* **(Right)** *Lateral radiograph shows a diastatic linear parietal skull fracture with a large overlying soft tissue hematoma in this 1 month old with numerous rib & metaphyseal fractures.*

Child Abuse

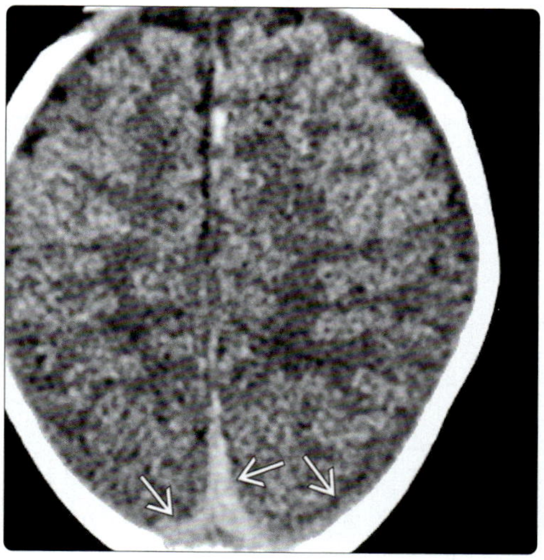

Child Abuse

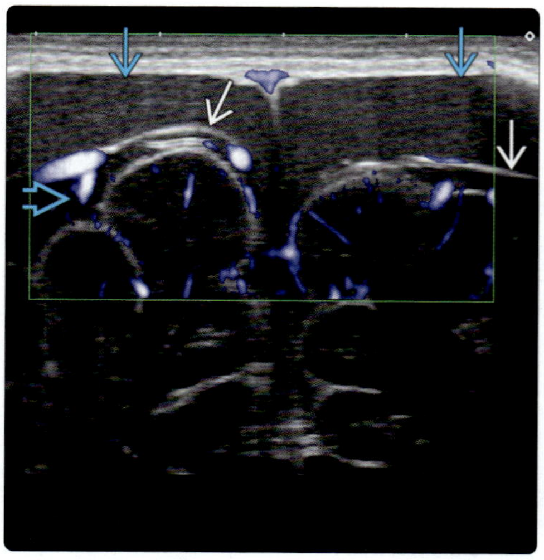

(Left) *Axial NECT shows hyperattenuating subdural blood overlying the occipital cortex in this 2 month old found to have > 15 fractures of varying ages.* **(Right)** *Coronal color Doppler US in a 2 month old with a bulging fontanelle shows large bilateral subdural collections with abnormal displacement of the arachnoid membrane from the dura. No traversing vessels are seen in the subdural spaces, only within the subarachnoid spaces . Numerous fractures were found upon further imaging.*

Birth Trauma

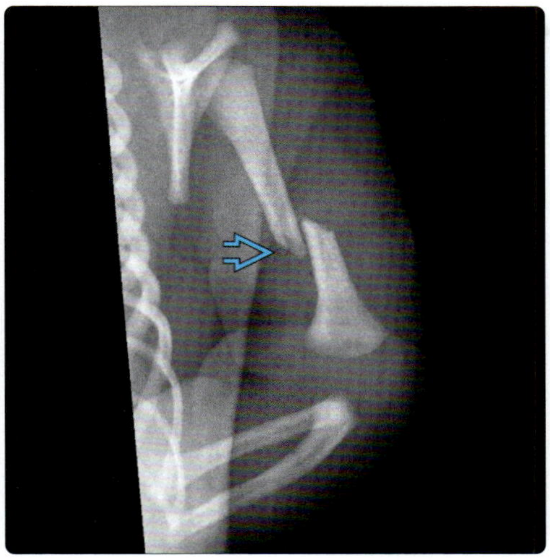

Birth Trauma

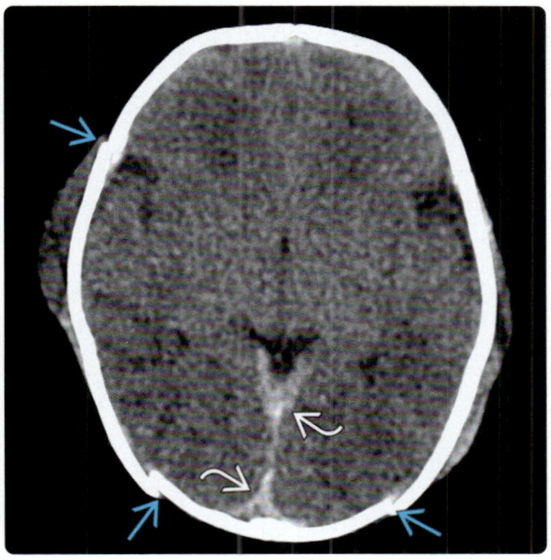

(Left) *Internal rotation radiograph in a 1 day old shows a displaced fracture of the left humeral diaphysis due to a birth injury.* **(Right)** *Axial NECT in a 1 day old shows small subdural hemorrhages & sutural diastasis. The delivery was difficult, requiring forceps & vacuum assistance.*

Benign Enlargement of Subarachnoid Spaces

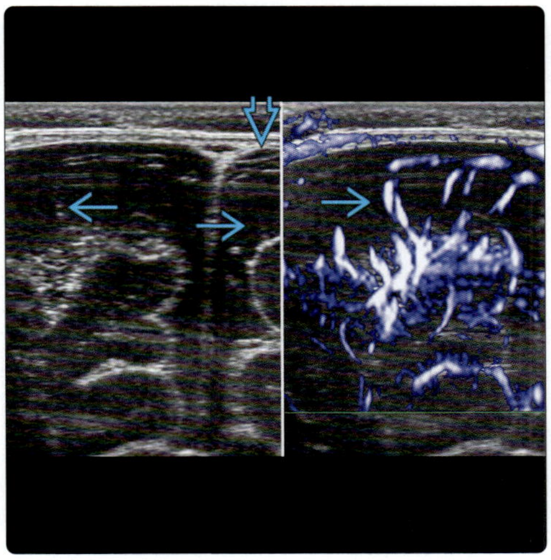

Benign Enlargement of Subarachnoid Spaces

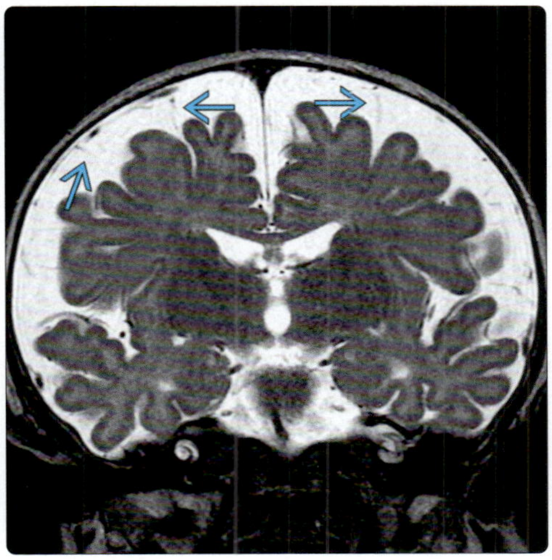

(Left) *Coronal grayscale & color Doppler US in a 2 month old with macrocrania show enlargement of the subarachnoid spaces, which are traversed by normal vessels. There is a tiny incidental subdural collection of doubtful significance.* **(Right)** *Coronal T2 MR in the same patient at 5 months of age shows continued moderate enlargement of the subarachnoid spaces. Normal vessels traverse the subarachnoid spaces, & no subdural collection is seen. There is no mass effect on the gyri.*

Periosteal Reaction of Other Causes

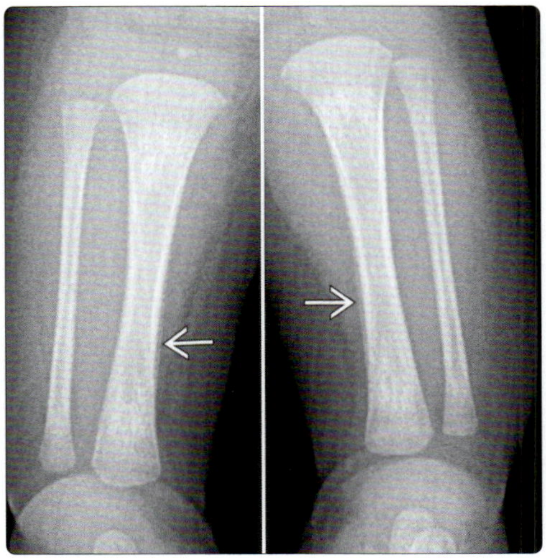

Normal Anatomic Variants

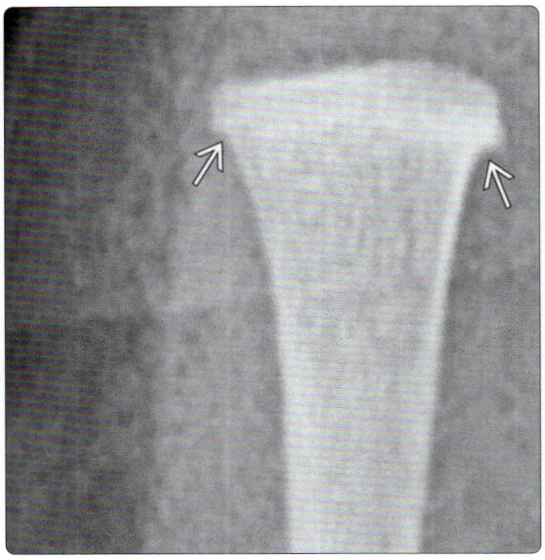

(Left) *AP radiographs of the bilateral lower legs in a 2 month old demonstrate physiologic periosteal reaction, which is thin, symmetric, & diaphyseal. This appearance is also commonly seen at the humeri & femurs between the ages of 1-6 months.* **(Right)** *PA radiograph of the distal radial metaphysis demonstrates a step-off at the junction of the cortex & subperiosteal bone collar. This is normal developmental anatomy & does not represent a fracture.*

(Left) *AP radiograph of the acromion shows a well-circumscribed ossicle at the anterior-inferior tip, consistent with a normal variant ➡, which could be mistaken for the acromion fracture (a high-specificity fracture for child abuse).* **(Right)** *Posterior 3D surface rendered CT from an 8 year old status post trauma depicts a large right accessory ossicle ➡ formed by connection of accessory sutures. There are multiple smaller intrasutural bones at the left lambdoid suture ➡.*

Normal Anatomic Variants

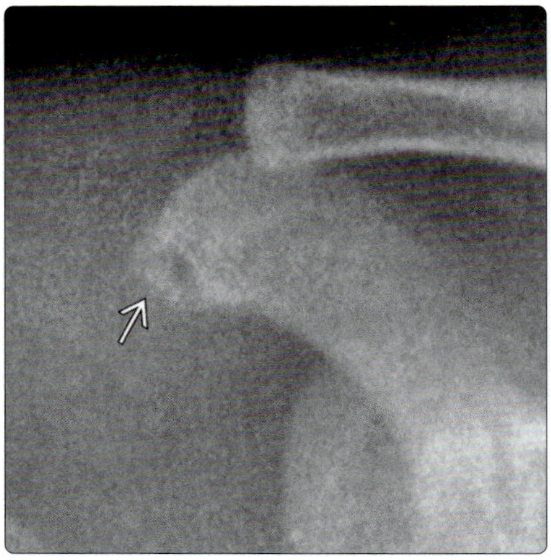

Wormian Bones & Accessory Sutures

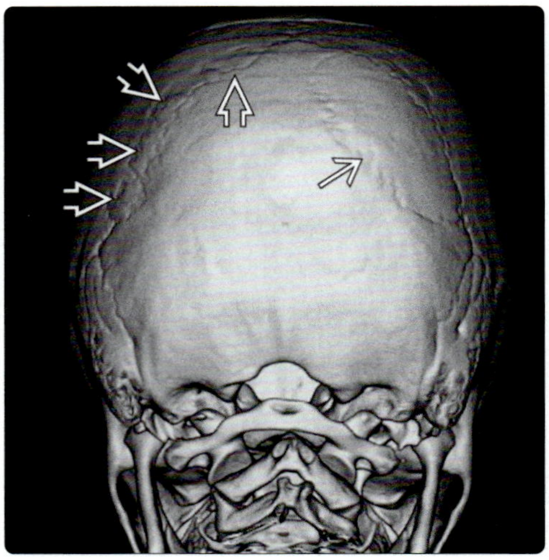

(Left) *Posterior 3D surface rendered CT of the skull in a term infant depicts a bipartite interparietal bone ➡ & mendosal sutures ➡, both of which are normal anatomic variants.* **(Right)** *Oblique radiograph demonstrates rounded densities overlying the left 4th-7th ribs ➡. These densities are the sternal ossification centers but could be mistaken for healing rib fractures.*

Wormian Bones & Accessory Sutures

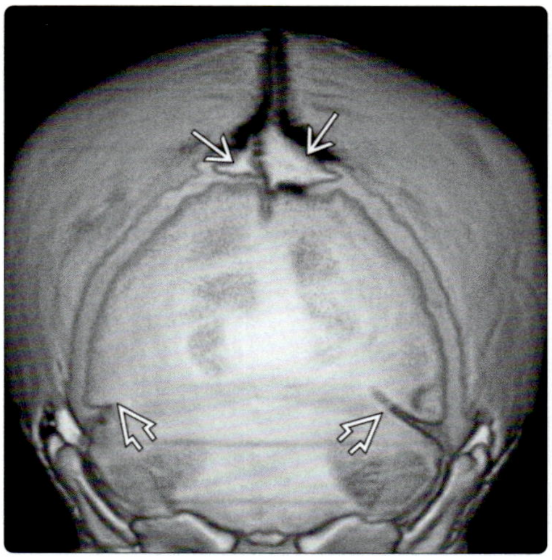

Artifacts

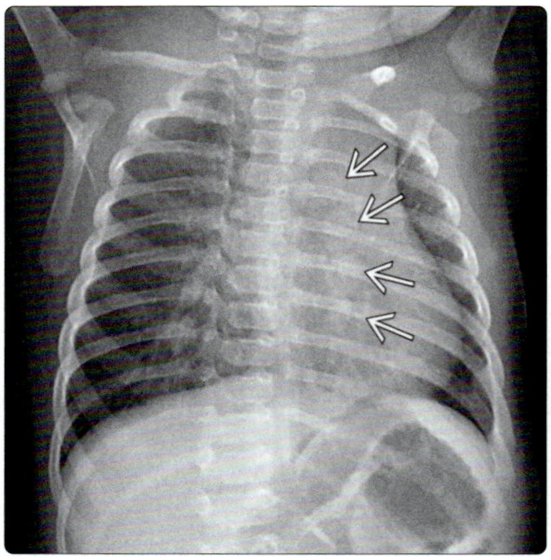

(Left) *PA radiograph of the wrist in a 4 year old with rickets depicts classic findings of the distal radius & ulna with metaphyseal cupping & fraying & loss of the ZPC.* **(Right)** *AP radiographs of the knees in the same patient with rickets demonstrates physeal widening with metaphyseal fraying, cupping, & flaring. Note that while fractures can be seen in rickets, they are typically in children with increased mobility (relative to young infants) & are not the high-specificity fractures seen in child abuse.*

Rickets

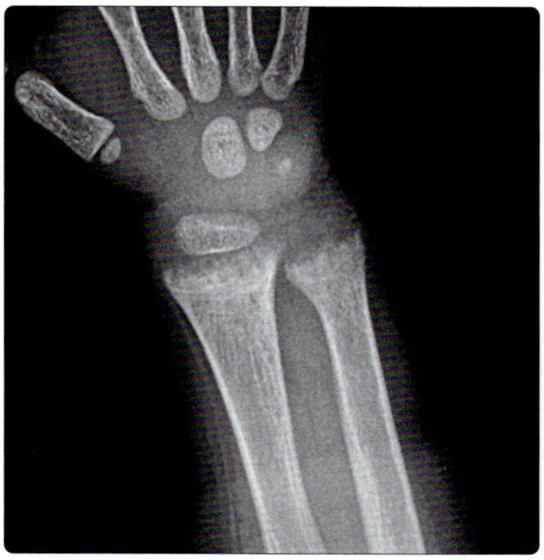

Rickets

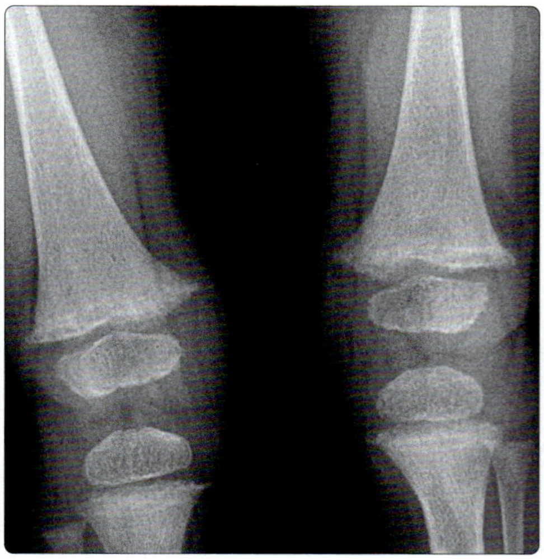

Osteogenesis Imperfecta

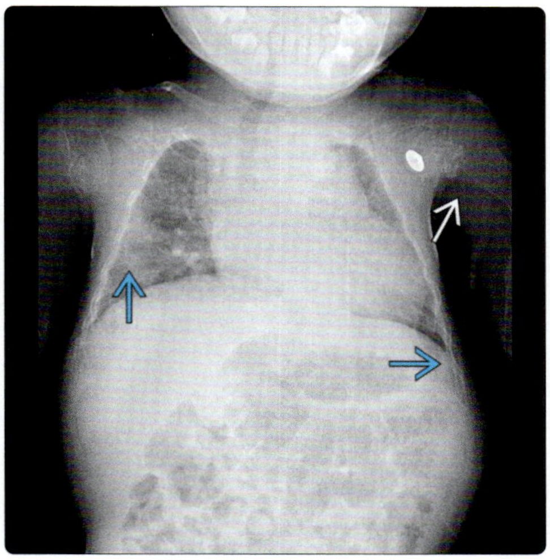

Osteogenesis Imperfecta

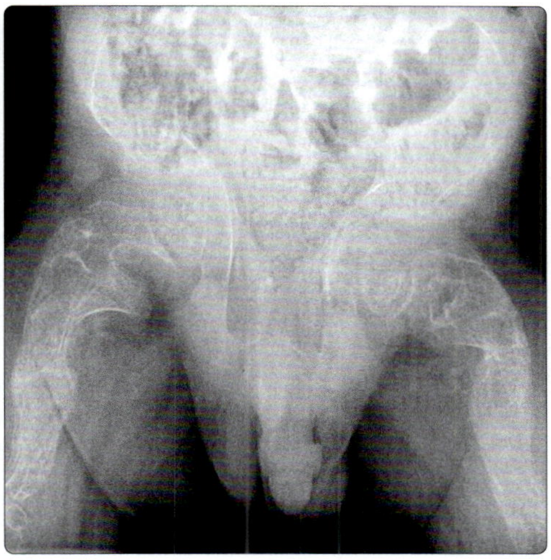

(Left) *Frontal radiograph of the chest in a 6 year old with osteogenesis imperfecta demonstrates diffuse osteoporosis. Remote fractures of the left humerus are partially visualized* ➡*, & the ribs are noted to have irregular undulations due to prior fractures* ⇨*.* **(Right)** *AP radiograph of the pelvis in the same patient with osteogenesis imperfecta shows severe deformities of the femurs secondary to multiple prior fractures with healing & remodeling.*

Osteogenesis Imperfecta

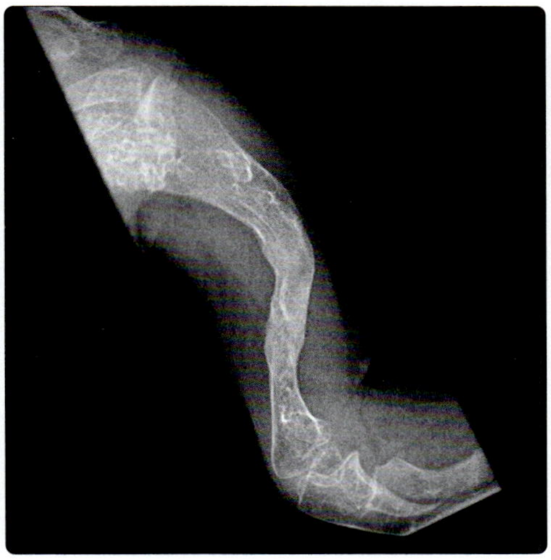

Congenital Syphilis

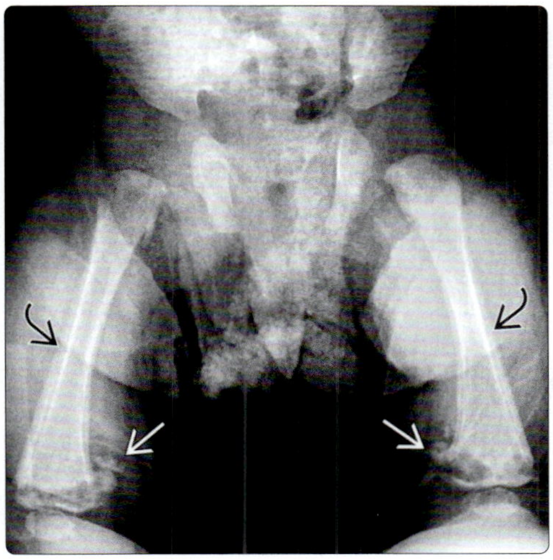

(Left) *External rotation radiograph shows severe deformity of the left humerus with evidence of healed fractures in the same patient with osteogenesis imperfecta. Similar changes are also partially visualized in the proximal forearm.* **(Right)** *Frontal radiograph shows a 10-week-old child with bilateral destructive metaphyseal lesions* ➡ *of the distal femurs with associated thick periosteal reaction* ⇨*. Serology confirmed congenital syphilis.*

Menkes Syndrome

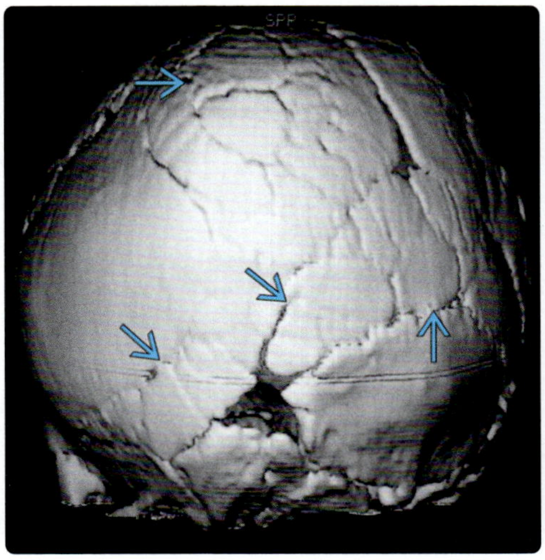

Menkes Syndrome

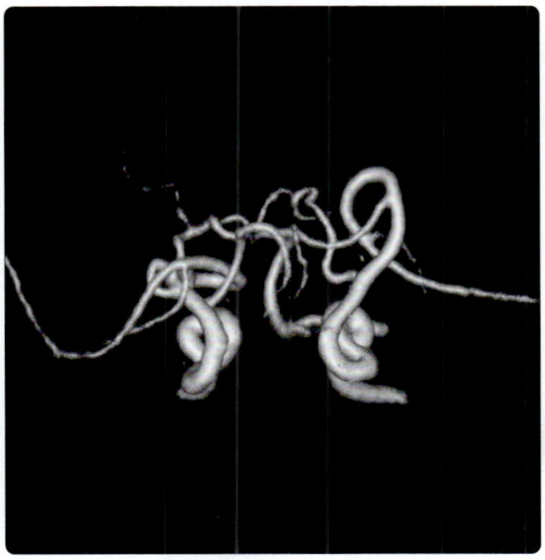

(Left) *Lateral surface rendered 3D CT of the skull in an 11 week old with seizures demonstrates numerous wormian bones* ⇨*.* **(Right)** *3D MRA from the same patient depicts marked tortuosity of the cervical & intracranial arteries, including the circle of Willis. This patient was confirmed to have Menkes syndrome, which can also demonstrate metaphyseal spurs & long bone fractures.*

SECTION 6

Brain

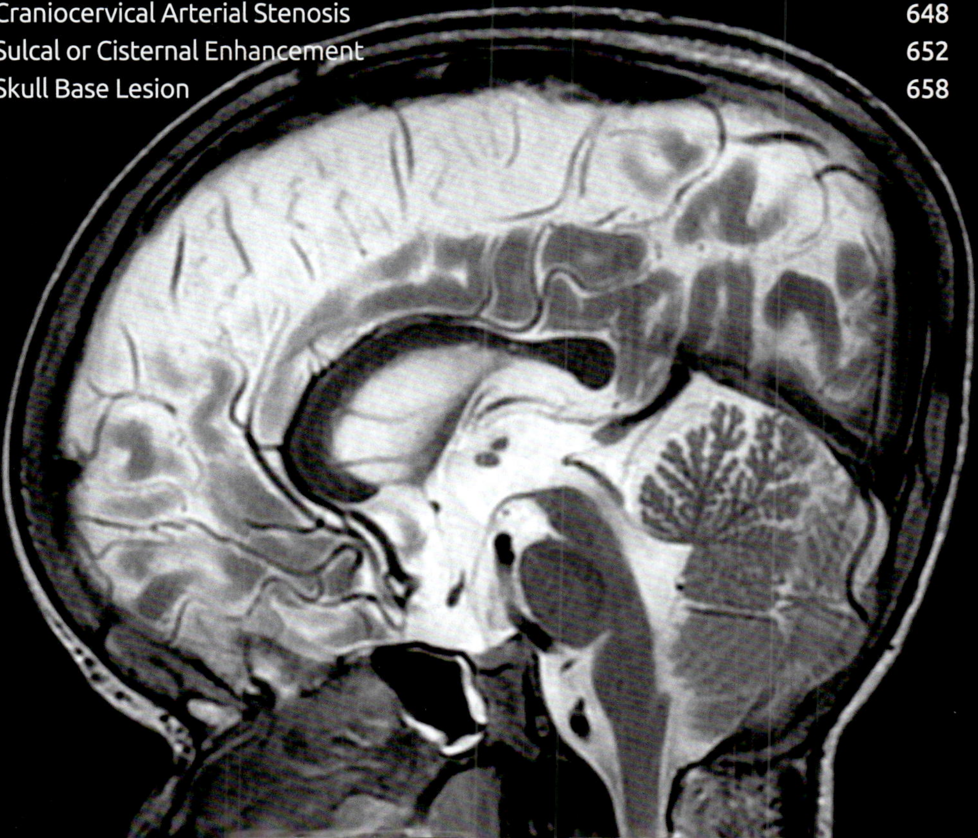

DIFFERENTIAL DIAGNOSIS

Common

- Secondary/Acquired From
  - Hypoxic-Ischemic Encephalopathy
  - Abusive Head Trauma
  - Shunted Severe Neonatal Hydrocephalus
  - Infectious Sequelae
    - TORCH Infections
    - Encephalitis
    - Meningitis
    - Neonatal Herpes Encephalitis

Less Common

- Primary/Genetic
  - Microcephaly With Simplified Gyral Pattern
  - Malformations of Cortical Development
    - Lissencephaly
    - Pachygyria
    - Polymicrogyria
  - Commissural Anomalies
    - Agenesis of Corpus Callosum
    - Callosal Dysgenesis
  - Holoprosencephaly

Rare but Important

- Craniosynostosis
- Pontocerebellar Hypoplasia
- Fetal Alcohol Syndrome
- Hypomyelination

ESSENTIAL INFORMATION

Key Differential Diagnosis Issues

- Clinical considerations
  - Review newborn head circumference
    - Small: Consider primary/genetic vs. intrauterine insult
    - Normal: Subsequent (i.e., postnatal) insult
  - Clinical history is key
    - Imaging sequelae of many postnatal insults (trauma, infection, ischemia, etc.) can look very similar
- Imaging considerations
  - ↓ craniofacial ratio on sagittal view suggests microcephaly
    - Confirm with head circumference measurement
  - Review prior imaging to help confirm etiology
  - Imaging patterns
    - Stenogyria → previously shunted severe hydrocephalus
    - Symmetric white matter Ca^{2+} → consider intrauterine infection
    - Brain malformations have specific anatomic abnormalities
    - Hypoxic ischemic encephalopathy → if symmetric, has typical imaging patterns
- Modality considerations
  - Fetal imaging (US & MR) may be very helpful in identifying etiology
  - NECT: Helpful to identify associated Ca^{2+}
  - MR: Best imaging tool
    - SWI: Helpful to identify Ca^{2+} & blood
    - 3D volumetric imaging with reconstructions for congenital malformations

Helpful Clues for Common Diagnoses

- **Hypoxic-Ischemic Encephalopathy**
  - Perinatal or birth asphyxia (asphyxia neonatorum)
  - Patterns helpful, even if no history
    - Profound: Atrophy, gliosis
      - Deep gray nuclei
      - Perirolandic cortex & cortical spinal tracts
    - Partial prolonged
      - Typical watershed encephalomalacia
    - Mixed or severe
      - Features of both
- **Abusive Head Trauma**
  - History is crucial
    - Majority of abuse occurs < 1 year of age
  - Early findings
    - Subdural hemorrhage over convexity, especially parasagittal
      - ± pollywog or lollipop sign of avulsed & thrombosed cortical vein
    - Brain parenchymal injury, often extensive, with edema
      - ± contusional tear/laceration/cleft
    - ± skull fracture
  - Chronic findings
    - ± chronic subdurals (with enhancing membranes)
    - Encephalomalacia in areas of prior parenchymal injury
- **Shunted Severe Neonatal Hydrocephalus**
  - Severe hydrocephalus results in overall brain parenchymal volume loss
    - Patients are usually macrocephalic initially; if shunted early in life, may become microcephalic
    - Stenogyria is typical in shunted patients with history of severe hydrocephalus
- **Infectious Sequelae**
  - **TORCH infections**
    - CMV, Zika, & rubella are most likely to cause microcephaly
    - Toxoplasmosis, CMV, HIV, Zika, & rubella may have intracranial Ca^{2+}
      - CMV: Parenchymal or periventricular Ca^{2+}
      - HIV: Basal ganglia & subcortical Ca^{2+}
      - Toxoplasmosis: Parenchymal or periventricular Ca^{2+}
    - Rubella, Zika, & herpes simplex virus: Lobar brain destruction/encephalomalacia
    - CMV: Cortical dysplasia, hypomyelination, temporal pole cysts, cerebellar anomalies
  - **Encephalitis**
    - Many viral & autoimmune encephalitides
    - Findings of diffusion restriction & hemorrhage often lead to significant brain atrophy → microcephaly
  - **Meningitis**
    - Early infancy: Group B *Streptococcus* is most damaging
      - Often profoundly affects deep gray matter due to small vessel vasculitis & resultant ischemia
      - Leptomeningeal involvement ± subdural empyema
  - **Neonatal herpes encephalitis**
    - Symptoms (e.g., seizures) occur 3-5 weeks after birth
    - Location quite variable; often extensive/multilobar

- Diffusion restriction is most sensitive for early disease
- Infection typically results in large areas of cystic encephalomalacia → microcephaly

Helpful Clues for Less Common Diagnoses

- **Primary/Genetic**
  - **Microcephaly with simplified gyral pattern**
    - Number of gyri/sulci are reduced, though gray-white matter interfaces are preserved
    - Numerous genetic causes, many of which have additional parenchymal malformations
      - Overlap with other categories
  - **Malformations of cortical development**
    - Lissencephaly
      - Severe malformation of cortical development
      - Absence of normal sulcation/gyration
      - Cerebral mantle is severely malformed with multiple abnormal layers of gray & white matter
    - Pachygyria
      - Abnormally thick cortex within broad, smooth gyri
    - Polymicrogyria
      - Irregular, nodular cortex & gray matter-white matter junction
      - Shallow sulci ± underlying white matter volume loss
      - Usually perisylvian in location but can occur anywhere
      - May be unilateral or bilateral (often symmetric)
      - Etiologies are diverse (CMV, syndromic, idiopathic, etc.)
  - **Commissural anomalies**
    - May be found with microcephaly, typically as part of underlying disorder rather than primary cause
    - Agenesis of corpus callosum
      - Look for absence of CC & cingulate gyrus
      - Parallel colpocephalic ventricles with high-riding 3rd ventricle
      - May be isolated or associated with other anomalies
    - Callosal dysgenesis
      - Small &/or malformed corpus callosum
      - Often associated with pericallosal lipoma
      - Usually associated with other brain malformations
  - **Holoprosencephaly**
    - Most severe forms typically have greatest degree of microcephaly
    - However, more severe forms will sometimes develop hydrocephalus & macrocephaly

Helpful Clues for Rare Diagnoses

- **Craniosynostosis**
  - It is rare for craniosynostosis to cause microcephaly
  - However, it is very common for patients with microcephaly from other causes to subsequently develop craniosynostosis
- **Pontocerebellar Hypoplasia**
  - Heterogeneous group of diseases
    - Many have associated supratentorial abnormalities causing microcephaly
  - Assess degree of deficiency
    - Presence of fastigial recess & primary fissure
    - Degree of vermian lobulation
    - Presence of elevated tegmentovermian angle (i.e., 4th ventricle appears open)
- **Fetal Alcohol Syndrome**
  - Often affects corpus callosum, cerebellar vermis, basal ganglia, & various parts of cerebrum
    - ↓ volume & altered microstructure
- **Hypomyelination**
  - White matter remains hyperintense on T2 MR beyond infancy
  - Many underlying disorders

SELECTED REFERENCES

1. Devakumar D et al: Infectious causes of microcephaly: epidemiology, pathogenesis, diagnosis, and management. Lancet Infect Dis. 18(1):e1-e13, 2018
2. von der Hagen M: Diagnostic approach to primary microcephaly. Neuropediatrics. 48(3):133-4, 2017
3. Gilmore EC et al: Genetic causes of microcephaly and lessons for neuronal development. Wiley Interdiscip Rev Dev Biol. 2(4):461-78, 2013
4. Basel-Vanagaite L et al: Clinical and brain imaging heterogeneity of severe microcephaly. Pediatr Neurol. 43(1):7-16, 2010

Hypoxic-Ischemic Encephalopathy

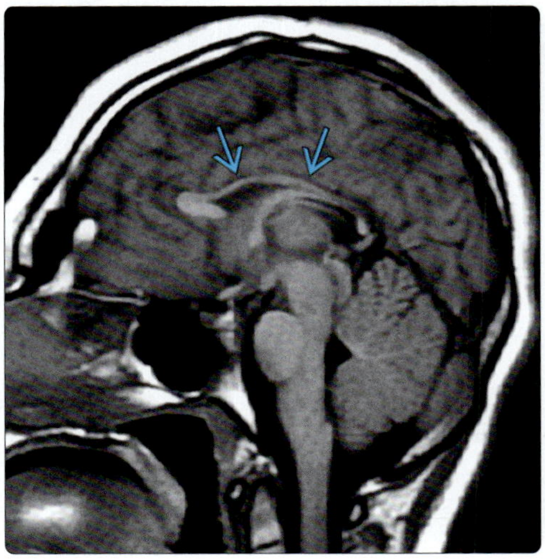

Hypoxic-Ischemic Encephalopathy

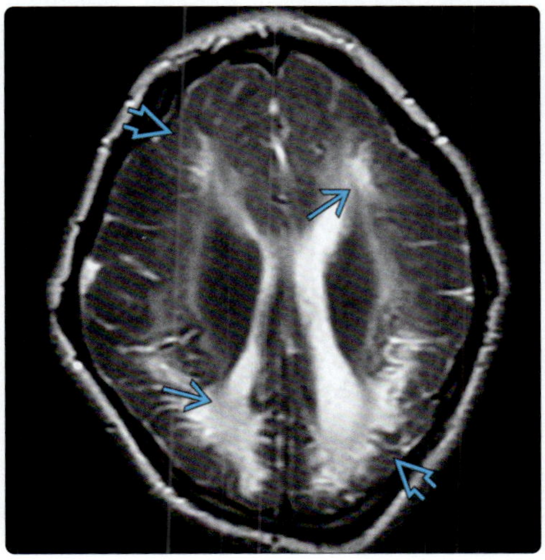

(Left) *Sagittal T1 MR in a 9 year old with microcephaly secondary to perinatal hypoxic-ischemic encephalopathy shows marked thinning of the corpus callosum ➙ as a consequence of severe bilateral encephalomalacia & leukomalacia.* **(Right)** *Axial T2 MR in the same patient shows extensive cortical encephalomalacia ➙ & severe leukomalacia ➙, resulting in microcephaly. Note the symmetric watershed distribution of injury, which is typical for moderate to severe partial-prolonged HIE.*

(Left) *Axial NECT in a 2 month old with severe abusive head trauma (AHT) shows a left-sided subdural hematoma with associated left cerebral hemisphere injury characterized by swelling & loss of deep & peripheral gray-white matter differentiation, resulting in marked subfalcine herniation.* **(Right)** *Follow-up coronal FLAIR MR in the same patient shows extensive foci of cystic & noncystic encephalomalacia, resulting in microcephaly.*

Abusive Head Trauma

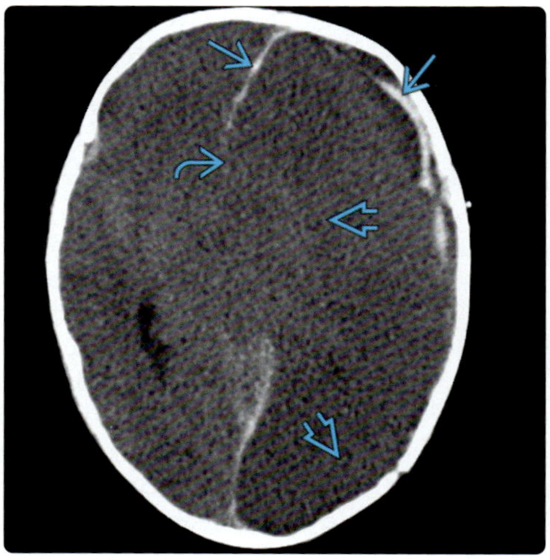

Abusive Head Trauma

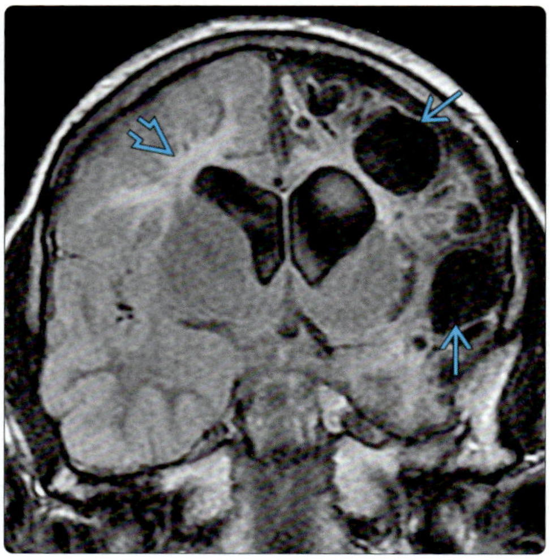

(Left) *Sagittal T2 MR in a neonate with severe hydrocephalus secondary to aqueductal stenosis shows marked enlargement of the lateral ventricles, which will require shunting.* **(Right)** *Sagittal T1 MR in the same patient at 3 years of age, after shunting, shows the relatively decreased size of the cerebrum in relation to the cerebellum. Note the thin, pencil-like parasagittal gyri (stenogyria). Also note the marked volume loss in the posterior corpus callosum due to the severe hydrocephalus.*

Shunted Severe Neonatal Hydrocephalus

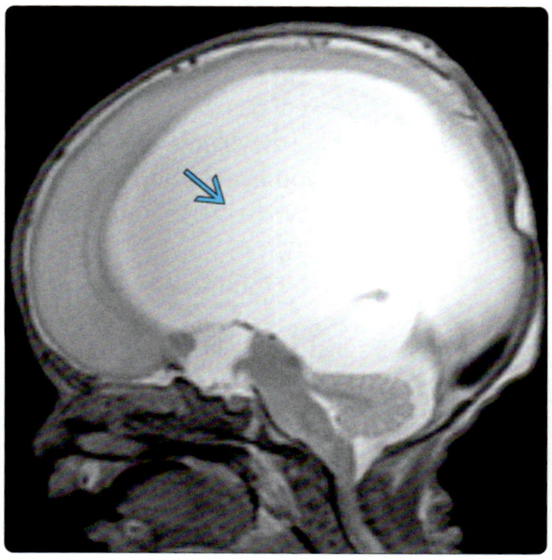

Shunted Severe Neonatal Hydrocephalus

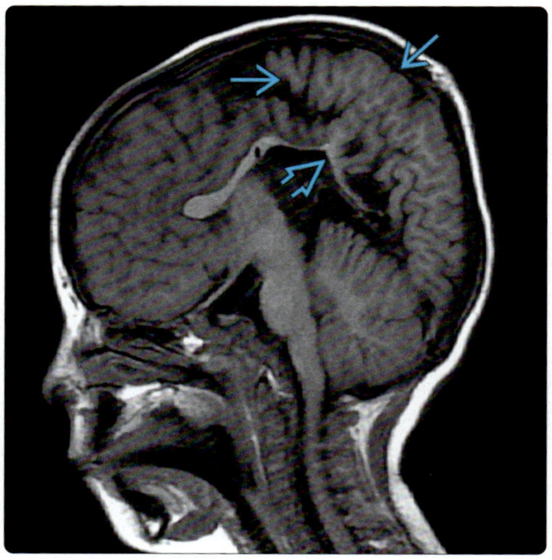

(Left) *Coronal NECT in a 3 year old with congenital CMV shows extensive periventricular Ca^{2+} & white matter gliosis. Look for associated findings of CMV, such as white matter changes, polymicrogyria, & anterior temporal cysts.* **(Right)** *Coronal NECT in an 8 year old with congenital toxoplasmosis shows nearly symmetric areas of cortical & subcortical Ca^{2+}, a common finding in congenital toxoplasmosis. When symmetric Ca^{2+} is present, consider congenital infection.*

TORCH Infections

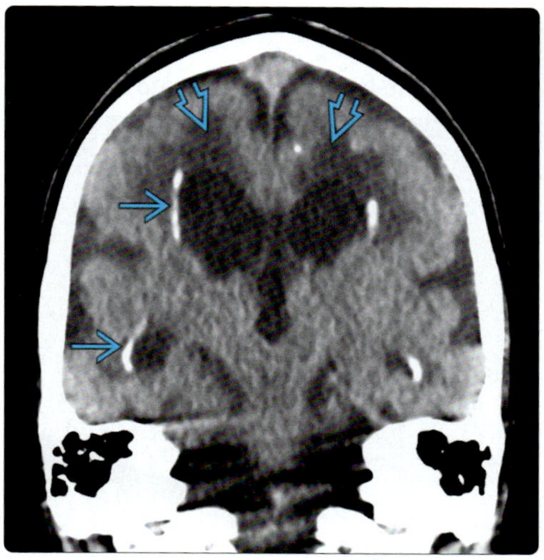

TORCH Infections

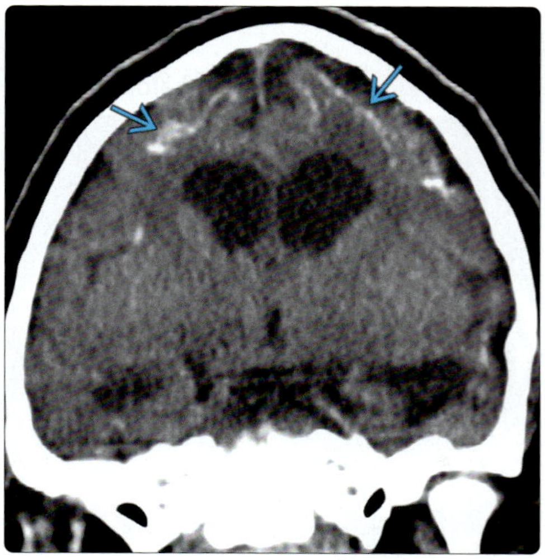

Encephalitis

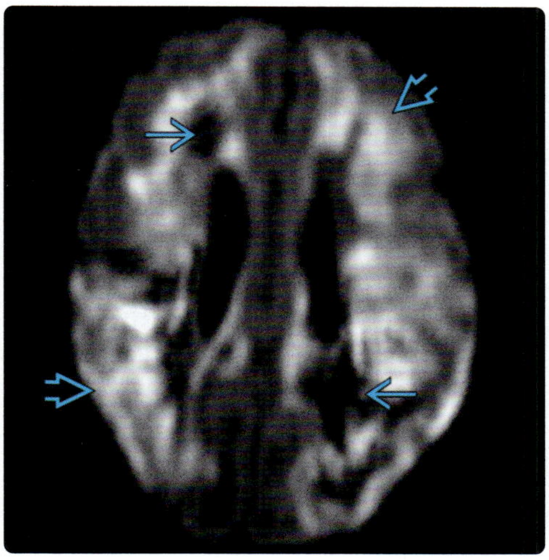

Encephalitis

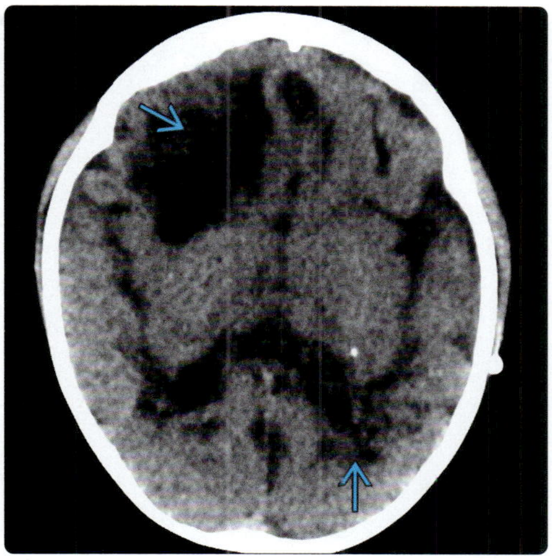

(Left) *Axial DWI MR in an 8 week old with necrotizing encephalitis shows nearly symmetric diffusion restriction → (↓ ADC, not shown) throughout both cerebral hemispheres. Areas of signal loss → corresponded to microhemorrhage on the SWI (not shown).* **(Right)** *Axial NECT in the same patient 6 years later shows multiple foci of encephalomalacia → & resultant brain parenchymal volume loss, contributing to microcephaly.*

Meningitis

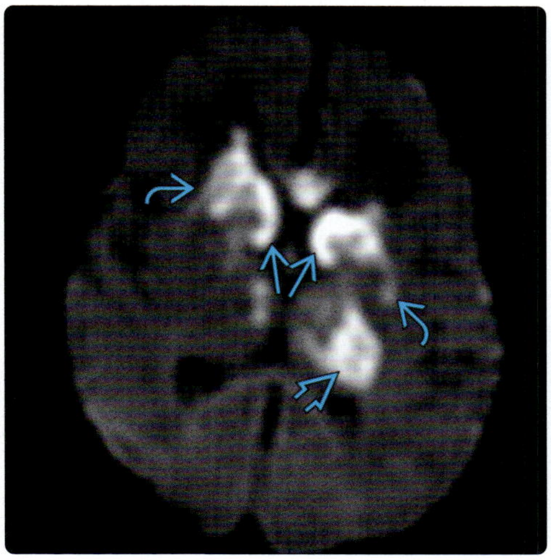

Meningitis

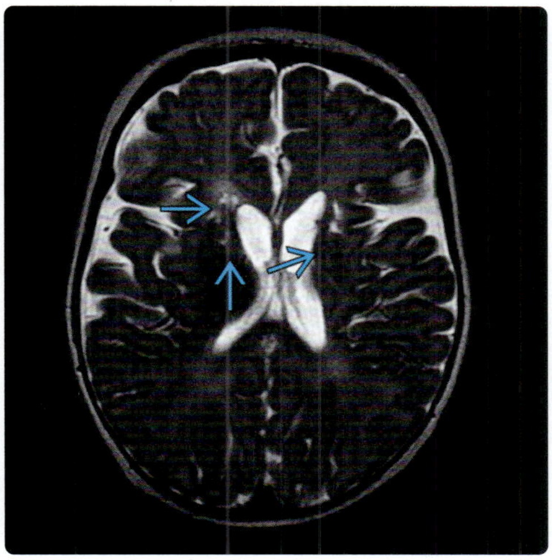

(Left) *Axial DWI MR in a 7 day old with group B streptococcal meningitis shows multiple foci of diffusion restriction (↓ ADC, not shown) in the bilateral caudate nuclei → & left thalamus → as well as external capsules →, likely secondary to small vessel vasculitis.* **(Right)** *Axial T2 MR in the same patient 2 years later shows encephalomalacic & volume loss in the previously affected areas →. Such processes leading to volume loss can result in microcephaly.*

Neonatal Herpes Encephalitis

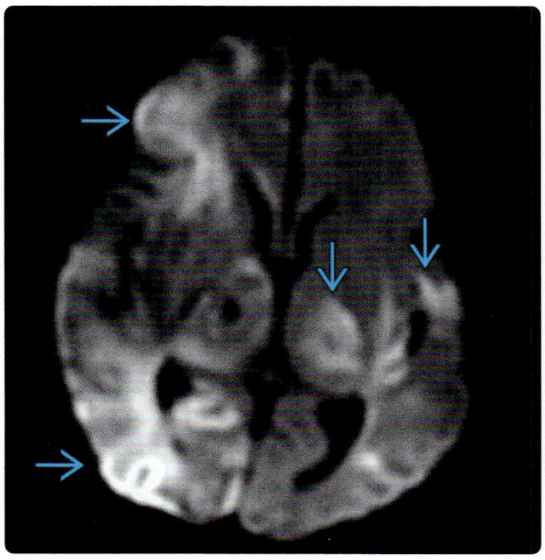

Neonatal Herpes Encephalitis

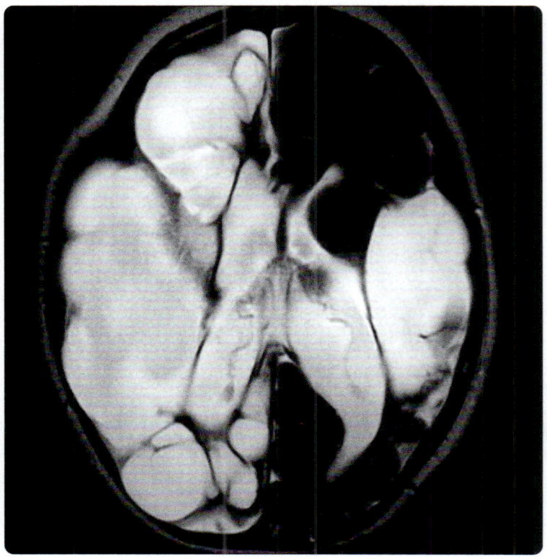

(Left) *Axial DWI MR in a 4 week old with neonatal herpes encephalitis shows extensive foci of diffusion restriction → (↓ ADC, not shown) in the bilateral (L > R) cerebral hemispheres & thalami, typical of herpes simplex virus type 2 in a neonate.* **(Right)** *Axial T2 MR in the same patient many months later shows large areas of cystic encephalomalacia at the sites previously affected on the 4-week MR exam. The degree of microcephaly depends upon whether the areas of cystic encephalomalacia expand or contract.*

(Left) *Axial T2 MR in a 3-week-old term infant with gyral simplification shows absence of the normal superior & middle frontal sulci in their expected locations →. The gray-white matter interfaces otherwise appear normal.* **(Right)** *Sagittal T1 MR in the same patient shows a smooth frontal lobe → & decreased craniofacial ratio in this patient with microcephaly.*

Microcephaly With Simplified Gyral Pattern

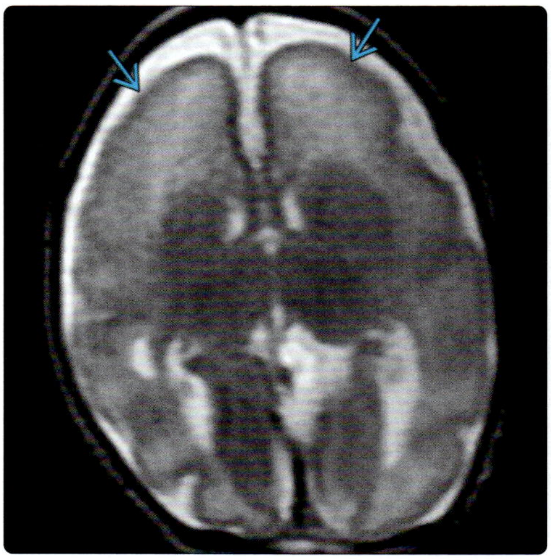

Microcephaly With Simplified Gyral Pattern

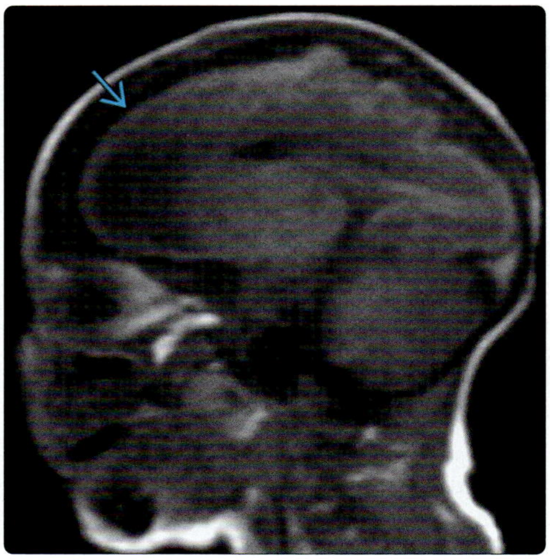

(Left) *Coronal T2 MR in a 1 year old shows a simplified gyral pattern with a markedly thickened cortex → in the frontal lobes, consistent with pachygyria.* **(Right)** *Coronal T2 MR in an 2 year old with polymicrogyria shows extensive symmetric cortical thickening with abnormally shallow sulci & nodular gyri →. Also note the enlargement of subarachnoid spaces → & ventricles →, secondary to the small brain parenchyma.*

Pachygyria

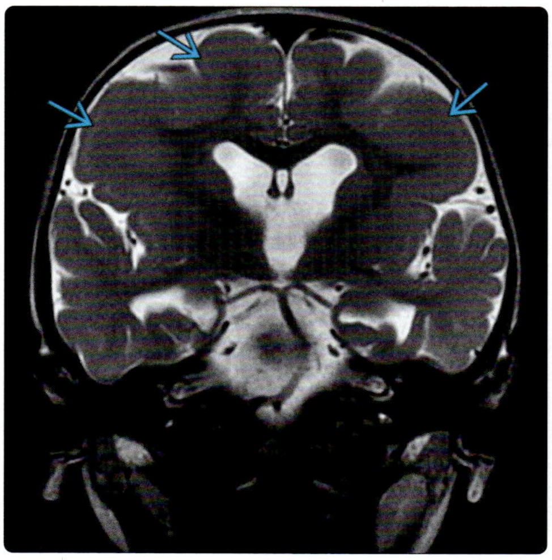

Polymicrogyria

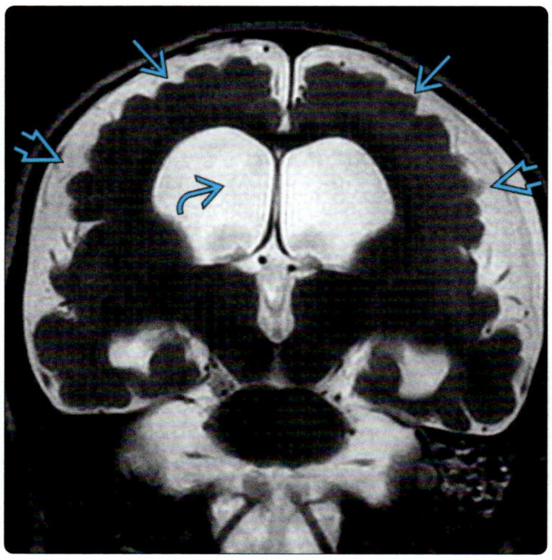

(Left) *Axial T2 MR in a neonate with lissencephaly shows a complete lack of sulcation with severe neuronal disorganization characterized by gray matter → extending from the periventricular zone to pia except for a small band of white matter → in the subcortical region.* **(Right)** *Sagittal T1 MR in a 5 month old with microcephaly & callosal dysgenesis shows a severely thinned & shortened corpus callosum →. No other malformations were identified.*

Lissencephaly

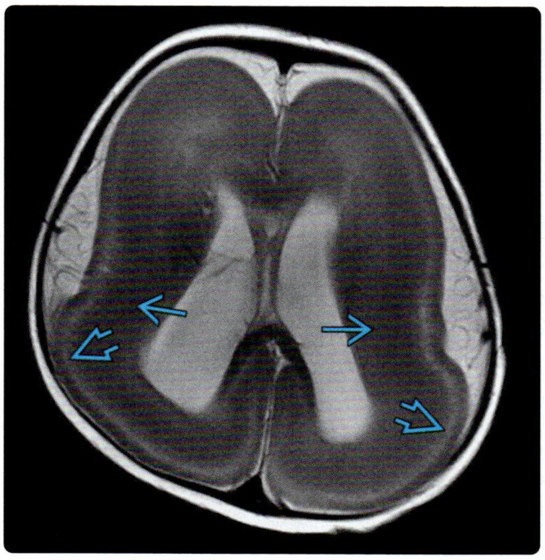

Callosal Dysgenesis

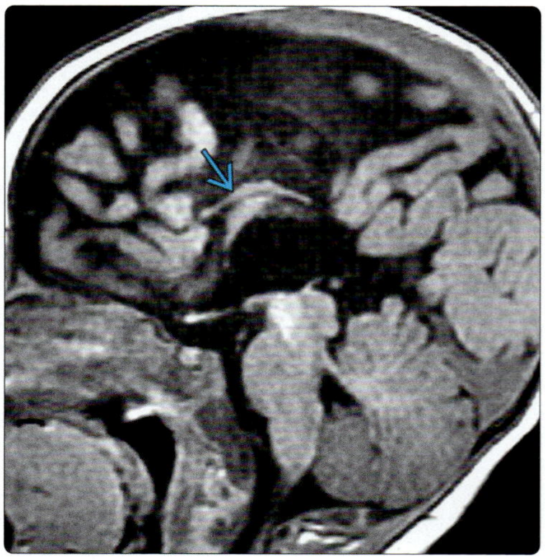

Agenesis of Corpus Callosum

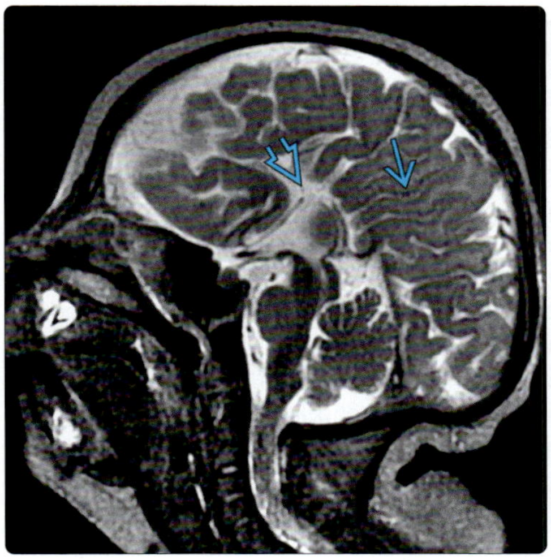

Agenesis of Corpus Callosum

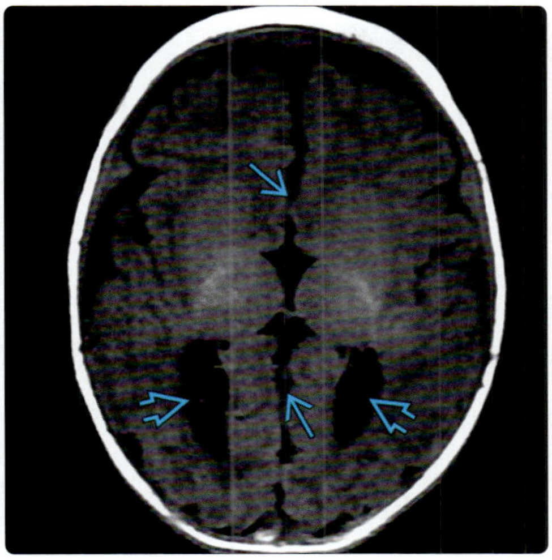

(Left) *Sagittal T2 MR in an 8 week old shows absence of the corpus callosum* ➡ *& cingulate gyrus with extension of parasagittal sulci* ➡ *to the deep midline. Note the small craniofacial ratio.* **(Right)** *Axial T1 MR in the same patient shows absence of the corpus callosum* ➡ *& mild dilation of the parallel lateral ventricles* ➡*, consistent with colpocephaly, a characteristic finding in callosal agenesis. Callosal agenesis may be solitary or associated with other anomalies.*

Holoprosencephaly

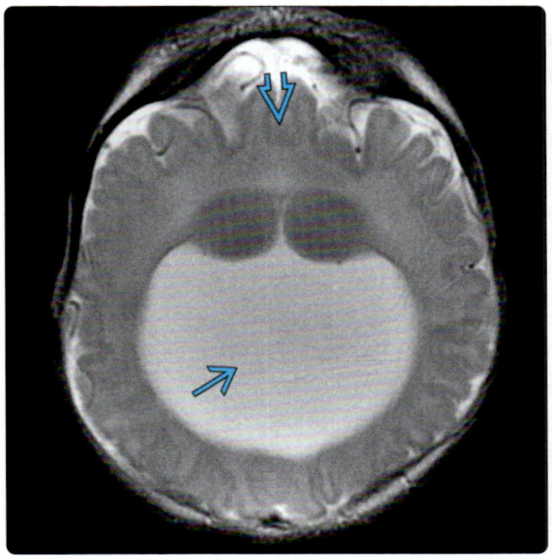

Holoprosencephaly

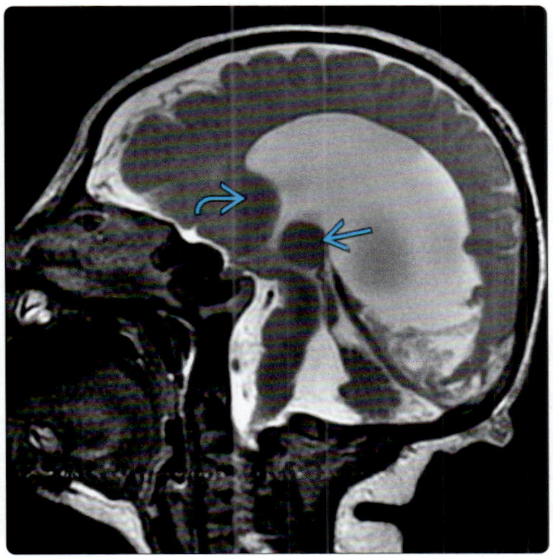

(Left) *Axial T2 MR in a neonate with alobar holoprosencephaly shows absence of the interhemispheric fissure* ➡ *due to a failure of division of the diencephalon into 2 cerebral hemispheres. Also note the characteristic large posterior monoventricle* ➡*.* **(Right)** *Sagittal T2 MR in the same patient with holoprosencephaly shows fused thalami* ➡ *& basal ganglia* ➡*. Note the decreased craniofacial ratio, consistent with microcephaly.*

Craniosynostosis

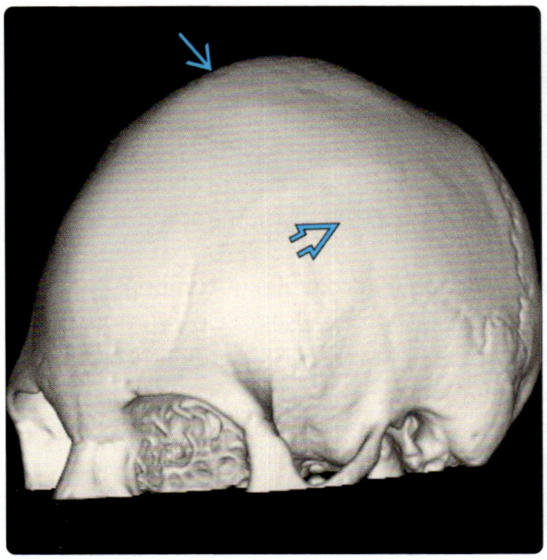

Pontocerebellar Hypoplasia

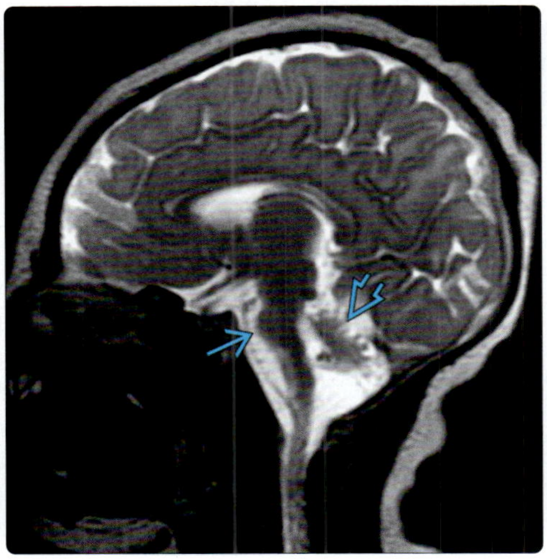

(Left) *CT 3D surface rendering of the skull in a 5 year old with gyral simplification shows premature fusion of the coronal* ➡ *& sagittal* ➡ *sutures. Craniosynostosis is more often a result of diseases causing microcephaly rather than the primary cause for microcephaly.* **(Right)** *Sagittal T2 MR in a neonate shows a small craniofacial ratio with very small size of the cerebellar vermis* ➡ *& pons* ➡*. Pontocerebellar hypoplasia is seen in a diverse array of diseases & genetic defects.*

Macrocrania/Macrocephaly

DIFFERENTIAL DIAGNOSIS

Common

- Benign Enlargement of Subarachnoid Spaces
- Hydrocephalus
  - Posthemorrhagic Hydrocephalus
  - Acute Infectious Hydrocephalus
  - Postinfectious Hydrocephalus
  - Aqueductal Stenosis
  - Obstructing Tumor
  - CSF Overproduction (Choroid Plexus Tumor)
- Chiari 2 Malformation
- Child Abuse (Abusive Head Trauma)

Less Common

- Neurofibromatosis Type 1
- Vein of Galen Aneurysmal Malformation
- Hemimegalencephaly
- Achondroplasia
- Dandy-Walker Malformation
- Hydranencephaly
- Holoprosencephaly

Rare but Important

- Glutaric Aciduria Type 1
- Alexander Disease
- Canavan Disease
- Vanishing White Matter Disease
- Megalencephalic Leukoencephalopathy With Subcortical Cysts

ESSENTIAL INFORMATION

Key Differential Diagnosis Issues

- Macrocrania = head circumference > 95th percentile
- Determinants of head circumference: Brain parenchyma, CSF spaces, calvarium, & scalp
- Clinical features to consider
  - Patients usually come to clinical attention during routine head circumference checks at well-child check-up
  - Age: Benign enlargement of subarachnoid spaces (BESS) develops in first 6-12 months & then plateaus
  - Normal or mild developmental delay suggests BESS
  - Focal neurologic signs, nausea/vomiting, ataxia, & seizures should prompt further work-up
- Imaging features to consider
  - Macrocephaly (large head) vs. megalencephaly (large brain)
    - Macrocephaly: Common, usually due to ↑ CSF spaces
    - Megalencephaly: Rare, due to brain overgrowth
  - Hydrocephalus
    - Obstructing hydrocephalus usually occurs at cerebral aqueduct, foramen of Monro, or 4th ventricle outlets
    - Communicating hydrocephalus results from CSF overproduction or poor CSF resorption
    - Some diseases have variable or mixed patterns
- Modality considerations
  - US: Important tool for initial evaluation of young infants with macrocephaly
    - Excellent visualization of paramidline CSF spaces
  - CT: Often 1st study with acute presentations & trauma
  - MR: Most definitive & comprehensive exam for determination of underlying cause of macrocephaly
    - Most sensitive for detecting previous Intraventricular hemorrhage (IVH) or infection

Helpful Clues for Common Diagnoses

- **Benign Enlargement of Subarachnoid Spaces**
  - a.k.a. benign hydrocephalus of infancy, external hydrocephalus, benign macrocrania of infancy
  - ↑ frontal/temporal subarachnoid spaces (SAS) ± mild ventriculomegaly
    - Will see normal veins traversing SAS, not displaced inward toward pial surface
  - Child is developmentally normal or has mild delay
  - Often with family history of macrocephaly
  - SAS usually normalize by ~ 2 years of age
- **Hydrocephalus**
  - Communicating: ↑ production or ↓ resorption of CSF
  - Obstructive: Flow of CSF is blocked by IVH, aqueductal stenosis, mass, etc.
  - Presents with enlarging head, crossing percentiles
    - May have signs of ↑ intracranial pressure
  - Often treated with shunting
  - **Posthemorrhagic hydrocephalus**
    - Most common in premature infants with IVH
    - Blood products/septations lead to obstruction of ventricular outlets &/or arachnoid granulations
    - Hemosiderin staining along ventricles/brainstem
      - □ SWI/GRE is most sensitive for detection of prior IVH
  - **Acute infectious hydrocephalus**
    - Increase in head size due to ↑ extraaxial spaces from meningitis &/or subdural/epidural empyema
  - **Postinfectious hydrocephalus**
    - Obstructing hydrocephalus may occur due to synechiae
    - Communicating hydrocephalus may occur due to arachnoid granulation dysfunction
  - **Aqueductal stenosis**
    - Congenital atresia/stenosis of cerebral aqueduct
    - Lateral & 3rd ventricular dilation with normal 4th
    - Narrowed/absent cerebral aqueduct on 3D SSFP MR
    - Lack of flow void within cerebral aqueduct on T2
  - **Obstructing tumor**
    - Can be secondary to small tumor in critical location
      - □ e.g., Subependymal giant cell astrocytoma (SEGA) at foramen of Monro, tectal plate glioma at cerebral aqueduct, ependymoma at 4th ventricular outlets
  - **CSF overproduction (choroid plexus tumors)**
    - CP papilloma/carcinoma causes CSF overproduction
      - □ Inability to resorb excess CSF → ↑ ventricular size
- **Chiari 2 Malformation**
  - Brain malformation due to spinal open neural tube defect (usually myelomeningocele)
  - Small posterior fossa, migration of cerebellum & brainstem into foramen magnum, elongated narrowed 4th ventricle, beaked tectum, dysplastic corpus callosum (CC), scalloped dorsal clivus, diminished extraaxial CSF spaces
  - Hydrocephalus requiring shunting occurs almost universally without in utero surgical repair

- May have microcephaly without hydrocephalus

- **Child Abuse (Abusive Head Trauma)**
  - Mechanism of injury: Shaking & impact
  - Subdural hemorrhages (SDHs), cytotoxic brain injury, ± skull fractures
    - Large SDHs may cause sudden increase in head size
  - Other findings: Bruising, burns, retinal hemorrhage

Helpful Clues for Less Common Diagnoses

- **Neurofibromatosis Type 1**
  - Café au lait macules, plexiform neurofibromas, & iris hamartomas
  - Nonenhancing lesions (often symmetric) in globus pallidus & cerebellum, large CC, optic pathway gliomas, & plexiform neurofibromas
- **Vein of Galen Aneurysmal Malformation**
  - Large posterior midline varix with phase-encoding pulsation artifact
    - Enlargement of venous sinuses & feeding arteries
    - Variable acute/chronic white matter (WM) damage
  - Secondary to direct communication between arterial network & median prosencephalic vein
    - Vein of Galen never forms
  - Ventricular enlargement may be due to
    - ↑ venous pressure → ↓ CSF resorption
    - Compression of ventricular outlets by varix
    - Parenchymal volume loss due to venous ischemia
- **Hemimegalencephaly**
  - Unilateral abnormal neuronal proliferation, migration, & differentiation → overgrowth of cerebral hemisphere (or lobe/lobes)
    - Elongated mildly enlarged ipsilateral ventricle
  - Neonate/infant: ↑ T1 & ↓ T2 signal in WM with blurred gray-WM junction
- **Achondroplasia**
  - Overgrowth of membranous calvarium → frontal bossing
  - ± hydrocephalus due to jugular foramen & foramen magnum stenosis
- **Dandy-Walker Malformation**
  - Vermian hypoplasia, large posterior fossa cyst communicating with 4th ventricle, lambdoid-torcular inversion
  - Often associated with hydrocephalus
- **Hydranencephaly**
  - In utero destruction of brain in internal carotid artery (ICA) territories
  - May cause poor CSF regulation & hydrocephalus requiring shunting
- **Holoprosencephaly**
  - Alobar subtype is often initially microcephalic; increasing size of monoventricle can lead to macrocrania
  - Typically treated with CSF shunting

Helpful Clues for Rare Diagnoses

- **Glutaric Aciduria Type 1**
  - Prominent sylvian fissures
  - ± basal ganglia signal abnormalities (↑ T2, ± diffusion restriction)
  - ± subdural collections, mimicking child abuse
- **Alexander Disease**
  - Frontal lobe demyelination & cysts, ventriculomegaly, & poor gray-WM differentiation
- **Canavan Disease**
  - Symmetric diffusion restriction in myelinated WM, elevated N-acetyl aspartate (NAA) on MR spectroscopy
- **Vanishing White Matter Disease**
  - Macrocephaly is less common but occurs secondary to expanding cystic CSF spaces that replace WM
  - Diffusely ↑ T2 in WM & thinning of CC without overall cerebral volume loss
- **Megalencephalic Leukoencephalopathy With Subcortical Cysts**
  - Diffuse expansion & ↑ T2 throughout WM with temporal & frontal cysts

SELECTED REFERENCES

1. Orrù E et al: The child with macrocephaly: differential diagnosis and neuroimaging findings. AJR Am J Roentgenol. 210(4):848-59, 2018

Benign Enlargement of Subarachnoid Spaces

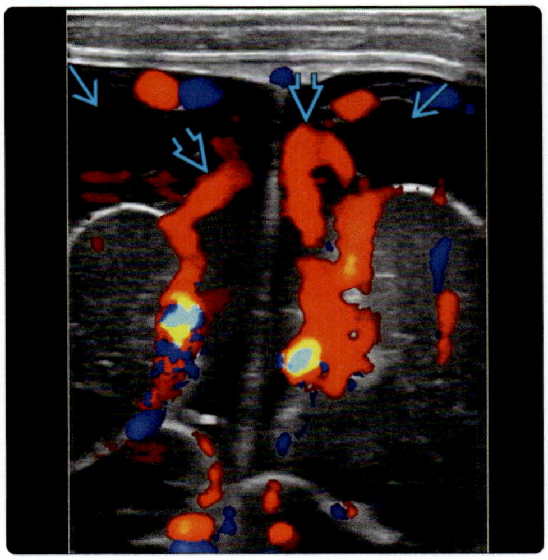

Benign Enlargement of Subarachnoid Spaces

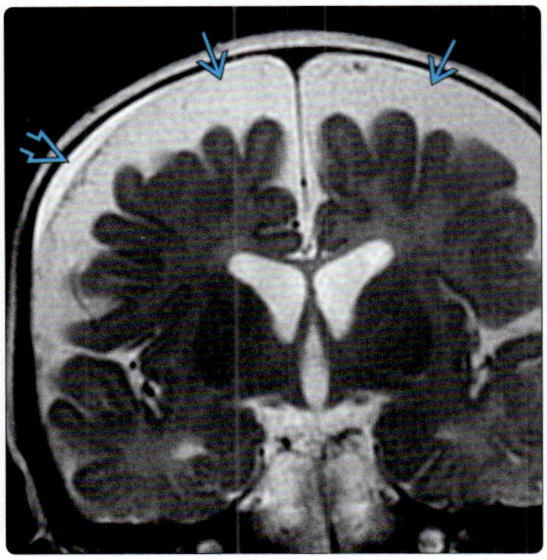

(Left) *Coronal color Doppler US in a 9 month old with benign enlargement of the subarachnoid spaces (BESS) shows vessels coursing through the CSF, consistent with prominent subarachnoid spaces.* **(Right)** *Coronal T2 MR in a developmentally normal 4 month old with BESS shows moderately enlarged subarachnoid spaces & a tiny, simple-appearing subdural collection on the right. Small, simple, subdural collections are associated with BESS & can be seen in as many as 10% of patients.*

(Left) *Sagittal T2 MR in a 1-month-old former premature infant with posthemorrhagic hydrocephalus shows marked enlargement of the lateral →, 3rd →, & 4th → ventricles. Note the dark hemosiderin → along the brainstem from prior intraventricular hemorrhage (IVH).* **(Right)** *Axial SWI MR in a 3-month-old former premature infant with posthemorrhagic hydrocephalus shows signal loss along the ependymal margins → of the ventricles & choroid plexus →, consistent with hemosiderin from prior IVH.*

Posthemorrhagic Hydrocephalus

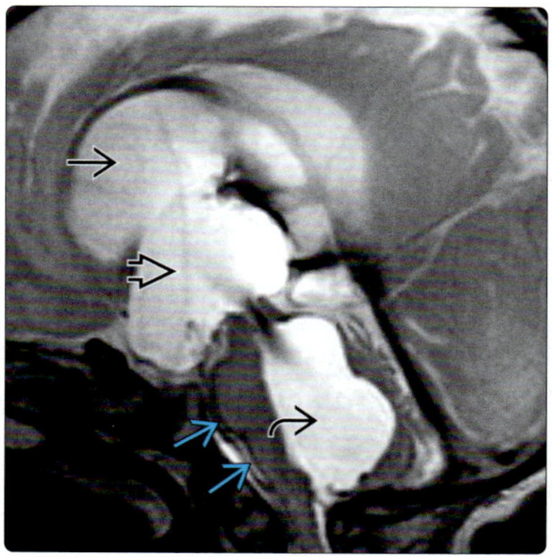

Posthemorrhagic Hydrocephalus

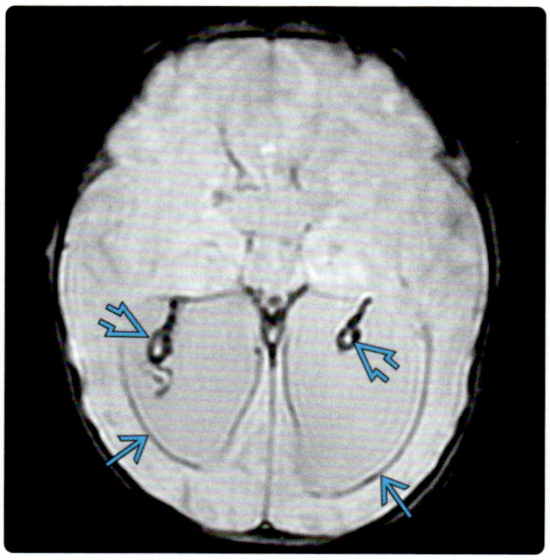

(Left) *Axial T1 C+ MR in a 7 year old with Haemophilus influenzae meningitis shows moderate expansion of the bifrontal subarachnoid spaces → & mild enlargement of the lateral ventricles →.* **(Right)** *Axial T1 C+ FS MR in an 8 month old with tuberculous meningitis shows extensive basilar leptomeningeal enhancement → & enlargement of the lateral ventricles →, resulting in macrocephaly. Granulomatous infections are more likely to result in hydrocephalus as compared to other bacterial meningitis.*

Acute Infectious Hydrocephalus

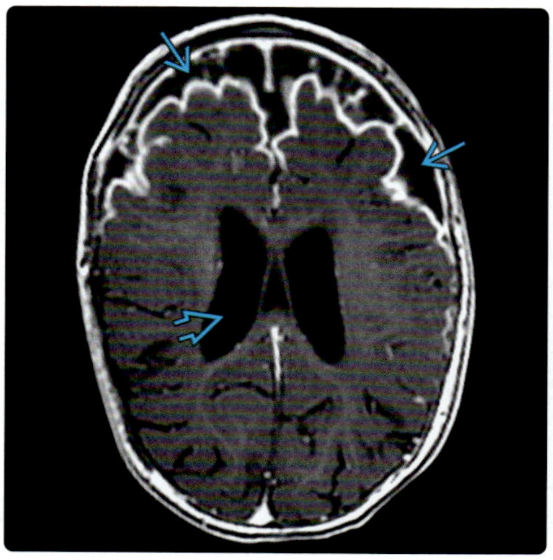

Postinfectious Hydrocephalus

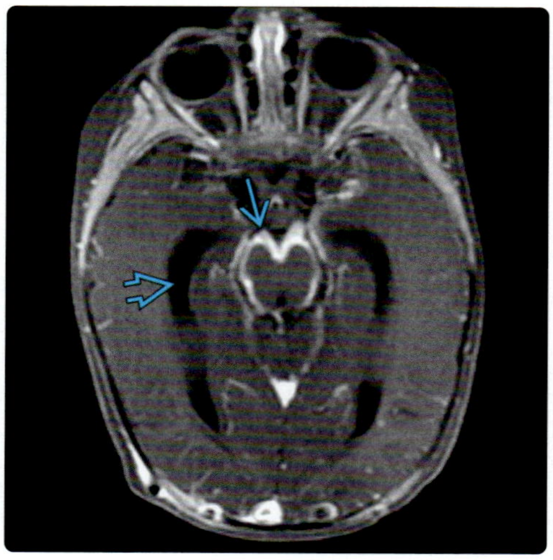

(Left) *Sagittal T2 MR in a neonate with aqueductal stenosis shows massive enlargement of the lateral ventricles → due to obstruction at the level of the cerebral aqueduct →.* **(Right)** *Sagittal FLAIR MR in a neonate shows a large obstructing & hemorrhagic posterior fossa mass (atypical teratoid-rhabdoid tumor) → causing enlargement of the lateral ventricles →. Note the markedly ↑ craniofacial ratio. Obstructing tumors in very young patients with open sutures may present with macrocephaly.*

Aqueductal Stenosis

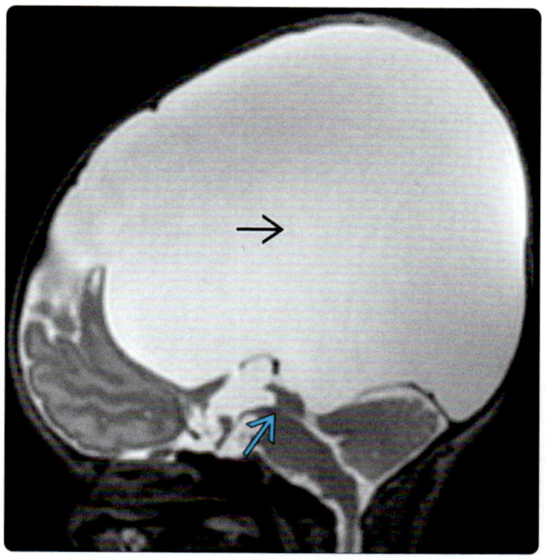

Obstructing Tumor

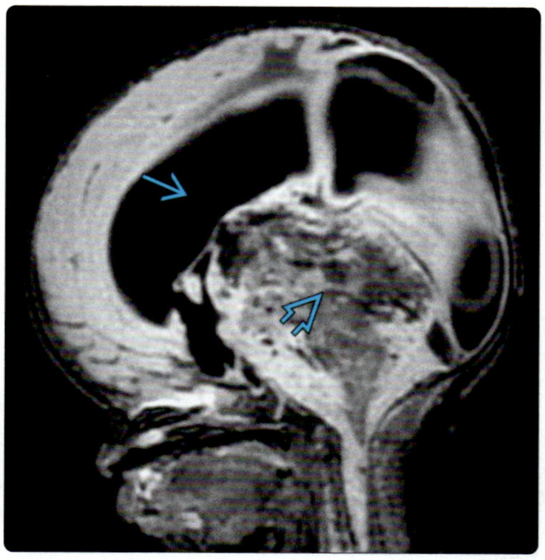

CSF Overproduction (Choroid Plexus Tumor)

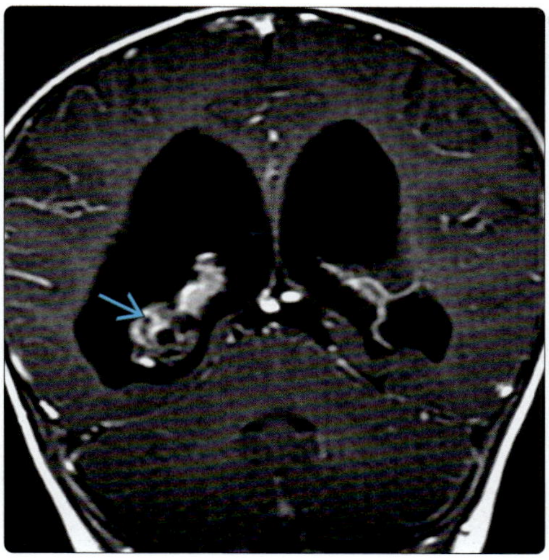

Chiari 2 Malformation

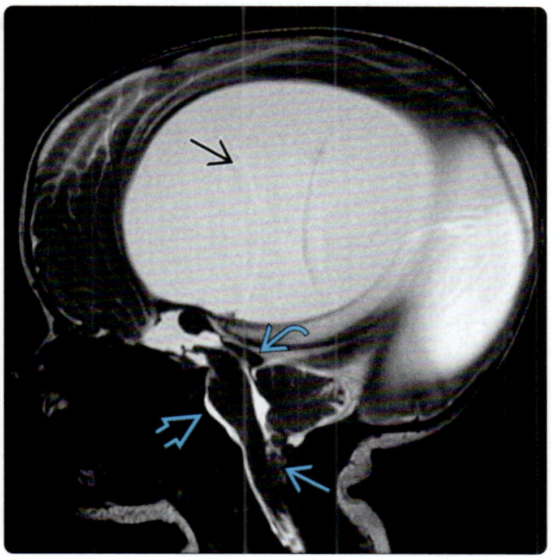

(Left) *Coronal T1 C+ MR in a 1 year old with an enhancing right choroid plexus papilloma* ⇨ *shows enlarged lateral ventricles but no evidence of obstruction. Hydrocephalus in this case is due to overproduction of CSF by the tumor.* **(Right)** *Sagittal 3D SSFP MR in a neonate with a myelomeningocele & Chiari 2 malformation shows marked enlargement of the lateral ventricles* ⇨ *& features of Chiari 2: Small posterior fossa, brainstem & tonsillar descent* ⇨*, beaked tectum* ⇨*, & scalloped clivus* ⇨*.*

Child Abuse (Abusive Head Trauma)

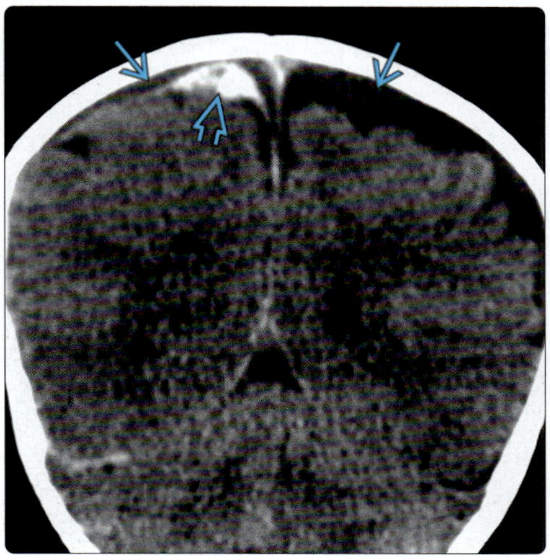

Child Abuse (Abusive Head Trauma)

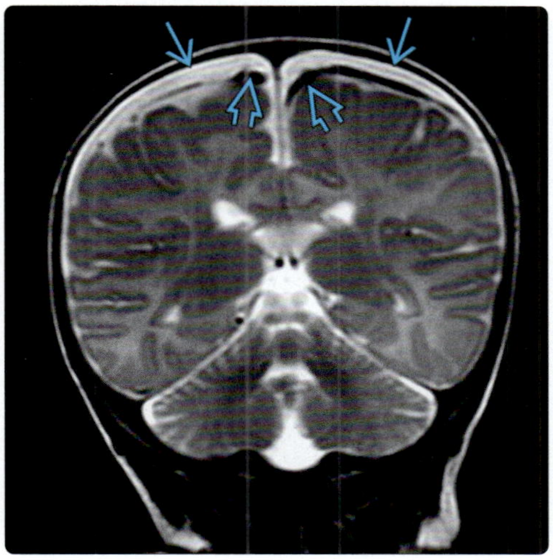

(Left) *Coronal NECT image in a 6 month old with abusive head trauma (AHT) shows bilateral subdural fluid collections* ⇨*, most of which are low in attenuation. The right parasagittal high attenuation* ⇨ *likely represents acute hemorrhage from a cortical vein avulsion, a finding highly associated with AHT.* **(Right)** *Coronal T2 MR in a 9 week old with AHT shows bilateral subdural fluid collections* ⇨ *with areas of hypointense signal* ⇨*, consistent with hemorrhage. Subdurals in AHT often cause an abrupt increase in head size.*

Neurofibromatosis Type 1

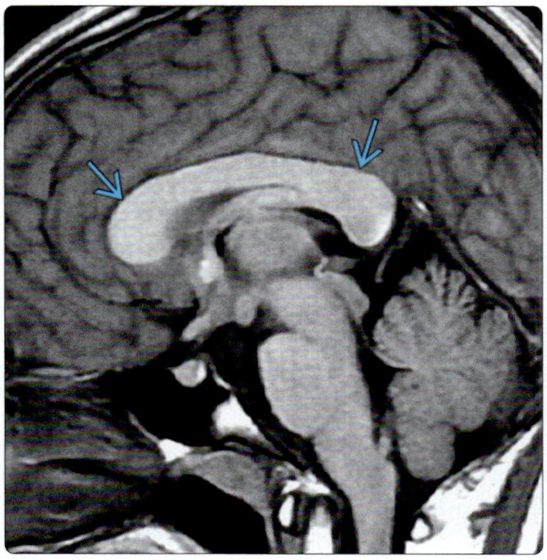

Vein of Galen Aneurysmal Malformation

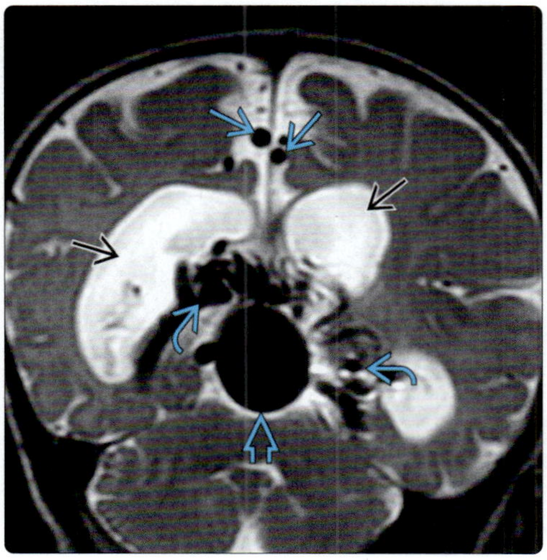

(Left) *Sagittal T1 MR in a teenager with neurofibromatosis type 1 (NF1) shows marked thickening of the corpus callosum* ⇨*. Some patients with NF1 will have mild macrocephaly due to megalencephaly.* **(Right)** *Coronal T2 MR in a neonate with a vein of Galen malformation has a large varix* ⇨ *with numerous enlarged choroidal* ⇨ *& pericallosal* ⇨ *feeding arteries. Note the enlarged ventricles* ⇨*, which are likely due to ↓ CSF resorption from ↑ venous pressures.*

Hemimegalencephaly

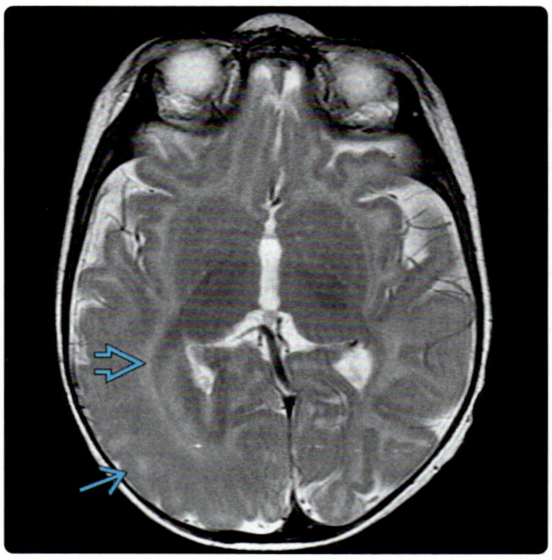

Hemimegalencephaly

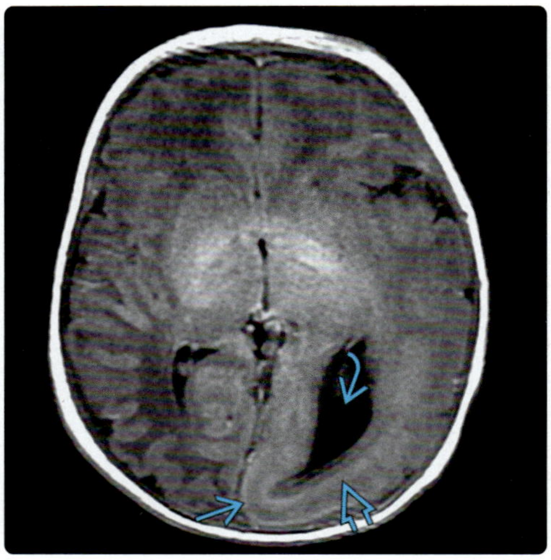

(Left) *Axial T2 MR in a 3 month old with hemimegalencephaly (HME) shows asymmetrically enlarged right temporal and occipital lobes with abnormal neuronal organization.* **(Right)** *Axial T1 MR in a neonate with seizures & HME shows ↑ size of the left parietal and occipital lobes with loss of normal sulcation & markedly abnormal neuronal organization. Also note the asymmetric enlargement of the left occipital horn, a common finding in HME.*

Achondroplasia

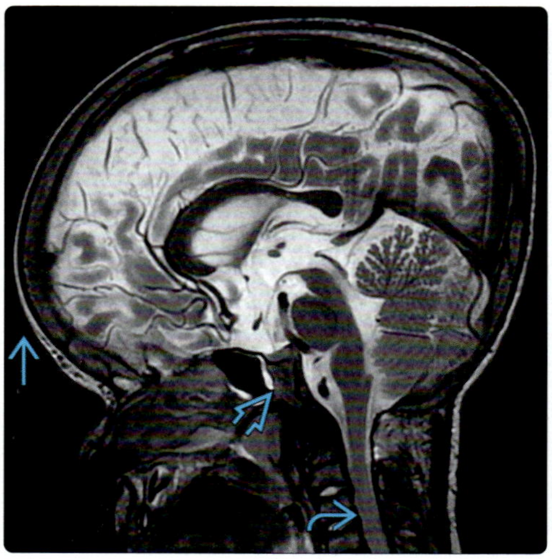

Dandy-Walker Malformation

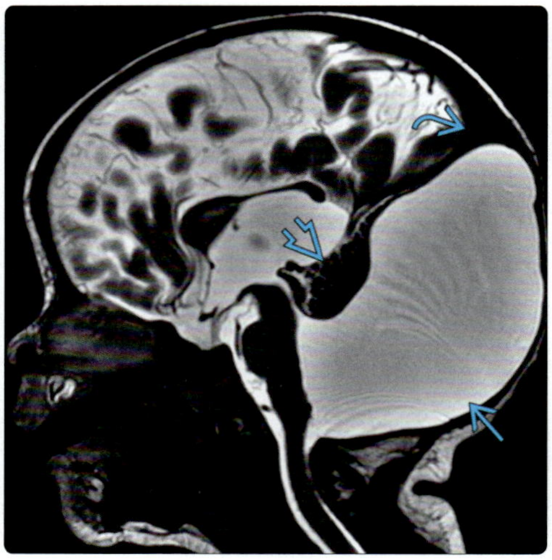

(Left) *Sagittal T2 MR in a 6 year old with achondroplasia shows characteristic features of the disease, including frontal bossing, a hypoplastic clivus, & narrowing of the upper cervical canal due to short pedicles.* **(Right)** *Sagittal 3D SSFP MR in a 2 month old shows a small cerebellar vermis & large posterior fossa cyst in continuity with the 4th ventricle, which elevates the tentorium & torcular Herophili, consistent with a classic Dandy-Walker malformation.*

Hydranencephaly

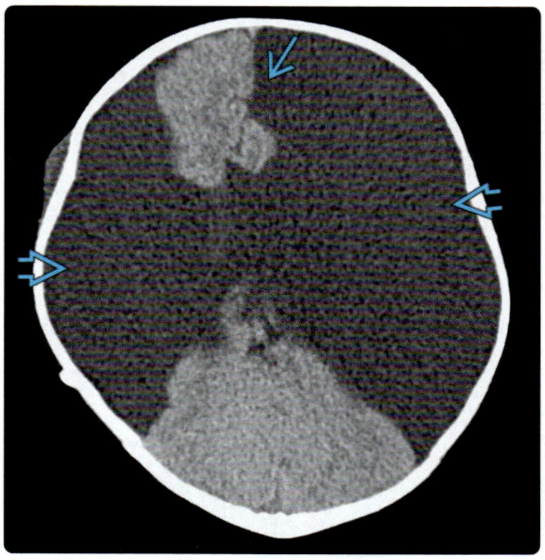

Holoprosencephaly

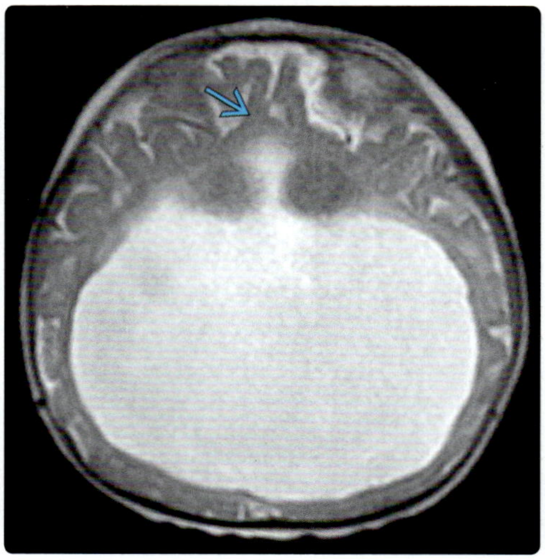

(Left) *Axial NECT in a 4 year old with hydranencephaly shows absence of brain parenchyma in the bilateral MCA & left ACA territories with an intact falx. Such patients become macrocephalic due to poor CSF regulation.* **(Right)** *Axial T2 MR in a 6 month old with holoprosencephaly shows marked enlargement of the monoventricle. Note the lack of cleavage of the anterior cerebrum. At birth, this patient was microcephalic but became macrocephalic over time due to increasing size of the monoventricle.*

Glutaric Aciduria Type 1

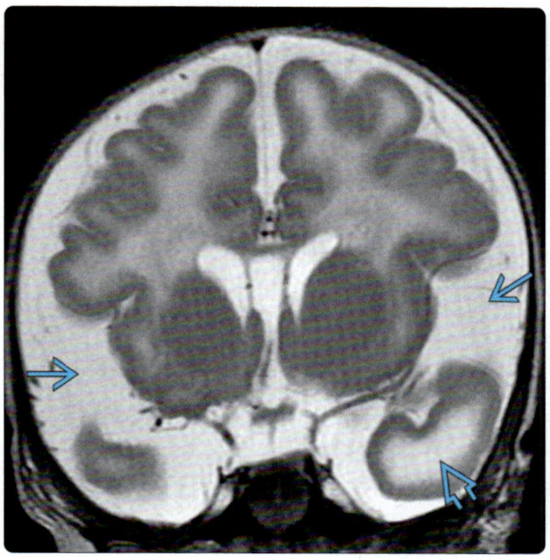

Alexander Disease

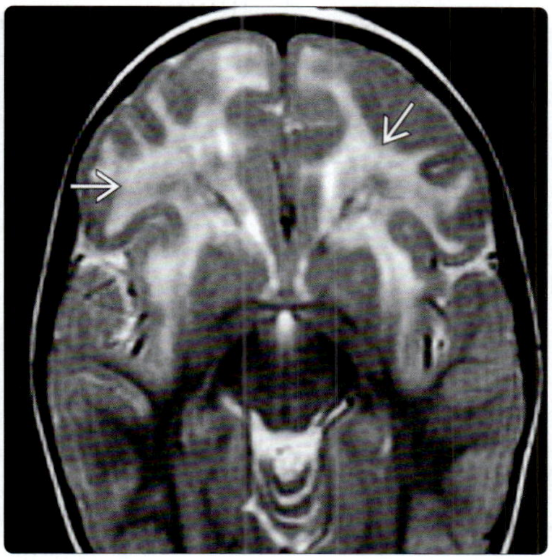

(Left) *Coronal T2 MR in a 6 week old with glutaric aciduria type 1 shows typical widening of the sylvian fissures → & cyst-like signal in the anterior left temporal lobe ⇒.* **(Right)** *Axial T2 MR shows abnormal ↑ signal due to demyelination in the bilateral frontal lobes ➡. On MR, Alexander disease is characterized by frontal lobe demyelination & cysts. Ventriculomegaly & poor gray-white matter (WM) differentiation can also be present.*

Canavan Disease

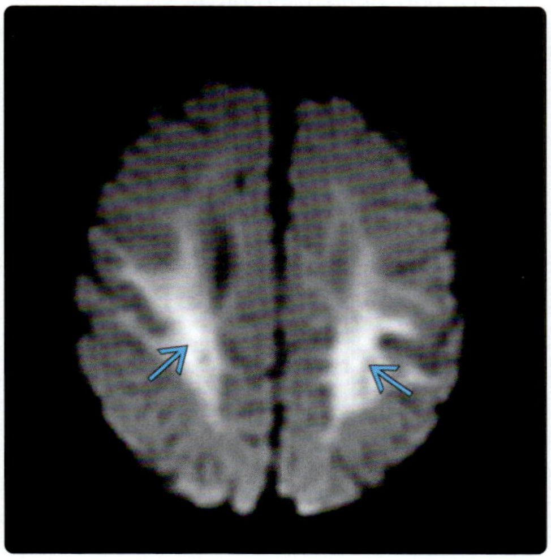

Canavan Disease

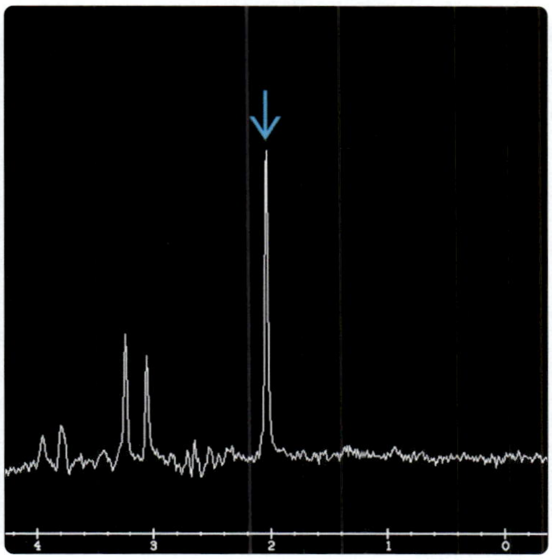

(Left) *Axial DWI MR in a 2 month old shows diffusion restriction (↓ ADC not shown) in areas of myelinated WM →, a common finding in Canavan disease. Canavan disease causes accumulation of N-acetyl aspartate (NAA) & neuronal swelling in the acute phase, leading to macrocephaly. Eventually, there is brain parenchymal volume loss.* **(Right)** *Long-echo MRS performed in the affected WM in the same patient shows a markedly elevated NAA peak →, a common finding in Canavan disease.*

Vanishing White Matter Disease

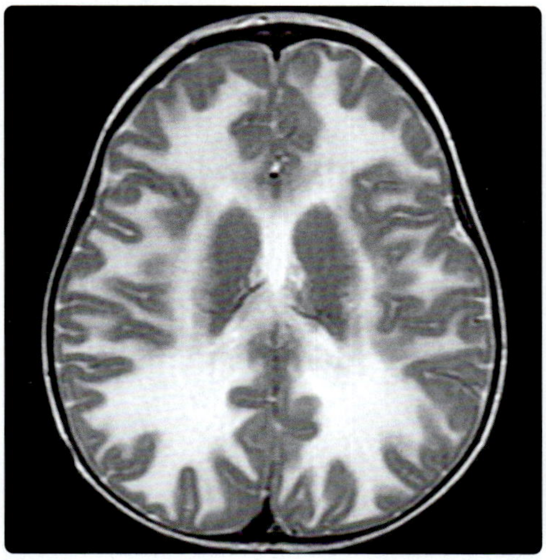

Vanishing White Matter Disease

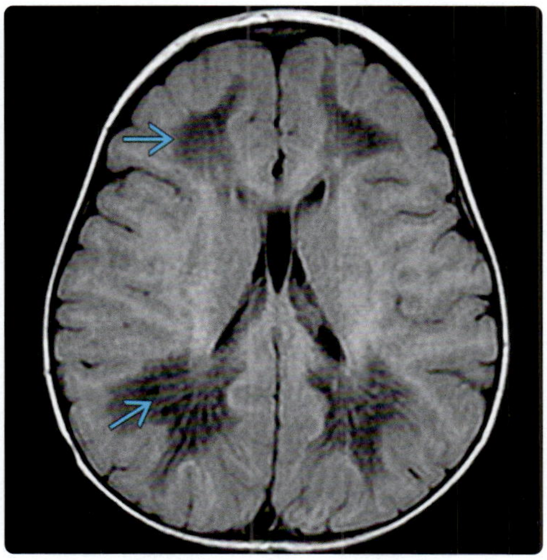

(Left) *Axial T2 MR in a 19 month old with tremor & vanishing WM disease (VWMD) shows diffusely ↑ T2 signal (= CSF) with expansion of the WM. In the acute phase of VWMD, patients can present with macrocephaly due to ↑ WM volume.* **(Right)** *Axial FLAIR MR in the same patient shows signal suppression of expanded WM → in the frontal & parietooccipital regions. This is a characteristic appearance for VWMD in contrast to other WM diseases in which WM is FLAIR hyperintense.*

DIFFERENTIAL DIAGNOSIS

Common

- Cavum Septum Pellucidum
- Mega Cisterna Magna
- Flow-Related MR Artifacts
- Enlarged Subarachnoid Spaces

Less Common

- Cavum Velum Interpositum
- Enlarged Optic Nerve Sheath

Rare but Important

- Blake Pouch Cyst
- Liliequist Membrane

ESSENTIAL INFORMATION

Key Differential Diagnosis Issues

- Normal variants have CSF density/intensity
- Important to recognize normal variants & differentiate from more ominous pathology

Helpful Clues for Common Diagnoses

- **Cavum Septum Pellucidum**
  - Elongated CSF collection between frontal horns of lateral ventricles
  - ± cavum vergae (posterior continuation between fornices)
  - Usually asymptomatic & incidental, even if mass effect is present
    - Absence in utero raises concern for other midline anomalies
- **Mega Cisterna Magna**
  - Enlarged cisterna magna communicates freely with normal 4th ventricle & basal cisterns
  - Normal cerebellum & vermis
  - Cistern is crossed by falx cerebelli, tiny veins
  - Occipital bone may appear scalloped
- **Flow-Related MR Artifacts**
  - CSF flow artifact is common in basal cisterns & ventricles
  - Commonly seen on T2 & FLAIR MR; reduced on SSFP
- **Enlarged Subarachnoid Spaces**
  - Idiopathic enlargement of subarachnoid spaces (SAS) during 1st year of life
    - Ventricles may be mildly enlarged
    - All modalities show veins coursing through SAS
    - Very rarely associated with small, nonhemorrhagic subdural collections
  - Increased head circumference (> 95%), typically in developmentally normal child
  - Resolves without therapy by 12-24 months

Helpful Clues for Less Common Diagnoses

- **Cavum Velum Interpositum**
  - Triangular-shaped CSF space between bodies of lateral ventricles, below fornices, & above 3rd ventricle
  - Often elevates & splays fornices, causing inferior displacement of internal cerebral veins & 3rd ventricle
- **Enlarged Optic Nerve Sheath**
  - May occur as normal variant
  - Often occurs in idiopathic intracranial hypertension (pseudotumor cerebri) or neurofibromatosis type 1

Helpful Clues for Rare Diagnoses

- **Blake Pouch Cyst**
  - Failed fenestration of normal Blake pouch (BP) & foramen of Luschka in utero results in persistent cyst that does not communicate with SAS
  - BP cyst remains continuous with inferior 4th ventricle & herniates into cisterna magna
  - Vermis is normal but rotated with elevated tegmento-vermian angle
  - Cyst wall is often not seen on imaging study
  - Enhancing choroid plexus lies along inferior surface of vermis in superior aspect of cyst wall
- **Liliequist Membrane**
  - Thin arachnoid membrane separates suprasellar, interpeduncular, & prepontine cisterns
  - May result in failure of 3rd ventriculostomy

Cavum Septum Pellucidum

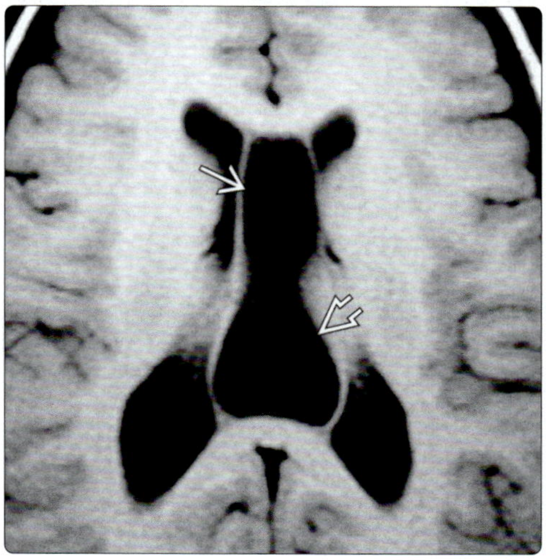

Mega Cisterna Magna

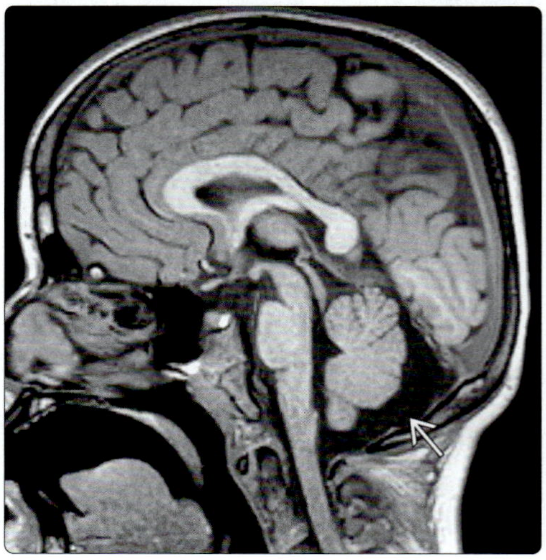

(Left) *Axial T1 MR shows a cavum septum pellucidum ➔ with posterior extension into a cavum vergae ➱, seen as an elongated CSF-signal intensity collection that lies between the bodies of the lateral ventricles.* **(Right)** *Sagittal T1 MR shows a prominent retrocerebellar CSF space ➔ due to a mega cisterna magna. This normal variant requires no treatment. Note the normal vermis & normal 4th ventricle.*

Mega Cisterna Magna

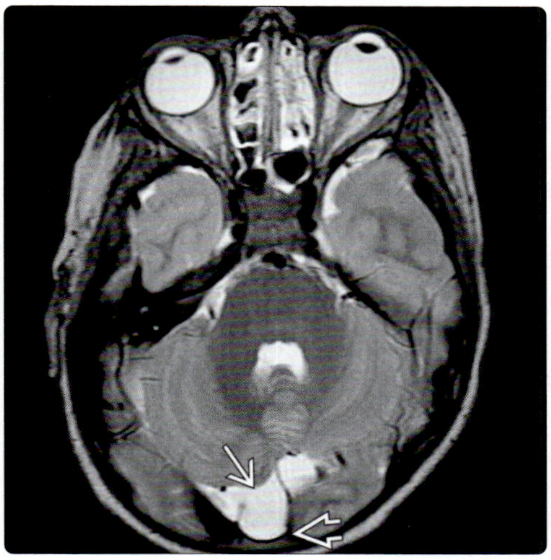

Flow-Related MR Artifacts

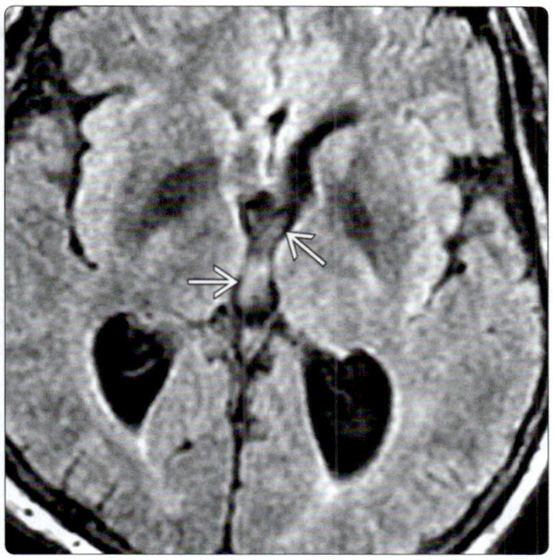

(Left) *Axial T2 MR shows a prominent retrocerebellar CSF space consistent with a mega cisterna magna ➡. Note the commonly associated remodeling of the adjacent occipital bone ➡ secondary to CSF pulsation.* **(Right)** *Axial FLAIR MR shows CSF flow artifact ➡ in the 3rd ventricle & foramen of Monro, which can mimic a mass or blood. This artifact is often seen on FLAIR MR & can be confirmed by its absence on SSFP sequences.*

Enlarged Subarachnoid Spaces

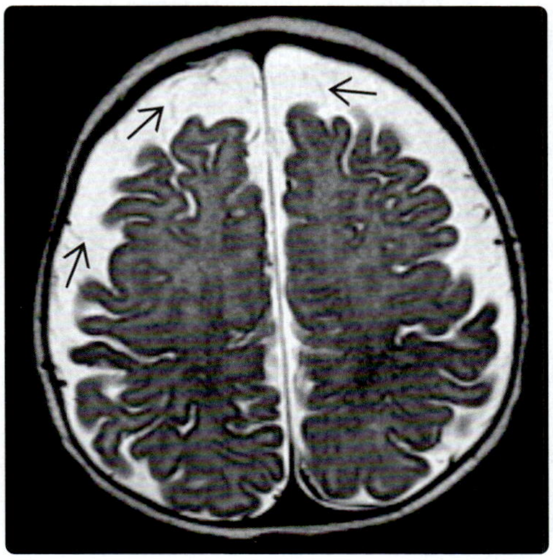

Cavum Velum Interpositum

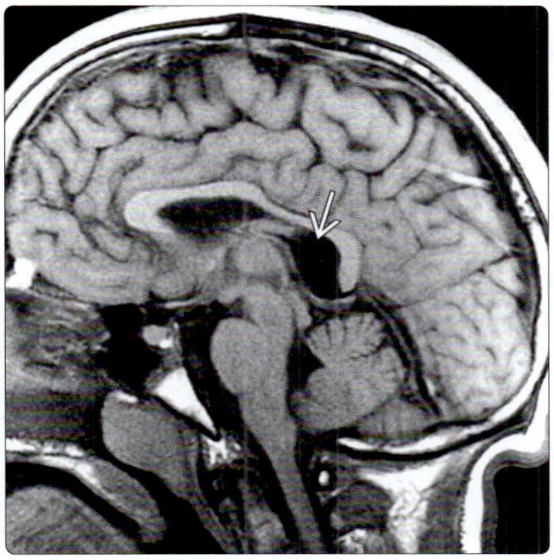

(Left) *Axial T2 MR shows marked enlargement of the bilateral frontal extraaxial CSF spaces. Curvilinear flow voids (due to traversing veins ⇨) confirm that these are enlarged subarachnoid spaces & not subdural or epidural collections. This condition typically resolves without therapy.* **(Right)** *Sagittal T1 MR shows a typical cavum velum interpositum ➡, ventral to the splenium. These CSF spaces typically elevate the fornices & inferiorly displace the internal cerebral veins (which are not well seen on this midline image).*

Enlarged Optic Nerve Sheath

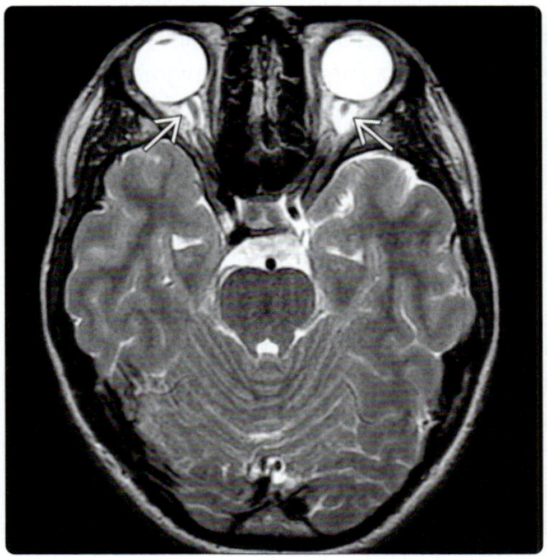

Blake Pouch Cyst

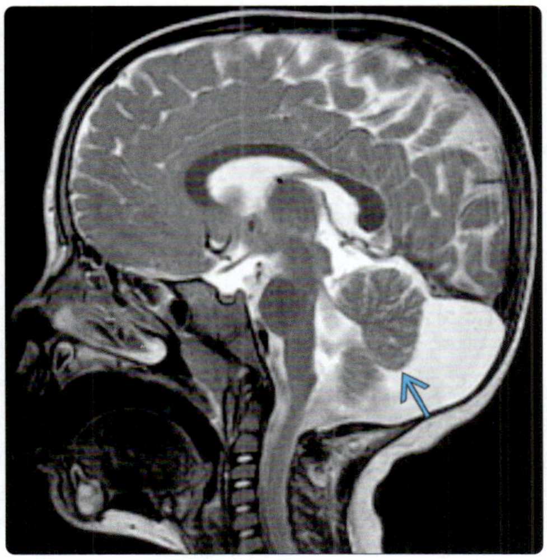

(Left) *Axial T2 MR in a teenager with a headache shows mild prominence of bilateral optic nerve sheath fluid ➡ without posterior scleral flattening. This patient did not have additional findings of idiopathic intracranial hypertension, & lumbar puncture opening pressure was normal, consistent with normal variant sheath enlargement.* **(Right)** *Sagittal T2 MR demonstrates retrocerebellar CSF collection that communicates with the 4th ventricle but not the SAS. This results in a rotated but otherwise normal vermis ⇨.*

DIFFERENTIAL DIAGNOSIS

Common

- Fetal Ventriculomegaly
- Benign Enlargement of Subarachnoid Spaces
- Chiari II Malformation
- Aqueductal Stenosis
- Acquired Hydrocephalus
  - Posthemorrhagic Hydrocephalus
  - Acute Infectious Hydrocephalus
  - Postinfectious Hydrocephalus
  - Obstructing Tumor
  - CSF Overproduction (Choroid Plexus Tumor)
- Brain Volume Loss
  - Hypoxic-Ischemic Encephalopathy
  - Arterial Ischemic Stroke
  - Periventricular Leukomalacia
  - Porencephaly
  - Metabolic Brain Disease

Less Common

- Hemimegalencephaly
- Vein of Galen Aneurysmal Malformation
- Dandy-Walker Malformation
- Hydranencephaly
- Holoprosencephaly

ESSENTIAL INFORMATION

Key Differential Diagnosis Issues

- 2 main causes of ventriculomegaly
  - ↑ CSF pressures → hydrocephalus
  - ↓ brain volume → passive ventricular enlargement
- Clinical features to consider
  - Head circumference is critical to interpreting significance of enlarged ventricles
    - ↑ head size: Hydrocephalus
    - ↓ head size: Brain parenchymal volume loss
  - Patients may come to clinical attention during prenatal screening or well-child check-ups
- Imaging features of hydrocephalus
  - Etiologies to consider
    - Obstruction usually occurs at cerebral aqueduct, foramen of Monro, or 4th ventricular outlets
    - Communicating hydrocephalus is due to CSF overproduction or poor CSF resorption
    - Some etiologies can cause either or mixed forms
  - Imaging signs of hydrocephalus
    - Macrocephaly: ↑ craniofacial ratio
    - Rounded margins of lateral ventricles, depressed floor of 3rd ventricle
    - Transependymal edema: Periventricular WM ↑ T2/FLAIR signal, greatest at frontal & occipital horns
    - Effacement of cerebral sulci & basilar cisterns
- Imaging features of volume loss
  - Etiologies to consider
    - Diffuse vs. focal cortical ischemia
    - Symmetric vs. focal white matter (WM) volume loss
  - Imaging signs of brain parenchymal volume loss
    - Microcephaly: ↓ craniofacial ratio
    - Angular margins of lateral ventricles
    - Prominent sulci & basilar cisterns
- Modality considerations
  - Fetal US for detection of in utero ventriculomegaly
    - Fetal MR imaging is excellent for underlying/associated anomalies
  - US is important tool for initial evaluation of neonates/infants with suspected ventriculomegaly
    - Requires open anterior fontanelle
  - CT is often 1st-line modality in acute presentations
  - MR imaging is most definitive test for determination of underlying cause of ventriculomegaly

Helpful Clues for Common Diagnoses

- **Fetal Ventriculomegaly**
  - Likelihood of normal neurologic development based on lateral ventricular size in utero
    - Mild (10-12 mm): > 90%
    - Moderate (13-15 mm): 80-93%
    - Severe (> 15 mm): ~ 62%
  - Underlying causes of fetal ventriculomegaly
    - Infectious (e.g., CMV), genetic (e.g., trisomy), & malformations (e.g., Chiari II)
      - CMV testing & amniocentesis typically performed
    - Obstructive causes considered separately
- **Benign Enlargement of Subarachnoid Spaces**
  - a.k.a benign hydrocephalus of infancy, benign macrocrania of infancy, external hydrocephalus
  - Enlarged subarachnoid spaces (SAS) ± mild ventriculomegaly
  - Findings develop in 1st few months of life & usually resolve by ~ 2 years of age
  - Normal development or mild developmental delay
  - Imaging: Prominent SAS over frontal & parietal convexities with normal vessels traversing SAS
    - No displacement of arachnoid membrane from dura (i.e., no subdural fluid)
- **Chiari II Malformation**
  - Brain malformation due to open neural tube defect (most commonly lumbosacral myelomeningocele)
  - Hydrocephalus requiring shunting occurs almost universally without in utero surgical repair
  - Imaging: Small posterior fossa, inferior migration of cerebellum/brainstem, beaked tectum, dysplastic corpus callosum, scalloping of dorsal clivus
- **Aqueductal Stenosis**
  - Congenital atresia/stenosis of cerebral aqueduct
  - Imaging: Lateral & 3rd ventricle dilation with normal 4th ventricle
    - Narrowed/absent cerebral aqueduct on 3D SSFP MR
    - Lack of flow void within cerebral aqueduct on T2
- **Acquired Hydrocephalus**
  - 2 main types: Communicating & noncommunicating
    - Communicating: ↑ production or ↓ resorption of CSF
    - Obstructive: Blockage of ventricular outlets
  - Depending on cause, may present enlarging head or signs of ↑ intracranial pressure
    - May have signs of ↑ intracranial pressure
  - **Posthemorrhagic hydrocephalus**
    - Most common in premature infants with germinal matrix/intraventricular hemorrhage (IVH)

- Look for hemosiderin along ventricles/brainstem
- SWI/GRE is most sensitive for detection of prior IVH
- **Acute infectious hydrocephalus**
  - During acute bacterial infection, ↑ head size may occur due to
    - ↑ extraaxial spaces from meningitis
    - Subdural/epidural empyema
- **Postinfectious hydrocephalus**
  - Obstruction may occur due to synechiae
  - Communicating hydrocephalus may occur due to arachnoid granulation dysfunction
- **Obstructing tumor**
  - Smaller tumors in critical locations may obstruct
    - e.g., subependymal giant cell astrocytoma (SEGA) at foramen of Monro, tectal plate glioma at cerebral aqueduct
  - Larger tumors anywhere in brain may obstruct
- **CSF overproduction (choroid plexus tumors)**
  - CP papilloma/carcinoma causes CSF overproduction
    - Inability to resorb excess CSF → ↑ ventricular size

- **Brain Volume Loss**
  - Brain volume loss results in ventricular enlargement
    - Focal (e.g., porencephaly, stroke)
    - Symmetric (e.g., periventricular leukomalacia, metabolic disease)
  - **Hypoxic-ischemic encephalopathy**
    - Often results in symmetric or asymmetric brain volume loss & associated ventricular enlargement
    - Look for characteristic patterns of injury (e.g., perirolandic or watershed)
  - **Arterial ischemic stroke**
    - Most often occurs in perinatal period or related to embolic phenomenon
    - Encephalomalacia develops in arterial territory with focal ventricular enlargement
  - **Periventricular leukomalacia**
    - Sequelae of WM injury of prematurity
    - Usually symmetric WM volume loss with little or no associated gliosis (↑ FLAIR signal)
  - **Porencephaly**
    - Most often results from grade 4 IVH but any insult early in development may cause porencephaly
    - Porencephaly develops rather than encephalomalacia as no astrocytic response occurs in very young brains
  - **Metabolic brain disease**
    - Numerous diseases cause significant brain volume loss, resulting in ventriculomegaly
    - Usually symmetric; may be
      - Frontal predominant (e.g., Alexander disease)
      - Posterior predominant [e.g., X-linked adrenoleukodystrophy (ALD)]
      - Diffuse (e.g., metachromatic leukodystrophy)

Helpful Clues for Less Common Diagnoses

- **Hemimegalencephaly**
  - Unilateral abnormal neuronal proliferation & migration
  - Neonate/infant: ↑ T1 & ↓ T2 in WM with blurred gray matter/WM junctions
  - Often shows enlarged ipsilateral ventricle
- **Vein of Galen Aneurysmal Malformation**
  - High-flow vascular malformation due to direct communication between arteries & median prosencephalic vein
  - Ventricular enlargement may occur due to
    - Mass effect of malformation on cerebral aqueduct
    - ↑ venous pressure & poor CSF resorption
    - Parenchymal insult with volume loss
- **Dandy-Walker Malformation**
  - Vermian hypoplasia with large posterior fossa cyst that communicates with 4th ventricle but not SAS
  - Lambdoid-torcular inversion
  - Often associated with hydrocephalus
- **Hydranencephaly**
  - In utero destruction of brain in internal carotid artery territories
  - May cause poor CSF regulation & hydrocephalus, requiring shunting
- **Holoprosencephaly**
  - Holoprosencephaly (alobar form) often develops ↑ size of monoventricle over time

Fetal Ventriculomegaly

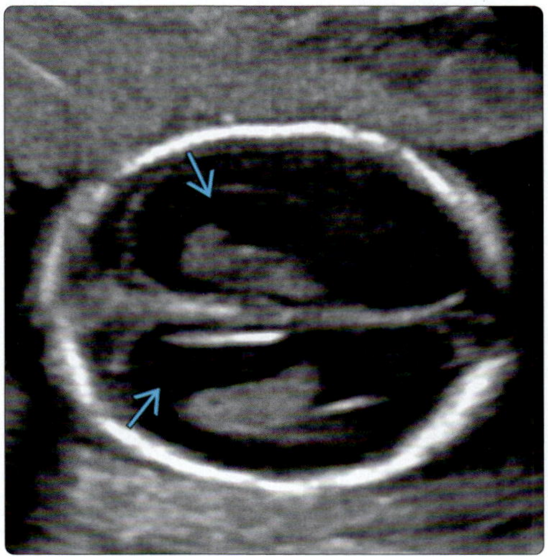

Fetal Ventriculomegaly

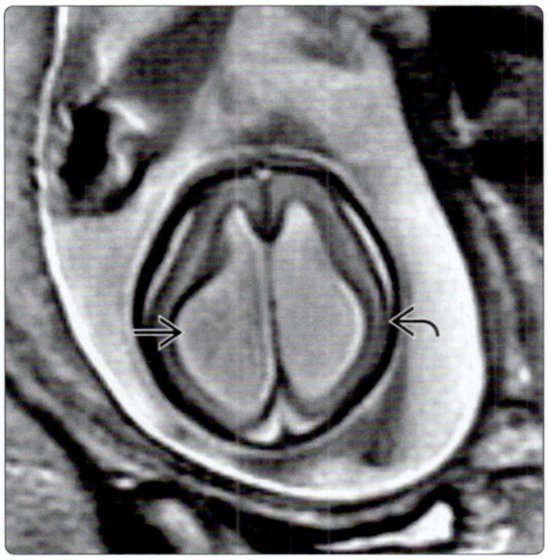

(Left) *Transverse oblique US in an 18-week fetus shows mild enlargement of the lateral ventricles* ➡ *(11 mm). If the ventriculomegaly worsens later in pregnancy, fetal or postnatal MR imaging should be obtained.* **(Right)** *Axial T2 SSFSE MR of a fetus shows marked enlargement (> 15 mm) of the lateral ventricles* ➡ *& thinning of the cerebrum* ↩*. With severe fetal ventriculomegaly (particularly in the setting of aqueductal stenosis), the septum pellucidum (& even the cerebral mantle) may become disrupted.*

(Left) *Coronal T2 MR in a 1 year old with macrocephaly shows mild enlargement of the lateral & 3rd ventricles with moderate enlargement of the bifrontal subarachnoid spaces (SAS), which are traversed by normal veins. Mild ventriculomegaly is often seen in benign enlargement of subarachnoid spaces (BESS).* **(Right)** *Coronal color Doppler US in a 9 month old with BESS shows normal vessels coursing through prominent fluid, an expected finding that helps differentiate the SAS from subdural collections.*

Benign Enlargement of Subarachnoid Spaces

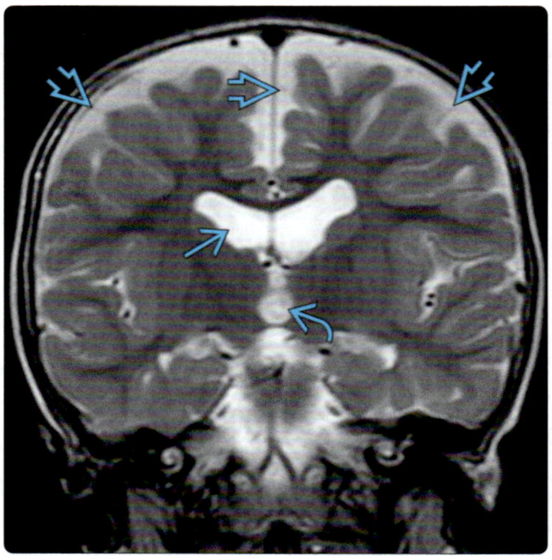

Benign Enlargement of Subarachnoid Spaces

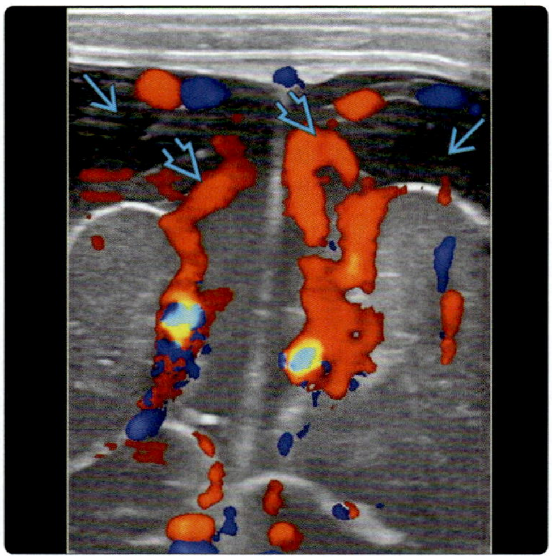

(Left) *Sagittal 3D SSFP MR in a neonate with a myelomeningocele shows marked enlargement of the lateral ventricles & characteristic features of a Chiari II malformation: Small posterior fossa, brainstem & cerebellar descent, tectal beaking, & a scalloped clivus.* **(Right)** *Sagittal T2 MR in a neonate shows massive enlargement of the lateral ventricles due to obstruction at the level of the cerebral aqueduct. The 3rd ventricle is also enlarged, but the 4th ventricle is normal, typical of this disorder.*

Chiari II Malformation

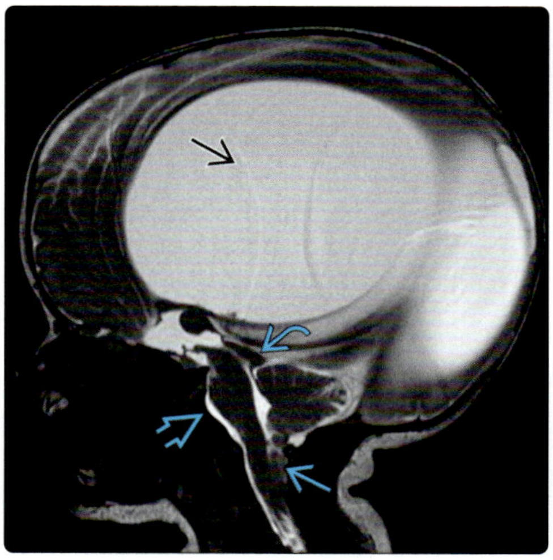

Aqueductal Stenosis

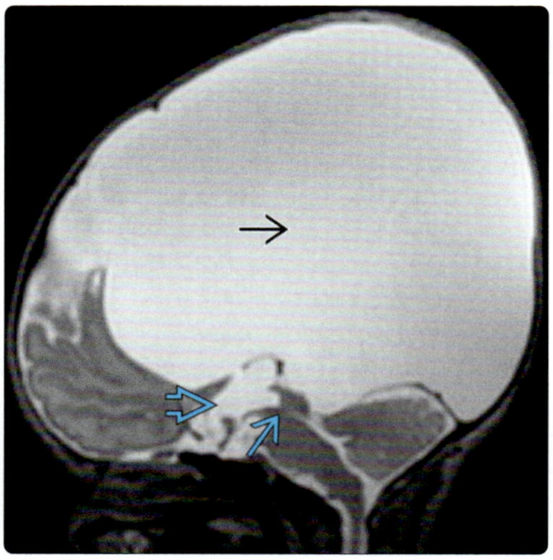

(Left) *Sagittal T2 MR in a 1-month-old former premature infant with posthemorrhagic hydrocephalus shows marked enlargement of the lateral, 3rd, & 4th ventricles. Note the dark hemosiderin lining the pial surface of brainstem from prior intraventricular hemorrhage (IVH).* **(Right)** *Axial SWI MR in a 3-month-old former premature infant with posthemorrhagic hydrocephalus shows signal loss along the ependymal margins of the ventricles & choroid plexus, consistent with prior IVH.*

Posthemorrhagic Hydrocephalus

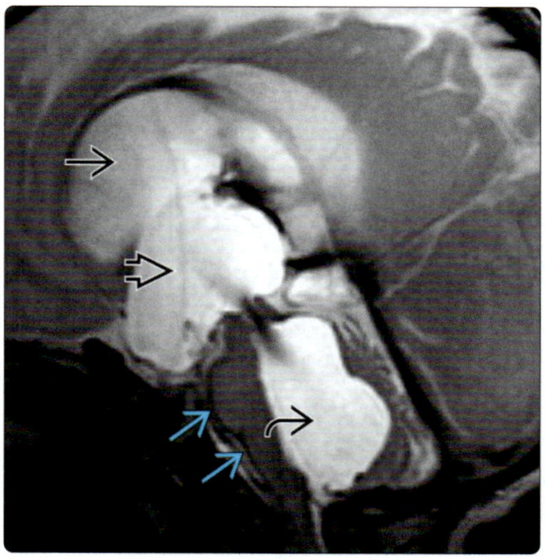

Posthemorrhagic Hydrocephalus

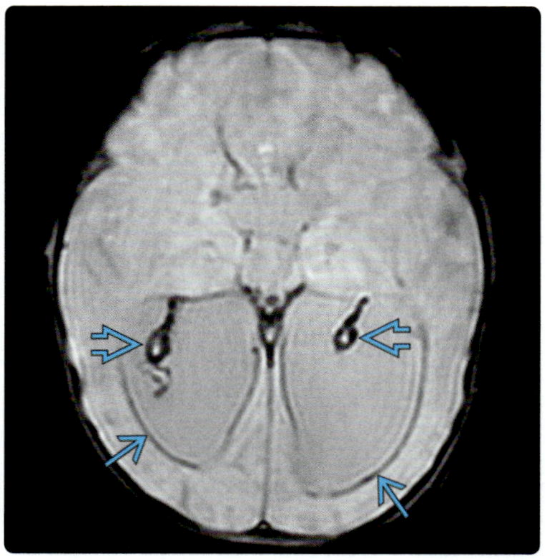

Acute Infectious Hydrocephalus

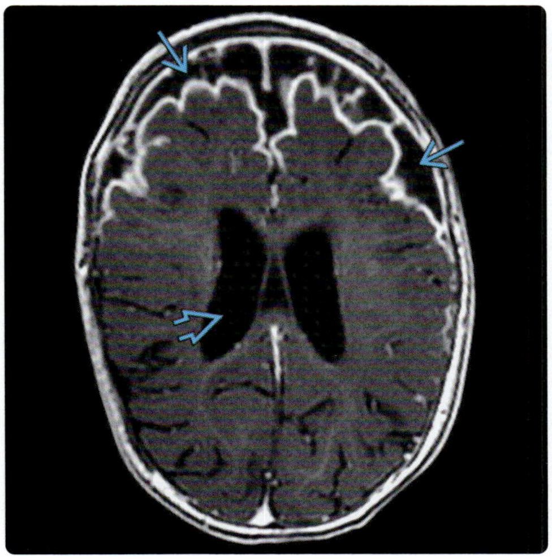

Postinfectious Hydrocephalus

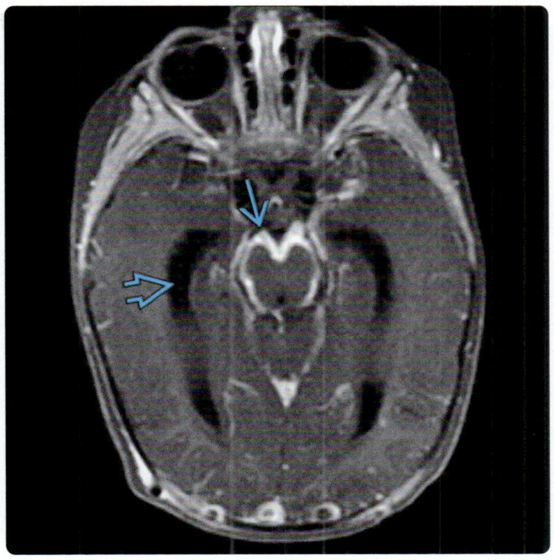

(Left) *Axial T1 C+ MR in a 7-year-old with Haemophilus influenzae meningitis shows marked expansion of the bifrontal subarachnoid spaces & mild enlargement of the lateral ventricles.* **(Right)** *Axial T1 C+ FS MR in an 8 month old with tuberculous meningitis shows extensive basilar leptomeningeal enhancement & enlargement of the lateral ventricles, resulting in macrocephaly. Granulomatous infections are more likely to result in hydrocephalus compared to other bacterial meningitis.*

Obstructing Tumor

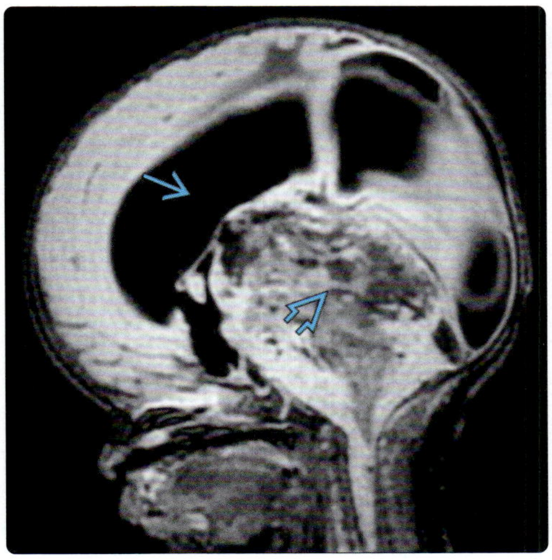

CSF Overproduction (Choroid Plexus Tumor)

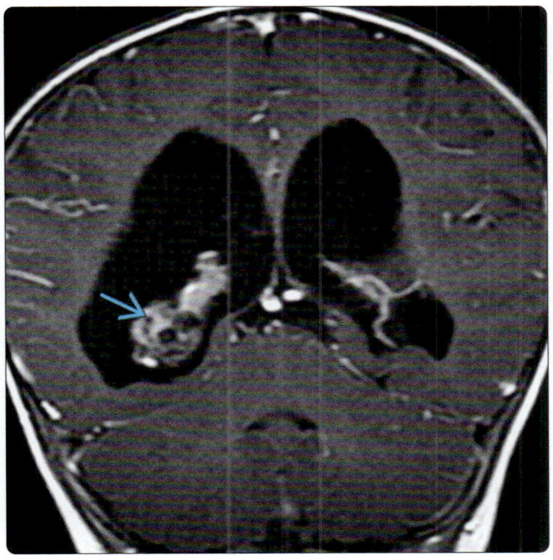

(Left) *Sagittal FLAIR MR in a neonate with a large obstructing hemorrhagic posterior fossa mass shows enlargement of the lateral ventricles & posterior fossa. Note the ↑ craniofacial ratio.* **(Right)** *Coronal T1 C+ MR in a 1 year old with a choroid plexus papilloma shows an enhancing mass in the right choroid plexus. The lateral ventricles are enlarged without evidence of obstruction. Hydrocephalus in this case is due to overproduction of CSF by the tumor.*

Hypoxic-Ischemic Encephalopathy

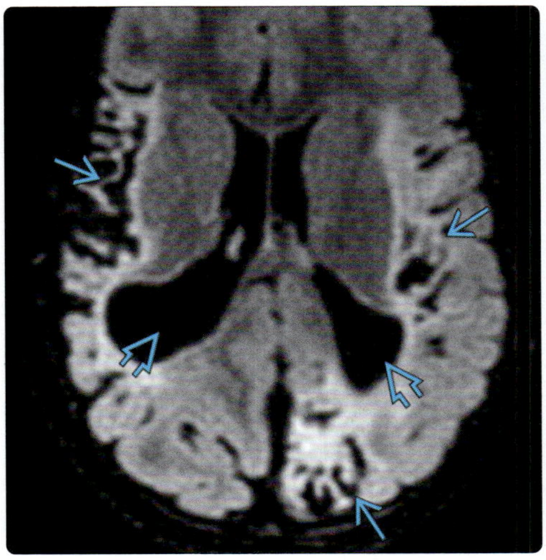

Hypoxic-Ischemic Encephalopathy

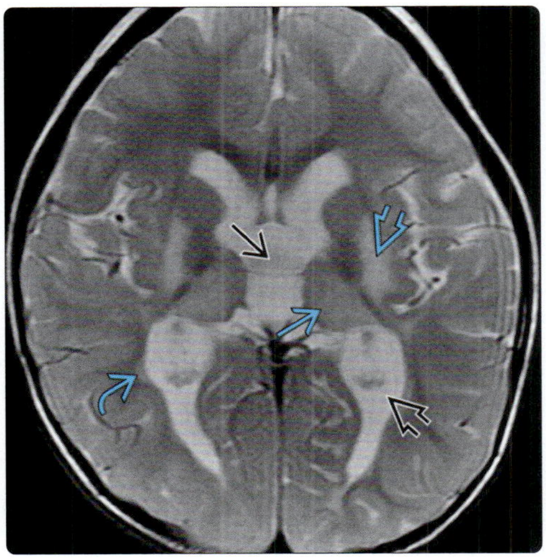

(Left) *Axial FLAIR MR in a 4 year old with a history of perinatal hypoxic-ischemic injury shows extensive areas of cortical encephalomalacia. Note the localized areas of ventriculomegaly due to overlying brain volume loss.* **(Right)** *Axial T2 MR in a 2 year old with a history of perinatal hypoxic-ischemic encephalopathy (HIE) shows symmetric areas of signal abnormality & volume loss involving the thalami, putamina, & periventricular white matter, resulting in enlargement of the lateral & 3rd ventricles.*

(Left) *Axial T2 MR in a 9 month old with previous infarction shows extensive cystic encephalomalacia → in right middle cerebral artery (MCA) territory with resultant asymmetric enlargement of the right lateral ventricle →.* **(Right)** *Axial FLAIR MR in a 7 year old with a history of extreme prematurity & periventricular leukomalacia (PVL) shows symmetric focal enlargement of the atria → with adjacent white matter volume loss. The relative lack of abnormal FLAIR signal compared to the degree of volume loss is typical of PVL.*

Arterial Ischemic Stroke

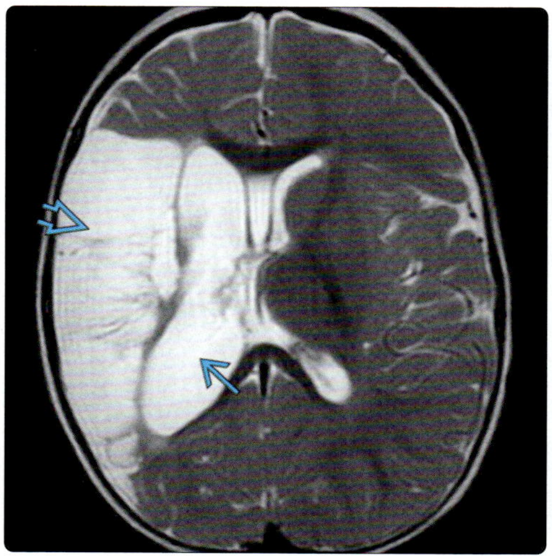

Periventricular Leukomalacia

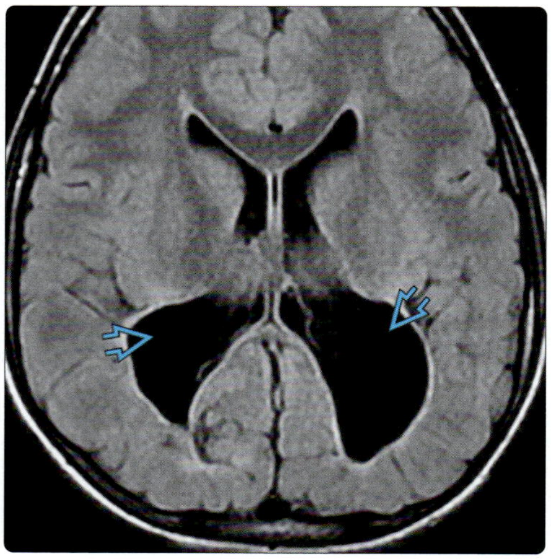

(Left) *Coronal US at 2 days of life in an extremely premature (23 weeks) infant shows a large right germinal matrix hemorrhage → with associated hemorrhagic venous infarction → in the right frontoparietal white matter.* **(Right)** *Coronal T2 MR in the same patient 3 months later shows the expected development of right parietal porencephaly & focal ventricular enlargement. Note the rim of T2 hypointensity →, consistent with hemosiderin. This hypointense rim will eventually resolve.*

Porencephaly

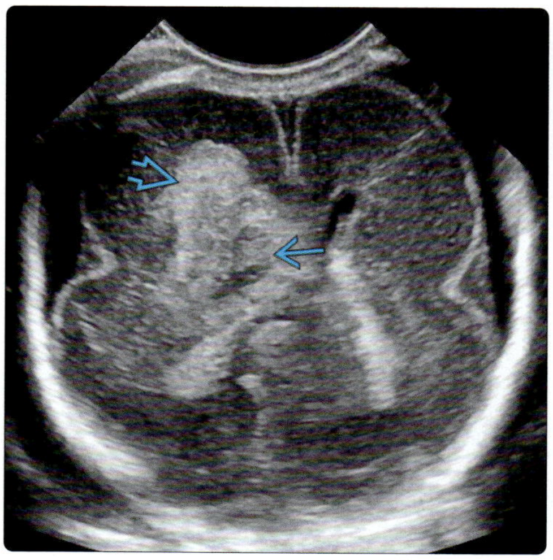

Porencephaly

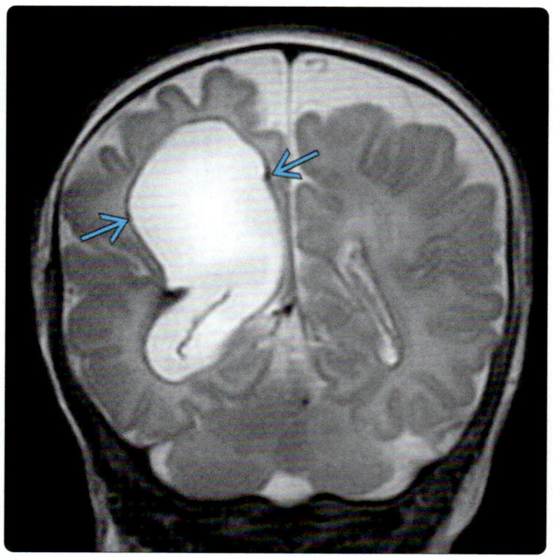

(Left) *Axial T2 MR in a teenager with metachromatic leukodystrophy shows ↑ signal & volume loss in the periventricular & deep white matter → with sparing of the subcortical white matter, characteristic of this disease. Note the enlargement of the lateral ventricles → & sulci → due to the brain volume loss.* **(Right)** *Axial T2 MR in a teenager with vanishing white matter disease shows extensive ↑ signal intensity & volume loss in the white matter → with associated enlargement of the lateral → & 3rd → ventricles & sulci →.*

Metabolic Brain Disease

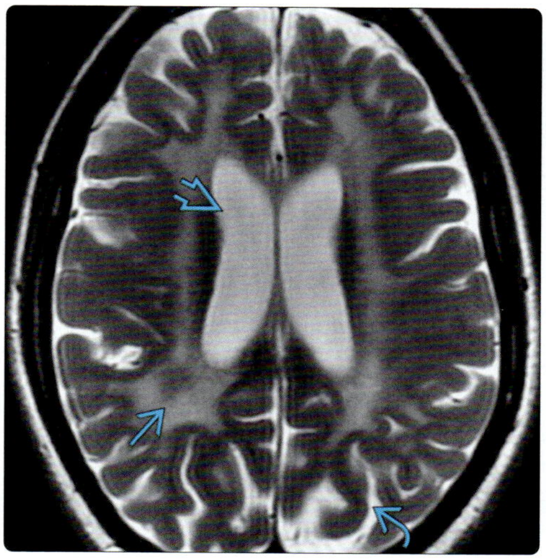

Metabolic Brain Disease

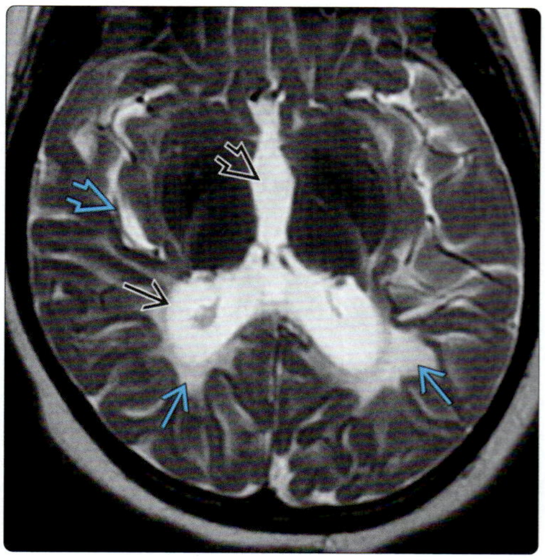

Hemimegalencephaly

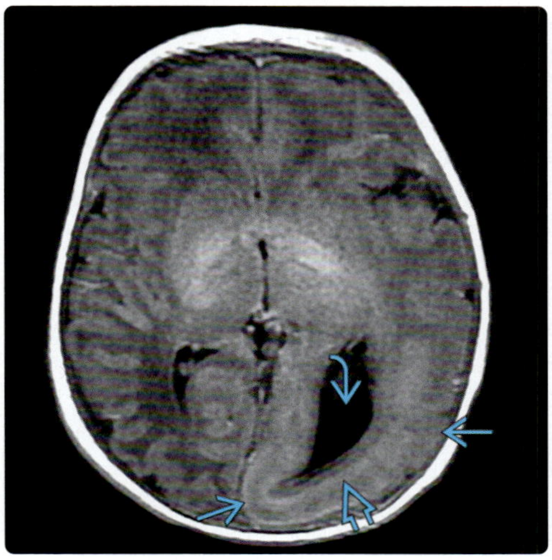

Hemimegalencephaly

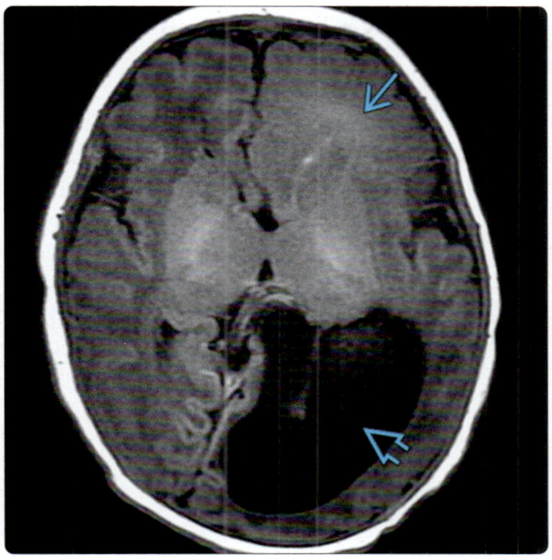

(Left) *Axial T1 MR in a neonate with seizures & hemimegalencephaly shows ↑ size of the left parietooccipital hemisphere with loss of normal sulcation & markedly abnormal neuronal organization. Also note enlargement of the ipsilateral occipital horn.* **(Right)** *Axial T1 MR in a 3-day-old with left hemimegalencephaly shows marked occipital horn enlargement. Note the abnormal white matter in the left frontal lobe. Enlargement of the ipsilateral occipital horn is common in this disease.*

Vein of Galen Aneurysmal Malformation

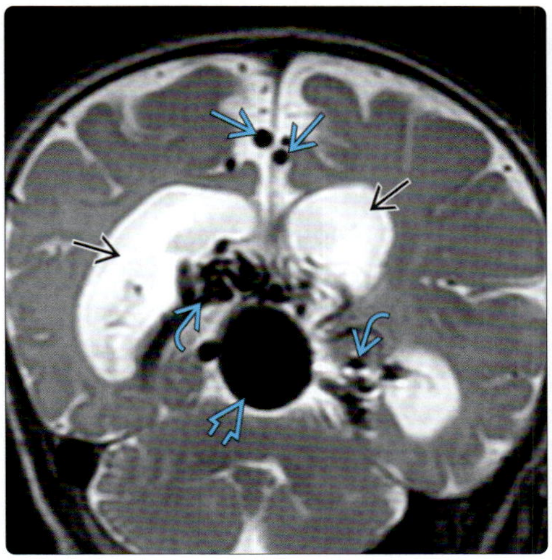

Dandy-Walker Malformation

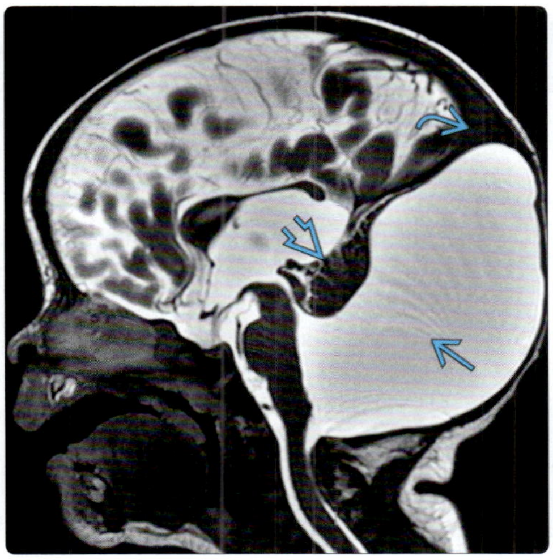

(Left) *Coronal T2 MR in a neonate with VGAM shows a markedly enlarged central vein with numerous enlarged choroidal & pericallosal feeding arteries. Note the enlarged ventricles, which are likely due to ↓ resorption of CSF due to ↑ venous pressures.* **(Right)** *Sagittal 3D SSFP MR in a 2 month old with Dandy-Walker malformation shows a small cerebellar vermis & large posterior fossa cyst that is continuous with the 4th ventricle. There is elevation of the tentorium & torcular Herophili.*

Hydranencephaly

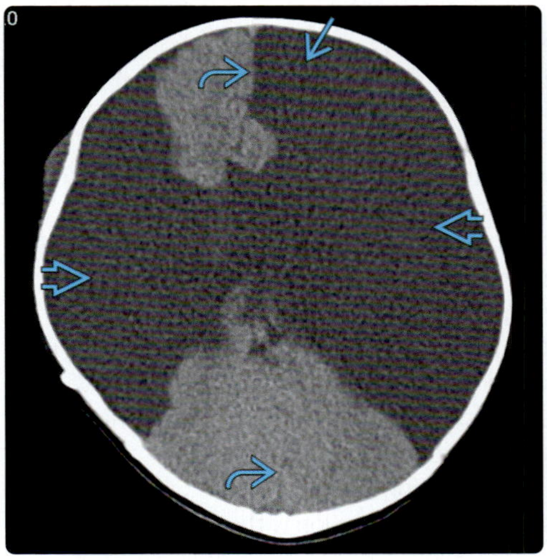

Holoprosencephaly

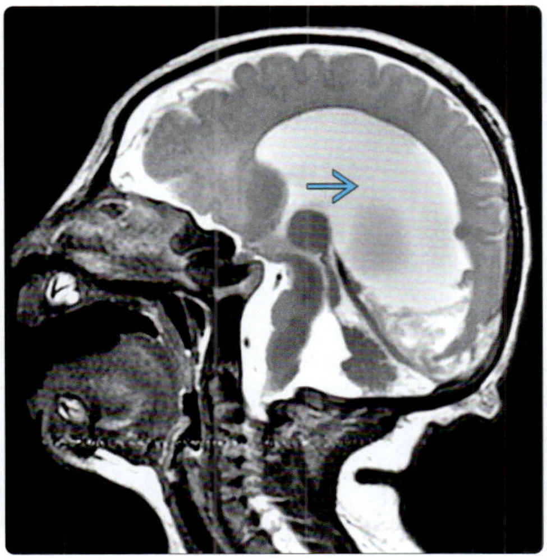

(Left) *Axial NECT in a 4 year old with hydranencephaly shows porencephaly in the bilateral MCA & left anterior cerebral artery (ACA) territories in continuity with the lateral ventricles. Note the intact falx. Patients with hydranencephaly typically become macrocephalic due to poor CSF regulation.* **(Right)** *Sagittal T2 MR in a neonate with holoprosencephaly shows an enlarged monoventricle. However, the patient is microcephalic overall due to the ↓ brain parenchymal volume.*

DIFFERENTIAL DIAGNOSIS

Common

- Germinal Matrix Hemorrhage
- Birth-Related Trauma
- Abusive Head Trauma

Less Common

- Venous Thrombosis & Infarction
- Arteriovenous Malformation
- Cavernous Malformation
- Cerebral Contusion
- Diffuse Axonal Injury
- Aneurysm

Rare but Important

- Hemorrhagic Neoplasms
- Subpial Hemorrhage
- Acute Hypertensive Encephalopathy, PRES
- Coagulopathies & Blood Dyscrasias
- Herpes Encephalitis

ESSENTIAL INFORMATION

Key Differential Diagnosis Issues

- Clinical features to consider
  - Age, history of present illness, past medical history
    - Preceding trauma may be obvious [e.g., motor vehicle accident (MVA)] or occult (e.g., child abuse), particularly in younger patients
  - Presenting signs/symptoms
    - Most common: Headache, focal neurologic signs, altered mental status
    - Less common: Seizures, fever, bulging fontanelle
- Modality considerations
  - US: Initial imaging in infants with open fontanelle (except for acute head trauma)
    - Excellent for detection of germinal matrix hemorrhage (GMH)/intraventricular hemorrhage (IVH) & ventriculomegaly
  - NECT: 1st line for virtually all other acute patients
    - Excellent depiction of acute/subacute hemorrhage, mass effect, Ca^{2+}
  - CTA: Allows for rapid diagnosis & characterization of underlying arteriovenous malformation (AVM) or aneurysm
    - Spontaneous hemorrhage without obvious clinical explanation → CTA to detect vascular lesion
  - MR: Most sensitive & specific for parenchymal lesions
    - May distinguish acute, subacute, & chronic stages of intraparenchymal hemorrhage
    - Useful after clot retraction to detect small AVMs or tumors that were compressed by acute hemorrhage

Helpful Clues for Common Diagnoses

- **Germinal Matrix Hemorrhage**
  - Affects neonates < 32-weeks gestation & < 1,500 g
  - Less common if > 34 weeks (without additional insult)
  - US: Initial imaging modality of choice
    - Grade 1: GMH alone, usually in caudothalamic groove
    - Grade 2: GMH + IVH
    - Grade 3: GMH + large IVH that enlarges ventricles
    - Grade 4: GMH + hemorrhagic venous infarct
- **Birth-Related Trauma**
  - Small (< 3-mm) posterior supra- & infratentorial subdural hemorrhage (SDH)
  - Occurs in ~ 50% of normal vaginal deliveries
  - Present for 4-6 weeks after birth
- **Abusive Head Trauma**
  - Inflicted head injury from (1) shaking (as alternating acceleration & deceleration forces lead to shearing injury) **or** (2) direct head impact
  - Most common cause of brain death < 2 years of age
  - Classic triad: SDH, skull fracture(s), parenchymal injury
    - SDH: Present in 90-98% of AHT cases
      - Note that collections of differing attenuations/signal intensities do not necessarily imply hemorrhage of different ages
      - Cortical vein avulsion → thrombosis of injured veins + adjacent perivascular clot → hyperdense parasagittal linear & globular foci (lollipop or tadpole sign, specific for AHT)
      - ± retinal hemorrhages on NECT or SWI MR
    - Skull fractures: Linear are common but not specific
    - Parenchymal injury
      - Cytotoxic edema: DWI MR is key to detection
      - Laceration/contusional tear: Hematocrit level in peripheral parenchymal cleft
      - DAI: Present in severe injury, not specific to AHT

Helpful Clues for Less Common Diagnoses

- **Venous Thrombosis & Infarction**
  - Cortical vein &/or dural sinus thrombosis → venous infarct → parenchymal hemorrhage of vascular territory
    - Cortical veins/sinuses → cortex
    - Internal cerebral veins → deep gray nuclei
    - Medullary/subependymal veins → periventricular/deep white matter
  - Hemorrhage within affected vascular territories
  - NECT: Hyperdense veins/sinuses in acute thrombosis
    - > 58 HU of sinus suggests clot
  - CTV/MRV: Areas of nonenhancing thrombus
  - MR: Signal change & ↑ DWI/↓ ADC of parenchyma → venous ischemia
    - Typically occurs when cortical veins are involved, not just large sinuses
- **Arteriovenous Malformation**
  - High-flow vascular malformation with AV shunting (due to absence of normal capillary bed)
  - NECT: Subtle replacement of parenchyma by tangle of abnormal vessels, ± Ca^{2+} & gliosis
    - No surrounding edema without acute hemorrhage
  - CTA/MRA: Used to identify AVM nidus as well as arterial supply & draining veins
    - Nidal aneurysm: Common source of hemorrhage
  - MR: ASL can help identify micro AVMs
- **Cavernous Malformation**
  - Benign low-flow vascular lesion with dilated sinusoids
  - Usually solitary unless part of familial multiple cerebral cavernous malformations
  - CT: Hyperdense lesion ± Ca^{2+}; 50% not visible
  - MR: Hemorrhages of different ages

- Popcorn ball appearance with cysts of varying signal, ± hematocrit levels; T2-hypointense hemosiderin rim
- Surrounding edema with recent hemorrhage
- Small punctate lesions may only be visible on SWI/GRE
- Minimal or no contrast enhancement of lesion
- Adjacent developmental venous anomaly in ~ 25%

- **Cerebral Contusion**
  - Posttraumatic superficial parenchymal hemorrhage
  - Anterior/inferior frontal & temporal lobes are common
    - Impact to irregular bony protuberance or dural fold
  - Adjacent vasogenic edema distinguishes from subarachnoid hemorrhage
  - ± associated scalp swelling, fracture, & other hemorrhages
  - Look for contrecoup injury opposite of impact site
- **Diffuse Axonal Injury**
  - Trauma-induced axonal shear injury; classically in corpus callosum, gray-white junction, & brainstem
  - Occurs exclusively in high-velocity injuries (e.g., motor vehicle accident)
  - NECT: Frequently normal; ± subtle microhemorrhages
  - MR: Best to detect full extent of shear injury
    - SWI/T2* GRE are highly sensitive for hemorrhage
- **Aneurysm**
  - Less common in children vs. adults
    - Idiopathic > trauma > vasculopathy > infection
  - 80% anterior circulation; 20% posterior circulation
  - Saccular > fusiform > pseudoaneurysm
  - DSA: Gold standard
  - CTA: > 95% sensitive for > 2 mm
  - MRA: > 90% sensitive for > 3 mm

Helpful Clues for Rare Diagnoses

- **Hemorrhagic Neoplasms**
  - Most pediatric high-grade tumors are at risk: Outgrow blood supply → necrosis → hemorrhage into tumor
  - MR: Areas of enhancing soft tissue suggest neoplasm
    - Large hemorrhage makes small underlying tumor hard to detect initially; follow-up MR is useful to detect persistent/enlarging mass
- **Subpial Hemorrhage**
  - Characteristic hemorrhage in neonates
  - Often occurs with normal labor & delivery
  - Seizures are most common presentation
  - Etiology is uncertain, possibly venous thrombosis
  - Most often occurs in temporal lobes
  - NECT: Superficial hemorrhage expanding sulci
  - MR: Adjacent parenchymal change, possibly with restricted diffusion & microhemorrhage
- **Acute Hypertensive Encephalopathy, PRES**
  - a.k.a. posterior reversible encephalopathy syndrome
  - Risk factors in children: Severe hypertension, immunosuppression with cyclosporine
  - Seizure, headache, encephalopathy are common
  - NECT: Findings often not visible; ~ 50% sensitive
  - MR: Scattered cortical/subcortical T2/FLAIR hyperintensities; hemorrhage is uncommon
    - Often bilateral, may not be posterior
    - Microhemorrhage often only visible on SWI/GRE
- **Coagulopathies & Blood Dyscrasias**
  - Hemolytic uremic syndrome, thrombotic thrombocytopenic purpura, disseminated intravascular coagulation, thrombocytopenia, vitamin K deficiency
    - Multifocal parenchymal hemorrhages are common
  - Anticoagulation complications
    - Mixed-density hemorrhage, ± fluid-fluid levels
    - Diligent search for hemorrhage in patients on ECMO
- **Herpes Encephalitis**
  - Neonatal HSV-2 most often presents at 2-5 weeks
  - Reactivation of HSV-1 may occur in children/adolescents
  - Presents with fever, seizures, encephalopathy
  - MR: Most sensitive for detection in early stages
    - HSV-2: Early diffusion changes
      - Temporal lobe most common but may occur anywhere; frequent deep gray involvement
      - Hemorrhage in ~ 50%, common in later stages
    - HSV-1: Limbic system, often bilateral (temporal lobes, insula, subfrontal area, cingulate gyri)

Germinal Matrix Hemorrhage

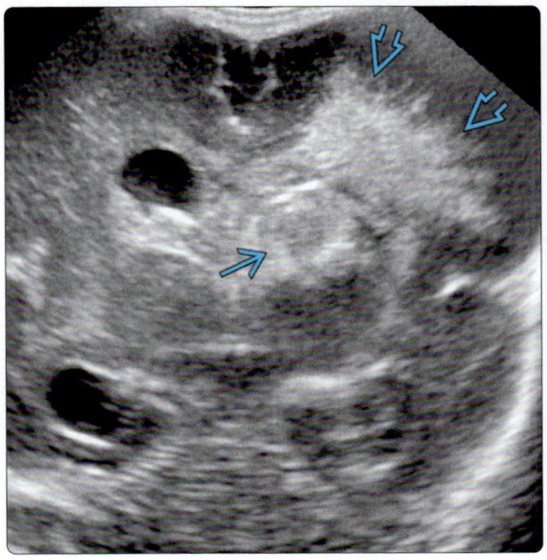

Germinal Matrix Hemorrhage

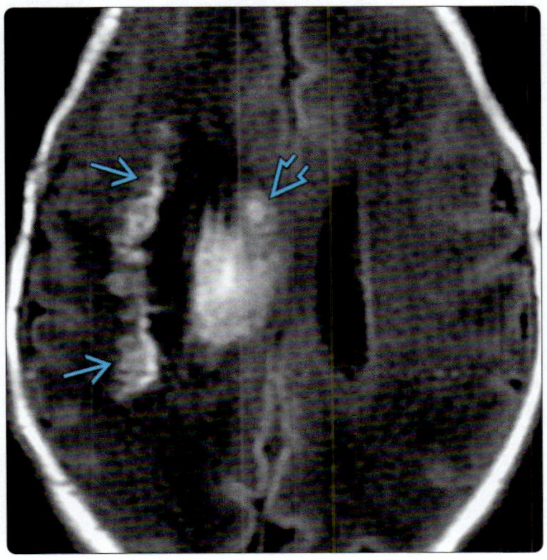

(Left) *Coronal US in a premature neonate shows a germinal matrix hemorrhage (GMH) in the left caudothalamic groove with fan-shaped increased echogenicity in the adjacent periventricular white matter, consistent with a hemorrhagic venous infarct (grade 4).* **(Right)** *Axial T1 MR in a premature infant with grade 4 GMH shows hyperintense hemorrhage in the right lateral ventricle with irregular intraparenchymal hemorrhage along the medullary veins.*

(Left) *Axial T1 MR in a neonate after a normal vaginal delivery shows a thin, bilateral, hyperintense subdural hemorrhage (SDH) → within the posterior fossa.* **(Right)** *Sagittal T1 MR in a neonate after vaginal delivery shows a small, hyperintense SDH → in the dependent supratentorial space. Such hemorrhages are seen in ~ 50% of neonates who have undergone routine delivery & should not cause alarm. They may be visible for a few weeks following delivery.*

Birth-Related Trauma

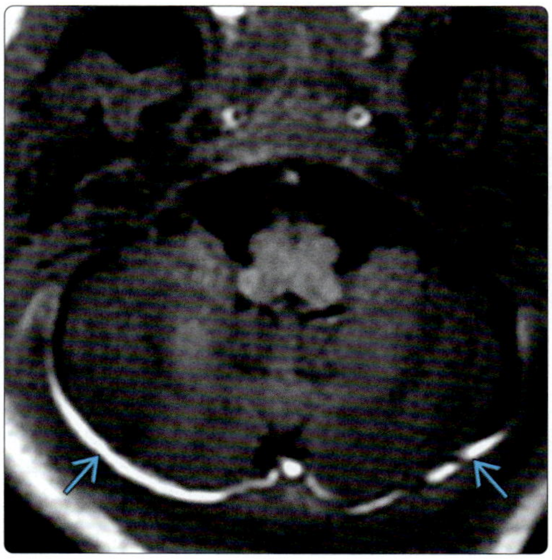

Birth-Related Trauma

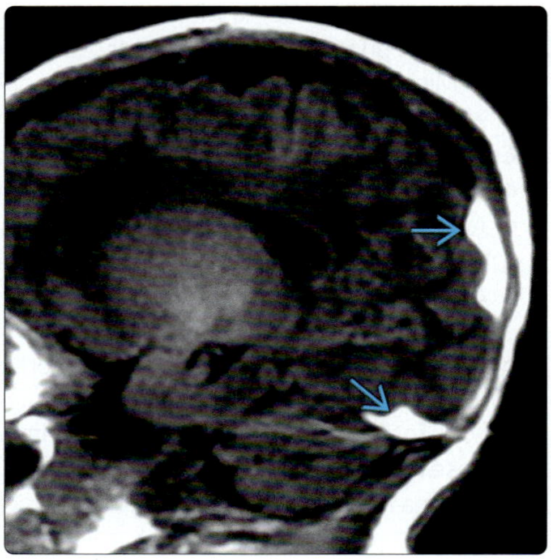

(Left) *Coronal NECT in a 3 month old with AHT shows bilateral mixed-attenuation subdural collections → with linear & globular foci of high attenuation → in the parasagittal regions, representing the tadpole or lollipop signs of bridging vein injuries.* **(Right)** *Axial SWI MR in a 6 week old with AHT shows multifocal areas of venous injury →, subdural fluid collections →, & a left frontal parenchymal laceration →. Parenchymal lacerations are characterized by parenchymal clefts or cysts with hematocrit levels.*

Abusive Head Trauma

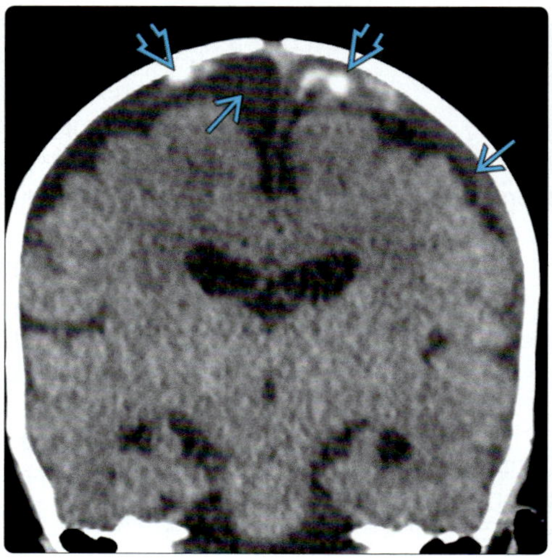

Abusive Head Trauma

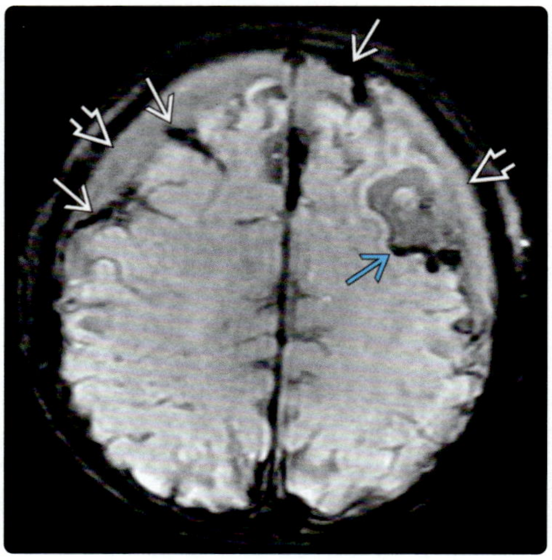

(Left) *Coronal NECT in a teenager with a left parietal hemorrhagic venous infarction → shows superficial tubular hyperdensities in the parasagittal region, corresponding to thrombosed cortical veins →.* **(Right)** *Coronal CT venogram in a 9 year old with a hemorrhagic venous infarct → in the left temporal lobe shows an empty delta sign in both the straight sinus → & left transverse sinus →, consistent with nearly occlusive thrombus.*

Venous Thrombosis & Infarction

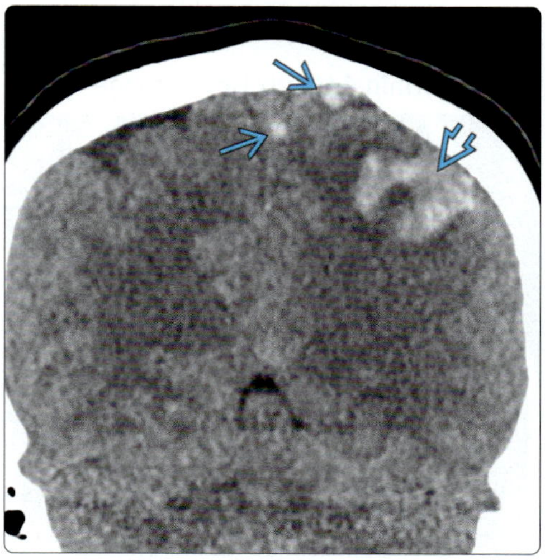

Venous Thrombosis & Infarction

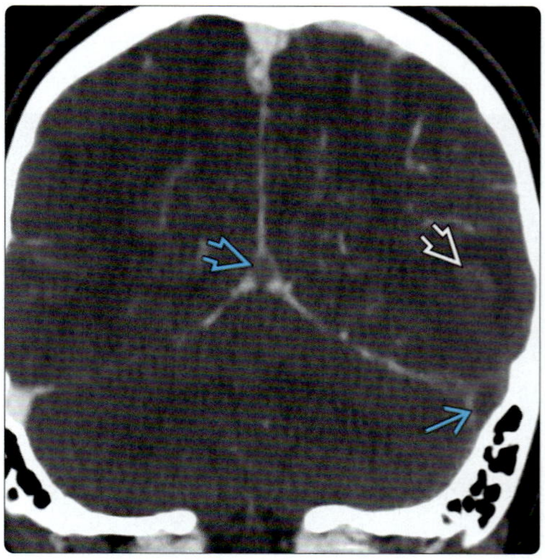

Arteriovenous Malformation

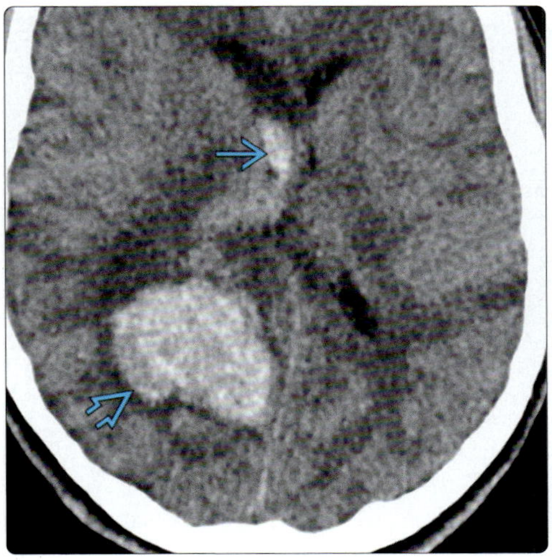

Arteriovenous Malformation

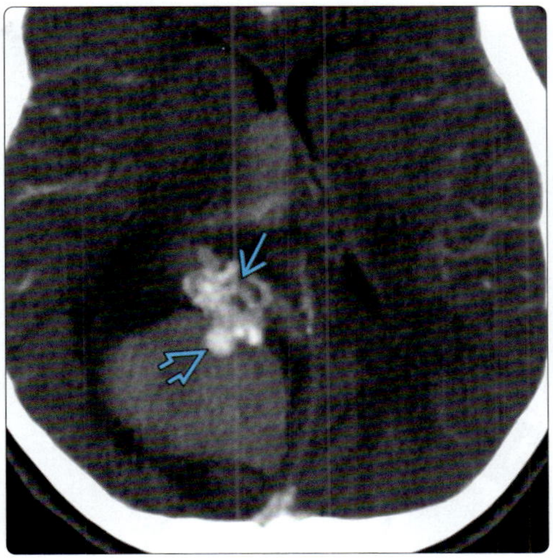

(Left) *Axial NECT in a young patient with a ruptured arteriovenous malformation (AVM) shows a right occipital hemorrhage ⇨ with extension into the right lateral ventricle →. Whenever such a hemorrhage is encountered, a CTA should be performed in an attempt to identify an underlying AVM or aneurysm.* **(Right)** *Axial CTA in the same patient shows a tangle of abnormal vessels corresponding to an AVM nidus → + a nidal aneurysm ⇨, which is the likely source of the hemorrhage.*

Cavernous Malformation

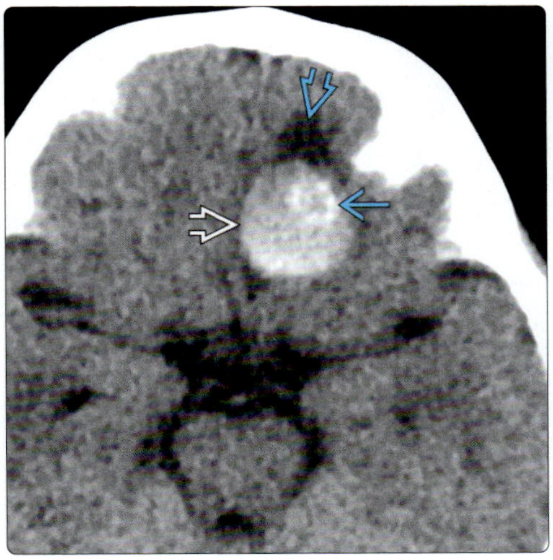

Cavernous Malformation

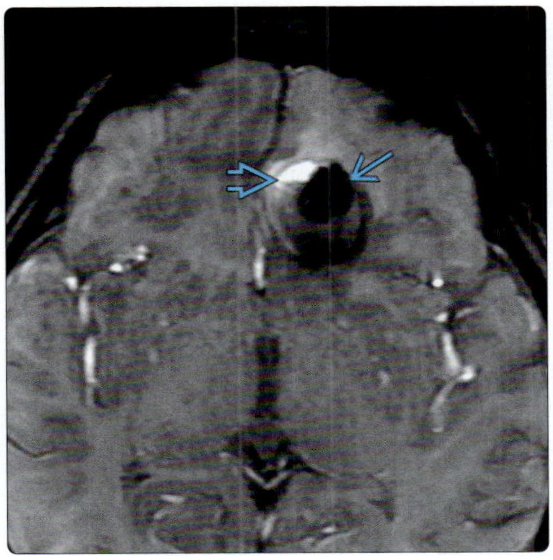

(Left) *Axial NECT in a 9 month old with an acute intraparenchymal hemorrhage ➡ shows a round, partially calcified, hyperdense lesion → of the left frontal lobe, suggesting a cavernous malformation (CM). Also note the vasogenic edema ⇨ anteriorly.* **(Right)** *Axial SWI MR in the same patient shows signal loss → in the region of the* Ca^{2+}*. There is also signal loss along the rim of the hemorrhagic cavity that contains a hematocrit level ⇨. These features are common with CMs.*

Cerebral Contusion

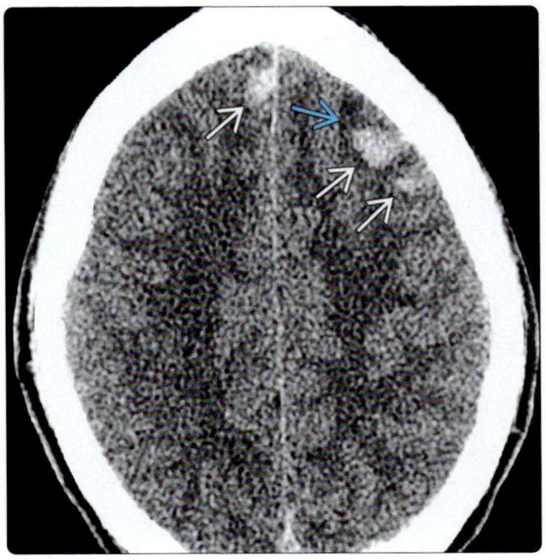

Cerebral Contusion

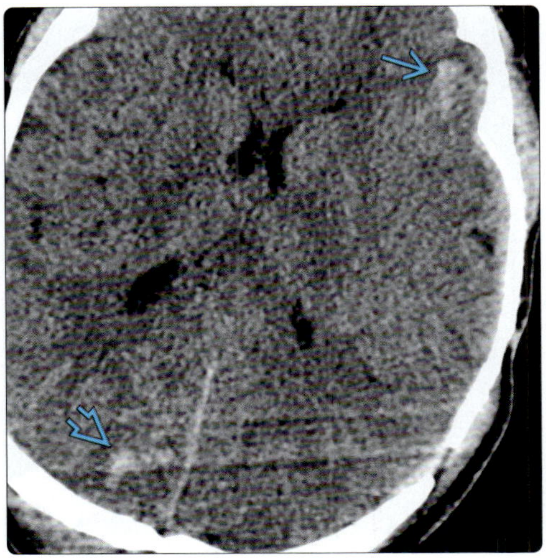

(Left) *Axial NECT shows multiple bilateral hemorrhagic frontal lobe contusions ➡ adjacent to the left frontal bone & anterior falx. Note the adjacent low-attenuation vasogenic edema →, a sign of intraaxial, rather than extraaxial, hemorrhage.* **(Right)** *Axial NECT in a teenager in an MVA shows a hemorrhagic contusion → in the left frontal lobe with associated contrecoup hemorrhage ⇨ in the right occipital lobe. Avoid satisfaction of search in traumatic ICH, as multifocality is common.*

(Left) *Parasagittal NECT in a 6 year old with diffuse axonal injury (DAI) from a motor vehicle accident shows areas of ↑ attenuation (due to hemorrhage) in the posterior body of the corpus callosum →, a common location for axonal shear injury.* **(Right)** *Axial SWI MR in a motor vehicle collision victim with DAI shows an extensive pattern of hemorrhagic shear injury within the corpus callosum → & right frontal lobe ⇒ at the gray-white matter junction. MR (with SWI or T2* GRE) shows a much greater extent of DAI vs. CT.*

Diffuse Axonal Injury

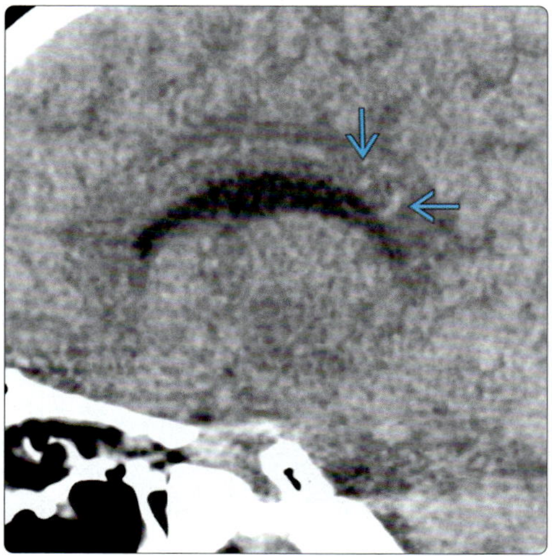

Diffuse Axonal Injury

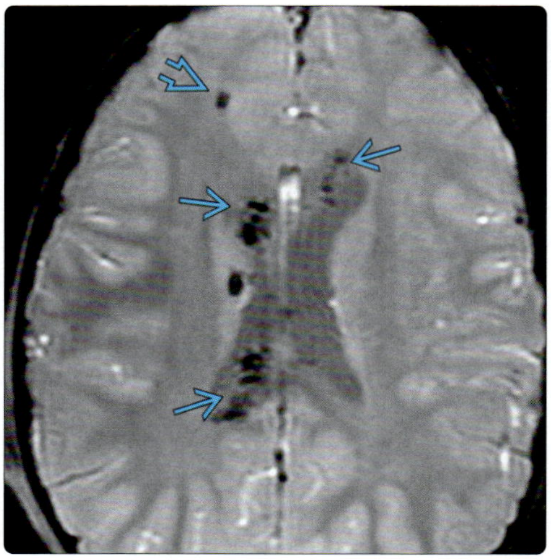

(Left) *Axial NECT in a teenager with recurrent ICH after the removal of a ventriculostomy catheter shows intraparenchymal hemorrhage → along the corpus callosum genu with adjacent vasogenic edema →.* **(Right)** *Lateral DSA in the same patient shows a round vascular outpouching → adjacent to a focal arterial narrowing, consistent with a pseudoaneurysm, the source of this patient's hemorrhage. While CTA & MRA will often detect aneurysms, DSA remains more sensitive.*

Aneurysm

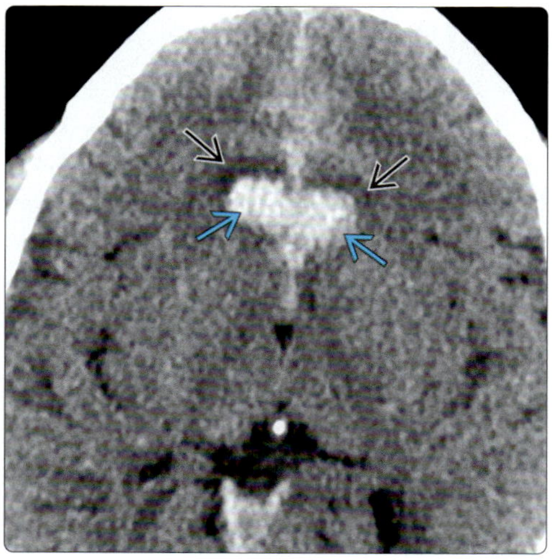

Aneurysm

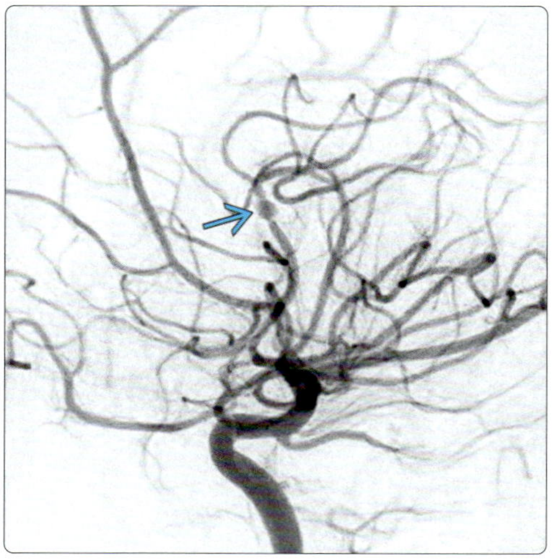

(Left) *Coronal NECT in a teenager with a hemorrhagic glioblastoma shows heterogeneous abnormal density → adjacent to the hyperdense hemorrhage ⇒, raising the possibility of an associated tumor. After a vascular lesion has been excluded by CTA, MR with contrast should be recommended.* **(Right)** *Axial T1 C+ MR in the same patient shows irregular rim enhancement of a necrotic lesion →, suggesting an underlying tumor. Pathology revealed glioblastoma.*

Hemorrhagic Neoplasms

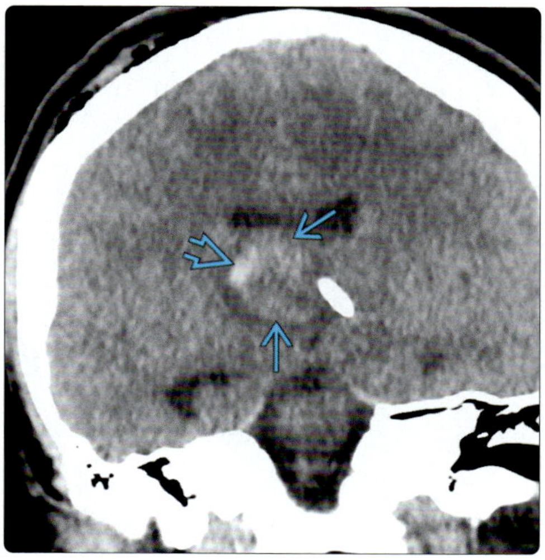

Hemorrhagic Neoplasms

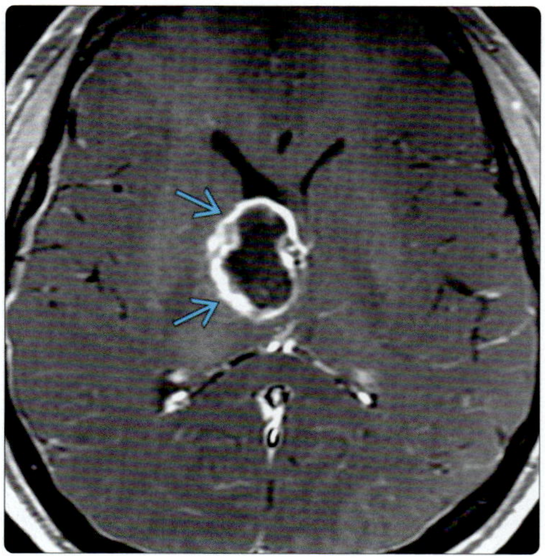

Subpial Hemorrhage

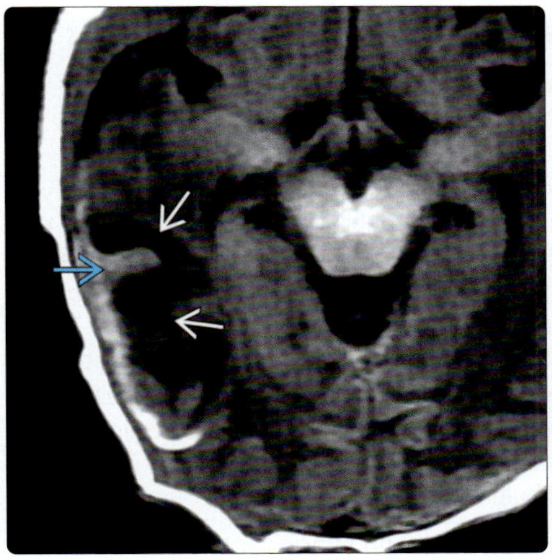

Subpial Hemorrhage

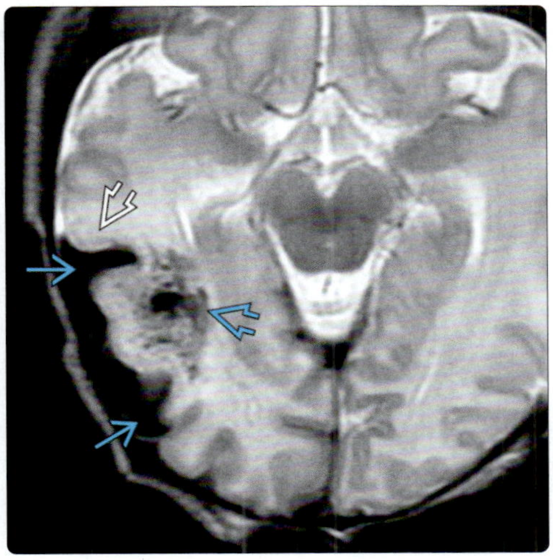

(Left) *Axial T1 MR in a neonate after a seizure shows a subpial hemorrhage. Note that the hemorrhage tracks into a sulcus* → *but, unlike subarachnoid hemorrhage (SAH), expands the affected sulcus & causes significant adjacent parenchymal changes* ➡. **(Right)** *Axial T2 MR in the same patient with subpial hemorrhage shows expanded sulci* → *with hemorrhagic changes* ⇨ *& loss of gray-white differentiation* ➡ *within the adjacent parenchyma.*

Coagulopathies & Blood Dyscrasias

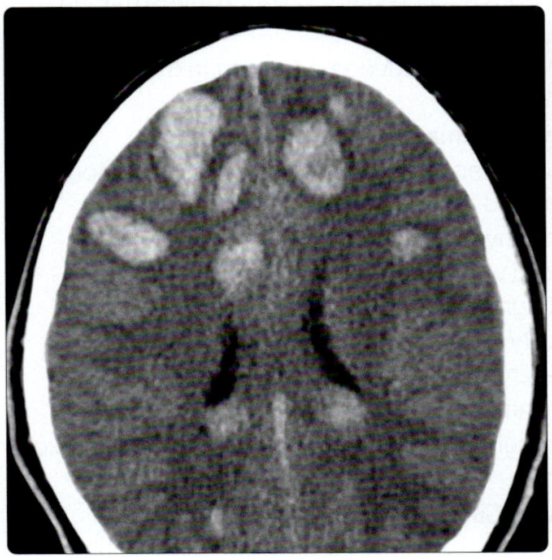

Coagulopathies & Blood Dyscrasias

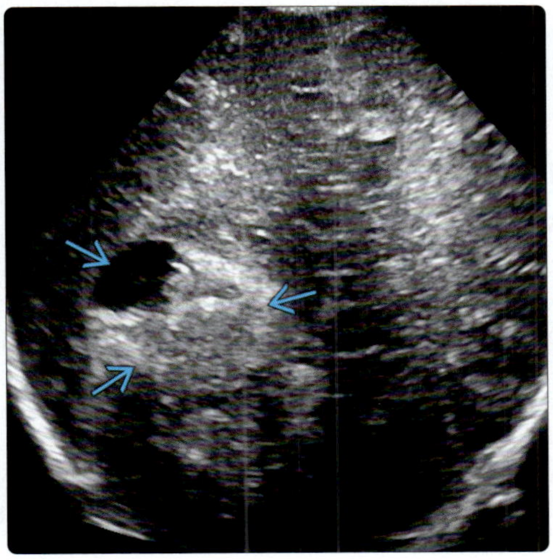

(Left) *Axial NECT in a teenager with hyperleukocytosis (WBC > 940K) shows multiple foci of intraparenchymal hemorrhage with rims of surrounding vasogenic edema. Multifocal intraparenchymal hemorrhage should suggest a coagulopathy.* **(Right)** *Coronal US in a 3 week old on ECMO shows a right occipital lobe hemorrhage with mixed echogenicity* →*. Look carefully for parenchymal & extraaxial hemorrhages in patients who are anticoagulated on ECMO.*

Herpes Encephalitis

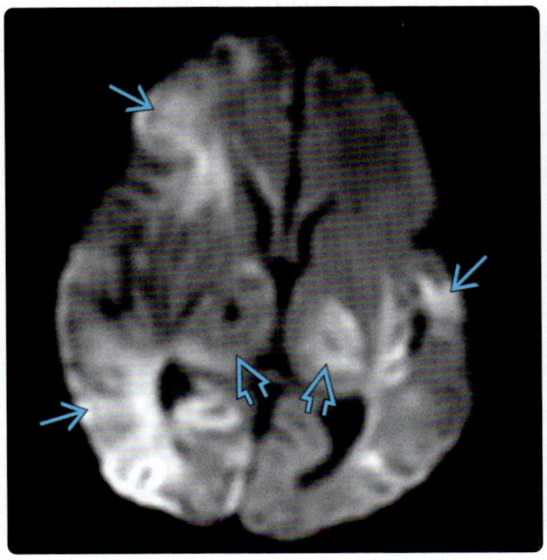

Herpes Encephalitis

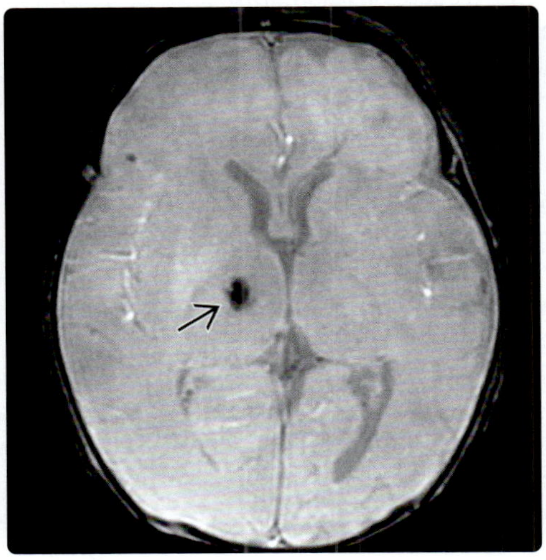

(Left) *Axial DWI MR in a 4 week old with seizures due to herpes encephalitis shows extensive asymmetric cytotoxic edema in the cerebral cortex* → *& deep gray nuclei* ⇨*, characteristic of herpes simplex virus type 2 (HSV-2). DWI is the key sequence for this diagnosis, as it shows abnormalities early in the disease course.* **(Right)** *Axial SWI MR in the same patient shows a focus of hemorrhage* → *in the right thalamus. Hemorrhage usually manifests more extensively in the subacute & late phases of herpes encephalitis.*

DIFFERENTIAL DIAGNOSIS

Common

- Pituitary Hyperplasia (Physiologic)
- Hypothalamic Glioma
- Optic Pathway Glioma
- Craniopharyngioma
- Germinoma
- Arachnoid Cyst
- Hydrocephalus (Mimic)

Less Common

- Pituitary Macroadenoma
- Hypothalamic Hamartoma
- Langerhans Cell Histiocytosis
- Rathke Cleft Cyst
- Teratoma
- Lipoma
- Dermoid Cyst
- Pituitary Stalk Anomalies

Rare but Important

- Retinoblastoma (Trilateral)
- Saccular Aneurysm
- Lymphocytic Hypophysitis

ESSENTIAL INFORMATION

Key Differential Diagnosis Issues

- Clinical features to consider
  - Associated syndromes
    - Neurofibromatosis type 1 (NF1): Optic pathway glioma
      - Typically more indolent than optic pathway gliomas in patients without NF1
    - *RB2* mutation: Trilateral retinoblastoma
  - Certain tumors are much more likely in young children
    - Teratoma, pilomyxoid astrocytoma
  - Certain tumors are much more likely in teenagers
    - Pituitary macroadenoma
  - Lesions highly associated with diabetes insipidus (DI)
    - Germinoma, Langerhans cell histiocytosis (LCH)
  - Gelastic seizures: Hypothalamic hamartoma
- Imaging feature to consider: Extra- vs. intraaxial
  - Extraaxial masses arise from pituitary/infundibulum, meninges, vessels
    - If extraaxial mass appears to arise from pituitary/infundibulum, determine origin of mass as precisely as possible
      - Pituitary gland: Think physiologic hyperplasia, hypophysitis, macroadenoma
      - Infundibular stalk: Germinoma, LCH, stalk anomalies
    - Nonpituitary extraaxial masses: Normal pituitary gland can usually be identified inferior to lesion
      - Craniopharyngioma
      - Hydrocephalus
      - Arachnoid cyst
      - Saccular aneurysm
  - Intraaxial masses arise from chiasm/hypothalamus
    - Pilocytic or pilomyxoid astrocytoma, tuber cinereum hamartoma
- Modality considerations
  - CT
    - Very helpful for identifying Ca^{2+} &/or hemorrhage
    - May show remodeling & enlargement of sella
  - MR
    - Precontrast sagittal T1: Critical sequence to identify posterior pituitary bright spot (neurohypophysis)
      - T1-hyperintense suprasellar mass should suggest craniopharyngioma, lipoma, dermoid, posterior pituitary ectopia
    - SWI/GRE: Helpful to identify Ca^{2+} & hemorrhage
    - DWI: Helpful in larger tumors to determine cellularity
    - High-resolution/3D SSFP: Helpful to determine origin of mass (e.g., continuity with optic nerves, infundibulum, etc.)

Helpful Clues for Common Diagnoses

- **Pituitary Hyperplasia (Physiologic)**
  - Up to 12-mm height with convex superior margin & homogeneous enhancement in young menstruating females
  - Consider with macroadenoma-appearing mass in teenage girl
- **Hypothalamic Glioma**
  - Majority are pilocytic astrocytomas (grade 1); minority are pilomyxoid astrocytomas (grade 2)
  - Centered in hypothalamus
  - Usually solid with intermediate to low T1 signal, high T2/FLAIR signal
  - Occasionally cystic but less likely to be cystic than pilocytic astrocytomas elsewhere in CNS
  - > 90% enhance to varying degrees
  - If hemorrhagic or in younger patient, suggest pilomyxoid astrocytoma
- **Optic Pathway Glioma**
  - Low-grade neoplasm of optic nerves, tracts, or chiasm
  - Best clue: Fusiform enlargement of optic nerves/chiasm in NF1 patient
    - Up to 60% have NF1; look for typical brain findings
  - Almost all are pilocytic astrocytomas, but imaging characteristics vary from other locations
    - Often nonenhancing & almost never cystic
- **Craniopharyngioma**
  - 90% have Ca^{2+} (globular, rim)
  - 90% are cystic (may have multiple)
    - Cyst contents are often hyperdense (CT) & T1 hyperintense (MR)
  - 90% enhance (usually at rim &/or nodule)
  - Centered in suprasellar region, but often extend into adjacent CSF spaces when large
- **Germinoma**
  - 30-40% of germinomas occur in suprasellar region
  - Unlike pineal region, M:F ratio is nearly equal in suprasellar germinoma
  - Often presents with DI
  - Often contains small cysts, especially when large
  - Solid components typically enhance & restrict diffusion
  - Look for leptomeningeal metastases (~ 25-40%)
- **Arachnoid Cyst**

- 1-5% are suprasellar
- Sharply marginated, thin-walled cyst ± mild bony remodeling
- Follows CSF on all sequences
- Mass effect on suprasellar structures → hydrocephalus & clinical symptoms (rare)

- **Hydrocephalus (Mimic)**
  - Enlarged 3rd ventricle (due to aqueductal stenosis or other distal obstruction) → anterior recess protrudes inferiorly
    - Mimics cystic lesion
  - May enlarge/remodel bony sella over time

Helpful Clues for Less Common Diagnoses

- **Pituitary Macroadenoma**
  - Very rare in 1st decade of life but one of most common suprasellar masses in late 2nd of decade
  - Figure 8 or snowman sign: Large sellar & suprasellar components separated by diaphragma sella
  - Correlation with pituitary hormone tests is helpful
- **Hypothalamic Hamartoma**
  - Isosexual precocious puberty is more common than gelastic seizures
  - Pedunculated ("collar button") or sessile mass between infundibular stalk & mammillary bodies
    - Can be tiny (1-2 mm) or giant (3-5 cm)
  - Hallmark features
    - Isointense to gray matter on all MR sequences (but often slightly hyperintense on T2/FLAIR)
    - No enhancement
- **Langerhans Cell Histiocytosis**
  - Often presents with DI
  - 10% of LCH cases involve stalk, pituitary gland ± hypothalamus
  - Look for solitary/multiple lytic bone lesions
- **Rathke Cleft Cyst**
  - Cyst arising between anterior & posterior pituitary
  - Rarely calcifies, does not enhance, variable MR signal
  - Intracystic nodule is virtually pathognomonic
- **Teratoma**
  - Optic chiasm > pineal locations
  - Ca^{2+}, cysts, soft tissue, & fat
- **Lipoma**
  - Fatty hypothalamic mass without soft tissue component
  - May have associated midline anomalies
- **Dermoid Cyst**
  - Fat-like mass ± fat droplets in CSF
    - Fat-suppression MR sequences confirm
  - 20% show Ca^{2+}
- **Pituitary Stalk Anomalies**
  - Posterior pituitary ectopia
    - Short stature ± endocrine deficiencies
    - Posterior pituitary "bright spot" is missing or ectopic
    - Stalk is small/absent
  - Duplicated pituitary gland/stalk
    - Endocrinologically normal
    - ± midline facial anomalies
    - Tuber cinereum/mammillary bodies are fused

Helpful Clues for Rare Diagnoses

- **Retinoblastoma (Trilateral)**
  - 3rd tumor in pineal or suprasellar region, often delayed compared to retinal tumors
  - 3D SSFP MR images help visualize small retinal lesions
- **Saccular Aneurysm**
  - Rare in children (< 2% of all saccular aneurysms)
  - Often large/bizarre, frequently with thrombus
  - Look for phase-encoding pulsation artifact on MR
- **Lymphocytic Hypophysitis**
  - Very rare in children, usually occurring in adolescents
  - Headache, vision impairment, & endocrine dysfunction are typical

SELECTED REFERENCES

1. Seeburg DP et al: Imaging of the sella and parasellar region in the pediatric population. Neuroimaging Clin N Am. 27(1):99-121, 2017
2. Yildiz AE et al: Suprasellar masses in children: characteristic MR imaging features. J Neuroradiol. 43(4):246-59, 2016

Pituitary Hyperplasia (Physiologic)

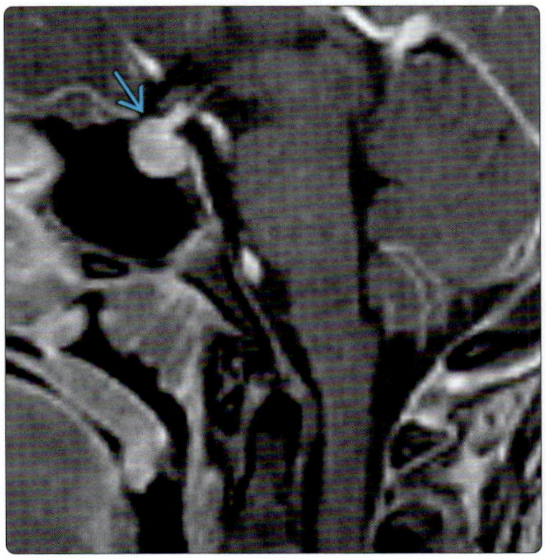

Pituitary Hyperplasia (Physiologic)

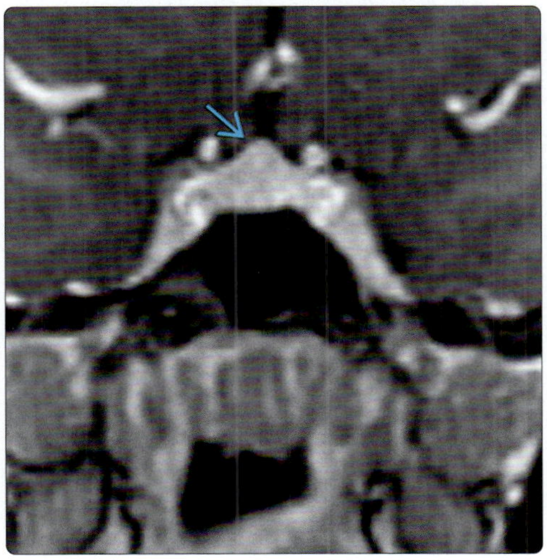

(Left) *Sagittal T1 C+ MR of a teenage girl with physiologic hyperplasia of the pituitary shows a convex superior pituitary margin ➡, which is commonly seen in this setting. Note the homogeneous pituitary enhancement, characteristic of physiologic hyperplasia.* **(Right)** *Coronal T1 C+ MR in the same patient shows superior convexity ➡ & homogeneous enhancement of the pituitary, characteristic of physiologic hyperplasia. Smooth midline bulging without deviation of the pituitary stalk is typical.*

Hypothalamic Glioma

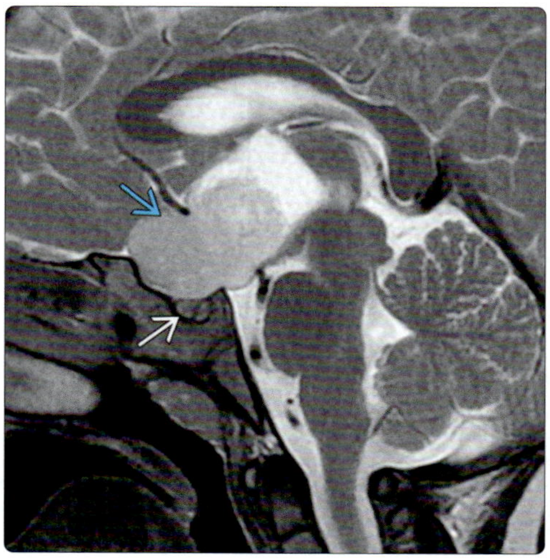

Hypothalamic Glioma

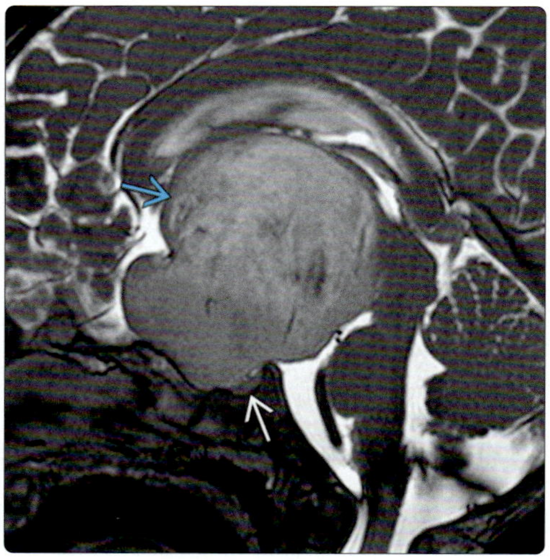

(Left) *Sagittal T2 MR in a 2 year old with a pilocytic astrocytoma (PA) shows a large mass → centered in the hypothalamus/optic chiasm. Note the preserved pituitary gland →, which helps distinguish this lesion from a mass arising from the sella/pituitary.* **(Right)** *Midline sagittal FIESTA MR in a 9 month old with a pilomyxoid astrocytoma (PMA) shows a large hypothalamic mass → with mass effect on the pituitary →. PMA is more likely to be hemorrhagic & occur in younger patients than PA.*

Optic Pathway Glioma

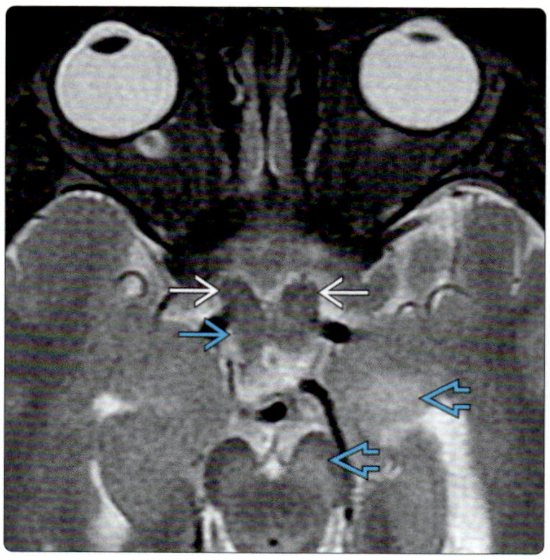

Optic Pathway Glioma

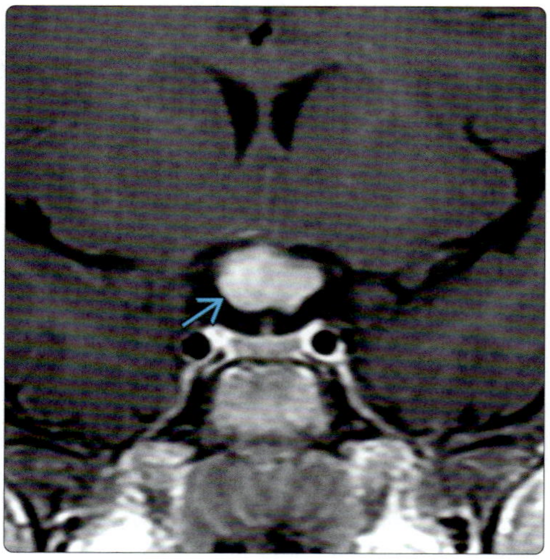

(Left) *Axial T2 MR in an neurofibromatosis type 1 (NF1) patient with an optic pathway glioma (OPG) shows fusiform thickening of the optic chiasm → & optic nerves →. When encountering an OPG, look closely for associated nonenhancing signal abnormalities → of the brain typical of NF1, as seen here.* **(Right)** *Coronal T1 C+ MR in a 2 year old with an OPG shows enlargement & avid enhancement of the optic chiasm → just superior to the pituitary. This enhancement extended into the optic nerves & optic tracts bilaterally.*

Craniopharyngioma

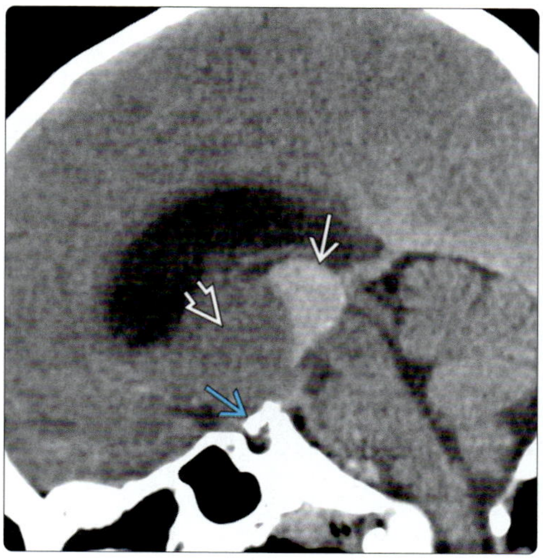

Craniopharyngioma

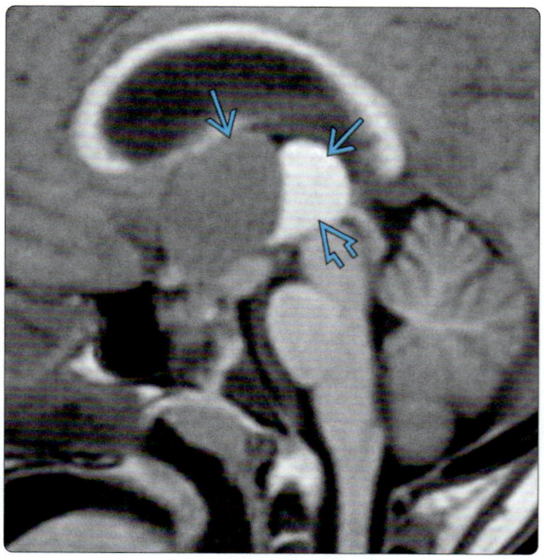

(Left) *Midline sagittal NECT in a 5 year old with a craniopharyngioma shows a suprasellar mass with cystic areas of relatively high → & low → attenuation. Also note the Ca^{2+} → along the inferior margin of the mass. The hyperdense cystic components & Ca^{2+} are pathognomonic for craniopharyngioma.* **(Right)** *Sagittal T1 MR in the same patient shows a multicystic suprasellar mass with components → of varying signal intensity, including T1 hyperintensity →, characteristic of a craniopharyngioma.*

Germinoma

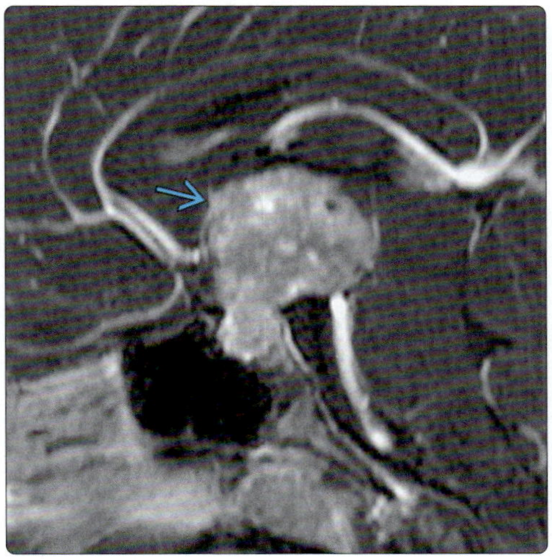

Germinoma

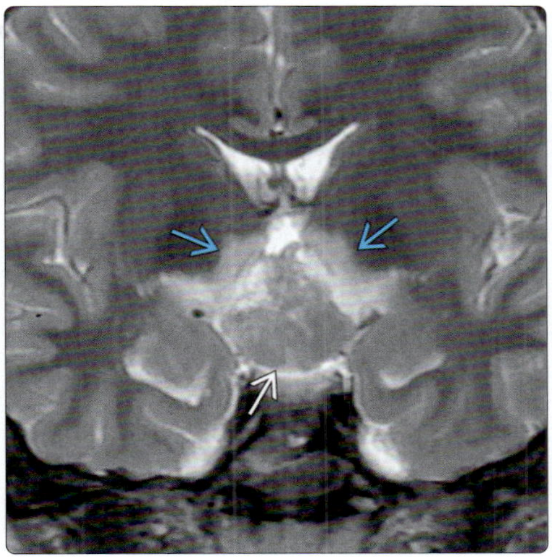

(Left) *Sagittal T1 C+ MR in an 11-year-old boy with a germinoma shows a large, heterogeneously enhancing sellar & suprasellar mass ➙. When large, germinomas often involve both the sellar & suprasellar regions but do not typically cause enlargement or remodeling of the sella.* **(Right)** *Coronal T2 MR in the same patient shows hypointense signal within the mass ➙. Note the extensive abnormal signal in the adjacent deep gray nuclei ➙, a characteristic finding in germinoma as compared to other suprasellar masses.*

Arachnoid Cyst

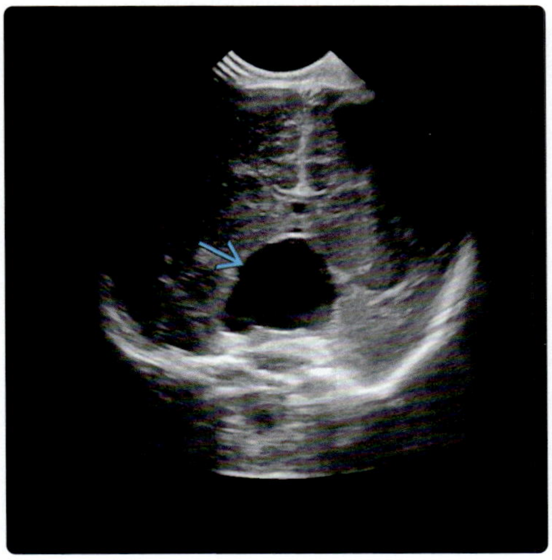

Arachnoid Cyst

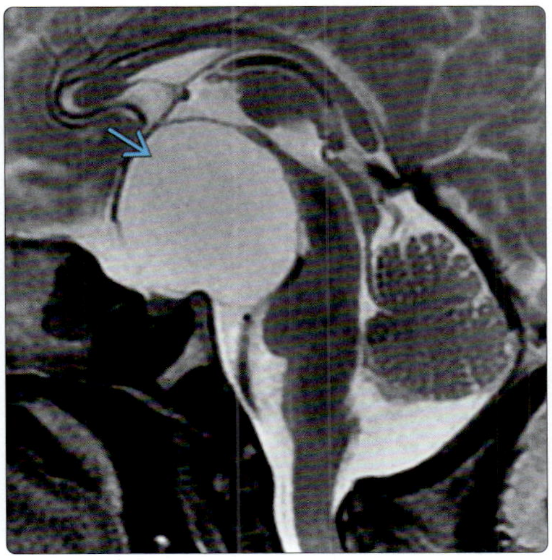

(Left) *Coronal US in a neonate with a prenatally identified mass shows an anechoic simple-appearing suprasellar lesion ➙, consistent with an arachnoid cyst.* **(Right)** *Sagittal T2 MR in the same neonate more completely characterizes the suprasellar arachnoid cyst ➙ & its mass effect on adjacent structures. Arachnoid cysts typically do not cause symptoms, except when located in the basilar cisterns where they may cause mass effect on critical structures & obstructive hydrocephalus, especially in younger patients.*

Hydrocephalus (Mimic)

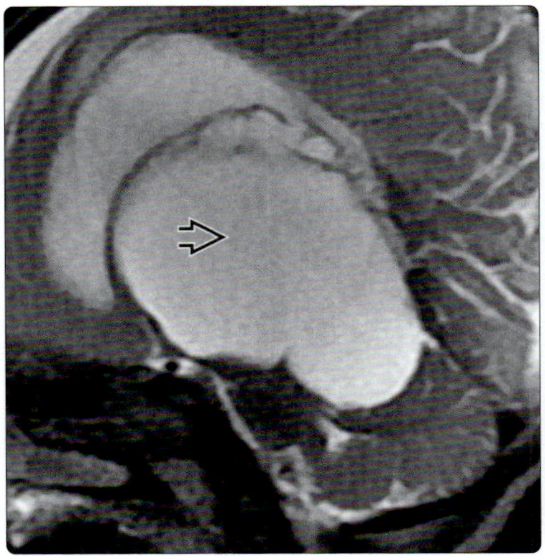

Hydrocephalus (Mimic)

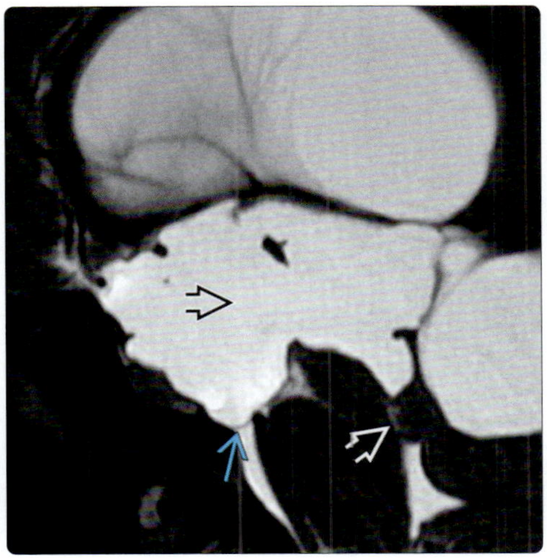

(Left) *Sagittal T2 MR in a 1 year old with multiloculated hydrocephalus shows marked enlargement of the 3rd ventricle ⇨. Expansion of the pineal recess causes mass effect on the cerebellum & brainstem.* **(Right)** *Sagittal FIESTA MR in a teenager with ventricular obstruction at the level of the cerebral aqueduct ➡ shows marked enlargement of the 3rd ventricle ⇨ with remodeling of the skull base & effacement of normal suprasellar structures. The floor of 3rd ventricle ➙ extends down to the basilar artery.*

(Left) *Midline sagittal CECT in a 12-year-old girl with prolactinemia shows an avidly enhancing mass arising from the sella turcica. Note the expansion of the sella, suggesting a relatively longstanding process. The findings are most suggestive of a pituitary macroadenoma.* **(Right)** *Sagittal T2 MR in the same patient demonstrates a mostly solid mass with a cyst containing a fluid-fluid level* → *. Hemorrhage is often identified in pituitary macroadenomas, especially larger tumors.*

Pituitary Macroadenoma

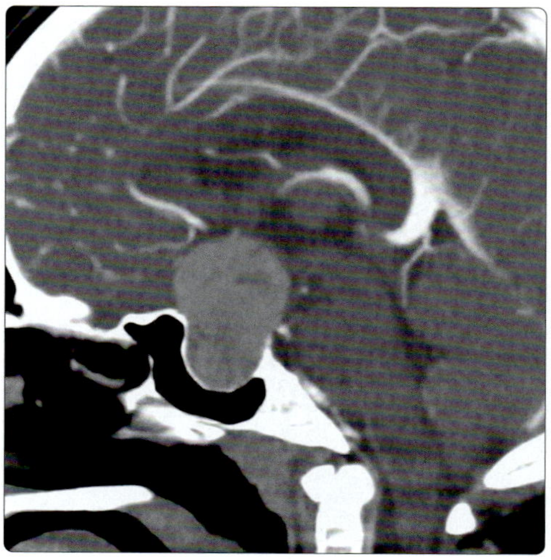

Pituitary Macroadenoma

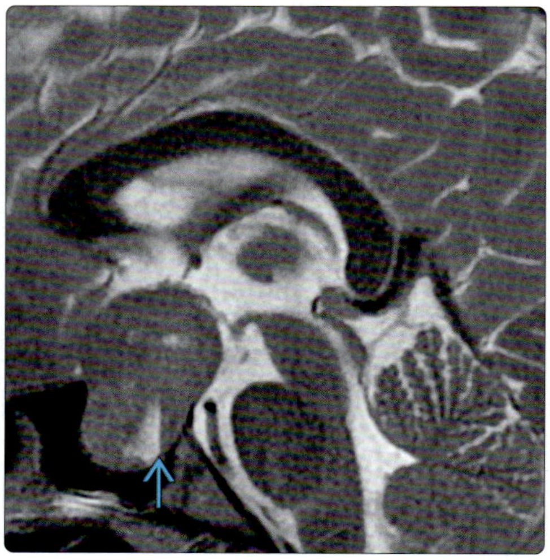

(Left) *Sagittal T2 MR in an 8 year old with precocious puberty shows a typical appearance of a hypothalamic hamartoma* → *, which is isointense to cortical gray matter.* **(Right)** *Sagittal T1 C+ MR images in a 4 year old with diabetes insipidus show an abnormally thick, enhancing pituitary infundibulum* → *. A lytic enhancing mass* ➡ *is also seen in the occipital bone. Biopsy confirmed Langerhans cell histiocytosis.*

Hypothalamic Hamartoma

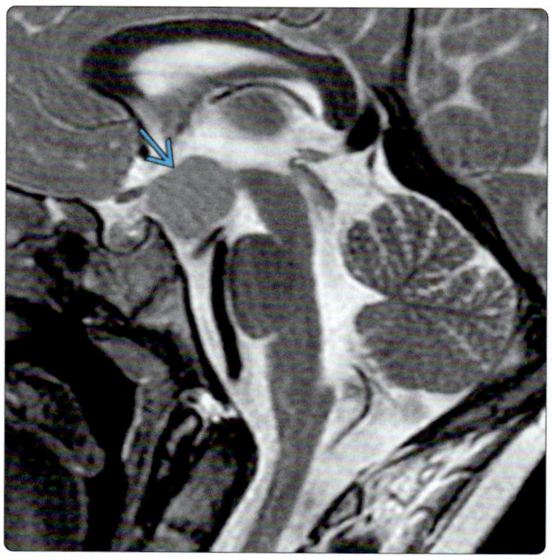

Langerhans Cell Histiocytosis

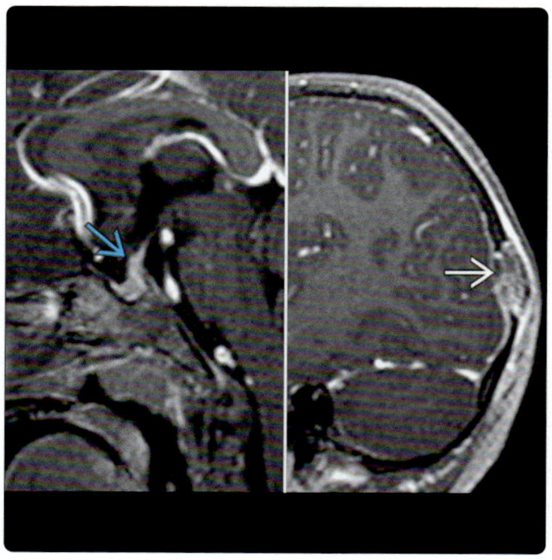

(Left) *Sagittal T1 MR in a 17 year old shows a T1-hyperintense cyst* → *located between the neurohypophysis & adenohypophysis, a typical location for a Rathke cleft cyst. The T1 signal intensity of these lesions is highly variable.* **(Right)** *Sagittal T2 MR in the same patient with a Rathke cleft cyst shows a characteristic T2-hypointense nodule* → *in the inferior aspect of the cyst.*

Rathke Cleft Cyst

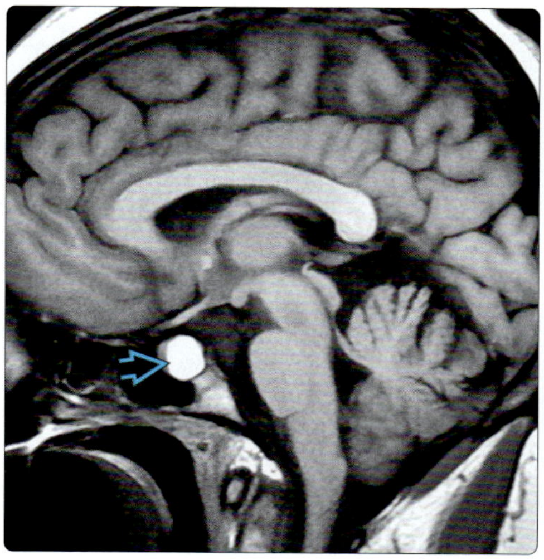

Rathke Cleft Cyst

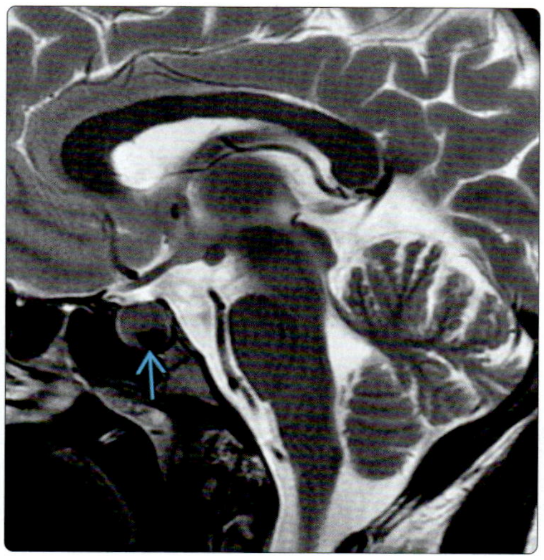

Teratoma

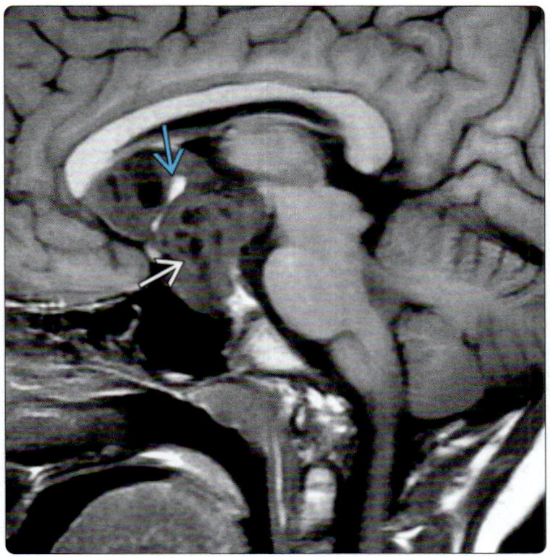

Lipoma

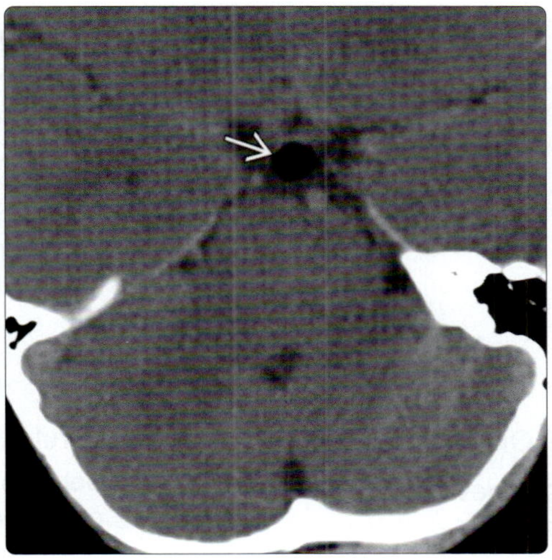

(Left) *Sagittal T1 MR in a 6-year-old girl with a mature cystic teratoma shows a large mixed solid & cystic mass in the sellar & suprasellar locations. Note the central linear focus of T1 shortening due to fat, a key finding to support the diagnosis of teratoma.* **(Right)** *Axial NECT in a 3-year-old boy with a suprasellar lipoma in a retrochiasmatic location is shown. The fat attenuation & lack of an associated soft tissue component are consistent with a lipoma, for which this is a common location.*

Pituitary Stalk Anomalies

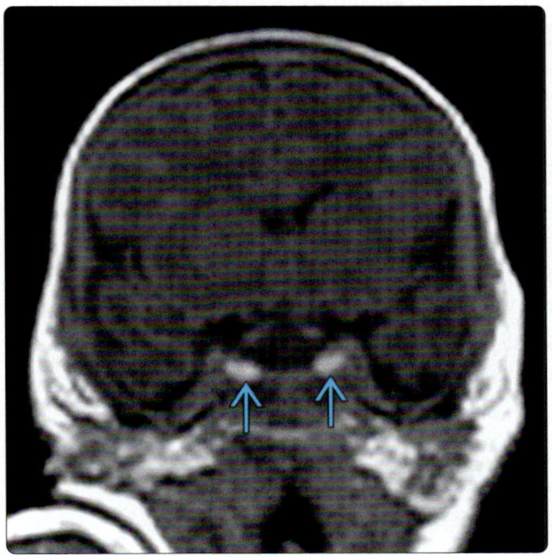

Retinoblastoma (Trilateral)

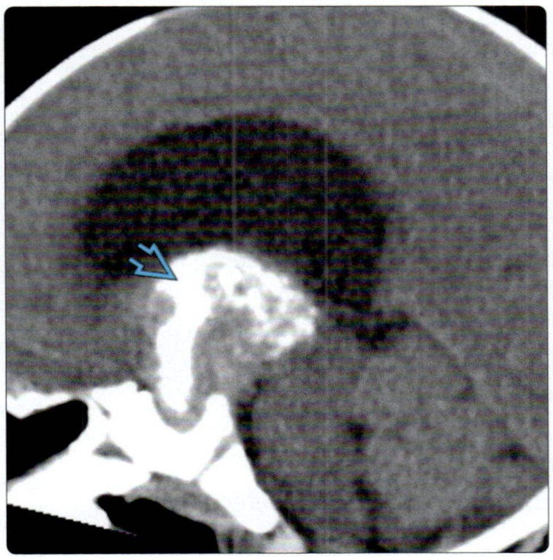

(Left) *Coronal reformatted MR from a volumetric T1 GRE acquisition in a newborn with an epignathus teratoma (not shown) demonstrates a duplicated pituitary gland. Note that the entire pituitary gland is typically bright on T1 MR images in neonates.* **(Right)** *Midline sagittal NECT in a 3 month old with trilateral retinoblastoma shows a heavily calcified sellar & suprasellar mass. Suprasellar retinoblastoma often has imaging features similar to the ocular tumors, including Ca^{2+} in a cellular enhancing tumor.*

Saccular Aneurysm

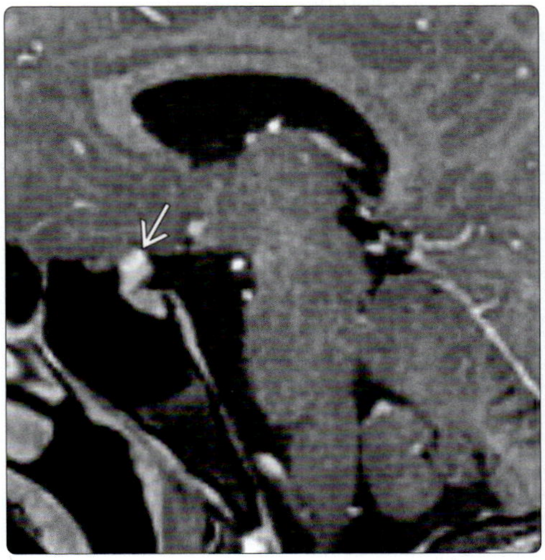

Saccular Aneurysm

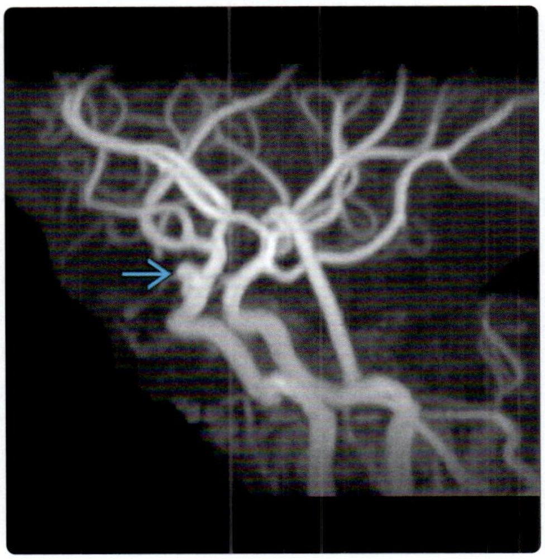

(Left) *Sagittal T1 C+ MR in an 11 year old with tuberous sclerosis shows a distal internal carotid aneurysm. Aneurysms are rarely mistaken for other suprasellar masses except when large & partially thrombosed. Look for clues, such as continuity with vessels & associated pulsation artifact.* **(Right)** *3D time-of-flight MRA in the same patient shows the distal ICA aneurysm. Time-of-flight MRA can be helpful to demonstrate flow within the lesion.*

DIFFERENTIAL DIAGNOSIS

Common

- Pineal Cyst

Less Common

- Germinoma
- Teratoma
- Other Germ Cell Tumors
- Pineoblastoma

Rare but Important

- Retinoblastoma
- Pineocytoma

ESSENTIAL INFORMATION

Key Differential Diagnosis Issues

- Clinical features to consider
  - Sex: Germ cell tumors (GCTs) are much more common in males
    - Include germinoma, teratoma, others (yolk sac, choriocarcinoma, embryonal carcinoma, mixed GCT)
  - Age: GCTs are most common in 2nd decade
  - Serum tumor markers: Elevated β-HCG, AFP, or placental alkaline phosphatase (PLAP) indicates GCT
- Modality considerations
  - MR
    - Imaging modality of choice
    - Allows for evaluation of tumor cellularity (DWI), Ca^{2+} morphology (GRE/SWI), & involvement of adjacent structures (e.g., thalami)
    - Most sensitive exam for leptomeningeal metastases
      - Image entire neuraxis for most pineal tumors
  - CT
    - Helpful to distinguish hemorrhage vs. Ca^{2+}
    - Helpful for identifying localized central vs. scattered pineal mass Ca^{2+}
    - Increased density indicates high tumor cellularity
    - Fat (e.g., mature teratoma) is often most conspicuous on CT
- Take home points
  - Clinical information (e.g., serum tumor markers) are very helpful in narrowing differential
  - Key imaging features: Tumor cellularity, Ca^{2+} morphology, & thalamic involvement

Helpful Clues for Common Diagnoses

- **Pineal Cyst**
  - Key facts
    - Intrapineal glial-lined cyst, nonneoplastic
    - Pineal cysts are very common in children (~ 50%) on high-resolution (i.e., 3D FIESTA) MR imaging
    - May increase or involute over time
    - Majority are 5-10 mm; may be > 20 mm
    - Rarely symptomatic: Hemorrhage, acute hydrocephalus, or Parinaud syndrome
  - Imaging
    - Well-defined, uni-/multiloculated cyst
    - Posterior to 3rd ventricle, above tectum, below internal cerebral veins
    - T1 & T2: Iso- to hyperintense to CSF
    - FLAIR: Usually hyperintense to CSF
    - DWI: Typically isointense to CSF
    - GRE/SWI: May rarely identify intracystic blooming if recent or old hemorrhage
      - Do not confuse pineal parenchymal Ca^{2+} for cyst hemorrhage
    - T1 C+: Thin (< 2-mm) rim of enhancement = compressed pineal tissue
      - Rarely nodular enhancement
      - If amount of pineal tissue is qualitatively increased, then recommend follow-up imaging
      - Avoid delayed postcontrast imaging, as it may show enhancement of cyst contents, making differentiation from tumors impossible

Helpful Clues for Less Common Diagnoses

- **Germinoma**
  - Key facts
    - Tumor of primordial germ cells (GCT)
    - Most common GCT (55-65% of all GCTs)
    - Most common pineal tumor in children
      - 30-40% of CNS germinomas occur in pineal region vs. 50-60% suprasellar & up to 15% in thalamus & basal ganglia
    - M > > F (15:1) in pineal region (vs. 1:1 in suprasellar region)
    - Presents with headache, hydrocephalus, & Parinaud syndrome (paralysis of upward gaze)
  - Imaging
    - Extension into thalami: Most specific finding for germinoma
    - Even small lesions may cause obstructive hydrocephalus due to infiltrative nature
    - Look carefully for subarachnoid metastases
    - CT
      - Iso-/hyperdense to gray matter
      - Localized (central or peripheral) pineal Ca^{2+}
    - MR
      - T1: Iso-/hypointense relative to gray matter
      - T2: Variable, ± hyperintense cysts
      - FLAIR: Iso- to hypointense relative to gray matter
      - DWI: Typically shows restricted diffusion or diffusion signal similar to gray matter
      - T1 C+: Avid contrast enhancement; often speckled pattern
      - GRE/SWI: Localized (central or peripheral) pineal Ca^{2+}
      - MRS: ↑ choline, ↓ NAA, ± lactate
- **Teratoma**
  - Key facts
    - Mature, immature, & malignant types
    - M > > F in pineal & suprasellar region
    - Presents with headache, hydrocephalus, & Parinaud syndrome (paralysis of upward gaze)
  - Imaging
    - Heterogeneous pineal region mass, usually with 3 tissue types: Fat, soft tissue, Ca^{2+}
    - Difficult to distinguish mature from immature
    - CT: Often best diagnostic tool because fat, soft tissue, & Ca^{2+} are so easily delineated

- MR: Must use variety of sequences to confirm 3 tissue types (as T1 may show ↑ signal from fat, variable signal from Ca^{2+})
  - T1/T2 with fat suppression confirms fat
  - SWI confirms Ca^{2+}
  - T1 C+ confirms enhancing soft tissue
- **Other Germ Cell Tumors**
  - Key facts
    - Tumor of primordial germ cells
    - Histologically & biochemically diverse tumors
      - Yolk sac, choriocarcinoma, embryonal carcinoma, mixed GCT
    - Serum markers & histology are important in determining tumor type
  - Imaging
    - Varied imaging findings
      - Often heterogeneous with multiple cysts
      - Usually have localized Ca^{2+}
      - Rarely extend into adjacent thalami (important to distinguish from germinoma)
- **Pineoblastoma**
  - Key facts
    - Embryonal tumor of pineal gland
    - Malignant: WHO grade 4
    - Children > adults
      - Up to 40% in infants
  - Imaging
    - Large (usually > 3-cm) pineal mass
    - Classic teaching: Scattered ("exploded") Ca^{2+}
    - Hydrocephalus from aqueductal obstruction
    - Often extends into 3rd ventricle
    - CT: Solid portion hyperdense
    - DWI: ↑ DWI & ↓ ADC signal due to high cellularity
    - T1: Solid portion is iso- to hyperintense to gray matter
    - T2: Solid portion is iso- to hyperintense to gray matter; frequent necrosis; occasional hemorrhage
    - Moderate heterogeneous enhancement
    - CSF spread in up to 40% at time of presentation

Helpful Clues for Rare Diagnoses

- **Retinoblastoma**
  - Key facts
    - Trilateral retinoblastoma = bilateral ocular retinoblastoma + midline intracranial tumor
      - Pineal (80%), suprasellar (20%)
    - Intracranial 3rd tumor usually presents 2-3 years after primary ocular tumors
    - Histologically identical to ocular tumors
  - Imaging
    - Enhancing pineal mass + bilateral ocular retinoblastoma
    - Differential diagnosis is metastatic retinoblastoma
- **Pineocytoma**
  - Key facts
    - Pineal parenchymal tumor
    - Rare in children; may occur at any age
      - Mean age: 35 years
    - M = F
    - Variable natural history from noninvasive & slow growing to aggressive with extensive metastases
  - Imaging
    - Well-defined, round, homogeneous mass
    - T1: Iso- to hypointense relative to gray matter
    - T2 & FLAIR: Iso- to hyperintense
    - Peripheral or central homogeneous enhancement
    - More uniform enhancement than pineoblastoma
    - May be similar to CSF on precontrast images, simulating simple cyst
    - Areas of necrosis are common in larger lesions

SELECTED REFERENCES

1. Tamrazi B et al: Pineal region masses in pediatric patients. Neuroimaging Clin N Am. 27(1):85-97, 2017
2. Awa R et al: Neuroimaging diagnosis of pineal region tumors-quest for pathognomonic finding of germinoma. Neuroradiology. 56(7):525-34, 2014
3. Dumrongpisutikul N et al: Distinguishing between germinomas and pineal cell tumors on MR imaging. AJNR Am J Neuroradiol. 33(3):550-5, 2012
4. Dhall G et al: Pineal region tumors in children. Curr Opin Neurol. 23(6):576-82, 2010

Pineal Cyst

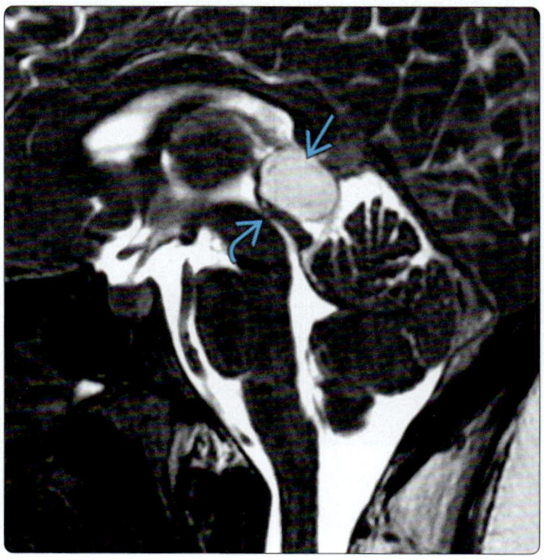

Pineal Cyst

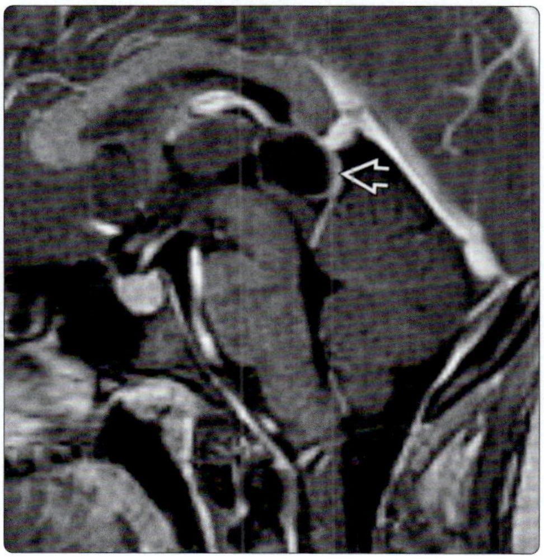

(Left) *Sagittal FIESTA MR in an 18 year old with headaches shows a cystic mass ➔ in the pineal gland. There is mass effect on the tectum with narrowing of the cerebral aqueduct ➔, but there is no obstructive hydrocephalus. In the absence of obstruction, even large pineal cysts are usually incidental.* **(Right)** *Sagittal T1 C+ MR in the same patient shows a thin rim ➔ of pineal tissue without nodularity. The total enhancing pineal volume appeared grossly normal, supporting the diagnosis of a simple cyst.*

(Left) *Axial NECT in a 15-year-old boy with difficulty walking shows a hyperdense pineal mass* ➡ *with localized central ("engulfed") pineal* Ca^{2+} → *, suggesting a germinoma. Also note the enlarged ventricles* ⇨*, consistent with obstructive hydrocephalus, a common finding in pineal region masses.* **(Right)** *Sagittal T1 C+ MR in the same patient shows an enhancing pineal mass* → *with a 2nd lesion* ➡ *within the septum pellucidum, consistent with leptomeningeal spread of disease.*

Germinoma

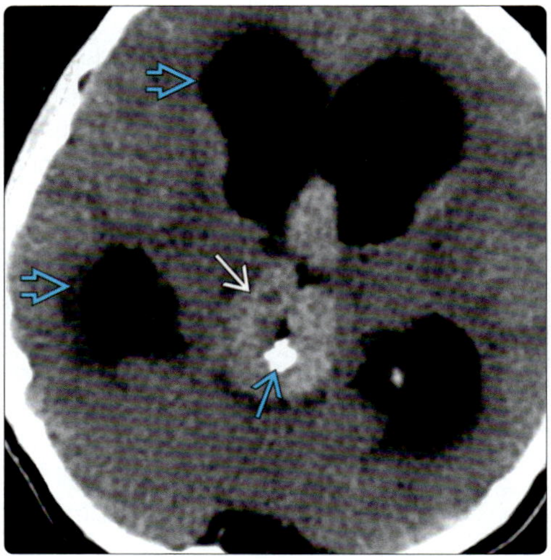

Germinoma

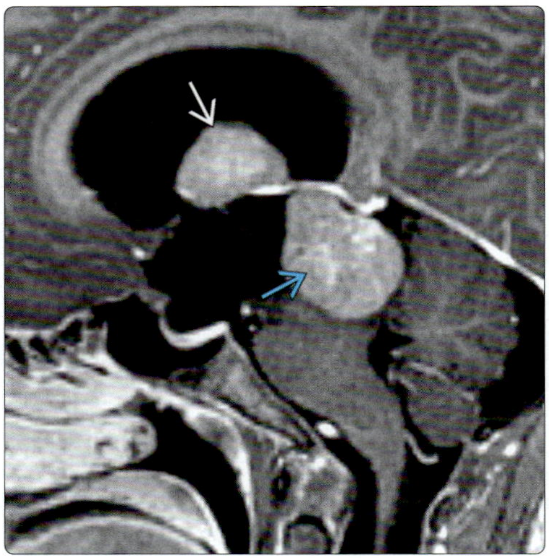

(Left) *Axial ADC MR in a 16-year-old boy with germinoma shows a pineal region mass* → *with decreased signal compared to brain parenchyma, consistent with a cellular tumor. Also note the facilitated diffusion* ➡ *(edema) in the adjacent thalami.* **(Right)** *Axial T1 C+ MR in the same patient shows a bilobed pineal region mass* →*. Extension into the bilateral thalamic nuclei with adjacent vasogenic edema (low T1 signal* ➡*) is a feature that is frequently seen in germinoma & is rare in other pineal region tumors.*

Germinoma

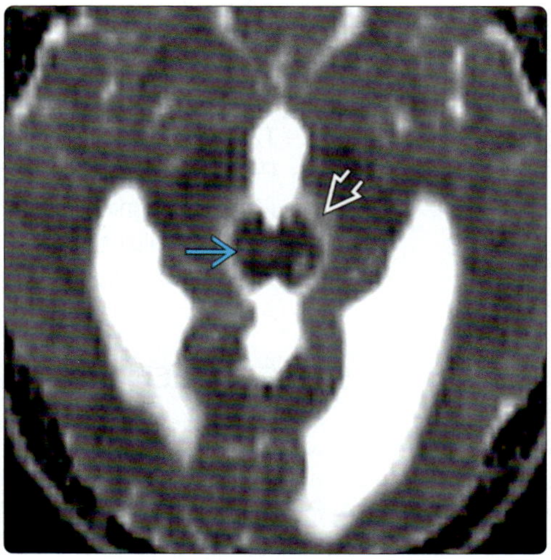

Germinoma

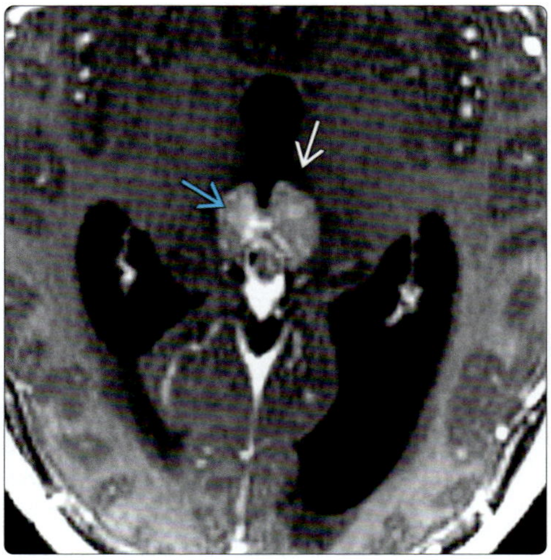

(Left) *Sagittal NECT in a 7-year-old boy with a mature teratoma shows all 3 characteristic tissue components: Fat* ➡*,* Ca^{2+} →*, & soft tissue* →*. These 3 components are often best demonstrated on CT.* **(Right)** *Axial T1 MR in the same patient shows intrinsic hyperintense signal* → *within the pineal lesion. When such a finding is encountered, fat saturation sequences should be employed to distinguish fat from hemorrhage or* Ca^{2+}*. Confirmation of fat is very helpful in narrowing the DDx.*

Teratoma

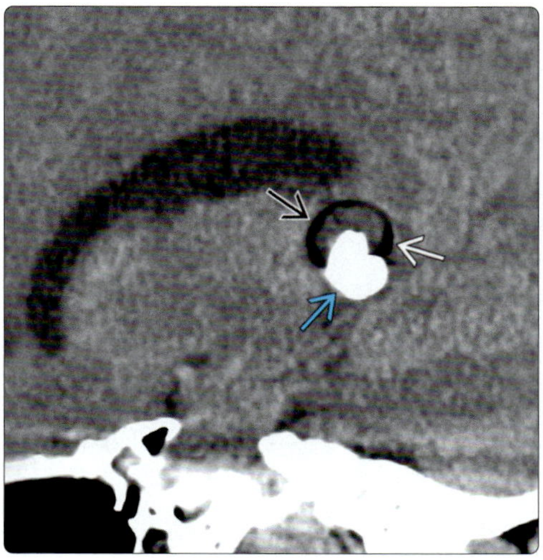

Teratoma

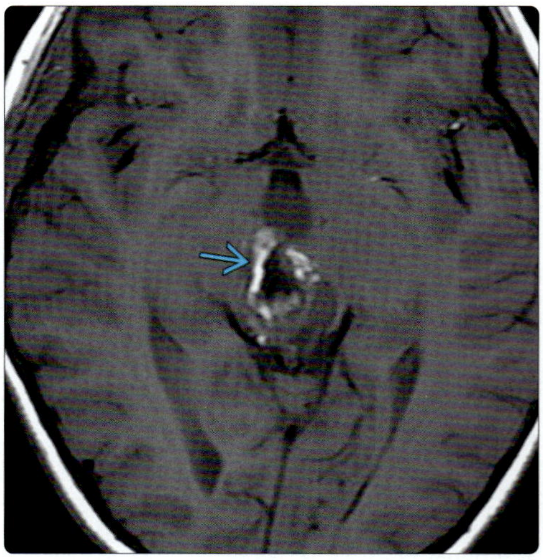

Other Germ Cell Tumors

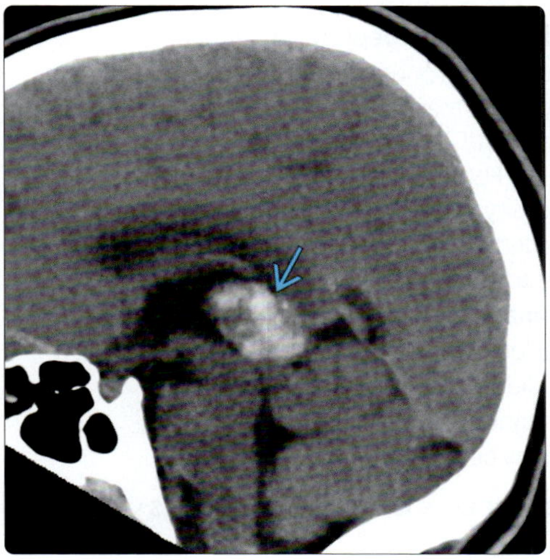

Other Germ Cell Tumors

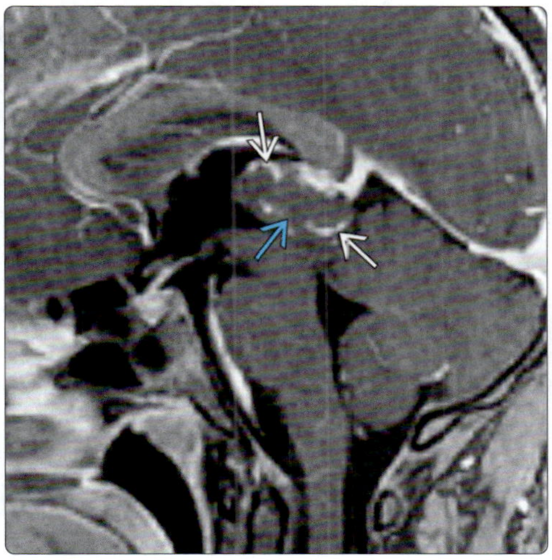

(Left) *Midline sagittal NECT in a 10-year-old boy with a choriocarcinoma shows a hemorrhagic pineal region mass* →. **(Right)** *Sagittal T1 C+ MR in the same patient with choriocarcinoma shows a mostly nonenhancing mass* → *with irregular peripheral enhancement* ➡. *Blood tests showed elevated β-HCG levels. Upon encountering a pineal region tumor, it is helpful to correlate with elevated hormone levels, which are pathognomonic for germ cell tumors (GCTs) (other) in this setting.*

Pineoblastoma

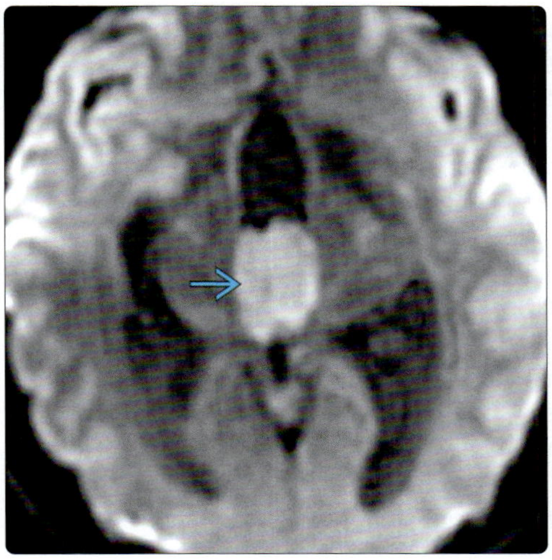

Pineoblastoma

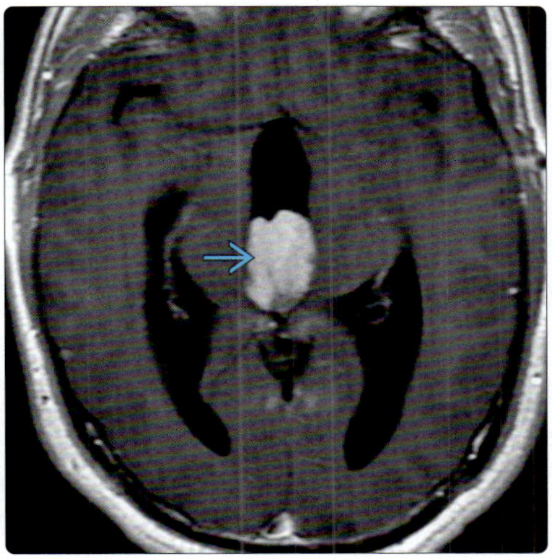

(Left) *Axial DWI MR shows a hyperintense pineal region mass* →. *ADC (not shown) demonstrated decreased signal intensity, consistent with a highly cellular tumor restricting diffusion. Pathology revealed a pineoblastoma.* **(Right)** *Axial T1 C+ MR in the same patient shows an avidly enhancing pineal region mass* → *without thalamic invasion. Absence of thalamic invasion by imaging makes germinoma less likely than pineoblastoma when a cellular pineal tumor is found.*

Retinoblastoma

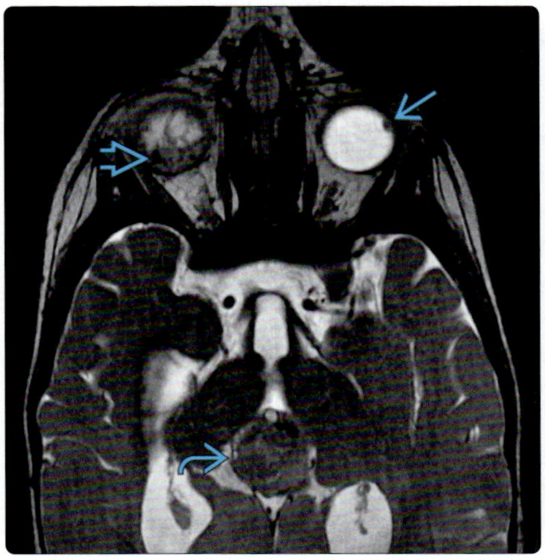

Pineocytoma

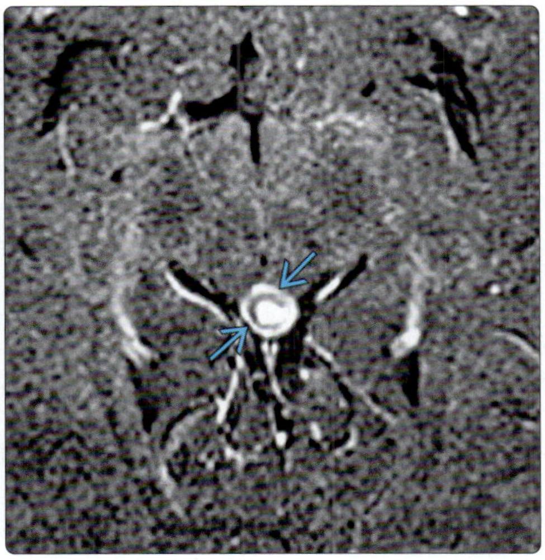

(Left) *Axial oblique FIESTA MR in a 19 month old shows masses within the right* ⇒ *& left* → *globes as well as the pineal gland* ↗, *consistent with trilateral retinoblastoma. The intracranial component classically occurs 2-3 years after the bilateral ocular tumors.* **(Right)** *Axial T1 C+ MR in a patient with a pineocytoma shows both peripheral & central enhancement of the small mass* →.

DIFFERENTIAL DIAGNOSIS

Common

- Dysembryoplastic Neuroepithelial Tumor
- Ganglioglioma

Less Common

- Pilocytic Astrocytoma
- Low-Grade Diffuse Astrocytoma
- Anaplastic Astrocytoma
- Germinoma
- Pleomorphic Xanthoastrocytoma
- Intraventricular Tumors (Mimic)
- Embryonal Tumor With Multilayered Rosettes
- Desmoplastic Infantile Tumors
- Supratentorial Ependymoma
- Glioblastoma
- Teratoma
- Pilomyxoid Astrocytoma
- Atypical Teratoid-Rhabdoid Tumor
- Abscess (Mimic)
- Demyelinating Disease (Mimic)
- Oligodendroglioma

Rare but Important

- Angiocentric Glioma
- Astroblastoma
- Primary CNS Lymphoma
- Metastases
- Neurocutaneous Melanosis
- Aneurysm (Mimic)

ESSENTIAL INFORMATION

Key Differential Diagnosis Issues

- Clinical features to consider
  - Some tumors are particularly epileptogenic
    - Ganglioglioma, dysembryoplastic neuroepithelial tumor, & angiocentric glioma
  - Neurofibromatosis type 1: Predisposition to astrocytic tumors
  - Some pediatric hemispheric tumors look like common adult tumors
    - Ganglioglioma (common in children) vs. oligodendroglioma (common in adults)
    - Embryonal tumor with multilayered rosettes (more common in children) vs. glioblastoma (common in adults)
- Imaging features to consider
  - CT
    - ↑ density suggests higher grade tumor
    - Also helps discriminate hemorrhage or Ca^{2+}
  - MR
    - Restricted diffusion suggests ↑ cellularity & higher grade tumor
      - Embryonal tumor with multilayered rosettes
      - Atypical teratoid-rhabdoid tumor
      - Glioblastoma
      - Germinoma
      - Primary CNS lymphoma
      - Desmoplastic infantile tumors (variable)
    - Exception: Low-grade desmoplastic infantile tumors

Helpful Clues for Common Diagnoses

- **Dysembryoplastic Neuroepithelial Tumor**
  - Almost all occur in patients < 20 years of age
  - Cortically based mass with bubbly or microcystic appearance on T2 MR
  - Ring sign on FLAIR MR: Well-defined outer rim of hyperintensity, complete or incomplete
  - No enhancement
  - May have adjacent cortical dysplasia
- **Ganglioglioma**
  - Temporal lobe is most common location (50%)
  - May be solid or mixed solid/cystic
  - ~ 50% enhance; 25-50% have Ca^{2+}
  - Margins may be sharp or indistinct

Helpful Clues for Less Common Diagnoses

- **Pilocytic Astrocytoma**
  - Very common in pediatric posterior fossa; cerebral hemisphere location is uncommon
    - Cerebellum > hypothalamus/optic pathway > brainstem > deep gray nuclei > cerebral hemispheres
  - Wide spectrum of imaging appearances
    - Mixed solid & cystic (~ 50%), cyst with mural nodule (~ 35%), solid (~ 15%)
  - Solid components typically have very hyperintense T2 & ADC signal on MR
  - ~ 95% have some enhancing component
  - Ca^{2+} in ~ 20%; hemorrhage is uncommon
- **Low-Grade Diffuse Astrocytoma**
  - Hemispheres, thalami (can be bithalamic), & brainstem
  - Poorly marginated
  - Hypointense on T1, hyperintense on T2 MR
  - No enhancement
- **Anaplastic Astrocytoma**
  - Infiltrating appearance with indistinct margins
  - Some enhancement is often present
  - May be bithalamic
  - More likely to be focal & show enhancement as compared to low-grade diffuse astrocytoma
- **Germinoma**
  - Most commonly suprasellar or pineal; 10-15% in basal ganglia
  - Best clue: Well-defined mass in basal ganglia with diffusion restriction
  - ± numerous small cysts, especially when large
- **Pleomorphic Xanthoastrocytoma**
  - Cortically based tumor, most commonly in temporal lobe
  - Enhancing, ill-defined mass + cyst
  - Dural reaction (tail sign)is common
- **Intraventricular Tumors (Mimic)**
  - Look for mass centered in ventricle, most often atrium of lateral ventricle
  - When large &/or infiltrative, may mimic intraaxial hemispheric mass
  - Most common large intraventricular tumors: Choroid plexus tumors & meningiomas
- **Embryonal Tumor With Multilayered Rosettes**
  - Formerly known as supratentorial primitive neuroectodermal tumor

- Large, bulky, complex hemispheric mass
- Diffusion restriction of solid components
- Ca^{2+}, hemorrhage, & necrosis are common
- Peritumoral edema is often sparse/absent

- **Desmoplastic Infantile Tumors**
  - Desmoplastic infantile ganglioglioma & desmoplastic infantile astrocytic variants
  - Peripheral supratentorial tumor with large cyst(s) & cortically based solid nodule/plaque in child < 2 years of age
  - Hemorrhage & Ca^{2+} are uncommon
- **Supratentorial Ependymoma**
  - Histologically similar but genetically distinct from posterior fossa ependymomas
  - Best clue: Large, heterogeneous, mixed solid/cystic mass with Ca^{2+} in cerebral hemisphere
- **Glioblastoma**
  - Solid components are typically cellular with diffusion restriction
  - Often contains areas of necrosis
  - May arise from low-grade astrocytoma (i.e., malignant transformation)
- **Teratoma**
  - Neonate with large, bulky midline mass
  - Ca^{2+}, soft tissue, cysts, fat
- **Pilomyxoid Astrocytoma**
  - Typically occurs in younger patients than pilocytic astrocytoma but imaging features are very similar
  - More commonly has intratumoral hemorrhage (~ 25%)
- **Atypical Teratoid-Rhabdoid Tumor**
  - Heterogeneous intracranial mass in child ≤ 3 years
    - Posterior fossa, cerebral hemisphere, intraventricular, or cranial nerve origin
  - Diffusion restriction of solid components
  - Hemorrhage & cysts are common
- **Abscess (Mimic)**
  - Central diffusion restriction with thin, enhancing, T2-hypointense rim
    - Marked central diffusion restriction is most specific finding
  - Usually arises from hematogenous spread when located in cerebral hemispheres
- **Demyelinating Disease (Mimic)**
  - Discontinuous rim enhancement with mass effect in acute phase
  - Look for additional white matter lesions
- **Oligodendroglioma**
  - Uncommon in children
  - Cortically based tumor with indistinct margins
  - ~ 50% enhance; 70-90% calcify; 20% show cystic degeneration

Helpful Clues for Rare Diagnoses

- **Angiocentric Glioma**
  - Indistinct nonenhancing cortical signal abnormality
  - May mimic focal cortical dysplasia
- **Astroblastoma**
  - Large, well-circumscribed hemispheric mass
  - Bubbly solid & cystic appearance
- **Primary CNS Lymphoma**
  - Usually solid with enhancement & diffusion restriction
  - May cross corpus callosum
- **Metastases**
  - Rare in children, particularly with brain as presenting site
  - Typically multiple, often centered at gray-white junction
  - Usually solid or centrally necrotic; cystic metastases rare
- **Neurocutaneous Melanosis**
  - Most common: Solitary or multifocal nonenhancing, T1-hyperintense lesions (especially at medial temporal lobe)
    - Focal melanosis is typically stable over time; malignant degeneration is rare
- **Aneurysm (Mimic)**
  - Partially thrombosed aneurysm may mimic mass
  - Look for continuity with arteries, pulsation artifact

SELECTED REFERENCES

1. Zamora C et al: Supratentorial tumors in pediatric patients. Neuroimaging Clin N Am. 27(1):39-67, 2017
2. Borja MJ et al: Conventional and advanced MRI features of pediatric intracranial tumors: supratentorial tumors. AJR Am J Roentgenol. 200(5):W483-503, 2013

Dysembryoplastic Neuroepithelial Tumor

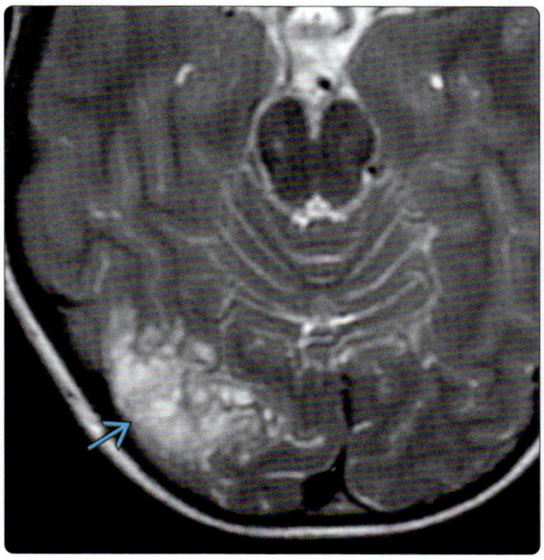

Dysembryoplastic Neuroepithelial Tumor

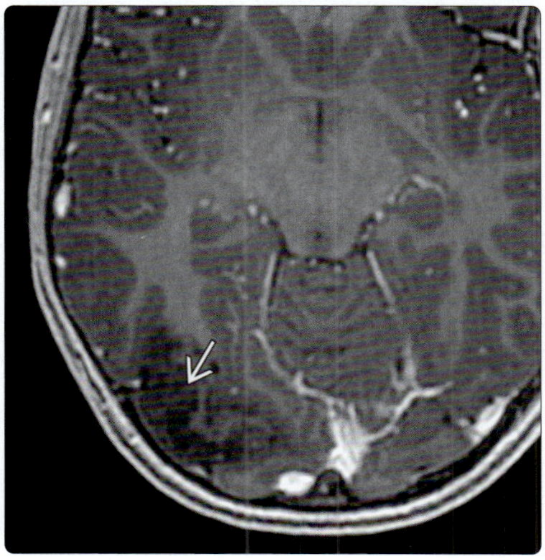

(Left) *Axial T2 MR in a 12 year old with seizures shows a cortically based, bubbly, infiltrative lesion ⇒ in the right lateral occipital lobe, a typical appearance for dysembryoplastic neuroepithelial tumor (DNET). This low-grade tumor often expands gyri, but there is usually little, if any, mass effect associated with a DNET.* **(Right)** *Axial T1 C+ MR in the same patient shows no enhancement in the cystic right occipital lobe lesion ➡, typical of a DNET.*

(Left) *Axial T2 MR shows a cortically based mass with solid → & cystic ➡ components in the left frontal lobe. There is minimal, if any, mass effect from this lesion, which is typical for DNET. The gyri are often preserved but appear infiltrated with this tumor.* **(Right)** *Axial FLAIR MR in the same patient shows the cortically based mass with solid → & cystic ➡ components. This case demonstrates the ring sign with suppression of central fluid signal of the cystic components & increased FLAIR signal along the periphery.*

Dysembryoplastic Neuroepithelial Tumor

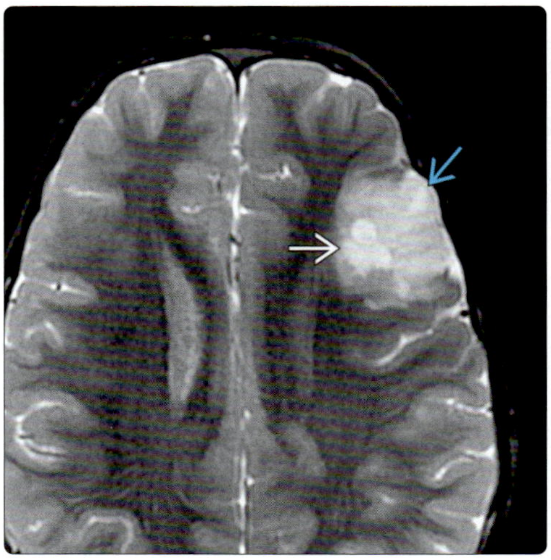

Dysembryoplastic Neuroepithelial Tumor

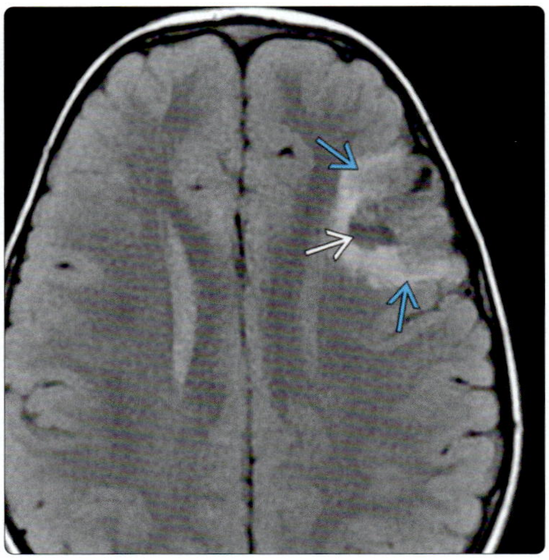

(Left) *Axial T2 MR in a teenager with seizures shows a well-defined, cortically based lesion → in the left superior temporal lobe. The margins of gangliogliomas vary from sharply defined to poorly defined. With the latter, an associated cortical dysplasia should be considered.* **(Right)** *Axial T1 C+ MR in the same patient shows enhancement → within the mass. Approximately 50% of gangliogliomas show some enhancement, & ganglioglioma should lead the differential diagnosis for an enhancing cortical mass.*

Ganglioglioma

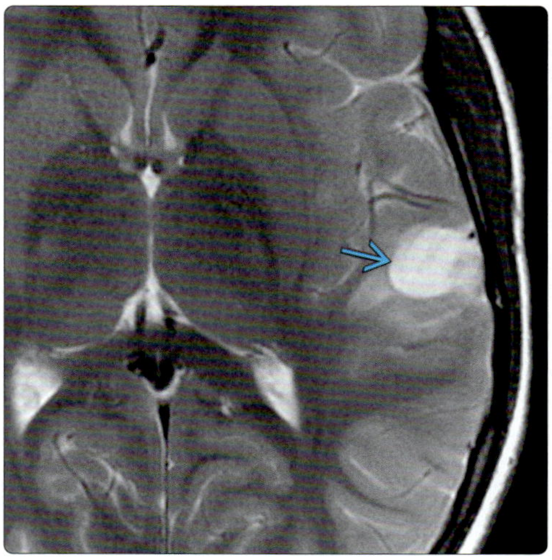

Ganglioglioma

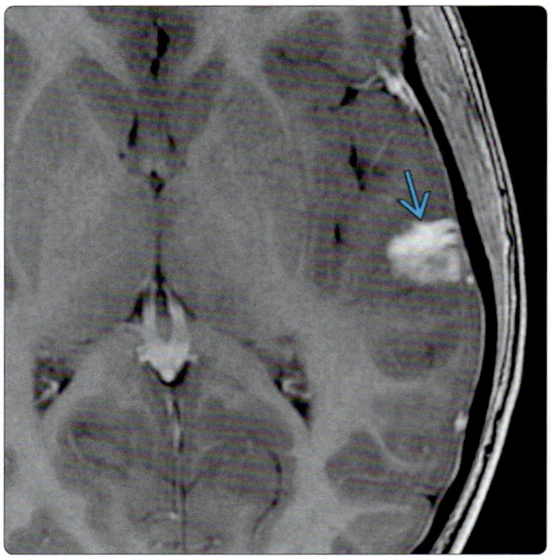

(Left) *Coronal T2 MR in a 5-year-old boy with seizures shows a well-defined, hyperintense, solid mass → in the right mesial temporal lobe causing enlargement of the hippocampus ➡. This is a common location & appearance for a ganglioglioma.* **(Right)** *Axial T1 C+ MR in the same patient shows a lack of contrast enhancement within the lesion ➡. Approximately 50% of gangliogliomas will demonstrate no enhancement.*

Ganglioglioma

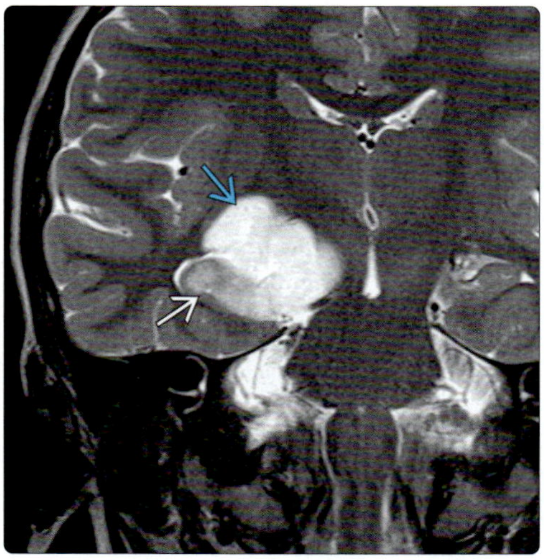

Ganglioglioma

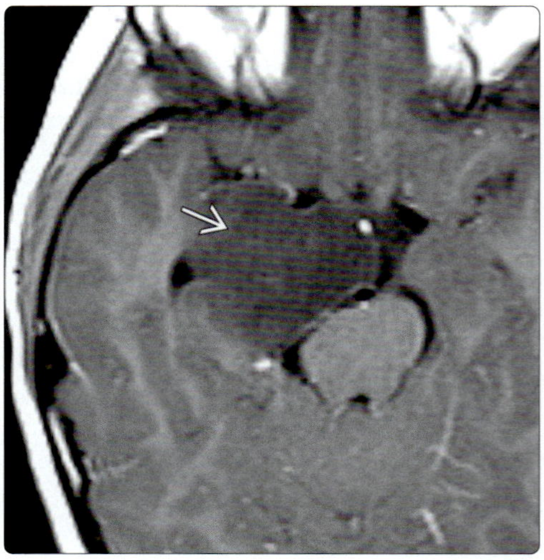

Low-Grade Diffuse Astrocytoma

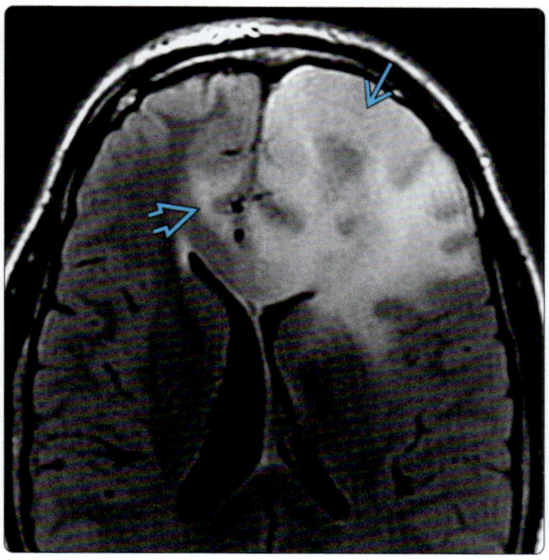

Anaplastic Astrocytoma

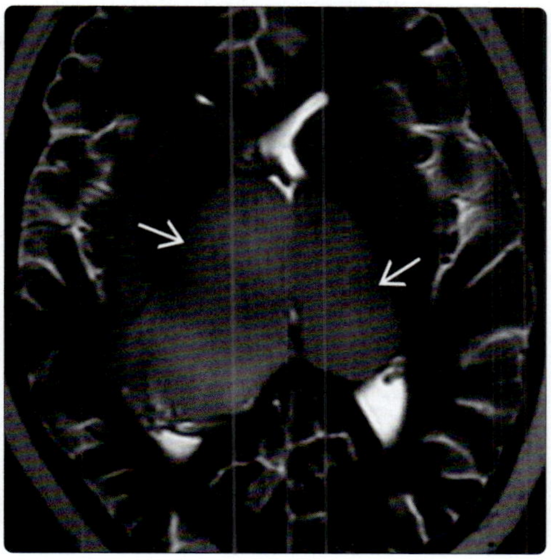

(Left) *Axial FLAIR MR in a 10 year old with a low-grade diffuse astrocytoma shows ill-defined signal in the left frontal lobe* ⇨ *with gyral expansion & mass effect on the left frontal horn. Note the extension into the right frontal lobe* ⇨. **(Right)** *Axial T2 MR in an 11 year old with anaplastic astrocytoma shows an infiltrative bithalamic tumor* ➡. *These findings are pathognomonic for infiltrating astrocytoma, either grade II (low-grade diffuse astrocytoma) or grade III (anaplastic). These can only be distinguished histologically.*

Germinoma

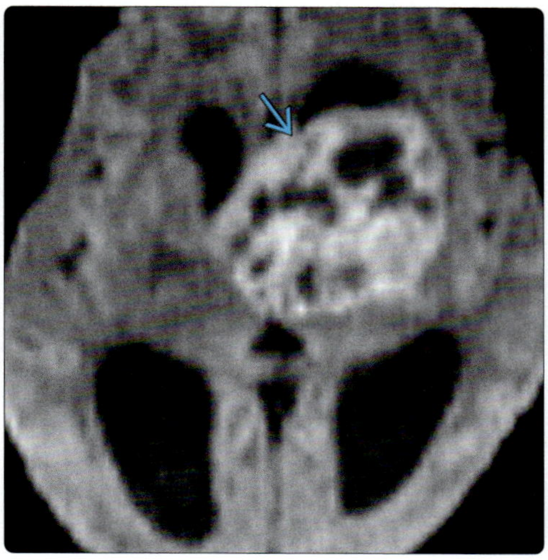

Intraventricular Tumors (Mimic)

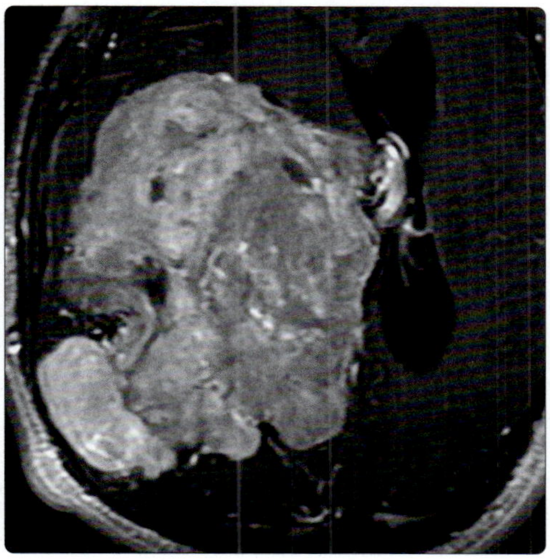

(Left) *Axial DWI MR in a 10 year old with a germinoma shows a large cellular mass* ⇨ *centered in the left basal ganglia. Multiple small intratumoral cysts are present. This is a typical appearance for germinoma.* **(Right)** *Axial T1 C+ MR in a 16 year old shows a heterogeneously enhancing intraventricular meningioma. When intraventricular tumors become very large, it can be difficult to determine whether they arose within the brain parenchyma or ventricle.*

Pleomorphic Xanthoastrocytoma

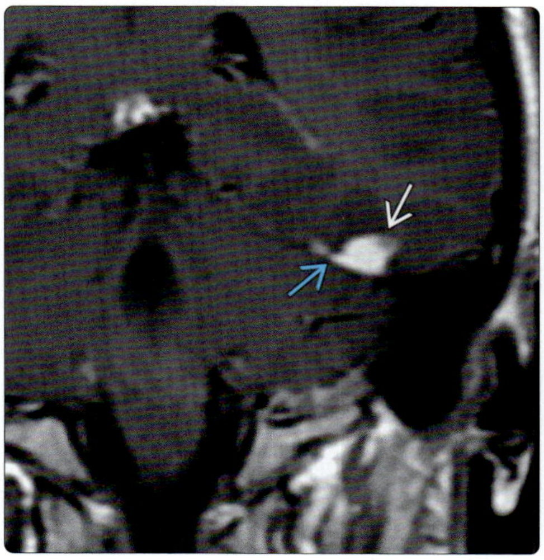

Embryonal Tumor With Multilayered Rosettes

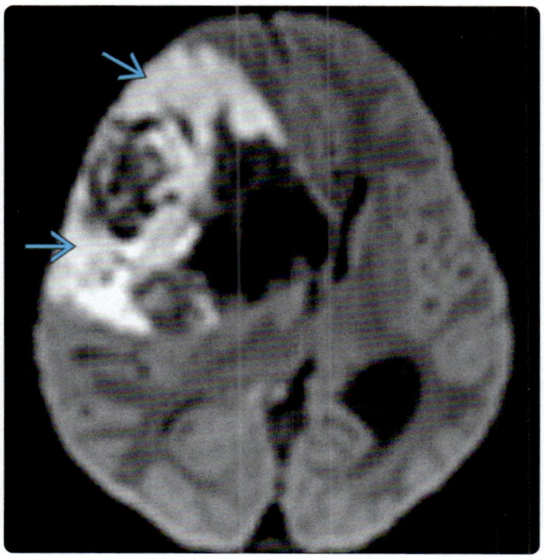

(Left) *Coronal T1 C+ MR in a teenager with a pleomorphic xanthoastrocytoma causing seizures demonstrates a well-defined, enhancing cortical lesion* ➡ *in the left temporal lobe with associated dural reaction* ⇨, *mimicking a dural tail.* **(Right)** *Axial DWI MR in a 2 year old with an embryonal tumor with multilayered rosettes (formerly primitive neuroectodermal tumor) shows a hemispheric mass with a heterogeneous highly cellular solid component* ⇨, *consistent with a high-grade tumor. CT showed areas of* Ca^{2+}.

(Left) *Axial T2 MR in a patient with a desmoplastic infantile ganglioglioma (DIG) shows a complex mixed solid & cystic mass → occupying most of the right temporal lobe. DIG should be considered in any complex hemispheric lesion in a young patient.* **(Right)** *Axial T2 MR in a 5 month old with a supratentorial ependymoma shows a heterogeneously mixed solid & cystic mass in the left cerebral hemisphere with surrounding vasogenic edema →. Note the central area of Ca^{2+} →.*

Desmoplastic Infantile Tumors

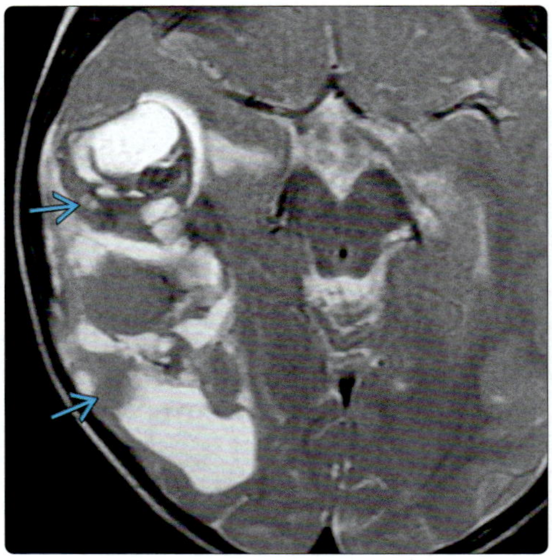

Supratentorial Ependymoma

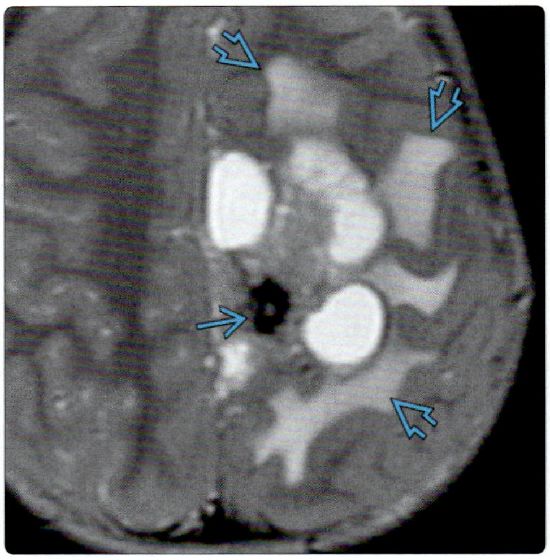

(Left) *Coronal T1 C+ MR in a patient with glioblastoma shows a centrally necrotic enhancing tumor → in the right insula. Clues that suggest a high-grade tumor are central necrosis & diffusion restriction of solid components (not shown).* **(Right)** *Axial NECT in an 11 week old with an immature teratoma shows a large, heterogeneous mass → in the left frontal region causing obstructive hydrocephalus →. The chunky Ca^{2+} → should prompt consideration of teratoma in the differential diagnosis.*

Glioblastoma

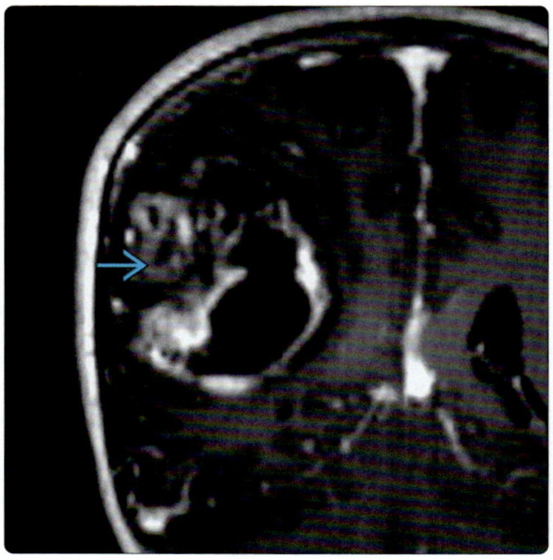

Teratoma

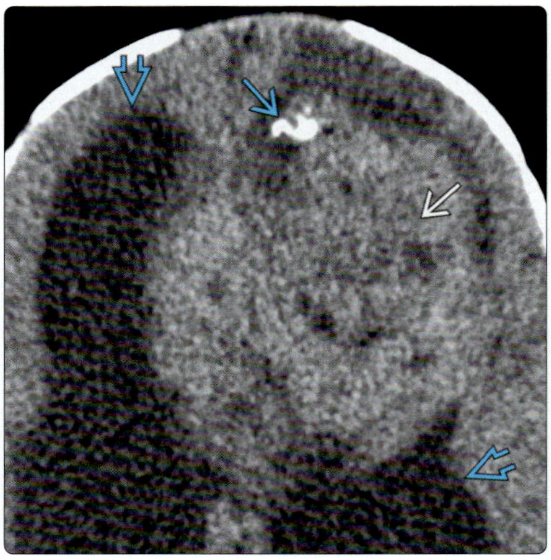

(Left) *Axial T1 C+ MR in a patient with a pilomyxoid astrocytoma shows a thick-rimmed mass → centered in the right basal ganglia. The thick, irregular rim is highly suggestive of tumor.* **(Right)** *Axial T1 C+ MR shows a lesion with a thin, smooth enhancing rim →, characteristic of an abscess. DWI (not shown) demonstrated central diffusion restriction, the most specific imaging feature for abscess.*

Pilomyxoid Astrocytoma

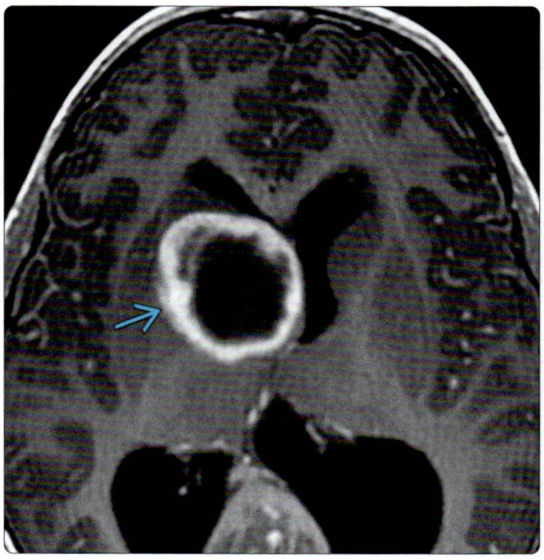

Abscess (Mimic)

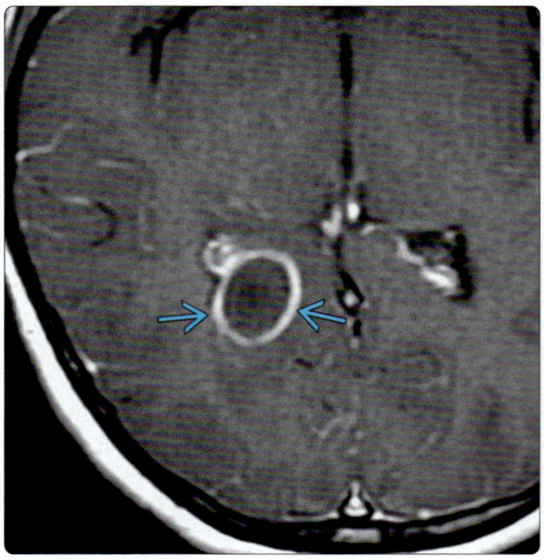

Demyelinating Disease (Mimic)

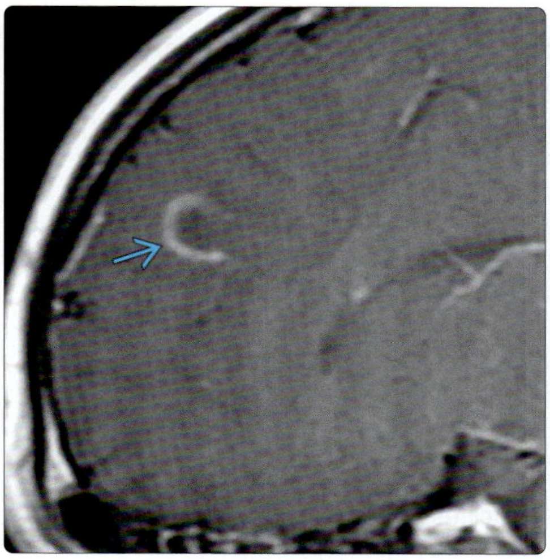

Oligodendroglioma

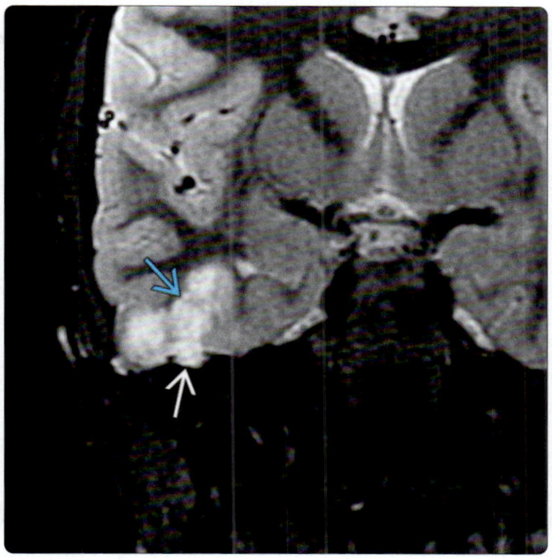

(Left) *Sagittal T1 C+ MR in a 13 year old with multiple sclerosis shows an incomplete ring of enhancement →, the classic appearance of demyelinating disease. In the acute phase, demyelinating lesions often show patchy or incomplete ring enhancement & diffusion restriction.* **(Right)** *Coronal T2 MR in a teenager with oligodendroglioma shows an ill-defined, cortically based mass → with minimal mass effect. There is suggestion of mild associated skull base remodeling →, a common feature. T1 C+ MR showed no enhancement.*

Primary CNS Lymphoma

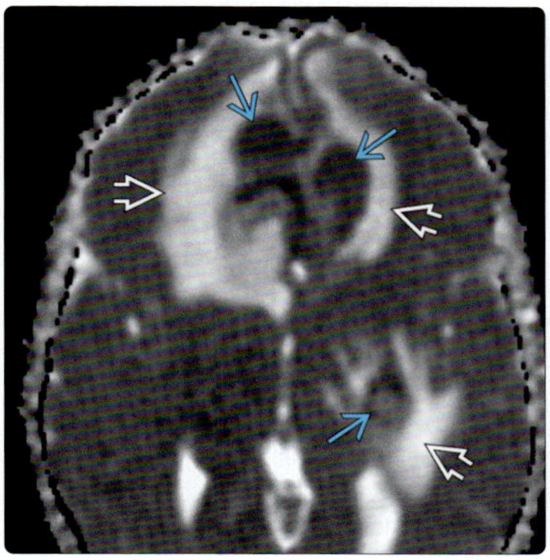

Metastases

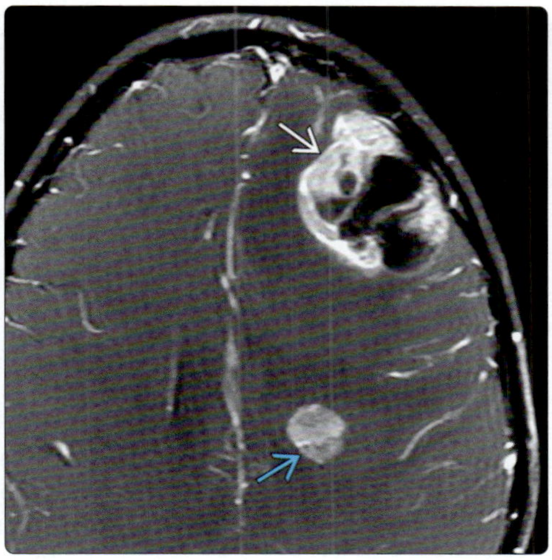

(Left) *Axial ADC MR in a patient with CNS lymphoma shows multiple peripheral hemispheric masses → with decreased signal, consistent with a cellular tumor. The adjacent hyperintense signal → represents peritumoral vasogenic edema.* **(Right)** *Axial T1 C+ MR in a 12 year old with Ewing sarcoma shows a heterogeneous peripheral left frontal lobe lesion → as well as a smaller, more homogeneous lesion →. Multiple lesions suggest metastases, although they are much less common in children than adults.*

Neurocutaneous Melanosis

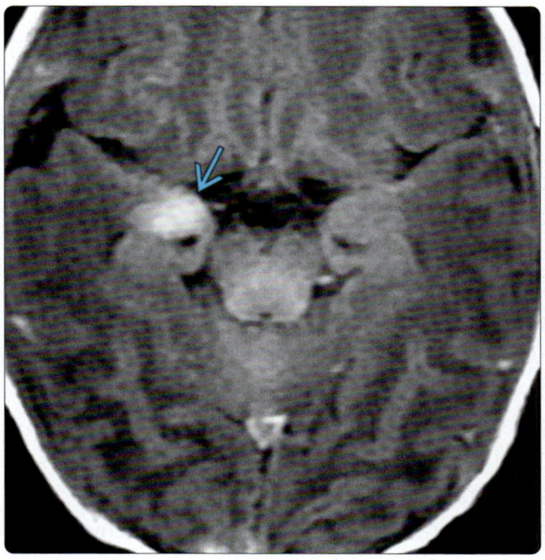

Aneurysm (Mimic)

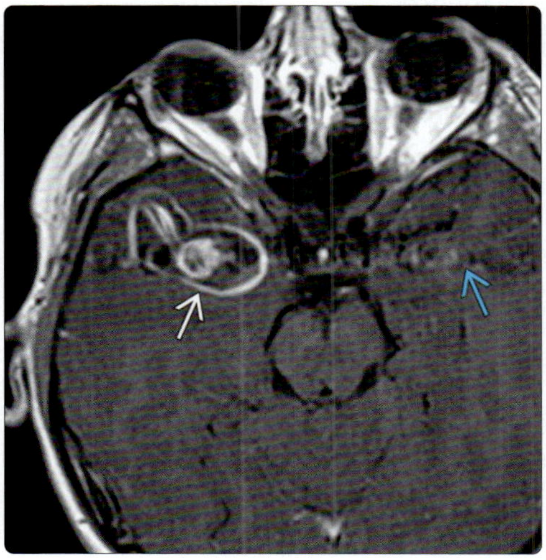

(Left) *Axial T1 MR in a newborn shows a hyperintense lesion → in the right medial temporal lobe/amygdala, typical of neurocutaneous melanosis (NCM) in a patient with a large melanocytic nevus.* **(Right)** *Axial T1 C+ MR in a teenager with a partially thrombosed fusiform aneurysm shows a tubular rim-enhancing lesion → with a smaller patent vessel centrally. Note the prominent pulsation artifact →, an important clue to an aneurysm.*

DIFFERENTIAL DIAGNOSIS

Common

- Intraventricular Hemorrhage
- Choroid Plexus Cyst

Less Common

- Subependymal Giant Cell Astrocytoma
- Choroid Plexus Papilloma
- Choroid Plexus Carcinoma
- Ependymal Cyst

Rare but Important

- Atypical Teratoid-Rhabdoid Tumor
- Choroid Plexus Enlargement of Sturge-Weber Syndrome
- Meningioma
- Ependymoma
- Choroid Plexus Xanthogranuloma
- Central Neurocytoma
- Subependymoma
- Langerhans Cell Histiocytosis

ESSENTIAL INFORMATION

Key Differential Diagnosis Issues

- Certain lesions are associated with specific syndromes
  - Subependymal giant cell astrocytoma (SEGA) in tuberous sclerosis complex (TSC)
  - Choroid plexus enlargement in Sturge-Weber syndrome (SWS)
  - Meningioma in neurofibromatosis type 2 (NF2)
- Modality considerations
  - MR: Imaging modality of choice
    - Especially helpful for cystic lesions (which are often not visible on CT)
    - Optimal anatomic localization helps narrow differential diagnosis
    - Most sensitive for leptomeningeal spread
  - CT: Usually 1st test for acute presentations
    - Rarely adds additional information to MR

Helpful Clues for Common Diagnoses

- **Intraventricular Hemorrhage**
  - Secondary to germinal matrix hemorrhage (GMH) of prematurity, trauma, vascular malformation, or tumor
  - Imaging findings
    - Intraventricular hemorrhage is initially hyperechoic (US) & hyperdense (CT)
    - Morphology is variable: Dependent layering fluid level in occipital horn &/or lobular clot adherent to choroid plexus, ± ventricular dilation
    - May cause ventriculitis & eventual posthemorrhagic hydrocephalus
    - Without obvious cause for intraventricular hemorrhage (e.g., prematurity with GMH), perform CTA to evaluate for arteriovenous malformation or aneurysm
- **Choroid Plexus Cyst**
  - Most common intraventricular lesion
    - Incidental choroid plexus cysts (CPCs) ↑ in incidence with age
      - Rarely large enough to cause obstructive hydrocephalus
      - Lateral ventricle > > 3rd ventricle
    - Fetal cysts should be differentiated from CPCs identified later in life
      - Fetal cysts have "soft" association with trisomy 18
      - If identified, look for other abnormalities to suggest aneuploidy
      - If other fetal abnormalities are absent, consider as incidental
      - Fetal cysts often resolve in 3rd trimester
  - Imaging findings
    - Cyst within or attached to choroid plexus
    - Enhancing choroid typically surrounds/lines cyst
    - Hyperintense FLAIR signal is common
    - ± irregular peripheral choroid plexus Ca^{2+}

Helpful Clues for Less Common Diagnoses

- **Subependymal Giant Cell Astrocytoma**
  - Essentially only identified in setting of TSC
    - Present in 15% of TSC patients
  - Classically resected; current 1st-line therapy is mTOR inhibitors
  - Imaging findings
    - Heterogeneously enhancing mass near foramen of Monro
    - Enhancement alone does not discriminate SEGA from subependymal nodule; growth suggests SEGA
    - ± Ca^{2+}
    - ± obstructive hydrocephalus
- **Choroid Plexus Papilloma**
  - 50% < 5 years of age; 26% < 1 year of age
  - Arises in lateral (60-70%) > 4th (20-30%) > 3rd (< 10%) ventricle in children
    - 4th ventricle most common in adults
  - Hydrocephalus may be secondary to obstruction, CSF overproduction by tumor, or hemorrhage (causing impaired CSF resorption)
  - Imaging findings
    - CT: Iso- or hyperattenuating in 75%
      - Ca^{2+} in 25%
    - MR: Variable signal characteristics & enhancement as either may show
      - Lbulated (frond-like) margins
      - Variable contrast enhancement, but classically very avid & homogeneous
      - Prominent vessel/flow void in mass
      - CSF dissemination (but less frequent in CPP than CPCa)
- **Choroid Plexus Carcinoma**
  - 75% < 5 years of age; 33% < 1 year of age
  - Usually presents with macrocrania, bulging fontanelle, vomiting, headache, ataxia
  - Imaging findings
    - Overlap in imaging features with CPP
      - Invasion of brain parenchyma with parenchymal edema is most helpful imaging finding to suggest CPCa over CPP
      - Cysts, hemorrhage, & necrosis are more common in CPCa
    - ± CSF metastasis

- **Ependymal Cyst**
  - Synonym: Neuroepithelial cyst
  - Congenital, benign, ependymal-lined cyst
  - Imaging findings
    - Lateral ventricle > > > 3rd & 4th ventricle
    - Nonenhancing, thin-walled cyst
    - Round or multiseptated
    - Similar to CSF on all imaging

Helpful Clues for Rare Diagnoses

- **Atypical Teratoid-Rhabdoid Tumor**
  - Malignant, grade IV, highly cellular embryonal tumor
  - Typically in very young patients (< 3 years)
  - Imaging findings
    - Diffusion restriction; less enhancement than CPP
- **Choroid Plexus Enlargement of Sturge-Weber Syndrome**
  - Imaging findings
    - Choroid plexus ipsilateral to cerebral atrophy & leptomeningeal angiomatosis shows asymmetric enlargement & ↑ enhancement
      - Likely due to alternate venous drainage pathways
- **Meningioma**
  - Uncommon in children; consider NF2
  - Lateral ventricular atrium is most common site; left > right
  - Imaging findings
    - Lobular, intensely enhancing intraventricular mass
    - ± Ca^{2+}, cysts, hemorrhage
    - Heterogeneity or indistinct margins favor higher degree of malignancy
- **Ependymoma**
  - 4th ventricle > > lateral ventricles
  - Usually in periventricular white matter when supratentorial
  - Imaging findings
    - Ca^{2+} common ± cysts, hemorrhage, necrosis
    - Variable enhancement of cyst walls & solid portion
- **Choroid Plexus Xanthogranuloma**
  - Benign lesion of choroid plexus containing macrophages, cellular debris, cholesterol, & hemosiderin
  - Uncertain etiology; often bilateral
  - Imaging findings
    - CT: Usually not visible
    - MR
      - DWI: Diffusion restriction from cellular debris
      - GRE/SWI: Signal loss from hemosiderin
- **Central Neurocytoma**
  - Arises from septum pellucidum
    - Primarily in young adults
  - Imaging findings
    - Bubbly mass with heterogeneous enhancement
    - Well-defined, lobulated mass
- **Subependymoma**
  - Very rare in children
  - Imaging findings
    - Nonenhancing mass
    - Frontal horns of lateral ventricles are most common
- **Langerhans Cell Histiocytosis**
  - CNS involvement
    - Active lesions: Pituitary infundibulum, dura, or choroid plexus
    - Delayed degenerative lesions: Parenchymal
      - May be paraneoplastic phenomenon
  - Imaging findings
    - Intense contrast enhancement of active lesions

SELECTED REFERENCES

1. Agarwal A et al: Intraventricular tumors. Semin Ultrasound CT MR. 37(2):150-8, 2016
2. Smith AB et al: From the radiologic pathology archives: intraventricular neoplasms: radiologic-pathologic correlation. Radiographics. 33(1):21-43, 2013
3. Naeini RM et al: Spectrum of choroid plexus lesions in children. AJR Am J Roentgenol. 192(1):32-40, 2009
4. Suh DY et al: Pediatric supratentorial intraventricular tumors. Neurosurg Focus. 10(6):E4, 2001

Intraventricular Hemorrhage

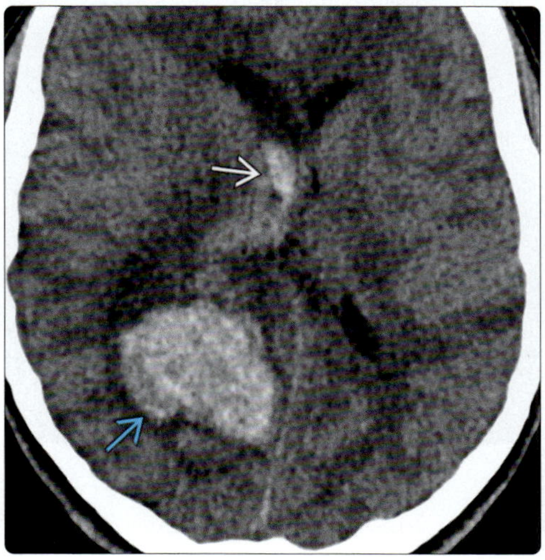

Intraventricular Hemorrhage

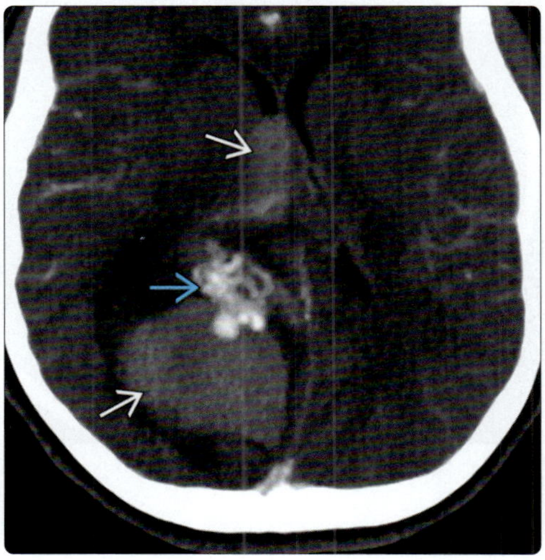

(Left) *Axial NECT in a 14 year old with acute IVH shows hyperattenuating material ➡ conforming to the ventricle. IVH is typically the result of intraparenchymal hemorrhage that has extended into the ventricle, as in this case of a right occipital lobe hemorrhage ➡.* **(Right)** *Axial CT angiogram in the same patient shows a right occipital arteriovenous malformation (AVM) ➡ as the source of hemorrhage ➡. In the setting of unexplained IVH, the primary cause (e.g., AVM, aneurysm, etc.) must be sought.*

(Left) *Axial T1 C+ MR in a 2 year old shows a cyst in the atrium of left lateral ventricle at the level of the choroid plexus. The thin rim of enhancing choroid* ➔ *surrounding the cyst is typical.* **(Right)** *Axial T1 C+ MR in a 7 year old with tuberous sclerosis complex (TSC) shows a heterogeneously enhancing mass* ➡ *in the left caudothalamic groove, a characteristic location for a SEGA. Also note the characteristic findings of TSC, including a subependymal nodule* ➔ *& migrational anomalies/dysplasias* ➡*.*

Choroid Plexus Cyst

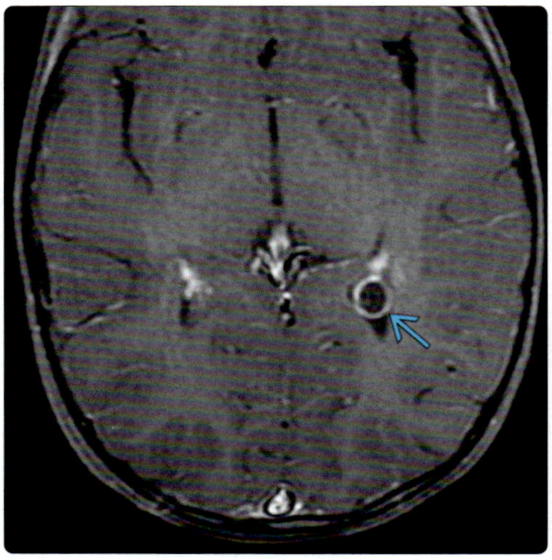

Subependymal Giant Cell Astrocytoma

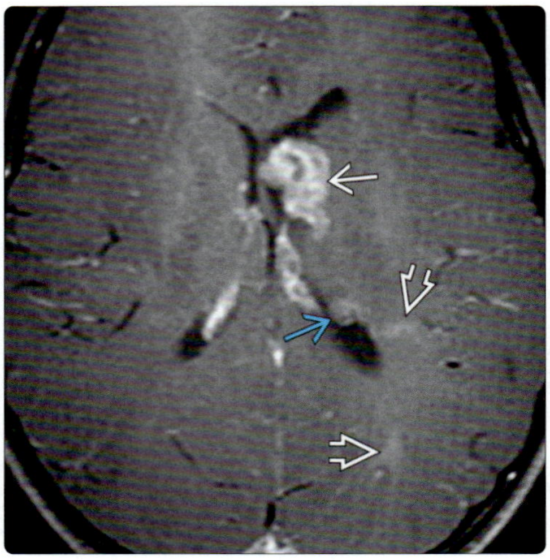

(Left) *Coronal T2 MR in a 2 year old with a choroid plexus papilloma shows a mass* ➡ *in the atrium of the left lateral ventricle, a common location for choroid plexus tumors. Note the lobular, frond-like margins* ➔ *of the mass, typical for choroid plexus tumors.* **(Right)** *Axial T1 C+ MR in the same patient shows only mild enhancement of this CPP* ➡*, much less than typically seen. While this patient has otherwise normal ventricles, many patients with choroid plexus tumors have enlarged ventricles due to CSF overproduction by the tumor.*

Choroid Plexus Papilloma

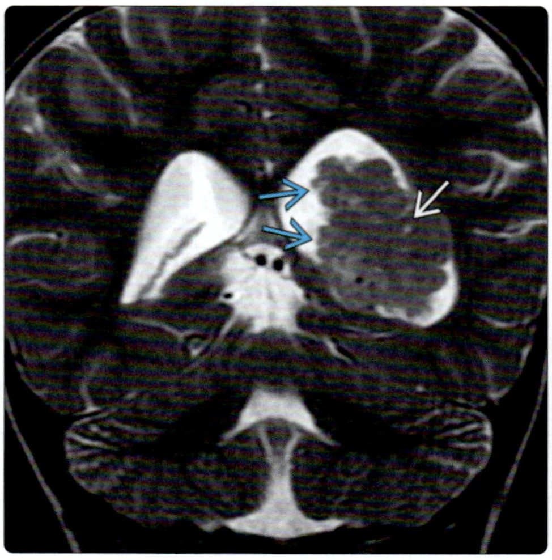

Choroid Plexus Papilloma

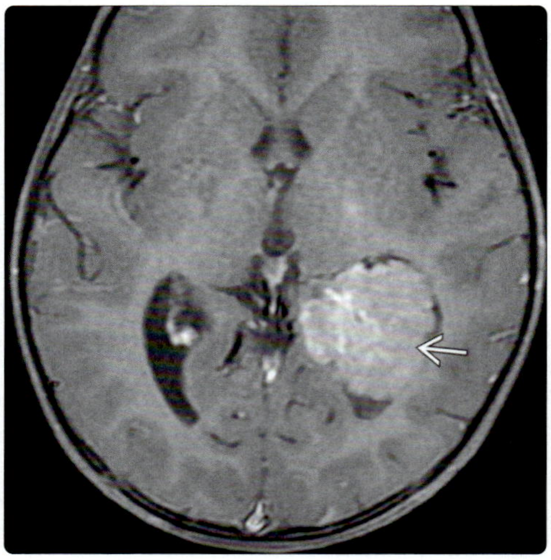

(Left) *Axial NECT in a 9 month old with a choroid plexus carcinoma (CPCa) shows a hyperattenuating mass* ➡ *in the atrium of the right lateral ventricle. The increased attenuation suggests higher cellularity & should prompt one to consider higher grade tumors, such as CPCa.* **(Right)** *Axial T2 MR in the same patient shows areas of parenchymal extension* ➔ *& adjacent increased white matter signal* ➔*. Parenchymal involvement should suggest the possibility of a CPCa.*

Choroid Plexus Carcinoma

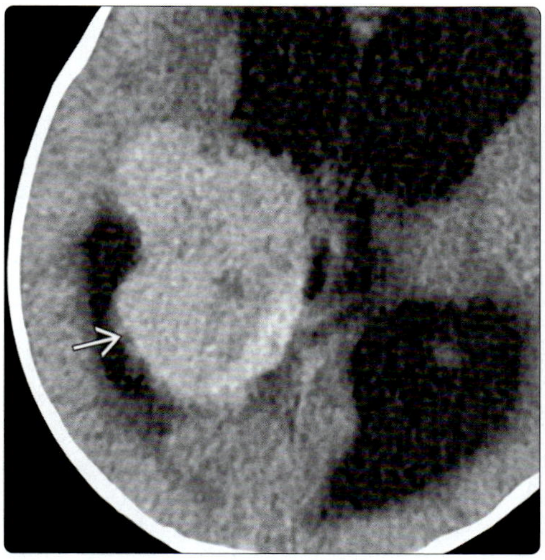

Choroid Plexus Carcinoma

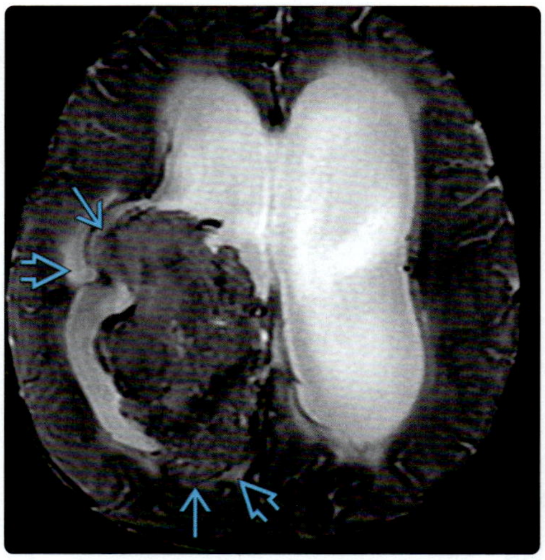

Atypical Teratoid-Rhabdoid Tumor

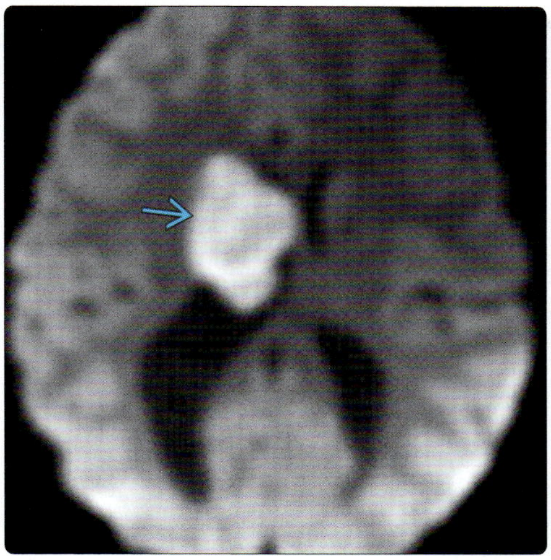

Choroid Plexus Enlargement of Sturge-Weber Syndrome

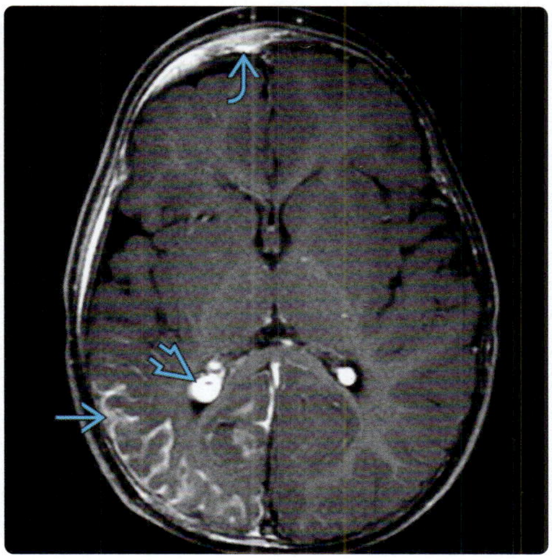

(Left) *Axial DWI MR in a child with a right lateral ventricular ATRT shows diffusion restriction in the mass, typical of high cellularity. ATRT should lead the differential diagnosis for a highly cellular intraventricular mass in a young child.* **(Right)** *Axial T1 C+ FS MR in a 14 month old with a forehead capillary malformation & seizures shows right cerebral atrophy with pial angiomatosis due to SWS. Note the enlargement & enhancement of the ipsilateral choroid plexus & calvarium due to alternate venous drainage pathways.*

Meningioma

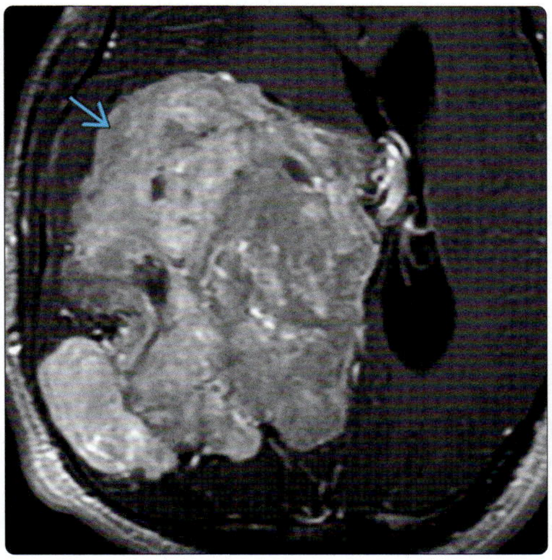

Meningioma

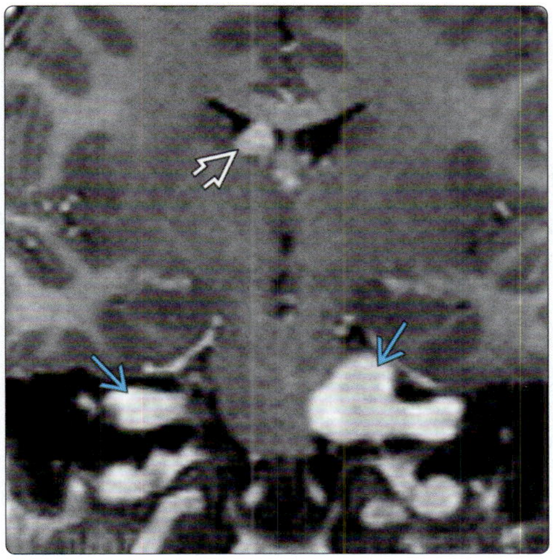

(Left) *Axial T1 C+ MR in a 16 year old with a meningioma shows a large, heterogeneously enhancing mass centered in the atrium of the right lateral ventricle with extension into the adjacent parenchyma.* **(Right)** *Coronal T1 C+ MR in a teenager with neurofibromatosis type 2 (NF2) shows a right ventricular meningioma. Note the bilateral vestibular schwannomas, consistent with NF2.*

Ependymoma

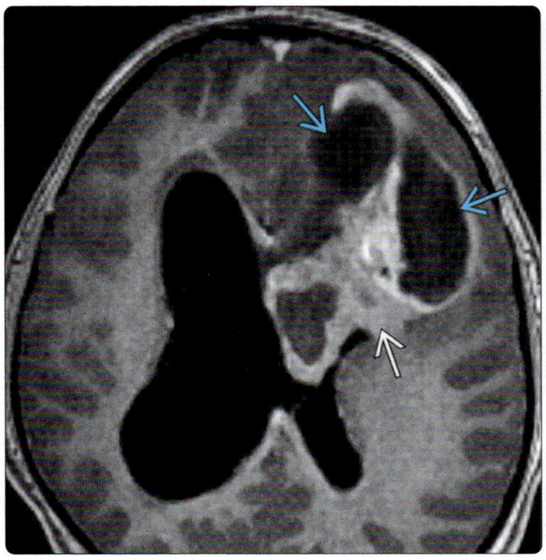

Central Neurocytoma

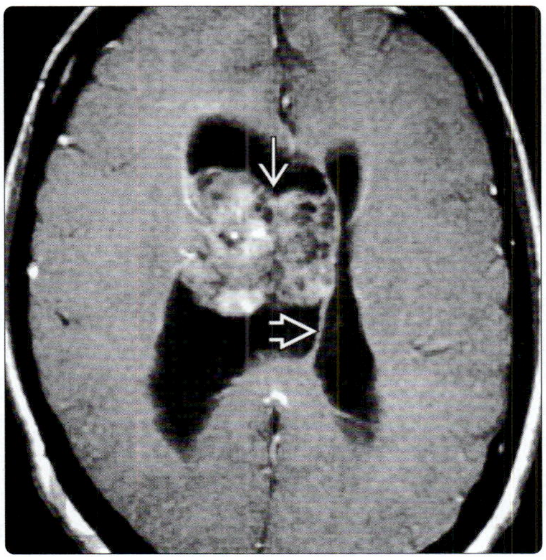

(Left) *Axial T1 C+ MR in an 11 year old with an ependymoma shows an intraventricular mass extending into the left frontal lobe. Mixed solid & cystic components are commonly seen in supratentorial ependymoma.* **(Right)** *Axial T1 C+ MR shows a bubbly, heterogeneously enhancing lateral ventricular mass with leftward bowing of the septum pellucidum. Attachment to the septum pellucidum is a key finding in the diagnosis of central neurocytoma.*

DIFFERENTIAL DIAGNOSIS

Common

- Pilocytic Astrocytoma
- Medulloblastoma
- Ependymoma
- Diffuse Intrinsic Pontine Glioma

Less Common

- Schwannoma
- Atypical Teratoid-Rhabdoid Tumor
- Ganglioglioma
- Meningioma, CPA-IAC
- Choroid Plexus Tumor
- Other Brainstem Gliomas
- High-Grade Astrocytoma
- Demyelinating Diseases (Mimic)
- Acute Cerebellitis (Mimic)

Rare but Important

- Hemangioblastoma
- Dysplastic Cerebellar Gangliocytoma
- Rosette-Forming Glioneuronal Tumor of 4th Ventricle
- Medulloepithelioma
- Abscess (Mimic)

ESSENTIAL INFORMATION

Key Differential Diagnosis Issues

- Clinical features to consider
    - Age
        - Posterior fossa tumors in children have very different diagnostic considerations vs. adults
        - Some tumors only occur in very young [e.g., atypical teratoid-rhabdoid tumor (ATRT)]
    - Tumors associated with syndromes
        - Neurofibromatosis type 2 (NF2): Schwannoma, meningioma
        - von Hippel-Lindau (VHL): Hemangioblastoma
- Imaging features to consider
    - Location
        - Cerebellum: Astrocytomas, ganglioglioma, medulloblastoma [Sonic Hedgehog (SHH) subtype]
        - 4th ventricle: Medulloblastoma, ependymoma, choroid plexus tumors
        - Brainstem: Diffuse intrinsic pontine glioma (DIPG) & other brainstem gliomas
        - Cerebellopontine angle (CPA): Schwannoma [internal auditory canal (IAC) involvement], meningioma
        - 4th ventricle + CPA: Ependymoma
- Modality considerations
    - MR: Best test for narrowing differential & detecting distant metastatic disease
        - DWI: Most helpful for tumor cellularity
            - Restricted diffusion (due to high cellularity): Medulloblastoma, ATRT, anaplastic ependymoma
        - T1 C+: Most sensitive to detect metastases
            - Must evaluate entire neuraxis in child with posterior fossa tumor prior to surgery
        - PWI: Helpful to distinguish pilocytic astrocytoma (PA) from hemangioblastoma
    - CT
        - Density of tumor reflects tumor cellularity
            - Hyperdense: Medulloblastoma, ATRT, anaplastic ependymoma
            - Hypodense: PA, ganglioglioma, DIPG
        - Ca^{2+} can be helpful
            - Fine, stippled Ca^{2+}: Ependymoma, choroid plexus tumors
            - Large, chunky Ca^{2+}: PA, ganglioglioma

Helpful Clues for Common Diagnoses

- **Pilocytic Astrocytoma**
    - Child or teen with enhancing cerebellar mass; ~ 50% have cystic component
    - Solid component has low cellularity: ↓ CT density; ↑ T2 signal, ↑ ADC signal on MR
    - PWI: ↓ signal (most helpful sequence to distinguish from hemangioblastoma)
    - 10% calcify, usually chunky
- **Medulloblastoma**
    - Young child with cellular posterior fossa mass
    - Location: 90% midline, 10% hemisphere/CPA
    - Location predicts molecular subtype
        - Hemispheric → SHH subtype
        - Midline → group 3 or 4 subtype, rarely SHH
        - CPA → wingless (WNT) subtype
    - Hypercellular: ↑ NECT density; ↓ T2, ↑ DWI/↓ ADC MR
- **Ependymoma**
    - Soft "plastic" tumor extending into/through 4th ventricular foramina
    - 50% with fine punctate Ca^{2+}
    - Increased cellularity suggests higher grade anaplastic ependymoma
- **Diffuse Intrinsic Pontine Glioma**
    - Mass centered in & expanding pons
    - Indistinct tumor margins (infiltrative appearance)
    - Expanded pons often surrounds basilar artery
    - Typically not cellular, showing ↑ ADC signal
    - Enhancement not common at diagnosis but more common after therapy

Helpful Clues for Less Common Diagnoses

- **Schwannoma**
    - IAC involvement is key diagnostic feature
    - Solid when small, often cystic when large
    - ↑ T2 signal & lack of dural tail (vs. meningioma)
    - Multiple in NF2
- **Atypical Teratoid-Rhabdoid Tumor**
    - Cellular tumor in young children that can occur anywhere along neuraxis (but often in posterior fossa)
    - Imaging similar to medulloblastoma but with ATRT
        - Patients are generally < 3 years old
        - Cysts, hemorrhage are more common
        - CPA involvement more is common
        - More frequent metastases at diagnosis
- **Ganglioglioma**
    - May occur in brainstem or cerebellum
    - Similar imaging features to supratentorial gangliogliomas
        - 50% enhance, often with indistinct margins

- Difficult to distinguish from more common PA by imaging alone
- **Meningioma, CPA-IAC**
  - Broad dural base, covers IAC
  - Variable signal, but ↓ T2 is common
  - ± hyperostosis, tumoral Ca^{2+}
- **Choroid Plexus Tumor**
  - 4th ventricle or CPA tumor with lobulated, frond-like margins
  - Avidly enhancing
  - Shares many other imaging features with ependymoma
  - Choroid plexus carcinoma is more likely than papilloma to show heterogeneous enhancement, necrosis, brain invasion, or CSF spread
- **Other Brainstem Gliomas**
  - Tectal plate glioma
    - Nonenhancing mass centered in tectum
    - Typically presents with obstructive hydrocephalus
  - Exophytic brainstem tumor
    - Tumor often protrudes dorsally into 4th ventricle
    - Imaging features are similar to PA with frequent enhancement
    - Common in neurofibromatosis type 1
- **High-Grade Astrocytoma**
  - Includes anaplastic astrocytoma & glioblastoma
  - Infiltrating mass involving predominantly white matter (WM)
  - Enhancement is variable
  - DWI: Isointense or hypointense ADC signal compared to brain parenchyma
- **Demyelinating Disease (Mimic)**
  - May mimic tumor in acute phase with mass effect
  - Discontinuous rim enhancement in acute phase
  - Look for additional WM lesions to support diagnosis
  - If centrally in brainstem, correlate with rapid history of Na^{+} correction
- **Acute Cerebellitis (Mimic)**
  - Usually bilateral cerebellar swelling but may mimic tumor when unilateral or asymmetric
  - T2/FLAIR signal changes, ± diffusion restriction, ± leptomeningeal enhancement

Helpful Clues for Rare Diagnoses

- **Hemangioblastoma**
  - Late teen or adult
  - Intraaxial (cerebellum > medulla, spinal cord)
    - Cyst with enhancing mural nodule > solid
    - Solid component shows flow voids, enhances avidly (similar to blood pool)
    - High perfusion in solid component
    - Multiple lesions are diagnostic of VHL
- **Dysplastic Cerebellar Gangliocytoma**
  - a.k.a. Lhermitte-Duclos
  - Diffuse or focal cerebellar hemispheric mass
  - Thick cerebellar folia with striated appearance
- **Rosette-Forming Glioneuronal Tumor of 4th Ventricle**
  - New in 2016 WHO CNS tumor classification
  - Solid or mixed solid/cystic mass arising from cerebellum with frequent protrusion into 4th ventricle
  - Shares many imaging features with PA & ganglioglioma
- **Medulloepithelioma**
  - Rare high-grade embryonal tumor, which may occur in eye & brain
  - Imaging features are that of high-grade tumor
  - Typically in very young patients (< 5 years), may arise prenatally
- **Abscess (Mimic)**
  - Rim-enhancing lesion with central diffusion restriction
    - Marked central diffusion restriction is most specific finding
  - Look for source of infection (e.g., mastoiditis)

SELECTED REFERENCES

1. Brandão LA et al: Posterior fossa tumors. Neuroimaging Clin N Am. 27(1):1-37, 2017
2. Dunham C: Uncommon pediatric tumors of the posterior fossa: pathologic and molecular features. Childs Nerv Syst. 31(10):1729-37, 2015
3. Raybaud C et al: Posterior fossa tumors in children: developmental anatomy and diagnostic imaging. Childs Nerv Syst. 31(10):1661-76, 2015

Pilocytic Astrocytoma

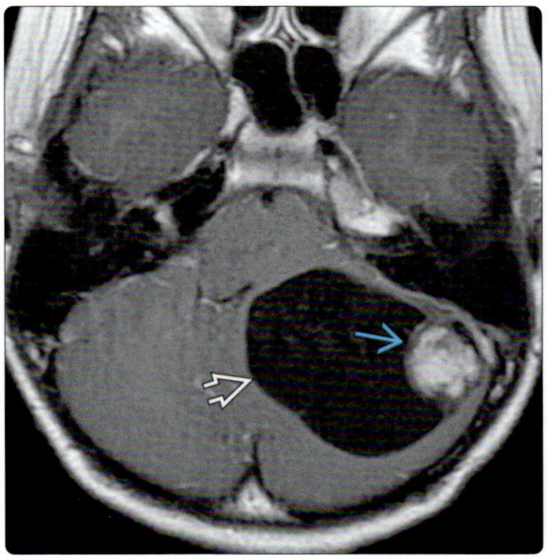

Pilocytic Astrocytoma

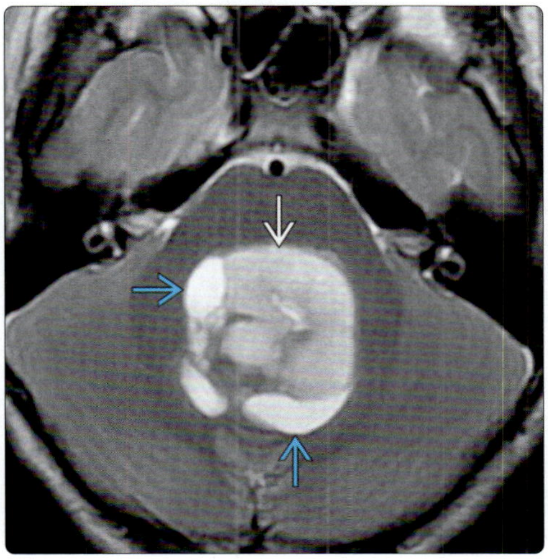

(Left) *Axial T1 C+ MR in a teenager with a pilocytic astrocytoma (PA) shows a cystic mass ➡ with an enhancing mural nodule ➡ in the cerebellar hemisphere. While this is a classic appearance for PA, only a minority will show such features.* **(Right)** *Axial T2 MR in a patient with a PA shows a predominantly solid midline mass ➡ with peripheral cysts ➡. While only 10% are midline, other typical imaging features (no diffusion restriction + bright T2 solid components) should keep PA as the primary consideration.*

(Left) *Sagittal T2 MR in a 4 year old shows a midline posterior fossa mass* ⇨ *to be similar in signal intensity to gray matter, typical for medulloblastoma. The mass also appears to arise from the roof of the 4th ventricle, a typical location for medulloblastoma.* **(Right)** *Axial DWI MR in the same patient with medulloblastoma shows increased signal in the mass* ⇨*. The ADC map (not shown) demonstrated corresponding decreased signal, consistent with true diffusion restriction due to the high cellularity of the tumor.*

Medulloblastoma

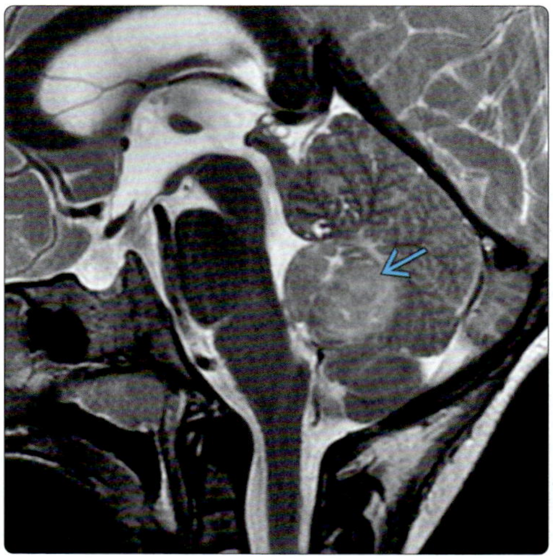

Medulloblastoma

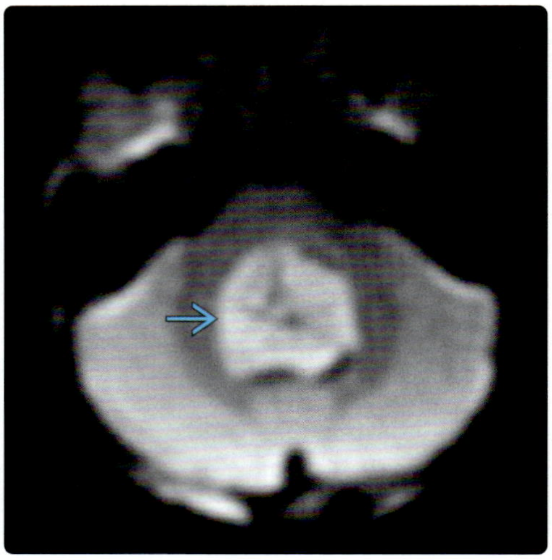

(Left) *Axial T2 MR in a 9 year old with medulloblastoma shows a mass in the right cerebellar hemisphere* ➡*. Approximately 10% of medulloblastomas occur in cerebellar hemispheres. This location is highly associated with SHH molecular subtype.* **(Right)** *Axial ADC MR in the same patient shows decreased ADC signal* ⇨ *in the mass due to high tumor cellularity, typical of a medulloblastoma (SHH subtype). In a younger (< 3 years old) patient, atypical teratoid-rhabdoid tumor (ATRT) should also be considered.*

Medulloblastoma

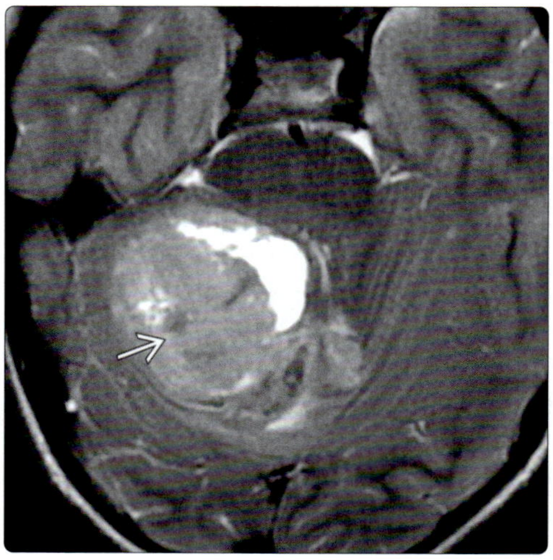

Medulloblastoma

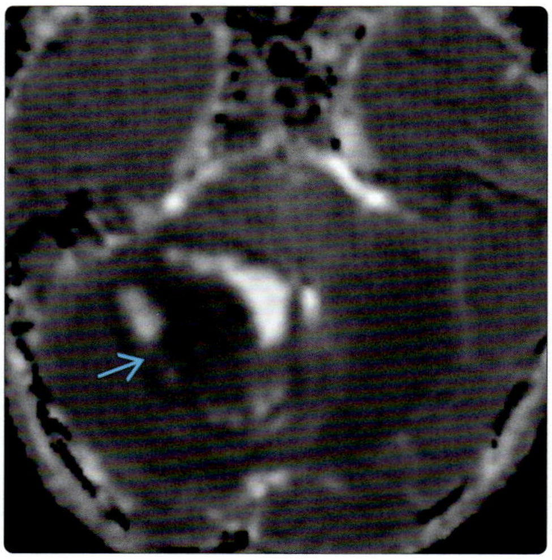

(Left) *Axial NECT shows a midline mass* ➡ *with stippled* Ca^{2+} ⇨*. Approximately 50% of all ependymomas show* Ca^{2+}*, typically fine & stippled rather than large & chunky (which is more characteristic of PA).* **(Right)** *Axial T1 C+ MR in a patient with ependymoma shows an avidly enhancing mass centered in the foramen of Luschka. The "plastic" nature of the tumor allows it to extend into the 4th ventricular foramina, which is the most characteristic imaging feature of ependymoma.*

Ependymoma

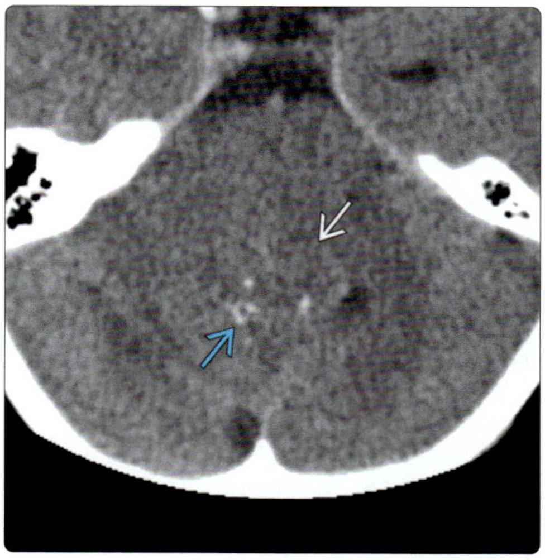

Ependymoma

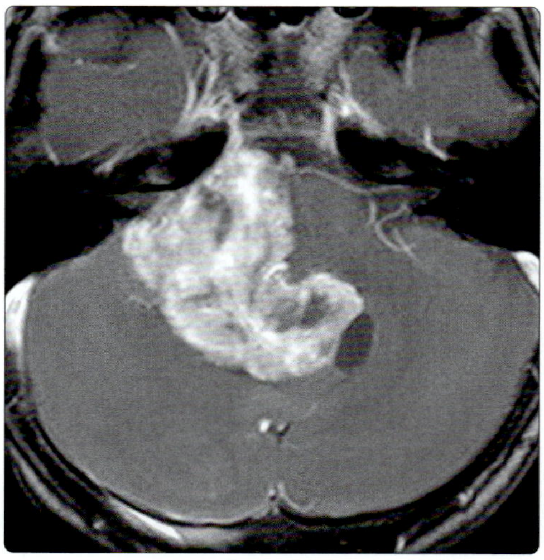

Diffuse Intrinsic Pontine Glioma

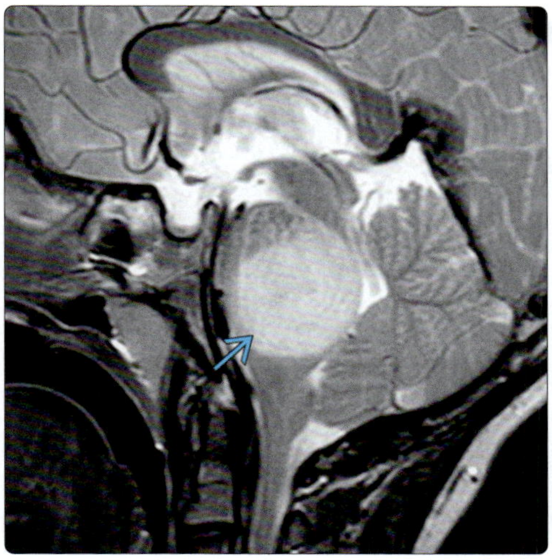

Diffuse Intrinsic Pontine Glioma

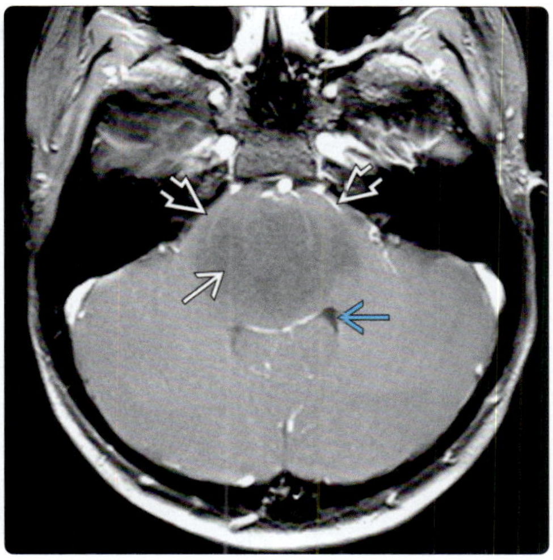

(Left) *Sagittal T2 MR in a 7 year old with nystagmus shows a mass ➡ centered in & expanding the pons. Location is the key diagnostic feature of diffuse intrinsic pontine glioma (DIPG).* **(Right)** *Axial T1 C+ MR in the same patient shows a nonenhancing, ill-defined mass ➡ centered in & expanding the pons with effacement of the adjacent 4th ventricle ➡ & basilar cisterns ➡. A lack of enhancement is typical for DIPG, although they often show some enhancement after initiating therapy.*

Schwannoma

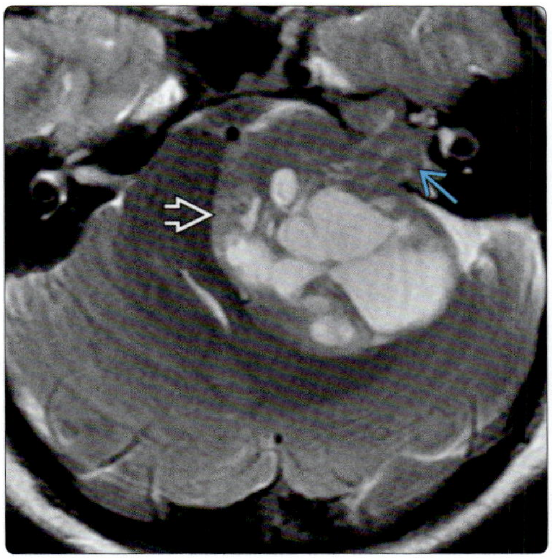

Schwannoma

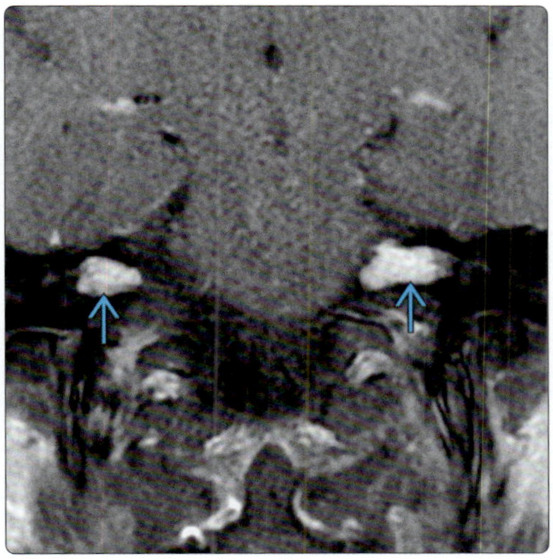

(Left) *Axial T2 MR in a 14 year old with a vestibular schwannoma shows a large mixed solid & cystic mass ➡ in the left cerebellopontine angle cistern. The key finding suggesting schwannoma is involvement of the IAC ➡. Large schwannomas are often partially cystic.* **(Right)** *Coronal T1 C+ MR in a 9 year old with NF2 & bilateral vestibular schwannomas shows enhancing masses ➡ in the IACs. Identifying a schwannoma or meningioma in a young patient should prompt careful evaluation for other signs of NF2.*

Atypical Teratoid-Rhabdoid Tumor

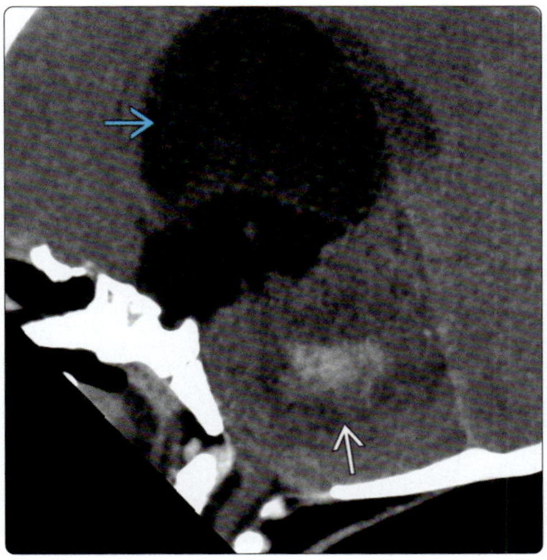

Atypical Teratoid-Rhabdoid Tumor

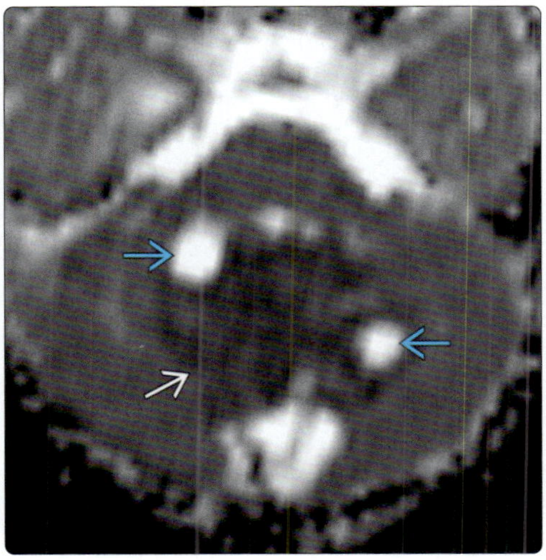

(Left) *Sagittal NECT in a 7 month old with an ATRT shows a hemorrhagic midline posterior fossa mass ➡ causing obstructive hydrocephalus ➡. Hemorrhage is common in ATRT, & the young age (< 3 years) is typical.* **(Right)** *Axial ADC MR in a 6 month old with ATRT shows a midline mass with peripheral cysts ➡ & hypointense solid components ➡, consistent with high cellularity. Any cellular posterior fossa tumor in a very young (< 3 years old) child should raise concern for ATRT.*

(Left) *Coronal FLAIR MR in a patient with a ganglioglioma shows a typical ill-defined focus of signal abnormality surrounding a cystic component . Both astrocytic tumors & ganglioglioma should be considered in this case.* **(Right)** *Axial T1 C+ MR in the same patient shows a nodular area of enhancement along the cyst. Approximately 50% of all gangliogliomas show contrast enhancement, making them difficult to distinguish from pilocytic astrocytoma.*

Ganglioglioma

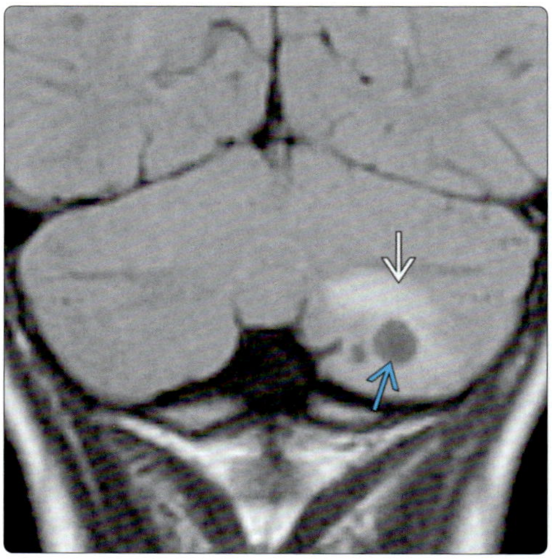

Ganglioglioma

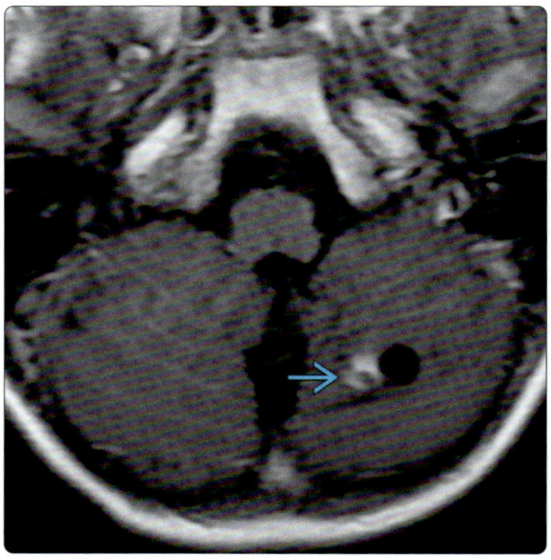

(Left) *Axial T1 C+ MR in a 12 year old with a meningioma shows a mass in the left CPA with extension into the left cavernous sinus & middle cranial fossa . Considerations for this mass would include both schwannoma & meningioma.* **(Right)** *Axial T1 C+ MR in a 4 year old with a choroid plexus papilloma shows an avidly enhancing mass centered in the 4th ventricle. The frond-like, lobulated margins help to distinguish choroid plexus tumors from ependymomas.*

Meningioma, CPA-IAC

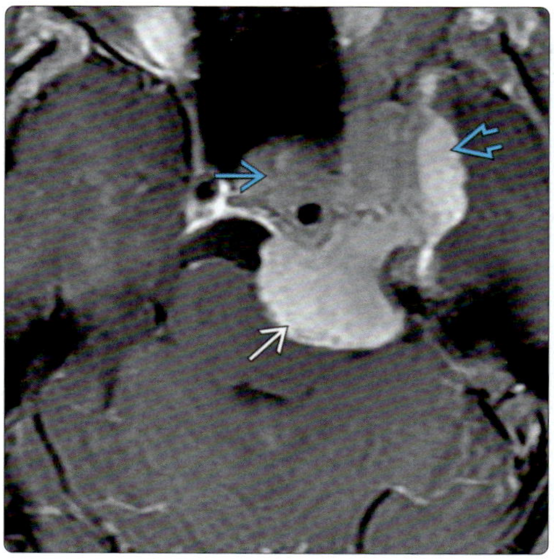

Choroid Plexus Tumor

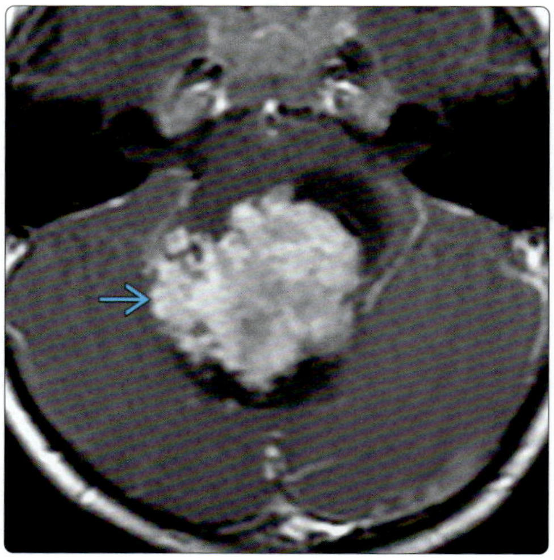

(Left) *Sagittal T1 C+ MR in an 11 year old with a brainstem PA shows an avidly enhancing dorsally exophytic tumor arising from the medulla. The exophytic appearance & contrast enhancement are typical for a non-DIPG brainstem tumor of the medulla.* **(Right)** *Axial T2 MR in an 11 year old with an anaplastic astrocytoma shows an ill-defined midline mass of the cerebellum. Indistinct margins, discontinuous poorly defined enhancement, & diffusion restriction favor a higher grade astrocytoma.*

Other Brainstem Gliomas

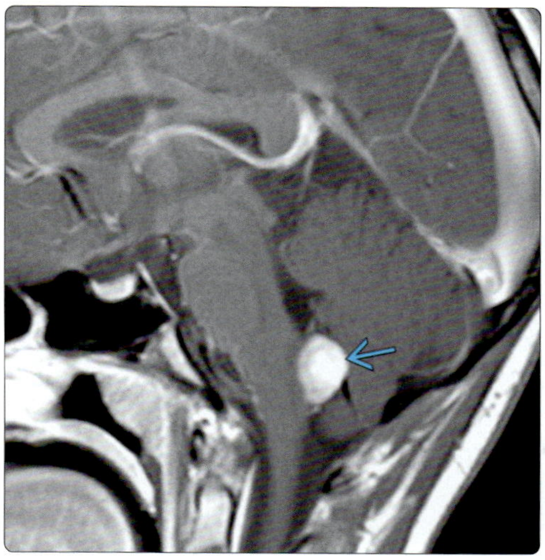

High-Grade Astrocytoma

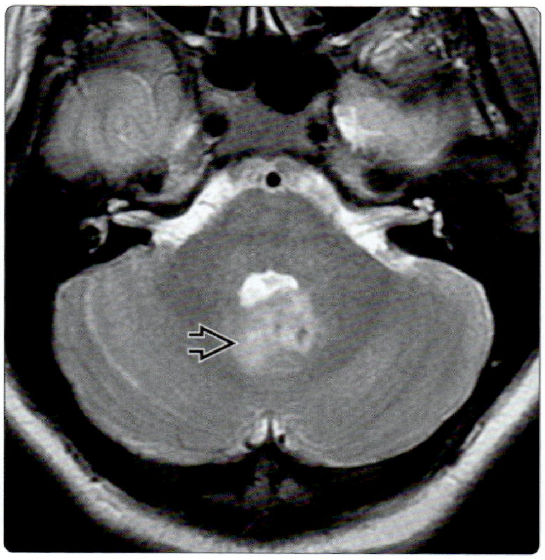

Demyelinating Diseases (Mimic)

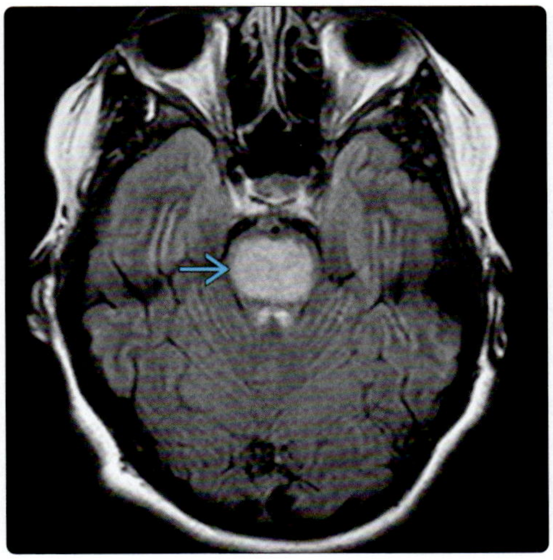

Acute Cerebellitis (Mimic)

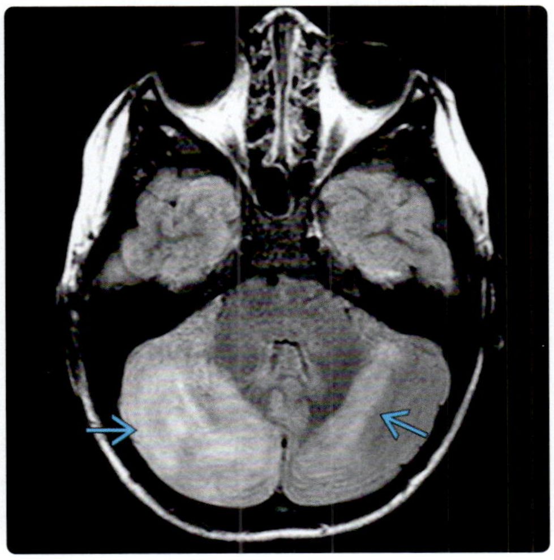

(Left) Axial FLAIR MR in an 18 year old with new-onset weakness, increased reflexes, & a positive Babinski sign after the rapid correction of a sodium deficit shows centrally increased signal with expansion of the pons → due to osmotic demyelination. **(Right)** Axial FLAIR MR in a 6 year old with headache & acute cerebellitis shows generalized cerebellar swelling with regions of increased signal →, more mass-like on the right. Mild restricted diffusion was also present in these regions.

Hemangioblastoma

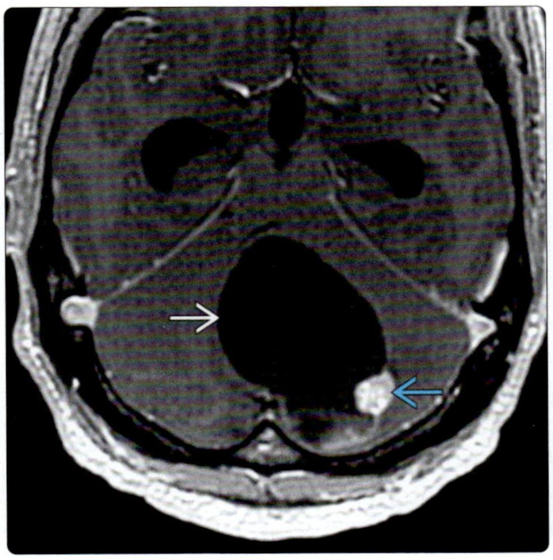

Dysplastic Cerebellar Gangliocytoma

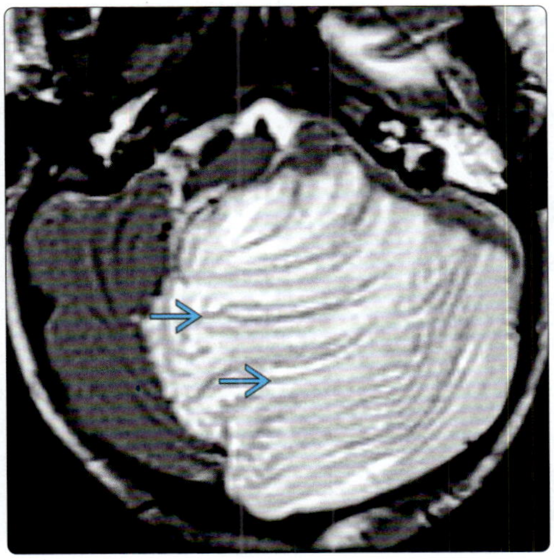

(Left) Axial T1 C+ MR in a patient with a hemangioblastoma shows a predominantly cystic mass ➡ with an enhancing mural nodule →. Imaging characteristics that would favor a hemangioblastoma rather than PA include increased perfusion in solid components (on PWI, not shown) & multiplicity of lesions. **(Right)** Axial T2 MR in a patient with a dysplastic cerebellar gangliocytoma shows a large mass expanding the cerebellar folia, creating a striated cerebellum pattern →.

Rosette-Forming Glioneuronal Tumor of 4th Ventricle

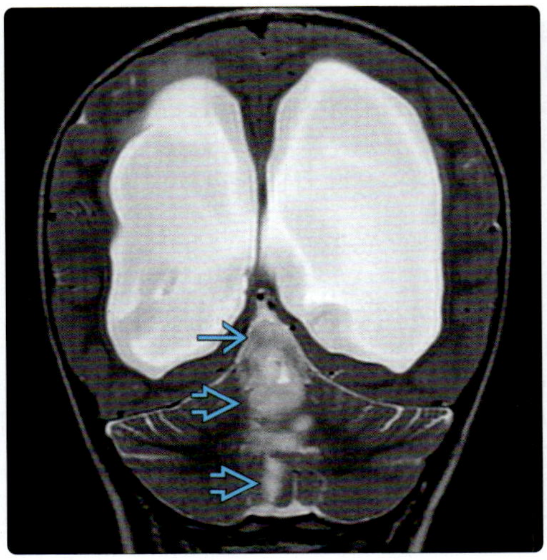

Abscess (Mimic)

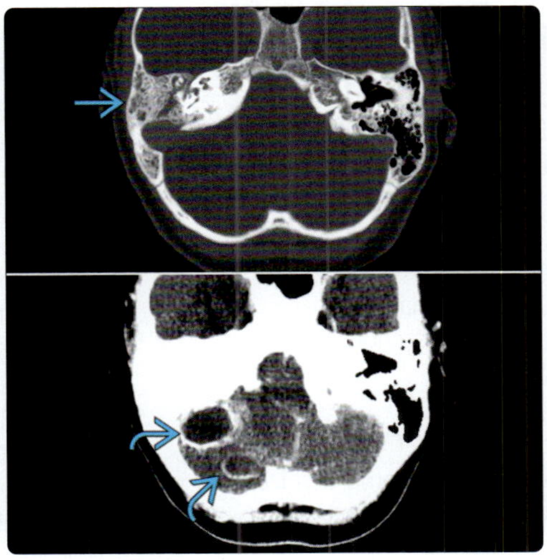

(Left) Coronal T2 MR in a 3 year old with swallowing difficulties shows an infiltrating lobulated mass → of the cerebellum extending superiorly though the 4th ventricle & superior cerebellar peduncles →. Lesion showed no enhancement or restricted diffusion. Rosette-forming glioneuronal tumor was found at biopsy. **(Right)** Axial CECT shows (bone windows, top) complete opacification → of the mastoid cells & middle ear cavity. Rim-enhancing abscesses → are visualized in the cerebellar parenchyma (brain windows, bottom).

DIFFERENTIAL DIAGNOSIS

Common

- Mega Cisterna Magna
- Arachnoid Cyst
- Pilocytic Astrocytoma
- Obstructive Hydrocephalus

Less Common

- Dandy-Walker Continuum
- Encephalocele
- Epidermoid Cyst
- Dermoid Cyst
- Syringobulbia
- Abscess

Rare but Important

- Schwannoma (Cystic)
- Chordoma
- Hemangioblastoma
- Ependymal Cyst
- Neuroglial Cyst
- Enlarged Perivascular Spaces
- Neurenteric Cyst
- Atypical Teratoid-Rhabdoid Tumor
- Neurocysticercosis

ESSENTIAL INFORMATION

Key Differential Diagnosis Issues

- Clinical features to consider
  - Common signs & symptoms: Macrocephaly, vomiting, cranial nerve deficits
    - Due to hydrocephalus or mass effect on brainstem
  - Most congenital malformations that are clinically significant present in utero or in infants
  - Arachnoid cysts (ACs) rarely grow larger or cause problems after ~ 5 years
- Imaging features to consider
  - Signal intensity: Cystic lesion relative to CSF
    - Follow CSF signal intensity **exactly** on all sequences
      - Mega cisterna magna (MCM), AC, Dandy-Walker continuum (DWC)
      - Trapped 4th ventricle, enlarged perivascular spaces (↑ PVSs), neuroglial or ependymal cyst
    - **Do not** follow CSF exactly
      - Congenital inclusion cysts: Dermoid, epidermoid, neurenteric cysts
      - Infection: Abscess, neurocysticercosis (NCC)
      - Neoplasm: Pilocytic astrocytoma, hemangioblastoma, metastasis, chordoma
  - Location: Intra- vs. extraaxial
    - Intraaxial
      - Trapped 4th ventricle (4th V), ↑ PVSs
      - Neoplasm [e.g., pilocytic astrocytoma, atypical teratoid-rhabdoid tumor (ATRT)], infection (abscess, NCC)
    - Extraaxial
      - MCM, AC, DWC, inclusion cyst, NCC, neoplasm (schwannoma, ATRT)
- Modality considerations
  - US: Many congenital cystic lesions are detected in utero or in neonates (with open anterior fontanelle)
  - MR: Greater contrast resolution & deeper spatial resolution
    - DWI: Key for distinguishing inclusion cyst (epidermoid/dermoid) & abscess from other cystic lesions
    - Contrast: Administer for any soft tissue components
    - 3D SSFP (e.g., FIESTA, CISS): Excellent spatial resolution (for thin cyst walls & relationship to cranial nerves) + absence of CSF flow artifact
  - CT: Helpful to detect Ca^{2+} in dermoid cysts or tumors
    - More readily available in emergent setting

Helpful Clues for Common Diagnoses

- **Mega Cisterna Magna**
  - Prominent midline retrocerebellar CSF space
  - Communicates freely with all CSF spaces
  - Normal tegmentovermian angle (< 5-10°)
  - Little, if any, mass effect
  - Difficult to distinguish from small AC in midline retrocerebellar space
    - However, neither is likely to be clinically significant
- **Arachnoid Cyst**
  - May occur anywhere in posterior fossa
  - Often has longstanding mass effect on cerebellum
  - ± hydrocephalus
  - Use FLAIR & DWI MR to exclude epidermoid
- **Pilocytic Astrocytoma**
  - Most PAs have cystic component
    - Cyst with imperceptible wall + mural nodule
    - Cyst with smooth enhancing wall + mural nodule
    - Cyst with irregular enhancing wall of varying thickness
    - Predominantly solid tumor with smaller cyst(s)
- **Obstructive Hydrocephalus**
  - Often sequelae of intraventricular hemorrhage
  - Blood products/septations obstruct outlets → 4th ventricle increases
    - Isolated enlargement if trapped
  - Maintains kidney bean configuration on axial images

Helpful Clues for Less Common Diagnoses

- **Dandy-Walker Continuum**
  - Prognosis of DWC is most affected by associated abnormalities
    - e.g., hydrocephalus, abnormal neuronal migration, etc.
  - "Classic" Dandy-Walker malformation
    - Hypoplastic, elevated, & rotated vermis
    - Cystic dilation of 4th ventricle fills enlarged posterior fossa (PF) → torcular-lambdoid inversion
  - Blake pouch cyst (BPC)
    - Embryonic BPC fails to fenestrate & herniates from inferior 4th ventricle into cisterna magna
    - Vermis is anatomically complete but rotated
- **Encephalocele**
  - Isolated encephalocele contains variable components of brain, meninges, & CSF ± venous sinuses, ventricle
    - Syndromic occipital encephalocele: Klippel-Feil, Meckel-Gruber, etc.

- Chiari 3 = Chiari 2 + cervical/occipito-cervical encephalocele containing cerebellum
- **Epidermoid Cyst**
  - Typically very similar to CSF on T1 & T2 MR but restricts diffusion & does not suppress completely on FLAIR
  - Most common location: Cerebellopontine angle
- **Dermoid Cyst**
  - Midline "fatty" mass
  - Fat droplets in CSF if mass has ruptured
  - Look for overlying dermal sinus & midline vertebral/skull anomalies
- **Syringobulbia**
  - Brainstem extension of syrinx (often from holocord syrinx in setting of Chari 1 or 2)
  - Follows CSF on all sequences
- **Abscess**
  - Thin-walled, rim-enhancing lesion with central diffusion restriction
  - T2-hypointense rim with surrounding edema

Helpful Clues for Rare Diagnoses

- **Schwannoma (Cystic)**
  - Enhancing mass arising in internal auditory canal along vestibular nerve with larger cisternal component ("ice cream on cone")
  - Vast majority are solid tumors but may become cystic
    - Cysts can be intratumoral or peritumoral
  - Look for other lesions of neurofibromatosis type 2 (additional schwannomas, meningiomas, ependymomas)
- **Chordoma**
  - Destructive clival mass with protruding lobulated T2-hyperintense components
  - Enhancement is variable
    - Classically honeycomb enhancement of internal septa
- **Hemangioblastoma**
  - Cyst with avidly enhancing mural nodule containing flow voids (due to high vascularity)
    - Enhances similar to blood pool
    - Very increased cerebral blood flow on perfusion imaging
  - Look for markers of von Hippel-Lindau (VHL)
    - Multiple hemangioblastomas of CNS
    - Visceral cysts, pancreatic tumors, renal cell carcinoma, pheochromocytoma
  - Rare in children without VHL
- **Ependymal Cyst**
  - Intra- or periventricular
  - Nonenhancing, follows CSF on all sequences
- **Neuroglial Cyst**
  - Intraparenchymal
  - Nonenhancing, follows CSF on all sequences
- **Enlarged Perivascular Spaces**
  - Very uncommon in pediatric posterior fossa, except for mucopolysaccharidosis
  - Follows CSF on all sequences
  - Most common posterior fossa site = dentate nuclei
- **Neurenteric Cyst**
  - Slightly hyperintense nonenhancing extraaxial cystic mass
  - Anterior pontomedullary & CPA cisterns
- **Atypical Teratoid-Rhabdoid Tumor**
  - Aggressive cellular tumor in young children
  - 50% are infratentorial (usually off midline)
  - Diffusion restriction in solid components
  - Intratumoral cysts & hemorrhage are common
- **Neurocysticercosis**
  - Cyst with internal "dot" (scolex); ± internal Ca^{2+} or surrounding edema (depending on stage)
  - Most commonly occurs in subarachnoid spaces, sulcal depths
  - Intraventricular cysts may be isolated
    - 4th ventricle is most common

SELECTED REFERENCES

1. Bosemani T et al: Congenital abnormalities of the posterior fossa. Radiographics. 35(1):200-20, 2015
2. Chapman T et al: Diagnostic imaging of posterior fossa anomalies in the fetus and neonate: part 2, posterior fossa disorders. Clin Imaging. 39(2):167-75, 2015

Mega Cisterna Magna

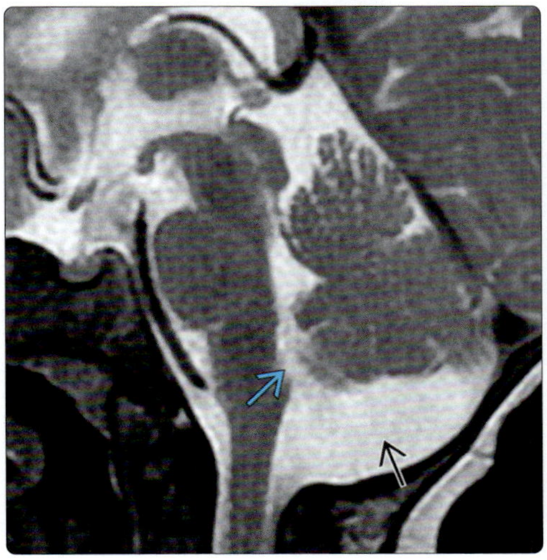

Mega Cisterna Magna

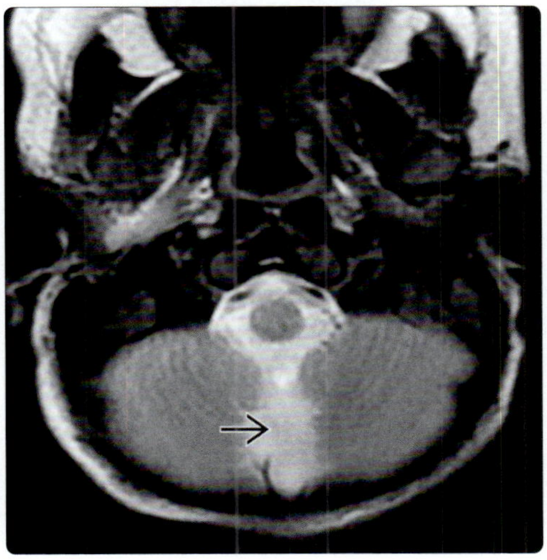

(Left) *Sagittal T2 MR in a 3 month old with a mega cisterna magna (MCM) shows a prominent CSF space ➡ inferior & posterior to the normal vermis. Note the normal tegmentovermian angle ➡ & lack of mass effect. A typical MCM is much more prominent on sagittal than axial images.* **(Right)** *Axial T2 MR in the same patient with a MCM shows that the prominent inferior CSF collection ➡ does not extend significantly beyond the midline & does not exert mass effect on adjacent structures.*

(Left) *Axial 3D SSFP MR in a 9 year old with an arachnoid cyst shows asymmetric expansion of right CP angle cistern with mild mass effect on right cerebellar hemisphere. Such a small cyst in an older child is almost always an incidental finding.* **(Right)** *Axial T2 FLAIR MR in an infant shows massive expansion of the left CP angle cistern by a large arachnoid cyst. There is shift & effacement of the 4th ventricle, resulting in obstructive hydrocephalus. Note the complete signal suppression on FLAIR.*

Arachnoid Cyst

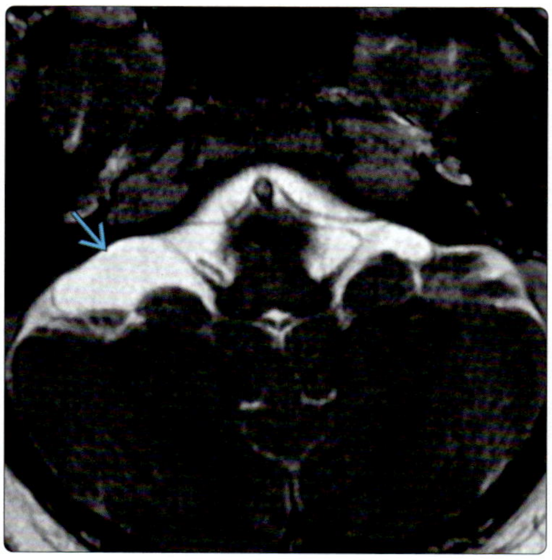

Arachnoid Cyst

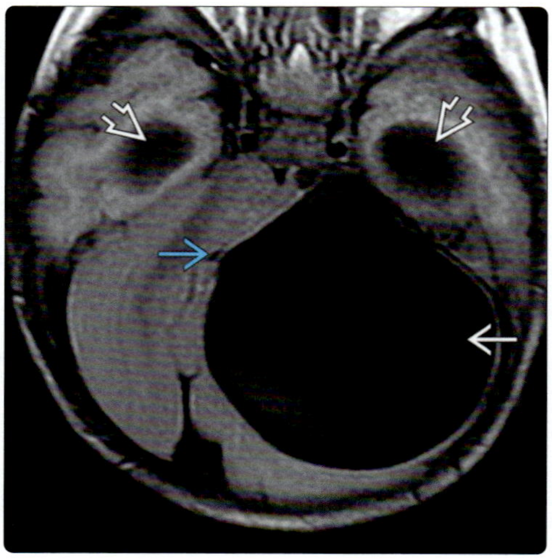

(Left) *Sagittal T2 MR in an 8 year old with a pilocytic astrocytoma (PA) shows a predominantly cystic mass with mural soft tissue, a classic appearance for JPA. A solid component is the best clue for a tumor when a cystic lesion is encountered in the posterior fossa.* **(Right)** *Axial T1 C+ MR in the same patient shows a thin rim of enhancement along the margin of the cyst with more focal nodular enhancing components. This is a typical appearance for PA.*

Pilocytic Astrocytoma

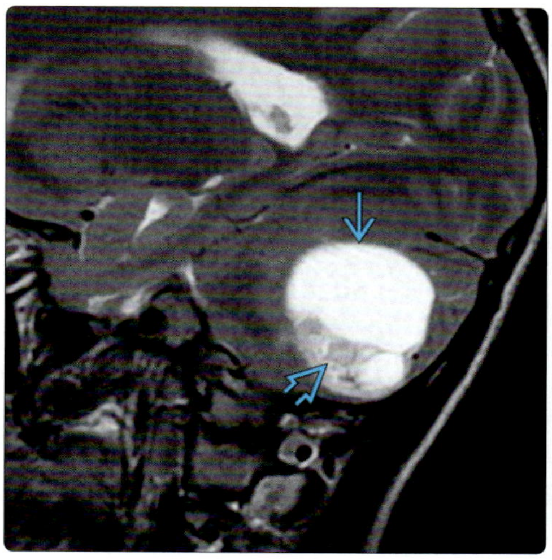

Pilocytic Astrocytoma

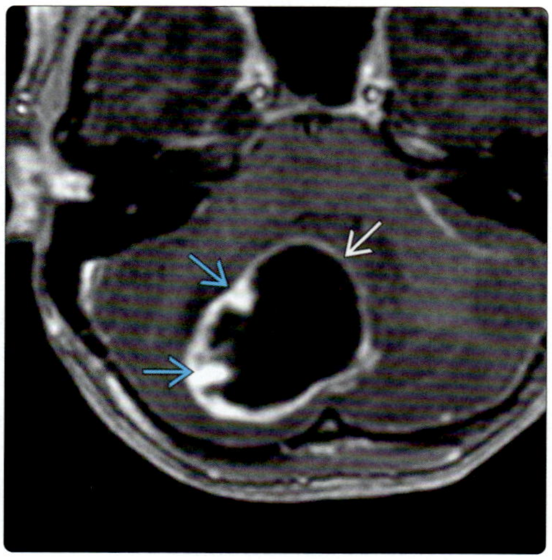

(Left) *Sagittal T2 MR in a 3 year old with a history of prematurity & intraventricular hemorrhage (IVH) shows posthemorrhagic hydrocephalus. The 4th ventricle is markedly enlarged due to obstruction at the level of the 4th ventricle outlets.* **(Right)** *Axial SWI MR in a 4 month old with isolated 4th ventricular enlargement shows multiple areas of hemosiderin deposition along the ventricle margins & brainstem. Prior IVH is the most likely etiology for isolated 4th ventricular hydrocephalus.*

Obstructive Hydrocephalus

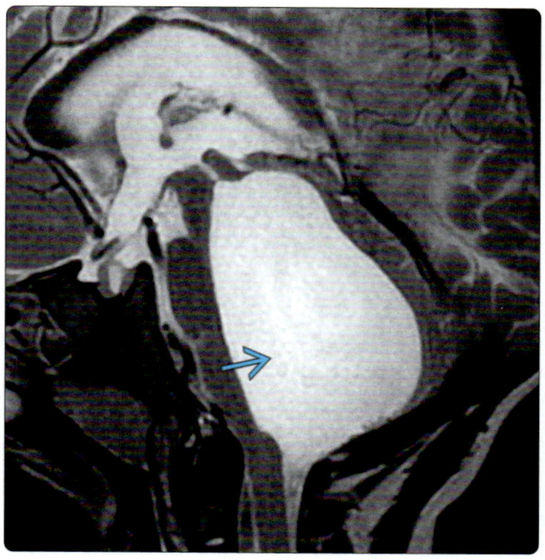

Obstructive Hydrocephalus

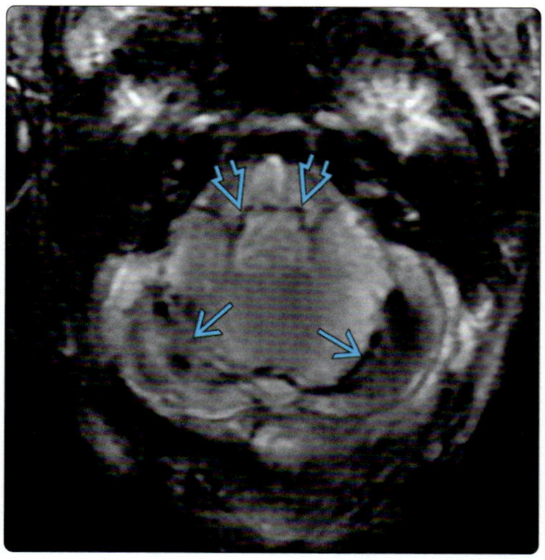

Dandy-Walker Continuum

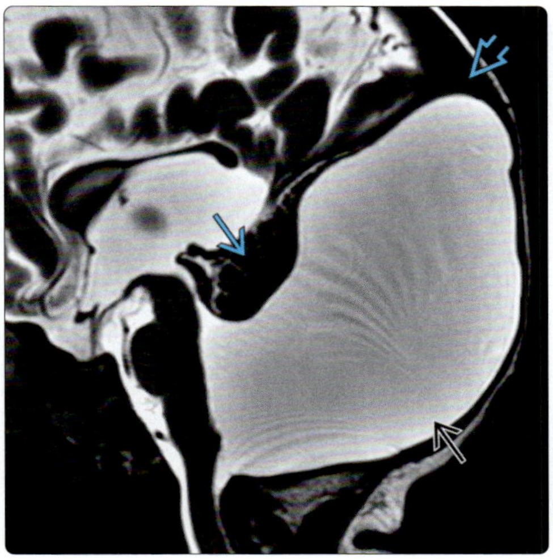

Dandy-Walker Continuum

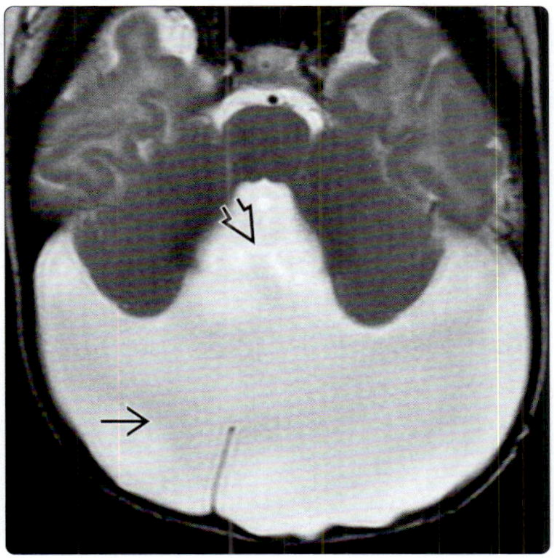

(Left) *Sagittal 3D SSFP MR in an infant with classic Dandy-Walker malformation (DWM) shows marked cystic enlargement ➔ of the posterior fossa in continuity with the 4th ventricle. There is a rotated hypogenetic vermis ➔ with elevation of the torcular Herophili ➔.* **(Right)** *Axial T2 MR in the same patient shows the marked cystic enlargement ➔ of the posterior fossa in continuity with the 4th ventricle ➔. While the posterior fossa cyst is striking, the prognosis is most related to associated findings (e.g., hydrocephalus).*

Encephalocele

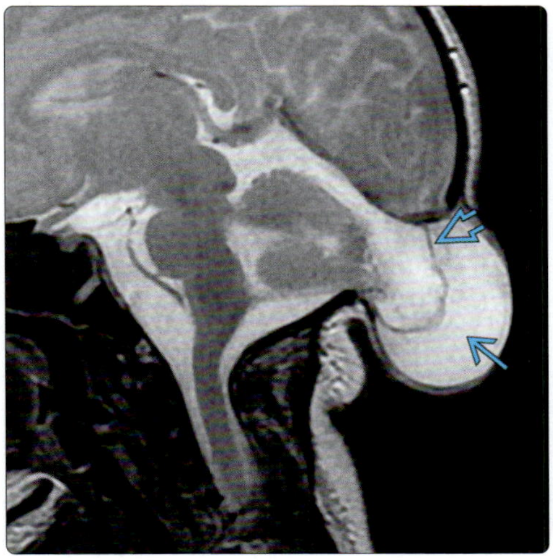

Encephalocele

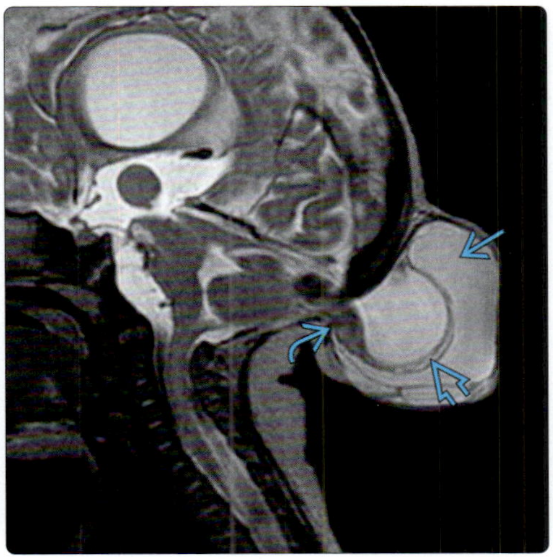

(Left) *Sagittal T2 MR in a neonate with an occipital cephalocele shows protrusion of CSF ➔ & meninges ➔ through an occipital osseous defect.* **(Right)** *Sagittal T2 MR in a neonate with an occipital encephalocele shows an osseous defect in the midline occipital bone with extension of CSF ➔, meninges ➔, & cerebellar tissue ➔ through the defect. Note the small posterior fossa & posteriorly tethered appearance of the cerebellum & brainstem, a common appearance in occipital encephaloceles.*

Epidermoid Cyst

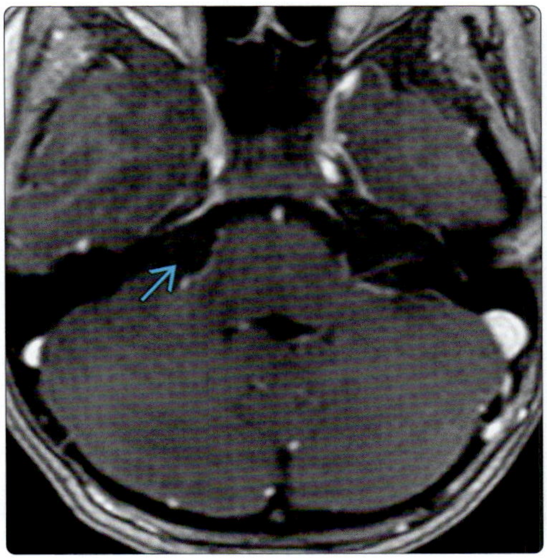

Epidermoid Cyst

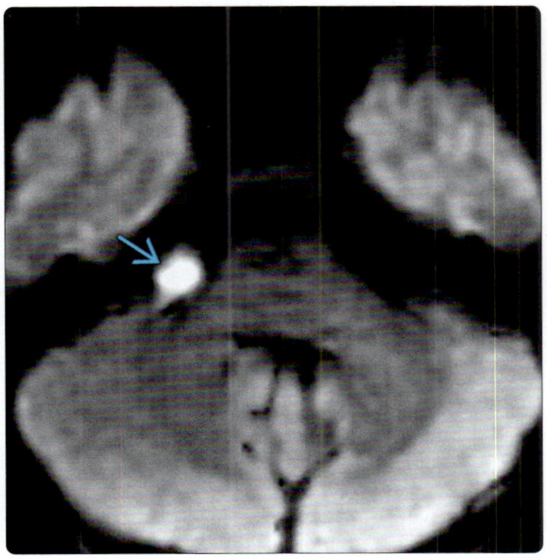

(Left) *Axial T1 C+ MR in a 9 year old with a right CP angle epidermoid cyst shows a small nonenhancing lesion ➔ with signal intensity similar to CSF. Epidermoid cysts are typically very inconspicuous on T1- & T2-weighted images.* **(Right)** *Axial DWI MR in the same patient shows a "light bulb bright" lesion ➔ in the right CP angle, a characteristic finding for an epidermoid cyst. Note that epidermoid cysts are often most conspicuous on DWI.*

Dermoid Cyst

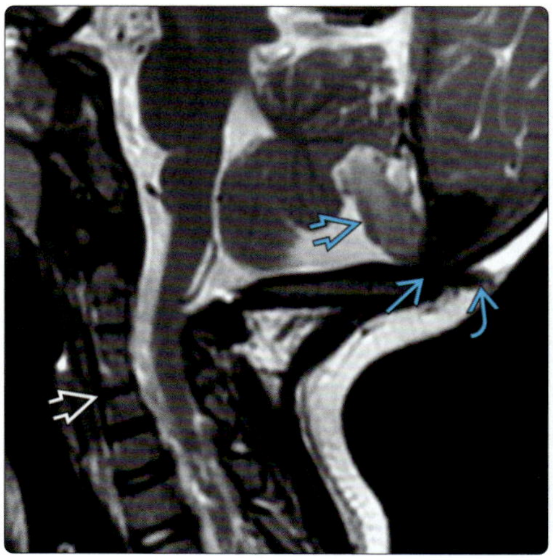

Dermoid Cyst

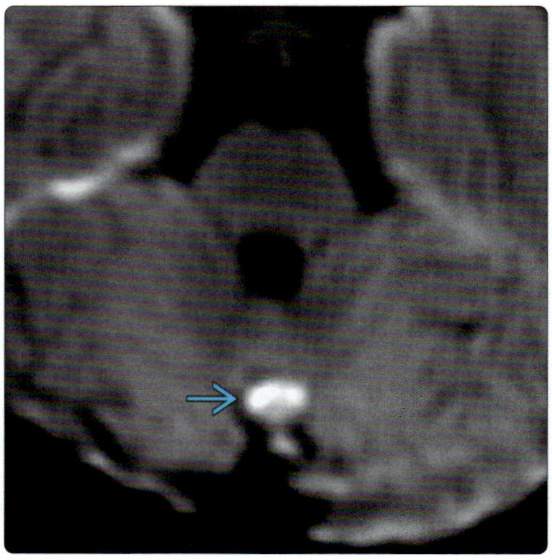

(Left) *Midline sagittal T2 MR in a 4 year old with a dermoid shows a lesion posterior to the cerebellum. It is associated with an occipital osseus defect & superficial dorsal dermal sinus tract. Also note the multiple segmentation anomalies in the upper cervical spine, consistent with Klippel-Feil syndrome (a common association).* **(Right)** *Axial DWI MR in the same patient shows diffusion restriction in the midline retrocerebellar lesion (which is more commonly seen with epidermoids than dermoids).*

Abscess

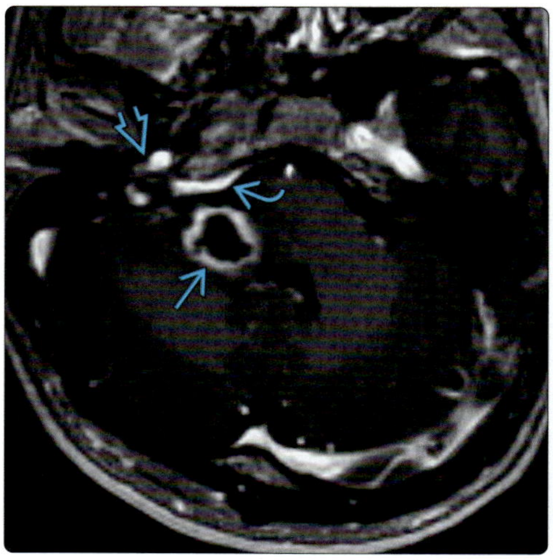

Abscess

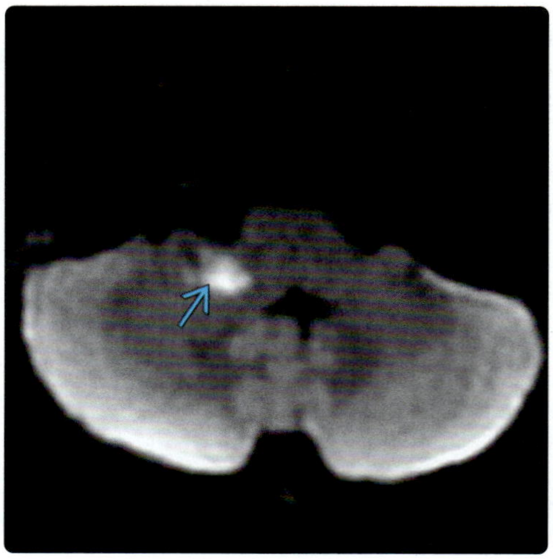

(Left) *Axial T1 C+ MR in a teenager with an abscess shows a rim-enhancing lesion centered in the right middle cerebellar peduncle. Also note the adjacent enhancing dura & internal auditory structures, suggesting a right temporal bone infection source.* **(Right)** *Axial DWI MR in the same patient shows central diffusion restriction associated with the lesion, which is the most specific imaging finding for cerebral abscess.*

Syringobulbia

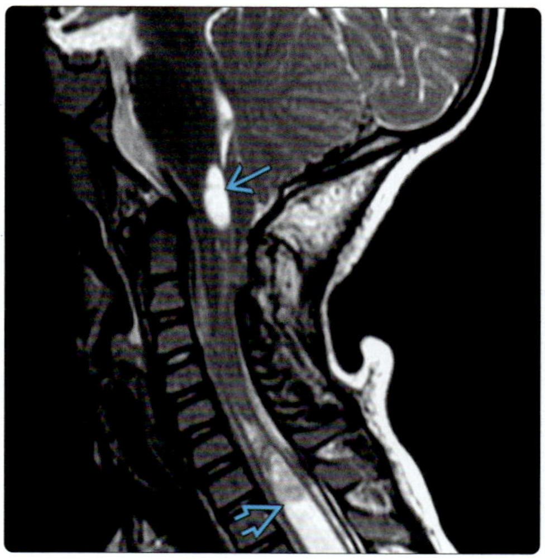

Schwannoma (Cystic)

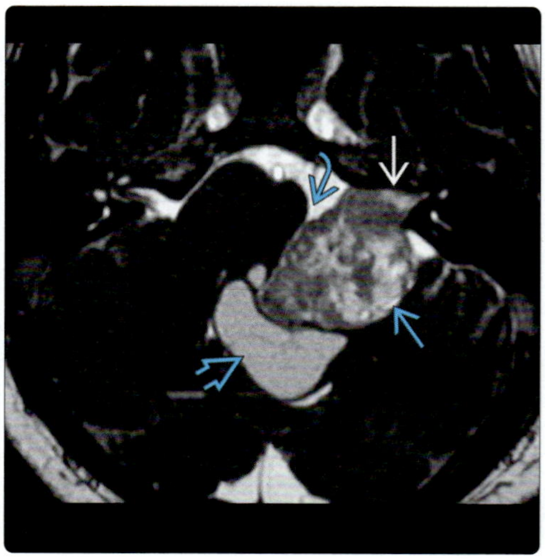

(Left) *Sagittal T2 MR in a patient with a Chiari 2 malformation & syringobulbia shows a cystic focus in posterior medulla that follows CSF. Note the associated cord syrinx, which is almost always present in syringobulbia.* **(Right)** *Axial 3D SSFP MR in a teenager with cystic schwannoma shows a mixed solid & cystic mass arising from an enlarged left internal auditory canal. The acute angle with brainstem & IAC involvement suggest that this is an extraaxial rather than intraaxial tumor.*

Chordoma

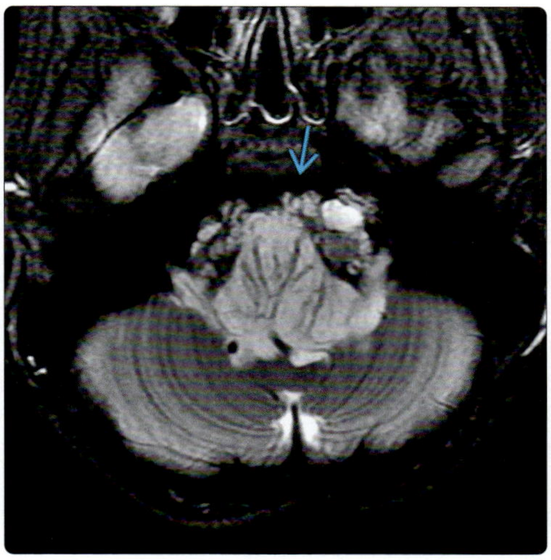

Hemangioblastoma

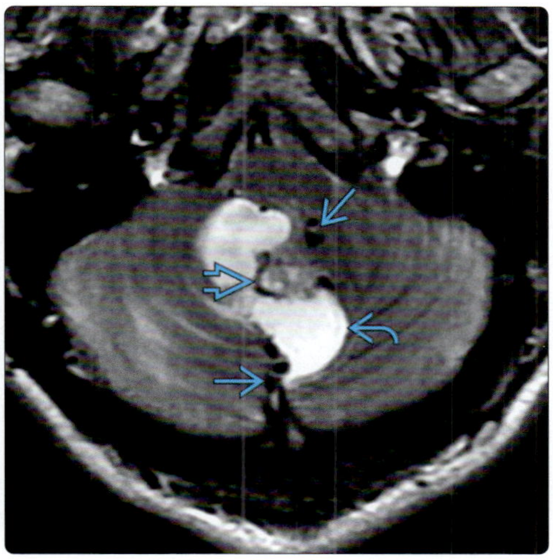

(Left) *Axial T2 MR in an 8 year old with a clival chordoma shows a lobulated T2-hyperintense lesion with multiple linear T2-hypointense striations, typical for chordoma. While chordomas are rarely cystic, they are frequently so bright on T2 that they may be mistaken for a cystic lesion.* **(Right)** *Axial T2 MR in a teenager with von Hippel-Lindau & hemangioblastoma (HB) shows a mixed solid & cystic lesion with multiple prominent flow voids, typical of HB.*

Hemangioblastoma

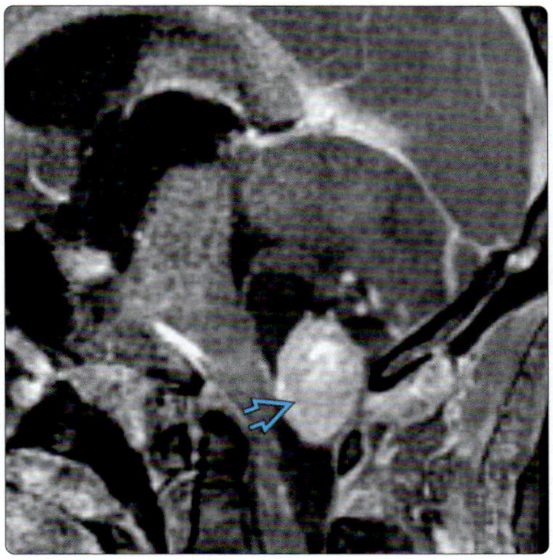

Enlarged Perivascular Spaces

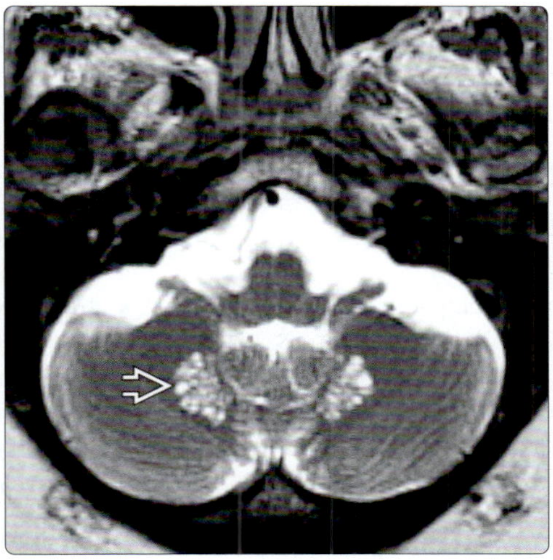

(Left) *Sagittal T1 C+ FS MR in the same patient shows an avidly enhancing solid component that is equal to blood pool, typical of HB. HBs in children occur almost exclusively in the setting of VHL. Look carefully for additional HBs or visceral findings (pancreatic cysts, renal cell carcinoma) to confirm VHL.* **(Right)** *Axial T2 MR shows clusters of tiny hyperintense foci in the dentate nuclei due to enlarged perivascular spaces. While rare in children, they are often seen in mucopolysaccharidosis.*

Atypical Teratoid-Rhabdoid Tumor

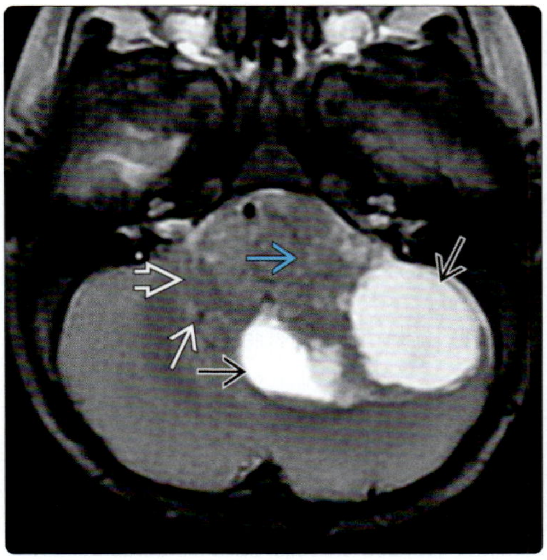

Atypical Teratoid-Rhabdoid Tumor

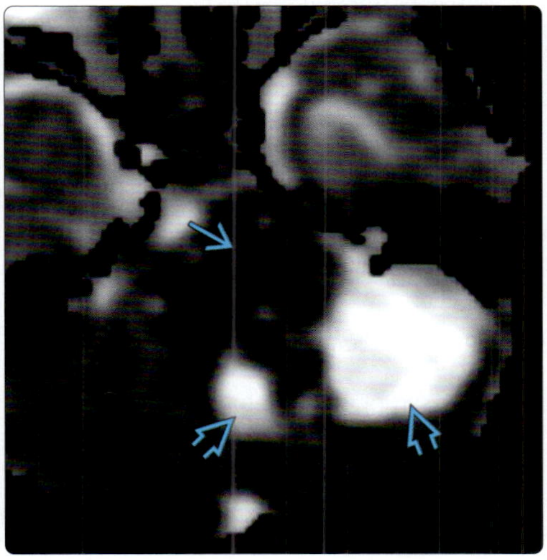

(Left) *Axial T2 MR in a 4 month old with an ATRT shows a mixed solid & cystic lesion centered in the left CP angle cistern. The lesion partially encases the basilar artery & causes marked mass effect on the brainstem & 4th ventricle.* **(Right)** *Axial ADC map MR in the same patient shows markedly hypointense signal in the solid portion of the lesion, consistent with a cellular tumor. Location, age, & cellularity are all highly suggestive of an ATRT. Note that the cysts show increased signal.*

DIFFERENTIAL DIAGNOSIS

Common

- Arachnoid Cyst
- Hematoma
- Empyema

Less Common

- Epidermoid Cyst
- Dermoid Cyst
- Lipoma
- Schwannoma
- Meningioma
- Atypical Teratoid-Rhabdoid Tumor
- Langerhans Cell Histiocytosis
- Metastatic Neuroblastoma

Rare but Important

- Chordoma
- Rhabdomyosarcoma
- Teratoma
- Infantile or Congenital Hemangioma
- Arteriovenous Fistula
- Giant Aneurysm
- Cranial Fasciitis

ESSENTIAL INFORMATION

Key Differential Diagnosis Issues

- Clinical features to consider
  - Trauma → hematoma; fever → empyema
  - Neurofibromatosis type 2 (NF2) → meningioma & schwannoma
  - Prior radiation therapy → meningioma
  - Multiple infantile hemangiomas → PHACE syndrome
- Imaging features to consider
  - Location
    - Extracranial: Rhabdomyosarcoma, cranial fasciitis, dermoid/epidermoid, teratoma
    - Osseus: Langerhans cell histiocytosis (LCH), metastatic neuroblastoma (NB), chordoma, dermoid/epidermoid, cranial fasciitis, hemangiopericytoma, meningioma (rare)
    - Extraaxial: Arachnoid cyst, hematoma, empyema, schwannoma, meningioma, lipoma, epidermoid/dermoid cyst
  - Diffusion restriction: Pus (empyema), blood products (hematoma), cellular debris (epidermoid), & cellular tumor [atypical teratoid-rhabdoid tumor (ATRT)]
- Modality considerations
  - US: May be initial exam in neonates/infants, especially with palpable lesion
  - CT: Excellent 1st-line test for acute symptoms, trauma, & infection
    - Best test to characterize calvarial involvement, if present
  - MR with contrast: Best test to characterize extraaxial lesions
    - T1 C+: Best sequence for evaluation of nontraumatic extraaxial lesions
      - Nonenhancement → epidermoid; dural tail → meningioma
    - DWI can be key discriminator for many lesions
    - 3D SSFP (FIESTA/CISS) can be helpful for extraaxial masses in basilar cisterns to define cranial nerve & vascular involvement
    - Perfusion (PWI): Markedly ↑ cerebral blood flow (CBF) of infantile/congenital hemangioma

Helpful Clues for Common Diagnoses

- **Arachnoid Cyst**
  - Best clue: Extraaxial lesion that follows CSF on all sequences
  - Most common locations are middle fossa & posterior fossa but can occur anywhere
  - Most likely symptomatic in suprasellar & basilar cisterns in fetus/infant
  - If necessary, can be treated with fenestration, microsurgical resection, or shunting
- **Hematoma**
  - Best clue: Hyperattenuating (CT) or mixed attenuation extraaxial collection
  - Epidural & subdural hematomas are most common overall but can be subpial in neonates
    - Epidural: Lentiform, constrained by sutures
    - Subdural: Crescentic, constrained by falx & tentorium
  - Almost always secondary to trauma
  - Look for associated fractures & parenchymal contusions
  - Always evaluate for mass effect leading to brain herniation, which will often prompt surgical evacuation
- **Empyema**
  - Best clue: Extraaxial rim-enhancing collection with central diffusion restriction
  - Look for source of infection (usually sinuses/mastoids)
  - Evaluate for underlying cerebritis
  - Typically treated with craniotomy & empyema washout

Helpful Clues for Less Common Diagnoses

- **Epidermoid Cyst**
  - Best clue: Nonenhancing cyst with marked diffusion restriction
  - May occur anywhere but often at sutures, midline, cerebellopontine (CP) angle
  - Nearly isointense to CSF on T1 & T2
  - Does not suppress on FLAIR
  - Often "light bulb bright" on DWI
- **Dermoid Cyst**
  - Best clue: Midline lesion, ± diffusion restriction
  - Often contains macroscopic fat → can rupture & cause chemical meningitis
  - Look for associated dermal sinus tract
- **Lipoma**
  - Best clue: Mass composed entirely of fat
  - Almost always midline (e.g., pericallosal, suprasellar)
  - CT: Can mimic gas on brain windows → adjust window/level to differentiate
  - MR: T1 hyperintense; use fat saturation to confirm fat
- **Schwannoma**
  - Best clue: Avidly enhancing lesion involving cranial nerves
  - Much less common in children vs. adults
  - Usually solid with uniform enhancement

- Large lesions may be heterogeneous ± cysts
- Look for other lesions (meningiomas) to suggest NF2

- **Meningioma**
  - Best clue: Avidly enhancing lesion with broad dural attachment & tail
  - Much less common in children vs. adults
  - Typically close to gray matter on all sequences with avid enhancement
    - Larger lesions may be more heterogeneous
  - Evaluate for additional lesions (schwannomas) to suggest NF2
- **Atypical Teratoid-Rhabdoid Tumor**
  - Best clue: Cellular extraaxial mass in infant
  - Grade IV cellular embryonal tumor
  - May be intra- or extraaxial in location
  - Heterogeneous (± hemorrhage & cysts) tumor with diffusion restriction
- **Langerhans Cell Histiocytosis**
  - Best clue: Enhancing, cellular lesion centered in bone
  - Lytic bone-centered tumor with extradural soft tissue component
  - Typically solid & cellular (↑ DWI/↓ ADC) mass
  - CT: "Punched-out" lesion with beveled edges
  - MR: Look for pituitary infundibulum involvement
- **Metastatic Neuroblastoma**
  - Best clue: Symmetric bifrontal/skull base osseous masses
  - Bone-centered mass with broad extradural soft tissue
  - CT: Look for typical osseous changes
    - Permeation, thinning, &/or irregular expansion of bone with radiating perpendicular spicules of new bone

Helpful Clues for Rare Diagnoses

- **Chordoma**
  - Best clue: T2-bright destructive mass arising from clivus
  - Enhancement patterns are highly variable but classically "honeycomb"
  - Often encases vertebral artery & cranial nerves
- **Rhabdomyosarcoma**
  - Best clue: Destructive head/neck mass with intracranial extension
  - Cellular tumor arising from paranasal sinuses/orbits/temporal bone
- **Teratoma**
  - Best clue: Heterogeneous mass of soft tissue, fat, & Ca^{2+}
  - May be intracranial, extracranial, or both
- **Infantile or Congenital Hemangioma**
  - Infantile: Small & localized to internal auditory canal (IAC) in setting of PHACE syndrome
    - Homogeneous, avid enhancement
    - Often shows prominent flow voids
    - Perfusion imaging shows markedly ↑ CBF
  - Congenital: Large heterogeneous mass with intracranial & extracranial components
    - May show hemorrhage & Ca^{2+}
    - Rapid involution vs. no involution; no proliferation
- **Arteriovenous Fistula**
  - Best clue: Large draining vein & enlarged arterial feeder
  - Arteriovenous malformations are typically intraaxial, while arteriovenous fistulas are typically extraaxial
- **Giant Aneurysm**
  - Best clue: Pulsation artifact in phase-encoding direction
  - Usually at least partially thrombosed
  - Rare in children
- **Cranial Fasciitis**
  - Best clue: Lytic calvarial lesion with frequent intracranial & dural involvement

SELECTED REFERENCES

1. Pinto PS et al: Magnetic resonance imaging features of meningiomas in children and young adults: a retrospective analysis. J Neuroradiol. 39(4):218-26, 2012
2. Al-Holou WN et al: Prevalence and natural history of arachnoid cysts in children. J Neurosurg Pediatr. 5(6):578-85, 2010
3. Zakhary MM et al: Prevalence and etiology of intracranial hemorrhage in term children under the age of two years: a retrospective study of computerized tomographic imaging and clinical outcome in 798 children. Acad Radiol. 16(5):572-7, 2009
4. Adame N et al: Sinogenic intracranial empyema in children: Pediatrics 2005, 116:e461-7

Arachnoid Cyst

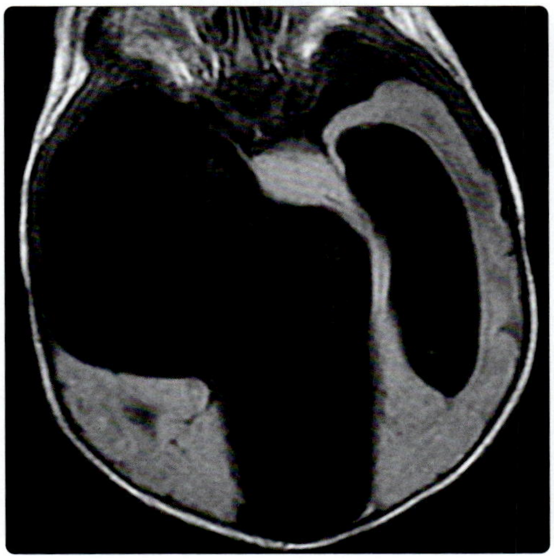

Arachnoid Cyst

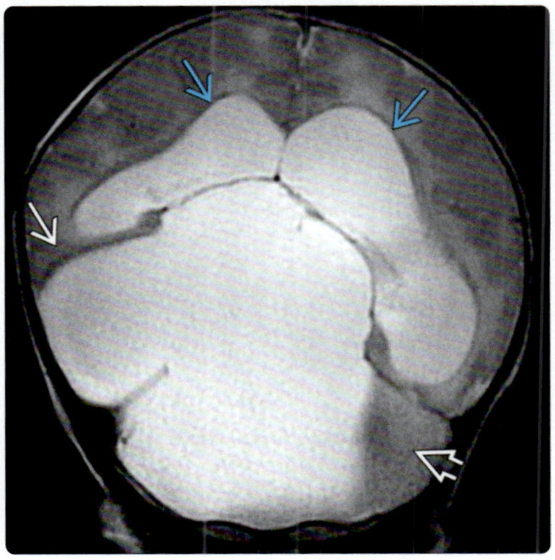

(Left) *Axial FLAIR MR in a 1 day old shows a large cystic mass occupying both the posterior fossa & right middle fossa. The contents of the mass are completely nulled on FLAIR, consistent with an arachnoid cyst.* **(Right)** *Coronal T2 MR in the same patient shows the extent of mass effect upon the cerebellum ➡ & right temporal lobe ➡. Note the enlarged lateral ventricles ➡, consistent with obstructive hydrocephalus.*

(Left) *Coronal NECT in a 3 year old with a subdural hematoma shows a large high-density crescentic collection that crosses sutures & is constrained by the falx. In the absence of a clear traumatic history, nonaccidental trauma should be considered.* **(Right)** *Axial NECT in a 7 year old with a traumatic epidural hematoma shows a typical lentiform high-density collection in the right frontal region that is constrained by the coronal suture. Note the subfalcine herniation.*

Hematoma

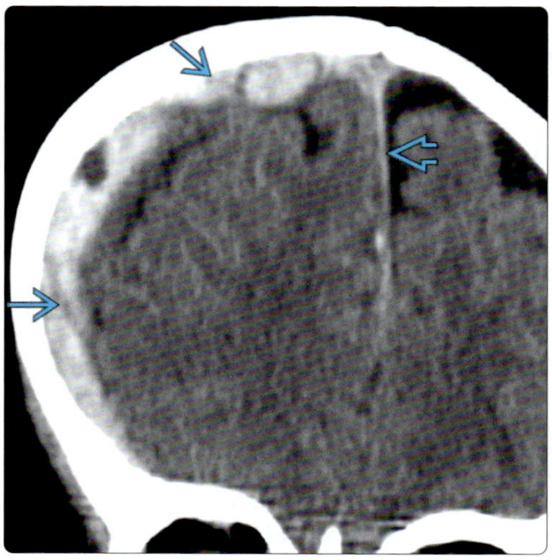

Hematoma

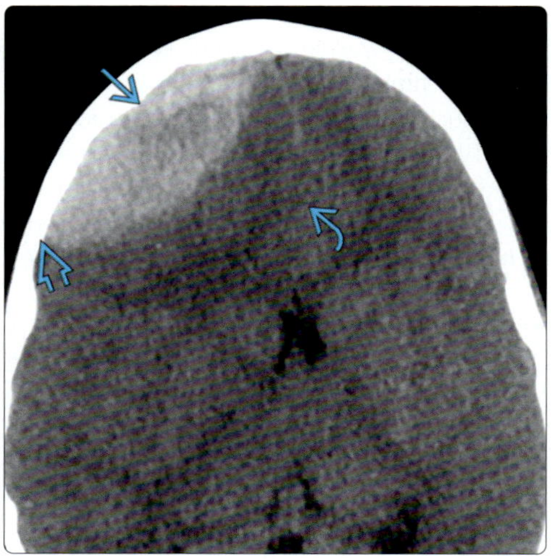

(Left) *Sagittal T2 MR in a 13 year old with an epidural empyema shows a collection with a fluid-fluid level. Restricted diffusion (not shown) was seen within the dependent material. Note the opacified paranasal sinuses, the source of the infection.* **(Right)** *Axial DWI MR in a 14 year old shows extraaxial empyemas with content that restricts diffusion. Note that the anterior lentiform epidural collection crosses the midline but is constrained by the sutures. The lateral crescentic collection was subdural in location.*

Empyema

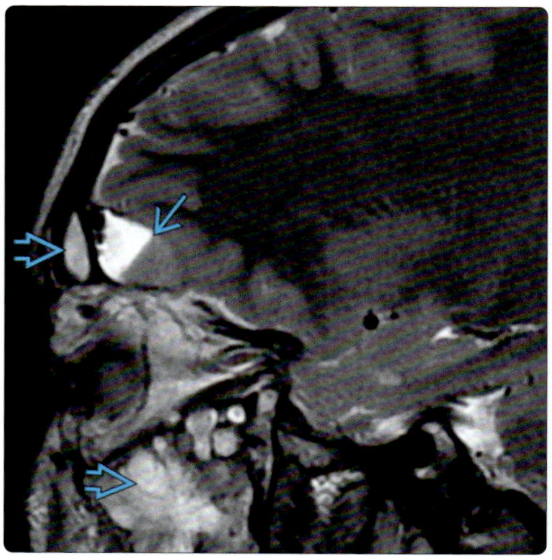

Empyema

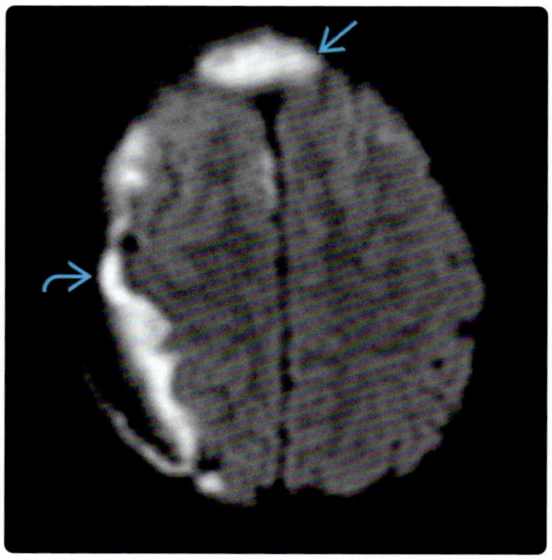

(Left) *Axial DWI MR in a 9 year old shows a "light-bulb bright" lesion in the right CP angle. This is a characteristic appearance & common location for an epidermoid cyst. The restricted diffusion is a reflection of the tightly packed squamous cells that constitute an epidermoid cyst.* **(Right)** *Axial T1 C+ MR in the same patient shows no enhancement within the lesion, typical of an epidermoid cyst.*

Epidermoid Cyst

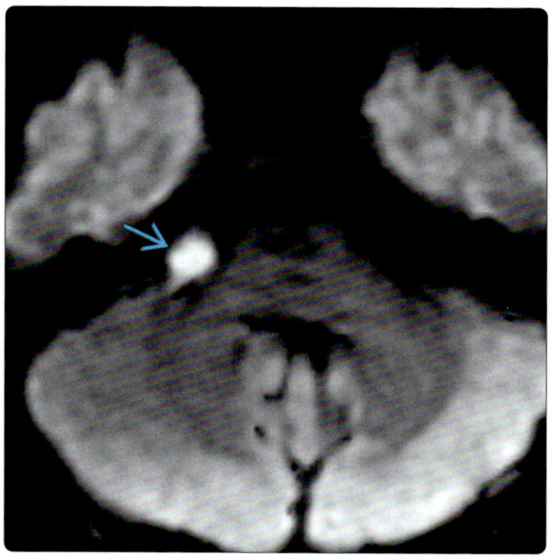

Epidermoid Cyst

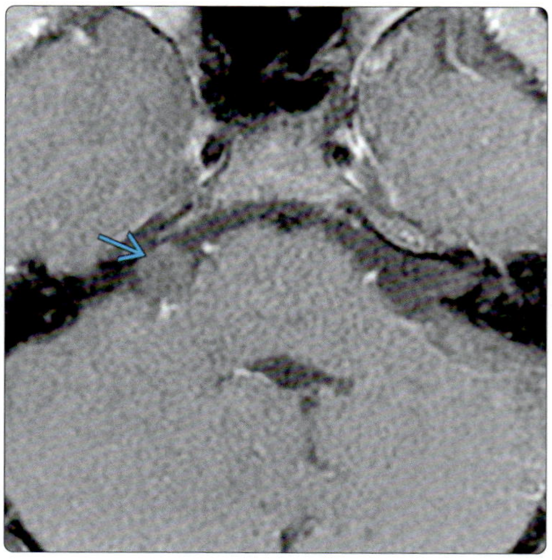

Dermoid Cyst

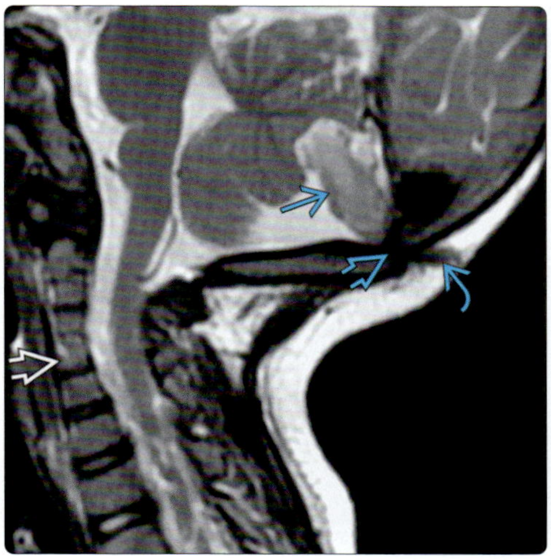

Dermoid Cyst

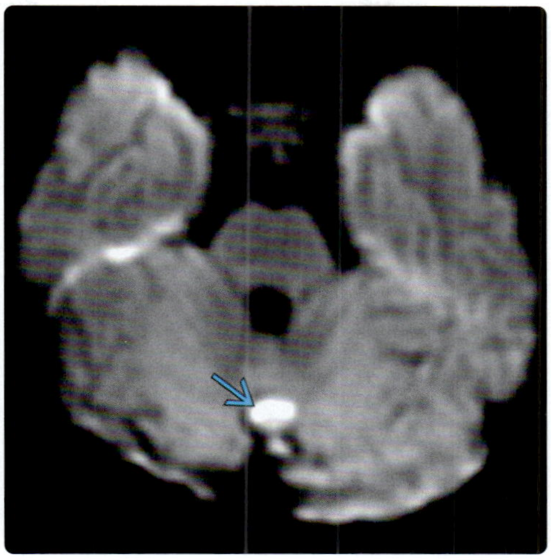

(Left) *Sagittal T2 MR in a patient with a dermoid cyst shows a midline lesion in the retrocerebellar space with an associated occipital bone defect & dermal sinus tract. Also note the multiple cervical segmentation anomalies, consistent with Klippel-Feil, a known association with dermoids.* **(Right)** *Axial DWI MR in the same patient shows diffusion restriction within the lesion. Diffusion restriction is not always present in dermoid cysts but is common due to the epidermal component of most dermoid cysts.*

Lipoma

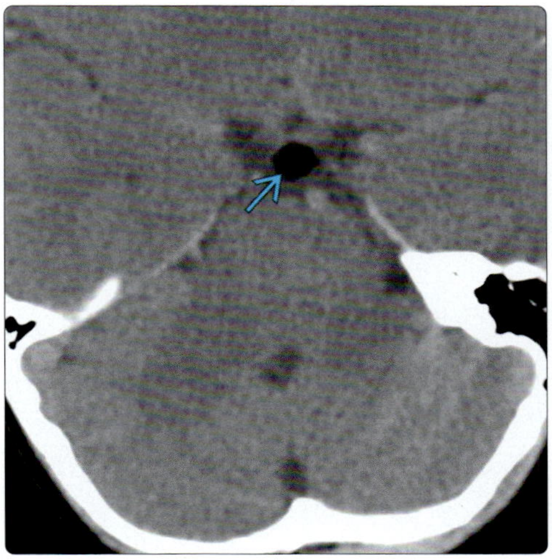

Lipoma

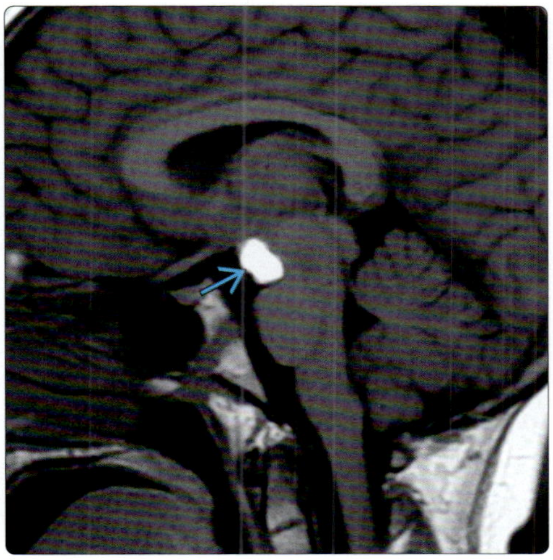

(Left) *Axial NECT in a 3 year old with an intracranial lipoma shows a midline fat-attenuation lesion centered in the suprasellar cistern just posterior to the optic chiasm.* **(Right)** *Sagittal T1 MR in a child with an intracranial lipoma shows a hyperintense lesion in the interpeduncular cistern. A T1 FS MR (not shown) demonstrated signal suppression, confirming a lipoma.*

Schwannoma

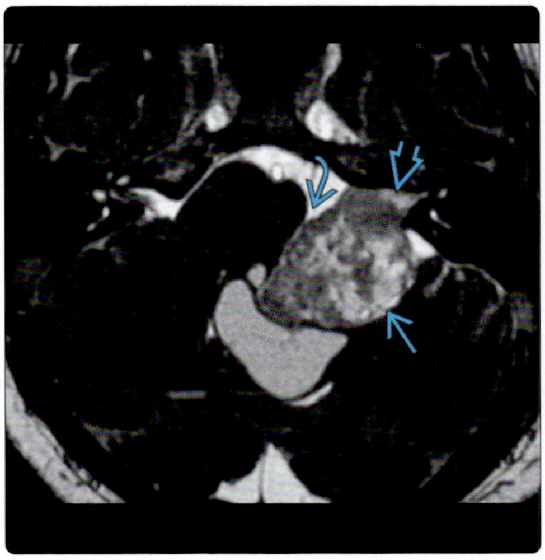

Schwannoma

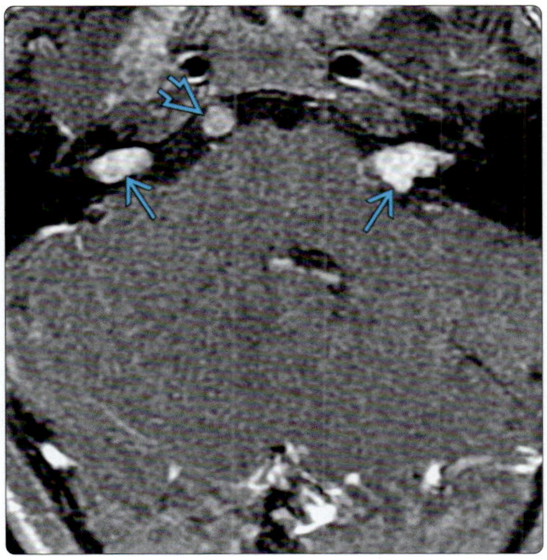

(Left) *Axial 3D FIESTA MR in a teenager with a schwannoma shows a mixed solid & cystic mass centered in the left cerebellopontine (CP) angle with involvement & expansion of the IAC. Note the acute angle between the mass & the brainstem, consistent with an extraaxial mass.* **(Right)** *Axial T1 C+ FS MR in a 10 year old with NF2 shows enhancing lesions in the bilateral IACs due to vestibular schwannomas. There is an additional cranial nerve schwannoma in the prepontine cistern.*

(Left) *Axial T1 C+ FS MR in a 6 year old with a history of radiation for a medulloblastoma shows a meningioma* → *& deformed 4th ventricle* ⇨ *from prior surgery. Meningiomas are uncommon in children & usually have an underlying risk factor, such as prior radiation or NF2.* **(Right)** *Axial T1 C+ FS MR in a 6 year old shows an enhancing lesion* → *in the right occipital periphery with a dural tail, typical of a meningioma. Also note the enhancing vestibular schwannoma* ⇨ *in the left IAC, consistent with NF2.*

Meningioma

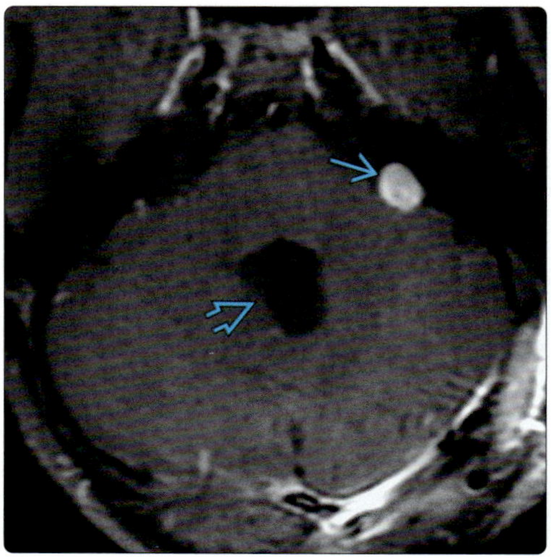

Meningioma

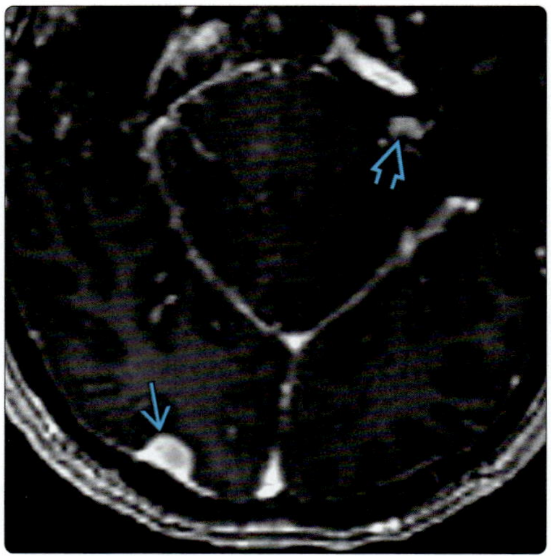

(Left) *Sagittal T2 FS MR in a child with Langerhans cell histiocytosis (LCH) shows a lytic lesion centered in the frontal bone with extradural* → *& scalp soft tissue components. Note the fluid-fluid levels* ⇨ *as well as the lack of any residual bone in the mass.* **(Right)** *Axial T1 C+ FS MR in a 9 year old with LCH shows an avidly enhancing lesion* ⇨ *centered in the calvarium with extradural extension abutting the superior sagittal sinus* →*. Enhancing soft tissue filling a well-circumscribed lytic lesion is typical of LCH.*

Langerhans Cell Histiocytosis

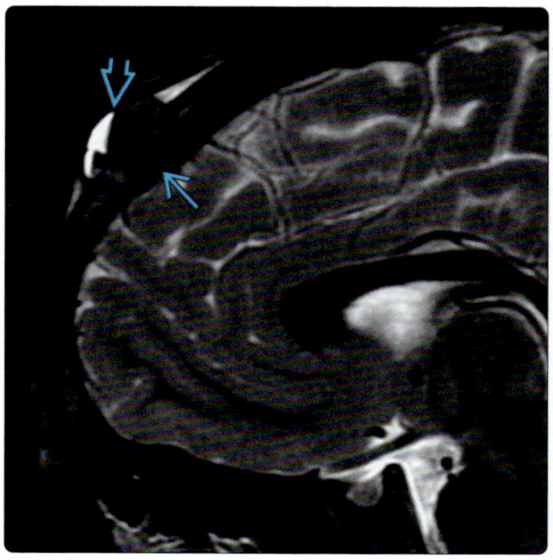

Langerhans Cell Histiocytosis

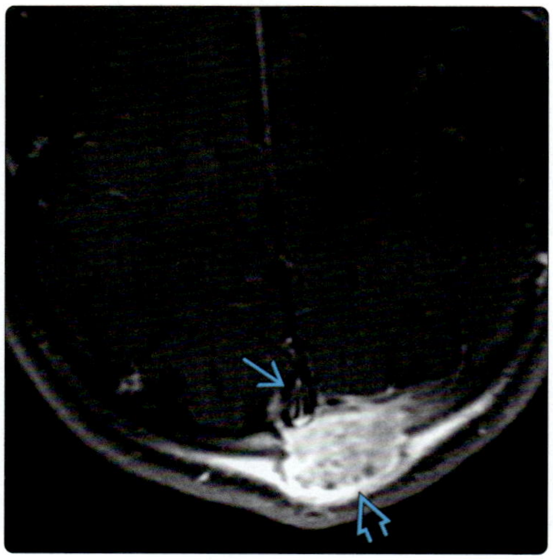

(Left) *Axial T1 C+ FS MR in a 4 month old with metastatic neuroblastoma (NB) shows enhancing lesions* → *centered in the bilateral frontal calvarium with extradural soft tissue components. The distribution & appearance are typical for metastatic NB.* **(Right)** *Coronal NECT in a 2 year old with metastatic NB shows irregular permeation* → *of the left parietal bone with spiculated bone growth* ⇨ *from the inner table of the calvarium, a common appearance for metastatic NB.*

Metastatic Neuroblastoma

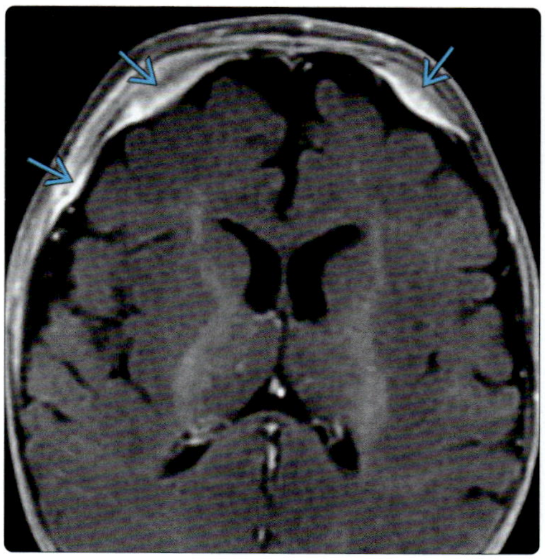

Metastatic Neuroblastoma

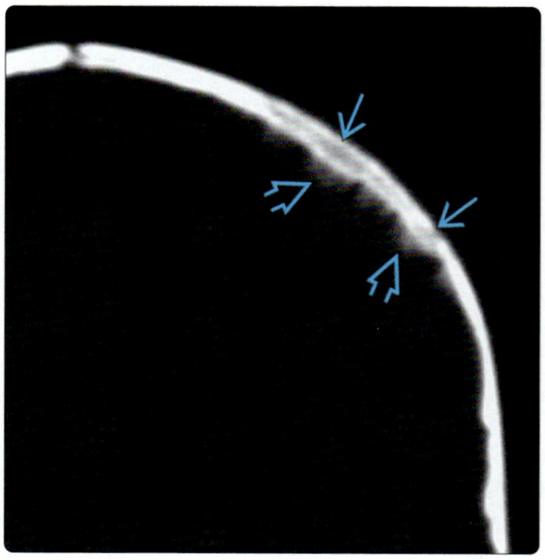

Chordoma

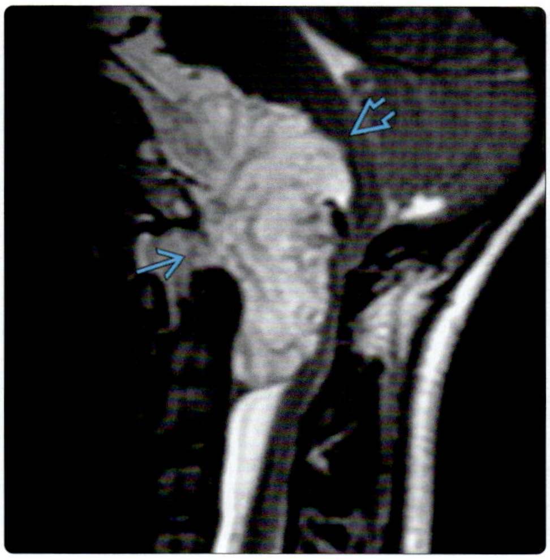

Teratoma

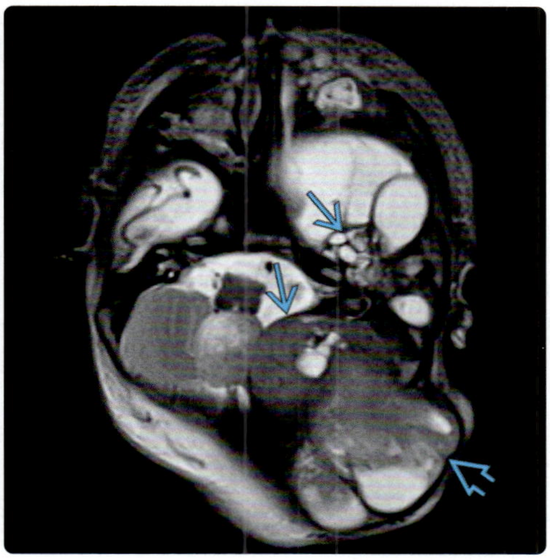

(Left) *Sagittal T2 MR in an 8 year old with a chordoma shows a large lobulated hyperintense extraaxial mass centered in the region of the clivodental interval →. Note the significant mass effect on the brainstem →.* **(Right)** *Axial T2 MR in a neonate with a congenital teratoma shows a large heterogeneous mass with both extracranial → & intracranial → components in the posterior fossa & middle fossa. Teratomas can be extracranial, intracranial, or both.*

Infantile or Congenital Hemangioma

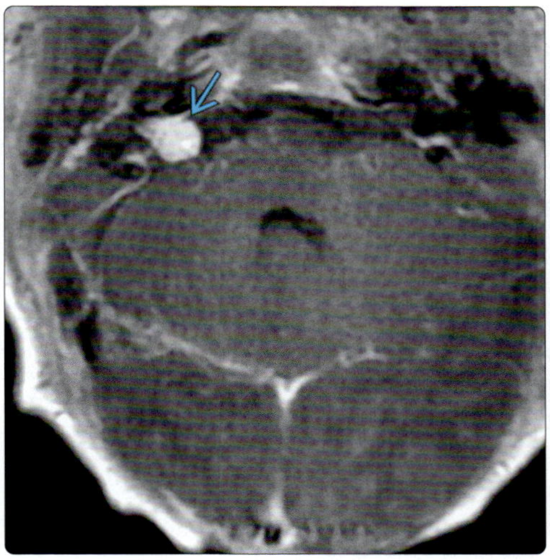

Infantile or Congenital Hemangioma

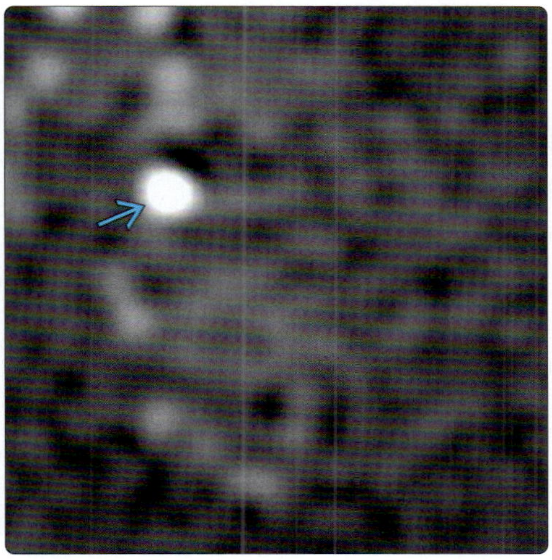

(Left) *Axial T1 C+ FS MR in a 5 week old with PHACE syndrome association shows an avidly enhancing infantile hemangioma → in the right CP angle with enhancement equal to blood pool.* **(Right)** *Axial ASL MR in the same patient shows markedly increased perfusion within the lesion →. Very pronounced increased cerebral blood flow is a characteristic finding for infantile hemangiomas in the proliferative phase. Look for associated arterial, posterior fossa, & eye abnormalities to suggest PHACES association.*

Arteriovenous Fistula

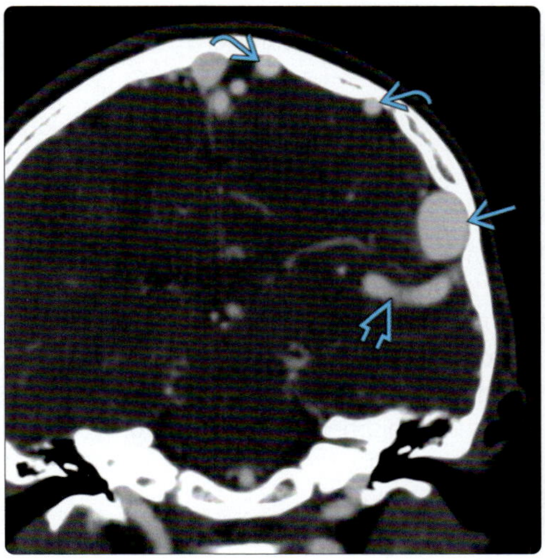

Cranial Fasciitis

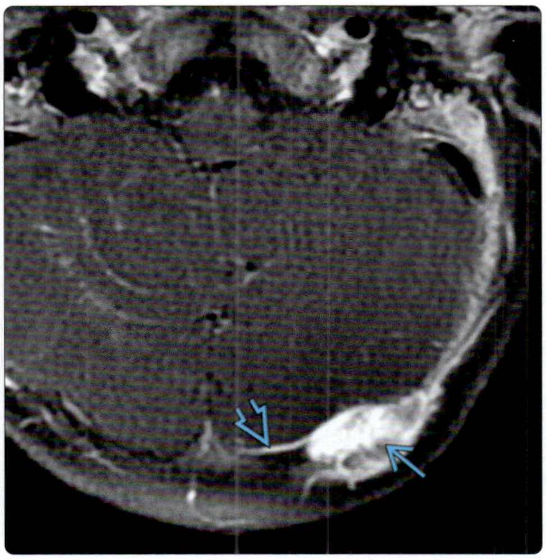

(Left) *Coronal CECT shows a large extraaxial varix → with an associated large feeding artery → & other dilated draining veins →. The findings are consistent with an arteriovenous fistula.* **(Right)** *Axial T1 C+ FS MR in a 10 month old with cranial fasciitis shows an avidly enhancing lesion → centered in the left occipital calvarium with extradural extension & associated dural thickening →. Cranial fasciitis is histologically identical to nodular fasciitis but is located in the calvarium.*

DIFFERENTIAL DIAGNOSIS

Common

- Atypical Teratoid-Rhabdoid Tumor
- Choroid Plexus Tumors (Papilloma/Carcinoma)
- Teratoma
- Supratentorial Ependymoma

Less Common

- Embryonal Tumor With Multilayered Rosettes
- Desmoplastic Infantile Tumors (Ganglioglioma/Astrocytoma)
- Medulloblastoma
- Anaplastic Astrocytoma
- Glioblastoma

Rare but Important

- Subependymal Giant Cell Astrocytoma
- Neurocutaneous Melanosis (Melanoma/Melanocytoma)
- Congenital Hemangioma
- Pineoblastoma
- Brainstem Glioma
- Medulloepithelioma
- Pilomyxoid Astrocytoma

ESSENTIAL INFORMATION

Key Differential Diagnosis Issues

- Presenting signs/symptoms
  - Most common: ↑ head circumference, bulging fontanelle, vomiting
  - Less common: Seizures, hemiparesis, cranial nerve palsy, nystagmus; congenital tumors may cause prolonged labor & difficult delivery due to large head size
- Imaging features
  - Supratentorial hemispheric tumors predominate in neonates/infants
  - Typically large, bulky, & heterogeneous
- Modality considerations
  - US: Initial imaging modality of choice in children < 6 months of age, as open anterior fontanelle creates acoustic window for brain visualization
    - Congenital tumors are often detected prenatally
  - CT: Often employed when neonates/infants present with acute neurologic signs & symptoms
    - Helpful for identification of hemorrhage & mineralization
  - MR: Modality of choice for complete neuraxis evaluation of CNS tumors in neonates/infants
    - Provides best information on tumor type & extent
      - DWI is helpful in predicting high- vs. low-grade tumor (as ↑ cellularity causes restricted diffusion)
    - Fetal MR provides excellent evaluation of CNS neoplasms initially detected on 2nd trimester US

Helpful Clues for Common Diagnoses

- **Atypical Teratoid-Rhabdoid Tumor**
  - High-grade tumor that can be intra- or extraaxial
    - Restricts diffusion due to high cellularity
    - Cysts & hemorrhage are common
    - Leptomeningeal metastasis are frequent at diagnosis
- **Choroid Plexus Tumors (Papilloma/Carcinoma)**
  - Imaging does not reliably discriminate choroid plexus papilloma (CPP) from choroid plexus carcinoma (CPCa)
  - Ventriculomegaly may result from obstruction (similar to other tumors) or CSF overproduction (unique feature)
  - CPP: Low-grade tumor; lateral > 4th > 3rd ventricles
    - NECT: Iso- to hyperdense
    - CECT/MR: Avidly enhancing with lobulated frond-like margins ± prominent internal vessel
  - CPCa: High-grade tumor arising from choroid plexus
    - More heterogeneous compared to CPP
    - Brain parenchymal invasion suggests CPCa
    - Poor prognosis: ~ 50% 5-year survival
- **Teratoma**
  - Large, heterogeneous tumor with chunky Ca^{2+}, cysts, &/or fat → fat is most discriminating finding
  - Most often midline & supratentorial; may involve multiple compartments (including extracranial components)
  - Look for associated congenital brain & face anomalies
- **Supratentorial Ependymoma**
  - Molecularly & genetically distinct from posterior fossa ependymoma
  - Large, heterogeneous solid & cystic cerebral tumor
    - Hemispheric > > intraventricular location
    - Cysts & hemorrhage are common; Ca^{2+} in ~ 50%
    - Surrounding vasogenic edema is typical

Helpful Clues for Less Common Diagnoses

- **Embryonal Tumor With Multilayered Rosettes**
  - Formerly supratentorial primitive neuroectodermal tumor
  - Large, complex hemispheric mass with diffusion restriction & little surrounding edema
    - Heterogeneous MR signal & enhancement
    - Irregular & stippled Ca^{2+} are common
    - Hemorrhage & necrosis are common
- **Desmoplastic Infantile Tumors (Ganglioglioma/Astrocytoma)**
  - Often have large cysts + elongated or nodular peripheral enhancing component with adjacent pial/dural enhancement
  - Solid components may restrict diffusion
- **Medulloblastoma**
  - ~ 90% in midline 4th ventricle; ~ 10% cerebellar hemisphere [sonic hedgehog (SHH) subtype]
  - Hypercellularity reflected on imaging
    - MR: Restricts diffusion; hypointense on T2
    - CT: Iso- to hyperdense to brain parenchyma
  - Enhancement is variable
  - Ca^{2+} & hemorrhage are uncommon
- **Anaplastic Astrocytoma**
  - Infiltrating minimally enhancing astrocytic tumor
  - Typically occurs in hemispheric white matter or bithalamic configuration
  - Ca^{2+} & hemorrhage are rare
  - Ring enhancement, hemorrhage, &/or necrosis favors glioblastoma (grade IV)
- **Glioblastoma**
  - Bulky, irregularly enhancing cellular tumor
  - Heterogeneous due to hemorrhage, necrosis, &/or cysts

- Diffusion restriction of solid components is common
- Peritumoral edema & significant mass effect are common

Helpful Clues for Rare Diagnoses

- **Subependymal Giant Cell Astrocytoma**
  - Enhancing mass near foramen of Monro
  - Found in tuberous sclerosis complex
  - Look for associated findings
    - Subependymal nodules with Ca^{2+} on SWI/GRE MR
    - Cortical/subcortical dysplastic tubers
      - T1 MR hyperintense in neonates/young infants
      - Become T1 hypointense & T2/FLAIR MR hyperintense as brain myelinates
- **Neurocutaneous Melanosis (Melanoma/Melanocytoma)**
  - Giant or multiple cutaneous melanocytic nevi
  - Parenchymal melanosis: Nonenhancing T1 MR hyperintense lesions, most often in medial temporal lobe
    - Most common finding in neurocutaneous melanosis (NCM) → good prognosis in isolation
  - Leptomeningeal melanosis/melanoma: Diffuse leptomeningeal enhancement
    - Uncommon finding in NCM: Poor prognosis
  - Parenchymal melanoma → enhancing mass
    - Rare finding in NCM → poor prognosis
- **Congenital Hemangioma**
  - Extraaxial mass, often extending through calvarium
  - Proliferation completed by birth; may rarely enlarge due to hemorrhage
  - Can be quite heterogeneous on imaging with variable internal vascularity
  - Rapidly involuting congenital hematoma (RICH) subtype regresses over 12-14 months
  - Partially involuting congenital hematoma (PICH) & noninvoluting congenital hematoma (NICH) subtypes cannot be differentiated from RICH by initial imaging
- **Pineoblastoma**
  - High-grade malignant pineal region mass
    - Usually scattered "exploded" Ca^{2+}, ± small cysts
    - Restricted diffusion due to high cellularity
  - Invades adjacent structures
    - Corpus callosum, thalamus, midbrain, vermis
- **Brainstem Glioma**
  - Prognosis depends on location, imaging appearance, & tumor type
  - Nonenhancing tectal plate mass
    - Typically pilocytic astrocytoma
    - Clinically indolent course (but may cause obstructive hydrocephalus)
  - Enhancing midbrain or medulla mass
    - Often exophytic with cystic component
    - Usually low-grade astrocytic tumor (e.g., pilocytic astrocytoma)
    - Intermediate clinical course depending on resectability
  - Diffuse intrinsic pontine glioma (DIPG)
    - Diffusely infiltrating glial neoplasm (usually of higher grades)
    - Poorly defined mass expanding pons with no/minimal enhancement
    - Poor prognosis
- **Medulloepithelioma**
  - Rare malignant embryonal brain tumor
  - Young children (< 5 years of age)
  - Histologic differentiation varies
    - Neuronal, astrocytic, ependymal, melanotic, etc.
  - Imaging appearance reflects variable differentiation
- **Pilomyxoid Astrocytoma**
  - Grade II myxoid variant of pilocytic astrocytoma
  - Most commonly occurs in infants & young children
  - Hypothalamus > cerebral hemispheres > cerebellum/brainstem
  - CSF dissemination is common

SELECTED REFERENCES

1. Shekdar KV et al: Brain tumors in the neonate. Neuroimaging Clin N Am. 27(1):69-83, 2017
2. Ghodsi SM et al: Brain tumors in infants. J Pediatr Neurosci. 10(4):335-40, 2015
3. Severino M et al: Congenital tumors of the central nervous system. Neuroradiology. 52(6):531-48, 2010

Atypical Teratoid-Rhabdoid Tumor

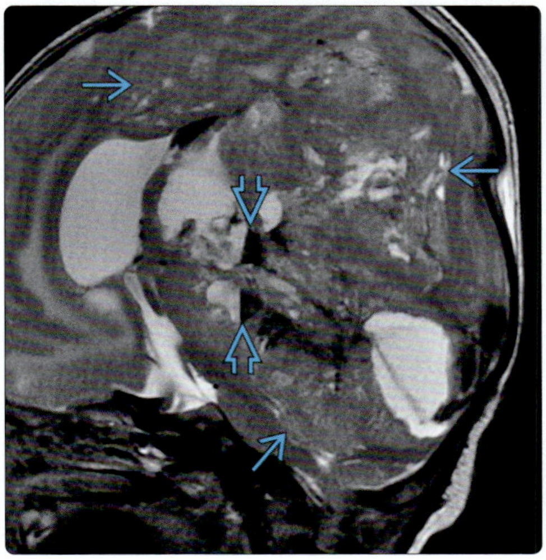

Atypical Teratoid-Rhabdoid Tumor

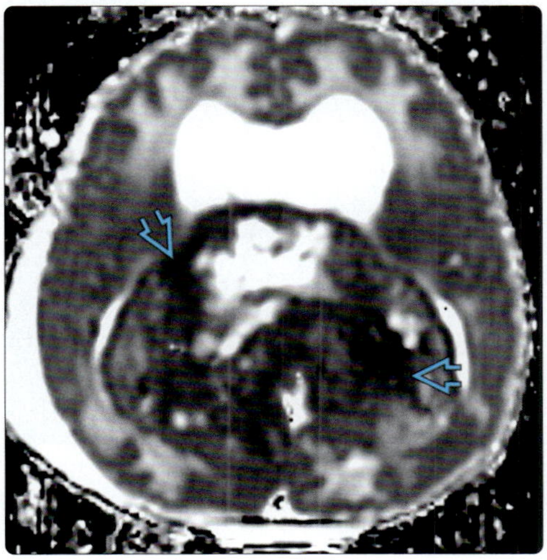

(Left) *Axial T2 MR in a 4 week old with a congenital atypical teratoid-rhabdoid tumor (ATRT) shows a large heterogeneous supra- & infratentorial mass ➡. Note the multiple cystic/necrotic foci with fluid levels ➡ due to hemorrhage. In the case of a cellular, cystic, & hemorrhagic CNS mass in a young child, ATRT should lead the DDx.* **(Right)** *Axial ADC MR (same patient) shows regions of ↓ ADC signal ➡ in the mass consistent with restricted diffusion & high cellularity. This suggests a high-grade tumor, such as ATRT.*

(Left) *Axial T1 C+ MR in a 7 month old shows a lobulated & avidly enhancing choroid plexus papilloma (in contrast to the normal right choroid plexus). Note the frond-like margins of the mass & associated ventriculomegaly typical for a choroid plexus papilloma.* **(Right)** *Axial T1 C+ MR in this 9 month old with a choroid plexus carcinoma shows a large, bulky, avidly enhancing left intraventricular tumor with invasion of the overlying brain. There are multiple intraventricular metastases.*

Choroid Plexus Tumors (Papilloma/Carcinoma)

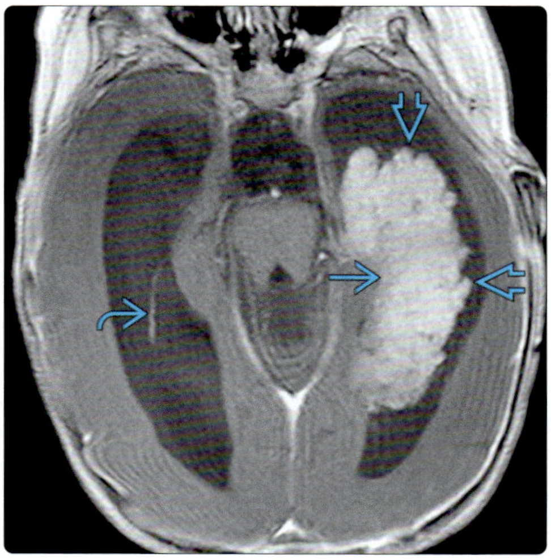

Choroid Plexus Tumors (Papilloma/Carcinoma)

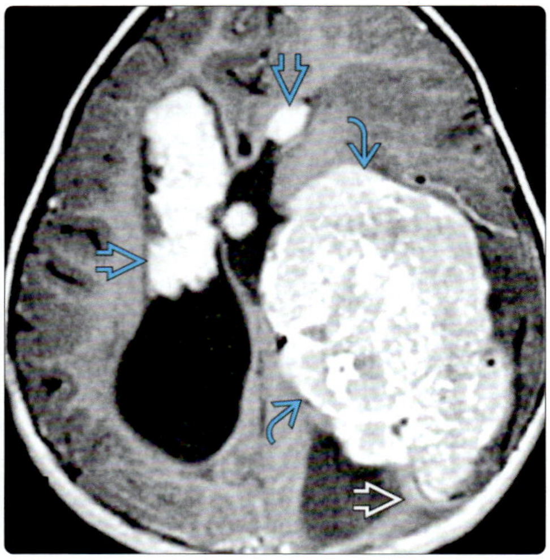

(Left) *Midline sagittal NECT in a 7 week old with an immature teratoma shows a large solid mass centered in the suprasellar region with scattered Ca^{2+}. Teratoma should be the primary consideration for a congenital midline mass with Ca^{2+}.* **(Right)** *Coronal SSFSE T2 MR in a 34-week fetus with a teratoma shows a predominantly solid mass with few cysts. The mass has both intracranial & extracranial components, a relatively unique feature of teratoma.*

Teratoma

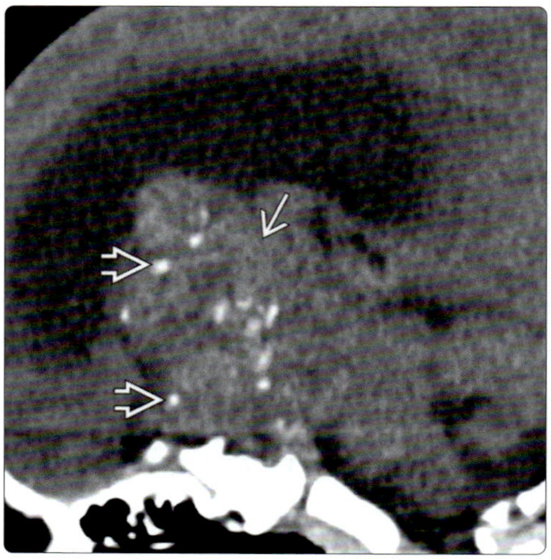

Teratoma

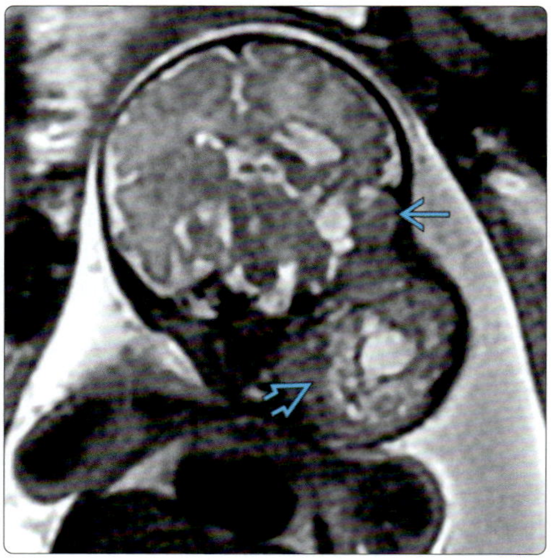

(Left) *Coronal T2 MR in a 10 month old with new-onset seizures & an atypical high-grade supratentorial ependymoma shows a mixed solid & cystic mass centered in the periphery of the cerebral hemisphere. The solid components are isointense to gray matter, suggesting high cellularity.* **(Right)** *Axial SWI MR in the same patient shows areas of signal hypointensity within the left parietal lobe, suggesting either Ca^{2+} or hemorrhage, both of which are common features of supratentorial ependymoma.*

Supratentorial Ependymoma

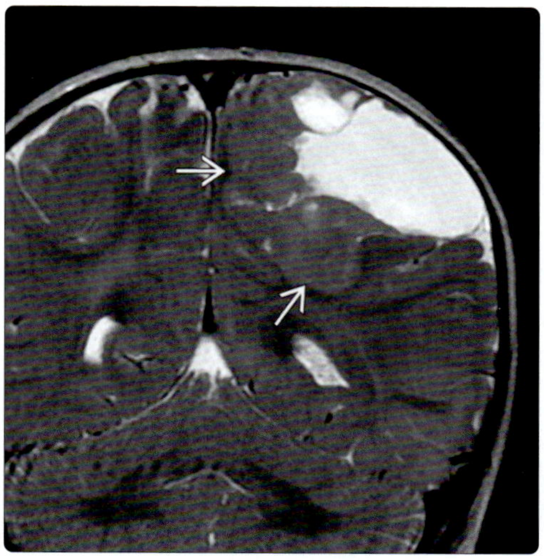

Supratentorial Ependymoma

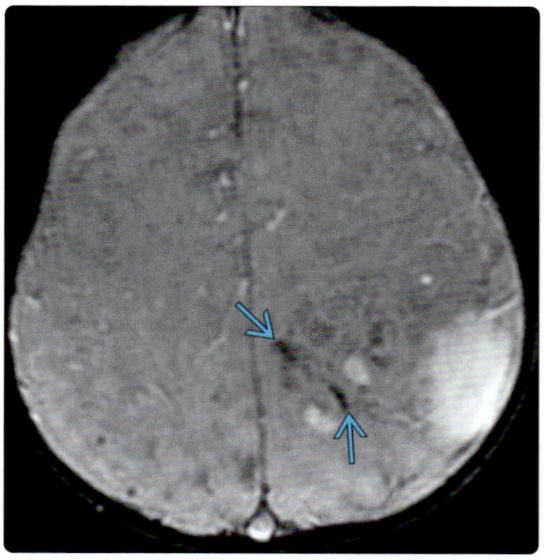

Embryonal Tumor With Multilayered Rosettes

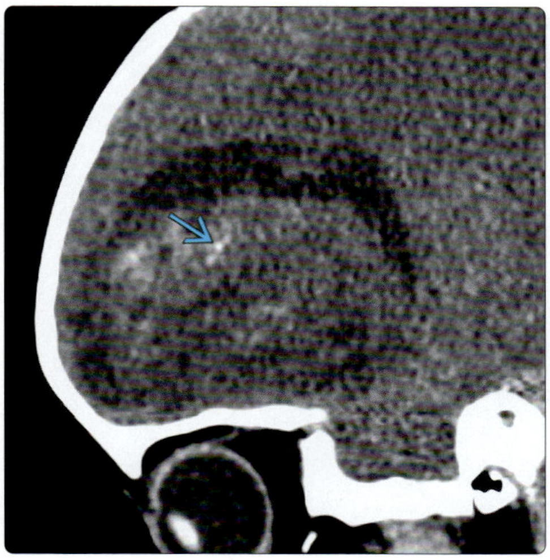

Embryonal Tumor With Multilayered Rosettes

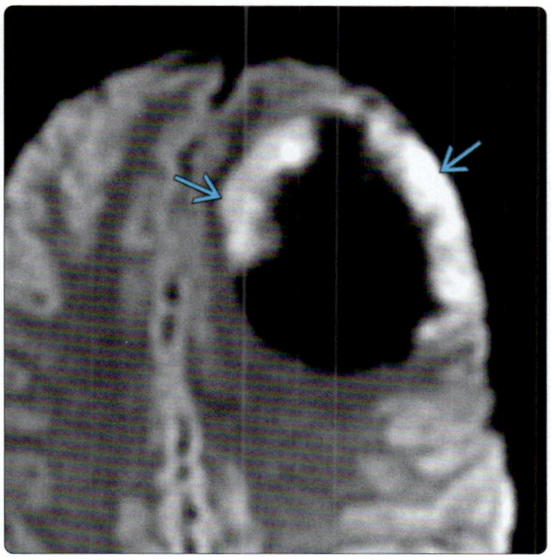

(Left) *Parasagittal NECT in a 1 year old with embryonal tumor with multilayered rosettes (ETMR) shows a large heterogeneous mass with scattered Ca^{2+} →. While nonspecific, Ca^{2+} & dense soft tissue components are frequently seen in ETMR.* **(Right)** *Axial DWI MR in a patient with ETMR shows a mixed solid & cystic lesion in the left frontal lobe. The solid portions → show diffusion restriction consistent with a highly cellular tumor. ETMR should be in the DDx of any highly cellular neonatal tumor.*

Desmoplastic Infantile Tumors (Ganglioglioma/Astrocytoma)

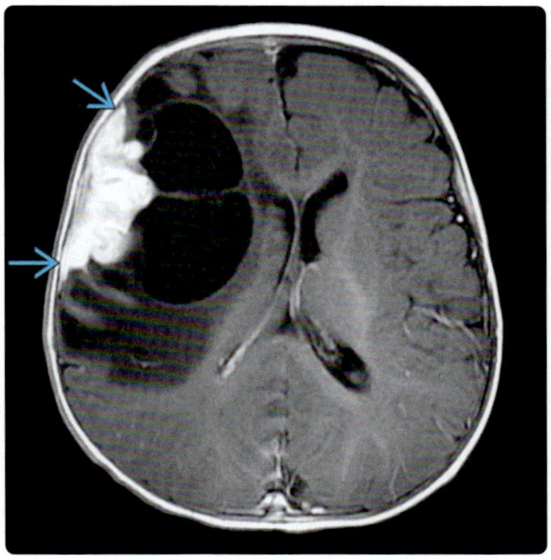

Desmoplastic Infantile Tumors (Ganglioglioma/Astrocytoma)

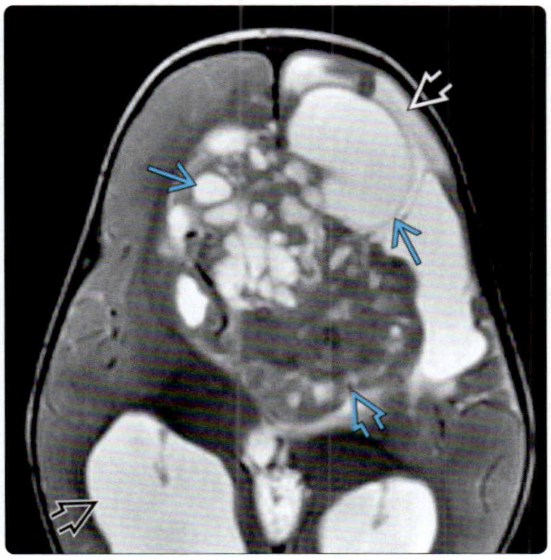

(Left) *Axial T1 C+ MR in a 5 month old with a desmoplastic infantile ganglioglioma (DIG) shows a peripheral mixed solid & cystic mass with an elongated enhancing superficial component →. The broad base of the enhancing component is typical of DIG.* **(Right)** *Axial T2 MR in a 1 year old with DIG shows a large mass ⇒ with numerous cysts → of varying sizes centered in the deep anterior cranial fossa. There is associated peritumoral edema ➡ & lateral ventricular obstruction ⇨.*

Medulloblastoma

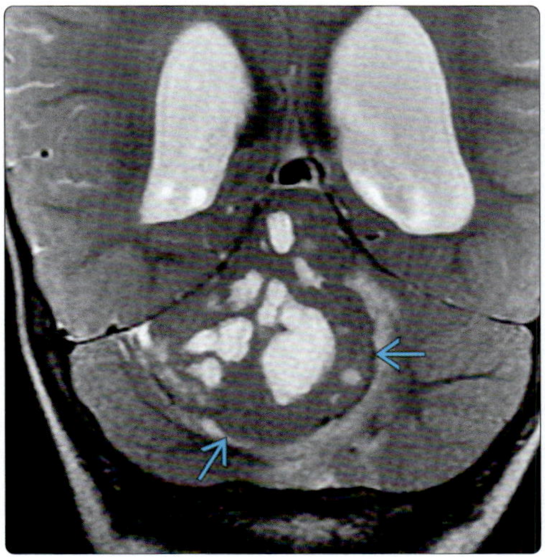

Medulloblastoma

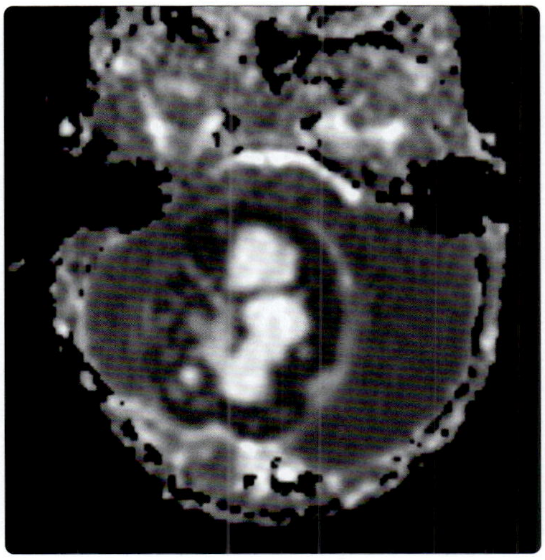

(Left) *Coronal T2 MR in a 14 month old with medulloblastoma (MB) shows a mixed solid & cystic lesion centered in the right cerebellar hemisphere. The relatively dark signal of solid components → is typical of MB, & the hemispheric location suggests the sonic hedgehog (SHH) molecular subtype.* **(Right)** *Axial ADC map MR in the same patient shows hypointense signal of diffusion restriction from the increased cellularity of this tumor. The primary considerations would include MB & ATRT.*

(Left) *Coronal CECT in this 7 month old with anaplastic astrocytoma shows obstructive hydrocephalus & a large, ill-defined midline mass with ring enhancement & central necrosis.* **(Right)** *Coronal T2 MR in the same patient shows the ill-defined margins of the mass, a characteristic appearance for infiltrating high-grade gliomas. Bithalamic & upper midbrain extension is typical for infiltrating gliomas, often causing obstructive hydrocephalus.*

Anaplastic Astrocytoma

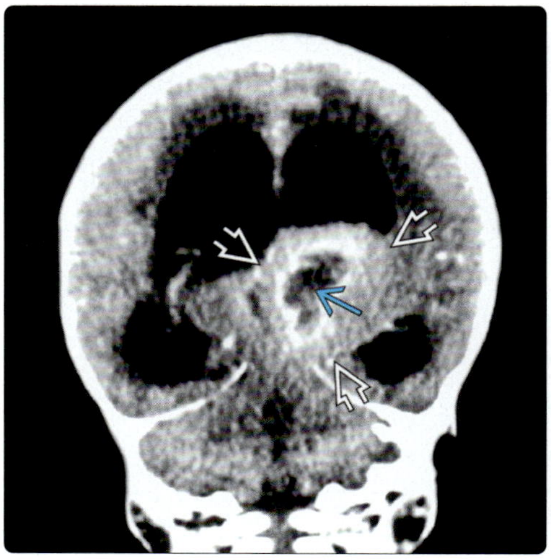

Anaplastic Astrocytoma

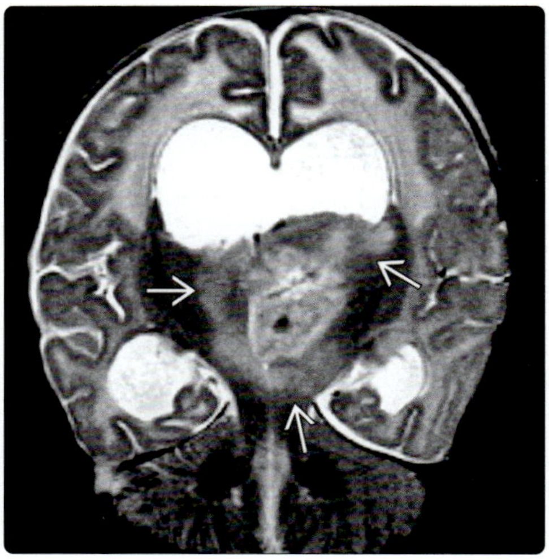

(Left) *Axial T2* GRE MR in a neonate with glioblastoma shows a large mass in the left cerebral hemisphere with multiple foci of decreased signal, suggesting blood products. Glioblastoma should be in the DDx for any large hemorrhagic neonatal CNS tumor.* **(Right)** *Longitudinal US shows a bulky subependymal giant cell astrocytoma at the foramen of Monro in this newborn with tuberous sclerosis complex. Foci of increased echogenicity in the cortex & subcortical white matter are consistent with tubers.*

Glioblastoma

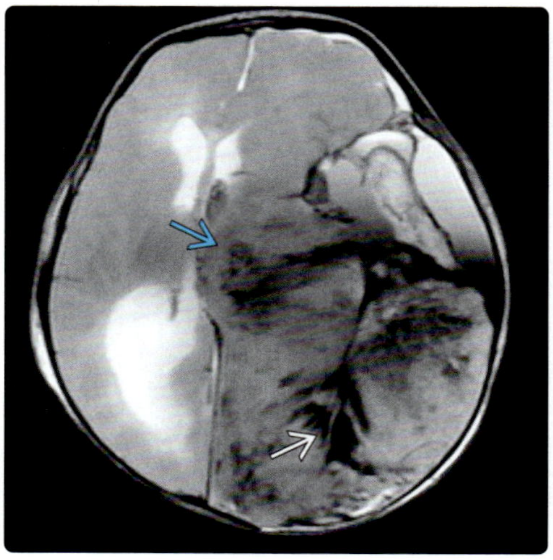

Subependymal Giant Cell Astrocytoma

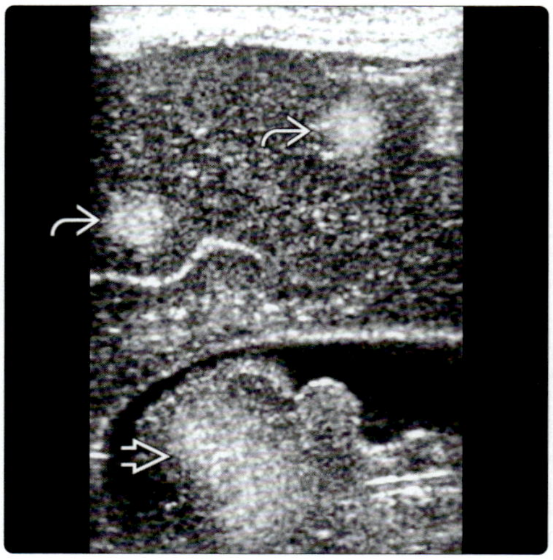

(Left) *Axial T1 MR in a 4 day old with a melanocytic nevus shows a T1-hyperintense lesion in the right amygdala region without significant mass effect. This is the most common location for isolated parenchymal melanosis. Such lesions are typically asymptomatic &, except in rare cases, stable over time.* **(Right)** *Coronal T1 C+ MR in another infant with neurocutaneous melanosis shows diffuse, smooth, thick leptomeningeal involvement, which is uncommon & portends a poor prognosis.*

Neurocutaneous Melanosis (Melanoma/Melanocytoma)

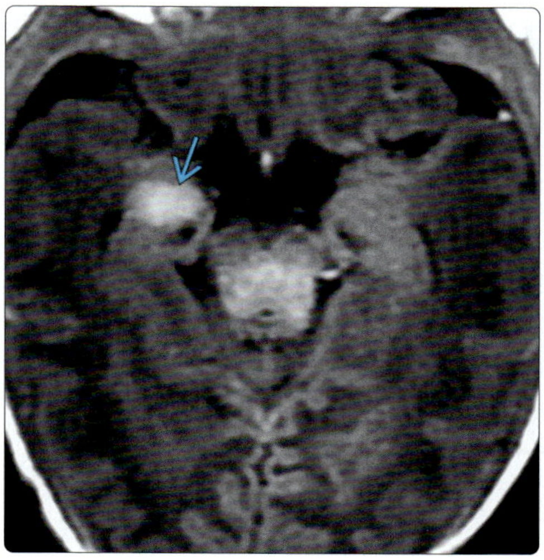

Neurocutaneous Melanosis (Melanoma/Melanocytoma)

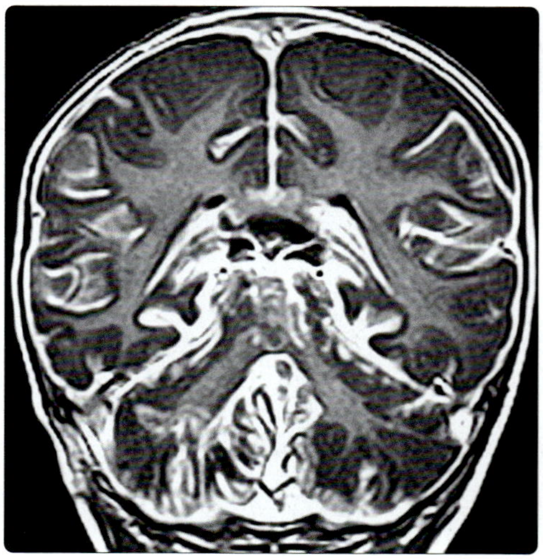

Congenital Hemangioma

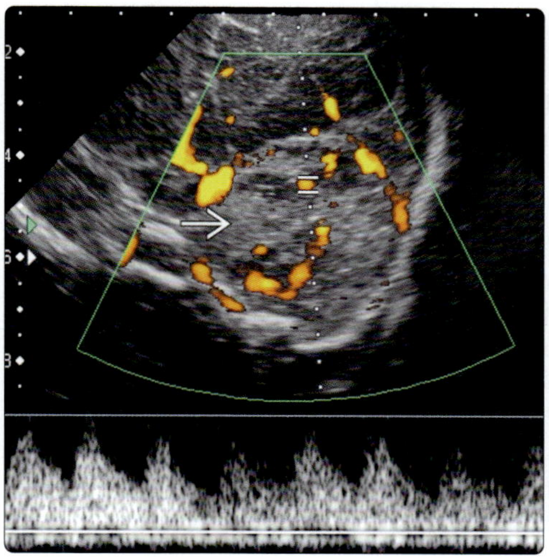

Congenital Hemangioma

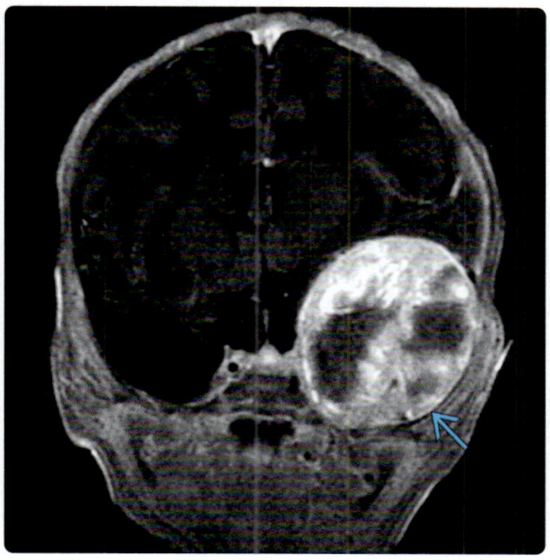

(Left) *Coronal Doppler US in a newborn with a congenital hemangioma demonstrates low-resistance arterial waveforms in this echogenic middle cranial fossa mass* ➡. *The patient also had an overlying cutaneous vascular lesion.* **(Right)** *Coronal T1 C+ FS MR in the same patient shows heterogeneous enhancement of the extraaxial mass* ⇨. *Given the cutaneous & imaging findings, the patient was treated conservatively, & the mass rapidly involuted over 8 months with near-complete resolution.*

Pineoblastoma

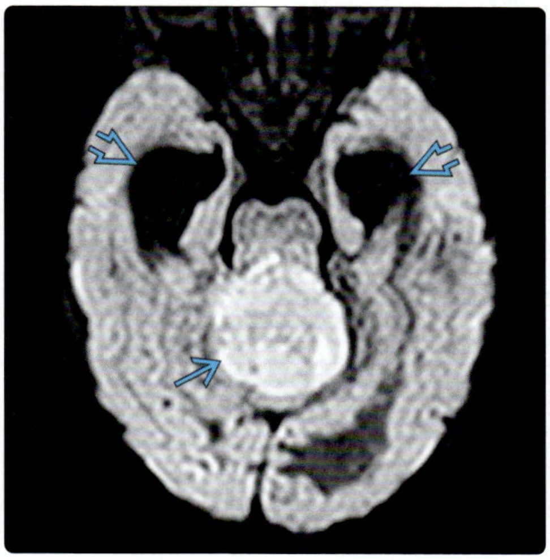

Brainstem Glioma

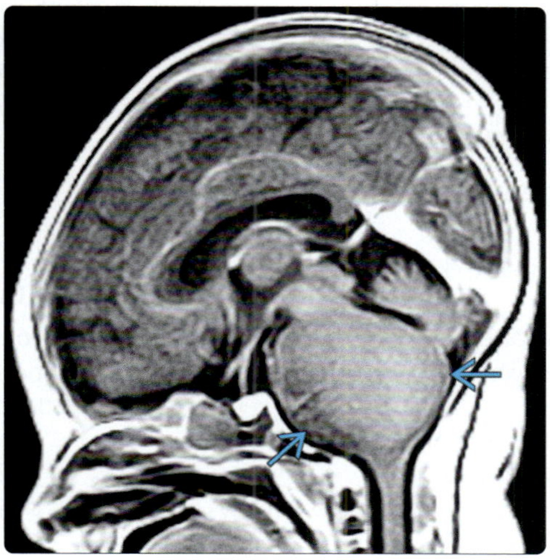

(Left) *Axial DWI MR in a 7 month old with pineoblastoma demonstrates a mass centered in the region of the pineal gland with marked diffusion restriction* ⇨ *typical of this high-grade tumor. Mass effect on the cerebral aqueduct led to obstructive hydrocephalus* ⇨ *& macrocephaly.* **(Right)** *Sagittal T1 C+ MR in a newborn with a diffuse intrinsic pontine glioma (DIPG) shows a nonenhancing mass* ⇨ *causing massive expansion of the pons & medulla.*

Medulloepithelioma

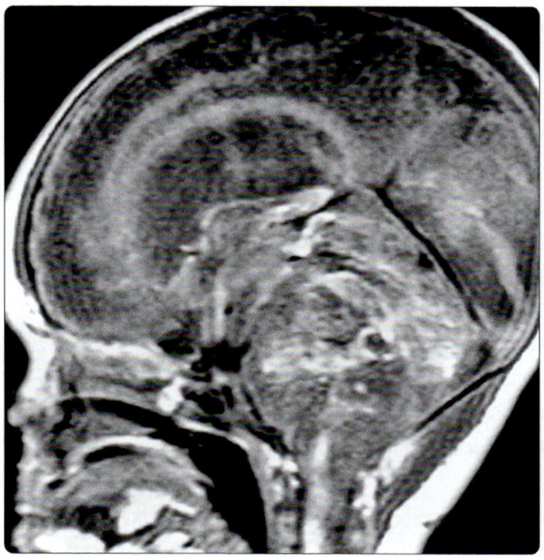

Pilomyxoid Astrocytoma

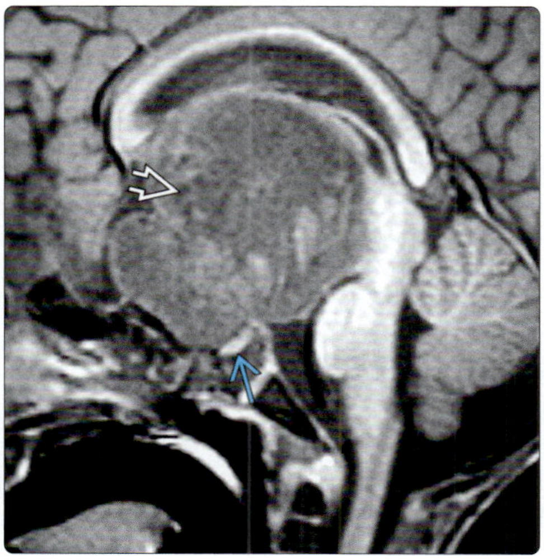

(Left) *Sagittal T1 MR in a neonate with medulloepithelioma shows a large hemorrhagic tumor replacing & expanding the brainstem, cerebellum, & upper cervical cord with upward transtentorial herniation.* **(Right)** *Sagittal T1 MR in a 9 month old with a pilomyxoid astrocytoma (PMA) shows a large hypothalamic mass* ➡ *that is separate from the pituitary* ⇨. *This is the most common location for PMA. PMA is a grade II variant of pilocytic astrocytoma that often occurs in younger patients.*

DIFFERENTIAL DIAGNOSIS

Common

- Cerebritis/Encephalitis
- Ischemia/Infarct

Less Common

- Tuberous Sclerosis Complex
- Focal Cortical Dysplasia
- Polymicrogyria
- Pachygyria
- Lissencephaly
- Hemimegalencephaly
- Cortically Based Neoplasms
  - DNET
  - Ganglioglioma
  - Angiocentric Glioma
  - Dysplastic Cerebellar Gangliocytoma

Rare but Important

- Hypomyelination (Pseudothick Cortex)
- Glioblastoma
- Gliomatosis Cerebri
- Meningioangiomatosis

ESSENTIAL INFORMATION

Key Differential Diagnosis Issues

- Clinical features to consider
  - Age: Infants may have pseudothickening due to incomplete myelination
  - Common presentation: Seizure
    - Correlation with EEG may help localize subtle cortical abnormalities
  - Tuberous sclerosis: Look for facial angiofibromas, forehead plaques, & shagreen patches
  - Polymicrogyria: Consider with congenital CMV & many genetic syndromes
- Imaging features to consider
  - Location
    - Focal: Focal cortical dysplasia (FCD), tumor, infarct
    - Bilateral/symmetric: Malformation of cortical development, encephalitis
  - CT: Associated Ca^{2+} suggests tumor or cortical tuber
  - MR: Best exam
    - DWI is critical for excluding acute abnormality
      - Infarct, MELAS, infection
    - T1/T2/FLAIR: Most malformations of cortical development follow gray matter (GM) signal
      - Tumors, infection, & ischemia typically are T2/FLAIR hyperintense & T1 hypointense to GM
    - T1 C+: Enhancement excludes cortical malformation & suggests tumor or acute process
- Imaging modality considerations
  - US may be 1st line in neonates/infants but is insensitive
  - CT is often used initially with acute presentation but is insensitive
  - MR is most sensitive for cortical abnormalities
    - Volumetric 3D T1 has excellent GM-white matter (WM) differentiation for detection of cortical thickening
    - 3D T2 FLAIR is helpful for detection of FCD
    - 3T is superior to 1.5T in detection of subtle FCD
  - PET & SPECT may be used to help identify subtle seizure focus

Helpful Clues for Common Diagnoses

- **Cerebritis/Encephalitis**
  - Cerebritis: Usually secondary to bacterial meningitis &/or subdural empyema
    - Predictable imaging evolution through stages of poorly defined cerebritis to well-defined abscess
  - Encephalitis: Usually viral or post viral [enterovirus, Epstein-Barr virus (EBV), human herpesvirus (HHV), influenza, herpes, etc.]; etiology not found in ~ 50%
    - Thickened hyperintense cortex on T2 & FLAIR
      - Loss of GM-WM distinction with restricted diffusion
      - ± enhancement or hemorrhage
    - Herpes: Usually manifests 2-5 weeks after birth
      - Cingulate gyrus, subfrontal cortex involvement is less common than older children or adults
      - Often bilateral, asymmetric
- **Ischemia/Infarct**
  - Global insult → watershed cortex; focal → arterial territory
  - Acute/subacute: Cortical swelling, loss of GM-WM distinction
  - Acute & early subacute: ↑ DWI/↓ ADC
  - Subacute: ± contrast enhancement
  - Chronic: Cortical volume loss with ↑ T2/FLAIR

Helpful Clues for Less Common Diagnoses

- **Tuberous Sclerosis Complex**
  - Tubers: Dysplastic cortical/subcortical lesions present from birth
    - Broad, thickened gyri with blurred GM-WM junction & T2/FLAIR hyperintense subcortical signal
      - Subcortical foci are often T1 hyperintense prior to brain myelination
    - Rarely can be calcified & involve entire mantle
  - Linear WM signal abnormalities (migration lines) & subependymal nodules are typical
- **Focal Cortical Dysplasia**
  - Focal malformation of cortical development
  - Type 2 is much more likely to have imaging abnormalities
    - Thickened cortex, often with subtle ↑ T2/FLAIR signal
      - May show ↑ T1 in unmyelinated brain
    - Blurred GM-WM junction
    - "Tail" of signal abnormality pointing towards ventricle
- **Polymicrogyria**
  - Associated with congenital CMV & many genetic syndromes
  - Numerous tiny gyri with shallow sulci
  - Nodular pial surface with irregular GM-WM junction
  - Density/signal intensity of affected cortex = GM
- **Pachygyria**
  - Thickened, dysplastic cortex (sometimes called incomplete lissencephaly)
  - Smooth pial surface & GM-WM junction differentiates from polymicrogyria
  - Affected areas usually have shallow or simplified gyral pattern

- **Lissencephaly**
  - Most severe form results in smooth brain (agyria)
  - 3 layers (outer to inner) on T2: Thin peripheral cellular (~ GM), thin cell sparse (↑ T2), & thick deep cellular (~ GM)
  - Hourglass configuration with shallow sylvian fissures in severe cases
  - May be associated with Miller-Dieker syndrome (*LIS1* mutation)
- **Hemimegalencephaly**
  - Hamartomatous overgrowth of hemisphere or portion
  - Enlarged hemisphere with thickened, often dysplastic cortex
  - Ipsilateral ventricle often enlarged & abnormally shaped
  - Abnormal WM signal intensity (↑ T1 in infants, ↑ T2 in older patients)
- **Cortically Based Neoplasms**
  - **DNET**
    - Epileptogenic cortically based mass in young patient
    - Well-demarcated, wedge-shaped, & cystic
    - Temporal lobe in > 50% but may occur in any cortex
    - Most have small cysts; minority are solid
    - Usually minimal mass effect given size
    - Often associated with adjacent cortical dysplasia
  - **Ganglioglioma**
    - Epileptogenic cortically based mass in child/young adult
    - Majority in temporal lobe but may occur anywhere
    - May be solid, solid with small cysts, or large cyst with mural nodule
    - ~ 25-50% have Ca^{2+}
    - ~ 50% show enhancement
  - **Angiocentric Glioma**
    - Low-grade cortically based epileptogenic tumor
    - Mimics imaging characteristics of FCD & tubers in tuberous sclerosis complex (TSC)
  - **Dysplastic Cerebellar Gangliocytoma**
    - Thickening & overgrowth of cerebellar folia
    - Gyriform layered or striated pattern
    - Can cause significant mass effect
    - Cowden-Lhermitte-Duclos (COLD) syndrome
      - Associated with *PTEN* mutation
      - Long-term cancer screening (breast, thyroid)

Helpful Clues for Rare Diagnoses

- **Hypomyelination (Pseudothick Cortex)**
  - Diminished/absent WM myelination for age
  - Lack of peripheral "arborization" blurs cortical-subcortical junction against otherwise extensive abnormal WM signal
- **Glioblastoma**
  - Infiltrative WHO grade IV tumor affecting WM > GM
  - Tumor infiltrates cortex with subpial extension
  - Hemorrhage, enhancement are common
  - Primary (older patient): 95% necrotic with thick irregular enhancing rim
  - Secondary (younger patient): Enhancing focus within lower grade tumor
- **Gliomatosis Cerebri**
  - Most are infiltrating WHO grade II or III diffuse astrocytomas
  - Tumor infiltrates but preserves underlying brain architecture of ≥ 3 lobes
    - T2-hyperintense expansion of cerebrum & basal ganglia
  - MRS shows elevated myoinositol (mI)
- **Meningioangiomatosis**
  - Perivascular proliferation of vessels in meninges & cortex → cortical mass with variable Ca^{2+}
  - Linear &/or gyriform enhancement
  - May infiltrate perivascular spaces, cause mass effect

SELECTED REFERENCES

1. Desikan RS et al: Malformations of cortical development. Ann Neurol. 80(6):797-810, 2016
2. Colombo N et al: Focal cortical dysplasia type IIa and IIb: MRI aspects in 118 cases proven by histopathology. Neuroradiology. 54(10):1065-77, 2012

Cerebritis/Encephalitis

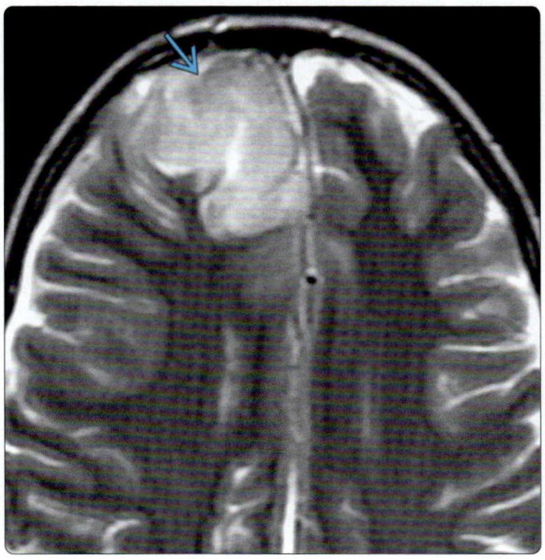

Cerebritis/Encephalitis

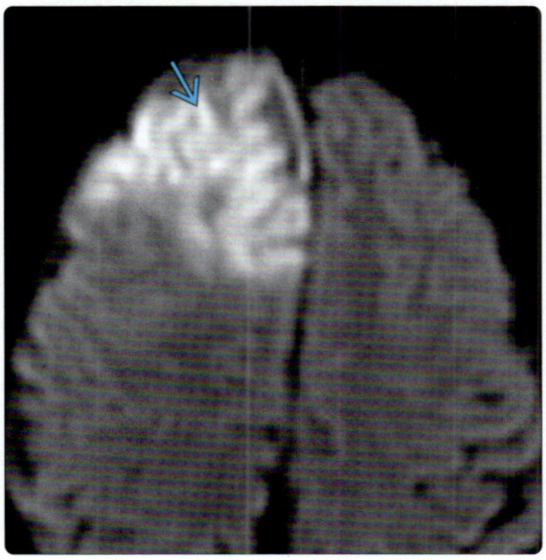

(Left) *Axial T2 MR in a 12 year old with right frontal cerebritis from group A Streptococcus shows focal cortical thickening & increased signal intensity* ⇒ *with loss of the normal gray matter (GM)-white matter (WM) junction.* **(Right)** *Axial DWI MR in the same patient shows diffusion restriction in the right frontal lobe* ⇒*, suggesting an acute process such as infection or infarction. The unilateral distribution that crosses arterial territories raises the possibility of infection/inflammation rather than an arterial infarct.*

(Left) *Axial T2 MR in a 4 week old with neonatal herpes encephalitis shows swelling of the right temporal lobe* → *with loss of GM-WM differentiation, a common location & appearance for herpes encephalitis.* **(Right)** *Axial DWI MR in the same patient shows diffusion restriction in the right temporal lobe. DWI is the most sensitive sequence for detection of early involvement by herpes encephalitis. Conventional sequences can remain normal for days after the onset of symptoms.*

Cerebritis/Encephalitis

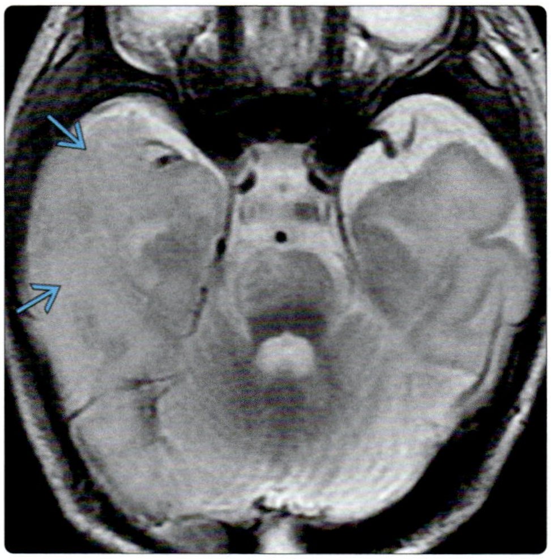

Cerebritis/Encephalitis

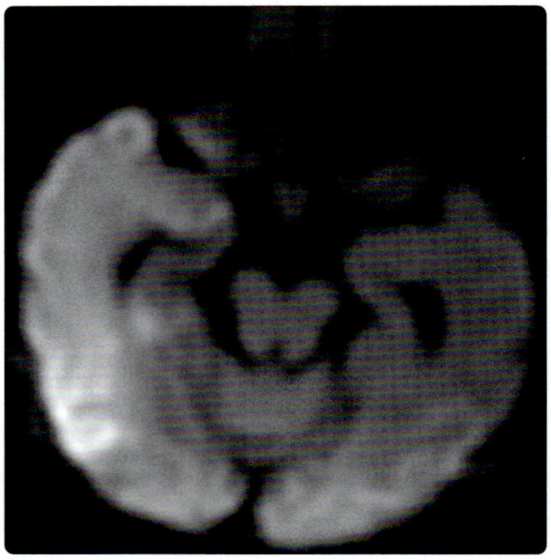

(Left) *Axial T2 MR in a 4 day old with seizures due to a perinatal arterial ischemic stroke (PAIS) shows swelling* → *of the entire left middle cerebral artery (MCA) territory with loss of GM-WM differentiation as well as signal abnormality within the deep gray nuclei* ⇨*.* **(Right)** *Axial DWI MR in the same patient shows diffusion restriction of the left MCA territory & deep gray nuclei, consistent with acute/subacute infarction. Note signal changes in corpus callosum* ➡*, consistent with secondary neuronal injury.*

Ischemia/Infarct

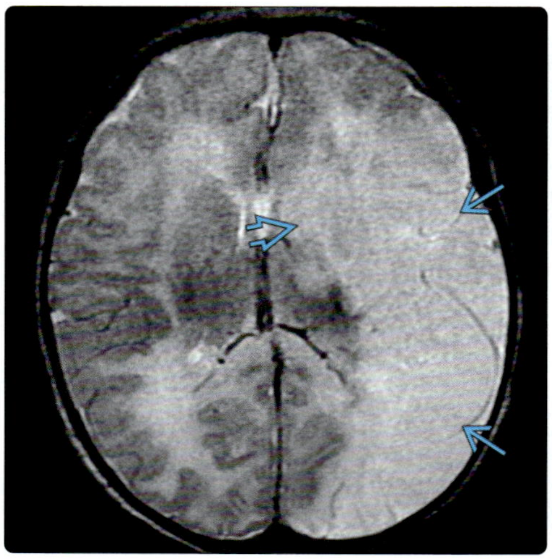

Ischemia/Infarct

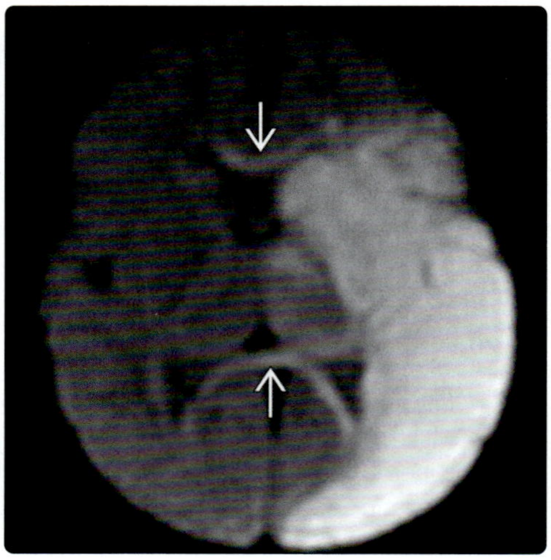

(Left) *Axial FLAIR MR in a 3-year-old boy with tuberous sclerosis complex (TSC) shows a moderate to severe burden of cerebral tubers* →*. These dysplastic lesions typically cause mild enlargement of the affected gyrus & may have cystic change* ⇨*.* **(Right)** *Axial NECT in a 1 year old with TSC shows an atypical, large, calcified tuber* → *involving the right frontal lobe with associated cortical thickening* ⇨*. Also note the calcified subependymal nodule* ↷ *in the left caudothalamic groove.*

Tuberous Sclerosis Complex

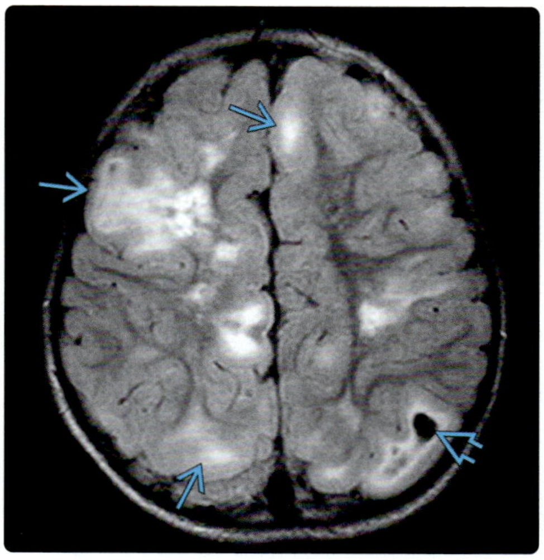

Tuberous Sclerosis Complex

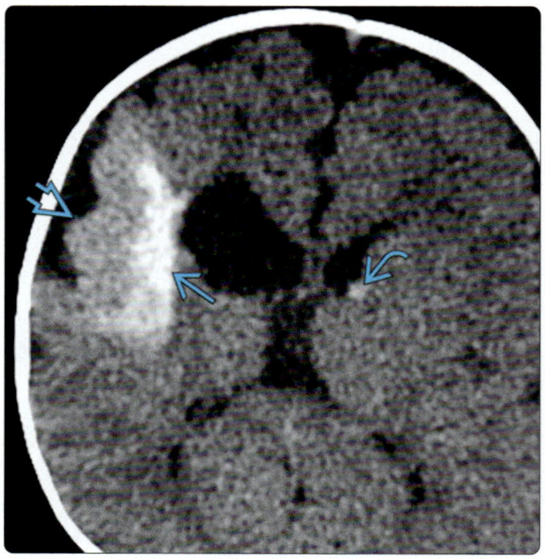

Focal Cortical Dysplasia

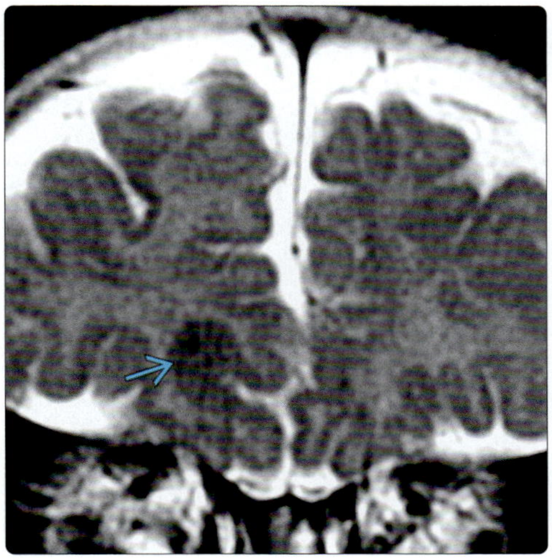

Focal Cortical Dysplasia

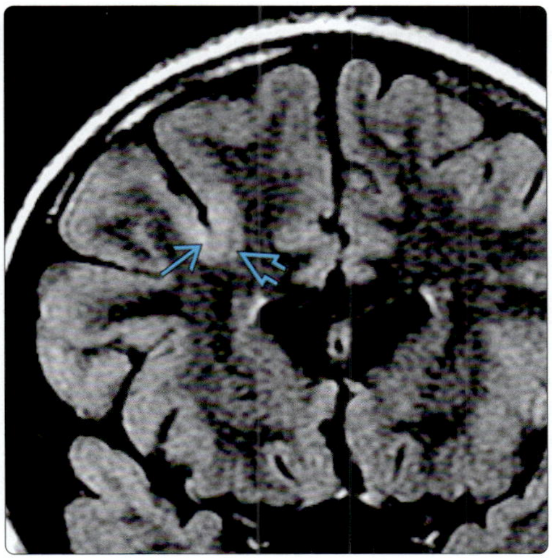

(Left) *Coronal T2 MR in a 4 month old with focal cortical dysplasia (FCD) demonstrates cortical thickening & decreased signal → in the right anteromedial frontal lobe. In an unmyelinated brain, FCD is T2 dark & T1 bright compared to adjacent parenchyma.* **(Right)** *Coronal FLAIR MR in a 16 year old with FCD shows an abnormally deep right superior frontal sulcus with thickening & hyperintense signal at the depth of the sulcus →. Also note the abnormal signal in the subcortical WM ⇨.*

Focal Cortical Dysplasia

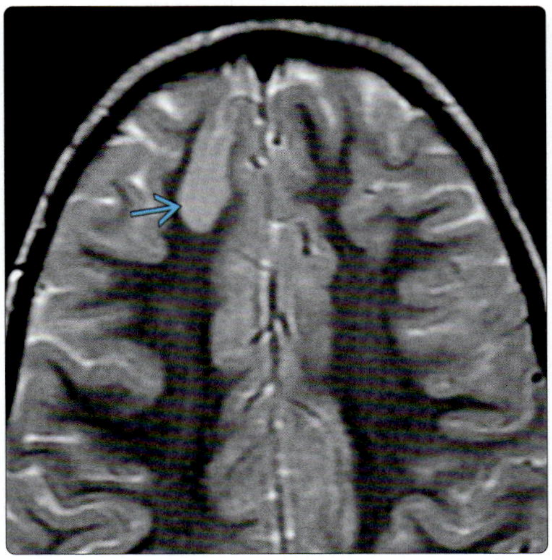

Focal Cortical Dysplasia

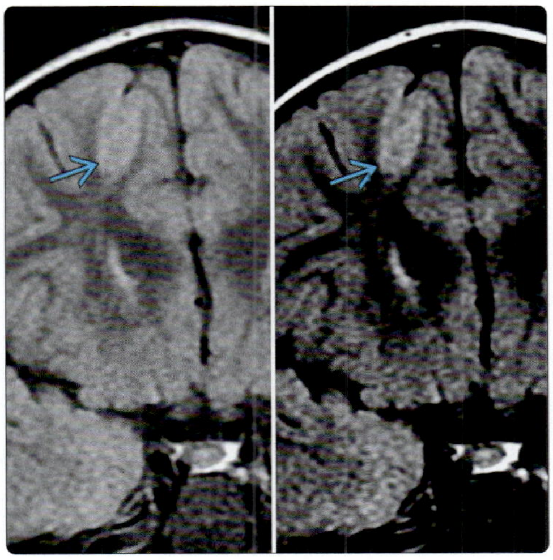

(Left) *Axial T2 MR in a 3 year old with seizures & FCD type 2B shows cortical thickening & slightly hyperintense signal along an abnormally deep sulcus →.* **(Right)** *Coronal FLAIR MR images in the same patient with FCD using routine (left) & narrowed (right) windowing & leveling shows how much more conspicuous the FCD lesion → becomes on narrowed windows. Such manipulation can be quite useful in the detection of these subtle lesions.*

Polymicrogyria

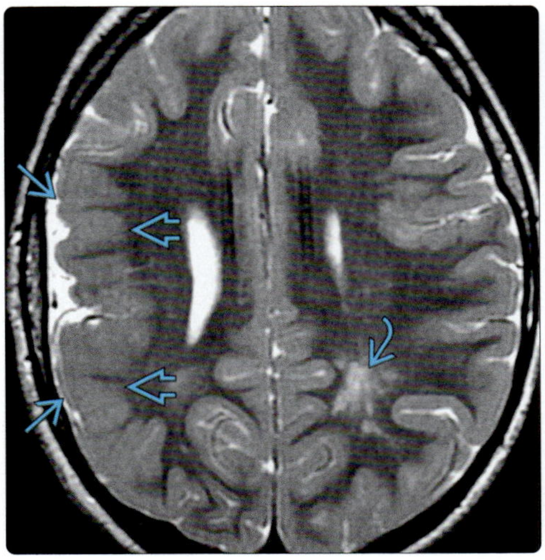

Polymicrogyria

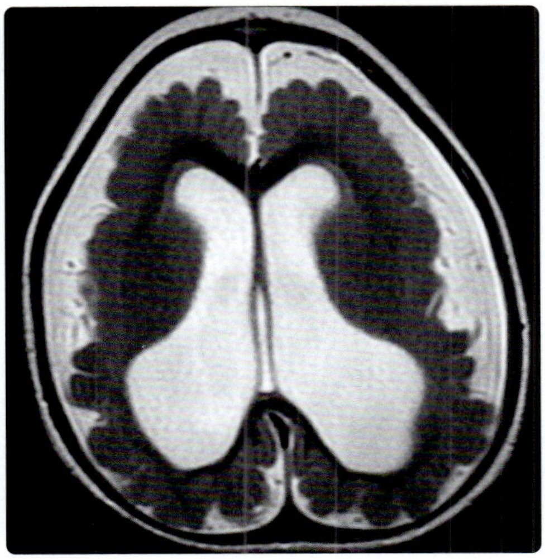

(Left) *Axial T2 MR in a 4 year old with CMV & right perisylvian polymicrogyria (PMG) shows thickening of the cortex with irregularity of the brain surface → & GM-WM junction ⇨. Also note the areas of WM signal abnormality ↷, often seen in CMV.* **(Right)** *Axial T2 MR in a 2 year old with microcephaly & extensive PMG shows thickening of both cerebral cortices with an irregular brain surface, most pronounced in the frontal lobes & insulae. PMG may be unifocal or bilateral (& can be symmetric).*

(Left) *Axial T1 MR in a 1 year old shows bilateral symmetric areas of smooth, decreased sulcation with cortical thickening , typical of pachygyria. In contrast to polymicrogyria, pachygyria has a smooth cortical surface & GM-WM junction.* **(Right)** *Coronal T2 MR in the same patient shows the marked cortical thickening of the bifrontal regions with decreased sulcation. Also note the generalized volume loss causing enlarged ventricles & microcephaly.*

Pachygyria

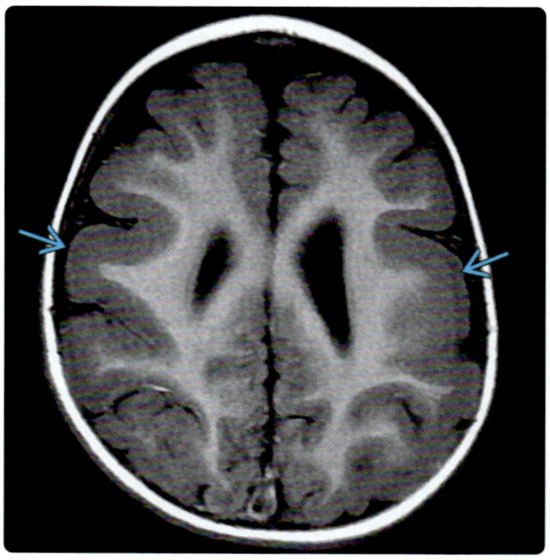

Pachygyria

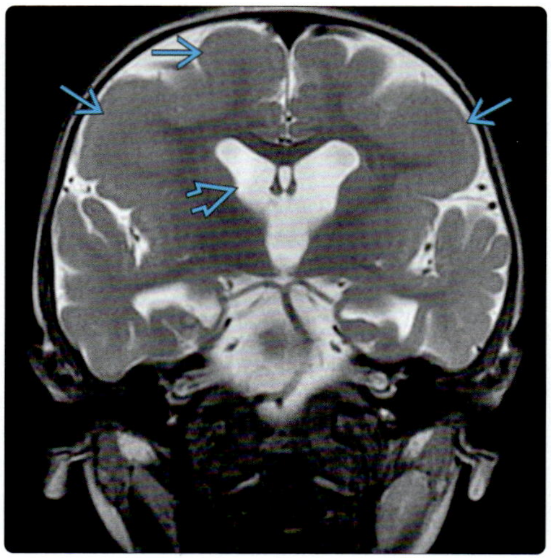

(Left) *Coronal T2 MR in a 6 month old with lissencephaly shows minimal sulcation with formation of the sylvian fissures & superior temporal sulci . Note the 3 layers: 1) thin outer cellular GM layer , 2) cell-sparse layer , & 3) thick, deep cellular GM layer .* **(Right)** *Axial T2 MR in the same patient with lissencephaly shows complete absence of gyri/sulci. Lissencephaly usually shows a 3-layered pattern: 1) thin outer cellular GM layer , 2) cell-sparse layer , & 3) thick, deep cellular GM layer .*

Lissencephaly

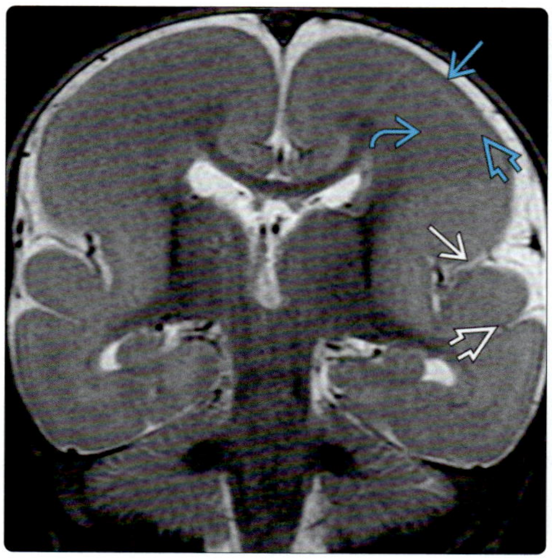

Lissencephaly

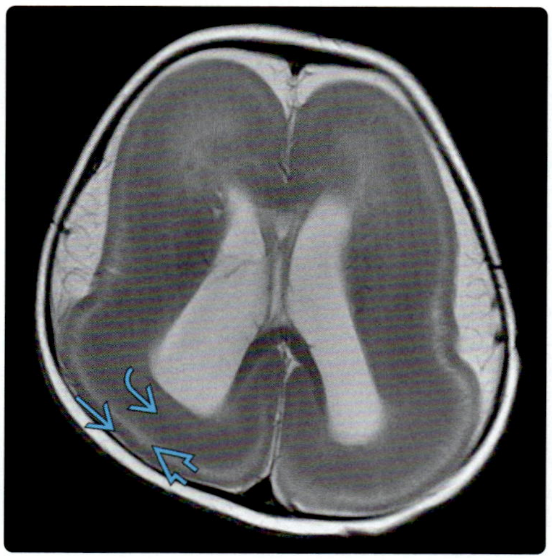

(Left) *Axial T1 MR in a neonate with hemimegalencephaly shows thickening & abnormal organization of the temporal-occipital cortex with poor sulcation. There is classically an increased size of the ipsilateral ventricle .* **(Right)** *Axial T2 MR in a 3 month old with seizures & hemimegalencephaly shows asymmetric enlargement & cortical thickening of the right temporal-occipital lobe with abnormal signal in the deep/periventricular WM & blurring of the GM-WM junction .*

Hemimegalencephaly

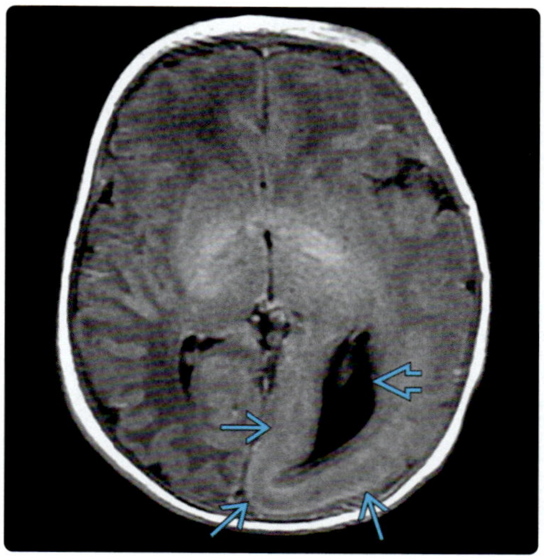

Hemimegalencephaly

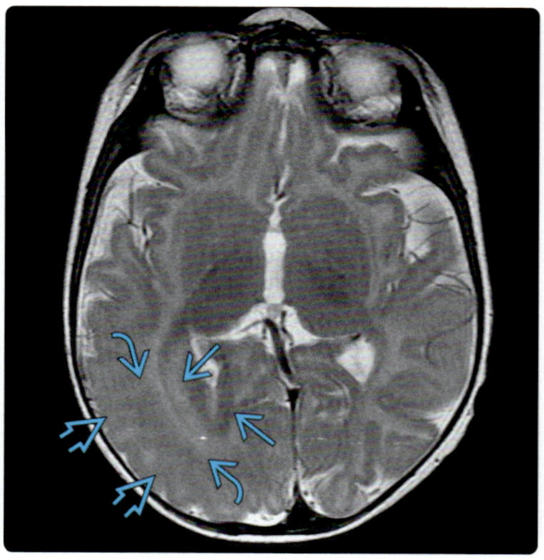

DNET

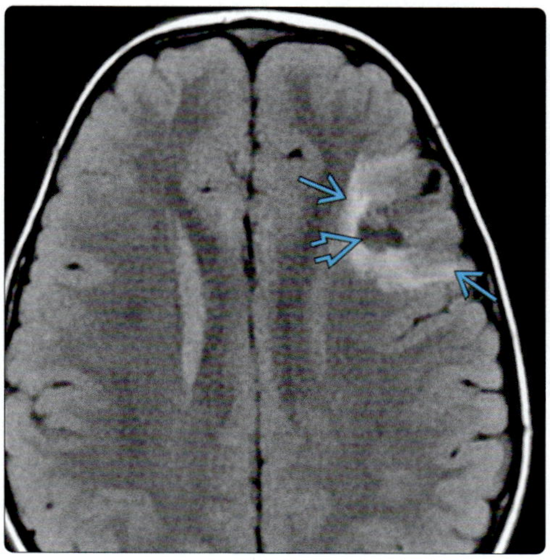

Ganglioglioma

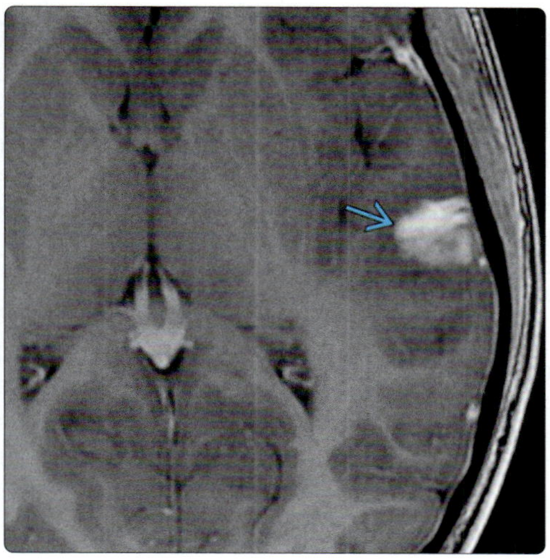

(Left) *Axial FLAIR MR in a 6-year-old boy with rapid eye movements & lip smacking shows a tumor with mixed solid & cystic components. Note the replacement of normal cortex with hyperintense tumor as well as the lack of mass effect.* **(Right)** *Axial T1 C+ MR shows a heterogeneously enhancing mass in the left superior temporal region. Approximately 50% of gangliogliomas will demonstrate associated enhancement.*

Angiocentric Glioma

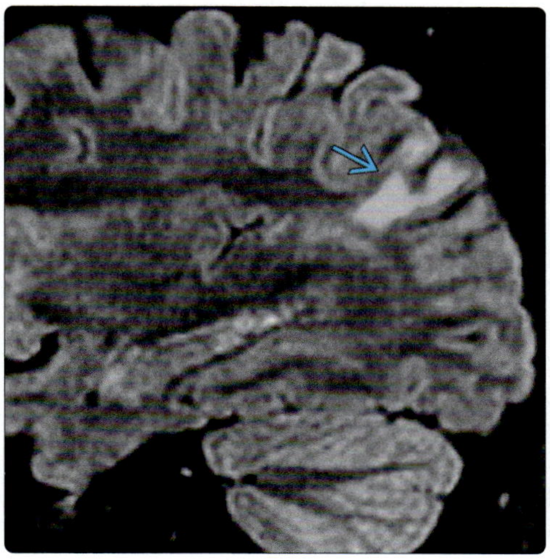

Dysplastic Cerebellar Gangliocytoma

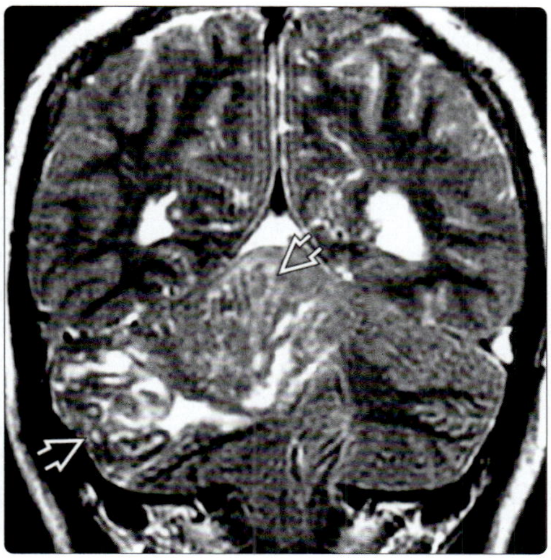

(Left) *Sagittal FLAIR MR in a patient with an angiocentric glioma shows a lesion in the parietal lobe involving the cortex & subcortical white matter. Angiocentric glioma often appears identical to focal cortical dysplasia & cortical tubers of TSC.* **(Right)** *Coronal T2 MR shows thickened, striated-appearing cerebellar folia in a patient with dysplastic cerebellar gangliocytoma (a.k.a. Lhermitte-Duclos disease). In this case, there was no association with Cowden syndrome.*

Gliomatosis Cerebri

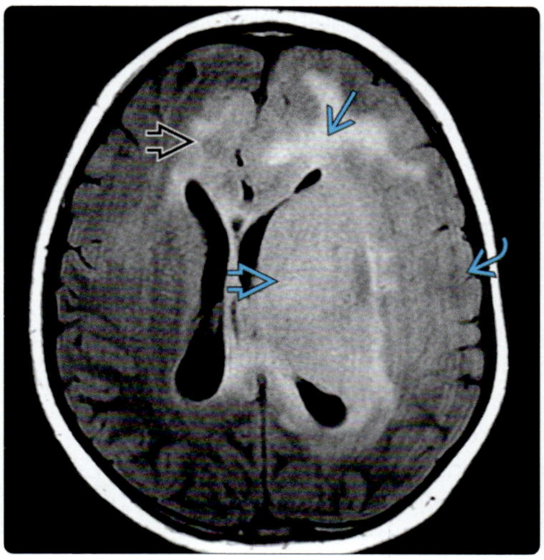

Meningioangiomatosis

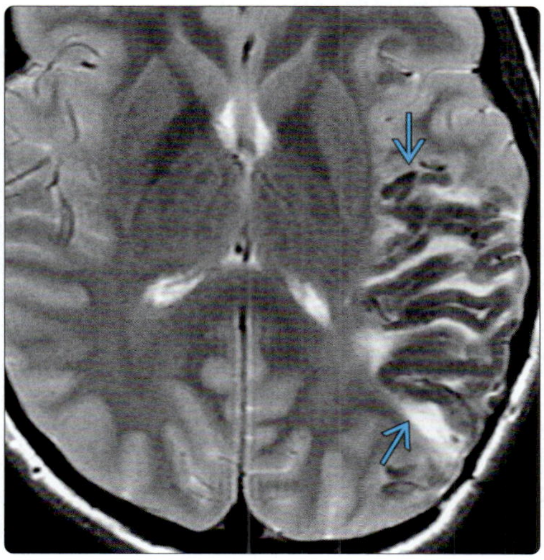

(Left) *Axial FLAIR MR in an 11 year old with gliomatosis cerebri shows enlargement & abnormal signal of the deep gray nuclei, WM, & cortex with effacement of left frontal sulci. The lesion crosses midline to the right frontal lobe. Note the preservation of the underlying brain architecture despite tumor infiltration.* **(Right)** *Axial T2 MR in a 14 year old with meningioangiomatosis shows decreased signal within the cortex & increased signal in the subcortical WM.*

Abnormal Shape/Configuration of Corpus Callosum

DIFFERENTIAL DIAGNOSIS

Common

- Normal Variant
- Thin Corpus Callosum
  - Periventricular Leukomalacia
  - Hypoxic-Ischemic Encephalopathy
  - Chronic Cerebral Infarction
  - Obstructive Hydrocephalus
  - Chemotherapy & Radiation Therapy
- Postsurgical Defects
  - Corpus Callosotomy
  - Ventricular Drainage Catheter Tract
  - Endoscopic 3rd Ventriculostomy

Less Common

- Callosal Agenesis
- Callosal Dysgenesis
  - Primary Callosal Dysgenesis
  - Chiari 2 Malformation
- Neoplasm
  - Glioblastoma
  - Lymphoma
- Pericallosal Lipoma
- Neurofibromatosis Type 1
- Holoprosencephaly

Rare but Important

- Hypomyelination
- Inherited Metabolic Leukodystrophies
  - Metachromatic Leukodystrophy
  - X-Linked Adrenoleukodystrophy
  - Alexander Disease
  - Krabbe Disease

ESSENTIAL INFORMATION

Key Differential Diagnosis Issues

- Clinical features to consider
  - Normal corpus callosum (CC) varies in thickness & shape
  - Associated anomalies portend worse prognosis
  - If not congenital anomaly, clinical history is crucial
    - Prior surgical history, prematurity etc.
- Imaging features to consider
  - Isolated callosal dysgenesis is not common → additional malformations in > 50%
    - Malformations of cortical development
    - Noncallosal midline anomalies
    - Abnormal brainstem or cerebellum
  - Look for parenchymal abnormalities to identify etiology
    - White matter (WM) volume loss, prior infarction, diffuse axonal injury
  - Ventricular abnormalities are common
    - Colpocephaly → CC agenesis/dysgenesis, Chiari 2
    - Enlarged, angular ventricles → periventricular leukomalacia
- Modality considerations
  - CT: Helpful to distinguish cellular vs. inflammatory
    - ↑ density → cellular mass, hemorrhage
    - ↓ density → edema, inflammation
  - MR: Best spatial & contrast resolution
    - Sagittal imaging is critical for evaluation of CC

Helpful Clues for Common Diagnoses

- **Normal Variant**
  - Immature CC is thin
    - Gradually thickens with progressive myelination
  - Size, shape, & thickness of normal CC vary
    - Splenium & genu are largest parts of CC
    - Normal narrowing at junction of body & splenium ("isthmus")
    - Dorsal surface of fully developed, normally myelinated CC is often "wavy"
- **Thin Corpus Callosum**
  - **Periventricular leukomalacia**
    - Premature infant is at greatest risk
    - Acute findings: US → ↑ periventricular WM echogenicity
      - MR: Diffusion restriction, ↑ T1, ↓ T2
    - Chronic findings: ↓ volume of periventricular WM
      - Thin posterior body & splenium are most common
      - Ventricular enlargement shows angular margins
  - **Hypoxic-ischemic encephalopathy**
    - Loss of cerebral WM → thin CC
    - May occur with profound or partial prolonged injury
    - Profound: Often perirolandic → posterior body CC
    - Partial prolonged: Watershed injury → entire CC
  - **Chronic cerebral infarction**
    - Axonal loss → focal/diffuse thinning of CC
  - **Obstructive hydrocephalus**
    - Look for obstructing lesion (e.g., tumor, aqueductal stenosis) or sequelae of prior hemorrhage/infection
    - Acute: CC stretched, bowed upward
    - Chronic: Thinned, irregular (sequela of CC impingement against falx & chronic WM injury from hydrocephalus)
  - **Chemotherapy & radiation therapy**
    - WM injury with volume loss
      - e.g., chronic methotrexate toxicity
- **Postsurgical Defects**
  - **Corpus callosotomy**
    - Surgical disruption for intractable epilepsy
      - Isolated callosotomy or part of functional hemispherotomy
      - Often imaged in postoperative setting to detect residual neuronal connections across midline
      - Best seen on sagittal or coronal MR
  - **Ventricular drainage catheter tract**
    - Small defect in paramidline CC
    - Typically with overlying WM parenchymal tract & postoperative skull focus
    - May see hypointense intracranial catheter ± hyperintense fluid-filled extracranial components
  - **Endoscopic 3rd ventriculostomy**
    - Small defect in CC represents scope tract, typically with overlying WM parenchymal tract & postoperative skull focus

Helpful Clues for Less Common Diagnoses

- **Callosal Agenesis**
  - Absent WM bridging cerebral hemispheres
  - Absent septum pellucidum

- Absent cingulate gyrus with vertically oriented parasagittal sulci radiating to high-riding 3rd ventricle
- Lateral ventricles: Colpocephaly, upturned frontal horns
  - Probst bundles (WM tracts that would have formed CC) lie along medial aspects of lateral ventricles

- **Primary Callosal Dysgenesis**
  - Absence of 1 or all segments
    - Rostrum & splenium are most likely to be deficient
    - Remnants vary in size, shape, configuration
  - Look for other associated malformations
  - "Micro" CC: Small but well formed, often syndromic
  - "Mega" CC: Megalencephalic (bulky WM) vs. small to normal brain (syndromic)
- **Chiari 2 Malformation**
  - Constellation of intracranial findings secondary to open neural tube defect (e.g., myelomeningocele)
    - Small posterior fossa, towering cerebellum that wraps around dorsal brainstem, small elongated 4th ventricle, vermian/tonsillar extension into upper cervical spine, "beaked" tectum, scalloped clivus
  - Degree of callosal dysgenesis is highly variable
    - Correlates with severity of hydrocephalus
- **Neoplasm**
  - **Glioblastoma**
    - Common in adults, uncommon in children
    - "Butterfly" glioma crosses CC
    - Central necrosis + thick, irregular rim enhancement
  - **Lymphoma**
    - NECT: Hyperdense
    - Strong, uniform enhancement
- **Pericallosal Lipoma**
  - 40-50% occur in interhemispheric fissure
  - Almost always located in subarachnoid space; blood vessels & cranial nerves course through lipoma
  - 2 morphologic types
    - Bulky, mass-like ("tubulonodular" type)
    - Thin, dorsal to body/splenium ("curvilinear" type)
  - Midline lipomas may be part of more general midline developmental disorder; CC is often deficient
- **Neurofibromatosis Type 1 (NF1)**
  - Patients with NF1 have ↑ CC volume
    - Sometimes markedly so & qualitatively evident
  - Nonenhancing lesions of NF1 can occur in CC
  - If focal lesions of CC enhance, suggest low-grade tumor
- **Holoprosencephaly**
  - Alobar
    - CC absent
    - "Pancake" anterior cerebral tissue
    - Monoventricle with large dorsal "cyst"
  - Semilobar
    - Frontal lobe fusion/hypoplasia; caudate head fusion
    - Splenium may be present
  - Lobar
    - Genu sometimes present; GM often crosses with genu
    - Absent anterior midline falx & fissure
  - Middle interhemispheric variant (a.k.a. syntelencephaly)
    - Splenium & genu present, body deficient
    - Middle CC body "dips"
    - GM crosses midline in expected location of CC body
    - ± bilateral perisylvian polymicrogyria

Helpful Clues for Rare Diagnoses

- **Hypomyelination**
  - Primary pathologic hypomyelination is rare
    - e.g., Pelizaeus-Merzbacher, *TUBB4A* disorders
- **Inherited Metabolic Leukodystrophies**
  - **Metachromatic leukodystrophy**
    - Entire CC affected, genu & splenium worst
  - **X-linked adrenoleukodystrophy**
    - Most commonly involves splenium
  - **Alexander disease**
    - Frontal lobe & genu involvement
  - **Krabbe disease**
    - Central WM + deep gray nuclei (especially thalamus)

SELECTED REFERENCES

1. Al-Hashim AH et al: Corpus callosum abnormalities: neuroradiological and clinical correlations. Dev Med Child Neurol. 58(5):475-84, 2016
2. Battal B et al: Corpus callosum: normal imaging appearance, variants and pathologic conditions. J Med Imaging Radiat Oncol. 54(6):541-9, 2010

Normal Variant

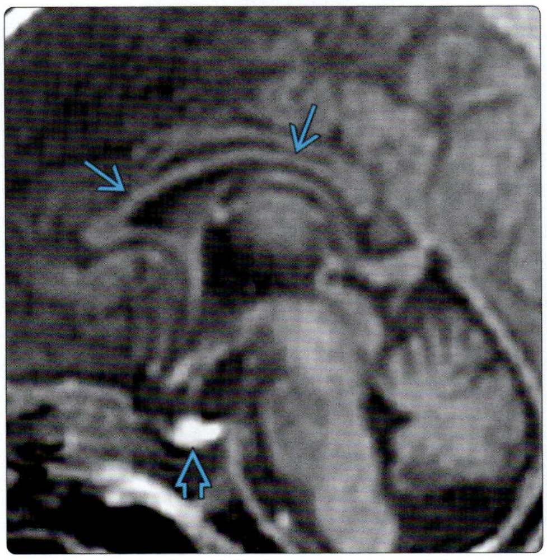

Normal Variant

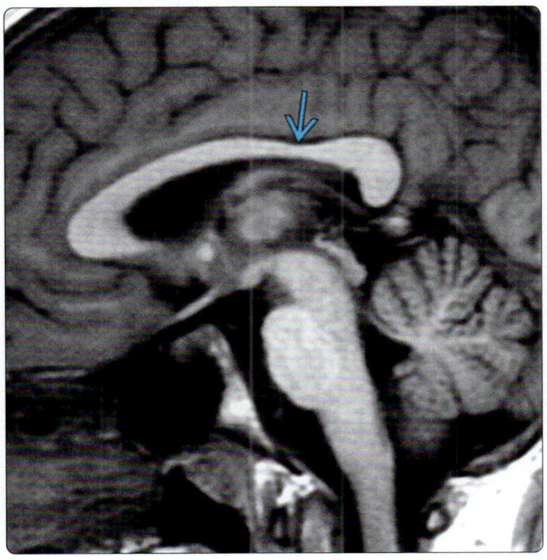

(Left) *Midline sagittal T1 MR in a normal term neonate shows a thin, unmyelinated corpus callosum (CC)* ➙*. The CC will gradually thicken as it myelinates from posterior to anterior. Note that the entire pituitary gland normally shows T1 shortening* ⇨ *in the 1st few weeks of life.* **(Right)** *Midline sagittal T1 MR in a 13 year old with headaches shows a normal variant morphology of the CC with relative thinning of the posterior body* ➙*. This should not be mistaken for a sign of white matter (WM) volume loss.*

(**Left**) *Axial FLAIR MR in a 7 year old with a history of prematurity & periventricular leukomalacia (PVL) shows severe WM volume loss with relatively little signal abnormality. Also note the angular margins of the expanded ventricular occipital horns, consistent with PVL related to extreme prematurity.* (**Right**) *Midline sagittal T1 MR in the same patient shows marked thinning of the posterior body & splenium of the CC due to WM volume loss. This is the most common area of CC involvement in PVL.*

Periventricular Leukomalacia

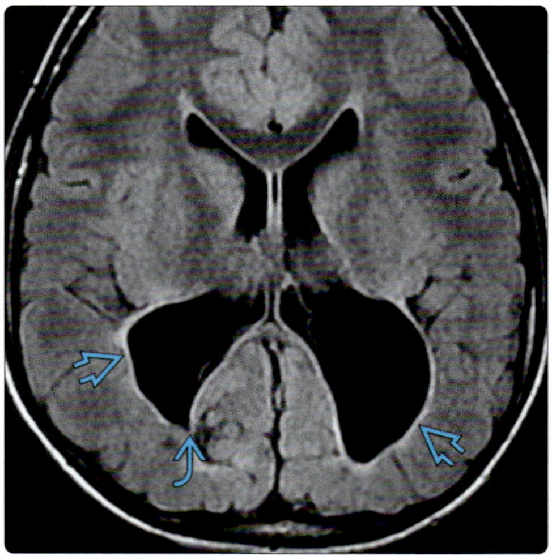

Periventricular Leukomalacia

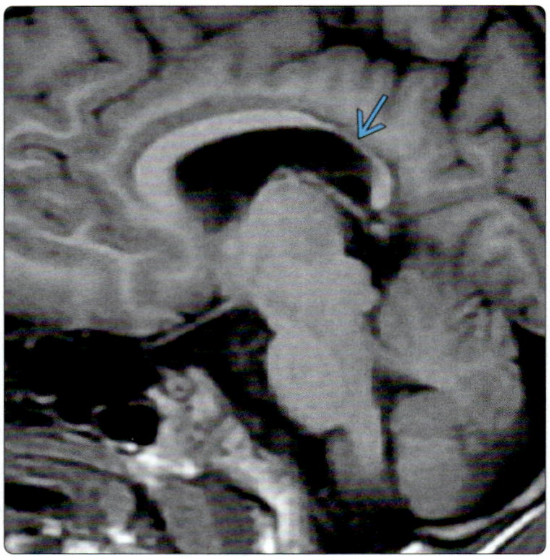

(**Left**) *Axial T2 MR in a 9 year old with a history of hypoxic-ischemic encephalopathy (HIE) at birth shows extensive gliosis & encephalomalacia causing WM volume & signal abnormality in a watershed distribution. This results in marked CC thinning.* (**Right**) *Midline sagittal T1 MR in the same patient shows marked thinning of the CC secondary to WM loss as a consequence of the remote HIE injury.*

Hypoxic-Ischemic Encephalopathy

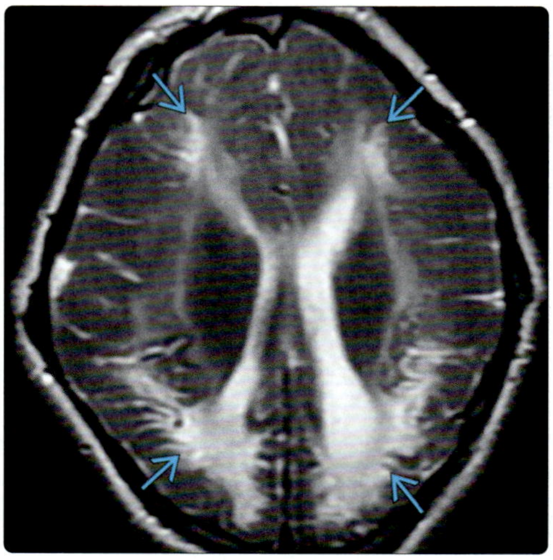

Hypoxic-Ischemic Encephalopathy

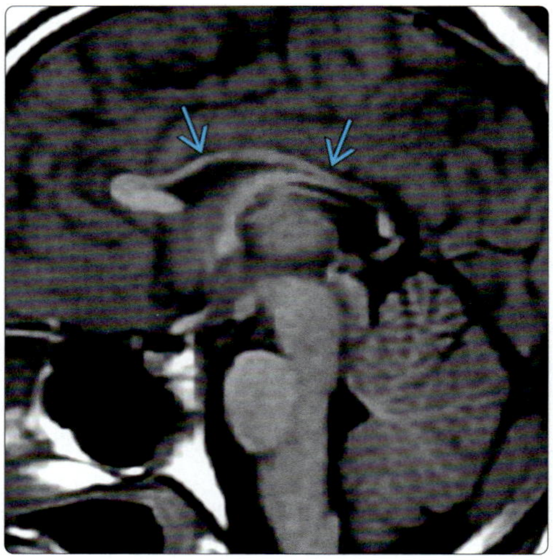

(**Left**) *Midline sagittal T2 MR in a neonate with posthemorrhagic hydrocephalus shows a stretched & thinned CC. Note the enlarged lateral, 3rd, & 4th ventricles as well as thin T2 hypointensity along the brainstem, consistent with hemosiderin deposition.* (**Right**) *Midline sagittal T1 MR in the same patient 1 year after shunting shows a thinned & dysmorphic CC as well as numerous thin, pencil-like gyri (stenogyria).*

Obstructive Hydrocephalus

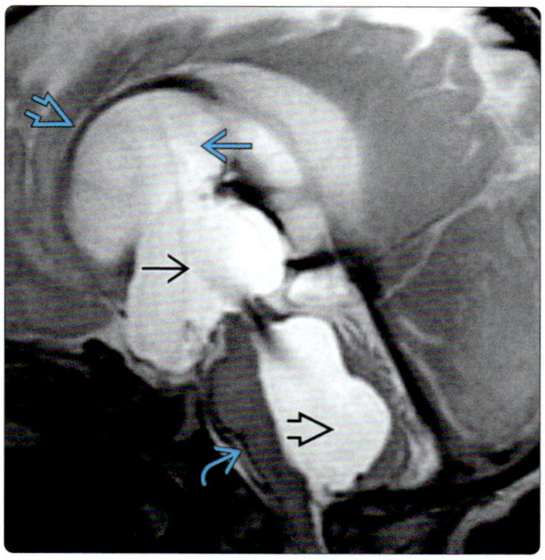

Obstructive Hydrocephalus

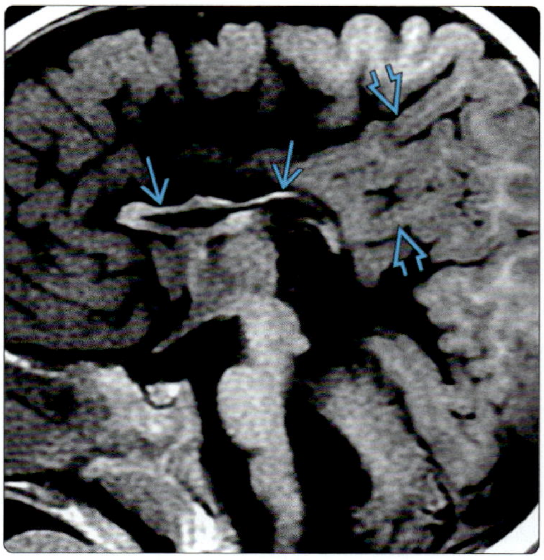

Corpus Callosotomy

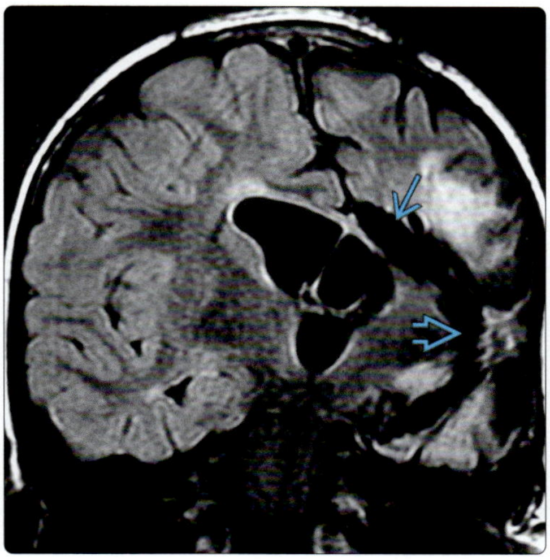

Corpus Callosotomy

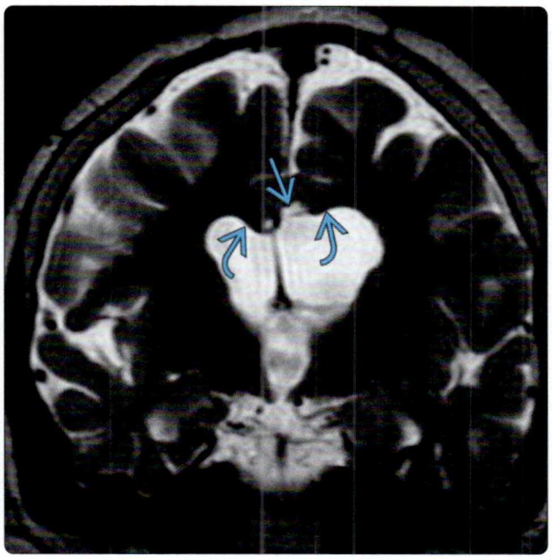

(Left) *Coronal FLAIR MR shows changes of a left functional hemispherotomy with a WM disconnection → & insular decortication ⇒. Corpus callosotomy may be performed in isolation or as part of a more extensive functional hemispherotomy, as in this patient.* **(Right)** *Coronal T2 MR shows absence of the midline CC → with persistent paramidline callosal tissue ↗, consistent with an isolated surgical callosotomy.*

Ventricular Drainage Catheter Tract

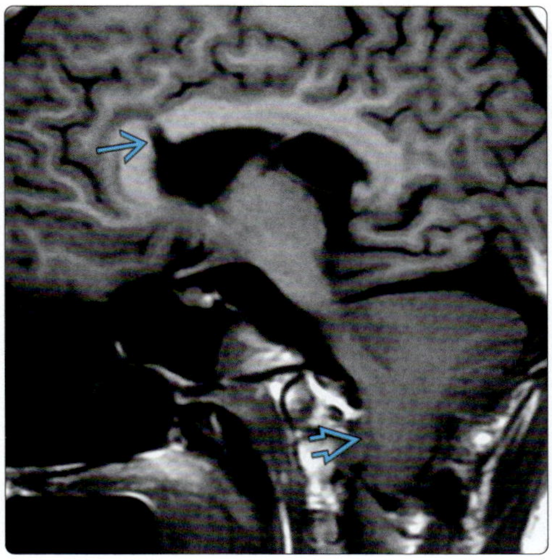

Endoscopic 3rd Ventriculostomy

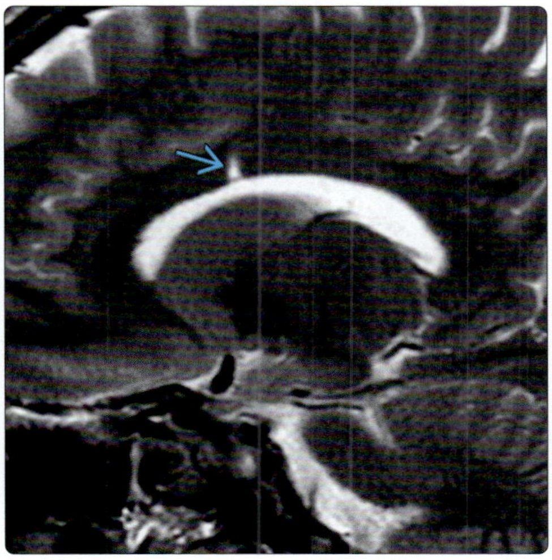

(Left) *Paramidline sagittal T1 MR in a 12 year old with Chiari 2 malformation shows a ventricular shunt catheter tract → in the anterior body of the CC. Note the caudal migration of the cerebellum & brainstem ⇒, consistent with Chiari 2.* **(Right)** *Paramidline sagittal T2 MR in a teenager with a history of a prior endoscopic 3rd ventriculostomy shows a linear defect → in the parasagittal body of the CC. The defect represents the site of surgical access for the scope to enter the 3rd ventricle.*

Callosal Agenesis

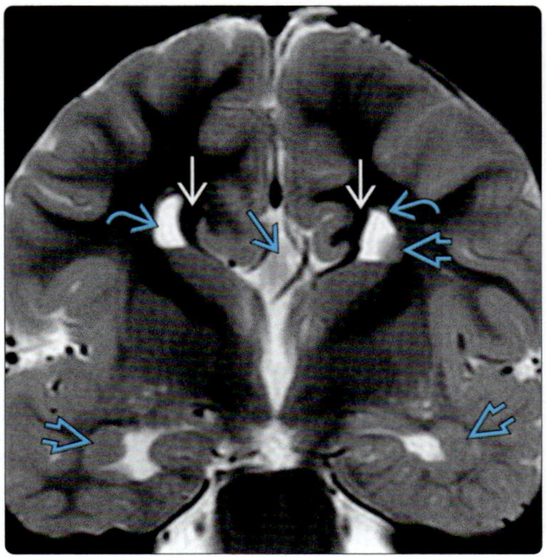

Callosal Dysgenesis

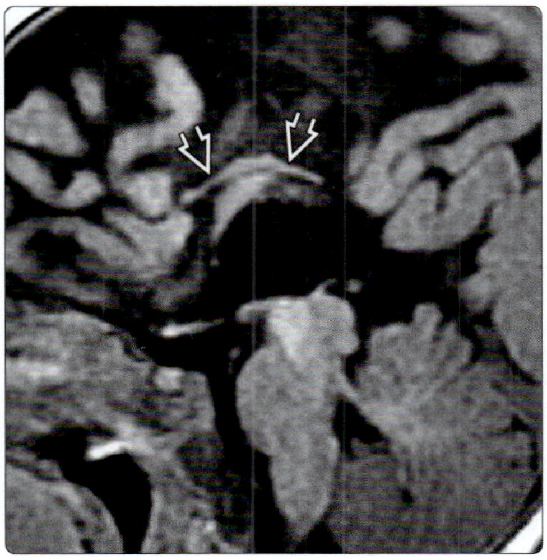

(Left) *Coronal T2 MR in a 4 year old with callosal agenesis shows widely spaced upturned lateral ventricular frontal horns ↗, a high-riding 3rd ventricle →, & bilateral Probst bundles ➡. Also note the extensive periventricular gray matter (GM) heterotopia ⇒.* **(Right)** *Midline sagittal T1 MR in a 5 month old with isolated callosal dysgenesis shows a very short & thin CC ➡ with no evident rostrum or splenium. Isolated callosal dysgenesis is uncommon. Associated anomalies should be carefully sought.*

(Left) *Midline sagittal T1 MR in a 7 year old with multiple anomalies shows a short, thin, & dysmorphic CC with a poorly formed splenium ➔ & rostrum ➔.* **(Right)** *Midline sagittal T2 MR in a child with a repaired myelomeningocele & Chiari 2 malformation (with beaked tectum ➔, small 4th ventricle ↗, & scalloped clivus ➔) shows a thinned & dysmorphic CC ➔.*

Callosal Dysgenesis

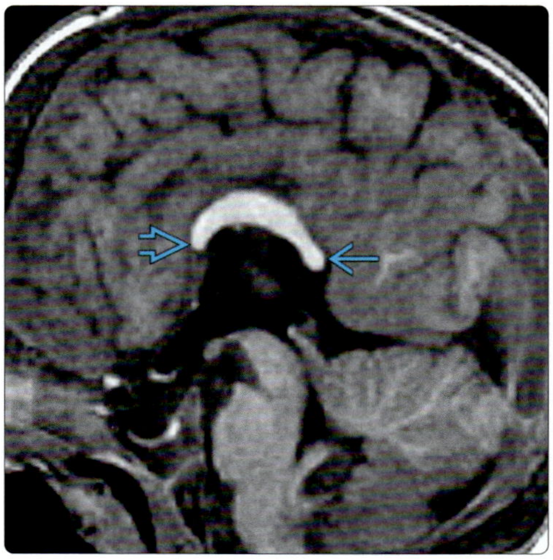

Chiari 2 Malformation

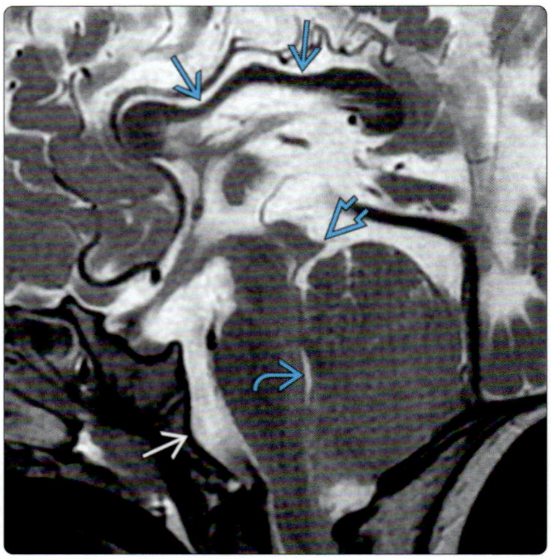

(Left) *Coronal T2 MR in a 10 year old with glioblastoma shows mass-like infiltrative signal ➔ crossing the midline through an expanded CC. Infiltrative high-grade glial neoplasms should be considered whenever such a finding is encountered, as they commonly spread along WM tracts, such as the CC.* **(Right)** *Midline sagittal T2 MR shows expansion & increased signal in the rostrum & anterior genu of the CC ➔, consistent with tumor infiltration/edema in this patient with CNS lymphoma.*

Glioblastoma

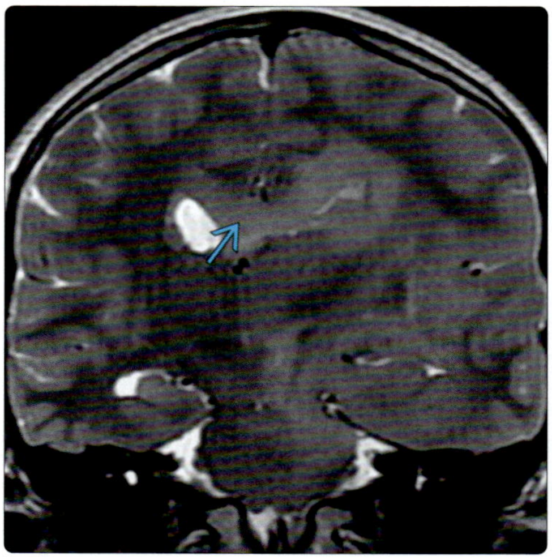

Lymphoma

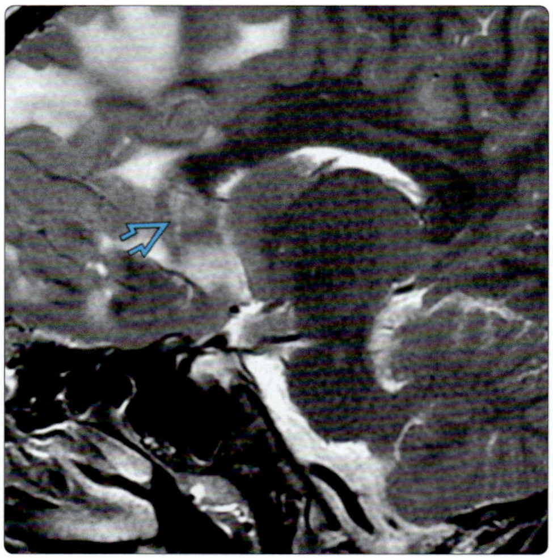

(Left) *Midline sagittal T1 MR in a 4 month old shows a T1-hyperintense lipoma ➔ along the dorsal CC with associated absence of the splenium ➔.* **(Right)** *Midline sagittal T1 MR in a 15 year old with neurofibromatosis type 1 (NF1) shows diffuse marked thickening of the entire CC, a finding that can be seen in NF1. Look for associated findings of NF1, such as nonenhancing signal abnormalities of the globus pallidus & medial cerebellum, optic pathway gliomas, & plexiform neurofibromas.*

Pericallosal Lipoma

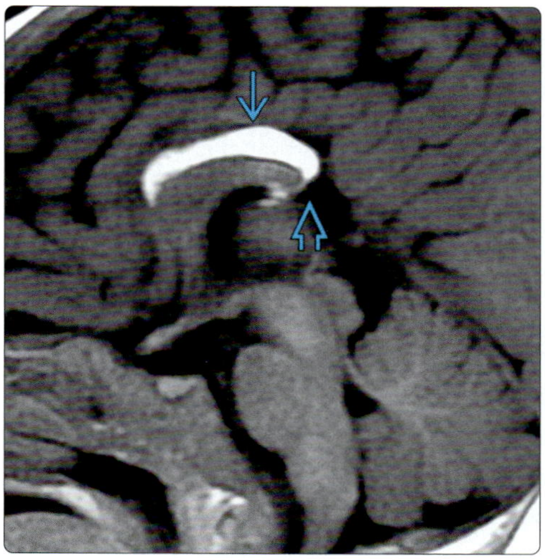

Neurofibromatosis Type 1

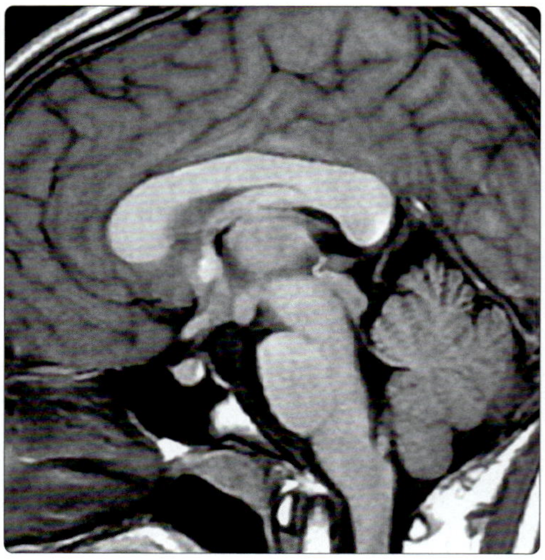

Holoprosencephaly

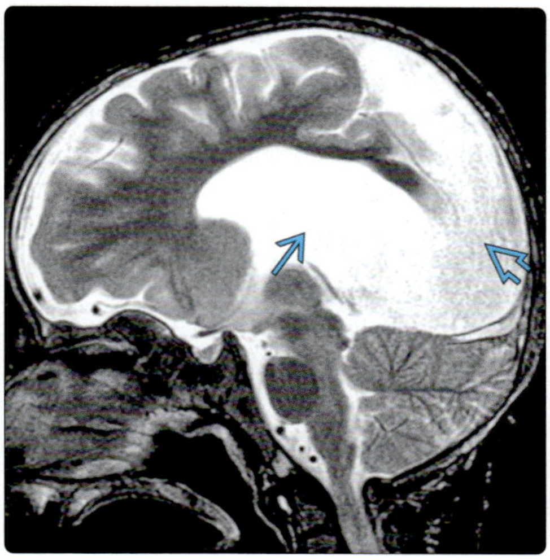

Holoprosencephaly

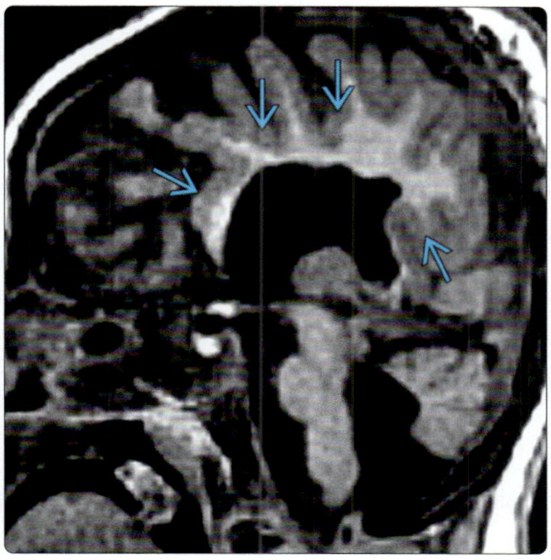

(Left) *Midline sagittal T2 MR shows absence of the CC in a patient with alobar holoprosencephaly. There is continuity of frontal WM & GM across the midline with a large dorsal cyst that communicates with a monoventricle. Note the lack of a vermian primary fissure due to associated rhombencephalosynapsis.* **(Right)** *Midline sagittal T1 MR in a 2 year old with semilobar holoprosencephaly shows absence of a normal CC & extension of cortical GM across the midline.*

Holoprosencephaly

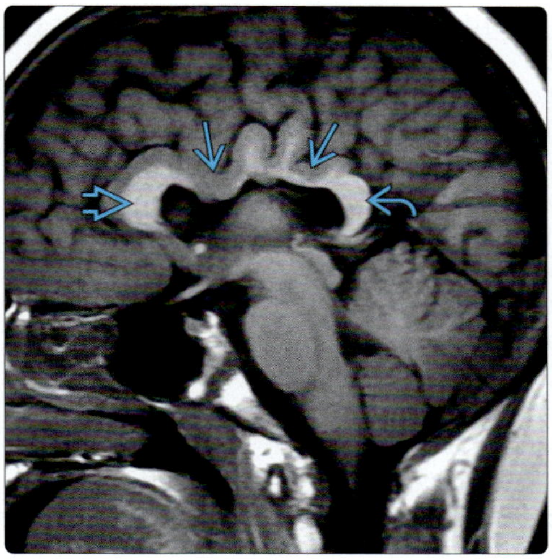

Holoprosencephaly

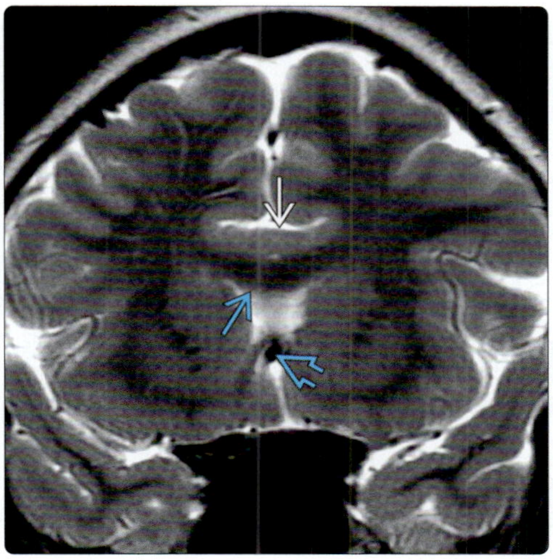

(Left) *Midline sagittal T1 MR in a teenager with the middle interhemispheric variant of holoprosencephaly shows an intact CC anteriorly & posteriorly but abnormal extension of GM across the midline in the expected location of the CC body. The abnormal body of the CC typically "dips" down toward the interthalamic adhesion.* **(Right)** *Coronal T2 MR in the same patient with syntelencephaly shows abnormal GM crossing the midline along the CC WM. Also note the azygous internal carotid artery (ICA).*

Metachromatic Leukodystrophy

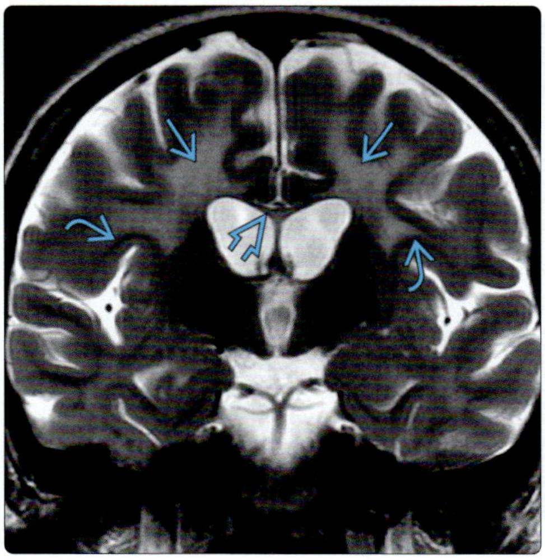

X-Linked Adrenoleukodystrophy

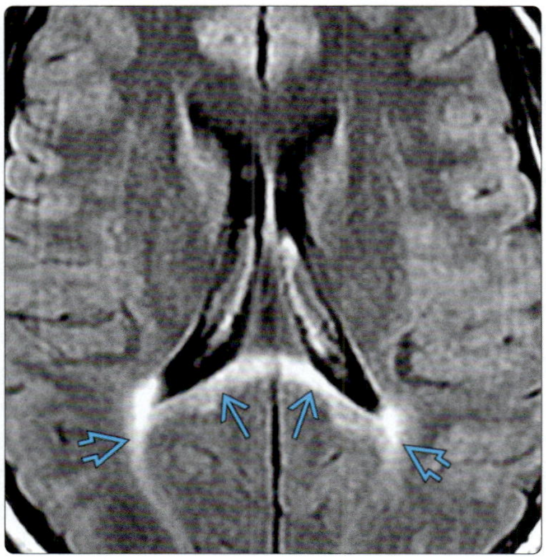

(Left) *Coronal T2 MR in a 13-year-old female patient with metachromatic leukodystrophy shows symmetric extensive WM signal abnormality with preservation of the subcortical WM. Note the marked thinning of the CC.* **(Right)** *Axial FLAIR MR in a 14-year-old male patient with X-linked adrenoleukodystrophy (ALD) shows symmetric increased FLAIR signal intensity that crosses the splenium of the CC. This is the most common distribution of signal abnormality in X-linked ALD.*

DIFFERENTIAL DIAGNOSIS

Common

- MR Artifact
- Postsurgical
  - Corpus Callosotomy
  - Endoscopic 3rd Ventriculostomy
  - Ventricular Drainage Catheter Tract
- Transependymal Edema (Obstructive Hydrocephalus)
- Multiple Sclerosis
- Diffuse Axonal Injury
- Hypoxic-Ischemic Encephalopathy

Less Common

- Neurofibromatosis Type 1
- Ischemia/Infarct
- Transient Cytotoxic Splenial Lesion
- Perivascular Spaces
- Acute Disseminated Encephalomyelitis

Rare but Important

- Neoplasm
  - Glioblastoma
  - Primary CNS Lymphoma
- Inherited Metabolic Leukodystrophies
  - Metachromatic Leukodystrophy
  - X-Linked Adrenoleukodystrophy
  - Alexander Disease
  - Krabbe Disease
  - Vanishing White Matter Disease

ESSENTIAL INFORMATION

Key Differential Diagnosis Issues

- Clinical features to consider
  - History of trauma: Diffuse axonal injury (DAI)
  - Seizure, infection: Transient cytotoxic splenial lesion
  - Prior surgical history: Corpus callosotomy, shunt placement, endoscopic 3rd ventriculostomy
  - Sex: Multiple sclerosis (MS) much more likely in female patients
  - Loss of developmental milestones: Leukodystrophies
- Modality considerations
  - CT: Helpful to distinguish cellular vs. inflammatory
    - ↑ density: Cellular mass, hemorrhage
    - ↓ density: Edema, inflammation
  - MR: Best imaging modality for evaluation of corpus callosum (CC)
    - Sagittal imaging is critical
    - 3D acquisitions allow multiplanar reconstructions

Helpful Clues for Common Diagnoses

- **MR Artifact**
  - Magic angle artifact occurs with combination of
    - Low TE sequences (e.g., T1, DWI)
    - Specific sites where neurons are
      - Densely unidirectional in orientation
      - Lying at certain angle to magnetic field
  - Splenium may appear dark on T1
  - Splenium & genu may be bright on DWI
- **Postsurgical**
  - **Corpus callosotomy**
    - Surgical disruption for intractable epilepsy
      - Isolated callosotomy or part of functional hemispherotomy
      - Often imaged to detect residual neuronal connections across midline
      - Best seen on sagittal or coronal MR
  - **Endoscopic 3rd ventriculostomy**
    - Small defect in CC represents scope tract
    - Linear tract through overlying parenchyma
  - **Ventricular drainage catheter tract**
    - Small defect in paramidline CC
    - Linear tract through overlying parenchyma
- **Transependymal Edema (Obstructive Hydrocephalus)**
  - ↑ T2/FLAIR signal along CC ventricular surface
    - Look for additional abnormal signal of frontal & occipital periventricular white matter (WM)
  - ↑ size of ventricles proximal to obstruction
    - Look for obstructing lesion
      - Most often at cerebral aqueduct
- **Multiple Sclerosis**
  - Demyelinating disease, usually multifocal & recurrent
  - F > M, 3-5:1
  - ↑ incidence in teenagers/adults, rare in children
  - 50-90% involve CC interface
    - Radiating linear/ovoid T2/FLAIR hyperintense lesions in/about CC: "Dawson fingers"
      - Enhancement with active lesions
  - Look for associated optic neuritis & spinal cord lesions
- **Diffuse Axonal Injury**
  - 20% involve CC
  - NECT: ↓ attenuation, ± hemorrhagic foci
  - MR: Much more sensitive for detection
    - Hemorrhagic DAI: Signal loss on SWI
    - Nonhemorrhagic DAI: ↑ T2/↓ T1, diffusion restriction
- **Hypoxic-Ischemic Encephalopathy**
  - Secondary neuronal injury may lead to ↑ DWI/ ↓ ADC on MR

Helpful Clues for Less Common Diagnoses

- **Neurofibromatosis Type 1**
  - Nonenhancing T2/FLAIR hyperintense lesions of neurofibromatosis type 1 (NF1) can occur in CC
    - Due to myelin vacuolization
    - Suggest low-grade tumor if enhancing
  - Look for associated lesions to confirm diagnosis
    - Nonenhancing signal abnormalities in deep gray nuclei (globus pallidus, thalami) & deep cerebellum
    - Optic pathway gliomas
    - Plexiform neurofibromas
    - Sphenoid wing dysplasia & lambdoid defects of skull
- **Ischemia/Infarct**
  - Diffusion restriction in CC is common in hemispheric infarctions
    - Unclear etiology; most likely due to neuronal damage of "acute wallerian degeneration"
  - Isolated focal infarction of CC is possible but uncommon
- **Transient Cytotoxic Splenial Lesion**
  - Round or boomerang-shaped diffusion restriction in CC splenium

- Typically associated with swelling & ↑ T1/↓ T2
- Diverse etiologies: Seizures (especially after cessation of antiepileptic medication), infection (especially viral, particularly influenza), chemotherapy, & trauma
- Imaging findings are typically reversible

- **Perivascular Spaces**
  - Cystic spaces that follow CSF on all sequences
  - CC is common location for prominent perivascular spaces
    - Small isolated perivascular spaces are most common
    - Large & numerous perivascular spaces occur almost exclusively in mucopolysaccharidosis
- **Acute Disseminated Encephalomyelitis**
  - Autoimmune postinfectious inflammation of brain & spinal cord
  - May mimic other demyelinating disease (e.g., MS)
    - CC involvement in acute disseminated encephalomyelitis (ADEM) < MS
    - Deep gray nuclei involvement in ADEM > MS
  - Usually single episode without recurrence
  - Complete or near-complete clinical recovery is common

Helpful Clues for Rare Diagnoses

- **Neoplasm**
  - **Glioblastoma**
    - Common in adults, uncommon in children
    - "Butterfly" glioma crossing through & expanding/distorting CC
      - Central necrosis + thick, irregular rim enhancement
  - **Primary CNS lymphoma**
    - More common in adults, very uncommon in children
    - NECT: Hyperdense lesions
    - Strong, uniform enhancement
    - MR: Diffusion restriction reflects high cellularity
- **Inherited Metabolic Leukodystrophies**
  - Any WM disease can cause signal abnormalities in CC
  - CC volume may be ↑ in acute phase & often ↓ in chronic phase
  - Findings are typically symmetric
  - **Metachromatic leukodystrophy**
    - Autosomal recessive lysosomal storage disorder
    - Entire CC, but genu & splenium are most pronounced
    - Look for "tigroid" WM & sparing of subcortical U fibers
  - **X-linked adrenoleukodystrophy**
    - X-linked recessive peroxisomal disorder
    - Most commonly involves CC splenium
    - Look for enhancing, diffusion-restricting margin in acute disease
  - **Alexander disease**
    - Autosomal dominant leukoencephalopathy
    - Frontal lobe & genu involvement
      - Signal abnormalities & ↑ WM volume
  - **Krabbe disease**
    - Autosomal recessive lysosomal storage disorder
    - Typically involves body of CC
    - Central WM + deep gray nuclei (especially thalamus)
    - Look for bithalamic Ca^{2+}
  - **Vanishing white matter disease**
    - Rare autosomal recessive WM disease of childhood
    - May have some waxing/waning of symptoms
    - Typically, normal CC size in acute phase with thinning in chronic phase
    - Diffuse WM signal abnormality eventually = to CSF on all sequences
    - Cerebellum often involved, especially vermis

SELECTED REFERENCES

1. Starkey J et al: Cytotoxic lesions of the corpus callosum that show restricted diffusion: mechanisms, causes, and manifestations. Radiographics. 37(2):562-76, 2017
2. Al-Hashim AH et al: Corpus callosum abnormalities: neuroradiological and clinical correlations. Dev Med Child Neurol. 58(5):475-84, 2016
3. Battal B et al: Corpus callosum: normal imaging appearance, variants and pathologic conditions. J Med Imaging Radiat Oncol. 54(6):541-9, 2010
4. Bourekas EC et al: Lesions of the corpus callosum: MR imaging and differential considerations in adults and children. AJR Am J Roentgenol. 179(1):251-7, 2002

MR Artifact

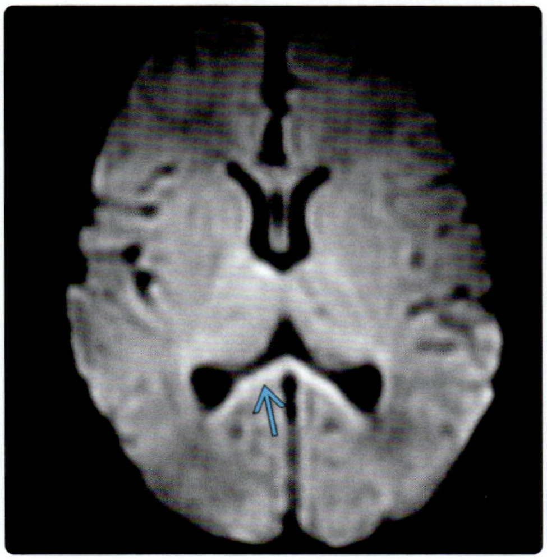

MR Artifact

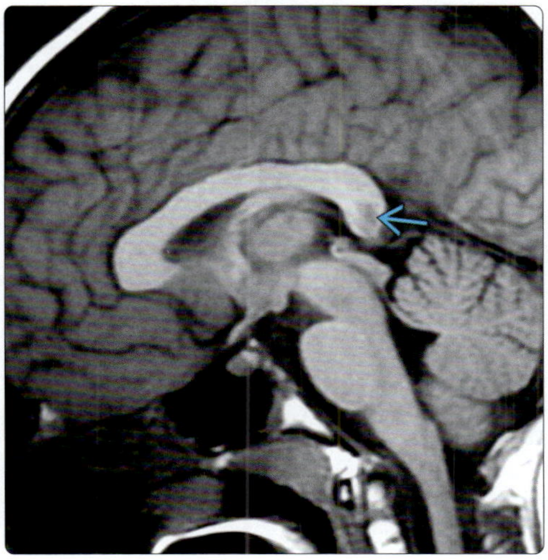

(Left) *Axial DWI MR in a neonate with an otherwise normal study shows ↑ signal in the splenium of the corpus callosum (CC) ⇒, suggesting magic angle artifact. Note the normal signal within the remainder of the brain parenchyma.* **(Right)** *Sagittal T1 MR in a 10 year old with headache shows an area of decreased signal intensity in the splenium ⇒ of the CC. All other sequences were normal in this region. This is an artifact that can occur with short-echo MR in areas of tightly packed unidirectional fibers.*

Corpus Callosotomy

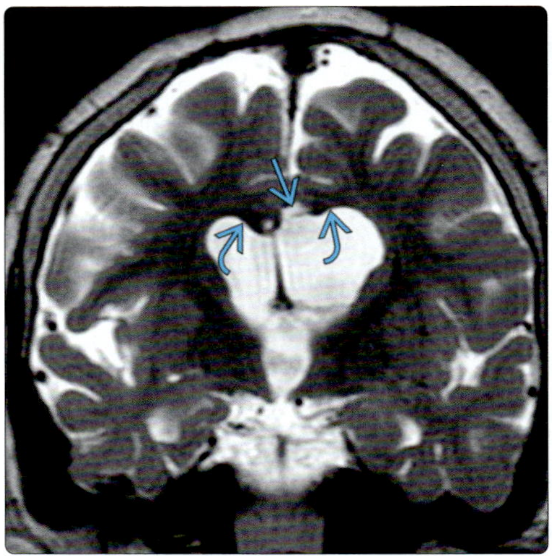

Corpus Callosotomy

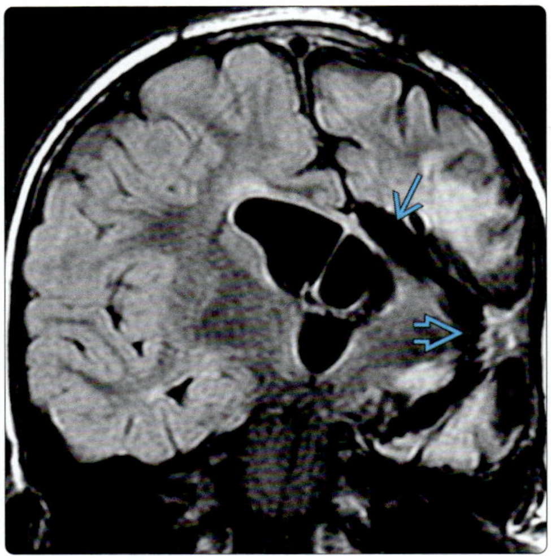

(Left) *Coronal T2 MR in a patient with a prior surgical callosotomy shows absence of the midline CC ➡ with callosal tissue still seen in the paramidline region ➡.* **(Right)** *Coronal FLAIR MR shows changes of a prior left functional hemispherotomy with a white matter (WM) disconnection ➡ & insular decortication ➡. Corpus callosotomy may be performed in isolation or as part of a more extensive functional hemispherotomy, as in this patient.*

Transependymal Edema (Obstructive Hydrocephalus)

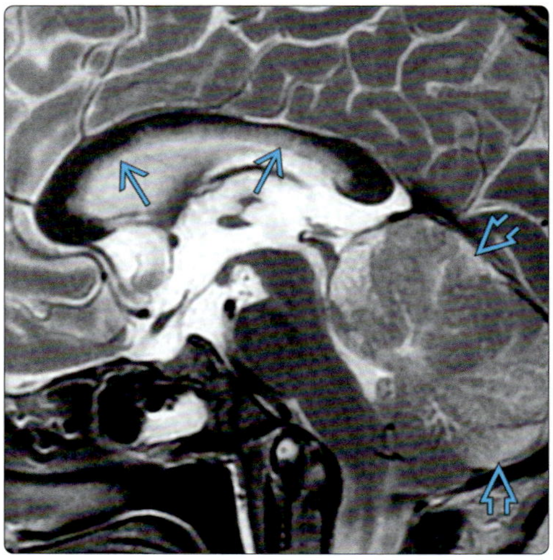

Transependymal Edema (Obstructive Hydrocephalus)

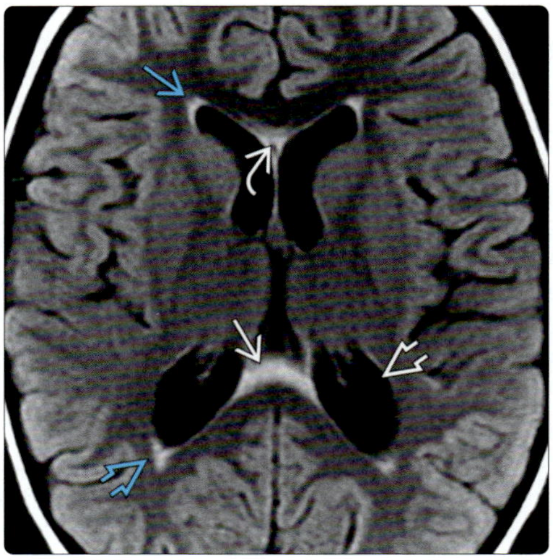

(Left) *Sagittal T2 MR in a 10 year old with acute cerebellitis causing obstructive hydrocephalus shows ↑ signal intensity ➡ along the ventricular surface of the CC. Note the hyperintense & swollen cerebellum ➡.* **(Right)** *Axial FLAIR MR in the same patient shows transependymal edema in the genu ➡ & splenium ➡ of the CC. Note the mild enlargement of the lateral ventricles ➡ & ↑ signal intensity in the frontal ➡ & occipital ➡ periventricular WM.*

Multiple Sclerosis

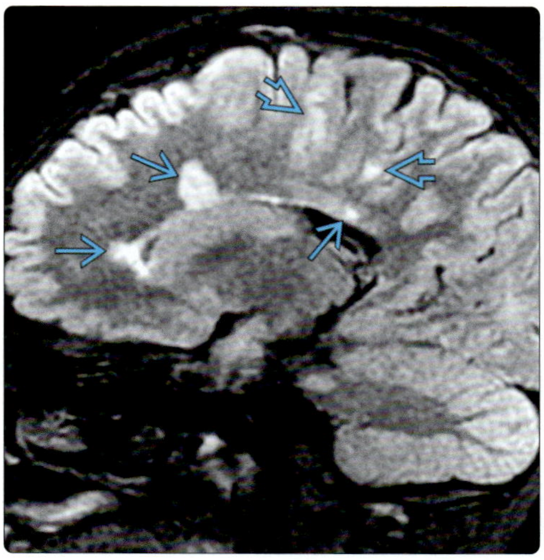

Multiple Sclerosis

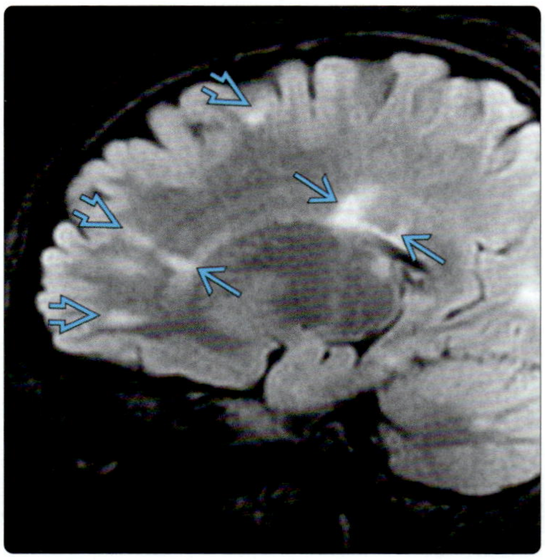

(Left) *Sagittal FLAIR MR in a 12 year old with multiple sclerosis (MS) shows multiple ovoid foci of hyperintense signal in the CC ➡. Such an appearance is often referred to as "Dawson fingers." Also note additional areas of subcortical WM involvement ➡.* **(Right)** *Sagittal FLAIR MR in a 14 year old with MS shows elongated foci of ↑ signal in the CC ➡ radiating away from the ventricle. Note additional areas of subcortical WM involvement ➡.*

Diffuse Axonal Injury

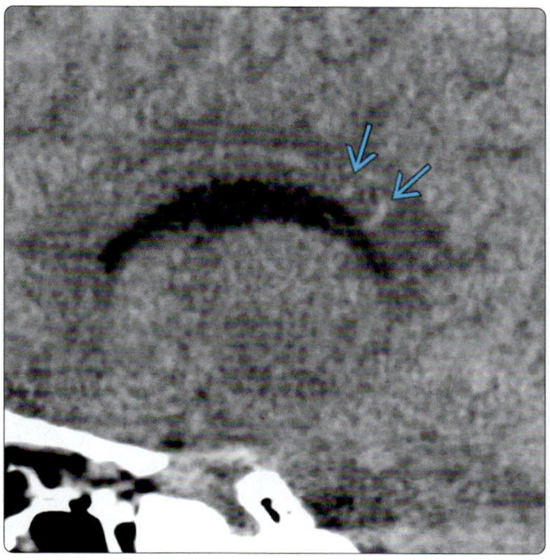

Diffuse Axonal Injury

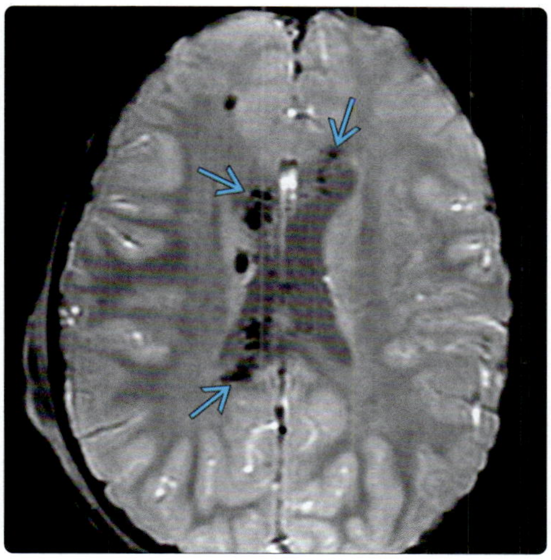

(Left) *Sagittal NECT in a 6 year old MVC victim with DAI shows small linear areas of ↑ attenuation ⇒ in the posterior body & splenium of the CC, consistent with hemorrhagic shear injury. Abnormalities on CT are typically the "tip of the iceberg," with MR usually showing more extensive injury.* **(Right)** *Axial SWI MR in the same patient shows more extensive areas of signal loss ⇒ in the CC, consistent with microhemorrhages. SWI is typically the most sensitive sequence for detecting the extent of injury.*

Diffuse Axonal Injury

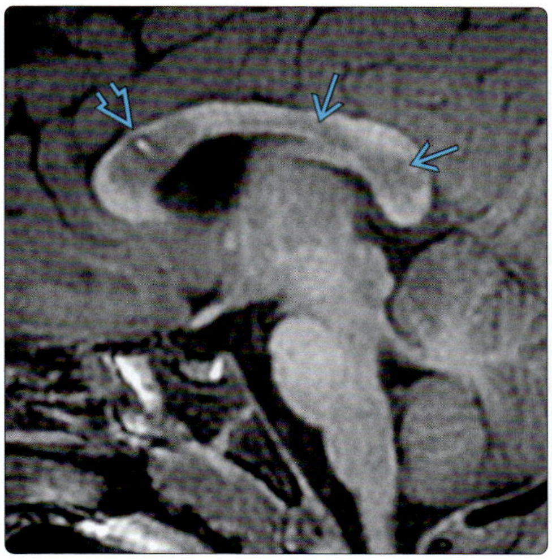

Diffuse Axonal Injury

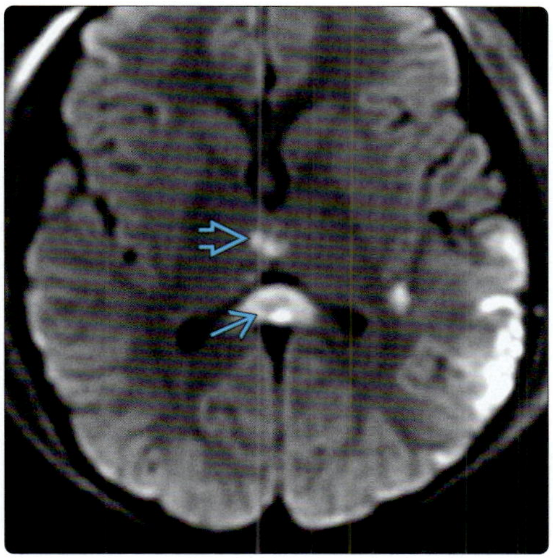

(Left) *Sagittal T1 MR in a 2 year old struck by a car shows areas of ↓ ⇒ & ↑ ⇒ signal in the CC due to DAI with hemorrhage.* **(Right)** *Axial DWI in a 6 year old who fell from a 2nd-story window shows diffusion restriction (↓ ADC not shown) in the splenium of the CC ⇒ & right thalamus ⇒. Nonhemorrhagic DAI is often most evident on the DWI sequence.*

Hypoxic-Ischemic Encephalopathy

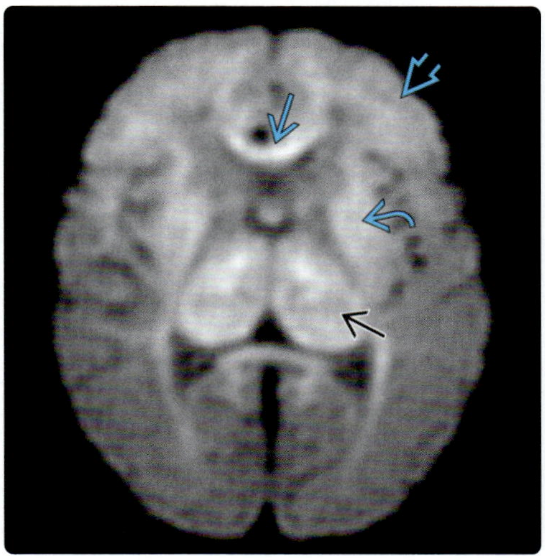

Hypoxic-Ischemic Encephalopathy

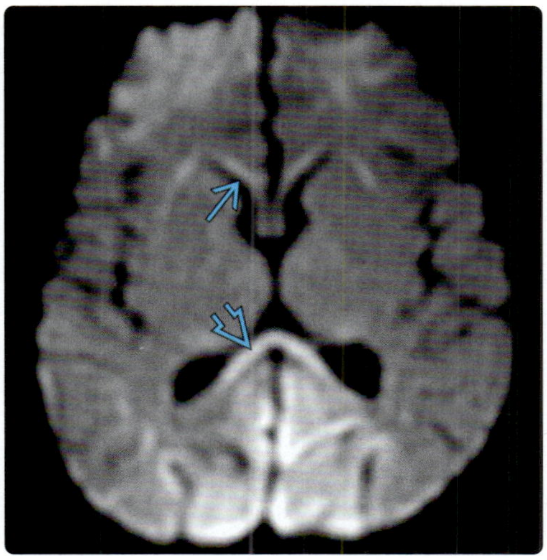

(Left) *Axial DWI MR in a 4 day old with hypoxic-ischemic encephalopathy (HIE) shows symmetric diffusion restriction (↓ ADC not shown) in the bifrontal regions ⇒, thalami ⇒, basal ganglia ⇒, & genu of the CC ⇒.* **(Right)** *Axial DWI MR in a 3 day old with HIE shows symmetric diffusion restriction (↓ ADC not shown) in the bilateral frontal & occipital watershed territories, consistent with ischemia. There is ↑ DWI signal in the genu ⇒ & splenium ⇒ of the CC, a finding thought to represent secondary neuronal injury.*

(Left) *Sagittal T2 MR in a 5 year old with neurofibromatosis type 1 (NF1) shows multiple foci of nonenhancing signal abnormality → in the body & splenium of the CC. Also note the hypothalamic mass ⇨. Look for similar signal changes in the globus pallidus, thalami, & deep cerebellum to confirm NF1.* **(Right)** *Axial DWI MR in a 2 year old with congenital heart disease shows a focal infarct in the right genu → of the CC. Restricted diffusion in the CC in children is more commonly secondary in the setting of cerebral infarctions.*

Neurofibromatosis Type 1

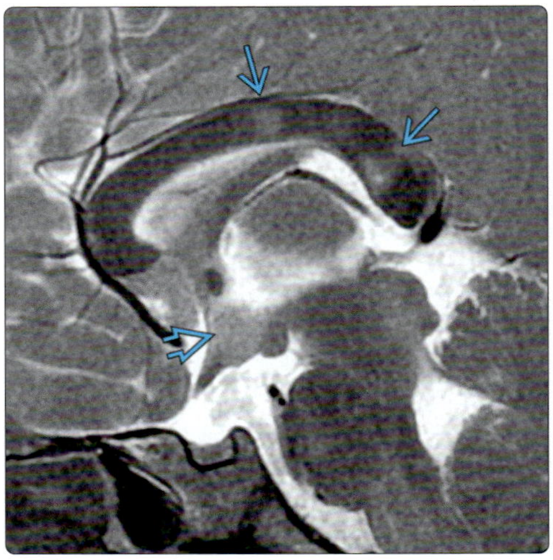

Ischemia/Infarct

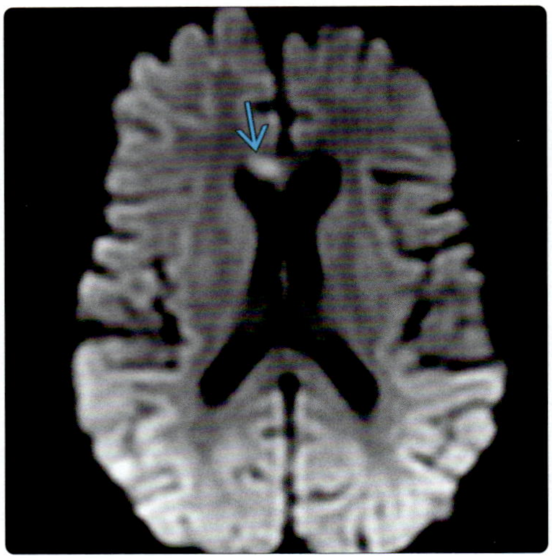

(Left) *Sagittal FLAIR MR in a 10 year old with seizures & recent withdrawal of medications for video EEG demonstrates a solitary finding of ↑ signal ⇨ in the splenium of the CC.* **(Right)** *Axial DWI MR in the same patient with a transient cytotoxic splenial lesion shows focal marked diffusion restriction (↓ ADC not shown) → in the CC splenium. Such findings typically will resolve over time without permanent imaging sequelae.*

Transient Cytotoxic Splenial Lesion

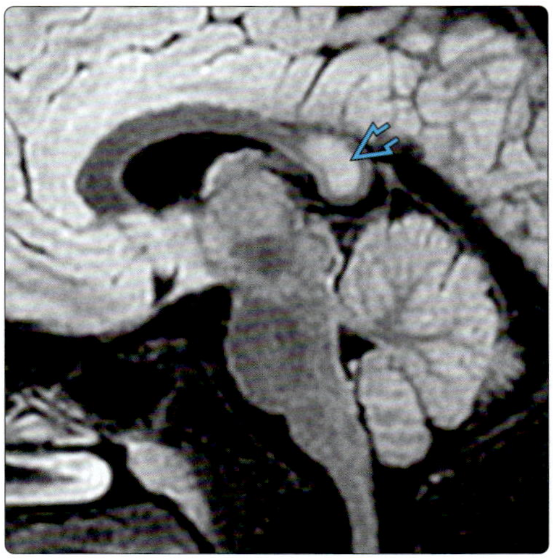

Transient Cytotoxic Splenial Lesion

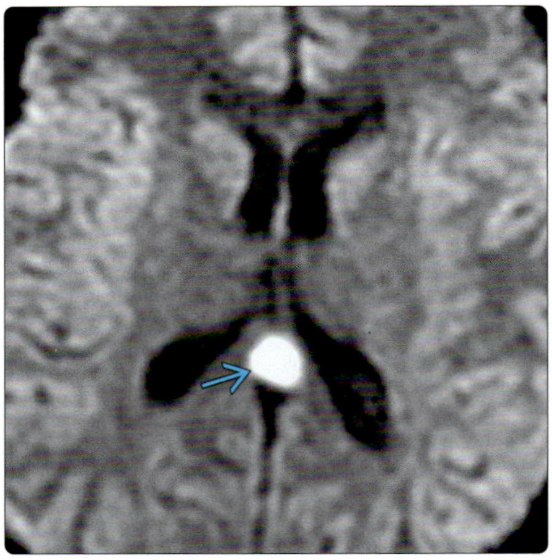

(Left) *Sagittal T2 MR in a 2 year old with Hurler syndrome shows multiple cystic spaces → within the CC & adjacent WM ⇨ due to prominent perivascular spaces. Such findings are common in the mucopolysaccharidoses.* **(Right)** *Axial FLAIR MR in the same patient shows complete suppression of the signal in the cystic spaces. Perivascular spaces should follow CSF signal on all sequences. Other than in the mucopolysaccharidoses, such findings are very rare in children.*

Perivascular Spaces

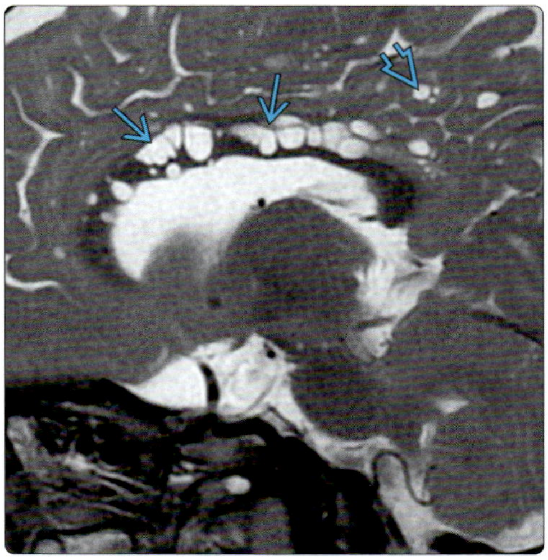

Perivascular Spaces

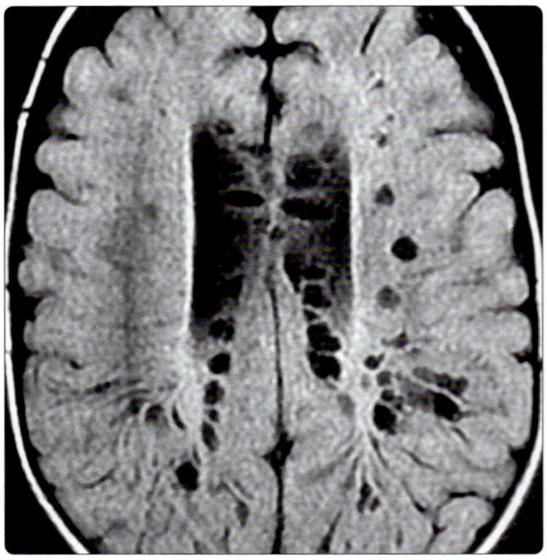

Acute Disseminated Encephalomyelitis

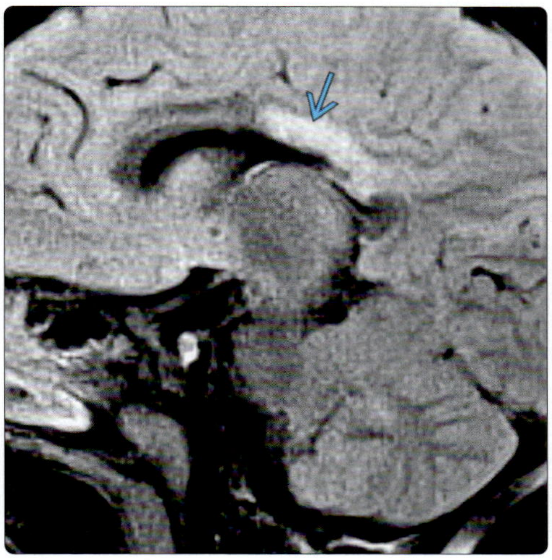

Acute Disseminated Encephalomyelitis

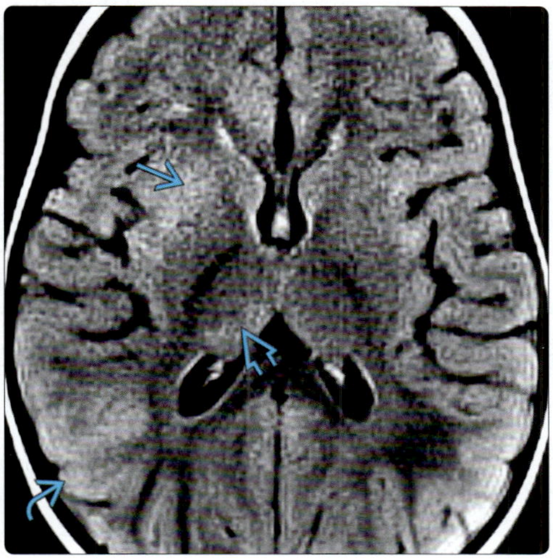

(Left) *Sagittal FLAIR MR in a 2 year old with acute disseminated encephalomyelitis (ADEM) shows confluent ↑ signal → in the posterior body of the CC. ADEM may mimic other demyelinating disorders, though involvement of the CC is much less common in ADEM as compared to MS.* **(Right)** *Axial FLAIR MR in the same patient with ADEM shows involvement of the right basal ganglia →, thalamus →, & cortical gray matter →. Gray matter involvement (often symmetric) is common in ADEM.*

Glioblastoma

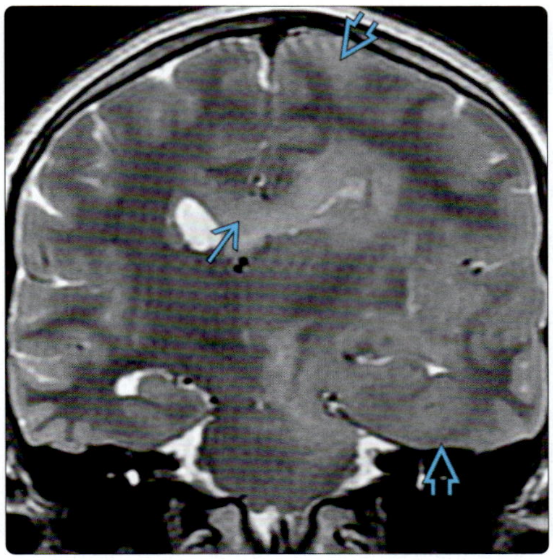

Primary CNS Lymphoma

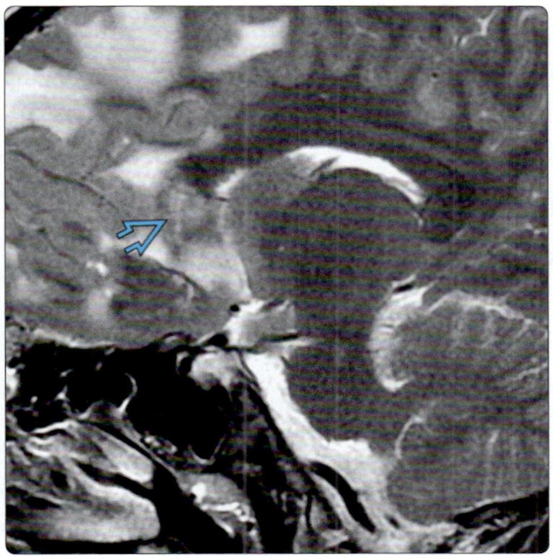

(Left) *Coronal T2 MR in a 10 year old with glioblastoma shows infiltrative & expansile ↑ signal → crossing the midline through the CC. There is involvement of most of the left cerebral hemisphere on this image, typical of gliomatosis →.* **(Right)** *Sagittal T2 MR shows expansion & ↑ signal in the rostrum & genu of the CC →, consistent with callosal infiltration/edema in this patient with CNS lymphoma.*

X-Linked Adrenoleukodystrophy

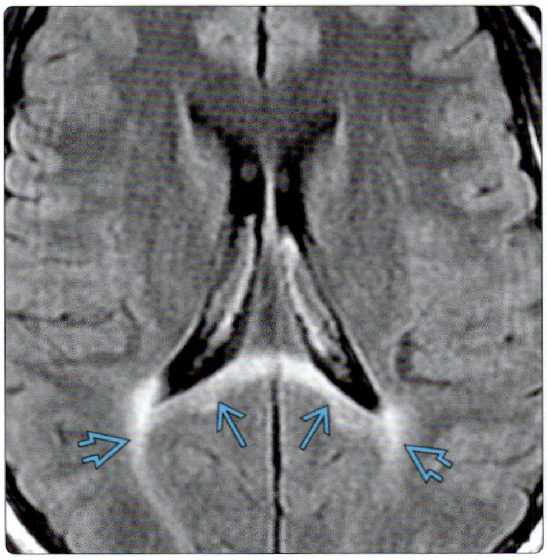

Vanishing White Matter Disease

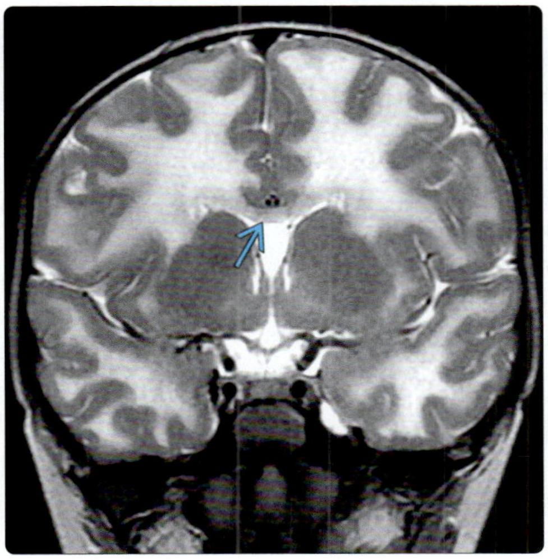

(Left) *Axial FLAIR MR in a 14-year-old boy with X-linked adrenoleukodystrophy shows symmetric posterior periventricular signal hyperintensity → that crosses the CC splenium →. This is the most common distribution of signal abnormality in X-linked adrenoleukodystrophy.* **(Right)** *Coronal T2 MR in a 19 month old with vanishing WM disease shows diffusely ↑ signal throughout the WM, including the CC →. In the acute phase, there should be no CC volume loss, though it will thin in the chronic phase.*

DIFFERENTIAL DIAGNOSIS

Common

- Brainstem Tumors
  - Diffuse Intrinsic Pontine Glioma
  - Pilocytic Astrocytoma
  - Tectal Plate Glioma

Less Common

- Tumor Mimics
  - Demyelinating Disease
  - Infection
- Dandy-Walker Malformation

Rare but Important

- Pontocerebellar Hypoplasia
- Molar Tooth Malformations/Joubert Syndrome & Related Disorders
- Pontine Tegmental Cap Dysplasia
- Congenital Muscular Dystrophy
  - Walker-Warburg Syndrome
  - Muscle-Eye-Brain Disease
  - Fukuyama Muscular Dystrophy
- Horizontal Gaze Palsy With Progressive Scoliosis
- Disconnection Syndrome
- Diencephalic-Mesencephalic Junction Dysplasia

ESSENTIAL INFORMATION

Key Differential Diagnosis Issues

- Clinical features to consider
  - Common symptoms: Cranial neuropathy, hypotonia, motor delay, nystagmus
  - Less common symptoms: Apnea, feeding difficulties, spasticity, seizures
  - Cognitive impairment is common but not universal
  - Structural eye abnormalities: Consider cobblestone malformations (e.g., muscle-eye-brain disease)
  - Specific clinical features are sometimes present
    - e.g., Joubert syndrome & related disorders (JSRD): Alternating tachypnea/apnea, polydactyly, coloboma, & renal/liver disease
  - Laboratory abnormalities may be present
    - ↑ creatine kinase: Congenital muscular dystrophies (CMDs)
  - Extreme prematurity can lead to small brainstem
- Imaging features to consider
  - Midline sagittal image is key for assessing size & morphology of brainstem
    - Allows comparison of brainstem to head/brain
    - Allows for recognition of specific morphologies
      - e.g., tegmental cap in pontine tegmental cap dysplasia (PTCD)
      - Enlargement, signal abnormality, & enhancement suggest tumor
  - Associated findings narrow differential & alter prognosis
    - Cerebellar malformations
    - Supratentorial findings
- Modality considerations
  - MR provides most detail of brainstem & associated anomalies
  - May be detected on fetal US & MR

Helpful Clues for Common Diagnoses

- **Brainstem Tumors**
  - **Diffuse intrinsic pontine glioma**
    - a.k.a. diffuse midline glioma
    - Poor prognosis (average survival ~ 1 year)
    - Centered in & expands pons; may encase basilar artery
    - CT: Pontine enlargement can be subtle
      - Effacement of cisterns & 4th ventricle
    - MR: Poorly defined ↑ T2/FLAIR signal expanding pons
      - T1 C+: Enhancement is uncommon, may be patchy
      - DWI: Diffusion restriction is rare, usually ↑ ADC
  - **Pilocytic astrocytoma**
    - Grade 1 astrocytic neoplasm
    - Usually located in medulla or ventral midbrain
    - Often exophytic
    - CT: Hypoattenuating lesion
    - MR: Well defined, ↑ T2, enhancing, ↑ ADC
  - **Tectal plate glioma**
    - Low-grade glial tumors (rarely biopsied) of tectal plate at dorsum of midbrain
    - Round mass vs. thickened tectum
    - CT: Tectal mass with obstructive hydrocephalus
    - MR: ↑ T2/FLAIR tectal mass, usually without enhancement
    - Typically indolent; treated with 3rd ventriculostomy

Helpful Clues for Less Common Diagnoses

- **Tumor Mimics**
  - **Demyelinating disease**
    - Multiple sclerosis, acute disseminated encephalomyelitis, neuromyelitis optica, osmotic demyelination
    - MR: May mimic tumors in acute phase with ↑ T2/FLAIR & mass effect
      - Suggestive features of demyelination: Incomplete faint rim enhancement; additional white matter (WM) lesions
  - **Infection**
    - Encephalitis > cerebritis, abscess
      - Encephalitis: Requires correlation with CSF analysis ± serial imaging
      - Abscess: May be associated with mastoiditis/skull base infection; look for rim enhancement with central ↑ DWI/↓ ADC on MR
- **Dandy-Walker Malformation**
  - Classic Dandy-Walker malformation is characterized by
    - Marked vermian hypoplasia
    - Elevation of tentorium/torcular Herophili
    - Dilated, cystic 4th ventricle
  - Hydrocephalus is common; ± other anomalies (including pontine hypoplasia)

Helpful Clues for Rare Diagnoses

- **Pontocerebellar Hypoplasia**
  - Heterogeneous group of inherited neurodegenerative disorders
  - ≥ 10 subtypes with various phenotypes & genotypes
    - Classified based on associated imaging findings, clinical features, gene mutations

- e.g., type 3: Optic atrophy (7q11-21)
- e.g., type 6: ↑ lactate in CSF
- e.g., type 9: Agenesis of corpus callosum

- Prematurity may cause pontocerebellar hypoplasia
  - Diagnosis made after excluding genetic cause

- **Molar Tooth Malformations/Joubert Syndrome & Related Disorders**
  - At least 6 subtypes of JSRD
    - Determined by clinical features & genotype
    - All are ciliopathies, resulting in extra-CNS disease
      - e.g., renal (nephronophthisis), hepatic fibrosis, ocular colobomas, & polydactyly
    - All share imaging phenotype
      - Horizontal, thickened, & elongated superior cerebellar peduncles
      - Vermian hypoplasia, rostral dysmorphic fastigium
      - Clefting of superior vermis
- **Pontine Tegmental Cap Dysplasia**
  - Sporadic malformation with unknown genotype
  - Clinical features: Hearing loss, facial paralysis, trigeminal anesthesia, difficulty swallowing
  - Imaging features: Elevated pontine tegmentum ("cap"), flat ventral pons, partial absence of middle cerebellar peduncles, vermian hypoplasia
- **Congenital Muscular Dystrophy**
  - Heterogeneous disorders characterized by dystrophic muscle
  - Subset of CMD have associated brain anomalies
  - Significant overlap in imaging findings between subtypes
    - Small & malformed brainstem
    - Cerebral cortical dysplasia
    - Cerebellar dysplasia ± subcortical cysts
  - **Walker-Warburg syndrome**
    - Myopathy ± eye disease
    - Imaging findings
      - Z-shaped brainstem
      - Type II ("cobblestone") lissencephaly
      - Cerebellar polymicrogyria ± subcortical cysts
  - **Muscle-eye-brain disease**
    - Myopathy + eye disease + brain malformations
    - Imaging findings
      - Pontine & vermian hypoplasia
      - Cerebral pachygyria/polymicrogyria (PMG)
      - Cerebellar polymicrogyria ± subcortical cysts
  - **Fukuyama disease**
    - Occurs almost exclusively in Japanese
    - Hypotonia & myopathy at birth
    - Imaging findings
      - Pontine hypoplasia
      - Type II ("cobblestone") lissencephaly
      - Cerebellar polymicrogyria ± subcortical cysts
- **Horizontal Gaze Palsy With Progressive Scoliosis**
  - Rare autosomal recessive disorder (mutation in *ROBO3)*
  - Absent horizontal eye movements + childhood scoliosis
  - Imaging findings
    - Hypoplastic pons with dorsal midline cleft
    - Butterfly-shaped medulla
    - Absent corticospinal tract decussation
- **Disconnection Syndrome**
  - Brainstem malformation of segmental dysgenesis
  - Imaging findings
    - Brainstem disconnection at pontomesencephalic or pontomedullary junctions
    - Usually with associated cerebellar hypoplasia
- **Diencephalic-Mesencephalic Junction Dysplasia**
  - Ill-defined junction between diencephalon & midbrain
  - ↓ rostrocaudal axis, ↑ dorsoventral axis of midbrain
  - Ventral cleft in midbrain contiguous with 3rd ventricle

SELECTED REFERENCES

1. Brandão LA et al: Posterior fossa tumors. Neuroimaging Clin N Am. 27(1):1-37, 2017
2. Bosemani T et al: Congenital abnormalities of the posterior fossa. Radiographics. 35(1):200-20, 2015
3. Chapman T et al: Diagnostic imaging of posterior fossa anomalies in the fetus and neonate: part 2, posterior fossa disorders. Clin Imaging. 39(2):167-75, 2015
4. Chapman T et al: Diagnostic imaging of posterior fossa anomalies in the fetus and neonate: part 1, normal anatomy and classification of anomalies. Clin Imaging. 39(1):1-8, 2015

Diffuse Intrinsic Pontine Glioma

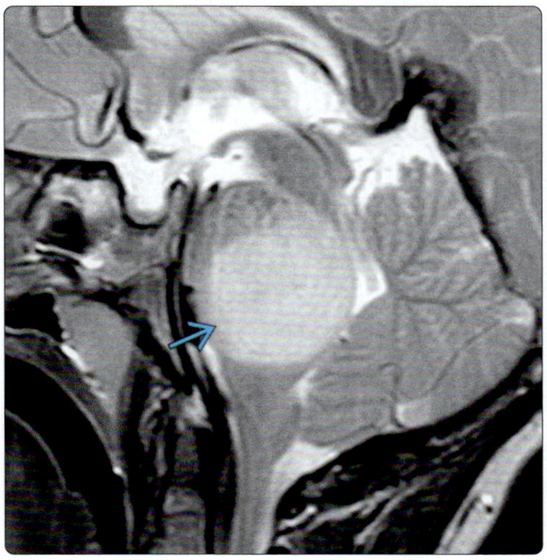

Pilocytic Astrocytoma

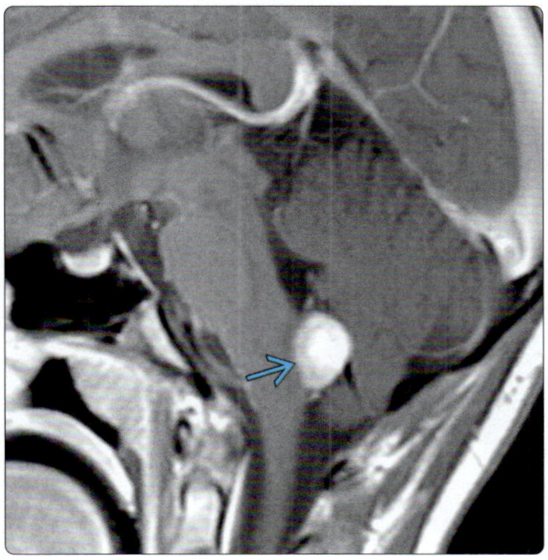

(Left) *Sagittal T2 MR in a 7 year old with a diffuse intrinsic pontine glioma shows an expansile hyperintense mass* ➔ *centered in the pons, a typical appearance for this tumor. There is typically little enhancement of this mass.* **(Right)** *Sagittal T1 C+ MR in an 11 year old with a pilocytic astrocytoma shows an avidly enhancing lesion* ➔ *extending exophytically from the dorsal medulla. The location & enhancement is typical for a pilocytic astrocytoma.*

(Left) *Sagittal T2 MR in a 16 year old with a tectal plate glioma shows a well-defined hyperintense lesion ➲ in the midbrain tectum (tectal plate). Such lesions typically cause obstructive hydrocephalus. They usually have an indolent course & are treated with endoscopic 3rd ventriculostomy.* **(Right)** *Axial T1 C+ FS MR in a 3 year old with demyelinating disease shows an expansile lesion ➲ of the right cerebral peduncle with an incomplete ring of enhancement. Always consider demyelination as a mimic for tumors.*

Tectal Plate Glioma

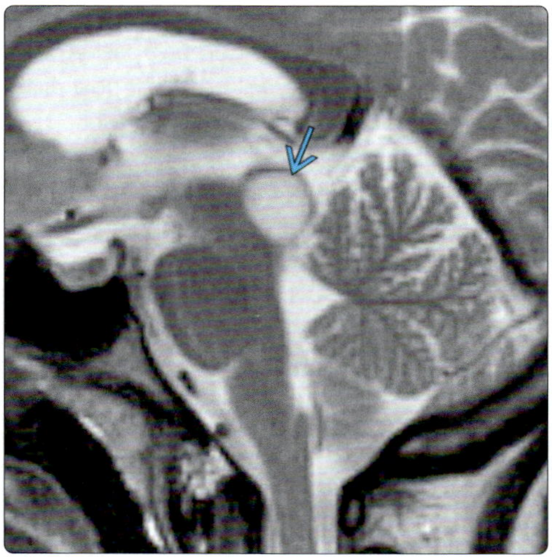

Demyelinating Disease

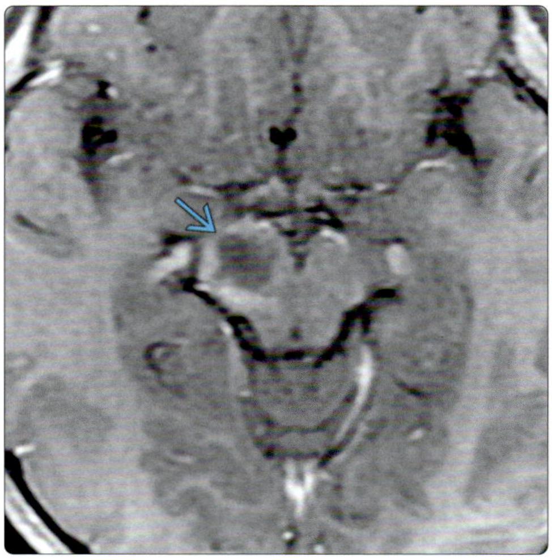

(Left) *Sagittal 3D SSFP MR in a neonate with Dandy-Walker malformation (DWM) shows a small pons ➲ with indentation of the dorsal pons ➲ & communication of the 4th ventricle with a large posterior fossa cyst ➡. Note the associated callosal agenesis ➲.* **(Right)** *Sagittal T1 MR in a 10 year old with a MAST1 gene mutation shows hypoplasia of the pons ➲ & cerebellum ➲. Note the associated thinning of the posterior corpus callosum ➲. Pontocerebellar hypoplasia is seen in many disorders.*

Dandy-Walker Malformation

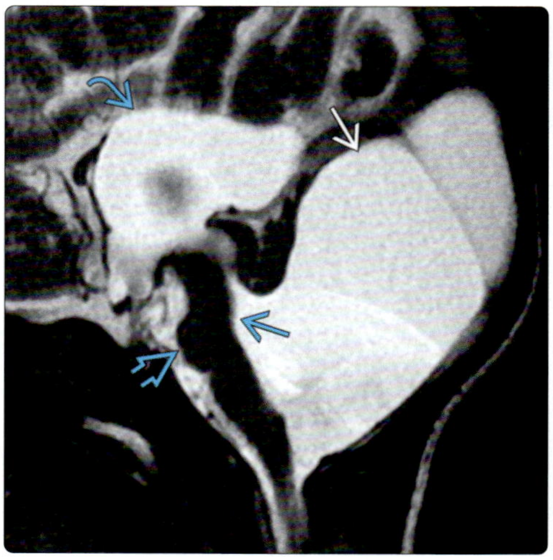

Pontocerebellar Hypoplasia

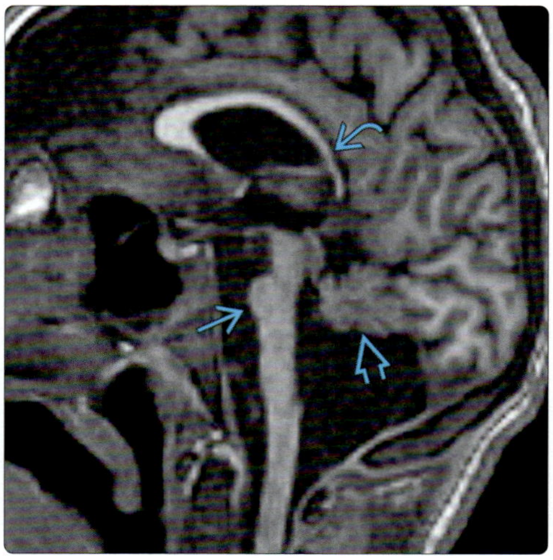

(Left) *Midline sagittal T2 MR in a 2 day old with a molar tooth sign (not shown) demonstrates rostral deviation of the 4th ventricle fastigium ➲, vermian hypoplasia ➲, & an abnormal pontomedullary junction ➲.* **(Right)** *Axial T2 MR in a 13 year old with a molar tooth sign shows typical horizontally oriented & thickened superior cerebellar peduncles ➲ with a prominent anterior midbrain cleft ➲. Also note the vermian hypoplasia. A more superior slice (not shown) demonstrated vermian clefting.*

Molar Tooth Malformations/Joubert Syndrome & Related Disorders

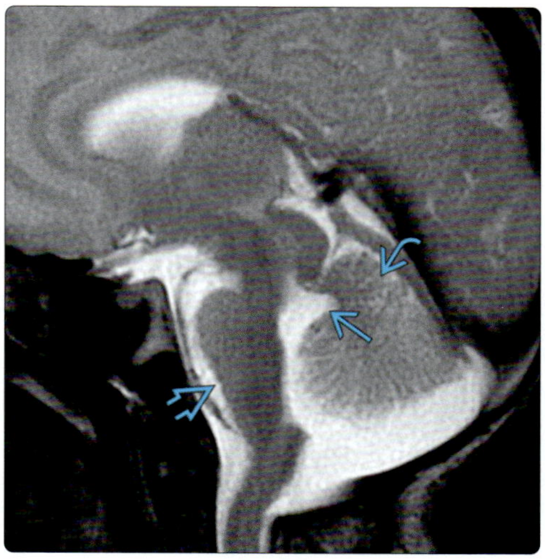

Molar Tooth Malformations/Joubert Syndrome & Related Disorders

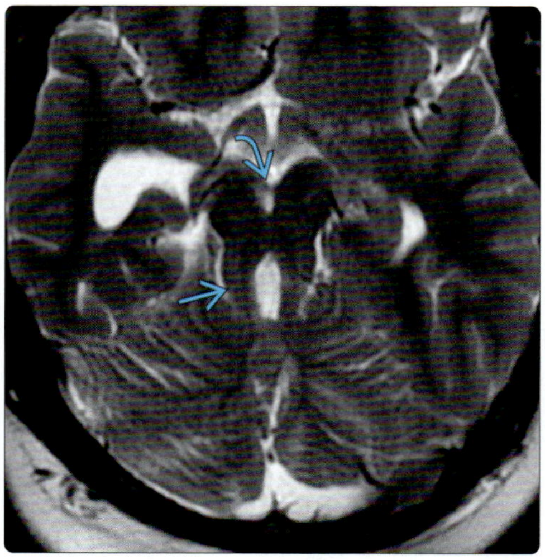

Pontine Tegmental Cap Dysplasia

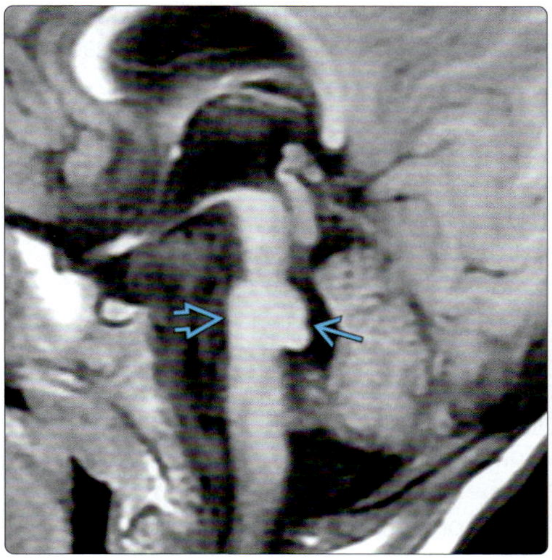

Congenital Muscular Dystrophy

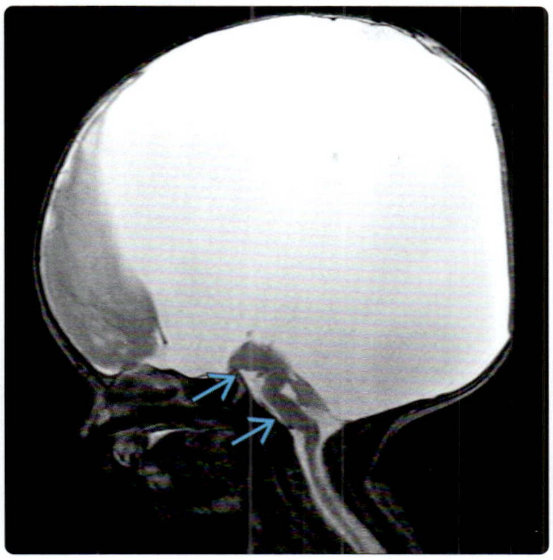

(Left) *Sagittal T1 MR in a 14 month old with swallowing difficulties shows an elevated pontine tegmentum ("cap") → & flattening of the ventral pons ⇨, a pathognomic appearance for pontine tegmental cap dyplasia (PTCD).* **(Right)** *Sagittal T2 MR in a 7 day old with the Walker-Warburg type of CMD shows the characteristic Z-shaped brainstem →. The cerebellar vermis is hypoplastic, & the ventricles are enlarged secondary to aqueductal stenosis. "Cobblestone" lissencephaly was seen on other images.*

Congenital Muscular Dystrophy

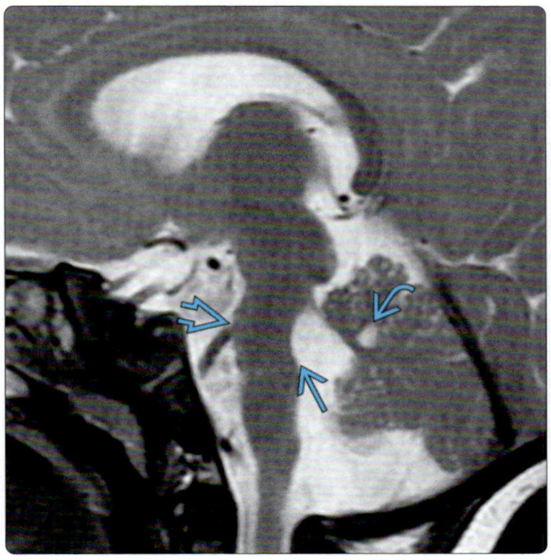

Congenital Muscular Dystrophy

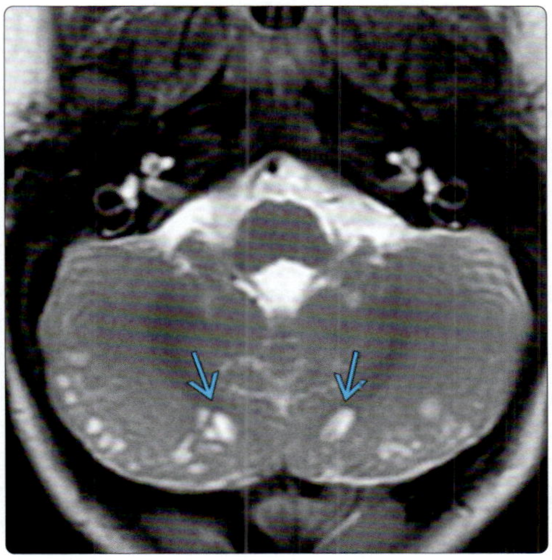

(Left) *Sagittal T2 MR in a 7 month old with suspected CMD shows marked pontine hypoplasia with flattening of the ventral pons ⇨ & a dorsal impression → in the pontine tegmentum. Note the small cerebellar cyst ↪.* **(Right)** *Axial T2 MR in the same patient shows nearly symmetric cerebellar cysts →. Cerebellar cysts may be the most specific imaging finding for CMD when the combination of an abnormal brainstem & cerebral cortical malformation is encountered.*

Congenital Muscular Dystrophy

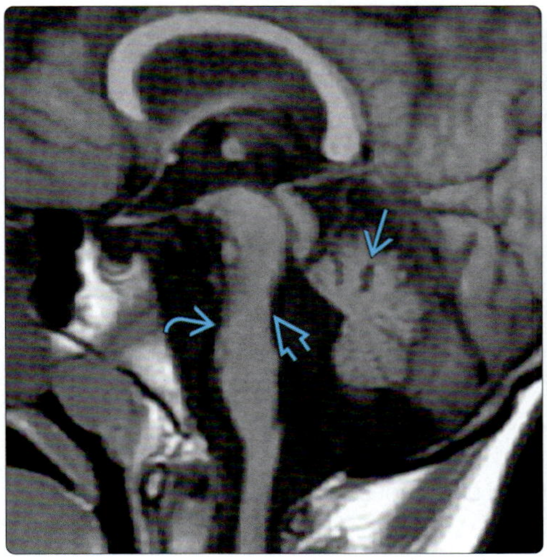

Congenital Muscular Dystrophy

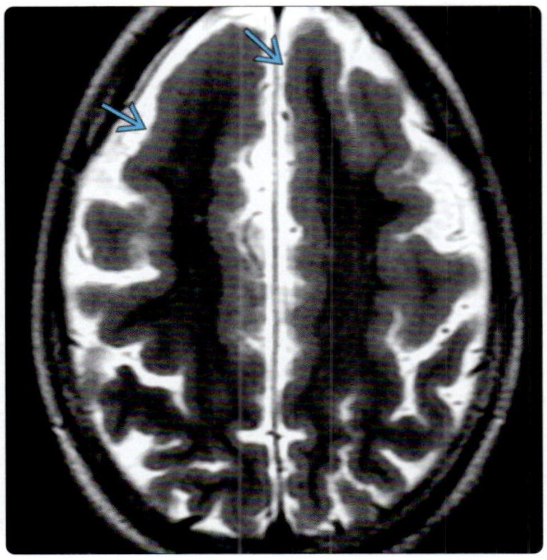

(Left) *Sagittal T1 MR in a 14 year old with muscle-eye-brain disease shows marked hypoplasia of the pons with a flat ventral pons ↪ & a dorsal impression ⇨. Note the small cerebellar cyst →. Pontine hypoplasia is a common finding among the CMDs with CNS involvement.* **(Right)** *Axial T2 MR in the same patient shows symmetric cortical micronodularity & thickening in the bilateral frontal lobes →, consistent with cobblestone lissencephaly (type II lissencephaly), a typical finding in CMD.*

DIFFERENTIAL DIAGNOSIS

Common

- Chiari 1 Malformation
- Chiari 2 Malformation

Less Common

- Cerebellar Hypoplasia
- Cerebellar Dysplasias (Unclassified)
- Dandy-Walker Continuum

Rare but Important

- Rhombencephalosynapsis
- Molar Tooth Malformations (Joubert Syndrome)
- Chiari 3 Malformation

ESSENTIAL INFORMATION

Helpful Clues for Common Diagnoses

- **Chiari 1 Malformation**
  - Caudal protrusion of pointed cerebellar tonsils below foramen magnum (FM)
    - Underdeveloped bony posterior fossa → downward hindbrain herniation
    - Rarely develops over time (rather than congenital); rarely resolves without treatment
  - Imaging: Cerebellar tonsils are low & pointed
    - CSF at FM is effaced
    - Small bony posterior fossa
    - ± syrinx, presyrinx edema, or ventriculomegaly
    - ± short clivus, dorsal tilt of dens, craniovertebral anomalies
- **Chiari 2 Malformation**
  - ~ 100% association with open neural tube defect (myelomeningocele > myelocele/myeloschisis)
  - Imaging: Caudal herniation of cerebellum & brainstem
    - "Cascade" or "waterfall" herniation of tissue downward, behind medulla
      - "Peg" = uvula/nodulus/pyramid of vermis
      - Cervicomedullary "kink" (70%)
      - "Towering" cerebellum through incisura → compressed midbrain, associated "beaked" tectum
      - 4th ventricle is small & elongated, without fastigium
    - Small posterior fossa
    - Low insertion of tentorium/torcular
    - Large funnel-shaped FM
    - ± syringohydromyelia (20-90%)
    - ± corpus callosum dysgenesis (90%)
    - ± posterior arch C1 anomalies, diastematomyelia, Klippel-Feil syndrome
    - ± aqueduct stenosis, gray matter (GM) heterotopia, absent septum pellucidum/fused forniceal columns, stenogyria
    - Lacunar skull (lückenschädel) = inner table calvarial undulations
      - Usually resolves by 6 months of age

Helpful Clues for Less Common Diagnoses

- **Cerebellar Hypoplasia**
  - Inherited or acquired; isolated or syndromic
    - Present in ~ 25% of patients with PHACE syndrome
  - Imaging: Isolated small cerebellar hemisphere(s) with normal fissures & interfoliate sulci
    - + brainstem hypoplasia = pontocerebellar hypoplasia
    - ± vermian hypoplasia, abnormal fissures, cortical dysplasia
    - ± Dandy-Walker spectrum, molar tooth syndromes, rhombencephalosynapsis, periventricular nodular heterotopia
    - Presence of gliosis suggests atrophy rather than congenital hypoplasia
      - Volume loss → enlarged cerebellar fissures/interfoliate sulci
- **Cerebellar Dysplasias (Unclassified)**
  - Focal or diffuse dysplasias of cerebellar hemispheres &/or vermis not associated with other known malformations or syndrome
    - Some may be related to tubulin mutations
  - Imaging: Variety of hemisphere &/or vermis abnormalities
    - Abnormal orientation of fissures & lobules
    - Disoriented foliation
    - Abnormal arborization of cerebellar white matter
    - Cerebellar GM heterotopia
    - Enlarged & vertically oriented fissures
    - Diffuse dysplasias are usually associated with supratentorial anomalies
      - Congenital muscular dystrophies
      - Lissencephalies
      - Polymicrogyria
- **Dandy-Walker Continuum**
  - Continuum (most severe to least) = "classic" Dandy-Walker malformation (DWM) > vermian hypoplasia > Blake pouch cyst (BPC) > mega cisterna magna (MCM)
    - Intelligence normal in up to 50% of "classic" DWM cases
    - Present in up to 10% of patients with PHACE syndrome
  - Imaging
    - "Classic" DWM
      - Cystic dilation of 4th ventricle → large posterior fossa, torcular-lambdoid inversion, superiorly rotated hypoplastic vermis
      - ± hydrocephalus
    - Vermian hypoplasia
      - ± upward rotation
      - Normal-sized posterior fossa & brainstem
    - BPC: Normal Blake pouch fails (along with foramen of Luschka) to fenestrate in utero → herniation of inferior 4th ventricle cyst into vallecula & retrovermian cistern
      - Enhancing choroid plexus along inferior surface of vermis in superior aspect of cyst wall
      - Elevated tegmento-vermian angle
      - Rotated but normal vermis
      - Cyst wall often not seen on imaging study
    - MCM
      - Cistern crossed by falx cerebelli
      - Enlarged cisterns communicate with basal subarachnoid spaces
      - Normal vermis/4th ventricle

- ± associated callosal anomalies, cortical dysplasia, GM heterotopia
- Imaging may have difficulty distinguishing mild DWM, BPC, & MCM

Helpful Clues for Rare Diagnoses

- **Rhombencephalosynapsis**
  - Congenital fusion of cerebellar hemispheres, dentate nuclei, & superior cerebellar peduncles
  - Imaging: Complete or partial fusion of hemispheres
    - Transversely oriented continuous folia on axial & coronal images
    - Continuous white matter tracts crossing midline
    - Absent primary fissure & no normal fastigial point
    - Small diamond- or keyhole-shaped 4th ventricle on axial images
    - Fused horseshoe-shaped dentate nuclei
    - Absent posterior cerebellar notch & vallecula
    - Absent or severely hypoplastic vermis
    - ± absent septum pellucidum, olivary hypoplasia, anomalies of limbic system, multiple cranial suture synostoses
    - ± corpus callosum dysgenesis, cerebral cortical dysplasia
    - ± aqueductal stenosis → hydrocephalus
- **Molar Tooth Malformations (Joubert Syndrome)**
  - Joubert anomaly is prototype
    - Joubert syndrome & related disorders (JSRD) considered as ciliopathy
      - > 20 causative genes discovered so far, all encoding proteins expressed in primary cilia & its apparatus
    - Classic Joubert syndrome patients present with episodic hyperpnea, abnormal eye movements, ataxia, & mental retardation
    - Identical imaging findings are seen in some patients without classic Joubert syndrome symptoms
      - ± renal or ocular anomalies, hepatic fibrosis/cysts, hypothalamic anomalies
  - Imaging
    - "Molar tooth" = large superior cerebellar peduncles on axial images
      - Also on axial images: Small dysplastic vermis → triangular mid-4th ventricle & "bat wing" superior 4th ventricle
    - Sagittal: Small, high cerebellar vermis
    - Coronal: "Split vermis" secondary to sagittal cleft
    - DTI: Superior cerebellar peduncles fail to decussate in mesencephalon
      - ± thinning of middle cerebellar peduncle, ventral pontocerebellar tracts
- **Chiari 3 Malformation**
  - Extremely rare; Chiari 2 malformation + high- to mid-cervical cephalocele, which contains cerebellum
    - Controversy: May actually be high cervical myelocystocele rather than Chiari malformation
  - Imaging: Craniocervical junction or high cervical cephalocele contains meninges, cerebellum ± brainstem, cisterns, 4th ventricle, &/or dural sinuses
    - ± hydrocephalus
    - ± intracranial Chiari 2 findings

SELECTED REFERENCES

1. Romaniello R et al: Tubulin-related cerebellar dysplasia: definition of a distinct pattern of cerebellar malformation. Eur Radiol. 27(12):5080-92, 2017
2. Cotes C et al: Congenital basis of posterior fossa anomalies. Neuroradiol J. 28(3):238-53, 2015
3. Oegema R et al: Recognizable cerebellar dysplasia associated with mutations in multiple tubulin genes. Hum Mol Genet. 24(18):5313-25, 2015
4. Poretti A et al: Cerebellar hypoplasia: differential diagnosis and diagnostic approach. Am J Med Genet C Semin Med Genet. 166(2):211-26, 2014
5. Sattar S et al: The ciliopathies in neuronal development: a clinical approach to investigation of Joubert syndrome and Joubert syndrome-related disorders. Dev Med Child Neurol. 53(9):793-8, 2011

Chiari 1 Malformation

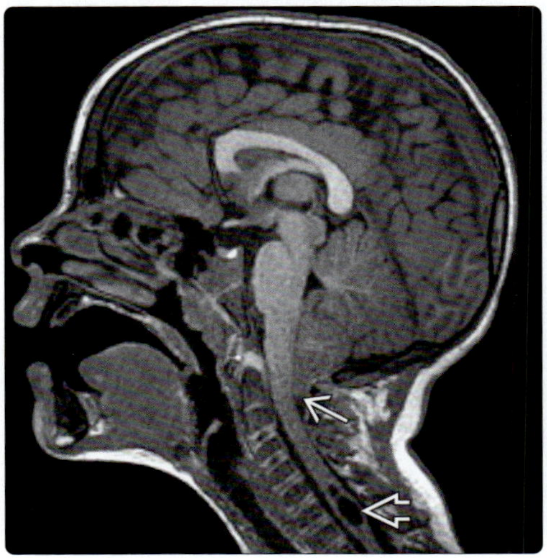

Chiari 1 Malformation

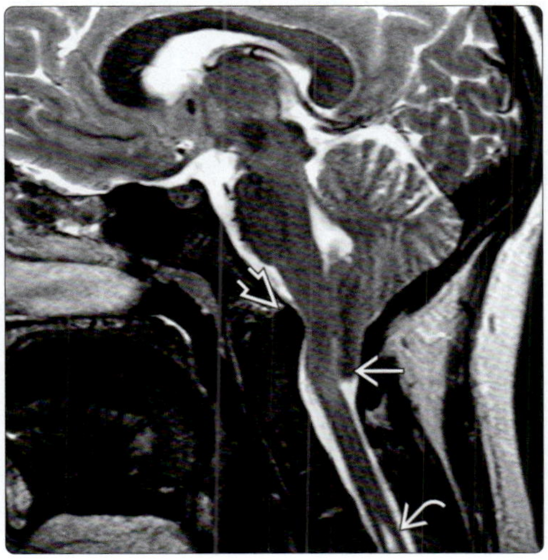

(Left) *Sagittal T1 MR in a 4 year old with seizures shows an unsuspected Chiari 1 malformation with significant inferior displacement & pointed configuration of the cerebellar tonsils ➡. There is associated effacement of CSF at the foramen magnum with a multiloculated cervicothoracic syrinx ➡.* **(Right)** *Sagittal T2 MR shows a pointed, low-lying cerebellar tonsil ➡, effacement of CSF at the foramen magnum, dorsally tilted dens ➡, small posterior fossa, & small lower cervical syrinx ➡.*

(Left) *Sagittal T1 MR in a child with prior myelomeningocele repair demonstrates classic features of Chiari 2 malformation, including a small posterior fossa with inferior herniation of the brainstem, cerebellum, & small 4th ventricle. There is also mild tectal beaking & severe crowding at the foramen magnum.* **(Right)** *Sagittal T2 MR shows a low-lying cerebellar "peg", "beaked" tectum, cervicomedullary "kink", small posterior fossa with low tentorial insertion, & dysplastic corpus callosum.*

Chiari 2 Malformation

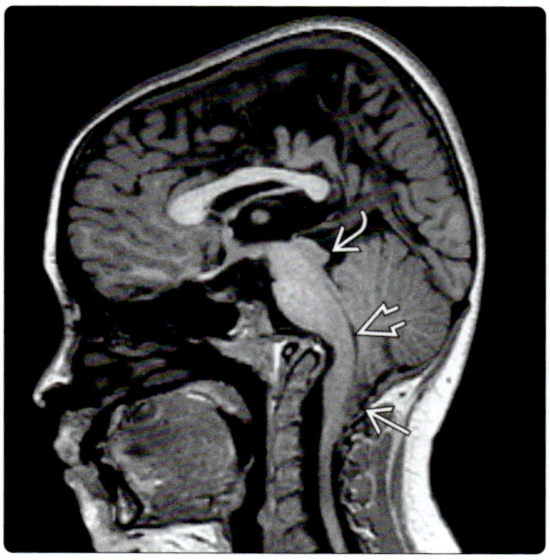

Chiari 2 Malformation

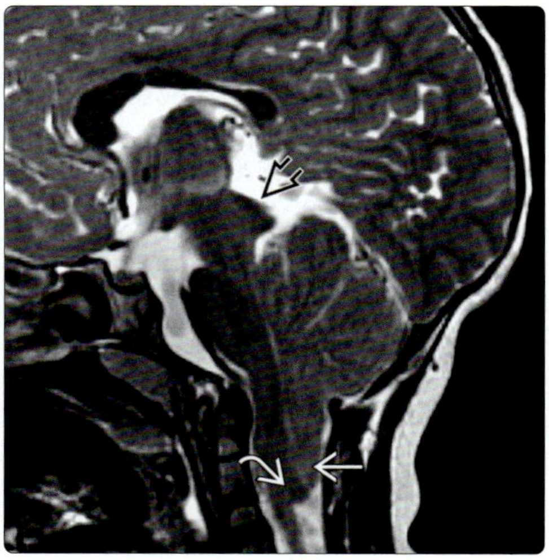

(Left) *Coronal T1 MR shows a small right cerebellar hemisphere secondary to congenital hypoplasia.* **(Right)** *Axial T1 C+ FS MR in a 1 year old with large facial infantile hemangiomas demonstrates right cerebellar hypoplasia & a right cerebellopontine angle/internal auditory canal infantile hemangioma, typical of a subset of children with PHACE syndrome.*

Cerebellar Hypoplasia

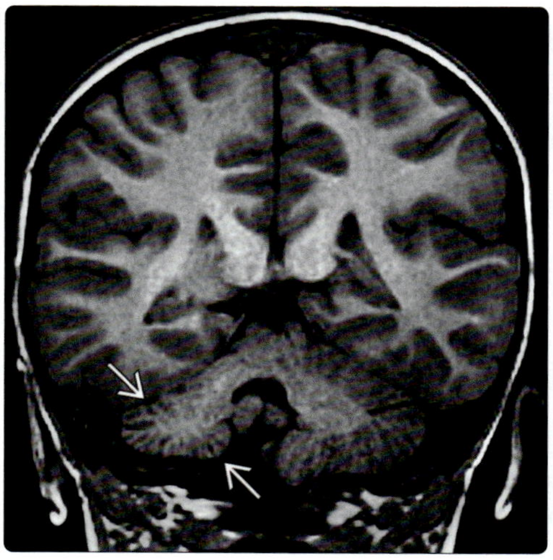

Cerebellar Hypoplasia

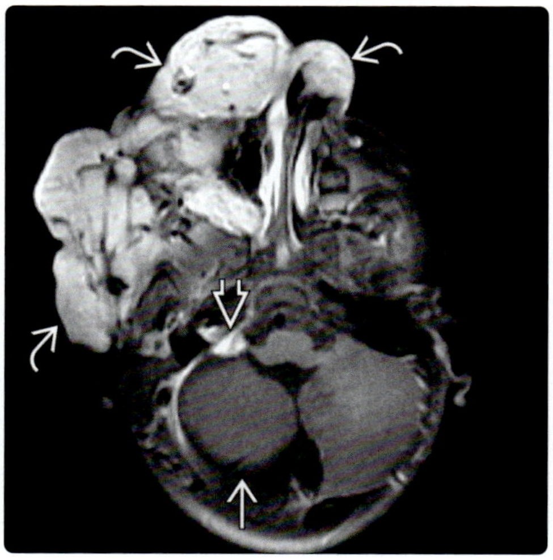

(Left) *Axial T2 MR shows a hypoplastic & dysplastic right cerebellar hemisphere with abnormal orientation of the cerebellar folia & irregular gray-white matter junctions.* **(Right)** *Sagittal T1 MR shows cystic dilation of the 4th ventricle with a markedly enlarged posterior fossa, torcular/lambdoid inversion, & a severely hypoplastic, superiorly rotated cerebellar vermis. The brainstem is compressed in this classic Dandy-Walker malformation.*

Cerebellar Dysplasias (Unclassified)

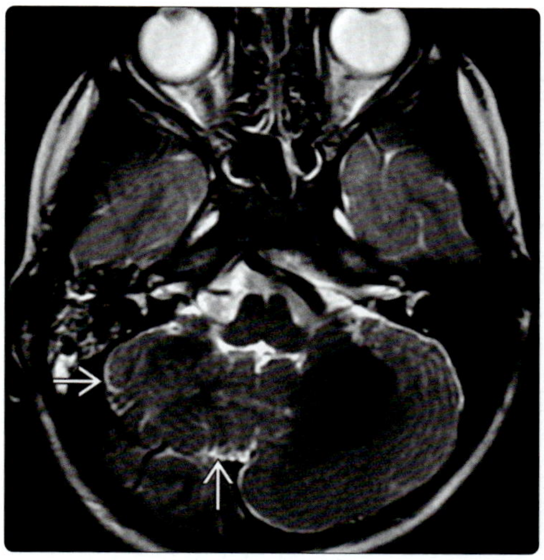

Dandy-Walker Continuum

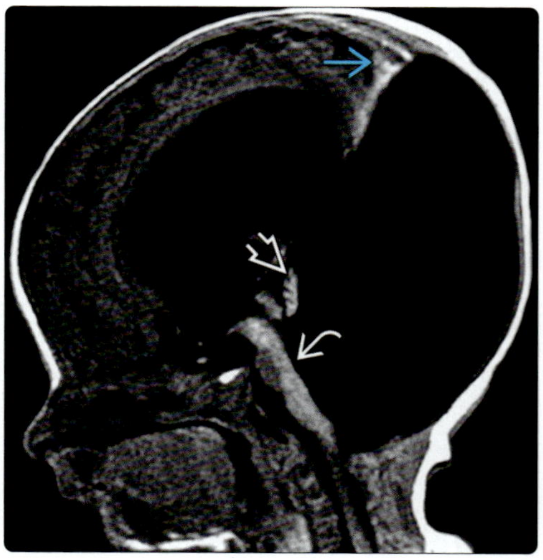

Dandy-Walker Continuum

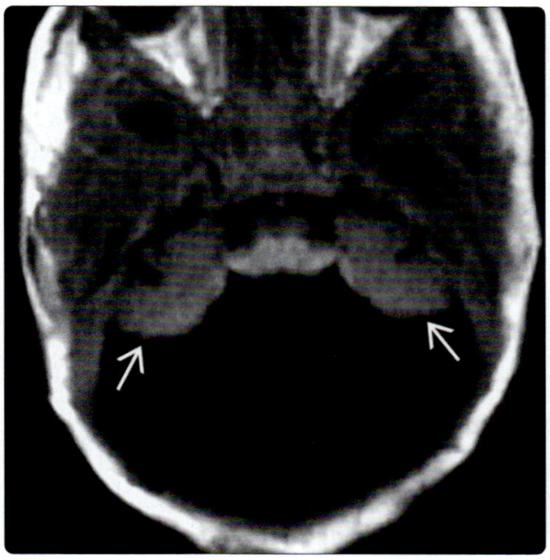

Dandy-Walker Continuum

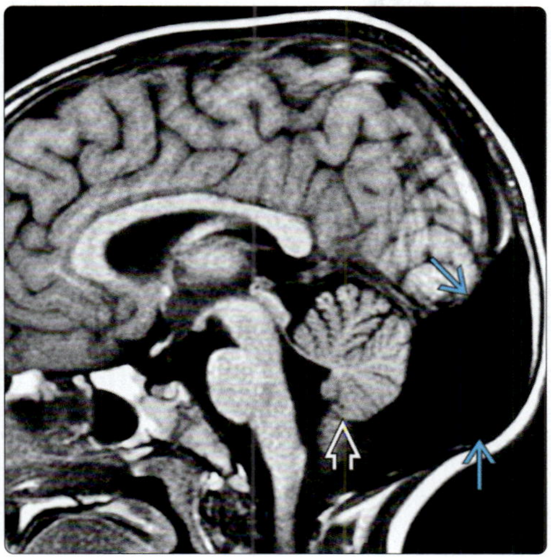

(Left) *Axial T1 MR in the same patient shows continuity of the cyst with the 4th ventricle. Note the hypoplastic cerebellar hemispheres pushed superiorly & laterally by the cyst.* **(Right)** *Sagittal T1 MR shows a prominent retrocerebellar CSF collection dorsal to a normal vermis with mild enlargement of the posterior fossa due to a mega cisterna magna (MCM) vs. arachnoid cyst. Subsequent cisternogram (not shown) demonstrated rapid communication of injected contrast, consistent with MCM.*

Rhombencephalosynapsis

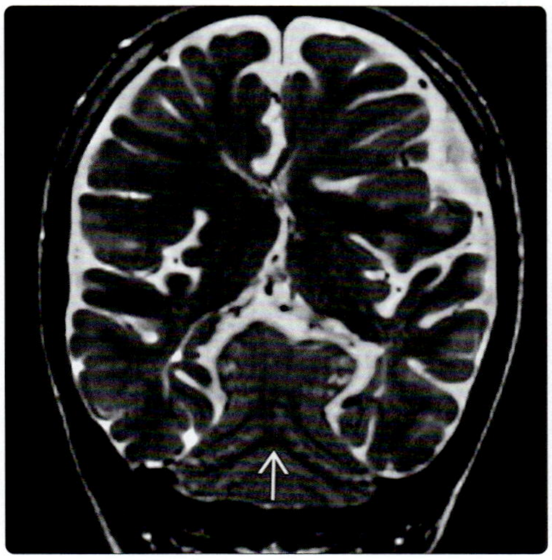

Rhombencephalosynapsis

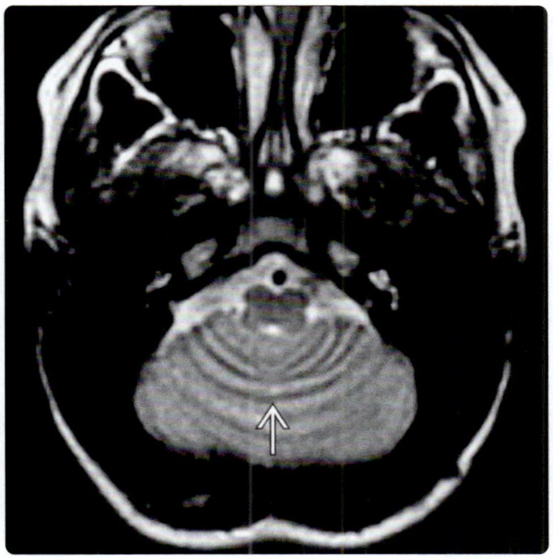

(Left) *Coronal T2 MR shows fusion of the cerebellar hemispheres with continuous white matter tracts crossing the midline without an intervening vermis.* **(Right)** *Axial T2 MR shows fusion of the cerebellar hemispheres with continuous white matter tracts crossing the midline. There is no intervening vermis. Note that the folia are horizontal. These patients typically have a small, keyhole-shaped 4th ventricle & may have associated callosal dysgenesis, cerebral cortical dysplasia, or hydrocephalus.*

Molar Tooth Malformations (Joubert Syndrome)

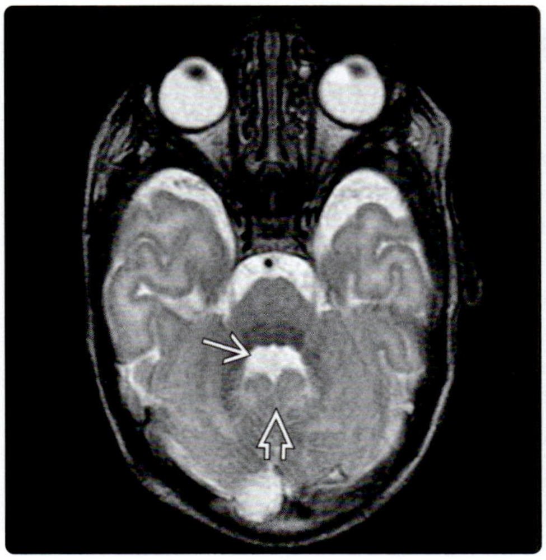

Molar Tooth Malformations (Joubert Syndrome)

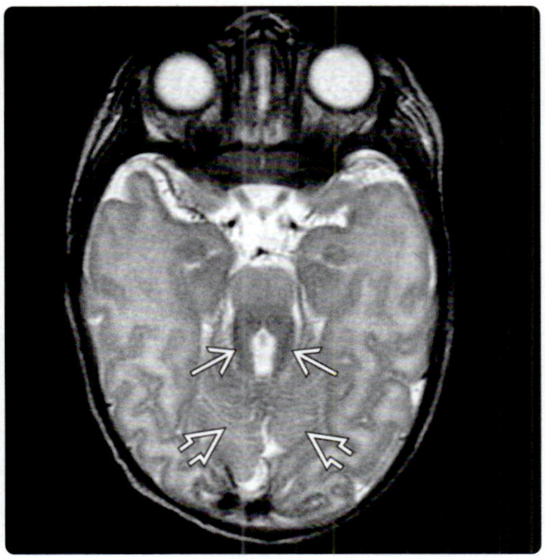

(Left) *Axial T2 MR in an infant with Joubert syndrome shows the classic "bat wing" 4th ventricle with a midline vermian sagittal cleft.* **(Right)** *Axial T2 MR in the same patient demonstrates the classic molar tooth appearance of the brainstem secondary to large superior cerebellar peduncles appearing as the molar roots. Note also the dysplastic, disorganized appearance of the cerebellum.*

DIFFERENTIAL DIAGNOSIS

Common

- Pineal Ca^{2+}
- Choroid Plexus Ca^{2+}
- Tuberous Sclerosis Complex

Less Common

- Congenital TORCH Infections
  - Congenital CMV
  - Congenital Toxoplasmosis
  - Congenital Herpes Encephalitis
  - Congenital HIV
  - Congenital Rubella
  - Other
- Postnatal Infections
  - Neurocysticercosis
  - Tuberculosis
  - Ventriculitis (Chronic)
- Vascular Malformations
  - Sturge-Weber Syndrome
  - Arteriovenous Malformations
  - Dural Arteriovenous Fistula
  - Cavernous Malformation
- Tumors
- Dural Ca^{2+}

Rare but Important

- Radiation & Chemotherapy
- Pseudo-TORCH
  - Aicardi-Goutières Syndrome
  - Coats Plus Syndrome

ESSENTIAL INFORMATION

Key Differential Diagnosis Issues

- Clinical features to consider
  - Seizures are common presentation
    - e.g., tuberous sclerosis complex (TSC), neurocysticercosis, polymicrogyria in CMV
- Imaging features to consider
  - Look for associations
    - Brain destruction → infection or ischemic complication
    - Cortical malformations → CMV
    - Mass effect → tumor
- Modality considerations
  - US: 1st-line exam in fetus & neonates
    - Look for echogenic foci with shadowing
  - CT: Best modality for confidently identifying Ca^{2+}
    - However, may be insensitive to developing parenchymal mineralization
  - MR: Sensitive modality (if SWI/GRE employed) for detection of Ca^{2+} but can be difficult to confidently distinguish hemorrhage & Ca^{2+}
    - SWI phase map to distinguish hemorrhage & Ca^{2+}
      - Still difficult with small foci
    - Best exam for identifying associated abnormalities

Helpful Clues for Common Diagnoses

- **Pineal Ca^{2+}**
  - Very common: ↑ prevalence with ↑ age
  - 8-14 years (39%), ≤ 10 years (8%), ≤ 6 years (1%)
- **Choroid Plexus Ca^{2+}**
  - Very common: ↑ prevalence with ↑ age
  - Present in > 25% by end of 1st decade of life
- **Tuberous Sclerosis Complex**
  - Classic triad: Intellectual disability, epilepsy, adenoma sebaceum
    - Note that full triad is only present in 1/3 of patients
  - Most subependymal nodules calcify
    - Variable-sized periventricular Ca^{2+}
  - Cortical tubers may also calcify but less commonly
    - ↑ Ca^{2+} of tubers with age

Helpful Clues for Less Common Diagnoses

- **Congenital TORCH Infections**
  - TORCH = toxoplasmosis, other, rubella, CMV, herpes, HIV
    - Caused by transplacental transmission of pathogens
    - All cause parenchymal Ca^{2+}
    - Most can cause lenticulostriate mineralization/vasculopathy (nonspecific radiating echogenic vessels in basal ganglia)
  - **Congenital CMV**
    - Most common cause of intrauterine infection in USA
    - Timing of infection predicts imaging findings (i.e., infections early in gestation result in most severe sequelae)
    - Classic cause of periventricular Ca^{2+} (though actually seen in minority of CMV cases)
    - Associated anomalies: Microcephaly, polymicrogyria, white matter (WM) gliosis, & anterior temporal cysts
  - **Congenital toxoplasmosis**
    - Periventricular & scattered Ca^{2+}
    - Hydrocephalus (colpocephaly-like)
  - **Congenital herpes encephalitis**
    - Meningitis, meningoencephalitis
    - Subsequent brain atrophy or cystic encephalomalacia
    - Ca^{2+} pattern varies in herpes simplex virus type 2 (HSV2)
      - Occurs in areas of hemorrhagic infarction
  - **Congenital HIV**
    - Basal ganglia Ca^{2+}, atrophy
  - **Congenital rubella**
    - Lobar destruction/encephalomalacia
    - Periventricular, scattered, & basal ganglia Ca^{2+}
    - Rarely "stone brain"
      - Extensive gliosis & gyral Ca^{2+}
    - Microinfarcts
  - **Other**
    - Includes Zika virus, syphilis
- **Postnatal Infections**
  - **Neurocysticercosis**
    - Usually involves convexity of subarachnoid space
      - Also gray-white junction &/or ventricles
    - Classic finding: "Dot inside cyst" (due to scolex); may show rim enhancement, surrounding vasogenic edema
    - Nodular calcified (healed) stage: Shrunken calcified nodule
  - **Tuberculosis**
    - Basal meningitis ± CNS tuberculoma

- ± localized Ca^{2+} in chronic phase
- Look for evidence of pulmonary tuberculosis
- **Ventriculitis (Chronic)**
  - Areas of prior hemorrhagic infarction are prone to dystrophic Ca^{2+}
- **Vascular Malformations**
  - **Sturge-Weber syndrome**
    - Cortical/subcortical gyriform Ca^{2+} in affected cerebrum
      - Typically associated with significant atrophy
    - ↑ with ↑ age & seizure burden
    - Early mineralization may be seen on SWI (MR) before NECT
    - Look for associated findings: Absent cortical veins, dilated medullary veins, leptomeningeal enhancement, ↑ ipsilateral choroid plexus size/enhancement
  - **Arteriovenous malformation**
    - Small Ca^{2+} may occur in arteriovenous malformation (AVM)
    - Parenchymal Ca^{2+} develops due to vascular steal or ↑ venous pressures (usually in setting of venous outflow stenosis)
  - **Dural arteriovenous fistula**
    - Parenchymal Ca^{2+} develops due to ↑ venous pressures
      - Usually in setting of venous outflow stenosis
    - Look for dilated venous sinuses
  - **Cavernous malformation**
    - Often occult on CT, especially when small; frequently mildly hyperdense
    - Characteristic MR findings include
      - "Popcorn" cluster of tiny cysts, ± fluid-fluid levels
      - ↓ T2 hemosiderin ring with blooming on SWI
      - Associated developmental venous anomaly (DVA) in ~ 25%
- **Tumors**
  - Many brain tumors have associated Ca^{2+}
    - Fine, stippled Ca^{2+}: Ependymoma, embryonal tumors, others
    - Large, chunky Ca^{2+}: Ganglioglioma, dysembryoplastic neuroepithelial tumor (DNET), oligodendroglioma, metastatic osteosarcoma, others
- **Dural Ca^{2+}**
  - Uncommon in children, present in < 1%
  - Multifocal dural Ca^{2+} → consider basal cell nevus syndrome
    - Keratocystic odontogenic tumors, basal cell carcinoma, medulloblastoma, bifid ribs

Helpful Clues for Rare Diagnoses

- **Radiation & Chemotherapy**
  - Mineralizing microangiopathy with history of previously treated intracranial tumor
- **Pseudo-TORCH**
  - **Aicardi-Goutières syndrome**
    - "Mendelian mimic of congenital infection"
    - Multifocal punctate Ca^{2+}
    - Variable locations including periventricular WM, basal ganglia, & dentate nuclei
    - Elevated CSF interferon
  - **Coats plus syndrome**
    - a.k.a. cerebroretinal microangiopathy with Ca^{2+} & cysts
    - Ocular Coats: Retinal telangiectasia & exudate
    - CNS small blood vessel Ca^{2+}
    - Extensive thalamic & gyral Ca^{2+}
    - Growth failure; defects of bone marrow & integument

SELECTED REFERENCES

1. Gumus K et al: Susceptibility-based differentiation of intracranial calcification and hemorrhage in pediatric patients. J Child Neurol. 30(8):1029-36, 2015
2. Whitehead MT et al: Physiologic pineal region, choroid plexus, and dural calcifications in the first decade of life. AJNR Am J Neuroradiol. 36(3):575-80, 2015
3. Grech R et al: Intracranial calcifications. A pictorial review. Neuroradiol J. 25(4):427-51, 2012

Pineal Ca^{2+}

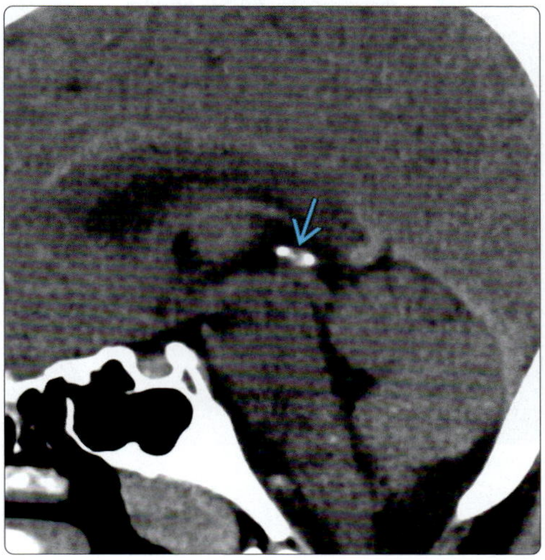

Choroid Plexus Ca^{2+}

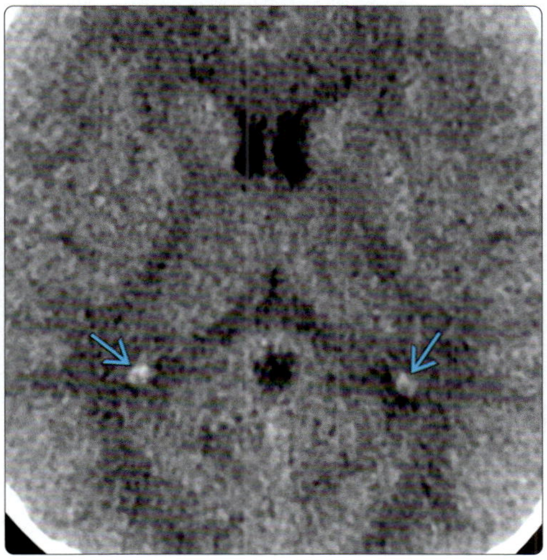

(Left) *Sagittal NECT in a 14 year old shows normal physiologic pineal Ca^{2+} ➡. Pineal Ca^{2+} are common in children & increase in prevalence with age (with 40% of early teens showing pineal Ca^{2+}).* **(Right)** *Axial NECT in a 4 year old shows Ca^{2+} within the bilateral choroid plexus glomus ➡. Such findings should not raise concern for pathology, as > 25% of children > 10 years of age will have choroid plexus Ca^{2+}.*

(**Left**) *Axial oblique NECT in a 23-month-old girl with tuberous sclerosis complex (TSC) shows multiple calcified subependymal nodules →. Note the location of nodules adheres to the distribution of the fetal germinal matrix (with a preponderance in the caudothalamic grooves).* (**Right**) *Coronal NECT in a 7-year-old girl with TSC shows prominent Ca^{2+} → in subcortical & deep white matter (WM) in association with cerebral tubers. A small percentage of tubers will calcify with increasing patient age.*

Tuberous Sclerosis Complex

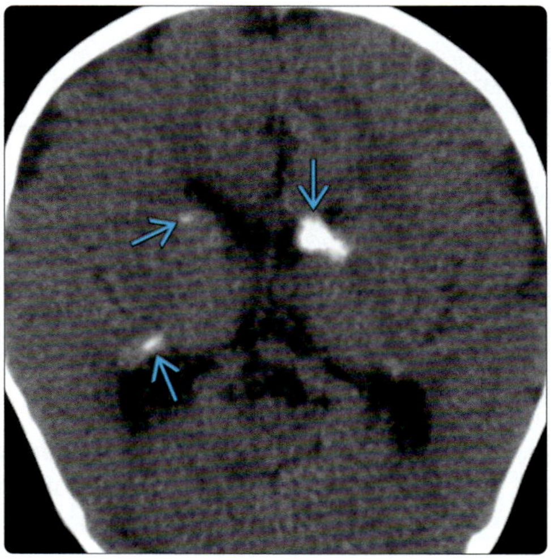

Tuberous Sclerosis Complex

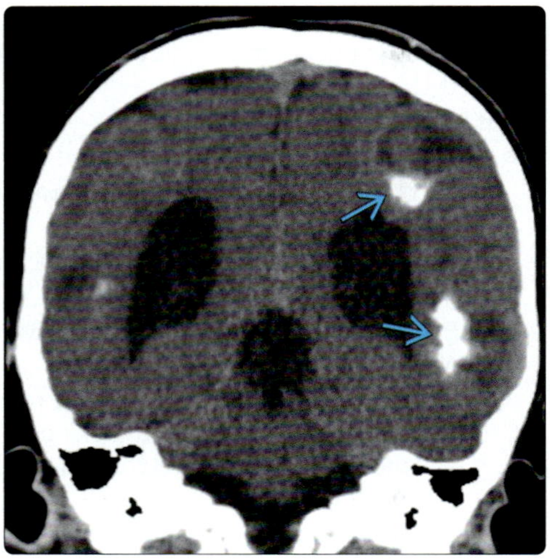

(**Left**) *Coronal NECT in a 3 year old shows nearly symmetric bilateral periventricular Ca^{2+} →, a typical distribution for CMV. Also note the enlarged ventricles → & WM gliosis →, common findings in congenital CMV.* (**Right**) *Coronal T2 MR in the same patient shows hypointense Ca^{2+} → & extensive WM abnormalities →. Also note the irregular cortical surface with shallow sulci →, consistent with polymicrogyria. This constellation strongly suggests congenital CMV.*

Congenital CMV

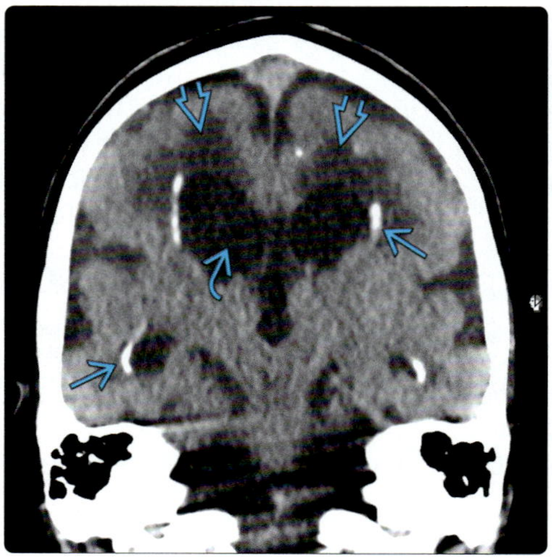

Congenital CMV

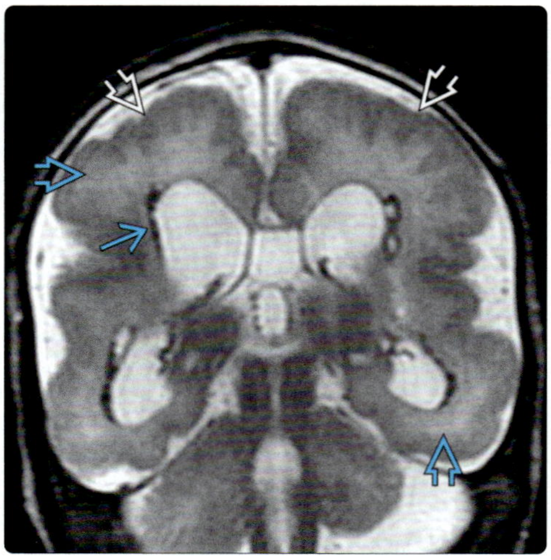

(**Left**) *Coronal NECT in an 8 year old shows cortical & subcortical Ca^{2+} →. Note that the distribution of Ca^{2+} in congenital toxoplasmosis is more variable than that of CMV.* (**Right**) *Axial NECT in the same patient shows the extent of peripheral cerebral Ca^{2+} → as well as bilateral (right > left) porencephaly → due to intrauterine injury. Note the colpocephalic morphology of the lateral ventricles, a common finding in congenital toxoplasmosis.*

Congenital Toxoplasmosis

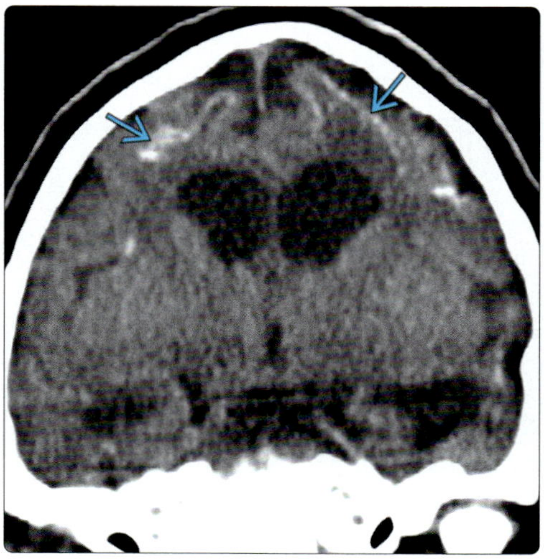

Congenital Toxoplasmosis

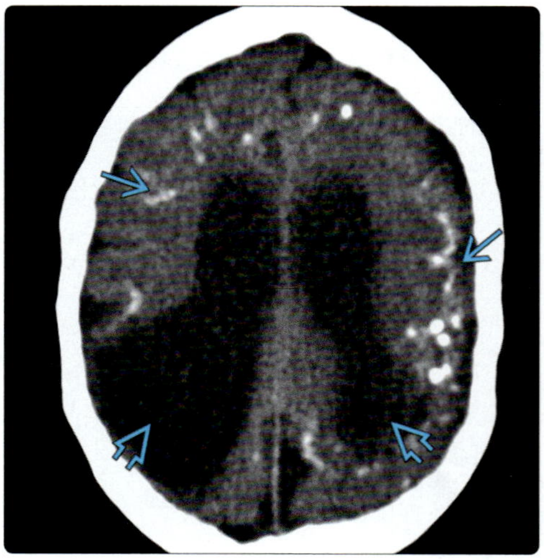

Congenital Herpes Encephalitis

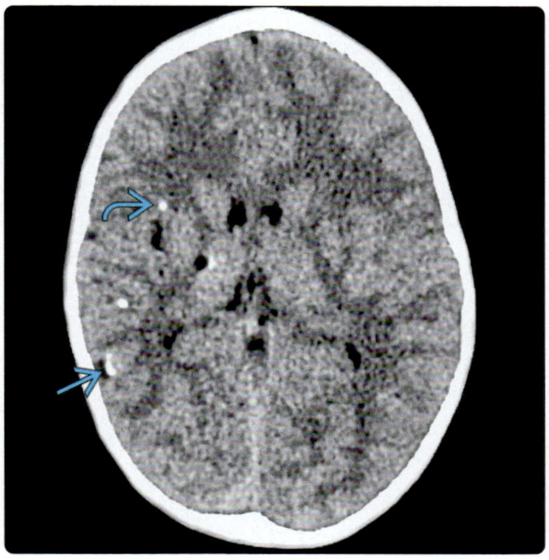

Congenital Herpes Encephalitis

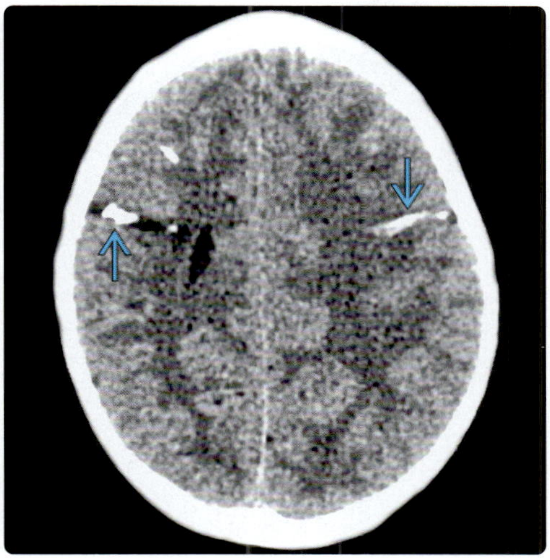

(Left) *Axial NECT in a child who survived congenital herpes encephalitis shows scattered small WM & cortical Ca^{2+}.* **(Right)** *Axial NECT in the same patient shows Ca^{2+} of the infarcted frontal perirolandic cortex. Ca^{2+} can be variable with congenital herpes simplex virus (HSV) but predominantly involve the damaged brain. Depending on the severity of infection, large areas of encephalomalacia are also often seen with this condition.*

Congenital HIV

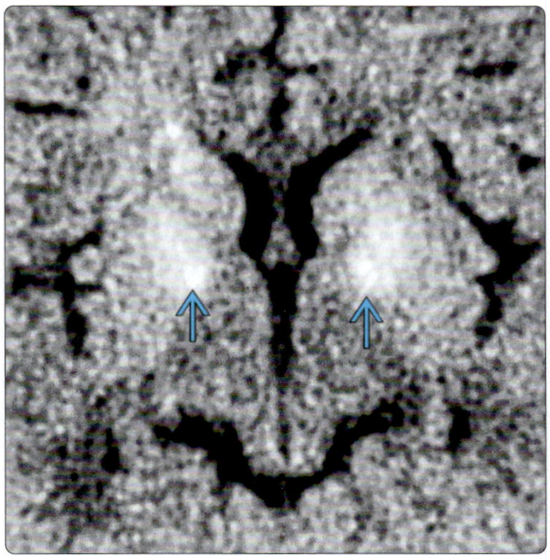

Congenital Rubella

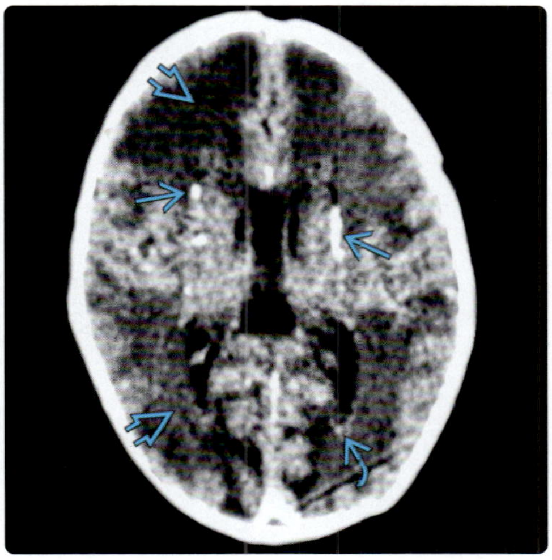

(Left) *Axial NECT in a 1 year old with congenital HIV shows hazy, symmetric basal ganglia Ca^{2+} with mildly prominent sulci & cisterns, consistent with volume loss. Basal ganglia mineralization is more common in HIV compared to other congenital TORCH infections.* **(Right)** *Axial NECT in a patient with congenital rubella shows basal ganglia Ca^{2+} & diffuse WM hypointensity. There are also faint bilateral subependymal Ca^{2+} lining the posterior horns.*

Neurocysticercosis

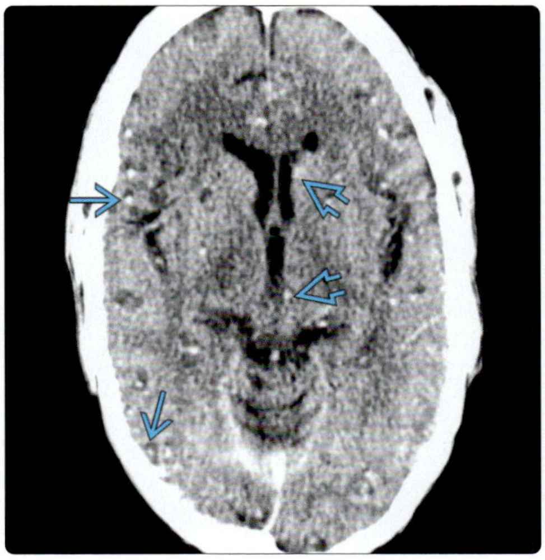

Neurocysticercosis

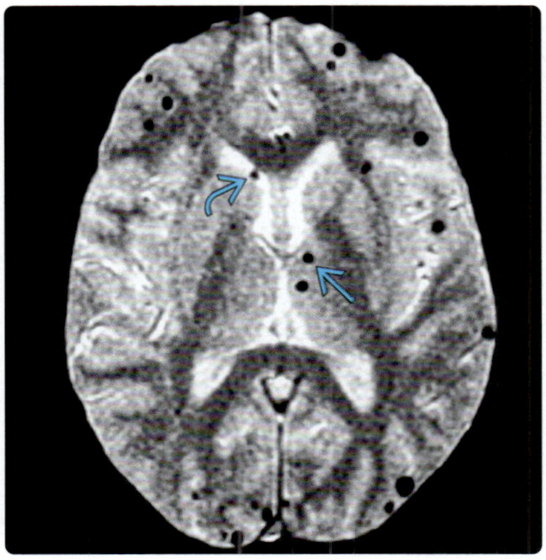

(Left) *Axial NECT shows the disseminated "miliary" form of neurocysticercosis (NCC). Note the numerous cysts, each with a hyperdense central "dot" representing a scolex. Innumerable small calcific foci, some of which are periventricular, cause the classic starry-sky appearance of healed NCC.* **(Right)** *Axial T2* GRE MR in a patient with NCC shows scattered Ca^{2+} throughout the brain. A few are in the deep gray structures, & one is intraventricular. GRE/SWI increases sensitivity for Ca^{2+} on MR imaging in chronic NCC.*

(Left) *Axial NECT in a 1 year old with Sturge-Weber syndrome (SWS) shows gyriform cortical/subcortical Ca^{2+} ➔ in the right frontal lobe with associated atrophy. The Ca^{2+} is thought to arise from a combination of venous insufficiency & chronic neuronal excitation from recurrent seizures.* **(Right)** *Axial T1 C+ FS MR in the same patient shows extensive leptomeningeal enhancement ➔ & enlargement of the medullary veins ⇨ in the atrophied cerebrum, classic findings of SWS.*

Sturge-Weber Syndrome

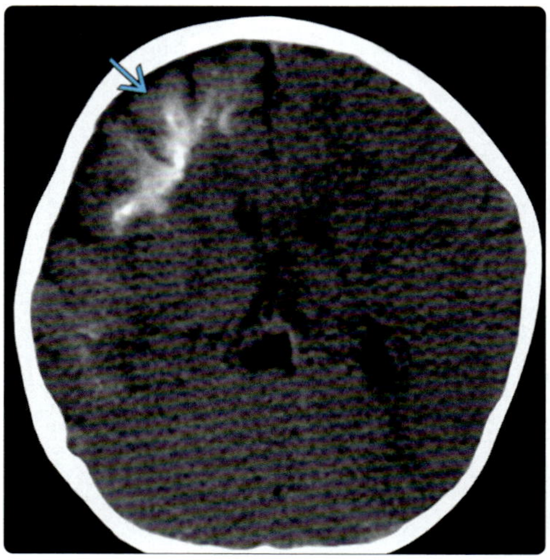

Sturge-Weber Syndrome

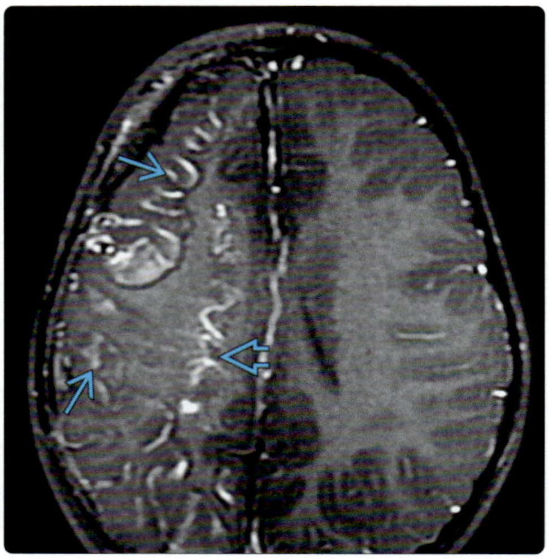

(Left) *Sagittal T1 C+ FS MR in a 10 month old with a high-flow dural arteriovenous fistula (AVF) with venous outflow stenosis shows markedly dilated dural venous sinuses ➔. The combination of a high-flow vascular malformation & venous outflow stenosis causes significant venous hypertension, which leads to brain parenchymal Ca^{2+}.* **(Right)** *Axial SWI MR in the same patient shows ↓ signal intensity throughout much of the bifrontal cortex ➔ & basal ganglia ↪, consistent with early Ca^{2+} deposition.*

Dural Arteriovenous Fistula

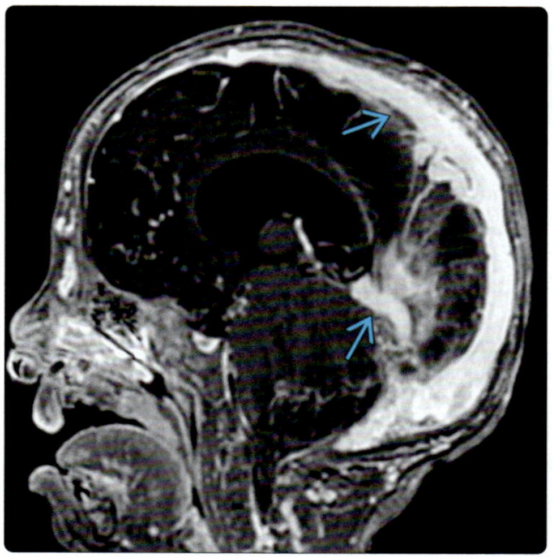

Dural Arteriovenous Fistula

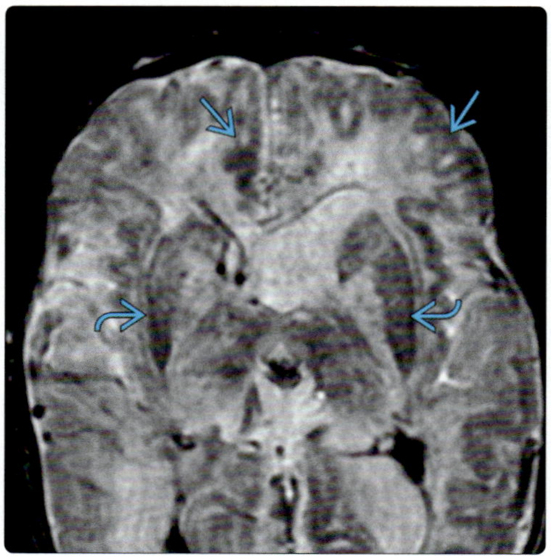

(Left) *Axial NECT in a 3 year old with a cavernous malformation shows irregular Ca^{2+} ➔ in the right frontal deep WM. This appearance is nonspecific & could reflect prior injury or tumor.* **(Right)** *Axial T2 MR in the same patient shows central hyperintense cystic foci ➔ with a rim of hypointensity, consistent with hemosiderin ⇨. This is a characteristic appearance for a cavernous malformation. There is no surrounding edema to suggest a recent hemorrhage.*

Cavernous Malformation

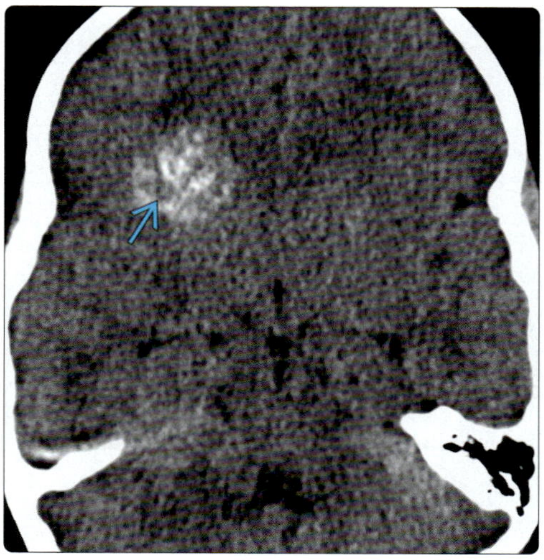

Cavernous Malformation

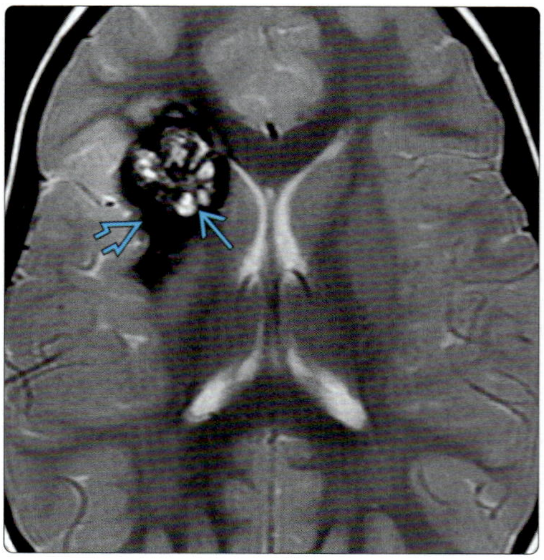

Tumors

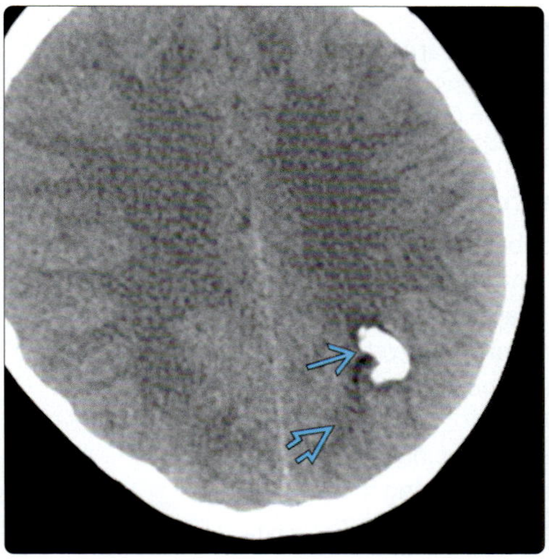

Tumors

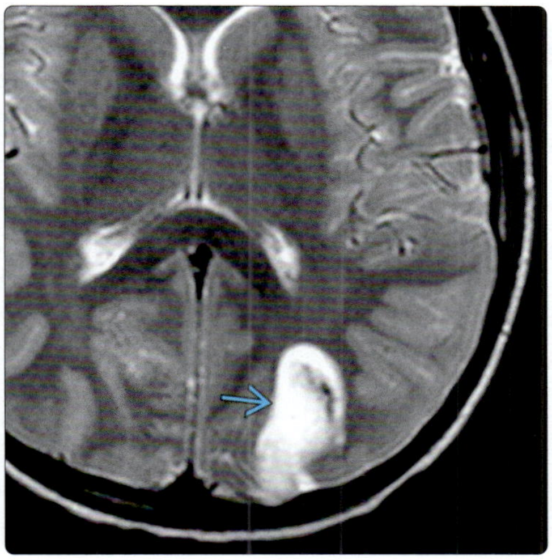

(Left) *Axial NECT in a 10-year-old boy with closed head trauma shows incidental findings of cortical & subcortical hypoattenuation with focal Ca^{2+}.* **(Right)** *Axial T2 MR in the same patient shows a hyperintense lesion associated with the Ca^{2+}, suggesting an underlying tumor. In this case, the pathology revealed a dysembryoplastic neuroepithelial tumor (DNET). Ca^{2+} is present in 6-36% of DNETs & is found even more commonly in other tumors, such as ganglioglioma & ependymoma.*

Radiation & Chemotherapy

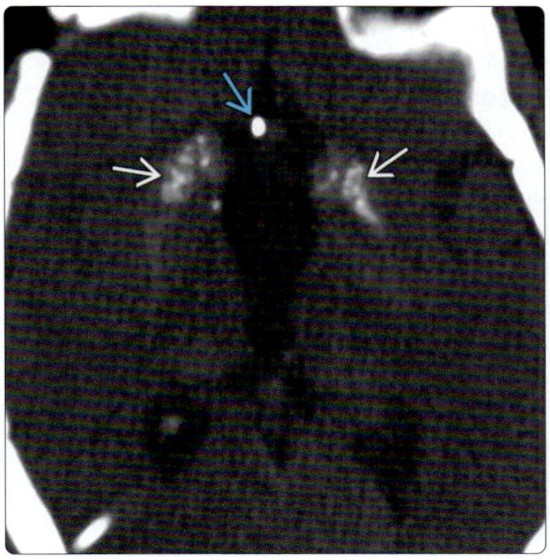

Radiation & Chemotherapy

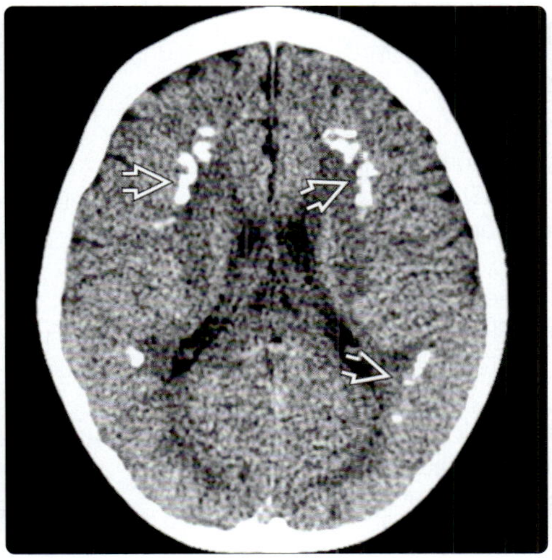

(Left) *Axial NECT in a 19 year old with a history of pilomyxoid astrocytoma & radiation (XRT) shows nearly symmetric Ca^{2+} in the bilateral basal ganglia. The central density is a shunt catheter. Ca^{2+} associated with chemotherapy & XRT can occur anywhere in the brain, including the deep gray nuclei & WM.* **(Right)** *Axial NECT shows bilateral symmetric Ca^{2+} at the gray-white junction due to mineralizing microangiopathy following RXT & chemotherapy.*

Aicardi-Goutières Syndrome

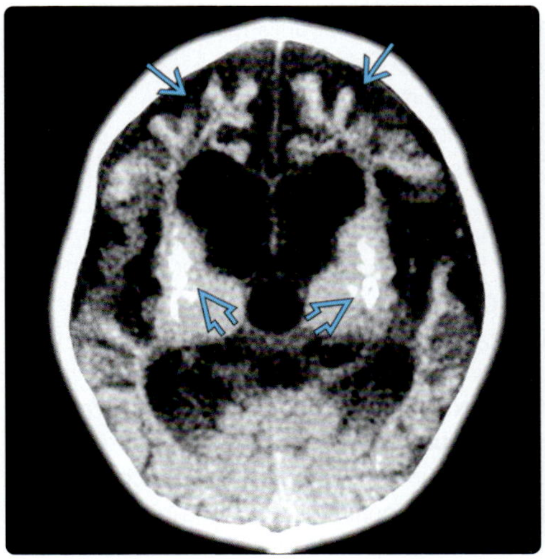

Coats Plus Syndrome

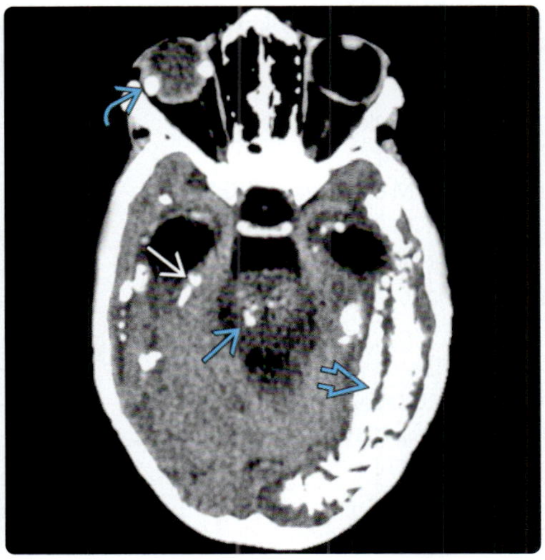

(Left) *Axial NECT in a patient with Aicardi-Goutieres syndrome shows marked bifrontal brain atrophy & bilateral symmetric Ca^{2+} in the basal ganglia. Extension into the corona radiata (not shown) was also present.* **(Right)** *Axial NECT in a patient with Coats plus syndrome shows extensive gyral, brainstem, & periventricular Ca^{2+}. The brainstem is also swollen & low in density. Note the postoperative change of the right globe.*

DIFFERENTIAL DIAGNOSIS

Common

- Incidental Subcortical White Matter Foci

Less Common

- Enlarged Perivascular Spaces
- Inflammatory Demyelinating Disorders
  - Multiple Sclerosis
  - Acute Disseminated Encephalomyelitis
  - Neuromyelitis Optica
- Posterior Reversible Encephalopathy Syndrome
- Tuberous Sclerosis Complex
- Neurofibromatosis Type 1
- Viral Encephalitis
- Diffuse Axonal Injury
- Metabolic Brain Disease
- Vasculitis

Rare but Important

- Lyme Disease

ESSENTIAL INFORMATION

Key Differential Diagnosis Issues

- Clinical features to consider
  - Sex: Demyelinating disease is more common in females, especially multiple sclerosis (MS)
  - Prior episodes of weakness, numbness, tingling → MS
  - Seizure, altered mental status, hypertension, immunosuppression → posterior reversible encephalopathy syndrome (PRES)
  - Fever, headache, seizure, altered mental status→ viral encephalitis
  - Stroke-like symptoms in leukemic patient receiving methotrexate → acute methotrexate toxicity
- Imaging features to consider
  - Location
    - Symmetric, bifrontal, subcortical white matter (WM) → usually incidental
    - Corpus callosum (CC) & subcortical WM → MS
    - Associated deep gray matter (GM) involvement → acute disseminated encephalomyelitis (ADEM), viral encephalitis
    - Broadened gyri, subependymal nodules → tuberous sclerosis complex (TSC)
    - Bilateral watershed subcortical WM & cortex → PRES
  - Morphology
    - Small, punctate → usually incidental
    - Varying sizes radiating away from CC ("Dawson fingers") → MS
  - Diffusion restriction
    - Acute demyelinating lesions, metabolic brain disease, vasculitides, encephalitides, & PRES may show diffusion restriction
  - Contrast enhancement
    - Helpful for establishing temporal heterogeneity in MS
      - Combination of enhancing (acute) & nonenhancing (chronic) lesions
- Modality considerations
  - CT: Insensitive for subtle or small WM lesions
  - MR: Best for detection & evaluation of WM disease
    - If demyelinating disease is suspected, perform dedicated orbit & spine imaging
    - DWI & contrast are important for determining acuity
      - Acute lesions: Often enhance, ± diffusion restriction (↓ ADC)
      - Chronic lesions: Usually do not enhance; ↑ ADC

Helpful Clues for Common Diagnoses

- **Incidental Subcortical White Matter Foci**
  - Typically small & round, < 10 in number
  - Typically bilateral with frontal predominance
  - Most common in subcortical WM but may occur deeper
  - Have been reported in literature with seizures, headaches, etc.
    - All are frequent indications for imaging
  - Do not require imaging follow-up

Helpful Clues for Less Common Diagnoses

- **Multiple Sclerosis**
  - Demyelinating disorder most commonly affecting female teens & young women
  - Typically presents with recurrent events of weakness, numbness, &/or tingling
  - Diagnosis made if both acute & chronic lesions are present on initial imaging
    - Or if new lesions are identified on subsequent exams
  - Demyelinating lesions may occur anywhere
    - CC & subcortical WM are typical
    - Lesions radiating along WM tracts of parasagittal CC are classic ("Dawson fingers")
  - T1 C+: Punctate, ring, or incomplete ring enhancement
    - Incomplete ring enhancement is most distinct pattern for demyelinating disease (vs. tumor or abscess)
  - DWI: Acute enhancing components may show diffusion restriction, but most lesions show ↑ ADC
- **Acute Disseminated Encephalomyelitis**
  - Para-/postinfectious immune-mediated inflammatory disorder of WM
  - Multifocal WM & deep GM lesions weeks after infection/immunization
    - WM involvement is almost universal
    - ~ 50% involve deep GM
    - ~ 25% involve spinal cord
  - CT: Initial CT is normal in ~ 40%
  - MR: T1 C+ shows punctate, ring, or incomplete ring enhancement
    - DWI: Enhancing areas may restrict diffusion; otherwise, lesions typically show ↑ ADC
- **Neuromyelitis Optica**
  - Idiopathic inflammatory demyelinating CNS disease with optic neuritis & long-segment myelitis
  - Serum marker: Neuromyelitis optica (NMO)-IgG, targets water channel aquaporin-4 (AQP4)
    - Seen in 70% of NMO patients: 99% specificity
  - Combination of additional clinical & MR criteria required for diagnosis depending on AQP4-IgG status
    - Optic neuritis
    - Longitudinally extensive transverse myelitis (LETM): Spinal cord MR lesion ≥ 3 vertebral segments

- Brain lesions with characteristic distribution: 3rd & lateral ventricle margins, dorsal brainstem, hypothalamus
  - ▫ Lesions tend to be parallel to ventricles
- **Posterior Reversible Encephalopathy Syndrome**
  - Cerebrovascular autoregulatory disorder, usually associated with hypertension
  - Encephalopathy, headache, & seizures are typical
  - CT: Often normal at presentation
  - MR: Symmetric ↑ cortical/subcortical FLAIR signal in watershed territories
    - T1 C+: ≤ 50% show subtle leptomeningeal/cortical enhancement
    - DWI: Diffusion restriction is uncommon (& can help distinguish from vasculitis)
- **Tuberous Sclerosis Complex**
  - Cortical/subcortical dysplastic lesions ("tubers")
  - Best clue: Multiple cortical/subcortical ↑ FLAIR lesions with calcified subependymal nodules
  - Most common symptom: Seizure
  - CT: Helpful to detect subependymal Ca^{2+}
  - MR: Most sensitive for tuber detection
    - FLAIR: ↑ subcortical signal ± tail toward ventricle
    - T1: Tubers show ↑ T1 in unmyelinated WM (infants)
- **Neurofibromatosis Type 1**
  - Phakomatosis with characteristic skin & eye lesions, axillary freckling, plexiform neurofibromas, scoliosis
  - MR: Foci of abnormal signal intensity (FASI) most commonly occur in globus pallidus & medial cerebellar hemispheres but may affect variety of locations
    - Represent myelin vacuolization
    - Typically do not enhance
    - Resolve by 3rd decade of life
  - Associated findings: Optic nerve glioma, plexiform neurofibroma, sphenoid wing dysplasia
- **Viral Encephalitis**
  - Acute brain inflammation secondary to viral infection
  - MR: May involve WM, GM, or both
    - May mimic ADEM & other demyelinating disorders
      - ▫ Findings are often more subtle & symmetric
      - ▫ May cause asymmetric gyral/lobar edema, enhancement, & restricted diffusion
- **Diffuse Axonal Injury**
  - Trauma-induced axonal stretch injury
  - Occurs exclusively in high-velocity injuries
  - Location: CC, WM, GM-WM junction, & brainstem
  - CT: Frequently normal or with subtle microhemorrhages
  - MR: SWI/T2* GRE is highly sensitive for extent of hemorrhagic injury
- **Metabolic Brain Disease**
  - Usually diffuse, symmetric WM involvement
  - Can show patchy multifocal WM abnormalities, especially early in course
- **Vasculitis**
  - Inflammatory vasculopathy with cerebral infarction
  - May affect WM; more commonly affects cortex & deep gray nuclei
  - MR: Multiple ischemic foci, showing diffusion restriction
  - MRA/CTA: Medium-vessel vasculitis may be evident
    - Angiography is often necessary for diagnosis

Helpful Clues for Rare Diagnoses

- **Lyme Disease**
  - Inflammatory tick-borne CNS disease caused by *Borrelia burgdorferi*
  - MR: Multifocal WM lesions + cranial nerve enhancement

SELECTED REFERENCES

1. Longoni G et al: White matter changes in paediatric multiple sclerosis and monophasic demyelinating disorders. Brain. 140(5):1300-15, 2017
2. Tenembaum SN: Pediatric multiple sclerosis: distinguishing clinical and MR imaging features. Neuroimaging Clin N Am. 27(2):229-50, 2017
3. Rostasy K et al: Differential diagnosis and evaluation in pediatric inflammatory demyelinating disorders. Neurology. 87(9 Suppl 2):S28-37, 2016
4. Fisch N et al: Incidental multifocal white matter lesions in pediatric magnetic resonance imaging. Pediatr Neurol. 47(1):7-12, 2012

Incidental Subcortical White Matter Foci

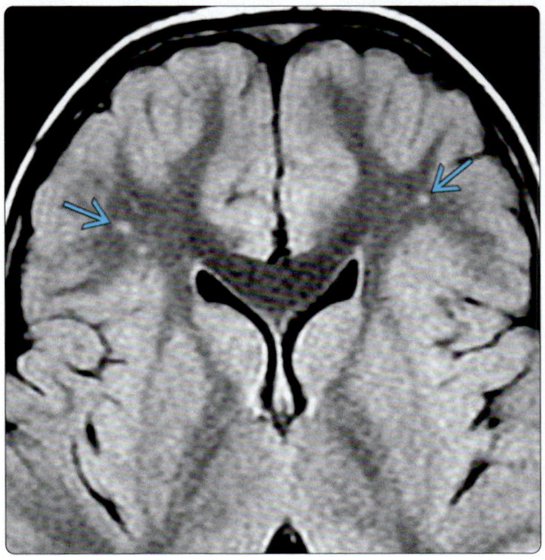

Incidental Subcortical White Matter Foci

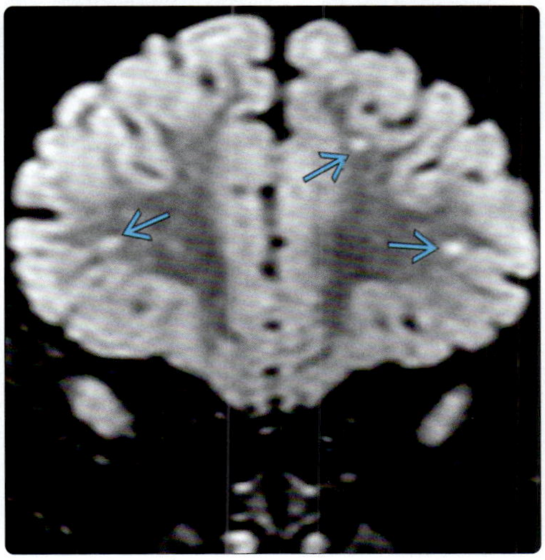

(Left) *Axial FLAIR MR a 7 year old with headaches shows punctate foci of increased signal intensity* ➔ *in the bifrontal subcortical white matter (WM). The location, size, number, & bilaterality are common. Such lesions are almost invariably stable over time & are typically considered incidental findings.* **(Right)** *Coronal FLAIR MR in a 2 year old with seizures shows small foci of increased signal intensity* ➔ *in the bifrontal subcortical WM. The multifocality, punctate size, & frontal location all suggest these are likely incidental.*

(Left) *Axial T2 MR in a 1 year old with Hurler syndrome shows multiple large, round to ovoid perivascular spaces in the hemispheric WM* ➔ *& corpus callosum* ➔*. Note the foci of more linear, but less pronounced, perivascular space enlargement* ➔*.* **(Right)** *Axial FLAIR MR in the same patient shows complete suppression of signal within the enlarged perivascular spaces. An abnormally large number & size of perivascular spaces is a common finding in the mucopolysaccharidoses.*

Enlarged Perivascular Spaces

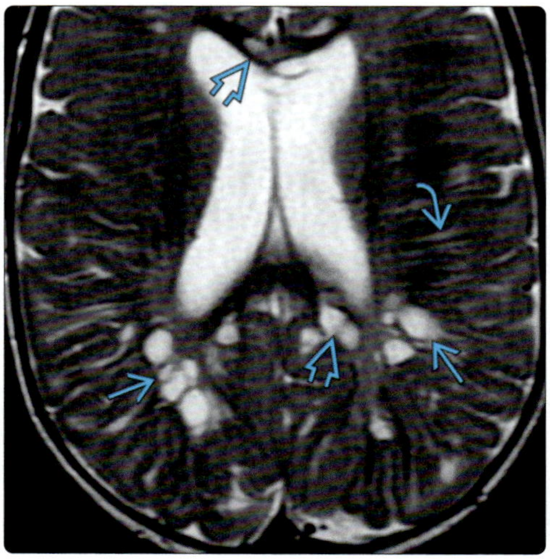

Enlarged Perivascular Spaces

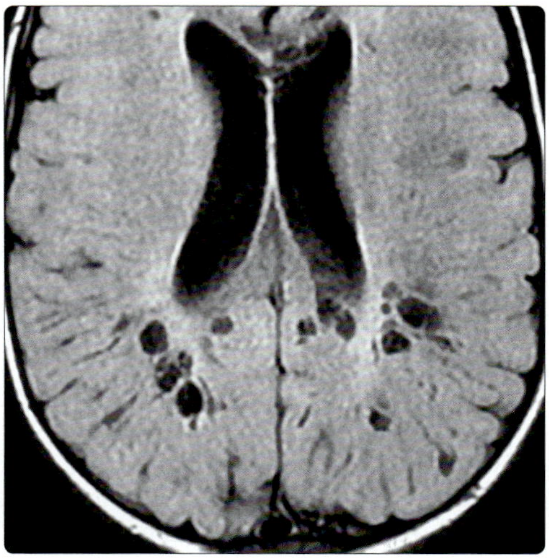

(Left) *Sagittal FLAIR MR in a 14-year-old girl with multiple sclerosis (MS) shows multiple radiating WM lesions involving the parasagittal corpus callosum* ➔ *& subcortical WM* ➔*, typical of MS.* **(Right)** *Sagittal FLAIR MR in a 12-year-old boy with MS shows similar classic findings of multiple radiating WM lesions involving the parasagittal corpus callosum* ➔ *("Dawson fingers") & subcortical WM* ➔*.*

Multiple Sclerosis

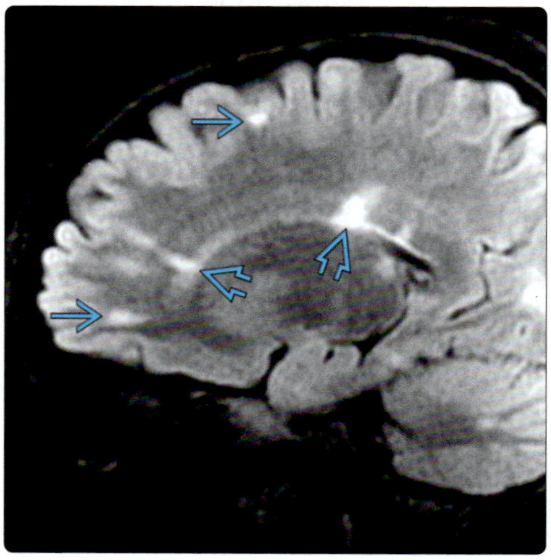

Multiple Sclerosis

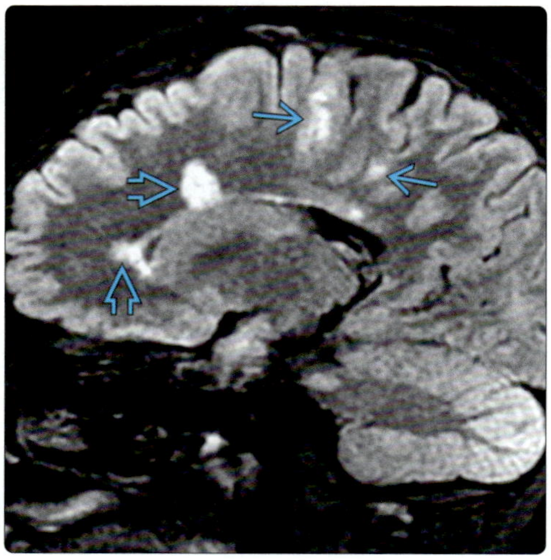

(Left) *Axial T1 C+ FS MR in a 15-year-old girl with MS, months of intermittent numbness & weakness, & newly decreased vision in the left eye shows short segment optic nerve enhancement* ➔*, consistent with optic neuritis.* **(Right)** *Sagittal T2 MR in the same patient shows multiple short-segment foci of increased signal* ➔*, consistent with demyelinating lesions. It is important to image the spine when brain findings concerning for demyelination are encountered (& vice versa).*

Multiple Sclerosis

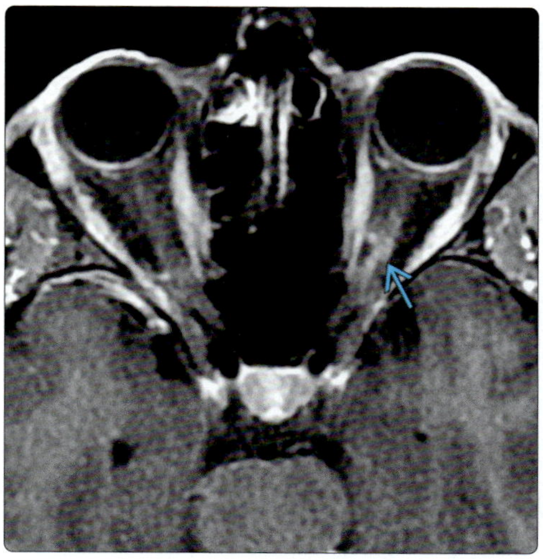

Multiple Sclerosis

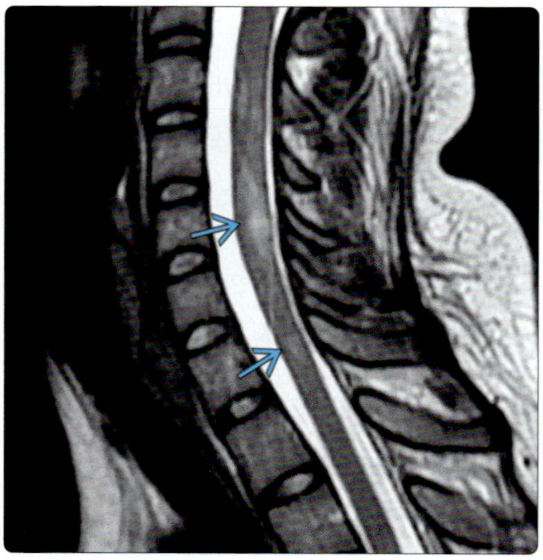

Acute Disseminated Encephalomyelitis

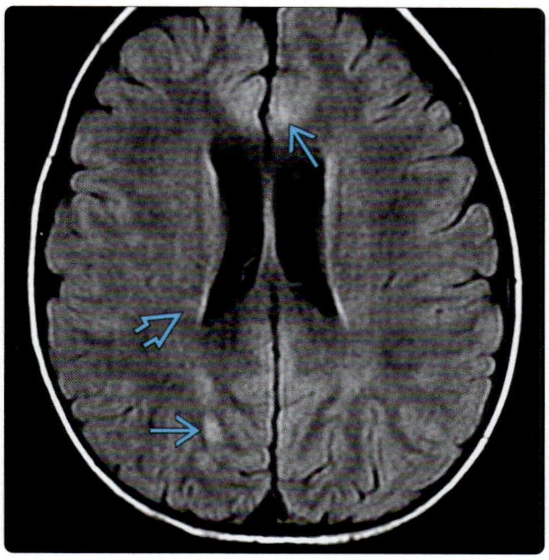

Acute Disseminated Encephalomyelitis

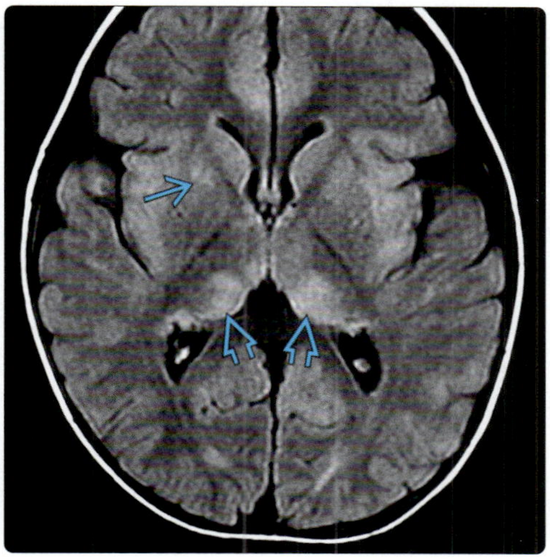

(Left) *Axial FLAIR MR in a 2 year old with encephalopathy weeks after a viral infection shows patchy bilateral subcortical → & periventricular ⇨ WM signal abnormalities, typical of acute disseminated encephalomyelitis (ADEM).* **(Right)** *Axial FLAIR MR in the same patient shows associated multifocal signal abnormalities in the bilateral thalami ⇨ & right putamen →. Gray matter (GM) involvement is seen more commonly in ADEM as compared to other demyelinating disorders.*

Neuromyelitis Optica

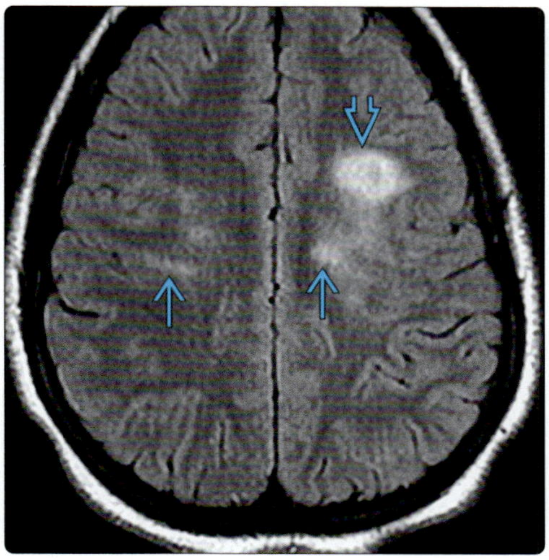

Neuromyelitis Optica

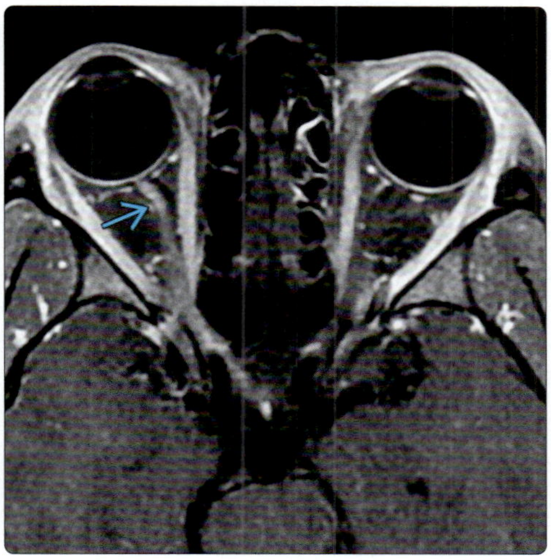

(Left) *Axial FLAIR MR in a 13 year old with neuromyelitis optica (NMO) shows signal abnormalities → within the bilateral WM, most pronounced in the left frontal centrum semiovale ⇨.* **(Right)** *Axial T1 C+ FS MR in the same patient shows enhancement throughout most of the right intraorbital optic nerve →, consistent with optic neuritis. Long-segment optic neuritis is typical of NMO. This patient had a positive NMO-IgG (aquaporin 4) test, which is very specific for a diagnosis of NMO.*

Neuromyelitis Optica

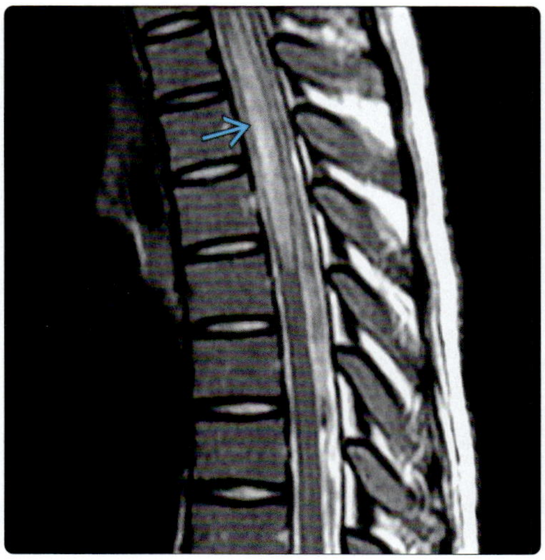

Posterior Reversible Encephalopathy Syndrome

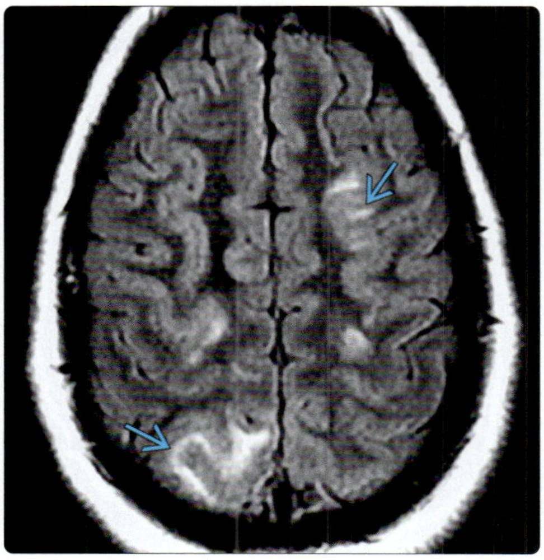

(Left) *Sagittal T2 MR in the same patient with NMO shows a long-segment (> 3 vertebral levels) spinal cord signal abnormality →. Long-segment myelitis is characteristic of NMO.* **(Right)** *Axial FLAIR MR in a 13 year old with hypertension & seizures shows bilateral frontoparietal subcortical WM signal abnormalities → in a watershed distribution. This is a classic history & characteristic distribution for posterior reversible encephalopathy syndrome (PRES).*

(Left) *Axial FLAIR MR of a 3-year-old boy with tuberous sclerosis complex (TSC) shows a number of subcortical WM lesions, consistent with cortical tubers. Cystic change is seen in one left parietal lobe tuber. Note the broadening of overlying gyri.* **(Right)** *Axial FLAIR MR in a 2 year old with TSC shows multiple bilateral WM signal abnormalities that extend from the cortex toward the ventricle, consistent with tubers. Note the subependymal nodule in the right caudothalamic groove.*

Tuberous Sclerosis Complex

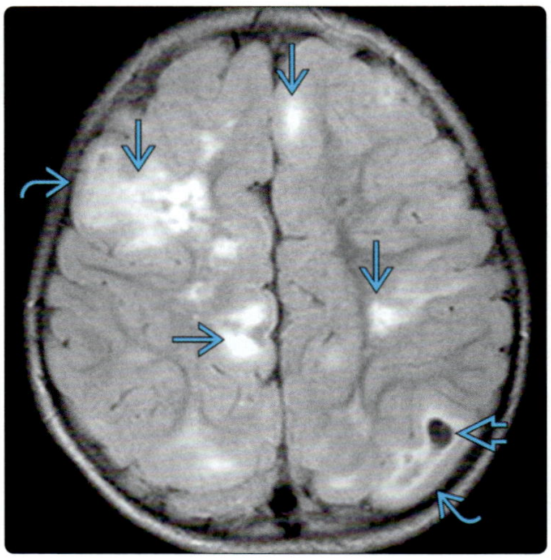

Tuberous Sclerosis Complex

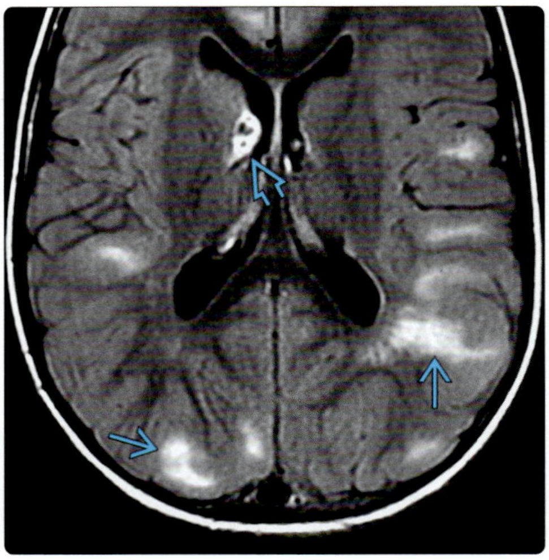

(Left) *Axial FLAIR MR in an 8 year old with NF1 shows a hyperintense lesion in the dorsal midbrain with mild mass effect. This is a common location for nonenhancing foci of NF1.* **(Right)** *Axial FLAIR MR in the same patient shows multiple foci of signal abnormality in the bilateral cerebellar WM, the most common location for such findings in NF1. These signal abnormalities fade with age & typically resolve by the late teenage years. Look also for additional findings of NF1 (e.g., optic glioma, plexiform neurofibroma).*

Neurofibromatosis Type 1

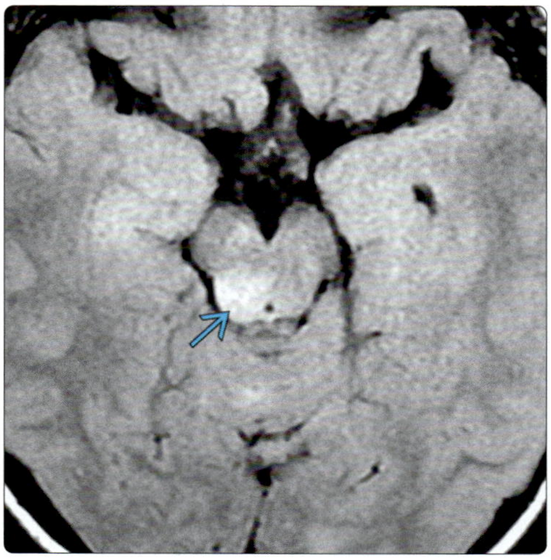

Neurofibromatosis Type 1

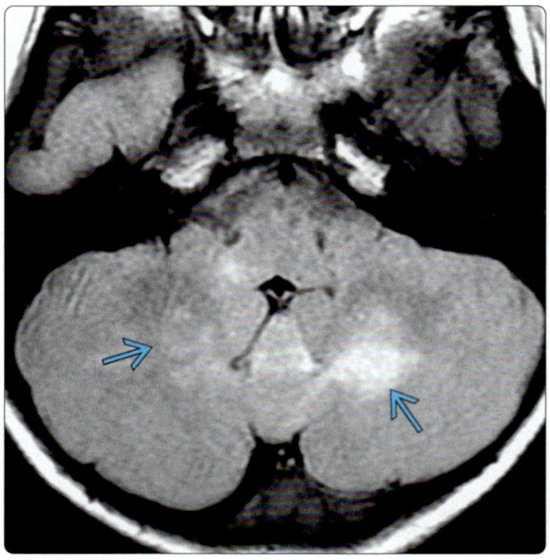

(Left) *Axial FLAIR MR in a 15 month old with human metapneumovirus encephalitis shows multifocal signal abnormalities scattered throughout the deep & subcortical WM.* **(Right)** *Axial DWI MR in the same patient shows areas of diffusion restriction (↓ ADC not shown) in the bilateral thalami. Deep GM involvement is typical in viral encephalitis but is also seen in ADEM. Clinical symptoms (e.g., fever) & history are important in distinguishing ADEM from viral encephalitis.*

Viral Encephalitis

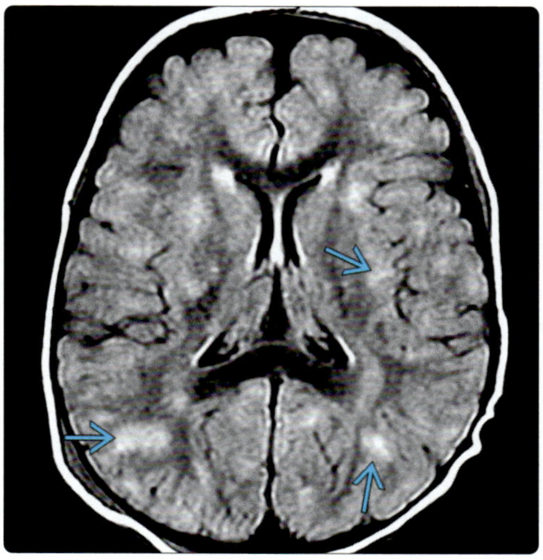

Viral Encephalitis

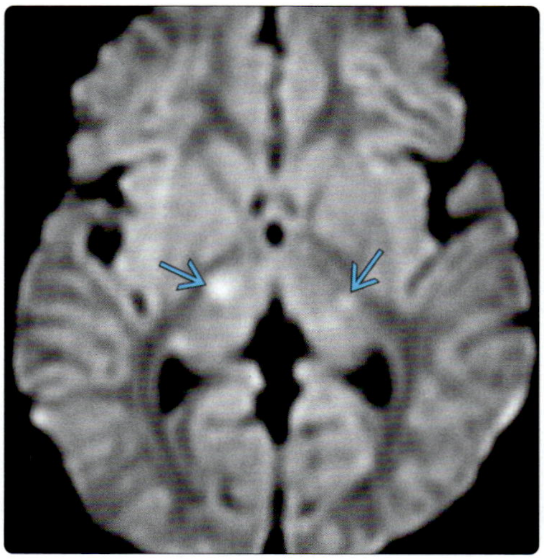

Diffuse Axonal Injury

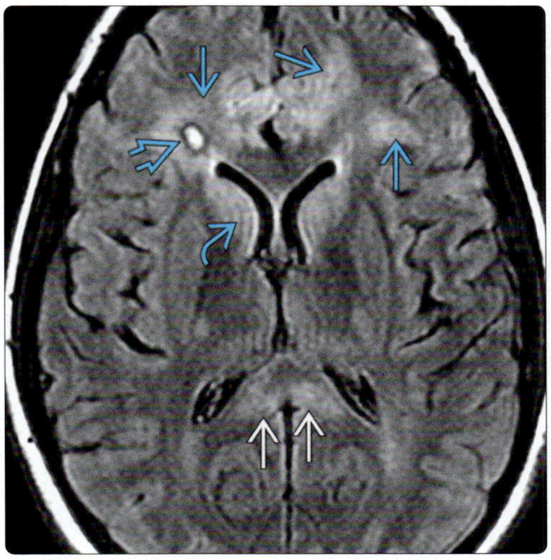

Diffuse Axonal njury

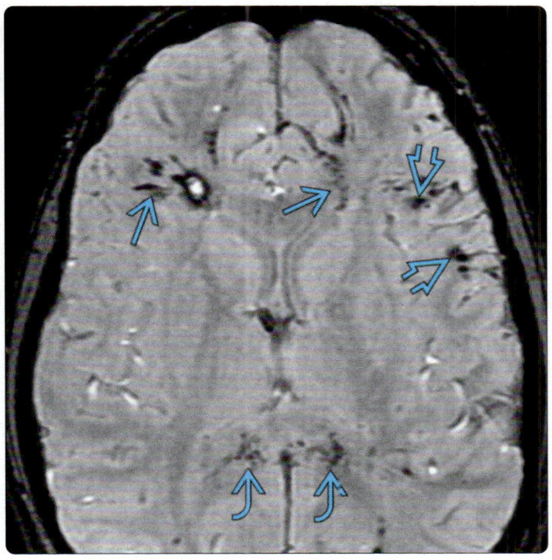

(Left) *Axial FLAIR MR in a 13-year-old MVA victim shows patchy foci of FLAIR hyperintensity within the bifrontal WM, caudate heads, & splenium of the corpus callosum. A round, hyperintense focus in the right frontal lobe corresponds to a small parenchymal hematoma.* **(Right)** *Axial SWI MR in the same patient shows radiating foci of signal loss in the areas of FLAIR abnormality within the WM, GM-WM junction, & corpus callosum, typical of diffuse axonal injury (DAI).*

Metabolic Brain Disease

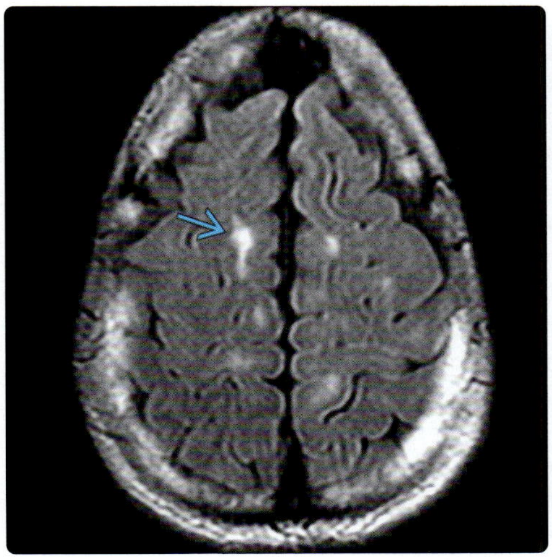

Metabolic Brain Disease

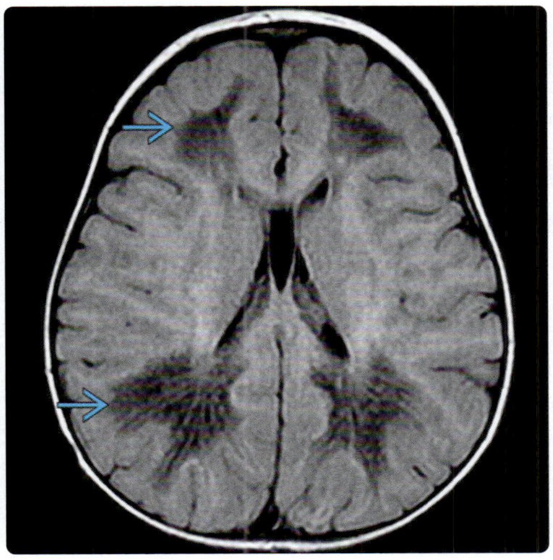

(Left) *Axial FLAIR MR in an 18 year old with Aicardi-Goutieres syndrome shows patchy areas of increased signal in the subcortical WM. Look for associated mineralization in the basal ganglia (especially globus pallidus) to suggest this particular diagnosis.* **(Right)** *Axial FLAIR MR in a 19 month old with tremor shows signal suppression of the expanded WM in the frontal & parietooccipital regions. This is a characteristic appearance for VWMD in contrast to other diseases in which the WM is hyperintense.*

Vasculitis

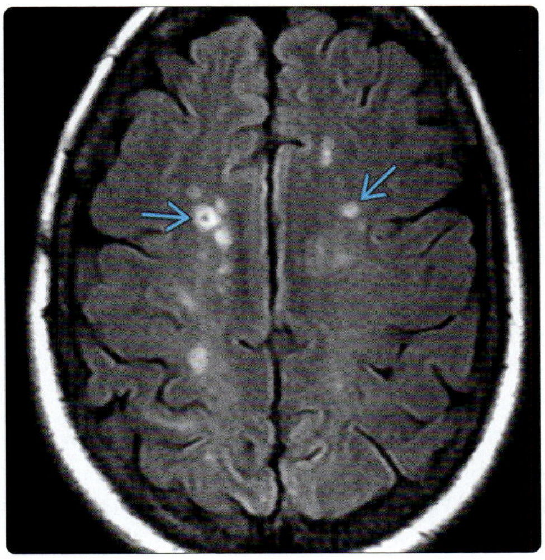

Vasculitis

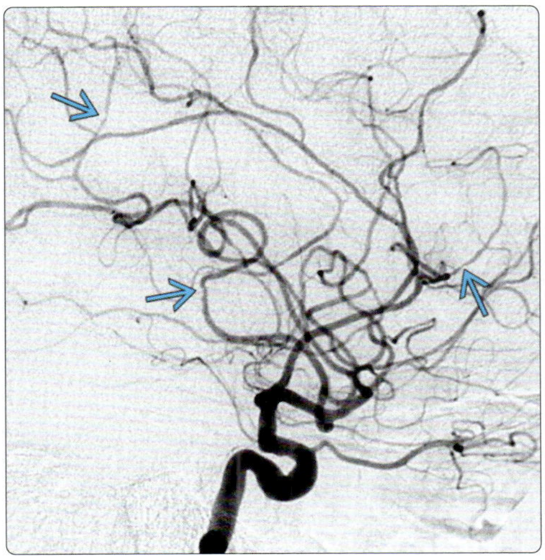

(Left) *Axial FLAIR MR in a patient with vasculitis shows multifocal bilateral WM lesions of variable size. DWI (not shown) demonstrated areas of diffusion restriction.* **(Right)** *Lateral view of an internal carotid artery (ICA) injection DSA shows foci of narrowing & irregularity in multiple small intracranial arteries, consistent with a small vessel vasculitis. It is unlikely that such findings would be evident on CTA or MRA.*

DIFFERENTIAL DIAGNOSIS

Common

- Leukodystrophies
  - X-Linked Adrenoleukodystrophy
  - Canavan Disease
  - Metachromatic Leukodystrophy
  - Krabbe Disease
  - Hypomyelination
  - Alexander Disease
  - Vanishing White Matter Disease

Less Common

- Mucopolysaccharidoses

Rare but Important

- Megalencephalic Leukoencephalopathy With Cysts
- Merosin Deficient Congenital Muscular Dystrophy
- Maple Syrup Urine Disease
- Nonketotic Hyperglycinemia
- Urea Cycle Disorders
- Giant Axonal Neuropathy
- Trichothiodystrophy
- Oculocerebrorenal (Lowe) Syndrome
- Hyperhomocysteinemia (Homocystinuria)

ESSENTIAL INFORMATION

Key Differential Diagnosis Issues

- Leukodystrophy definition
  - Inborn errors of metabolism → abnormal growth or development of myelin sheath → progressive degeneration of white matter (WM)
    - Historically classified as hypomyelinating, demyelinating, dysmyelinating, & myelinolytic diseases
    - Recent proposed classification: Myelin disorders, astrocytopathy, leuko-axonopathies, microgliopathies, & leuko-vasculopathies
- Symmetric involvement of subcortical or deep WM ± gray matter (GM)
- Macrocephaly: Canavan, Alexander, & megalencephalic leukoencephalopathy (MLC)
- Initial periventricular WM involvement: Metachromatic leukodystrophy (MLD), Krabbe [globoid cell leukodystrophy (GLD)], X-linked adrenoleukodystrophy (X-ALD)
- Initial subcortical WM involvement: MLC, vanishing WM
- Many lead to diffuse WM disease & atrophy
- MRS: Majority show ↓ NAA; Canavan shows ↑ NAA

Helpful Clues for Common Diagnoses

- **X-Linked Adrenoleukodystrophy**
  - Most common in boys 5-12 years old
  - Disorder of peroxisome metabolism secondary to impaired β oxidation of very long chain fatty acids (VLCFA)
  - Immune-mediated inflammation at active zones of demyelination → enhancement
    - 80% splenium → peritrigonal WM → corticospinal tracts/fornix/commisural fibers/visual & auditory pathways
    - 15% frontal pattern, genu, anterior/genu internal capsule ± cerebellar WM
  - Spares subcortical U-fibers
  - ± Ca^{2+}
  - MRS: ↓ NAA; ↑ choline, myoinositol, lactate; abnormal peaks between 0.9 & 1.4 ppm (probably VLCFA macromolecules)
- **Canavan Disease**
  - Macrocephaly
  - ↑ T2 of subcortical U-fibers, thalamus, & globus pallidus
  - MRS: ↑ NAA
- **Metachromatic Leukodystrophy**
  - Autosomal recessive lysosomal disorder 2° to *ARSA* gene mutation → arylsulfatase A deficiency → accumulation of sulfatides → demyelination
  - Most common form is late-infantile variant, presenting in 2nd year of life
    - Juvenile & adult-onset forms are less common
  - Favors frontal & posterior WM
  - Symmetric, confluent, nonenhancing ↑ T2 of periventricular WM in butterfly pattern
  - ± radial stripes/tigroid pattern due to relative sparing of perivenular myelin
  - Atrophy with subcortical U-fibers involved late
  - MRS: ↑ choline, ± ↑ myoinositol
- **Krabbe Disease**
  - NECT: Symmetric, bilateral high attenuation in thalami on early CT (3-6 months old)
  - ↑ T2: Thalami, basal ganglia, cerebellar nuclei, periventricular WM, corticospinal & pyramidal tracts
  - ± optic nerve enlargement
  - ± enhancement at junction of normal & abnormal WM
  - ± lumbar nerve root enhancement
  - MRS: ↑ choline, myoinositol; ↓ NAA
- **Hypomyelination**
  - T2 hypointensity of myelin normally lags behind T1 hyperintensity by 4-8 months
  - Myelination on T2 should be complete by 3 (but usually by 2) years of age
  - Primary hypomyelination syndromes are 2° to chromosome deletions & mutations
    - Pelizaeus-Merzbacher disease (PMD)
    - Spastic paraplegia type 2 (SPG2)
    - Hypomyelination with atrophy of basal ganglia & cerebellum (H-ABC)
    - 18q- syndrome
    - Jacobsen syndrome (11q-)
    - Hypomyelination with congenital cataracts (*DRCTNNB1A*)
    - Hypomyelination + trichothiodystrophy
- **Alexander Disease**
  - Astrocytopathy 2° to mutations in astrocyte-specific glial fibrillary acidic protein (GFAP) gene
  - Macrocephaly
  - Infantile form most common: Developmental delay, spasticity, seizures
  - ↑ T2 in bifrontal WM; caudate heads > putamina, thalami
  - Enhancement in periventricular frontal lobe WM in infantile form
  - Enhancement in cerebellum & medulla in juvenile form
  - ± enhancement in thalami, brainstem, dentate nuclei, cerebellar cortex, optic chiasm, fornix

- ± obstructive hydrocephalus 2° to periaqueductal disease
- **Vanishing White Matter Disease**
  - a.k.a. childhood ataxia with diffuse CNS hypomyelination or childhood ataxia with central hypomyelination (CACH)
  - Caused by mutations in genes encoding 5 subunits of eukaryotic translation initiation factor 2B (eIF2B)
  - Considered astrocytopathy: Loss of essential astrocytic functions & gain of detrimental functions → degeneration of WM
  - Bilateral symmetric, nonenhancing, diffuse hypointense T1/FLAIR & hyperintense T2 signal in cerebral WM
    - Begins in central cerebral WM
  - WM eventually becomes isointense to CSF → cystic degeneration
  - ± optic atrophy

Helpful Clues for Less Common Diagnoses

- **Mucopolysaccharidoses**
  - Hunter & Hurler syndrome are most common
  - Enlarged Virchow-Robin spaces, filled with glycosaminoglycans
  - Mild periventricular WM disease

Helpful Clues for Rare Diagnoses

- **Megalencephalic Leukoencephalopathy With Cysts**
  - a.k.a. van der Knaap disease
  - Most commonly caused by recessive mutations in *MLC1* or *GLIALCAM* genes
  - Macrocephaly
  - Peripheral WM swollen with enlarged gyri due to chronic WM edema
  - Less severe involvement of cerebellar WM
  - Subcortical cysts in posterior frontal & anterior temporal lobes
- **Merosin Deficient Congenital Muscular Dystrophy**
  - Hypomyelination of central cerebral WM
  - ± cerebellar vermis & pontine hypoplasia
- **Maple Syrup Urine Disease**
  - Acute phase: Edema & restricted diffusion in areas where normal neonatal WM should be myelinated
    - Deep cerebellar & perirolandic WM, dorsal brainstem, cerebral peduncles, posterior limb internal capsule ± globus pallidus
- **Nonketotic Hyperglycinemia**
  - Delayed myelination & edema in frontal cortex & subcortical WM
  - Long-echo MRS: Abnormal peak at 3.56 ppm probably represents glycine
- **Urea Cycle Disorders**
  - Multiple different enzyme deficiencies
  - Severe edema in cortex, subcortical WM, & basal ganglia
- **Giant Axonal Neuropathy**
  - Due to defects in gigaxonin that maintains neuroaxonal cytoskeletal integrity & transport (leuko-axonopathy) as well as proper intermediate filament degradation in astrocytes (astrocytopathy)
  - ↑ T2 signal in cerebral & cerebellar WM, sparing subcortical U-fibers
- **Trichothiodystrophy**
  - Galactosemia: Delayed myelination in subcortical WM on T2 with normal T1; ± cerebral & cerebellar atrophy
  - Cockayne syndrome: ↑ T2 periventricular WM, basal ganglia, cerebellar dentate nuclei
- **Oculocerebrorenal (Lowe) Syndrome**
  - X-linked recessive
  - Multiple CSF cysts in subcortical WM
  - Confluent areas of ↑ T2 in WM, sparing subcortical U-fibers
- **Hyperhomocysteinemia (Homocystinuria)**
  - Myelin destruction & ↓ volume of deep cerebral WM, sparing internal capsule, peripheral WM, & subcortical U-fibers

SELECTED REFERENCES

1. van der Knaap MS et al: Leukodystrophies: a proposed classification system based on pathological changes and pathogenetic mechanisms. Acta Neuropathol. 134(3):351-82, 2017
2. Parikh S et al: A clinical approach to the diagnosis of patients with leukodystrophies and genetic leukoencephelopathies. Mol Genet Metab. 114(4):501-15, 2015
3. Patay Z et al: Neurometabolic diseases of childhood. Pediatr Radiol. 45 Suppl 3:S473-84, 2015

X-Linked Adrenoleukodystrophy

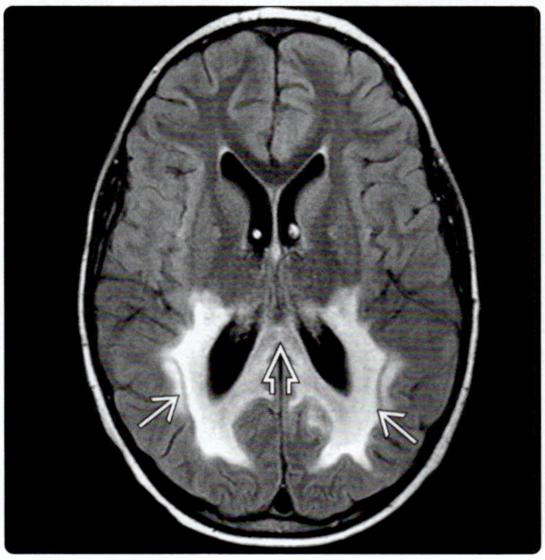

Canavan Disease

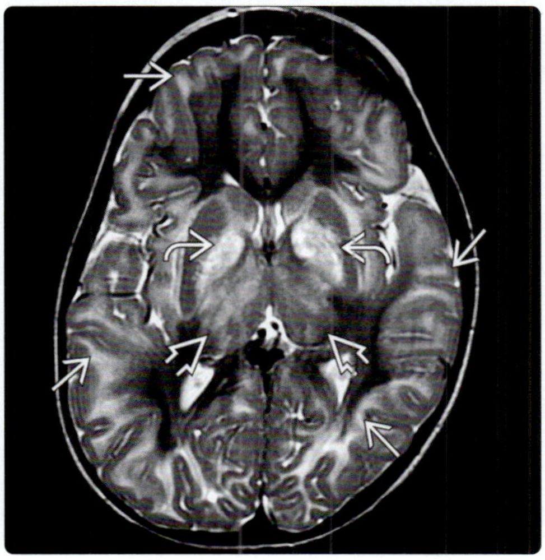

(Left) *Axial FLAIR MR in an 8-year-old boy shows symmetric, bilateral confluent areas of hyperintense signal abnormality in the parietooccipital white matter (WM) ➡ & corpus callosum splenium ➡, a classic distribution of demyelination in X-linked adrenoleukodystrophy.* **(Right)** *Axial T2 MR shows symmetric, bilateral, hyperintense signal in the subcortical U-fibers ➡, thalamus ➡, & globus pallidus ➡ bilaterally in a macrocephalic 3 year old with Canavan disease.*

(Left) *Axial T2 MR shows bilateral, symmetric hyperintense signal in the parietal & frontal lobe deep WM →, sparing the subcortical U-fibers ⇨.* **(Right)** *Axial T2 MR shows the typical radial stripes or tigroid appearance → of metachromatic leukodystrophy, which is secondary to relative sparing of the perivenular myelin. Also note sparing of the subcortical U-fibers ⇨, which are not involved until late in the disease.*

Metachromatic Leukodystrophy

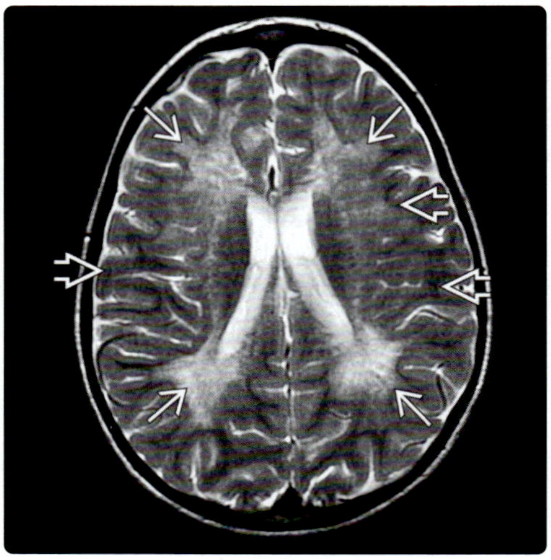

Metachromatic Leukodystrophy

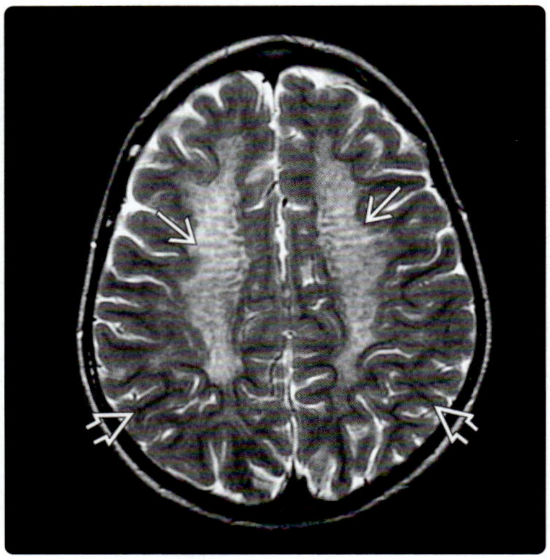

(Left) *Axial NECT shows hyperdense foci → in the bilateral thalami. The CT findings of hyperdensity may be present as early as 3-6 months of age & can precede abnormalities on MR in patients with Krabbe disease (also known as globoid cell leukodystrophy).* **(Right)** *Axial T2 MR shows symmetric increased signal in the posterior periventricular WM →, corticospinal tracts ⇨, & thalami ↷. Postcontrast images may show enhancement at the junction of normal & abnormal WM & in lumbar nerve roots.*

Krabbe Disease

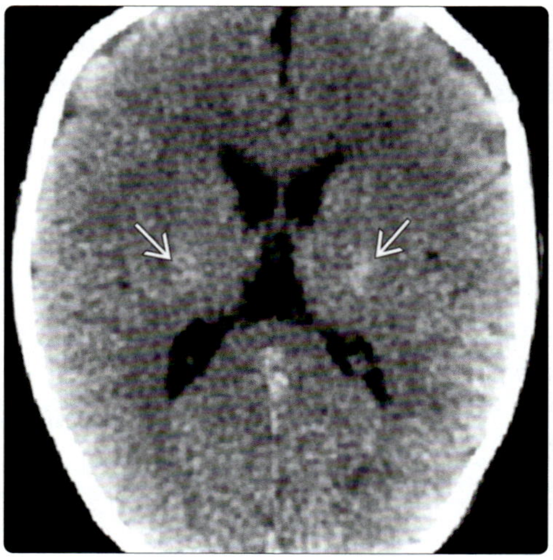

Krabbe Disease

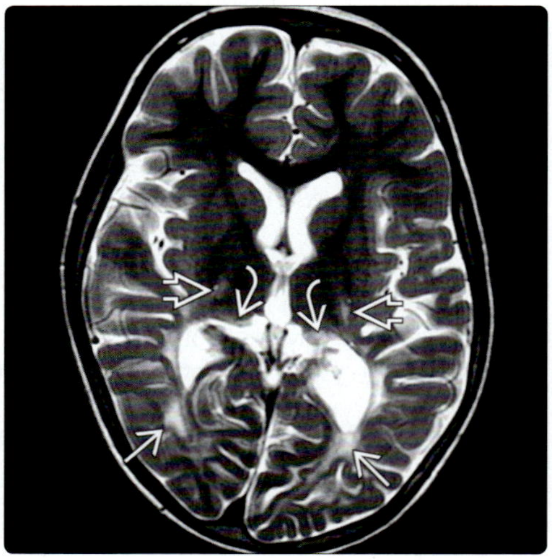

(Left) *Axial T2 MR in a 2 year old shows a diffuse lack of hypointense myelin in the deep WM of both cerebral hemispheres →, the corpus callosum ⇨, & the internal capsules ↷. Nearly all of the WM structures should be myelinated (hypointense on T2 MR) at this age.* **(Right)** *Axial T1 C+ MR shows abnormal symmetric hypointensity in the frontal lobe WM → as well as periventricular contrast enhancement ⇨, a typical distribution of Alexander disease in children.*

Hypomyelination

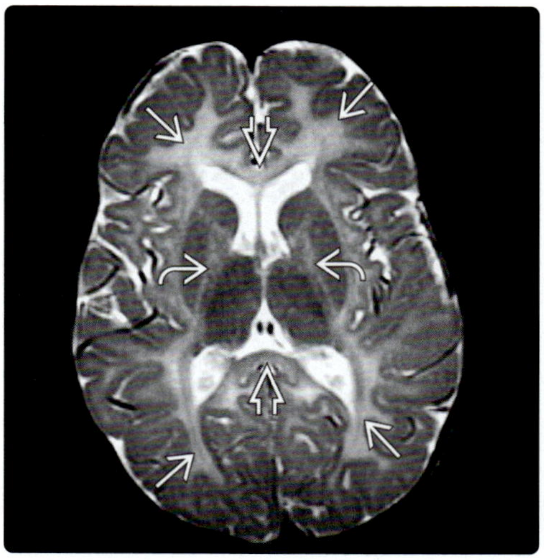

Alexander Disease

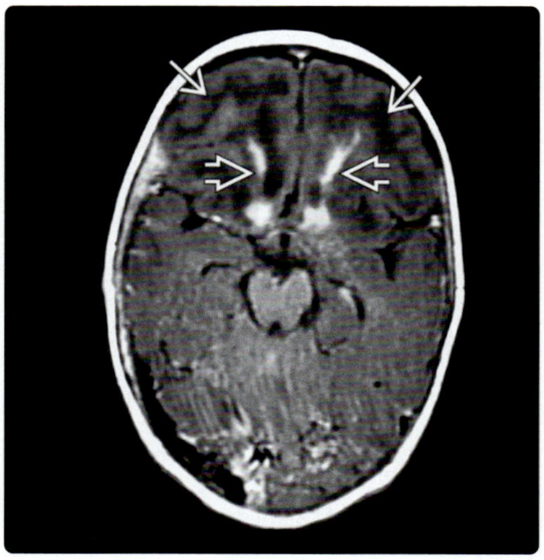

Vanishing White Matter Disease

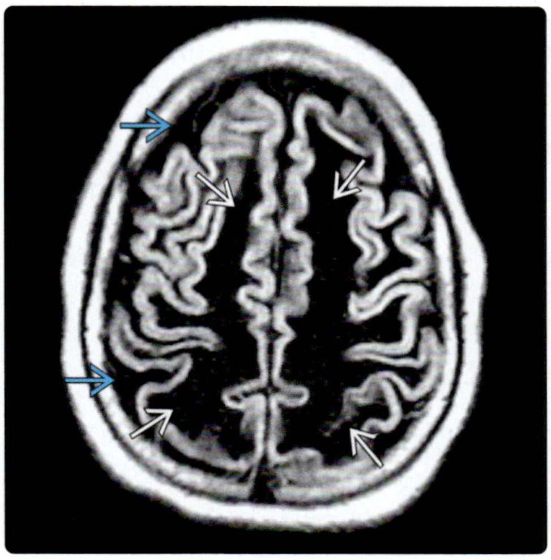

Mucopolysaccharidoses

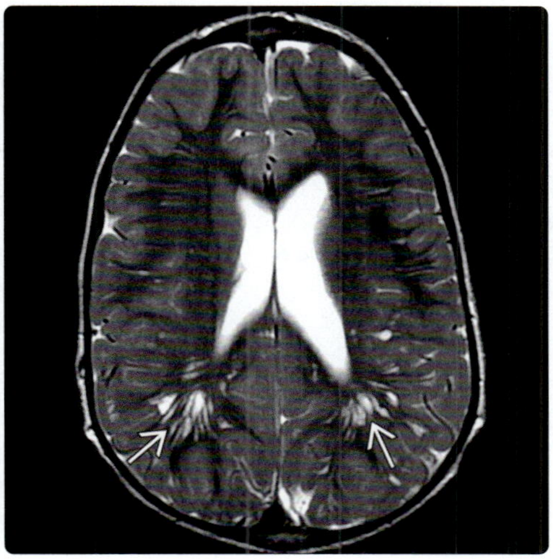

(Left) *Axial FLAIR MR shows diffusely abnormal WM that is isointense to CSF in a child with vanishing WM disease, also known as childhood ataxia with central hypomyelination (CACH).* **(Right)** *Axial T2 MR shows enlarged Virchow-Robin perivascular spaces in the bilateral parietal lobe WM in a child with Hurler syndrome. The enlarged spaces are thought to be filled with glycosaminoglycans.*

Megalencephalic Leukoencephalopathy With Cysts

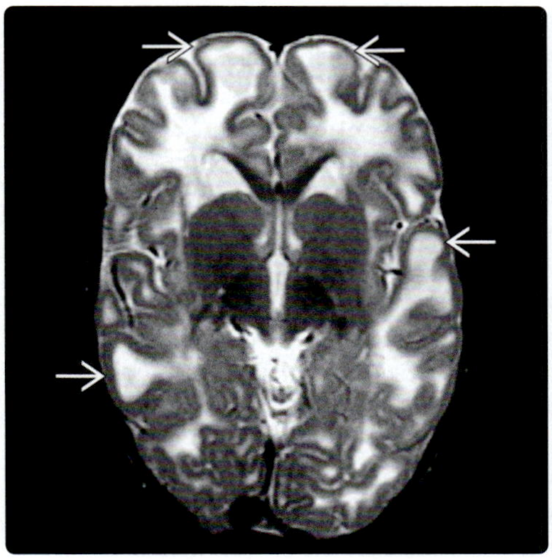

Megalencephalic Leukoencephalopathy With Cysts

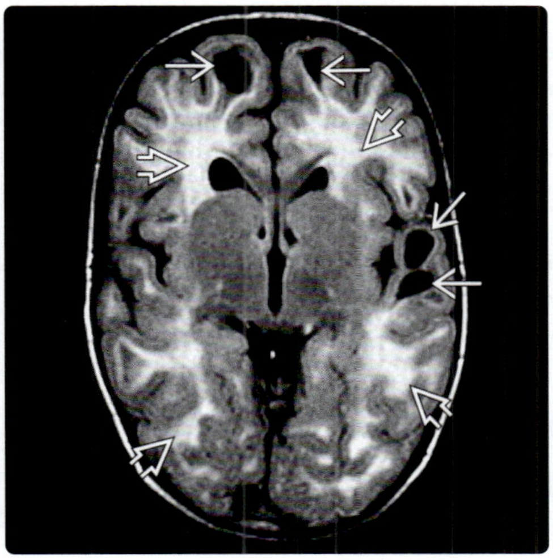

(Left) *Axial T2 MR shows abnormal, symmetric hyperintensity throughout the WM of both cerebral hemispheres. The frontal & temporal lobe WM appears swollen with enlarged gyri.* **(Right)** *Axial FLAIR MR in the same patient better differentiates the cysts from the adjacent abnormal, hyperintense, noncystic WM. The location of cysts in the frontal & anterior temporal lobes is typical. Patients with megalencephalic leukoencephalopathy may also have involvement of the cerebellar WM.*

Merosin Deficient Congenital Muscular Dystrophy

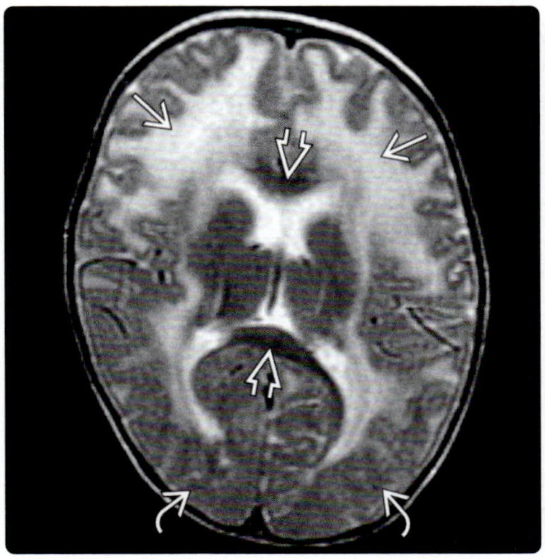

Maple Syrup Urine Disease

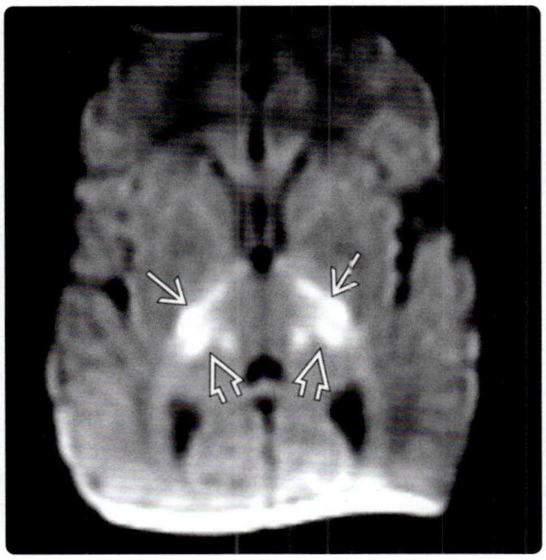

(Left) *Axial T2 MR shows diffusely abnormal hyperintense WM throughout both cerebral hemispheres in this 2 year old. The corpus callosum is spared & the subcortical U-fibers are partially spared.* **(Right)** *Axial DWI MR in a 10 day old with hypotonia & a newborn screen positive for MSUD shows marked diffusion restriction in the bilateral posterior limbs of the internal capsules & lateral thalami. Similar findings were also noted in the cerebellar WM & dorsal brainstem, typical areas of myelination in newborns.*

DIFFERENTIAL DIAGNOSIS

Common

- Prematurity

Rare but Important

- Primary Hypomyelination Syndromes
  - Pelizaeus-Merzbacher Disease
  - *TUBB4A*-Related Hypomyelinating Disorder
  - Hypomyelination With Atrophy of Basal Ganglia & Cerebellum
  - 18q- Syndrome
  - Gangliosidosis
  - Hypomyelination With Congenital Cataracts
  - Oculodentodigital Dysplasia
  - Fucosidosis
  - Trichothiodystrophy
  - Congenital Glycosylation Disorder
- Dysmyelination Syndromes
  - Mucopolysaccharidoses
  - Leukodystrophies
    - Merosin-Deficient Congenital Muscular Dystrophy
    - Metachromatic Leukodystrophy
    - Maple Syrup Urine Disease
    - Aicardi-Goutieres Syndrome
    - Neuronal Ceroid Lipofuscinosis
    - Vanishing White Matter Disease
    - Canavan Disease
    - Globoid Cell Leukodystrophy (Krabbe Disease)
  - Therapy-Related White Matter Changes
    - Chronic Methotrexate Toxicity
    - Radiation Therapy

ESSENTIAL INFORMATION

Key Differential Diagnosis Issues

- Clinical features to consider
  - Most common symptoms: Developmental delay (DD)/regression, hypotonia, & spasticity
    - Less common: Nystagmus, seizure, & ataxia
  - Primary hypomyelination (HM) disorders typically present in 1st year of life with DD
    - Most are autosomal recessive (AR) or sporadic; M ~ F
  - Dysmyelination disorders present at varying ages with developmental regression
  - Note that some disorders could potentially be classified into either category
- Imaging features to consider
  - Critical to understand normal MR pattern of myelination during first 2 years of life
    - T1 is most helpful < 12 months (as myelination is generally complete on T1 by ~ 12 months in term infant)
    - T2 is most helpful > 12 months (as myelination is generally complete on T2 by ~ 24-30 months if term)
    - FLAIR is not generally helpful until myelination is complete on T2
  - Degree of HM varies from marked to subtle
    - Many primary HM disorders are subtle
      - □ Near normal on T1 but abnormal on T2 & FLAIR
    - Many have overlapping imaging features
  - Dysmyelination disorders usually have more severe imaging findings
    - Abnormal on T1, T2, & FLAIR
    - Many dysmyelination disorders have specific imaging features, at least early in disease course
- Modality considerations
  - CT: Will show ↓ attenuation in more severe cases
  - MR: Routine brain sequences are mainstay of diagnosis
    - DWI/DTI: Most HM & dysmyelination syndromes lead to ↑ ADC, ↓ FA, & ↑ RD
    - MRS: Some specific patterns in certain leukodystrophies

Helpful Clues for Common Diagnoses

- **Prematurity**
  - Critical to know gestational age at birth when interpreting infant MR
    - If patient is premature & this is not accounted for, one will interpret as delayed myelination
      - □ e.g., 24-week gestation premature infant will have myelination pattern of term newborn at 4 months

Helpful Clues for Rare Diagnoses

- **Primary Hypomyelination Syndromes**
  - **Pelizaeus-Merzbacher disease**
    - X-linked with nystagmus & dystonia
    - Homogeneous HM on T1 & T2; late atrophy
      - □ T1 looks like FLAIR & FLAIR looks like T1 (beyond time when myelination is expected to be complete)
  - **TUBB4A-related hypomyelinating disorder**
    - DD, hypotonia, nystagmus, spastic paresis
    - Isolated HM
  - **HM with atrophy of basal ganglia & cerebellum**
    - DD, hypotonia, nystagmus, extrapyramidal movement disorder
    - Homogeneous HM, atrophy of putamen
  - **18q- syndrome**
    - Abnormal facies, sensorineural hearing loss, hypotonia, seizures, nystagmus
    - Homo- or heterogeneous HM, cerebellar atrophy
  - **Gangliosidosis**
    - Rare lysosomal disorder with multiple subtypes (e.g., Tay-Sachs)
    - Progressive neuromotor deterioration, hypotonia, seizures
    - Symmetric diffuse HM; ↑ T1 & ↓ T2 in deep gray nuclei
  - **HM with congenital cataracts**
    - Cataracts, motor delay
    - Heterogeneous HM, periventricular ↓ T1 ↑ T2, atrophy
  - **Oculodentodigital dysplasia**
    - Abnormal dentition, eyes, hands; ataxia, seizures
    - Homogeneous HM, cerebellar atrophy, ↓ T2 of globus pallidus
  - **Fucosidosis**
    - Rare disorder due to α-L-fucosidase deficiency
    - Progressive neurologic deterioration, coarse facies, skin abnormalities, intrauterine growth restriction
    - Symmetric diffuse HM + deep gray nuclei abnormalities

- Trichothiodystrophy
  - Coarse & brittle hair, ichthyosis, short stature, abnormal facies
  - Homogeneous HM on T1 & T2, cerebellar atrophy
- Congenital glycosylation disorder
  - Hypotonia, liver & renal disease, facial dysmorphism
  - Homo- or heterogeneous HM, cerebellar atrophy

- **Dysmyelination Syndromes**
  - **Mucopolysaccharidoses**
    - e.g., Hunter, Hurler syndromes
    - Lysosomal storage disorders
    - Normal at birth; develop coarse facies, myelopathy
    - Symmetric white matter (WM) signal abnormality, prominent perivascular spaces, craniocervical junction stenosis, hydrocephalus
  - **Merosin-deficient congenital muscular dystrophy**
    - Hypotonia, weakness, near-normal intelligence
    - Diffuse symmetric WM signal abnormality
  - **Metachromatic leukodystrophy**
    - Lysosomal storage disease due to arylsulfatase A deficiency
    - Spasticity, ataxia, intellectual disability
    - Symmetric periventricular & deep WM with sparing of subcortical WM; classic "tigroid" WM
      - Cranial nerve enhancement
  - **Maple syrup urine disease**
    - Disorder of branched-chain amino acid metabolism
    - Presents at 4-10 days with ketoacidosis, hyperammonemia
    - Affects myelinated brain
    - MRS: Broad peak at chemical shift of 0.9 ppm
  - **Aicardi-Goutieres syndrome**
    - Inherited leukodystrophy (multiple genes)
    - Variable clinical course, spasticity
    - Diffuse symmetric WM abnormalities, atrophy, brain Ca^{2+} from microangiopathy
  - **Neuronal ceroid lipofuscinosis**
    - a.k.a. Batten disease
    - Lysosomal storage disease (lipofuscin deposition)
    - Neuromotor deterioration, blindness, seizures
    - Diffuse symmetric WM abnormality, cerebral & cerebellar cortical atrophy, ↓ T2 in thalami
  - **Vanishing WM disease**
    - Poorly understood leukoencephalopathy of childhood
    - Rapid neuromotor deterioration after trauma/illness
    - Diffuse WM abnormalities follow CSF signal
  - **Canavan disease**
    - Progressive AR spongiform leukodystrophy
    - Hypotonia, macrocephaly, seizures
    - Involves both WM & deep gray nuclei
    - ↑ T2 & diffusion restriction in areas of involvement
      - Diffusion restriction may persist for years
    - MRS: ↑ NAA
  - **Globoid cell leukodystrophy (Krabbe disease)**
    - Progressive AR degenerative leukodystrophy
    - Spasticity, ataxia, seizures, & peripheral neuropathy
    - Diffuse symmetric cerebral & cerebellar WM abnormalities
    - Frequent involvement of deep gray nuclei
      - Ca^{2+} on CT, ↓ T2/SWI on MR
    - Peripheral nerve root enhancement

- **Therapy-Related White Matter Changes**
  - **Chronic methotrexate (MTX) toxicity**
    - Permanent WM injury related to high-dose intravenous (IV) or intrathecal MTX (vs. acute reversible form)
    - Symmetric ↑ T2 in WM that typically progresses slowly
  - **Radiation therapy (XRT)**
    - Whole-brain XRT can rarely lead to diffuse WM injury
    - Delayed onset, often years after XRT
    - Usually spares subcortical WM
    - Disseminated necrotizing leukoencephalopathy: Rare complication of whole-brain XRT + chemotherapy

SELECTED REFERENCES

1. Barkovich AJ et al: Hypomyelinating disorders: An MRI approach. Neurobiol Dis. 87:50-8, 2016

Prematurity

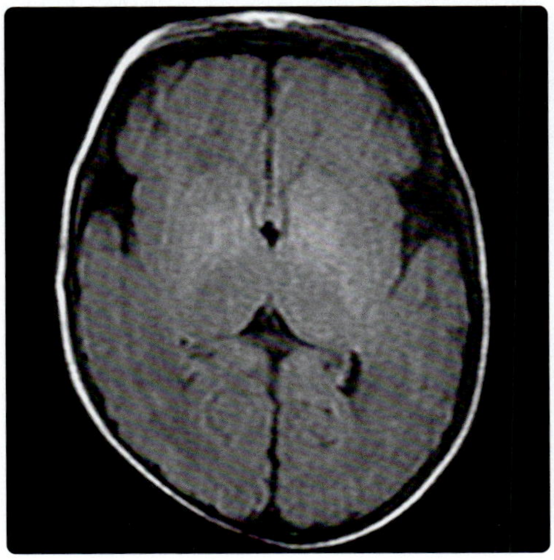

Prematurity

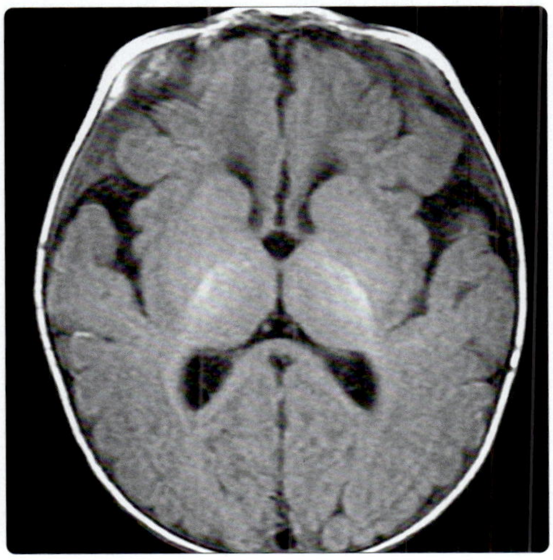

(Left) *Axial T1 MR in a 3 month old born at 25-weeks gestation shows expected myelination for a 37-week infant. If, however, this is interpreted without the clinical history of prematurity, one would incorrectly suggest delayed myelination or hypomyelination.* **(Right)** *Axial T1 MR in a 6 month old born at 24-weeks gestation shows expected myelination for a 2 month old. If this is study is interpreted as a 6-month-old term infant, one would incorrectly suggest delayed myelination or hypomyelination.*

(Left) *Axial T1 MR shows a 26 month old with nystagmus & head titubation, diagnosed with Pelizaeus-Merzbacher disease. The homogeneous absence of myelin deposition causes this T1 MR to mimic a normal FLAIR MR in a mature brain.* **(Right)** *Conversely, this axial FLAIR MR in a 6 year old with Pelizaeus-Merzbacher disease resembles a normal T1 MR with hyperintense signal of the white matter (WM) relative to gray matter throughout.*

Pelizaeus-Merzbacher Disease

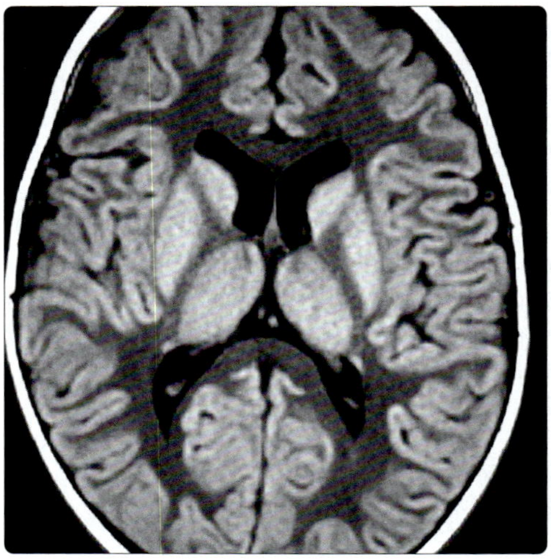

Pelizaeus-Merzbacher Disease

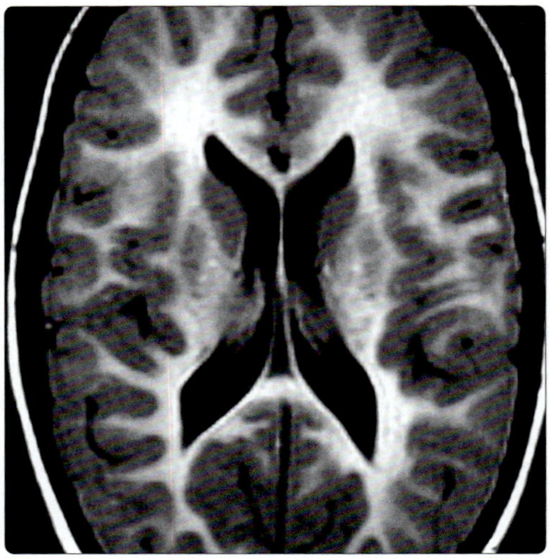

(Left) *Coronal T2 MR in a 14 year old shows hypomyelination & atrophy of the basal ganglia & cerebellum (H-ABC). Note the absence of any visible caudate nuclei ➔ & corpus callosum in addition to the abnormal hyperintense signal of unmyelinated WM.* **(Right)** *Axial T1 MR in a 9 month old with 18q- syndrome shows only faint T1 shortening that is limited to the internal capsules & optic radiations. At 9 months, only the most distal rami of WM should be without bright T1 signal.*

Hypomyelination With Atrophy of Basal Ganglia & Cerebellum

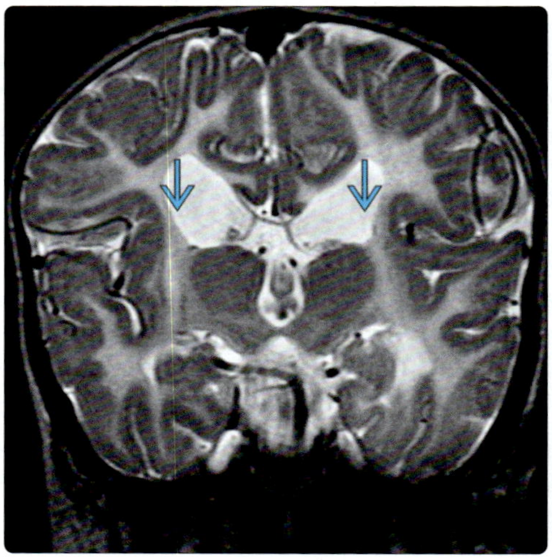

18q- Syndrome

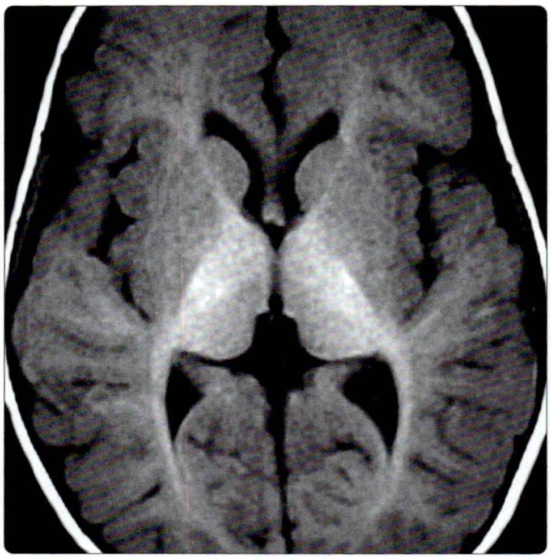

(Left) *Axial T1 MR in a 7 month old with GM1 gangliosidosis shows absence of normal hyperintensity in the anterior limb of the internal capsule ➔ & optic radiations ➯, areas that should be myelinated at this age.* **(Right)** *Sagittal T1 MR in the same patient shows a thin corpus callosum & no myelination in areas that should show bright signal at this age (e.g., dorsal brainstem ➯, mid corpus callosum ➔, etc.), consistent with hypomyelination.*

Gangliosidosis

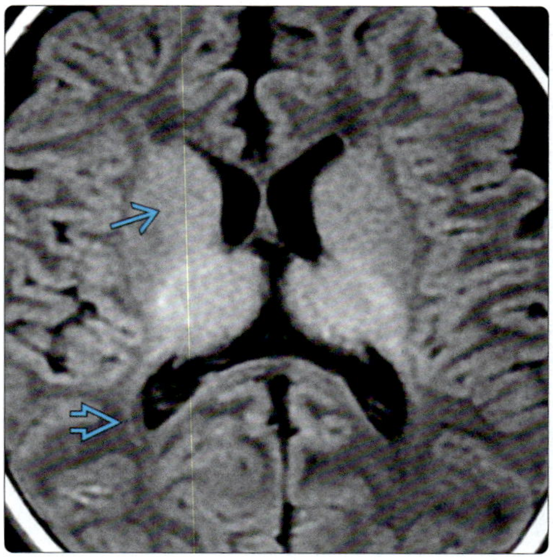

Gangliosidosis

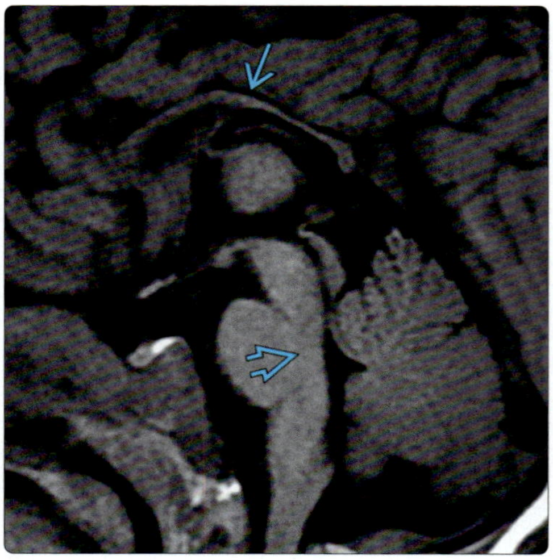

Oculodentodigital Dysplasia

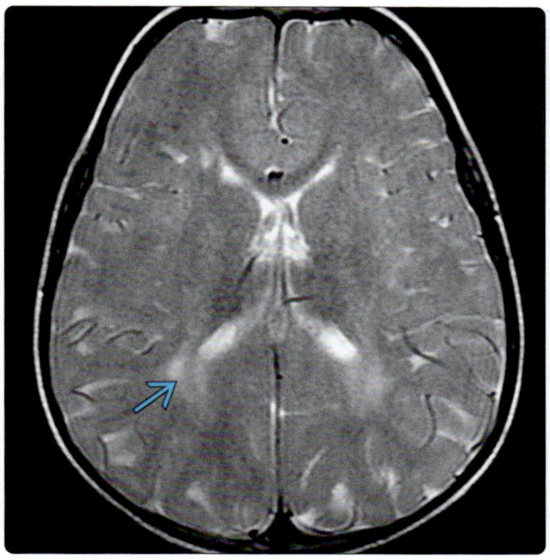

Fucosidosis

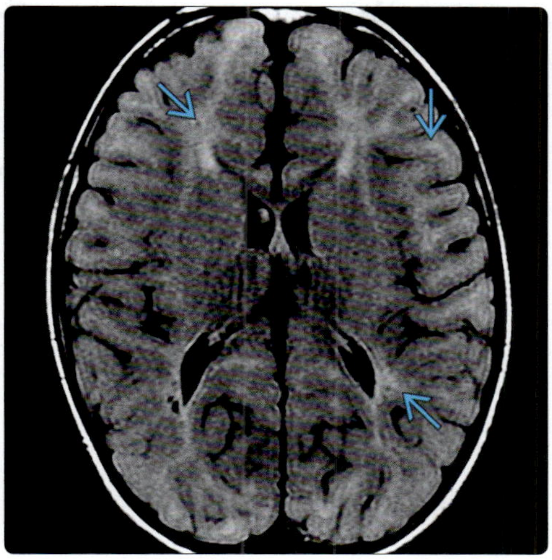

(Left) *Axial T2 MR in a 4 year old with oculodentodigital dysplasia shows hyperintense signal in the periventricular WM → with poor delineation of cortical gray matter & subcortical WM, consistent with hypomyelination.* **(Right)** *Axial FLAIR MR in a 3 year old with fucosidosis shows increased signal throughout the WM → at an age when myelination should be nearly complete (i.e., WM should be of decreased FLAIR signal intensity).*

Trichothiodystrophy

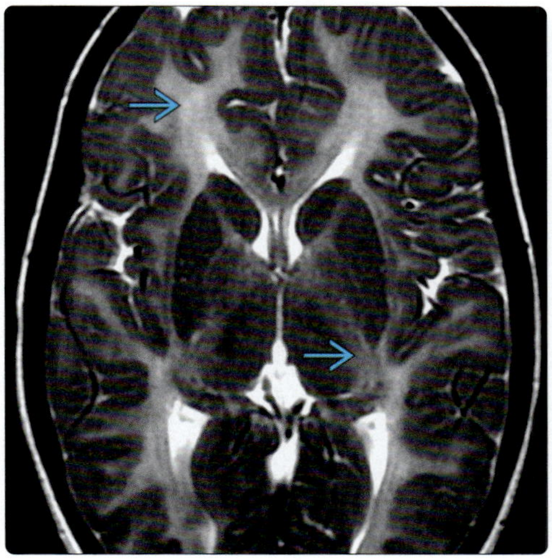

Congenital Glycosylation Disorder

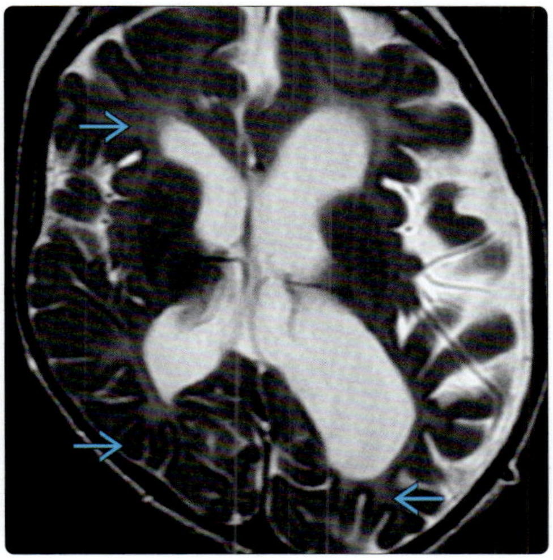

(Left) *Axial T2 MR in a 12 year old with trichothiodystrophy shows a near-complete absence of myelination throughout the brain →. Examination of the hair under polarized light demonstrated characteristic "tiger-tail" bands, & radiographs showed central osteosclerosis.* **(Right)** *Axial T2 MR in a 9 year old with a congenital disorder of glycosylation shows a small volume of WM with increased signal involving the periventricular, deep, & subcortical WM →.*

Mucopolysaccharidoses

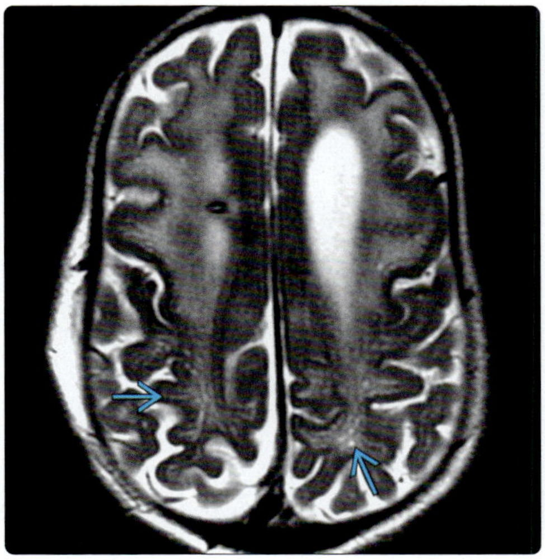

Merosin-Deficient Congenital Muscular Dystrophy

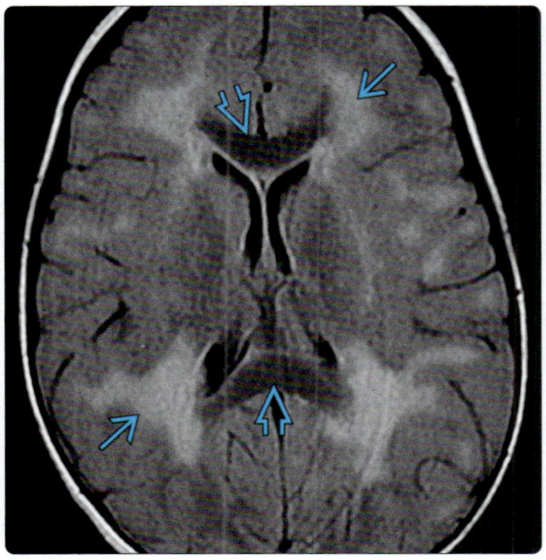

(Left) *Axial T2 MR in a 5 year old with type 1 mucopolysaccharidosis (Hurler syndrome) shows increased signal throughout the WM. Also note the linear areas of fluid signal → in the subcortical WM, consistent with prominent perivascular spaces, a common finding in this disorder.* **(Right)** *Axial FLAIR MR in a 2 year old with merosin-deficient congenital muscular dystrophy shows symmetric hyperintensity → throughout the WM with sparing of the corpus callosum →.*

Metachromatic Leukodystrophy

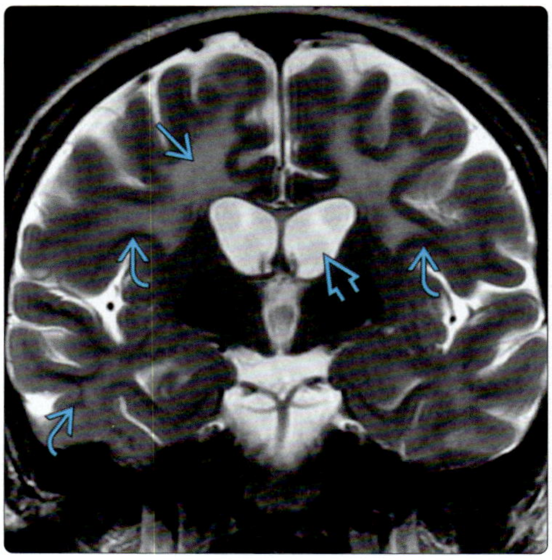

Metachromatic Leukodystrophy

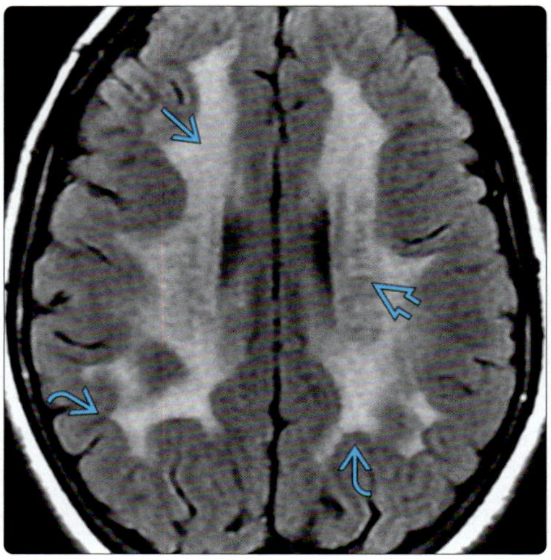

(Left) *Coronal T2 MR in a 13 year old with metachromatic leukodystrophy (MCL) shows centrally increased WM signal → with sparing of the immediate subcortical WM →. There is associated volume loss with ex vacuo ventriculomegaly →, which is typically progressive in this disease.* **(Right)** *Axial FLAIR MR in the same patient shows WM hyperintense signal → with sparing of the immediate subcortical WM →. Also note the linear hypointense foci in the centrum semiovale (tigroid pattern) →, a common finding in MCL.*

Maple Syrup Urine Disease

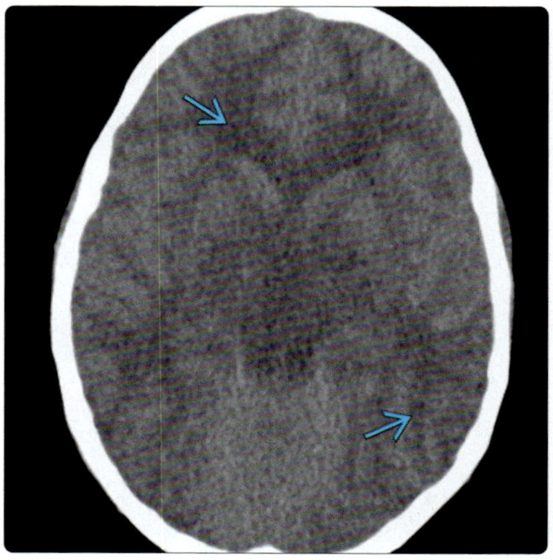

Maple Syrup Urine Disease

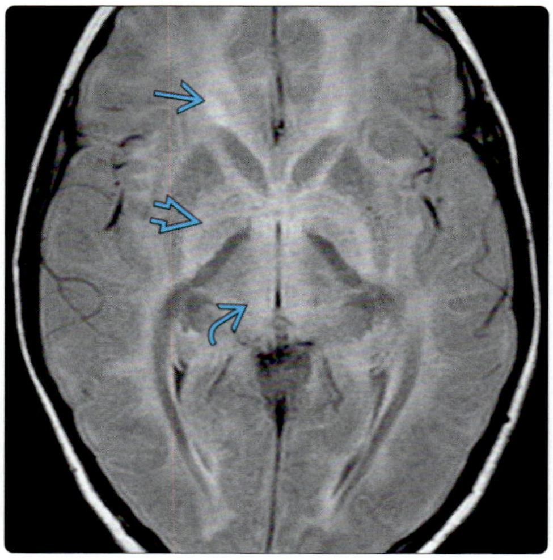

(Left) *Axial NECT in a 9 year old with maple syrup urine disease (MSUD) shows decreased attenuation throughout the WM →. This disease, when uncontrolled, causes permanent injury to myelinated WM.* **(Right)** *Axial FLAIR MR in the same patient shows hyperintense signal throughout much of the WM → as well as globus pallidus → & thalamus →. This appearance is nonspecific but should prompt consideration of this diagnosis.*

Aicardi-Goutieres Syndrome

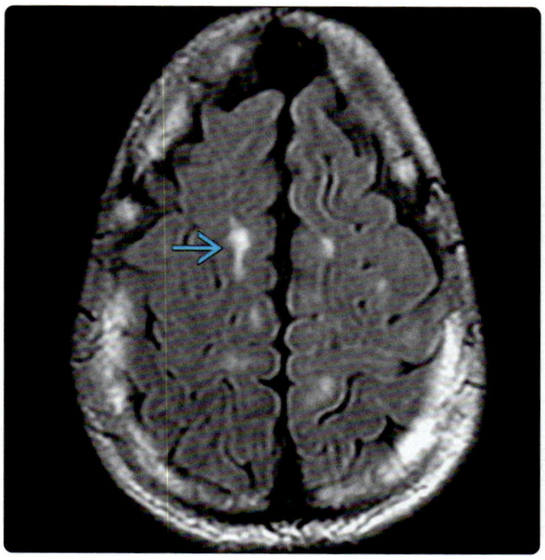

Aicardi-Goutieres Syndrome

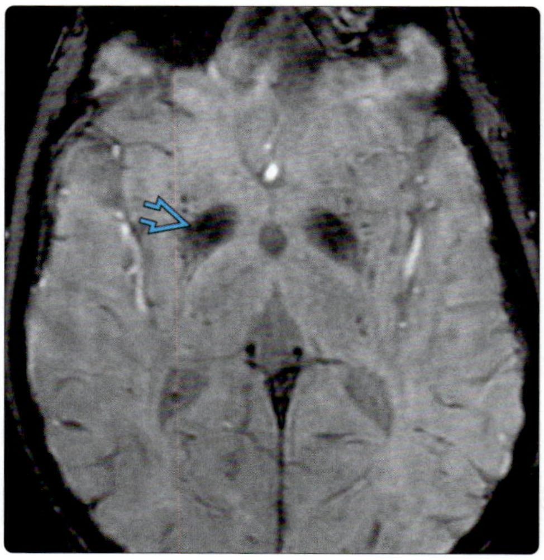

(Left) *Axial FLAIR MR in an 18 year old with Aicardi-Goutieres syndrome shows patchy areas of increased signal → in the subcortical WM. Look for associated mineralization in the basal ganglia (especially globus pallidus) to suggest this particular diagnosis.* **(Right)** *Axial SWI MR in the same patient shows symmetric marked signal loss in the bilateral globus pallidus nuclei →, suggesting mineralization.*

Vanishing White Matter Disease

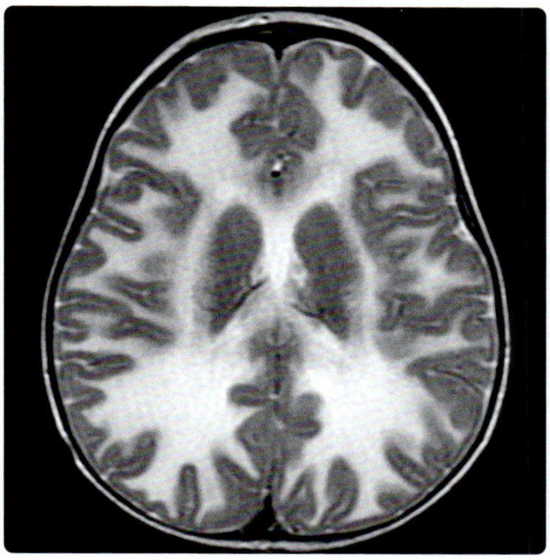

Vanishing White Matter Disease

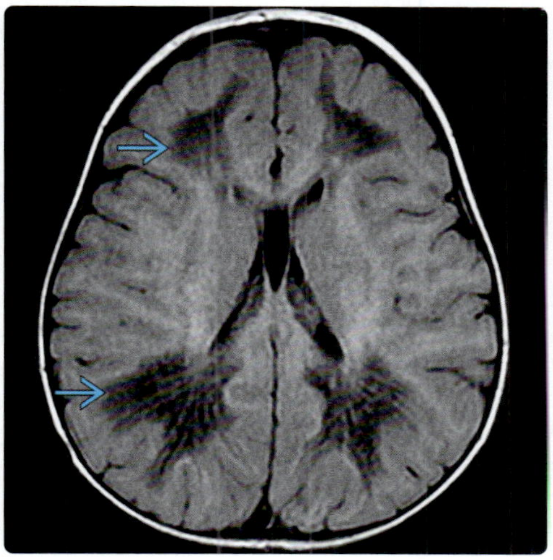

(Left) *Axial T2 MR in a 19 month old with vanishing WM disease (VWMD) shows markedly increased signal & increased volume of the WM diffusely. In this disease, the WM signal follows CSF on nearly all sequences.* **(Right)** *Axial FLAIR MR in a 19 month old with VWMD shows markedly increased signal & volume of the WM. Since the WM signal follows CSF signal on nearly all sequences in this disorder, suppression of the affected WM signal on FLAIR is a characteristic finding.*

Canavan Disease

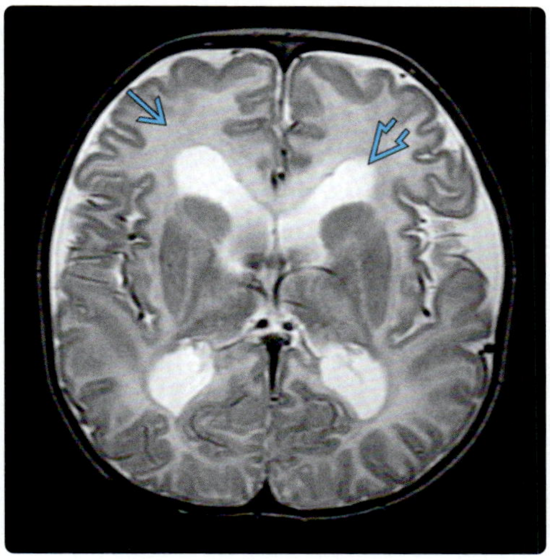

Canavan Disease

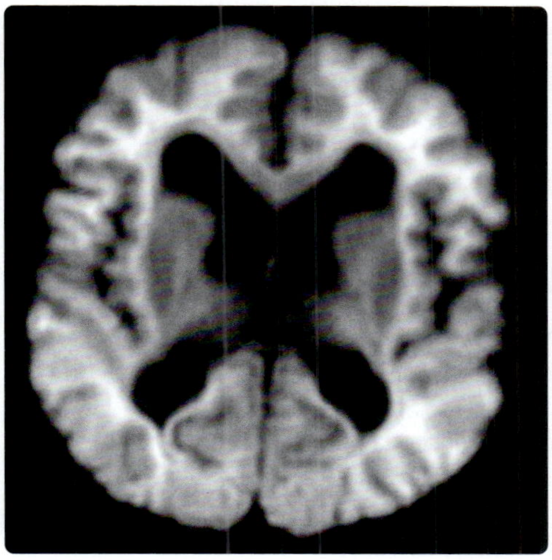

(Left) *Axial T2 MR in a 3 year old with macrocephaly due to Canavan disease shows increased signal throughout the WM with lateral ventricular enlargement.* **(Right)** *Axial DWI MR in the same patient shows diffusion restriction (↓ ADC not shown) throughout the WM, a finding that can persist for years. Markedly increased NAA on MR spectroscopy can also help to distinguish it from other dysmyelinating leukodystrophies.*

Chronic Methotrexate Toxicity

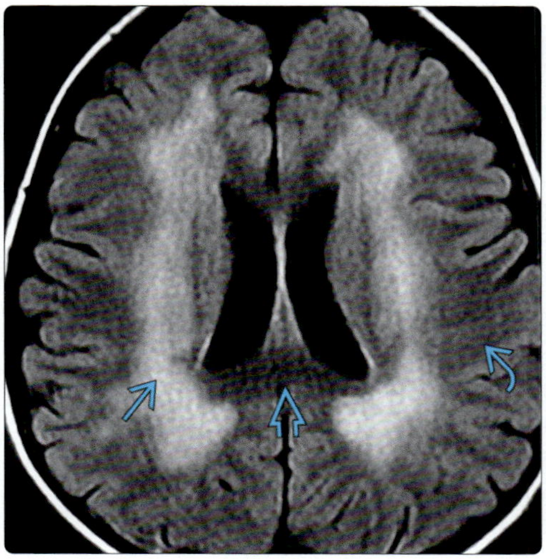

Chronic Methotrexate Toxicity

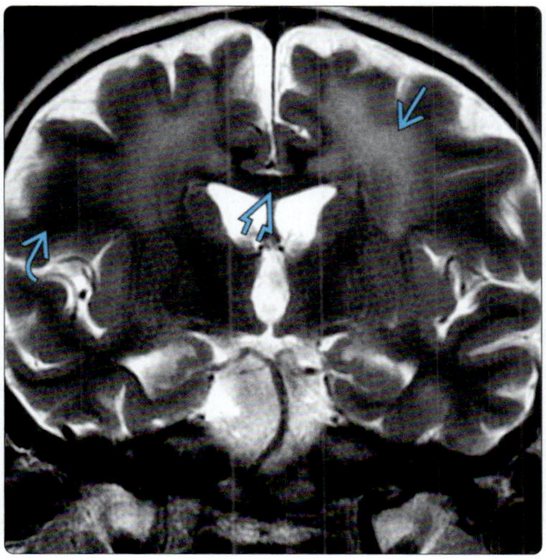

(Left) *Axial FLAIR MR in a 4 year old with acute lymphoblastic leukemia, previously treated with intrathecal methotrexate (MTX), shows symmetric signal hyperintensity in the periventricular & deep WM with sparing of the corpus callosum & subcortical WM.* **(Right)** *Coronal T2 MR in the same patient shows symmetric signal hyperintensity in the periventricular & deep WM with sparing of the corpus callosum & subcortical WM.*

Deep Gray Nuclei Abnormalities

DIFFERENTIAL DIAGNOSIS

Common

- Hypoxic-Ischemic Encephalopathy
- Gadolinium Deposition
- Neurofibromatosis Type 1

Less Common

- Venous Ischemia
- Arterial Infarct
- Leigh Syndrome
- Low-Grade Glioma
- Bithalamic Glioma
- Germinoma
- Neonatal Herpes Encephalitis
- Group B Streptococcal Meningitis
- Acute Disseminated Encephalomyelitis

Rare but Important

- Hemolytic Uremic Syndrome
- Carbon Monoxide Intoxication
- Kernicterus
- Wilson Disease
- Nonalcoholic Wernicke Encephalopathy
- Juvenile Huntington Disease
- Krabbe Disease
- Pantothenate Kinase-Associated Neurodegeneration
- Creutzfeldt-Jakob Disease

ESSENTIAL INFORMATION

Key Differential Diagnosis Issues

- Many diagnoses have characteristic history
  - Low Apgar scores, apnea, bradycardia, & seizures or cardiac arrest: Hypoxic-ischemic encephalopathy (HIE)
  - Gadolinium (Gd) deposition (many prior MR scans with contrast)
  - Classic skin lesions, Lisch nodules, plexiform neurofibromas: Neurofibromatosis type 1 (NF1)
  - Fever & seizure in neonate: Herpes encephalitis vs. group B streptococcal meningitis
  - Wilson disease (liver failure)
  - Kernicterus (hyperbilirubinemia)
  - Nonalcoholic Wernicke encephalopathy [chronic total parenteral nutrition (TPN)]
  - Juvenile Huntington disease (rigidity, bradykinesia, ataxia)
- Symmetry is main imaging feature to consider
  - Unilateral: Low-grade glioma, germinoma, infection, arterial/venous ischemia
  - Bilateral: HIE, toxic/metabolic/degenerative, infection, bithalamic glioma, venous ischemia
- Modality considerations
  - CT: Many diagnoses are not visible
    - Helps identify Ca^{2+} (Krabbe disease)
    - Acute vascular thrombus is often most conspicuous on NECT
  - MR: Most sensitive exam for deep gray abnormalities
    - DWI: Aids in distinguishing acute & chronic abnormalities
    - SWI: Helpful to identify thrombosis & associated Ca^{2+}

Helpful Clues for Common Diagnoses

- **Hypoxic-Ischemic Encephalopathy**
  - MR: Symmetric diffusion restriction in deep gray nuclei ± cortex hours to days after hypoxic-Ischemic (HI) event
    - Neonatal brain often shows alterations in T1 & T2 signal ~ 2-3 days after insult
  - CT: Loss of gray-white differentiation
  - Deep gray involvement suggests "profound" injury due to complete or near-complete lack of blood flow/oxygen
    - e.g., placental abruption in neonate or cardiac arrest
  - Deep gray structures are often preserved by cerebrovascular autoregulation in partial or less severe HI episodes
- **Gadolinium Deposition**
  - MR: Symmetric ↑ T1 in globus pallidus & dentate nuclei due to multiple previous contrasted exams
  - Typically seen in patients with history of tumor, tuberous sclerosis complex, NF1, & multiple sclerosis
- **Neurofibromatosis Type 1**
  - MR: Nonenhancing signal abnormalities are most common in globus pallidi (GP) & thalami
    - Look for other signs of NF1
      - Additional nonenhancing lesions in brainstem & deep cerebellum
      - Optic pathway glioma, orbital/facial plexiform neurofibroma, moyamoya arteriopathy, sphenoid wing dysplasia

Helpful Clues for Less Common Diagnoses

- **Venous Infarction**
  - MR: Uni- or bilateral deep gray signal abnormalities ± diffusion restriction with deep venous thrombosis
    - Internal cerebral veins & straight sinus are most commonly affected
    - Use GRE/SWI to look for blooming in deep veins
  - NECT: ↑ density in acutely thrombosed vessels
- **Arterial Infarction**
  - Deep gray structures are often involved in proximal middle cerebral artery/posterior cerebral artery ischemia
    - Due to occlusion of thalamostriate & anterior choroidal arteries
    - Usually in association with cortical ischemia
    - Look for underlying cause: Proximal branch vessel thrombus, moyamoya, or embolic phenomenon
- **Leigh Syndrome**
  - MR: Symmetric ↑ T2/↓ T1 & diffusion restriction in deep gray nuclei due to precipitating illness superimposed on mitochondrial defect
    - Putamen most common but often multiple nuclei
  - Correlate with ↑ brain, CSF, & serum lactate
- **Low-Grade Glioma**
  - Unilateral, mass-like expansion of deep gray nuclei
  - Heterogeneous appearance depending on solid vs. cystic components
  - Majority of low-grade gliomas show enhancement
- **Bithalamic Glioma**
  - Nearly symmetric bithalamic enlargement (often massive)
  - Usually due to grade III astrocytoma
  - Typically shows no enhancement
- **Germinoma**

- ~ 10% arise in deep gray (putamen > thalami)
- Enhancing, cellular (↑ DWI/↓ ADC MR) mass, ± small cysts
- **Neonatal Herpes Encephalitis**
  - Deep gray involvement is common in herpes simplex virus 2 but rarely in isolation
    - Almost always has associated cortical involvement (especially temporal)
  - DWI MR is most sensitive for early detection & full extent
- **Group B Streptococcal Meningitis**
  - Infectious vasculitis causes ischemia within arterial territories & often affects deep gray nuclei
  - Diffusion restriction ± abnormal signal in involved areas
- **Acute Disseminated Encephalomyelitis**
  - Autoimmune demyelination of brain & spinal cord
  - Multifocal white matter & deep gray matter lesions occur days to weeks after infection or vaccination
  - Thalami & basal ganglia involvement are common, usually symmetric

Helpful Clues for Rare Diagnoses

- **Hemolytic Uremic Syndrome**
  - Hemolytic anemia/thrombocytopenia + renal failure
    - Caused by Shiga-toxin producing *Escherichia coli* O157:H7
  - CNS complications occur in minority of cases
  - ↑ FLAIR MR signal with patchy diffusion restriction in deep gray nuclei
    - Often with hemorrhagic component
- **Carbon Monoxide Intoxication**
  - CO impairs RBC capacity to carry oxygen → HI injury
  - Acute phase: ↑ T2 MR + diffusion restriction in GP
  - Chronic phase: ↑ T2 MR + volume loss in GP
  - May affect white matter & cortex (especially temporal) in severe cases
- **Kernicterus**
  - Brain injury secondary to hyperbilirubinemia
  - Acute: ↑ T1 MR in globus pallidus, hippocampi
  - Chronic: ↑ T2 MR in globus pallidus, hippocampi
- **Wilson Disease**
  - Autosomal recessive (AR) copper metabolism disorder resulting in copper accumulation in liver & brain (basal ganglia)
  - MRI: Symmetric ↑ T2, ↓ T1 in all deep gray nuclei
    - ↑ DWI/↓ ADC in acute phase; ↑ ADC in chronic phase
- **Nonalcoholic Wernicke Encephalopathy**
  - Thiamine (vitamin B1) deficiency or chronic TPN in children
  - MR: Symmetric ↑ T2 FLAIR + ↑ DWI/↓ ADC in medial thalami, hypothalamus, mammillary bodies, & tectum
- **Juvenile Huntington Disease**
  - Rare childhood onset of Huntington disease
  - CT/MR: Volume loss in caudate & putamen
  - MR: Symmetric ↑ T2, ↓ T1 in caudate & putamen
- **Krabbe Disease**
  - a.k.a. globoid cell leukodystrophy
  - Progressive AR degenerative leukodystrophy
  - CT: Symmetric Ca^{2+} in thalami, basal ganglia, corona radiata, & cerebellum
  - MRI: ↓ T1 & ↓ T2 in thalami & basal ganglia; ↓ T1 & ↑ T2 in white matter
- **Pantothenate Kinase-Associated Neurodegeneration**
  - Most common form of neurodegeneration with brain iron accumulation (NBIA)
  - Eye of tiger sign → rim of ↓ T2 (iron) with central ↑ T2 (gliosis) in GP
- **Creutzfeldt-Jakob Disease**
  - Prion brain disease causing rapid-onset dementia
    - Very rare in children
  - MR: Symmetric ↑ T2 FLAIR + ↑ DWI/↓ ADC in posteromedial thalami, caudate, & putamen

SELECTED REFERENCES

1. Lyons DA et al: Non-alcoholic Wernicke encephalopathy. Pediatr Neurol. 56:94-5, 2016
2. Bekiesinska-Figatowska M et al: Basal ganglia lesions in children and adults. Eur J Radiol. 82(5):837-49, 2013
3. Hegde AN et al: Differential diagnosis for bilateral abnormalities of the basal ganglia and thalamus. Radiographics. 31(1):5-30, 2011
4. Ho VB et al: Bilateral basal ganglia lesions: pediatric differential considerations. Radiographics. 13(2):269-92, 1993

Hypoxic-Ischemic Encephalopathy

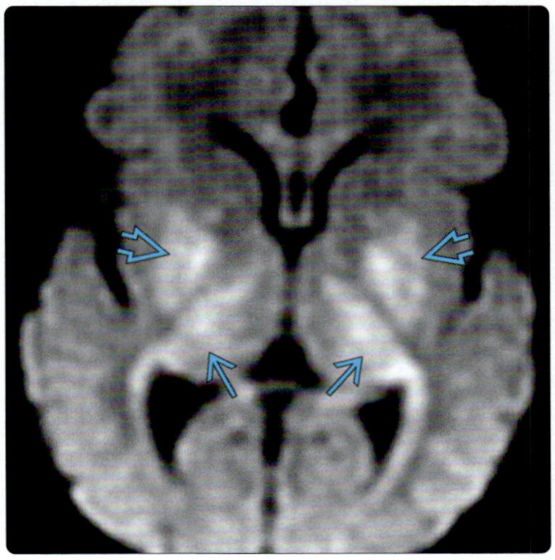

Hypoxic-Ischemic Encephalopathy

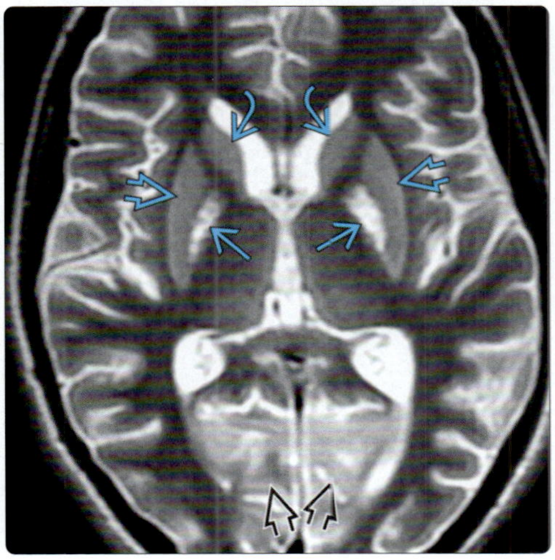

(Left) *Axial DWI MR in a 5 day old with hypoxic-ischemic encephalopathy (HIE) shows symmetric high signal in the thalami* → *& posterior putamina* ⇒. *Approximately 5 days after a birth-related HI event is the optimum time for detecting DWI changes.* **(Right)** *Axial T2 MR in a teenager who had a profound HI event 1 month ago shows severe signal changes in the globus pallidus nuclei* → *& mild to moderate signal changes in the putamina* ⇒ *& caudate heads* ↗. *Also note the injury to the bilateral occipital lobes* ⇒.

(Left) *Axial T1 MR in a 13 year old with gadolinium (Gd) deposition who was diagnosed with anaplastic ependymoma > 10 years ago & has undergone > 25 contrast-enhanced MR exams shows symmetric hyperintense signal → in the globus pallidus nuclei.* **(Right)** *Axial T1 MR in the same patient shows symmetric hyperintense signal in the bilateral dentate nuclei → of the cerebellum. The combination of hyperintense T1 signal in the GP & dentate nuclei is strongly suggestive of Gd deposition.*

Gadolinium Deposition

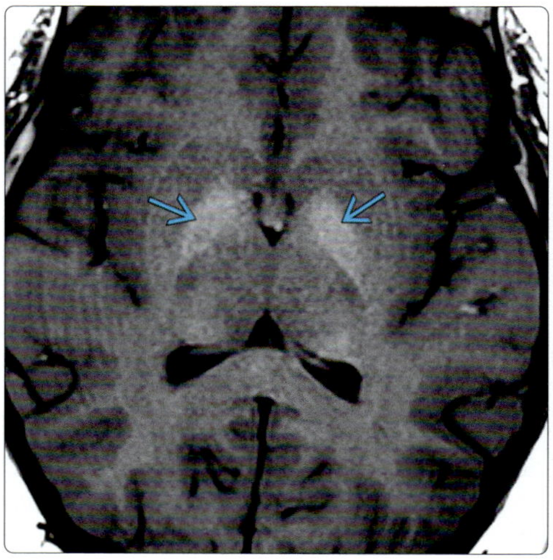

Gadolinium Deposition

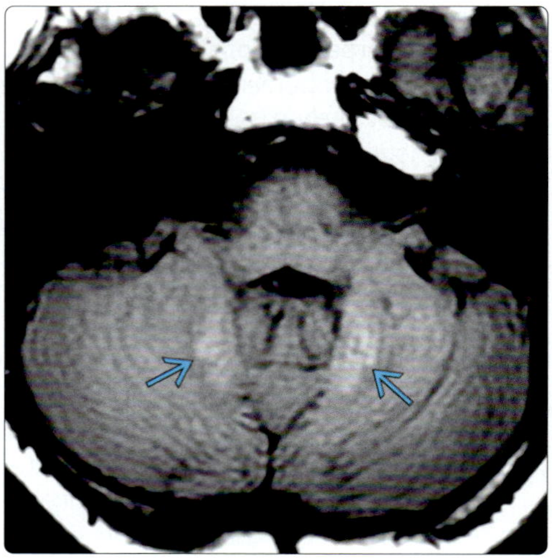

(Left) *Axial FLAIR MR in an 8 year old with NF1 shows globular signal hyperintensities → in the bilateral nuclei of the globus pallidus, a characteristic location for nonenhancing lesions associated with NF1. When such findings are encountered, look for similar lesions in the dentate nuclei as well as optic pathway gliomas & orbital plexiform neurofibromas.* **(Right)** *Axial T2 FS MR in the same patient shows thickened & tortuous optic nerves → & a small left orbital plexiform neurofibroma ⇒.*

Neurofibromatosis Type 1

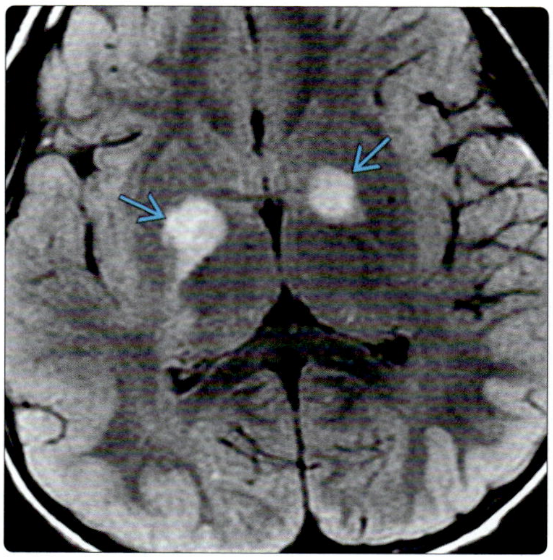

Neurofibromatosis Type 1

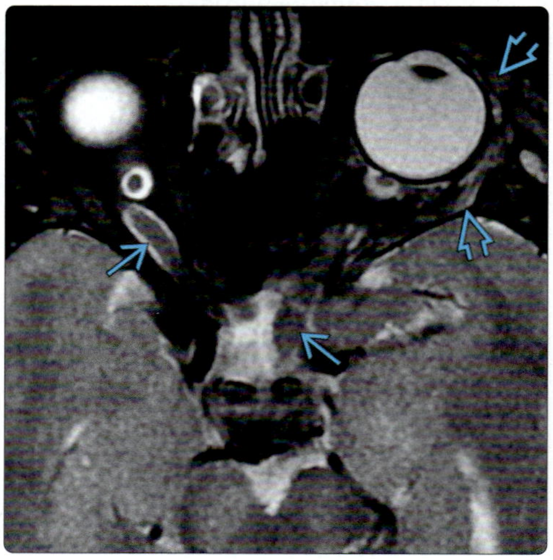

(Left) *Axial NECT in a 1 year old with venous ischemia shows an area of expanded hypoattenuation in the right thalamus ⇒. Also note the key finding of associated hyperattenuation within the internal cerebral veins → & vein of Galen →, consistent with thrombosis.* **(Right)** *Axial DWI MR in the same patient shows small, patchy areas of diffusion restriction (↓ ADC not shown) in the right thalamus → & caudate head ⇒. In venous ischemia, the area of diffusion restriction is < the total area of FLAIR signal abnormality.*

Venous Ischemia

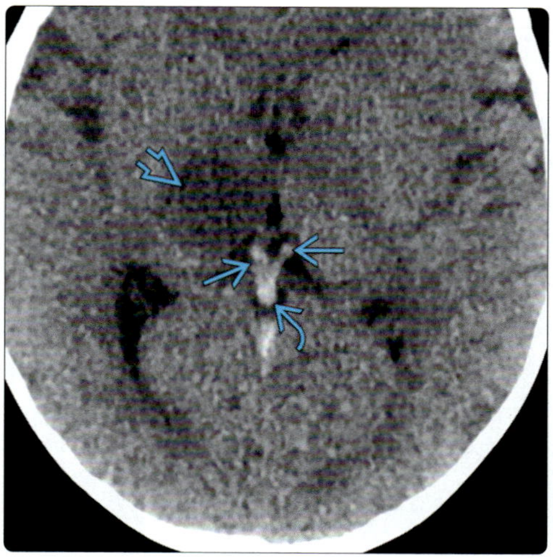

Venous Ischemia

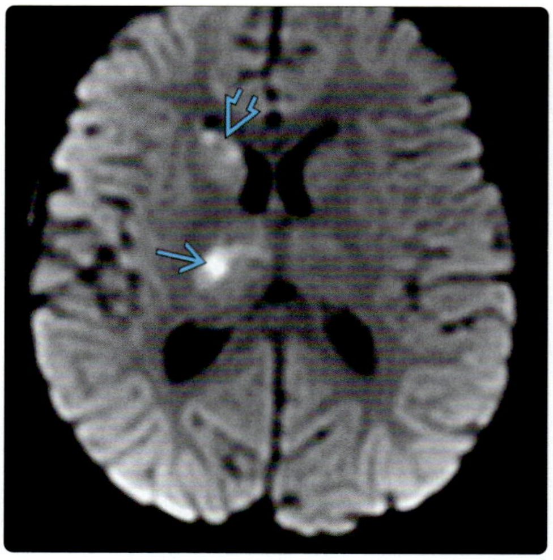

Arterial Infarct

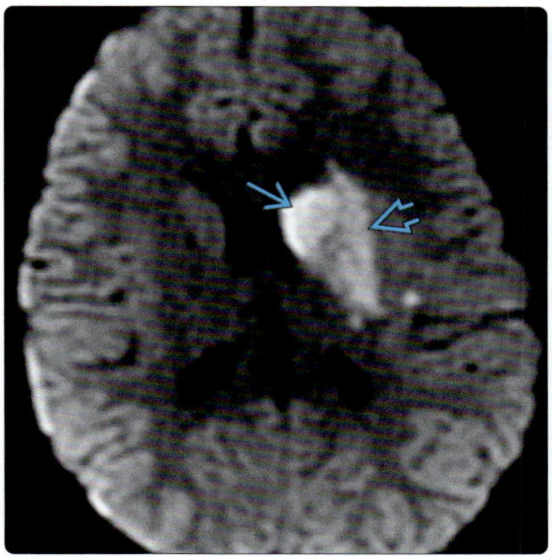

Arterial Infarct

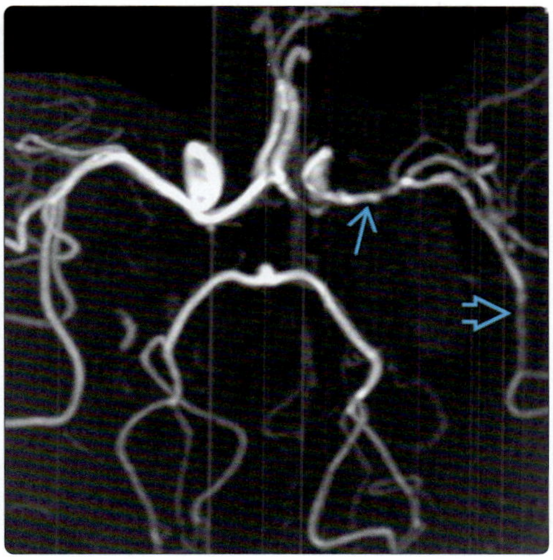

(Left) *Axial DWI MR in a 6 year old with an arterial infarct shows diffusion restriction (↓ ADC not shown) in the left caudate head → & putamen ⇨. Whenever an area of diffusion restriction is identified in the basal ganglia (especially when unilateral), MRA & MRV should be performed to identify a vascular etiology.* **(Right)** *3D MRA in the same patient shows multiple foci of irregular arterial narrowing, including the left M1 segment → & more distal middle cerebral artery branches ⇨, typical of vasculitis.*

Leigh Syndrome

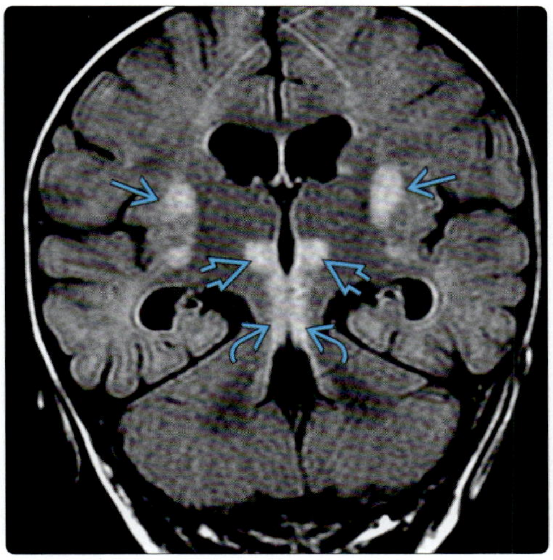

Leigh Syndrome

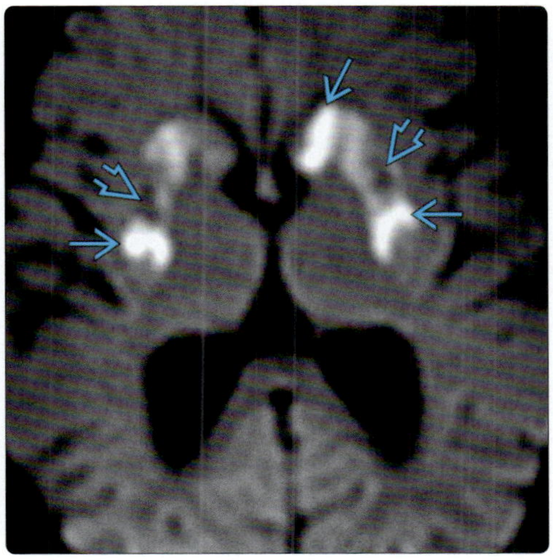

(Left) *Coronal FLAIR MR in an 11 month old with seizures & lactic acidosis shows nearly symmetric areas of signal abnormality in the bilateral putamina →, medial thalami ⇨, & periaqueductal gray matter ↪.* **(Right)** *Axial DWI MR in the same patient shows patchy areas of diffusion restriction → (↓ ADC not shown) due to cytotoxic edema. Note that some foci within the injured putamina show no diffusion restriction ⇨ because they are chronic, likely from a prior exacerbation.*

Low-Grade Glioma

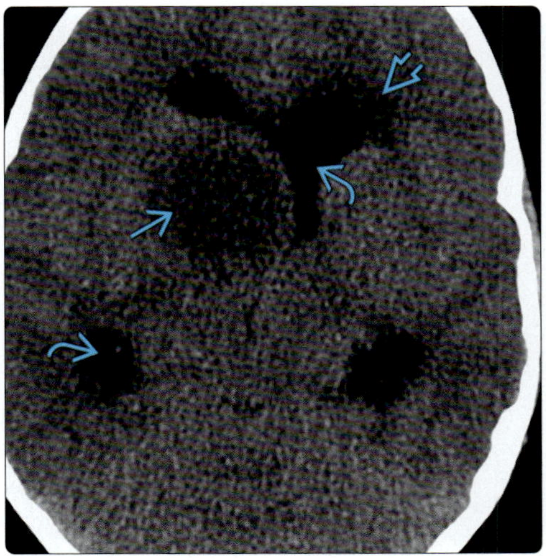

Low-Grade Glioma

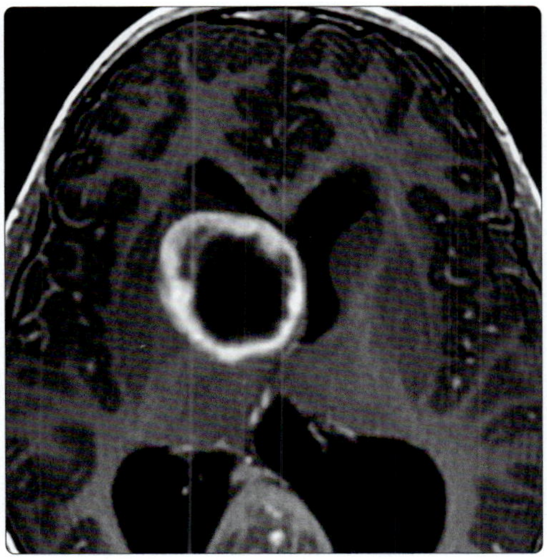

(Left) *Axial NECT in a 9 year old with a low-grade glioma (pilomyxoid astrocytoma) shows a low-attenuation mass → centered in the right deep gray nuclei. Note the increased size of the lateral ventricles ↪ with transependymal edema ⇨ due to obstruction at the foramina of Monro.* **(Right)** *Axial T1 C+ MR in the same patient shows thick, irregular rim enhancement of the mass, typical of a tumor. The central portion showed no evidence of diffusion restriction to suggest an abscess.*

(Left) *Axial FLAIR MR in a 6 year old with intractable vomiting shows marked mass-like enlargement & signal abnormality within the bilateral (R > L) thalami with extension of abnormal signal into the right caudate head. Note the associated obstructive hydrocephalus, a common finding in bithalamic gliomas.* **(Right)** *Axial T1 C+ MR in the same patient shows no significant enhancement, characteristic of a bithalamic glioma. The punctate foci of enhancement in the lesion are due to vessels.*

Bithalamic Glioma

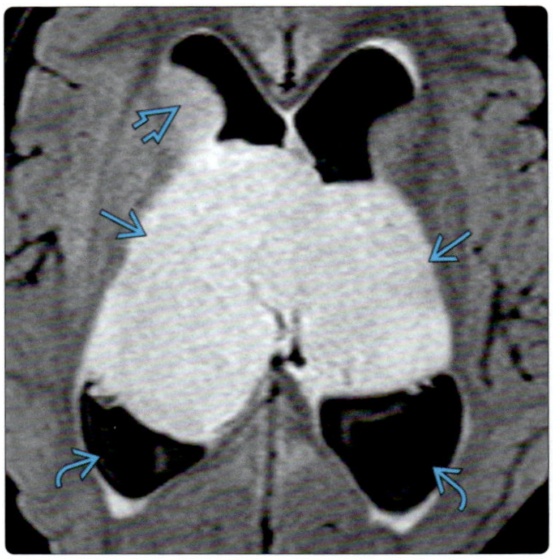

Bithalamic Glioma

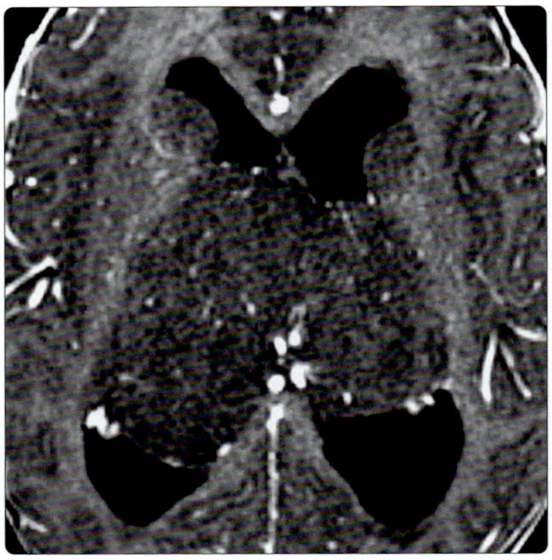

(Left) *Axial T2 MR in a 10 year old shows a large mass centered in the left basal ganglia. The dark solid components & numerous small intratumoral cysts are typical of germinoma. Approximately 5-10% of germinomas occur in the deep gray nuclei (basal ganglia > thalami).* **(Right)** *Axial DWI MR in the same patient shows diffusion restriction (↓ ADC not shown) within the solid components of the tumor, consistent with a cellular tumor, such as germinoma.*

Germinoma

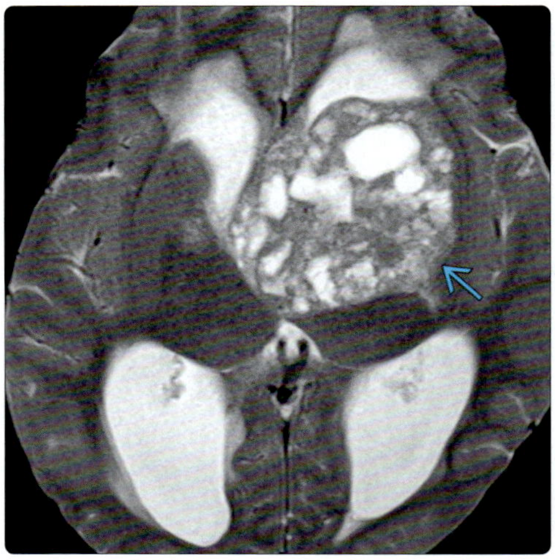

Germinoma

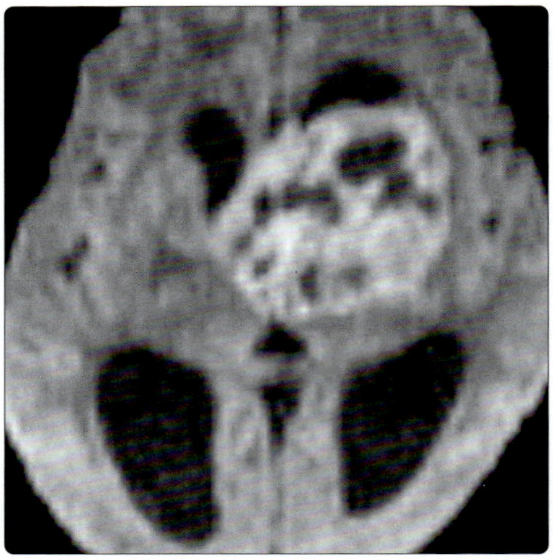

(Left) *Axial DWI MR in a 5 week old with seizures & herpes encephalitis shows extensive diffusion restriction within both thalami as well as much of the cerebral cortex. The focus of signal loss in the right thalamus corresponded to hemorrhage on SWI (not shown).* **(Right)** *Axial T2 MR in the same patient several months later shows extensive cystic encephalomalacia within the regions of previously seen restricted diffusion. Such an evolution of injury is typical for neonatal herpes simplex virus.*

Neonatal Herpes Encephalitis

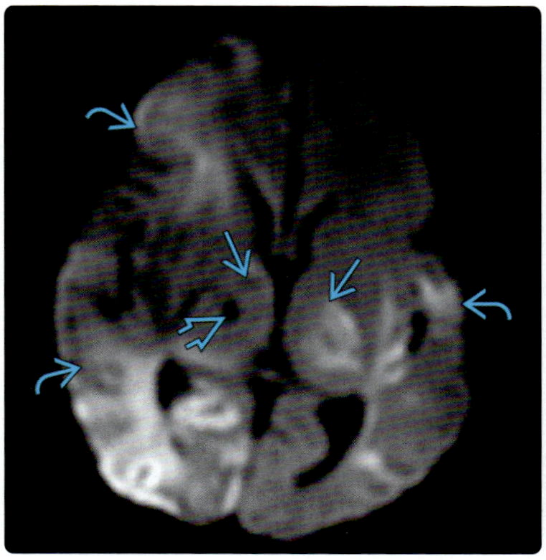

Neonatal Herpes Encephalitis

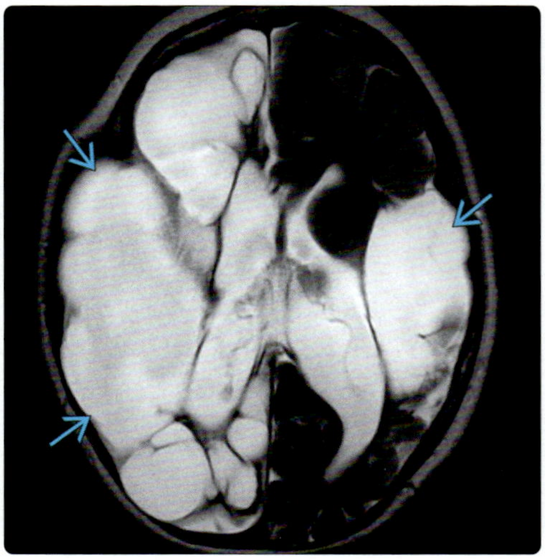

Group B Streptococcal Meningitis

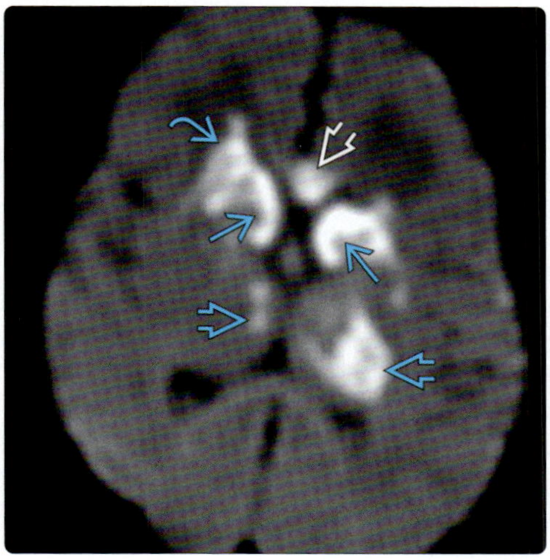

Group B Streptococcal Meningitis

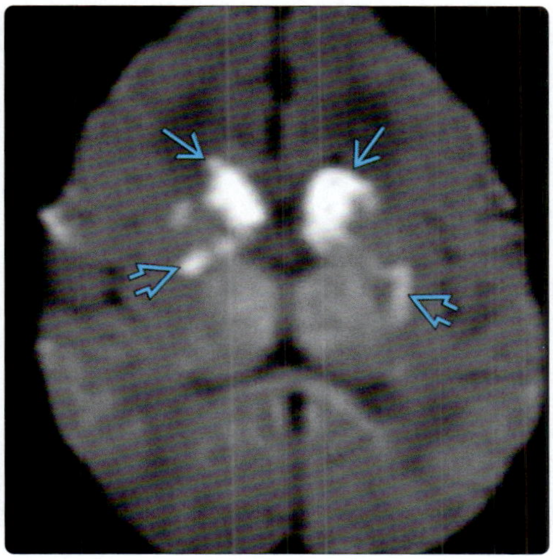

(Left) *Axial DWI MR in a 7 day old with group B streptococcal meningitis shows diffusion restriction of the bilateral caudate heads → & thalami → as well as white matter → & corpus callosum → (↓ ADC not shown). Deep gray nuclei involvement is thought to be due to vasculitis of the deep perforating vessels in this disease.* **(Right)** *Axial DWI MR in a 5 day old with group B streptococcal meningitis shows nearly symmetric diffusion restriction (↓ ADC not shown) in the bilateral caudate heads → & putamina →.*

Acute Disseminated Encephalomyelitis

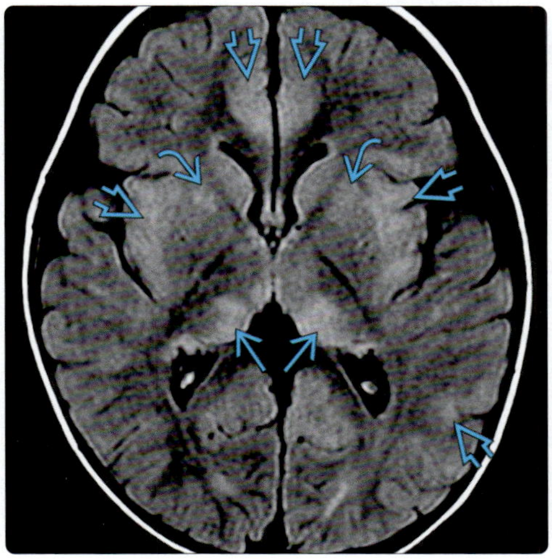

Hemolytic Uremic Syndrome

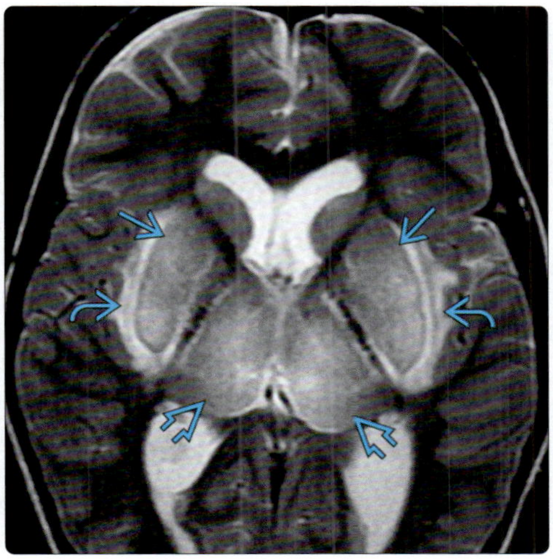

(Left) *Axial FLAIR MR in a 2 year old with ADEM shows nearly symmetric hyperintensities in the medial thalami →, anterior putamina →, & scattered cortical/subcortical locations →.* **(Right)** *Axial T2 MR in a 4 year old with anemia, renal failure, & diarrhea due to hemolytic uremic syndrome (HUS) shows symmetric swelling & increased signal within the basal ganglia → & thalami → as well as the adjacent insular white matter →. Involvement of the deep gray nuclei is typical for complicated HUS.*

Kernicterus

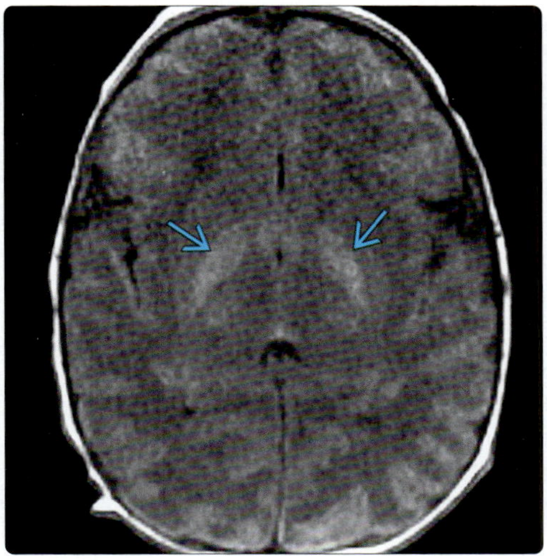

Krabbe Disease

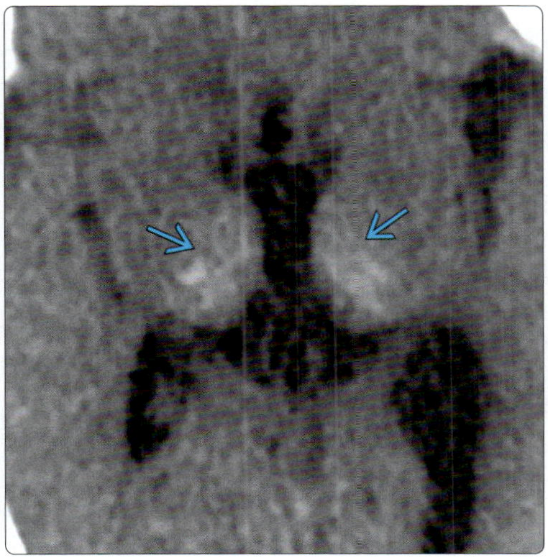

(Left) *Axial T1 MR in an 8 day old with severe hyperbilirubinemia & kernicterus shows symmetric increased signal in the bilateral globus pallidus nuclei →. Such findings can be seen in the acute phase of kernicterus.* **(Right)** *Axial NECT in a 2 month old with Krabbe disease shows small areas of mineralization → within both thalami, a finding often seen in Krabbe disease when patients are young. This finding may resolve later in life.*

DIFFERENTIAL DIAGNOSIS

Common

- Abscess
- Pilocytic Astrocytoma

Less Common

- Demyelinating Disease
  - Acute Disseminated Encephalomyelitis
  - Multiple Sclerosis
- Subacute Cerebral Infarction
- Subacute Intracerebral Hematoma
- Neurocysticercosis
- Other Neoplasms
  - Pilomyxoid Astrocytoma
  - Hemangioblastoma
  - Ganglioglioma
  - Glioblastoma
  - Parenchymal Metastases
  - Primary CNS Lymphoma

Rare but Important

- Aneurysm (Thrombosed)
- Other Infections
  - Tuberculosis
  - Fungal Diseases
  - Acquired Toxoplasmosis
  - Lyme Disease

ESSENTIAL INFORMATION

Key Differential Diagnosis Issues

- Clinical features to consider
  - Signs/symptoms of infection helps narrow differential
  - Many infections have extra CNS manifestations
  - CNS metastases are rare in children vs. adults
  - Relative frequency of infection vs. tumor depends on practice location
    - Developing world: Infection > > tumor
    - Developed world: Tumor & demyelination > infection
- Imaging features to consider
  - Multiplicity: Common in infection, demyelination, & metastases
  - Type of rim enhancement
    - Smooth/thin: More likely infectious or low-grade tumor
    - Irregular/thick: More likely tumor (with central necrosis)
    - Incomplete: Demyelination or infarct; abscess in neonate/infant
  - Diffusion-weighted imaging (DWI)
    - Central diffusion restriction: Abscess
    - Diffusion restriction of enhancing rim: Tumor & demyelination
  - Susceptibility-weighted imaging (SWI)
    - Smooth, complete hypointense rim: Abscess
    - Double-rim sign: Abscess
      - ◻ T2-hypointense outer + hyperintense inner rims
    - Irregular, incomplete hypointense rim with internal foci of signal loss: Higher grade tumor

Helpful Clues for Common Diagnoses

- **Abscess**
  - Pyogenic > fungal, granulomatous, or parasitic
  - Single or multiple lesions
  - Relatively thin & smooth rim contrast enhancement (CE)
  - Thin T2 outer hypointense rim
  - Restricted diffusion centrally
  - Early capsule stage: Moderate vasogenic edema & mass effect
  - Late capsule stage: Edema & mass effect ↓
  - ± ventriculitis &/or meningitis
  - ± sinusitis or mastoiditis as cause; if none, suggest central hematogenous source
- **Pilocytic Astrocytoma**
  - May occur anywhere in CNS
    - 60% infratentorial, 40% supratentorial
  - Peak: 5-15 years of age
  - Variable appearance
    - Nonenhancing cyst + CE mural nodule
    - CE cyst wall + CE mural nodule
    - Solid + homogeneous CE

Helpful Clues for Less Common Diagnoses

- **Demyelinating Disease**
  - **Acute disseminated encephalomyelitis**
    - Autoimmune-mediated demyelination: Brain & spinal cord
    - Typically monophasic, 10-14 days after viral infection or vaccination
    - Multifocal hyperintense T2 & FLAIR signal lesions of white matter (WM) & basal ganglia (BG) > gray matter (GM); cerebrum > cerebellum & brainstem
    - Bilateral lesions are common but asymmetric
    - Punctate or ring-like enhancement (complete or incomplete)
  - **Multiple sclerosis**
    - Autoimmune-mediated demyelination in genetically susceptible individuals
    - Imaging may be identical to acute disseminated encephalomyelitis
    - Multifocal lesions of periventricular WM (PVWM), subcortical U-fibers, brachium pontis, brainstem, & spinal cord
    - Perivenular extension along path of deep medullary veins: Dawson fingers
      - ◻ T2/FLAIR: Linear ↑ signal radiating from ventricles
    - Infratentorial: Children > adults
    - Nodular or ring CE, occasionally semilunar CE or large tumefactive enhancing rings
- **Subacute Cerebral Infarction**
  - Swelling & signal abnormality in vascular territory
  - Rarely imaged with contrast
    - Gyriform > ring-like CE
  - Single vascular territory due to vessel occlusion/injury
  - Multiple vascular territories due to central embolic source
- **Subacute Intracerebral Hematoma**
  - Rarely imaged with contrast
  - History of trauma or coagulopathy

- Look for evidence of blood products centrally (e.g., blooming on SWI/GRE)
- Look for other evidence of trauma (e.g., axonal shear injury, contusions)
- History & prior imaging most helpful in narrowing DDx

- **Neurocysticercosis**
  - Pork tapeworm: *Taenia solium*
  - 5- to 20-mm cyst; ± 1- to 4-mm eccentric scolex
  - Single or multiple lesions
  - Cisterns/sulci > parenchyma > intraventricular
  - Postcontrast appearance depends on developmental stage & host response
    - Vesicular stage: No rim CE, ± scolex CE
    - Colloidal stage: Cyst wall CE ± scolex CE
    - Granular nodular stage: Nodular or ring CE
    - Nodular calcified stage: Minimal or no CE
  - ± surrounding edema; frequent during colloidal stage
  - Ca^{2+} frequently occurs in final nodular calcified stage
- **Other Neoplasms**
  - **Pilomyxoid astrocytoma**
    - Difficult to distinguish from pilocytic astrocytoma (PA) but more likely to have hemorrhage
  - **Hemangioblastoma**
    - Almost exclusively occurs in von Hippel-Lindau syndrome in children
    - Small lesions have enhancing nodules; larger lesions show cystic lesion with mural nodule
    - Look for flow voids & ↑ perfusion in solid component to distinguish from PA
  - **Ganglioglioma**
    - Solid, cystic, or mixed; usually cortical-based lesion, without surrounding edema
    - Ca^{2+} in ~ 50%
    - Variable degree of CE: Diffuse or ring-like
    - Larger & more cystic lesions in infants
      - Intense nodular meningeal CE along cysts of desmoplastic infantile ganglioglioma
  - **Glioblastoma**
    - Irregular rim CE
    - ↓ ADC signal in rim & ↑ ADC signal centrally
    - Internal SWI signal loss
  - **Parenchymal metastases**
    - Rare in children compared to adults
    - Usually multiple in number
    - Often located at gray-white junction
  - **Primary CNS lymphoma**
    - Ring enhancement in immunocompromised patients
    - Often crosses corpus callosum

Helpful Clues for Rare Diagnoses

- **Aneurysm (Thrombosed)**
  - Partially or completely thrombosed
  - Laminated appearance of thrombus
  - Appearance depends on aneurysm type
    - Round: Saccular aneurysm
    - Tubular: Fusiform aneurysm
  - If not completely thrombosed, look for pulsation artifact
- **Other Infections**
  - **Tuberculosis:** *Mycobacterium tuberculosis* infection
    - CNS tuberculosis (TB) patients usually have pulmonary TB
    - Thick basilar meningitis
    - ± dural-based tuberculomas
    - ± parenchymal tuberculomas
    - Multiple > solitary tuberculomas
    - Solid CE or necrotic center
  - **Fungal diseases**: Rare, usually in immunocompromised patients
    - Nocardia, blastomycosis, candidiasis, coccidiomycosis, histoplasmosis
    - Multiple > single lesions; solid CE or necrotic center
  - **Acquired toxoplasmosis**: Single or multiple lesions; nodular or ring CE; immunocompromised patients, especially HIV(+)
  - **Lyme disease**: Multifocal PVWM lesions ± CE; cranial nerve CE common; rash & flu-like symptoms

Abscess

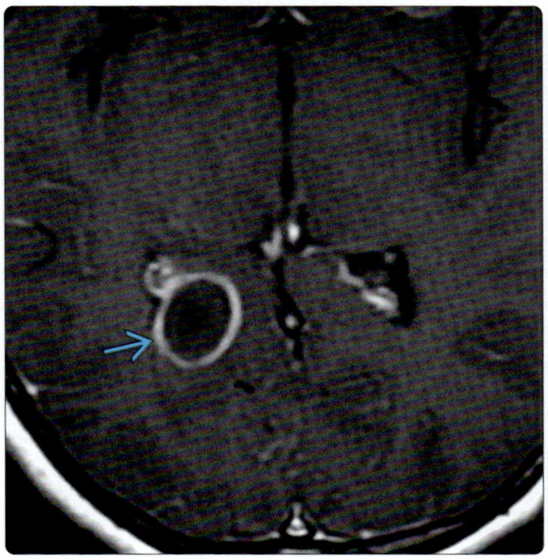

Abscess

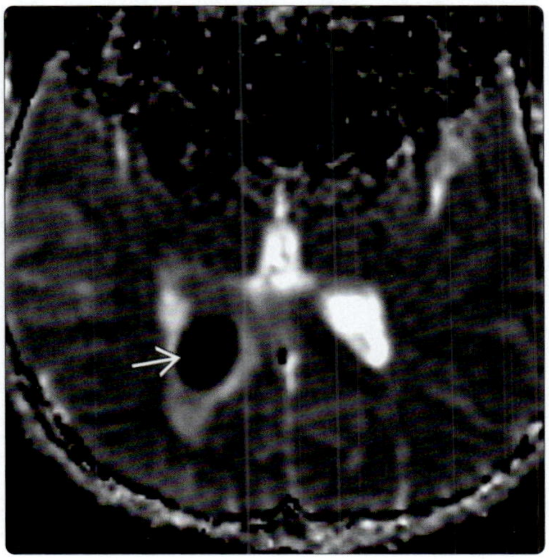

(Left) *Axial T1 C+ MR in a patient with a cerebral abscess shows a rim-enhancing lesion with a thin, smooth rim ⇨, characteristic of abscess. Compared to tumors, abscesses typically have a thinner & smoother rim of enhancement.* **(Right)** *Axial ADC map MR in the same patient with a cerebral abscess shows marked diffusion restriction of the central nonenhancing fluid ➡. No imaging finding is more specific for cerebral abscess than central diffusion restriction.*

Pilocytic Astrocytoma

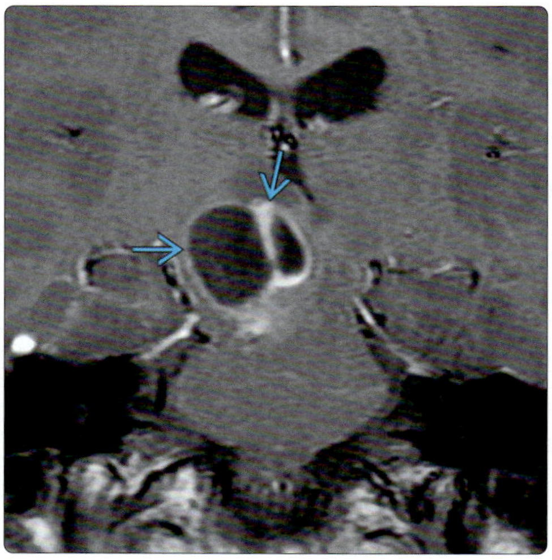

Pilocytic Astrocytoma

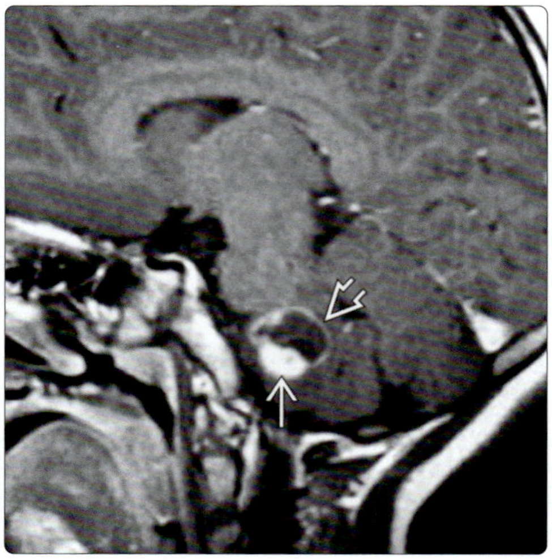

(Left) *Coronal T1 C+ MR in a 9 year old with a pilocytic astrocytoma (PA) shows a bilobed rim-enhancing lesion in the right cerebral peduncle. Note the varying thickness of the cyst walls →. The internal cyst contents did not restrict diffusion.* **(Right)** *Sagittal T1 C+ MR shows an intensely enhancing solid mural nodule ➡ & rim-enhancing cystic component ➡ in the medulla. While the imaging spectrum of PA is broad, a thin rim of enhancement with solid enhancing mural nodule is the most specific pattern.*

Multiple Sclerosis

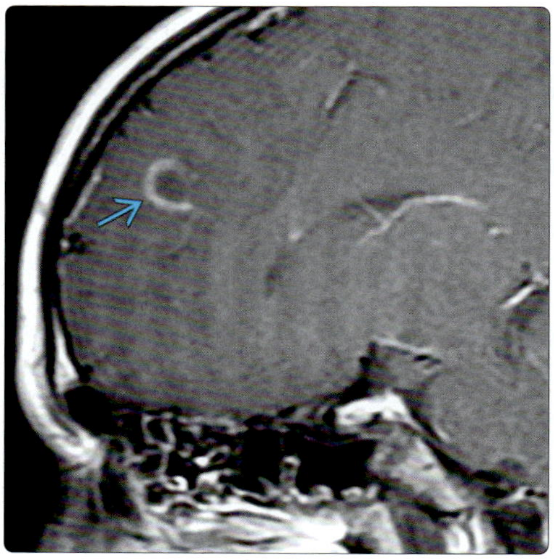

Subacute Cerebral Infarction

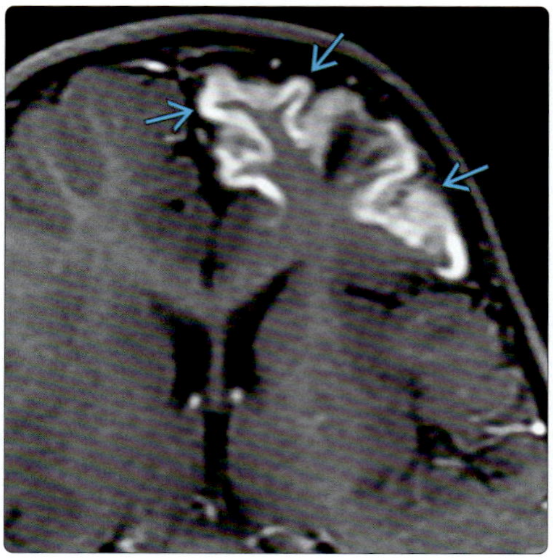

(Left) *Sagittal T1 C+ MR in a 13 year old with multiple sclerosis shows an incomplete rim of enhancement →, which is the classic appearance of demyelinating disease. In the acute phase, demyelinating lesions typically show patchy or incomplete ring enhancement with diffusion restriction.* **(Right)** *Axial T1 C+ MR in a 2 year old with arteriopathy & a left frontal infarct ~ 1 week prior to imaging shows contiguous rim enhancement → of the cortical ribbon, a typical appearance for subacute infarct.*

Subacute Intracerebral Hematoma

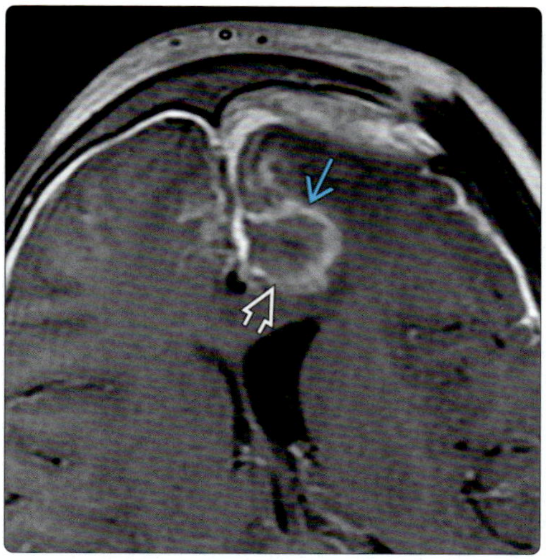

Neurocysticercosis

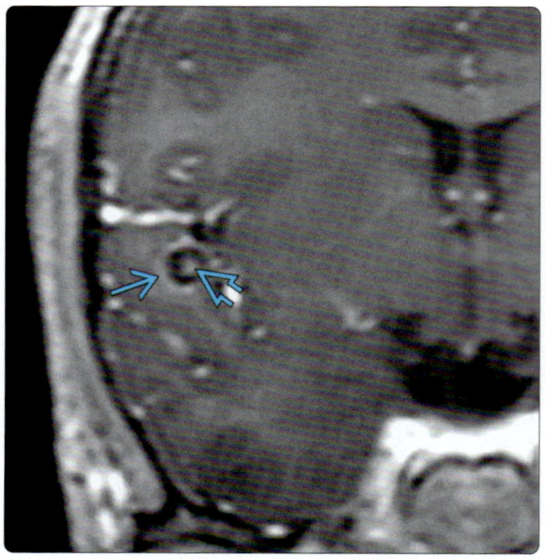

(Left) *Axial T1 C+ MR in a patient with a penetrating wound 2 months prior shows a thin, somewhat irregular rim of enhancement → surrounding a resolving subacute intraparenchymal hematoma ➡.* **(Right)** *Coronal T1 C+ MR in a 13 year old with seizures & solitary neurocysticercosis shows a small lesion → with thin, smooth rim enhancement & a central nodule ➡, consistent with a scolex.*

Pilomyxoid Astrocytoma

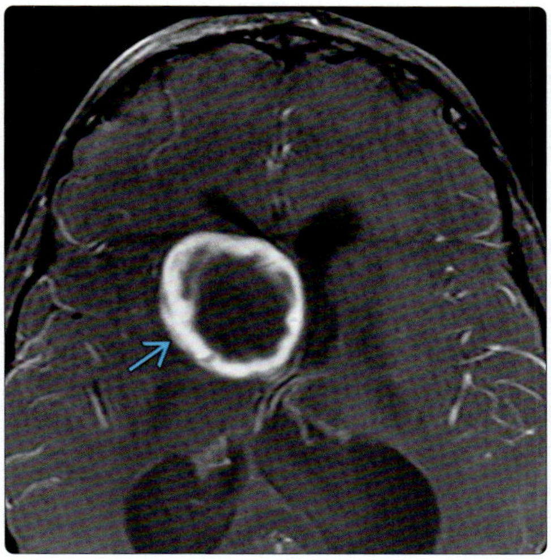

Ganglioglioma

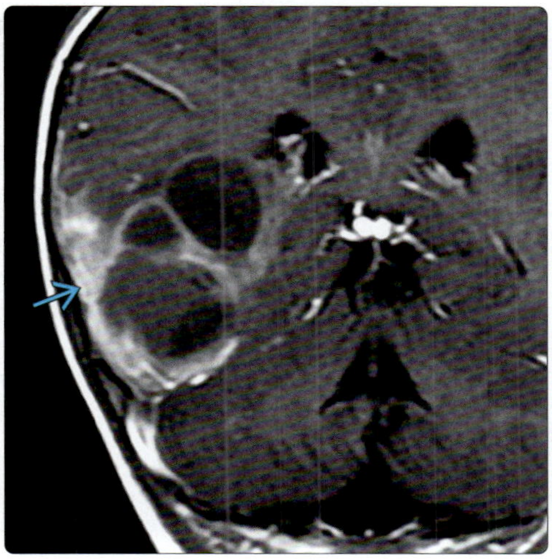

(Left) *Axial T1 C+ MR in a patient with a pilomyxoid astrocytoma shows a thick-rimmed mass → centered in the medial right basal ganglia. The thick, irregular rim is highly suggestive of tumor. DWI showed no central diffusion restriction.* **(Right)** *Coronal T1 C+ MR in a patient with a desmoplastic infantile ganglioglioma (DIG) shows a complex multicystic mass → occupying most of the right temporal lobe. DIG should be considered in any multicystic lesion in a young patient.*

Glioblastoma

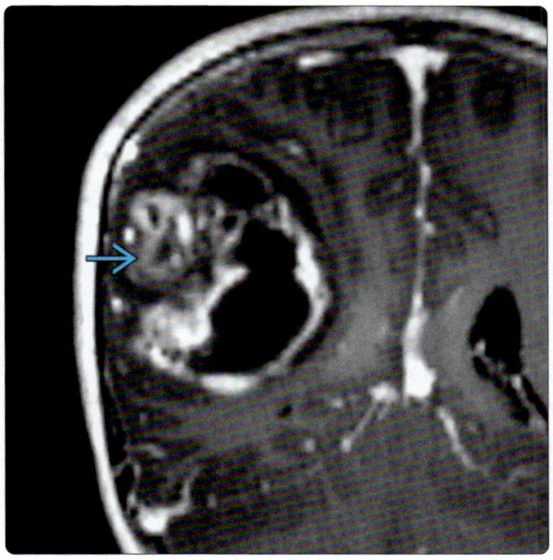

Parenchymal Metastases

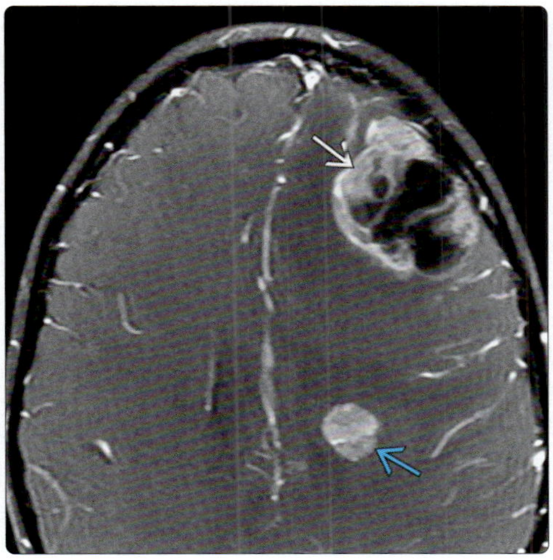

(Left) *Coronal T1 C+ MR in a patient with a glioblastoma shows a centrally necrotic enhancing tumor → in the right insula. Clues that suggest a high-grade tumor are central necrosis & diffusion restriction of solid components.* **(Right)** *Axial T1 C+ MR in a 12 year old with Ewing sarcoma shows a left frontal lesion ➡ with rim enhancement of varying thickness, typical of tumor. Multiple lesions → are typical of metastases, though metastases are much less common in children than adults.*

Primary CNS Lymphoma

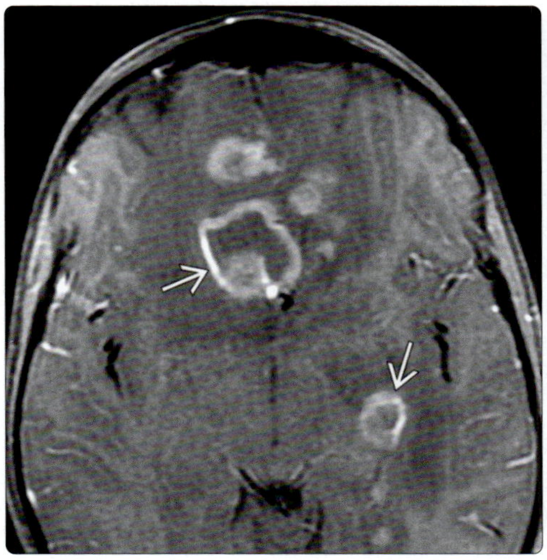

Aneurysm (Thrombosed)

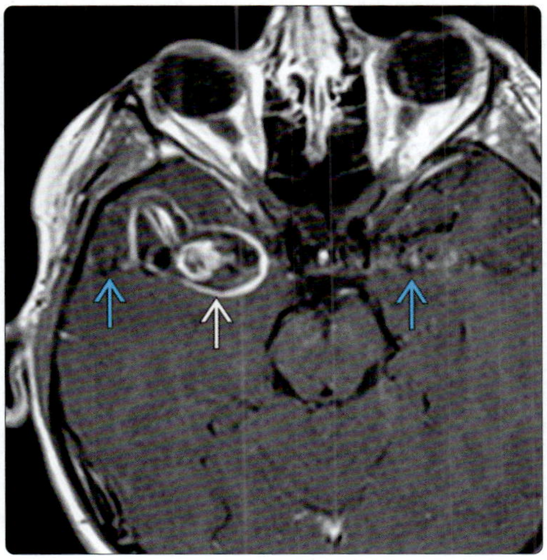

(Left) *Axial T1 C+ MR in an 11 year old with CNS lymphoma shows multiple lesions, the largest of which show rim enhancement ➡. As with other cellular tumors, areas of enhancement should show diffusion restriction in the setting of lymphoma.* **(Right)** *Axial T1 C+ MR in a teenager with a partially thrombosed fusiform aneurysm shows a tubular rim-enhancing lesion ➡ surrounding a smaller patent vessel centrally. Note the prominent pulsation artifact →, an important clue to an aneurysm.*

DIFFERENTIAL DIAGNOSIS

Common

- Vasospasm

Less Common

- Moyamoya Arteriopathy
- Arterial Dissection
- Focal Cerebral Arteriopathy-Inflammatory Type

Rare but Important

- Multifocal CNS Vasculitis
- Fibromuscular Dysplasia
- Reversible Cerebral Vasoconstriction Syndrome

ESSENTIAL INFORMATION

Key Differential Diagnosis Issues

- Risk factors/clinical markers
  - Arterial dissection: Trauma, connective tissue diseases, such as Ehlers-Danlos (EDS) type IV, Marfan syndrome, fibromuscular dysplasia (FMD)
  - Moyamoya syndrome
    - Common: Sickle cell disease (SCD), trisomy 21, neurofibromatosis type 1 (NF1), prior radiation therapy (XRT)
    - Uncommon: Alagille syndrome, morning glory syndrome, tuberculous meningitis, & others
  - Reversible cerebral vasoconstriction syndrome (RCVS): Rare in children, common in middle-aged women
- Imaging features to consider
  - Infarcts (especially with trauma) in single arterial territory → arterial dissection
  - Infarcts of various ages → moyamoya
  - Involvement of distal internal carotid artery (ICA) & proximal middle cerebral artery (MCA)/anterior cerebral artery (ACA) vessels → moyamoya & focal cerebral arteriopathy-inflammatory type (FCA-i)
  - Distal small branch vessels → small vessel vasculitis
- Modality considerations
  - CTA: Excellent test for large & medium vessel narrowing
    - Especially helpful in trauma to evaluate dissection
      - Petrous temporal bone fracture → recommend CTA
    - Helpful in clarifying questionable MR findings
  - MR: Excellent brain parenchymal assessment
    - DWI: Key sequence to detect ischemia/infarct
    - MRA: Excellent test for follow-up exams
    - Perfusion imaging: Allows detection of altered perfusion due to arterial stenoses & may guide clinical management
      - Arterial spin labeling (ASL): Noncontrast technique
      - Dynamic susceptibility contrast (DSC) perfusion: Bolus tracking T2* technique
    - Axial T1 FS: ↑ T1 in wall due to hematoma
    - Arterial wall imaging (AWI): Thinner slice T1 C+ FS spin-echo-based images (i.e., fast-flowing blood is dark)
      - Etiologic associations with specific patterns are not yet established in children
  - 3D & MIP reconstructions
    - Very helpful in CTA & MRA to identify areas of stenosis
    - Should not supplant careful evaluation of source images
  - Digital subtraction angiography (DSA)
    - Most sensitive & specific test for vessel evaluation
    - Small & medium vessel vasculitis is most evident on DSA
    - Carries risk of infarct & vessel injury

Helpful Clues for Common Diagnoses

- **Vasospasm**
  - Temporary narrowing/irregularity of vessel due to irritation; may be due to
    - Process outside vessel: Inflammation, subarachnoid hemorrhage (SAH), trauma
    - Endothelial irritation: Catheter, injection
  - Time to resolution depends upon etiology
    - External irritation typically lasts longer
  - May lead to devastating ischemic complications if severe
    - e.g., vasospasm days after basilar cistern SAH
  - Can be difficult to distinguish vasospasm from dissection in setting of trauma

Helpful Clues for Less Common Diagnoses

- **Moyamoya Arteriopathy**
  - Chronic progressive arteriopathy with characteristic sites of narrowing/occlusion resulting in abundant tiny collateral vessels ("puff of smoke")
    - Distal ICA, proximal MCA/ACA are most common
  - Moyamoya disease: Idiopathic moyamoya
    - Higher incidence in Asian population
  - Moyamoya syndrome: Moyamoya secondary to underlying disease
    - Common: SCD, trisomy 21, NF1, XRT
    - Uncommon: Alagille syndrome, morning glory syndrome, tuberculous meningitis, & others
  - MR: Infarcts of varying ages
    - Attenuated major vessel flow voids in basilar cisterns on T2
      - May see numerous tiny flow voids in deep gray structures
    - Leptomeningeal enhancement due to dilated pial vessels vs. collateral formation
      - Ivy sign of high signal in sulci on unenhanced FLAIR or T1 C+
  - CTA/MRA: Stenosis/occlusion of affected vessels
    - "Puff of smoke" lenticulostriate collaterals
  - Perfusion imaging
    - ASL: ↓ CBF in affected territories
    - DSC: ↓ rCBV & ↑ MTT in affected territories
  - Treatment
    - Pial synangiosis: Most common in children
    - Superficial temporal artery bypass: More common in adults
- **Arterial Dissection**
  - Vessel wall injury is most often due to trauma
    - May be secondary to predisposing disease
      - EDS type IV, Marfan syndrome, FMD
  - Denver blunt cerebrovascular injury (BCVI) scale
    - Grade 1: Irregularity, narrowing, intramural hematoma (IH) with ≤ 25% luminal narrowing

- Grade 2: Intraluminal thrombus, intimal flap, or ≥ 25% luminal narrowing
- Grade 3: Pseudoaneurysm
- Grade 4: Vessel occlusion
- Grade 5: Vessel transection
- CTA: Look for narrowing or irregularity
  - Intimal flap in large & medium-sized vessels
- MR
  - DWI: Infarcts in single arterial territory
  - Ax T1 FS: ↑ T1 in wall = IH
  - MRA: Vessel narrowing/irregularity
- Treatment
  - Antiplatelet agent (e.g., aspirin, clopidogrel)
  - Stenting or vessel sacrifice if severe (e.g., pseudoaneurysm)

- **Focal Cerebral Arteriopathy-Inflammatory Type**
  - a.k.a. transient cerebral arteriopathy
  - Acute, monophasic inflammatory/infectious arteriopathy
    - Unilateral stenosis (usually of anterior circulation)
    - May be due to viral infection (e.g., varicella)
    - ↑ inflammatory markers (e.g., CRP & serum amyloid A)
  - May be progressive over days/weeks
  - ↑ risk of recurrent stroke (up to 25% within 1 year)
  - CTA/MRA: Unilateral proximal MCA/ACA narrowing/irregularity
  - MR AWI: Enhancement of affected vessel wall
  - Treatment: Steroids

Helpful Clues for Rare Diagnoses

- **Multifocal CNS Vasculitis**
  - Inflammatory arteritis of multiple small-medium cerebral arteries, usually bilateral
  - Less common in children vs. adults
  - May present with ischemia or hemorrhage
  - CT: May be normal or show areas of ↓ attenuation
    - ± intraparenchymal or SAH
  - MR: Multifocal white matter (WM) &/or cortical lesions
    - Diffusion restriction is helpful to suggest diagnosis
  - CTA/MRA: Often normal
  - DSA: Best for small-medium artery narrowing
- **Fibromuscular Dysplasia**
  - Noninflammatory arteriopathy, most commonly affecting renal arteries
  - Predisposes to arterial dissection
  - Extracranial carotid disease occurs in < 25% of children
  - CTA/MRA: String-of-beads pattern is less common in children; focal, stenotic arteriopathy is more likely
- **Reversible Cerebral Vasoconstriction Syndrome**
  - Transient vasculopathy associated with severe headaches & stroke
    - Rare in children
  - Predisposing conditions: Illicit drugs, pregnancy, trauma
  - CT/MR: SAH over cerebral convexities
  - CTA/MRA: Usually occult
  - DSA best to detect narrowing of peripheral cerebral artery
  - Treatment: Ca^{2+} channel blocker, usually with good recovery

SELECTED REFERENCES

1. Dlamini N et al: Arterial wall imaging in pediatric stroke. Stroke. 49(4):891-8, 2018
2. Wintermark M et al: Clinical and imaging characteristics of arteriopathy subtypes in children with arterial ischemic stroke: results of the VIPS study. AJNR Am J Neuroradiol. 38(11):2172-9, 2017
3. Fullerton HJ et al: Risk of recurrent arterial ischemic stroke in childhood: a prospective international study. Stroke. 47(1):53-9, 2016
4. Ibrahimi DM et al: Moyamoya disease in children. Childs Nerv Syst. 26(10):1297-308, 2010
5. Braun KP et al: The course and outcome of unilateral intracranial arteriopathy in 79 children with ischaemic stroke. Brain. 132(Pt 2):544-57, 2009

Vasospasm

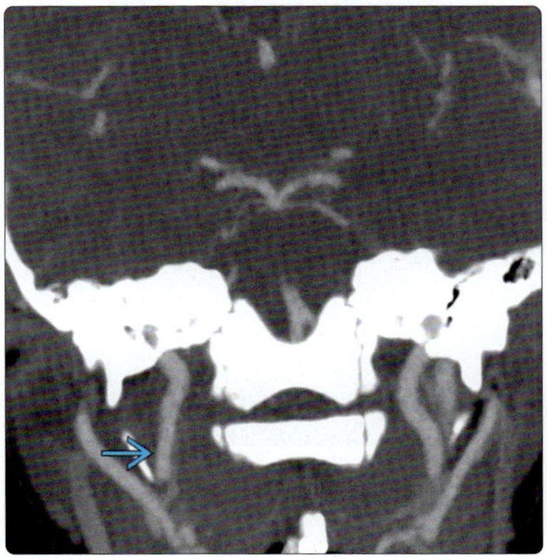

Vasospasm

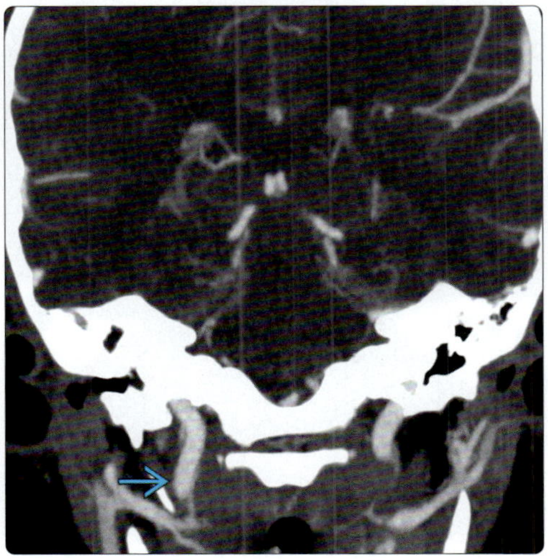

(Left) *Coronal CTA MIP in a 5 year old involved in a bicycle vs. car accident shows mild (< 25%) irregular narrowing* ➡ *of the right distal cervical internal carotid artery (ICA) with adjacent soft tissue swelling. The differential for this finding is vasospasm vs. dissection.* **(Right)** *Coronal CTA MIP in the same patient performed 3 days later shows resolution of the narrowing* ➡*, confirming vasospasm rather than a dissection.*

(Left) *Axial T2 MR in a 21 year old with sickle cell disease & moyamoya arteriopathy shows absence of the normal terminal ICA & proximal middle cerebral artery (MCA) flow voids in the suprasellar cistern. Note multiple small tortuous flow voids ⇒ representing collateral vessels.* **(Right)** *Axial MRA in the same patient at the level of the deep gray nuclei shows multiple lenticulostriate collaterals ⇒ in the bilateral basal ganglia, a typical location for collateral formation in moyamoya arteriopathy.*

Moyamoya Arteriopathy

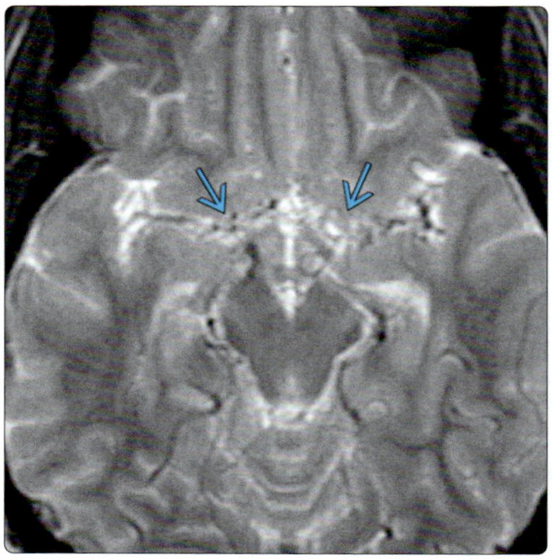

Moyamoya Arteriopathy

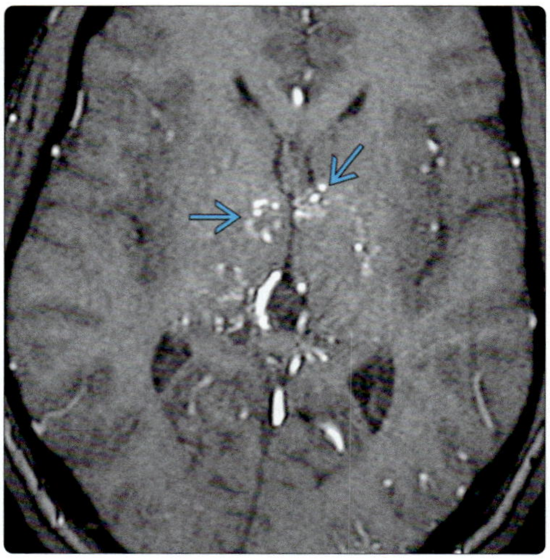

(Left) *Lateral 3D view of an MRA in the same patient shows severe narrowing of the bilateral carotid termini ⇒ with pronounced lenticulostriate collaterals ⇒ that form the "puff of smoke" after which the disease is named.* **(Right)** *Axial T1 C+ MR in the same patient shows ↑ sulcal leptomeningeal enhancement ⇒ over the right cerebral convexity due to dilated pial vessels &/or leptomeningeal collaterals, a common finding in moyamoya that is referred to as the ivy sign on unenhanced FLAIR or T1 C+ MR images.*

Moyamoya Arteriopathy

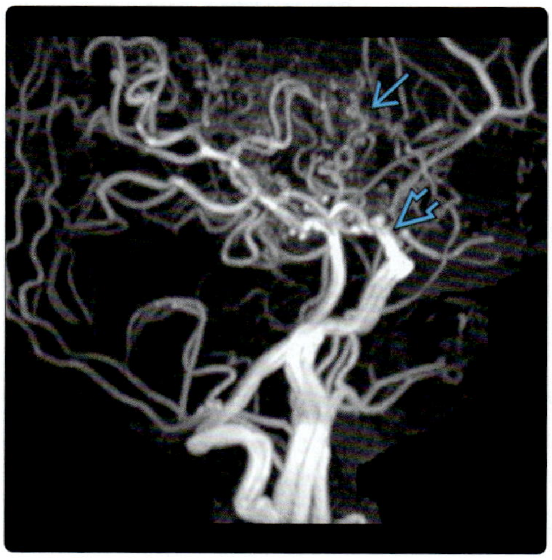

Moyamoya Arteriopathy

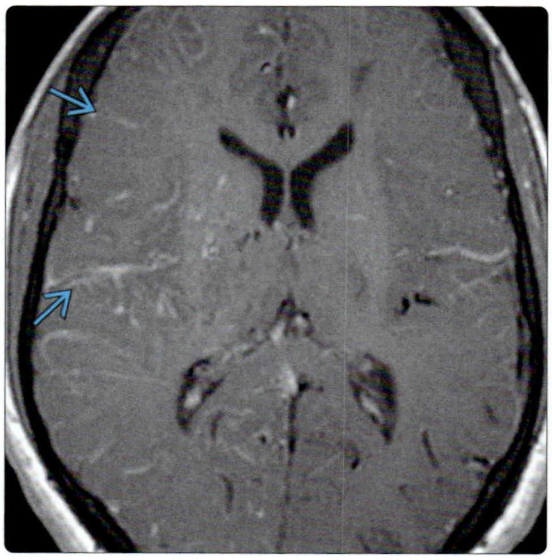

(Left) *Axial CTA in a 6 year old with a traumatic right ICA dissection shows ~ 50% luminal narrowing of the right supraclinoid ICA ⇒ as compared to the normal left ICA ⇒. Focal narrowing may be the only finding on CTA to suggest a dissection.* **(Right)** *Axial CTA in a 13 year old with a petrous temporal bone fracture after an MVA shows a left cavernous ICA dissection flap ⇒. CTA should be performed in the setting of petrous fractures to evaluate for carotid arterial injuries.*

Arterial Dissection

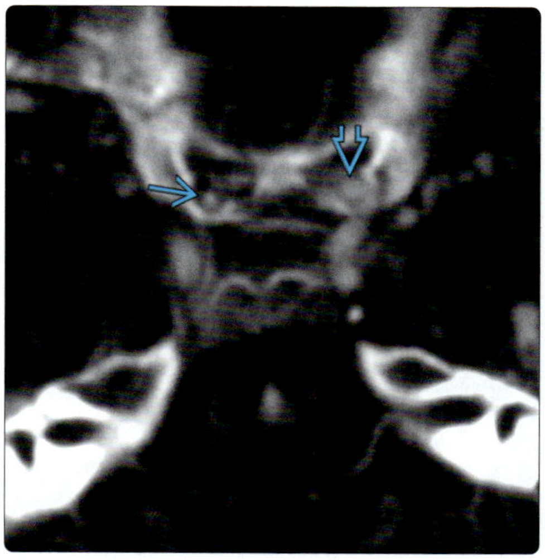

Arterial Dissection

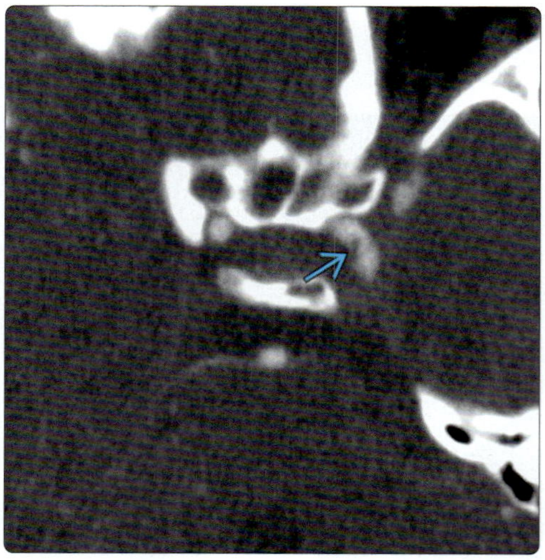

Arterial Dissection

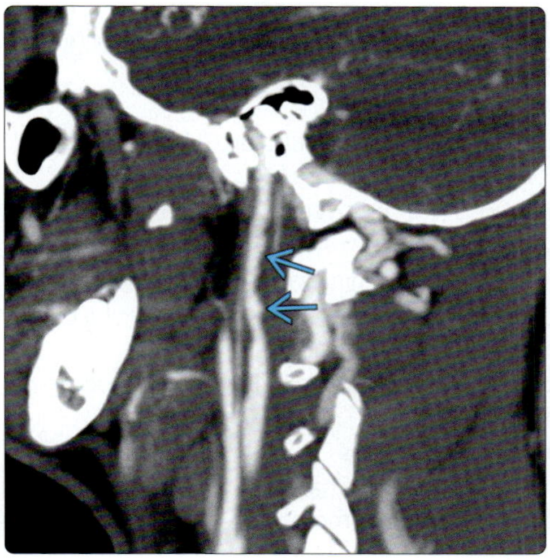

Arterial Dissection

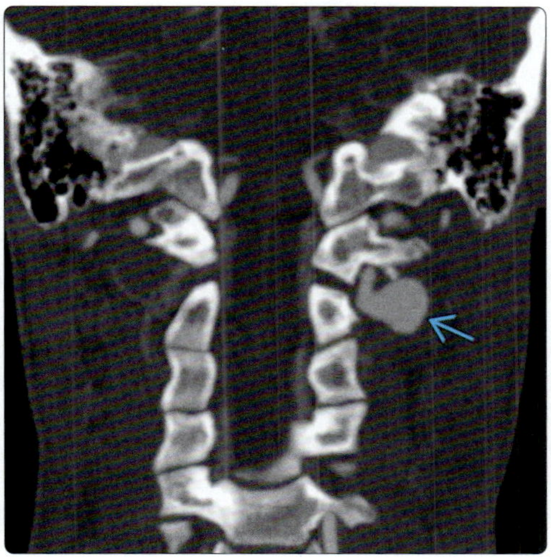

(Left) *Sagittal CTA MIP in a 21-year-old man involved in an MVA shows a long segment of cervical ICA irregularity & narrowing ➔. MIPs reconstructed along the length of an artery can be helpful in visualizing a long segment of vessel & improve detection of arterial narrowing.* **(Right)** *Coronal CTA MIP in a 16 year old with a gunshot wound 3 weeks prior shows a left vertebral pseudoaneurysm ➔, which is a frequent complication of arterial injury.*

Focal Cerebral Arteriopathy-Inflammatory Type

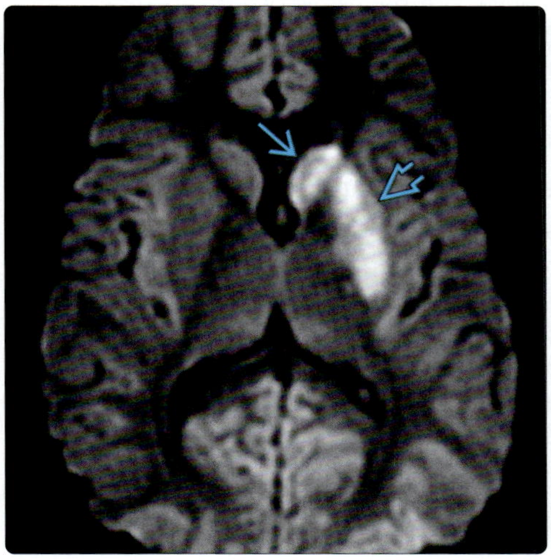

Focal Cerebral Arteriopathy-Inflammatory Type

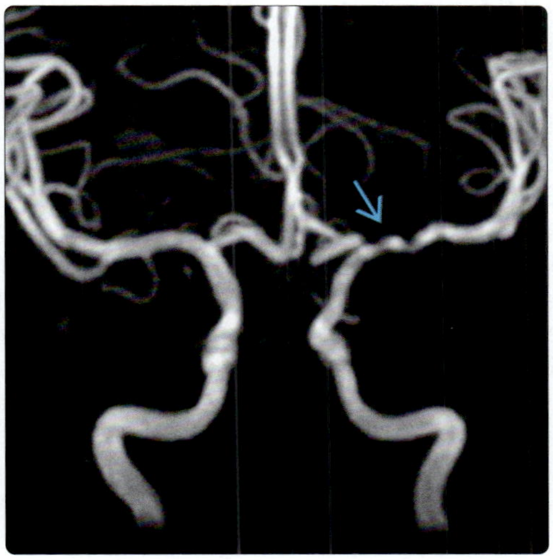

(Left) *Axial DWI MR in a 5 year old with focal cerebral arteriopathy-inflammatory type (FCA-i) shows diffusion restriction (↓ ADC not shown) in the left putamen ➔ & caudate head ➔, consistent with infarction.* **(Right)** *Frontal 3D projection of an MRA in the same patient shows irregularity & narrowing of the M1 segment ➔ of the left MCA. The proximal MCA & anterior cerebral artery (ACA) vessels are the most commonly affected in FCA-i, & inflammatory markers are typically elevated.*

Multifocal CNS Vasculitis

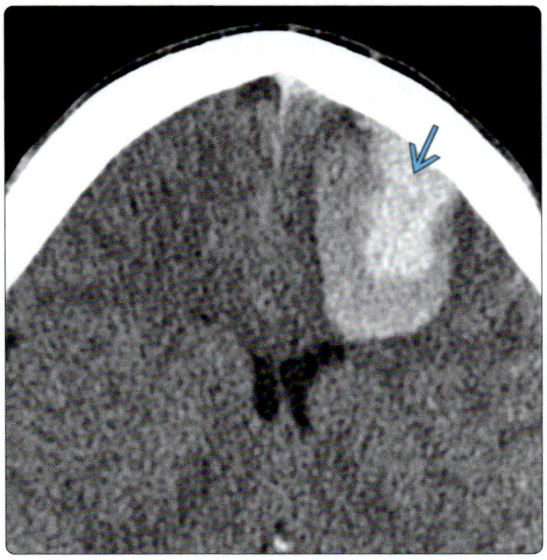

Multifocal CNS Vasculitis

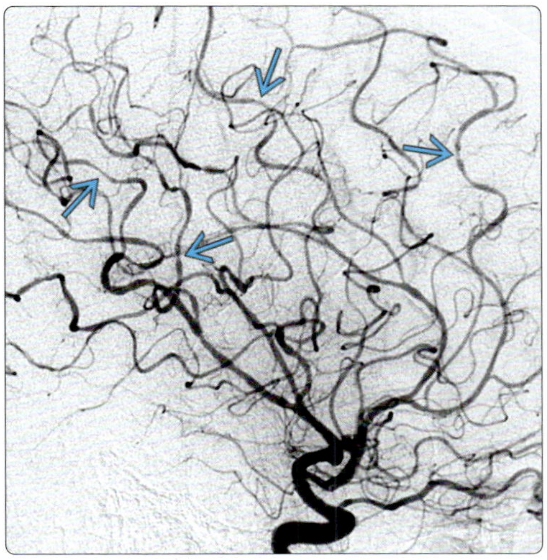

(Left) *Axial NECT in a young woman with multifocal CNS vasculitis who presented with an acute onset of headache shows an acute intraparenchymal hemorrhage ➔ in the left frontal lobe. CTA was performed & was normal.* **(Right)** *Lateral projection of a DSA after ICA injection in the same patient shows numerous foci of irregularity & narrowing ➔ of the small peripheral vessels. This peripheral location & multifocality is typical of small vessel vasculitis & may only be evident on DSA.*

DIFFERENTIAL DIAGNOSIS

Common

- Bacterial Meningitis
- Leptomeningeal Metastases

Less Common

- Moyamoya Arteriopathy
- Sturge-Weber Syndrome
- Tuberculous Meningitis
- Posterior Reversible Encephalopathy Syndrome

Rare but Important

- Leukemia
- Fungal Meningitis
- Diffuse Leptomeningeal Glioneuronal Tumor
- Neurocysticercosis
- Meningioangiomatosis
- Neurocutaneous Melanosis
- Neurosarcoid

ESSENTIAL INFORMATION

Key Differential Diagnosis Issues

- Clinical features to consider
  - Fever, neck pain, headache → meningitis
  - CNS or systemic neoplasm → leptomeningeal metastases
  - Facial port-wine stain → Sturge-Weber syndrome (SWS)
  - Sickle cell disease (SCD), neurofibromatosis type 1 (NF1), trisomy 21, prior radiation (XRT) → moyamoya
  - Hypertension, renal disease, transplant, chemotherapy → posterior reversible encephalopathy syndrome (PRES)
  - Large cutaneous melanocytic nevi → neurocutaneous melanosis (NCM)
- Imaging features to consider
  - Nodular enhancement → metastases or sarcoid
  - Associated findings
    - Loculated collections with ↑ DWI/↓ ADC → meningitis + empyema
    - Dominant intracranial mass → leptomeningeal metastasis
    - Prominent transmedullary veins → SWS
    - Associated infarcts → moyamoya or vasculitic meningitis
    - Atrophy with ongoing enhancement → SWS, moyamoya
    - Watershed distribution of subcortical signal → PRES
    - Parenchymal rim-enhancing lesions → infection (e.g., meningitis, neurocysticercosis)
- Modality considerations
  - NECT: Insensitive for leptomeningeal processes
    - May show associated abnormalities (e.g., Ca^{2+} in SWS or neurocysticercosis)
  - CECT: May show leptomeningeal enhancement but less sensitive than MR
  - MR: Best test for detection & characterization of leptomeningeal enhancement
    - Spin-echo-based are classically more sensitive than GRE-based sequences
      - Adding FLAIR postcontrast can ↑ sensitivity
    - SWI helpful to identify associated hemorrhage or Ca^{2+}
    - MRA if concern for associated vascular disease
    - Volumetric T1 C+ or 3D SSFP (FIESTA/CISS) may best show small lesions along cranial nerves

Helpful Clues for Common Diagnoses

- **Bacterial Meningitis**
  - Diagnosis is made by lumbar puncture (LP); imaging is typically performed to evaluate for
    - Complications (e.g., empyema/cerebritis)
    - Contraindications to LP
  - Mild: Thin linear leptomeningeal enhancement
  - Moderate: Leptomeningeal enhancement with loculated subarachnoid spaces & diffusion restriction
  - Severe: Leptomeningeal enhancement with associated empyema ± cerebritis
- **Leptomeningeal Metastases**
  - Occur in many pediatric primary CNS tumors (e.g., medulloblastoma, ependymoma, etc.)
    - Rare in pediatric extra-CNS tumors
  - Morphology: Scattered nodular enhancement; may see discrete masses
  - Location: Anywhere, but basilar cisterns are most common
  - MR: Best seen on T1 C+, but DWI is helpful in high-grade tumors
    - Perform spine MR to fully evaluate extent

Helpful Clues for Less Common Diagnoses

- **Moyamoya Arteriopathy**
  - Moyamoya disease: Idiopathic arteriopathy (especially in Asian population)
  - Moyamoya syndrome: Arteriopathy in setting of predisposing disease (e.g., SCD, NF1, trisomy 21, XRT)
  - MR: Leptomeningeal enhancement is due to dilated pial vessels vs. collateral formation
    - Ivy sign of high signal in sulci on unenhanced FLAIR or T1 C+
    - Look for attenuated major vessel flow voids in basilar cisterns on T2
      - May see numerous tiny flow voids in deep gray structures
    - MRA best shows vessel narrowing & collateral lenticulostriate & thalamoperforating arteries
      - Look for external carotid (e.g., meningeal artery) collaterals
  - ± infarcts of varying ages
- **Sturge-Weber Syndrome**
  - Syndrome of abnormal cortical venous development
  - Sulcal enhancement represents leptomeningeal angiomatosis (collateral vessels) due to insufficient cortical venous drainage
  - CT: Atrophy ± gyral/subcortical Ca^{2+}
  - MR: Atrophy & leptomeningeal enhancement
    - Abundant medullary & deep draining veins
    - Ipsilateral choroid plexus glomus enlargement
    - ± choroidal angioma in posterior globe, expanded calvarial/skull base venous drainage
- **Tuberculous Meningitis**
  - Risk factors: Endemic area, HIV, immunosuppression
  - MR: Thick, confluent enhancement within basilar cisterns
    - Often accompanied by hydrocephalus

- Look for infarcts from associated arteritis
- May present with cranial neuropathies

- **Posterior Reversible Encephalopathy Syndrome**
  - Cerebrovascular autoregulatory disorder occurring in numerous disease states (but usually accompanied by hypertension)
  - Most often affects cortex & subcortical white matter in watershed distributions; can affect deep gray, brainstem, & cerebellum
  - MR: Some degree of enhancement in ~ 50%
    - May be leptomeningeal only but often has associated small patchy cortical enhancement
    - Enhancement does not indicate more severe disease or poorer prognosis

Helpful Clues for Rare Diagnoses

- **Leukemia**
  - Meningeal disease, usually with acute lymphoblastic leukemia
  - MR: Cranial nerve involvement, plus
    - Osseous metastatic disease
      - Well circumscribed or poorly defined diffuse
      - Spin-echo-based T1 is better at lesions in fatty marrow than GRE-based T1
    - Dural & extracranial myeloid sarcoma lesions
- **Fungal Meningitis**
  - Caused by *Cryptococcus, Coccidioidomycosis, Candida*
    - *Cryptococcus*: Parenchymal gelatinous pseudocysts
    - *Coccidioidomycosis*: Abscesses, vasculitis
    - *Candida*: Parenchymal microabscesses
  - Rarely occur in absence of systemic disease manifestations
- **Diffuse Leptomeningeal Glioneuronal Tumor**
  - Officially identified in 2016 WHO CNS tumor update
  - MR: Thick nodular leptomeningeal enhancement with predilection for basilar cisterns & posterior fossa
    - Specific but inconsistent finding: Small subpial cysts in areas of leptomeningeal enhancement
    - No dominant or primary intracranial tumor
- **Neurocysticercosis**
  - Intracranial parasitic infection by *Taenia solium*
  - Cisterns > parenchyma > ventricles
  - MR: Cisternal neurocysticercosis may appear racemose (multilobulated, grape-like) & typically lacks scolex
    - Complications: Meningitis, hydrocephalus, vasculitis
- **Meningioangiomatosis**
  - Hamartomatous cortical/leptomeningeal malformation
  - Often seen in association with NF2
  - CT/MR: Cortical gyriform enhancement with Ca^{2+} (± cysts)
- **Neurocutaneous Melanosis**
  - Congenital phakomatosis with giant or multiple cutaneous melanocytic nevi (CMN) + benign & malignant melanotic CNS lesions
  - Leptomeningeal enhancement is uncommon manifestation of NCM (~ 10%)
  - MR: Diffuse or focal leptomeningeal enhancement may extend into parenchyma along perivascular spaces
    - Look for parenchymal melanosis (foci of precontrast ↑ T1 signal, most often in medial temporal region)
- **Neurosarcoid**
  - Leptomeningeal disease is seen in ~ 40% of neurosarcoid
  - Predilection for basilar cisterns, often involving cranial nerves & pituitary infundibulum
  - MR: May extend into brain along perivascular spaces
  - Look for systemic disease with chest radiograph; correlate with ACE serum levels

SELECTED REFERENCES

1. Sublett JM et al: Pediatric primary diffuse leptomeningeal primitive neuroectodermal tumor: a case report and literature review. Pediatr Neurosurg. 52(2):114-21, 2017
2. Ahmad A et al: Differentiation of leptomeningeal and vascular enhancement on post-contrast FLAIR MRI sequence: role in early detection of infectious meningitis. J Clin Diagn Res. 9(1):TC08-12, 2015
3. Matsumura M et al: Leptomeningeal melanomatosis associated with neurocutaneous melanosis: an autopsy case report. Pathol Int. 65(2):100-5, 2015
4. Mugikura S et al: Cortical microvascularization and leptomeningeal collaterals in moyamoya disease. Eur Neurol. 73(5-6):351-2, 2015

Bacterial Meningitis

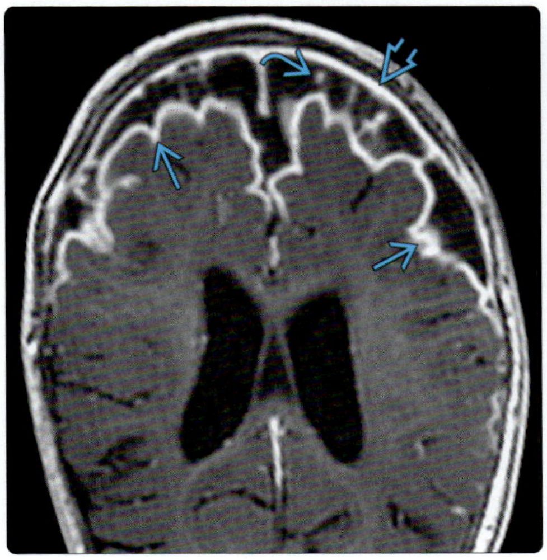

Bacterial Meningitis

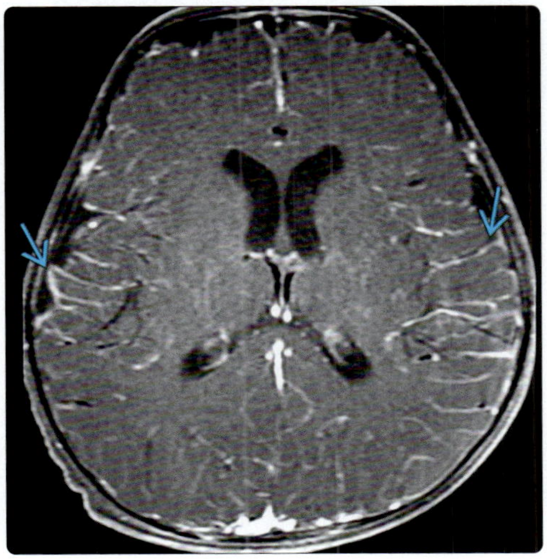

(Left) *Axial T1 C+ MR in a 7 month old with Haemophilus influenzae meningitis shows extensive smooth leptomeningeal enhancement ➡. Also note the prominent vessels ➡ coursing through the subarachnoid spaces & the smooth dural enhancement ➡.* **(Right)** *Axial T1 C+ FS in a 4 month old with pneumococcal meningitis shows thin smooth leptomeningeal enhancement ➡ of both frontoparietal regions, consistent with uncomplicated meningitis.*

(Left) *Axial T1 C+ MR in a 3 year old with metastatic medulloblastoma shows thick nodular enhancement along the brainstem & left trigeminal nerve. Note the enlarged 4th ventricle status post tumor resection.* **(Right)** *Sagittal T1 C+ MR in the same patient shows the extent of leptomeningeal disease along the upper cervical cord, brainstem, hypothalamus, & ependyma.*

Leptomeningeal Metastases

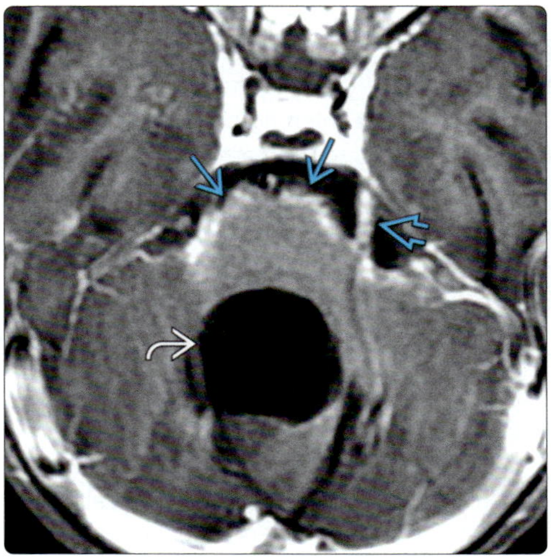

Leptomeningeal Metastases

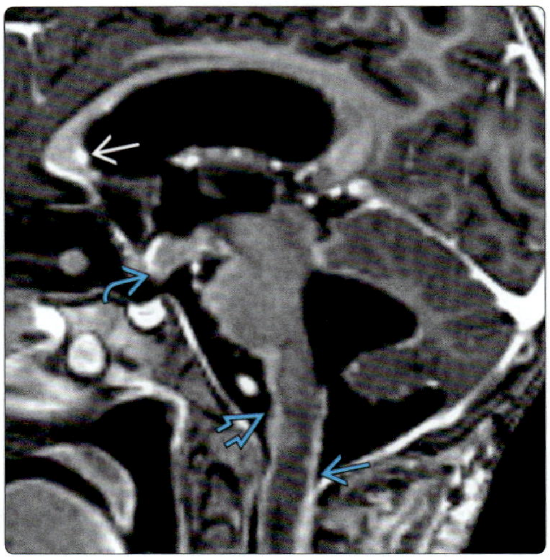

(Left) *Axial T1 C+ MR in a teenager with sickle cell disease & moyamoya arteriopathy shows thin leptomeningeal enhancement over the right cerebral hemisphere as well as prominent vessels in the right basal ganglia. This finding is secondary to slow flow in collateral vessels.* **(Right)** *Lateral oblique 3D MRA in the same patient shows severe narrowing at the terminal internal carotid arteries with extensive collateral vessels in the basal ganglia.*

Moyamoya Arteriopathy

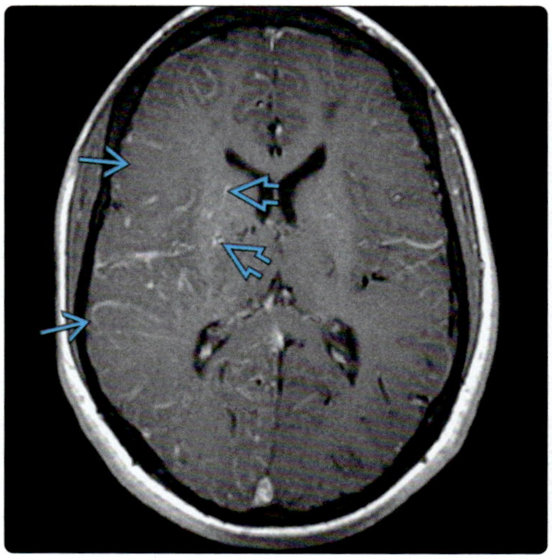

Moyamoya Arteriopathy

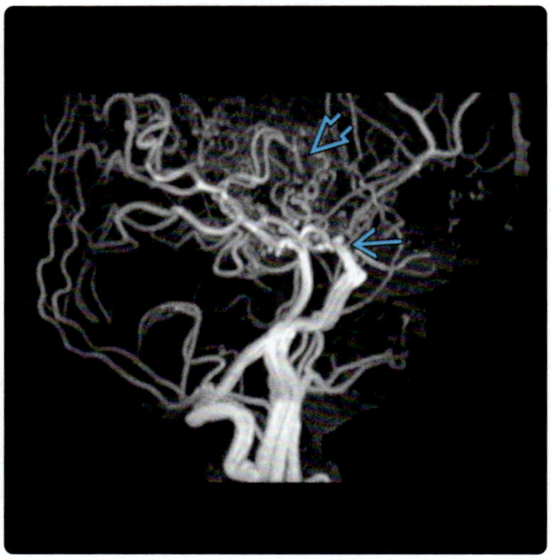

(Left) *Coronal NECT in a 3 year old with Sturge-Weber syndrome (SWS) shows the development of cortical & subcortical Ca^{2+}. Such a finding is rarely present at birth but becomes increasingly common with age & is usually accompanied by parenchymal volume loss.* **(Right)** *Axial T1 C+ FS MR in a 1 year old with SWS shows leptomeningeal enhancement in the right parietal region, corresponding to leptomeningeal angiomatosis.*

Sturge-Weber Syndrome

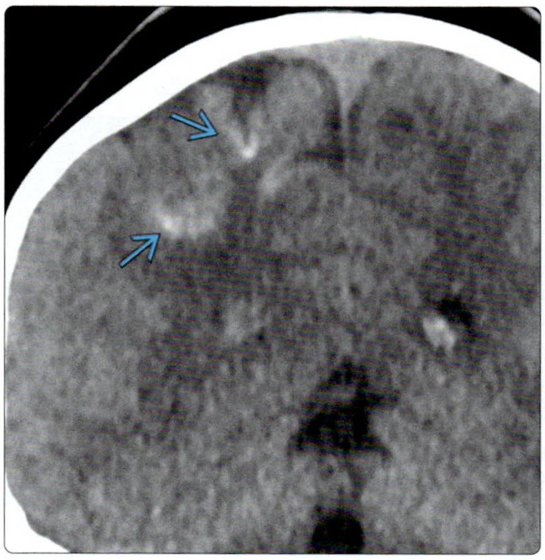

Sturge-Weber Syndrome

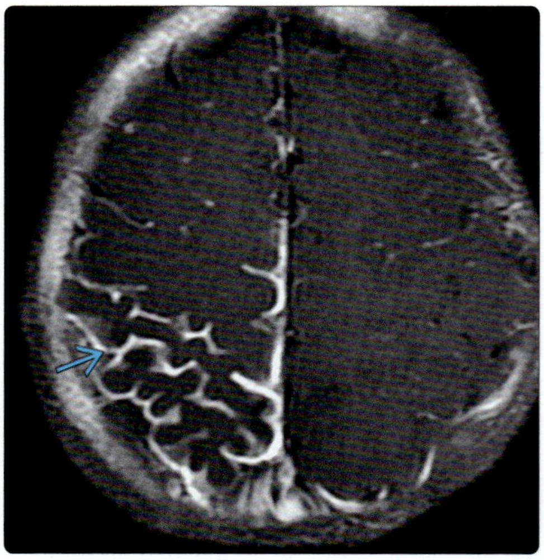

Sturge-Weber Syndrome

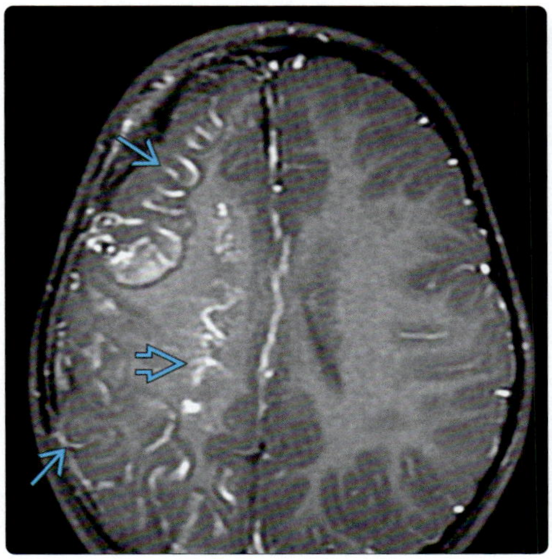

Sturge-Weber Syndrome

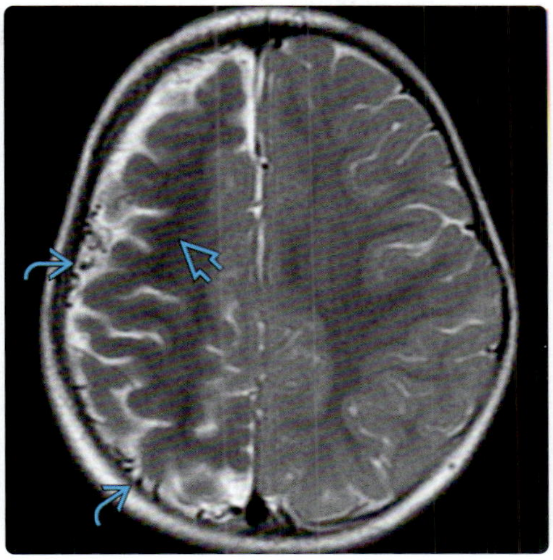

(Left) *Axial T1 C+ FS MR in a 1 year old with SWS shows extensive right cerebral hemisphere leptomeningeal enhancement with frontal atrophy, consistent with leptomeningeal & pial angiomatosis. Also note the enlarged medullary veins providing collateral venous drainage.* **(Right)** *Axial T2 MR in the same patient with SWS at 16 months old shows marked atrophy of the right cerebral hemisphere, decreased white matter signal, & dilated tortuous vessels in the right convexity subarachnoid spaces.*

Tuberculous Meningitis

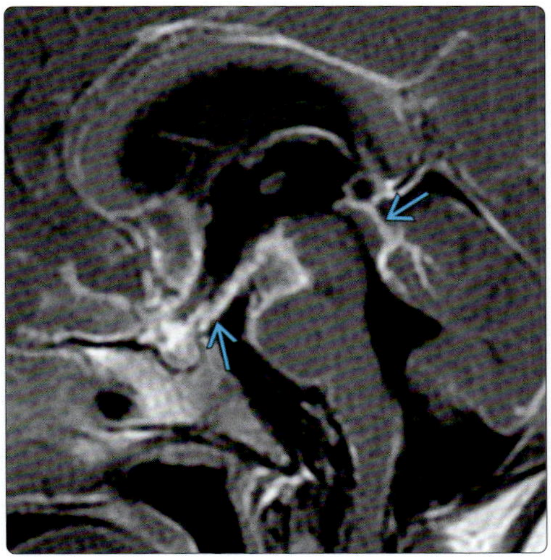

Tuberculous Meningitis

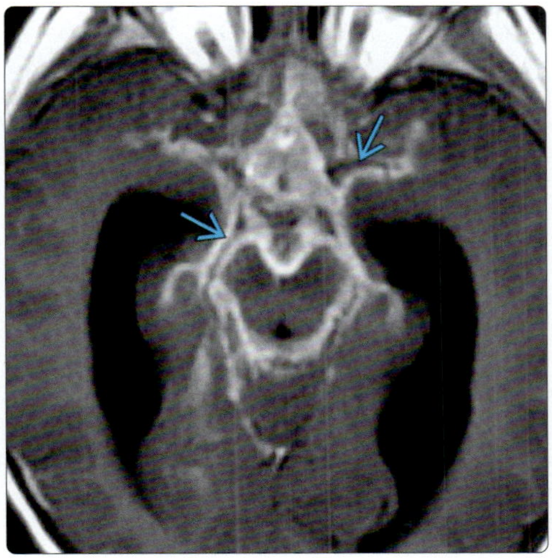

(Left) *Sagittal T1 C+ MR in a 2 year old with tuberculous meningitis shows thick, micronodular leptomeningeal enhancement predominantly affecting the basilar cisterns.* **(Right)** *Axial T1 C+ MR in the same patient shows extensive thick basilar enhancement with preservation of the leptomeninges over the cerebral convexities. This predilection for basilar involvement is typical of tuberculous meningitis. The patient's chest radiographs showed right paratracheal lymphadenopathy*

Posterior Reversible Encephalopathy Syndrome

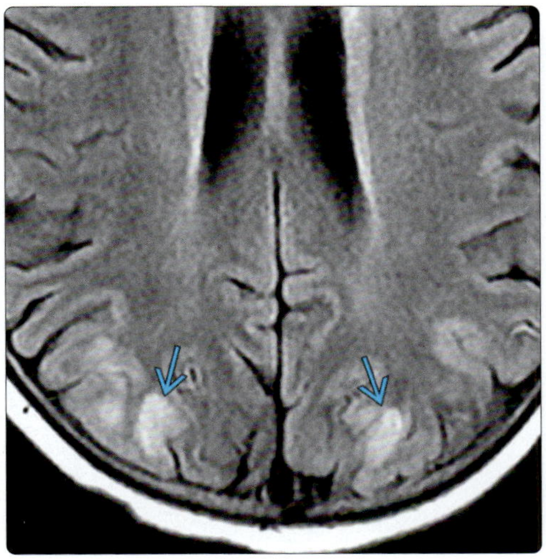

Posterior Reversible Encephalopathy Syndrome

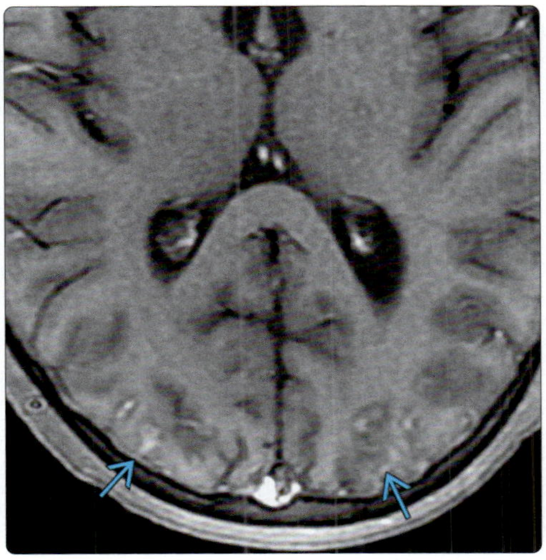

(Left) *Axial FLAIR MR in an 8 year old with leukemia, seizures, & hypertension shows nearly symmetric signal abnormalities in the bilateral parietooccipital watershed cortex, typical for posterior reversible encephalopathy syndrome (PRES).* **(Right)** *Axial T1 C+ FS MR in the same patient shows subtle leptomeningeal enhancement adjacent to the areas of cortical involvement. Enhancement is seen in ~ 50% of PRES patients, although usually subtle. Patchy cortical enhancement may also occur.*

(Left) *Axial T1 C+ MR in a patient with acute lymphoblastic leukemia with a blast crisis shows leptomeningeal enhancement along the cerebellar folia. CSF demonstrated blast cells.* **(Right)** *Axial T1 C+ FS MR in a 7 year old with leukemia shows symmetric enlargement & enhancement of the extraocular muscles & the bilateral trigeminal nerves, representing leukemic infiltration. History & identification of associated findings are key to making this diagnosis.*

Leukemia

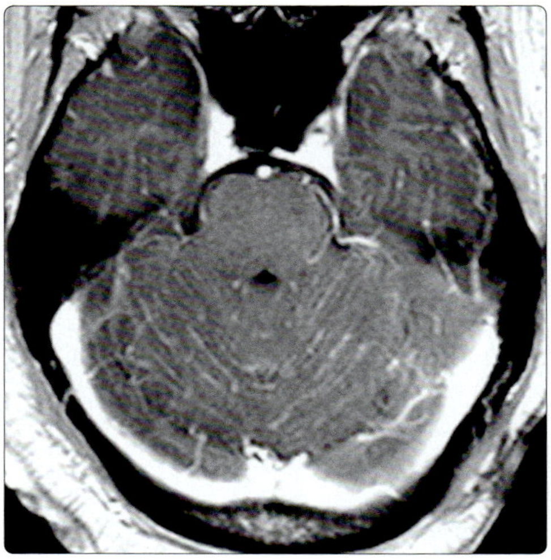

Leukemia

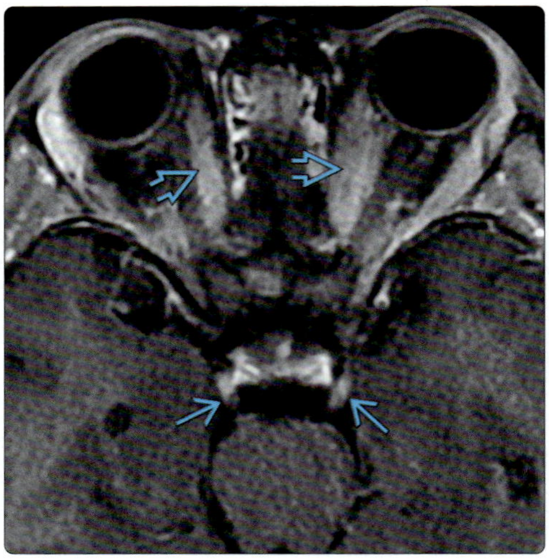

(Left) *Axial T1 C+ MR in a patient with coccidioidomycosis shows very thick enhancement of the basal cisterns with sparing of the cerebral hemispheres. Fungal meningitis has a very similar appearance to tuberculous meningitis.* **(Right)** *Axial T1 C+ MR in a patient with coccidioidomycosis meningitis shows extensive leptomeningeal enhancement in the suprasellar & ambient cisterns. Note the early hydrocephalus with prominence of temporal horns, a common complication of fungal meningitis.*

Fungal Meningitis

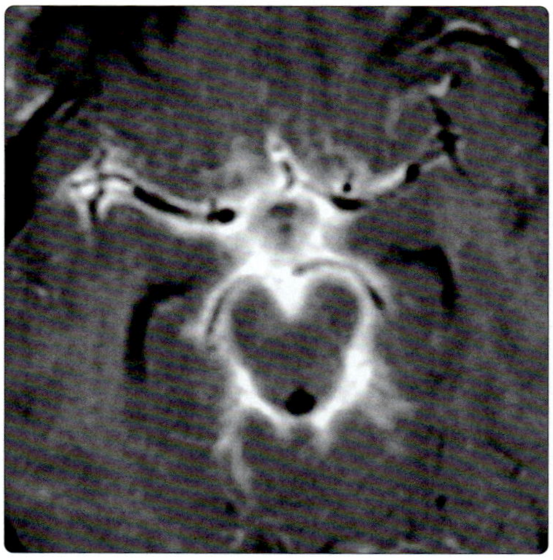

Fungal Meningitis

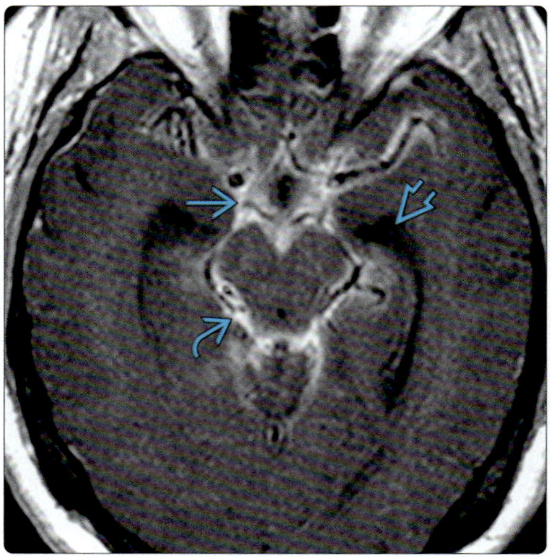

(Left) *Axial T1 C+ FS MR in a 3 year old with cranial nerve palsies due to a diffuse leptomeningeal glioneuronal tumor shows multiple nodular leptomeningeal deposits within the suprasellar & ambient cisterns.* **(Right)** *Sagittal T1 C+ MR in the same patient shows extensive leptomeningeal nodular enhancement throughout the posterior fossa cisterns. While other conditions can rarely cause nodular enhancement, tumor should be the primary consideration in such cases.*

Diffuse Leptomeningeal Glioneuronal Tumor

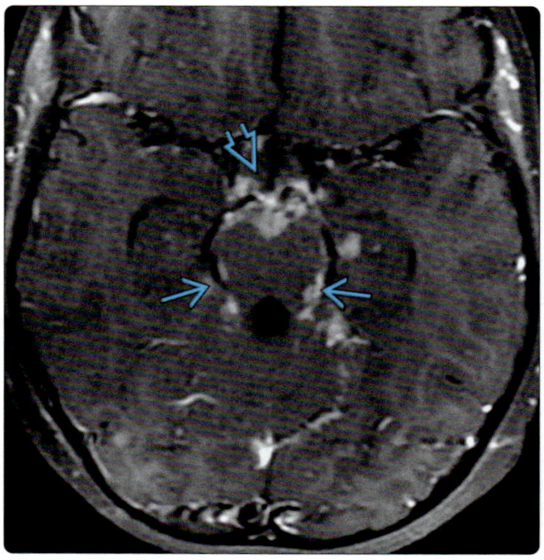

Diffuse Leptomeningeal Glioneuronal Tumor

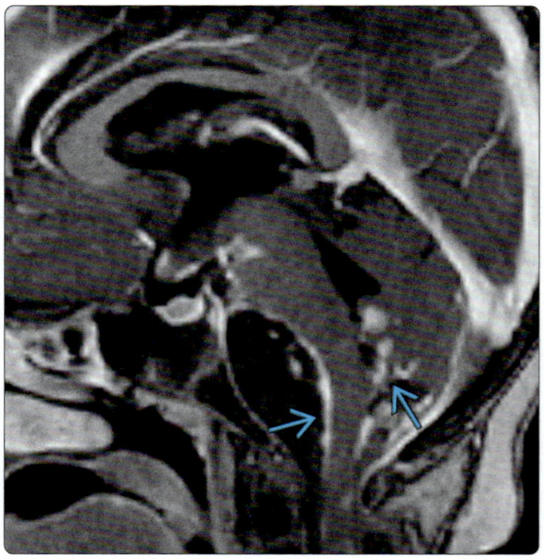

Meningioangiomatosis

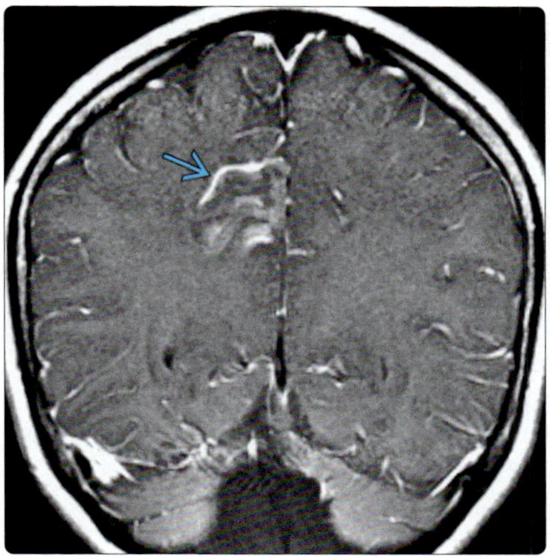

Meningioangiomatosis

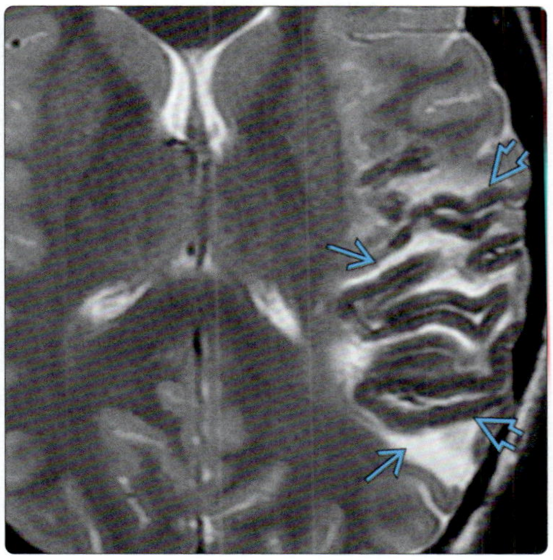

(Left) *Coronal T1 C+ MR in a patient with meningioangiomatosis shows smooth leptomeningeal enhancement → in the right medial parietal lobe. The NECT (not shown) demonstrated associated cortical* Ca^{2+}. **(Right)** *Axial T2 MR in a 14 year old with meningioangiomatosis shows decreased signal within the affected cortex → & increased signal in the underlying white matter →, consistent with gliosis. The hypointense T2 signal in the cortex is a key finding to make this diagnosis.*

Neurocutaneous Melanosis

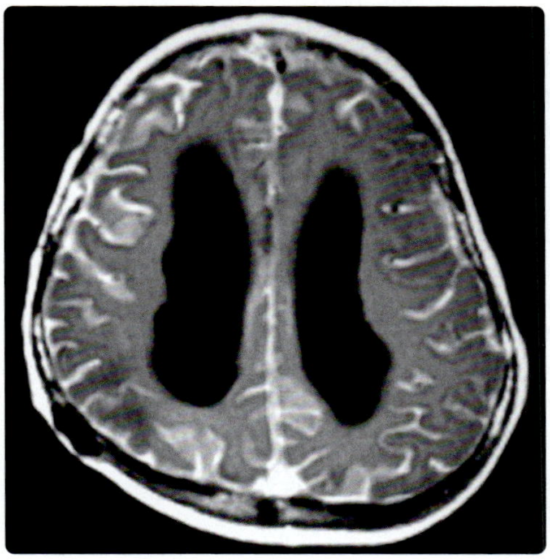

Neurocutaneous Melanosis

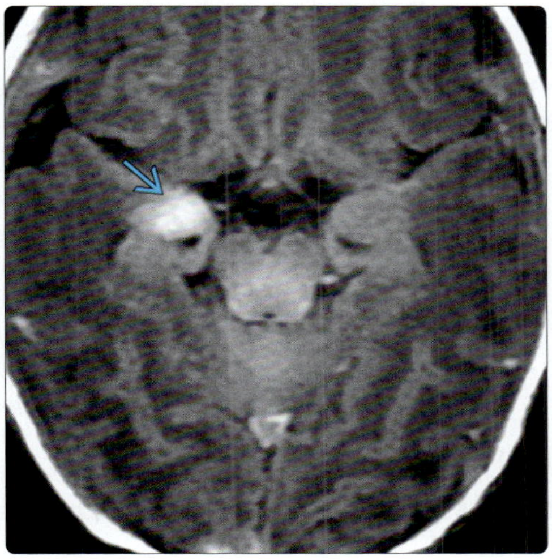

(Left) *Axial T1 C+ MR in a patient with neurocutaneous melanosis (NCM) shows leptomeningeal enhancement of the entire brain. Note the associated communicating hydrocephalus. Leptomeningeal melanosis is a rare manifestation of NCM (< 10%).* **(Right)** *Axial T1 MR in a neonate with multiple large congenital cutaneous nevi shows a single focus of hyperintense signal → in the right medial temporal lobe, a classic location for parenchymal melanosis (most common NCM manifestation).*

Neurosarcoid

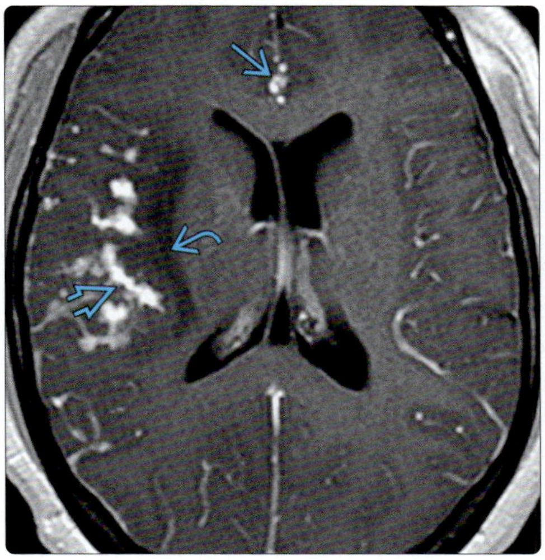

Neurosarcoid

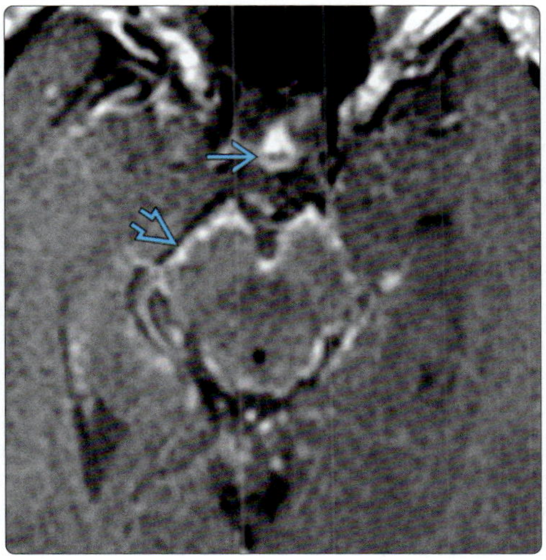

(Left) *Axial T1 C+ MR in a patient with neurosarcoid demonstrates nodular leptomeningeal enhancement in the anterior interhemispheric fissure → & right sylvian fissure →. Note the vasogenic edema → in the adjacent right perisylvian brain parenchyma.* **(Right)** *Axial T1 C+ FS MR shows linear & nodular coating of the midbrain → due to neurosarcoid. Note the thickening of the infundibular stalk →. Correlation with chest radiographs & ACE levels can be helpful in establishing this diagnosis.*

DIFFERENTIAL DIAGNOSIS

Common

- Incomplete/Arrested Pneumatization of Sphenoid Sinus

Less Common

- Dermoid/Epidermoid
- Craniopharyngioma
- Juvenile Angiofibroma
- Pituitary Macroadenoma
- Cholesteatoma
- Nasopharyngeal Carcinoma
- Chordoma
- Fibrous Dysplasia
- Cephalocele/Encephalocele
- Langerhans Cell Histiocytosis
- Plexiform Neurofibroma
- Osteomyelitis With Abscess
- Teratoma
- Rhabdomyosarcoma
- Schwannoma
- Metastatic Disease
  - Neuroblastoma
  - Myeloid Sarcoma/Osseus Leukemic Involvement
  - Other Metastatic Disease

Rare but Important

- Lymphatic Malformation
- Meningioma
- Ewing Sarcoma
- Esthesioneuroblastoma
- Enchondroma
- Osteosarcoma

ESSENTIAL INFORMATION

Key Differential Diagnosis Issues

- Clinical features to consider
  - Age
    - Infants: Teratoma, neuroblastoma (NB)
    - Adolescents: Juvenile angiofibroma (JAF) nasopharyngeal carcinoma (NPC), esthesioneuroblastoma
    - Adults (rare in children): Meningioma
  - Sex: JAF occurs almost exclusively in males
  - Skin lesions: Nasal dermoid, plexiform neurofibroma (PN), fibrous dysplasia (FD)
  - Hormonal abnormalities: Pituitary macroadenoma
  - Multifocal lesions: Langerhans cell histiocytosis (LCH), FD, leukemia, metastases, enchondromas, lymphatic malformation (LM)
- Imaging features to consider
  - Location
    - Anterior skull base: Dermoid/epidermoid, esthesioneuroblastoma
    - Middle skull base: Incomplete/arrested pneumatization of sphenoid sinus, craniopharyngioma, JAF, pituitary macroadenoma, cholesteatoma
    - Posterior skull base: Chordoma, NPC
    - Others can occur in any skull base location
  - Modalities
    - CT: Best at cortical involvement, bone response (destruction vs. remodeling), & calcified matrix
    - MR: Best for evaluating marrow & soft tissue disease, lesions with noncalcified matrix

Helpful Clues for Common Diagnoses

- **Incomplete/Arrested Pneumatization of Sphenoid Sinus**
  - Well-defined lucent lesion in sphenoid body with fat &/or cystic-appearing components
  - Common in 1st & early 2nd decades
  - Frequently misdiagnosed as fibroosseous lesion

Helpful Clues for Less Common Diagnoses

- **Dermoid/Epidermoid**
  - Congenital ectodermal inclusion cyst, often occurring as foramen cecum mass with nasal dermoid
  - CT: Smooth enlargement of foramen cecum
  - MR: Nonenhancing, ± diffusion restriction
- **Craniopharyngioma**
  - Sellar & suprasellar mass with cysts & Ca^{2+}
  - CT: Cystic mass with Ca^{2+}, ± sellar remodeling
  - MR: Mixed solid & cystic mass with foci of ↓ SWI (Ca^{2+}); often contain cysts with T1 shortening
- **Juvenile Angiofibroma**
  - Benign, vascular, locally invasive mass of posterior nasal cavity occurring in teenage male with epistaxis
  - CT: Avidly enhancing mass near sphenopalatine foramen ± osseous remodeling or destruction
  - MR: Enhancing nasal mass with obliteration of normal sphenopalatine fat & adjacent fat planes
- **Pituitary Macroadenoma**
  - Can extend beyond sellar margins as enhancing figure 8-shaped mass
  - CT: Sellar expansion with large sellar/suprasellar mass
  - MR: Enhancing sellar mass ± cysts/hemorrhage
- **Cholesteatoma**
  - Locally destructive mass in middle ear/mastoid due to acquired or congenital epidermal inclusion cyst
  - CT: Osseous erosion of ossicles & adjacent bone
  - MR: Nonenhancing mass with ↑ DWI/ ↓ ADC
- **Nasopharyngeal Carcinoma**
  - Mucosal tumor associated with Epstein-Barr virus (EBV) in adolescents
  - May invade middle skull base (sphenoid)
- **Chordoma**
  - Notochordal remnant arising from clivus
  - CT: Destructive mass centered in clivus
  - MR: Marked ↑ T2 signal mass, variable enhancement
- **Fibrous Dysplasia**
  - Fibroosseous expansile lesion commonly in skull base
  - CT: Ground-glass matrix (think frosted or smudged glass); may have lytic & sclerotic components
  - MR: Fibrous matrix may have ↓ T2, but active lesions can show ↑ T2 & avid enhancement
- **Cephalocele/Encephalocele**
  - Protrusion of meninges ± brain through osseous defect
  - CT: Smoothly remodeled osseous defects in skull base
  - MR: Continuity of CSF ± brain into defect
- **Langerhans Cell Histiocytosis**
  - Systemic or localized proliferation of specific histiocytes

- CT: Sharply marginated ("punched-out") lytic lesion(s)
- MR: Cellular (↑ DWI/↓ ADC) enhancing mass fills defect
- **Plexiform Neurofibroma**
  - Lobulated masses with target appearance: ↓ T2 center, ↑ T2 periphery
  - ± other findings of neurofibromatosis type 1 (NF1)
- **Osteomyelitis With Abscess**
  - Extension of paranasal sinus infection to skull base
  - CT: Rim-enhancing epidural fluid ± bone destruction
  - MR: Abnormal marrow signal/enhancement with abscess (which often shows ↑ DWI/↓ ADC) & soft tissue edema; ± intracranial complications
- **Teratoma**
  - Large solid & cystic congenital germ cell tumor; may have intracranial, oral cavity, or cervical origin
  - CT: Skull base remodeling/invasion ± fat, Ca^{2+} in mass
  - MR: Large solid & cystic tumor ± fat
- **Rhabdomyosarcoma**
  - Most common soft tissue malignancy in children; can arise from many different sites about head & neck
  - CT/MR: Variable heterogeneity & enhancement; ↑ DWI/↓ ADC
- **Schwannoma**
  - Enhancing benign neoplasm of peripheral/cranial nerves; often centered in neural foramina
  - Multifocal lesions in neurofibromatosis type 2 (NF2) + meningiomas & ependymomas
- **Metastatic Disease**
  - **Neuroblastoma**
    - Multifocal permeative lesions in child < 5 years of age; particularly fond of orbits/facial bones
    - CT: Mildly expansile permeative lesions; "hair-on-end" radiating spicules of new bone within soft tissue mass
    - MR: Discrete & sharply circumscribed against normal marrow fat (best seen on spin echo-based T1) vs. diffuse confluent replacement of fatty marrow; cellular (↑ DWI/↓ ADC) & enhancing
  - **Myeloid sarcoma/osseus leukemic involvement**
    - Solitary or multifocal leukemic lesions
    - CT: Osteoporosis with scattered permeation; focal lucency at metaphyseal equivalents (lucent bands)
    - MR: Similar to neuroblastoma
  - **Other metastatic disease**
    - Typically from sarcomas; various combinations of above features
    - More commonly lytic than sclerotic

Helpful Clues for Rare Diagnoses

- **Lymphatic Malformations**
  - Generalized lymphatic anomaly (GLA) or Gorham-Stout disease (GSD)
    - GLA: Multifocal cystic lesions of skeleton without frank cortical destruction; splenic & pleural involvement are common
    - GSD: Aggressive destruction of multiple adjacent bones by microcystic LM
  - ± patchy ↑ fat signal of bone
- **Meningioma**
  - Uncommon benign neoplasm in children; look for NF2 or remote history of radiation treatment
  - CT: ± Ca^{2+}, hyperdensity
  - MR: Heterogeneous/intermediate/low T2; vigorous enhancement with broad base & dural tail
- **Ewing Sarcoma**
  - Soft tissue or bone origin
  - Destructive, permeative mass; ↑ DWI/↓ ADC on MR
- **Esthesioneuroblastoma**
  - Neural crest tumor arising in olfactory neuroepithelium
  - CT: Destructive mass of cribriform plate
  - MR: Enhancing dumbbell-shaped mass with intracranial & ethmoid sinus extension; peripheral cysts
- **Enchondroma**
  - Rare lesion arising in petrooccipital fissure; most common in enchondromatosis
  - MR: Lobulated ↑ T2 lesion with ↓ T2 septations; rim & nodular enhancement of cartilage lobules
- **Osteosarcoma**
  - Destructive skull base mass with osteoid matrix

Incomplete/Arrested Pneumatization of Sphenoid Sinus

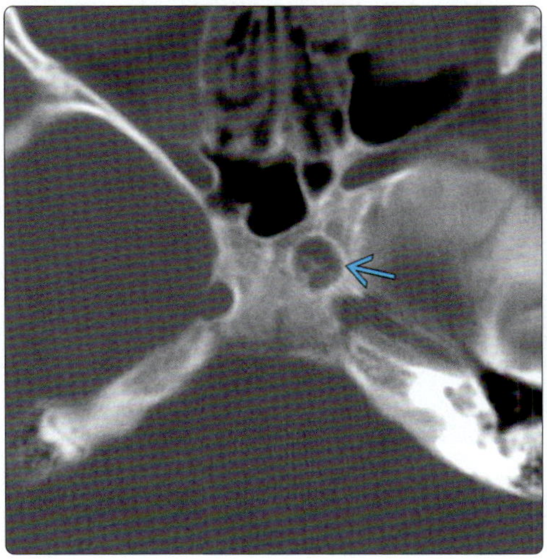

Incomplete/Arrested Pneumatization of Sphenoid Sinus

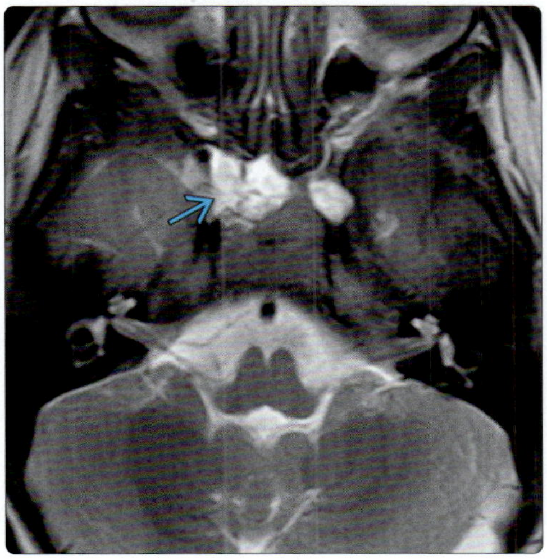

(Left) *Axial NECT in a 5 year old with incomplete pneumatization of the sphenoid sinus shows an apparent lytic lesion ➡ in the left sphenoid body. Soft tissue windows showed fat attenuation within the lesion.* **(Right)** *Axial T2 MR in a 7 year old shows heterogeneously hyperintense signal in the right sphenoid body ➡, a characteristic location & appearance for incomplete pneumatization of the sphenoid sinus. This is a "do-not-touch" lesion & should not be mistaken for a lesion of clinical concern.*

(Left) *Sagittal T2 MR in a 9 year old with a nasal pit shows a hyperintense epidermoid cyst ➔ in the anterior cranial fossa with extension into an expanded foramen cecum ➔ & sinus tract ➔ that extends into the nose.* **(Right)** *Axial DWI MR in the same patient shows the intracranial portion of the mass ➔ to restrict diffusion (↓ ADC not shown), characteristic for an epithelial inclusion cyst, such as an epidermoid cyst. DWI is an important component of any skull base mass evaluation.*

Dermoid/Epidermoid

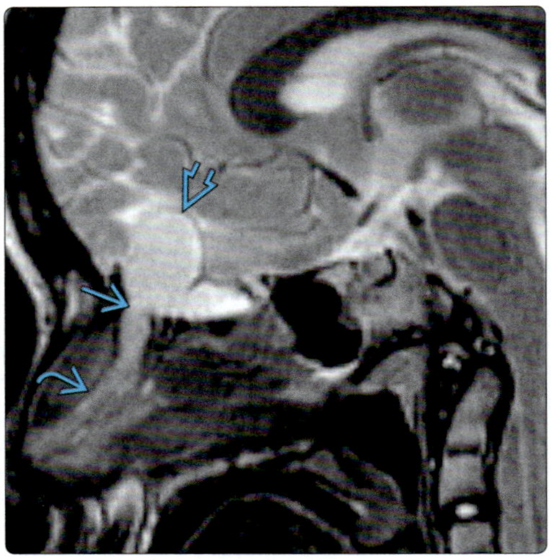

Dermoid/Epidermoid

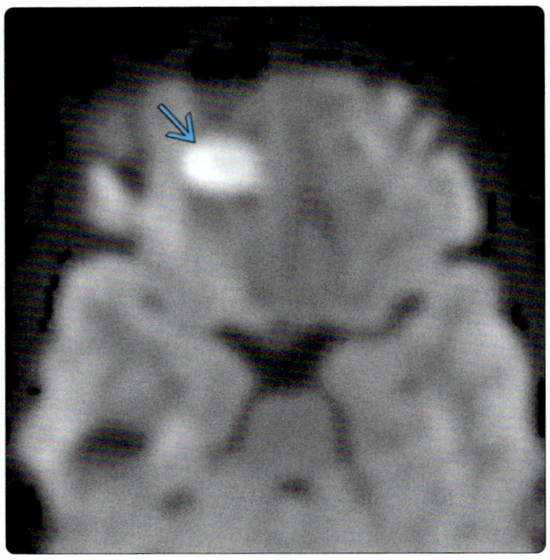

(Left) *Sagittal NECT in a 5 year old shows a mixed solid & cystic mass ➔ involving the sella & suprasellar regions. Note the peripheral Ca^{2+} ➔, typical for craniopharyngioma. The mass causes significant remodeling & enlargement of the sella turcica ➔.* **(Right)** *Axial CECT in a 15-year-old boy with recurrent epistaxis shows an enhancing mass ➔ in the left posterior nasal cavity arising from the left sphenopalatine foramen ➔. This location is typical for juvenile angiofibroma (JAF).*

Craniopharyngioma

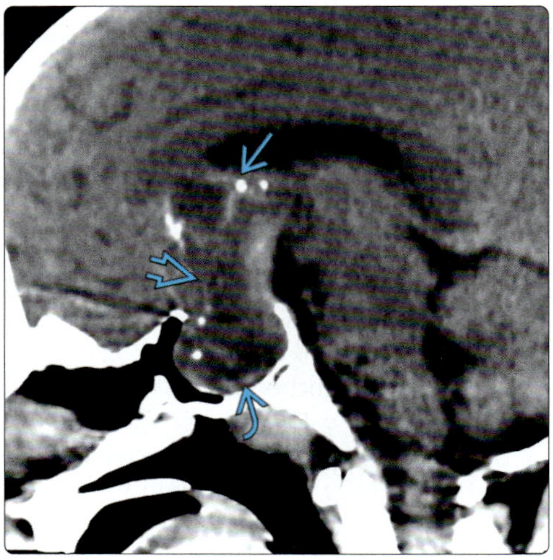

Juvenile Angiofibroma

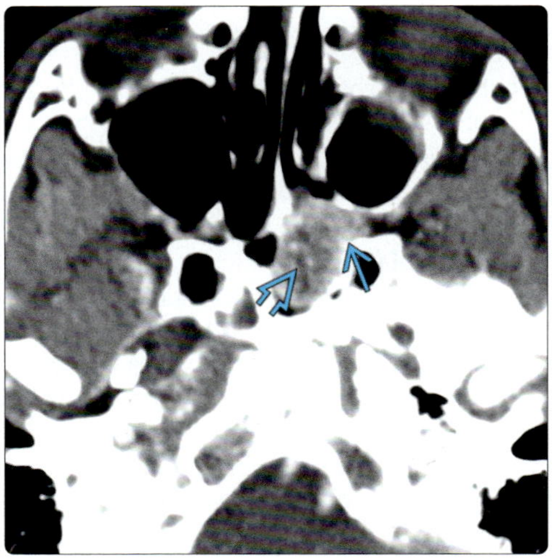

(Left) *Axial T1 MR in a 13-year-old boy shows a mass ➔ in the left posterior nasal cavity with obliteration of the normal fat in the left sphenopalatine foramen ➔, typical of JAF. Postcontrast images (not shown) will typically demonstrate early & intense enhancement of a JAF.* **(Right)** *Axial T2 MR in a 10-year-old boy with elevated prolactin demonstrates a large sellar mass ➔ with invasion of the cavernous sinus & encasement of the carotid arteries ➔, consistent with a pituitary macroadenoma.*

Juvenile Angiofibroma

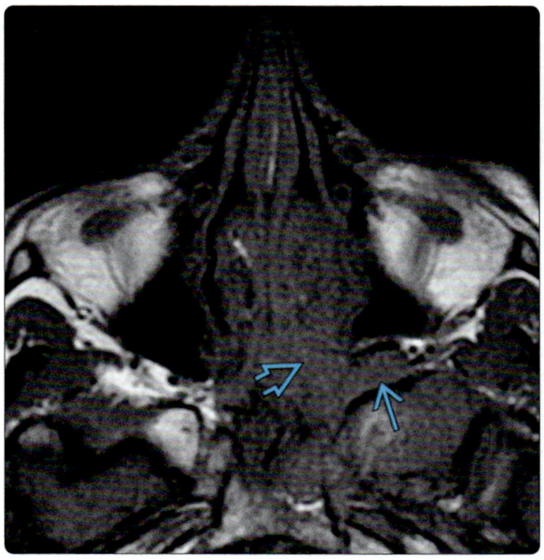

Pituitary Macroadenoma

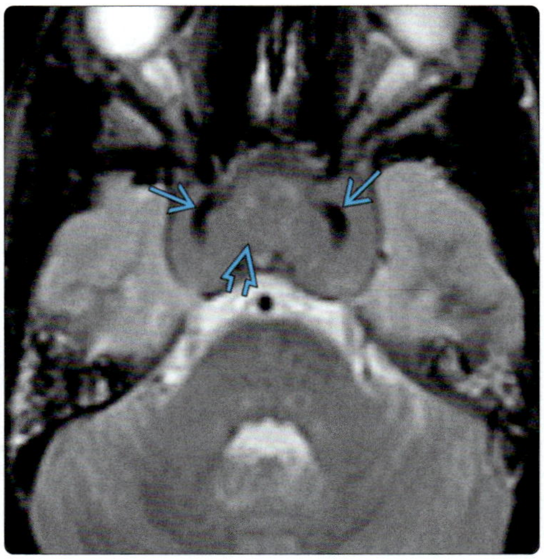

Nasopharyngeal Carcinoma

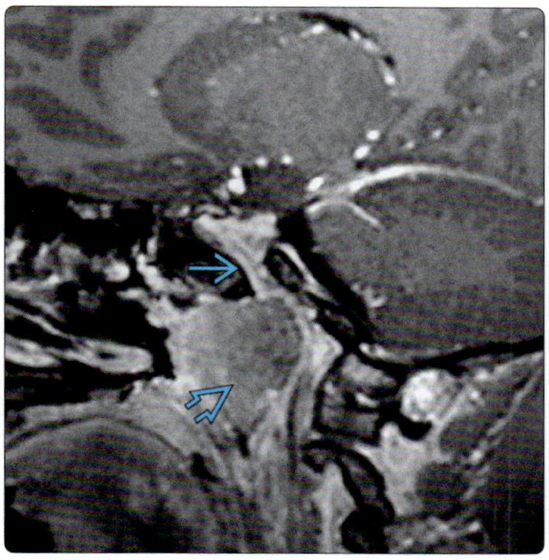

Chordoma

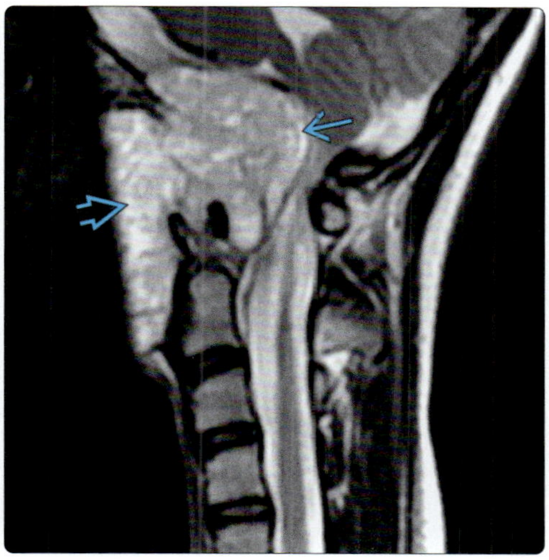

(Left) *Sagittal T1 C+ FS MR in an 18 year old with nasopharyngeal carcinoma shows an enhancing nasopharyngeal mass ⇒ extending into the carotid canal → & cavernous sinus.* **(Right)** *Sagittal T2 MR in a 15 year old with tongue deviation shows a heterogeneously hyperintense mass centered in the inferior clivus with large anterior prevertebral ⇒ & posterior intracranial → components. This is a typical location & appearance for chordoma.*

Fibrous Dysplasia

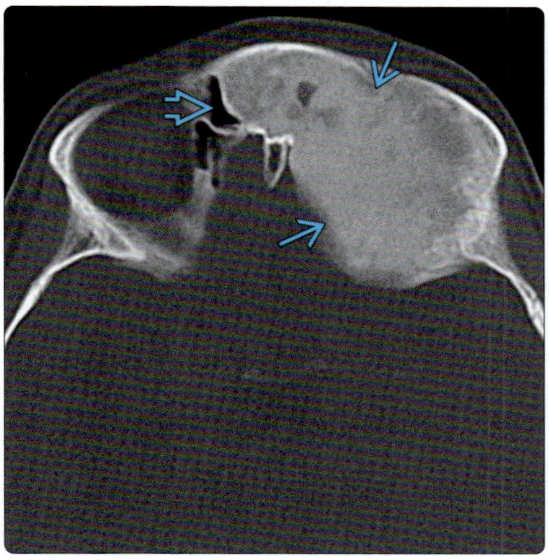

Fibrous Dysplasia

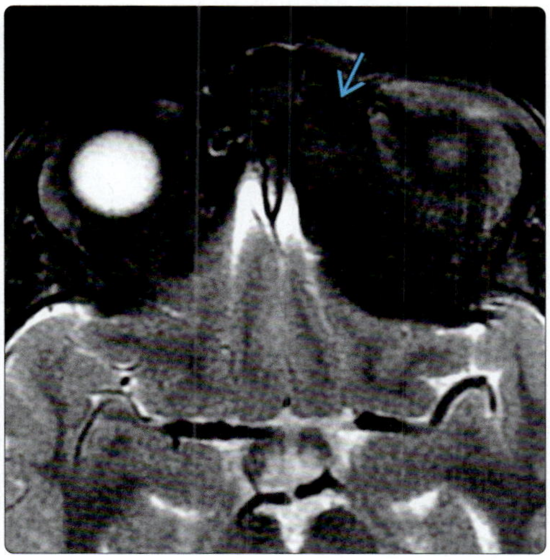

(Left) *Axial NECT in a 13 year old shows an expansile lesion → of the left frontal bone with nearly homogeneous ground-glass matrix, typical of fibrous dysplasia (FD). Note the partial obliteration of the frontal sinuses ⇒.* **(Right)** *Axial T2 FS MR in the same patient shows the expansile lesion → to be homogeneously hypointense, though active FD lesions may by hyperintense & show enhancement. Skull base FD may result in severe deformities with neuroforaminal narrowing.*

Cephalocele/Encephalocele

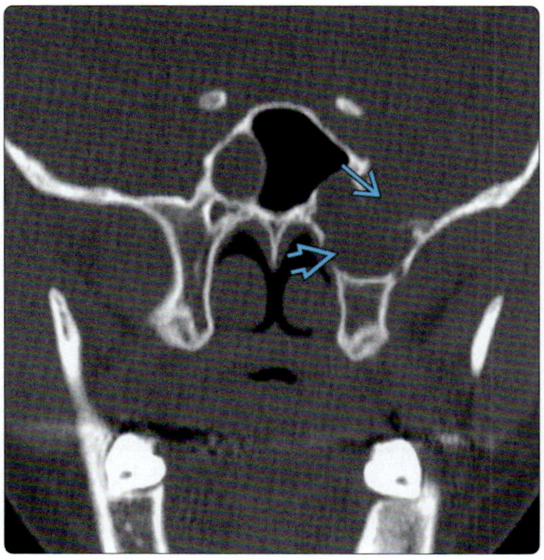

Cephalocele/Encephalocele

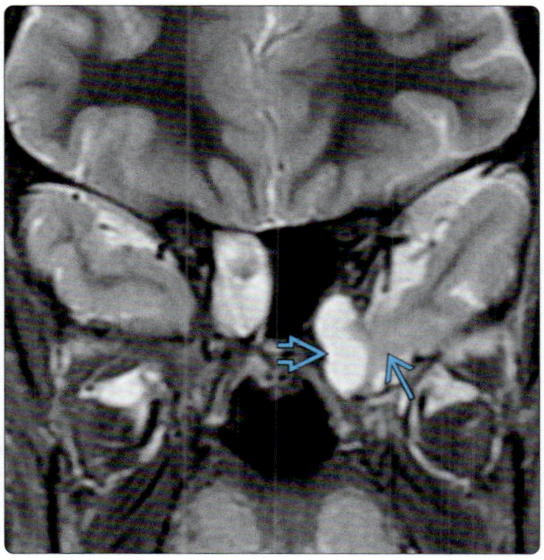

(Left) *Coronal NECT in a 10 year old with an encephalocele shows a lucent lesion ⇒ in the left sphenoid body with an osseous defect → between the lesion & the left middle cranial fossa. Confirmation of an encephalocele can be made with MR imaging.* **(Right)** *Coronal T2 FS MR in the same patient shows gliotic brain parenchyma → & CSF ⇒ filling the lesion, confirming an encephalocele. Cephaloceles may be congenital or occur secondary to surgery or a lytic lesion.*

(Left) *Axial NECT in a 2 year old shows multifocal lytic lesions involving the right sphenoid greater wing & bilateral mastoids . Note the complete loss of bone at these levels with sharp margins, typical for Langerhans cell histiocytosis (LCH).* **(Right)** *Axial T1 C+ FS MR in the same patient shows avidly enhancing lesions involving most of the sphenoid & bilateral mastoids . LCH typically enhances diffusely & demonstrates some degree of diffusion restriction due to high cellularity.*

Langerhans Cell Histiocytosis

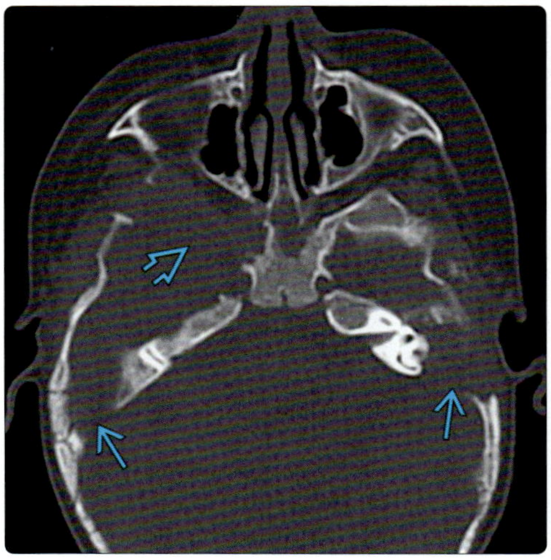

Langerhans Cell Histiocytosis

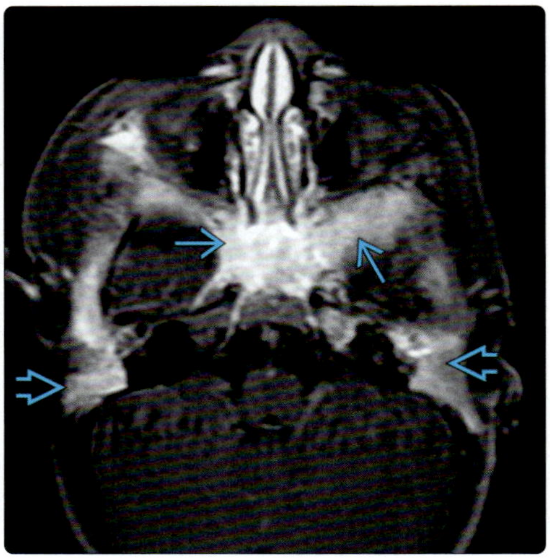

(Left) *Sagittal T2 MR in an 8 year old with acute sinusitis & clival osteomyelitis shows abnormal marrow signal with subperiosteal abscesses along the caudal & dorsal clivus. Note the relatively dark purulent material in the sphenoid sinus .* **(Right)** *Coronal SSFSE T2 MR of a 34-week gestation fetus with a cervical teratoma shows a large mixed solid & cystic mass centered in the floor of the left middle cranial fossa with large extracranial & smaller intracranial components.*

Osteomyelitis With Abscess

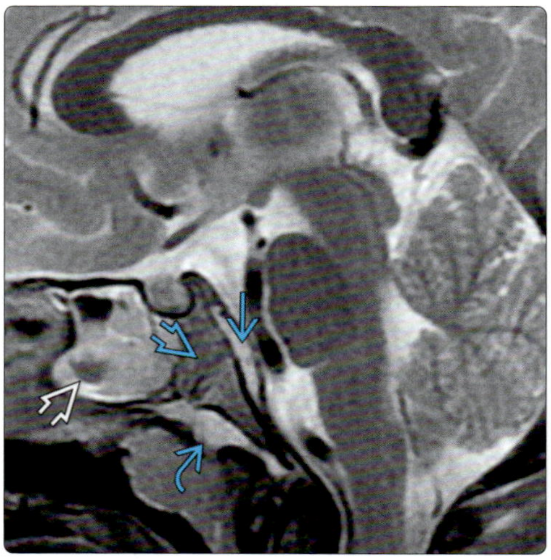

Teratoma

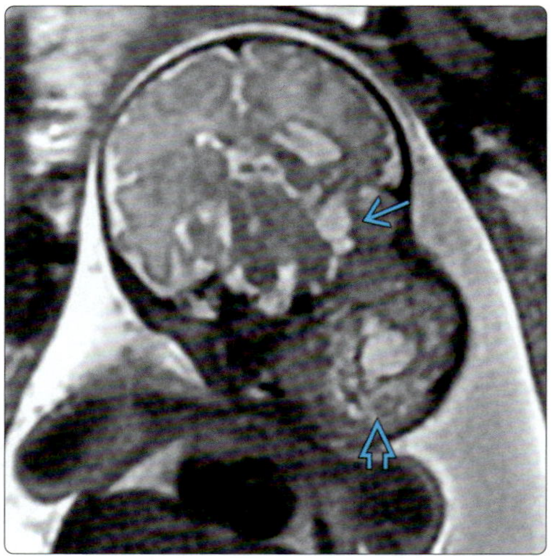

(Left) *Axial T1 C+ FS MR in a 5 year old with neurofibromatosis type 2 shows a large homogeneously enhancing schwannoma centered in the left cavernous sinus. Also note the small vestibular schwannomas in the bilateral internal auditory canals.* **(Right)** *Axial T1 C+ FS MR in a 15 year old with myeloid sarcoma shows an enhancing mass centered in the left sphenoid greater wing with soft tissue components extending into the left orbit , middle cranial fossa , & infratemporal fossa .*

Schwannoma

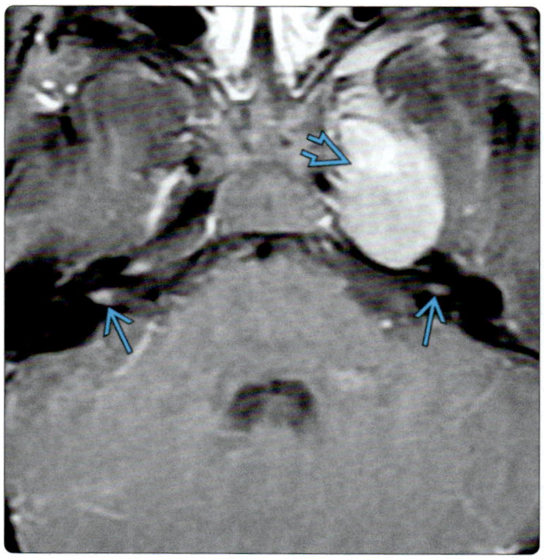

Myeloid Sarcoma/Osseus Leukemic Involvement

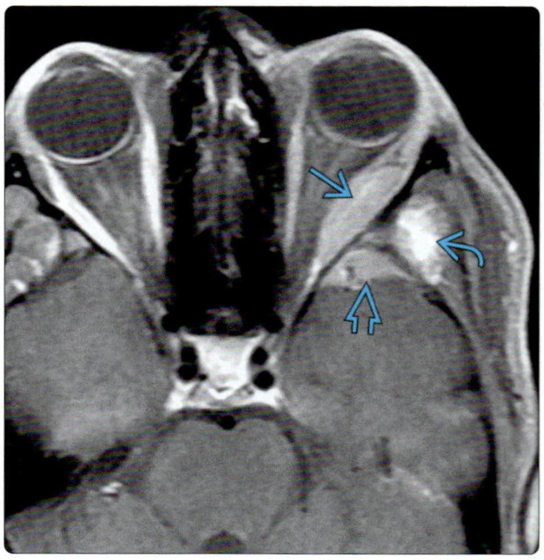

Other Metastatic Disease

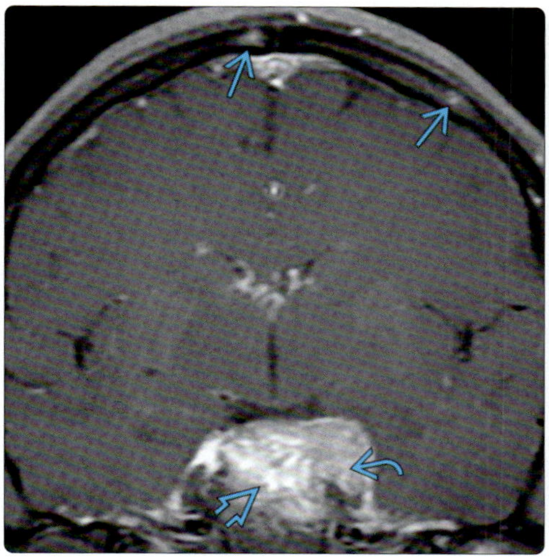

Lymphatic Malformation

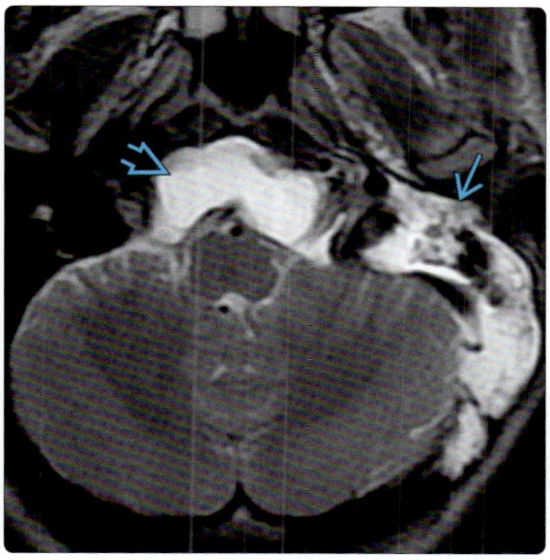

(Left) *Coronal T1 C+ FS MR in a teenager with a lower extremity sarcoma shows a large enhancing metastatic lesion centered within the sphenoid body with extension into the left cavernous sinus. Note the additional sites of calvarial metastatic disease.* **(Right)** *Axial T2 FS MR in a patient with generalized lymphatic anomaly shows expansile fluid signal intensity lesions throughout the left temporal bone & clivus. Postcontrast images (not shown) demonstrated only rim enhancement.*

Meningioma

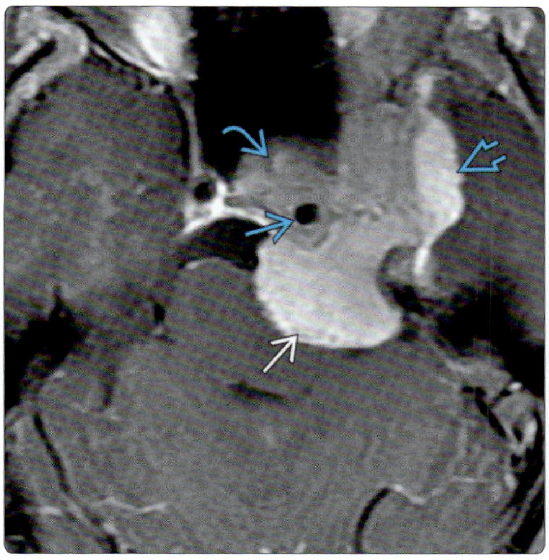

Esthesioneuroblastoma

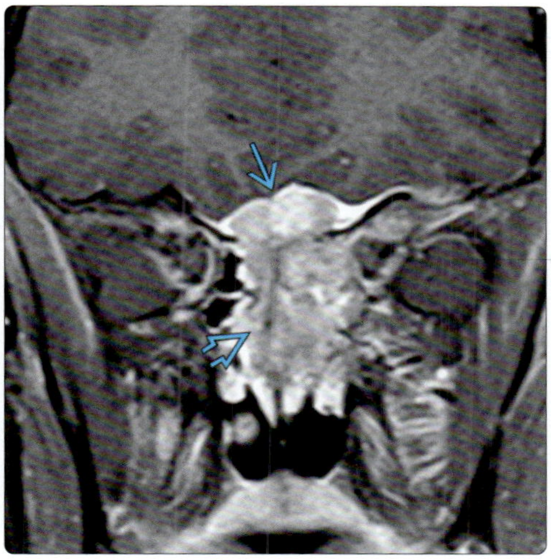

(Left) *Axial T1 C+ FS MR in a 12 year old with a meningioma shows a large mass centered in the left cavernous sinus with extension into the left middle cranial fossa, cerebellopontine angle, & sphenoid sinus with encasement of the left internal carotid artery.* **(Right)** *Coronal T1 C+ FS MR in an 11 year old with esthesioneuroblastoma shows a homogeneously enhancing mass centered at the cribriform plate with intracranial & ethmoid/nasal components.*

Enchondroma

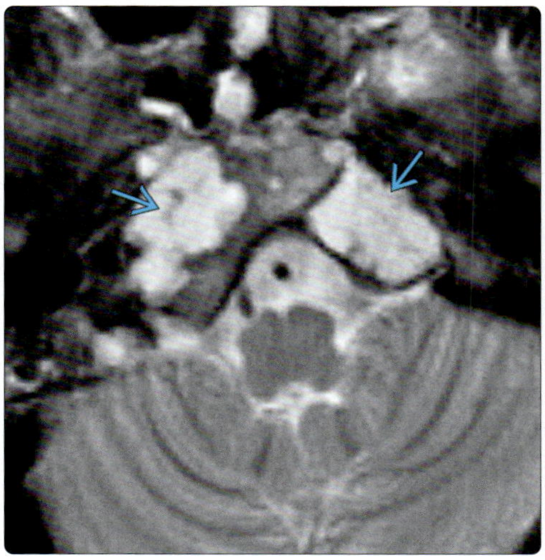

Osteosarcoma

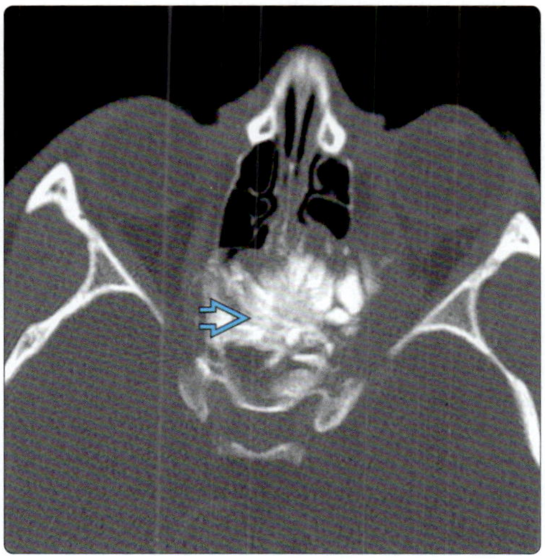

(Left) *Axial T2 MR in a patient with Maffucci syndrome shows T2-hyperintense enchondromas (with typical low-signal internal septa) of the bilateral petrooccipital fissures, a characteristic location for chondral lesions.* **(Right)** *Axial NECT in a 13 year old with osteosarcoma shows a large mass centered in the posterior nasal cavity with involvement of the anterior cranial fossa & left orbit. Note the osteoid matrix, which can be seen in osteomas & osteosarcomas.*

SECTION 7

Head and Neck

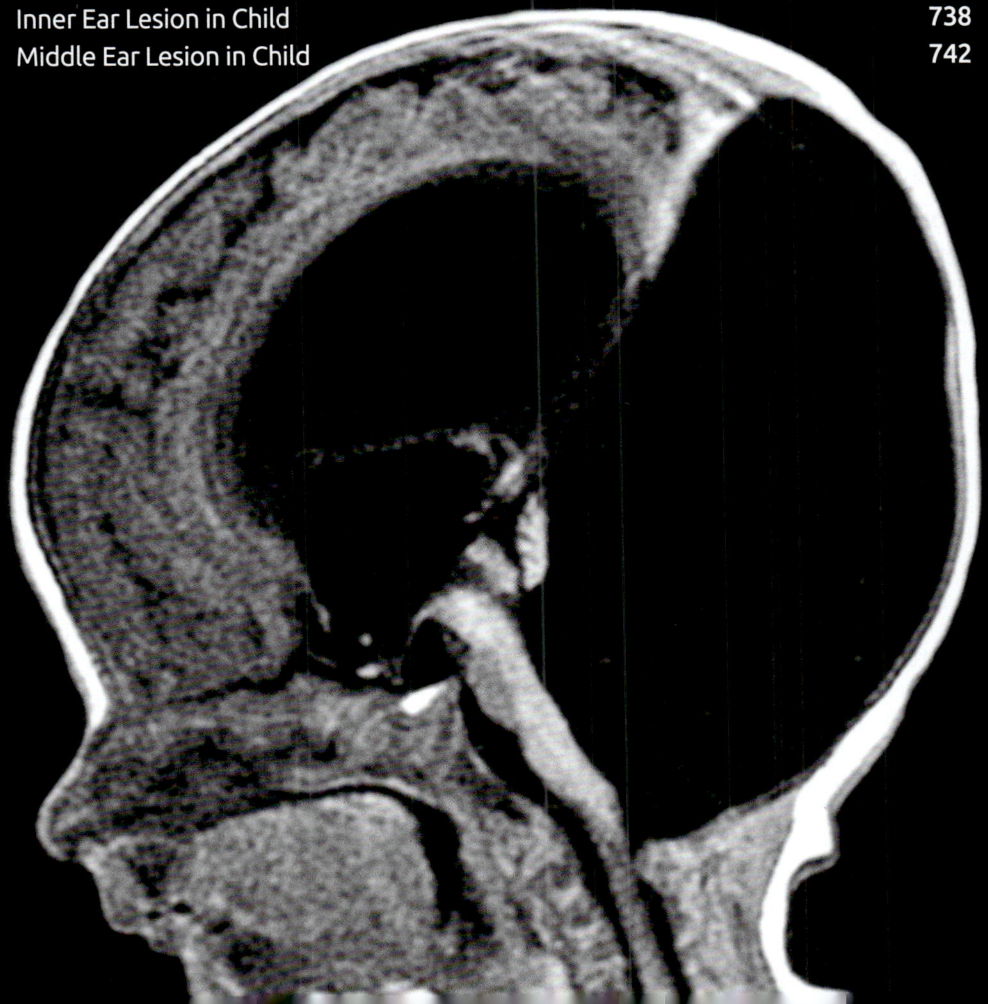

DIFFERENTIAL DIAGNOSIS

Common

- Laryngomalacia
- Croup
- Foreign Body, Esophagus

Less Common

- Subglottic Hemangioma
- Bacterial Tracheitis
- Innominate Artery Compression Syndrome
- Tracheal Stenosis, Congenital
- Tracheal Stenosis, Iatrogenic
- Vocal Cord Paralysis

Rare but Important

- Epiglottitis
- Right Arch With Aberrant Left Subclavian Artery
- Foreign Body, Trachea
- Papillomatosis

ESSENTIAL INFORMATION

Key Differential Diagnosis Issues

- Stridor: High-pitched respiratory sound caused by turbulent airflow around partial airway obstruction
  - Timing of stridor in respiratory cycle loosely corresponds to location of obstruction
    - Inspiratory: Supraglottis or glottis
    - Expiratory: Below thoracic inlet
    - Biphasic: Subglottis to thoracic inlet
  - Timing of stridor onset may suggest etiology
    - Acute onset: Most commonly of infectious origin
      - Less often: Esophageal foreign body (FB), hemangioma, or tracheal FB
    - Chronic: Most common cause is laryngomalacia
      - Less often: Vocal cord paralysis, tracheal stenosis, airway papillomas, vascular rings

Helpful Clues for Common Diagnoses

- **Laryngomalacia**
  - Congenitally abnormal (floppy) supraglottis in infant leading to chronic stridor, difficulty feeding, apnea, etc.
  - Symptoms typically worsen in first few months of life; most cases resolve by 20 months of age
  - Diagnosis made by scope, not imaging
- **Croup**
  - Viral inflammation of upper airway → symmetric subglottic edema → stridor + barky cough
  - Most common age: 6 months to 3 years; peak at 1 year
  - Imaging
    - AP radiograph: Symmetric subglottic tracheal narrowing → loss of normal shouldering of subglottic trachea → steeple sign
      - Pencil tip or inverted V appearance
    - Lateral radiograph: Ill-defined AP narrowing of subglottic airway, ± hypopharyngeal distension
    - Radiographs obtained to exclude other causes
- **Foreign Body, Esophagus**
  - Most likely to lodge at thoracic inlet >> level of arch/carina > distal esophagus
  - If FB is not passed, may lead to edema anterior to esophagus & around trachea → stridor
  - Coins are most common radiopaque FB in esophagus
  - Button batteries require emergent removal to prevent severe esophageal injury ± mediastinitis, aortic injury
  - Imaging
    - Food or plastic toys are not typically radiodense
    - Metallic coins & button batteries will typically be seen en face on AP view & in tangent on lateral view
      - Coins are relatively uniform in density
      - Button batteries have double-layered metallic edge en face, edge step-off in tangent
    - ± thickening of tissue between esophagus & trachea
    - ± anterior bowing/narrowing of trachea at level of FB

Helpful Clues for Less Common Diagnoses

- **Subglottic Hemangioma**
  - Benign vascular neoplasm, **not** vascular malformation
  - Patients usually < 6 months of age
  - Cutaneous hemangiomas in up to 50% of patients
  - 7% of patients with PHACE syndrome affected
  - Imaging
    - Asymmetric subglottic narrowing on radiographs
    - Enhancing soft tissue mass on CT or MR
- **Bacterial Tracheitis**
  - Purulent infection can lead to tracheal exudates that may slough & occlude airway
  - Usually older patients than with viral croup
    - Mean age 5 years, peak age 3-8 years
  - Synonyms: Exudative tracheitis, membranous or pseudomembranous croup, membranous laryngotracheobronchitis, membranous tracheitis
  - Imaging
    - Subglottic tracheal narrowing
    - ± linear soft tissue densities (membranes) in trachea
    - ± tracheal wall irregularities (plaques)
    - ± hazy or indistinct margins of tracheal air column
- **Innominate Artery Compression Syndrome**
  - Infantile trachea lacks rigidity
  - Increased incidence with esophageal atresia
    - Dilated esophageal pouch deviates trachea forward & innominate artery compresses anterior trachea
  - Airway symptoms usually resolve as child grows
  - Imaging
    - Anterior tracheal narrowing at crossing innominate artery below thoracic inlet
- **Tracheal Stenosis, Congenital**
  - Secondary to complete cartilaginous rings
  - ± associated anomalies (e.g., pulmonary artery sling, bronchial branching anomalies)
  - Imaging
    - Small caliber, round trachea (rather than horseshoe-shaped) on cross-sectional imaging
    - Focal or diffuse stenosis possible
    - ± inverted T-shaped carina on conventional radiograph or coronal reformatted CT images
    - ± left pulmonary artery sling
- **Tracheal Stenosis, Iatrogenic**
  - History of prior endotracheal tube (ET) intubation, tracheostomy, or other injury

- Imaging
  - Subglottic tracheal narrowing at level of prior ET tube or tracheostomy tube
  - Smooth focal narrowing (ET tube) or irregular longer narrowing (tracheostomy secondary to granulation tissue ± structural damage to tracheal rings)
- **Vocal Cord Paralysis**
  - Etiologies: Birth trauma, iatrogenic, neurologic, idiopathic
  - Presents with stridor, abnormal cry, feeding difficulty
  - Classically diagnosed by scope, not imaging
    - Recent descriptions of ultrasound use

Helpful Clues for Rare Diagnoses

- **Epiglottitis**
  - Edema of epiglottis & supraglottic structures potentially leading to rapid airway occlusion
  - Classically due to *Haemophilus influenzae*
    - Incidence markedly decreased due to vaccination
  - Classic symptoms of infectious epiglottitis: Abrupt-onset stridor, dysphagia, high fever, sore throat, dysphonia, hoarseness, & drooling
    - Airway obstruction worsens when recumbent: Perform lateral radiograph in upright position
  - Other causes include
    - Angioedema, mucositis (from chemotherapy), viral, granulomatous
    - May not have same classic presentation or urgency
  - Imaging
    - Enlargement of epiglottis (thumb sign, not thumbprint) & thickening of aryepiglottic folds on upright lateral radiograph
    - ± symmetric subglottic tracheal narrowing on frontal radiograph, present in up to 25%
- **Right Arch With Aberrant Left Subclavian Artery**
  - May be asymptomatic; however, vascular ring with left ligamentum arteriosum may lead to stridor, apnea, cyanosis, chronic cough
  - Posterior esophageal indentation by aberrant left subclavian artery (SCA) may cause dysphagia or feeding difficulties in infants
  - Imaging
    - Esophagram: Posterior esophageal indentation by aberrant left SCA/diverticulum of Kommerell; leftward deviation of trachea from right arch
    - CT/MR: Aberrant left SCA coursing posterior to esophagus
- **Foreign Body, Trachea**
  - Bronchial FB much more common than tracheal FB
  - Aspiration incident usually not witnessed
  - Imaging
    - Most airway FBs are not radiopaque
      - Majority due to food (e.g., peanuts, carrots)
    - If FB is not radiopaque, look for secondary signs
      - Hyperinflation, air-trapping, regional oligemia, atelectasis, pneumomediastinum, pneumothorax
- **Papillomatosis**
  - Recurrent respiratory papillomatosis: Benign tumors of aerodigestive tract caused by infection with HPV
    - Perinatal transmission of HPV from mother to child
    - 95% caused by HPV-6 & HPV-11
  - Larynx most common site; other sites include trachea, bronchi, & lung parenchyma
  - Mean age at diagnosis = 4 years
  - Remission can occur spontaneously at any stage
  - At risk for long term malignant transformation to squamous cell carcinoma
  - Imaging
    - Nodular distortion of airway lumen
      - May not be evident on airway radiographs
    - ± multiple solid &/or cavitary lung nodules

SELECTED REFERENCES

1. Pugmire BS et al: Imaging button battery ingestions and insertions in children: a 15-year single-center review. Pediatr Radiol. 47(2):178-85, 2017
2. Darras KE et al: Imaging acute airway obstruction in infants and children. Radiographics. 35(7):2064-79, 2015
3. Salamone FN et al: Bacterial tracheitis reexamined: is there a less severe manifestation? Otolaryngol Head Neck Surg. 131(6):871-6, 2004

Croup

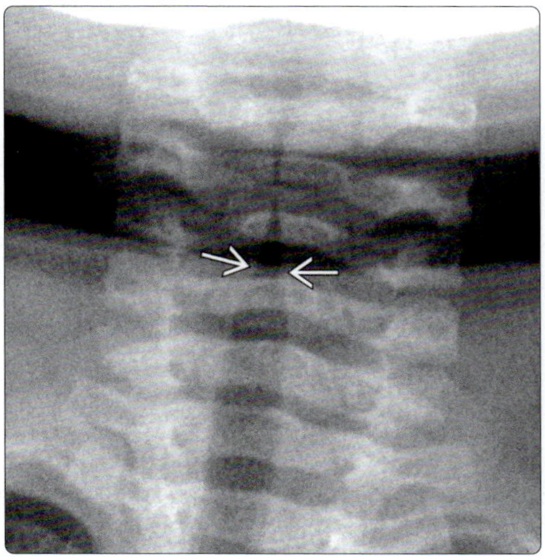

Croup

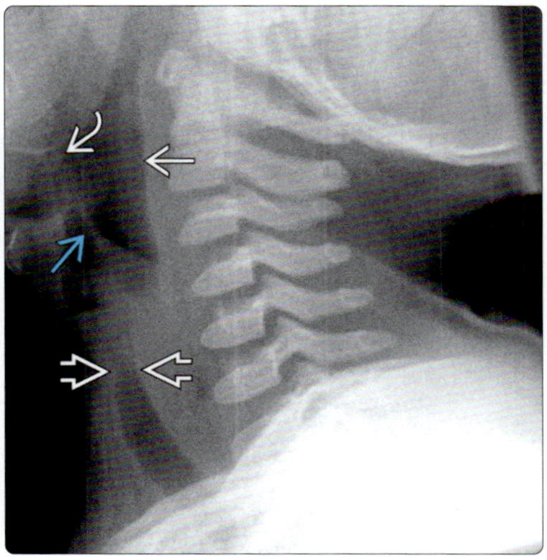

(Left) *AP radiograph shows loss of normal shouldering in the subglottic airway, producing a steeple sign ➡. This is the typical appearance of subglottic edema in a child with viral croup. This appearance is less commonly seen in other diseases such as bacterial tracheitis & epiglottitis (though usually with other findings).* **(Right)** *Lateral radiograph in a child with stridor shows mild hypopharyngeal distention ➡ & a narrow subglottic airway ➡. Note the normal, thin appearance of the epiglottis ➡ & aryepiglottic folds ➡.*

(Left) *Lateral radiograph shows a metallic coin in the esophagus, a dilated proximal esophagus, & circumferential tracheal narrowing at the level of the coin. Note the soft tissue swelling between the coin & the trachea, which can predict a difficult removal of the coin.* (Right) *Axial CECT demonstrates a small, intensely enhancing subglottic mass in a child with stridor but no cutaneous hemangiomas. On endoscopy, an infantile hemangioma of the submucosal airway was visible.*

Foreign Body, Esophagus

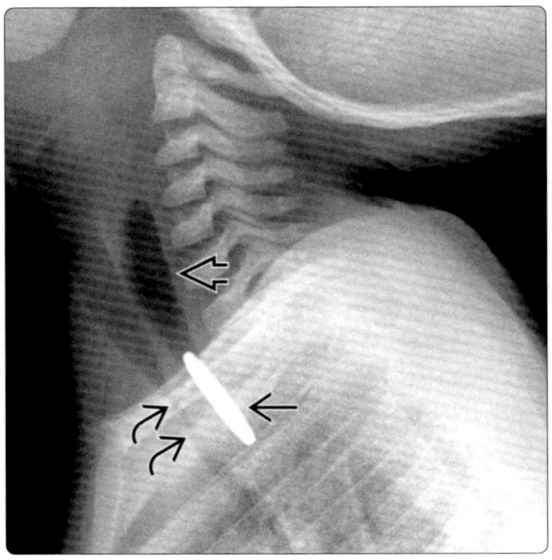

Subglottic Hemangioma

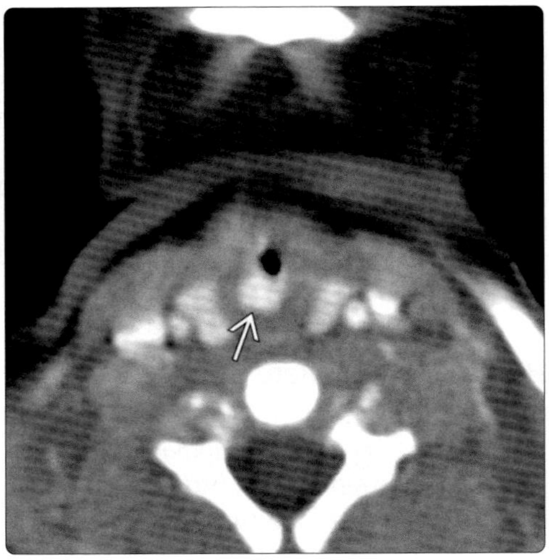

(Left) *Sagittal CECT in the same patient shows the posterior enhancing mass, resulting in focal tracheal narrowing. Airway hemangiomas causing respiratory symptoms are typically treated with propranolol, steroids, &/or laser to prevent further growth in this critical location.* (Right) *Lateral airway radiograph in a 9 year old with respiratory distress & stridor shows linear, irregular intraluminal filling defects in the subglottic trachea, consistent with exudative bacterial tracheitis.*

Subglottic Hemangioma

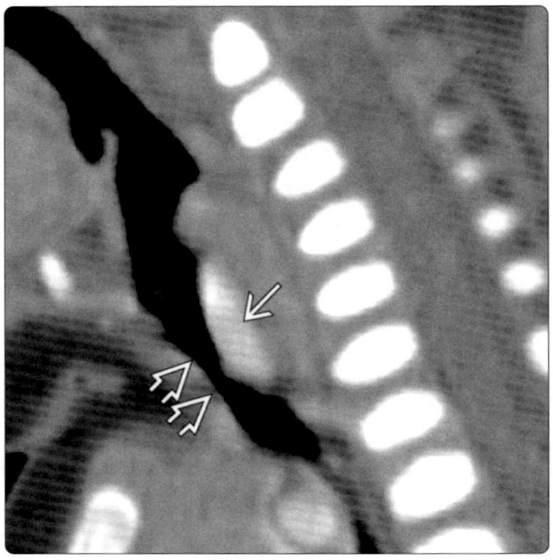

Bacterial Tracheitis

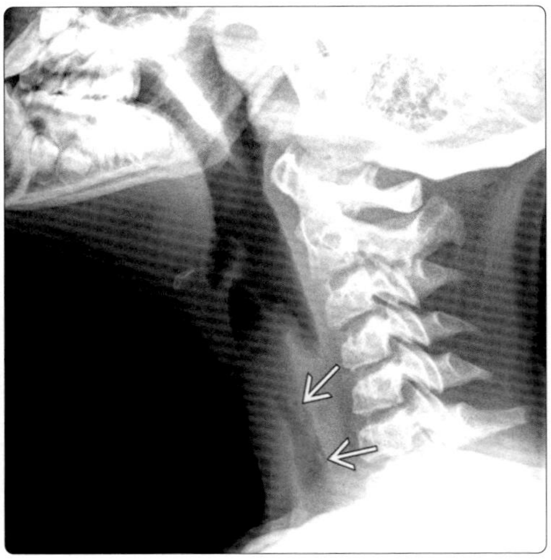

(Left) *Axial CECT reveals moderate AP narrowing of the trachea at the level of the crossing innominate artery in this infant with stridor. A pH probe is also seen in the upper thoracic esophagus.* (Right) *Lateral esophagram shows anterior tracheal compression at the level of a crossing innominate artery. Also noted is a small esophageal stricture in this patient with prior esophageal atresia repair. There is an increased incidence of innominate artery compression syndrome in these children.*

Innominate Artery Compression Syndrome

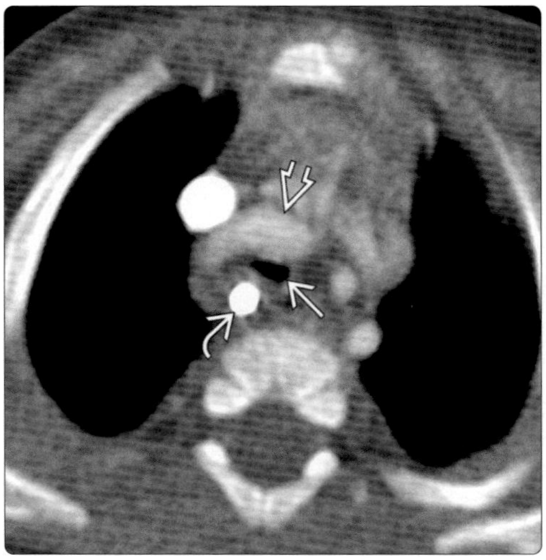

Innominate Artery Compression Syndrome

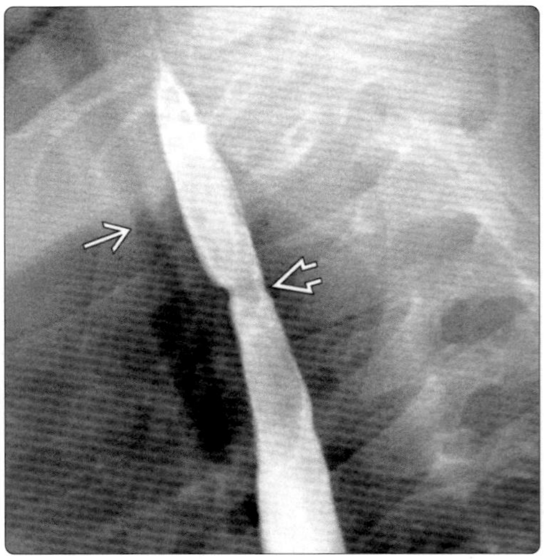

Tracheal Stenosis, Congenital

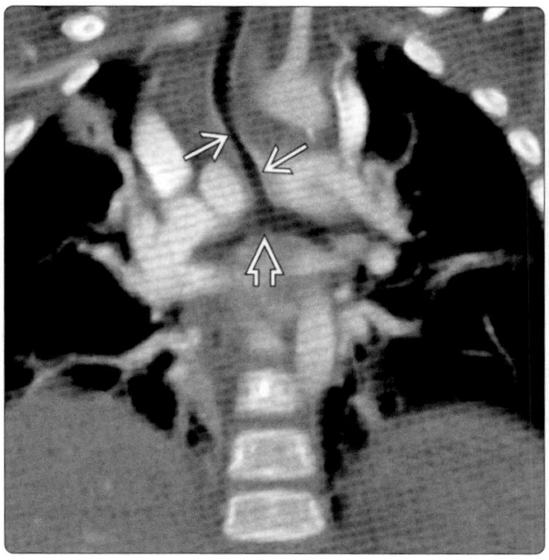

Tracheal Stenosis, Iatrogenic

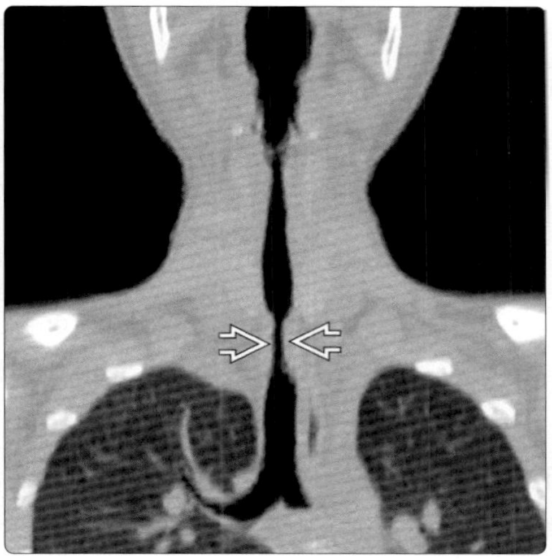

(Left) *Coronal CECT shows distal intrathoracic tracheal narrowing ➔ with a nearly 180° angle between the main bronchi, resulting in an inverted-T appearance of the carina ⇨. Axial images through the area of narrowing (not shown) demonstrated a small-caliber, round (rather than horseshoe-shaped) trachea.* **(Right)** *Coronal bone CT demonstrates an abrupt shelf that causes > 50% luminal tracheal narrowing at the level of the thoracic inlet ⇨. This child had a prior history of prolonged endotracheal intubation.*

Epiglottitis

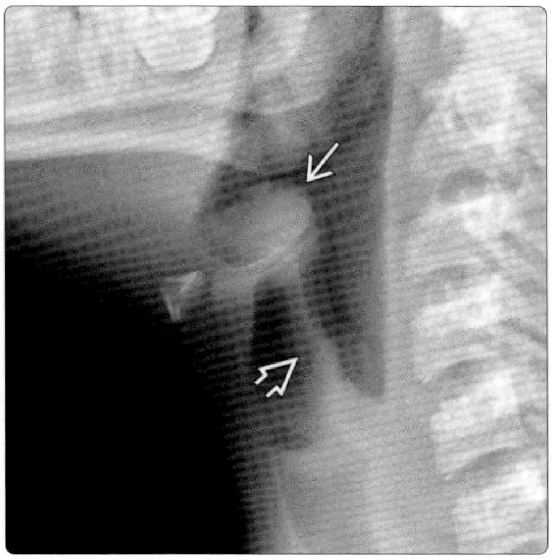

Right Arch With Aberrant Left Subclavian Artery

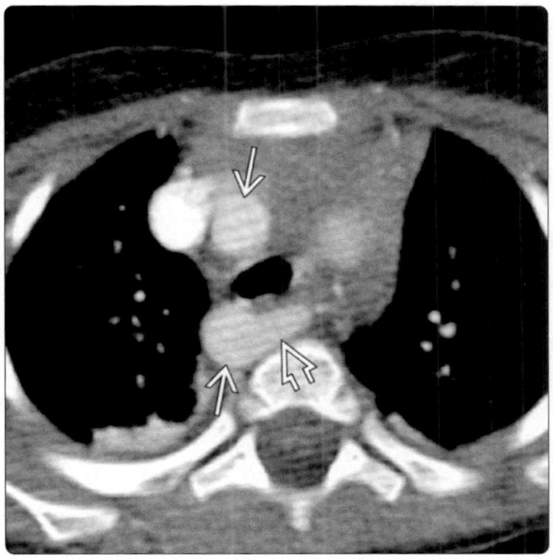

(Left) *Lateral airway radiograph shows a markedly swollen epiglottis ➔ & mildly thickened aryepiglottic folds ⇨, diagnostic of epiglottitis in a toxic child with respiratory distress & difficulty handling secretions. The differential diagnosis of epiglottic enlargement includes angioedema, mucositis, & caustic or thermal injury.* **(Right)** *Axial CECT shows a congenital right aortic arch ➔ associated with an aberrant left subclavian artery (& diverticulum of Kommerell ⇨) coursing posterior to the trachea.*

Foreign Body, Trachea

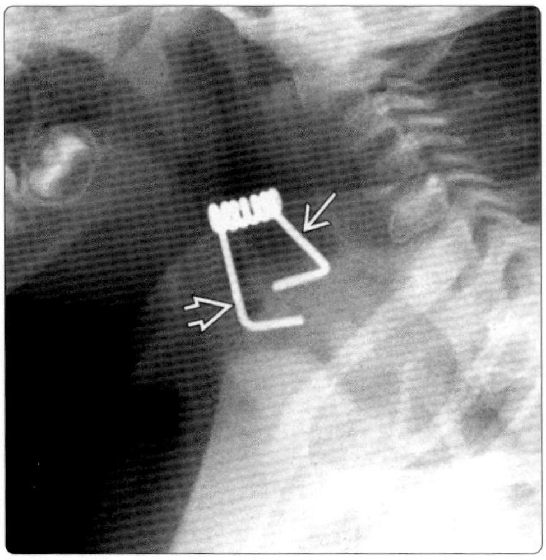

Papillomatosis

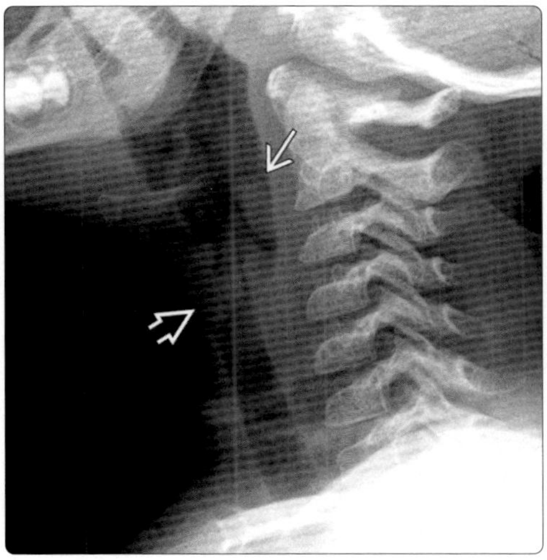

(Left) *Lateral radiograph reveals a radiopaque spring from a wooden clothes pin in the hypopharynx ➔ & larynx ⇨.* **(Right)** *Lateral radiograph in a nearly 3 year old with stridor demonstrates multiple intraluminal soft tissue masses in the posterior hypopharynx ➔ & ventral subglottic trachea ⇨. While a single lesion might raise the question of an airway hemangioma, multiple lesions in a small child should raise concern for respiratory papillomatosis, which was proven in this patient.*

DIFFERENTIAL DIAGNOSIS

Common

- Epiglottitis
- Ω Epiglottis (Normal Variant)
- Enlarged Lingual Tonsils
- Thyroglossal Duct Cyst

Less Common

- Foreign Body

Rare but Important

- Vallecular Mass
- Vascular Malformation
- Infantile Hemangioma

ESSENTIAL INFORMATION

Key Differential Diagnosis Issues

- Age, duration of symptoms, medical history, & vaccination status help direct considerations

Helpful Clues for Common Diagnoses

- **Epiglottitis**
    - Acute airway obstruction secondary to inflammation of epiglottis & surrounding tissues
    - Affected mean age has increased from 3.5 years to 14.6 years since *Haemophilus influenzae* vaccine was introduced
    - Etiologies: Bacterial, viral, angioneurotic edema, mucositis, trauma/burns, caustic ingestion, & allergic reactions
        - Consider *H. influenzae* in unvaccinated child
    - Lateral radiographs: Marked thickening of epiglottis & aryepiglottic folds
        - Epiglottis with thumbprint appearance (rounded ± poorly defined margins)
        - Aryepiglottic folds become convex superiorly
- **Ω Epiglottis (Normal Variant)**
    - Lateral folds of epiglottis appear more prominent due to greater curvature
    - May appear as hitchhiker's thumb, not thumbprint
    - Epiglottis maintains sharp central posterior margin
- **Enlarged Lingual Tonsils**
    - Round, mildly lobulated mass at posterior tongue base; may fill vallecula & displace epiglottis
    - Patients with prior tonsillectomy & adenoidectomy may be predisposed
- **Thyroglossal Duct Cyst**
    - Remnant of thyroglossal duct between foramen cecum at tongue base & thyroid
    - Typically lies in midline at/about hyoid bone but may protrude posteriorly from tongue base into vallecula

Helpful Clues for Less Common Diagnoses

- **Foreign Body**
    - Consider with chronic or sudden onset of symptoms in young afebrile child
    - Radiopaque or nonradiopaque foreign body may lodge in vallecula or hypopharynx
    - Suggested by straight margins or unusual shapes on radiographs

Helpful Clues for Rare Diagnoses

- **Vallecular Mass**
    - Congenital vallecular cyst: Arises from lingual surface of epiglottis
    - Foregut duplication cysts: Enteric or bronchogenic cysts
    - Rarely, malignant neoplasms, such as sarcoma
- **Vascular Malformation**
    - Low-flow lesions (such as lymphatic malformation) commonly involve tongue & deep neck soft tissues
    - US is typically diagnostic of macrocystic lymphatic malformations; MR best determines extent
- **Infantile Hemangioma**
    - Vascular neoplasm, most common in subglottic location
    - Typically presents < 6 months of age
    - Asymmetric airway narrowing on radiographs; hyperenhancing mass on CECT

Epiglottitis

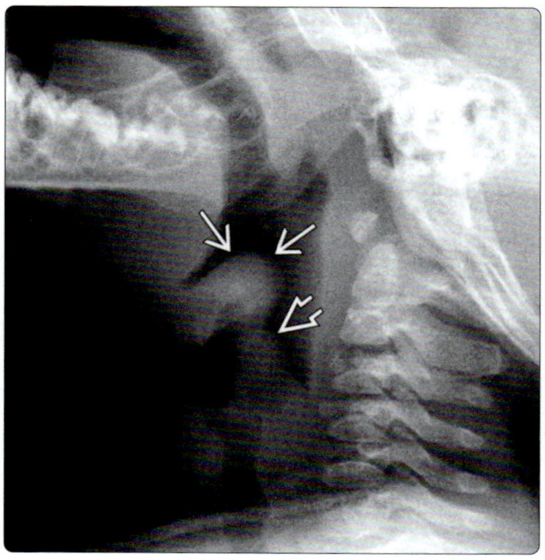

Enlarged Lingual Tonsils

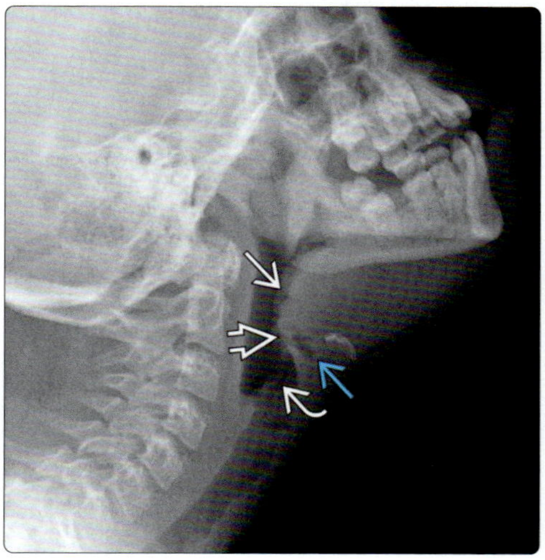

(Left) *Lateral radiograph in a 6 month old with fever & difficulty breathing shows marked thickening of the epiglottis ➔ & aryepiglottic folds ➔, typical of epiglottitis.* **(Right)** *Lateral radiograph of the neck in a 10 year old with obstructive sleep apnea depicts enlarged & mildly lobulated lingual tonsils ➔ at the tongue base. The epiglottis ➔ & aryepiglottic folds ➔ are thin & well defined. A small amount of normal air is seen in the vallecula ➔ between the lingual tonsils & epiglottis.*

Thyroglossal Duct Cyst

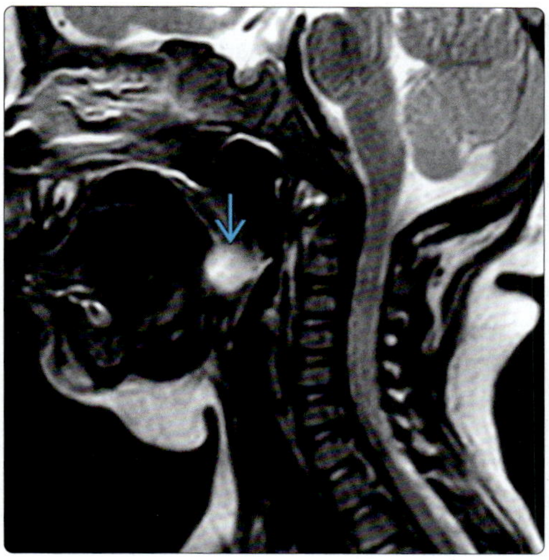

Vallecular Mass

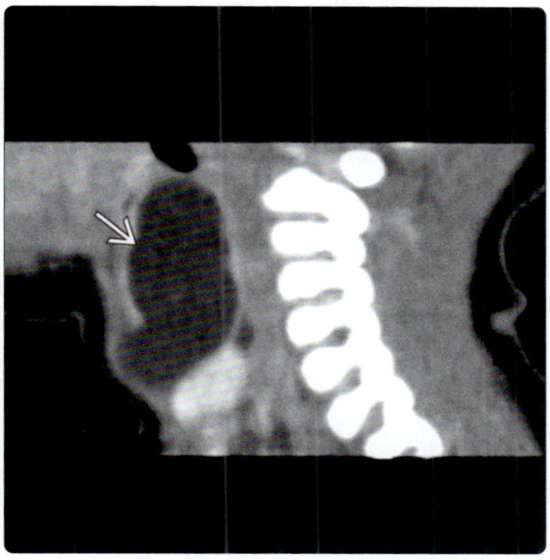

(Left) *Sagittal T2 MR of a 7 month old with abnormal breathing demonstrates a 9 mm, round thyroglossal duct cyst at the tongue base.* **(Right)** *Right parasagittal CECT in a 3 day old with a neck mass, cyanosis, & stridor demonstrates a large, rim-enhancing cystic mass that fills the hypopharynx. There was leftward deviation & effacement of the trachea (not shown). A bronchogenic cyst was found at resection.*

Vallecular Mass

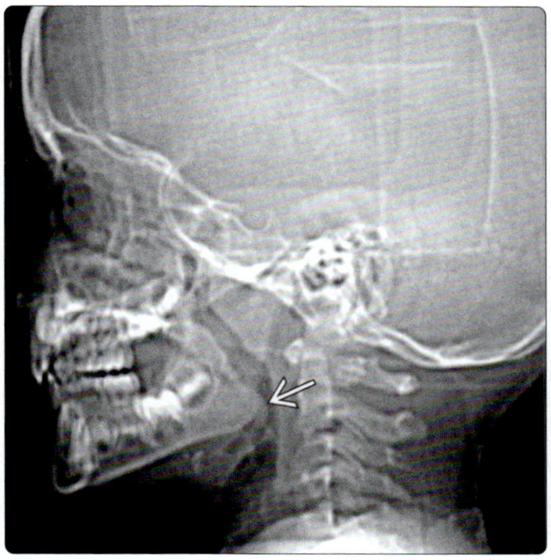

Vallecular Mass

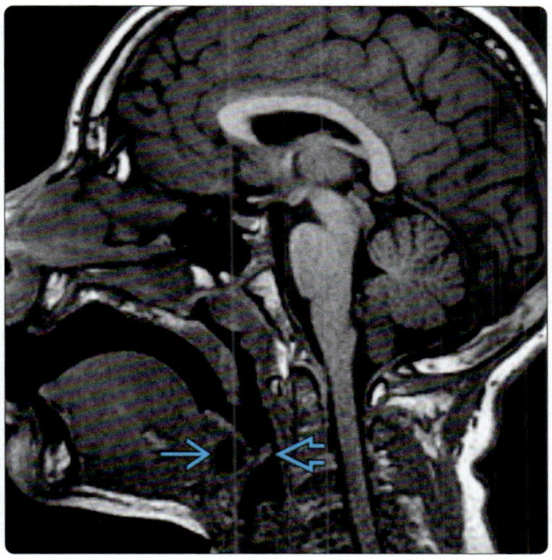

(Left) *Scout image from a CT of a 5 year old with stridor demonstrates a round mass at the tongue base that was found to be a vallecular cyst upon resection.* **(Right)** *Sagittal T1 MR in a 12 year old shows a round, fluid signal intensity mass centered in the vallecula with mild mass effect on the epiglottis. A vallecular cyst was confirmed upon resection.*

Vallecular Mass

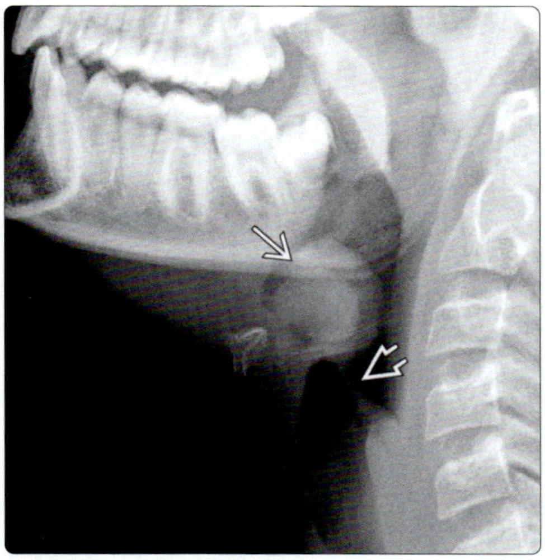

Vascular Malformation

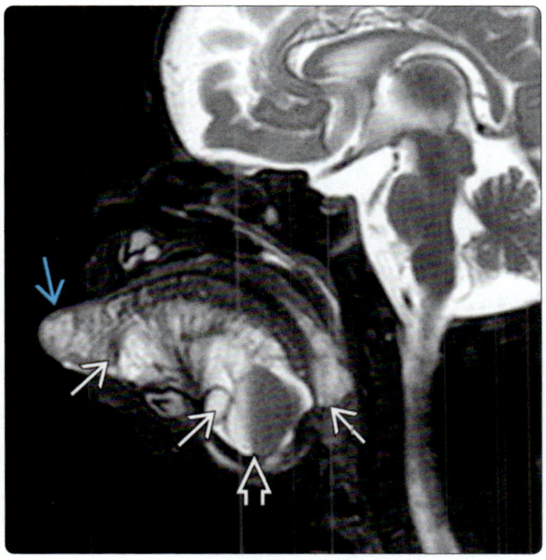

(Left) *Lateral radiograph in a 12 year old shows a bulbous mass in the vallecula without a visible epiglottis. The aryepiglottic folds are normal. This mass proved to be a synovial sarcoma of the vallecula, not epiglottitis.* **(Right)** *Sagittal T2 FS MR of a 15 day old with facial swelling demonstrates extensive fluid signal tubular & cystic foci in the floor of the mouth & tongue, typical of a lymphatic malformation. An internal fluid-fluid level suggests hemorrhage. Note the associated macroglossia.*

DIFFERENTIAL DIAGNOSIS

Common

- Pseudothickening
- Retropharyngeal Edema
- Retropharyngeal Adenopathy
- Retropharyngeal Abscess
- Cervical Spine Injury

Less Common

- Mass

Rare but Important

- Retropharyngeal Course of Internal Carotid Artery

ESSENTIAL INFORMATION

Key Differential Diagnosis Issues

- General features
  - AP thickness of normal retropharyngeal soft tissues on lateral radiograph is typically no more than 1 vertebral body width
  - Normal step-off is typically visible at junction of hypopharynx & esophagus
- Clinical presentations
  - Infection: Fever, dysphagia, stridor, drooling, sore throat
  - Trauma: Motor vehicle accident (MVA) or fall
  - Mass: Palpable abnormality, dysphagia
  - Any of these can present with pain & limited range of motion or torticollis

Helpful Clues for Common Diagnoses

- **Pseudothickening**
  - Typically due to expiratory timing ± inadequate neck extension on lateral radiograph in infant
  - Easily clarified on real-time fluoroscopic imaging in lateral position using image hold/last image capture
    - Minimal radiation required
- **Retropharyngeal Edema**
  - Fluid infiltration of retropharyngeal space without well-defined rim enhancement
  - Secondary to infection (cellulitis), inflammation, allergic reaction, burns, venous thrombosis, or trauma
- **Retropharyngeal Adenopathy**
  - Retropharyngeal infection → lymphadenopathy ± necrosis/suppuration with adjacent cellulitis
    - Hyperemic enlarged lymph node = adenitis; hypodense/hypoechoic lymph node with loss of vascularity = necrosis
- **Retropharyngeal Abscess**
  - Extranodal, rim-enhancing, low-density collection
  - May see gas within abscess
  - Patient may be toxic or septic-appearing
- **Cervical Spine Injury**
  - Clear history of trauma
  - Prevertebral soft tissue swelling that is indistinguishable from retropharyngeal tissues on lateral radiograph
  - Radiographs/CT: Look for bone abnormalities, including malalignment/disruption of spinal lines &/or vertebral fracture/height loss
  - MR: Soft tissue edema with ligamentous injury ± marrow edema, cord injury

Helpful Clues for Less Common Diagnoses

- **Mass**
  - Duplication cyst: Well-circumscribed, round or ovoid low-attenuation mass along esophagus, trachea, &/or paraspinal region
  - Lymphatic malformation: Transspatial multicystic mass; more commonly involves anterior neck, floor of mouth/tongue
  - Plexiform neurofibromas: Lobulated solid lesions of nerves with target sign in cross section on T2/STIR
    - Pathognomonic for neurofibromatosis type 1

Helpful Clues for Rare Diagnoses

- **Retropharyngeal Course of Internal Carotid Artery**
  - Normal anatomic variant
  - Important to recognize to avoid injury during procedures/surgery
  - Enhancing arteries course paramidline in retropharyngeal space

Pseudothickening

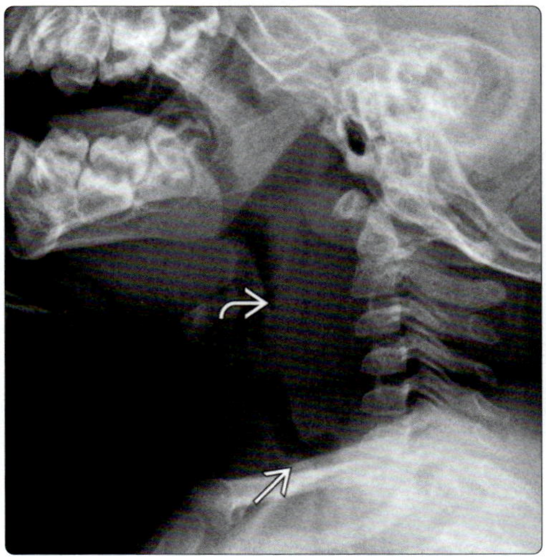

Pseudothickening

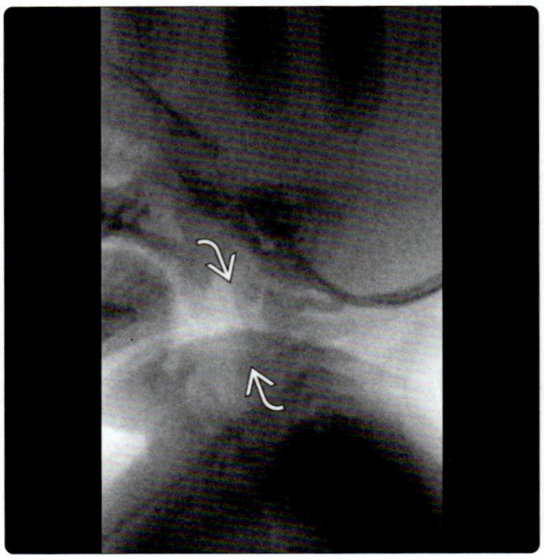

(Left) *Lateral radiograph of the neck demonstrates marked buckling of the trachea at the thoracic inlet. The retropharyngeal soft tissues appear thickened. Fluoroscopy can be used to better evaluate the retropharyngeal soft tissues in young children if adequate extension & inspiration cannot be obtained during radiography.* **(Right)** *Lateral airway fluoroscopy was performed in the same patient & demonstrates normal thickness of the retropharyngeal soft tissues during inspiration.*

Retropharyngeal Edema

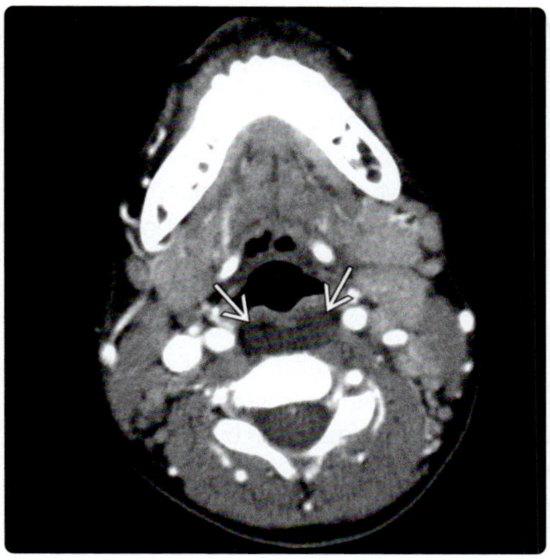

Retropharyngeal Abscess

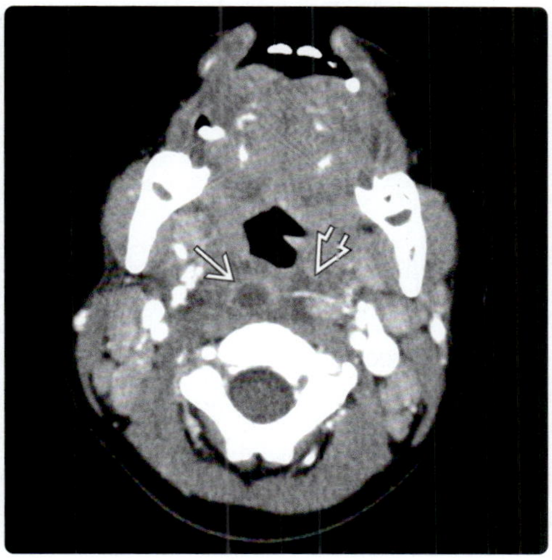

(Left) *Axial CECT shows poorly defined fluid/edema expanding the retropharyngeal space in this 3 year old with fever & sore throat. While not specific, this appearance is most commonly due to infection/cellulitis.* **(Right)** *Axial CECT from the same patient shows a rim-enhancing, low-density collection, consistent with a retropharyngeal abscess. Ill-defined fluid was also identified, due to retropharyngeal edema/cellulitis.*

Retropharyngeal Abscess

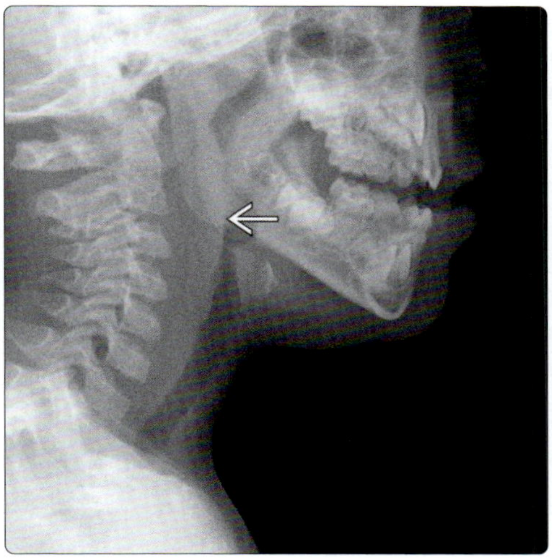

Cervical Spine Injury

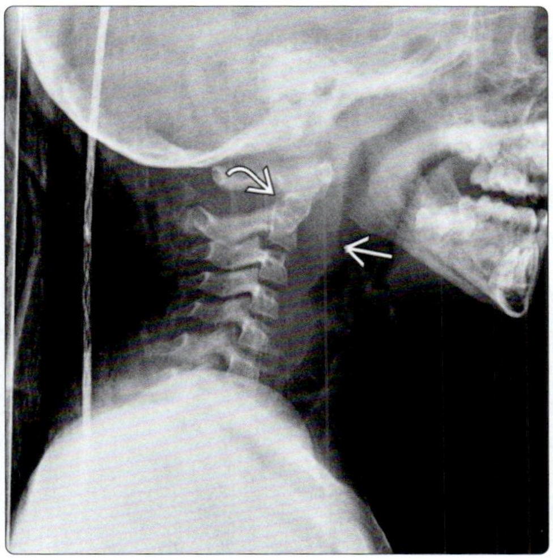

(Left) *Lateral radiograph of a 3 year old with fever & neck pain shows retropharyngeal soft tissue swelling despite adequate neck extension. This patient is beyond the typical age where pseudothickening is often seen, suggesting a true inflammation.* **(Right)** *Lateral radiograph from a 5 year old status post MVA demonstrates focal thickening & convexity of soft tissues at C2. There is associated abnormal angulation of the dens. CT & MR confirmed a C2 synchondrosis fracture with ligamentous injury.*

Mass

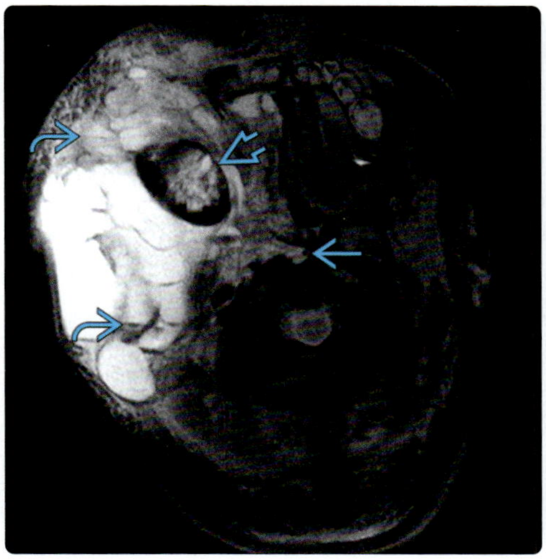

Retropharyngeal Course of Internal Carotid Artery

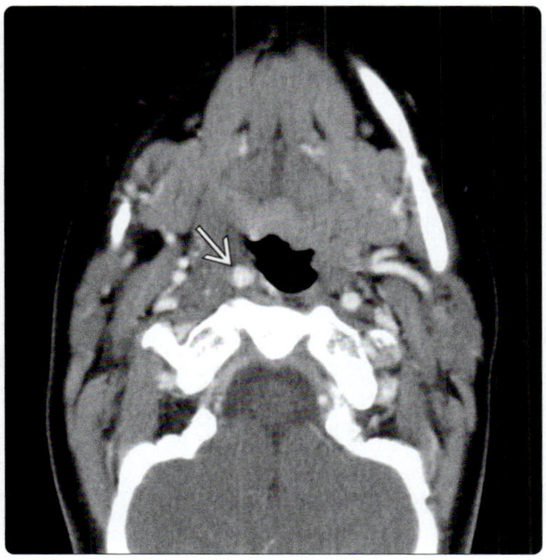

(Left) *Axial T2 FS MR in a newborn with a large soft right neck mass shows confluent thin-walled cysts extending throughout the right neck soft tissues. Layering levels of blood products & foci of clot retraction are noted. The features are typical of a lymphatic malformation. Extension into the retropharyngeal space is noted.* **(Right)** *Axial CECT demonstrates a medial course of the right internal carotid artery into the retropharyngeal space.*

Enlarged Lymph Nodes in Neck

DIFFERENTIAL DIAGNOSIS

Common

- Reactive Lymph Nodes
- Suppurative Lymph Nodes
- Hodgkin Lymphoma
- Non-Hodgkin Lymphoma
- Nontuberculous *Mycobacterium*
- Cat-Scratch Disease

Less Common

- Metastatic Neuroblastoma
- Posttransplant Lymphoproliferative Disorder
- Differentiated Thyroid Carcinoma

Rare but Important

- Systemic Metastases
- Langerhans Cell Histiocytosis

ESSENTIAL INFORMATION

Helpful Clues for Common Diagnoses

- **Reactive Lymph Nodes**
  - "Reactive" implies benign
    - Usually response to infection/inflammation
  - Acute or chronic
  - Any head/neck nodal group may be affected
  - Imaging: Enlarged, well-defined, oval-shaped nodes
    - Variable contrast enhancement, usually mild & homogeneous
    - Typically retain normal nodal architecture with fatty hilum & radiating vessels on ultrasound/Doppler
    - ± stranding of adjacent fat (cellulitis)
      - Common with bacterial infection
      - Usually absent in nontuberculous *Mycobacterium* (NTM)
    - ± edema in adjacent muscles (myositis)
    - ± necrosis/suppuration in other nodes: Bacterial, NTM, & cat-scratch disease
- **Suppurative Lymph Nodes**
  - Pus within node = intranodal abscess
  - If untreated, rupture may lead to extranodal soft tissue abscess
  - Potential clinical predictors of drainable adenitis: Absence of pharyngitis, WBC > 15,000/mm³, age ≤ 3 years, largest conglomerate of palpable nodes > 3 cm, prior antibiotic treatment > 24 hours
  - Any nodal H&N group may be affected
    - Jugulodigastric, retropharyngeal, submandibular are most common
  - Imaging: Thick enhancing walls + central hypodensity suggests drainable abscess (though phlegmon may have similar appearance)
    - US: Central decreased echogenicity with increased through transmission
      - Swirling internal debris upon compression confirms drainable fluid
      - Color Doppler shows increased peripheral vascularity without internal vascularity
    - Restricted diffusion on DWI MR
    - May be seen normally
    - Associated cellulitis: Common in bacterial infection, absent in NTM
    - Associated nonsuppurative adenopathy common
    - ± thickening of muscles (myositis)
    - ± internal carotid artery narrowing = vasospasm
      - Usually self-limited; most common in children
- **Hodgkin Lymphoma**
  - B-cell origin; histology shows Reed-Sternberg cells
  - Most commonly involves cervical & mediastinal nodes
  - Extranodal disease is uncommon
  - Imaging: Round nodal masses with variable contrast enhancement
    - Single or multiple nodal chains
      - Cannot distinguish Hodgkin lymphoma (HL) from non-Hodgkin lymphoma (NHL) by imaging
    - May be hypoechoic on US
    - ± necrotic center
    - Ca^{2+} is uncommon (unless treated)
    - FDG PET scans for staging & evaluating response to treatment
- **Non-Hodgkin Lymphoma**
  - Extranodal disease is more common in NHL than HL
  - Burkitt lymphoma is aggressive B-cell form of NHL, usually in children ≤ 15 years of age
  - Imaging: Single dominant node or multiple enlarged nonnecrotic nodes
    - Nonnodal lymphatic disease: Palatine, lingual, or adenoid tonsils
    - Nonnodal extralymphatic disease: Paranasal sinus, skull base, & thyroid gland
- **Nontuberculous Mycobacterium**
  - Most often *Mycobacterium avium* complex
    - *M. avium* & *M. intracellulare*
  - Usually nontender lymphadenopathy
  - Imaging: Rim-enhancing/necrotic lymphadenopathy is common
    - Lack of surrounding cellulitis in most cases
    - Normal chest radiograph
- **Cat-Scratch Disease**
  - *Bartonella henselae* is typical pathogen
  - Classic presentation: Regional adenopathy + fever 1-3 weeks after scratch or bite
    - Single lymph node involvement is most common
    - Disseminated disease in up to 15%
      - Hepatic &/or splenic involvement, conjunctivitis, retinitis, encephalopathy, osteomyelitis, endocarditis, pneumonia
  - Imaging: Homogeneous or necrotic lymphadenopathy

Helpful Clues for Less Common Diagnoses

- **Metastatic Neuroblastoma**
  - < 5% of primary neuroblastomas occur in neck
  - Most cervical involvement with neuroblastoma is metastatic adenopathy
  - Imaging: Large lymph nodes, rarely necrotic
    - Bilateral skull base/orbital metastases are common
      - Enhancing masses with aggressive bone permeation & expansion with "hair on end" spiculated periosteal reaction
    - MIBG uptake in 90% of neuroblastomas

- **Posttransplant Lymphoproliferative Disorder**
  - Spectrum: Benign reactive hyperplasia → lymphoma in posttransplant, immunosuppressed patients
    - Children > > adults
    - May affect abdomen, chest, allograft, H&N, CNS
  - Most common in patients who are EBV seronegative prior to transplant
  - More common after heart or lung transplant than after kidney transplant
  - Imaging: Large nodal masses or clusters of normal-sized nodes
    - Frequently with nonenhancing necrosis & debris
    - ± adenotonsillar hypertrophy; may lead to upper airway obstruction
    - Increased FDG uptake on PET/CT
- **Differentiated Thyroid Carcinoma**
  - Nodal spread is common in papillary type; distant spread is common in follicular type
  - Presents in 3rd & 4th decade; occasionally in adolescents, rare in young children
    - 3x more common in women than men
  - Imaging
    - Variable: Small to large nodes; homogeneous or heterogeneous; hemorrhagic or cystic necrosis
    - Focal Ca^{2+} & solid foci of enhancement may be present
    - Microcalcifications on US
    - T1 shortening on MR prior to contrast
    - Note: If thyroid cancer is known/suspected, neck & chest CT scans should be performed without IV contrast
      - Iodinated IV contrast will interfere with further iodine uptake by tumor, potentially delaying therapy for weeks

Helpful Clues for Rare Diagnoses

- **Systemic Metastases**
  - In children, primary malignancy is usually known
    - Neuroblastoma is most common; other primary malignancies include nasopharyngeal carcinoma, rhabdomyosarcoma, testicular carcinoma, hepatoblastoma, renal cell carcinoma
    - Supraclavicular metastasis suggests chest or abdominal primary
  - Imaging: Single or multiple enlarged nodes ± necrosis
- **Langerhans Cell Histiocytosis**
  - Spectrum of diseases caused by neoplastic clonal proliferation of dendritic cells
    - Singe system (uni- or multifocal) vs. multisystem disease
      - Unifocal > > multifocal
    - Skeletal & skin involvement are most most common; adenopathy occurs with systemic disease
    - Acute disseminated form (Letterer-Siwe) occurs in children < 2 years of age
  - Imaging: Diffuse lymphadenopathy in disseminated form
    - Plus hepatosplenomegaly, skin rash, marrow failure, & pulmonary disease

SELECTED REFERENCES

1. Kimia AA et al: Predictors of a drainable suppurative adenitis among children presenting with cervical adenopathy. Am J Emerg Med. 37(1):109-13, 2018
2. Heyes R et al: Posttransplant lymphoproliferative disorder: otolaryngological manifestations and management. Otolaryngol Head Neck Surg. 157(5):750-59, 2017
3. Katabathina V et al: Complications of immunosuppressive therapy in solid organ transplantation. Radiol Clin North Am. 54(2):303-19, 2016
4. Sharp SE et al: MIBG in neuroblastoma diagnostic imaging and therapy. Radiographics. 36(1):258-78, 2016
5. *Robson CD et al: Nontuberculous mycobacterial infection of the head and neck in immunocompetent children: CT and MR findings. AJNR Am J Neuroradiol. 20(10):1829-35, 1999

Reactive Lymph Nodes

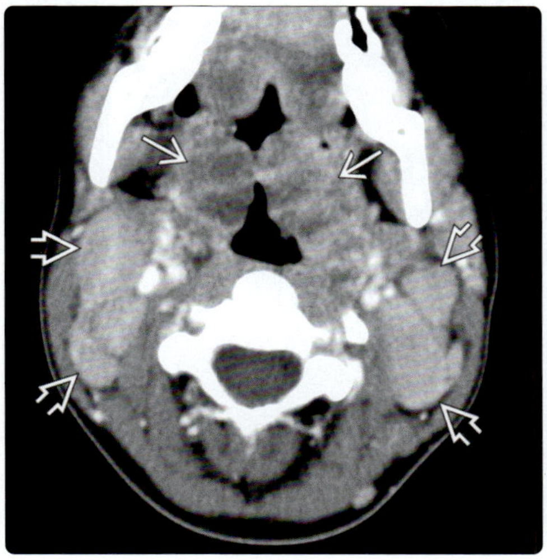

Reactive Lymph Nodes

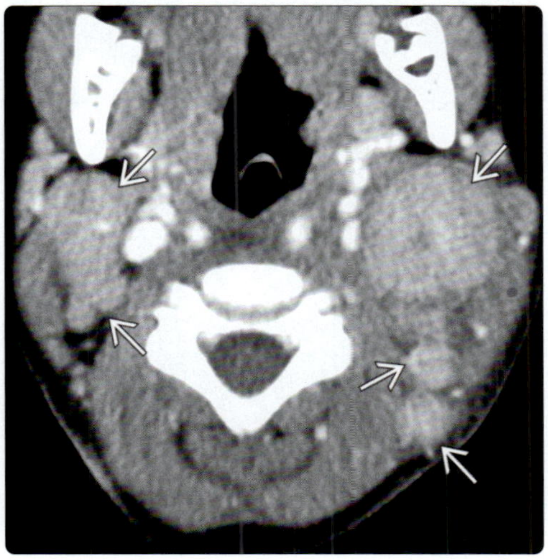

(Left) *Axial CECT shows enlarged palatine tonsils ➡ & bilaterally enlarged reactive cervical lymph nodes ➡ in a teenager. This constellation of findings should raise the possibility of mononucleosis, & this patient did test positive for EBV.* **(Right)** *Axial CECT demonstrates left larger than right nonsuppurative cervical adenopathy ➡ in a child with a throat swab positive for beta-hemolytic Streptococcus. Note also the loss of fat planes on the left secondary to mild soft tissue edema/cellulitis.*

(Left) *Axial CECT in a 9 month old with congestion, cough, fever, & neck swelling shows a well-defined, enlarged, low-attenuation left lateral retropharyngeal lymph node with minimal rim enhancement ➡ that surgically proved to contain drainable pus. Note the multiple other nonsuppurative lymph nodes ➡ & adjacent left internal carotid artery narrowing ➡.* **(Right)** *Axial CECT shows a well-defined, rim-enhancing, low-attenuation intranodal abscess ➡ with surrounding soft tissue edema ➡.*

Suppurative Lymph Nodes

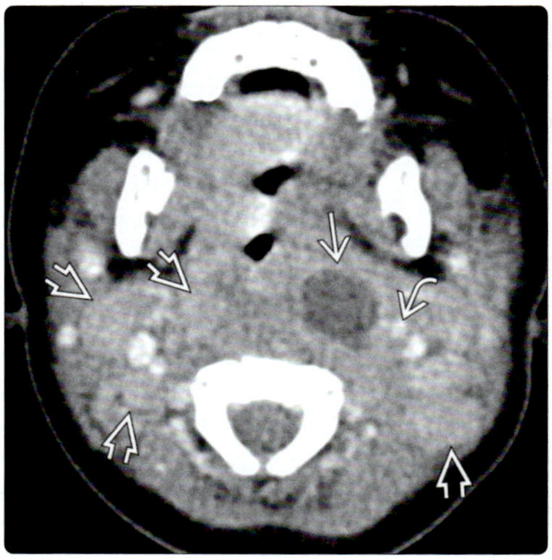

Suppurative Lymph Nodes

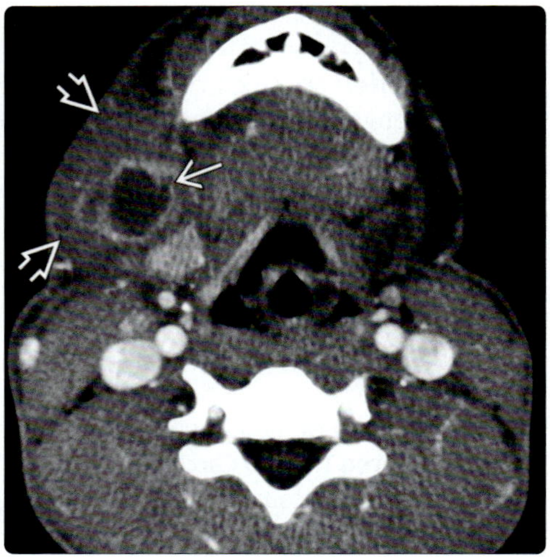

(Left) *Axial CECT in a 9 year old with Hodgkin lymphoma demonstrates large bilateral level IV lymph nodes ➡. There is mass effect on the dorsal aspect of the right jugular vein ➡. Note the lack of surrounding soft tissue edema.* **(Right)** *Axial CECT demonstrates marked enlargement of the relatively low-attenuation right cervical lymph nodes ➡ in a teenager with Hodgkin lymphoma.*

Hodgkin Lymphoma

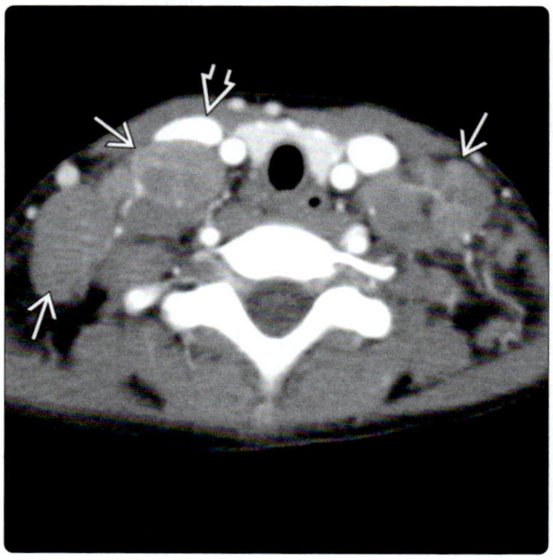

Hodgkin Lymphoma

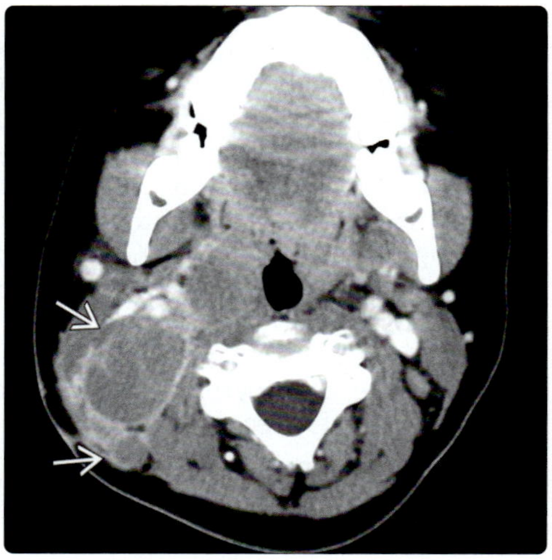

(Left) *Axial STIR MR in a child with Burkitt lymphoma shows marked enlargement of bilateral level IIA lymph nodes ➡. There is no significant surrounding edema. Note that imaging cannot distinguish between non-Hodgkin & Hodgkin-type lymphomas.* **(Right)** *Axial CECT shows left-sided necrotic cervical lymph nodes ➡ without edema of the adjacent fat. This toddler presented with a left neck mass without fever or elevated white blood cell count. Mycobacterium avium intracellulare was isolated from the excision specimen.*

Non-Hodgkin Lymphoma

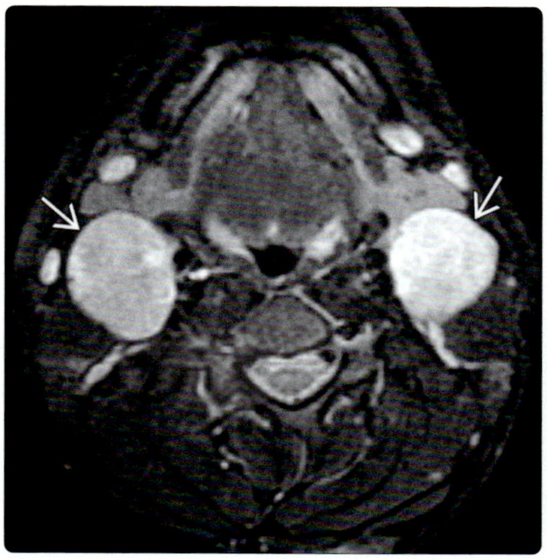

Nontuberculous *Mycobacterium*

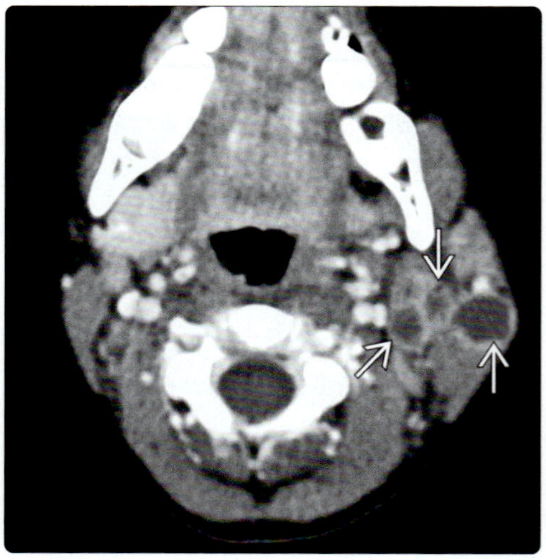

Cat-Scratch Disease

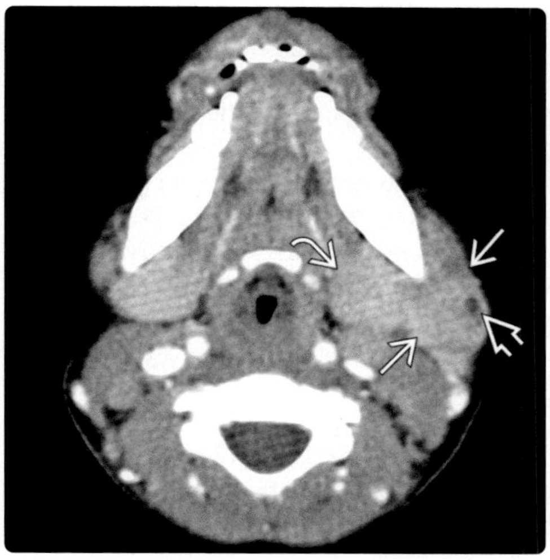

Metastatic Neuroblastoma

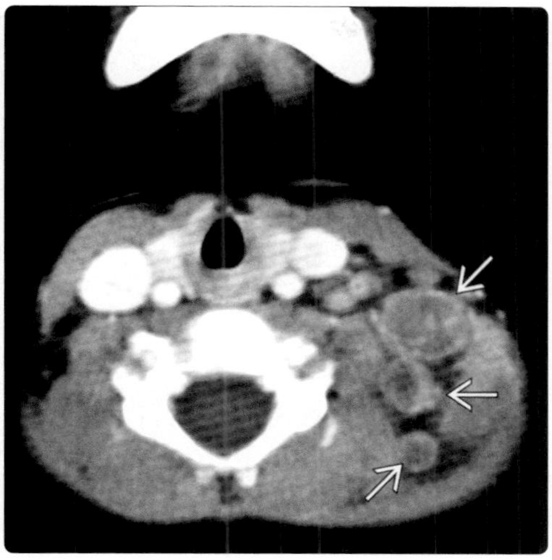

(Left) *Axial CECT shows an ill-defined nodal mass ➡ with a small central area of necrosis ➡ adjacent to the left submandibular gland ➡. There is no significant surrounding soft tissue edema, which is a common appearance of cat-scratch adenopathy.* **(Right)** *Axial CECT demonstrates several low-attenuation left cervical lymph nodes ➡ due to metastatic neuroblastoma.*

Posttransplant Lymphoproliferative Disorder

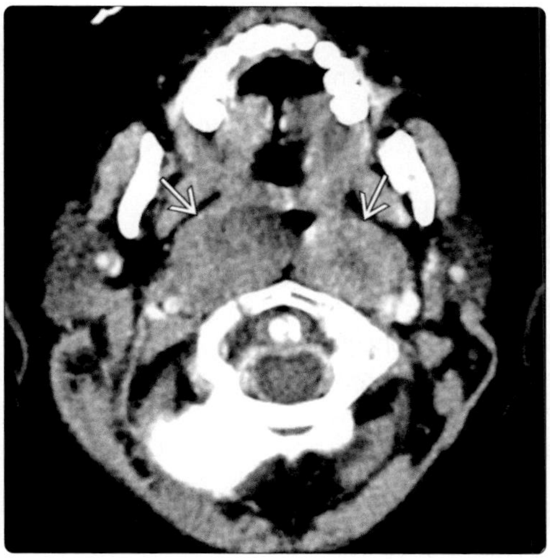

Differentiated Thyroid Carcinoma

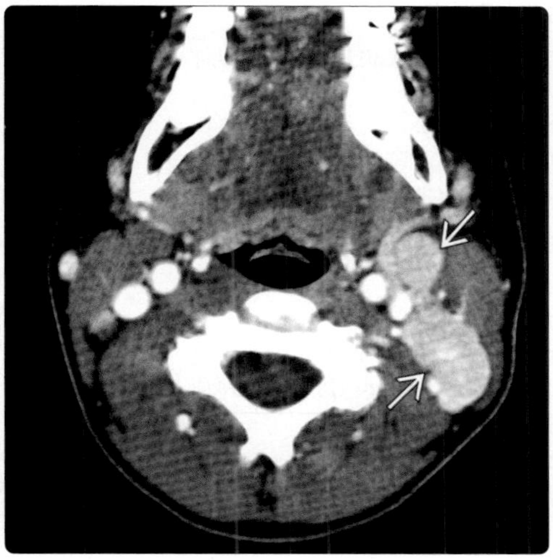

(Left) *Axial CECT in a child with a history of bone marrow transplant demonstrates massively enlarged bilateral retropharyngeal lymph nodes ➡ with ill-defined, low-attenuation foci centrally but without surrounding cellulitis. This patient also had other enlarged cervical lymph nodes (not shown).* **(Right)** *Axial CECT shows diffusely enhancing left-sided level II cervical lymph nodes ➡ in a teenager who presented with a left neck mass that proved to be metastatic thyroid carcinoma.*

Systemic Metastases

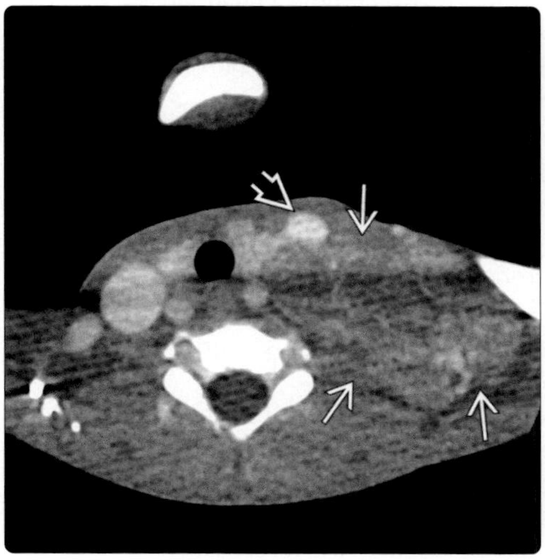

Langerhans Cell Histiocytosis

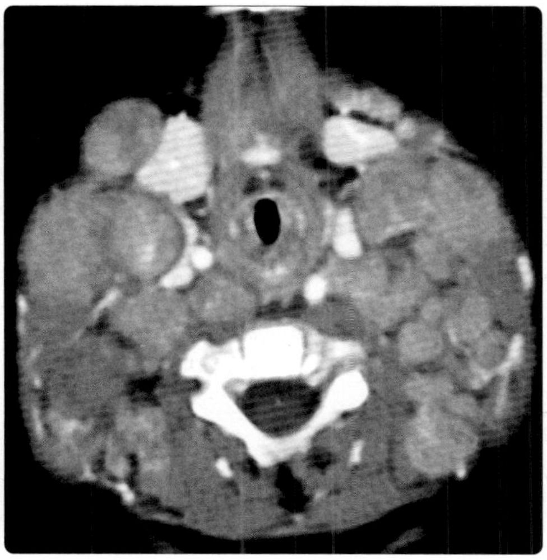

(Left) *Axial CECT in a child with known renal cell carcinoma shows a large, heterogeneous left supraclavicular metastatic nodal mass ➡ causing rightward deviation of the thyroid & airway as well as anterior deviation of the left jugular vein ➡.* **(Right)** *Axial CECT reveals massively enlarged, bilateral, nonnecrotic anterior & posterior cervical lymph nodes (too numerous to count) in a child with disseminated Langerhans cell histiocytosis.*

DIFFERENTIAL DIAGNOSIS

Common

- Reactive Lymph Nodes
- Infantile Hemangioma (IH)
- Fibromatosis Colli

Less Common

- Teratoma
- Metastatic Neuroblastoma
- Neurofibromatosis Type 1 (NF1)
- Cervical Thymus

Rare but Important

- Other Fibrous Lesions
- Congenital Hemangioma (CH)
- Langerhans Cell Histiocytosis
- Primary Cervical Neuroblastoma
- Lipoblastoma

ESSENTIAL INFORMATION

Key Differential Diagnosis Issues

- Ultrasound is 1st-line imaging modality & can be highly specific for top 3 common considerations
- MR may be required to assess deeper extent & relationship to critical structures (e.g., airway, orbit, etc.)
  - CECT may be used more acutely

Helpful Clues for Common Diagnoses

- **Reactive Lymph Nodes**
  - "Reactive" implies benign etiology
    - Most common: Response to infection/inflammation
    - May be acute or chronic & involve any nodal group
  - Imaging: Enlarged, oval-shaped lymph nodes
    - Variable enhancement, usually mild
    - ± enlargement of tonsillar tissues
    - ± stranding of adjacent fat (cellulitis)
    - ± edema in adjacent muscles (myositis)
    - ± suppurative nodes or abscess
- **Infantile Hemangioma (IH)**
  - Benign vascular neoplasm, **not** vascular malformation
    - Most common soft tissue tumor of childhood
  - Predictable clinical course
    - Usually absent at birth
    - Rapid growth during 1st few weeks/months of life (proliferating phase)
    - Spontaneous regression over subsequent months to years (involuting phase)
  - Mass remains soft throughout clinical course
  - Classic cutaneous, round or lobulated "cherry red" or "strawberry" mark if IH is superficial vs. blue or no skin discoloration if in IH lies in deeper tissues
  - GLUT1-positive staining on histology in all phases
  - Imaging: Solid, lobulated, avidly enhancing mass
    - Internal high-flow vessels in proliferative phase
      - > 5 vessels/cm^2 on Doppler ultrasound with abundant low-resistance arteries
      - Bright on arterial spin labeled MR
    - Fatty infiltration during involution
      - May leave residual fatty mass
    - Typically involves subcutaneous fat; may occupy & replace entire parotid gland
      - Deeper lesions (e.g., intraorbital, airway) are more common with PHACE syndrome: Posterior fossa anomalies, IHs, arterial anomalies, cardiovascular defects, eye anomalies, sternal clefts
- **Fibromatosis Colli**
  - a.k.a., sternocleidomastoid (SCM) tumor of infancy, congenital muscular torticollis
  - Self-limited, painless, benign mass in SCM muscle, thought to be due to scar-like reaction
    - History of breech presentation &/or difficult delivery is common
  - Presents with neck mass ± torticollis, usually within first 2-4 weeks of life
  - Imaging: Heterogeneous mass within & expanding SCM
    - Variable echogenicity, attenuation, & signal intensity; heterogeneous enhancement on CT/MR
      - Muscular edema of SCM may be noted around T2-hypointense mass
      - No extramuscular extension of mass
    - Variable internal & surrounding vascularity
    - Right > left, rarely bilateral
    - No associated adenopathy

Helpful Clues for Less Common Diagnoses

- **Teratoma**
  - Contains all 3 germ cell layers
  - Mature or immature; rarely malignant in neonate
  - Imaging: Large, heterogeneous unilateral cervical mass; may be exophytic
    - Solid & cystic components
    - Frequently shows fat & Ca^{2+}
    - May rarely demonstrate intracranial extension
    - May rarely arise in midline from palate (epignathus)
- **Metastatic Neuroblastoma**
  - Most cervical neuroblastomas are metastatic from retroperitoneal primary lesion
    - Most common in children > 1 year of age
  - Imaging: Large lymph nodes, rarely necrotic
    - Skull metastasis are common: Enhancing masses with aggressive osseous permeation/erosion &/or expansion, radiating spicules of new bone, & intracranial/intraorbital extension
- **Neurofibromatosis Type 1 (NF1)**
  - Localized, diffuse, or plexiform subtypes
    - Plexiform is classic form associated with NF1
  - Single or multiple; may involve any space but commonly involve carotid space, perivertebral space, brachial plexus
  - Imaging
    - Localized: Well-circumscribed, smooth, solid masses with variable enhancement
    - Diffuse: Plaque-like thickening of skin with poorly defined linear branching lesion in subcutaneous fat
    - Plexiform: Lobulated, rope-like expansions of major nerves creating tangle of worms appearance; cross section of any lobule shows target sign
      - Hypointense center/hyperintense periphery on T2 FS/STIR MR
      - Enhancing center/nonenhancing periphery on T1 C+ FS MR

- Localized & plexiform neurofibromas frequently show low attenuation on pre- & postcontrast CT
  - May mimic slow-flow vascular malformation
- **Cervical Thymus**
  - Mass-like solid thymic remnant along path of thymopharyngeal duct
    - Contiguous extension of normal mediastinal thymic tissue into lower neck is much more common but is typically found incidentally on imaging
  - Imaging: Mildly enhancing soft tissue mass closely associated with anterior carotid sheath
    - Small dot-dash echoes on ultrasound, similar to mediastinal thymus
    - ± associated cystic component

Helpful Clues for Rare Diagnoses

- **Other Fibrous Lesions**
  - Aggressive infantile fibromatosis, infantile myofibroma/myofibromatosis, infantile fibrosarcoma, fibrous hamartoma
  - Imaging: Well-defined vs. poorly defined infiltrative mass
    - May be quite heterogeneous with significant regions of T2 hypointensity due to fibrous tissue &/or Ca^{2+}
    - Variable enhancement
    - ± erosion or bizarre remodeling of adjacent bone
    - Specific lesion characteristics
      - Fibrosarcoma often has cystic components
      - Fibrous hamartoma often has streaks of fat
      - Myofibromatosis frequently shows relatively symmetric lytic & expansile metadiaphyseal lesions of skeleton
- **Congenital Hemangioma (CH)**
  - Benign vascular neoplasm, fully developed by birth
    - Lesion may rarely enlarge after birth due to hemorrhage, not cellular proliferation
  - 3 variants based on biological behavior
    - RICH: Rapidly involuting, usually by 14 months
    - PICH: Partially involuting
    - NICH: Noninvoluting
  - GLUT1 negative on histology
  - Imaging: Solid, heterogeneous, less well-defined mass (compared to IH)
    - ± Ca^{2-}, hemorrhage, necrosis
    - Variable internal vascularity on Doppler ultrasound
    - No fatty replacement during involution of RICH
- **Langerhans Cell Histiocytosis**
  - Spectrum of diseases caused by neoplastic clonal proliferation of dendritic cells
  - Singe system (uni- or multifocal) vs. multisystem disease
    - Acute disseminated form (Letterer-Siwe) occurs in children < 2 years of age
    - Acute onset of hepatosplenomegaly, rash, lymphadenopathy, marrow failure
    - Skeletal involvement may be absent
  - Imaging: Large, nonspecific cervical lymph nodes
    - Hepatosplenomegaly
- **Primary Cervical Neuroblastoma**
  - < 5% of neuroblastomas are primary cervical lesions
  - May present with opsoclonus-myoclonus syndrome
  - Imaging: Solid mass closely associated with carotid sheath/space
    - ± Ca^{2+} (much more common in adrenal primary)
    - Mild to moderate contrast enhancement
    - ± foraminal or intraspinal extension (rarely)
- **Lipoblastoma**
  - Benign, well-defined neoplasm of immature fat cells
    - Lipoblastomatosis: Infiltrative form
  - Primarily in extremities, rarely in H&N
  - Almost all found in infancy & early childhood
  - Imaging: Complex fatty mass with septations & nodules isointense to muscle on MR; variable enhancement

SELECTED REFERENCES

1. Bansal AG et al: US of pediatric superficial masses of the head and neck. Radiographics. 38(4):1239-63, 2018
2. Quintanilla-Dieck L et al: Congenital neck masses. Clin Perinatol. 45(4):769-85, 2018
3. Brown RE et al: Diagnostic imaging of benign and malignant neck masses in children-a pictorial review. Quant Imaging Med Surg. 6(5):591-604, 2016

Reactive Lymph Nodes

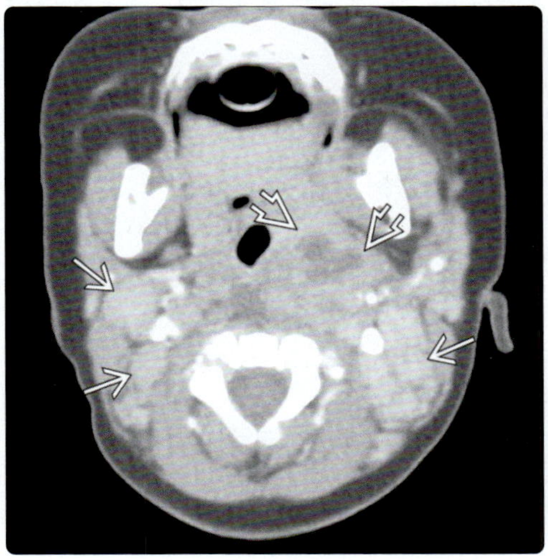

Infantile Hemangioma (IH)

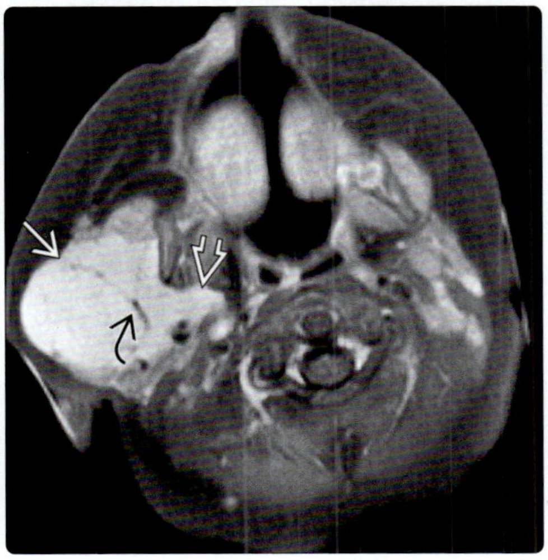

(Left) *Axial CECT shows bilateral, nonsuppurative cervical lymph nodes ➡ & a large necrotic inflammatory mass in the left lateral retropharyngeal space ➡ in a 4-month-old boy.* **(Right)** *Axial T1 C+ FS MR shows diffuse enlargement & intense enhancement of the right parotid gland, typical of an infantile hemangioma. Note that the lesion is holoparotid, involving both the superficial ➡ & deep ➡ lobes, & contains high-flow intralesional vessels ➡.*

(Left) *Axial T2 FS MR in a 2 week old with a left neck mass shows diffuse enlargement & abnormal hyperintensity of the left sternocleidomastoid (SCM) muscle. Note the normal size & shape of the right SCM muscle.* **(Right)** *Longitudinal ultrasound demonstrates the classic findings of fibromatosis colli with mildly heterogeneous expansion of the central SCM muscle without extramuscular extension.*

Fibromatosis Colli

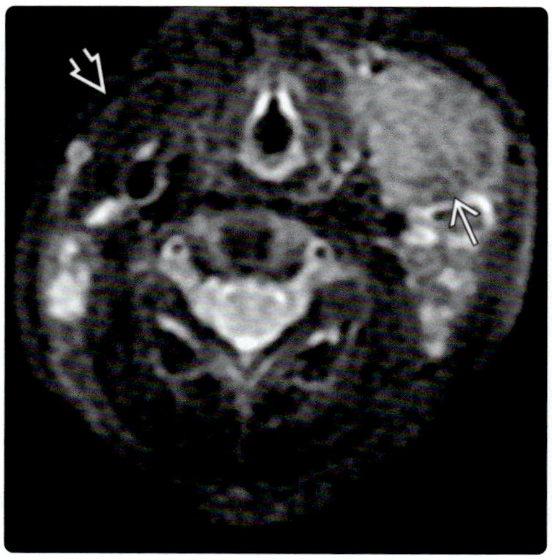

Fibromatosis Colli

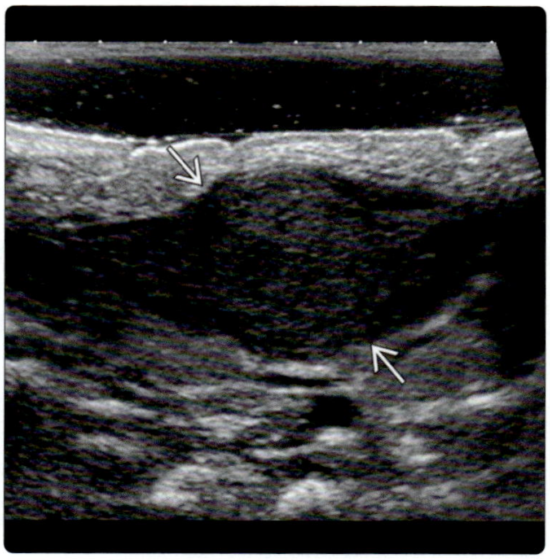

(Left) *Axial T1 C+ FS MR in a 1 day old shows a large, heterogeneous mass involving the anterior & posterior left neck with moderately enhancing solid components & nonenhancing cystic components. Note the significant deviation of the supraglottic airway.* **(Right)** *Axial CECT shows a large, heterogeneous transspatial neck mass in a 6-day-old infant. Some areas are cystic, while others are more solid. There are also small foci of Ca^{2+}, consistent with a congenital teratoma.*

Teratoma

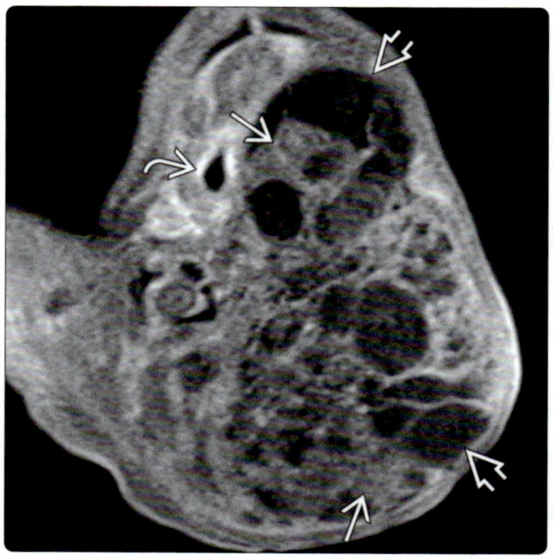

Teratoma

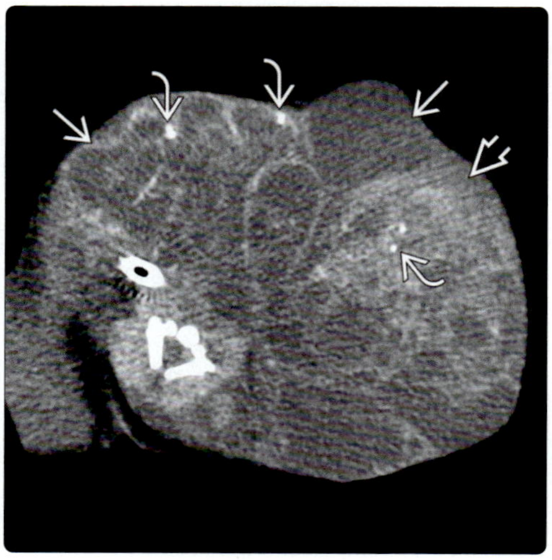

(Left) *Axial CECT shows a conglomeration of metastatic left cervical lymph nodes in a girl with a primary adrenal neuroblastoma. The left jugular vein is displaced anteriorly, & the left carotid artery is deviated posteromedially.* **(Right)** *Axial T2 MR in a child with neurofibromatosis type 1 depicts the classic appearance of bilateral, hyperintense plexiform neurofibromas that extend medially from the carotid sheaths into the retropharyngeal space. The left lesion shows decreased signal intensity centrally.*

Metastatic Neuroblastoma

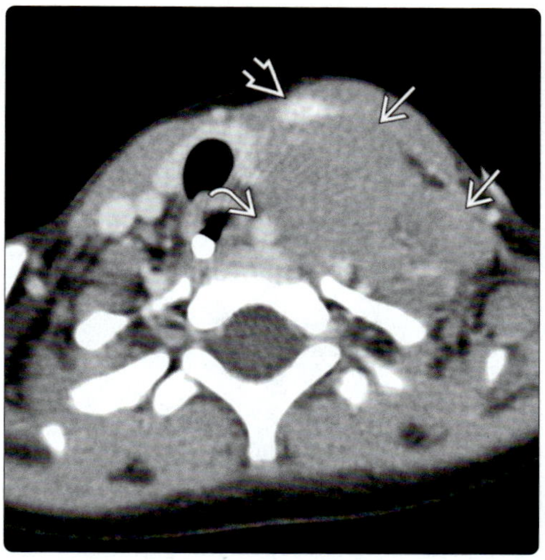

Neurofibromatosis Type 1 (NF1)

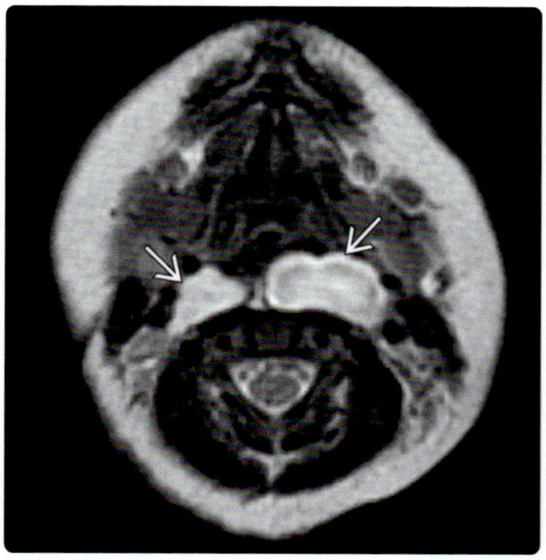

Cervical Thymus

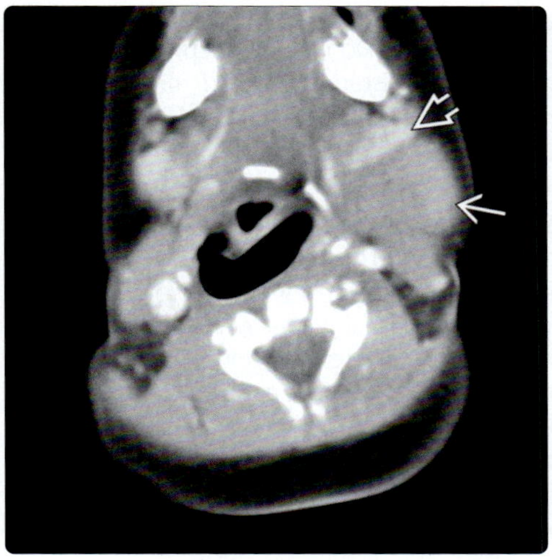

Other Fibrous Lesions

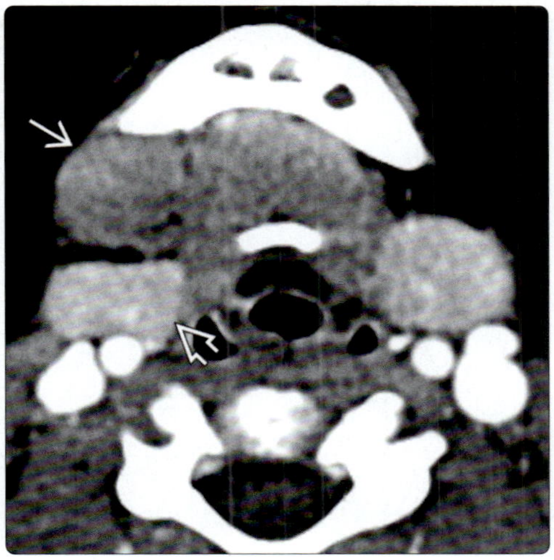

(Left) *Axial CECT shows a well-defined, intermediate-attenuation left anterior neck mass ➡ in a 3 month old with a pathologically proven cervical thymus remnant. The left submandibular gland ➡ is flattened & displaced anteriorly.* **(Right)** *Axial CECT shows a palpable right neck mass ➡ compressing the submandibular gland ➡. There is smooth bone remodeling & no aggressive periosteal reaction. Fibromatosis was found at biopsy.*

Congenital Hemangioma (CH)

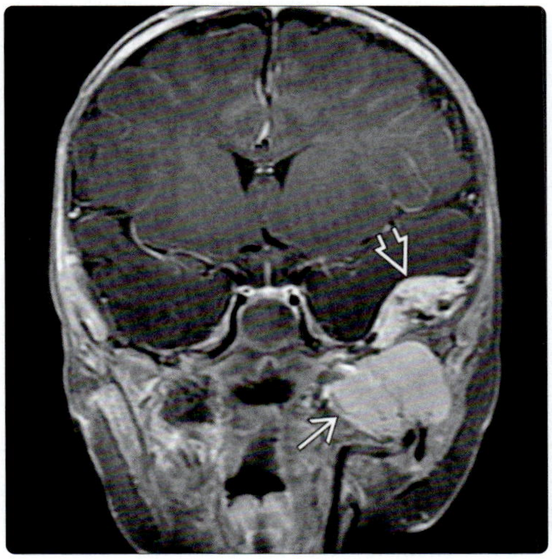

Langerhans Cell Histiocytosis

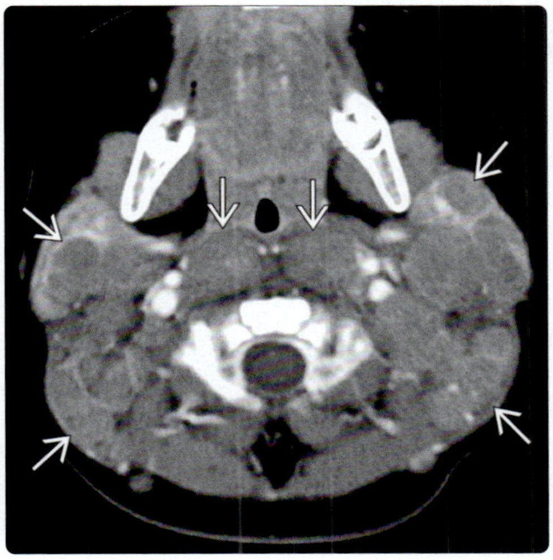

(Left) *Coronal T1 C+ FS MR in a newborn shows a homogeneously enhancing mass in the left infratemporal fossa ➡ & a more intensely enhancing mass in the left middle cranial fossa ➡. Both were contiguous via temporal bone destruction (not shown) but demonstrated rapid involution over several months.* **(Right)** *Axial CECT shows massive bilateral cervical adenopathy in all nodal groups ➡ in an 8-month-old boy with an acute disseminated form of Langerhans cell histiocytosis.*

Primary Cervical Neuroblastoma

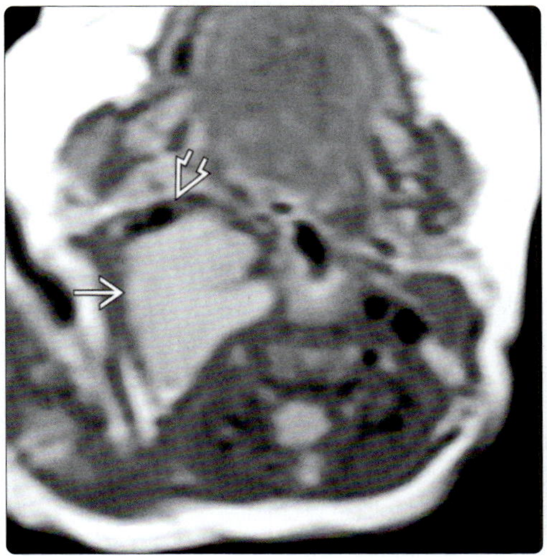

Lipoblastoma

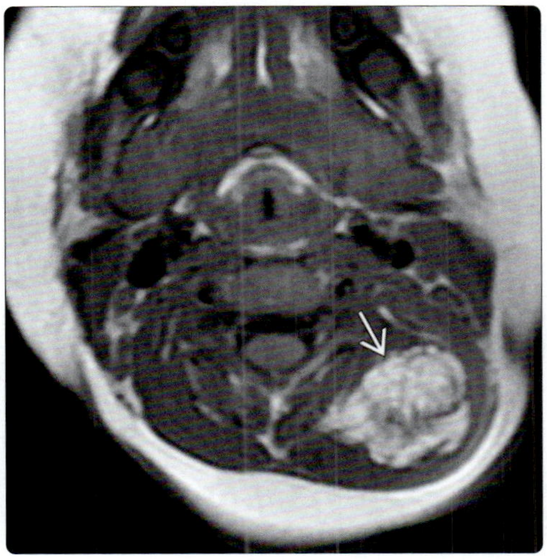

(Left) *Axial PD MR reveals a well-defined right carotid sheath primary cervical neuroblastoma ➡ without intraspinal extension. Note the anterior displacement of the carotid artery & internal jugular vein ➡.* **(Right)** *Axial T1 MR in an infant with a growing neck mass shows a fairly well-defined, hyperintense mass ➡ interspersed between the right posterior paraspinal muscles. With the exception of mild, wispy internal enhancement (not shown), the mass was isointense to fat on all sequences.*

DIFFERENTIAL DIAGNOSIS

Common

- Reactive Lymph Nodes
- Hodgkin Lymphoma
- Infantile Hemangioma
- Neurofibromatosis Type 1
- Non-Hodgkin Lymphoma

Less Common

- Metastatic Neuroblastoma
- Pilomatrixoma
- Rhabdomyosarcoma
- Cervical Thymus
- Lipoma

Rare but Important

- Differentiated Thyroid Carcinoma
- Squamous Cell Carcinoma
- Primary Cervical Neuroblastoma

ESSENTIAL INFORMATION

Helpful Clues for Common Diagnoses

- **Reactive Lymph Nodes**
  - "Reactive" implies benign etiology
    - Most common: Response to infection/inflammation
    - May be acute or chronic & involve any nodal group
  - Imaging: Enlarged oval-shaped lymph nodes
    - Variable enhancement, usually mild
    - ± enlarged tonsillar tissue
    - ± stranding of adjacent fat (cellulitis)
    - ± edema in adjacent muscles (myositis)
    - ± suppurative nodes or abscess
- **Hodgkin Lymphoma**
  - Cervical & mediastinal nodes are common location; Waldeyer ring or extranodal in < 1%
  - B-cell origin; histology shows Reed-Sternberg cells
    - Tumors EBV(+) in up to 50%
  - Imaging: Cannot distinguish Hodgkin lymphoma (HL) from non-Hodgkin lymphoma (NHL)
    - Single vs. multiple contiguous nodal groups
    - Homogeneous lobulated nodal masses
    - Variable contrast enhancement
    - Necrotic center may be present
    - May be hypoechoic on ultrasound
- **Infantile Hemangioma**
  - Benign vascular neoplasm, **not** vascular malformation
    - Most common soft tissue tumor of childhood
  - Predictable clinical course
    - Usually absent at birth
    - Rapid growth over first few weeks/months of life (proliferating phase)
    - Spontaneous regression over subsequent months to years (involuting phase)
  - Mass remains soft throughout clinical course
  - Classic cutaneous round or lobulated "cherry red" or "strawberry" mark if infantile hemangioma (IH) is superficial vs. blue or no skin discoloration if in IH lies in deeper tissues
  - GLUT1(+) staining on histology in all phases
  - Imaging: Solid, lobulated, avidly enhancing mass
    - Intralesional high-flow vessels during proliferative phase
      - > 5 vessels/cm² on Doppler ultrasound with abundant low-resistance arteries
      - Bright on arterial spin labeled MR
    - Fatty infiltration during involution
      - May leave residual fatty mass
    - Typically involves subcutaneous fat; may occupy & replace entire parotid gland
      - Deeper lesions (e.g., intraorbital, airway) are more common with PHACE syndrome: Posterior fossa abnormalities, IHs, arterial abnormalities, cardiovascular defects, eye abnormalities, sternal clefts
- **Neurofibromatosis Type 1**
  - Localized, diffuse, or plexiform subtypes; plexiform is classic form associated with NF1
  - Single or multiple; may involve any space
    - Carotid space, perivertebral space, & brachial plexus are common
  - Imaging
    - Localized: Well-circumscribed, smooth, solid masses with variable enhancement
    - Diffuse: Plaque-like thickening of skin with poorly defined linear branching lesion in subcutaneous fat
    - Plexiform: Lobulated, tortuous, rope-like expansions of major nerves creating tangle of worms appearance; cross-section of any lobule shows target sign
      - Hypointense center/hyperintense periphery on T2 FS/STIR MR
      - Enhancing center/nonenhancing periphery on T1 C+ FS MR
    - Localized & plexiform neurofibromas frequently show low attenuation on pre- & postcontrast CT
      - May mimic slow flow vascular malformation
- **Non-Hodgkin Lymphoma**
  - All nodal chains can be involved in nodal form
  - Extranodal in 30%: Lymphatic tissue (tonsils) or extralymphatic (paranasal sinuses, skull base, & thyroid)
  - Imaging: Single dominant node or multiple nonnecrotic enlarged nodes
    - Imaging cannot distinguish NHL from HL

Helpful Clues for Less Common Diagnoses

- **Metastatic Neuroblastoma**
  - Most cervical neuroblastomas are metastatic
    - Primary cervical in < 5%
  - Imaging: Large lymph nodes, rarely necrotic
    - Skull metastasis are common: Enhancing masses with aggressive osseous permeation/erosion &/or expansion, radiating spicules of new bone, & intracranial/intraorbital extension
- **Pilomatrixoma**
  - a.k.a. calcifying epithelioma of Malherbe
  - Benign tumor of hair follicle in children
  - Imaging: Small, round, well-defined subcutaneous mass that is adherent to skin; ± Ca^{2+}
    - Ultrasound: Internal reticulations, hypoechoic rim, mildly increased echogenicity of surrounding tissues; variable flow on color Doppler

- **Rhabdomyosarcoma**
  - Most common pediatric soft tissue malignancy
    - Neck mass may be primary lesion or metastatic adenopathy
  - Most common location in H&N is parameningeal (i.e., middle ear, paranasal sinus, nasopharynx)
    - Intracranial extension in up to 55% of parameningeal lesions
  - Imaging: Well-circumscribed soft tissue mass
    - Intermediate to high T2 signal intensity & variable enhancement (often only mild)
      - Restricted diffusion common due to cellularity
    - ± bone erosion or nonaggressive bone remodeling
    - ± metastatic cervical adenopathy
- **Cervical Thymus**
  - Mass-like solid thymic remnants along path of thymopharyngeal duct
    - Contiguous extension of normal mediastinal thymic tissue into lower neck is much more common but is typically found incidentally on imaging
  - Imaging: Mildly enhancing soft tissue mass closely associated with anterior carotid sheath
    - ± associated cystic component
- **Lipoma**
  - Benign fatty mass
  - 15% occur in H&N
    - Can involve any space; may be transspatial
    - Posterior cervical, submandibular, anterior cervical, & parotid spaces are most common
  - Occasionally are residua of involuted IH
  - Lipoblastoma is more heterogeneous (but benign) fatty tumor, typically in young children
  - Imaging: Well-circumscribed homogeneous fat attenuation/signal mass on CT/MR without significant enhancement
    - 75% hyperechoic, 25% iso-/hypoechoic vs. muscle on ultrasound
    - Any significant matrix in older child raises concern for liposarcoma (though fat-poor myxoid liposarcoma is more common in children)

Helpful Clues for Rare Diagnoses

- **Differentiated Thyroid Carcinoma**
  - Nodal spread is common in papillary; distant spread is common in follicular
  - 3x more common in women
    - Usually 3rd & 4th decades; occasionally in adolescents, rare in young children
  - Imaging: Small to large nodes, may be "reactive" in appearance vs. heterogeneous, hemorrhagic, &/or cystic (from necrosis)
    - ± mirco Ca^{2+}, T1 shortening
    - Look for primary thyroid mass
- **Squamous Cell Carcinoma**
  - Unknown primary is rare in children
  - Nasopharyngeal carcinoma (NPC) with adenopathy may occur in teenagers
  - Imaging: Nonspecific enlarged round nodes
    - May be heterogeneous ± multiple confluent nodes
    - Look for lateral pharyngeal recess mass of NPC with skull base invasion
- **Primary Cervical Neuroblastoma**
  - < 5% of neuroblastomas are primary cervical lesions
  - Range from immature neuroblastoma to mature benign ganglioneuroma
  - Imaging: Well-defined, solid mass closely associated with carotid sheath, typically in posterior carotid space
    - Intraspinal extension is rare
    - ± Ca^{2+} (much more common in adrenal primary)
    - Mild to moderate enhancement; restricts diffusion

SELECTED REFERENCES

1. Bansal AG et al: US of pediatric superficial masses of the head and neck. Radiographics. 38(4):1239-63, 2018
2. Brown RE et al: Diagnostic imaging of benign and malignant neck masses in children-a pictorial review. Quant Imaging Med Surg. 6(5):591-604, 2016
3. Bulman JC et al: Pilomatricoma of childhood: a common pathologic diagnosis yet a rare radiologic one. AJR Am J Roentgenol. 206(1):182-8, 2016
4. Friedman ER et al: Imaging of pediatric neck masses. Radiol Clin North Am. 49(4):617-32, v, 2011

Reactive Lymph Nodes

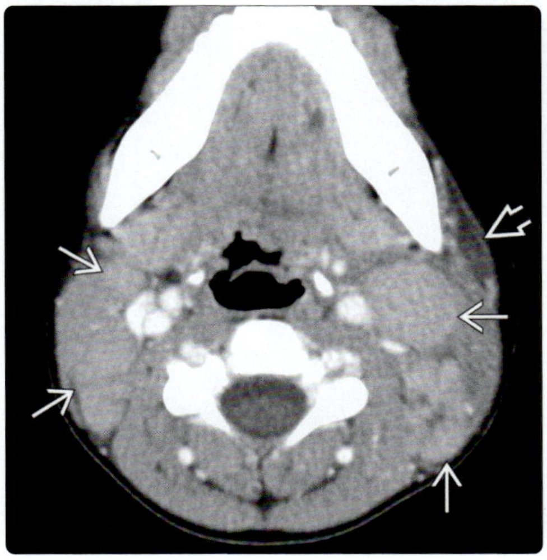

Hodgkin Lymphoma

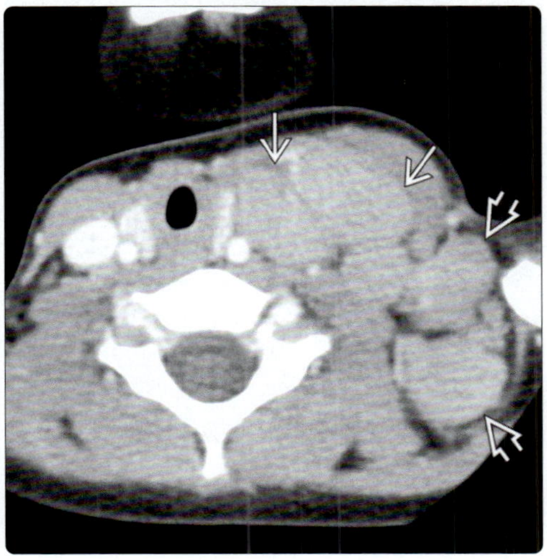

(Left) *Axial CECT shows left greater than right reactive cervical adenopathy ➡ & mild overlying soft tissue edema/cellulitis ➡ in a toddler with an elevated white blood cell count. Note the lack of necrosis in this case.* **(Right)** *Axial CECT demonstrates asymmetric enlargement of cervical lymph nodes in a 4 year old with Hodgkin lymphoma. Both the internal jugular ➡ & spinal accessory ➡ chain nodes are involved. Note the lack of surrounding inflammation or internal necrosis.*

(Left) *Axial T1 C+ FS MR shows right greater than left enhancing parotid space masses. The right mass completely replaces the parotid gland, & the left is superficial to an otherwise normal-appearing parotid gland. Note the absence of a right internal carotid artery flow void in this child with PHACE syndrome.* **(Right)** *Axial T1 C+ FS MR in a child with PHACE syndrome shows multiple enhancing infantile hemangiomas in the right parotid gland, right sublingual space, & left subcutaneous fat.*

Infantile Hemangioma

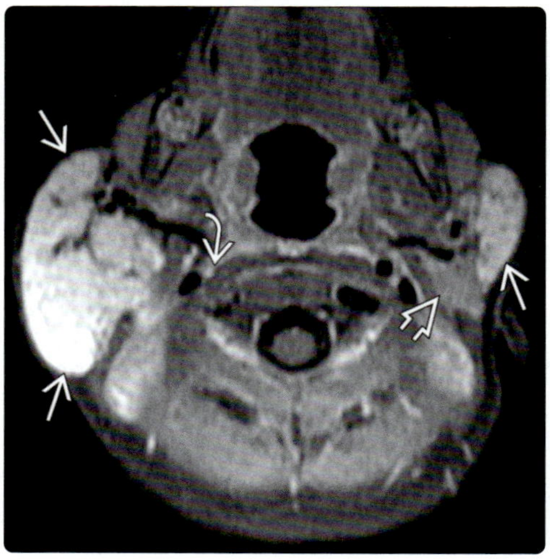

Infantile Hemangioma

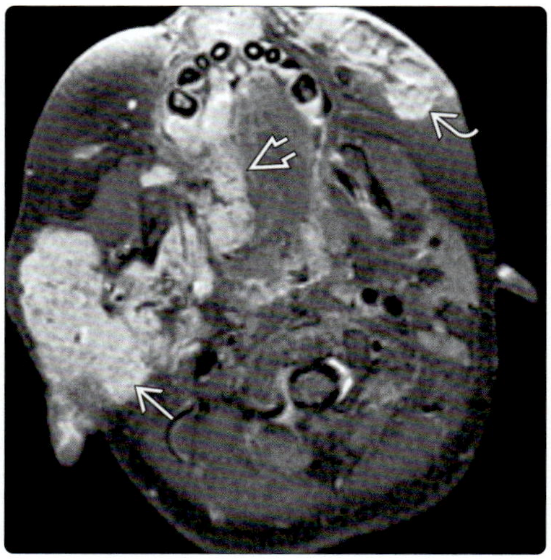

(Left) *Axial STIR MR in a child with NF1 demonstrates numerous hyperintense, nodular lesions throughout all spaces of the neck, including the carotid, retropharyngeal, submandibular, sublingual, & posterior paraspinal spaces. Many of the lesions have the typical target appearance of plexiform neurofibromas with a hypointense center & hyperintense periphery.* **(Right)** *Axial CECT reveals mild enlargement of multiple bilateral internal jugular chain lymph nodes in a teenager with T-cell lymphoblastic lymphoma.*

Neurofibromatosis Type 1

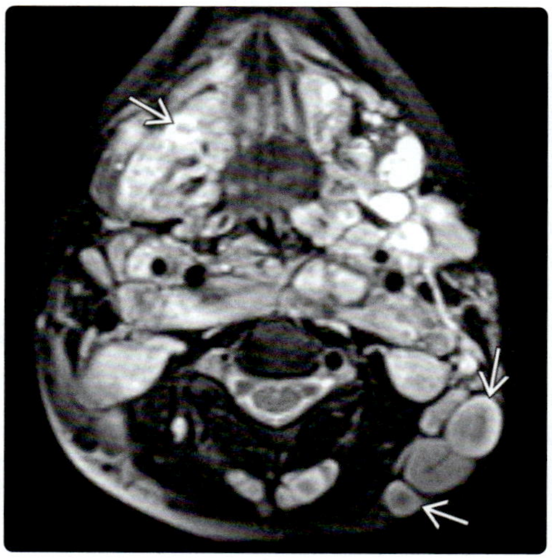

Non-Hodgkin Lymphoma

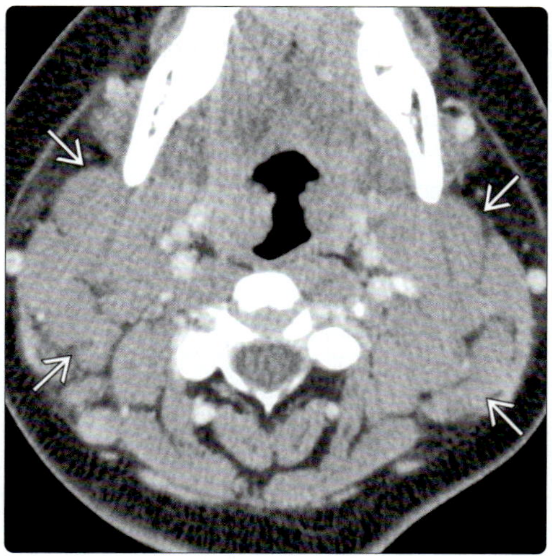

(Left) *Axial CECT in a child with a known primary adrenal neuroblastoma reveals multiple partially necrotic metastatic left spinal accessory lymph nodes without intrinsic Ca^{2+} or associated overlying cellulitis.* **(Right)** *Axial CECT in a 9 year old with a neck mass for 1 year shows a well-defined lesion in the subcutaneous tissues of the right neck. The mass is partially calcified & inseparable from the overlying skin, typical of a pilomatrixoma.*

Metastatic Neuroblastoma

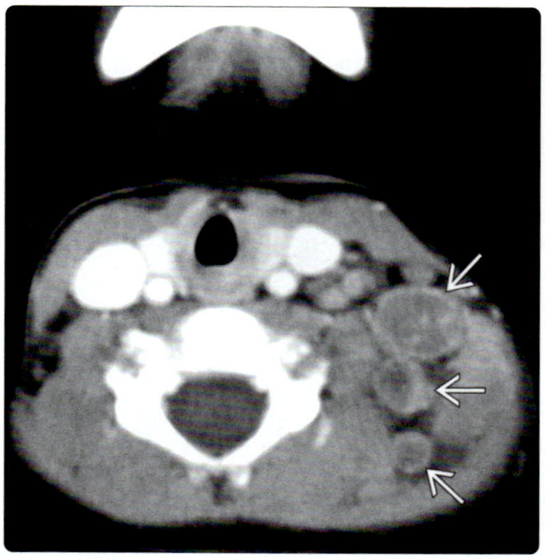

Pilomatrixoma

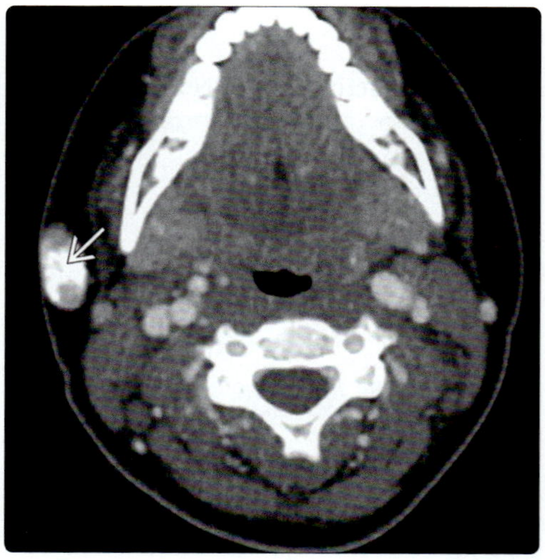

Rhabdomyosarcoma

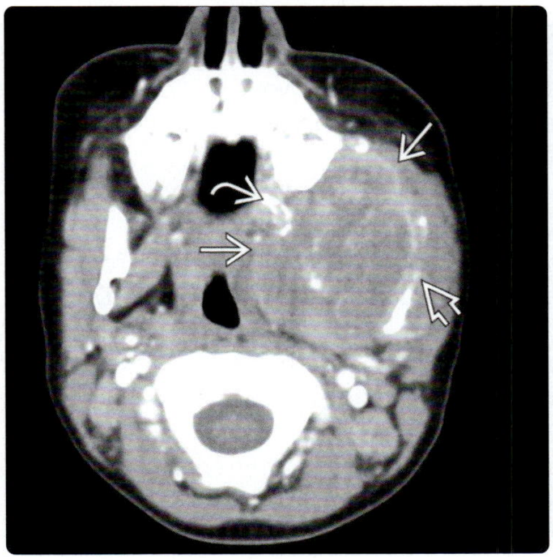

Cervical Thymus

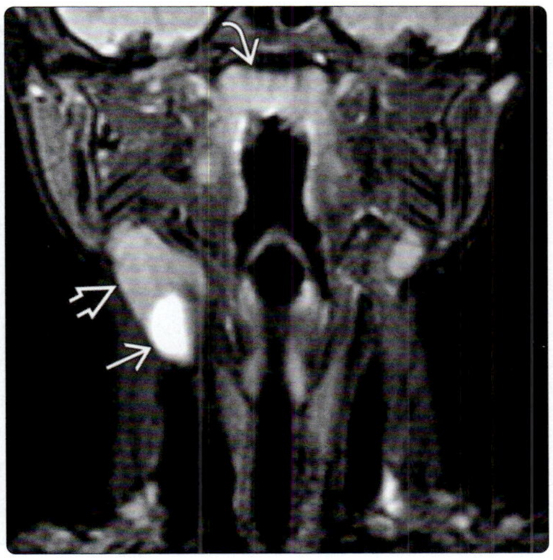

(Left) *Axial CECT in a 3 year old reveals a large heterogeneous left masticator space rhabdomyosarcoma ➔. Note the aggressive osseous destruction of the left mandibular ramus ➔ & pterygoid plate ➔.* **(Right)** *Coronal STIR MR shows a mixed cystic ➔ & solid ➔ neck mass that is similar in signal characteristics to adenoid tonsil tissue ➔. Axial images (not shown) demonstrated that the mass was posterior to the submandibular gland & closely associated with the anterior carotid space.*

Lipoma

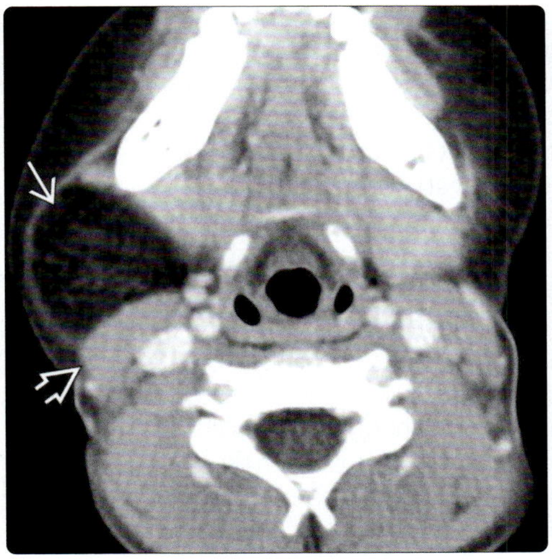

Differentiated Thyroid Carcinoma

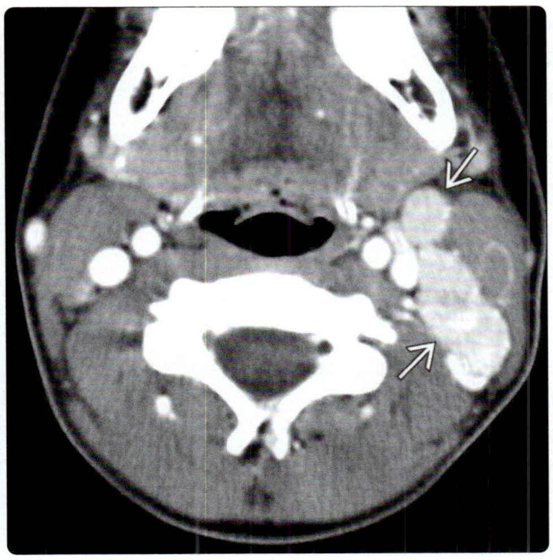

(Left) *Axial CECT in a 5 year old shows a well-defined fat attenuation mass ➔ anterior to the right sternocleidomastoid muscle ➔ without significant solid components, typical of a focal lipoma.* **(Right)** *Axial CECT demonstrates high-attenuation, partially calcified papillary thyroid carcinoma nodal metastases ➔. Solid enhancing, cystic, or calcified components in the neck nodes of a teenager suggest a differentiated thyroid carcinoma primary tumor.*

Squamous Cell Carcinoma

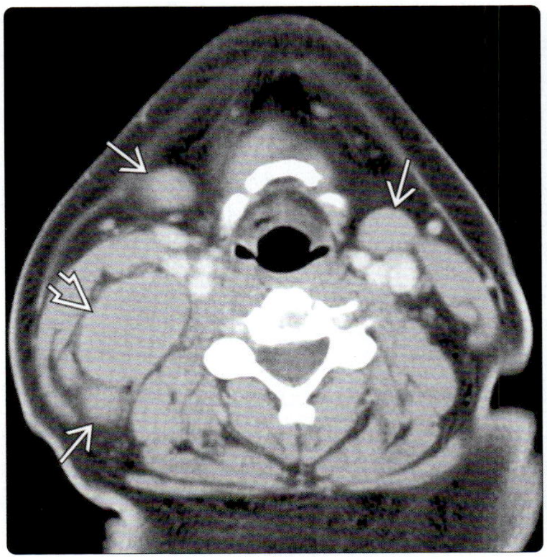

Primary Cervical Neuroblastoma

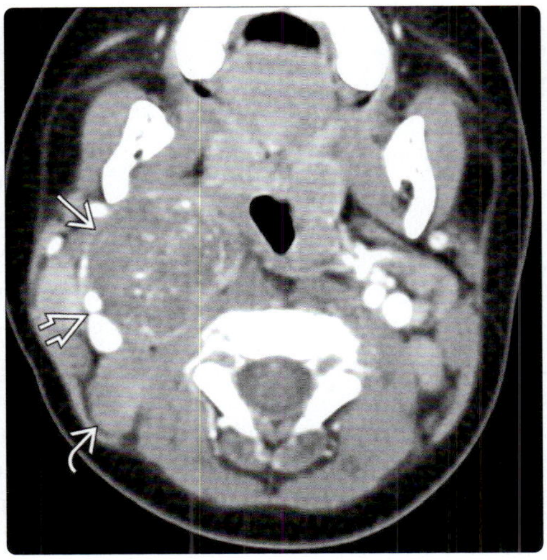

(Left) *Axial CECT shows multiple enlarged nonnecrotic cervical lymph nodes ➔. The largest ➔ is deep to the sternocleidomastoid muscle at the level of the hyoid bone in this teenager with metastatic nasopharyngeal carcinoma.* **(Right)** *Axial NECT reveals a well-defined round mass ➔ with speckled intrinsic Ca^{2+} that deviates the carotid space laterally ➔. Biopsy showed a ganglioneuroblastoma, which is a more mature mixture of neuroblastoma & ganglioneuroma. Note also the nodal metastasis ➔.*

DIFFERENTIAL DIAGNOSIS

Common

- Suppurative Lymph Nodes
- Abscess
- Thyroglossal Duct Cyst
- Lymphatic Malformation
- 2nd Branchial Cleft Cyst

Less Common

- 1st Branchial Cleft Cyst
- Ranula
- Cervical Thymic Cyst

Rare but Important

- Dermoid & Epidermoid
- Teratoma
- Foregut Duplication Cyst

ESSENTIAL INFORMATION

Helpful Clues for Common Diagnoses

- **Suppurative Lymph Nodes**
  - Pus in lymph node = intranodal abscess
    - If untreated → rupture → extranodal soft tissue abscess
  - Can affect any nodal H&N group
    - Jugulodigastric, retropharyngeal (RP), & submandibular are most common
  - Imaging: Thick, enhancing nodal wall with central hypodensity; phlegmon may have similar appearance
    - Edema in surrounding fat (cellulitis)
      - Common in bacterial infection; usually absent in non-TB *Mycobacterium*
    - ± thickening of muscles (myositis)
    - Associated nonsuppurative adenopathy
- **Abscess**
  - Conglomeration of suppurative nodes or rupture of node → extranodal abscess
  - Superficial abscesses: Anterior cervical, posterior cervical, & submandibular space are most common
  - RP, parapharyngeal, or tonsillar/peritonsillar abscesses may grow rapidly → airway compromise
  - If anterior to left thyroid lobe, think of 4th branchial apparatus anomaly
  - Exclude dental infection & salivary gland calculus as underlying cause
  - Imaging
    - Radiograph: Wide prevertebral soft tissues = RP cellulitis/edema ± frank abscess
      - False-positive: RP thickening in infants due to redundant soft tissues (if image is taken without inspiration &/or adequate extension)
    - US: Central decreased echogenicity with increased through transmission
      - Compression demonstrating swirling internal echoes confirms drainable fluid
      - Color Doppler shows increased peripheral vascularity without central vascularity
    - CECT/MR: Rim-enhancing mass with nonenhancing center; majority will contain drainable pus
      - Variable thickness & irregularity of enhancing wall
      - Restricted diffusion on DWI MR
      - Occasionally air in abscess cavity
      - Edema in surrounding fat (cellulitis)
      - ± thickening of muscles (myositis)
      - Effacement of adjacent internal jugular vein is common
      - ± internal carotid artery narrowing = vasospasm
- **Thyroglossal Duct Cyst**
  - Remnant of thyroglossal duct, anywhere from foramen cecum at base of tongue to thyroid bed in infrahyoid neck
    - At hyoid > suprahyoid = infrahyoid
  - Treatment: Resect cyst, tract, & midline hyoid bone (Sistrunk procedure)
  - Imaging: Round cyst with minimal rim enhancement
    - Most in suprahyoid neck are midline; may be paramidline in infrahyoid neck (embedded in strap muscles)
    - May contain hyperechoic debris without hemorrhage or infection
    - Increased enhancement & surrounding inflammatory change when infected
    - ± nodularity or calcifications if thyroid carcinoma has developed (adults)
      - Rare; present histologically in > 3.2%
- **Lymphatic Malformation**
  - Subtype of congenital slow-/low-flow vascular malformation due to error in lymphatic vessel formation
  - Variably sized cystic foci
    - Macrocyst > 1 cm, microcyst < 1 cm
  - Present at birth, grows with child
  - Sudden increase in size with minor trauma (hemorrhage), infection, or times of hormonal stimulation
  - Imaging: Typically multilocular with thin septations, extending across tissue planes; only cystic lesion to commonly involve bilateral neck
    - Macrocystic: Enhancement limited to rim & septations
      - Lack high-flow vessels (unless normal vessel is encased by abnormal lymphatics)
      - Fluid-fluid levels are common, typically due to hemorrhage
      - Soft & compressible by US with internal swirling debris
      - Protein, blood products, or chyle/fat may cause bright T1 signal intensity on MR
    - Microcystic: May be poorly defined & solid-appearing
      - ± diffuse enhancement
- **2nd Branchial Cleft Cyst**
  - Cystic remnant of cervical sinus
  - Characteristic location
    - Posterolateral to submandibular gland
    - Lateral to carotid space
    - Anteromedial to sternocleidomastoid muscle (SCM)
  - Uncommon locations: Parapharyngeal space, beaking in between internal & external carotid artery, or anterior surface of infrahyoid carotid space
  - Imaging: Well-defined unilocular cyst in typical location with no significant contrast enhancement
    - If infected, wall is thicker & enhances with surrounding soft tissue cellulitis

Helpful Clues for Less Common Diagnoses

- **1st Branchial Cleft Cyst**
  - Remnant of 1st branchial apparatus
  - In or superficial to parotid gland, around pinna or external auditory canal; may extend to angle of mandible
  - Proximity to facial nerve important for surgical planning
  - Imaging: Well-defined, nonenhancing cyst
    - ± enhancing wall with surrounding inflammation if infected
- **Ranula**
  - Sublingual gland or sublingual space (SLS) minor salivary gland retention cyst
    - Result of salivary gland trauma or inflammation or congenitally imperforate duct
  - Simple = true cyst with epithelial lining
  - Diving = extravasation pseudocyst when ranula ruptures out of SLS into submandibular space (SMS)
  - Imaging
    - Simple: Well-defined, obliquely oriented, elongated cyst in SLS
      - Unilateral oval or bilateral horseshoe shape
    - Diving: Comet-shaped unilocular cyst in SLS & SMS
      - "Body" in SMS & "tail" in SLS
      - Tail sign = collapsed SLS portion
- **Cervical Thymic Cyst**
  - Cystic remnant of thymopharyngeal duct
    - 3rd pharyngeal pouch remnant
    - Wall contains Hassall corpuscles
  - Imaging: Cystic mass along course of thymopharyngeal duct, ± solid enhancing thymic tissue
    - Closely associated with carotid sheath
      - May splay carotid artery & jugular vein
    - Usually in lateral infrahyoid neck
      - Rarely ruptures into parapharyngeal space
    - May be connected to mediastinal thymus

Helpful Clues for Rare Diagnoses

- **Dermoid & Epidermoid**
  - Cystic mass resulting from congenital epithelial inclusion or rest
  - Dermoid: Epithelial elements + dermal substructure, including dermal appendages
  - Epidermoid: Epithelial elements only
  - Imaging
    - Epidermoid: Well-defined cyst filled with fluid
    - Dermoid: Well-defined cyst with fluid, fatty material, &/or Ca^{2+}
    - Often restrict diffusion
- **Teratoma**
  - All 3 germ cell lines; mature vs. immature
  - Imaging: Mixed cystic & solid mass, usually involving anterior neck or oral cavity
    - Fat, calcium, cystic, & solid components
- **Foregut Duplication Cyst**
  - Most occur in thorax & abdomen; rare in neck
  - Imaging: Well-defined midline cyst posterior to trachea

SELECTED REFERENCES

1. Kimia AA et al: Predictors of a drainable suppurative adenitis among children presenting with cervical adenopathy. Am J Emerg Med. 37(1):109-13, 2018
2. Merrow AC et al: 2014 Revised classification of vascular lesions from the International Society for the Study of Vascular Anomalies: radiologic-pathologic update. Radiographics. 36(5):1494-516, 2016
3. LaPlante JK et al: Common pediatric head and neck congenital/developmental anomalies. Radiol Clin North Am. 53(1):181-96, 2015
4. Wassef M et al: Vascular anomalies classification: recommendations from the International Society for the Study of Vascular Anomalies. Pediatrics. 136(1):e203-14, 2015
5. Gaddikeri S et al: Congenital cystic neck masses: embryology and imaging appearances, with clinicopathological correlation. Curr Probl Diagn Radiol. 43(2):55-67, 2014

Suppurative Lymph Nodes

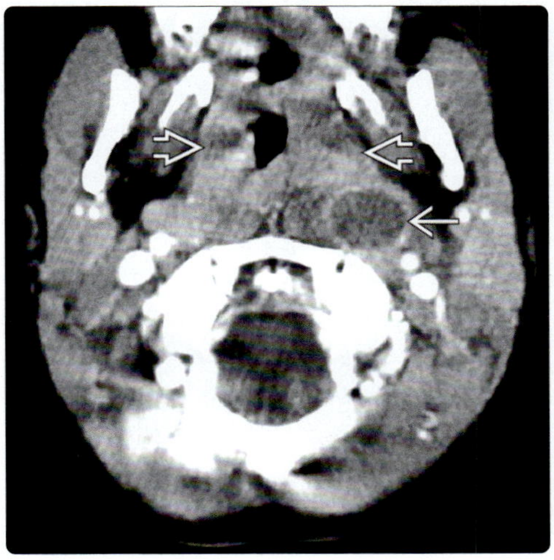

Suppurative Lymph Nodes

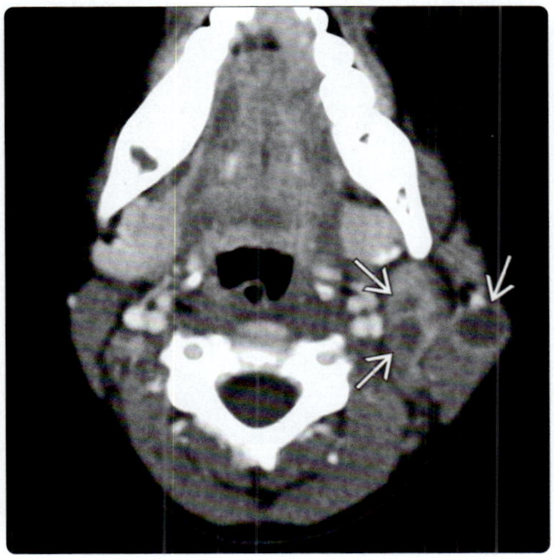

(Left) *Axial CECT demonstrates a well-defined, rim-enhancing, suppurative left lateral retropharyngeal lymph node ➔ in a patient with pharyngitis. Note the associated mildly swollen palatine tonsils ⇨.* **(Right)** *Axial CECT in a 2 year old with lymphadenitis unresponsive to antibiotics shows multiple necrotic left-sided cervical lymph nodes ➔. The lack of associated inflammatory changes in the adjacent fat is typical of Mycobacterium avium-intracellulare.*

(Left) *Axial CECT reveals a large, multiloculated abscess with a fairly well-defined rim of enhancement in the left parapharyngeal ➡, deep parotid ➡, & oropharyngeal mucosal ➡ spaces in a 10 month old with a persistent mass despite oral antibiotics.* **(Right)** *Axial CECT in a child with mononucleosis & persistent sore throat demonstrates a well-defined, low-attenuation collection ➡ that deviates the left palatine tonsil ➡ anteriorly & inferiorly, consistent with a peritonsillar abscess.*

Abscess

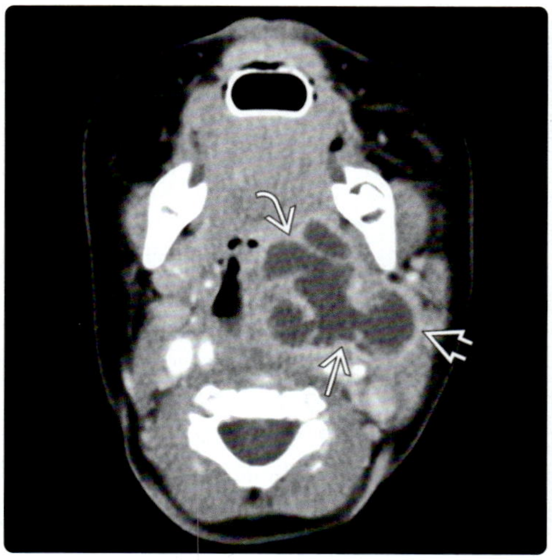

Abscess

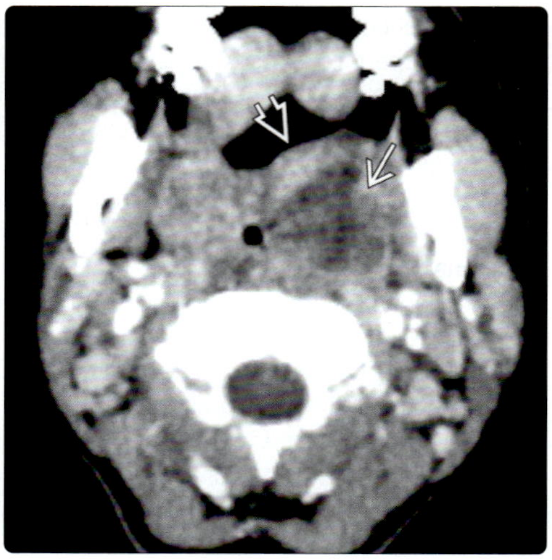

(Left) *Axial CECT shows a sharply marginated, nonenhancing infrahyoid thyroglossal duct cyst ➡ embedded in the left strap muscles. The paramedian location of infrahyoid thyroglossal duct cysts is characteristic.* **(Right)** *Axial T2 FS MR reveals dependently layering blood products within 2 locules of a multiseptated macrocystic lymphatic malformation ➡.*

Thyroglossal Duct Cyst

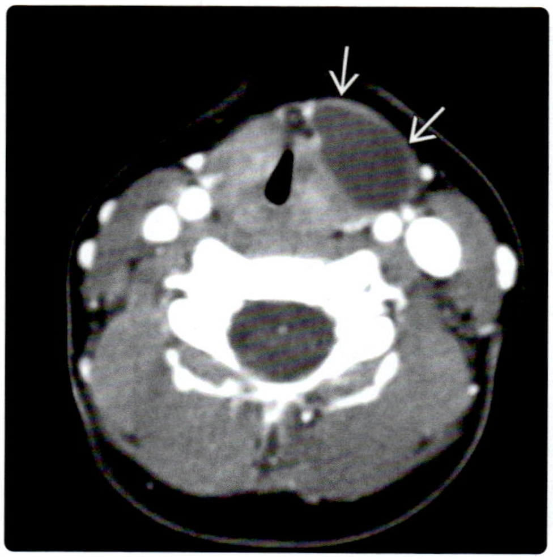

Lymphatic Malformation

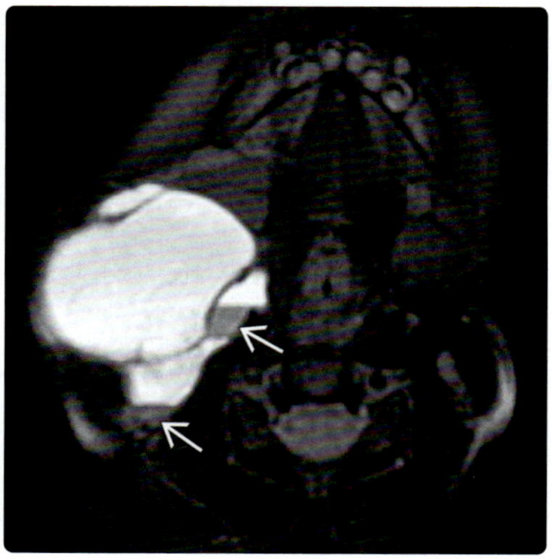

(Left) *Axial CECT in a teenager with a tender neck mass shows a well-defined, low-attenuation cyst ➡ with surrounding edema in the typical location of a 2nd branchial cleft cyst: Posterior to the submandibular gland ➡, anterior to the sternocleidomastoid muscle (SCM) ➡, & lateral to the carotid artery ➡.* **(Right)** *Axial CECT shows a low-attenuation, nonenhancing cyst within the left parotid gland in a child with an intraparotid 1st branchial apparatus cyst ➡.*

2nd Branchial Cleft Cyst

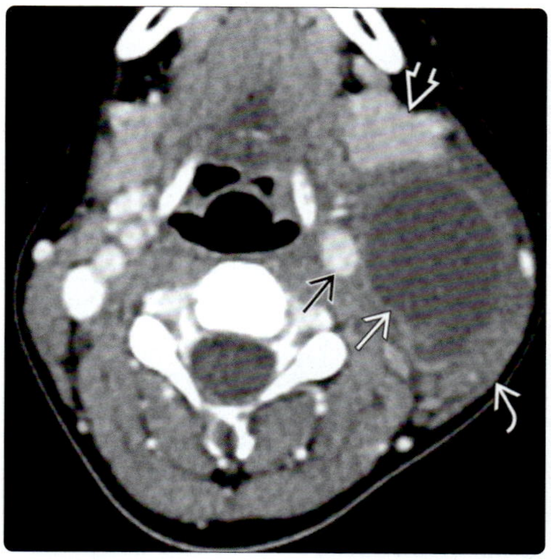

1st Branchial Cleft Cyst

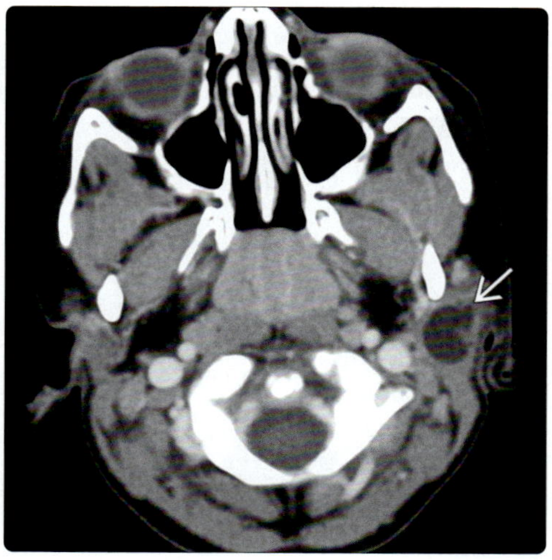

Ranula

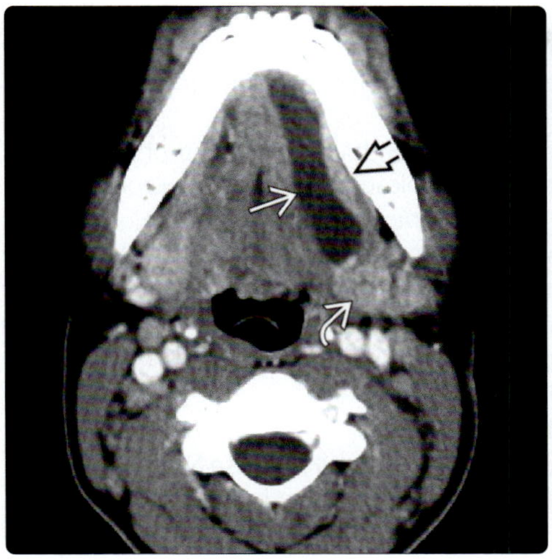

Ranula

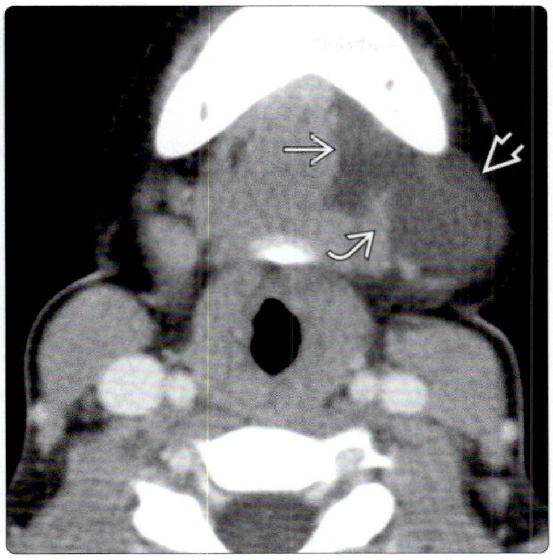

(Left) *Axial CECT in a patient with a sublingual mass shows an elongated low-attenuation, nonenhancing ranula in the left sublingual space. This is a simple ranula as it is confined to the sublingual space. Note also the submandibular gland & mylohyoid muscle.* **(Right)** *Axial CECT in a child with a plunging ranula demonstrates a low-attenuation, nonenhancing mass spanning the left sublingual & submandibular spaces, extending through a defect in the mylohyoid muscle.*

Cervical Thymic Cyst

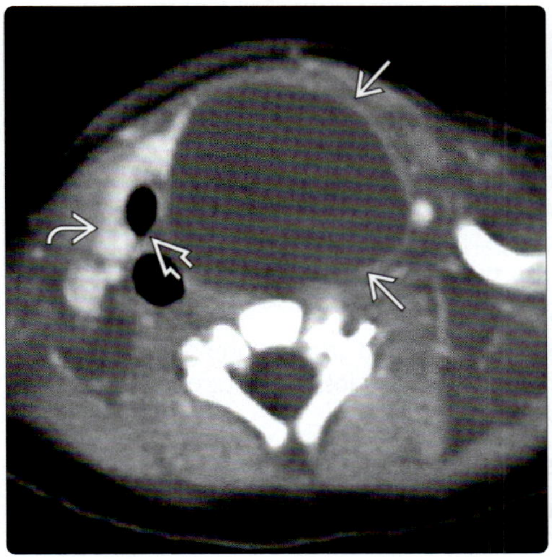

Dermoid & Epidermoid

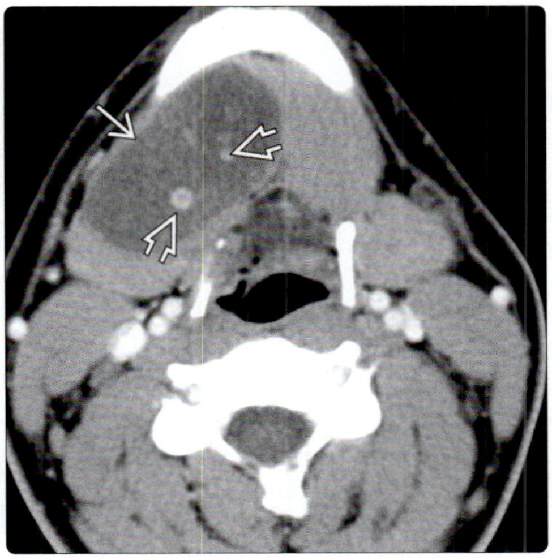

(Left) *Axial CECT demonstrates a large, simple thymic cyst in the left anterior neck, significantly deviating the airway & thyroid gland to the right. In this patient, the cyst extended from the skull base to the upper mediastinum.* **(Right)** *Axial CECT in a 14 year old demonstrates a well-defined, low-attenuation mass with internal Ca^{2+}. On coronal images, the mass deviated the mylohyoid muscle inferiorly, causing the mass to appear clinically as submandibular in origin.*

Teratoma

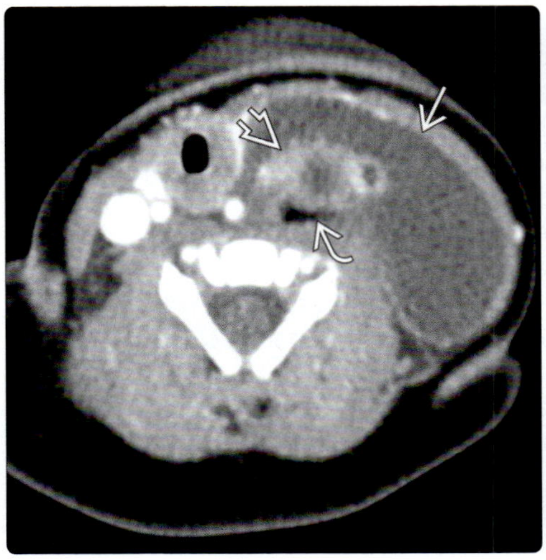

Foregut Duplication Cyst

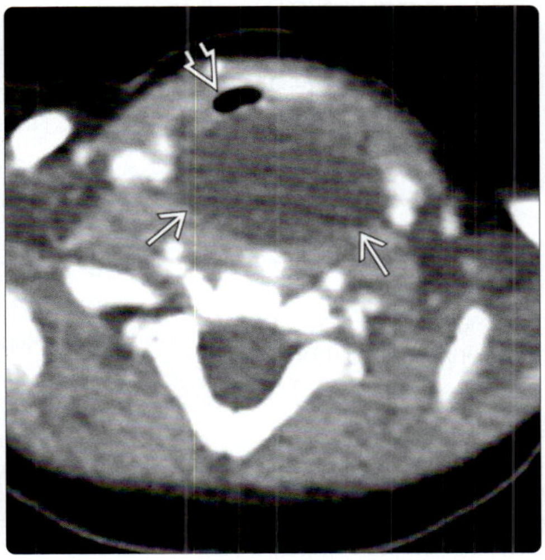

(Left) *Axial CECT in a 6 year old shows a heterogeneous mass deep to the left SCM & deviating the airway to the right. The mass is primarily hypoattenuating with scattered areas of enhancement & fat attenuation, consistent with a teratoma.* **(Right)** *Axial CECT in a 6 month old with a progressive increase in noisy breathing demonstrates a large, nonenhancing, low-attenuation midline cyst causing significant anterior deviation & flattening of the trachea.*

DIFFERENTIAL DIAGNOSIS

Common

- Abscess
- Lymphatic Malformation
- Venous Malformation
- Neurofibromatosis Type 1

Less Common

- Rhabdomyosarcoma
- Infantile Hemangioma
- Cervical Thymic Cyst
- 4th Branchial Anomaly

Rare but Important

- Lipoma
- Teratoma
- Fibrous Masses

ESSENTIAL INFORMATION

Key Differential Diagnosis Issues

- Transspatial: Extending across tissue planes into adjacent compartments

Helpful Clues for Common Diagnoses

- **Abscess**
  - Occurs in superficial &/or deep soft tissues of neck
  - Typically presents with new onset swelling, redness, tenderness, fever (i.e., signs/symptoms of infection)
    - ± dysphagia, stridor
  - Imaging: Necrotic/phlegmonous collection vs. walled-off drainable fluid; ± gas in abscess
    - US: Heterogeneous mass with surrounding hyperemia but no internal vascularity
      - Internal swirling debris confirms fluid
    - CECT: Rim-enhancing, low-attenuation collection
      - 75% are drainable pus; 25% are necrotic/phlegmonous (nondrainable)
      - May extend via danger space into mediastinum
    - MR: Restricted diffusion on DWI
      - Fluid levels suggest blood rather than pus
    - Adenopathy & edema of surrounding fat/muscles
    - ± internal carotid artery narrowing = vasospasm
      - Usually self-limited, most common in children
- **Lymphatic Malformation**
  - Congenital low-flow lesion due to abnormal lymphatic development
  - Often presents as cystic ("squishy") mass in utero, at birth, or later in life
    - Grows commensurate with patient but may rapidly enlarge due to hemorrhage, infection, or hormonal stimulation
  - Imaging: Multilocular cystic mass; numerous thin septations
    - Typically involves anterior neck, chest wall, mediastinum; often crosses midline
    - Macrocystic (cysts > 1 cm): Enhancement is limited to rim & septations
      - Compressible by US with internal swirling debris
      - Blood products may cause T1 MR hyperintense fluid &/or layering fluid-fluid levels
    - Microcystic (cysts < 1 cm): May be poorly defined, appearing solid; ± diffuse enhancement
    - May encase normal arteries/veins
- **Venous Malformation**
  - Congenital low-flow lesion due to abnormal venous development
  - Mass increases in size with Valsalva, crying, or bending over (due to communication with normal venous system)
  - Imaging: Tend to be more tubular/elongated in morphology than lymphatic malformation (LM)
    - Often contain fluid levels due to stagnant blood
    - Typically show gradual enhancement
    - Phleboliths are virtually diagnostic
- **Neurofibromatosis Type 1**
  - Soft tissue masses include
    - Localized neurofibroma (NF), diffuse NF, plexiform NF, or malignant peripheral nerve sheath tumor (MPNST)
  - Imaging
    - Localized: Well-circumscribed, fusiform, solid mass with moderate enhancement; ± dumbbell-shaped extension into neural foramina
    - Diffuse NF: Plaque-like subcutaneous lesion with poorly defined infiltrating margins with moderate enhancement
    - Plexiform NF: Lobulated, tortuous, rope-like enlargement in major nerve distribution; resembles tangle of worms
      - Cross section of individual lesion shows target sign: Peripheral hyperintensity & central hypointensity on T2/STIR
    - MPNST
      - Favor if ≥ 5 cm, rapid growth, intensely enhancing with infiltrative margins, loss of target sign, PET SUV > 3.5

Helpful Clues for Less Common Diagnoses

- **Rhabdomyosarcoma**
  - Up to 40% occur in H&N
    - Parameningeal (middle ear, paranasal sinus, nasopharynx, masticator space, pterygopalatine fossa, parapharyngeal space), orbit, other sites
  - Imaging: Solid firm round to ovoid soft tissue mass with variable contrast enhancement (often mild to moderate)
    - ± bone erosion or nonaggressive bone remodeling
    - ± cervical metastatic adenopathy
    - Coronal T1 C+ MR is best to evaluate for intracranial extension
- **Infantile Hemangioma**
  - Benign vascular neoplasm
  - Presents in 1st weeks of life; usually not present at birth
    - Rapid growth in 1st weeks/months of life (proliferating phase)
    - Spontaneous regression over months to years (involuting phase)
  - Imaging: Lobulated soft mass, often mildly elongated
    - Isolated lesions are typically well circumscribed & subcutaneous
      - Multifocal & transspatial lesions are more likely in PHACE syndrome
    - US: Patchy regions of increased & decreased echogenicity

        - > 5 vessels/cm² on Doppler with numerous low resistance arterial waveforms
    - CECT/MR: Avid homogeneous enhancement
        - Scattered flow voids/high flow vessels
        - Increased perfusion on ASL MR
        - Gradual fatty involution
- **Cervical Thymic Cyst**
    - Imaging: Cystic remnant along course of embryologic thymopharyngeal duct
        - ± solid, enhancing thymic tissue
        - Closely associated with carotid sheath
            - May splay carotid artery & jugular vein
        - May be connected to mediastinal thymus directly or by fibrous cord
        - Rarely extends to skull base; may rupture into parapharyngeal space
- **4th Branchial Anomaly**
    - Sinus tract extending from apex of pyriform sinus to lower anterior neck
    - Leads to recurrent thyroiditis or anterior neck abscess
    - Imaging: Abscess (or cyst) anterior to left thyroid lobe with associated thyroiditis
        - Barium swallow (± subsequent CT) may show sinus tract extending from apex of pyriform sinus to anterior lower neck

Helpful Clues for Rare Diagnoses

- **Lipoma**
    - Benign neoplasm of mature fat
    - 15% occur in H&N
    - Imaging: Typically simple & homogeneous in appearance
        - Margins may be difficult to define against normal subcutaneous fat
        - US: 75% hyperechoic, 25% iso-/hypoechoic vs. muscle
        - CECT/MR: Well-circumscribed homogeneous mass of fat attenuation/signal intensity without significant enhancement
            - Minority of lesions will have nonfatty soft tissue component
        - Other fatty masses to consider
            - Lipoblastoma: Consider with heterogeneous fatty mass in young child
            - Fibrous hamartoma: Often has streaks of fat
            - Hibernoma: Nonspecific tumor of brown fat
            - Liposarcoma: Essentially nonexistent in first 5-8 years of life; more likely to be fat poor in 2nd decade
- **Teratoma**
    - Tumor of all 3 germ cell lines
    - Mature >> immature, malignant subtypes
    - Imaging: Heterogeneous mixed solid & cystic mass; ± fat & Ca^{2+}
        - Tends to be more bulbous, solid, & exophytic than infiltrative cystic LM
- **Fibrous Masses**
    - Various lesions, both benign & malignant varieties
        - Desmoid fibromatosis, lipofibromatosis, infantile myofibromatosis, infantile fibrosarcoma
        - Even benign types are often locally aggressive/invasive
    - Imaging: Well-defined or poorly marginated mass
        - May have T2-hypointense nonenhancing fibrous components (inactive) &/or T2-hyperintense enhancing components (active)
        - ± cysts, Ca^{2+}
        - ± bone erosion, remodeling, or invasion

SELECTED REFERENCES

1. Merrow AC et al: 2014 revised classification of vascular lesions from the International Society for the Study of Vascular Anomalies: radiologic-pathologic update. Radiographics. 36(5):1494-516, 2016
2. Sargar KM et al: Pediatric fibroblastic and myofibroblastic tumors: a pictorial review. Radiographics. 36(4):1195-214, 2016
3. Thomas B et al: Revisiting imaging features and the embryologic basis of third and fourth branchial anomalies. AJNR Am J Neuroradiol. 31(4):755-60, 2010

Abscess

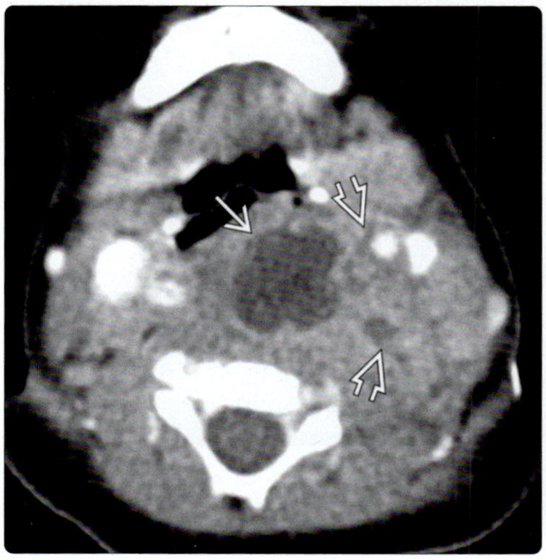

Lymphatic Malformation

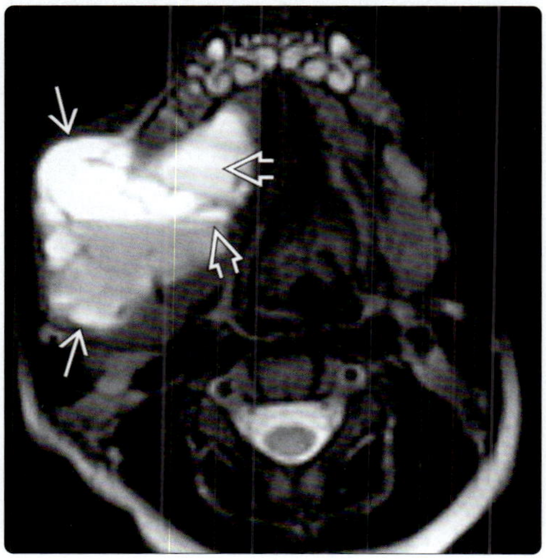

(Left) *Axial CECT in a young child shows an irregular, low-attenuation abscess with minimal rim enhancement ➡ in the left lateral retropharyngeal space. Irregular fluid collections also extend laterally ➡, deviating the carotid sheath anteriorly.* **(Right)** *Axial T2 FS MR shows the typical appearance of a transspatial lymphatic malformation. The lesion is characterized by multiple thin-walled cysts ➡, many of which contain fluid-fluid levels ➡ due to layering blood products.*

(Left) *Axial T1 C+ FS MR reveals a lobulated, heterogeneously enhancing venous malformation involving the left masseter & medial pterygoid muscles. Note the focal signal voids secondary to phleboliths in both the deep & superficial components.* **(Right)** *Axial CECT shows a lobulated, heterogeneously enhancing venous malformation in the left cheek with multiple variably sized phleboliths & hypertrophy of the adjacent fat.*

Venous Malformation

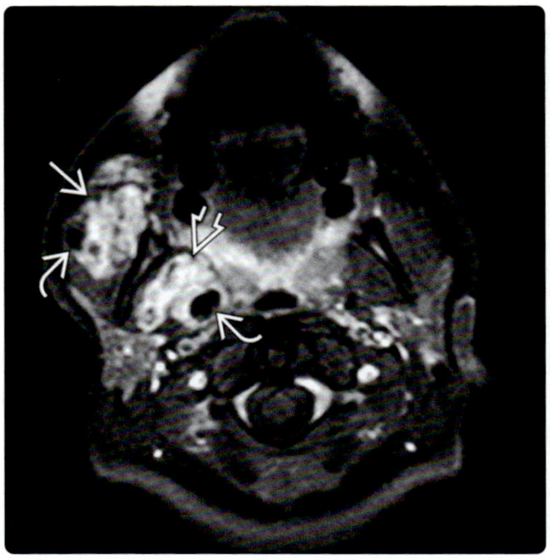

Venous Malformation

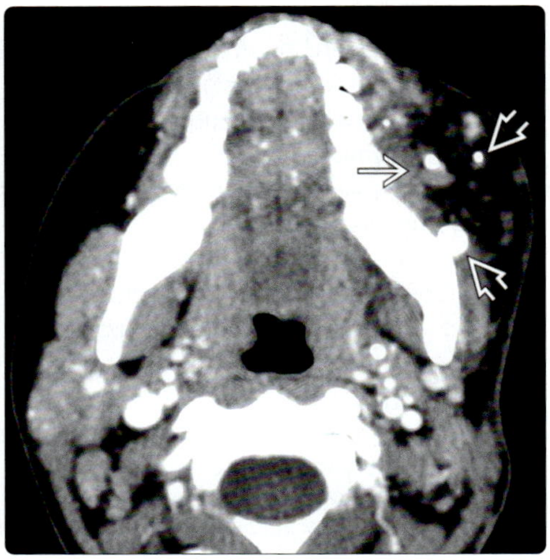

(Left) *Axial CECT shows an infiltrative low-attenuation plexiform neurofibroma involving the retropharyngeal space & left carotid space. The mass extends between the left pyriform sinus & hyoid bone.* **(Right)** *Axial STIR MR in the same patient reveals an infiltrative hyperintense plexiform neurofibroma involving the retropharyngeal space, left carotid space, & parapharyngeal space. Some of the lesions show the typical target sign in cross section.*

Neurofibromatosis Type 1

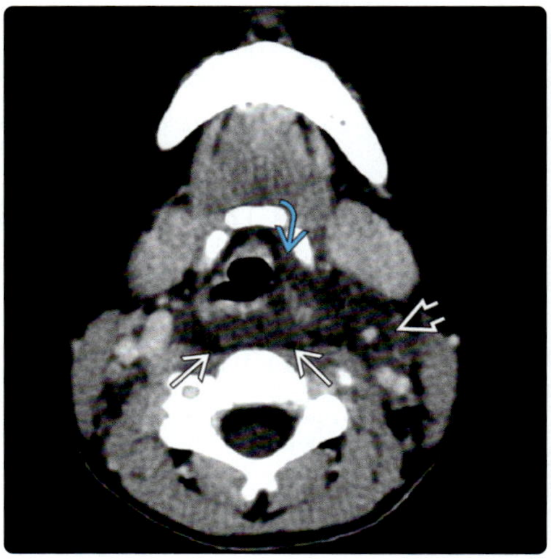

Neurofibromatosis Type 1

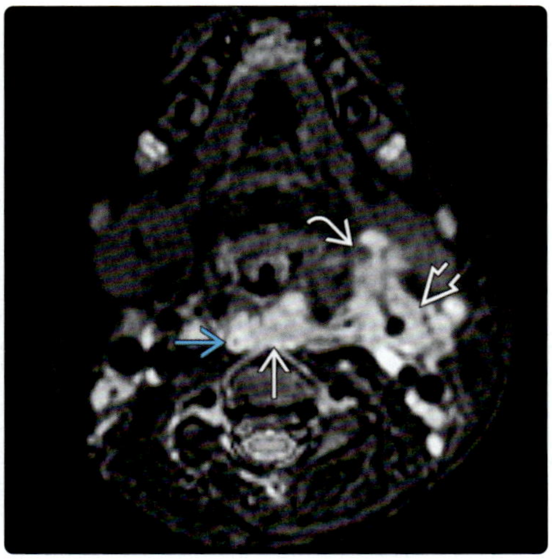

(Left) *Axial T1 C+ FS MR shows a large, heterogeneously enhancing rhabdomyosarcoma involving the left masticator space & deep parotid space. Note how the rhabdomyosarcoma erodes & remodels the mandible.* **(Right)** *Axial T1 C+ FS MR demonstrates a homogeneously enhancing lobulated infantile hemangioma involving the left carotid, posterior cervical, & left submandibular spaces. These lesions showed increased flow on ASL sequences (not shown).*

Rhabdomyosarcoma

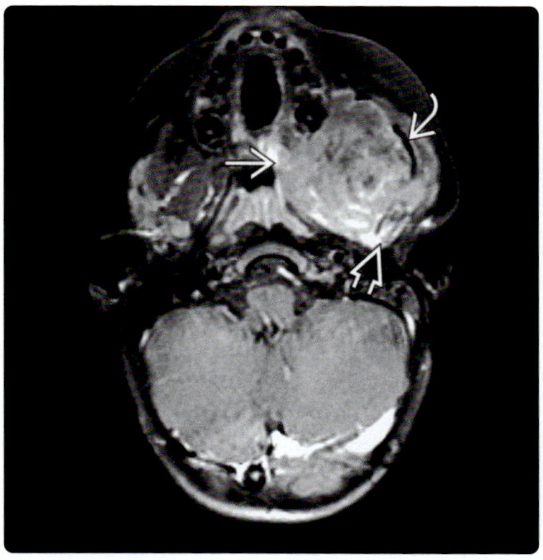

Infantile Hemangioma

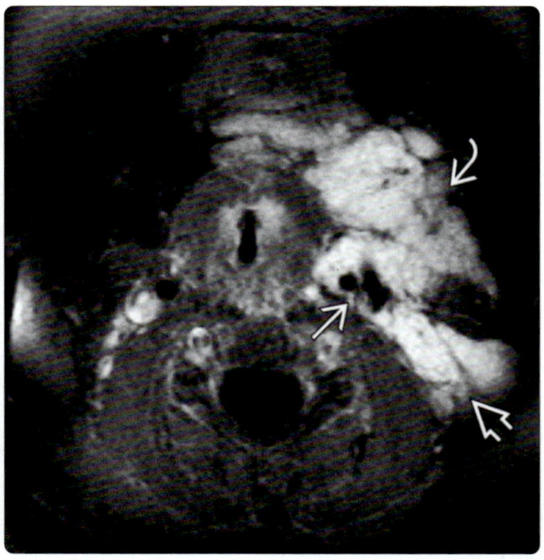

Cervical Thymic Cyst

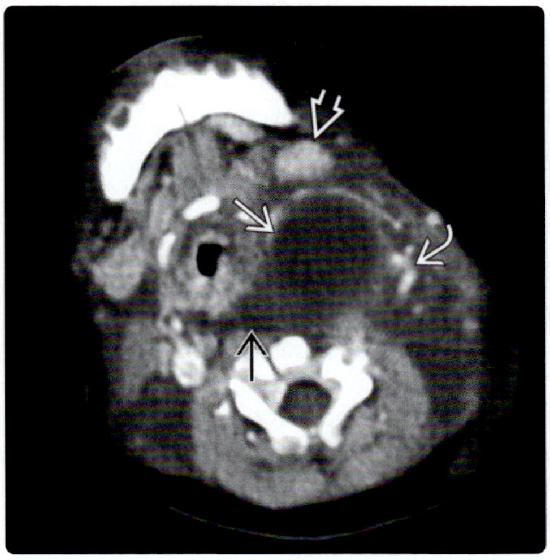

Cervical Thymic Cyst

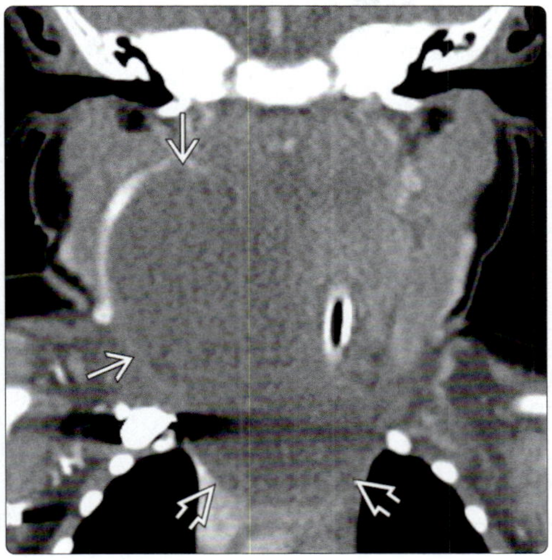

(Left) *Axial CECT reveals a large thymic cyst → posterior to the left submandibular gland →, anteromedial to the carotid vessels →, & extending to the retropharyngeal space →.* **(Right)** *Coronal CECT in an infant demonstrates a large, nonenhancing mass in the right neck → with inferior extension into the mediastinum →. This is the typical appearance of a cervical thymic cyst.*

4th Branchial Anomaly

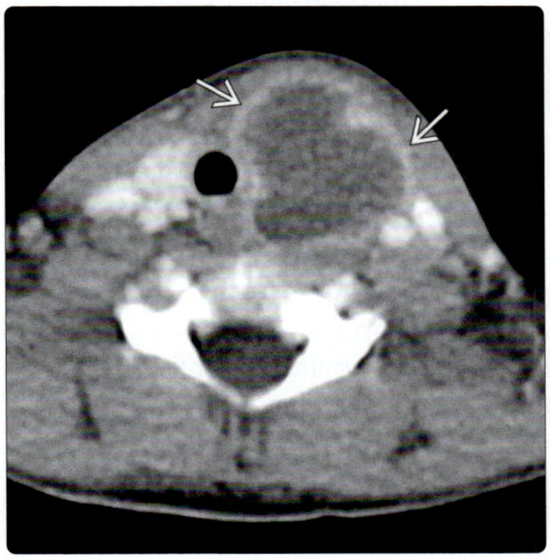

Lipoma

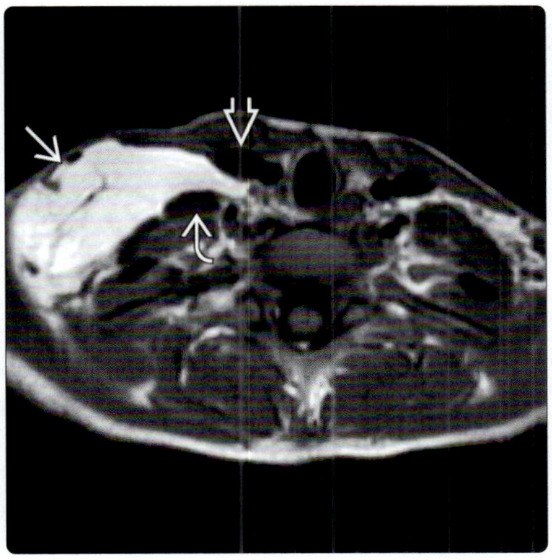

(Left) *Axial CECT in a child with an anterior neck mass demonstrates a left-sided, rim-enhancing abscess → replacing the left thyroid lobe. Inflammation extended to the left pyriform sinus (not included), & a sinus tract was proven at endoscopy.* **(Right)** *Axial T1 MR demonstrates a well-defined right posterior cervical space lipoma → insinuating between the internal jugular vein → & anterior scalene muscle →, resulting in mild leftward deviation of the trachea.*

Teratoma

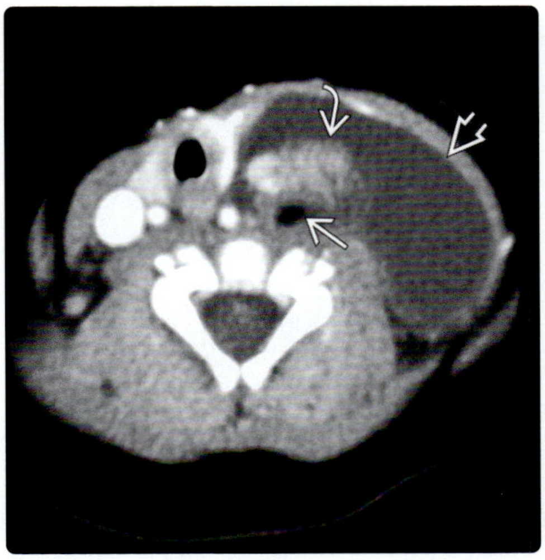

Fibrous Masses

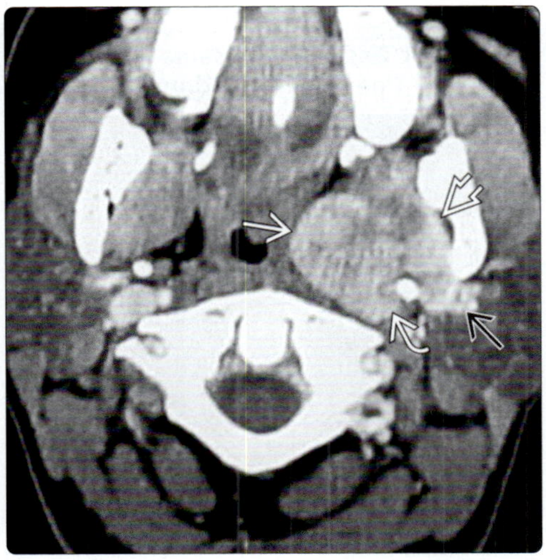

(Left) *Axial CECT shows a low-attenuation benign teratoma that contains fat → as well as cystic → & solid → components. The visceral, carotid, & posterior cervical spaces are all affected.* **(Right)** *Axial CECT reveals an enhancing mass of the left parapharyngeal space →, masticator space →, carotid space →, & deep parotid space →. A pathologic diagnosis of fibromatosis was made in this patient with Gardner syndrome.*

DIFFERENTIAL DIAGNOSIS

Common

- Soft Tissue Emphysema From Pneumomediastinum
- Trauma
- Retropharyngeal Abscess

Less Common

- Oral Cavity Abscess
- 4th Branchial Apparatus Anomaly

Rare but Important

- Laryngocele
- Esophagopharyngeal Diverticulum
- Lateral Cervical Esophageal Diverticulum

ESSENTIAL INFORMATION

Helpful Clues for Common Diagnoses

- **Soft Tissue Emphysema From Pneumomediastinum**
  - Forced Valsalva (during coughing, bronchospasm, or vomiting) → alveolar rupture → gas tracks in peribronchovascular interstitium to mediastinum → gas tracks along fascial planes into neck
  - Spontaneous pneumomediastinum (SPM) may be primary (with no known lung disease) or secondary (due to lung disease) but is typically self-limited
  - Imaging: Linear gas collections along fascial planes in mediastinum or neck; more irregular in chest wall
    - Esophagram generally not indicated for SPM
- **Trauma**
  - Internal or external penetrating injury may affect any portion of upper aerodigestive tract
    - May be accidental (e.g., fall on foreign body), inflicted (e.g., child abuse), or iatrogenic (e.g., traumatic intubation)
  - Blunt trauma may also lead to SPM
  - Imaging: Extraluminal air in neck tracking in fascial planes
    - ± laryngeal, hyoid, or facial fractures
    - Esophagram not indicated in blunt trauma without other chest findings (i.e., fractures, effusion, etc.)
- **Retropharyngeal Abscess**
  - Lies posterior to pharyngeal mucosal space & anterior to prevertebral space
  - Imaging: Extranodal fluid with rim enhancement & surrounding edema
    - ± gas in or adjacent to fluid collection
      - Gas is uncommon despite frequency of retropharyngeal abscess (RPA)
    - ± extension to mediastinum

Helpful Clues for Less Common Diagnoses

- **Oral Cavity Abscess**
  - Imaging: Rim-enhancing fluid collection, most commonly from dental infection
    - Look for bone defect around tooth
  - If gas is present, consider preceding intervention, gas-forming organisms, or necrotizing fasciitis (particularly if transspatial)
- **4th Branchial Apparatus Anomaly**
  - 4th pharyngeal pouch remnant
    - Extends from apex of pyriform sinus to lower neck, anterior to left thyroid lobe
    - Presents with recurrent thyroiditis or neck abscess
  - Imaging: Abscess anterior to left thyroid lobe
    - ± inflammatory change in ipsilateral thyroid lobe
    - Inflamed, airless pyriform sinus apex
    - May see fluid or air-filled sinus tract extending from pyriform apex to abscess

Helpful Clues for Rare Diagnoses

- **Laryngocele**
  - Imaging: Air-filled dilated laryngeal saccule (i.e., outpouching of laryngeal ventricle), ± air-fluid level
- **Esophagopharyngeal Diverticulum**
  - a.k.a., Zenker diverticulum
  - Imaging: Air-filled pouch posterior to esophagus; usually extends left of esophagus
    - Contrast filled on esophagram
- **Lateral Cervical Esophageal Diverticulum**
  - Imaging: Air-filled pouch lateral to cervical esophagus, usually left sided

Soft Tissue Emphysema From Pneumomediastinum

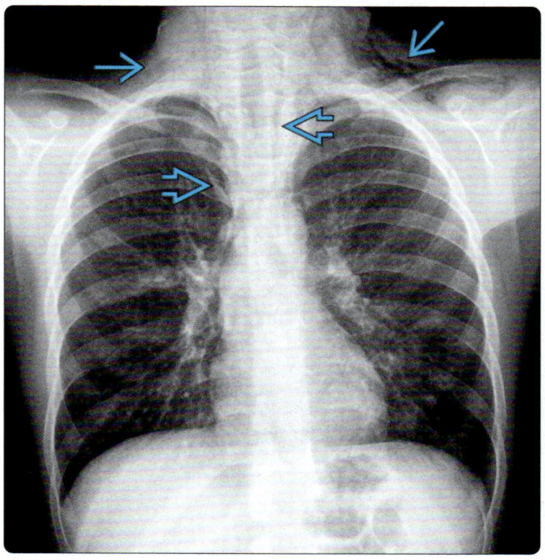

Soft Tissue Emphysema From Pneumomediastinum

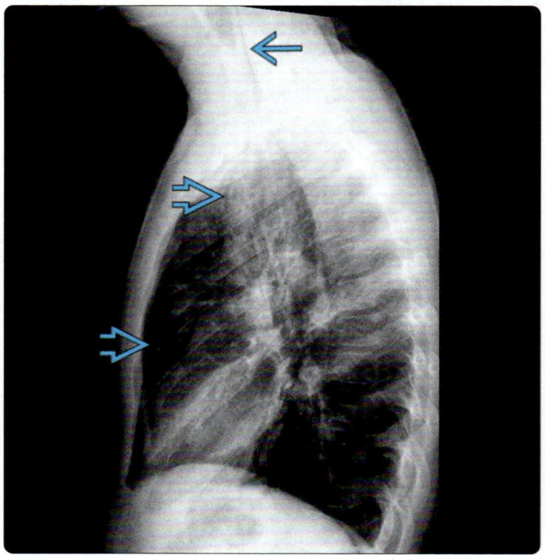

(Left) *AP chest radiograph in an 8 year old with neck swelling & chest pain after coughing shows linear foci of pneumomediastinum* ➯ *tracking into the neck & upper chest wall* ➔. **(Right)** *Lateral radiograph in the same patient shows pneumomediastinum* ➯ *tracking superiorly into the prevertebral soft tissues* ➔. *Spontaneous pneumomediastinum is typically self-limited.*

Trauma

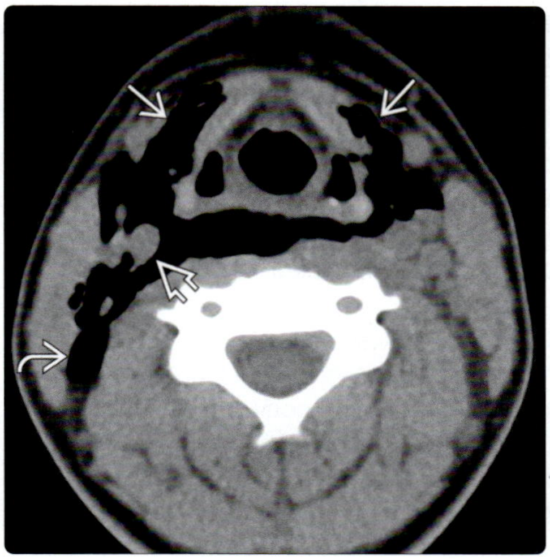

Retropharyngeal Abscess

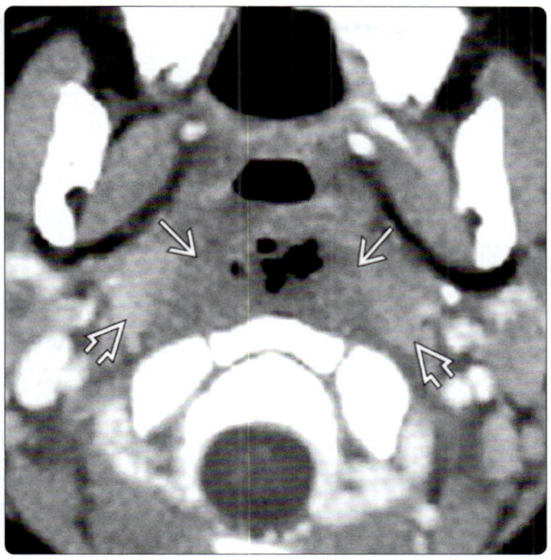

(Left) *Axial NECT in a child who was thrown from a horse shows extensive air throughout the neck, surrounding the larynx & right carotid vessels & extending into the posterior triangle.* **(Right)** *Axial CECT shows locules of gas within edematous retropharyngeal soft tissues secondary to a retropharyngeal space abscess (RPA). Note the ill-defined fat planes between this collection & the adjacent lateral retropharyngeal lymph nodes.*

Oral Cavity Abscess

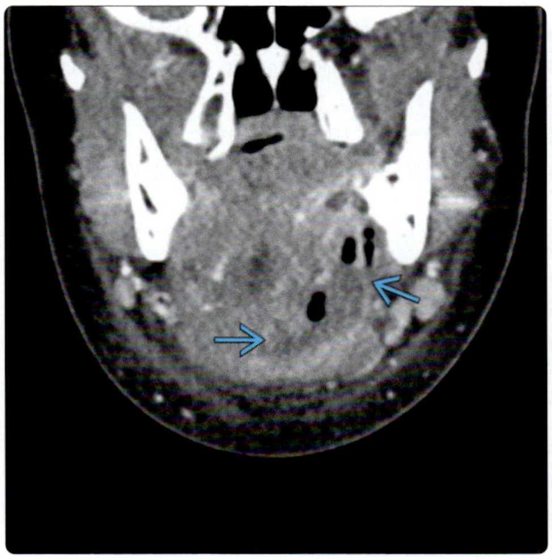

4th Branchial Apparatus Anomaly

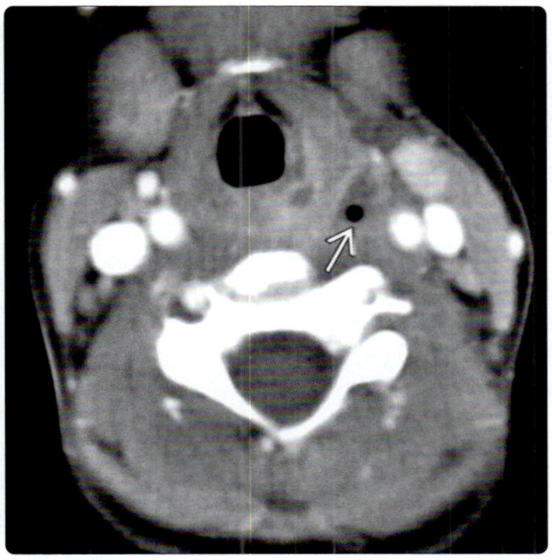

(Left) *Coronal CECT of the neck in a 12 year old with a recent root canal & new neck swelling shows a rim-enhancing, gas-containing abscess in the submandibular & sublingual spaces.* **(Right)** *Axial CECT in a 10 year old shows the superior extent of a gas-containing abscess that involved the left thyroid lobe (not shown). This abscess was due to a 4th branchial remnant sinus tract.*

Laryngocele

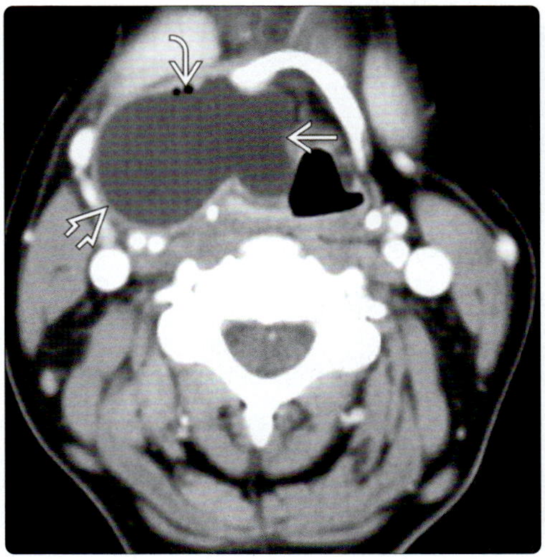

Lateral Cervical Esophageal Diverticulum

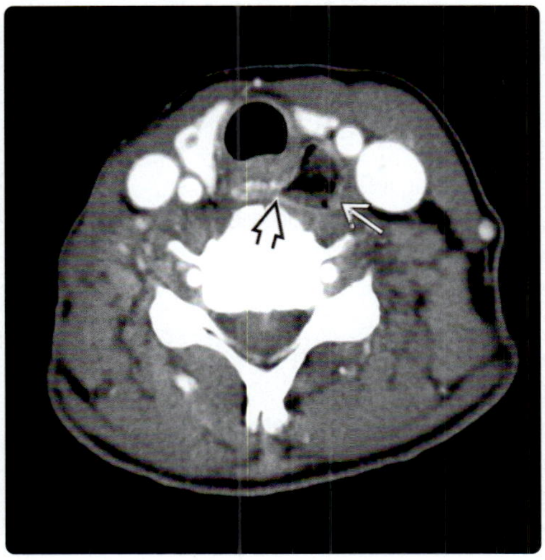

(Left) *Axial CECT shows a mixed laryngocele involving both the paraglottic space & the anterior neck, causing significant leftward deviation of the airway. The mass is primarily fluid filled but contains small bubbles of gas anteriorly.* **(Right)** *Axial CECT demonstrates a connection between the lateral esophageal wall & a lateral cervical diverticulum. The diverticulum is filled with air & debris. Both the esophagopharyngeal & lateral cervical esophageal diverticula are much more common in adults than children.*

DIFFERENTIAL DIAGNOSIS

Common

- Retinoblastoma
- Retinal Detachment

Less Common

- Retinopathy of Prematurity
- Coloboma
- Persistent Hyperplastic Primary Vitreous
- Coats Disease

Rare but Important

- Congenital Cataract
- Toxocariasis
- Ocular Melanoma
- Medulloepithelioma
- Retinal Dysplasia

ESSENTIAL INFORMATION

Key Differential Diagnosis Issues

- Leukocoria: White pupillary reflex
  - Due to abnormality between lens & retina preventing normal red pupillary reflex
  - Differential diagnosis is quite extensive

Helpful Clues for Common Diagnoses

- **Retinoblastoma**
  - Key facts: Primary retinal malignancy of primitive neuroectodermal tumor type
    - Most common childhood intraocular malignancy
    - Mean age of 18 months; > 90% by 5 years of age
    - 60% sporadic; 40% inherited
  - Imaging
    - Punctate, speckled, or flocculent Ca^{2+} in > 90%
    - Strong enhancement
    - Retinal detachment is not unusual
    - Unilateral in 75%
    - Look for coincident contralateral, suprasellar, or pineal tumor in patients with inherited disease
      - Trilateral: Bilateral ocular tumors + midline intracranial tumor (pineal > > suprasellar)
- **Retinal Detachment**
  - Key facts: Separation between inner sensory retina & outer pigmented epithelium
    - Many etiologies, including vascular, inflammatory, neoplastic, congenital, traumatic, & other processes
    - 3 mechanisms: Rhegmatogenous (tear), tractional (adhesions), & exudative (tumor or inflammation)
  - Imaging
    - Detached retina bulges toward vitreous with underlying biconvex collection
    - Leaves of retina converge at optic disc → V contour
    - Signal varies depending on content
      - Often bloody or proteinaceous fluid
      - Hyperintense on most MR sequences
      - Hyperdense on CT
    - May see evidence of treatment
      - Intraocular gas tamponade, scleral buckling procedure, encircling silicone sponge

Helpful Clues for Less Common Diagnoses

- **Retinopathy of Prematurity**
  - Key facts: Fibrovascular proliferation of immature retina, related to hyperoxia of extrauterine NICU environment
    - Synonym: Retrolental fibroplasia
  - Imaging
    - Microphthalmia + shallow anterior chamber
    - Retinal detachment is common
    - ± blood-fluid levels
    - Ca^{2+} is rare except in advanced stages (phthisis bulbi)
- **Coloboma**
  - Key facts: Incomplete closure of embryonic choroidal fissure
    - May involve iris, lens, ciliary body, retina, choroid, sclera, or optic nerve
    - Syndromic associations
      - CHARGE, trisomy 13 & trisomy 18, Aicardi syndrome, & branchiooculofacial syndrome
  - Imaging
    - Defect of posterior globe wall → vitreous outpouching
    - ± microphthalmia &/or secondary cyst
- **Persistent Hyperplastic Primary Vitreous (PHPV)**
  - Key facts: Failure of embryonic hyaloid vasculature to regress
    - Normally regresses at 7 months gestation
    - Bilateral is typically syndromic, e.g., Norrie-Warburg
  - Imaging
    - Microphthalmia
    - Enhancing retrolental hyaloid remnant + linear Cloquet canal (extending from dorsal lens to optic disc) resembles martini glass
      - Hyperdense on CT
      - ↓ T1 & T2 on MR
    - ± retinal detachment
    - ± vitreous hemorrhage
- **Coats Disease**
  - Key facts: Retinal telangiectasia
    - Subretinal exudate: Cholesterol crystals & lipid-laden macrophages → retinitis & detachment
    - M > F; peak age: 6-8 years
    - Unilateral in up to 90%
  - Imaging
    - Normal or small globe
    - Retinal detachment is sine qua non
    - Hyperdense exudate on CT
    - Hyperintense on T1& T2
    - Occasionally calcifies (~ 10%)

Helpful Clues for Rare Diagnoses

- **Congenital Cataract**
  - Key facts: Lens opacification from birth to 6 months of age
    - Bilateral cataracts are often syndromic
      - Genetic, metabolic, infectious, gestational, etc.
    - Best seen with direct visualization
  - Imaging
    - Small, hyperdense lens
      - Or absent lens after lens extraction
    - Lens may be spherical in shape (spherophakia), differentiating from acquired cataract

- **Toxocariasis**
  - Key facts: Immunoallergic reaction to antigens following larval death → sclerosing endophthalmitis with small eosinophilic abscess
    - Ocular disease months to years after initial ingestion of larvae, which then migrate from intestine to eye
      - *Toxocara canis/cati* (dog/cat roundworm)
  - Imaging
    - Enhancing granulomatous nodule posteriorly in eye with inflammatory & postinflammatory features
    - Uveoscleral thickening & nodularity
    - Subretinal exudate at site of larval infiltration, variable hyperintensity
- **Ocular Melanoma**
  - Key facts: Most common primary ocular malignancy in adults but uncommon in children
    - 85% of pediatric cases occur in 2nd decade of life
    - Uveal tract origin
      - Choroid > > ciliary body > iris
  - Imaging
    - US for initial evaluation & surveillance
      - Hypoechoic mass without Ca^{2+}
    - MR or CT to assess retrobulbar invasion
    - ↑ T1, ↓ T2 but depends on degree of pigmentation
      - Less intrinsic T1 signal when amelanotic
    - Lenticular, mound- or mushroom-shaped mass with moderate enhancement
    - Retinal detachment is common
- **Medulloepithelioma**
  - Key facts: Nonhereditary unilateral congenital neoplasm derived from primitive neuroepithelium
    - Most commonly involves ciliary body
      - Rarely optic nerve & retina
    - Malignant histology
      - Distant metastasis & mortality rare
    - Usually diagnosed in 1st decade, rarely in adults
  - Imaging
    - Mixed cystic & enhancing solid components ± dystrophic Ca^{2+}
    - Occasionally associated with PHPV
- **Retinal Dysplasia**
  - Key facts: Reduction or absence of retinal ganglion cells, nerve fibers, & blood vessels
    - Associated with syndromes, especially when bilateral
      - Trisomy 13, Walker-Warburg, Norrie disease
  - Imaging
    - Retinal detachment, hyperintense fluid
    - Variably enhancing dysplastic tissue

Alternative Differential Approaches

- Ca^{2+}
  - Present
    - Retinoblastoma (> 90%)
    - Late inflammatory or traumatic changes
  - Absent
    - Retinopathy of prematurity
    - Coloboma
    - PHPV
    - Coats disease
    - Toxocariasis
- Globe size
  - Normal
    - Retinoblastoma, except bulky tumor
    - Retinal detachment
    - Coats disease
    - Toxocariasis
  - Small
    - Retinopathy of prematurity
    - PHPV
    - Coloboma, with microphthalmia
    - Phthisis bulbi: Calcified, small globe (end-stage damage to globe) from any cause

SELECTED REFERENCES

1. Jansen RW et al: MR imaging features of retinoblastoma: association with gene expression profiles. Radiology. 288(2):506-15, 2018
2. Vachha BA et al: Imaging of pediatric orbital diseases. Neuroimaging Clin N Am. 25(3):477-501, 2015
3. Brennan RC et al: US and MRI of pediatric ocular masses with histopathological correlation. Pediatr Radiol. 42(6):738-49, 2012

Retinoblastoma

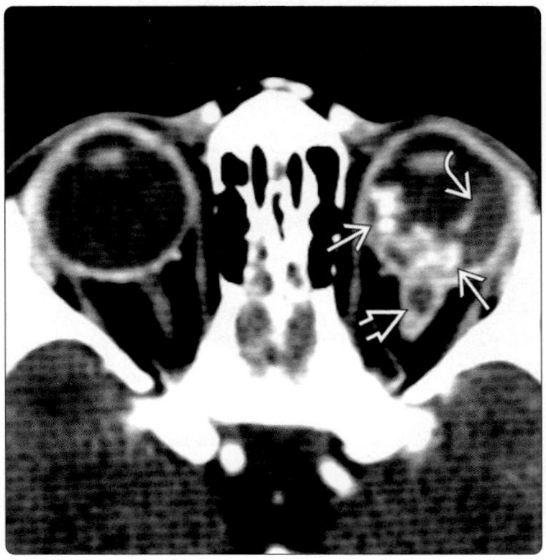

Retinoblastoma

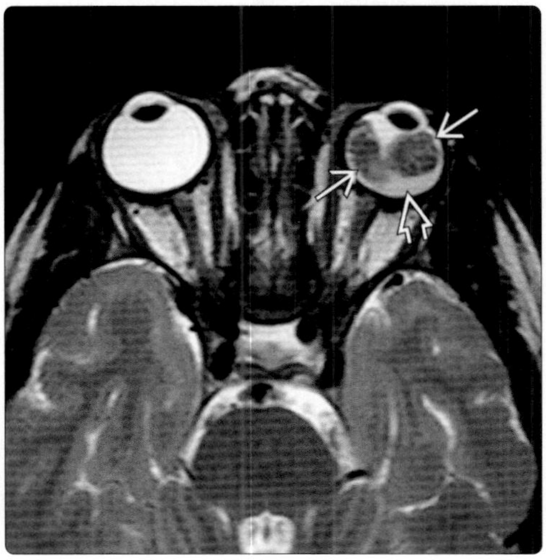

(Left) *Axial CECT in a young child with leukocoria demonstrates a heterogeneously calcified left intraocular mass ➡, characteristic of retinoblastoma. Note also the extraocular extension ➡ & associated retinal detachment ➡.* **(Right)** *Axial T2 MR in a 2 year old with leukocoria shows a large, lobulated left intraocular retinoblastoma ➡ with typical T2 hypointensity due to Ca^{2+} &/or dense cellularity. Mildly hyperintense T2 signal in the posterior globe ➡ represents retinal detachment.*

(**Left**) *Graphic shows a detached retina in the right eye →. The retinal attachment at the optic nerve head results in the characteristic V shape. By comparison, choroidal detachment typically has a lenticular contour, as demonstrated in the left eye →.* (**Right**) *Axial FLAIR MR in a child with retinal detachment demonstrates elevated inner retinal layers → & hyperintense signal within the hemorrhagic material.*

Retinal Detachment

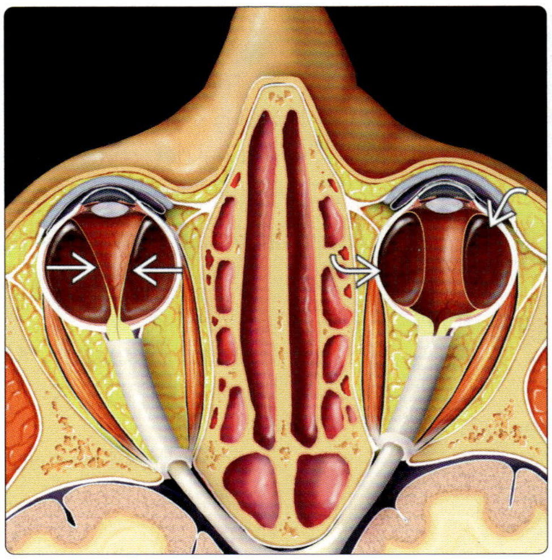

Retinal Detachment

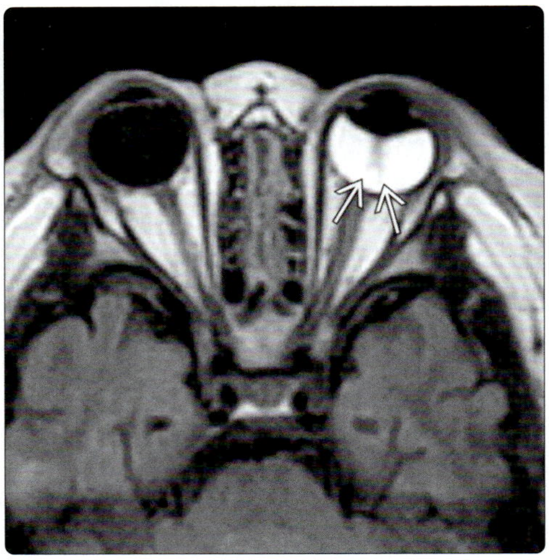

(**Left**) *Axial T2 FS MR shows bilateral microphthalmia with heterogeneous signal, including a blood-fluid level on the right →. Peripheral low signal → on the left represents Ca^{2+} from advanced disease.* (**Right**) *Axial T2 FS MR in a former premature infant shows bilateral microphthalmia. There is right choroidal detachment →. The linear signal on the left is due to apposed layers of nasal & temporal retinal detachment →. Complicated signal in each globe is due to blood products.*

Retinopathy of Prematurity

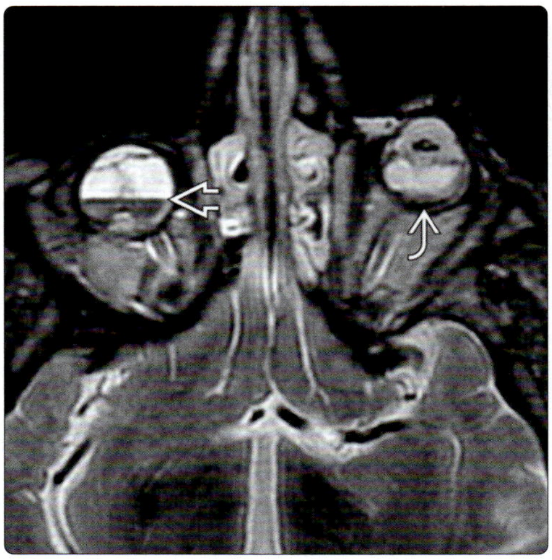

Retinopathy of Prematurity

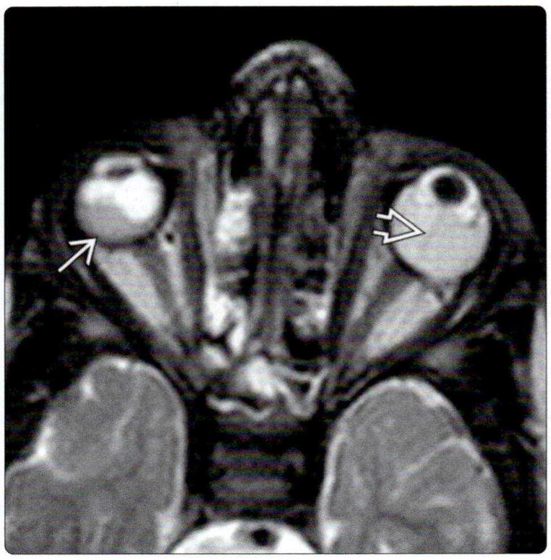

(**Left**) *Axial NECT shows an optic disc coloboma →, which is seen as dehiscence of the posterior globe through a broad defect centered at the location of the optic nerve head.* (**Right**) *Axial T1 C+ MR shows triangular retrolental enhancing tissue → & a stalk-like hyaloid remnant →, representing failure of involution of embryonic fibrovascular tissue. The contour of this tissue has been described as resembling a martini glass.*

Coloboma

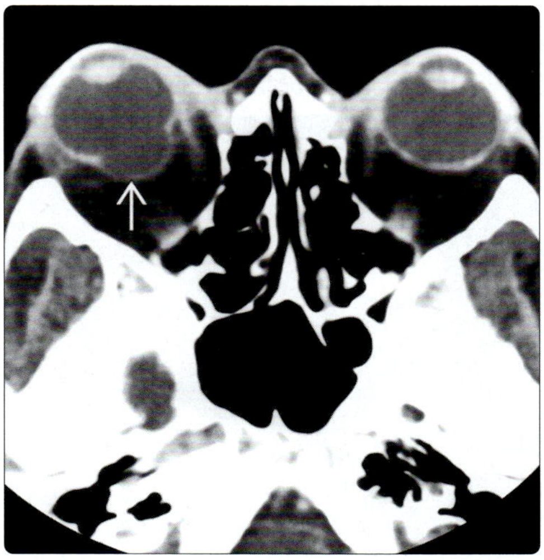

Persistent Hyperplastic Primary Vitreous

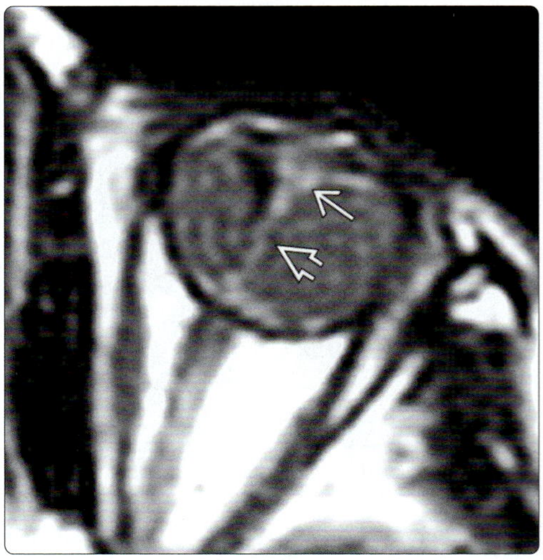

Coats Disease

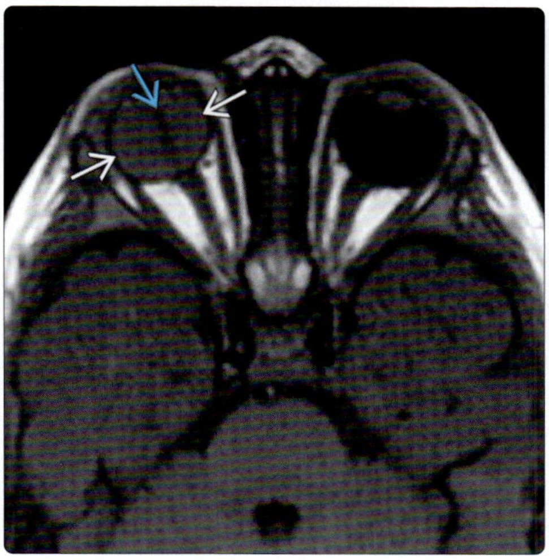

Congenital Cataract

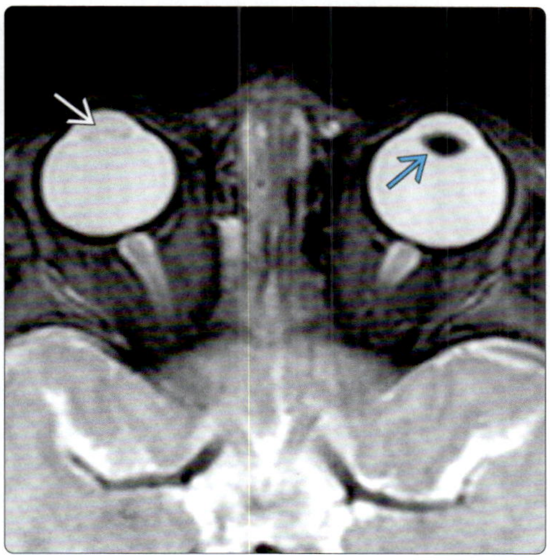

(Left) *Axial T1 MR in a child suspected clinically to have diffuse retinoblastoma shows mildly hyperintense subretinal exudates →, complete retinal detachment with inner layers opposed in the midline → (simulating PHPV), & decreased size of the involved globe, typical of Coats disease.* **(Right)** *Axial T2 MR in a 6 month old with a congenital cataract shows a typical postoperative appearance of the globe with an absent right lens → after extraction. Note the normal appearance of the contralateral left lens →.*

Toxocariasis

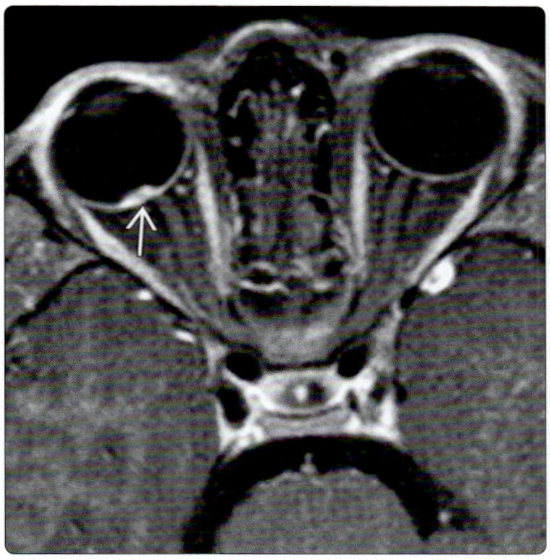

Ocular Melanoma

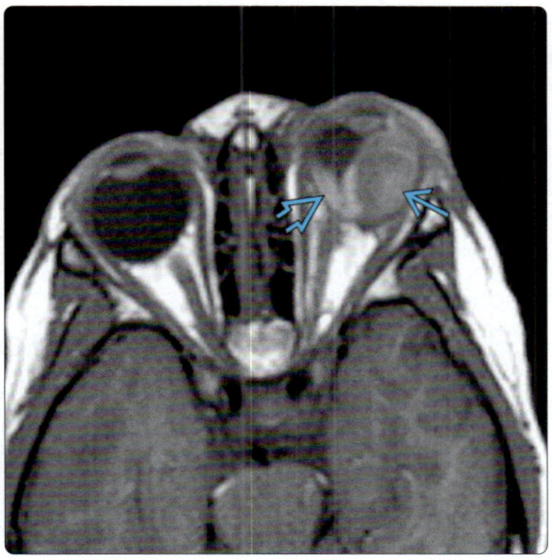

(Left) *Axial T1 C+ FS MR shows ocular toxocariasis manifesting as uveoscleral nodularity in the posterior aspect of the right globe →.* **(Right)** *Axial T1 MR in a 4 year old who presented with proptosis secondary to ocular melanoma shows a large, intraocular mass in the left globe with faint, hyperintense foci →. Overall, the lesion is not as hyperintense as the V-shaped, hemorrhagic retinal detachment →.*

Medulloepithelioma

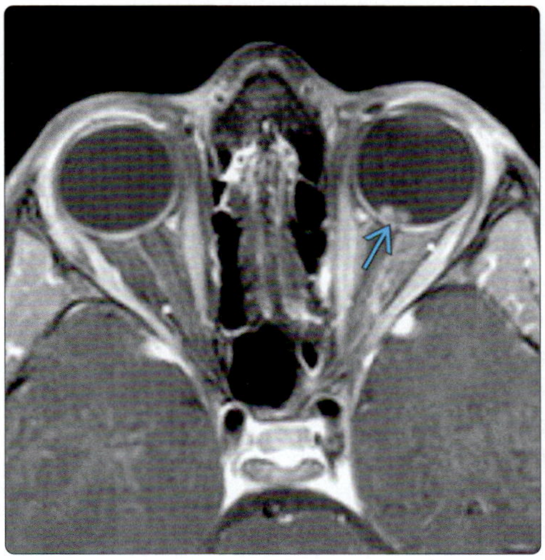

Retinal Dysplasia

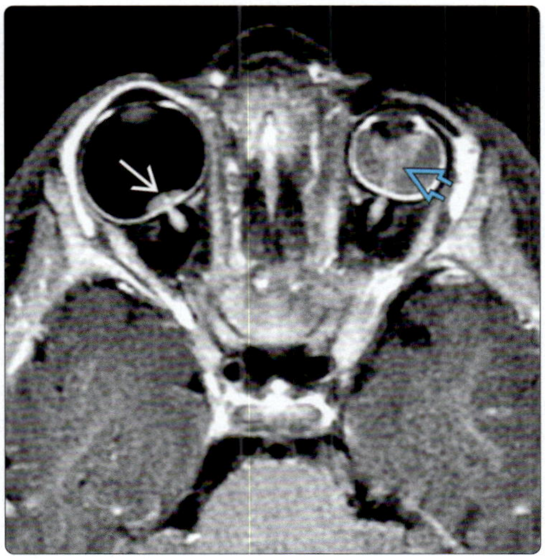

(Left) *Axial T1 C+ FS MR in a 6-year-old boy shows a lobulated, enhancing mass → at the level of the left optic disc, histologically proven to be medulloepithelioma. This is a rare lesion & most often involves the ciliary body.* **(Right)** *Axial T1 C+ FS MR in a child demonstrates right macrophthalmia with an enhancing tuft of dysplastic retinal tissue → overlying the optic disc. Note also the typical imaging appearance of the PHPV → involving the microphthalmic left globe.*

DIFFERENTIAL DIAGNOSIS

Common

- Retinoblastoma
- Persistent Hyperplastic Primary Vitreous
- Retinopathy of Prematurity
- Congenital Cataract

Less Common

- Coats Disease
- Coloboma
- Toxocariasis
- Microphthalmos

Rare but Important

- Retinal Astrocytoma
- Norrie Disease
- Walker-Warburg Syndrome

ESSENTIAL INFORMATION

Helpful Clues for Common Diagnoses

- **Retinoblastoma**
  - Key facts: Malignant tumor arising from neuroectodermal cells of retina
    - Classified as primitive neuroectodermal tumor
    - Most common intraocular tumor of childhood
    - Most common cause of leukocoria
    - Rare trilateral or quadrilateral forms: ~ 5-15% of familial lesions
      - Trilateral: Bilateral intraocular lesions + pineal
      - Quadrilateral: Bilateral intraocular lesions + pineal + suprasellar tumor
  - Imaging
    - Unilateral (70-75%)
    - CT: Punctate or speckled, calcified intraocular mass
      - CECT: Moderate to significant enhancement
    - MR: Mildly T1 hyperintense, moderately T2 hypointense
      - Moderate to marked heterogeneous enhancement
      - Extension of mass: Endophytic into vitreous or exophytic into subretinal space
    - Look for choroidal, scleral, & optic nerve involvement
- **Persistent Hyperplastic Primary Vitreous**
  - Key facts: Congenital lesion due to incomplete regression of embryonic vitreous & blood supply; normally regresses at 7-months gestation
    - 2nd most common cause of leukocoria
    - Most are unilateral & can involve anterior or posterior segments (~ 25%) or both (~ 50-80%)
    - Bilateral disease is typically syndromic
  - Imaging
    - Hyperdense or hyperintense small globe, no Ca^{2+}
    - Retrolental, enhancing soft tissue, classically with martini glass shape
      - Central linear tissue stalk of hyaloid remnant in vitreous
    - Vitreous may enhance
      - Ciliary body & lens may enhance in anterior form
    - Associated retinal detachments & vitreous hemorrhage are common
- **Retinopathy of Prematurity**
  - Key facts: Occurs due to prolonged exposure to supplemental oxygen in premature infants
    - Premature birth interrupts normal vasculogenesis → incomplete vascularization of retina → hypoxia → abnormal neovascularization
    - Incidence is ~ 20% in USA
    - Female, low birth weight, & gestational age are predictive of retinopathy of prematurity (ROP)
      - ~ 30% with weight birth weight of 750-1,000 g
  - Imaging: Usually bilateral
    - Hyperdense globe
    - Ocular detachments are common
    - Early: Microphthalmia + shallow anterior chamber
    - Advanced: Small, calcified globe (phthisis bulbi)
    - More severe ROP: ↓ myelination in optic radiations, internal & external capsules
- **Congenital Cataract**
  - Key facts: Lens opacification from birth to 6 months
    - Most are sporadic & unilateral
    - ~ 20% familial
    - ~ 17% associated with systemic disease or syndrome: Trisomy 21, craniofacial syndromes, diabetes, etc.
    - May occur with congenital rubella infection (TORCH)
    - Best seen with direct visualization
  - Imaging
    - Small lens
      - Or absent lens after lens extraction
    - Lens may assume spherical shape (spherophakia), differentiating from acquired cataract

Helpful Clues for Less Common Diagnoses

- **Coats Disease**
  - Key facts: Primary retinal vascular anomaly with retinal telangiectasis & exudative retinal detachment
    - Unilateral in 80-90%
    - Most patients are young males
  - Imaging
    - Advanced stages may appear to obliterate vitreous
    - CT: Mild diffusely & homogeneously hyperdense vitreous without Ca^{2+}
    - MR: Retinal detachment with nonenhancing T1 & T2 hyperintense subretinal exudate
    - Coats plus = cerebroretinal microangiopathy with Ca^{2+} & cysts
      - Rare syndrome of exudative retinopathy, leukodystrophy, Ca^{2+}, & parenchymal cysts
- **Coloboma**
  - Key facts: Defect in ocular tissue involving structures of embryonic cleft
    - Bilateral > unilateral
    - Posterior may involve optic disc or paramacular areas (chorioretinal)
    - Anterior may involve ciliary body, iris, lens, or eyelid
  - Imaging
    - Focal defect of posterior globe → vitreous outpouch
    - Defect at optic nerve head insertion with funnel-shaped excavation
    - Isodense or isointense to vitreous on CT & MR
    - May have retrobulbar cysts

- Related but distinct anomalies
  - ◻ Morning glory disc anomaly: Central, enhancing glial tissue in defect, isointense to white matter
  - ◻ Peripapillary staphyloma: Scleral defect at optic nerve head encircles optic disc
- **Toxocariasis**
  - Key facts: Eosinophilic granuloma caused by infection of larval nematode *Toxocara cani* or *cati*
  - Imaging
    - CT: Diffuse hyperdensity in vitreous ± discrete mass; no Ca^{2+}
    - MR: Enhancing, variable T1-hypo/isointense, T2-iso/hyperintense retrolental or vitreous mass
- **Microphthalmos**
  - Key facts: Corneal diameter of < 11 mm & anteroposterior diameter of globe < 20 mm at birth
    - Isolated or associated with craniofacial anomalies, coloboma, persistent hyperplastic primary vitreous (PHPV), ROP
  - Imaging
    - Overall volume & dimension of globe < unaffected side
    - Simple microphthalmia, i.e., structurally normal but small eye, vs. complex with associated findings

Helpful Clues for Rare Diagnoses

- **Retinal Astrocytoma**
  - Key facts: Retinal astrocytic hamartoma is ocular manifestation of tuberous sclerosis complex
  - Imaging
    - Enhancing exophytic juxtapapillary or epipapillary retinal mass
    - Mass may be multifocal ± bilateral
    - Rarely may occur in isolation without tuberous sclerosis complex
- **Norrie Disease**
  - Key facts: X-linked recessive syndrome of retinal malformation, deafness, & mental retardation
  - Imaging
    - Bilateral hyperdense vitreous, small anterior chamber
    - Small lens without Ca^{2+}
    - May have associated retrolental mass, retinal detachment, microphthalmia, optic nerve atrophy
- **Walker-Warburg Syndrome**
  - Key facts: Muscle, brain, & eye abnormalities
    - a.k.a HARD+E = **h**ydrocephaly, **a**gyria, **r**etinal **d**etachment ± **e**ncephalocele
    - a.k.a cerebroocular dysplasia-muscular dystrophy syndrome
  - Imaging
    - Ocular abnormalities are variable
      - ◻ PHPV, microphthalmia, retinal dysplasia, coloboma, buphthalmos, glaucoma
      - ◻ ± retinal detachment, vitreous hemorrhage
    - Associated hydrocephalus, agyria/dysgenesis of cerebral & cerebellar gray & white matter
    - Z-shaped or kinked brainstem

SELECTED REFERENCES

1. Dimaras H et al: Retinoblastoma, the visible CNS tumor: A review. J Neurosci Res. 97(1):29-44, 2018
2. Ludwig CA et al: The epidemiology of retinopathy of prematurity in the United States. Ophthalmic Surg Lasers Imaging Retina. 48(7):553-62, 2017
3. Hodgson N et al: Ophthalmic manifestations of tuberous sclerosis: a review. Clin Exp Ophthalmol. 45(1):81-86, 2017
4. Whitehead MT et al: Normal developmental globe morphology on fetal MR imaging. AJNR Am J Neuroradiol. 37(9):1733-7, 2016
5. Grosso A et al: Pearls and pitfalls in diagnosis and management of coats disease. Retina. 35(4):614-23, 2015
6. Vachha BA et al: Imaging of pediatric orbital diseases. Neuroimaging Clin N Am. 25(3):477-501, 2015
7. Burns NS et al: Diagnostic imaging of fetal and pediatric orbital abnormalities. AJR Am J Roentgenol. 201(6):W797-808, 2013
8. Chung EM et al: From the archives of the AFIP: Pediatric orbit tumors and tumorlike lesions: neuroepithelial lesions of the ocular globe and optic nerve. Radiographics. 27(4):1159-86, 2007

Retinoblastoma

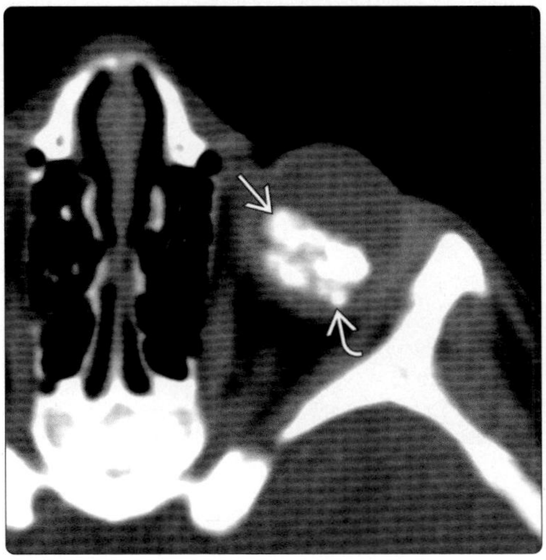

Retinoblastoma

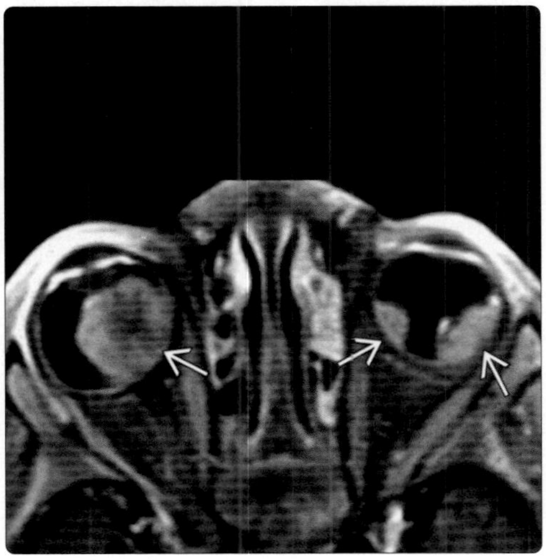

(Left) *Axial NECT in an infant with leukocoria shows coarse Ca^{2+} ➡ typical of retinoblastoma in the posterior segment of the right globe. These involve the vitreous body as well as the choroidal-retinal layers ➡.* **(Right)** *Axial T1 C+ FS MR in an infant with bilateral leukocoria shows enhancing bilateral retinal masses ➡ extending into the vitreous. There is no evidence of extension beyond the sclera into the optic nerve or intraconal orbit. Bilateral lesions are usually inherited.*

Persistent Hyperplastic Primary Vitreous

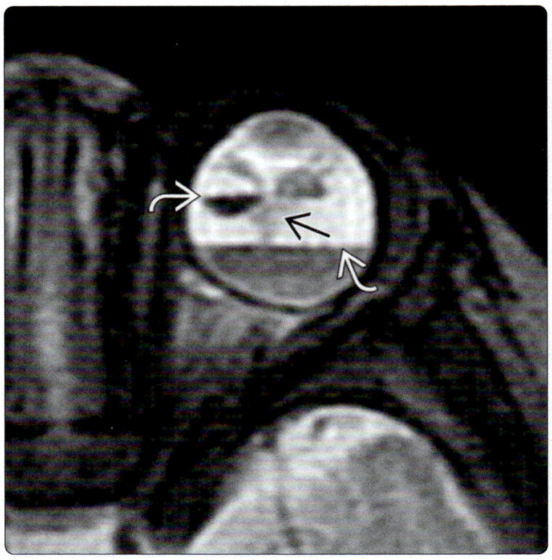

Persistent Hyperplastic Primary Vitreous

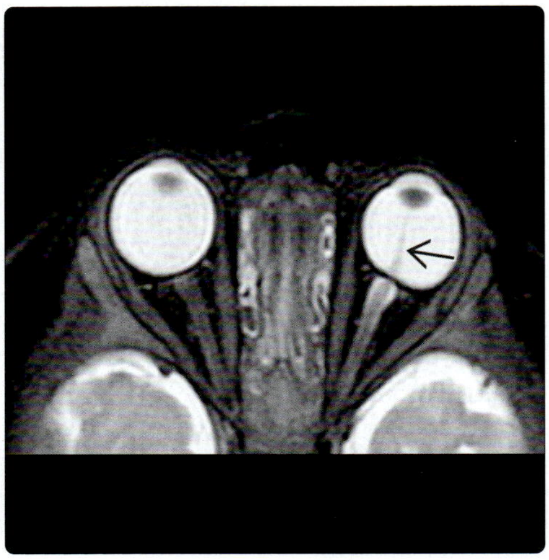

(Left) *Axial T2 FS MR reveals a hypointense, retrolental, martini glass-shaped mass with associated fluid-fluid levels in the vitreous, consistent with persistent hyperplastic primary vitreous (PHPV). This diagnosis can be difficult to make in a globe complicated by ocular detachments.* **(Right)** *Axial T2 FS MR shows a linear soft tissue band extending from the posterior aspect of the lens capsule to the optic disc. This corresponds to the hyaloid channel. The globe is small, as is usually seen in patients with PHPV.*

Retinopathy of Prematurity

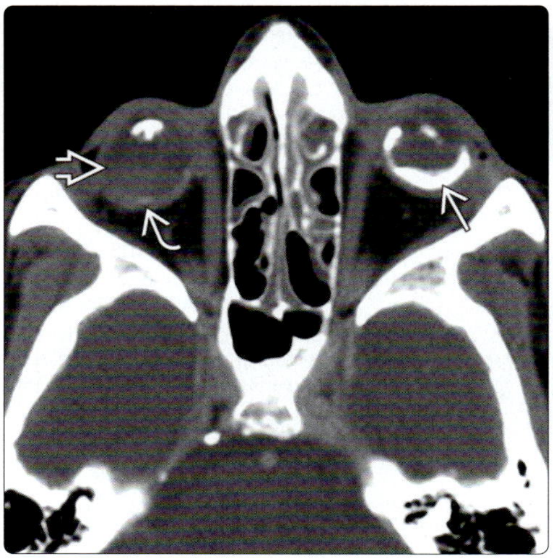

Retinopathy of Prematurity

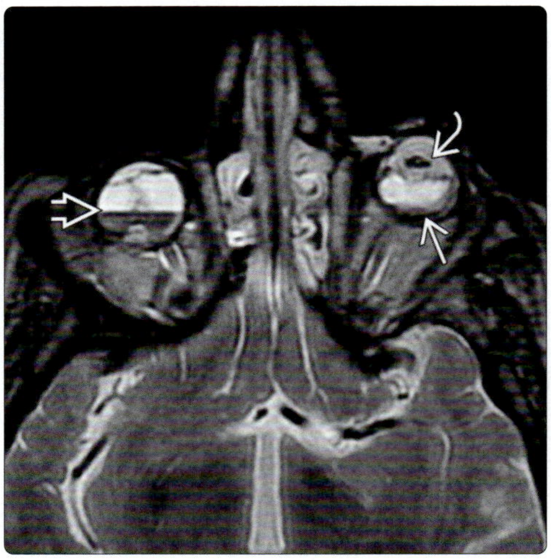

(Left) *Axial CECT in a formerly premature infant shows bilateral microphthalmia. The left globe contains dense peripheral Ca^{2+}. The right globe shows more punctate, scattered Ca^{2+} & a fluid-fluid level, indicating vitreous hemorrhage.* **(Right)** *Axial T2 MR in the same patient reveals a fluid-fluid level & peripheral low signal intensity from dense Ca^{2+}. Note the deformed, low signal intensity calcified lens.*

Congenital Cataract

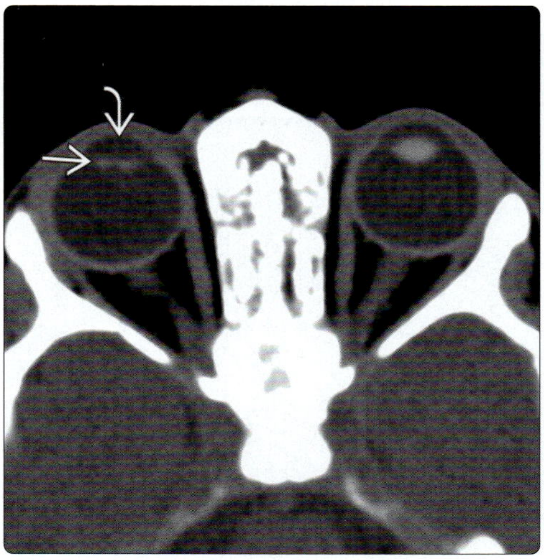

Coats Disease

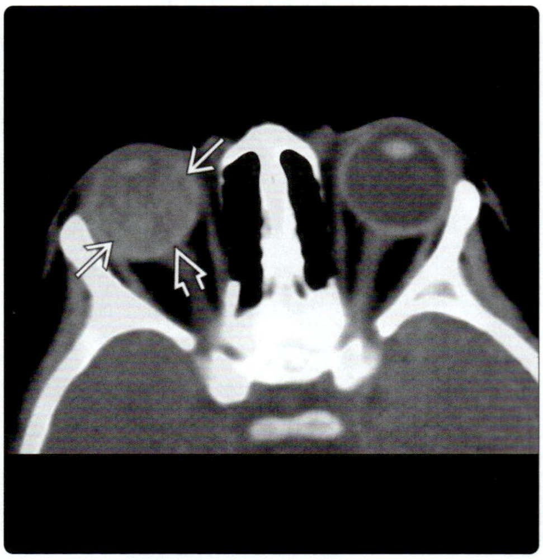

(Left) *Axial NECT in a child with leukocoria shows significant thinning & loss of density of the right lens with increased depth of the anterior chamber compared to the opposite normal left globe.* **(Right)** *Axial NECT in a young male patient without trauma or surgery shows medial & lateral hyperdensities, suggesting vitreous hemorrhage. However, the central linear hypodensity represents the apposed inner layers of retina in the midline secondary to subretinal hemorrhage. Note the absence of Ca^{2+}.*

Coloboma

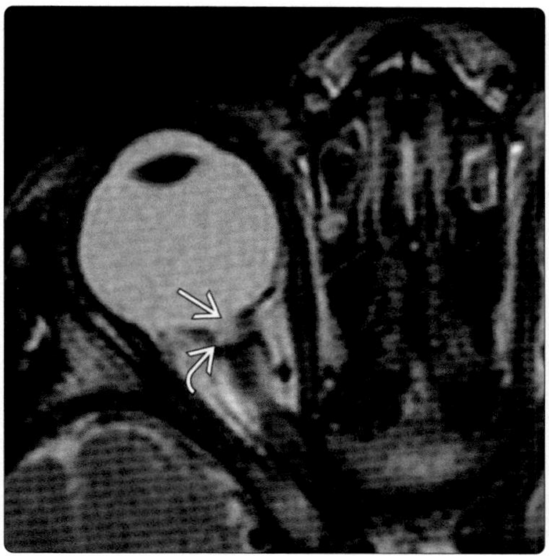

Toxocariasis

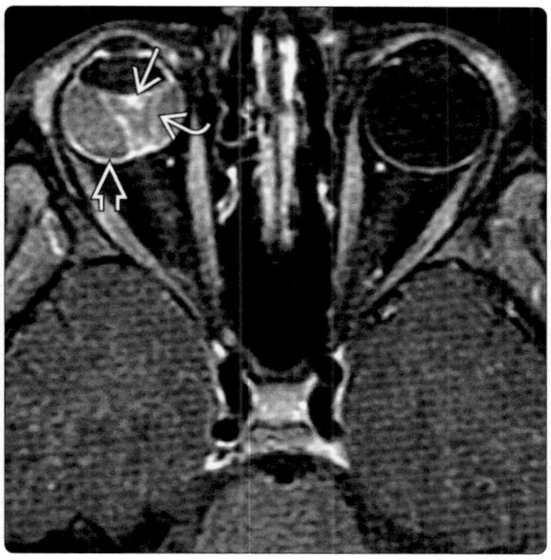

(Left) **(Left)** *Axial T2 MR shows a defect of the posterior sclera ➡ with posterior extension of the vitreous ➡. The defect & associated vitreous outpouching are oriented along the long axis of the globe, typical of a coloboma.* **(Right)** *Axial T1 C+ FS MR demonstrates hyperintensity of the small right globe vitreous with an enhancing retrolental mass ➡, retinal detachments ➡, & hypointense retinal & scleral nodules ➡. Noncalcified nodules & retinal detachments are typical of this granulomatous infection.*

Microphthalmos

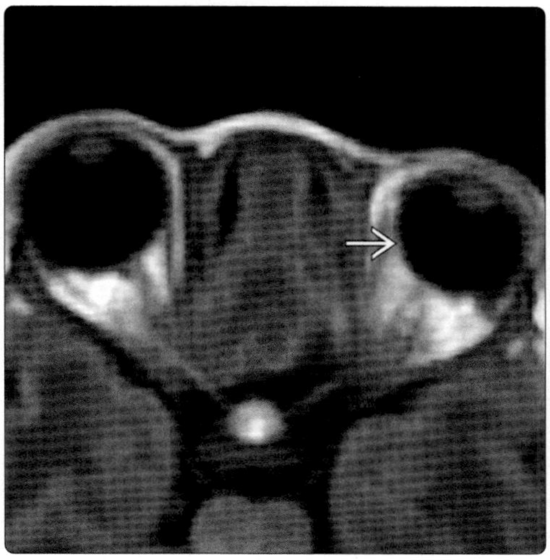

Retinal Astrocytoma

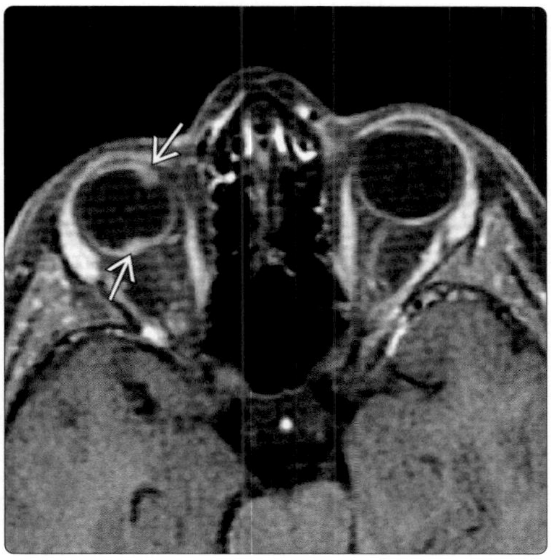

(Left) *Axial T1 MR shows a normal right globe & a microphthalmic left globe ➡ with an otherwise normal lens, vitreous body, & choroidal-retinal layers.* **(Right)** *Axial T1 C+ FS MR reveals a microphthalmic right globe with enhancing nodular retinal astrocytomas ➡ in a child with tuberous sclerosis. In the absence of tuberous sclerosis, multifocal retinoblastoma could have a similar appearance (though the globe size is usually normal).*

Norrie Disease

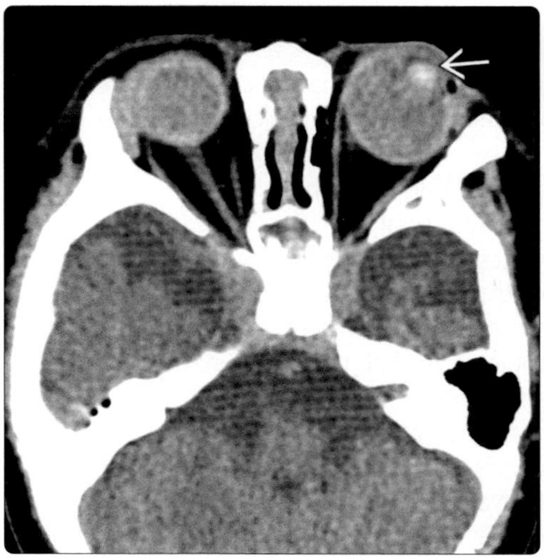

Walker-Warburg Syndrome

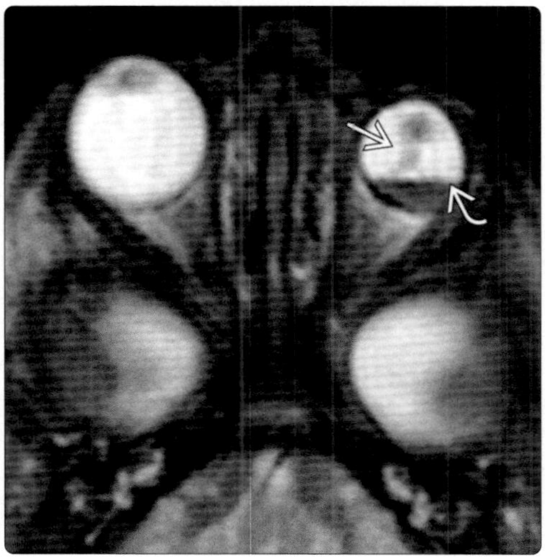

(Left) *Axial NECT shows a bilateral abnormal increase in globe density. The left globe & orbit are enlarged with a decrease in size of the anterior chamber ➡. Norrie disease is diagnosed clinically when grayish-yellow fibrovascular masses are found in the globes of an infant.* **(Right)** *Axial T2 MR in an infant with Walker-Warburg syndrome shows a microphthalmic left eye, a linear retrolental T2-hypointense structure (that represents PHPV) ➡, & a fluid-fluid level secondary to vitreous hemorrhage ➡.*

DIFFERENTIAL DIAGNOSIS

Common

- Orbital Trauma
- Retinopathy of Prematurity
- Ocular Detachment
- Coloboma

Less Common

- Persistent Hyperplastic Primary Vitreous
- Congenital Microphthalmos

Rare but Important

- Toxocariasis
- Other Orbital Infections

ESSENTIAL INFORMATION

Key Differential Diagnosis Issues

- Knowledge of globe anatomy is crucial
- Anterior segment of globe = anterior to anterior margin of vitreous
  - Ciliary body, suspensory ligaments, & lens
  - Anterior & posterior chambers
  - Iris & cornea
- Posterior segment of globe
  - Vitreoretinal portion of eye & its layers
    - Vitreous chamber, retina, choroid, sclera
- Anterior chamber
  - Major chamber of anterior segment
  - Between cornea & iris
  - Filled with aqueous humor for nutrition & structure
- Posterior chamber
  - Small potential space posterior to iris & anterior to lens/ligament complex
  - Contiguous with anterior chamber through pupil
- Vitreous chamber
  - Large chamber that fills posterior segment
  - Filled with viscoelastic transparent gel
- Tunicae
  - Tunica interna (retina), vasculosa (uvea), fibrosa (sclera)

Helpful Clues for Common Diagnoses

- **Orbital Trauma**
  - Key facts
    - Blunt or penetrating injury may lead to ocular damage
  - Imaging
    - Hyperdensity in vitreous body or at level of hemorrhagic ocular detachment
    - ± globe rupture, intraocular gas, shattered or dislocated lens
    - ± foreign body
      - BB is common; wood may be similar to air or of intermediate attenuation
    - Posterior scleral rupture may cause deep anterior chamber
- **Retinopathy of Prematurity**
  - Key facts
    - Vasculoproliferative disorder in low-birth-weight premature infants secondary to prolonged exposure to supplemental oxygen
      - Premature birth interrupts normal vasculogenesis → incomplete vascularization of retina → hypoxia → abnormal neovascularization
  - Imaging
    - Bilateral microphthalmos, hyperdense globes
    - Noncalcified, retrolental mass = retinal detachment
    - ± Ca^{2+} as late finding
- **Ocular Detachment**
  - Key facts
    - 3 potential spaces/ocular detachments
      - Posterior hyaloid (between posterior hyaloid membrane & inner sensory retina)
      - Subretinal (between inner sensory retina & outer retinal pigmented epithelium)
      - Posterior choroidal (between choroid & sclera)
    - Many causes: Traumatic, spontaneous, persistent hyperplastic primary vitreous (PHPV), retinopathy of prematurity, ocular masses, Coats disease, or infection
  - Imaging
    - Posterior hyaloid = posterior C-shaped density crossing midline
    - Retinal = V-shaped density converging at optic disc
      - Total retinal detachment may simulate PHPV
    - Choroidal = lenticular-shaped peripheral opacities
      - Usually nasal or temporal aspect of globe
    - ± microphthalmos
- **Coloboma**
  - Key facts
    - Gap or defect of ocular tissue; may involve any structures of embryonic cleft
      - Commonly familial & may occur with other congenital malformations
    - 2 types of posterior coloboma
      - Optic disc coloboma: Confined to optic disc
      - Chorioretinal coloboma: Separate from or extends beyond disc, arises from globe wall
    - 2 distinct entities frequently confused with coloboma
      - Morning glory disc anomaly: Funnel-shaped excavation in posterior globe that incorporates optic disc; central tuft of glial tissue within defect; usually sporadic, may be associated with other congenital anomalies
      - Peripapillary staphyloma: Congenital scleral defect at optic nerve head; nearly all unilateral
  - Imaging
    - Focal outpouching of vitreous
    - Bilateral or unilateral
    - Usually occurs with microphthalmos, rarely with macrophthalmos
    - ± optic tract & chiasm atrophy
    - ± retrobulbar cyst that may communicate with globe
    - Sclera enhances
    - Rarely has dystrophic Ca^{2+} at margins
    - ± other abnormalities if associated with syndromes (Meckel, Walker-Warburg, Aicardi, CHARGE), basal cephaloceles, midline facial clefting

Helpful Clues for Less Common Diagnoses

- **Persistent Hyperplastic Primary Vitreous**
  - Key facts

- Remnants of primary vitreous & primitive hyaloid artery (failure of involution) occur along course of Cloquet canal: Anterior, posterior, or both (most common)
- 2nd most common cause of leukocoria after retinoblastoma
- Unilateral is usually sporadic; bilateral is more common with syndromes (Walker-Warburg, Norrie)
  - Imaging
    - Noncalcified, tubular, cylindrical, or triangular-shaped enhancing tissue within vitreous compartment
    - Microphthalmos; retinal detachment ± ↑ attenuation of entire vitreous body is common
    - Small dysplastic lens & shallow anterior chamber with anterior Cloquet canal involvement
- **Congenital Microphthalmos**
  - Key facts
    - Microphthalmos: Eye < 2/3 normal size or < 16-mm axial dimension
      - Associated with coloboma in fetal alcohol syndrome, ring 14 & 14q terminal deletion syndromes, & many other genetic abnormalities
    - Anophthalmia: Complete absence of globe or only vestigial remnant
    - Genetic basis is now identifiable in up to 30%
  - Imaging
    - Small globe; unilateral or bilateral
    - ± intracranial structural abnormalities
      - More common in bilateral microphthalmos
    - ± coloboma or cyst

Helpful Clues for Rare Diagnoses

- **Toxocariasis**
  - Key facts
    - Inflammatory response to nematode *Toxocara canis* causes chorioretinitis
    - Granulomatous inflammation surrounds dead larvae
    - May appear as focal posterior or peripheral retinal granuloma
    - Most commonly unilateral
  - Imaging
    - Focal or diffuse thickening & enhancement of globe
    - Retinal detachment may be associated
    - ↑ attenuation/intensity of vitreous is possible
- **Other Orbital Infections**
  - Key facts
    - Viral [herpes simplex, herpes zoster, CMV, rubella, rubeola, mumps, Epstein-Barr virus (EBV)]
    - Bacterial (syphilis, Lyme, brucellosis, cat-scratch disease, *Escherichia coli*)
    - Fungal (candidiasis) or parasitic (*T. canis*)
    - Most patients are not imaged
    - Most are treated without sequelae of microphthalmos
  - Imaging
    - Thickened, enhancing sclera (scleritis)
    - Thickened, enhancing uvea (uveitis)
    - ↑ attenuation/signal of vitreous secondary to ↑ protein; ± uveitis, ± ocular detachment in endophthalmitis
    - Endophthalmitis: Intraocular infectious or inflammatory process involving vitreous cavity or anterior chamber

Other Essential Information

- End-stage damage to globe from any cause may lead to phthisis bulbi (calcified, small globe)

SELECTED REFERENCES

1. Nguyen VD et al: Demystifying orbital emergencies: a pictorial review. Radiographics. 37(3):947-62, 2017
2. Plaisancie J et al: Genetic advances in microphthalmia. J Pediatr Genet. 5(4):184-8, 2016
3. Vachha BA et al: Imaging of pediatric orbital diseases. Neuroimaging Clin N Am. 25(3):477-501, 2015
4. Williamson KA et al: The genetic architecture of microphthalmia, anophthalmia and coloboma. Eur J Med Genet. 57(8):369-80, 2014

Orbital Trauma

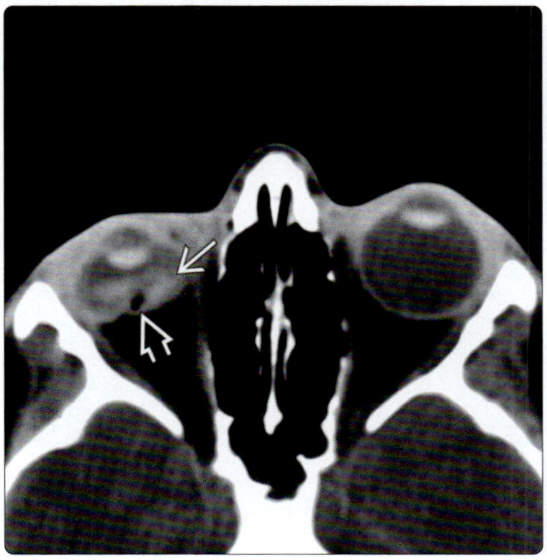

Orbital Trauma

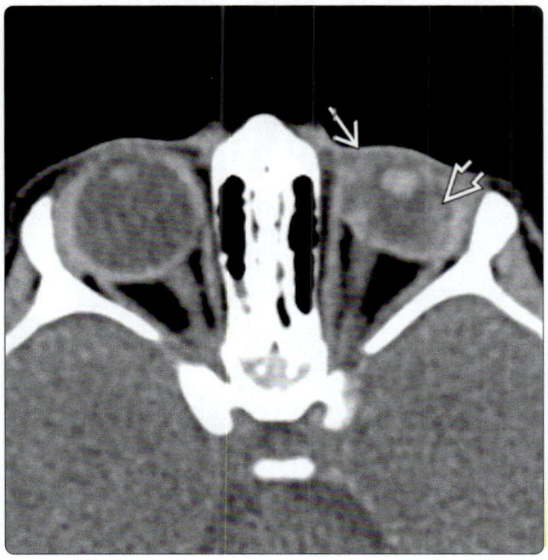

(Left) *Axial NECT shows posttraumatic rupture of the right globe with a decreased volume of the vitreous cavity & high-attenuation vitreous hemorrhage ➡. Note also a small posterior bubble of intraocular gas ➡ in this child with prior penetrating injury.* **(Right)** *Axial NECT in a 2 year old accidentally struck with a plastic projectile demonstrates a ruptured, small-volume left globe ➡ with a high-attenuation vitreous hemorrhage ➡ & a mildly rotated ocular lens.*

(Left) *Axial T2 MR in an infant born prematurely demonstrates bilateral, right > left microphthalmos with hyperintense proteinaceous fluid nearly obliterating each vitreous cavity.* **(Right)** *Axial NECT demonstrates right microphthalmos with a crescent-shaped posterior hyaloid detachment* → *secondary to hemorrhage between the posterior hyaloid membrane & the inner sensory layer of retina.*

Retinopathy of Prematurity

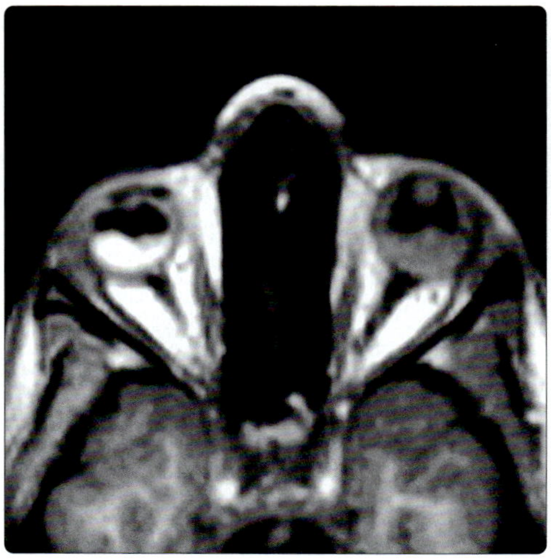

Ocular Detachment

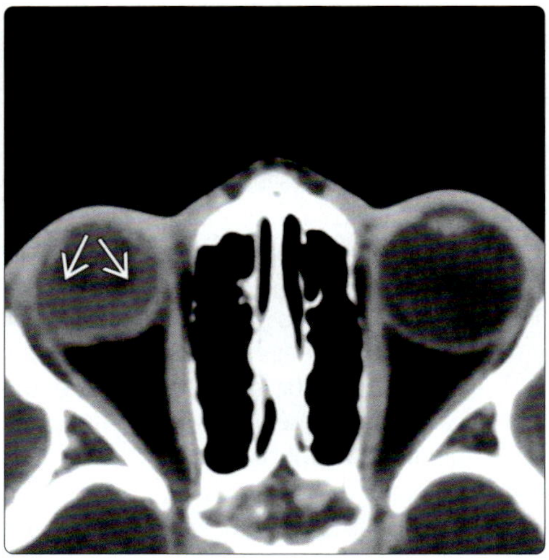

(Left) *Axial FLAIR MR reveals a small, hyperintense right globe with near-complete retinal detachment* →*, obliterating the vitreous cavity. Retinal detachment occurs between the inner sensory & outer pigmented layers of retina.* **(Right)** *Axial NECT shows a small misshapen left globe with the typical appearance of nasal & temporal areas of posterior choroidal detachment* → *secondary to hemorrhage between the choroid & sclera.*

Ocular Detachment

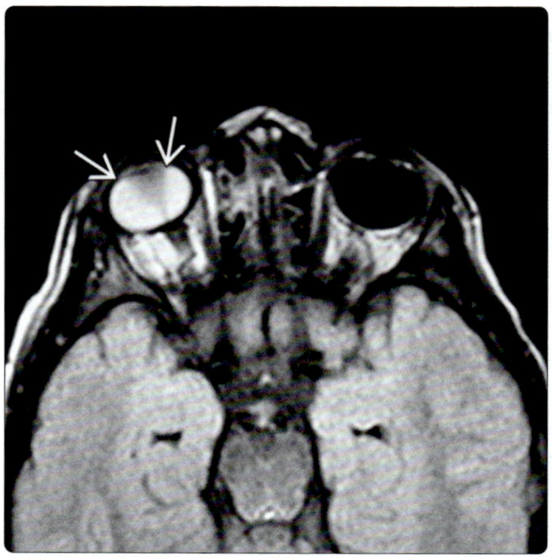

Ocular Detachment

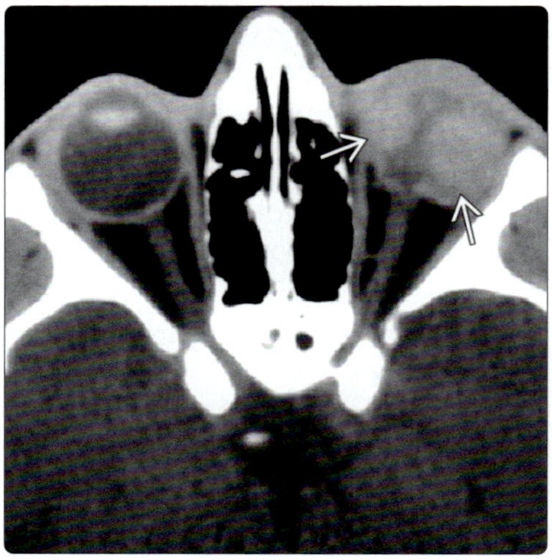

(Left) *Axial NECT shows bilateral microphthalmos with bilateral optic disc colobomas* →*. Note the large, left-sided retrobulbar colobomatous cyst* →*.* **(Right)** *Axial T1 C+ FS MR demonstrates a small left globe with a Y-shaped enhancing tuft* → *representing the hyaloid remnant & hyperintense, nonenhancing fluid in layers of near-complete retinal detachment* →*. Note also the right macrophthalmos with posterior enhancement* → *that by clinical exam was thought to represent retinal dysplasia.*

Coloboma

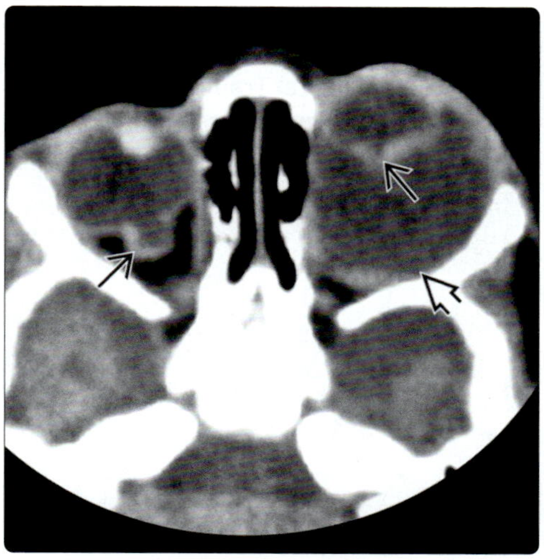

Persistent Hyperplastic Primary Vitreous

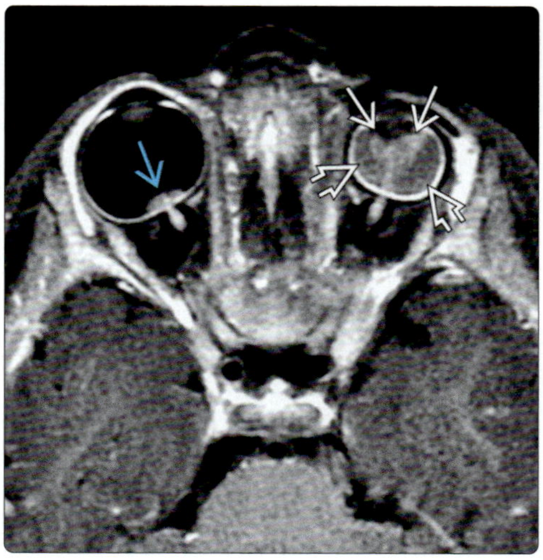

Congenital Microphthalmos

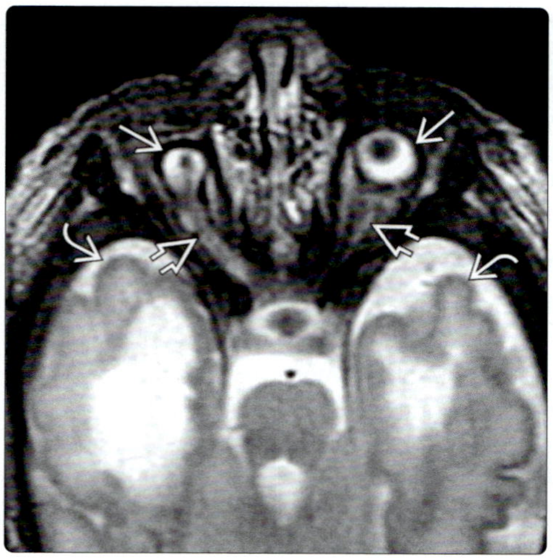

Congenital Microphthalmos

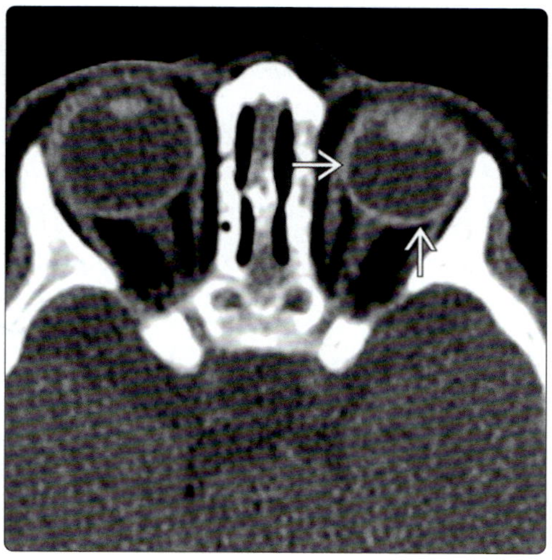

(Left) *Axial T2 MR in an infant with multiple congenital anomalies shows severe bilateral microphthalmos ➡, right > left, with only diminutive remnants of globes, a diminutive right-sided lens, & left > right optic nerve hypoplasia ➡. Note also the diffuse bilateral cortical migration anomalies ➡ & ventriculomegaly.* **(Right)** *Axial NECT in a 7-month-old child demonstrates moderate left-sided congenital microphthalmos ➡.*

Congenital Microphthalmos

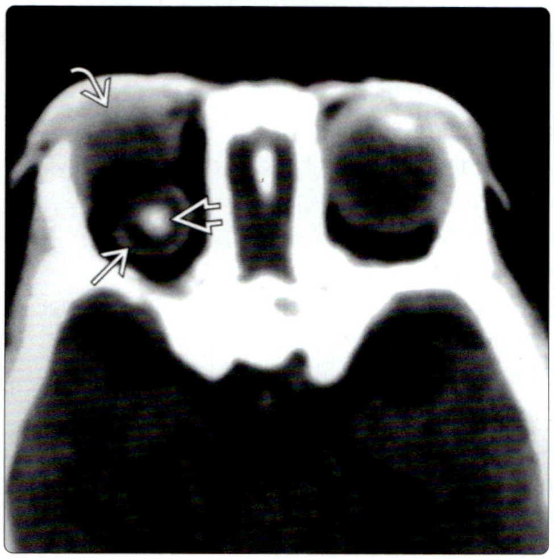

Congenital Microphthalmos

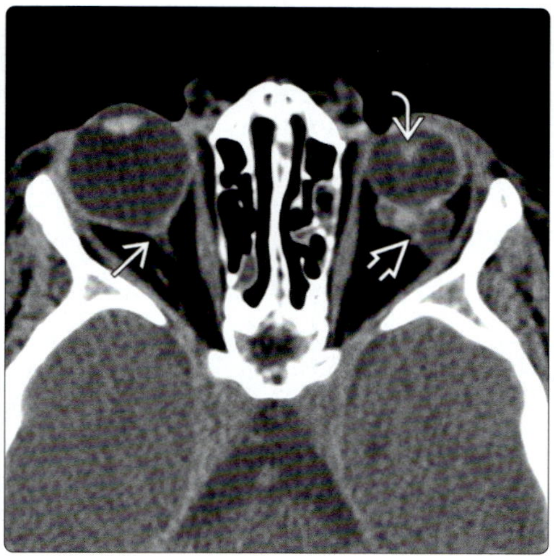

(Left) *Axial NECT reveals a small microphthalmic right globe ➡ with a malpositioned lens ➡ & a large anterior cyst ➡ in a child with unilateral congenital microphthalmos.* **(Right)** *Axial NECT demonstrates a deformed right globe with a small optic disc coloboma ➡. There is also a microphthalmic left globe with multiple small posterior colobomatous cysts ➡. Note also the small left lens ➡.*

Toxocariasis

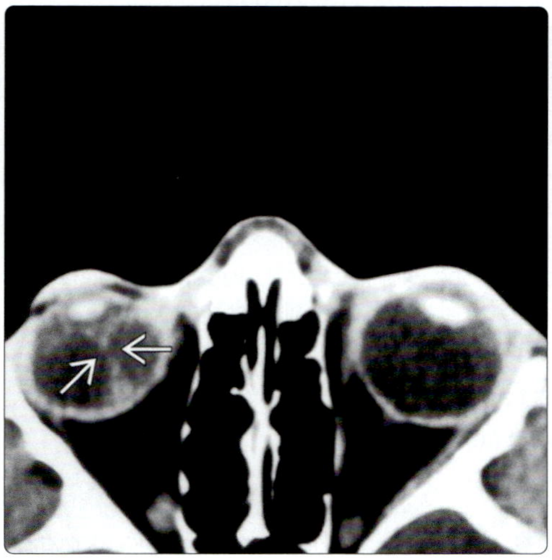

Other Orbital Infections

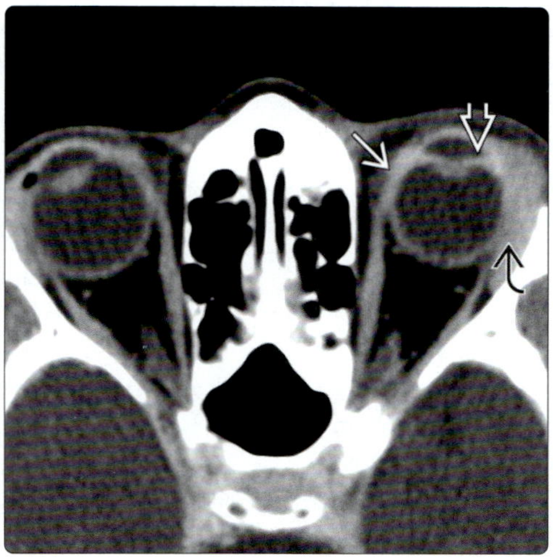

(Left) *Axial NECT shows a small right globe with complete retinal detachment ➡ secondary to toxocariasis. Layers of the inner retina are apposed near the midline, simulating a persistent hyperplastic primary vitreous.* **(Right)** *Axial CECT shows a thick, enhancing sclera ➡ & ciliary body ➡ in association with a mild decrease in the size of the left globe. There is also enlargement of the left lacrimal gland ➡ in this patient with nonspecific scleritis & uveitis.*

DIFFERENTIAL DIAGNOSIS

Common

- Congenital Glaucoma
- Neurofibromatosis Type 1

Less Common

- Sturge-Weber Syndrome
- Staphyloma

Rare but Important

- Acquired Glaucoma
- Congenital Myopia
- Intraocular Mass
- Congenital Cystic Eye
- Coloboma With Macrophthalmia

ESSENTIAL INFORMATION

Key Differential Diagnosis Issues

- Elongated globe in anteroposterior (AP) dimension
  - May be secondary to myopia (nearsightedness), staphyloma, or coloboma
- Diffuse enlargement of globe in AP & transverse dimension = buphthalmos ("ox eye" or "cow eye")
  - May be present in neurofibromatosis type 1 (NF1), Sturge-Weber syndrome (SWS), or congenital vs. acquired glaucoma

Helpful Clues for Common Diagnoses

- **Congenital Glaucoma**
  - Key facts
    - Incidence 1:5,000-1:10,000 live births
    - Boys > > girls
    - Bilateral in majority
    - Usually diagnosed within 1st year of life
    - Clinical: Large eyes, excessive tearing, cloudy cornea, & light sensitivity
    - Obstruction to flow of aqueous humor from anterior chamber → elevated intraocular pressure → enlargement of globe & deep anterior chamber
      - □ Normal mean anterior chamber depth = 3.0 mm
      - □ Congenital glaucoma mean anterior chamber depth = 6.3 mm
  - Imaging
    - Enlarged AP dimension of globe
    - Deep anterior chamber
    - ± optic nerve atrophy &/or subluxated lens
    - ± surgically placed treatment device
- **Neurofibromatosis Type 1**
  - Key facts
    - Congenital neurocutaneous syndrome
    - Mutation of gene on chromosome 17
    - Orbitofacial abnormalities are typically unilateral
    - Plexiform neurofibroma (PNF) is diagnostic
    - Up to 50% of patients with facial & eyelid involvement have ipsilateral glaucoma
  - Imaging
    - Buphthalmos
    - Thickening of uveal & scleral layer; remodeling & thickening of anterior orbital rim
    - PNF of orbit & skull base + sphenoid bony dysplasia → enlargement of osseous orbit, orbital foramina, & middle cranial fossa → intracranial contents herniate into posterior orbit → pulsatile exophthalmos
    - ± enlargement, tortuosity, &/or enhancement of associated optic nerve glioma
    - ± nonenhancing (often symmetric) hyperintense T2/FLAIR foci in cerebellar white matter, deep gray matter structures, & brainstem are typical of NF1

Helpful Clues for Less Common Diagnoses

- **Sturge-Weber Syndrome**
  - Key facts
    - Sporadic disorder of fetal cortical vein development
    - Intracranial imaging features result from progressive venous occlusion, recruitment of alternate drainage pathways, & chronic venous ischemia
    - 50-95% have facial port-wine stain (from capillary malformation)
      - □ Classically in V1 segment
    - Glaucoma in 30-70% related to anterior chamber malformations & elevated episcleral venous pressure
      - □ Choroidal angioma (alternate drainage pathway) → glaucoma &/or exudative retinal detachment
  - Imaging
    - Ocular findings
      - □ Contrast enhancement at site of choroidal angioma
      - □ Buphthalmos
      - □ ± retinal detachment
    - Extraocular imaging abnormalities
      - □ Serpentine leptomeningeal enhancement of pial angiomatosis (80% unilateral)
      - □ Enlarged ipsilateral choroid plexus
      - □ Gyral/subcortical Ca^{2+} (may be tram-track appearance) + parenchymal volume loss
      - □ ± calvarial thickening & sinus hyperpneumatization
- **Staphyloma**
  - Key facts
    - Thinning & stretching of scleral-uveal (outer) layer of globe
      - □ Uveal (middle globe layer) tissue protrudes through weak point in outer scleral-uveal layer
    - Progressive myopia → posterior staphyloma
      - □ Due to glaucoma, connective tissue disorders, scleritis, necrotizing infection, or trauma
    - Corneal thinning → anterior staphyloma
      - □ Infection & inflammation are most common causes
  - Imaging
    - Elongated globe with focal protrusion/outpouch
    - Thinning of posterior > > > anterior walls
    - Unilateral or bilateral

Helpful Clues for Rare Diagnoses

- **Acquired Glaucoma**
  - Key facts
    - Acquired glaucoma, without associated NF1 or SWS, is leading cause of blindness in African Americans & 2nd leading cause of blindness worldwide in all age groups
    - Risk factors

    - African American, > 60 years, family member with glaucoma, Hispanic, Asian, high myopia, diabetes mellitus, hypertension, trauma
    - In children, most commonly secondary to surgery or trauma
  - Primary open-angle > > angle closure (also called closed-angle) glaucoma
  - Diagnosis made by
    - Tonometry: Measures intraocular pressure
    - Ophthalmoscopy: May show evidence of optic nerve atrophy
    - Visual field tests: Lose peripheral vision 1st
    - Gonioscopy: Measures angle between iris & cornea
  - Treatment may include glaucoma drainage implants
- Imaging
  - Most patients are not imaged to assess for glaucoma; secondary globe findings may be recognized on brain imaging for other clinical reasons
  - Less plasticity in adult globe; therefore, buphthalmos & deep anterior chamber are uncommon
  - ± glaucoma drainage implants, Ahmed valve
    - ± small fluid collections/bleb surrounding device

- **Congenital Myopia**
  - Key facts
    - Idiopathic globe enlargement in AP dimension → convergence of light anterior to retina → nearsightedness
  - Imaging
    - May see increased AP dimension of oval-shaped globe
    - Unilateral or bilateral
- **Intraocular Mass**
  - Large intraocular mass may enlarge globe
    - Advanced retinoblastoma is most common cause in children
    - Rarely melanoma
  - Smaller intraocular masses may lead to glaucoma → enlarged globe
- **Congenital Cystic Eye**
  - Key facts
    - Synonym: Anophthalmos with cyst
    - Secondary to failure of involution of primary optic vesicle early in embryologic development
      - Cyst formation rather than globe
    - Cyst filled with proliferating glial tissue, may become complex cyst
  - Imaging
    - Large malformed cyst within orbit
    - No identifiable ocular lens
    - ± complex solid-appearing components
    - Remnants of extraocular muscles & optic nerve are variable
    - Unilateral is much more common than bilateral
    - ± midline intracranial anomalies
- **Coloboma With Macrophthalmia**
  - Key facts
    - Coloboma (gap or defect of ocular tissue), usually with microphthalmia, rarely with macrophthalmia
    - Colobomatous macrophthalmia with microcornea syndrome
      - Autosomal dominant inheritance
      - Gene linked to region of 2p23-p16
      - Myopia & microcornea
      - ± glaucoma
  - Imaging
    - Axial enlargement of globe
    - Inferonasal iris coloboma
    - Chorioretinal coloboma

SELECTED REFERENCES

1. Anderson DM et al: Magnetic resonance imaging characteristics of a baerveldt glaucoma implant. J Glaucoma. 26(6):534-40, 2017
2. Mantelli F et al: Ocular manifestations of Sturge-Weber syndrome: pathogenesis, diagnosis, and management. Clin Ophthalmol. 10:871-8, 2016
3. Vachha BA et al: Imaging of pediatric orbital diseases. Neuroimaging Clin N Am. 25(3):477-501, 2015
4. Burns NS et al: Diagnostic imaging of fetal and pediatric orbital abnormalities. AJR Am J Roentgenol. 201(6):W797-808, 2013
5. Singer JR et al: Congenital cystic eye in utero: novel prenatal magnetic resonance imaging findings. JAMA Ophthalmol. 131(8):1092-5, 2013

Congenital Glaucoma

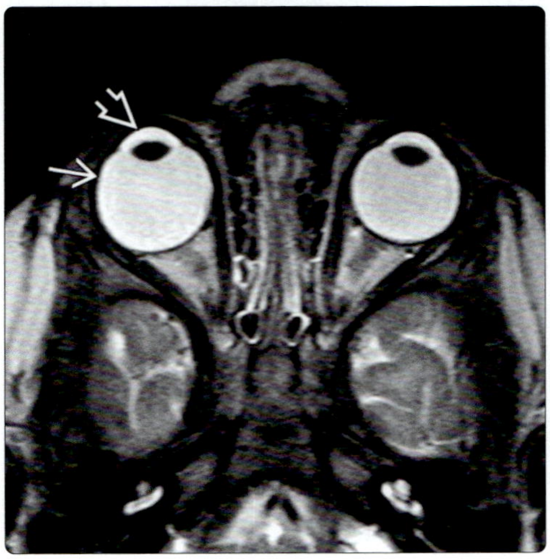

Neurofibromatosis Type 1

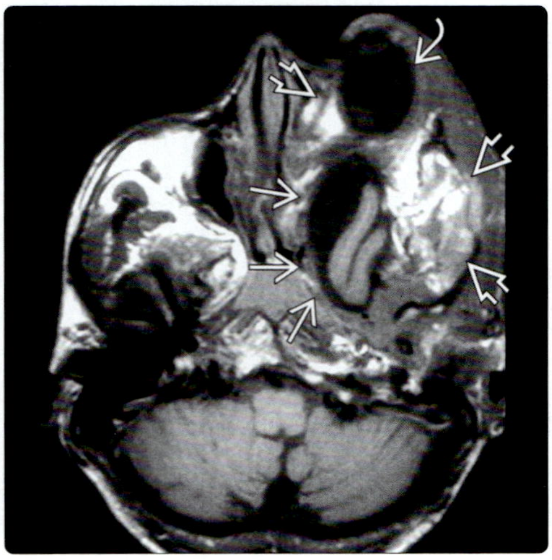

(Left) *Axial T2 MR in a young child with congenital glaucoma shows diffuse enlargement of the right globe ➔, including mild increased depth of the right anterior chamber ➔.* **(Right)** *Axial T1 C+ MR shows severe left sphenoid dysplasia/hypoplasia ➔, extensive plexiform neurofibromas ➔, marked proptosis, & buphthalmos ➔. Additional intracranial abnormalities (not shown) might include hyperintense T2 foci in the cerebellar white matter & basal ganglia + optic pathway gliomas.*

(**Left**) *Axial T2 MR demonstrates right sphenoid wing dysplasia ➡ & infiltrative nodular hyperintense plexiform neurofibromas ➡ causing distortion of the orbit. There is also proptosis & buphthalmos ➡ in this patient with neurofibromatosis type 1 (NF1).* (**Right**) *Axial CECT shows right buphthalmos ➡, a dysplastic right sphenoid bone ➡, & plexiform neurofibromas that involve the right cavernous sinus ➡ in a child with NF1.*

Neurofibromatosis Type 1

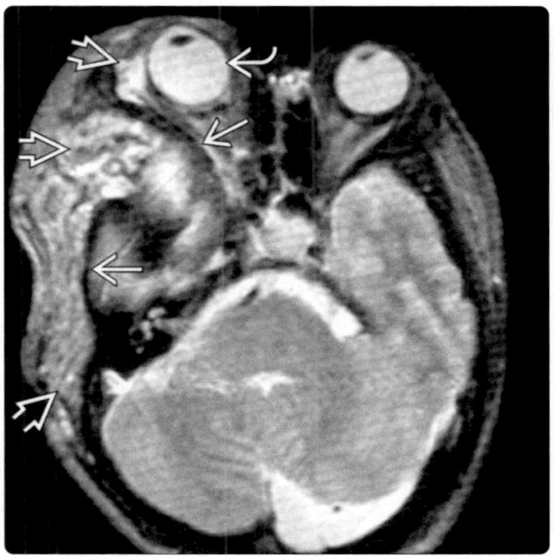

Neurofibromatosis Type 1

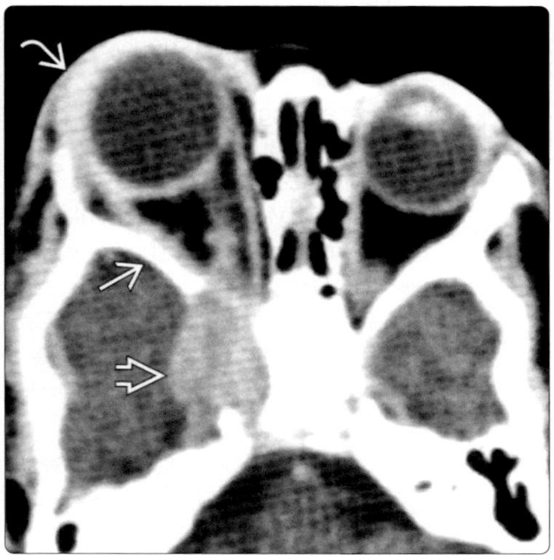

(**Left**) *Axial T1 C+ MR in a child with Sturge-Weber syndrome shows smooth contrast enhancement of choroidal angiomas ➡ without retinal detachment. Note also the diffuse enlargement of the right > left globes secondary to glaucoma, which can be very difficult to treat in these patients.* (**Right**) *Coronal T1 C+ MR in the same child shows 2 right-sided & 1 left-sided Ahmed valves ➡, placed for the treatment of glaucoma.*

Sturge-Weber Syndrome

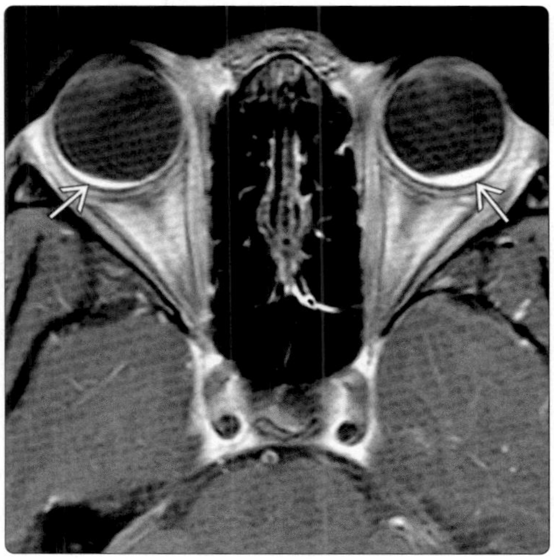

Sturge-Weber Syndrome

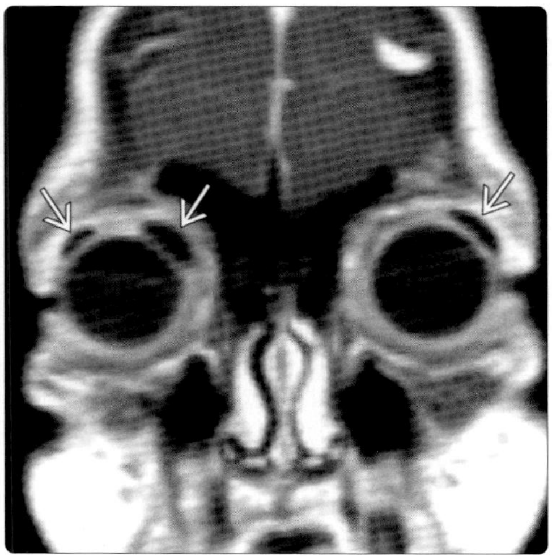

(**Left**) *Axial T2 MR in a patient with bilateral glaucoma secondary to Sturge-Weber syndrome demonstrates a bilateral increase in depth of the anterior chambers ➡. The right globe is slightly larger than the left as well. These findings are typical in children with glaucoma, as the globe walls are still pliable.* (**Right**) *Axial T2 MR shows bilateral longitudinal elongation of the globes ➡ caused by degenerative weakness of each posterior globe.*

Sturge-Weber Syndrome

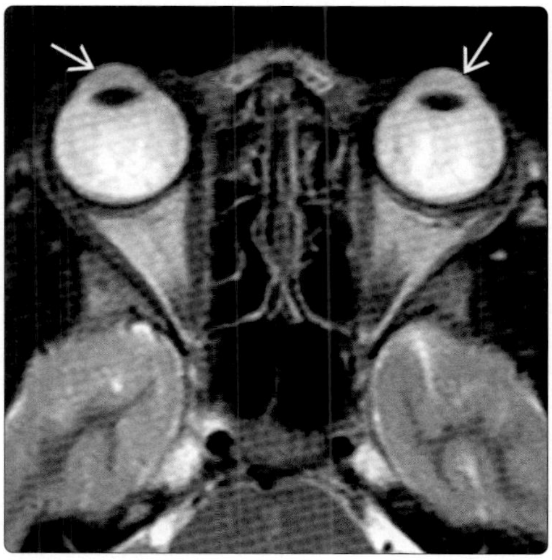

Staphyloma

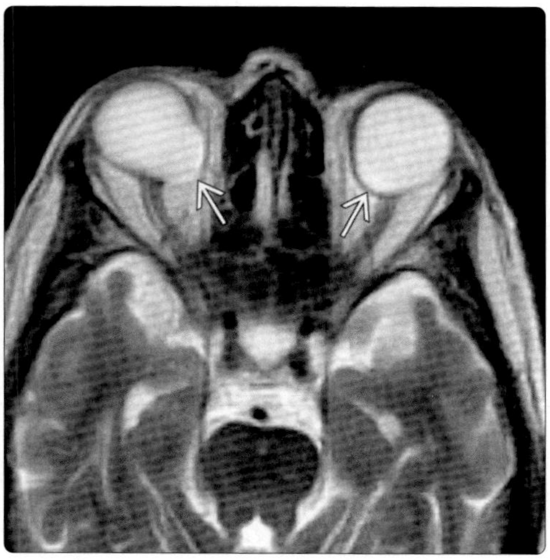

Staphyloma

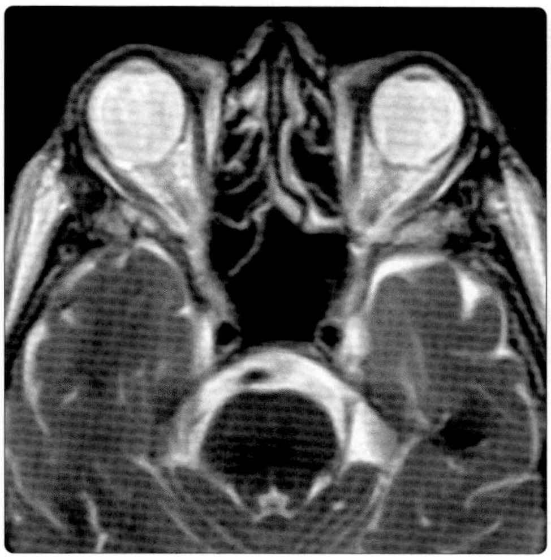

Staphyloma

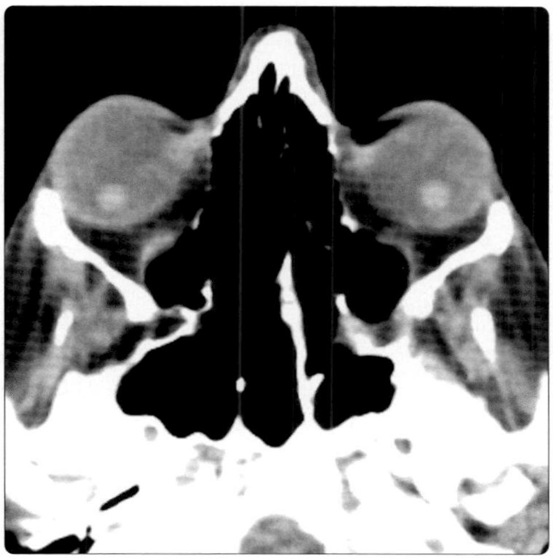

(Left) *Axial T2 MR demonstrates mild elongation of both globes in a patient with staphyloma. This entity is caused by thinning & stretching of the scleral-uveal layer of the globe, typically in adults.* **(Right)** *Axial NECT reveals mild enlargement of the right globe with bilateral lens dislocations in an adult with Marfan syndrome. The incidence of glaucoma is also increased in Ehlers-Danlos syndrome, ± staphyloma.*

Congenital Myopia

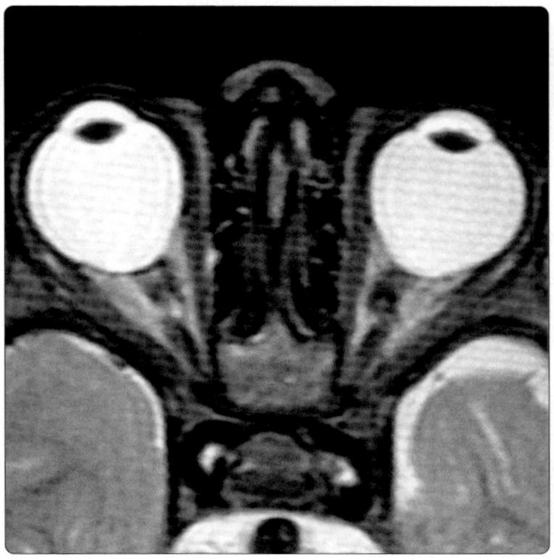

Intraocular Mass

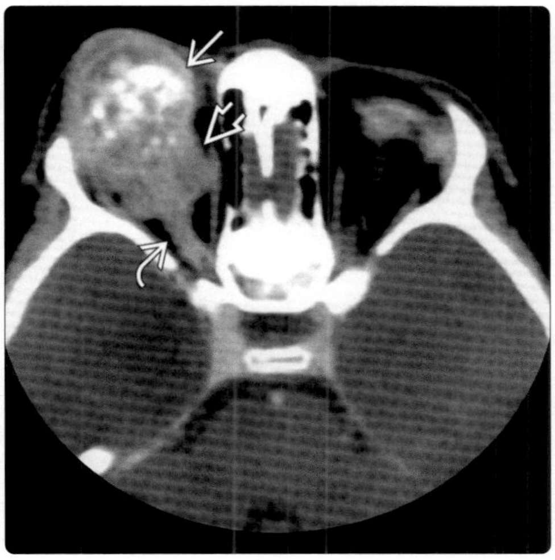

(Left) *Axial T2 MR shows AP enlargement of both globes in a patient with congenital myopia (which results in convergence of light anterior to the retina, causing nearsightedness). This appearance is similar to that noted in older patients with posterior staphyloma.* **(Right)** *Axial CECT in a young child shows right macrophthalmos due to a large retinoblastoma with extraocular extension. The optic nerve is thickened due to tumor spread along the nerve sheath. The patient was previously treated for left-sided disease.*

Congenital Cystic Eye

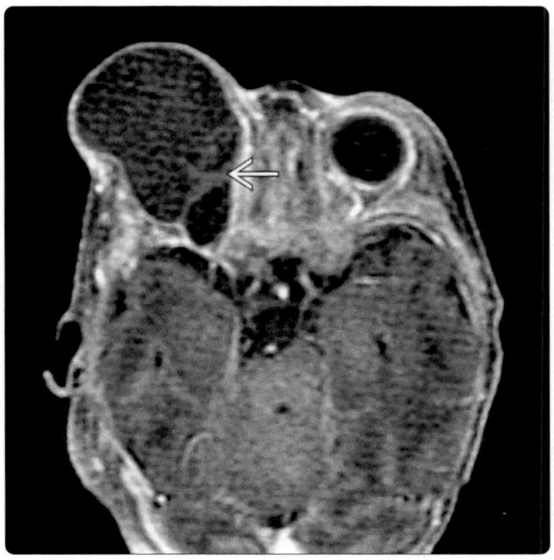

Coloboma With Macrophthalmia

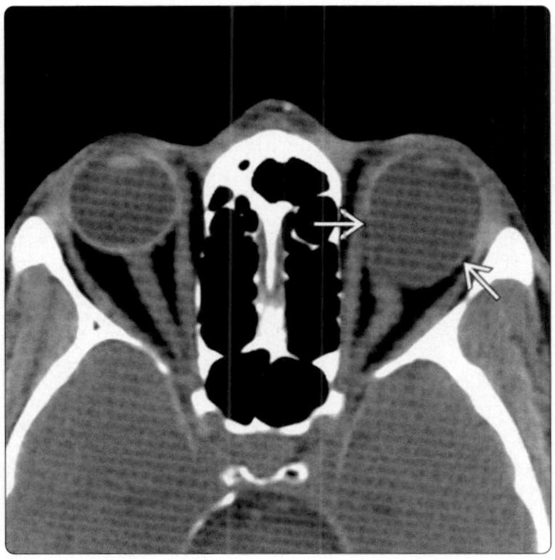

(Left) *Axial T1 C+ FS MR shows a large cystic mass in the right orbit with complex elements posteromedially but no identifiable lens. A cyst forms rather than a true globe secondary to failure of involution of the primary optic vesicle.* **(Right)** *Axial NECT reveals a broad-based coloboma defect involving a large left globe. The globe enlargement is greater in the AP than transverse dimensions. This is a rare genetic abnormality, as most colobomas are associated with microphthalmos.*

Optic Nerve or Nerve Sheath Lesion

DIFFERENTIAL DIAGNOSIS

Common

- Optic Pathway Glioma
- Optic Neuritis

Less Common

- Optic Nerve Sheath Meningioma
- Idiopathic Perineuritis
- Orbital Sarcoid

Rare but Important

- Lymphoproliferative Lesions
- Infectious Optic Neuritis

ESSENTIAL INFORMATION

Helpful Clues for Common Diagnoses

- **Optic Pathway Glioma**
  - Key facts: Benign tumor in children
    - 30-40% of patients have neurofibromatosis type 1 (NF1)
    - Malignant variant is rare
  - Imaging: Fusiform mass ± enhancement
    - Kinking or buckling is common
    - May involve nerve, chiasm, tract, or central pathways
    - Look for findings of NF1
      - Foci of increased T2/FLAIR signal intensity in medial cerebellar hemispheres & globus pallidus
      - Cervicomedullary gliomas
      - Carotid terminus occlusion
      - Plexiform neurofibromas
- **Optic Neuritis**
  - Key facts: Acute vision loss
    - Inflammatory or autoimmune etiology
    - High prevalence of multiple sclerosis
    - Bilateral is more typical in neuromyelitis optica
  - Imaging: Unilateral in 70%
    - Diffuse enhancement without mass
    - T2 hyperintensity is usually also present
    - Look for lesions of periventricular white matter & cervical cord

Helpful Clues for Less Common Diagnoses

- **Optic Nerve Sheath Meningioma**
  - Key facts: Slow-growing, benign tumor
    - Painless progressive vision loss
  - Imaging: Uniform nerve enhancement
    - Ca^{2+} in 30-50%
    - Tram-track appearance outlines sheath
    - Perioptic cyst behind optic nerve head
- **Idiopathic Perineuritis**
  - Key facts: Subtype of idiopathic orbital inflammatory disease (pseudotumor)
    - Myositic, tumefactive, & lacrimal forms are more common than optic nerve sheath involvement
  - Imaging: Nerve involvement may be isolated or occur with other lesions
- **Orbital Sarcoid**
  - Key facts: Systemic disease is common
  - Imaging: Nerve involvement may be isolated or occur with other central nervous system lesions

Helpful Clues for Rare Diagnoses

- **Lymphoproliferative Lesions**
  - Key facts: MALT-type lymphoma
  - Imaging: Solid tumor anywhere in orbit
    - Pliable tumor molds to normal structures
- **Infectious Optic Neuritis**
  - Key facts: Acute vision loss
    - CMV, HIV, herpes, other viruses
    - Tuberculosis, Lyme disease, syphilis, toxoplasmosis
  - Imaging: Diffuse enhancement of optic nerves

Alternative Differential Approaches

- Entities concomitant lesions elsewhere in orbit
  - Optic pathway glioma (with NF1)
  - Idiopathic perineuritis (pseudotumor)
  - Sarcoidosis
  - Lymphoproliferative lesions

Optic Pathway Glioma

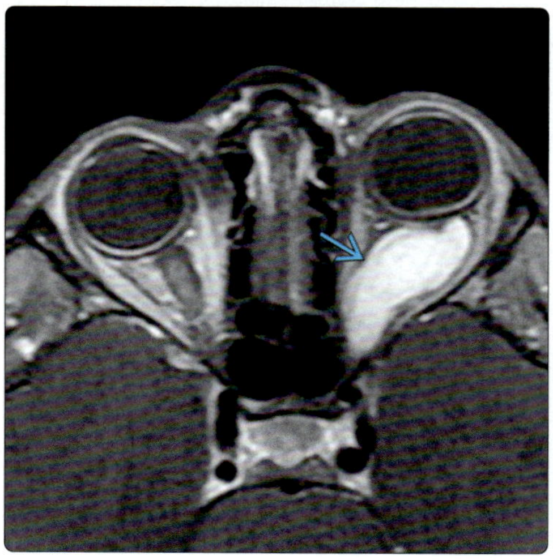

Optic Neuritis

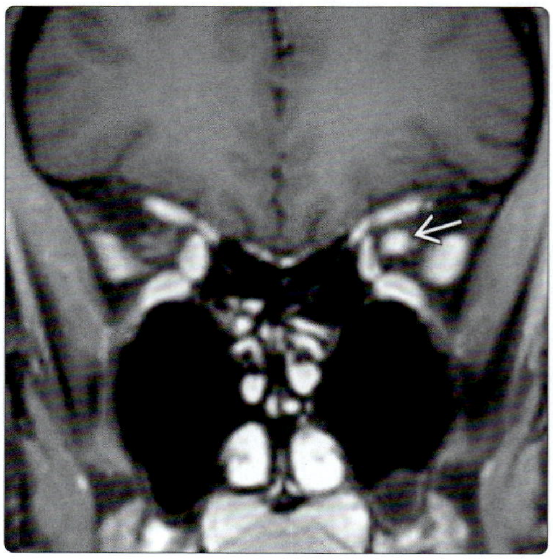

(Left) *Axial T1 C+ FS MR shows fusiform enlargement & enhancement of the left optic nerve ➡, consistent with an optic nerve glioma in this patient with neurofibromatosis type 1 (NF1).* **(Right)** *Coronal T1 C+ FS MR shows enhancement (without enlargement) of the left optic nerve ➡, consistent with optic neuritis in this patient with acute vision loss. Additional periventricular white matter FLAIR hyperintensities were present in this patient with multiple sclerosis (not shown).*

Optic Neuritis

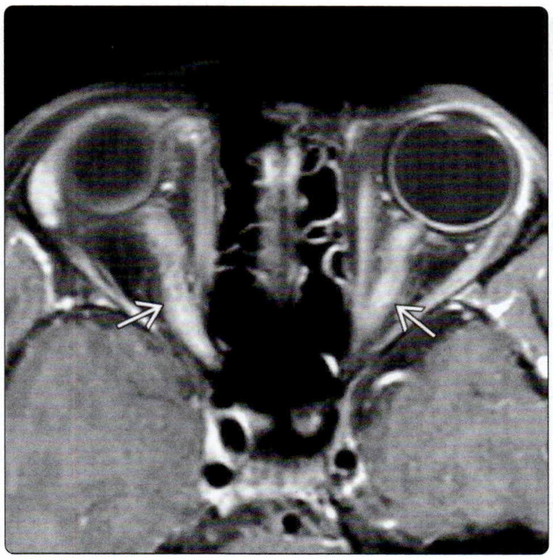

Optic Nerve Sheath Meningioma

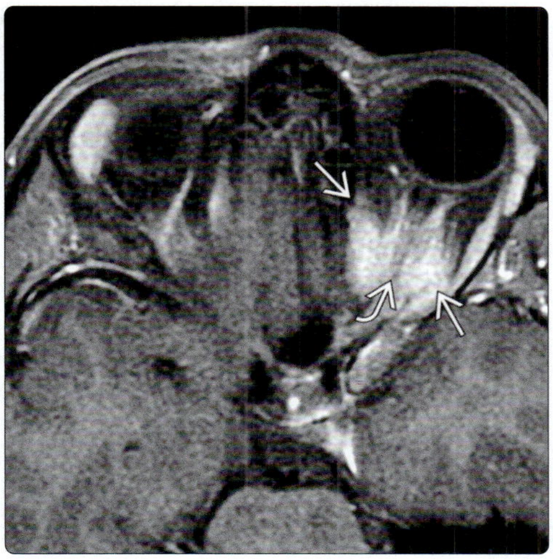

(Left) *Axial T1 C+ FS MR in a 10-year-old child with acute onset of vision loss demonstrates abnormal enhancement of the left > right intraorbital optic nerves* →. *The margins of the nerves are poorly defined with adjacent fat stranding.* **(Right)** *Axial T1 C+ FS MR in a teenager with a 3-month history of declining vision & 6 weeks of diplopia shows a moderately enhancing mass* → *arising from the optic nerve sheath & surrounding intraorbital optic nerve* →. *The tram-track appearance is typical of meningioma.*

Idiopathic Perineuritis

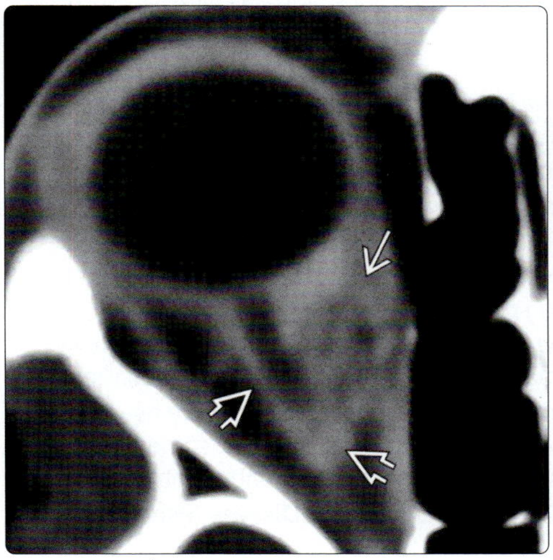

Idiopathic Perineuritis

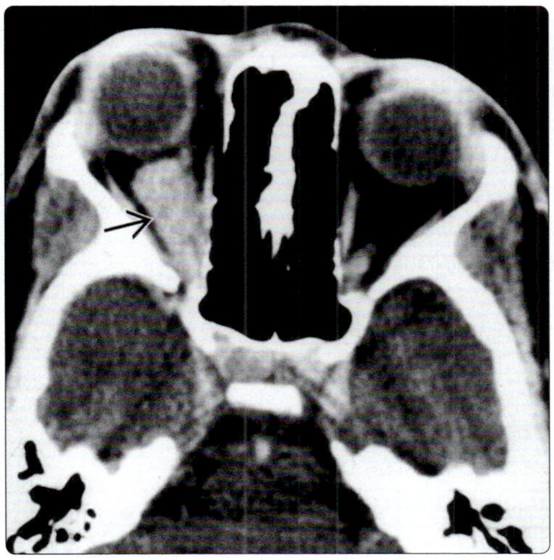

(Left) *Axial CECT in a child with right orbital pain & vision loss shows a tumefactive form of idiopathic orbital pseudotumor as an intraconal mass* → *with perineuritic spread along the optic nerve sheath* →. **(Right)** *Axial CECT shows a homogeneously enhancing intraconal mass* → *that is indistinguishable from the optic nerve sheath complex. This example of idiopathic orbital inflammatory disease (pseudotumor) demonstrates isolated optic nerve involvement.*

Orbital Sarcoid

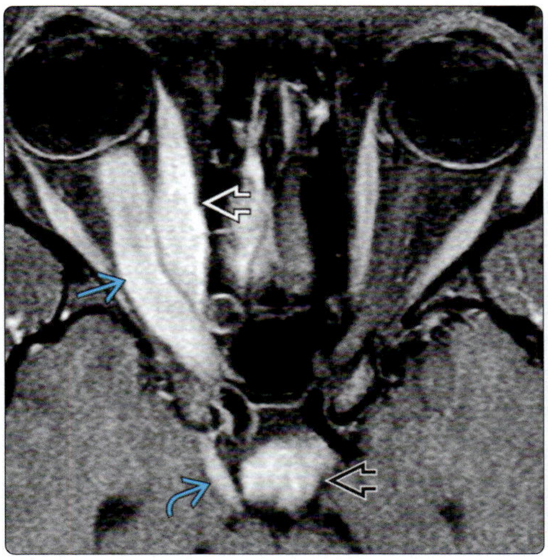

Lymphoproliferative Lesions

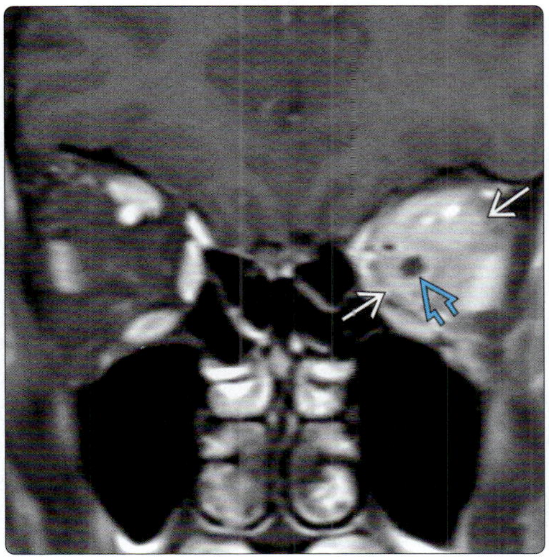

(Left) *Axial T1 C+ FS MR shows marked diffusely thickening & enhancement of the right optic nerve* →. *Oculomotor enhancement due to neuritis* → *is evident as well as medial rectus* → *& suprasellar* → *involvement from sarcoid.* **(Right)** *Coronal T1 C+ FS MR demonstrates a diffuse enhancing mass* → *in the left intraconal space. This pliable mass surrounds the optic nerve* → *& vasculature without significant mass effect, a common imaging characteristic of non-Hodgkin lymphoma.*

DIFFERENTIAL DIAGNOSIS

Common

- Subperiosteal Abscess
- Infantile Hemangioma
- Lymphatic Malformation

Less Common

- Trauma
- Idiopathic Orbital Inflammatory Disease (Pseudotumor)
- Rhabdomyosarcoma
- Langerhans Cell Histiocytosis
- Metastatic Neuroblastoma

Rare but Important

- Lymphoproliferative Lesions
- Carotid-Cavernous Fistula

ESSENTIAL INFORMATION

Helpful Clues for Common Diagnoses

- **Subperiosteal Abscess**
  - Key facts
    - Pus between orbital wall & periosteum
      - Medial > superior orbital walls, usually due to adjacent to ethmoid > frontal sinusitis
  - Imaging (CECT)
    - Lentiform, rim-enhancing extraconal fluid collection, typically overlying adjacent sinusitis
      - Usually with deviation of adjacent extraocular muscle (EOM)
    - ± air-fluid level in collection (which confirms drainable pus)
    - ± edematous intraconal or extraconal fat, enlargement of EOMs (myositis)
    - ± superior ophthalmic vein (SOV) thrombosis
    - Brain MR is performed if intracranial complication of sinusitis is suspected
- **Infantile Hemangioma**
  - Key facts
    - Benign vascular neoplasm, **not** malformation
    - Not present at birth; becomes apparent within 1st few weeks of life
    - Rapidly grows (proliferates) over 1st months/year of life, then slowly involutes over several years
    - Superficial components often have characteristic cutaneous stigmata
    - Mass remains soft clinically
  - Imaging (CECT/MR)
    - Proliferating phase: Solid, intensely enhancing mass with internal flow voids; high flow on ASL MR
      - Abundance of low-resistance arterial flow on Doppler
    - Involuting phase: Fatty infiltration, decreasing size
    - May be part of PHACE syndrome: Posterior fossa abnormalities, infantile hemangiomas, arterial anomalies, cardiovascular defects, eye abnormalities
- **Lymphatic Malformation**
  - Key facts
    - Congenital, low-flow vascular malformation composed of abnormal lymphatic channels of varying sizes
      - Subtypes: Macrocystic, microcystic, & mixed
    - Present at birth, grows commensurate with child
      - Hemorrhage, infection, or hormonal stimulation may cause sudden increase in size
  - Imaging (CECT/MR)
    - Uni- or multilocular; macrocystic (> 1 cm) or microcystic (< 1 cm) components
    - Transspatial: Intraconal &/or extraconal location
    - Thin septal enhancement only (unless mixed with venous components or presenting with associated infection or hemorrhage); microcystic may appear more solid and ill-defined
    - Fluid-fluid levels of internal hemorrhage

Helpful Clues for Less Common Diagnoses

- **Trauma**
  - Key facts
    - Orbital fracture ± retrobulbar hematoma/gas
    - Suspect penetrating injury with occult orbital foreign body (FB) in pediatric orbital trauma
  - Imaging (NECT)
    - FB, bone fragments, &/or adjacent hematoma/gas → proptosis
      - Metallic FBs are most dense
      - Glass is more dense than bone
      - Wood is very low density (~ air) initially; gradually absorbs water to become intermediate attenuation
      - Living plant material is soft tissue density
    - ± globe deformity, anterior chamber enlargement, lens fragmentation or dislocation, intracranial injury
    - Posterior tenting of globe at optic nerve head is associated with decreased visual outcomes; necessitates emergent surgical intervention
- **Idiopathic Orbital Inflammatory Disease (Pseudotumor)**
  - Key facts
    - Benign inflammatory process with fibrosis → painful proptosis
  - Imaging (CECT/MR)
    - Myositic: Most common subtype
      - Diffuse enlargement & enhancement of EOMs, involves tendinous insertions
    - Lacrimal: Enlargement & enhancement
    - Anterior: Thickening & enhancement of sclera ± choroid, ± involvement of retrobulbar fat, nerve, or sheath
    - Diffuse: Intra- ± extraconal, may be mass-like, usually without globe deformity or bone erosion
    - Apical: Enhancing orbital apex mass, extension through fissures
- **Rhabdomyosarcoma**
  - Key facts
    - Most common soft tissue sarcoma in children < 15 years of age
    - Arises from primitive mesenchymal tissue, not directly from EOMs
    - Head & neck (H&N) sites: Orbit > parameningeal (middle ear, paranasal sinus, nasopharynx) > all other H&N sites

  - Orbital primary presents with proptosis, rarely metastatic spread (given early presentation)
- Imaging
  - Well-circumscribed soft tissue mass with variable enhancement
    - Rarely shows abundant internal vascularity
  - Bone erosion is frequently not present
    - When present, may lead to intracranial extension
  - Diffusion restriction is common on MR

- **Langerhans Cell Histiocytosis**
  - Key facts
    - In H&N: Orbit, maxilla, mandible, temporal bone, cervical spine, calvarium
    - Staging: Unifocal, single system (most common) vs. multifocal, single system vs. multifocal, multisystem
    - Orbital involvement is usually unifocal
    - Pituitary infundibular involvement presents with diabetes insipidus
  - Imaging (CECT/MR)
    - Enhancing soft tissue mass filling & extending from well-circumscribed lytic lesion
      - Lacks spiculated periosteal reaction, expansion
    - Typically at superior or superolateral orbit
    - ± other bone lesions or thickened pituitary infundibulum/absent posterior pituitary bright spot on T1 MR
- **Metastatic Neuroblastoma**
  - Key facts
    - Most common malignancy in children < 1 year of age
    - Primary tumors arise at sites of sympathetic ganglia
      - Majority of primary tumors are adrenal origin
      - Primary cervical origin in < 5%
    - Metastatic disease to orbits may cause periorbital ecchymosis ("racoon eyes")
  - Imaging (CECT/MR)
    - Soft tissue mass arising from bone with aggressive bone permeation & spiculated periosteal reaction
    - Frequently involves lateral orbital walls
      - ± intracranial extension

Helpful Clues for Rare Diagnoses

- **Lymphoproliferative Lesions**
  - Key facts
    - Includes non-Hodgkin lymphoma & lymphoid hyperplasia (benign polyclonal reactive hyperplasia & indeterminate atypical hyperplasia)
    - Can be primary to orbit (typically MALT lymphoma) or systemic (typically diffuse large B-cell lymphoma)
  - Imaging (CECT/MR)
    - Diffuse or focal masses, unilateral or bilateral
    - Homogeneously enhancing soft tissue mass anywhere in orbit
    - Low ADC values (i.e., restricted diffusion) on MR
- **Carotid-Cavernous Fistula**
  - Key facts
    - Direct fistula of cavernous internal carotid artery (ICA) to cavernous sinus (CS)
    - Presents with pulsating exophthalmos, orbital edema/erythema, ↓ vision, bruit, glaucoma, headache
    - Most present days to weeks after trauma
  - Imaging (CTA or MRA/MRV)
    - Large SOV with abnormal flow, dilated CS, & enlarged EOMs
    - "Dirty" orbital fat related to venous congestion
    - DSA to confirm
      - Early filling of CS + outflow pathways, including retrograde filling of SOV, angular, & facial veins
      - Reduced or absent antegrade flow in ICA beyond fistula, depending on size of ICA tear

SELECTED REFERENCES

1. Merrow AC et al: 2014 Revised classification of vascular lesions from the International Society for the Study of Vascular Anomalies: radiologic-pathologic update. Radiographics. 36(5):1494-516, 2016
2. Vachha BA et al: Imaging of pediatric orbital diseases. Neuroimaging Clin N Am. 25(3):477-501, 2015
3. Herwig MC et al: Langerhans cell histiocytosis of the orbit: five clinicopathologic cases and review of the literature. Surv Ophthalmol. 58(4):330-40, 2013

Subperiosteal Abscess

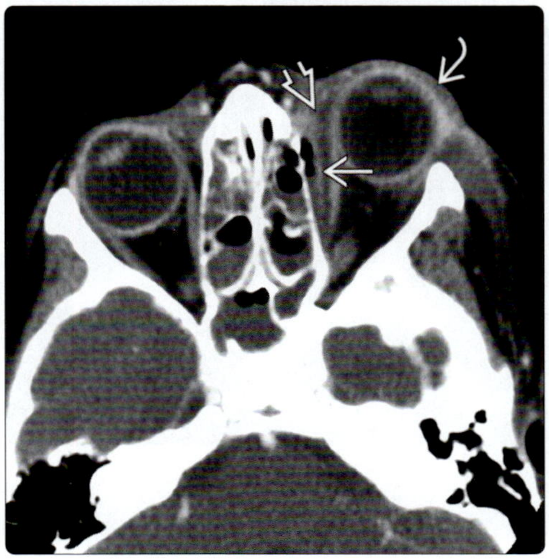

Subperiosteal Abscess

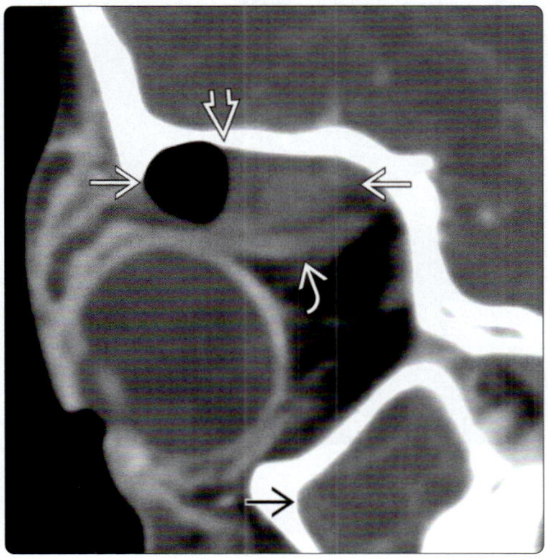

(Left) *Axial CECT shows an elliptical subperiosteal abscess with an air-fluid level ➡ in the medial left orbit with extraconal edema ➡, medial rectus muscle deviation, proptosis, & preseptal soft tissue edema ➡. Note the causative adjacent ethmoid & sphenoid sinusitis.* **(Right)** *Sagittal CECT shows a lentiform fluid collection ➡ with an air-fluid level ➡ causing mass effect upon the superior rectus complex ➡, compatible with subperiosteal abscess. The causative sinusitis is partially seen in the left maxillary sinus ➡.*

(Left) *Axial T1 C+ FS MR shows a large infantile hemangioma involving the right orbit, face, & nose with postseptal extension, resulting in proptosis. The homogeneous intense enhancement & high-flow vessels indicate that the lesion is in the proliferating phase.* (Right) *Axial T1 C+ FS MR defines the preseptal & postseptal intraconal & extraconal extension of an infantile hemangioma.*

Infantile Hemangioma

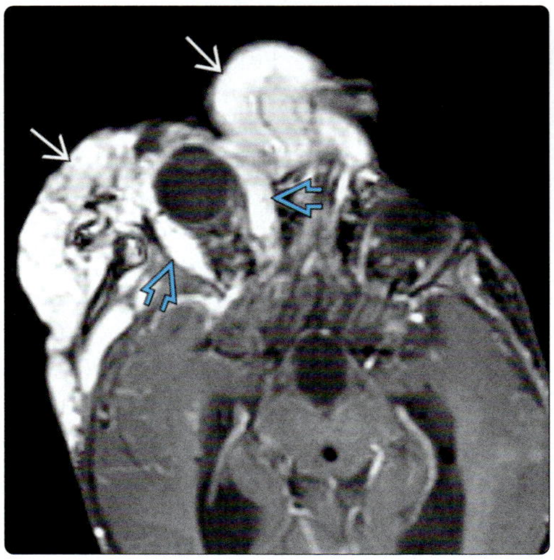

Infantile Hemangioma

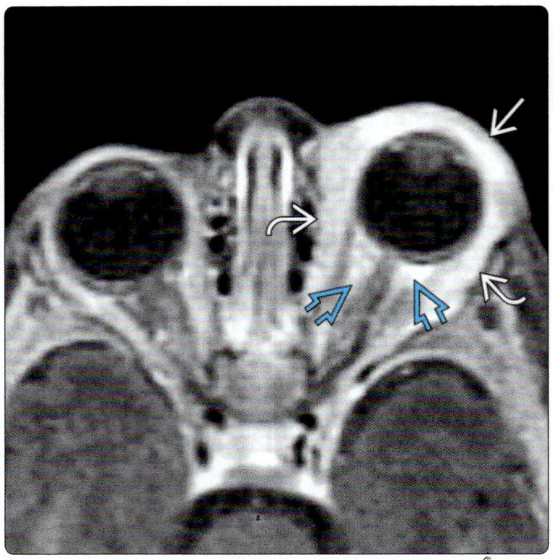

(Left) *Axial T1 FS MR in a patient with the acute onset of right eye proptosis shows hyperintense blood products layering within an intraconal macrocystic lymphatic malformation.* (Right) *Axial T2 MR in the same patient shows hyperintense fluid signal in the mass with layering fluid-fluid levels secondary to intralesional hemorrhage. Note the smaller extraconal component anteromedially.*

Lymphatic Malformation

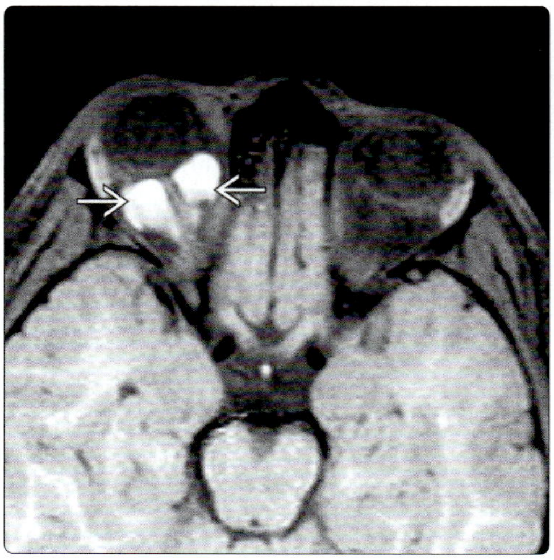

Lymphatic Malformation

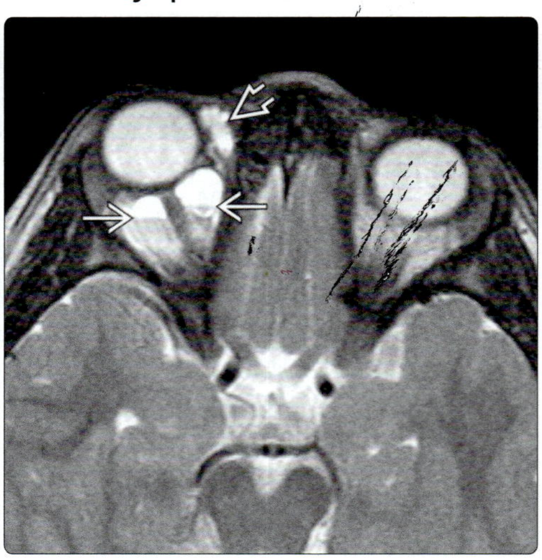

(Left) *Axial NECT reveals mild right proptosis secondary to the penetration of the medial extraconal space by an air-containing twig from a tree branch. Care must be taken not to confuse retained wooden foreign bodies with air or fat.* (Right) *Axial NECT shows depressed lateral wall fracture fragments & orbital hemorrhage, leading to severe proptosis & near-complete traumatic enucleation of the small right globe, which contains fragments of a shattered lens.*

Trauma

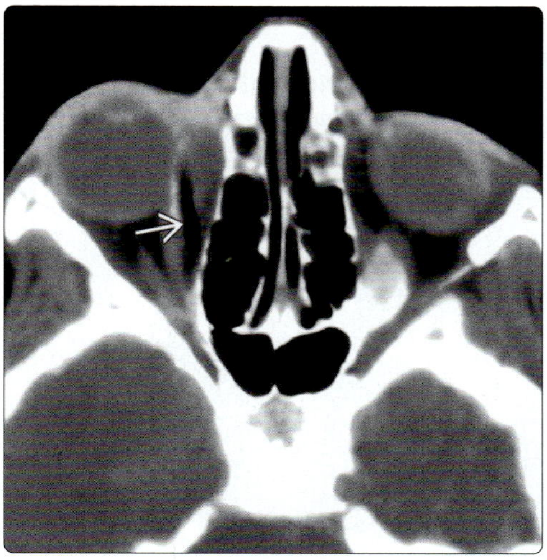

Trauma

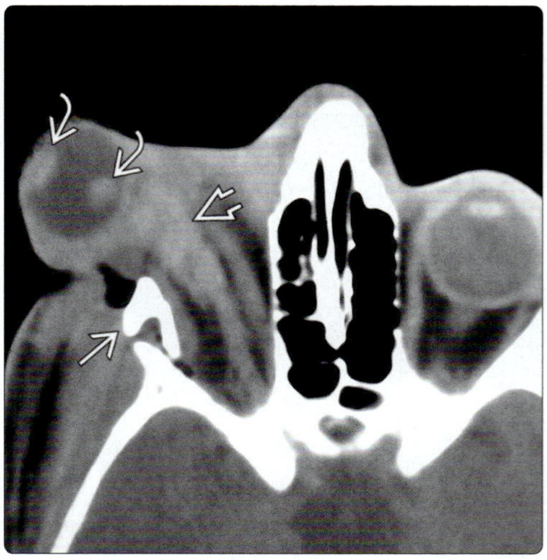

Idiopathic Orbital Inflammatory Disease (Pseudotumor)

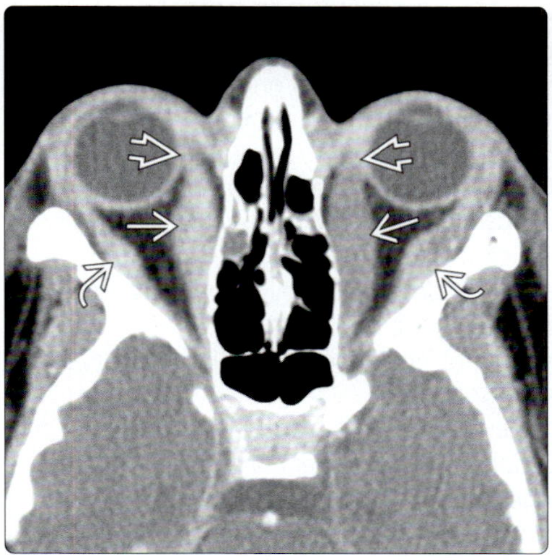

Rhabdomyosarcoma

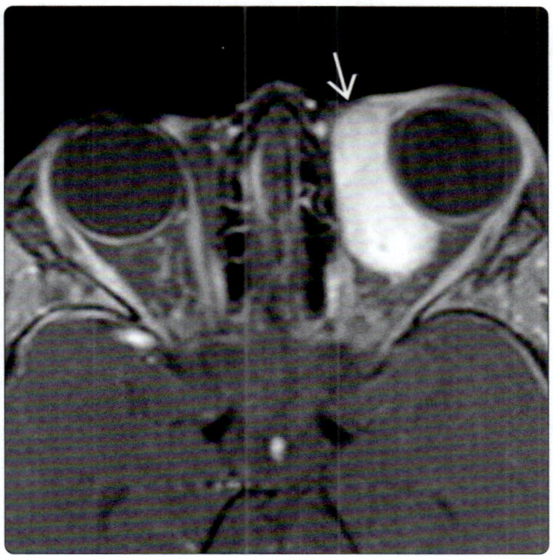

(Left) *Axial CECT shows diffuse enlargement of bilateral medial ➡ > lateral ➡ rectus muscles, including the tendinous insertions ➡. This child presented with painful proptosis, & biopsy showed idiopathic orbital inflammatory disease.* **(Right)** *Axial T1 C+ FS MR shows an enhancing soft tissue mass ➡ in the medial left orbit due to rhabdomyosarcoma (RMS). While this imaging appearance could be seen with infantile hemangioma, RMS rarely occurs in the first 1-3 months of life.*

Langerhans Cell Histiocytosis

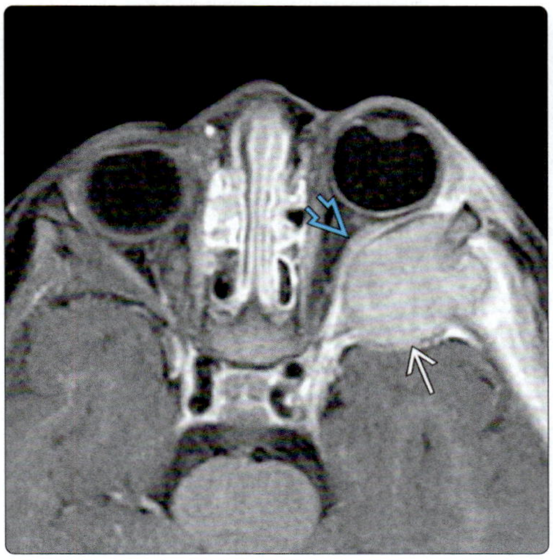

Metastatic Neuroblastoma

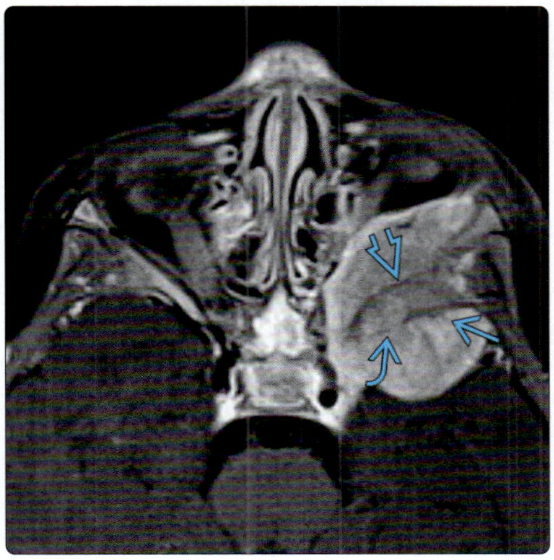

(Left) *Axial T1 C+ FS MR in a child with proptosis shows a large, well-defined, moderately enhancing mass arising from & destroying the sphenoid wing with orbital ➡ & intracranial ➡ extension. Note the absence of any residual bone at the center of the mass. Biopsy showed Langerhans cell histiocytosis.* **(Right)** *Axial T1 C+ FS MR in a 15 month old with neuroblastoma (NB) shows the typical features of bony orbital NB metastases, including permeation ➡, mild expansion ➡, & spiculated periosteal reaction ➡.*

Lymphoproliferative Lesions

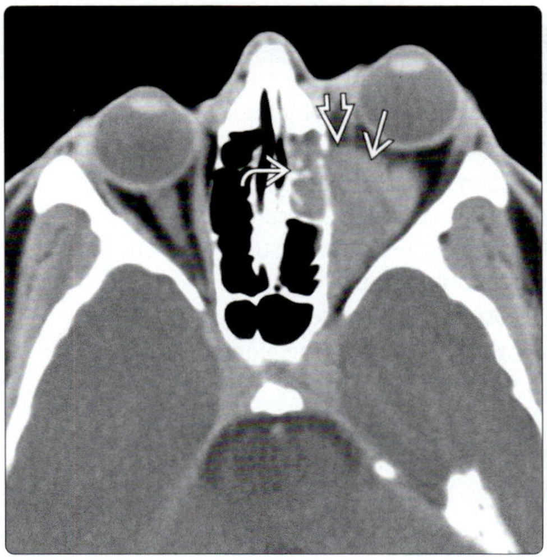

Carotid-Cavernous Fistula

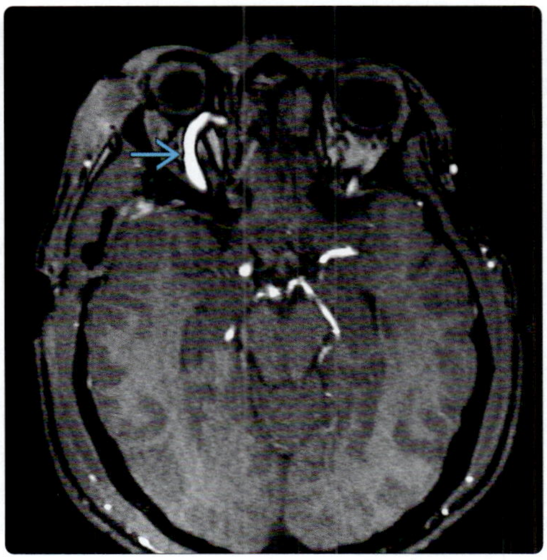

(Left) *Axial CECT demonstrates an intraconal ➡ & extraconal ➡ solid left orbital mass with ethmoid extension ➡ due to non-Hodgkin lymphoma.* **(Right)** *Axial 3D TOF MRA in a teenager with a history of skull base fractures shows engorgement & abnormal flow of the right superior ophthalmic vein ➡ due to a carotid-cavernous fistula. Expansion & abnormal flow was also visualized in the right cavernous sinus (not shown).*

DIFFERENTIAL DIAGNOSIS

Common

- Adenoid Tonsil Hypertrophy
- Sinonasal Polyposis
- Solitary Sinonasal Polyp
- Allergic Fungal Sinusitis
- Pyogenic Granuloma

Less Common

- Infantile Hemangioma
- Juvenile Angiofibroma
- Non-Hodgkin Lymphoma
- Rhabdomyosarcoma
- Nasopharyngeal Carcinoma

Rare but Important

- Esthesioneuroblastoma

ESSENTIAL INFORMATION

Helpful Clues for Common Diagnoses

- **Adenoid Tonsil Hypertrophy**
  - Adenoid tonsils are rarely visible before 6 months of age
    - Proliferate rapidly & reach maximal size by 2-10 years of age
    - Acute enlargement is usually inflammatory, rarely neoplastic
    - Chronic enlargement may lead to obstructive sleep apnea (OSA)
      - Adenoid tonsil regrowth is common cause of recurrent OSA following palatine tonsillectomy & adenoidectomy (T&A)
    - If there is associated palatine tonsil enlargement & cervical adenopathy, think EBV infection
  - Imaging
    - Symmetric soft tissue fullness of posterior wall of nasopharynx (NP); > 12-mm thickness on lateral
    - Homogeneous enhancement, unless mucous retention cyst or tumor is present
    - MR cine sleep studies performed for persistent/recurrent OSA
- **Sinonasal Polyposis**
  - Most common in children with cystic fibrosis or allergies
    - Nonneoplastic, inflammatory swelling of sinonasal mucosa → buckling to form "polyps"
  - Imaging
    - Multiple bilateral nasal cavity & paranasal sinus polypoid masses
      - Predominately along lateral nasal wall & roof of nasal cavity
    - Variable attenuation & signal intensity, dependent on water content
      - Hypodense CT/hyperintense T2 MR due to high water content
      - Hyperdense CT/hypointense T2 MR as mucus becomes dessicated
    - MR complimentary to CT for assessing
      - Intraorbital & intracranial extension
      - Differentiation of sinonasal polyposis (SNP) from neoplasm
- **Solitary Sinonasal Polyp**
  - Inflammatory polyp secondary to edematous hypertrophy of respiratory epithelium
    - Most common type: Antrochoanal polyp
    - Other types named by site of origin → termination: Sphenochoanal, ethmoidochoanal, nasochoanal
  - Imaging
    - Nonenhancing polyp of maxillary antrum → enlarged maxillary ostium or accessory ostium → nasal cavity
      - Large lesions → choana → NP
    - May have ↑ CT density centrally depending on chronicity ± fungal colonization
    - Hypointense T1/hyperintense T2 MR secondary to high water content
      - Variable signal intensity with chronicity
    - Thin, peripheral enhancement of mucosa
- **Allergic Fungal Sinusitis**
  - Severe form of chronic rhinosinusitis with polyposis
    - Allergic response to fungal antigens characterized by eosinophilic mucin & noninvasive fungal hyphae
    - Considered minority subtype of SNP
  - Imaging
    - Multiple expanded sinuses filled with inspissated material
      - Bony remodeling ± erosion
    - Centrally hyperdense & peripherally hypodense on CT
    - Hypointense on T2 MR, may mimic air
- **Pyogenic Granuloma**
  - a.k.a. lobular capillary hemangioma
    - Benign vascular tumor
    - Soft, red-blue anterior nasal mass, most common along anterior nasal septum
      - Other locations: Nasal vestibule, inferior turbinate > middle turbinate > uncinate process
  - Imaging
    - Well-circumscribed, small, intensely enhancing mass vs. central nodular areas of enhancement; T2 MR hyperintense
    - ± iso- to hypodense CT "cap" of variable thickness
    - ± bone erosion or remodeling

Helpful Clues for Less Common Diagnoses

- **Infantile Hemangioma**
  - Benign vascular neoplasm, not vascular malformation
    - Most common soft tissue tumor of childhood
    - Usually absent at birth, rapid growth in 1st few weeks/months of life (proliferating phase), spontaneous regression over subsequent months to years (involuting phase)
    - GLUT-1 positive in all phases
    - In nasal cavity, most common along anterior nasal septum
  - Imaging
    - Avidly enhancing submucosal mass
      - ± intralesional flow voids, frequently absent in small lesions
    - T2 MR hyperintense
    - Multiple &/or segmental distribution → think PHACE syndrome
- **Juvenile Angiofibroma**
  - Adolescent male with nasal obstruction &/or epistaxis

- Imaging
  - Vascular mass with flow voids & avid enhancement
  - Centered at sphenopalatine foramen with spread into pterygopalatine fossa, nasal cavity, & NP
  - ± bone erosion of pterygoid plates, floor of sphenoid sinus, ethmoid sinus, middle cranial fossa
- **Non-Hodgkin Lymphoma**
  - Sinonasal disease, most common in older adults
    - Nasal cavity > paranasal sinuses
    - Skull base lesions may extend into NP
  - Imaging
    - Homogeneously hypointense T2 MR, moderately enhancing
    - Bone remodeling &/or bone destruction
    - May be difficult to differentiate from rhabdomyosarcoma on imaging
- **Rhabdomyosarcoma**
  - Most common childhood soft tissue sarcoma
    - Most common location in H&N: Parameningeal (middle ear, paranasal sinus, NP)
      - Intracranial extension in up to 55%
  - Imaging
    - Soft tissue mass with variable contrast enhancement
    - Bone destruction more common when occurs in skull base &/or NP
      - Usually without aggressive bone destruction if arising in nose/nasal ala
    - May be difficult to differentiate from non-Hodgkin lymphoma on imaging
    - ± cervical metastatic adenopathy
- **Nasopharyngeal Carcinoma**
  - Most common cancer in Asian male patients
    - Associated with EBV
    - Triad of symptoms: Neck mass (metastatic adenopathy), serous otitis media, bloody nasal discharge
    - Pediatric patients tend to present late
  - Imaging
    - Mass centered in lateral pharyngeal recess
    - Simulates asymmetric adenoid tonsil hypertrophy
    - Central skull base invasion, widening of petroclival fissure; extends into parapharyngeal space, pterygopalatine fossa, & masticator space
    - Unilateral or bilateral cervical adenopathy

Helpful Clues for Rare Diagnoses

- **Esthesioneuroblastoma**
  - Malignant neuroectodermal tumor arising from olfactory neuroepithelium in superior nasal cavity
  - 2 incidence peaks (2nd & 6th decades)
  - Imaging
    - Destructive mass in upper nasal cavity/ethmoids
    - Avidly enhancing, dumbbell-shaped mass with "waist" at cribriform plate
    - Cysts at intracranial tumor-brain interface; orbital invasion is common

SELECTED REFERENCES

1. Peckham ME et al: Intranasal esthesioneuroblastoma: ct patterns aid in preventing routine nasal polypectomy. AJNR Am J Neuroradiol. 39(2):344-9, 2018
2. Rodriguez DP et al: Masses of the nose, nasal cavity, and nasopharynx in children. Radiographics. 37(6):1704-30, 2017
3. Koeller KK: Radiologic features of sinonasal tumors. Head Neck Pathol. 10(1):1-12, 2016
4. Merrow AC et al: 2014 Revised classification of vascular lesions from the International Society for the Study of Vascular Anomalies: Radiologic-Pathologic Update. Radiographics. 36(5):1494-516, 2016
5. Raz E et al: Fungal sinusitis. Neuroimaging Clin N Am. 25(4):569-76, 2015
6. Szymańska A et al: Invasive growth patterns of juvenile nasopharyngeal angiofibroma: radiological imaging and clinical implications. Acta Radiol. 55(6):725-31, 2014
7. Robson CD: Imaging of head and neck neoplasms in children. Pediatr Radiol. 40(4):499-509, 2010
8. Stambuk HE et al: Nasopharyngeal carcinoma: recognizing the radiographic features in children. AJNR Am J Neuroradiol. 26(6):1575-9, 2005

Adenoid Tonsil Hypertrophy

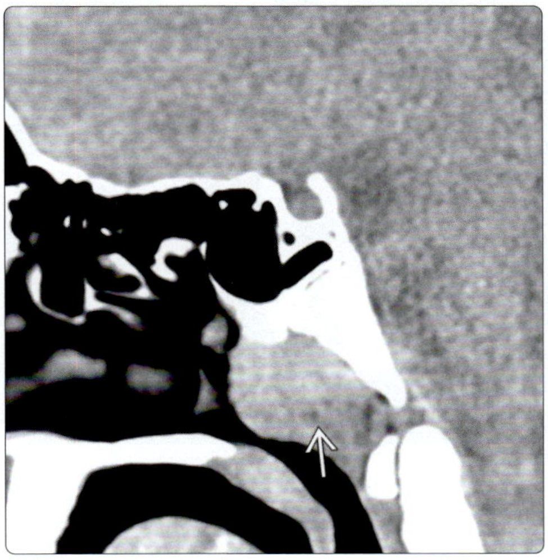

Adenoid Tonsil Hypertrophy

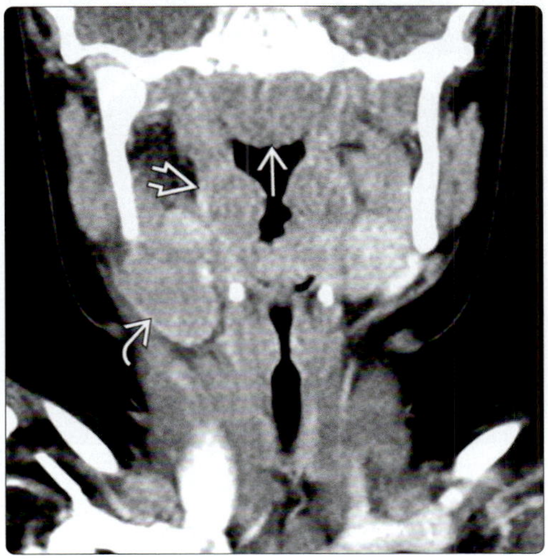

(Left) *Sagittal NECT in a teenager with sleep apnea demonstrates moderate prominence of the adenoids ➔ with subtotal occlusion of the nasopharyngeal airway.* **(Right)** *Coronal CECT in a teenager with fever & sore throat shows enlarged adenoids ➔, enlarged palatine tonsils ➔, & associated cervical adenopathy ➔, secondary to EBV.*

Sinonasal Polyposis

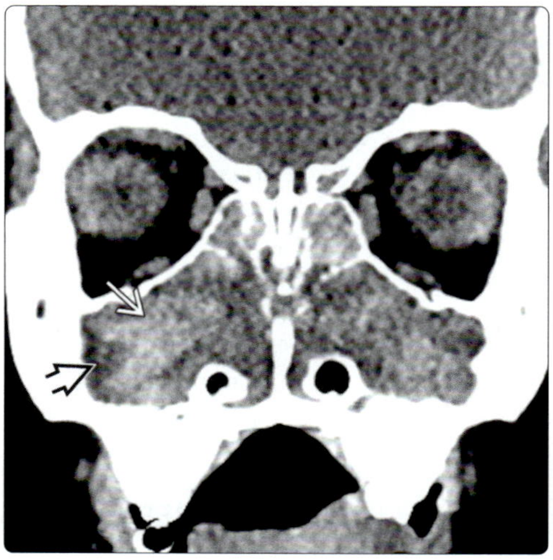

Solitary Sinonasal Polyp

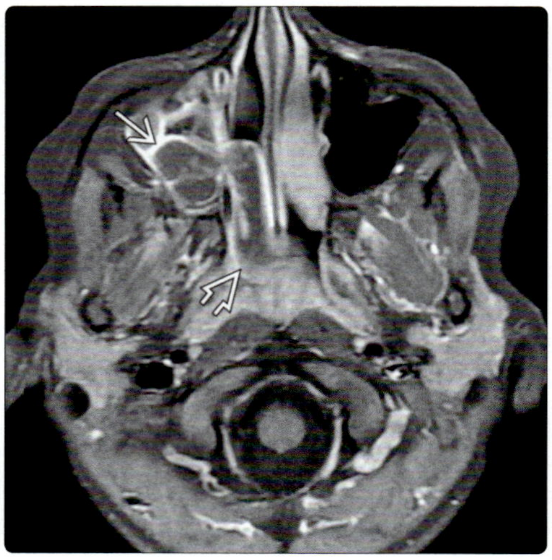

(Left) *Coronal NECT of the sinuses in a child with cystic fibrosis demonstrates typical findings of sinonasal polyposis with complete filling of the bilateral ethmoid & maxillary sinuses & the bilateral nasal cavities. Note the typical central hyperdensity* ➔ *& peripheral hypodensity* ⇨. **(Right)** *Axial T1 C+ FS MR in a teenager with nasal obstruction shows a hypointense polyp extending from the right maxillary antrum* ➔ *into the right nasal cavity & choana* ⇨ *via the maxillary ostium, typical of an antrochoanal polyp.*

Allergic Fungal Sinusitis

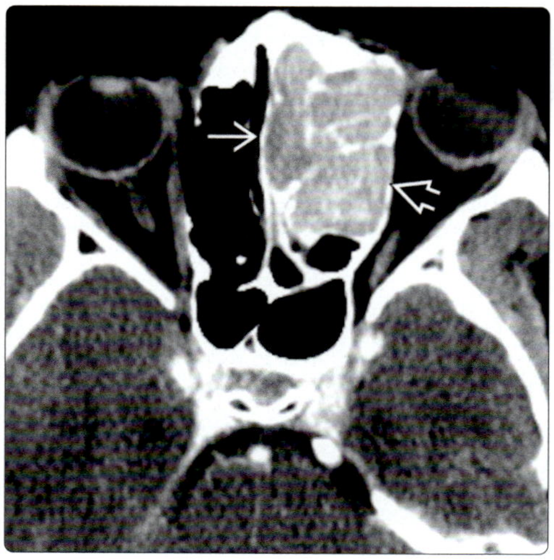

Allergic Fungal Sinusitis

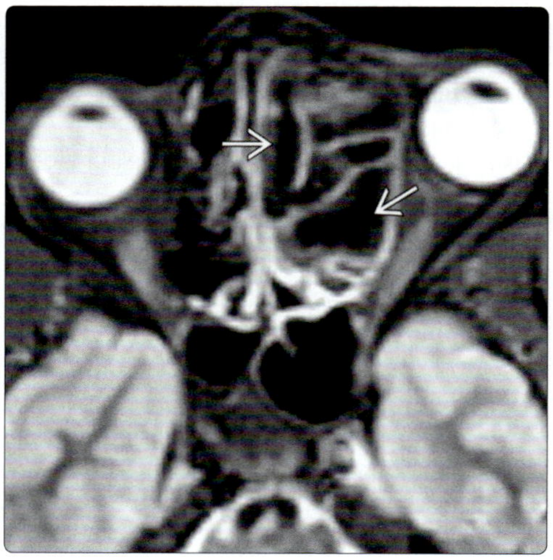

(Left) *Axial CECT in a child with proptosis demonstrates diffuse opacification & expansion of the left ethmoid air cells* ➔ *with encroachment on the left orbit* ⇨*, resulting in mild left proptosis.* **(Right)** *Axial T2 FS MR in the same patient demonstrates diffuse hypointense signal throughout the expanded left ethmoid air cells* ➔*, nearly void of signal & corresponding to the opacification on the CT, simulating air. This appearance is typical of allergic fungal sinusitis.*

Pyogenic Granuloma

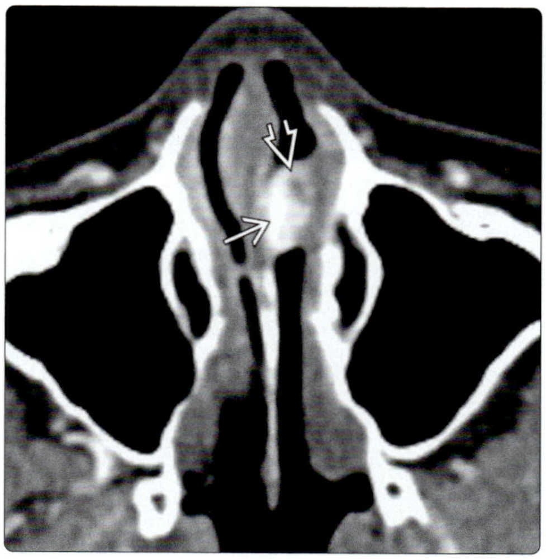

Infantile Hemangioma

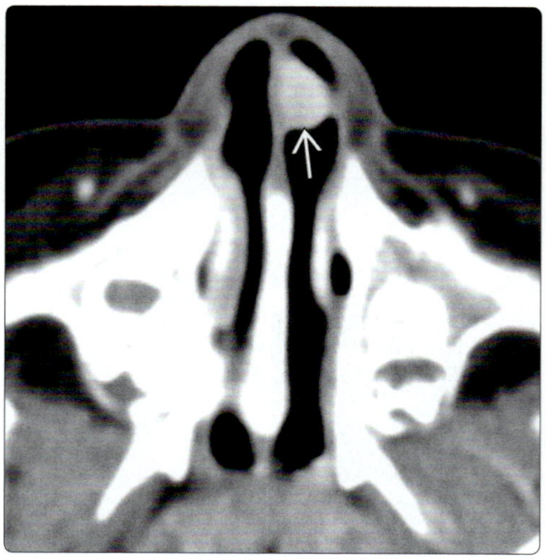

(Left) *Axial CECT in an older child with nasal obstruction demonstrates an ovoid, enhancing mass* ➔ *occluding the left nasal cavity. There is a small hypodense cap* ➔*, a finding not uncommon in pyogenic granuloma.* **(Right)** *Axial CECT in an 8 month old with a nasal mass shows an intensely enhancing mass* ➔ *attached to the nasal septum, nearly occluding the left naris. Intranasal infantile hemangiomas are usually small & frequently lack the typical intralesional flow voids seen on MR in larger lesions.*

Juvenile Angiofibroma

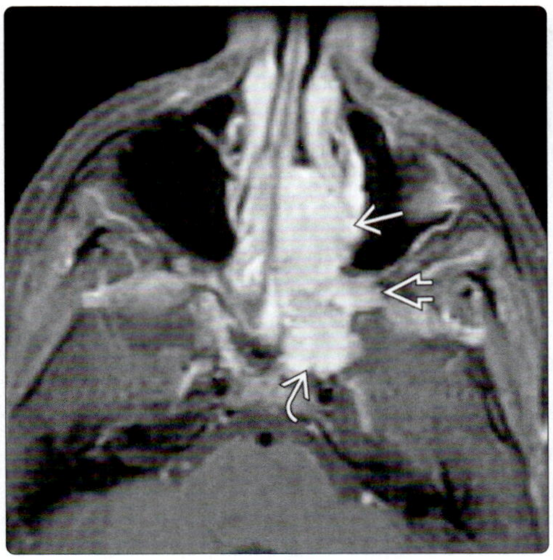

Non-Hodgkin Lymphoma

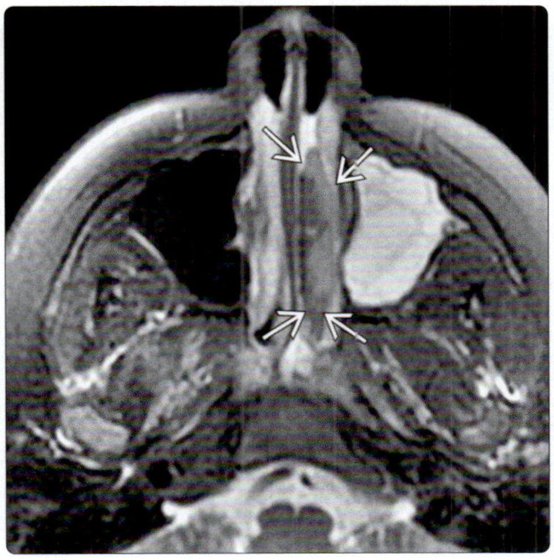

(Left) *Axial T1 C+ FS MR in a teenage boy with nasal obstruction & epistaxis demonstrates an intensely enhancing mass filling the posterior 1/2 of the left nasal cavity with extension into the left maxillary sinus ➔. There is also extension of the mass into the widened left pterygopalatine fossa ➔ & left sphenoid base ➔.* **(Right)** *Axial T2 FS MR in a 10 year old with nasal obstruction demonstrates an oblong, hypointense mass occluding the left nasal cavity ➔, proven to be non-Hodgkin lymphoma.*

Rhabdomyosarcoma

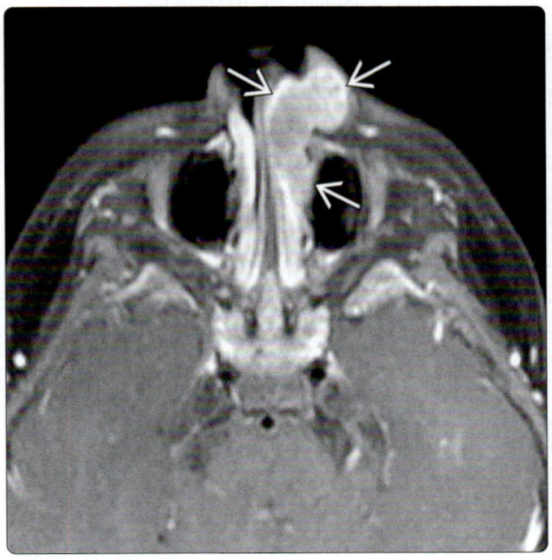

Nasopharyngeal Carcinoma

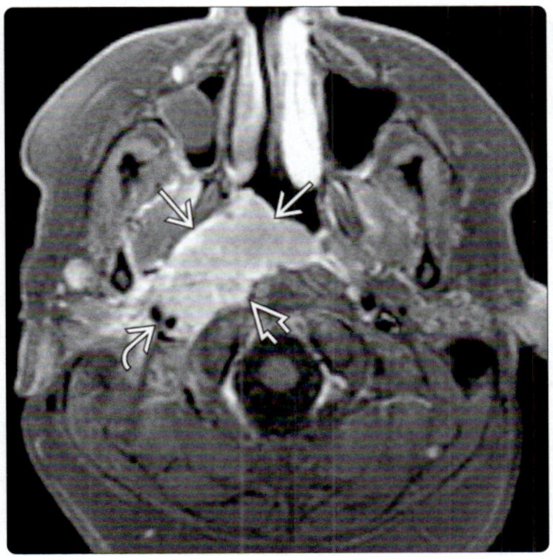

(Left) *Axial T1 C+ FS MR in a young child with a left nasal mass shows a heterogeneously enhancing mass ➔ involving the left naris. The mass occludes the left nasal cavity without significant bone destruction.* **(Right)** *Axial T1 C+ FS MR in a teenager shows a moderately enhancing nasopharyngeal mass ➔ with invasion of the right longus coli muscle ➔ & posterior displacement of the carotid sheath vessels ➔. This appearance, simulating asymmetric adenoids, is typical of nasopharyngeal carcinoma.*

Nasopharyngeal Carcinoma

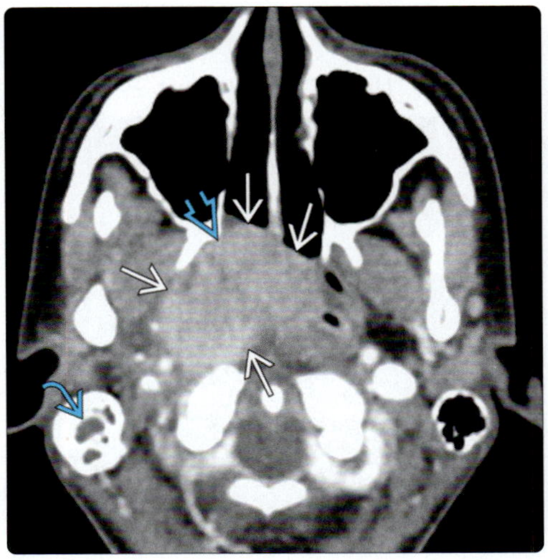

Esthesioneuroblastoma

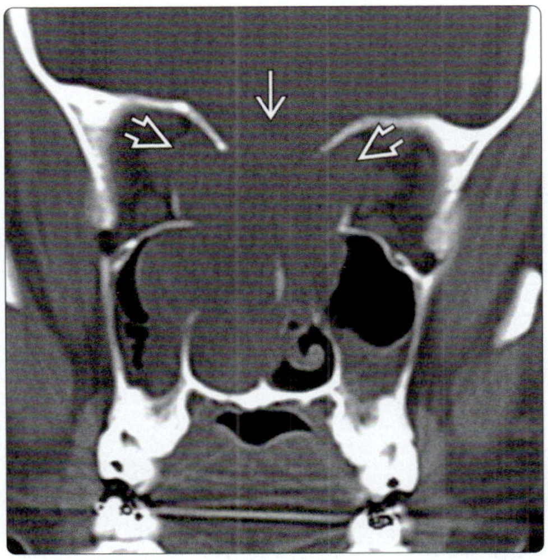

(Left) *Axial CECT in a teenager with jaw pain demonstrates a large, moderately enhancing mass occluding the nasopharynx ➔, R > L, & eroding the medial right pterygoid plate ➔. The mass is obstructing the right eustachian tube, which has resulted in right mastoid air cell opacification ➔.* **(Right)** *Coronal bone CT in a young adult with esthesioneuroblastoma shows a large mass filling the nasal cavity. There is destruction of the floor of the anterior fossa ➔, ethmoid air cells, & medial orbital walls ➔ bilaterally.*

DIFFERENTIAL DIAGNOSIS

Common

- Nasal Dermal Sinus
- Choanal Atresia
- Pyriform Aperture Stenosis

Less Common

- Frontoethmoidal Cephalocele

Rare but Important

- Nasal Glioma

ESSENTIAL INFORMATION

Key Differential Diagnosis Issues

- Nasal dermal sinus & cephalocele: Important to identify intracranial extension & associated cysts at imaging
- MR: Best imaging tool to evaluate extent of dermal sinuses & cephaloceles
- CT: Modality of choice to evaluate bony narrowing in choanal atresia & pyriform aperture stenosis

Helpful Clues for Common Diagnoses

- **Nasal Dermal Sinus**
  - Clinical clue: Pit or nasoglabellar mass may be present along nasal dorsum
  - CT/MR: Fluid tract may anywhere from nasal tip to anterior skull base at foramen cecum
    - Bifid crista galli or enlarged foramen cecum may be present
    - May see epidermoid or dermoid cyst
    - Intracranial extension of nasal dermal sinus in 20%
    - Craniofacial anomalies in 15%
- **Choanal Atresia**
  - Congenital obstruction of posterior nasal apertures, unilateral or bilateral
  - Clinical clue: Respiratory distress in newborn if bilateral; later presentation if unilateral
  - CT: Membranous or bony; unilateral or bilateral; thickened posterior vomer & medial bowing of posterior maxilla
    - Unilateral > > bilateral
      - Other anomalies are common in bilateral
- **Pyriform Aperture Stenosis**
  - Congenital bony stenosis of anterior nasal aperture
  - Clinical clue: Respiratory distress in newborn, especially when feeding (similar to choanal atresia)
  - CT: Narrow bony nasal inlet with small, triangle-shaped hard palate
    - Solitary median maxillary central incisor in 75%
      - Frequently with midline intracranial abnormalities

Helpful Clues for Less Common Diagnoses

- **Frontoethmoidal Cephalocele**
  - Clinical clue: Nasoglabellar or intranasal mass that may change in size with crying
  - MR: Extension of meninges, CSF, &/or brain tissue through defect in anterior skull base between frontal & nasal bones
  - Other intracranial abnormalities in up to 80%

Helpful Clues for Rare Diagnoses

- **Nasal Glioma**
  - Dysplastic neural tissue at nasal dorsum or in nasal cavity without connection to brain
    - Glioma is misnomer: Not neoplastic
  - Clinical clues: Subcutaneous blue or red mass on nasal dorsum (extranasal type); polypoid submucosal mass (intranasal type)
  - MR: Intra- or extranasal soft tissue mass
    - MR signal typically is **not** similar to brain parenchyma

SELECTED REFERENCES

1. Ginat DT et al: CT and MRI of congenital nasal lesions in syndromic conditions. Pediatr Radiol. 45(7):1056-65, 2015
2. Saettele M et al: Congenital midline nasofrontal masses. Pediatr Radiol. 42(9):1119-25, 2012

Nasal Dermal Sinus

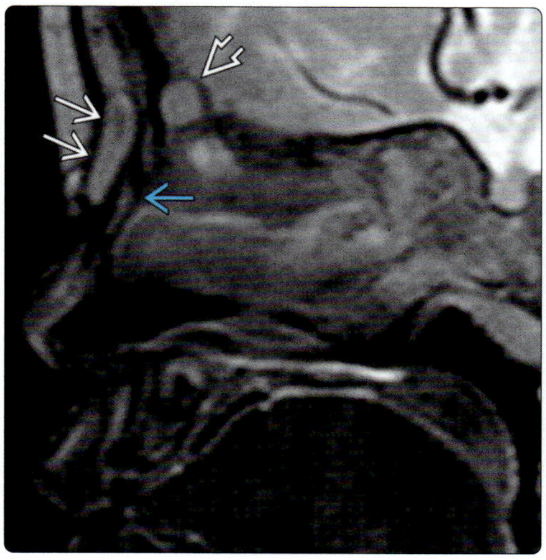

Nasal Dermal Sinus

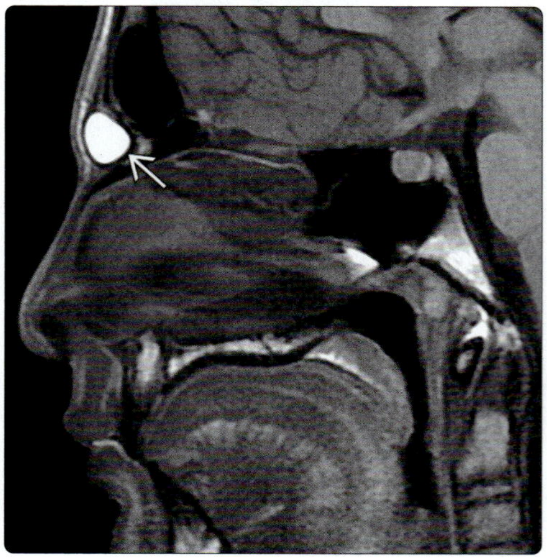

(Left) *Sagittal T2 MR in a 1 year old with a bump at the nasal bridge → shows the classic appearance of prenasal → & intracranial → dermoid cysts without an obvious connection. The intracranial component is situated at the enlarged foramen cecum. Both components demonstrated diffusion restriction (not shown).* **(Right)** *Sagittal T1 MR shows a homogeneously hyperintense lesion → superficial to the nasal bridge & frontal sinus, typical of a dermoid arising from a nasal dermal sinus tract.*

Choanal Atresia

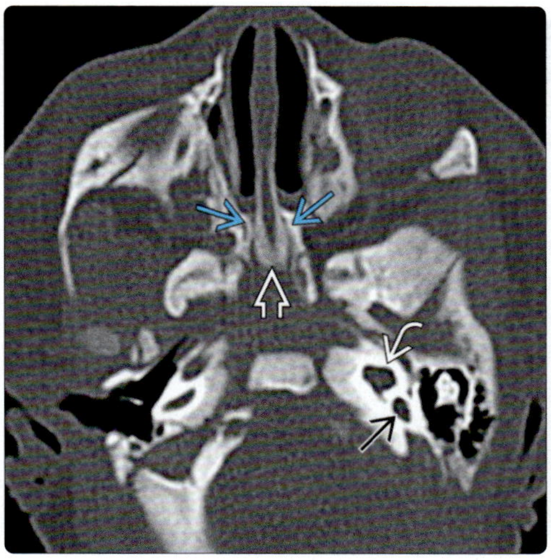

Choanal Atresia

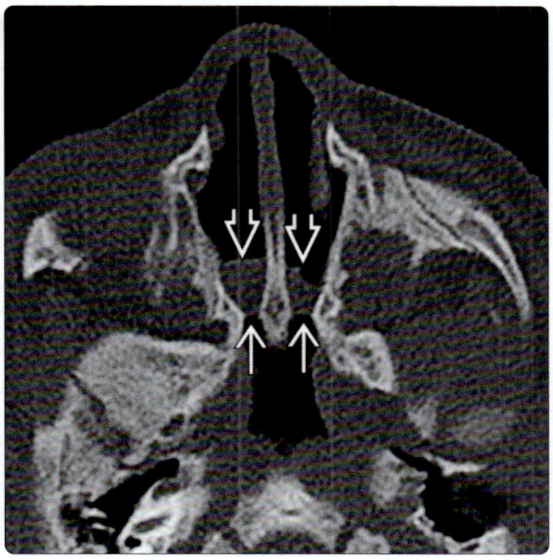

(Left) *Axial bone CT in an infant shows bilateral bony choanal atresia with bilateral medialization of the maxillae → & a large vomer ⇨. Also note the dysplastic cochlea ↪ & diminutive vestibule →. The semicircular canals were also absent, a characteristic finding in CHARGE syndrome.* **(Right)** *Axial bone CT demonstrates bilateral narrowing of the choanae secondary to bony stenosis & membranous atresia →. Note the typical fluid levels ⇨ of retained secretions in the nasal cavities anterior to the obstructing membranes.*

Pyriform Aperture Stenosis

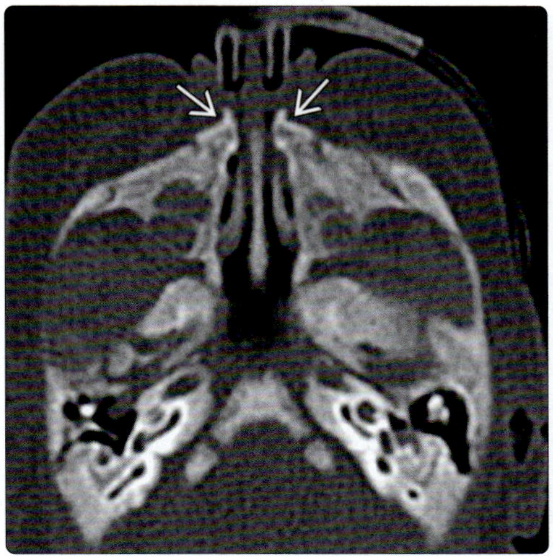

Pyriform Aperture Stenosis

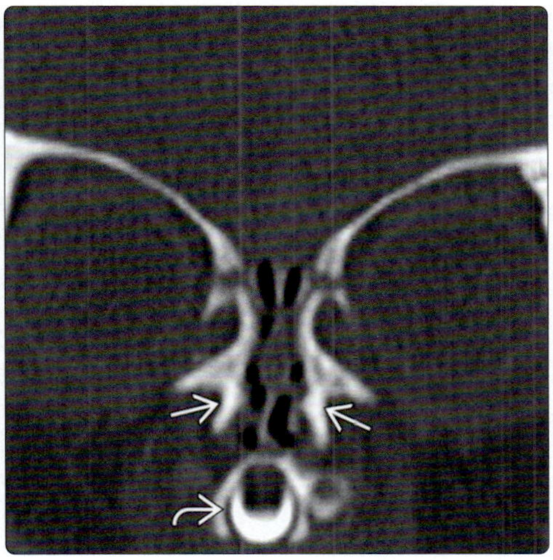

(Left) *Axial bone CT in a newborn demonstrates thickening of the anterior maxillae & nasal processes →, resulting in narrowing of the anterior nasal aperture. A solitary median maxillary central incisor & associated intracranial abnormalities were also present (not shown).* **(Right)** *Coronal bone CT shows pyriform aperture stenosis with narrowing of the anterior nasal cavities →. In this case, a single central megaincisor ↪ is seen in the midline maxilla.*

Frontoethmoidal Cephalocele

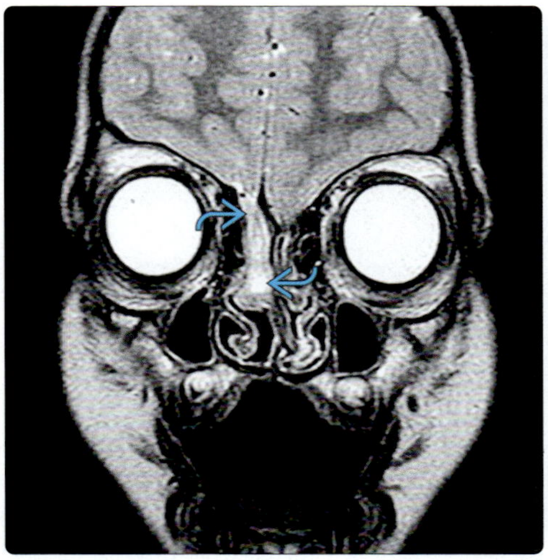

Nasal Glioma

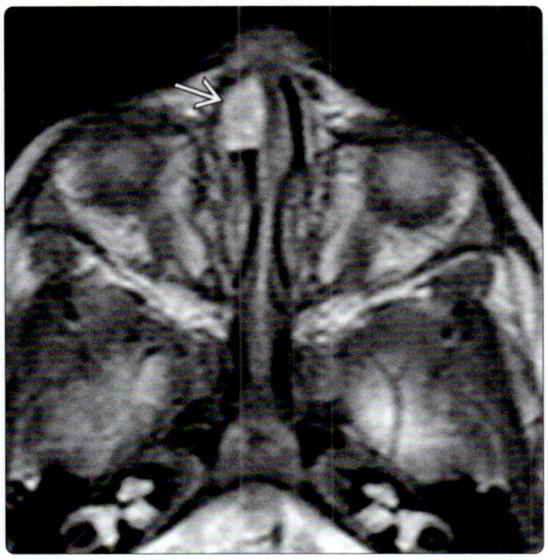

(Left) *Coronal T2 MR shows a cephalocele ↪ extending from the anterior cranial fossa through a skull base defect into the right nasal cavity. The cephalocele contains CSF & dysplastic brain tissue.* **(Right)** *Axial T2 MR in a 1 year old with nasal obstruction shows a nonspecific, mildly heterogeneous mass → in the right nasal cavity. There was no intracranial or nasolacrimal duct extension. An intranasal type of nasal glioma was ultimately confirmed.*

DIFFERENTIAL DIAGNOSIS

Common

- Nasolacrimal Duct Mucocele
- Choanal Atresia

Less Common

- Nasal Dermal Sinus
- Frontoethmoidal or Basal Cephalocele
- Nasal Glioma

Rare but Important

- Pyriform Aperture Stenosis
- Infantile Hemangioma
- Rhabdomyosarcoma

ESSENTIAL INFORMATION

Key Differential Diagnosis Issues

- Newborns are obligate nose breathers; therefore, bilateral nasal cavity lesions produce respiratory distress
  - Unilateral lesions may present later in childhood
- Imaging modality considerations
  - CT for osseous abnormalities
  - MR for intracranial components of congenital frontonasal masses & tumor characterization

Helpful Clues for Common Diagnoses

- **Nasolacrimal Duct Mucocele**
  - Well-defined, cystic medial canthal mass contiguous with nasolacrimal duct (NLD)
  - Cystic protrusion of NLD below inferior turbinate → nasal obstruction
  - Associated enlargement of bony nasolacrimal canal
  - More commonly unilateral than bilateral
- **Choanal Atresia**
  - Bony narrowing ± soft tissue membrane/plug obstructs posterior nasal passage
    - Thick vomer, medial bowing of posterior maxilla & pterygoid plate; stenosis more common than atresia
  - Unilateral in up to 75%; right > left
  - Bilateral in up to 25%; 75% have other anomalies
    - CHARGE association, craniosynostosis

Helpful Clues for Less Common Diagnoses

- **Nasal Dermal Sinus**
  - Fluid-filled cyst or sinus tract anywhere in midline septum from foramen cecum (at floor of anterior cranial fossa) to nasal tip
  - ± large foramen cecum, bifid crista galli, intracranial cyst
- **Frontoethmoidal or Basal Cephalocele**
  - Extracranial extension of intracranial contents
    - Contains variable amounts of meninges, CSF, & brain
  - Numerous subtypes named by course of extension; can potentially fill any portion of nasal airway
  - May enlarge with crying or jugular vein compression
- **Nasal Glioma**
  - "Nasal glial heterotopia" (**not** true neoplasm)
    - Dysplastic tissue without intracranial connection
  - Extranasal (at nasal dorsum) or intranasal
  - MR: Mixed to low T1, iso- to hyperintense T2; no enhancement

Helpful Clues for Rare Diagnoses

- **Pyriform Aperture Stenosis**
  - Symmetric bony narrowing of anterior nasal passageway
  - 75% also have solitary median maxillary central incisor ± midline intracranial anomalies
- **Infantile Hemangioma**
  - Benign vascular neoplasm typically arising after birth
  - Intensely enhancing nasal cavity mass, most common along anterior nasal septum
  - MR: T2 hyperintense ± flow voids; increased perfusion on ASL sequence
- **Rhabdomyosarcoma**
  - Most common childhood soft tissue sarcoma; rare in newborns
  - Often well-circumscribed; contrast enhancement is quite variable but usually < infantile hemangioma

Nasolacrimal Duct Mucocele

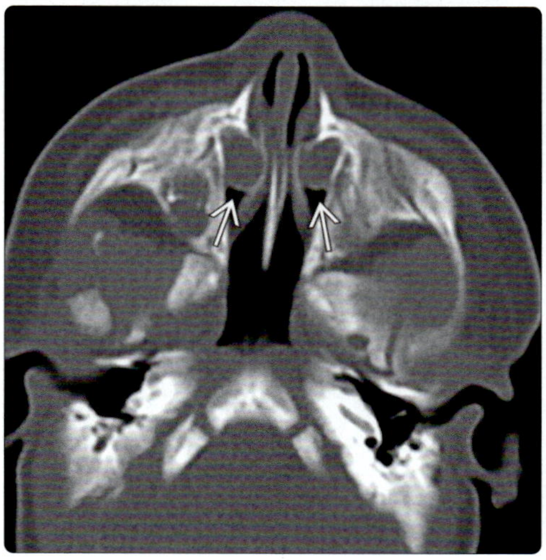

Choanal Atresia

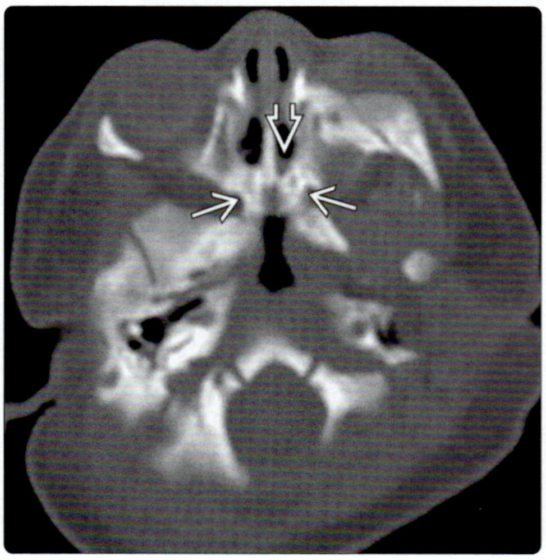

(Left) *Axial bone CT demonstrates low-density masses extending from the nasolacrimal ducts into the inferior meatus bilaterally, compatible with nasolacrimal duct mucoceles ➡. This newborn did have respiratory distress due to the bilateral masses.* **(Right)** *Axial bone CT shows bilateral osseous choanal atresia ➡ with a small amount of fluid layering in the posterior left nasal cavity ➡. This child required intubation immediately after birth.*

Nasal Dermal Sinus

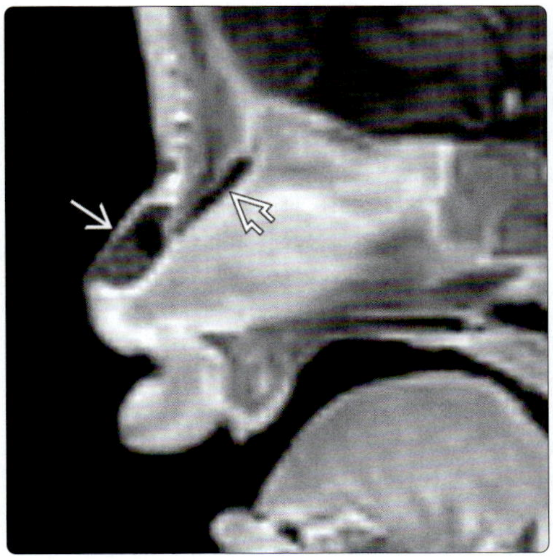

Frontoethmoidal or Basal Cephalocele

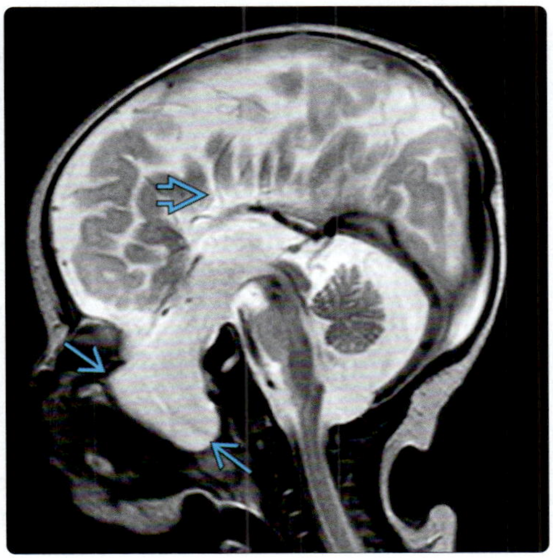

(Left) *Sagittal T1 C+ FS MR in an infant shows a heterogeneous dermoid cyst* ➔ *with a deeper sinus tract* ⇨ *extending toward the foramen cecum.* **(Right)** *Sagittal T2 MR in a 1 week old shows a large sphenoethmoidal subtype of basal cephalocele* ➔*. This mass obstructs the nasopharynx & oropharynx as it traverses a palatal cleft. There is also complete agenesis of the corpus callosum with sulci radiating* ⇨ *from the high-riding 3rd ventricle.*

Nasal Glioma

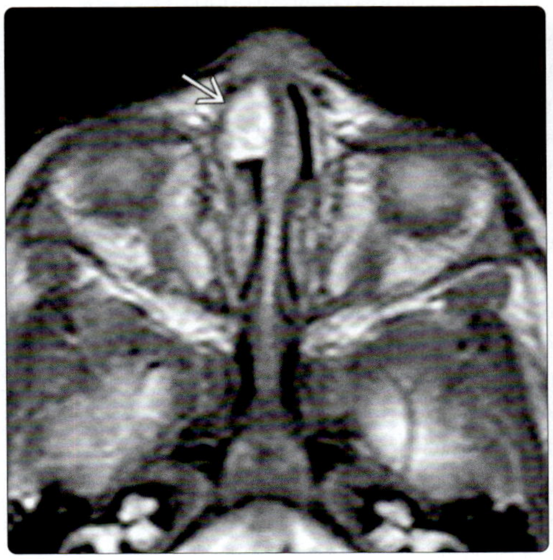

Pyriform Aperture Stenosis

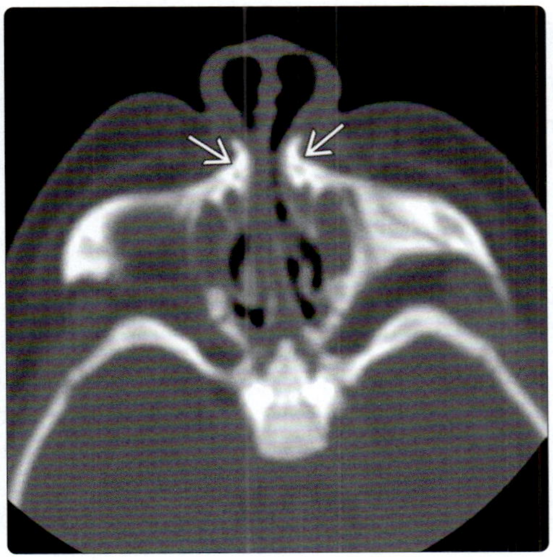

(Left) *Axial T2 MR in a 3 month old shows a nonspecific hyperintense mass obstructing the right nostril* ➔*. The mass was without intracranial connection & was pathologically proven to be heterotopic glial tissue/nasal glioma.* **(Right)** *Axial bone CT in a 2 day old with desaturation spells during feeding shows bilateral stenosis of the anterior nasal inlet* ➔ *consistent with pyriform aperture stenosis. Additional images demonstrated a solitary median maxillary central incisor (not shown).*

Infantile Hemangioma

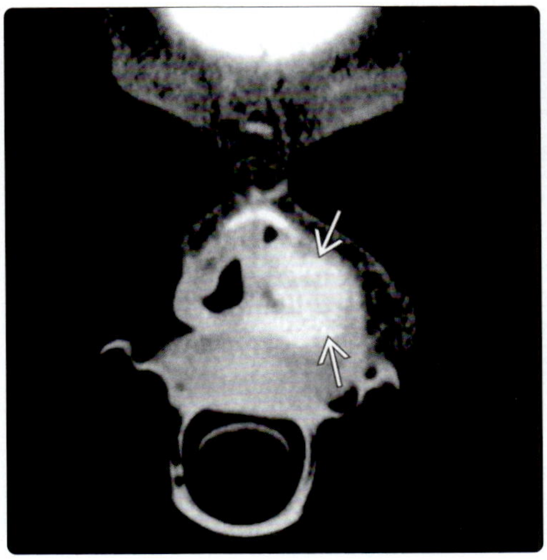

Rhabdomyosarcoma

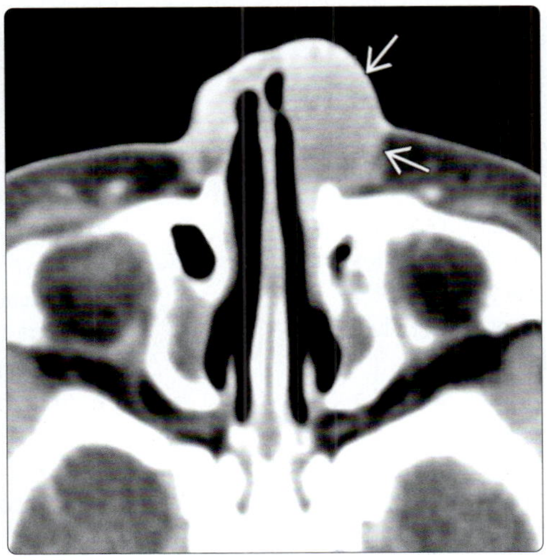

(Left) *Coronal CECT in a 2 month old with an enlarging left nasal cavity mass demonstrates a lobulated, markedly enhancing mass* ➔ *occluding the left nostril. The appearance is typical for an infantile hemangioma.* **(Right)** *Axial CECT in an 1 month old shows a mildly heterogeneous mass involving the left nasal ala* ➔*, causing mild narrowing of the left nasal cavity. The lack of significant enhancement is much more typical of rhabdomyosarcoma than infantile hemangioma.*

DIFFERENTIAL DIAGNOSIS

Common

- Internal Jugular Vein Asymmetry
- Jugular Bulb Diverticulum
- Chiari 1
- Chiari 2

Less Common

- Neurofibromatosis Type 1
- Aberrant Internal Carotid Artery
- Persistent Stapedial Artery
- Sphenoid Migration of Carotid Artery
- Agenesis of Internal Carotid Artery

Rare but Important

- Craniostenoses
- 4th Occipital Sclerotome Anomalies
- Medial Basal Canal (Basilaris Medianus)
- Persistent Craniopharyngeal Canal
- Chiari 3

ESSENTIAL INFORMATION

Helpful Clues for Common Diagnoses

- **Internal Jugular Vein Asymmetry**
  - Most commonly seen normal variant: Right internal jugular vein (IJV) is dominant in 68-75%
  - Imaging: Right sigmoid sinus, jugular bulb, & IJV are larger than left
    - Increased signal of left IJV on MR due to slow flow in left brachiocephalic vein from compression during respiratory cycle
- **Jugular Bulb Diverticulum**
  - Asymptomatic normal variant
  - Imaging: Coronal plane best (bone CT, MRV, or T1 C+ MR)
    - "Pouch" projects from jugular bulb, usually superiorly behind internal auditory canal
    - High signal on MR may simulate mass
- **Chiari 1**
  - Mismatch between posterior fossa size & cerebellar tissue
  - Imaging: Low-lying, pointed (not rounded), peg-like cerebellar tonsils
    - Tonsils project below (≥ 5 mm) or are impacted in foramen magnum
    - Effacement of CSF spaces at foramen magnum
    - 4th occipital sclerotome (OS) anomalies in > 50% → small occipital enchondral skull
    - ± retroflexed odontoid, horizontal clivus, basilar invagination, C1 assimilation, syrinx
- **Chiari 2**
  - ~ 100% with open neural tube defect
  - Imaging: Small bony posterior fossa with downward herniation of cerebellum & caudal brainstem through enlarged, funnel-shaped foramen magnum
    - "Towering" cerebellum with elongated 4th ventricle & flattened fastigium
    - Low-lying tentorium/torcular
    - "Scalloped" petrous pyramid & "notched" clivus
    - Associated intracranial abnormalities: Tectal beaking, ventriculomegaly, large massa intermedia, callosal agenesis/dysgenesis

Helpful Clues for Less Common Diagnoses

- **Neurofibromatosis Type 1**
  - Most common neurocutaneous disorder
    - Autosomal dominant; only small percentage have acquired skull base abnormalities
    - Characterized by diffuse neurofibromas, intracranial hamartomas, & benign & malignant neoplasms
  - Imaging: Sphenoid wing dysplasia, usually with adjacent plexiform neurofibroma; middle cranial fossa is expanded anteriorly
    - Enlarged optic foramina & fissures
    - Foramen magnum, skull base, & lambdoid defects
- **Aberrant Internal Carotid Artery**
  - Courses through middle ear
  - Imaging: Enters posterior middle ear through enlarged inferior tympanic canaliculus
    - Courses anteriorly across cochlear promontory
    - Joins horizontal carotid canal through dehiscent carotid plate
    - Absent carotid foramen & vertical segment of petrous internal carotid artery (ICA)
    - ± associated persistent stapedial artery (PSA) in 30%
- **Persistent Stapedial Artery**
  - Embryologic stapedial artery persists
    - PSA becomes middle meningeal artery
  - Imaging: Enlarged CNVII canal
    - Small canal leaving carotid canal at genu of vertical & horizontal petrous ICA
    - Absent ipsilateral foramen spinosum
- **Sphenoid Migration of Carotid Artery**
  - Seen in skull base syndromes involving enchondral bone
    - Achondroplasia, branchiootorenal syndrome, bicoronal synostoses (Apert, Pfeiffer, Crouzon)
  - Imaging: Medial migration of bony carotid artery canals at level of sphenoid
- **Agenesis of Internal Carotid Artery**
  - Isolated or syndromic (PHACE, morning glory disc anomaly, Goldenhar, clefting syndromes)
  - Imaging: Absent or hypoplastic vertical & horizontal petrous portions of ICA

Helpful Clues for Rare Diagnoses

- **Craniostenoses**
  - Early fetal fusion of 6 occipital bone ossification centers → premature obliteration of sutures
    - Syndromic (fibroblastic growth factor, *TWIST1*, & *MSX2* mutations)
    - Nonsyndromic
  - Imaging: Early fusion of occipital sutures surrounding foramen magnum
    - Enchondral skull base: Achondroplasia, syndromic bicoronal synostoses, kleeblattschädel
- **4th Occipital Sclerotome Anomalies**
  - Synonym: Proatlas anomalies
  - Normal development
    - Hypocentrum of 4th OS → anterior clival tubercle

    - Centrum of 4th OS → apical cap of dens & apical ligament
    - Ventral portion of neural component of 4th OS → anterior margin of foramen magnum & occipital condyle
    - Caudal portion of neural component of 4th OS → lateral C1 masses & superior posterior arch of C1
  - Imaging: 4th OS anomalies
    - Short clivus & atlas assimilation
    - Craniovertebral bony anomalies
- **Medial Basal Canal (Basilaris Medianus)**
  - Notochord remnant of cephalic terminus
  - Rarely leads to meningitis
  - Imaging: Midline clivus is site of anomaly
    - Lucency posterior to sphenooccipital synchondrosis
    - Currarino types A-F denote completeness & location of defect
    - Tortuous canal may indent superior or inferior aspect of clivus
    - ± nasopharyngeal cyst (rarely)
- **Persistent Craniopharyngeal Canal**
  - Tract from nasopharyngeal roof to pituitary fossa
  - Imaging: Lucency anterior to sphenooccipital synchondrosis, variable in appearance
    - Small incidental canal
    - Medium-sized canal with ectopic adenohypophysis
    - Large canal containing cephalocele
- **Chiari 3**
  - Occipitocervical cephalocele
    - Occipital squama defect may involve upper cervical vertebrae
  - Imaging
    - Low occipital or high cervical cephalocele contains cerebellum ± brainstem, meninges, vessels, CSF
    - Intracranial bony features of Chiari 2 also present

SELECTED REFERENCES

1. Khairy S et al: Canalis basalis medianus with cerebrospinal fluid leak: rare presentation and literature review. Br J Neurosurg. 1-2, 2017
2. Blaser SI et al: Skull base development and craniosynostosis. Pediatr Radiol. 45 Suppl 3:S485-96, 2015
3. Abele TA et al: Craniopharyngeal canal and its spectrum of pathology. AJNR Am J Neuroradiol. 35(4):772-7, 2014

Internal Jugular Vein Asymmetry

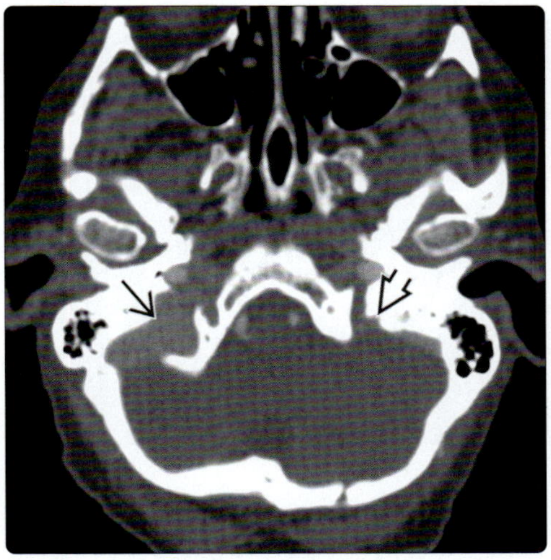

Internal Jugular Vein Asymmetry

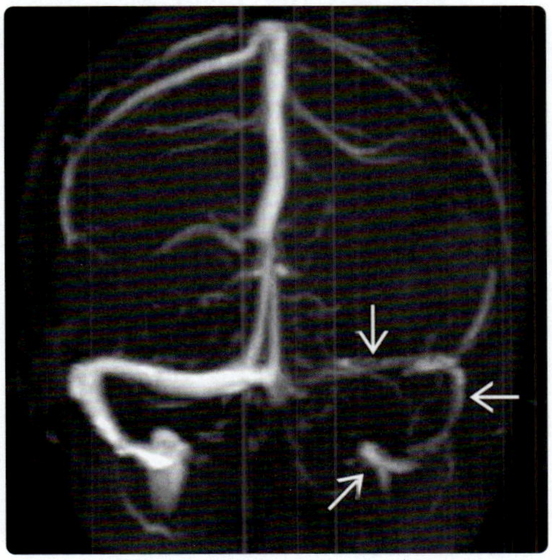

(Left) *Axial CT angiogram at the skull base shows asymmetry of the sigmoid sinus & jugular foramen, both larger on the right ⇨ than the left ⇨.* **(Right)** *Coronal MIP of a 2D TOF MR venogram shows normal-variant hypoplasia of the left transverse & sigmoid sinuses as well as the proximal internal jugular vein ➔. This is the most common variant with the majority of patients showing a dominant right venous system. This normal variant should not be confused with thrombosis (which can be excluded with a volumetric T1 C+ GRE sequence).*

Jugular Bulb Diverticulum

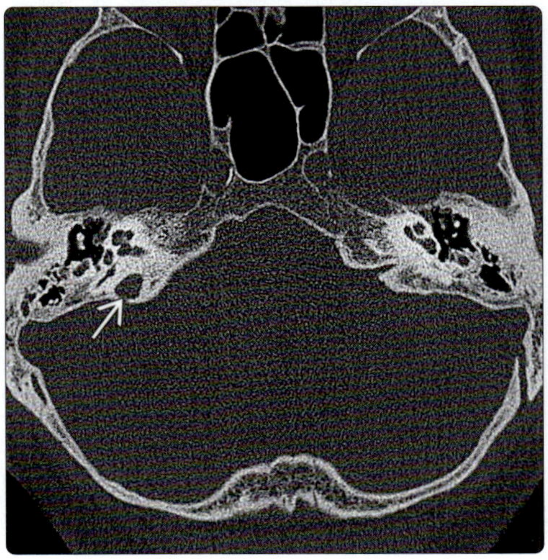

Jugular Bulb Diverticulum

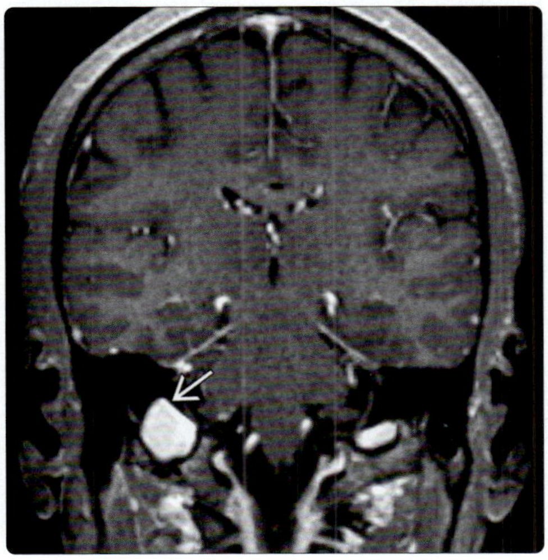

(Left) *Axial bone CT shows a well-circumscribed lucency ➔ of the right temporal bone, posterior to the membranous labyrinth. Continuity with the jugular foramen prevents misinterpretation as an enlarged vestibular aqueduct.* **(Right)** *Coronal T1 C+ MR shows outpouching of the superior aspect of the jugular bulb, consistent with a diverticulum ➔. CT is useful to detect dehiscence of the sigmoid plate into the middle ear cavity. "High riding" occurs when the bulb roof is superior to the floor of the internal auditory canal.*

(Left) *Sagittal T1 MR shows peg-like cerebellar tonsils extending below the foramen magnum with inferior displacement of the obex & a syrinx in the cervical cord. Note the mild scalloping of the dorsal surface & flattening of the angle of the clivus.* **(Right)** *Sagittal SSFSE T2 MR shows a small posterior fossa with a low torcular Herophili, herniated dysplastic cerebellar tonsils, & elongated 4th ventricle of Chiari 2. Note the hypoplastic corpus callosum splenium, scalloped clivus, & tectal beaking.*

Chiari 1

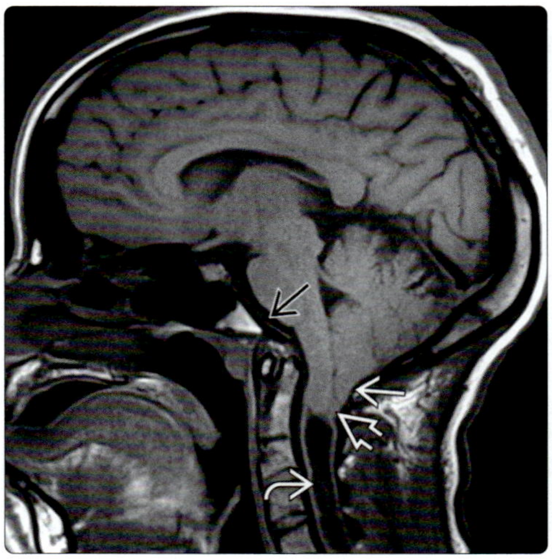

Chiari 2

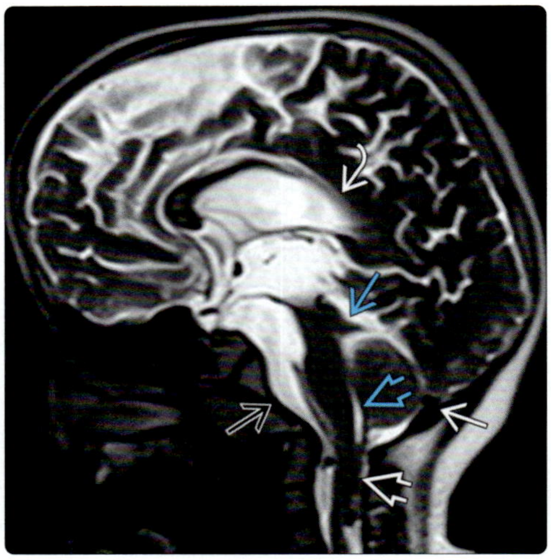

(Left) *Axial T1 C+ FS MR in a child with neurofibromatosis type 1 (NF1) shows hypoplasia/dysplasia of the right sphenoid wing with a diffuse, mildly enhancing preseptal & postseptal extraconal plexiform neurofibroma & moderate enlargement of the right globe (buphthalmos).* **(Right)** *Anterior 3D surface-rendered CT in the same patient shows diffuse enlargement of the right bony orbit with smooth, diffuse enlargement of the superior & inferior orbital fissures.*

Neurofibromatosis Type 1

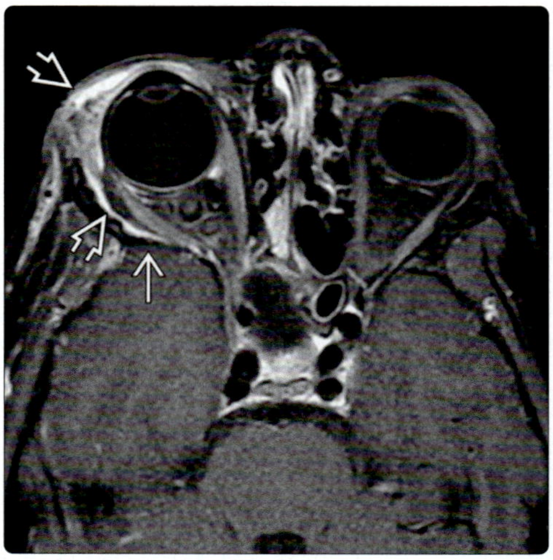

Neurofibromatosis Type 1

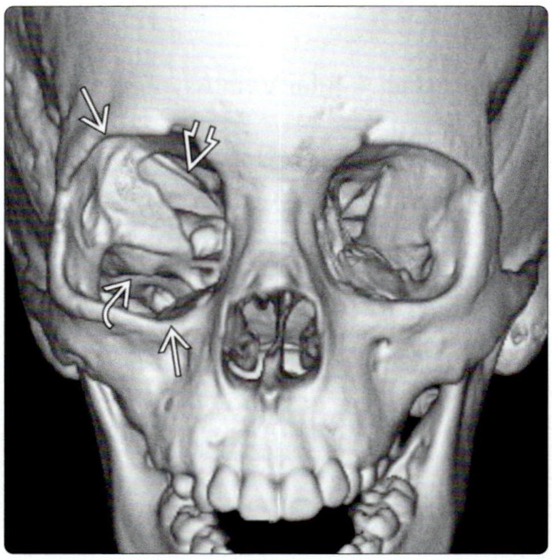

(Left) *Coronal T2 FS MR shows thinning/dysplasia of the right greater sphenoid wing to the level of the pterygoid plate with accompanying inferior herniation of the right temporal lobe & CSF. This is frequently also associated with anterior herniation of CSF into the posterior orbit, which causes pulsatile exophthalmos in these patients.* **(Right)** *Axial temporal bone CT shows a round soft tissue mass within the middle ear adjacent to the cochlear promontory. Note the hypoplastic petrous carotid canal.*

Neurofibromatosis Type 1

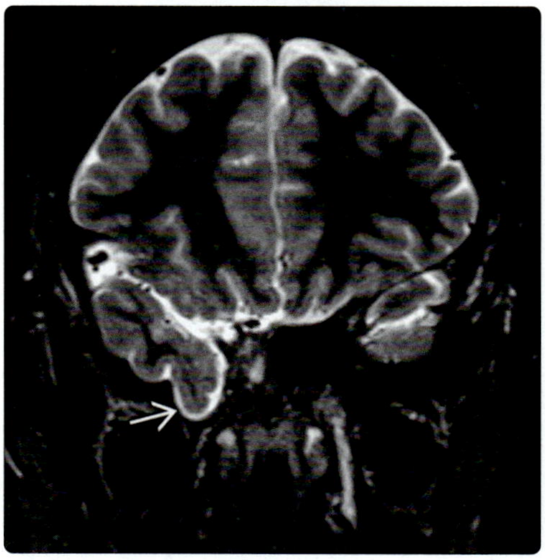

Aberrant Internal Carotid Artery

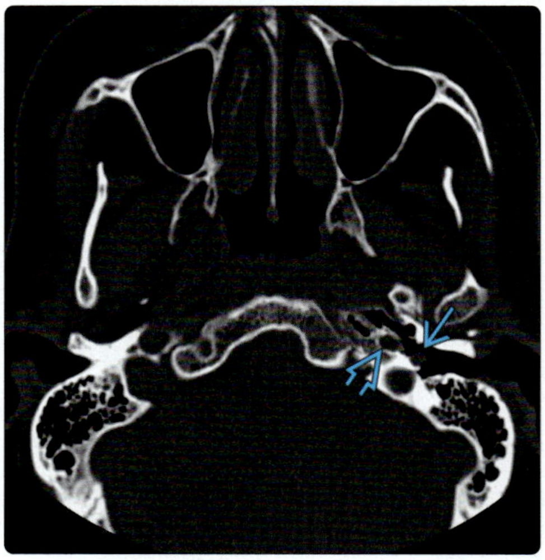

Aberrant Internal Carotid Artery

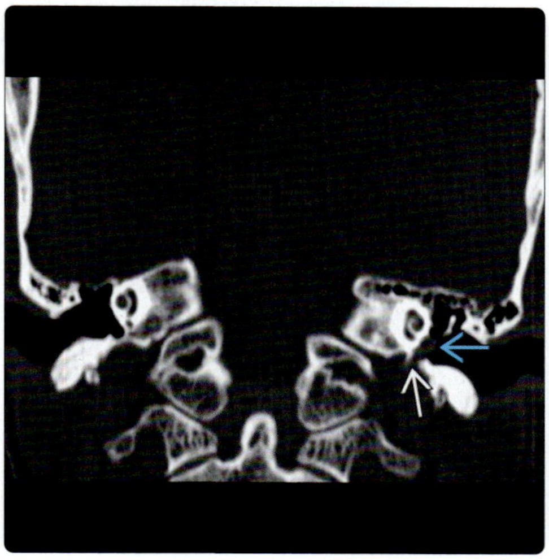

Aberrant Internal Carotid Artery

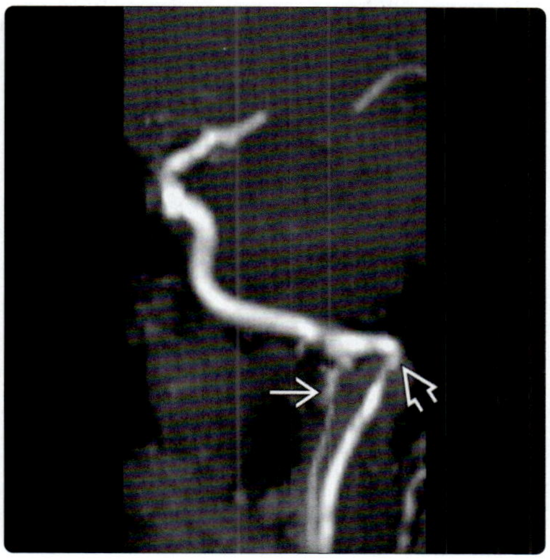

(Left) *Coronal temporal bone CT in the same patient shows that the soft tissue mass in the middle ear adjacent to the cochlear promontory is connected to an enlarged inferior tympanic canaliculus, consistent with an aberrant internal carotid artery.* **(Right)** *3D MIP of the left internal carotid artery from a TOF MRA in the same patient shows a hypoplastic conventional internal carotid artery that joins a larger aberrant internal carotid segment traveling through the middle ear.*

Persistent Stapedial Artery

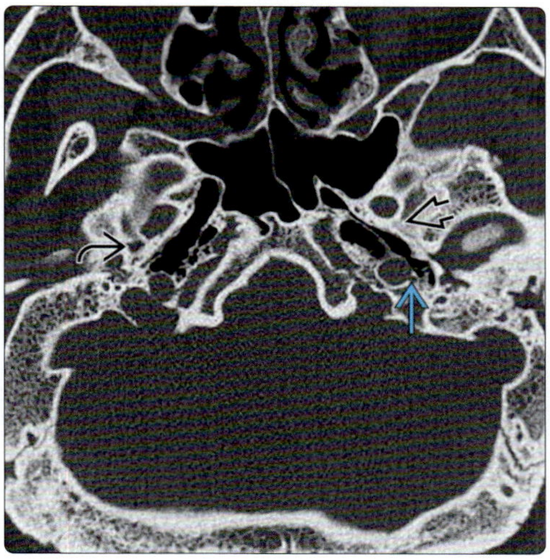

Persistent Stapedial Artery

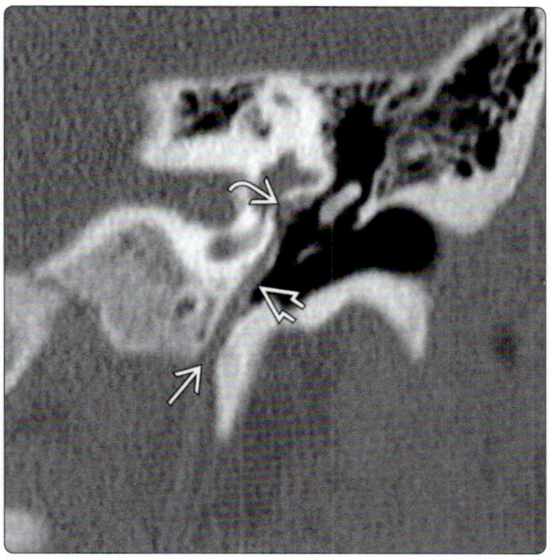

(Left) *Axial temporal bone CT show a small canal exiting the left petrous carotid canal. Note the absent left but normal right foramen spinosum.* **(Right)** *Coronal bone CT shows the persistent stapedial artery arising off the genu of the petrous internal carotid artery & ascending along the posterior cochlear promontory, passing over the oval window on its way to join the tympanic segment of the facial nerve canal.*

Sphenoid Migration of Carotid Artery

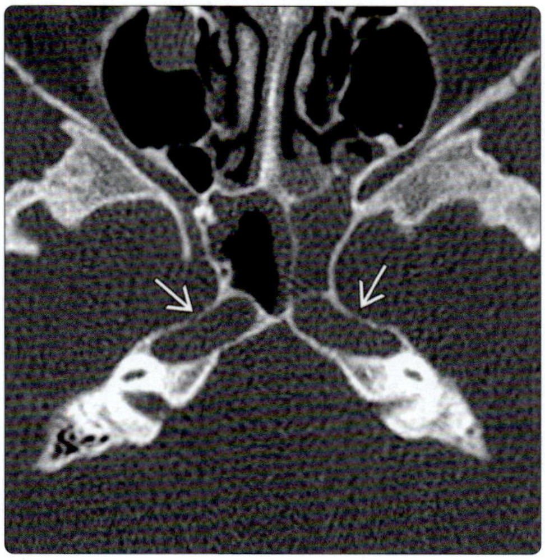

Agenesis of Internal Carotid Artery

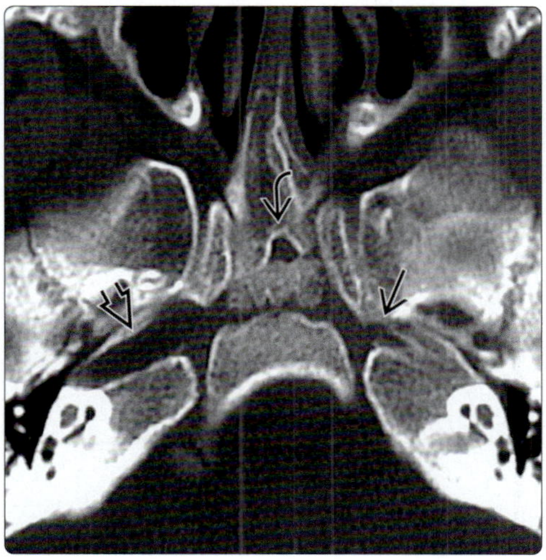

(Left) *Axial bone CT in a child with achondroplasia shows marked medial deviation of the internal carotid arteries, sometimes referred to as "kissing" in the midline. The internal carotid arteries remain covered by bone but indent the posterior walls of the sphenoid sinuses.* **(Right)** *Axial bone CT reveals a normal-sized right petrous internal carotid artery canal but an atretic left carotid canal. Note the prominent craniopharyngeal canal in this child with morning glory syndrome.*

(Left) *Axial bone CT in a young child with achondroplasia shows the typical transverse narrowing of the foramen magnum ➡ related to faulty enchondral ossification. Note also the elongation of the external auditory canals ➡ & narrowed central skull base, resulting in closely positioned carotid canals ➡.* **(Right)** *Axial bone CT 3D reconstruction in a normal newborn shows patency of the anterior ➡ & posterior ➡ intraoccipital sutures. The foramen ovale ➡ are symmetric.*

Craniostenoses

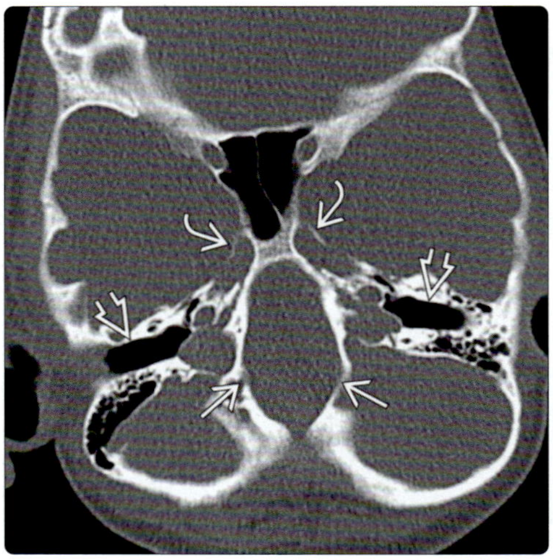

Craniostenoses

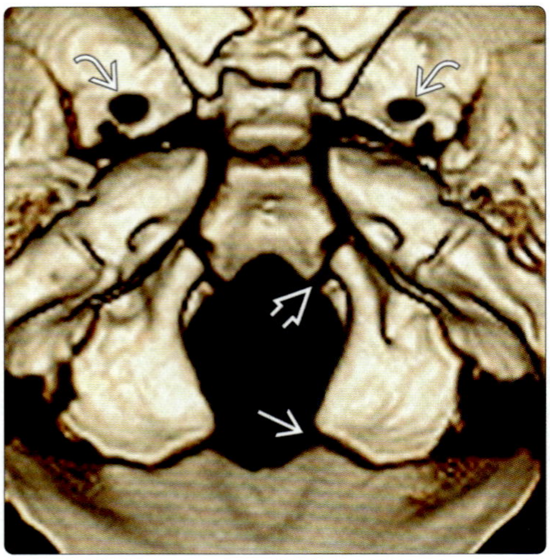

(Left) *Axial bone CT 3D reconstruction in a newborn with a disorder of enchondral ossification shows a deformed foramen magnum due to fusion of the sutures. There is hypertrophy of the internal occipital crest ➡. Note also the distortion of the left foramen ovale ➡.* **(Right)** *Axial CECT demonstrates absence of the clivus ➡ & an anomalous odontoid ➡ in an infant with severe anomalies of the skull base.*

Craniostenoses

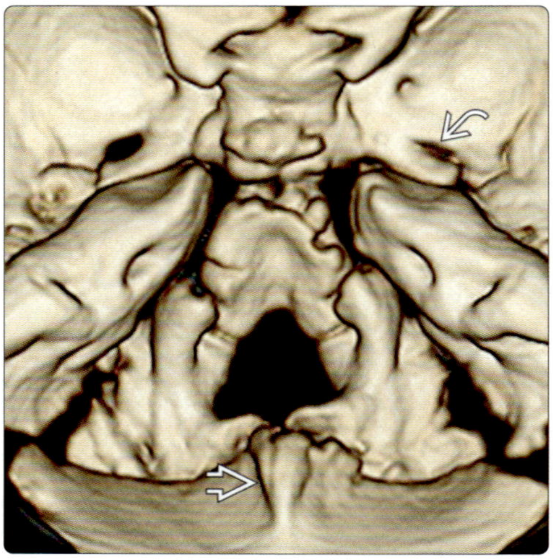

4th Occipital Sclerotome Anomalies

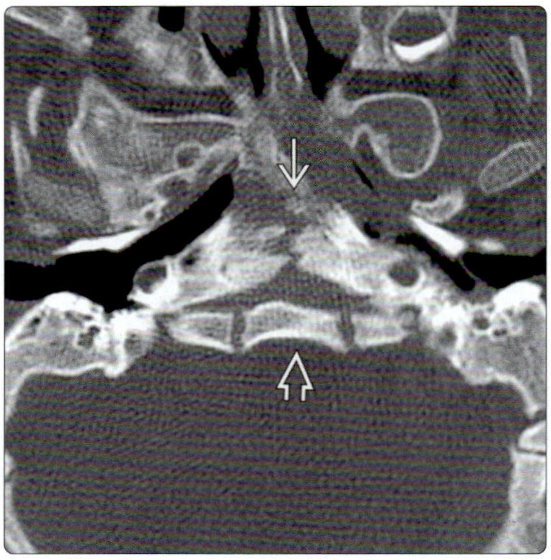

(Left) *Coronal reformatted bone CT demonstrates complete assimilation of the bilateral lateral masses of C1 with the occiput ➡ plus a hypoplastic dens ➡.* **(Right)** *Axial bone CT in the same patient demonstrates anomalous, bilateral, well-corticated clefts ➡ in the clivus.*

4th Occipital Sclerotome Anomalies

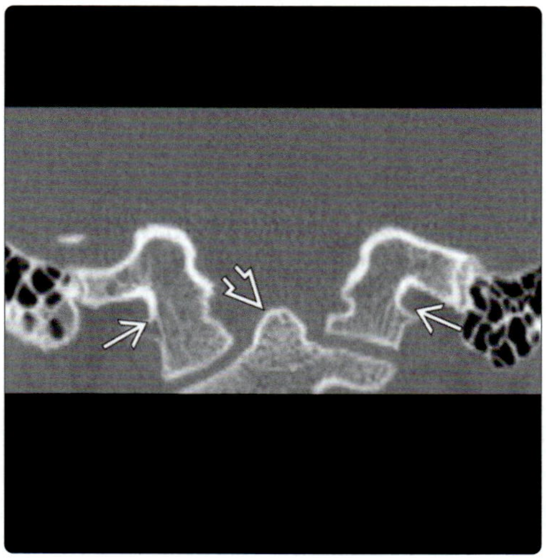

4th Occipital Sclerotome Anomalies

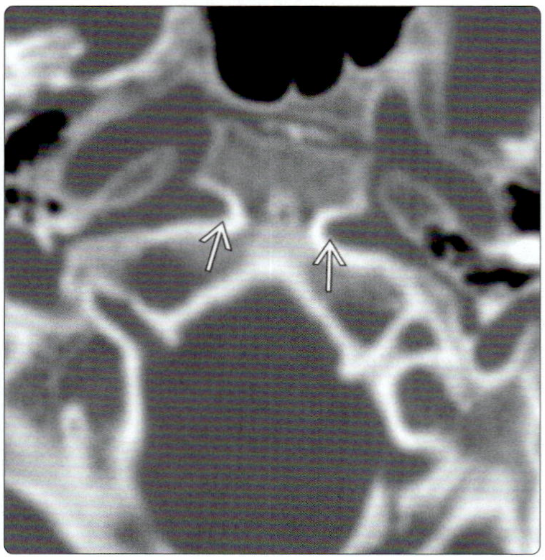

Medial Basal Canal (Basilaris Medianus)

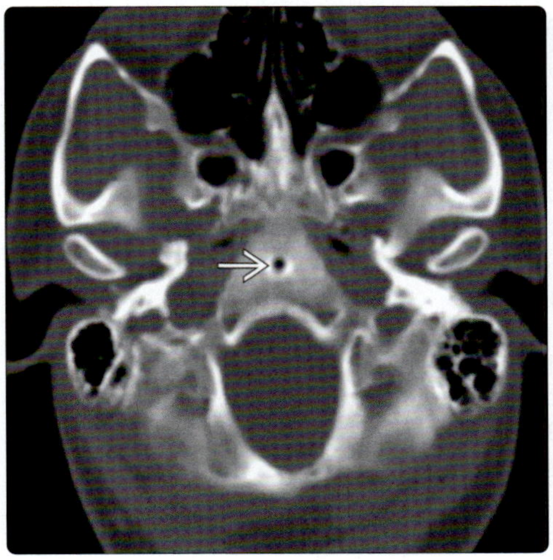

Medial Basal Canal (Basilaris Medianus)

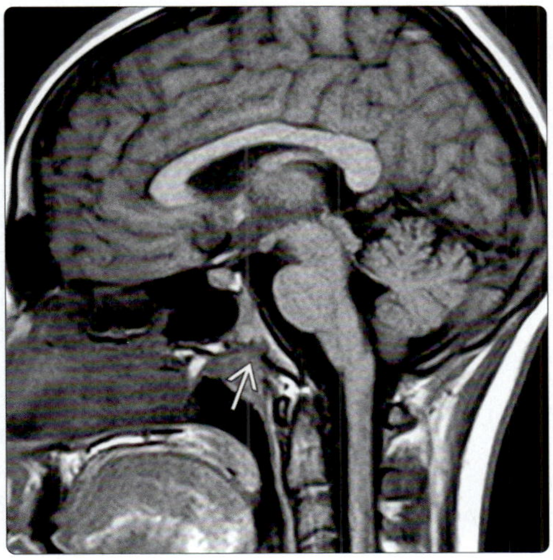

(Left) *Axial CT through the skull base shows a well-circumscribed, corticated midline lucency in the clivus ➡. This midline variant may indent the cortical margin of the clivus or be a complete remnant with a well-defined, through-&-through lucency.* **(Right)** *Sagittal T1 MR shows a ventral defect in the clivus ➡, which appears to include nasopharyngeal mucosal tissue. This cleft overlies the expected location of a Tornwaldt cyst, also a notochord remnant.*

Persistent Craniopharyngeal Canal

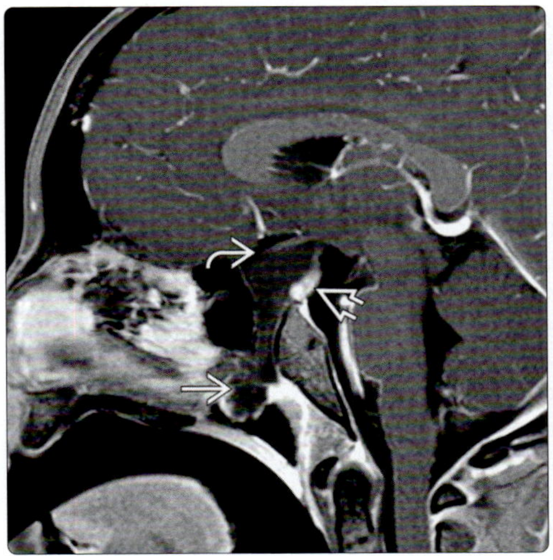

Persistent Craniopharyngeal Canal

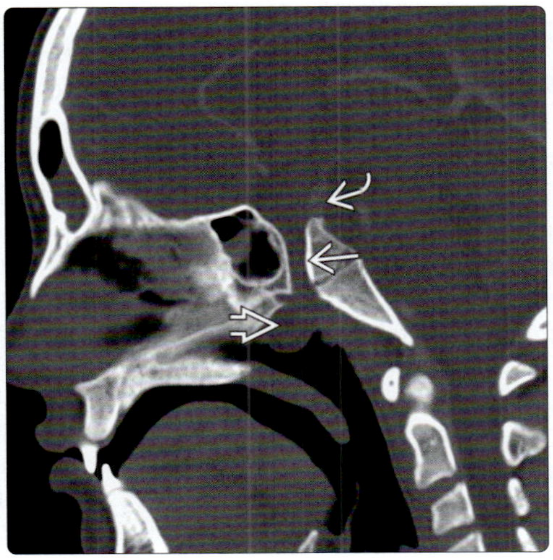

(Left) *Sagittal T1 C+ FS MR demonstrates a nonenhancing cyst ➡ within the large persistent craniopharyngeal canal. There is mass effect on the underlying nasopharynx, pituitary gland ➡, & suprasellar structures ➡.* **(Right)** *Sagittal CECT in bone windows shows a well-corticated channel ➡ communicating from the nasopharynx to the floor of the sella. Note the excess soft tissue of the nasopharynx ➡ as well as the superiorly & posteriorly displaced enhancing pituitary ➡.*

Chiari 3

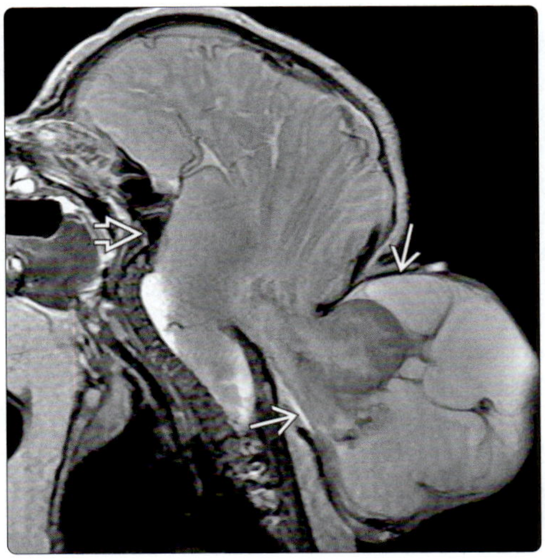

Chiari 3

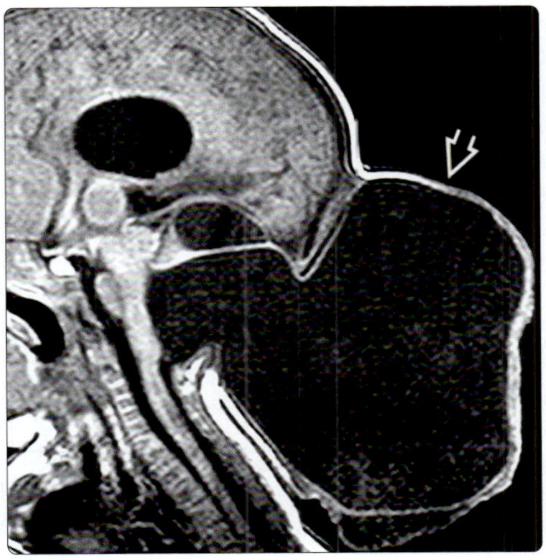

(Left) *Sagittal T2 MR shows a large occipitocervical encephalocele ➡ containing CSF, dysplastic cerebellum, & dysplastic occipital lobe. There is also ill-defined dysplastic parenchyma extending into the widened upper cervical canal, & the brainstem is difficult to discern as a separate structure. Note also the hypoplastic clivus ➡.* **(Right)** *Sagittal T1 MR in a newborn shows a large posterior cephalocele ➡ involving the foramen magnum & occipital bone. The opisthion & upper cervical spine are typically involved.*

DIFFERENTIAL DIAGNOSIS

Common

- Large Endolymphatic Sac Anomaly (IP-II)
- Temporal Bone Fractures
- Semicircular Canal Malformation
- Labyrinthine Ossificans

Less Common

- Labyrinthitis
- Cochlear Nerve & Cochlear Nerve Canal Aplasia-Hypoplasia
- Cystic Cochleovestibular Malformation (IP-I)
- CPA-IAC Lipoma

Rare but Important

- Vestibular Schwannoma
- Intralabyrinthine Schwannoma
- Facial Nerve Schwannoma in CPA-IAC
- Common Cavity Malformation
- Cochlear Aplasia
- Labyrinthine Aplasia

ESSENTIAL INFORMATION

Key Differential Diagnosis Issues

- History is important
  - **Congenital sensorineural hearing loss (SNHL)**
    - Failed newborn screening hearing test
    - Look for inner ear anomalies with CT &/or MR
      - If unilateral, look for cochlear nerve & cochlear nerve canal (CNC) hypoplasia/aplasia
  - **Fluctuating or "cascading" SNHL** in child (without history of meningitis)
    - Look for large vestibular aqueduct (LVA) ± cochlear malformation & modiolar deficiency on CT
    - Look for large endolymphatic sac/duct ± cochlear malformation & modiolar deficiency on MR
  - **Trauma**
    - Look for fracture involving inner ear structures ± pneumolabyrinth on CT
  - **Associated genetic disorders**
    - CHARGE, trisomy 21, Waardenburg, or Apert syndromes: Look for semicircular canal (SCC) malformations
  - **Prior meningitis**
    - CT: Look for labyrinthine ossification
    - T1 C+ MR: Labyrinthine enhancement during meningitis (acute phase)
    - T2/3D bSSFP MR: Normal high-intensity fluid replaced with low intensity (fibrosis or ossification) in membranous labyrinth
- Best imaging tool
  - Thin-section temporal bone CT for congenital inner ear anomalies, labyrinthine ossificans, fractures
  - High-resolution T2 &/or 3D bSSFP (FIESTA-C, CISS, etc.) MR for large endolymphatic sac, cochlear malformation, cochlear nerve aplasia/hypoplasia
  - T1 C+ MR best for schwannoma & other tumors, acute labyrinthitis, & autoimmune labyrinthitis (delayed enhancement)

Helpful Clues for Common Diagnoses

- **Large Endolymphatic Sac Anomaly (IP-II)**
  - Most common congenital anomaly of inner ear found by imaging
  - Axial CT: Vestibular aqueduct (VA) ≥ 2 mm at operculum or ≥ 1 mm at midpoint
  - Associated with incomplete cochlear partition type II (IP-II), modiolar deficiency, vestibule &/or SCC malformation
  - Additional prognostic information
    - Avoid contact sports or other activities that may lead to head trauma
    - Up to 40% of all patients with LVA & IP-II will have pendrin gene (*SLC26A4*) mutation → Pendred syndrome with thyroid organification defect ± goiter
- **Temporal Bone Fractures**
  - Transverse, longitudinal, or complex fractures may cross inner ear structures, ± pneumolabyrinth
  - Otic capsule violating vs. otic capsule sparing
- **Semicircular Canal Malformation**
  - Spectrum of abnormalities: ≥ 1 SCC is malformed, hypoplastic, or aplastic
  - Unilateral or bilateral (e.g., syndromic cases)
  - Most common is short, dilated lateral SCC & vestibule forming single cavity or with small bone island
  - ± cochlear malformation, oval window atresia, &/or ossicular anomalies
  - CHARGE syndrome
    - Bilateral hypoplasia or absence of all SCCs
    - Associated anomalies: Small vestibule, absent cochlear nerve aperture ("isolated cochlea"), oval window atresia (± overlying tympanic segment of CNVII), ± choanal atresia, ± coloboma
  - Lateral SCC is last to form embryologically; anomalies most frequently affect lateral SCC
    - Unless it is obliterated by labyrinthine ossificans or malformed in Waardenburg, branchiootorenal, & Alagille syndromes
- **Labyrinthine Ossificans**
  - Synonyms: Labyrinthitis ossificans, labyrinthine ossification, chronic labyrinthitis, ossifying labyrinthitis
  - Acute inflammatory response → fibrous then osseous replacement of membranous labyrinth over weeks or years
    - May involve cochlea ± vestibule ± SCCs
  - Bilateral in meningogenic form (meningitis) & in hematogenic form (blood-borne infections)
  - Unilateral in tympanogenic form (middle ear infection)
  - Temporal bone CT: High-attenuation bone deposition in formerly fluid-filled membranous labyrinth
    - Areas of ossification are crucial to identify when planning cochlear implantation
  - T2/bSSFP MR: Focal or diffuse low intensity replaces high-intensity fluid, with apparent "enlargement" of modiolus if cochlea is involved
  - T1 C+ MR: Enhancement of involved membranous labyrinth structures in early stage, may persist into ossifying stages

Helpful Clues for Less Common Diagnoses

- **Labyrinthitis**
  - Sudden onset of SNHL, vertigo, &/or tinnitus

- Bacterial, posttraumatic, or autoimmune causes
- Viral disease: Imaging usually not indicated
- Subacute inflammation of fluid-filled inner ear structures
- Temporal bone CT: Normal in early phases, may progress to labyrinthine ossificans
- T2/bSSFP MR: Low intensity replaces normal high-intensity fluid within membranous labyrinth structures
- T1 C+ MR: Mild to moderate enhancement
  - Enhancement may persist after symptoms resolve

- **Cochlear Nerve & Cochlear Nerve Canal Aplasia-Hypoplasia**
  - Temporal bone CT: Small IAC & CNC
  - MR: Fluid in CNC is completely or partially replaced by low-signal bone
  - Cochlear nerve diminutive or absent (with CNC aplasia)
- **Cystic Cochleovestibular Malformation (IP-I)**
  - Cystic, featureless cochlea + dilated vestibule & horizontal SCC
    - Cochlea: Absent internal septation & absent modiolus (IP-I), cochlea & vestibule form bilobed cyst
    - Vestibule: Dilated, large, communicates with cochlea
    - SCC: Dilated horizontal + vestibule → common cavity
  - IAC: Small or dilated, defective fundus
  - VA: Usually normal
- **CPA-IAC Lipoma**
  - Congenital fatty lesion of CPA ± IAC ± inner ear
  - Caveat: If T1 C+ MR is done without fat saturation, may be mistaken for vestibular schwannoma

Helpful Clues for Rare Diagnoses

- **Vestibular Schwannoma**
  - Enhancing lesion in IAC or "ice cream" on cone-shaped mass aligned with CPA-IAC
  - Hypointense on T2 MR
- **Intralabyrinthine Schwannoma**
  - Rare in children
  - Intracochlear: Schwannoma within cochlea
  - Intravestibular: Schwannoma within vestibule
  - Vestibulocochlear: Involves both vestibule & cochlea
  - Transmodiolar: Crosses modiolus; cochlea to IAC fundus
  - Transmacular: Crosses from vestibule into IAC fundus
  - Transotic: Crosses entire inner ear from IAC fundus to middle ear
- **Facial Nerve Schwannoma in CPA-IAC**
  - Rare in children
  - SNHL with associated facial neuropathy
  - Enhancing, well-circumscribed mass in CPA-IAC; extends into labyrinthine segment of CNVII
- **Common Cavity Malformation**
  - Featureless common cavity represents rudimentary cochlea, vestibule, & lateral SCC
  - Posterior & superior SCC: Absent, normal, or malformed
  - IAC: Often small with defective fundus ± anomalous course & small or absent CNVIII components
  - Middle ear space & ossicles: Normal or anomalous stapes & stenotic oval window
  - VA: Normal or absent
- **Cochlear Aplasia**
  - Absent cochlea with variable deformity of vestibule & SCCs
  - Absent/flattened cochlear promontory helps differentiate from labyrinthine ossificans
  - Absent CNC & nerve
  - Hypoplastic IAC
  - Normal VA & normal-sized middle ear cavity
  - Normal or malformed stapes
- **Labyrinthine Aplasia**
  - Absent cochlea, vestibule, & SCCs
  - Absent/flattened cochlear promontory
  - IAC aplasia/hypoplasia
  - Absent vestibular & cochlear nerves
  - Normal or malformed ossicles/middle ear
  - Normal or absent carotid canal
  - Old synonym: Michel anomaly

SELECTED REFERENCES

1. Prosser JD et al: Diagnostic evaluation of children with sensorineural hearing loss. Otolaryngol Clin North Am. 48(6):975-82, 2015

Large Endolymphatic Sac Anomaly (IP-II)

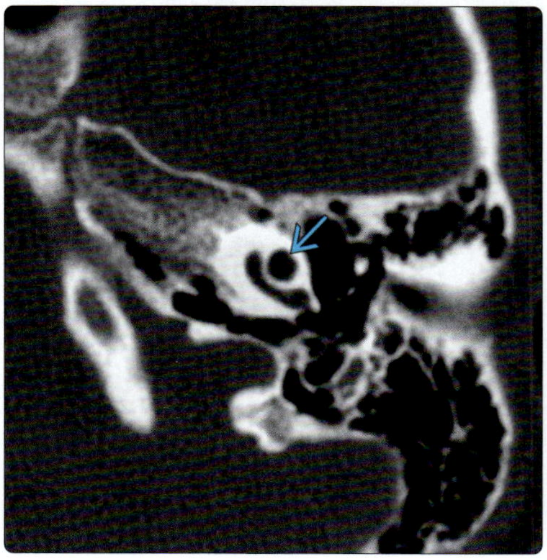

Large Endolymphatic Sac Anomaly (IP-II)

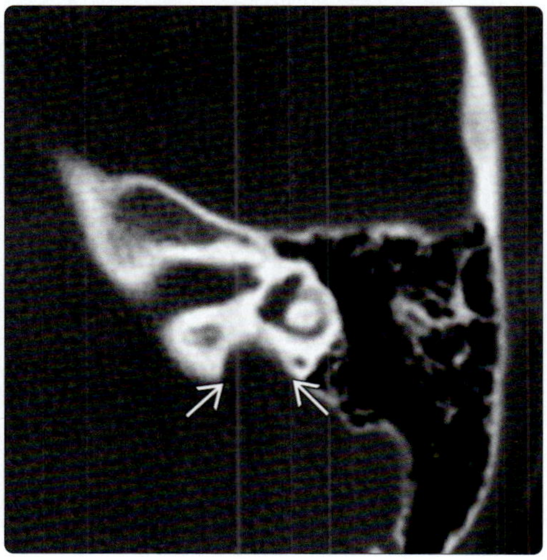

(Left) *Axial bone CT in an 8 year old with severe bilateral sensorineural hearing loss (SNHL) shows incomplete partitioning between the middle & apical turns of the left cochlea ⇨, typical of IP-II morphology.* **(Right)** *Axial bone CT in the same patient shows a markedly enlarged left vestibular aqueduct ➡, much larger than 2 mm at the operculum.*

(Left) *Axial 3D FIESTA MR in a 3 year old with SNHL shows enlargement of the bilateral endolymphatic sacs, incomplete cochlear partitioning, & mildly dysmorphic vestibules. An SCL26A4 mutation/Pendred syndrome analysis returned negative.* **(Right)** *Axial bone CT in a 14 year old involved in a dirt bike accident reveals a horizontal, otic capsule-violating right temporal bone fracture crossing the vestibule. Note the air in the vestibule & cochlea as well as multiple skull base & orbital fractures.*

Large Endolymphatic Sac Anomaly (IP-II)

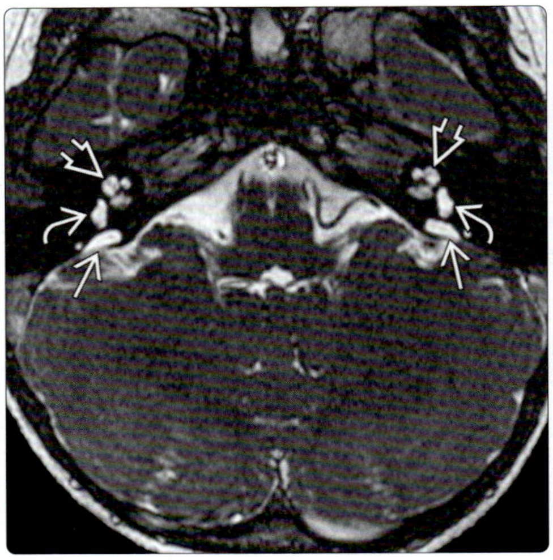

Temporal Bone Fractures

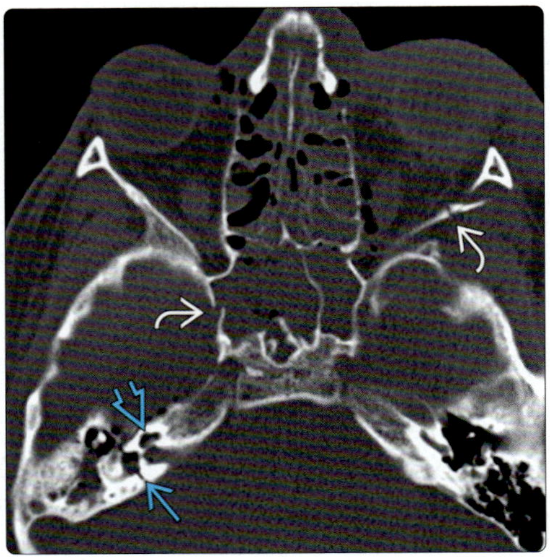

(Left) *Axial bone CT in a 6 year old demonstrates a short, dilated lateral semicircular canal (SCC) forming a single cavity with the vestibule, a common type of SCC anlage malformation.* **(Right)** *Axial bone CT in a 3 year old with a history of bilateral choanal atresia & hearing loss demonstrates diminutive vestibules & absence of the SCCs bilaterally, which is a characteristic appearance for the labyrinth in children with CHARGE syndrome.*

Semicircular Canal Malformation

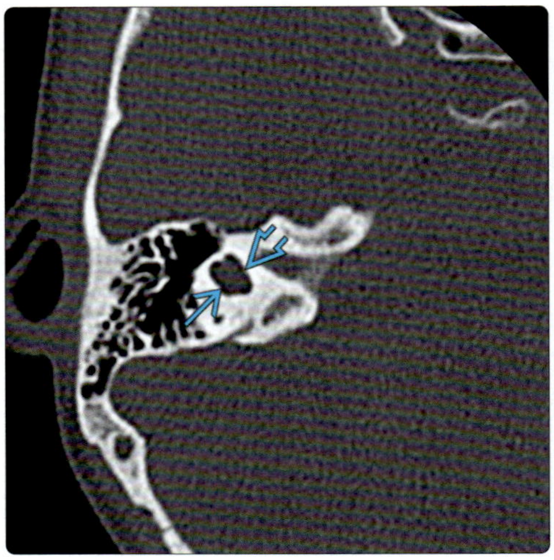

Semicircular Canal Malformation

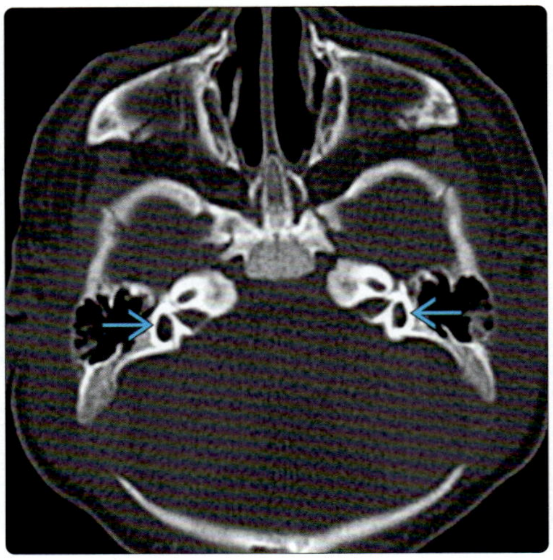

(Left) *Axial bone CT shows a relatively normal-caliber posterior limb of the left superior SCC, aplasia of the anterior limb of the superior SCC, & aplasia of the posterior SCC. In the presence of a normal lateral SCC (in other images), these findings are typical of Alagille syndrome.* **(Right)** *Axial bone CT in a patient with prior meningitis & subsequent rapid-onset hearing loss shows near-complete osseous replacement of the posterior & the lateral aspects of lateral SCCs & left cochlea.*

Semicircular Canal Malformation

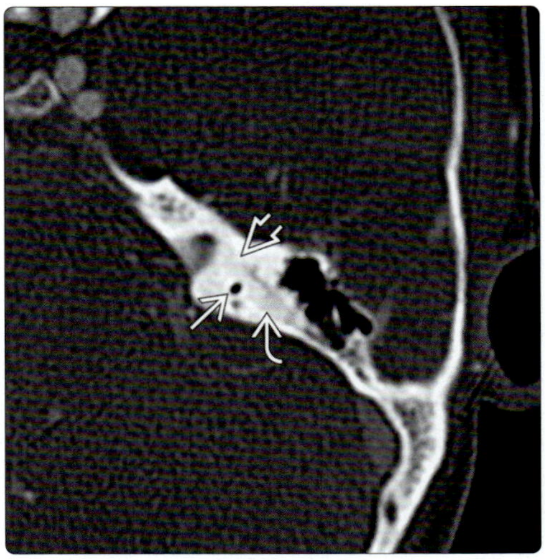

Labyrinthine Ossificans

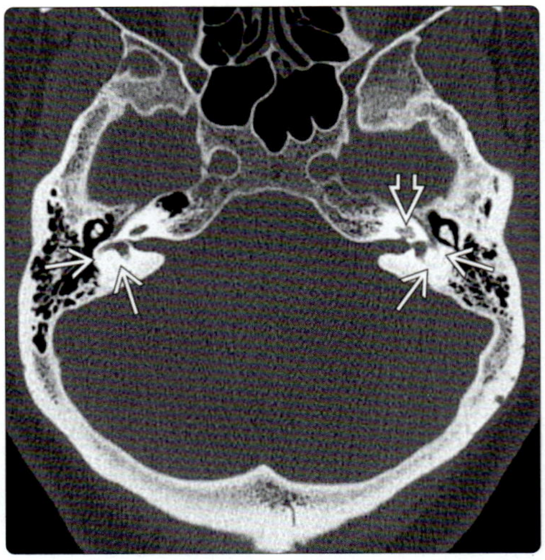

Labyrinthine Ossificans

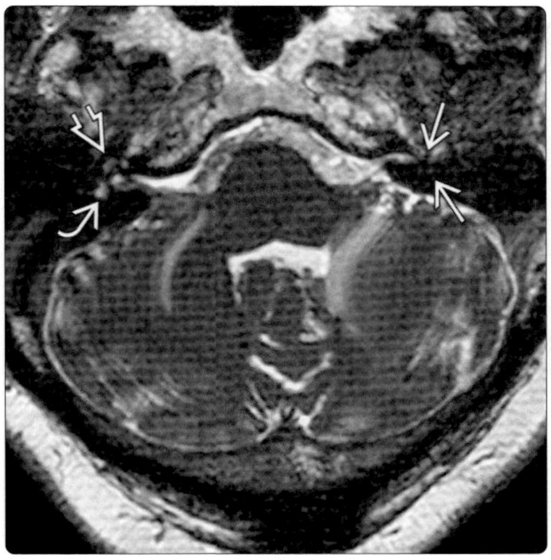

Labyrinthine Ossificans

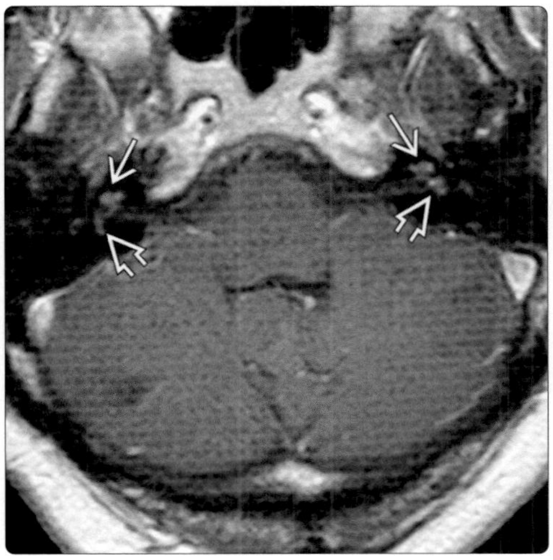

(Left) *Axial high-resolution CISS MR in a patient with prior meningitis & known partial labyrinthine ossification shows a lack of normal fluid signal in the left membranous labyrinth . There is also decreased fluid signal in the right cochlea & vestibule , which are barely visible.* **(Right)** *Axial T1 C+ MR in the same patient shows mild, patchy, abnormal enhancement of the cochlea & vestibule bilaterally.*

Labyrinthitis

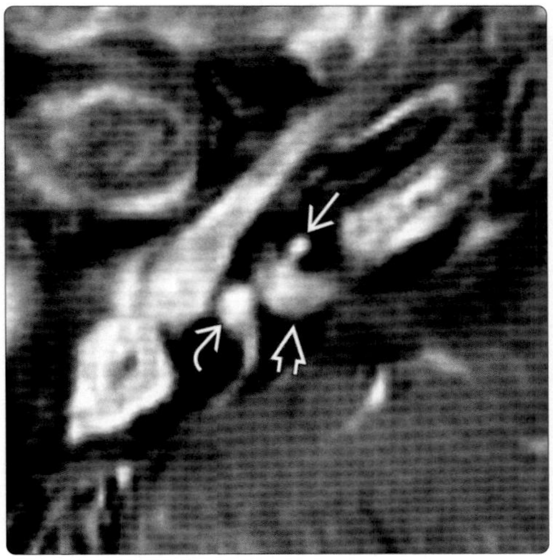

Labyrinthitis

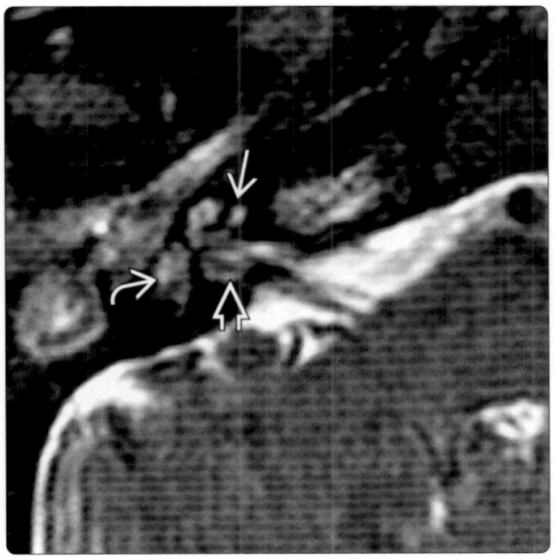

(Left) *Axial T1 C+ FS MR shows abnormal enhancement in the middle ear, mastoid, cochlea , vestibule , & IAC secondary to actinomycosis labyrinthitis.* **(Right)** *Axial 3D FIESTA MR shows corresponding loss of hyperintense fluid signal in the cochlea , vestibule , & IAC .*

Cochlear Nerve & Cochlear Nerve Canal Aplasia-Hypoplasia

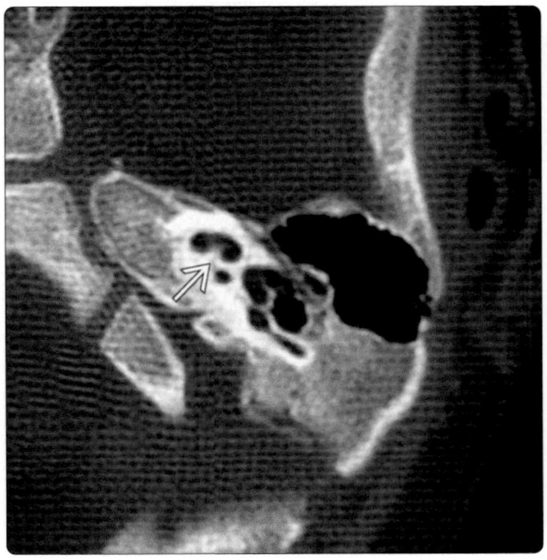

Cochlear Nerve & Cochlear Nerve Canal Aplasia-Hypoplasia

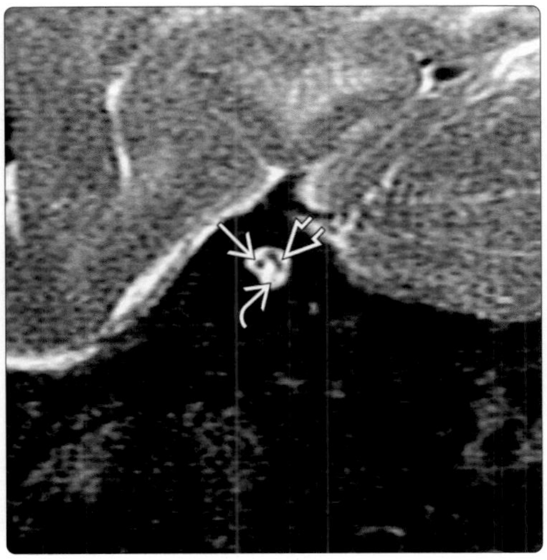

(Left) *Axial bone CT in a 3 year old with unilateral SNHL who failed her newborn hearing test shows an absent cochlear nerve canal , sometimes referred to as an "isolated" or "detached" cochlea.* **(Right)** *Sagittal oblique T2 MR at the level of the left IAC shows a normal-appearing facial nerve , superior/inferior vestibular nerve complex , & diminutive left cochlear nerve .*

(**Left**) *Axial 3D FIESTA MR shows absence of a definable right cochlear nerve* → *within the right IAC. There is also lack of a cochlear nerve canal & hypoplasia of the right modiolus* →. (**Right**) *Sagittal oblique T2 MR through the right IAC in the same child shows absence of the cochlear nerve* → *at its expected location. The cochlear nerve should normally be at least as large as the facial nerve* → *on sagittal oblique images through the IAC.*

Cochlear Nerve & Cochlear Nerve Canal Aplasia-Hypoplasia

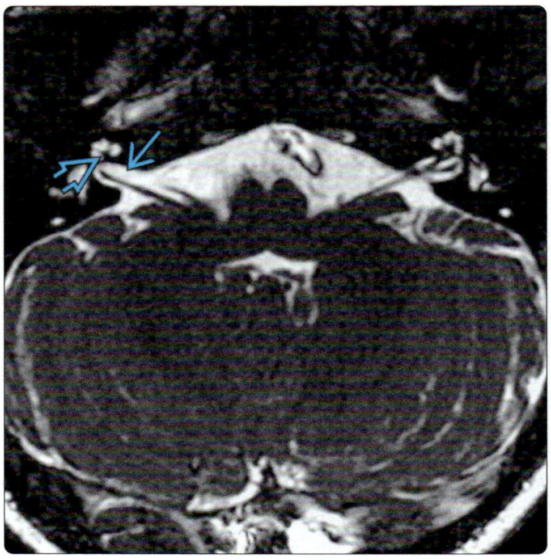

Cochlear Nerve & Cochlear Nerve Canal Aplasia-Hypoplasia

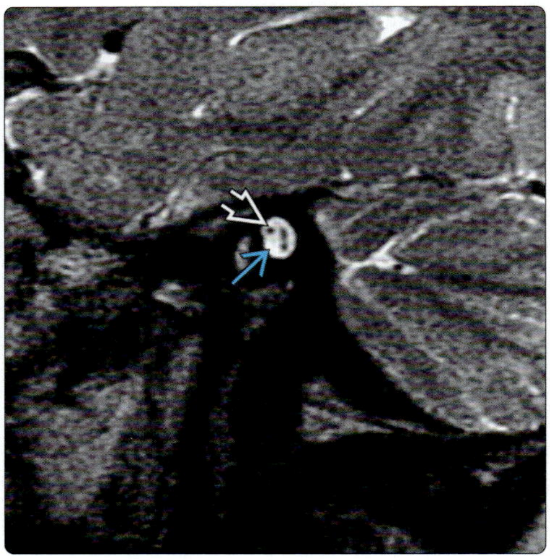

(**Left**) *Axial bone CT shows the typical appearance of a cystic cochleovestibular anomaly. The vestibule is globular* →. (**Right**) *Axial bone CT in the same patient reveals a featureless cochlea* → *without a definable modiolus, also termed an IP-I anomaly.*

Cystic Cochleovestibular Malformation (IP-I)

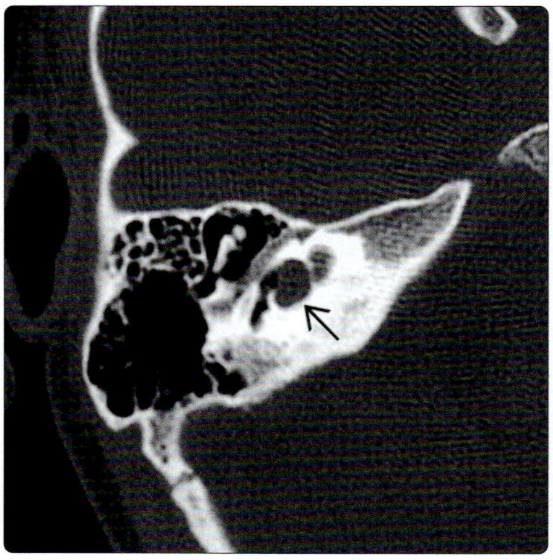

Cystic Cochleovestibular Malformation (IP-I)

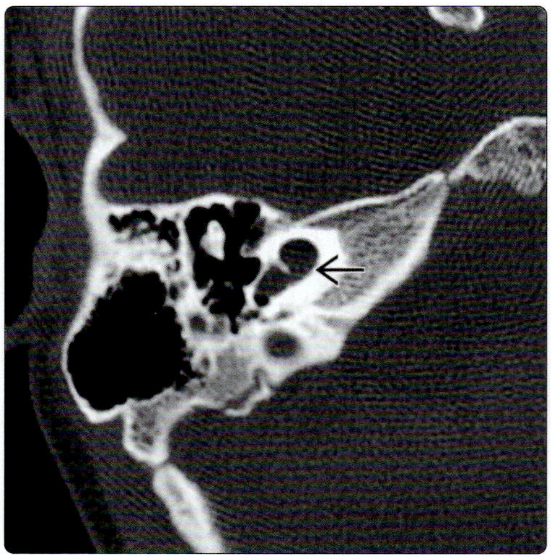

(**Left**) *Axial NECT shows focal low attenuation from a small lipoma in the left CPA cistern* →. (**Right**) *Coronal T1 MR shows a hyperintense lipoma in the left CPA cistern* →.

CPA-IAC Lipoma

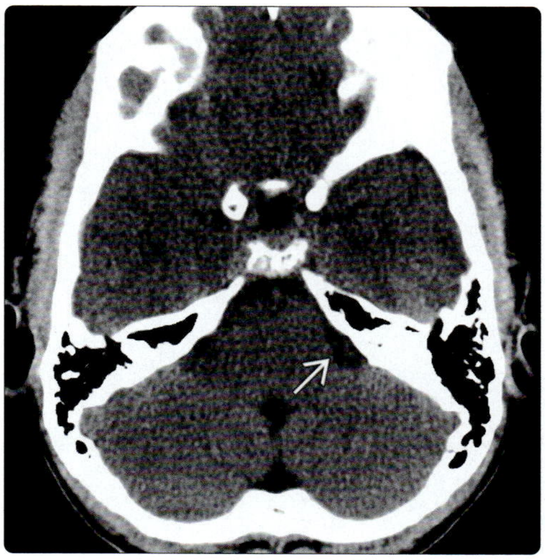

CPA-IAC Lipoma

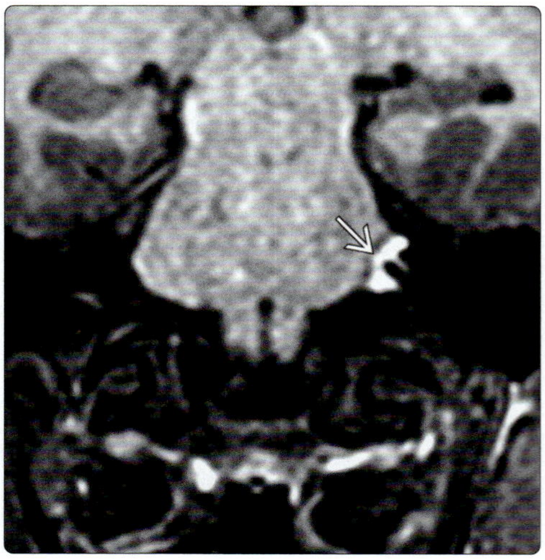

Vestibular Schwannoma

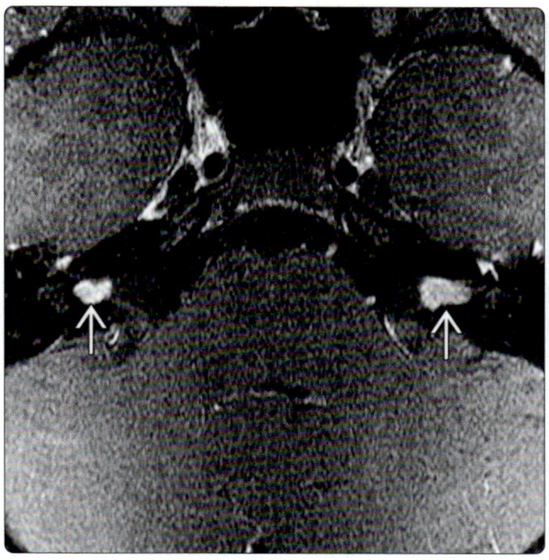

Vestibular Schwannoma

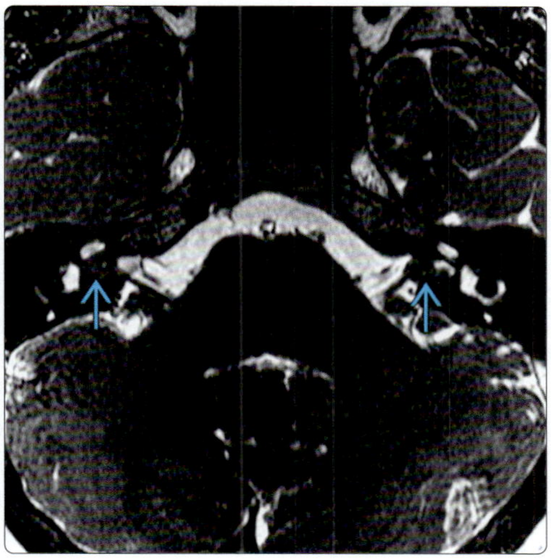

(Left) *Axial T1 C+ FS MR in a 2-year-old boy with neurofibromatosis type 2 shows enhancing masses* → *within the bilateral IACs, inseparable from the CNVII/CNVIII complexes.* **(Right)** *Axial 3D FIESTA MR in the same patient demonstrates hypointense IAC masses* → *replacing the normal hyperintense fluid signal, typical of schwannomas.*

Intralabyrinthine Schwannoma

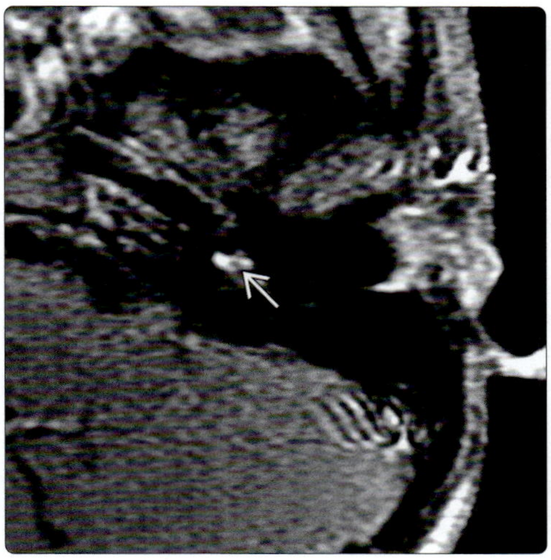

Common Cavity Malformation

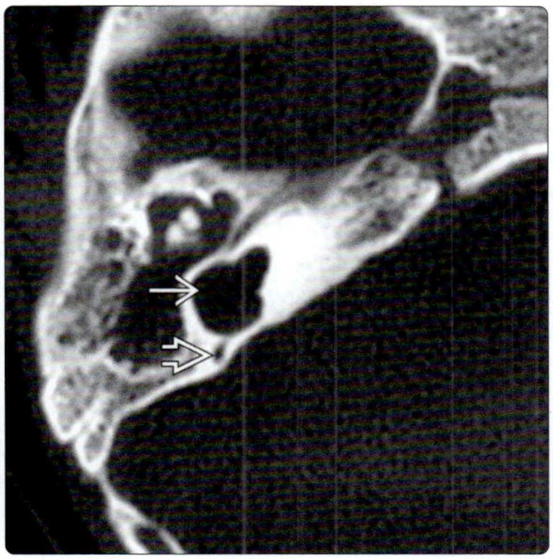

(Left) *Axial T1 C+ FS MR in a 15-year-old girl with unilateral SNHL shows an enhancing mass* → *in the middle turn of the cochlea. The tumor enlarged over time & was subsequently resected, confirming an intracochlear schwannoma.* **(Right)** *Axial bone CT demonstrates a common cavity anomaly with the globular cystic structure representing the vestibule, rudimentary cochlear bud, & horizontal semicircular canal* →*. There is a relatively normal-appearing posterior semicircular canal* →*.*

Cochlear Aplasia

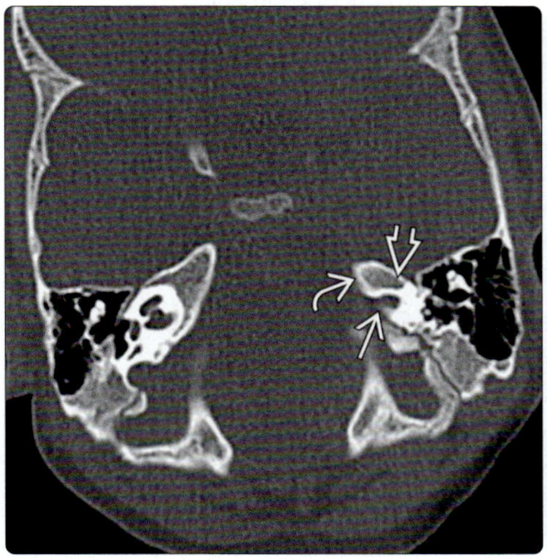

Labyrinthine Aplasia

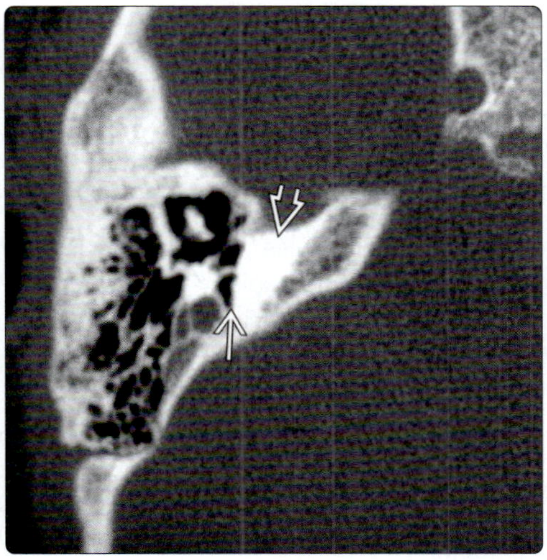

(Left) *Axial bone CT in a 1 year old with SNHL demonstrates a small left IAC* → *& absence of the left cochlea* →*. Note also the mild hypoplasia of the left petrous apex* →*.* **(Right)** *Axial bone CT shows that the otic capsule is featureless* → *& without definable labyrinthine structures. The lateral wall is flat* →*, indicating congenital absence rather than acquired ossificans.*

DIFFERENTIAL DIAGNOSIS

Common

- Cochlear Cleft Pseudolesion
- Subarcuate Canaliculus Pseudolesion
- Pseudoenlarged Vestibular Aqueduct
- Temporal Bone Fracture Involving Inner Ear
- Cochlear Incomplete Partition Type II (IP-2)
- Labyrinthine Ossificans

Less Common

- Labyrinthitis
- Intralabyrinthine Hemorrhage

Rare but Important

- CHARGE Syndrome
- Cystic Cochleovestibular Malformation (IP-I)
- Cochlear Nerve & Cochlear Nerve Canal Aplasia-Hypoplasia
- Common Cavity Malformation
- Cochlear Aplasia
- X-Linked Stapes Gusher
- Branchiootorenal Syndrome
- Osteogenesis Imperfecta
- Labyrinthine Aplasia

ESSENTIAL INFORMATION

Key Differential Diagnosis Issues

- Congenital deafness has imaging abnormality in < 50% of cases
  - Large vestibular aqueduct (LVA) is most common
    - Vestibular aqueduct (VA) is CT correlate of endolymphatic sac (ELS) on MR
- Imaging protocols for childhood sensorineural hearing loss (SNHL)
  - Temporal bone axial CT with coronal short-axis oblique (Pöschl) & long-axis oblique (Stenver) reformations for ideal evaluation of all structures
  - High-resolution T2 MR imaging in axial & oblique sagittal planes to define internal auditory canal (IAC) size, integrity of cochlear nerve aperture/cochlear nerve canal (CNC), & presence of cochlear nerve

Helpful Clues for Common Diagnoses

- **Cochlear Cleft Pseudolesion**
  - Common CT finding, disappears with age
    - Nonosseous otic capsule space in children → pericochlear lucency
  - CT: Thin C-shaped lucency in bilateral otic capsules
    - Anterior to oval window, adjacent to middle & apical > basal cochlear turns
- **Subarcuate Canaliculus Pseudolesion**
  - Asymptomatic normal variant that disappears in first 2 years of life
    - Synonym: Petromastoid canal
  - CT/MR: Lucent/hyperintense T2 canal inferior to superior semicircular canal (SCC) arch
- **Pseudoenlarged Vestibular Aqueduct**
  - Infants < 3 months: Immature, unossified area adjacent to VA on CT
  - Older child or adult: High-riding jugular bulb may simulate LVA
  - CT: Coronal & oblique reformats best distinguish unossified area & jugular bulb from VA
    - Infant: Normal VA medial to unossified area of petrous bone
    - Older child/adult: High-riding jugular bulb mistaken for LVA on axial images
- **Temporal Bone Fracture Involving Inner Ear**
  - Complex temporal bone fractures may involve inner ear structures
    - Otic capsule violating vs. otic capsule sparing
  - CT: Fracture line crosses inner ear; ± pneumolabyrinth
- **Cochlear Incomplete Partition Type II (IP-2)**
  - Most common congenital imaging abnormality found with SNHL
    - Cascading hearing loss pattern in child or young adult
  - CT: Deficient interscalar septum (ISS) between middle & apical cochlear turns
    - Flattening of interscalar ridge (anchor point) between upper basal & upper middle cochlear turns
    - Usually with enlarged bony VA
  - MR: Deficient ISS between middle & apical cochlear turns
    - Usually with ELS/duct
    - New literature suggests dysplastic osseous spiral lamina-basilar membrane neural complex may mimic ISS on high-resolution 3D cisternographic MR images → underdiagnosed IP-2 anomalies
      - Reformat images parallel to lateral SCC to measure distance X (distance between osseous spiral lamina-basilar membrane complex of upper basal turn & 1st linear signal void anterior to basilar membrane)
      - When first linear signal void = normal ISS, distance X < 1.2 mm
      - When first linear signal void = dysplastic osseous spiral lamina-basilar membrane neural complex, distance X ≥ 1.2 mm
- **Labyrinthine Ossificans**
  - Profound SNHL after episode of meningitis or middle ear infection
    - Healing suppurative labyrinthitis may lead to osteoneogenesis within inner ear fluid spaces
    - Requires urgent/emergent CT imaging to assess for ossification (as this may inhibit placement of cochlear implant)
  - CT: Ossific plaques impinge on inner ear fluid spaces; may occur within weeks of insult
    - Define as cochlear & noncochlear for cochlear implant evaluation
  - MR: High-resolution T2 images show encroachment on membranous labyrinthine fluid spaces

Helpful Clues for Less Common Diagnoses

- **Labyrinthitis**
  - Acute-onset vertigo & hearing loss ± facial nerve paralysis
  - CT: Normal in acute phase
  - MR: Normal or diffuse enhancement of inner ear fluid spaces
- **Intralabyrinthine Hemorrhage**
  - Etiologies: Idiopathic, anticoagulant therapy, posttraumatic, sickle cell disease
  - CT: Normal unless associated with trauma
  - MR: High T1 signal in inner ear fluid

Helpful Clues for Rare Diagnoses

- **CHARGE Syndrome**
  - **C**oloboma, **h**eart defects, choanal **a**tresia, **r**etardation (mental/growth), **g**enitourinary & **e**ar abnormalities
  - CT: Absent bilateral SCCs, small vestibules, oval window atresia, CNC atresia
  - MR: Same as CT + cochlear nerve hypoplasia or absence
- **Cystic Cochleovestibular Malformation (IP-I)**
  - CT/MR: Cochlea + vestibule have "figure 8 contour"
    - Cochlea: Lacks internal septation & modiolus
    - Vestibule & horizontal SCC: Dilated
    - CNVIII: Nerves are hypoplastic or absent
    - VA/ELS are usually normal
- **Cochlear Nerve & Cochlear Nerve Canal Aplasia-Hypoplasia**
  - CT: Complete or partial bony narrowing of base of CNC
  - MR: Fluid in CNC is completely or partially replaced by low-signal bone
    - Cochlear nerve is absent or hypoplastic
- **Common Cavity Malformation**
  - CT/MR: Cochlea & vestibule are cystic → inner ear looks like single cyst (of variable size)
    - Posterior & superior SCC: Usually absent or malformed
    - VA/ELS are not dilated but may be absent
    - IAC: Small or absent CNVIII components ± anomalous course of CNVII
- **Cochlear Aplasia**
  - CT: Cochlea absent + variable deformity of vestibule & SCCs
  - MR: Absent cochlea & cochlear nerve
- **X-Linked Stapes Gusher**
  - a.k.a. X-linked deafness type 2 (DFNX2)
  - Open communication between IAC cerebrospinal fluid & cochlear fluid creates perilymphatic hydrops
    - "Gusher" results if stapes is disturbed
  - Found in male children with bilateral mixed conductive & sensorineural hearing loss
  - CT: Corkscrew cochlear morphology
    - Absent ISS
    - CNC is enlarged with no modiolus
    - Labyrinthine & anterior tympanic facial nerve canal may be enlarged
- **Branchiootorenal Syndrome**
  - Auricular deformity, prehelical pits, mixed hearing loss, branchial fistulae, & renal abnormalities
    - 40% with clinical manifestations have mutations of *EYA1* gene on chromosome 8q13.3
  - CT: Hypoplastic apical turn of cochlea, medial deviation facial nerve, funnel-shaped IAC, patulous eustachian tube
- **Osteogenesis Imperfecta**
  - Mild form develops deafness by 40 years of age
  - Blue sclera in some forms
  - CT: Active disease shows lucent foci in otic capsule surrounding cochlea
  - MR: Active disease shows enhancing foci in otic capsule
- **Labyrinthine Aplasia**
  - CT/MR: Inner ear structures & IAC absent

SELECTED REFERENCES

1. Freeman SR et al: Management of cochlear nerve hypoplasia and aplasia. Adv Otorhinolaryngol. 81:81-92, 2018
2. Talenti G et al: High-resolution 3 T magnetic resonance findings in cochlear hypoplasias and incomplete partition anomalies: a pictorial essay. Br J Radiol. 91(1089):20180120, 2018
3. Conte G et al: MR Imaging in sudden sensorineural hearing loss. Time to talk. AJNR Am J Neuroradiol. 38(8):1475-79, 2017
4. D'Arco F et al: Do measurements of inner ear structures help in the diagnosis of inner ear malformations? A review of literature. Otol Neurotol. 38(10):e384-e92, 2017
5. Sennaroğlu L et al: Classification and current management of inner ear malformations. Balkan Med J. 34(5):397-411, 2017
6. DeMarcantonio M et al: Radiographic evaluation of children with hearing loss. Otolaryngol Clin North Am. 48(6):913-32, 2015
7. Giesemann A et al: Some remarks on imaging of the inner ear: options and limitations. Clin Neuroradiol. 25 Suppl 2:197-203, 2015

Cochlear Cleft Pseudolesion

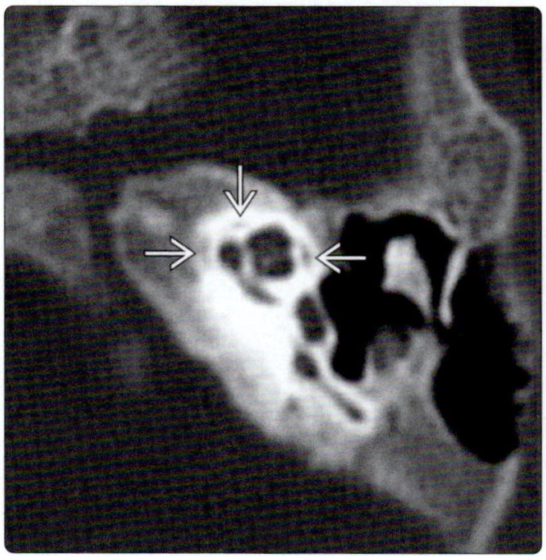

Subarcuate Canaliculus Pseudolesion

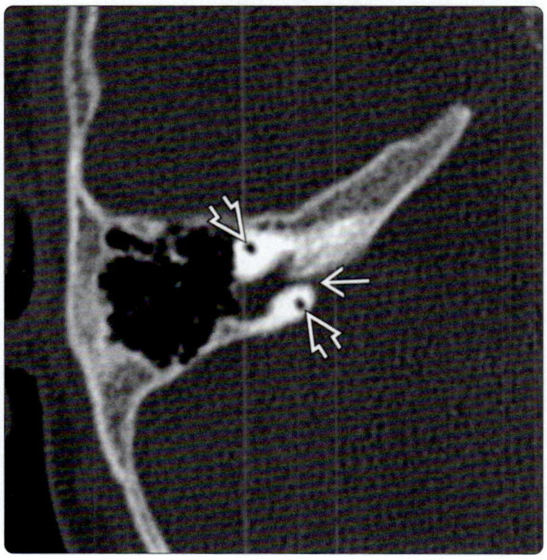

(Left) *Axial bone CT of the left ear demonstrates a cochlear cleft lucency ➡, which was found incidentally in an infant. This is a benign developmental variant that will become less conspicuous with age & ultimately disappear.* **(Right)** *Axial bone CT of the right ear shows a prominent but normal subarcuate artery canal ➡ (& associated subarachnoid space) passing under the superior semicircular canal arch ➡. This normal dural-lined subarachnoid space will involute but remain visible as a thin line with sclerotic margins in older children.*

(**Left**) *Axial bone CT in a 6 day old shows normal variant concave lucencies at the dorsal aspects of the petrous bones ➔, inferolateral to the vestibular aqueducts, which are not included on this image. These foci will ossify & no longer be visible within a few months.* (**Right**) *Axial bone CT in a teenager involved in a motocross accident demonstrates an otic capsule-violating fracture ➔ with associated pneumolabyrinth in the vestibule ➔ & cochlea ➔. Also note the small amount of intracranial air ➔.*

Pseudoenlarged Vestibular Aqueduct

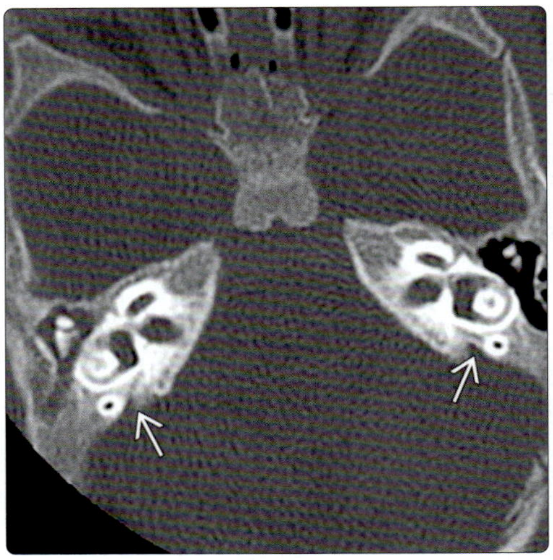

Temporal Bone Fracture Involving Inner Ear

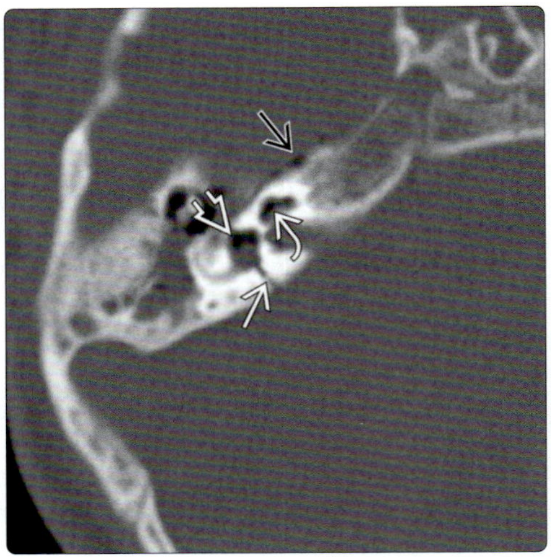

(**Left**) *Axial T2 MR reveals a large endolymphatic sac ➔ associated with a significant cochlear malformation ➔ that is characterized by modiolar absence & the lack of a well-defined interscalar septum.* (**Right**) *Axial bone CT in a child with a prior history of meningitis demonstrates labyrinthine ossificans as subtotal ossification of the left cochlea, with remnant basal ➔ & middle/apical ➔ turns remaining barely visible.*

Cochlear Incomplete Partition Type II (IP-2)

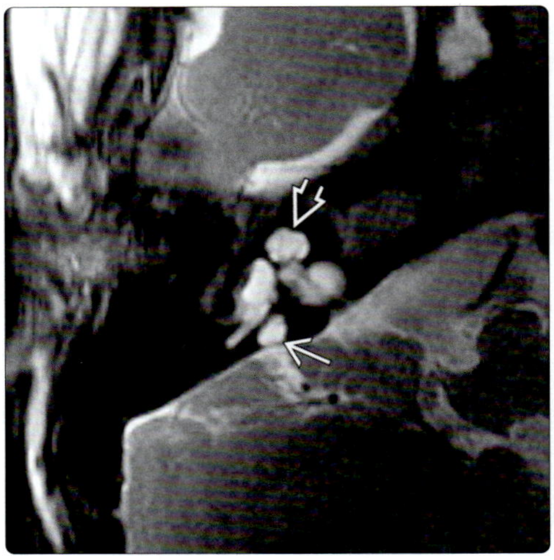

Labyrinthine Ossificans

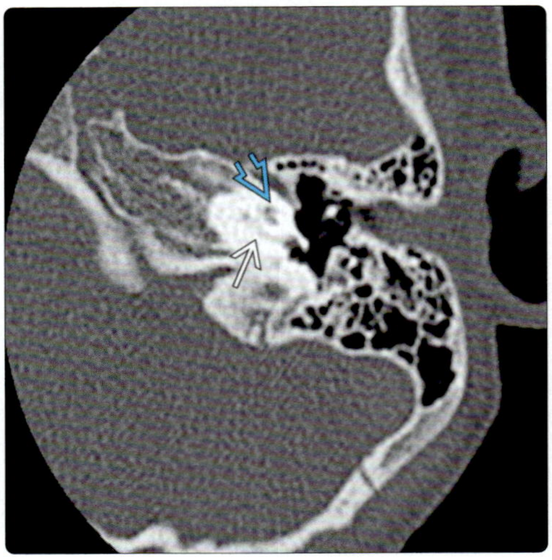

(**Left**) *Axial T1 C+ FS MR in an 11 year old with sudden-onset deafness shows abnormal, diffuse enhancement of the cochlea bilaterally ➔. There was also abnormal enhancement of the bilateral vestibules (not shown) with corresponding loss of T2 hyperintensity in the inner ear fluid spaces (not shown).* (**Right**) *Axial 3D time-of-flight MRA source image shows T1 shortening of blood in the vestibular ➔ & cochlear ➔ fluid spaces. Acute sensorineural hearing loss & vertigo heralded this intralabyrinthine bleed.*

Labyrinthitis

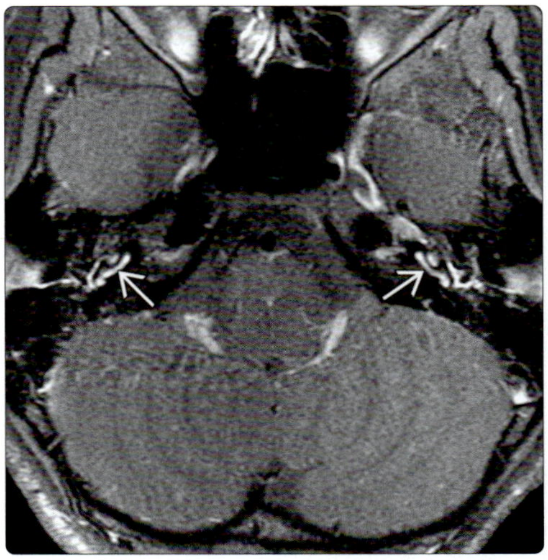

Intralabyrinthine Hemorrhage

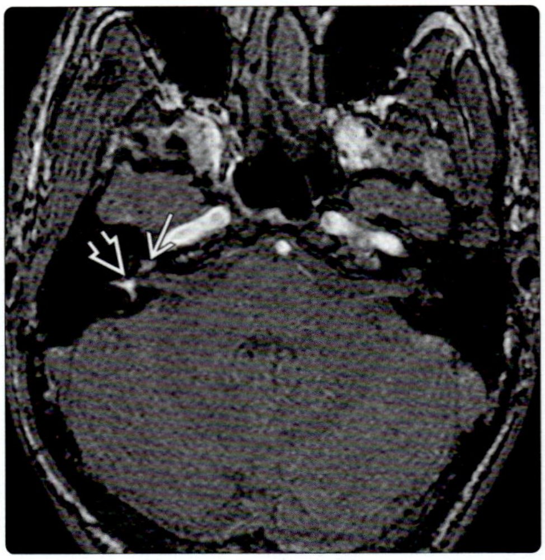

CHARGE Syndrome

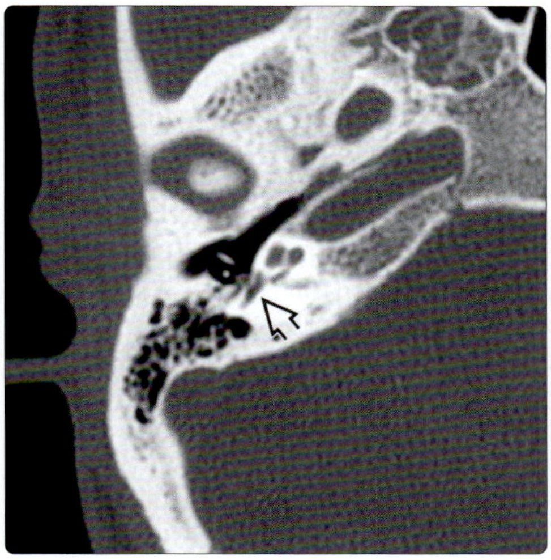

Cystic Cochleovestibular Malformation (IP-I)

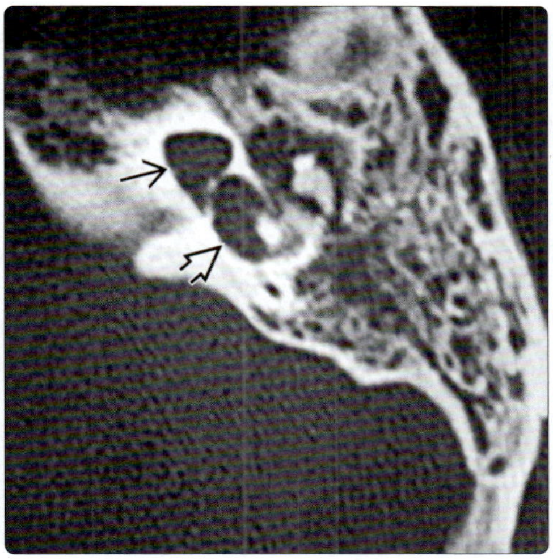

(Left) *Axial bone CT shows CHARGE-related absence of the semicircular canals associated with oval window atresia. The "bare vestibule" has a characteristic small, slightly elongated shape ⇨.* **(Right)** *Axial bone CT shows a grossly abnormal inner ear. Both the cochlea ⇨ & the vestibule ⇨ are cystic, hence the name cystic cochleovestibular anomaly; however, they maintain some separation, secondary to developmental arrest at the 5th gestational week (vs. the 4th gestational week in the common cavity deformity).*

Cochlear Nerve & Cochlear Nerve Canal Aplasia-Hypoplasia

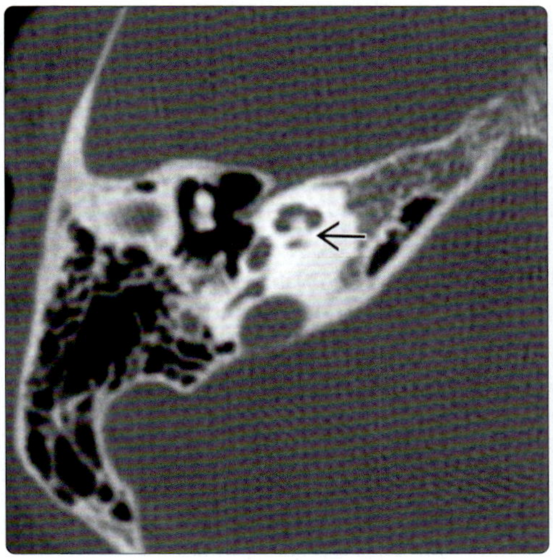

Common Cavity Malformation

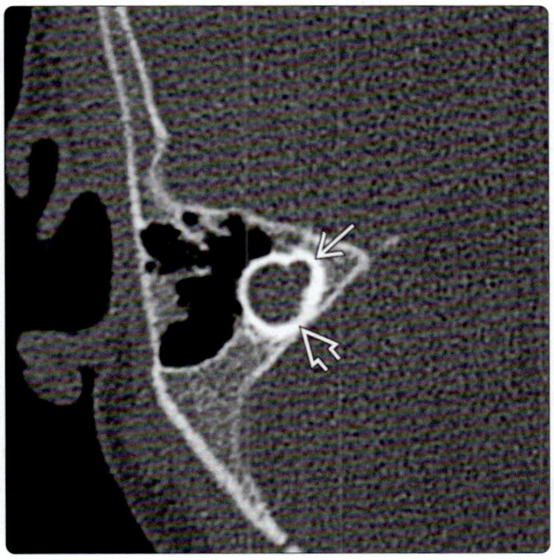

(Left) *Axial bone CT demonstrates a bony bar ⇨ across the cochlear base, separating it from the internal auditory canal fundus. Given that the cochlear nerve canal is absent, no visible cochlear nerve would be present on MR in this lesion (not shown).* **(Right)** *Axial bone CT shows the single cyst of an inner ear common cavity deformity due to an undifferentiated cochlea, vestibule, & horizontal semicircular canal with large vestibular ➡ & small cochlear ➡ components.*

Cochlear Aplasia

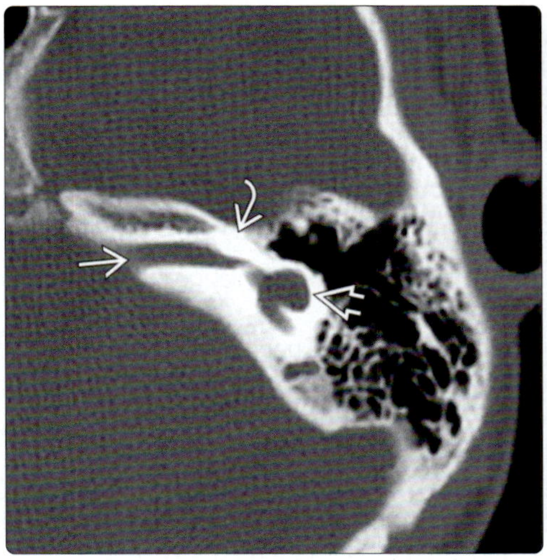

X-Linked Stapes Gusher

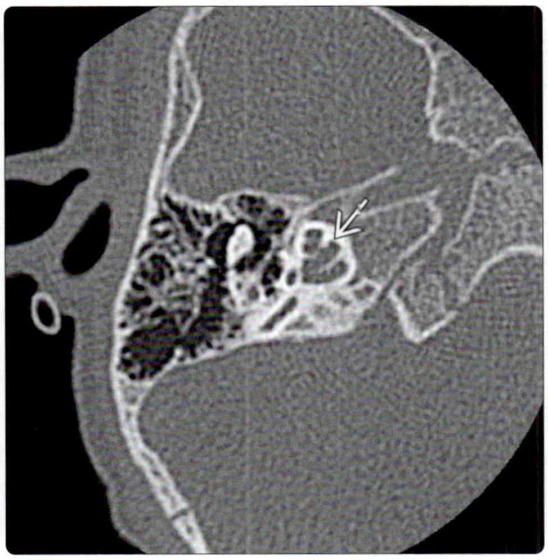

(Left) *Axial bone CT reveals a small internal auditory canal ➡, malformed vestibule-semicircular canals ➡, & an absent cochlea ➡. An absent cochlea implies an absent cochlear nerve.* **(Right)** *Axial bone CT shows absence of the cochlear modiolus with the typical corkscrew appearance ➡ of the cochlea in a patient with an X-linked stapes gusher (DFNX2) anomaly. These patients present with mixed hearing loss. They are at risk of a perilymph/CSF "gusher" during stapedectomy/cochleostomy.*

DIFFERENTIAL DIAGNOSIS

Common

- Chronic Otitis Media
- Acquired Cholesteatoma of Pars Flaccida
- Acute Coalescent Otomastoiditis

Less Common

- Congenital Cholesteatoma
- Acquired Cholesteatoma of Pars Tensa
- Chronic Otomastoiditis With Tympanosclerosis
- Dehiscent Jugular Bulb

Rare but Important

- Langerhans Cell Histiocytosis
- Rhabdomyosarcoma
- Cephalocele
- Cholesterol Granuloma
- Chronic Otomastoiditis With Ossicular Erosions
- Aberrant Internal Carotid Artery
- Osseous Lymphatic Malformation

ESSENTIAL INFORMATION

Key Differential Diagnosis Issues

- Otoscopic findings often provide critical clues to precise diagnosis of middle ear (ME) lesions in children
  - Presence or absence of tympanic membrane (TM) rupture or retraction pocket is important
    - Pars tensa-acquired cholesteatoma: Ruptured TM
    - Pars flaccida-acquired cholesteatoma: Retracted, bulging, or ruptured TM
    - Congenital cholesteatoma: Intact TM
  - Color & location of retrotympanic mass may be key to imaging diagnosis

Helpful Clues for Common Diagnoses

- **Chronic Otitis Media**
  - Otoscopy: Thickened TM
  - CT: Underpneumatized mastoid air cells with surrounding sclerosis
    - ± ME/mastoid opacification
- **Acquired Cholesteatoma of Pars Flaccida**
  - Otoscopy: Ruptured or bulging TM or retraction pocket affecting pars flaccida portion of TM
  - CT: Nondependent soft tissue filling Prussak space with erosion of ossicles & scutum
    - ± inferomedial ossicular displacement
    - Possible complications: Dehiscent tegmen tympani, lateral semicircular canal, &/or facial nerve canal
- **Acute Coalescent Otomastoiditis**
  - Otoscopy: Bulging, inflamed TM
  - CT: Complete ME/mastoid opacification + mastoid trabecular & cortical erosion
    - Must check soft tissue windows for postauricular abscess, epidural abscess, brain abscess, &/or venous thrombosis

Helpful Clues for Less Common Diagnoses

- **Congenital Cholesteatoma**
  - Otoscopy: White mass behind intact TM in patient without history of otitis media, otorrhea, or surgery
  - CT: Smooth, round, well-circumscribed soft tissue mass in ME; often medial to ossicular chain
    - Variant: Rounded opacity in hypotympanum; easily overlooked
    - Ossicles: Erosion is often absent; with increasing size, ossicles are eroded & displaced laterally
    - Mastoid pneumatization is often normal
- **Acquired Cholesteatoma of Pars Tensa**
  - Otoscopy: Ruptured pars tensa portion of TM
  - CT: Meso- & hypotympanic soft tissue mass
    - Often extends posteriorly or medially; ± ossicular erosion & lateral ossicular displacement
- **Chronic Otomastoiditis With Tympanosclerosis**
  - Otoscopy: Opaque, calcified TM
  - CT: Postinflammatory Ca^{2+}
    - May affect TM, ossicles, stapedius/tensor tympani muscles, ossicle ligaments, &/or mastoid air cells
- **Dehiscent Jugular Bulb**
  - Otoscopy: "Blue" lesion behind posteroinferior quadrant of TM
  - CT: Dehiscent sigmoid plate projects jugular bulb into posteroinferior ME cavity

Helpful Clues for Rare Diagnoses

- **Langerhans Cell Histiocytosis**
  - Otoscopy: Postauricular mass is common; may present with otorrhea
  - CT: Unilateral or bilateral (30%) sharply marginated lytic bone lesions
    - Soft tissue mass may extend into ME space
    - Mastoid & squamous temporal bone are more commonly affected than petrous apex & ME
  - MR: Variable signal on T2; moderate homogeneous enhancement
- **Rhabdomyosarcoma**
  - Otoscopy: External auditory canal (EAC) "polyp"
  - CT: Destructive ME mass
    - Often affects EAC, ossicles, surrounding bones, overlying dura
    - Petrous apex & ME are more commonly affected than mastoid
  - MR: Usually low signal on T2; variable enhancement
- **Cephalocele**
  - Otoscopy: Mass may be occult if it lies above level of TM; presents with conductive hearing loss (CHL) ± CSF leakage
  - CT: Congenital or acquired defect in tegmen tympani with CSF ± brain herniating into ME space
  - MR: CSF signal ± temporal lobe herniating into ME space
- **Cholesterol Granuloma**
  - Otoscopy: Blue-black material behind intact TM
  - CT: ME soft tissue mass with minimal bony erosion
  - MR: Material in ME is hyperintense on T2 & FS T1
    - Old blood in cholesterol granuloma creates T1 shortening
- **Chronic Otomastoiditis With Ossicular Erosions**
  - Otoscopy: Thickened TM without normal ossicle impressions
  - CT: Linear ME & mastoid air cell opacifications with partial ossicle absence

- Incus lenticular process & stapes hub are most commonly affected
- **Aberrant Internal Carotid Artery**
  - Otoscopy: Reddish mass
    - Passes across inferior 1/2 of TM
  - CT: Tubular structure passes into posteroinferior ME cavity through enlarged inferior tympanic canaliculus
    - Aberrant internal carotid artery (ICA) passes out of ME cavity anteromedially by accessing posterolateral margin of horizontal petrous ICA
- **Osseous Lymphatic Malformation**
  - Otoscopy: Mass may be occult; presents with CHL ± other evidence of osseous lymphatic malformation
  - CT: "Lacy" lytic lesion may involve ossicles
  - MR: High signal on T2; nonenhancing

Other Essential Information

- Best imaging tool for ME lesion in child
  - Temporal bone CT without contrast
  - Thin-section FS MR used for further evaluation of larger lesions involving inner ear, floor of middle cranial fossa, or sigmoid sinus & posterior fossa
- Tumor or tumor-like lesions to consider in ME of child: Rhabdomyosarcoma & Langerhans cell histiocytosis
  - May be difficult to distinguish
  - Langerhans cell histiocytosis
    - Sharply defined, "punched-out" lytic bone destruction
    - Contrast-enhancing soft tissue mass (usually with moderate or vigorous enhancement)
    - Centered around ME cavity, especially in mastoid
      - Mastoid temporal bone > petrous apex & ME
    - May present as postauricular mass or otorrhea
    - May be bilateral
  - Rhabdomyosarcoma
    - Unilateral; permeative, lytic bone destruction
    - Contrast-enhancing soft tissue mass (variable in degree)
    - Centered in or extending into ME cavity
      - Petrous apex & ME > mastoid temporal bone
    - May present with EAC "polyp"

SELECTED REFERENCES

1. Galiay L et al: Temporomandibular joint anomalies in pediatric craniofacial Gorham-Stout disease. J Craniomaxillofac Surg. 46(8):1179-84, 2018
2. Chevallier KM et al: Differentiating pediatric rhabdomyosarcoma and Langerhans cell histiocytosis of the temporal bone by imaging appearance. AJNR Am J Neuroradiol. 37(6):1185-9, 2016
3. Gluth MB: Rhabdomyosarcoma and other pediatric temporal bone malignancies. Otolaryngol Clin North Am. 48(2):375-90, 2015
4. Atmaca S et al: High and dehiscent jugular bulb: clear and present danger during middle ear surgery. Surg Radiol Anat. 36(4):369-74, 2014
5. Neilan RE et al: Langerhans cell histiocytosis of the temporal bone. Otol Neurotol. 33(4):e31-2, 2012
6. Psarommatis IM et al: Algorithmic management of pediatric acute mastoiditis. Int J Pediatr Otorhinolaryngol. 76(6):791-6, 2012
7. Baráth K et al: Neuroradiology of cholesteatomas. AJNR Am J Neuroradiol. 32(2):221-9, 2011
8. Schwartz KM et al: The utility of diffusion-weighted imaging for cholesteatoma evaluation. AJNR Am J Neuroradiol. 32(3):430-6, 2011
9. Freling NJ et al: Imaging findings in craniofacial childhood rhabdomyosarcoma. Pediatr Radiol. 40(11):1723-38; quiz 1855, 2010
10. Sauvaget E et al: Aberrant internal carotid artery in the temporal bone: imaging findings and management. Arch Otolaryngol Head Neck Surg. 132(1):86-91, 2006

Chronic Otitis Media

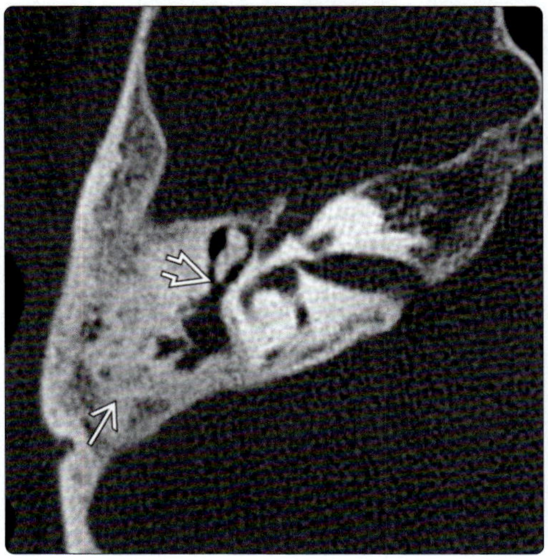

Acquired Cholesteatoma of Pars Flaccida

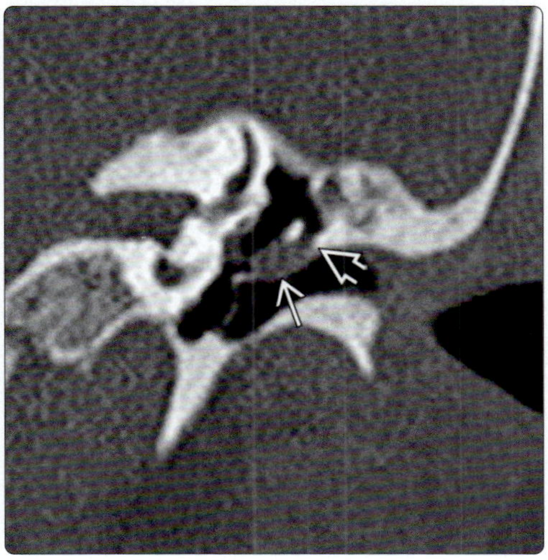

(Left) *Axial bone CT shows inflammatory debris in the posterior epitympanum ➡ & mastoid antrum with underpneumatization & sclerosis of the mastoid ➡, consistent with sequelae of chronic otitis media.* **(Right)** *Coronal bone CT in a teenager with a history of recurrent otitis media & tympanic membrane perforation shows a soft tissue mass ➡ abutting the truncated scutum ➡ & surrounding the demineralized/eroded portion of the incus body.*

(Left) *Axial CECT in a child with left ear proptosis, fever, & otitis media shows a well-defined, rim-enhancing subperiosteal abscess ➡ overlying the left mastoid. On bone window images, frank lateral mastoid cortex dehiscence was identified.* **(Right)** *Coronal bone CT in a 4 year old presenting with a white retrotympanic mass, without a history of otitis media or tympanic membrane perforation, shows a well-defined, round middle ear mass ➡ without adjacent ossicular erosion.*

Acute Coalescent Otomastoiditis

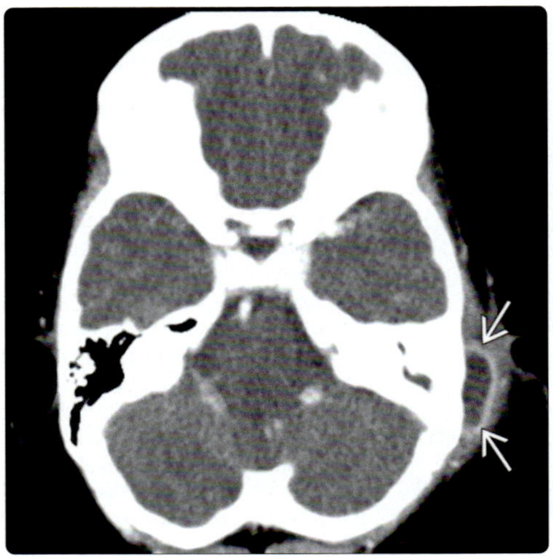

Congenital Cholesteatoma

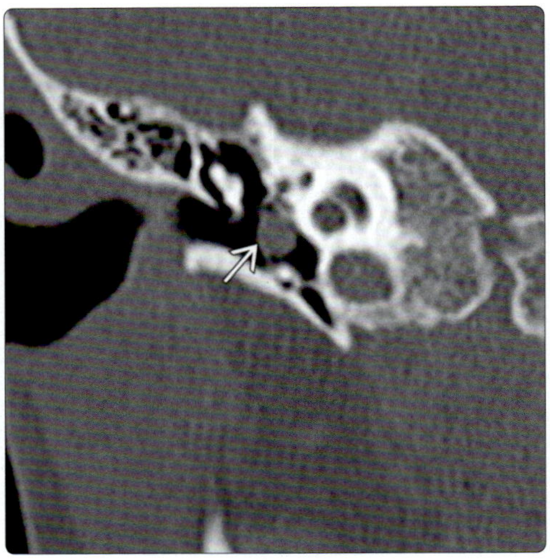

(Left) *Axial bone CT shows a middle ear soft tissue mass ➡ medial to the ossicles with incus short process erosion & sparing of the Prussak space ➡. Otoscopy showed perforation in the pars tensa portion of the tympanic membrane.* **(Right)** *Axial bone CT reveals multiple calcified foci ➡ in the inflammatory debris surrounding the ossicles. Mastoid underpneumatization is a common sequela of chronic otitis media.*

Acquired Cholesteatoma of Pars Tensa

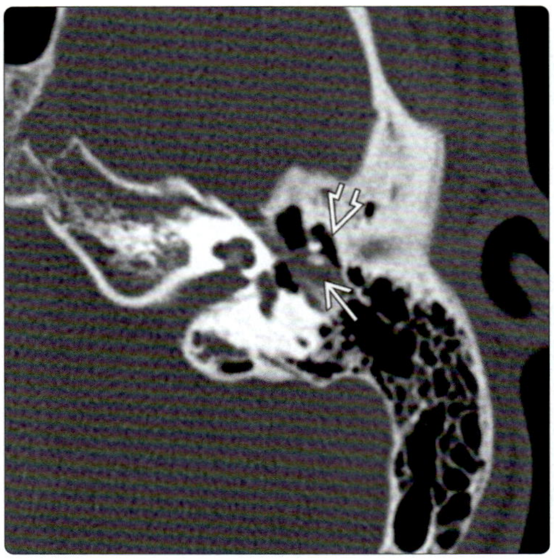

Chronic Otomastoiditis With Tympanosclerosis

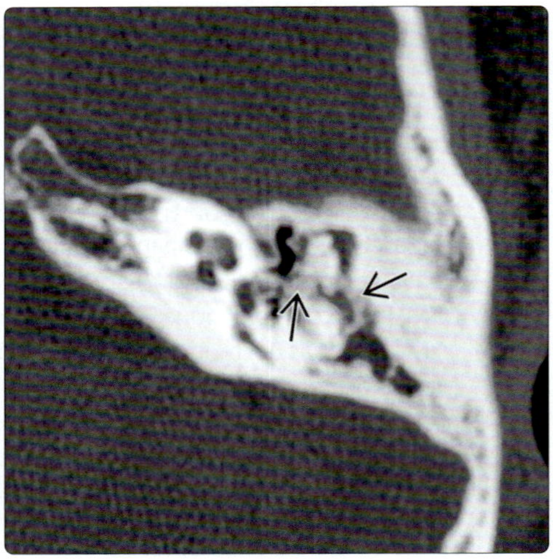

(Left) *Axial bone CT in a child with a history of inadvertent right jugular bulb injury during tympanostomy tube placement demonstrates dehiscence of the contralateral left jugular bulb ➡ with protrusion of the bulb ➡ into the mesotympanum.* **(Right)** *Axial CECT in a 1 year old with a right ear mass shows a large, moderately enhancing mass ➡ with complete lysis of the affected right mastoid temporal bone, floor of the middle cranial fossa, & sigmoid plate. Note a smaller lesion on the left ➡.*

Dehiscent Jugular Bulb

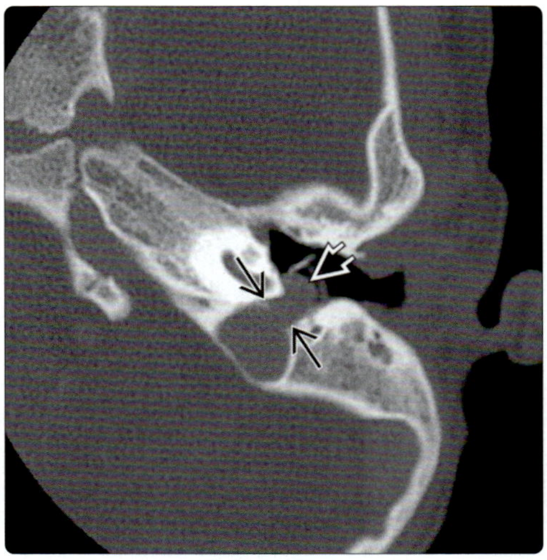

Langerhans Cell Histiocytosis

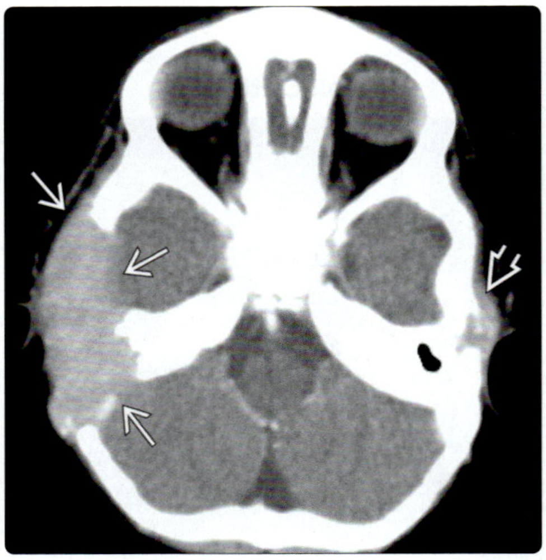

Rhabdomyosarcoma

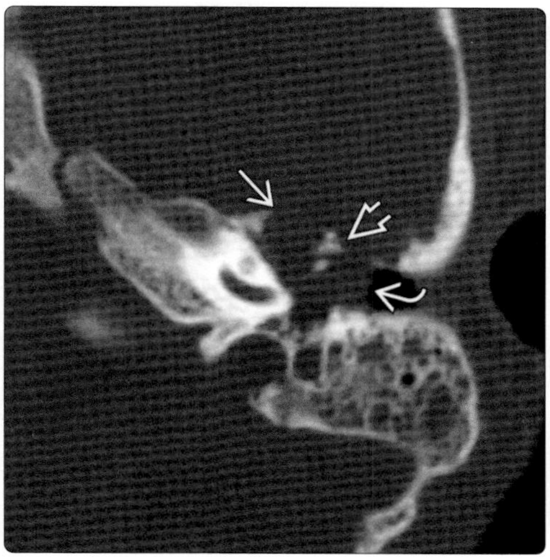

Cephalocele

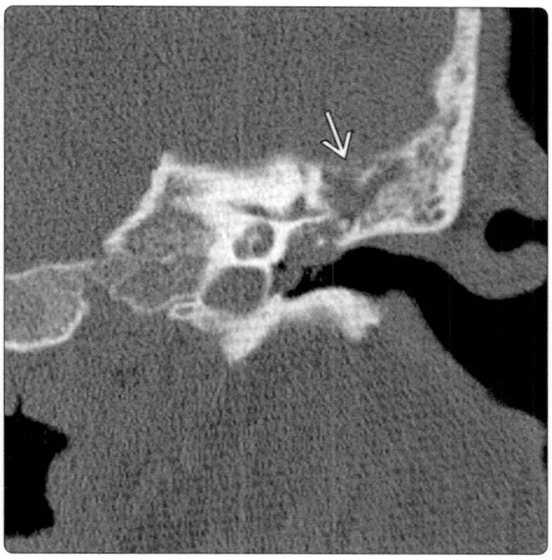

(Left) *Axial bone CT demonstrates a destructive mass in the middle ear with erosion of the anterior bony wall of the middle ear cavity ➡ & the ossicular chain ➡. Otoscopic exam showed an external auditory canal "polyp" ➡ in this case of rhabdomyosarcoma.* **(Right)** *Coronal bone CT shows focal dehiscence of the anterior tegmen tympani ➡ at the site of a temporal lobe cephalocele (confirmed on MR) with opacification of the middle ear cavity & mastoids secondary to a CSF leak.*

Cholesterol Granuloma

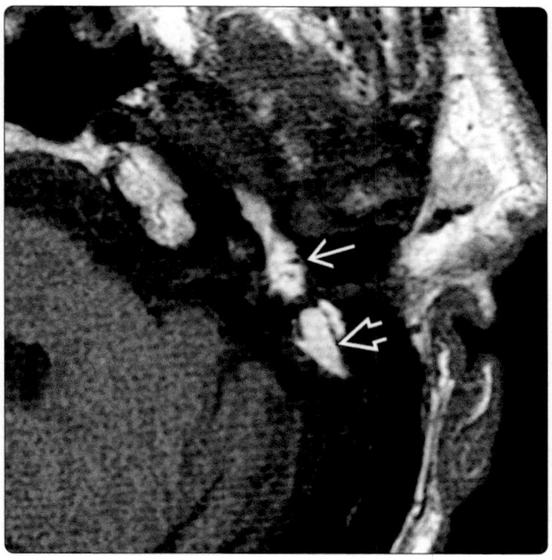

Chronic Otomastoiditis With Ossicular Erosions

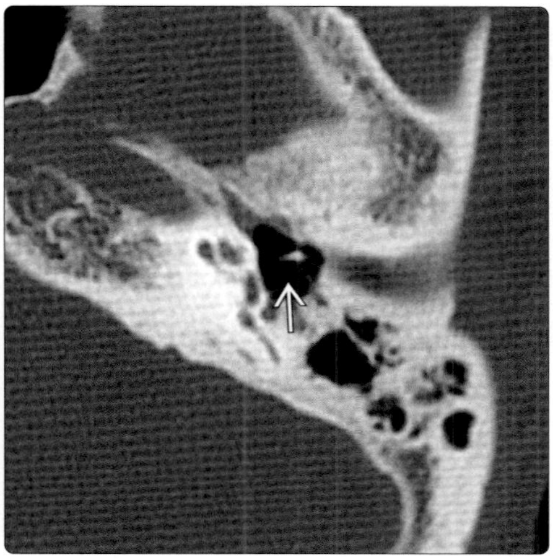

(Left) *Axial T1 MR shows high-signal material in the middle ear ➡ & mastoid ➡ cavities. T1 shortening in a cholesterol granuloma is due to a mixture of old blood & high protein.* **(Right)** *Axial bone CT shows absence of the distal incus lenticular process as well as the hub of the stapes ➡. Note also the linear stranding in the middle ear cavity from chronic otomastoiditis.*

Aberrant Internal Carotid Artery

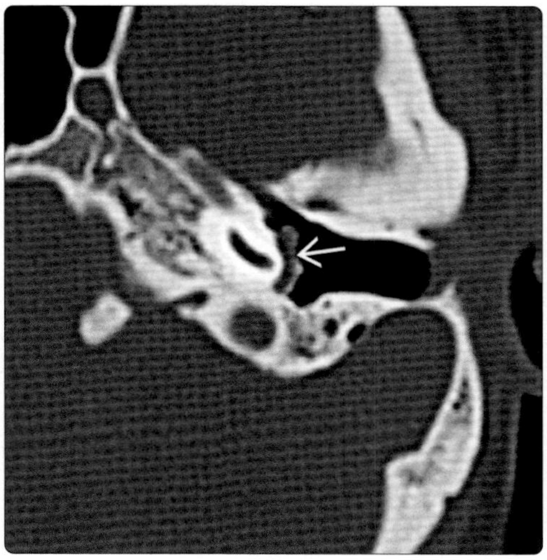

Osseous Lymphatic Malformation

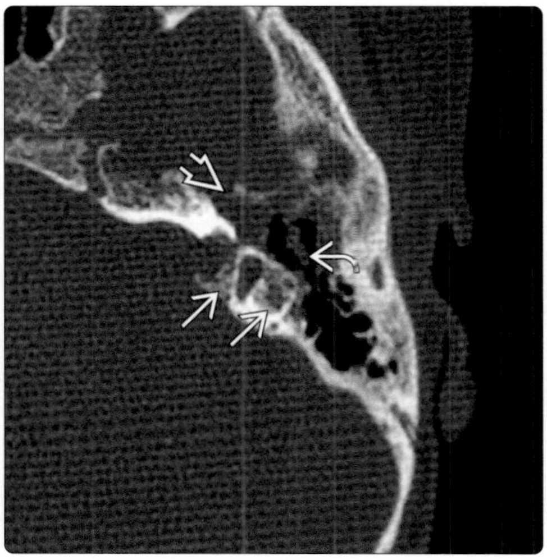

(Left) *Axial bone CT shows an aberrant internal carotid artery (ICA) ➡ along the cochlear promontory in the middle ear. The tubular appearance & connection to the ICA horizontal petrous segment are key for differentiation from a paraganglioma.* **(Right)** *Axial bone CT reveals "lacy" bone destruction involving the otic capsule bone ➡ around the vestibule, IAC, & semicircular canal. There is a defect in the anterior epitympanum ➡, & a "ghost" of the ossicles is seen ➡. Biopsy revealed Gorham-Stout disease.*

SECTION 8
Spine

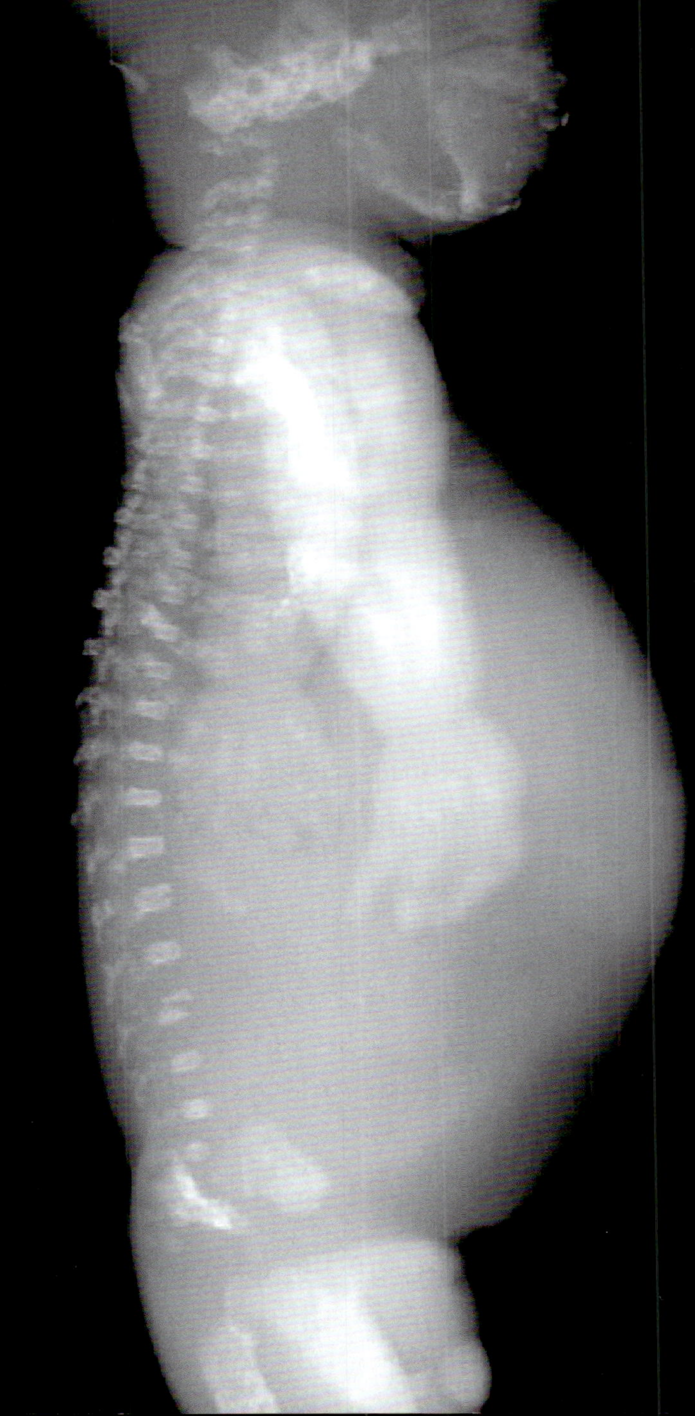

DIFFERENTIAL DIAGNOSIS

Common

- Idiopathic Scoliosis
  - Infantile: Diagnosed from birth to 3 years
  - Juvenile: Diagnosed from 4-9 years
  - Adolescent: Diagnosed from 10-18 years
  - Adult: Diagnosed ≥ 18 years
- Neuromuscular Scoliosis
  - Cerebral Palsy
  - Muscular Dystrophy
  - Chiari I
  - Friedrich Ataxia
  - Poliomyelitis
  - Hemiparesis/Hemiplegia
  - Paraparesis/Paraplegia
- Congenital Scoliosis From Abnormally Formed Vertebrae
  - Vertebral Segmentation & Fusion Anomalies
  - Klippel-Feil Spectrum
  - VACTERL Association
- Chest Wall Abnormality
  - Rib Anomaly
  - Sprengel Deformity
- Trauma
  - Lateral Compression Fracture, Lumbar
  - Lateral Compression Fracture, Thoracic
  - Lateral Flexion Injury, Cervical
- Infection
  - Paraspinal Abscess
  - Pyogenic Osteomyelitis
  - Granulomatous Osteomyelitis
- Limb Length Inequality

Less Common

- Tumor
  - Osteoid Osteoma
  - Osteoblastoma
  - Pathologic Vertebral Fracture
- Congenital Syndromes With Normal Segmentation
  - Connective Tissue Disorders
  - Neurofibromatosis Type 1
  - Osteogenesis Imperfecta
  - Mucopolysaccharidoses
  - Fibrous Dysplasia
  - Fetal Alcohol Syndrome
  - Proteus Syndrome
  - Tethered Spinal Cord
- Pleural or Pulmonary Abnormality
  - Empyema
  - Pneumonectomy
  - Fibrothorax
- Radiation Therapy

ESSENTIAL INFORMATION

Helpful Clues for Common Diagnoses

- Painful scoliosis
  - Trauma, tumor, infection
- Short-curve scoliosis
  - Congenital anomaly, tumor, infection, trauma, degenerative, postoperative
- Balanced S-curve scoliosis
  - Idiopathic, connective tissue disorders
- C-curve scoliosis
  - Neuromuscular, osteogenesis imperfecta
- Consider MR imaging with clinical features suggesting neuropathy
  - Left thoracic, double thoracic, triple major, short-segment, or long right thoracic curves
  - Wide spinal canal or wide neural foramina
  - Severe curvature, which develops after skeletal maturity

SELECTED REFERENCES

1. Scoliosis Research Society. https://www.srs.org/professionals/online-education-and-resources. Reviewed April 29, 2019. Accessed April 29, 2019.
2. Kim H et al: Scoliosis imaging: what radiologists should know. Radiographics. 30(7):1823-42, 2010

Idiopathic Scoliosis

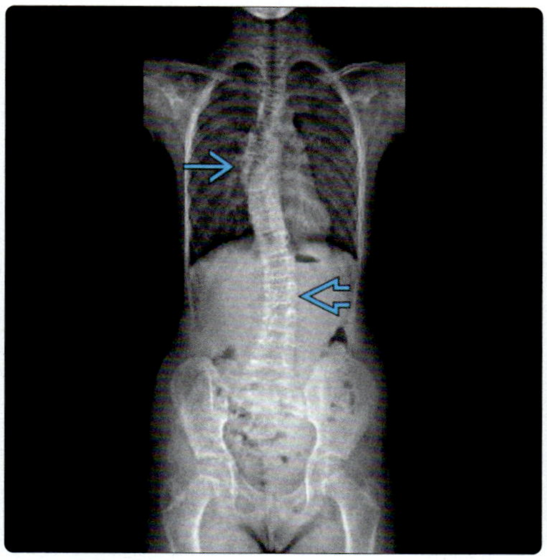

Neuromuscular Scoliosis

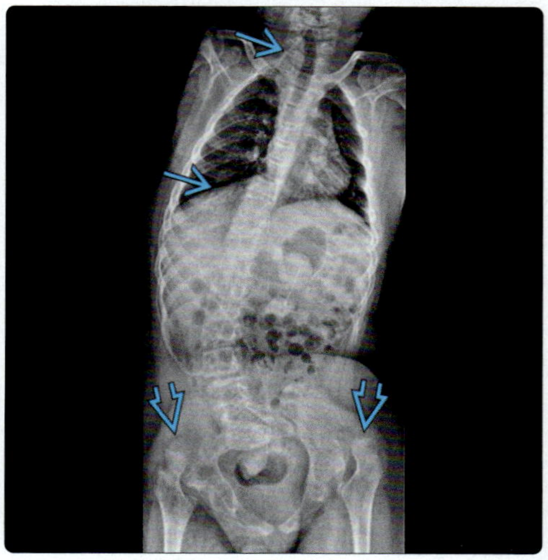

(Left) *Frontal radiograph in a 9-year-old girl with juvenile idiopathic scoliosis shows a typical S-shaped spinal curve with a thoracic dextrocurvature ➔ & lumbar levocurvature ⇨.* **(Right)** *Frontal radiograph in a 13 year old with hydranencephaly & shunted hydrocephalus (note the ventriculoperitoneal shunt ➔) shows an associated C-shaped dextrocurvature of the thoracolumbar spine, typical of neuromuscular scoliosis. There is also bilateral coxa valga with bilateral hip dislocations ⇨.*

Vertebral Segmentation & Fusion Anomalies

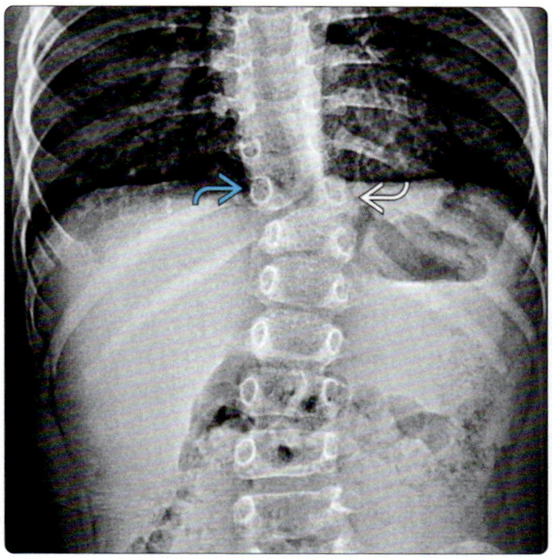

Vertebral Segmentation & Fusion Anomalies

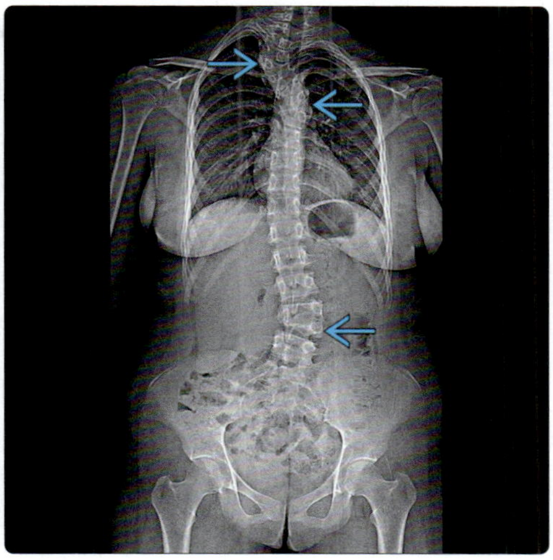

(Left) *AP radiograph shows a left T11 hemivertebra fused to T12 & a right T11 hemivertebra fused to T10, resulting in a congenital scoliosis.* **(Right)** *Frontal radiograph in a 14-year-old girl with congenital scoliosis shows multiple vertebral segmentation anomalies within the thoracic & lumbar spine.*

Vertebral Segmentation & Fusion Anomalies

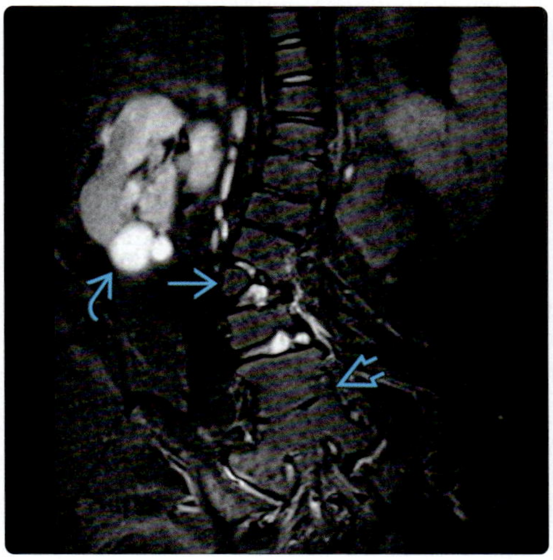

Rib Anomaly

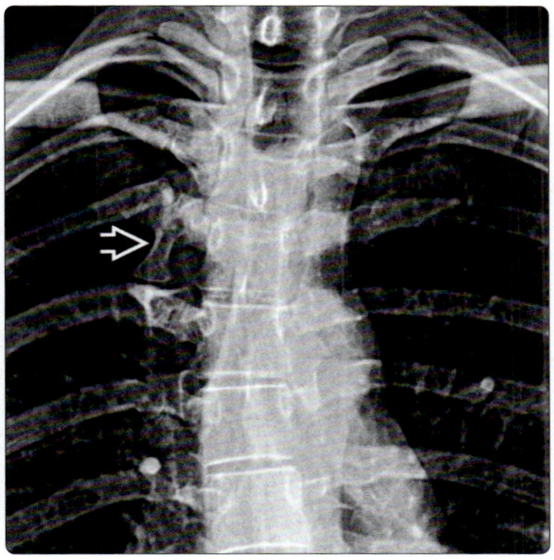

(Left) *Coronal T2 FS MR in a 10-year-old girl shows vertebral segmentation anomalies, including a lumbar hemivertebra & fusion of L5 to a dysplastic sacrum. The patient has a solitary dysplastic right kidney with multiple cysts. Note the absence of a kidney in the left renal fossa in this patient with VACTERL association.* **(Right)** *AP radiograph shows dextroscoliosis related to a rib anomaly that has caused separation of the right 4th & 5th ribs.*

Tumor

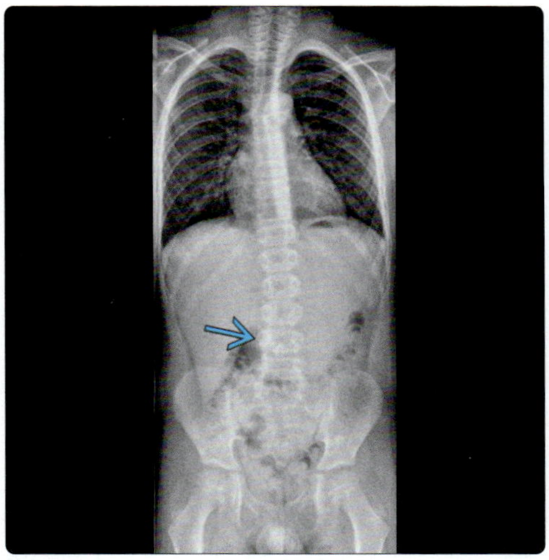

Tumor

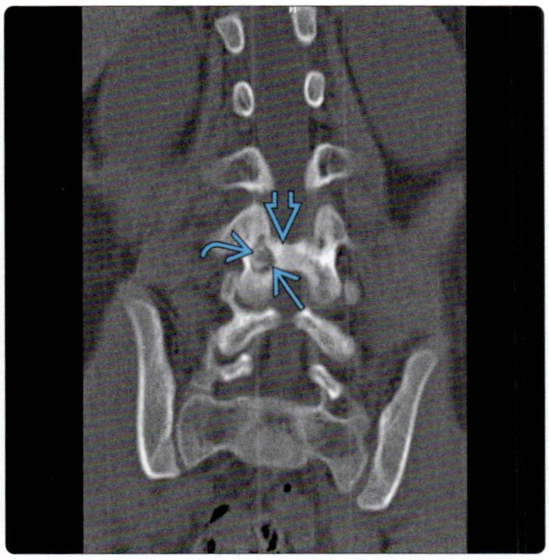

(Left) *Frontal radiograph in an 8-year-old boy with painful scoliosis shows mild dextrocurvature of the thoracic & mild levocurvature of the lumbar spine. There is very subtle increased sclerosis of the right pedicle of the L4 vertebral body.* **(Right)** *Coronal reformatted image from a NECT scan in the same child shows a focal lucent lesion in the right L4 lamina with a central partially sclerotic nidus. There is surrounding sclerosis. The findings are typical of an osteoid osteoma, which was confirmed at pathology.*

Kyphosis

DIFFERENTIAL DIAGNOSIS

Common

- Normal Infantile
- Idiopathic
- Traumatic
  - Compression
    - Normal Mineralization
    - Osteoporosis
  - Burst Fracture
  - Chance Fracture
- Neuromuscular Scoliosis
- Scheuermann Disease
- Congenital
  - Failure of Vertebral Segmentation
    - Klippel-Feil Spectrum
  - Failure of Vertebral Body Formation
  - Tethered Spinal Cord
  - Caudal Regression Syndrome

Less Common

- Neurofibromatosis Type 1
- Skeletal Dysplasias
  - Achondroplasia
  - Mucopolysaccharidoses
- Tumor
  - Langerhans Cell Histiocytosis
  - Osteoid Osteoma
  - Osteoblastoma
  - Aneurysmal Bone Cyst
  - Ewing Sarcoma
  - Leukemia/Lymphoma
- Infectious/Inflammatory
  - Pyogenic Osteomyelitis
  - Chronic Recurrent Multifocal Osteomyelitis
  - Granulomatous Osteomyelitis
  - Postoperative Infection
- Connective Tissue Disorders
- Postoperative Spinal Complications

Rare but Important

- Prior Radiation
- Diastematomyelia

ESSENTIAL INFORMATION

Key Differential Diagnosis Issues

- MR may be useful in certain cases
  - Painful scoliosis: Tumor, infection
  - Atypical curve: Short segment, hyperkyphotic, rapidly progressing, other radiographic abnormalities; often have underlying bony, neural, or paraspinal abnormalities
  - Congenital scoliosis: Assess full extent of anomalies
- CT is useful for bone detail in congenital scoliosis

Helpful Clues for Common Diagnoses

- Lumbar kyphosis is normal in infants
  - Lumbar lordosis develops upon sitting upright
- Idiopathic: Vertebral morphology shows normal to mild anterior wedging & normal endplates
  - No underlying cause is identified; may be of infantile, juvenile, or adolescent (most common) onset
- Traumatic: Common with falls & motor vehicle collisions
  - Compression fractures are common in osteoporosis without abnormal stress on bone
    - Most commonly seen with steroid administration, such as with Duchenne muscular dystrophy
- Neuromuscular scoliosis: Due to disorders of brain, spinal cord, & muscular system; infantile kyphosis may persist
- Scheuermann kyphosis presents in adolescence & may be misdiagnosed as fracture
  - Involves multiple adjacent levels with marked undulation &/or Schmorl nodes of endplates
- Congenital: Various bone anomalies cause kyphosis; curve may progress rapidly, especially if it includes unfused hemivertebrae
- Infectious: Pyogenic is typically centered at disc/endplates; granulomatous classically spares disc
- Inflammatory: Chronic recurrent multifocal osteomyelitis (CRMO) can cause vertebra plana like Langerhans cell histiocytosis & other tumors

Traumatic

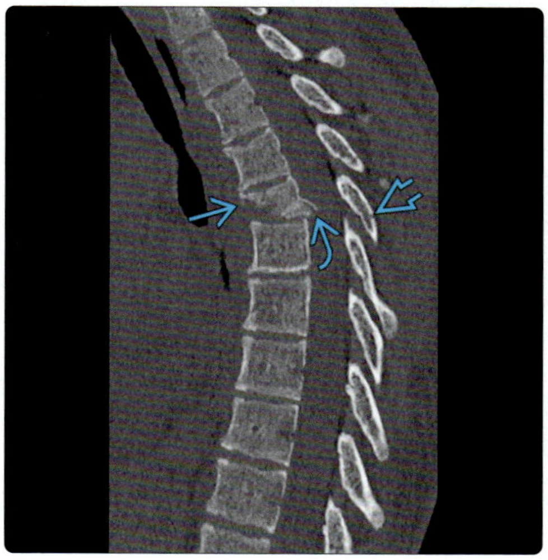

Neuromuscular Scoliosis

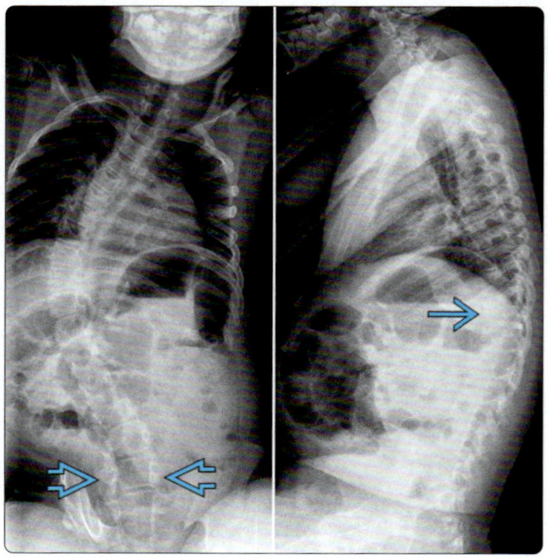

(Left) *Sagittal bone CT in a 17 year old after a motor vehicle collision shows a fracture of T5 with anterior height loss, fragment retropulsion into the spinal canal, & extension into the posterior elements. There is a secondary kyphosis.* **(Right)** *Frontal & lateral radiographs in a 9 year old with a history of myelomeningocele show a long C-shaped curve of the thoracolumbar spine, typical of neuromuscular causes. There is short segment kyphosis. Note the lumbosacral dysraphism.*

Scheuermann Disease

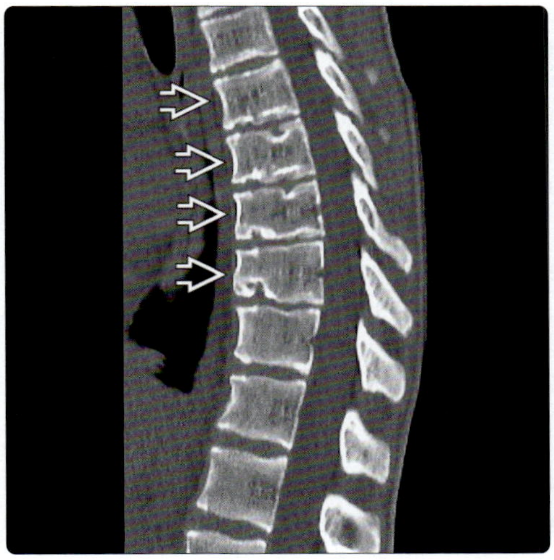

Congenital

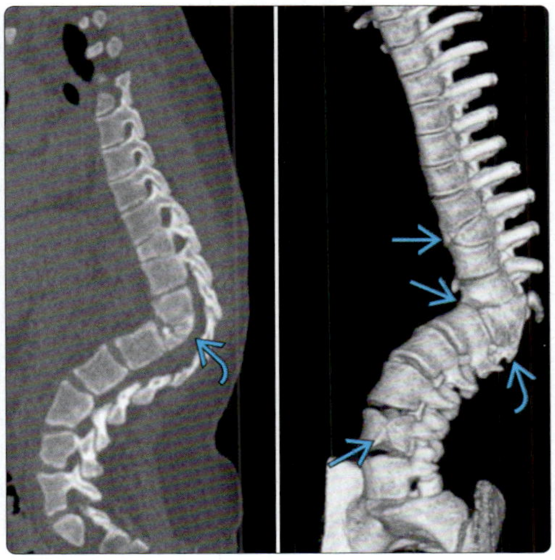

(Left) *Sagittal bone CT shows kyphosis due to accentuated vertebral wedging ➔. Note the undulating endplates & Schmorl nodes at 4 contiguous levels, typical of Scheuermann disease (though it can be more extensive).* **(Right)** *Sagittal (left) & 3D surface rendered (right) images from a bone CT in a 2-year-old girl show vertebral segmentation anomalies at multiple levels ➔ with severe kyphosis ➔.*

Congenital

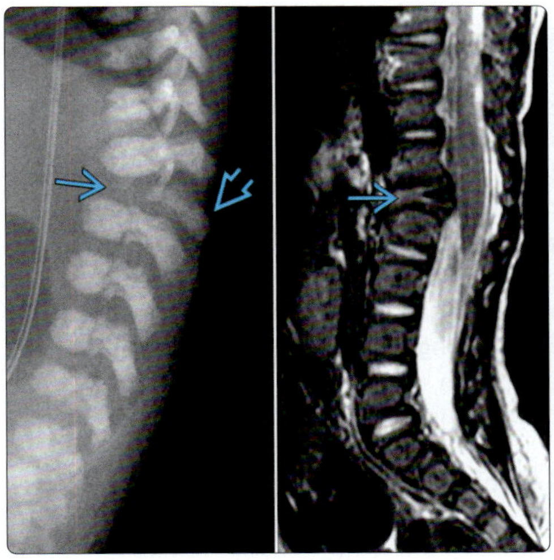

Infectious/Inflammatory

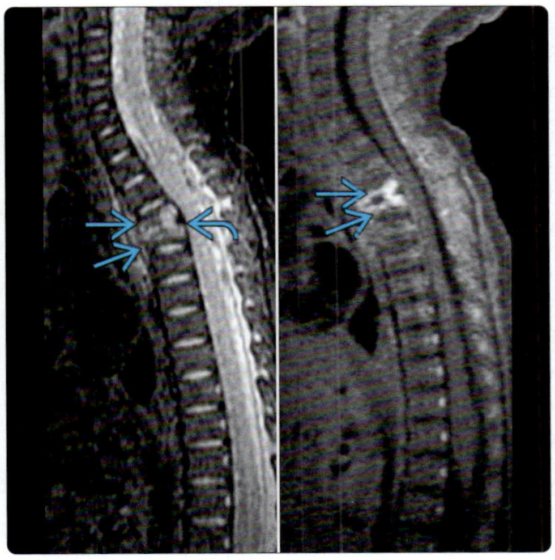

(Left) *Lateral radiograph (left) & sagittal T2 MR (right) in an infant show an absence of a normal L1 vertebral body ➔ despite the presence of hypoplastic posterior elements ➔, creating a focal kyphosis. No normal discs are seen at this level.* **(Right)** *Sagittal STIR (left) & T1 C+ FS (right) MR images in a 1 month old with osteomyelitis & discitis show flattening of the T3 & T4 vertebral bodies with endplate irregularity, disc destruction, & hyperenhancement ➔. Focal kyphosis is noted ➔.*

Tumor

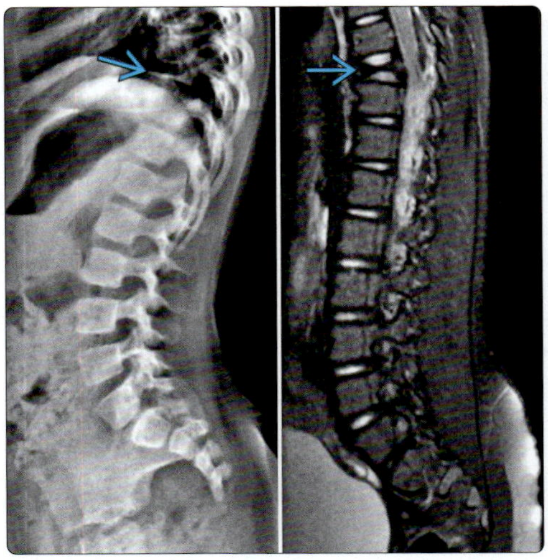

Tumor

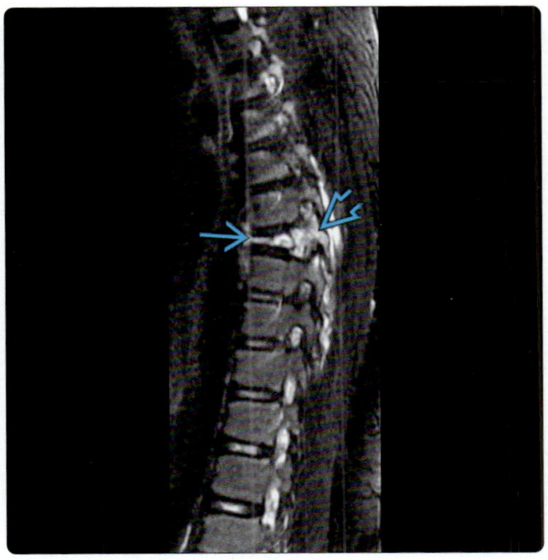

(Left) *Lateral radiograph (left) & sagittal STIR MR (right) in a 3 year old with back pain show complete flattening of the T10 vertebral body (vertebra plana) ➔ due to Langerhans cell histiocytosis (LCH). Note that the adjacent discs are preserved, which helps to distinguish LCH from typical pyogenic infection.* **(Right)** *Sagittal STIR MR shows near-complete height loss at the T5 vertebral body ➔ with associated kyphosis. Note the diffusely ↑ signal intensity throughout the T5 vertebra, including posterior elements ➔. Biopsy showed lymphoma.*

Bullet-Shaped Vertebra/Anterior Vertebral Body Beaking

DIFFERENTIAL DIAGNOSIS

Common

- Normal Developmental Vertebral Changes
- Anterior Vertebral Compression Fractures

Less Common

- Skeletal Dysplasias
  - Achondroplasia
  - Pseudoachondroplasia
- Radiation-Induced Growth Deformities

Rare but Important

- Mucopolysaccharidoses
  - Hurler Syndrome
  - Morquio Syndrome
- Other Metabolic Disorders With Dysostosis Multiplex
- Hypothyroidism (Congenital)

ESSENTIAL INFORMATION

Helpful Clues for Common Diagnoses

- **Normal Developmental Vertebral Changes**
  - Ring apophyses at superior/inferior endplates
    - Before ossification is complete, anterior vertebral margins may appear rounded or deficient ± notching
  - Mild physiologic wedging (especially midthoracic)
    - Superior & inferior endplates slope mildly towards each other from posterior to anterior
      - Smooth, symmetric, without focal indentation
    - Adjacent levels typically share this morphology
- **Anterior Vertebral Compression Fractures**
  - Focal endplate interruption &/or height loss; often asymmetric between superior & inferior endplates
  - Typically disproportionate to adjacent levels

Helpful Clues for Less Common Diagnoses

- **Skeletal Dysplasias**
  - Achondroplasia
    - Rhizomelic dwarfism
    - Bullet-shaped vertebrae with posterior scalloping, spinal stenosis, inferiorly decreased interpediculate distances, exaggerated lumbosacral lordosis
  - Pseudoachondroplasia
    - Rhizomelic dwarfism
    - C1-2 subluxation, accentuated lumbar lordosis, early osteoarthritis, short thick tubular bones
- **Radiation-Induced Growth Deformities**
  - Regional osteoporosis ± scoliosis

Helpful Clues for Rare Diagnoses

- **Mucopolysaccharidoses**
  - Heterogeneous group of lysosomal storage diseases
  - Dysostosis multiplex: Constellation of bone dysplasia features seen variably in mucopolysaccharidosis (MPS)
  - MPS I-H: Hurler syndrome
    - Anterior inferior vertebral body beaking
    - Mental retardation, short stature, coarse facial features, macrocephaly, & abnormal sella
    - Small iliac bones with inferior tapering, steep acetabuli, abnormal femoral heads, thickened tubular bones, contractures
  - MPS IV: Morquio syndrome
    - Anterior central vertebral body beaking
    - Short stature, macrocephaly, odontoid hypoplasia, ↑ lumbar lordosis, paddle-shaped ribs
    - Flared iliac wings, inferiorly tapering iliac bones, steep acetabuli, coxa valga
- **Other Metabolic Disorders With Dysostosis Multiplex**
  - May have anterior beaking (e.g., mucolipidoses, Niemann-Pick, gangliosidosis, fucosidosis, mannosidosis)
- **Hypothyroidism (Congenital)**
  - Mental retardation, delayed skeletal maturation, stippled epiphyses, short thick bones

SELECTED REFERENCES

1. Jaremko JL et al: Common normal variants of pediatric vertebral development that mimic fractures: a pictorial review from a national longitudinal bone health study. Pediatr Radiol. 45(4):593-605, 2015

Normal Developmental Vertebral Changes

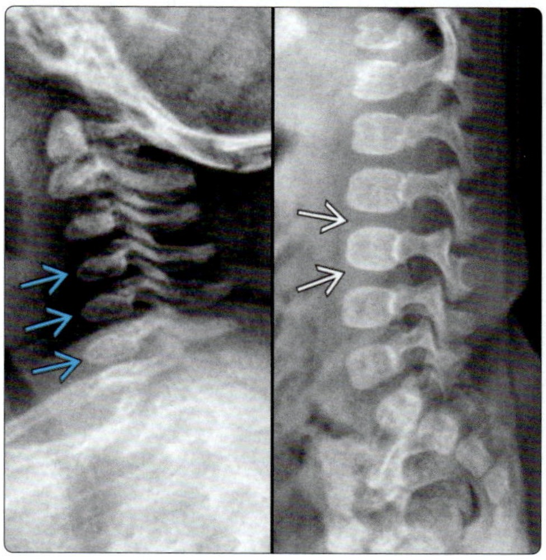

Normal Developmental Vertebral Changes

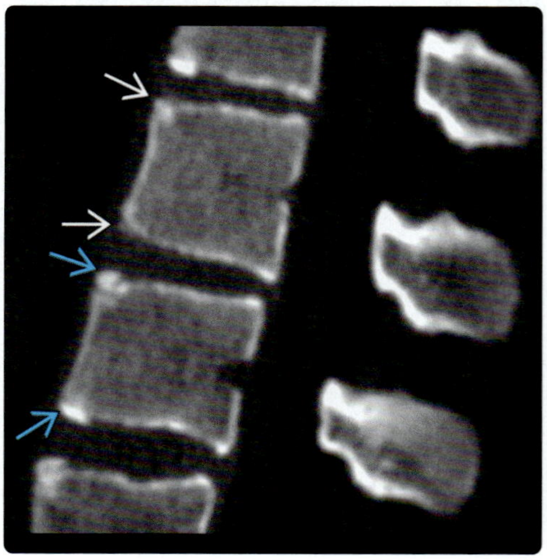

(Left) *Lateral radiographs of the spine in a 6 month old show a rounded appearance of the cervical* → *& lumbar* ➡ *vertebrae anteriorly. This normal rounding is due to the unossified ring apophyses superiorly & inferiorly. The appearance could mimic compression fractures or anterior beaking.* **(Right)** *Sagittal bone CT of normal lumbar vertebrae in a 15 year old shows ossified ring apophyses* → *at the superior & inferior margins of L2. Ring apophyses at L1 are less ossified* ➡*, giving a wedged appearance at L1 anteriorly.*

Anterior Vertebral Compression Fractures

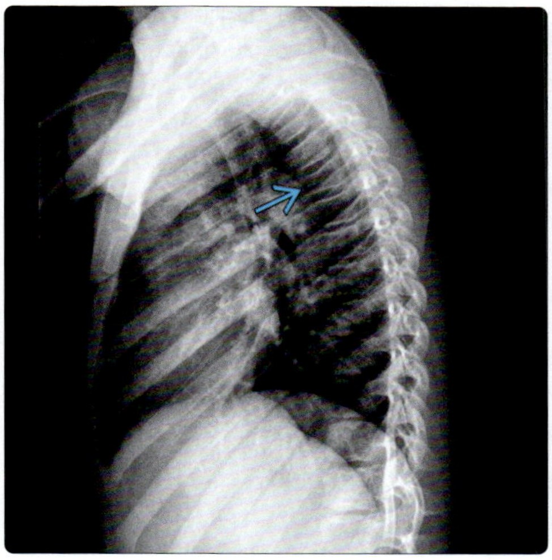

Achondroplasia

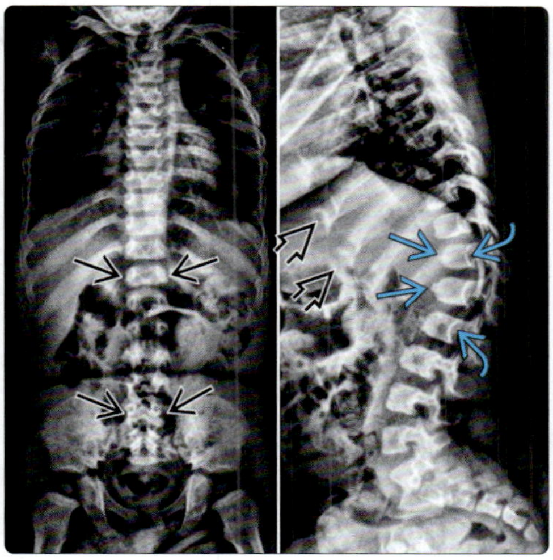

(Left) *Lateral radiograph in an 8 year old with acute upper back pain after a fall onto the neck shows a mild compression fracture of the T4 vertebra* →*.* **(Right)** *Frontal & lateral radiographs in a 2-year-old boy with achondroplasia show central anterior beaking of the vertebral bodies* →*, creating a bullet shape. Other findings of achondroplasia include posterior vertebral body scalloping* ↗*, short pedicles, inferior narrowing of the interpedicular distances* →*, flared anterior ribs* ⇒*, squared iliac bones, & horizontal acetabula.*

Pseudoachondroplasia

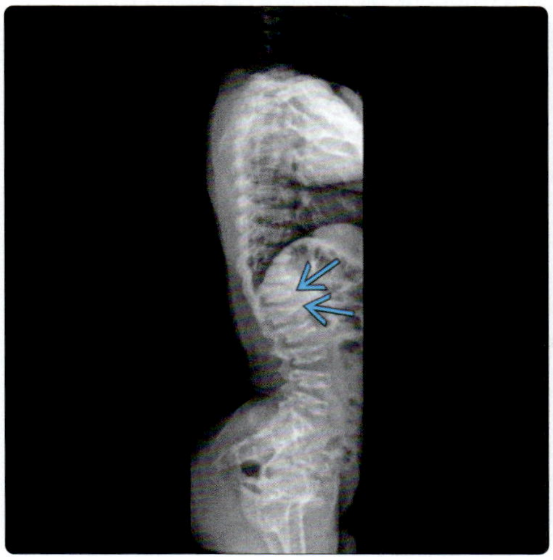

Radiation-Induced Growth Deformities

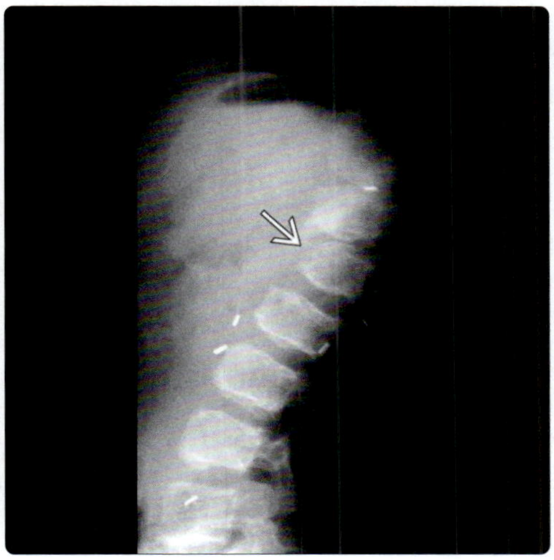

(Left) *Lateral radiograph of the spine in a 17-year-old boy with pseudoachondroplasia shows mild platyspondyly & anterior vertebral body beaking* →*.* **(Right)** *Lateral radiograph shows a hypoplastic, almost bullet-shaped L1 vertebra* ➡ *in a child who was radiated 1 year earlier for a Wilms tumor. Radiation therapy to a growing bone slows or stops growth due to vascular damage.*

Hurler Syndrome

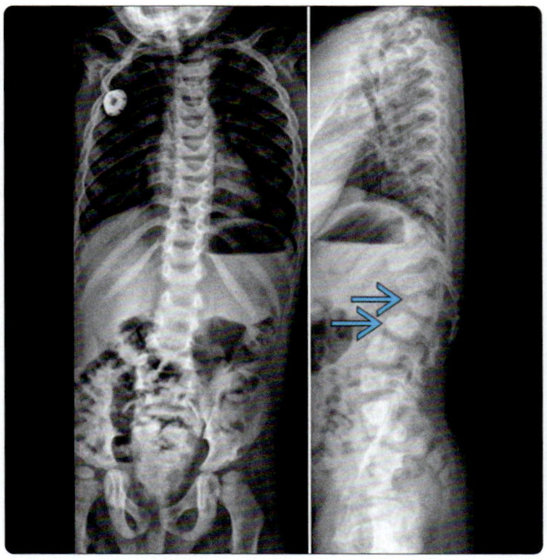

Morquio Syndrome

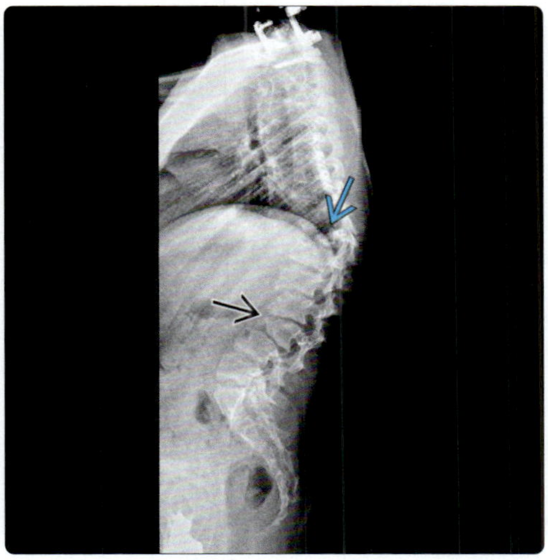

(Left) *Spine radiographs in a 2-year-old boy with mucopolysaccharidosis (MPS) I-H (Hurler syndrome) show superior notches & inferior beaks in the anterior aspects of the L2 & L3 vertebral bodies* → *with an associated thoracolumbar gibbus deformity. Also note the steep acetabula.* **(Right)** *Lateral spine radiograph in a 17-year-old girl with MPS IV (Morquio syndrome) shows central beaking of L3* →*. T11 is also markedly hypoplastic with anterior central beaking* →*, resulting in an associated kyphosis.*

Scalloped Vertebral Bodies

DIFFERENTIAL DIAGNOSIS

Common

- Vertebral Segmentation Failure

Less Common

- Achondroplasia
- Mucopolysaccharidoses
- Dural Dysplasia

Rare but Important

- Spinal Dysraphism
- Syringomyelia
- Intraspinal Mass

ESSENTIAL INFORMATION

Key Differential Diagnosis Issues

- May be due to congenital or developmental disorder of bony elements &/or meninges vs. slowly expanding lesion in spinal canal
- Depending on underlying abnormality, scalloping may occur focally at each affected vertebra vs. more broadly over several vertebral levels

Helpful Clues for Common Diagnoses

- **Vertebral Segmentation Failure**
  - May affect 1 or more pairs of vertebral elements
  - Typically creates hourglass configuration of vertebral bodies centered at hypoplastic disc
    - Narrowed AP dimension of vertebral bodies
    - Various configurations of posterior elements

Helpful Clues for Less Common Diagnoses

- **Achondroplasia**
  - Bullet-shaped vertebra with anterior beaking/blunting, short pedicles, & posterior scalloping
  - Spinal stenosis secondary to degenerative disease + congenitally short pedicles
  - Lumbosacral hyperlordosis, thoracolumbar kyphoscoliosis
  - ± craniocervical junction stenosis, rarely C1-2 instability
- **Mucopolysaccharidoses**
  - Inherited lysosomal storage disorders; Hurler syndrome [mucopolysaccharidosis (MPS IH)] is most common
  - Anterior vertebral beaking, thoracolumbar gibbus ± spinal stenosis, posterior vertebral scalloping
  - Narrow foramen magnum, short posterior C1 arch, odontoid hypoplasia
- **Dural Dysplasia**
  - a.k.a. dural ectasia
  - Patulous dural sac + posterior vertebral body scalloping
    - ± neurofibromas or other spinal neoplasms in neurofibromatosis type 1 (NF1)
    - ± arterial dissection or aneurysm in Marfan & Ehlers-Danlos syndromes
    - Osteoporosis in homocystinuria

Helpful Clues for Rare Diagnoses

- **Spinal Dysraphism**
  - Myelomeningocele: Open neural tube defect with wide osseous dysraphism ± syrinx or kyphoscoliosis
    - ~ 100% have Chiari 2 malformation
    - Increasing frequency of in utero repair may affect long-term bone changes
  - Lipomyelocele or lipomyelomeningocele: Skin-covered (i.e., closed) dysraphism with neural placode/lipoma complex extending through osseous dysraphic defect
  - Diastematomyelia: Split cord malformation with fibrous, osteocartilaginous, or osseous spur, intersegmental vertebral fusion, thick filum, &/or tethered cord
- **Syringomyelia**
  - ± wide canal
  - Typically secondary to spinal dysraphism, Chiari 1, or neoplasm
- **Intraspinal Mass**
  - Slow-growing intramedullary or extramedullary mass → enlargement of canal &/or vertebral scalloping

(Left) *Sagittal T2 MR (left) & NECT (right) images show an hourglass configuration of vertebral bodies at the C6-7 & T1-2 levels where there is failed segmentation in the setting of Klippel-Feil anomaly.* **(Right)** *Lateral radiographic (left) & sagittal T2 MR (right) images in an 18 month old with achondroplasia show characteristic vertebral changes with anterior beaking, posterior scalloping, short pedicles, canal stenosis, & exaggerated lumbosacral lordosis.*

Vertebral Segmentation Failure

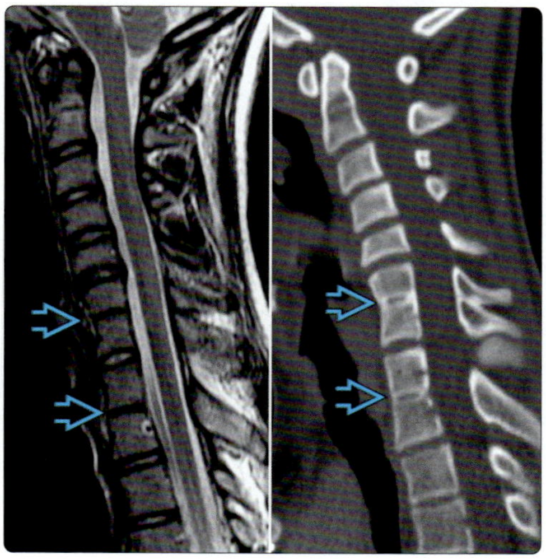

Achondroplasia

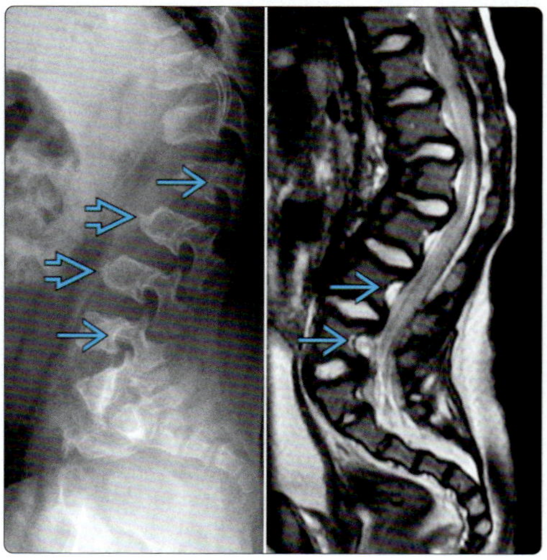

Mucopolysaccharidoses

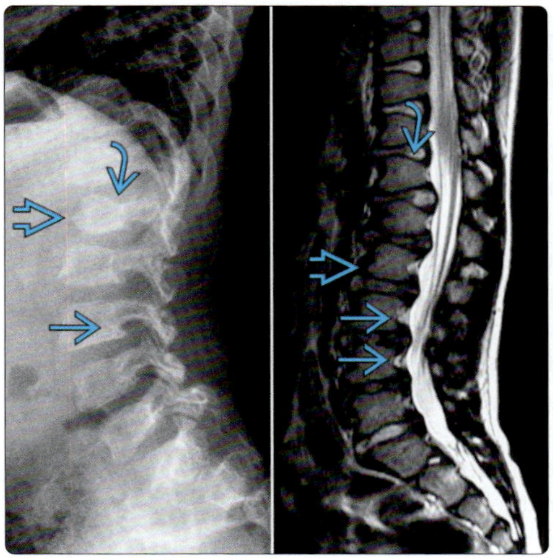

Dural Dysplasia

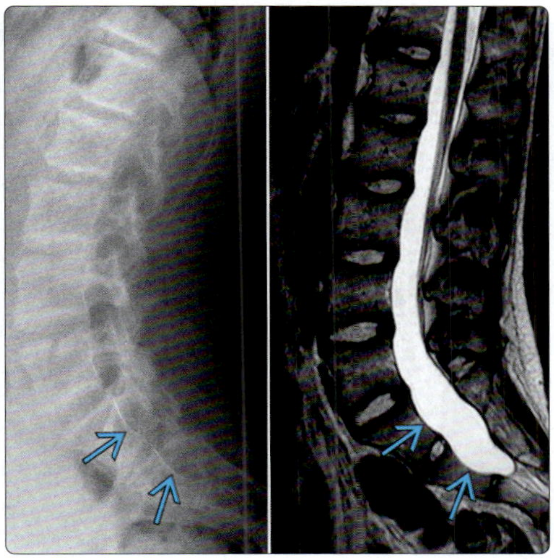

(Left) *Lateral radiographic (left) & sagittal T2 MR (right) images in a 9 year old with Hurler syndrome MPS IH show characteristic vertebral changes with posterior scalloping, anterior beaking, & sloped posterior endplates.* **(Right)** *Lateral radiographic (left) & sagittal T2 MR (right) images in a 13 year old with Marfan syndrome show mild posterior vertebral body scalloping secondary to dural ectasia.*

Dural Dysplasia

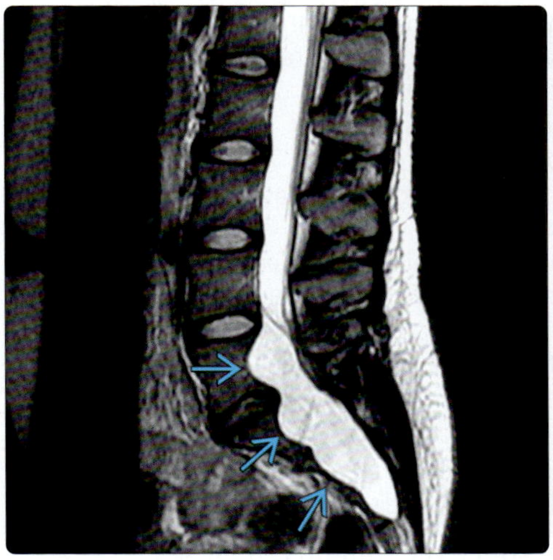

Dural Dysplasia

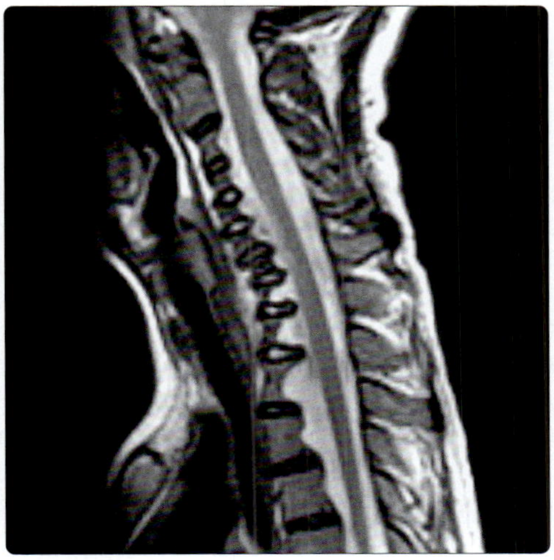

(Left) *Sagittal T2 MR in a 17 year old with back pain shows marked posterior vertebral body scalloping secondary to dural ectasia. The patient was subsequently diagnosed with the hypermobile form of Ehlers-Danlos syndrome.* **(Right)** *Sagittal T2 MR in a 10 year old with neurofibromatosis type 1 (NF1) shows severe posterior cervical vertebral body scalloping secondary to dural dysplasia. Only minimal bone is remaining at most cervical vertebral bodies.*

Intraspinal Mass

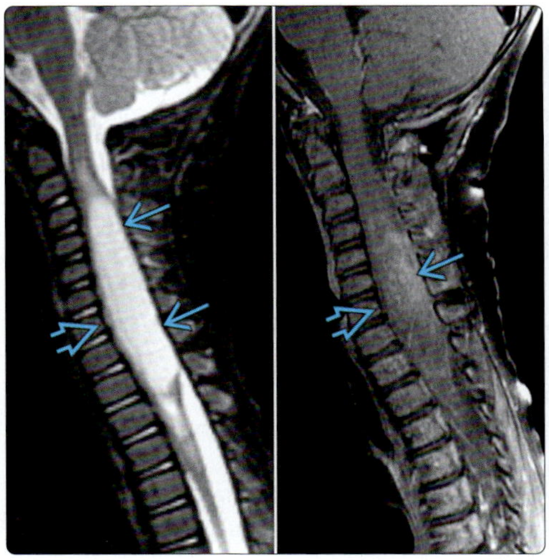

Intraspinal Mass

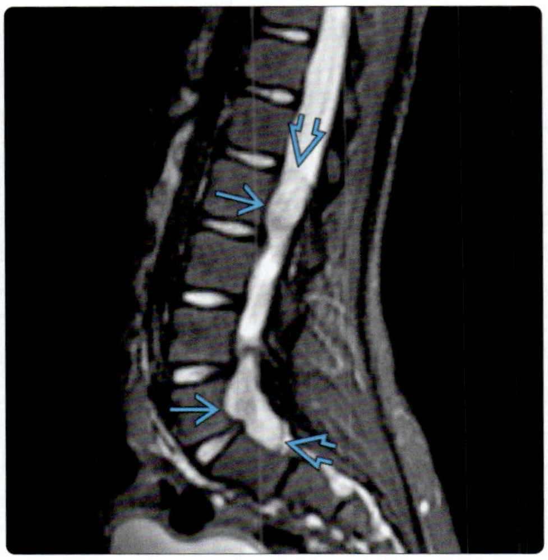

(Left) *Sagittal STIR (left) & T1 C+ FS (right) MR images in a 15 month old show an expansile mass of the cervicothoracic spinal cord with minimal enhancement. Surgery confirmed an astrocytoma. Note the widening of the spinal canal by the tumor with subtle broad scalloping of the posterior vertebral bodies.* **(Right)** *Sagittal STIR MR in an 11 year old with NF1 shows posterior vertebral body scalloping at the L2 & L5 levels secondary to intraspinal plexiform neurofibromas.*

DIFFERENTIAL DIAGNOSIS

Common

- Fracture Without Underlying Lesion
- Langerhans Cell Histiocytosis
- Leukemia
- Chronic Recurrent Multifocal Osteomyelitis
- Bone Tumor
- Infection

Less Common

- Skeletal Dysplasias
- Radiation Induced

Rare but Important

- Hypophosphatasia
- Idiopathic Juvenile Osteoporosis

ESSENTIAL INFORMATION

Key Differential Diagnosis Issues

- Platyspondyly: Flattening of vertebral body
  - Generalized: Involving all vertebra
  - Multiple: Involving some vertebrae
  - Localized: Involving only 1 vertebrae
    - Some authors consider localized platyspondyly = vertebra plana
  - Definitions can vary but typically refers to vertebral flattening with preserved endplates
    - Endplate configurations remain relatively parallel
- Vertebra plana: Near-complete collapse of vertebral body
  - Original definition: Only 1 vertebral level + ↑ sclerosis
- Both terms are used liberally for any vertebral flattening
- Differentiating features of vertebral height loss
  - Vertebrae involved: Localized (1), multiple, or diffuse
  - Congenital vs. acquired
    - Congenital: Typically due to skeletal dysplasia, rarely reported with other causes (e.g., congenital Cushing)
    - Acquired localized: Trauma, Langerhans cell histiocytosis (LCH), infection, malignancy
    - Acquired diffuse: Metabolic, endocrine, diffuse marrow process
  - Tumors, LCH, & chronic recurrent multifocal osteomyelitis (CRMO) may show multiple scattered enhancing vertebral lesions without collapse

Helpful Clues for Common Diagnoses

- **Fracture Without Underlying Lesion**
  - Typically does not fit exact definitions for platyspondyly/vertebra plana
    - Usually not complete collapse (e.g., anterior wedging)
    - Typically associated with endplate deformity & irregularity
  - May be solitary or multifocal (often adjacent)
  - Trauma history is typically apparent; if not, consider
    - Abnormal underlying bones
      - Diffuse osteoporosis [i.e., steroid use, metabolic bone disease, osteogenesis imperfecta (OI)]
      - Malignancy (metastatic disease or primary tumor)
    - Nonaccidental trauma
- **Langerhans Cell Histiocytosis**
  - Most common cause of true vertebra plana in children
  - Solitary > multifocal
  - May reconstitute during healing
  - Skeletal survey or PET may detect other lesions
    - "Punched-out" lytic skull lesion & mandibular "floating tooth" are classic LCH lesions where bone is completely gone but filled with enhancing soft tissue
  - MR is most sensitive in spine
- **Leukemia**
  - May be solitary or multifocal
  - Variable presentations
    - Generalized osteoporosis, diffuse collapse
    - Metaphyseal bands (lucent, dense, or alternating)
    - Focal lesion(s) with permeative destruction, periostitis, soft tissue mass
- **Chronic Recurrent Multifocal Osteomyelitis**
  - May be solitary or multifocal
  - Spine lesions may be very similar to LCH
  - Skeletal survey or whole-body MR
    - Lesions may be bubbly, aggressively lytic, or sclerotic
    - Pelvis, long bones, & clavicles are frequently involved
    - Lesions are often periphyseal (with metaphyseal & epiphyseal involvement but relative physeal sparing) & relatively symmetric
    - No fluid collections are seen
- **Bone Tumor**
  - Metastatic disease (e.g., neuroblastoma, rhabdomyosarcoma)
    - Typically multifocal or diffuse lesions; may be discrete lesions or confluent marrow replacement
  - Primary bone tumors of vertebral body (e.g., Ewing sarcoma) can mimic vertebral plana of LCH
  - ± soft tissue mass
- **Infection**
  - Vertebral endplates are typically involved with process centered at narrowed disc space; ± soft tissue abscess

Helpful Clues for Less Common Diagnoses

- **Skeletal Dysplasias**
  - Many cause varying degrees of platyspondyly
  - Platyspondyly is present at birth in some dysplasias but develops during childhood in others
  - **Achondroplasia**
    - More common heterozygous form shows minimal vertebral flattening; homozygous form has severe diffuse congenital platyspondyly
    - Classic vertebral findings otherwise include
      - Bullet-shaped vertebral bodies
      - Narrowed lumbar interpediculate distances
      - Posterior vertebral body scalloping
      - Accentuated lumbosacral lordosis
      - Craniocervical junction stenosis
    - Numerous other classic skeletal findings
  - **Pseudoachondroplasia**
    - Primarily spinal, metaphyseal, & epiphyseal changes
    - Vertebrae: Normal at birth, changes seen by 2-4 years
      - Diffuse platyspondyly + anterior tongue
  - **Thanatophoric dysplasia**
    - Most common lethal bone dysplasia (1:10,000 births)
    - Respiratory failure due to small thorax

- Diffuse severe platyspondyly at birth
- Markedly short, curved limbs
- **Spondyloepiphyseal dysplasia**
  - Primarily involve vertebrae & proximal epiphyses
  - Congenital (evident at birth) & tarda (presents at 5-10 years) forms
- **Mucopolysaccharidoses (MPS)**
  - Heterogeneous group of lysosomal storage diseases due to deficiency of glycosaminoglycan-degrading enzymes
  - Includes: Hurler (MPS I-H), Hunter (MPS II), & Morquio (MPS IV) syndromes
  - Dysostosis multiplex (DM): Constellation of bone dysplasia features seen variably in MPS
  - DM group: Includes all storage diseases leading to skeletal dysplasia (MPS, mucolipidoses, Gaucher, etc.)
  - Congenital presentation
  - Spine: Thoracolumbar gibbus (sharply angled kyphosis) with anteriorly beaked vertebral bodies
  - Ribs: Oar-shaped (thin proximally, wide distally)
  - Pelvis: Ilia small & tapered inferiorly, steep acetabular roofs, coxa valga, ± femoral head avascular necrosis (AVN) & subluxation
- **Osteogenesis Imperfecta**
  - Group of clinically heterogeneous genetic disorders caused by type I collagen abnormalities
  - ↑ bone fragility → frequent fractures → malunion & bowing
  - Range of severity based on type of OI (mild → severe)
    - Type I < IV < VI < VII < III < II (most severe)
  - Generalized osteoporosis + fractures of axial & appendicular skeleton
  - Spine: Kyphoscoliosis, biconcave or flattened vertebral bodies (platyspondyly), compression fractures
    - Solitary, multiple, or diffuse vertebral involvement
- **Metatropic dysplasia**
  - Metatropic: Changing
    - Early life: Short limb, normal trunk
    - Later life: Relative ↑ of limbs vs. trunk with severe kyphoscoliosis
  - Diffuse severe platyspondyly at birth
    - Infancy: "Dense, wafer-thin" vertebral bodies
    - Later: Vertebrae fill in but platyspondyly persists
- **Kniest dysplasia**
  - Skeletal dysplasia, retinal detachment, & deafness
  - Delayed, irregular epiphyseal ossification
  - Vertebrae: Coronal clefts (birth), platyspondyly + endplate irregularity (later)
- **Short rib-polydactyly syndrome type I**
  - Lethal dwarfism with short ribs & polydactyly
  - Diffuse platyspondyly & irregular vertebrae at birth
- **Radiation Induced**
  - Regional osteoporosis
  - May affect only 1 side of vertebra; ± scoliosis

Helpful Clues for Rare Diagnoses

- **Hypophosphatasia**
  - Defective gene for alkaline phosphatase → deficient mineralization of cartilage & osteoid
  - Perinatal (most severe), infantile, childhood, & adult (least severe) forms
  - Perinatal form: Severe lack of mineralization of skeleton
    - Skull base may be mineralized, calvarium is not
    - Mineralization of remainder of skeleton is variable
    - Diffuse vertebral collapse
  - Variable degree & number of collapsed vertebra with later presentations
- **Idiopathic Juvenile Osteoporosis**
  - Axial & appendicular osteoporosis
    - Complicated by fractures
    - Spine involvement is solitary, multifocal, or diffuse
  - May mimic mild OI
  - Resolves after puberty

SELECTED REFERENCES

1. Zaveri J et al: More than just Langerhans cell histiocytosis: a radiologic review of histiocytic disorders. Radiographics. 34(7):2008-24, 2014

Fracture Without Underlying Lesion

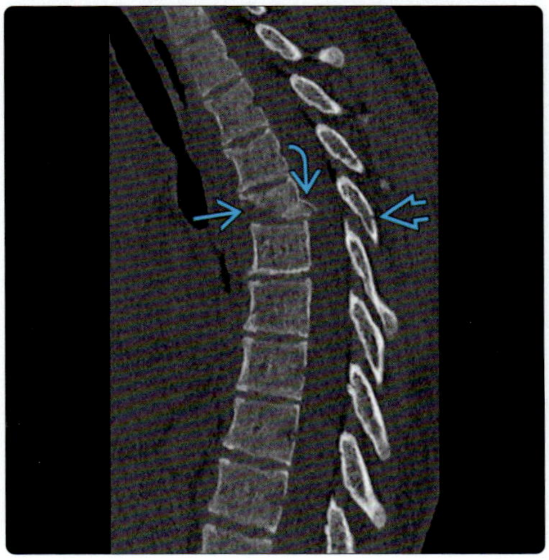

Fracture Without Underlying Lesion

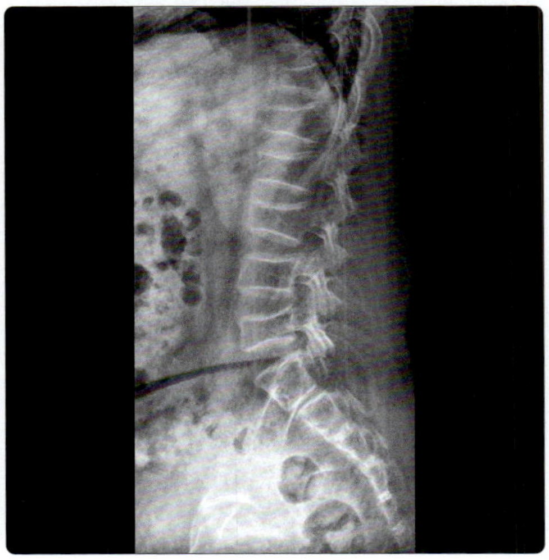

(Left) *Sagittal bone CT in a 17 year old after an MVC shows a fracture of T5 with anterior height loss ➡, a retropulsed fracture fragment ➡, & fracture extension into the posterior elements ➡, consistent with a 3-column Chance fracture.* **(Right)** *Lateral radiograph of the lumbar spine in a 15-year-old girl shows diffuse osteoporosis with mild to moderate anterior height loss of all lumbar vertebral bodies from compression fractures. This girl had been on chronic steroid treatment for lupus.*

(Left) *Lateral radiograph (left) & sagittal T2 FS MR (right) in a 3-year-old girl with back pain show complete flattening of the T10 vertebral body. The adjacent disc spaces are preserved.* **(Right)** *Coronal STIR MR of the bilateral femurs (left) & sagittal SSFP MR sequence of the brain (right) in the same child show additional lesions in the proximal left femur & calvarium. Additional Langerhans cell histiocytosis (LCH) lesions can be sought with a skeletal survey, PET scan, or whole-body MR.*

Langerhans Cell Histiocytosis

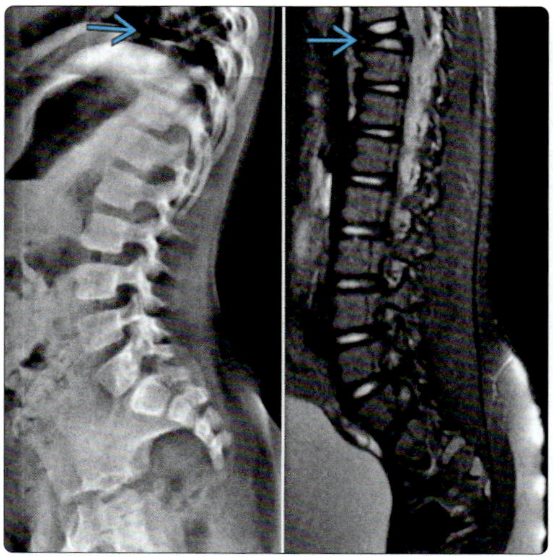

Langerhans Cell Histiocytosis

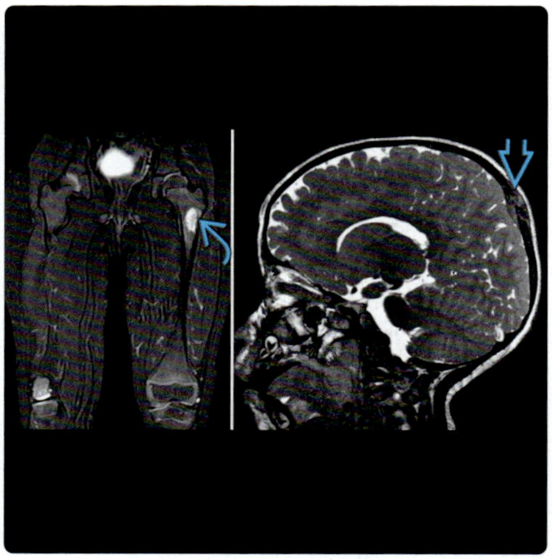

(Left) *Sagittal T1 MR (left) & STIR MR (right) in a 15-year-old boy with acute lymphocytic leukemia (ALL) & back pain show diffusely decreased T1 & mildly increased STIR signal intensity throughout the vertebral bodies. Vertebral height loss from compression fractures is present at multiple levels.* **(Right)** *Sagittal reformatted chest CT of a 17-year-old boy with acute myeloid leukemia (AML) shows loss of height of multiple thoracic vertebral bodies from compression fractures.*

Leukemia

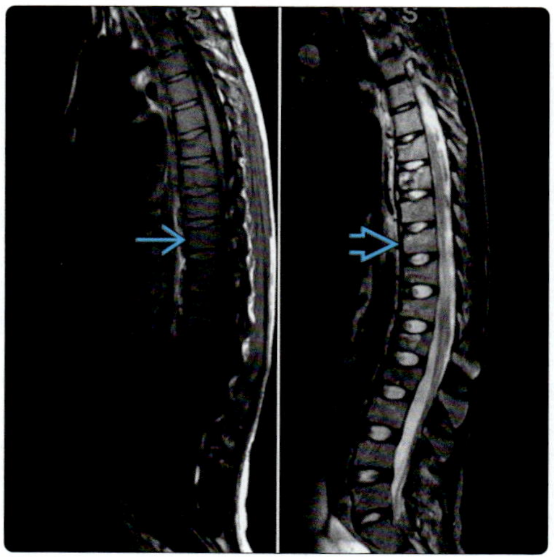

Leukemia

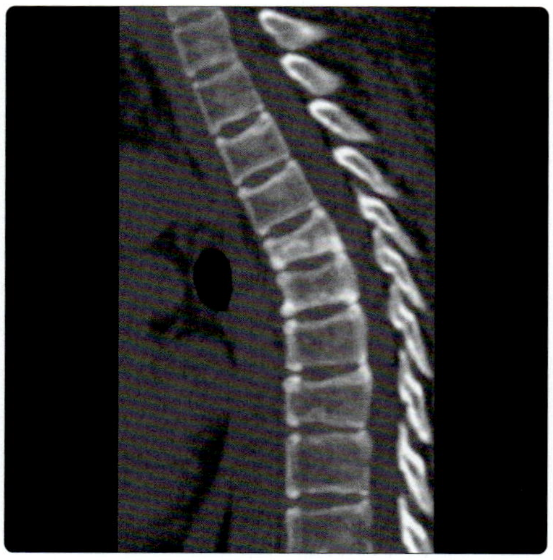

(Left) *Frontal (left) & lateral (right) radiographs of the thoracic spine in a 14 year old with back pain show marked height loss of the T5 vertebral body. This was initially suspected to be due to LCH.* **(Right)** *Sagittal STIR MR in the same patient shows near-complete height loss at the T5 vertebral body. Also note the diffusely increased signal intensity in the T5 posterior elements. Biopsy showed lymphoma.*

Bone Tumor

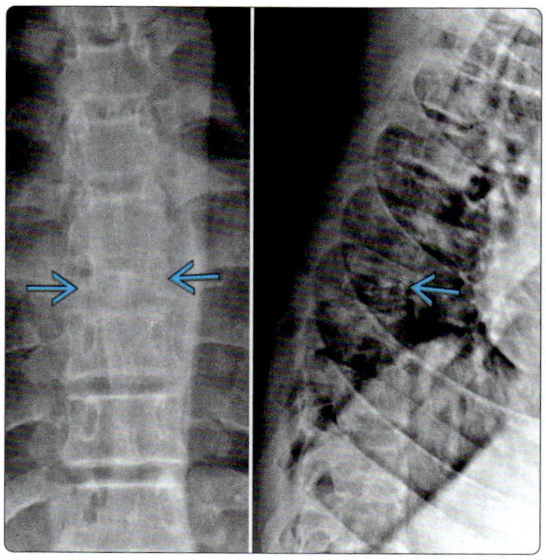

Bone Tumor

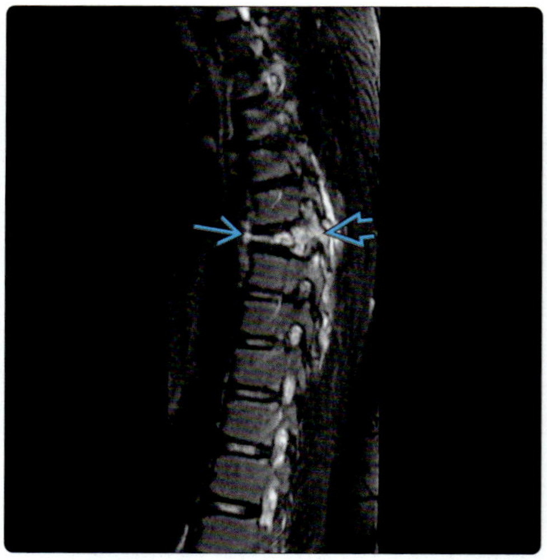

Bone Tumor

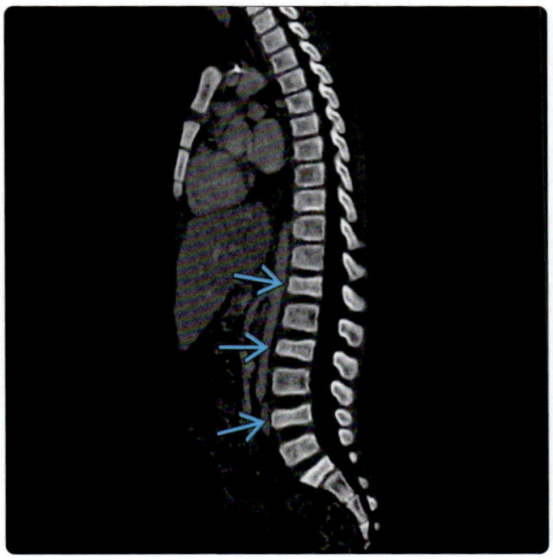

Infection

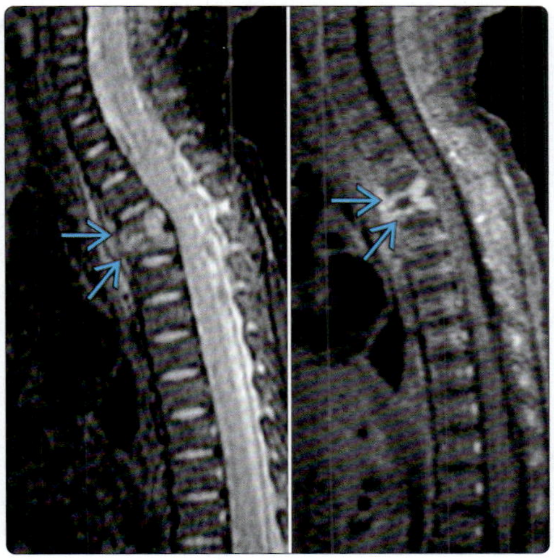

(Left) *Sagittal CECT of the chest, abdomen, & pelvis in an 8-year-old boy with metastatic neuroblastoma shows patchy areas of increased sclerosis throughout the spine (due to metastatic disease) with multiple levels of vertebral height loss from pathologic fractures* →. **(Right)** *Sagittal STIR MR (left) & T1 C+ FS MR (right) in a 1 month old with osteomyelitis/discitis show flattening of the T3 & T4 vertebral bodies with endplate irregularity & hyperenhancement* →. *The normal intervening disc signal & morphology are lost.*

Skeletal Dysplasias

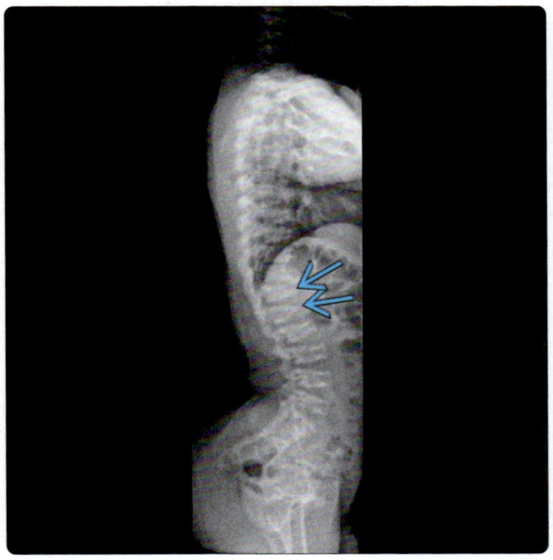

Skeletal Dysplasias

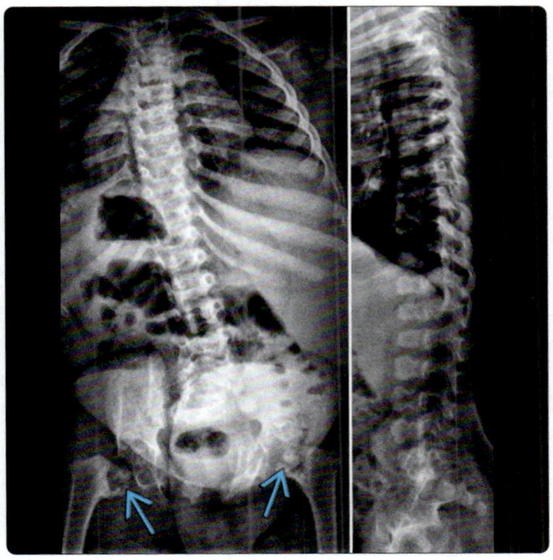

(Left) *Lateral radiograph of the spine in a 17-year-old boy with pseudoachondroplasia shows diffuse mild platyspondyly & anterior vertebral body beaking* →. **(Right)** *Frontal & lateral spine radiographs in a 4-year-old boy with spondyloepiphyseal dysplasia show flattening & irregularity of the vertebral bodies diffusely. Additionally, the femoral heads* → *are hypoplastic & markedly irregular.*

Skeletal Dysplasias

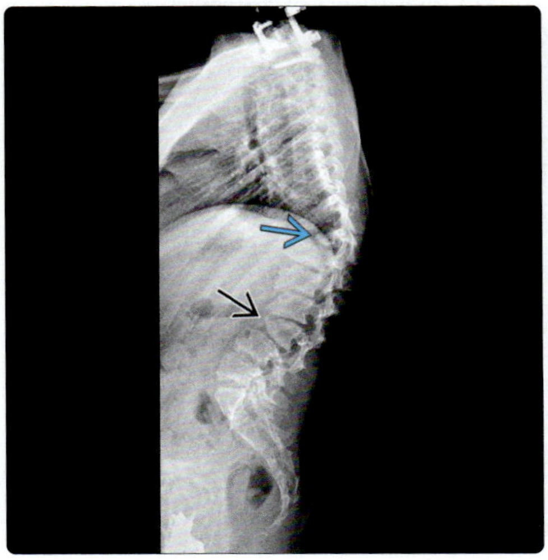

Skeletal Dysplasias

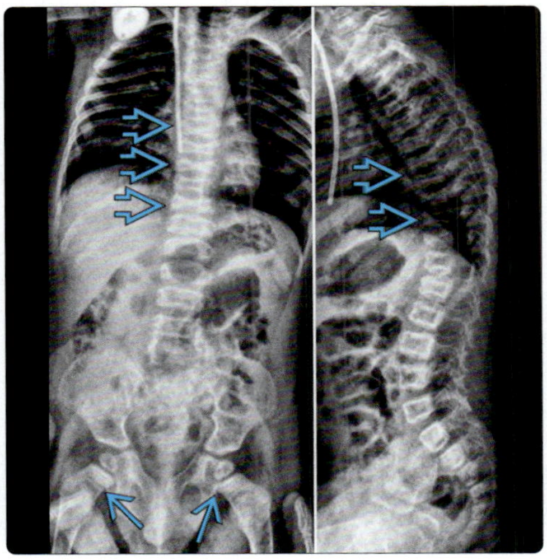

(Left) *Lateral spine radiograph in a 17-year-old girl with mucopolysaccharidoses (MPS) IV (Morquio syndrome) shows central beaking of L3* →. *T11 is also markedly hypoplastic with anterior central beaking* →, *resulting in an associated kyphosis.* **(Right)** *Frontal & lateral radiographs of the spine in a 1-year-old boy with osteogenesis imperfecta (OI) show height loss of multiple thoracic vertebral bodies from compression fractures* →. *Also note the sclerotic metaphyseal bands paralleling the growth plates* → *from bisphosphonate treatments.*

DIFFERENTIAL DIAGNOSIS

Common

- Spondylolysis
- Scoliosis
- Fracture
- Scheuermann Disease

Less Common

- Pyogenic Osteomyelitis/Discitis
- Sacroiliitis
- Chronic Recurrent Multifocal Osteomyelitis
- Congenital Spinal Stenosis
- Syringomyelia
- Neoplasm
  - Langerhans Cell Histiocytosis
  - Aneurysmal Bone Cyst
  - Osteoid Osteoma/Osteoblastoma
  - Neuroblastic Tumor
  - Ewing Sarcoma
  - Leukemia/Lymphoma
  - Hematogenous Metastases
  - CNS Neoplasm
  - CSF Disseminated Metastases

Rare but Important

- Intervertebral Disc Herniation
- Guillain-Barré Syndrome
- Transverse Myelitis
- Tuberculous Osteomyelitis

ESSENTIAL INFORMATION

Key Differential Diagnosis Issues

- In school age children, low back pain is most commonly
  - Musculoskeletal in nature without identifiable etiology
  - Self-limited
- Initial imaging evaluation: Almost always radiographs
- Specific "red flags" warranting MR imaging
  - Pain that is constant, at night, radicular, or lasting > 4 weeks
  - Fever or chills
  - Point tenderness
  - Neurologic findings

Helpful Clues for Common Diagnoses

- **Spondylolysis**
  - Unilateral or bilateral fracture of pars interarticularis; L5 > > L4 > others
    - Stress reaction may occur before cortical break
    - Spondylolisthesis: Spondylolysis leading to anterior subluxation of superior relative to inferior vertebra
  - Oblique radiographs add little sensitivity beyond lateral
  - CT highly sensitive & specific; can be targeted
  - STIR or T2 FS MR is particularly helpful to visualize marrow edema as cortical disruption may be missed on MR
  - Bone scintigraphy is sensitive for detecting stress reaction prior to pars fracture
    - Combined SPECT/CT shows anatomic correlate
- **Scoliosis**
  - 80% due to adolescent idiopathic scoliosis (AIS)
    - F > > M; age > 10 years
    - AIS is classically not associated with pain
      - Painful scoliosis traditionally triggers further imaging work-up due to higher association with treatable underlying cause (e.g., tumor, syrinx)
      - Newer literature suggests pain may be 2x as common in AIS compared to normal; more common if curve > 50°
- **Fracture**
  - Falls & motor vehicle accidents are most common causes
    - Type of fracture varies by mechanism
  - Look for multicolumn extension or spinal canal intrusion
    - Chance-type fractures have high association with bowel/mesentery & aortic injuries
  - Isolated compression fractures may be subtle; look at superior endplate for
    - Wedging out of proportion to adjacent levels
    - Focal indentation
    - Asymmetry of superior endplate on AP view
- **Scheuermann Disease**
  - "Osteochondrosis" of adolescent spine
  - Involves 3 or more adjacent vertebrae with anterior wedging & endplate irregularity causing kyphosis

Helpful Clues for Less Common Diagnoses

- **Pyogenic Osteomyelitis/Discitis**
  - Hematogenous spread of organisms to vascularized growth plates superiorly & inferiorly → extension into disc space → narrowing of disc space ± irregularity of adjacent endplates
  - Abnormal signal intensity of disc & surrounding vertebral marrow ± paraspinal or epidural inflammation/abscess
- **Sacroiliitis**
  - May be due to infection (rarely) or subtype of juvenile idiopathic arthritis (JIA), particularly enthesitis-related
    - ± concurrent inflammatory bowel disease in JIA
  - Contrast & DWI MR are sensitive but may not be necessary (beyond T2 FS) for noninfectious causes
  - Radiographic widening & irregularity are seen late
- **Chronic Recurrent Multifocal Osteomyelitis**
  - Patchy foci of marrow involvement ± vertebral collapse
  - No adjacent abscess
  - Look for typical lucent lesions of metaphysis or clavicle, ultimately leading to sclerosis
- **Congenital Spinal Stenosis**
  - Reduced diameter of central spinal canal
  - Pedicles are short & thick, may have narrowed interpediculate distance on AP view
- **Syringomyelia**
  - Chiari 1 is most common association in children
  - Consider contrast administration to exclude neoplasm if
    - Syrinx has no clear etiology
    - Nodularity is detected
- **Neoplasm**
  - **Langerhans Cell Histiocytosis**
    - Benign clonal proliferation of specific dendritic cells
    - Classic etiology of severe vertebra plana
    - Look for additional "punched-out" lytic lesions of flat & long bones filled with enhancing tissue
      - PET may be preferred for determining extent

- **Aneurysmal Bone Cyst**
  - Expansile bubbly lucent lesion with multiple locules & layering fluid-fluid levels, rim enhancement
- **Osteoid Osteoma/Osteoblastoma**
  - Osteoid osteoma: Lucent nidus (± central Ca^{2+}, early intense enhancement), surrounding edema & sclerosis
  - Osteoblastoma: Larger with diffuse enhancement
  - Pain is classically worst at night
  - Symptoms alleviated with NSAIDs
- **Neuroblastic Tumor**
  - Neuroblastoma usually paraspinal
    - Median age of 15-17 months
    - Older patients are more likely to have increased differentiation (ganglioneuroblastoma, ganglioneuroma)
  - Frequently surrounds vessels & invades vital structures (including spinal canal)
- **Ewing Sarcoma**
  - Typically found in adolescents
  - Aggressive permeative lesion, often with osteoporosis & some degree of expansion
  - Pelvic lesions often have large soft tissue masses
- **Leukemia/Lymphoma**
  - Varying degrees of marrow replacement ± aggressive periosteal reaction, focal destruction
- **Hematogenous Metastases**
  - Neuroblastoma & leukemia are most likely to cause extensive marrow replacement in young children
    - May also cause multifocal, well-defined lesions of marrow, along with various sarcomas
- **CNS Neoplasm**
  - Astrocytoma > ependymoma > ganglioglioma
    - Intramedullary tumor expands cord
  - Myxopapillary ependymoma is uncommon in children but is classically associated with
    - Low back pain
    - Enhancing mass at or below conus medullaris
- **CSF Disseminated Metastases**
  - Most pediatric CNS neoplasms (particularly > WHO grade I) can cause drop metastases
    - Also leukemia
  - T2 MR hypointense (to CSF) enhancing nodular masses (often with restricted diffusion) along surface of cord & nerve roots, accumulating in distal thecal sac

Helpful Clues for Rare Diagnoses

- **Intervertebral Disc Herniation**
  - Diagnostic criteria identical to adults
- **Guillain-Barré Syndrome**
  - Acute inflammatory demyelinating polyneuropathy (AIDP)
  - Acute onset of ascending weakness, diminished reflexes
  - Smooth, linear enhancement of cauda equina & conus
    - Ventral > dorsal nerve roots
    - Mild enlargement & increased T2 signal of nerves may continue into paraspinal tissues (& beyond)
- **Transverse Myelitis**
  - Idiopathic or secondary inflammation of spinal cord
  - Symmetric bilateral motor & sensory deficits
  - Central cord lesion extends > 2 vertebral segments; variable enhancement
- **Tuberculous Osteomyelitis**
  - ± disc sparing between involved vertebrae
  - Anterior collapse of involved vertebra(e) leading to kyphosis (Gibbus deformity)
  - Large psoas abscesses later calcify

SELECTED REFERENCES

1. Calloni SF et al: Back pain and scoliosis in children: when to image, what to consider. Neuroradiol J. 30(5):393-404, 2017
2. Expert Panel on Pediatric Imaging:. et al: ACR Appropriateness Criteria® Back Pain-Child. J Am Coll Radiol. 14(5S):S13-S24, 2017
3. MacDonald J et al: Musculoskeletal low back pain in school-aged children: a review. JAMA Pediatr. 171(3):280-7, 2017
4. Patel DR et al: Evaluation and management of lower back pain in young athletes. Transl Pediatr. 6(3):225-35, 2017
5. Randall RM et al: Review of pediatric spondylolysis and spondylolisthesis. Sports Med Arthrosc Rev. 24(4):184-7, 2016
6. Trout AT et al: Spondylolysis and beyond: value of SPECT/CT in evaluation of low back pain in children and young adults. Radiographics. 35(3):819-34, 2015

Spondylolysis

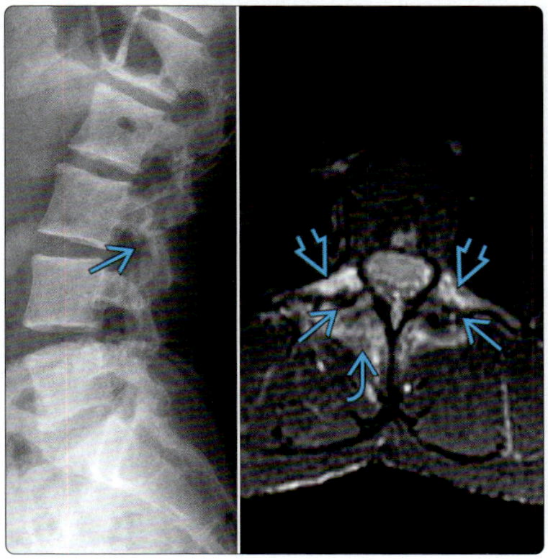

Spondylolysis

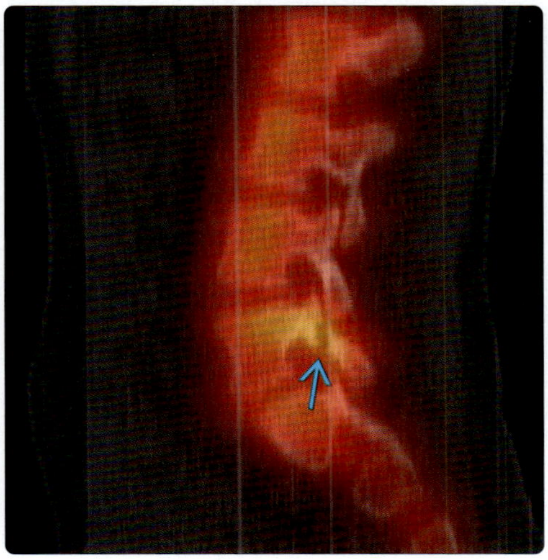

(Left) *Lateral radiograph & subsequent axial STIR MR in a 15 year old with back pain show spondylolysis at L3 with adjacent marrow & soft tissue edema.* **(Right)** *Sagittal Tc-99m MDP SPECT/CT in a 12 year old with back pain shows a focal pars interarticularis defect with increased radiotracer activity, consistent with spondylolysis.*

Spondylolysis

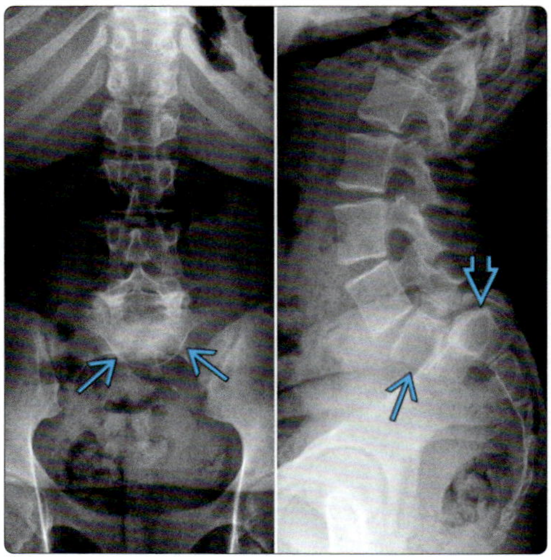

Scoliosis

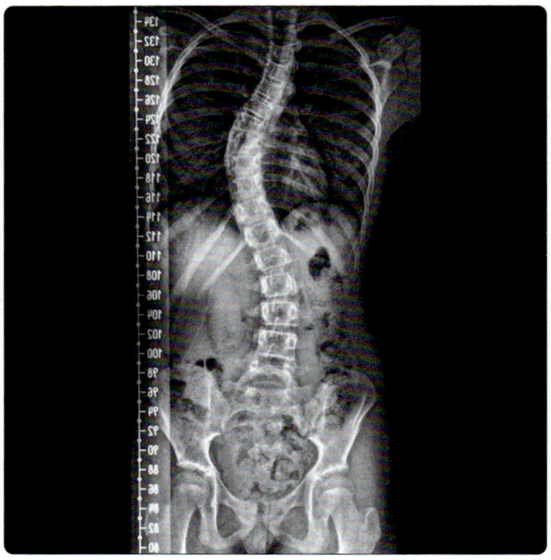

(Left) *AP (left) & lateral (right) radiographs of the lumbar spine in a 12 year old with lower back stiffness for 6 months show a grade 3-4 spondylolisthesis of L5 → on S1 ⇒.* **(Right)** *Frontal radiograph in a female adolescent shows an S-shaped idiopathic thoracic dextroscoliosis with compensatory lumbar levoscoliosis.*

Fracture

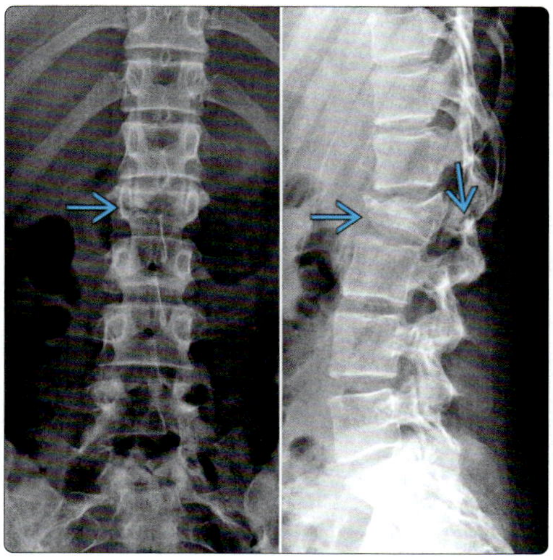

Scheuermann Disease

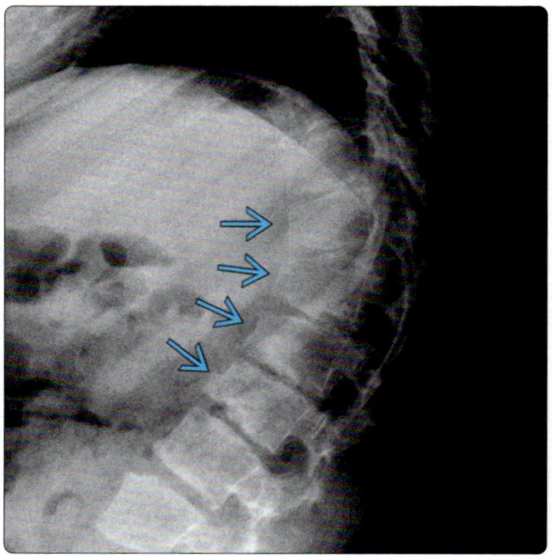

(Left) *Frontal (left) & lateral (right) radiographs in a 14 year old with pain after a sledding accident show a Chance fracture of the L2 vertebra with loss of the vertebral body height & a fracture plane → that extends through the 3 columns.* **(Right)** *Lateral radiograph in a 15 year old with back pain & worsening kyphosis shows multiple contiguous vertebral levels of anterior wedging, endplate irregularity, & disc space narrowing →, resulting in kyphosis. This is typical of Scheuermann disease.*

Pyogenic Osteomyelitis/Discitis

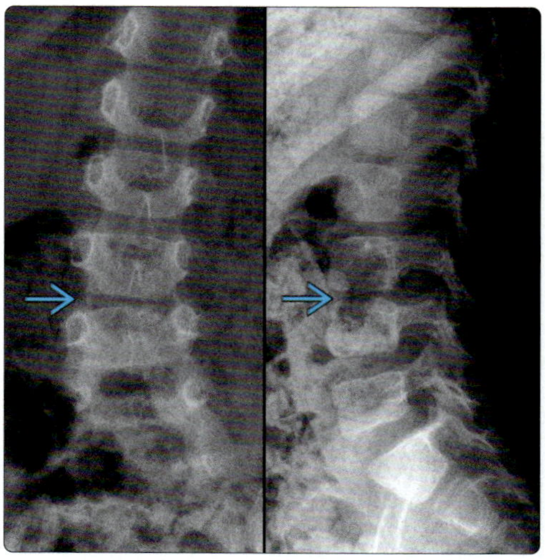

Pyogenic Osteomyelitis/Discitis

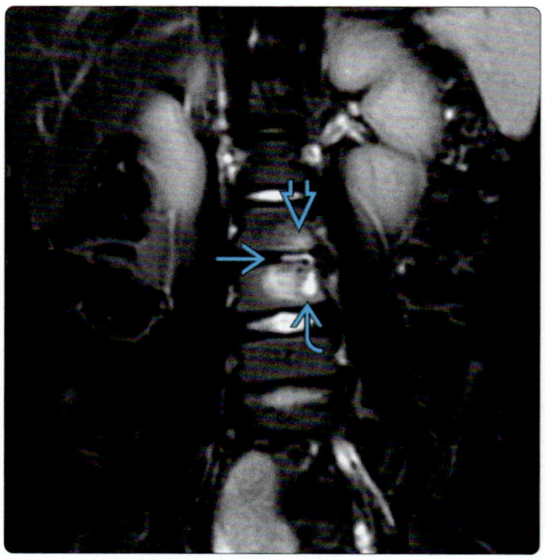

(Left) *Frontal (left) & lateral (right) radiographs in a 4 year old with fever, pain, & refusal to walk show narrowing of the disc space → with mild endplate irregularities at the L4-L5 level, typical of discitis-osteomyelitis. (Note that the patient has 6 non-rib-bearing vertebrae.)* **(Right)** *Coronal T2 FS MR in the same patient shows decreased disc space height with a fluid collection extending from the vertebral body ↗ into the disc →. There is surrounding marrow edema ⇒. The appearance is typical of pediatric pyogenic discitis-osteomyelitis.*

Sacroiliitis

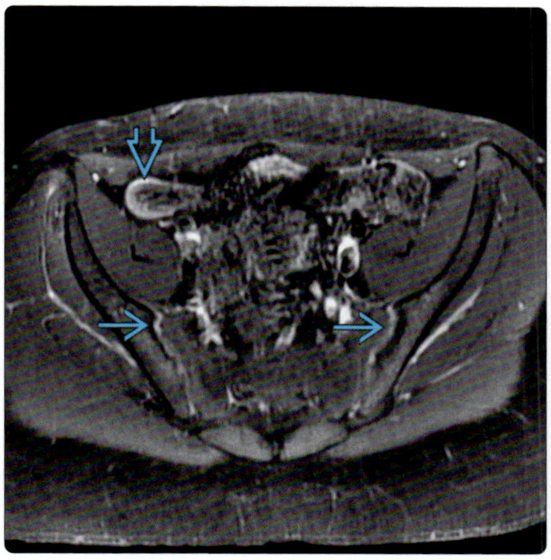

Chronic Recurrent Multifocal Osteomyelitis

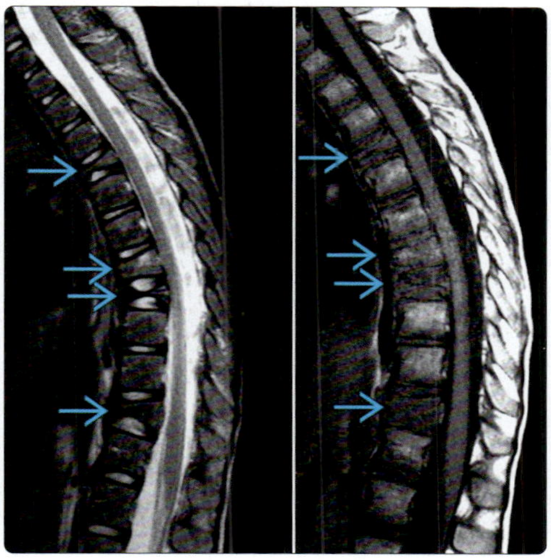

(Left) *Axial T1 C+ FS MR in a 9 year old with presumed enthesitis-related juvenile idiopathic arthritis shows abnormal increased enhancement of the bilateral sacroiliac joints ⇨. There is also wall thickening & mural stratification of the terminal ileum ⇨, suggesting Crohn disease.* **(Right)** *Sagittal T2 FS (left) & T1 (right) MR images of the thoracic spine in a 4 year old with recurrent fevers & leg pain show collapse & marrow signal abnormalities at multiple vertebral levels ⇨. Biopsy confirmed CRMO.*

Congenital Spinal Stenosis

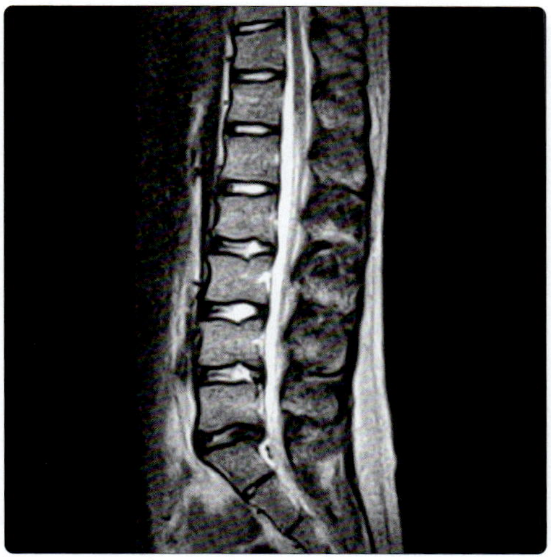

Syringomyelia

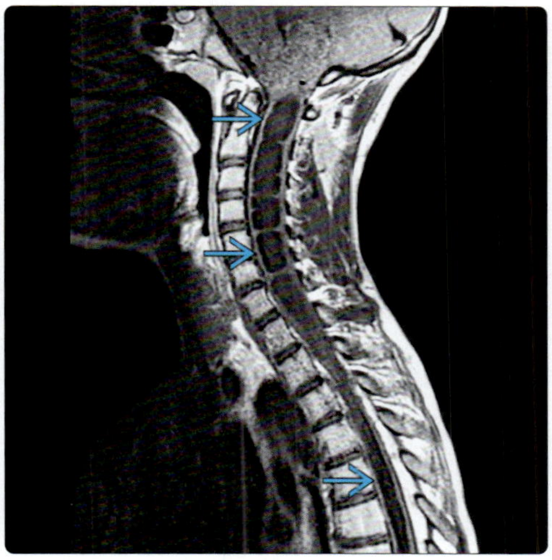

(Left) *Sagittal T2 MR demonstrates marked narrowing of the lumbar spinal canal anteroposterior diameter. The anteroposterior canal diameter should normally increase rather than decrease in the lower lumbar spine.* **(Right)** *Sagittal T1 MR in a patient with Chiari 1 malformation shows a large cervical & thoracic syrinx ⇨. Despite this sacculated appearance, the syrinx is usually continuous & would likely respond to a single drain.*

Langerhans Cell Histiocytosis

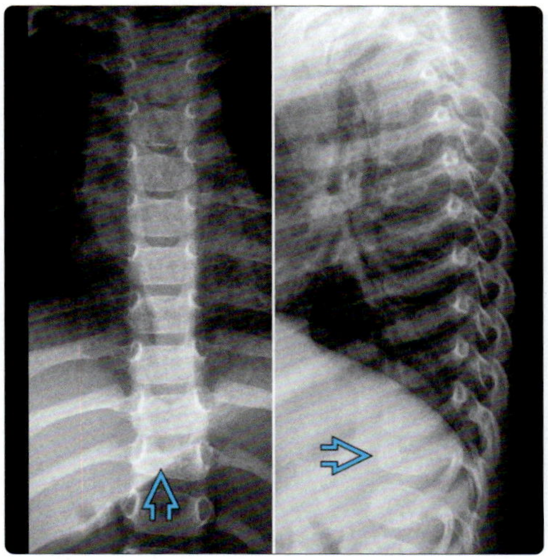

Langerhans Cell Histiocytosis

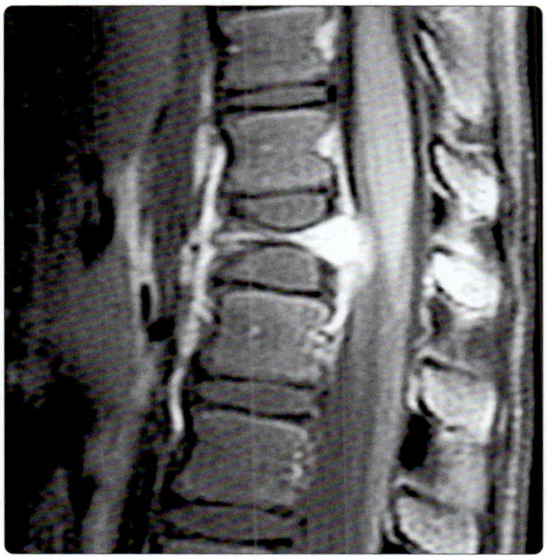

(Left) *Frontal (left) & lateral (right) thoracic spine radiographs in a 2 year old with back pain show partial collapse of the T11 vertebral body ⇨. A lytic tibial lesion was biopsied, confirming Langerhans cell histiocytosis (LCH).* **(Right)** *Sagittal T1 C+ FS MR depicts complete collapse of the T12 vertebra (vertebra plana). The vertebral body shows marked enhancement following gadolinium administration. These features are typical of LCH.*

(Left) *Lateral radiograph (left) of the sacrum in a 16 year old with pain & perineal numbness shows a lytic lesion of the S3 posterior elements. Sagittal STIR MR (right) reveals a multiloculated cystic lesion containing fluid-fluid levels, typical of an aneurysmal bone cyst.* **(Right)** *Axial bone CT of the cervical spine demonstrates a well-circumscribed, round, lucent lesion in the expanded right pedicle with a partially calcified central nidus, typical of an osteoid osteoma.*

Aneurysmal Bone Cyst

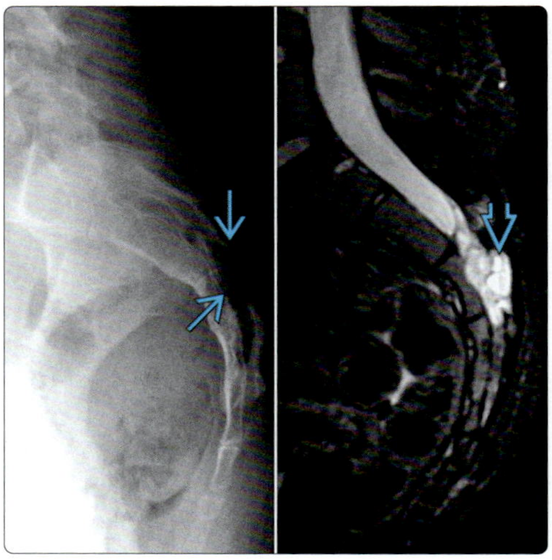

Osteoid Osteoma/Osteoblastoma

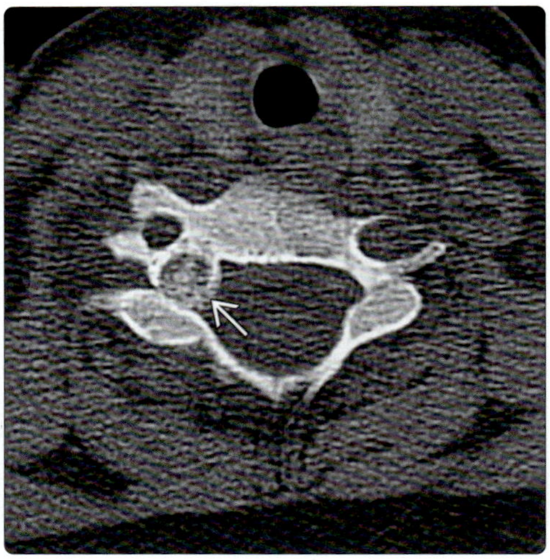

(Left) *Frontal radiograph in a 13 year old with back pain shows absence of a normal left pedicle at the L4 level. Note that normal pedicles are seen at the right L4 level as well as other levels bilaterally.* **(Right)** *Axial T1 C+ FS MR in the same patient shows an enhancing mass replacing the left L4 pedicle & extending into the vertebral body. Note the marked surrounding vertebral marrow & soft tissue edema. An osteoblastoma was confirmed at resection.*

Osteoid Osteoma/Osteoblastoma

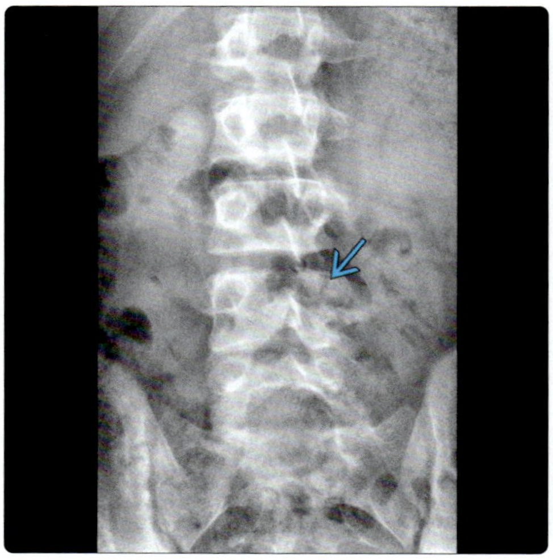

Osteoid Osteoma/Osteoblastoma

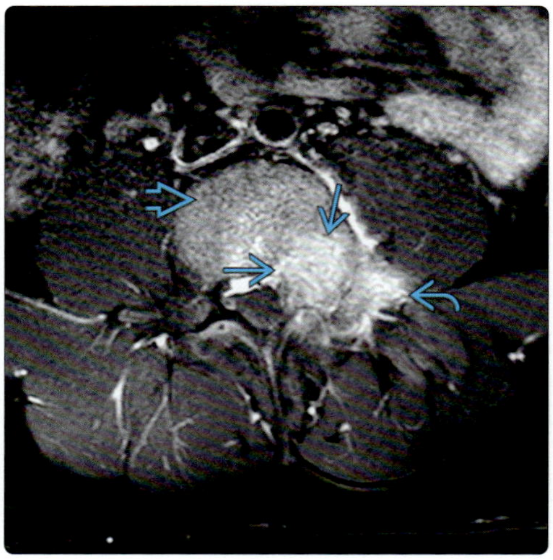

(Left) *Frontal radiograph in a 6 year old with back pain shows an abnormal appearance of the left L2 vertebral elements, including osteoporosis, flattening & broadening of the vertebral body, & expansion of the pedicle.* **(Right)** *Coronal T1 MR in the same patient shows a mass expanding & permeating the left L2 pedicle & extending into the adjacent soft tissues. This Ewing sarcoma extends through the marrow into the right L2 pedicle as well.*

Ewing Sarcoma

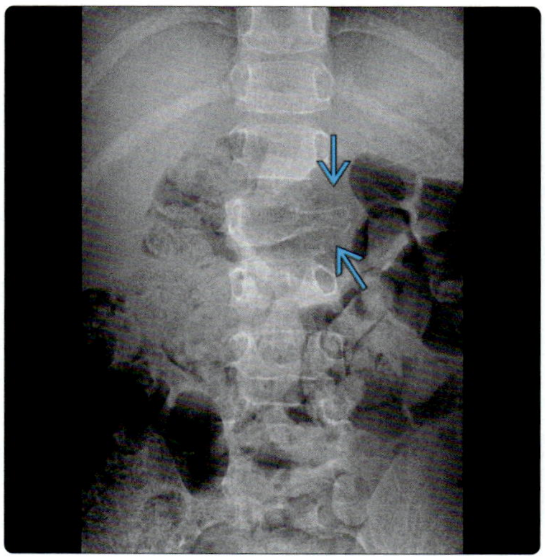

Ewing Sarcoma

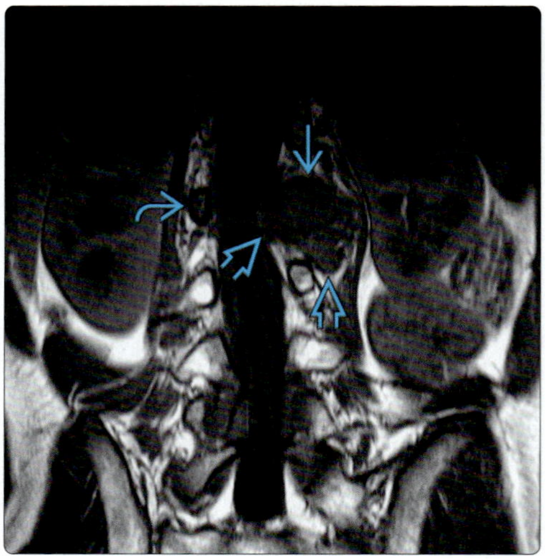

Leukemia/Lymphoma

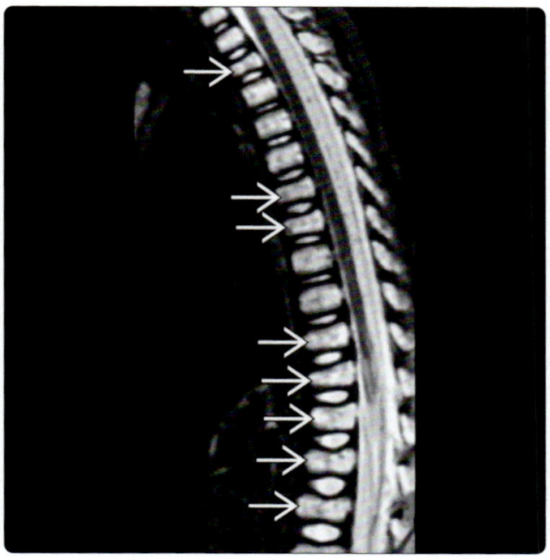

Hematogenous Metastases

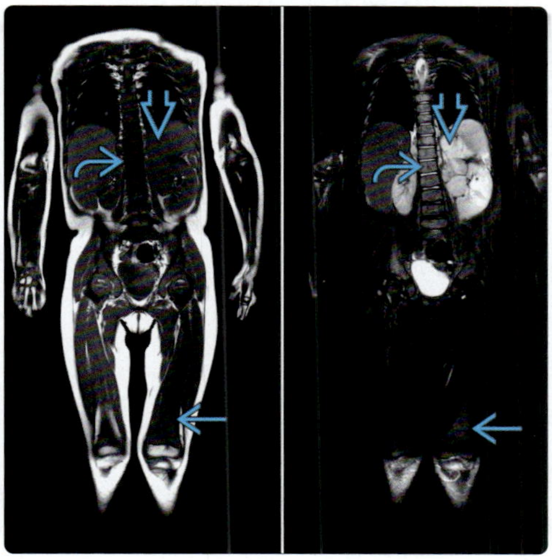

(Left) *Sagittal STIR MR in a patient with lymphoma reveals diffusely abnormal hyperintense marrow signal & numerous vertebral compression fractures.* **(Right)** *Coronal whole-body T1 (left) & STIR (right) MR images in a 3 year old with back pain & refusal to walk shows extensive marrow replacement (most pronounced in the left femoral metadiaphysis & vertebral bodies) due to a metastatic neuroblastoma.*

CNS Neoplasm

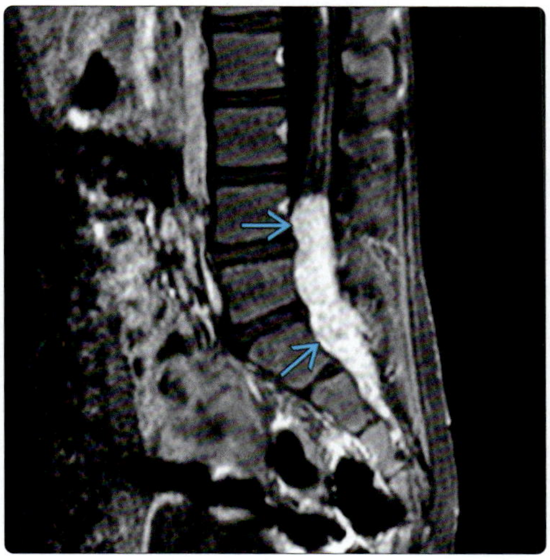

Guillain-Barré Syndrome

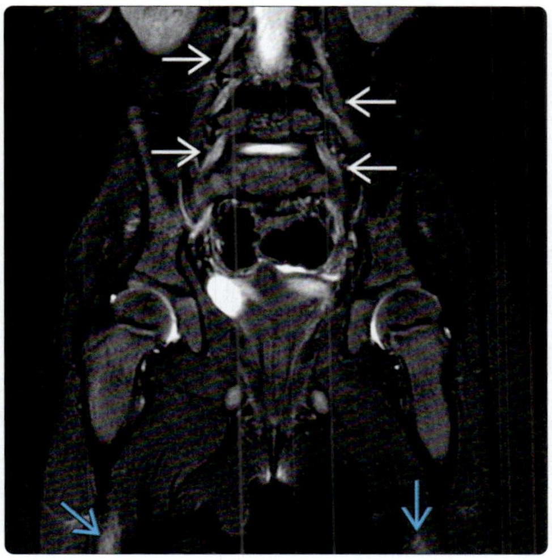

(Left) *Sagittal T1 C+ FS MR in an 8 year old with back pain for 1 year shows a homogeneously enhancing mass in the distal thecal sac. Biopsy confirmed a myxopapillary ependymoma, though drop metastases could appear similar.* **(Right)** *Coronal STIR MR in a 21 month old with hip & back pain + lower extremity areflexia shows enlargement & increased signal intensity of all nerve roots as well as the sciatic nerves. The lumbar puncture showed elevated protein, confirming Guillain-Barre syndrome.*

Transverse Myelitis

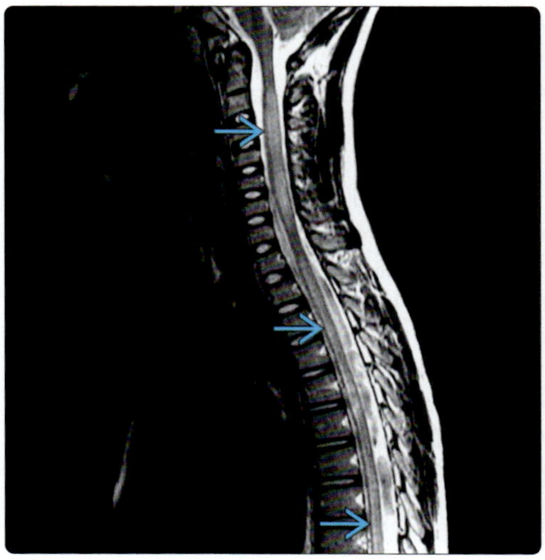

Tuberculous Osteomyelitis

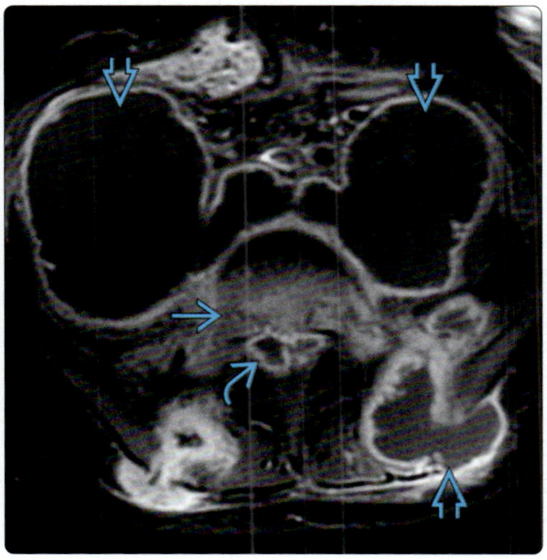

(Left) *Sagittal T2 MR in a 12 year old with lower extremity weakness, neck pain, difficulty walking, & urinary retention shows extensive abnormal signal throughout the central spinal cord with cervical cord expansion. Elevated protein & pleocytosis on the lumbar puncture confirmed transverse myelitis.* **(Right)** *Axial T1 C+ FS MR of the lumbar spine in a patient with known disseminated tuberculosis shows massive paraspinal abscesses with adjacent vertebral infection & an epidural abscess.*

DIFFERENTIAL DIAGNOSIS

Common

- Incomplete Fusion of Posterior Elements
- Myelomeningocele
- Lipomyelocele/Lipomyelomeningocele

Less Common

- Diastematomyelia
- Dorsal Dermal Sinus

Rare but Important

- Dorsal Spinal Meningocele
- Terminal Myelocystocele
- Segmental Spinal Dysgenesis

ESSENTIAL INFORMATION

Key Differential Diagnosis Issues

- Spina bifida: Incomplete closure of posterior bony elements
- Spina bifida aperta = spina bifida cystica: Protrusion of spinal canal elements through posterior bony defect
  - Simple meningocele: Dura & arachnoid, no neural elements; skin covered
  - Myelocele: Midline plaque of exposed neural tissue, flush with skin surface
  - Myelomeningocele (MMC): Myelocele protrudes beyond skin surface with expansion of subarachnoid space (SAS)
    - Bulging sac consists of neural placode (distal nonneurulated segment of cord) & arachnoid
    - Nerve roots extend back through sac to exit neural foramina
- Occult (closed) spinal dysraphism develops beneath intact skin surface
  - Meningocele, diastematomyelia, split notochord syndrome, dorsal dermal sinus, fibrolipoma of filum terminale, spinal lipoma, lipomyelocele (LM)/lipomyelomeningocele (LMM), lumbosacral hypogenesis, segmental spinal dysgenesis, myelocystocele

Helpful Clues for Common Diagnoses

- **Incomplete Fusion of Posterior Elements**
  - Spina bifida occulta is old terminology
  - Incomplete fusion of posterior elements is preferred
  - Usually asymptomatic
  - Occasionally associated with skin dimple on midline back
  - Imaging
    - Incomplete fusion of spinous process/lamina
    - No abnormal neural, dural, or lipomatous tissue within posterior osseous defect
  - Lumbosacral junction (L5 > S1) > > cervical (C1 > C7) > thoracic
- **Myelomeningocele**
  - Open neural tube defect, lacks skin covering
  - Level of dysraphism determines neurological deficit
  - In utero repair of MMC has lead to increasing use of preoperative fetal MR imaging
  - In absence of prenatal repair, preoperative postnatal MR imaging is rarely obtained (as MMC requires urgent repair due to risk of infection)
  - Postoperative spinal imaging is obtained with neurological decline despite adequate treatment of hydrocephalus or if neurologic exam suggests additional underlying lesions
  - Imaging
    - CSF sac & neural elements protrude through wide osseous dysraphism
    - Abnormal low-lying cord extends into defect
    - Postoperative: Neural placode inserts dorsally, deep to skin-covered postoperative repair
    - Associated abnormalities
      - Chiari 2 malformation (~ 100%), hydrocephalus; ± gray matter heterotopia
      - Kyphoscoliosis, segmentation anomalies, SCM, dorsal dermal sinus, syrinx, intraspinal dermoid/epidermoid, orthopedic abnormalities
- **Lipomyelocele/Lipomyelomeningocele**
  - Skin-covered spinal dysraphism
    - Neural placode of elongated spinal cord attaches to lipomatous mass
  - Cutaneous stigmata in up to 50%
    - Hemangioma, dimple, dermal sinus, skin tag, or hairy patch
  - Imaging
    - LM: Neural placode-lipoma complex is contiguous with subcutaneous fat through dysraphic defect, attaching to & tethering spinal cord
    - LMM: Thinned, elongated conus is tethered dorsally to lipoma
      - Tethered cord, SAS, & meninges extend dorsally through dysraphic posterior elements (LM + meningocele)
      - Spinal SAS expands ventrally
    - Dorsal & ventral nerve roots exit from ventral surface of placode
    - ± segmentation anomalies, sacral anomalies, syrinx, diastematomyelia, anorectal & genitourinary abnormalities

Helpful Clues for Less Common Diagnoses

- **Diastematomyelia**
  - a.k.a. split cord malformation (SCM)
  - Majority occur between T9 & S1
  - Most common cutaneous stigmata is "fawn's tail" patch of hair
  - Imaging
    - SCM: Sagittal division of spinal cord into 2 hemicords, each with 1 central canal, dorsal horn, & ventral horn
      - ± fibrous, osteocartilaginous, or osseous spur
      - Hemicords may be symmetric or asymmetric
    - Pang type 1 SCM: Separate dural sac & SAS around each hemicord, separated by fibrous/osseous spur
    - Pang type 2 SCM: Single dural sac & SAS without spur ± adherent fibrous bands tethering cord
    - Nearly all reunite below split
    - ± thick filum, tethered cord, or syringohydromyelia in 1 or both hemicords
      - Hemimyelomeningocele = 1 hemicord has MMC
    - ± intersegmental laminar fusion (pathognomonic for diastematomyelia)
    - ± other vertebral segmentation anomalies

- **Dorsal Dermal Sinus**
  - Sinus tract lined by stratified squamous epithelium; extends from skin surface toward spinal canal
  - Midline or rarely paramedian dimple or pinpoint ostium ± pigmented patch, hairy nevus, or cutaneous hemangioma
  - Differentiate from simple sacral dimple (< 2.5 cm from anus, no tract) & pilonidal sinus (low ostium, tract extends inferiorly toward coccyx & does not enter spine)
  - High suspicion for sinus if dimple lies above intergluteal fold
  - Imaging
    - Hypointense curvilinear tract through subcutaneous fat
    - Tract extends deep, for variable distance
      - May end in subcutaneous tissue, fascia/muscle, vertebra, epidural space, SAS, or, rarely, intramedullary within spinal cord
      - If extends into canal, may terminate in conus medullaris, SAS, filum terminale, nerve root, fibrous nodule on surface of cord, or dermoid/epidermoid
    - Dorsal dural "tenting" at point of dural penetration
    - Lumbosacral > occipital > thoracic > cervical spine
      - ± cord tethering in lumbosacral lesions
    - ± varying degrees of dysraphism, from incomplete posterior element fusion to multilevel dysraphism
    - ± dermoid/epidermoid (anywhere along tract), abscess, or arachnoiditis

Helpful Clues for Rare Diagnoses

- **Dorsal Spinal Meningocele**
  - Skin covered dysraphic defect
  - Usually neurologically normal
  - Lumbosacral junction, sacral > > cervical, thoracic
  - Imaging
    - CSF signal intensity dural sac protrudes through posterior dysraphic defect into subcutaneous fat
    - Cord tethering & syrinx are rare
    - ± filum terminale or nerve roots within defect
      - Simple: No neural tissue in sac
      - Complex: Neural tissue in sac
- **Terminal Myelocystocele**
  - Large skin-covered mass, usually sacral/coccygeal
  - Often associated with OEIS/cloacal exstrophy
  - Imaging
    - Hydromyelic low-lying tethered cord extends through osseous defect into meningocele sac & attaches to subcutaneous fat
    - Cyst-within-cyst appearance of distal cord dilated central canal surrounded by meningocele
    - Fluid in distal spinal cord does not communicate with surrounding SAS in meningocele sac
- **Segmental Spinal Dysgenesis**
  - Focal dysmorphic/hypoplastic vertebrae, meninges, & spinal cord with normal spine above & below
  - Imaging
    - Localized segmental lumbar or thoracolumbar vertebral & spinal cord dysgenesis or agenesis
    - Congenital acute angle kyphosis or kyphoscoliosis at level of dysplastic vertebrae
    - Thecal sac narrows & then terminates; spinal cord narrows & disappears rostral to thecal sac
      - Thecal sac reappears below dysplastic segments
      - Cord reappears below reappearance of thecal sac

SELECTED REFERENCES

1. Valeur NS et al: Cervicothoracic cystic dysraphism. Pediatr Radiol. 46(10):1471-81, 2016
2. Egloff A et al: Magnetic resonance imaging evaluation of fetal neural tube defects. Semin Ultrasound CT MR. 36(6):487-500, 2015
3. Schwartz ES et al: Congenital spine anomalies: the closed spinal dysraphisms. Pediatr Radiol. 45 Suppl 3:S413-9, 2015
4. Sewell MJ et al: Neural tube dysraphism: review of cutaneous markers and imaging. Pediatr Dermatol. 32(2):161-70, 2015
5. Kole MJ et al: Currarino syndrome and spinal dysraphism. J Neurosurg Pediatr. 13(6):685-9, 2014
6. Pang D et al: Terminal myelocystocele: surgical observations and theory of embryogenesis. Neurosurgery. 70(6):1383-404; discussion 1404-5, 2012

Incomplete Fusion of Posterior Elements

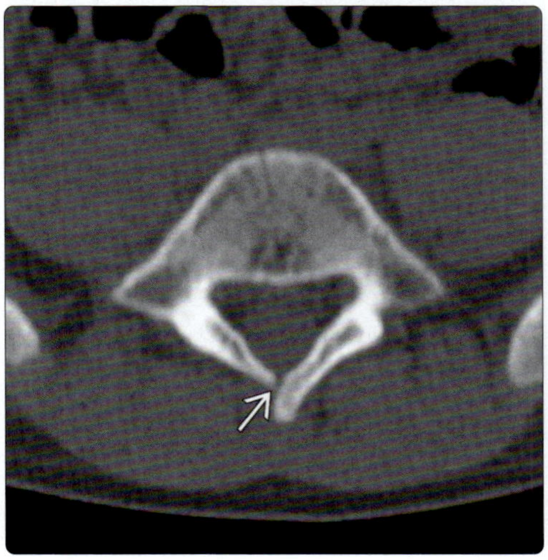

Myelomeningocele

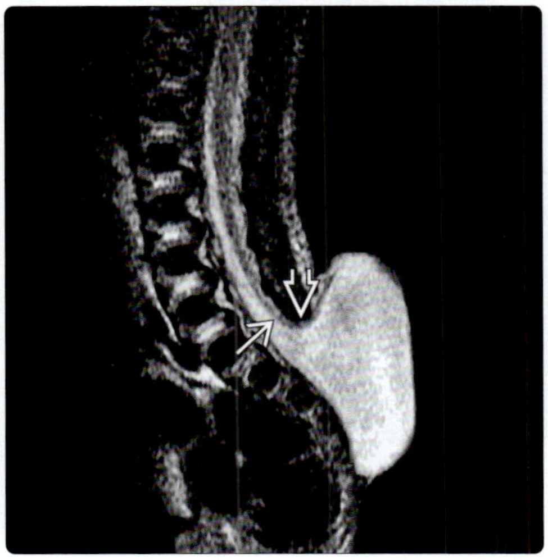

(Left) *Axial NECT in a 13 year old shows the typical appearance of an incidental asymptomatic incomplete midline fusion of the L5 spinous process ➡ (spina bifida occulta).* **(Right)** *Sagittal T2 MR shows an elongated spinal cord ➡ coursing through a dysraphic defect ➡ in the upper sacrum. The overlying CSF-filled sac wall represents the bulging neural placode & arachnoid, which are not covered by skin.*

(Left) *Sagittal SSFP MR in a 22-week fetus shows a bulging myelomeningocele (MMC) sac at the lumbosacral junction. Note the typical posterior fossa & craniocervical junction features of a Chiari 2 malformation.* **(Right)** *Sagittal T1 MR in a patient with a repaired lumbosacral MMC shows elongation of the spinal cord with the placode extending to the dorsal aspect of the widened thecal sac at the level of the dysraphism. Note also a small thoracic syrinx, not uncommon in these children.*

Myelomeningocele

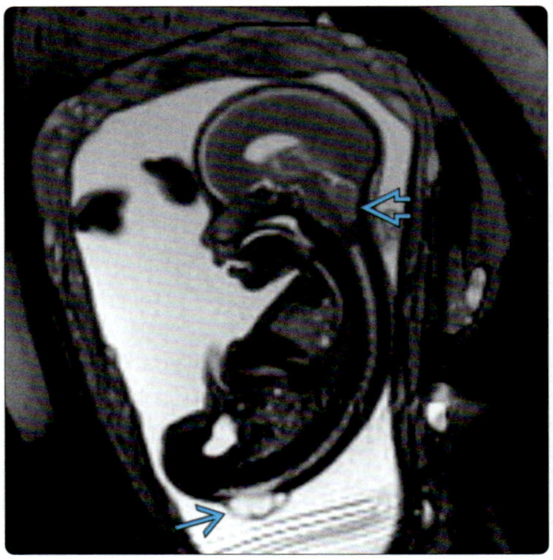

Myelomeningocele

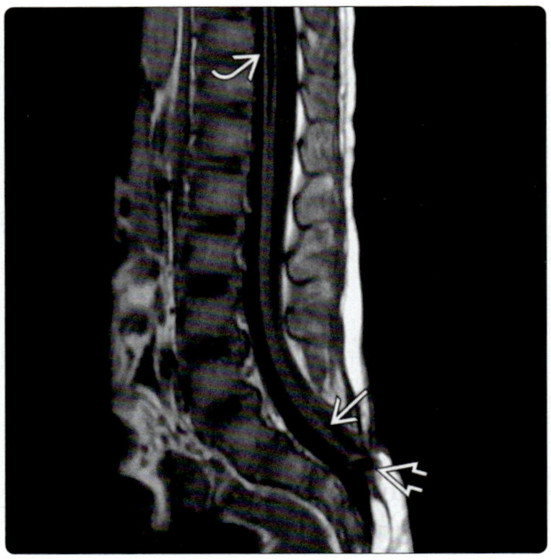

(Left) *Longitudinal US in a 10 day old with a sacral skin tag shows elongation of the spinal cord into an echogenic fatty mass, both of which blend with the subcutaneous fat through dorsal osteocartilaginous defects.* **(Right)** *Sagittal T1 MR of the same patient at 3 months of age shows the elongated spinal cord & hyperintense lipomatous mass. The mass blended with the subcutaneous fat through an osteocartilaginous defect on an adjacent image (not shown), consistent with lipomyelocele (LM).*

Lipomyelocele/Lipomyelomeningocele

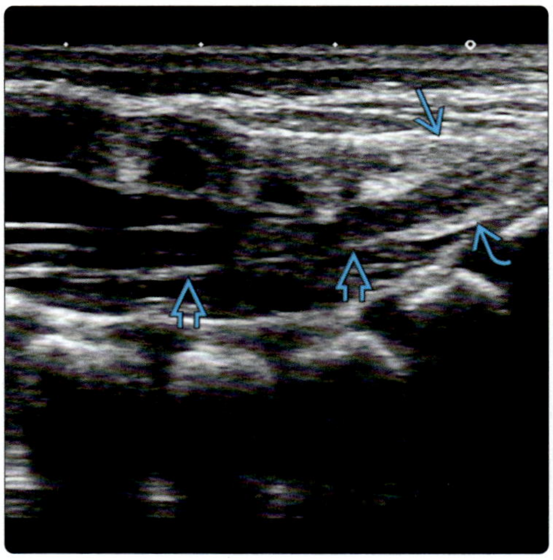

Lipomyelocele/Lipomyelomeningocele

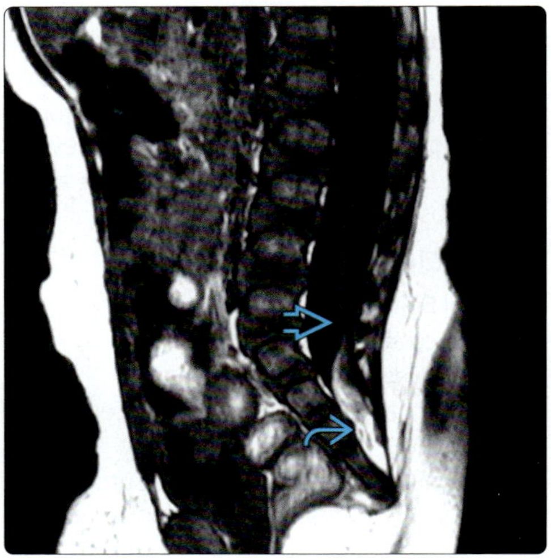

(Left) *Sagittal T1 MR in an infant shows a tethered cord & continuity of a placode/lipoma complex with the subcutaneous fat through an osseous defect. This LM shows no extension of CSF beyond the defect.* **(Right)** *Sagittal T1 MR shows a low-lying cord, neural elements, & an intraspinal lipoma extending through a lumbar dysraphic defect with a small CSF sac in the subcutaneous lipomatous mass, consistent with LMM. The intraspinal lipoma is continuous with subcutaneous fat.*

Lipomyelocele/Lipomyelomeningocele

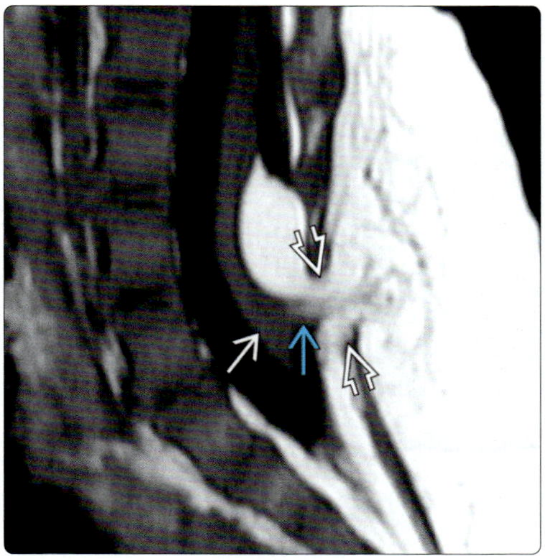

Lipomyelocele/Lipomyelomeningocele

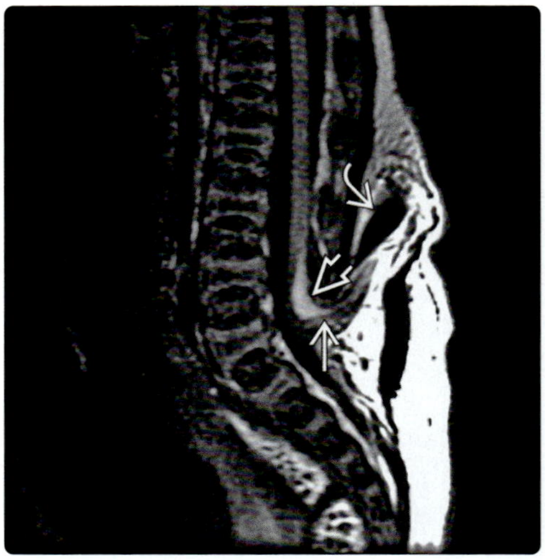

Diastematomyelia

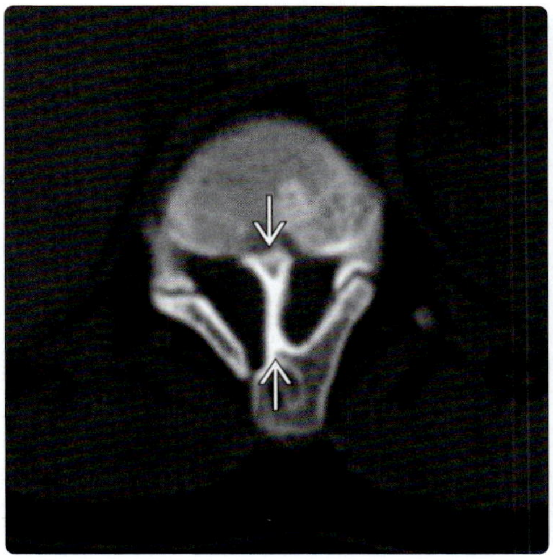

Diastematomyelia

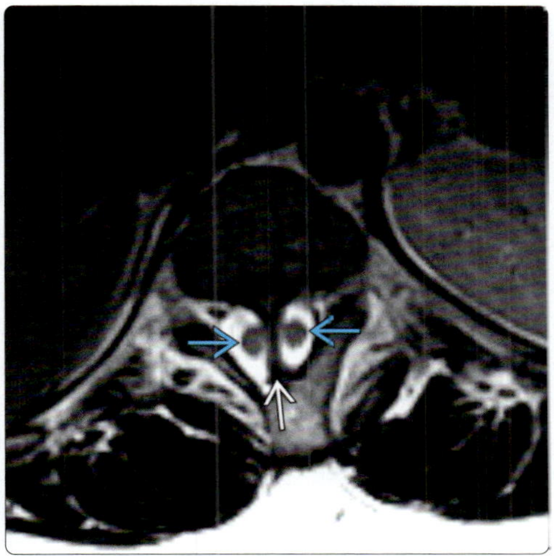

(Left) *Axial bone CT in a 12 year old with a limb discrepancy shows a bone spur dividing the spinal canal.* **(Right)** *Axial T2 MR in the same patient shows separation of the 2 relatively symmetric hemicords by the bone spur. Rarely, one of the hemicords may terminate as a hemimyelomeningocele with an open dysraphism of only 1/2 of the spinal canal.*

Dorsal Dermal Sinus

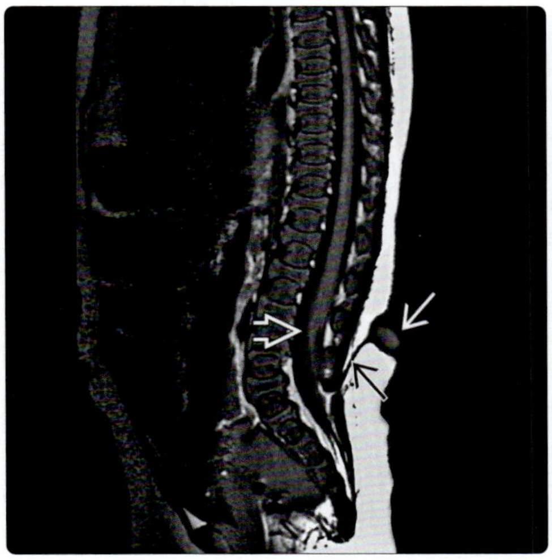

Dorsal Dermal Sinus

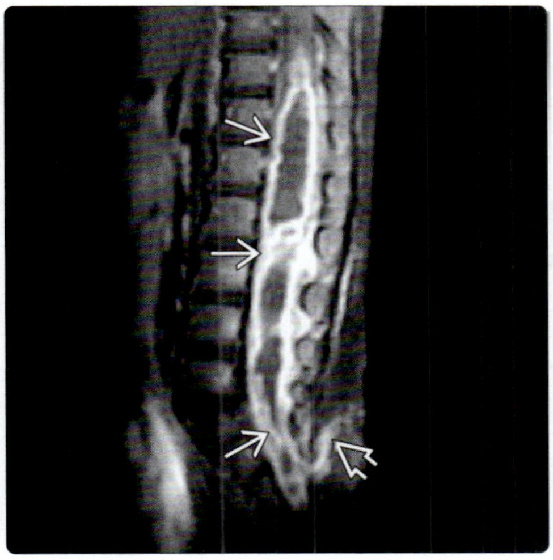

(Left) *Sagittal T1 MR shows a vitamin E capsule at the cutaneous opening of a dermal sinus. The dermal sinus traverses the subcutaneous fat & enters the dorsal canal at the LS junction. Note the associated low-lying spinal cord.* **(Right)** *Sagittal T1 C+ FS MR in a 1 year old with fever & urinary retention demonstrates a large intramedullary abscess within a tethered cord. Note the infected, enhancing dorsal dermal sinus extending through the subcutaneous fat to the dorsal aspect of the thecal sac.*

Dorsal Spinal Meningocele

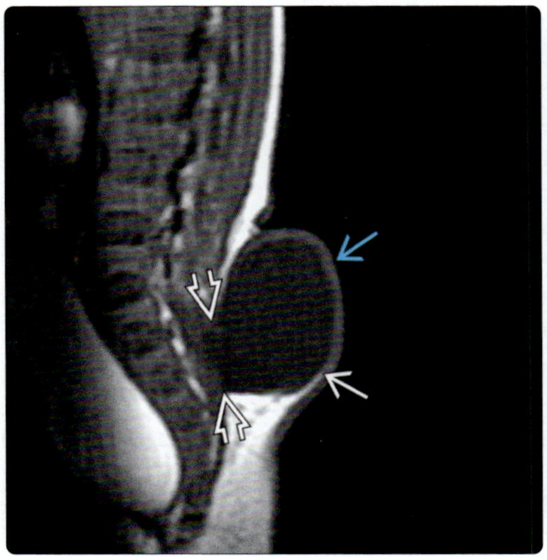

Terminal Myelocystocele

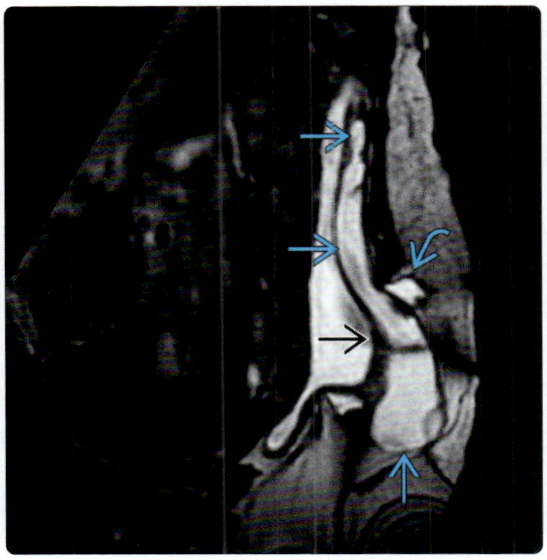

(Left) *Sagittal T1 MR in an infant shows a large CSF-filled meningocele protruding through a dorsal dysraphic defect without visible neural elements. Note the thickened sac wall, typical of a closed dysraphism (i.e., covered with skin).* **(Right)** *Sagittal 3D SSFP MR in a 3 week old with OEIS complex shows elongation of the spinal cord & meninges through a dorsal dysraphic defect. A large syrinx is present, & the meninges & neural elements are covered by fat & skin, typical of a terminal myelocystocele.*

Presacral or Sacrococcygeal Mass

DIFFERENTIAL DIAGNOSIS

Common

- Sacrococcygeal Teratoma
- Venolymphatic Malformation
- Myelomeningocele

Less Common

- Plexiform Neurofibroma
- Postoperative Changes (Mimic)
- Lymphoma
- Rhabdomyosarcoma
- Neuroblastoma
- Ewing Sarcoma

Rare but Important

- Presacral Abscess
- Osteosarcoma
- Other Extragonadal Germ Cell Tumors
- Anterior Sacral Meningocele
- Epidermoid Cysts
- Terminal Myelocystocele
- Enteric Cyst
- Tailgut Cyst
- Vascular Neoplasms
- Chordoma

ESSENTIAL INFORMATION

Key Differential Diagnosis Issues

- Age, exact location/extent, & cystic content are particularly helpful in focusing DDx
  - Perineal mass in newborn: Sacrococcygeal teratoma (SCT) > vascular malformation or neoplasm
  - Dorsal lumbosacral cyst in newborn: Myelomeningocele >> terminal myelocystocele
  - Invasive solid presacral mass from infancy up to adolescence: Neuroblastoma, germ cell tumors, soft tissue sarcomas
  - Preadolescence & beyond: Sarcomas (bone & soft tissue)
- Many presacral masses will present with pain, nerve-related symptoms of extremities, &/or bowel/bladder dysfunction
- Malignant neoplasms will typically restrict diffusion & show heterogeneous T2 signal/enhancement on MR
- Critical to assess mass relationships to bone, nerves, spinal canal, vessels, bowel, & bladder
- Currarino triad: Sacral anomaly, anorectal malformation, & presacral mass (teratoma, anterior meningocele or lipomyelomeningocele)

Helpful Clues for Common Diagnoses

- **Sacrococcygeal Teratoma**
  - Mixed solid & cystic presacral/perineal mass in newborn
  - Most commonly exophytic with variable internal (abdominopelvic) components
    - Purely internal lesions are more likely to be diagnosed after newborn period
      - Higher rate of malignancy if purely internal
    - ± spinal canal invasion &/or bowel/bladder obstruction
  - Very heterogeneous mass; may contain fat &/or Ca^{2+}
  - Often detected on 2nd trimester obstetric ultrasound
    - ↑ risk of fetal demise with
      - Solid/vascular SCT leading to hydrops
      - Large exophytic tumor leading to rupture
    - Rarely: Maternal mirror syndrome with preeclampsia
  - Majority (> 80%) are benign & cured with surgery
    - Coccyx must be resected to prevent recurrence
- **Venolymphatic Malformation**
  - Low-flow congenital error of vascular development
  - Generally grows commensurate with patient; rapid enlargement may occur with
    - Internal hemorrhage or infection
    - Periods of hormonal stimulation (e.g., puberty)
  - Infiltrating fluid signal intensity mass extending into multiple compartments
    - Clusters of cysts (lymphatics) &/or tubular foci (veins)
    - Both components often have
      - Fluid-fluid levels due to stagnant blood products
      - T1-hyperintense foci due to fat, hemorrhage/protein, or thrombi
    - Lymphatic components show
      - Discrete cysts with thin internal septations
      - Intermixed solid appearing microcystic foci
      - Enhancement of septations or microcystic foci
    - Venous components show
      - Sheet-like muscular infiltration
      - Round calcified phleboliths
      - Patchy, gradual enhancement
- **Myelomeningocele**
  - Most common open neural tube defect, typically in dorsal lumbosacral region
  - Abnormally elongated conus medullaris extends through posterior dysraphic elements
    - Bulging neural placode appears as thin-walled sac over skin/bone defect; size of sac is quite variable
    - Extent/location of dysraphism is quite variable
      - Involved levels predict neurologic deficits
  - Almost all result in intracranial Chiari 2 malformation

Helpful Clues for Less Common Diagnoses

- **Plexiform Neurofibroma**
  - Occurs in neurofibromatosis type 1 (NF1)
  - Lobulated T2/STIR-hyperintense lesions of nerves
    - Target appearance is classic for cross-section of lobule: T2-hypointense center that enhances
    - Extensive lesions: Rope-like or "bag of worms"
    - Patients usually have typical cutaneous & CNS lesions
- **Postoperative Changes (Mimic)**
  - Patients with prior surgery for anorectal malformations or Hirschsprung disease
  - Anterior displacement of rectum away from sacrum on lateral radiograph or contrast enema
    - Secondary to surgical intervention
- **Lymphoma**
  - Bulky relatively homogeneous nodal masses with frequent bowel & solid organ involvement
    - Multiple round solid renal masses in child older than 5 years are particularly suggestive
  - Often large &/or diffuse at diagnosis
- **Rhabdomyosarcoma**
  - Soft tissue malignancy with frequent bone invasion
  - May arise from GU or musculoskeletal systems

- Lobulated, solid, & heterogeneous
- **Neuroblastoma**
  - Malignant tumor arising from primitive neural crest cells of sympathetic chain
    - Paraspinal location is typical; < 5% arise in pelvis
  - Most common solid extracranial malignancy in children; median age of 15-17 months
  - Lobulated predominantly solid mass
    - Frequent Ca^{2+}; often engulfs vessels, invades spine
  - Typically produces catecholamines → MIBG avid
- **Ewing Sarcoma**
  - Classically occurs from ages 5-25 years
  - More frequently arises from other pelvic bones
  - May permeate/expand entire bone with osteoporosis, lysis, & aggressive periosteal reaction
  - Associated soft tissue mass is often quite large

Helpful Clues for Rare Diagnoses

- **Presacral Abscess**
  - Fever with elevation of serum inflammatory markers
  - Secondary to vertebral osteomyelitis/discitis, perirectal abscess from inflammatory bowel disease, or iatrogenic
  - Fluid (± gas) collection with irregular rim enhancement
    - Adjacent bones or colon may be abnormal
- **Osteosarcoma**
  - Aggressive lesion occurring around adolescence
  - Osteoid matrix essentially confirms diagnosis
- **Other Extragonadal Germ Cell Tumors**
  - Yolk sac tumors: ↑ α-fetoprotein
  - Choriocarcinoma: ↑ β-human chorionic gonadotropin
  - Others: Mixed, embryonal carcinoma, germinoma
  - Frequently invade spine & bone
- **Anterior Sacral Meningocele**
  - Cyst continuity with thecal sac through enlarged neural foramen or sacral defect is diagnostic
  - Follows CSF signal on all sequences
    - Fatty component continuous into spinal canal to elongated cord suggests lipomyelocele/lipomyelomeningocele
- **Epidermoid Cysts**
  - Consider congenital dermal sinus tract or prior intervention at site
  - Contains fat &/or squamous debris
  - Diffusion restriction is common
- **Terminal Myelocystocele**
  - Closed neural tube defect (skin covered)
  - Elongated spinal cord extends through dorsal dysraphism into cyst within cyst appearance
    - Distal dilation of central canal extending into dilated subarachnoid space (meningocele)
  - High association with OEIS/cloacal exstrophy
  - Rarely results in Chiari 2 intracranial findings
- **Enteric Duplication Cyst**
  - < 5% of GI duplication cysts are retrorectal
  - May be tubular or round; ± communication with bowel
  - "Gut signature" of wall on ultrasound
- **Tailgut Cyst**
  - a.k.a. retrorectal hamartoma
  - Nonspecific small cystic lesion
- **Vascular Neoplasms**
  - Infantile & congenital hemangiomas are common but not in sacral region
    - Look for LUMBAR syndrome: Anomalies of arteries, anus/rectum, GU tract, spine
  - Kaposiform hemangioendothelioma rarely occurs here
    - Associated with Kasabach-Merritt coagulopathy
  - Look for avid enhancement, ↑ vascularity
- **Chordoma**
  - Malignant tumor of notochordal remnant
  - Much more common at skull base in children (vs. adults)
  - May present with skin ulceration
  - Lobulated very high T2 signal mass destroying & extending out of sacrum
    - Numerous internal hypointense septations
    - Variable enhancement

SELECTED REFERENCES

1. AbouZeid AA et al: The Currarino triad: what pediatric surgeons need to know. J Pediatr Surg. 52(8):1260-8, 2017

Sacrococcygeal Teratoma

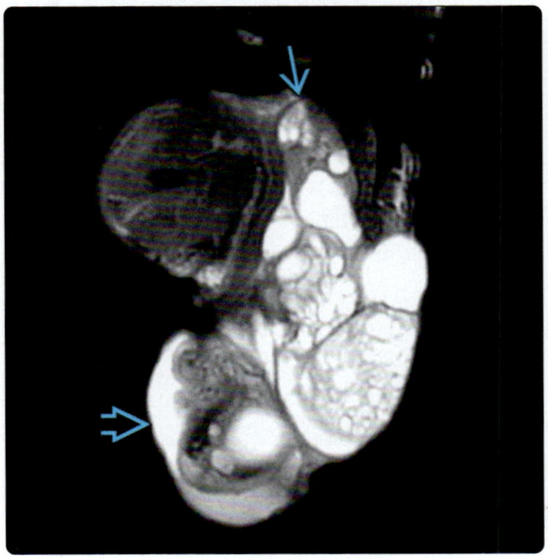

Sacrococcygeal Teratoma

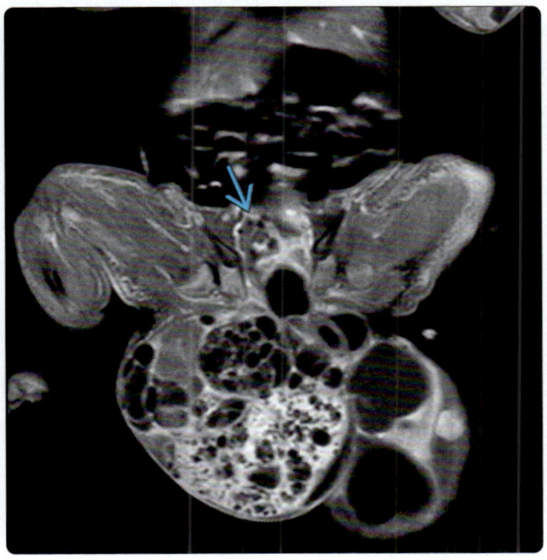

(Left) *Sagittal T2 FS MR in a newborn with a prenatally detected sacrococcygeal teratoma (SCT) shows a mixed cystic & solid mass with large presacral* ➡ *& exophytic* ➾ *components. There is no intraspinal extension.* **(Right)** *Coronal T1 C+ FS MR in the same patient shows heterogeneous enhancement of the mixed cystic & solid mass with moderate intrapelvic extension* ➡ *of this lesion. Immature components were found at resection.*

Sacrococcygeal Teratoma

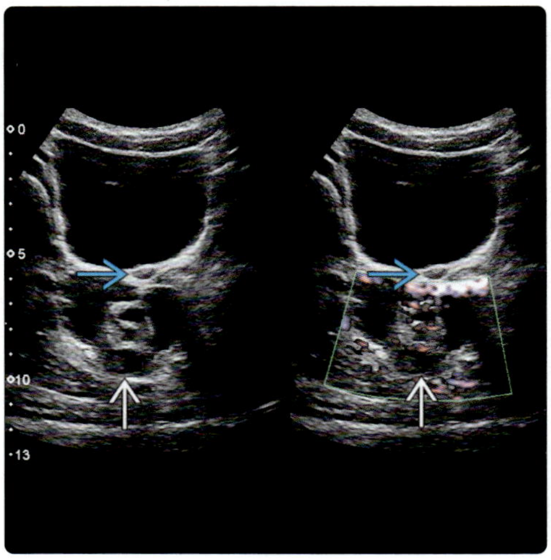

Sacrococcygeal Teratoma

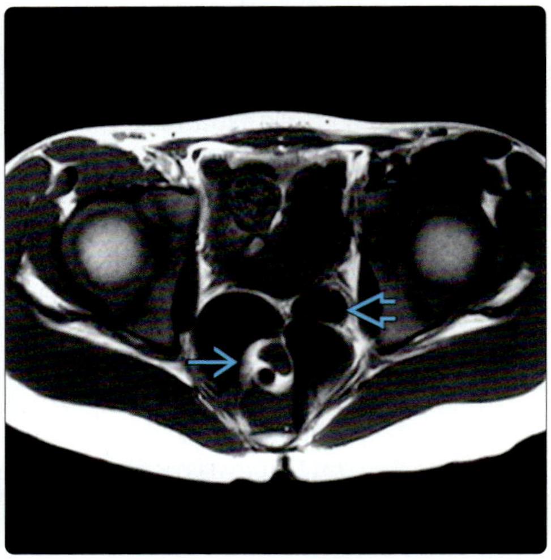

(Left) *Transverse grayscale & color Doppler ultrasound images in a 6-year-old girl show a mixed cystic & solid mass ➡ posterior to the urinary bladder & uterus ⇨. **(Right)** Axial T1 MR in the same patient shows fat ⇨ within the solid components of the mostly cystic mass. The rectum is displaced anteriorly ⇨. A mature cystic teratoma was confirmed upon resection. Completely internal teratomas (as seen here) are more likely to present beyond infancy & have malignant components.*

Venolymphatic Malformation

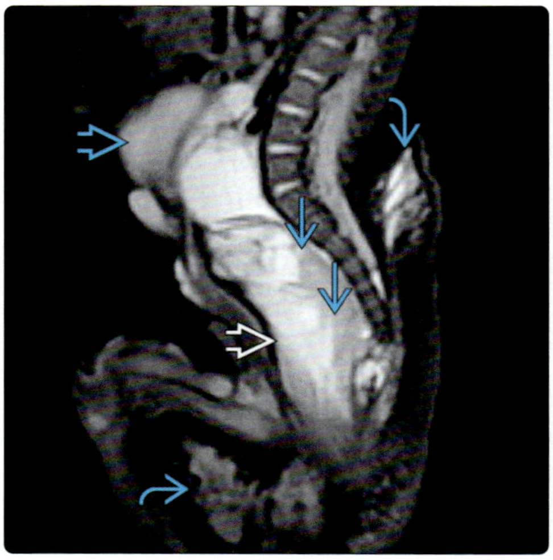

Venolymphatic Malformation

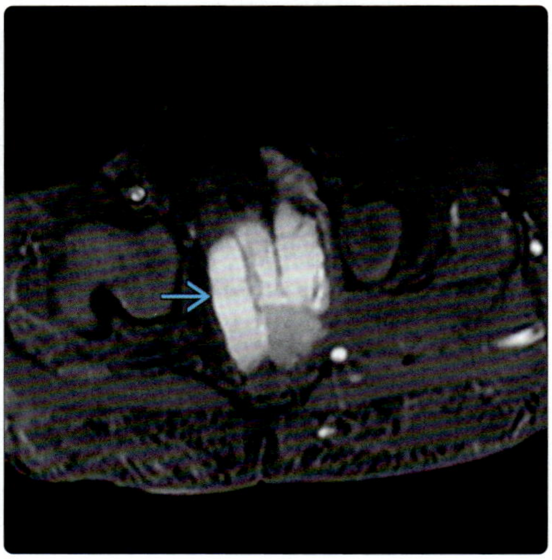

(Left) *Sagittal STIR MR in a 3 month old with a large capillary-venolymphatic malformation shows numerous cystic foci involving the presacral ➡, mesenteric ⇨, & superficial ⇨ soft tissues. Many fluid-fluid levels are noted ⇨ in the lesion. These findings are typical of a low-flow vascular malformation.* **(Right)** *Axial T1 FS MR in the same patient shows T1 shortening throughout much of the lesion ⇨ due to internal hemorrhage &/or proteinaceous content.*

Myelomeningocele

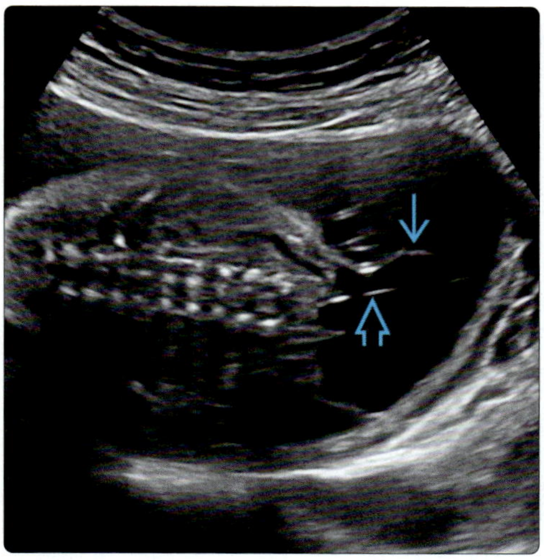

Plexiform Neurofibroma

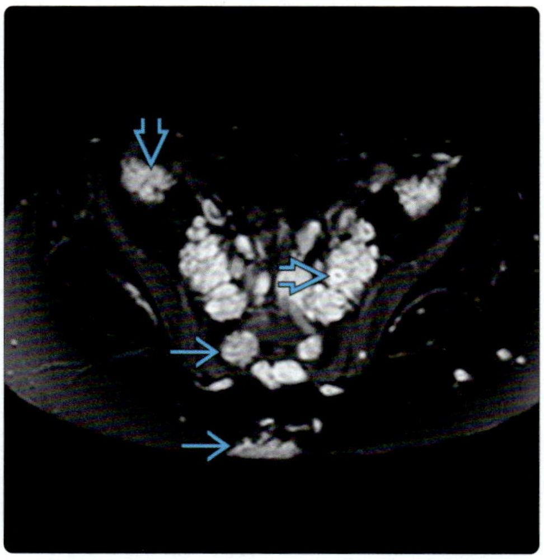

(Left) *Coronal ultrasound in a 22-week fetus shows a large thin-walled cystic lesion ⇨ emanating from a sacral spinal dysraphism & containing neural elements ⇨, consistent with a myelomeningocele.* **(Right)** *Axial T2 FS MR in a 9 year old with neurofibromatosis type 1 shows typical lobulated fluid signal intensity masses along the course of many superficial & deep nerves ⇨. In cross section, many of these lesions show the classic target sign of plexiform neurofibromas with a hypointense center ⇨.*

Postoperative Changes (Mimic)

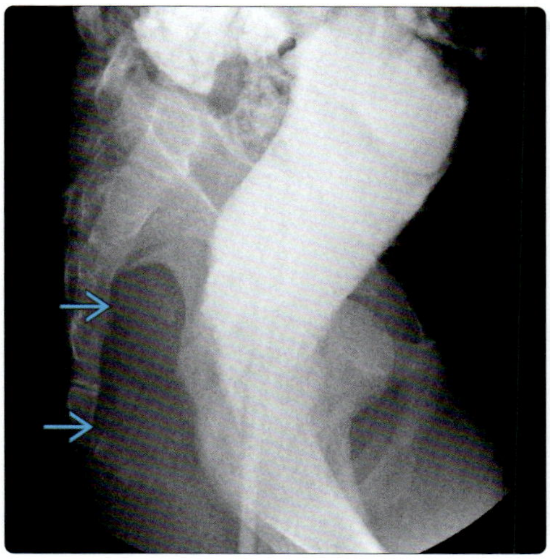

Lymphoma

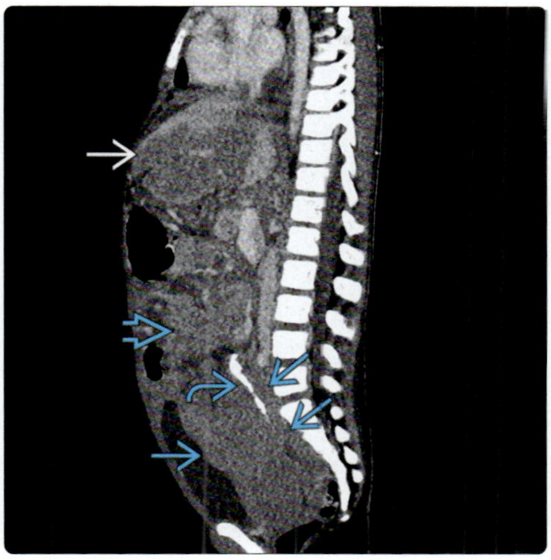

(Left) *Lateral contrast enema in a 14 year old with a remote history of a posterior sagittal anorectoplasty (PSARP) for an anorectal malformation shows postsurgical thickening of the presacral soft tissues, displacing the rectum anteriorly.* **(Right)** *Sagittal CECT in a 7 year old with pain & abdominal distention shows numerous homogeneous soft tissue masses infiltrating the pelvic & mesenteric tissues as well as the liver. Note the narrowing of the contrast-filled rectum. Burkitt lymphoma was found upon biopsy.*

Rhabdomyosarcoma

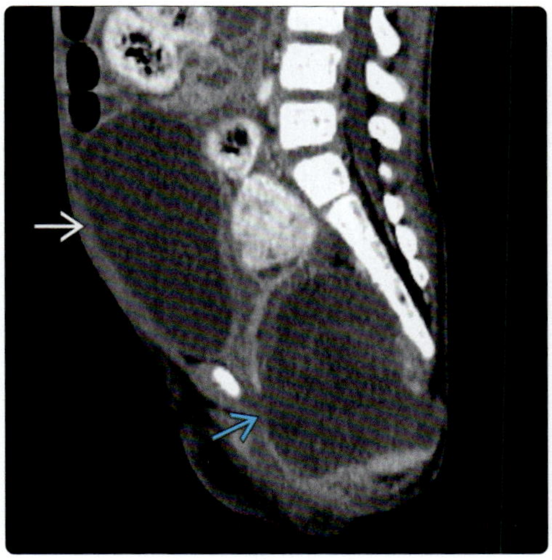

Rhabdomyosarcoma

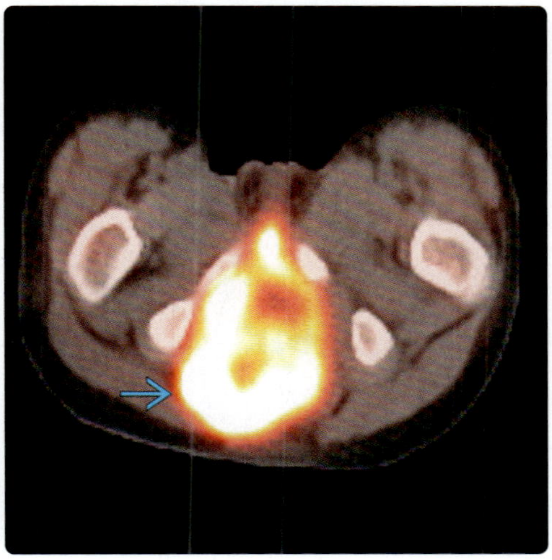

(Left) *Sagittal CECT in a 5 year old with urinary retention shows elevation of the bladder by a heterogeneous presacral mass.* **(Right)** *Axial FDG PET CT in the same patient shows increased metabolic activity in the mass. Embryonal rhabdomyosarcoma was found upon biopsy. Note that rhabdomyosarcoma in the pelvis may arise from the soft tissues or genitourinary organs.*

Neuroblastoma

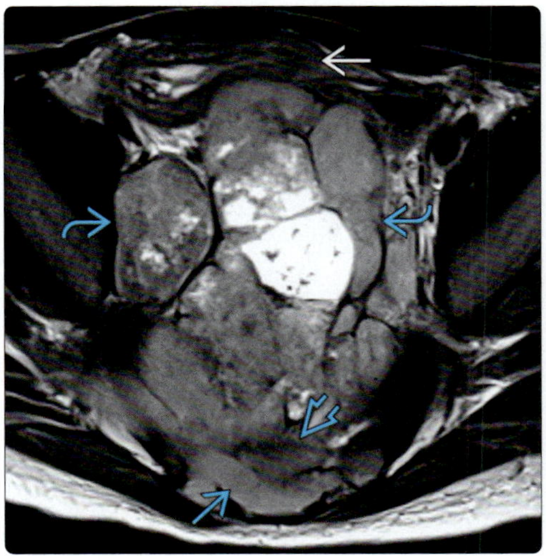

Neuroblastoma

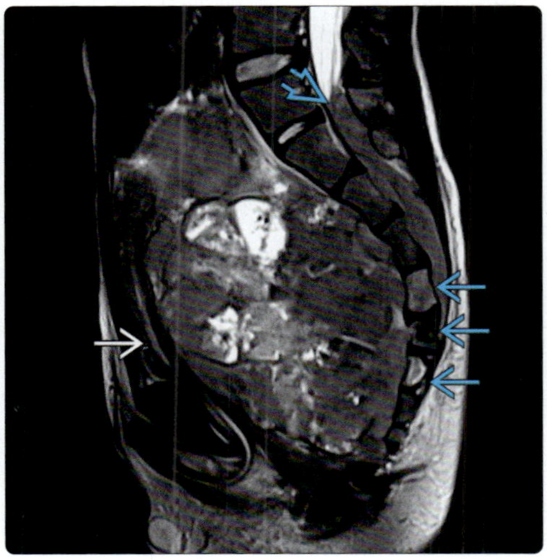

(Left) *Axial T2 MR in a 7 year old with back pain, constipation, & urinary retention shows a large lobulated cystic & solid mass of the presacral soft tissues. There is invasion of the sacrum & neural foramina. The urinary bladder is displaced anteriorly.* **(Right)** *Sagittal T2 MR in the same patient shows the large mass displacing the urinary bladder & invading the sacrum & spinal canal.*

(Left) *Sagittal CECT in a 4 year old with fever status post reoperation for Hirschsprung disease shows a rim-enhancing gas & fluid collection displacing the residual distal colon anteriorly. The findings are consistent with a presacral abscess.* **(Right)** *Axial T1 C+ FS MR in a 16 year old with right sciatica shows a destructive heterogeneous mass arising from the right sacrum. Osteosarcoma was found upon biopsy.*

Presacral Abscess

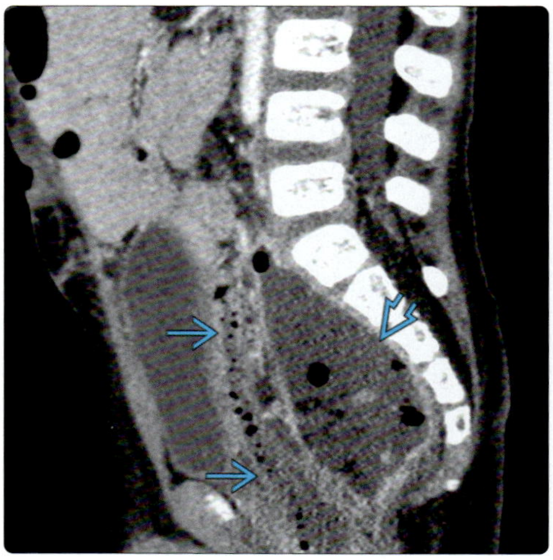

Osteosarcoma

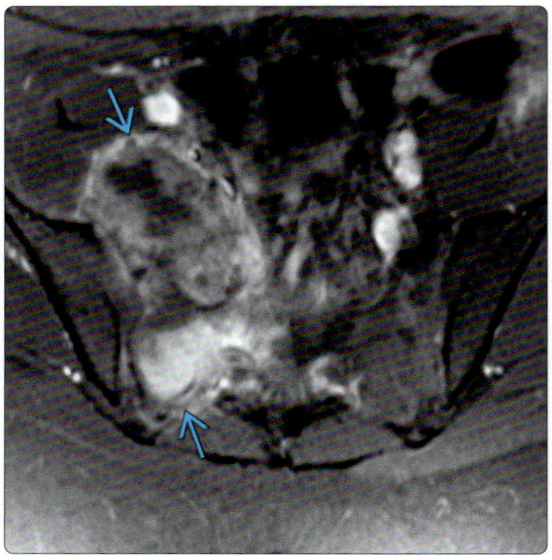

(Left) *AP radiograph in a 3 year old with a limp & right leg atrophy shows a large pelvic soft tissue mass displacing bowel. There is a vertebra plana appearance of the L4 & L5 vertebral bodies.* **(Right)** *Sagittal T1 (left) & T1 C+ FS (right) MR images in the same patient show L4 & L5 vertebra plana secondary to invasion by an adjacent soft tissue mass. Intraspinal extension is also noted. A yolk sac tumor was found at biopsy.*

Other Extragonadal Germ Cell Tumors

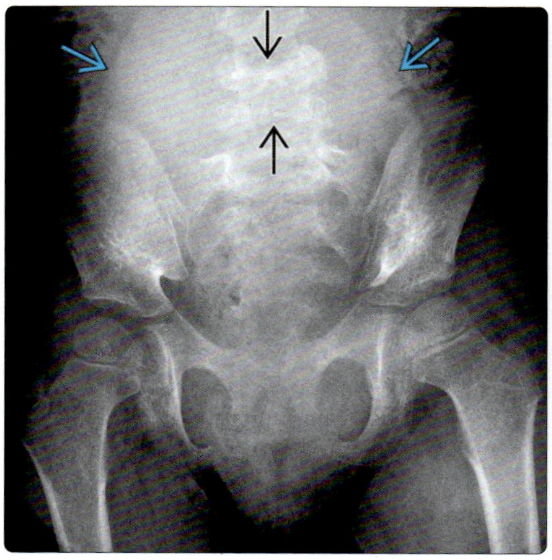

Other Extragonadal Germ Cell Tumors

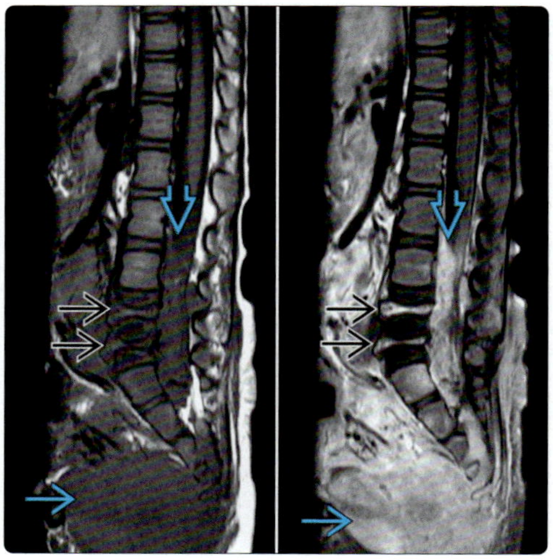

(Left) *Coronal STIR MR in the same patient shows the presacral yolk sac tumor with pathologic fractures of L4 & L5 as well as multiple liver metastases.* **(Right)** *Sagittal T2 FS MR in a 6-year-old girl with a history of an anorectal malformation shows a fluid-filled cystic lesion bulging anteriorly through an abnormal sacrum. The cyst communicates with the thecal sac, consistent with an anterior meningocele in the Currarino triad.*

Other Extragonadal Germ Cell Tumors

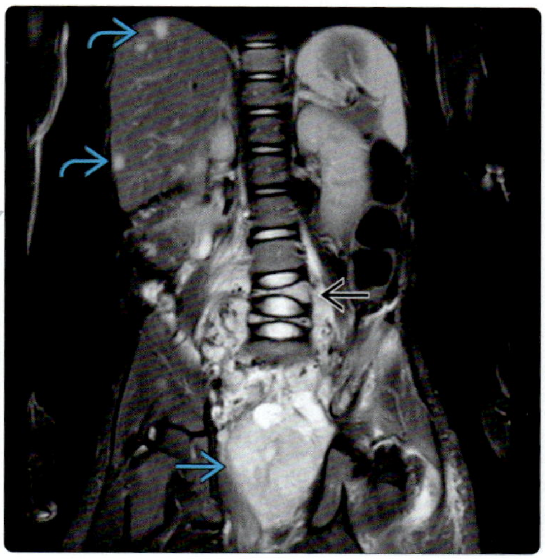

Anterior Sacral Meningocele

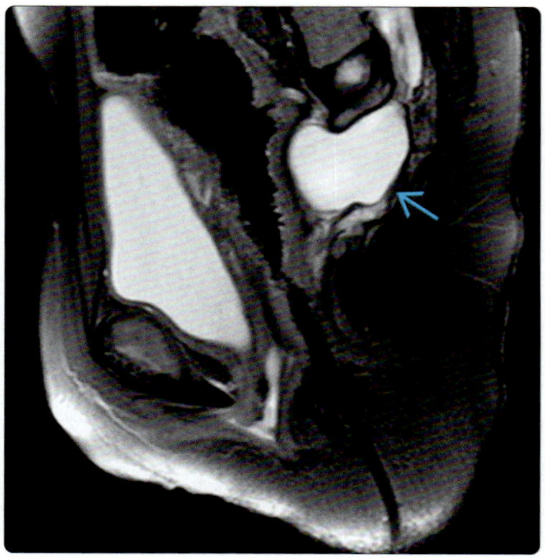

Anterior Sacral Meningocele

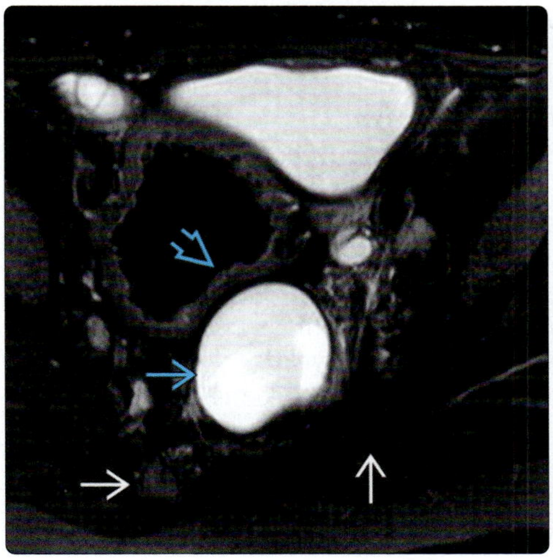

Epidermoid Cysts

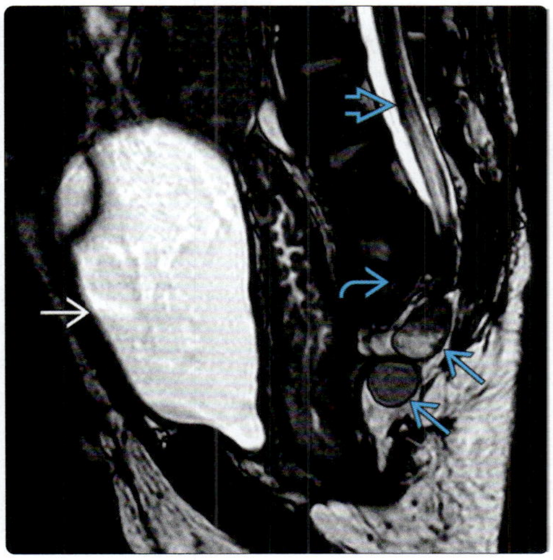

(Left) *Axial T2 FS MR in the same patient shows mass effect on the rectum by the anterior meningocele. Note the inferior portions of the bifid sacrum.* **(Right)** *Sagittal 3D bSSFP MR in a 1 year old shows sacral agenesis with elongation of the spinal cord toward the osseous defect. Several small masses are seen inferior to the sacrum. Note the towering configuration of the neurogenic bladder.*

Epidermoid Cysts

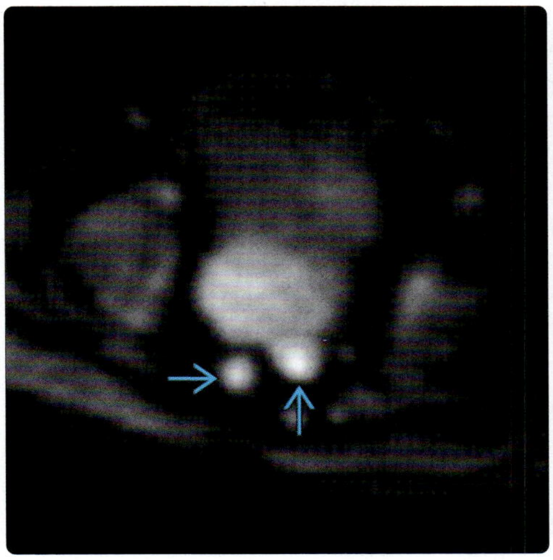

Terminal Myelocystocele

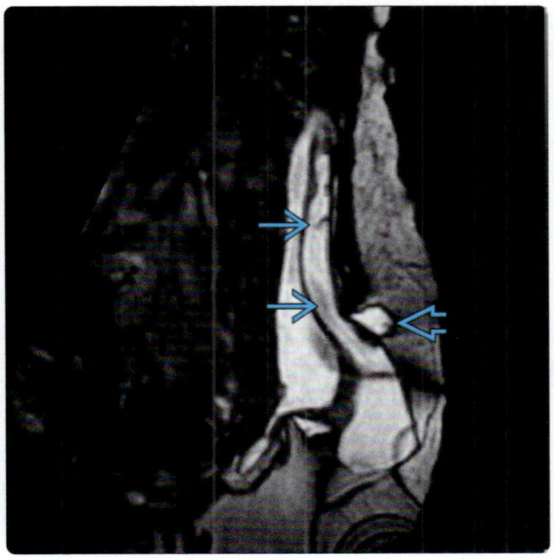

(Left) *Axial DWI MR in the same patient shows restricted diffusion (confirmed on the ADC map) within these lesions, typical of dermoid/epidermoid cysts (which were proven at resection).* **(Right)** *Sagittal 3D bSSFP MR in a 3-month-old infant with OEIS (omphalocele, cloacal exstrophy, imperforate anus, & spinal anomalies) shows the classic associated closed spinal dysraphism of a terminal myelocystocele with the dilated central canal extending into a bulging skin-covered sac.*

Tailgut Cyst

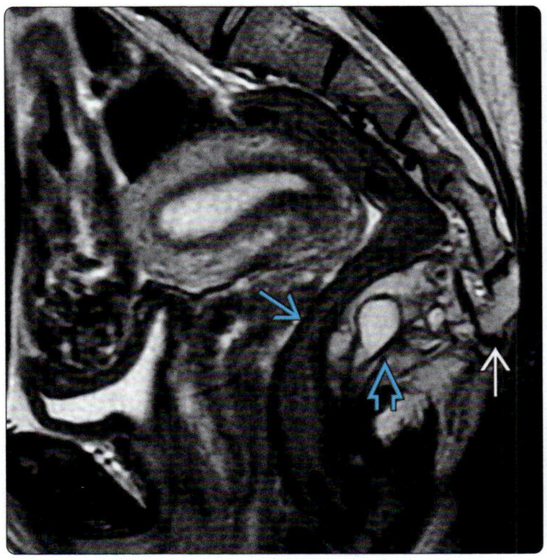

Tailgut Cyst

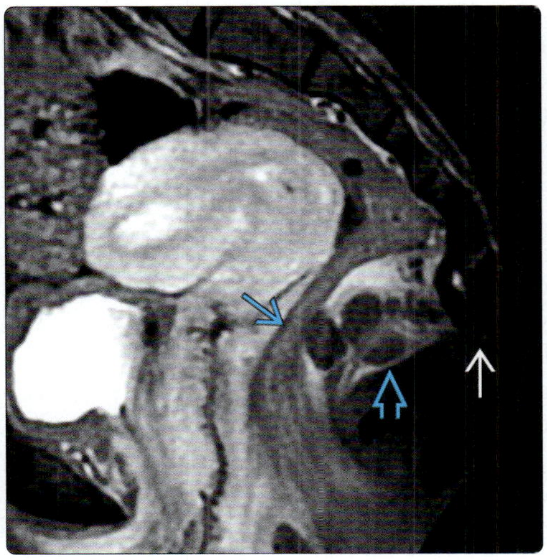

(Left) *Sagittal T2 MR in a 19 year old with pelvic pain shows a multicystic mass between the rectum & a dysplastic coccyx.* **(Right)** *Sagittal T1 C+ FS MR in the same patient shows enhancement of the cyst margins in the lesion that extends between the dysplastic coccyx & the compressed rectum. A tailgut cyst was found upon resection. These cysts are often much smaller & incidental.*

Intramedullary Spinal Cord Lesion

DIFFERENTIAL DIAGNOSIS

Common

- Syrinx
- Acute Disseminated Encephalomyelitis
- Idiopathic Acute Transverse Myelitis
- Acute Transverse Myelopathy

Less Common

- Contusion/Hematoma
- Multiple Sclerosis
- Astrocytoma
- Ependymoma

Rare but Important

- Abscess
- Dermoid & Epidermoid Tumors
- Cavernous Malformation
- Spinal Cord Infarction
- Hemangioblastoma

ESSENTIAL INFORMATION

Key Differential Diagnosis Issues

- Tumor vs. demyelinating disease
  - Tumors tend to be ovoid in shape & enlarge cord; ± cysts
  - Demyelinating disease tends to be flame-shaped white matter (WM) lesion(s) without cord enlargement or cyst
  - Differentiation may require follow-up
- Adult vs. pediatric spinal cord tumors
  - Intramedullary tumors tend to be more rostral in children: 50% are cervical or cervicothoracic in children
  - Astrocytoma is most common cord tumor in children; ependymoma is most common cord tumor in adults
- Hemorrhagic foci: Contusion, ependymoma, cavernoma, hemangioblastoma

Helpful Clues for Common Diagnoses

- **Syrinx**
  - Hydromyelia: Cystic central canal
    - Syringomyelia: Cystic cord cavity, not contiguous with central canal
    - Syringohydromyelia: Features of both syringomyelia & hydromyelia
    - Syringobulbia: Brainstem syrinx extension
    - "Presyrinx state": Reversible spinal cord edema secondary to altered CSF flow dynamics
  - Imaging findings
    - Expanded cord + nonenhancing, elongated central cyst or dilated central canal
    - Tubular, beaded, or sacculated in morphology
    - ± widened spinal canal, vertebral scalloping
    - ± hydrocephalus, Chiari 1, Chiari 2, dysraphism, tethered cord, or scoliosis
    - ± adjacent gliosis or myelomalacia
    - Contrast is not required (to rule out tumor) if there is
      - Known predisposing cause (e.g., Chiari 1)
      - No solid nodular component
      - No surrounding cord signal abnormality
- **Acute Disseminated Encephalomyelitis**
  - Typically, monophasic, self-limited, para-/postinfectious immune-mediated inflammatory disorder of WM
    - Antibodies to pathogens exhibit cross immunoreactivity with myelin basic protein
    - Brain > spinal cord involvement
  - Imaging findings
    - Increased T2 signal ± enhancement
    - Flame-shaped lesions with slight cord swelling
    - May see gray matter involvement
    - Almost always associated with brain lesions in deep cerebral hemispheres, subcortical WM, basal ganglia, thalamus, brainstem, &/or cerebellum
- **Idiopathic Acute Transverse Myelitis**
  - Autoimmune phenomenon with formation of antigen-antibody complexes
    - Small vessel vasculopathy, cord ischemia, demyelinating process
  - Imaging findings
    - Normal in up to 50%
    - Increased T2 signal with variable enhancement
    - Mild fusiform cord enlargement in acute phase; cord atrophy in late stage
    - Usually central, > 2/3 cross-sectional area of cord
    - ≥ 2 vertebral segments in length, usually 3-4 segments
    - Lacks associated intracranial lesions
    - Variable enhancement: Absent in up to 50% cases
- **Acute Transverse Myelopathy**
  - Secondary to collagen vascular disease, viral infection, post vaccination or post irradiation, paraneoplastic syndrome, or chronic ischemia/venous stasis from AVM
  - Imaging findings: Same as idiopathic acute transverse myelitis

Helpful Clues for Less Common Diagnoses

- **Contusion/Hematoma**
  - Traumatic axonal injury, cord edema, &/or hemorrhage
    - In children, high-velocity mechanism most common
  - Imaging findings
    - Acute: Edema or hematoma, cord swelling
    - Transection: Best identified on T1 MR
    - Chronic: Gliosis, atrophy ± cyst, syringomyelia, hemosiderin scar
    - ± fracture, subluxation, ligamentous injuries, traumatic disc herniation
- **Multiple Sclerosis**
  - Multiphasic demyelinating disease of CNS
  - Imaging findings
    - Increased T2 signal ± patchy or confluent enhancement during acute or subacute phase
    - Multiple lesions showing variable enhancement
    - Cervical cord is most common site
    - Usually < 2 vertebral segments in length; < 1/2 cross-sectional area of spinal cord
    - Wedge-shaped on axial MR with apex directed centrally
    - Cord enlargement is uncommon
    - Majority of patients have associated brain lesions: Periventricular, callosal, brainstem, or cerebellar WM
- **Astrocytoma**
  - Most common spinal cord tumor in children (60%)
    - Tumor margins often extend beyond enhancement

- Majority are pilocytic (WHO grade I) or fibrillary (grade II); 10-15% are anaplastic (grade III)
- Cervical > thoracic > lumbar
- Imaging findings
  - Fusiform enlargement of cord with infiltrative margins of T2 hyperintensity
  - Mild to moderate enhancement
  - More eccentric & less enhancing than ependymomas
  - Peritumoral cysts in up to 40%
    - Fluid is slightly T1 hyperintense to CSF
  - ± expansion of canal, scoliosis
- **Ependymoma**
  - 2nd most common cord tumor in children (30%)
  - Imaging findings
    - Heterogeneous expansile mass with heterogeneous enhancement
    - Circumscribed, usually centrally located in cord
      - Tumor margin usually equals margin of enhancement
    - Hemorrhagic foci are common in or at margins
      - Hemosiderin (cap sign) at superior & inferior borders in 20%
    - Peritumoral cysts in up to 80%
    - ± widened canal, scoliosis, scalloping

Helpful Clues for Rare Diagnoses

- **Abscess**
  - Typically occurs as direct extension from dysraphism in children; idiopathic or hematogenous spread in adults
  - Imaging findings
    - Irregular ring enhancement + cord expansion; ± restricted diffusion
    - Abscess arising from dysraphism usually shows soft tissue inflammation
- **Dermoid & Epidermoid Tumors**
  - Benign tumor
    - Intramedullary (40%), extramedullary (60%), extradural (rare)
    - From cells that produce skin, hair follicles, sweat, & sebaceous glands
  - Imaging findings
    - Similar to CSF on T1 & T2 MR; ± T1-hyperintense fat in dermoid
    - Epidermoid may be hyperintense on DWI, slightly hyperintense on FLAIR
    - ± mild ring enhancement
    - Suspect infection with abundant enhancement
- **Cavernous Malformation**
  - 3-5% occur in spinal cord
    - Thoracic > cervical > > conus medullaris
  - Imaging findings
    - Heterogeneous due to varying ages of blood products
      - "Blooming" of internal components or rim on SWI/GRE secondary to hemosiderin
    - ± speckled or popcorn appearance, fluid-fluid levels
    - Absent or minimal enhancement
    - Surrounding edema if hemorrhage is recent
- **Spinal Cord Infarction**
  - Sudden onset of symptoms
  - Imaging findings
    - Hyperintense T2/DWI in cord: Central owl's eye pattern; ± patchy enhancement in subacute phase
    - ± cord expansion
    - ± hemorrhagic conversion
    - Length usually > 1 vertebral body
- **Hemangioblastoma**
  - Extremely rare in children
  - Imaging findings
    - Cyst with enhancing nodule in dorsal cord
    - Often multiple (including posterior fossa)
    - Look for findings of von Hippel-Lindau syndrome

SELECTED REFERENCES

1. Wendebourg MJ et al: Magnetic resonance imaging in immune-mediated myelopathies. J Neurol. ePub, 2019
2. Baruah D et al: A simplified algorithm for diagnosis of spinal cord lesions. Curr Probl Diagn Radiol. 44(3):256-66, 2015
3. Karikari IO et al: Impact of tumor histology on resectability and neurological outcome in primary intramedullary spinal cord tumors: a single-center experience with 102 patients. Neurosurgery. 76 Suppl 1:S4-13; discussion S13, 2015

Syrinx

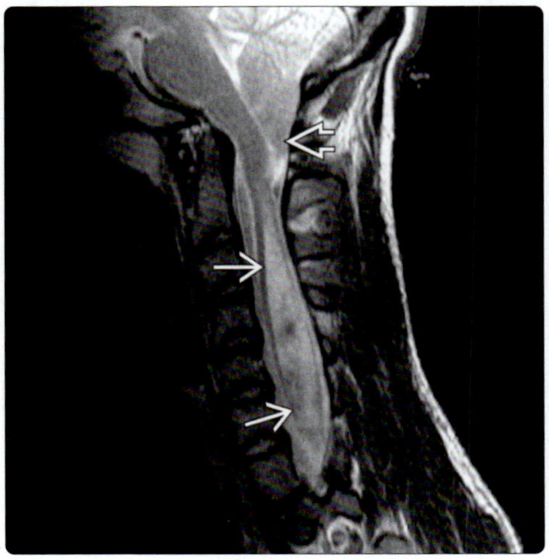

Acute Disseminated Encephalomyelitis

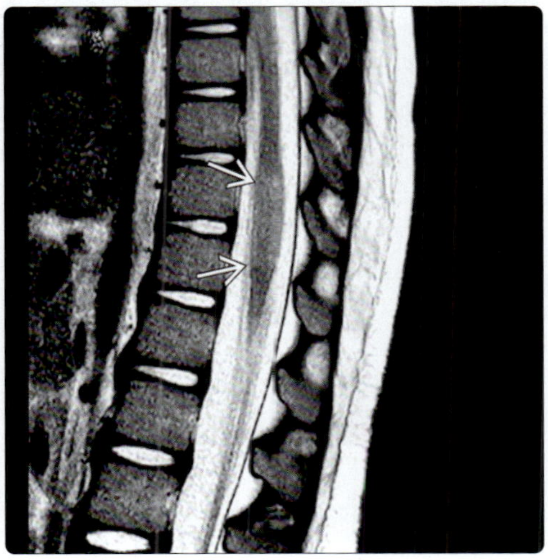

(Left) *Sagittal T2 MR in a teenager presenting with scoliosis shows a large cervical syrinx ➡ in a patient with inferiorly positioned & pointed cerebellar tonsils ➡ with associated effacement of CSF at the foramen magnum, consistent with Chiari 1.* **(Right)** *Sagittal T2 MR in a child with intracranial lesions typical of acute disseminated encephalomyelitis (ADEM) shows a hyperintense intramedullary lesion ➡ with slight swelling of the distal cord.*

(Left) Sagittal T2 MR in a child with weakness & decreased rectal tone shows fusiform enlargement of the cervical & upper thoracic cord with hyperintense signal ➡ spanning > 4 vertebral segments in length. There was no appreciable enhancement on postcontrast images, & no demyelinating lesions were identified in the brain. **(Right)** *Axial T2* GRE MR demonstrates 2 focal areas of intramedullary hemorrhage ➡ in a child who suffered cervical vertebral body ➡ & lamina ➡ fractures in a diving accident.*

Idiopathic Acute Transverse Myelitis

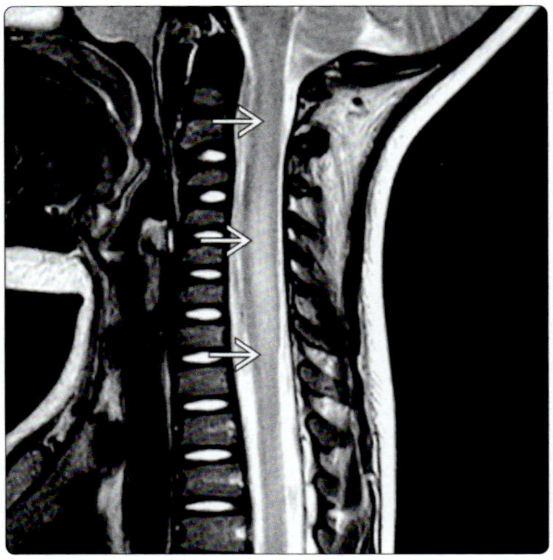

Contusion/Hematoma

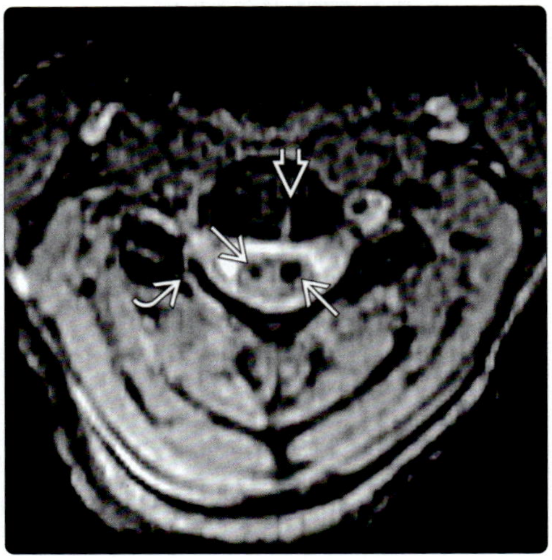

(Left) *Sagittal T2 MR shows multiple small, hyperintense intramedullary lesions ➡ in the cervical cord without significant cord enlargement, typical of multiple sclerosis. Note the similar lesions in the brainstem ➡.* **(Right)** *Sagittal T2 MR in a teenager with weakness, numbness, & tingling in the trunk & legs demonstrates a fusiform focus of hyperintense intramedullary T2 signal abnormality ➡ in the upper thoracic cord, spanning < 2 vertebral segments.*

Multiple Sclerosis

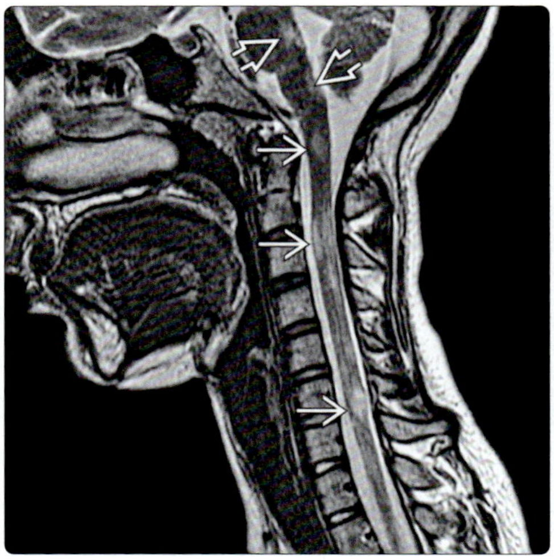

Multiple Sclerosis

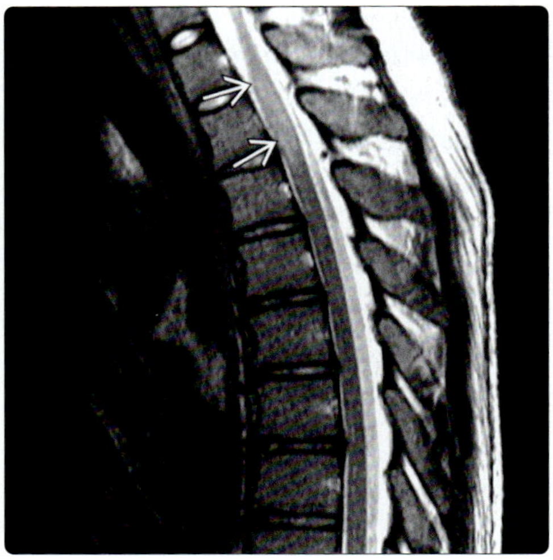

(Left) *Sagittal T2 MR shows a well-defined, hyperintense intramedullary lesion expanding the cervicothoracic cord ➡. Note the ill-defined, flame-shaped areas of hyperintensity ➡ along the margins of the expansile tumor, which may be due to edema or tumor infiltration. Only subtle, patchy enhancement was noted in the lesion (not shown).* **(Right)** *Sagittal T1 C+ MR shows cord enlargement by a solid, enhancing tumor ➡ that is capped by nonenhancing cysts ➡, typical of ependymoma.*

Astrocytoma

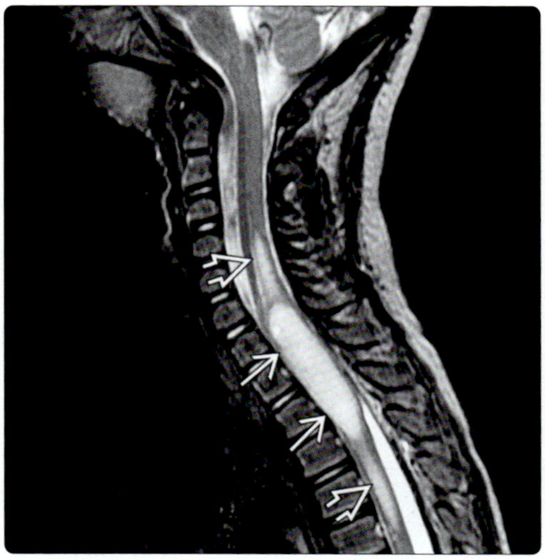

Ependymoma

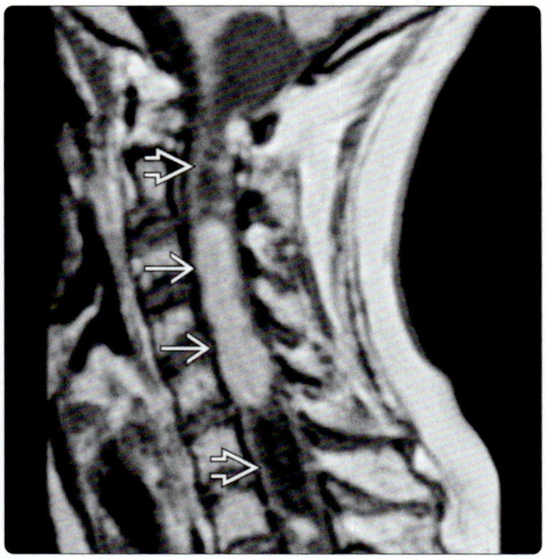

Abscess

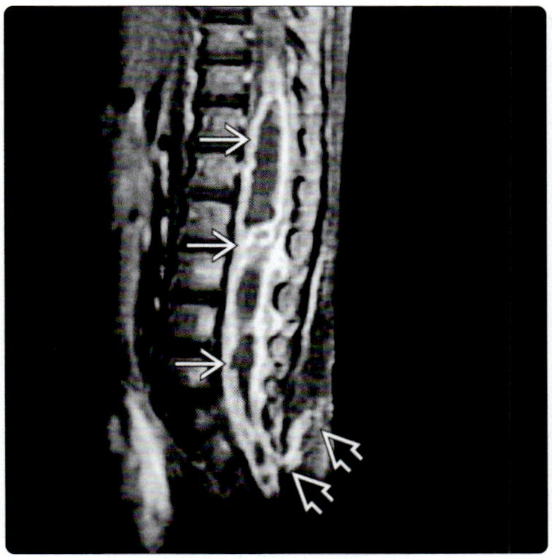

Dermoid & Epidermoid Tumors

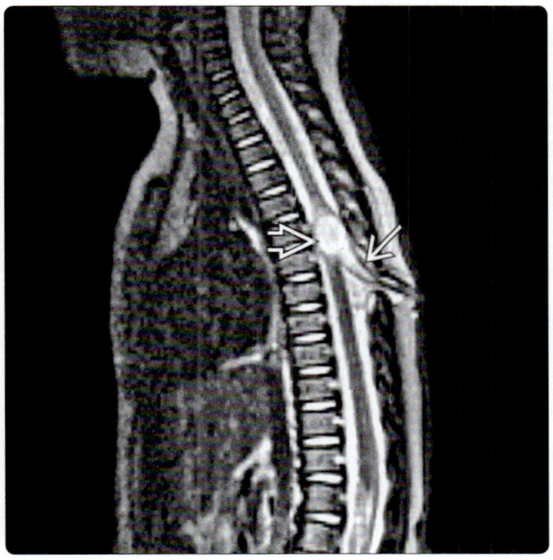

(Left) *Sagittal T1 C+ FS MR shows a large, peripherally enhancing intramedullary abscess within a tethered cord. There is also enhancement of the dorsal dermal sinus that connects the skin surface to the tethered cord.* **(Right)** *Sagittal T2 MR shows a hyperintense intramedullary dermoid that is contiguous with an extramedullary component into a sinus tract to the skin surface.*

Cavernous Malformation

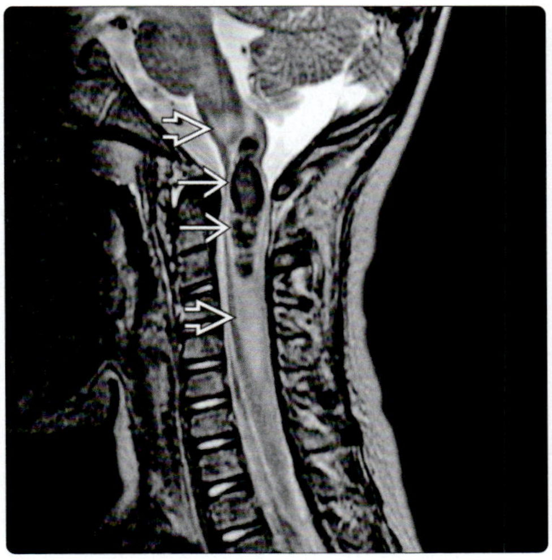

Spinal Cord Infarction

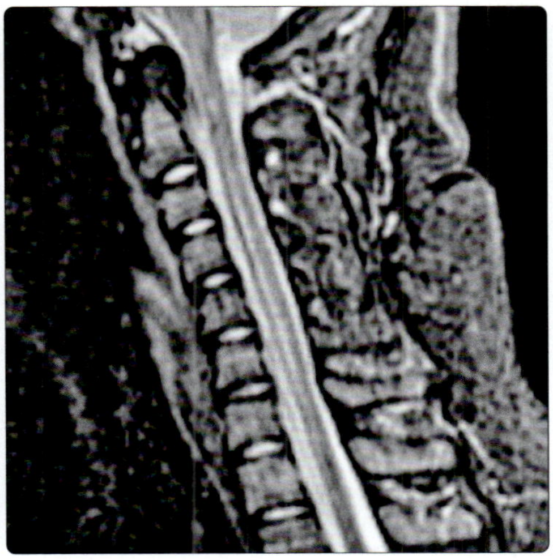

(Left) *Sagittal T2 MR shows hypointense intramedullary hemorrhage & surrounding edema in the cervicomedullary junction secondary to a cavernous malformation.* **(Right)** *Sagittal T2 MR shows a long segment of central hyperintense cord signal abnormality in a teenager who developed progressive quadriplegia after an aggressive back massage.*

Spinal Cord Infarction

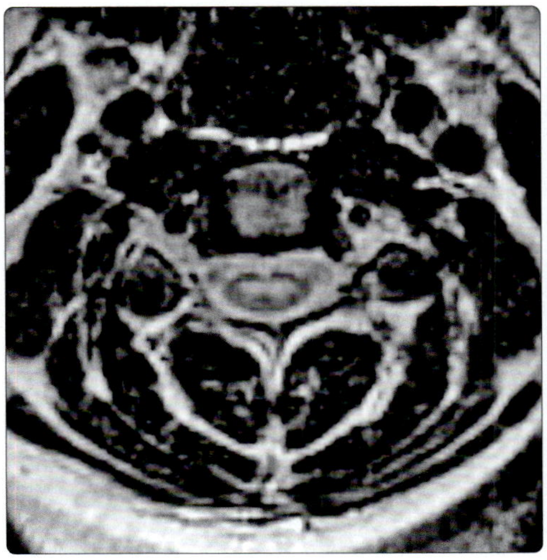

Hemangioblastoma

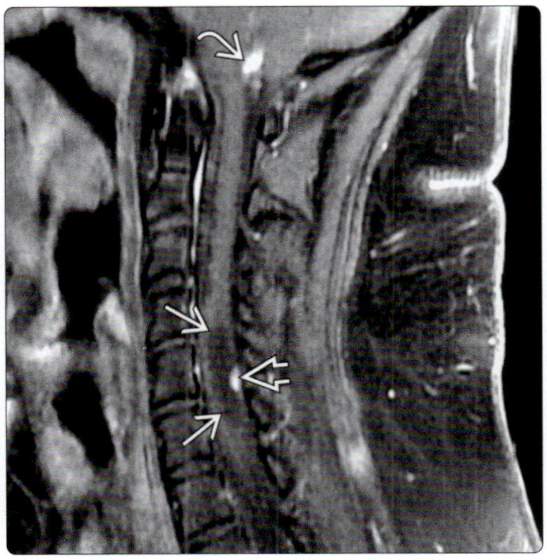

(Left) *Axial T2 MR shows central gray matter hyperintensity in the same patient, creating a central owl's eye pattern that is typical of spinal cord infarction.* **(Right)** *Sagittal T1 C+ FS MR in a child with von Hippel-Lindau syndrome shows an oblong cystic lesion with an enhancing peripheral nodule in the lower cervical cord, typical of a hemangioblastoma. Note also the enhancing nodule in the posterior fossa in this child with multiple intracranial lesions.*

INDEX

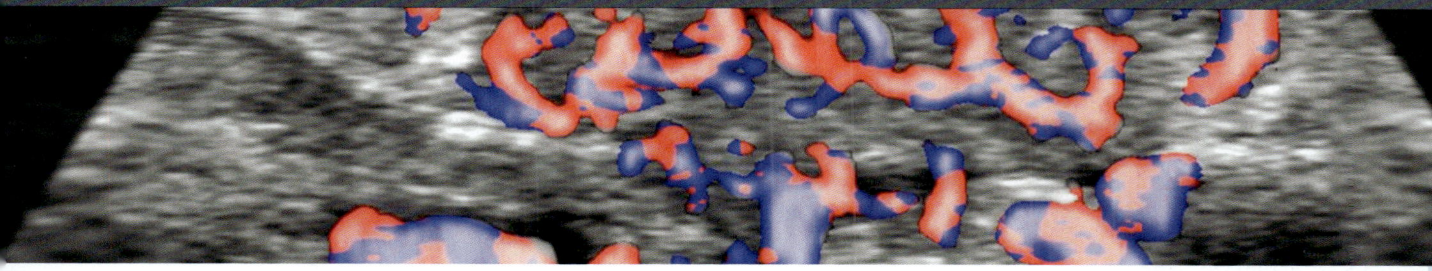

A

INDEX

INDEX

INDEX

B

INDEX

C

INDEX

INDEX

INDEX

D

E

INDEX

F

G

INDEX

H

INDEX

INDEX

I

INDEX

J

K

INDEX

L

INDEX

M

INDEX

INDEX

N

INDEX

O

P

R

S

INDEX

T

U

V

W

X

Y